KU-411-441

KELLEY'S
Textbook of
Rheumatology

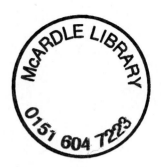
McARDLE LIBRARY
0151 604 7223

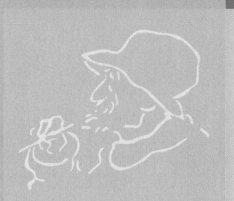

VOLUME
II

KELLEY'S
Textbook of
Rheumatology

EIGHTH EDITION

Gary S. Firestein, MD

Professor of Medicine
Chief, Division of Rheumatology, Allergy,
  and Immunology
Dean, Translational Medicine
University of California, San Diego, School of Medicine
La Jolla, California

Ralph C. Budd, MD

Professor of Medicine
Director, Immunobiology Program
University of Vermont College of Medicine
Burlington, Vermont

Edward D. Harris, Jr., MD

George DeForest Barnett Professor of Medicine, Emeritus
Stanford University School of Medicine
Academic Secretary to Stanford University, Emeritus
Stanford University
Stanford, California

Iain B. McInnes, PhD, FRCP

Professor of Experimental Medicine
Honorary Consultant Rheumatologist
Centre for Rheumatic Diseases, Faculty of Medicine
University of Glasgow
Glasgow, United Kingdom

Shaun Ruddy, MD

Professor Emeritus, Department of Internal Medicine,
  Division of Rheumatology, Allergy, and Immunology
Virginia Commonwealth University School of Medicine
  at the Medical College of Virginia
Richmond, Virginia

John S. Sergent, MD

Professor of Medicine
Vice Chair for Education and Residency Program Director
Vanderbilt University School of Medicine
Nashville, Tennessee

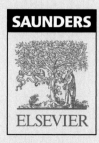

SAUNDERS

ELSEVIER

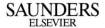

SAUNDERS
ELSEVIER

1600 John F. Kennedy Blvd.
Ste 1800
Philadelphia, PA 19103-2899

ISBN: 978-1-4160-3285-4 (Expert Consult)
978-1-4160-4842-8 (Expert Consult Premium Ed.)

KELLEY'S TEXTBOOK OF RHEUMATOLOGY

Copyright © 2009, 2005, 2001, 1997, 1993, 1989, 1985, 1981 by Saunders, an imprint of Elsevier Inc.

All rights reserved. No part of this publication may be reproduced or transmitted in any form or by any means, electronic or mechanical, including photocopying, recording, or any information storage and retrieval system, without permission in writing from the publisher. Permissions may be sought directly from Elsevier's Rights Department: phone: (+1) 215 239 3804 (US) or (+44) 1865 843830 (UK); fax: (+44) 1865 853333; e-mail: healthpermissions@elsevier.com. You may also complete your request on-line via the Elsevier website at http://www.elsevier.com/permissions.

Notice

Knowledge and best practice in this field are constantly changing. As new research and experience broaden our knowledge, changes in practice, treatment, and drug therapy may become necessary or appropriate. Readers are advised to check the most current information provided (i) on procedures featured or (ii) by the manufacturer of each product to be administered, to verify the recommended dose or formula, the method and duration of administration, and contraindications. It is the responsibility of the practitioner, relying on experience and knowledge of the patient, to make diagnoses, to determine dosages and the best treatment for each individual patient, and to take all appropriate safety precautions. To the fullest extent of the law, neither the Publisher nor the Editors assume any liability for any injury and/or damage to persons or property arising out of or related to any use of the material contained in this book.

The Publisher

Library of Congress Cataloging-in-Publication Data
Kelley's textbook of rheumatology / [edited by] Gary S. Firestein ... [et al.]. -- 8th ed.
    p. ; cm.
  Includes bibliographical references and index.
  ISBN 978-1-4160-3285-4
  1. Rheumatology. 2. Rheumatism. 3. Arthritis. I. Firestein, Gary S. II. Kelley, William N., 1939-
III. Title: Textbook of rheumatology.
  [DNLM: 1. Rheumatic Diseases. 2. Arthritis. WE 544 K29 2009]
  RC927.T49 2009
  616.7'23--dc22

               2007048387

Acquisitions Editor: Kimberly Murphy
Developmental Manager: Cathy Carroll
Developmental Editor: Angela Norton
Publishing Services Manager: Linda Van Pelt
Project Manager: Francisco Morales
Design Direction: Ellen Zanolle
Cover Design: Ellen Zanolle

Printed in Canada

Last digit is the print number: 9 8 7 6 5 4 3 2 1

Working together to grow libraries in developing countries

www.elsevier.com | www.bookaid.org | www.sabre.org

ELSEVIER   BOOK AID International   Sabre Foundation

Sincerest thanks to my wonderful wife, Linda, and our children,
David and Cathy, for their patience and support.
Also, the editorial help of our two Cavalier King Charles puppies,
Winston and Humphrey, was invaluable.
Gary S. Firestein

Sincere thanks for the kind mentoring
from Edward D. Harris Jr.,
H. Robson MacDonald, and C. Garrison Fathman,
as well as for the support of my wife, Lenore,
and my children, Graham and Laura.
Ralph C. Budd

Many thanks to my mentor, Steve Krane,
and for the support of the Harris boys,
Ned, Tom, and Chandler, and Eileen . . .
and for the happy smiles of the grandkids—
Andrew, Eliza, Maeve, and Liam.
Ted Harris

To my wife, Karin, for her patience,
understanding, and love and to our wonderful girls,
Megan and Rebecca, who continue to enlighten me.
Iain B. McInnes

To my wife, Millie; our children, Christi and Candace;
and our grandchildren, Kevin, Matthew, and Katharine.
Shaun Ruddy

To Carole and our children, Ellen and Katie,
and to our grandchildren, Kathryn, Henry,
Emmaline, and Romy.
John S. Sergent

CONTRIBUTORS

Steven B. Abramson, MD
Professor of Medicine and Pathology
New York University School of Medicine
New York, New York
  *Neutrophils and Eosinophils; Pathogenesis of
  Osteoarthritis*

Leyla Alparslan, MD
Instructor in Orthopaedic Radiology
Uppsala University Faculty of Medicine
Staff Radiologist, Akademiska Hospital
Uppsala, Sweden
  Imaging Modalities in Rheumatic Disease

Thomas P. Andriacchi, PhD
Professor
Department of Mechanical Engineering
Stanford University School of Engineering
Department of Orthopaedics
Stanford University School of Medicine
Stanford
VA Palo Alto Research & Development, Bone and Joint
  Research Center
Palo Alto, California
  *Joint Biomechanics: The Role of Mechanics in Joint
  Pathology*

John P. Atkinson, MD
Samuel B. Grant Professor of Medicine and Professor of
  Molecular Microbiology
Washington University in St. Louis School of Medicine
Physician, Barnes-Jewish Hospital
St. Louis, Missouri
  Complement System

Stefan Bachmann, MD
FMH Specialist in Internal Medicine and Rheumatology
FMH Specialist in Physical Medicine and Rehabilitation
Leitender Artz/Chefarzt-Stellvertreter
Klinik für Rheumatologie und Rehabilitation des
  Bewegungsapparates
Valens, Switzerland
  Introduction to Physical Medicine and Rehabilitation

Leslie R. Ballou, PhD
Professor of Medicine and Molecular Sciences, Department
  of Rheumatology
University of Tennessee College of Medicine
Research Chemist, VA Medical Center and UT Health
  Science Center
Memphis, Tennessee
  Nonsteroidal Anti-inflammatory Drugs

Stanley P. Ballou, MD
Associate Professor of Medicine
Case Western Reserve University School of Medicine
Director of Rheumatology
MetroHealth Medical Center
Cleveland, Ohio
  *Acute-Phase Reactants and the Concept of
  Inflammation*

Walter G. Barr, MD
Professor of Medicine
Northwestern University Feinberg School of Medicine
Chicago, Illinois
  *Mycobacterial Infections of Bones and Joints; Fungal
  Infections of the Bones and Joints*

Dorcas Eleanor Beaton, BScOT, MSc, PhD
Assistant Professor, Department of Health Policy,
  Management and Evaluation
University of Toronto Faculty of Medicine
Scientist and Director, Mobility Program Clinical Research
  Unit
St. Michael's Hospital
Toronto, Ontario, Canada
  Assessment of Health Outcomes

Robert M. Bennett, MD, FRCP, MACR
Professor of Medicine and Nursing Research
Oregon Health & Science University School of Medicine
  and School of Nursing
Portland, Oregon
  Overlap Syndromes

Francis Berenbaum, MD, PhD
Professor of Rheumatology
Pierre and Marie Curie University (UPMC—Paris
  Universitas) Faculty of Medicine
Hospital Saint-Antoine
Paris, France
  Clinical Features of Osteoarthritis

Johannes W.J. Bijlsma, MD, PhD
Professor and Chair, Department of Rheumatology
  & Clinical Immunology
University Medical Center Utrecht
Utrecht, The Netherlands
  Glucocorticoid Therapy

Linda K. Bockenstedt, MD
Harold W. Jockers Professor of Medicine
Department of Internal Medicine, Section of Rheumatology
Yale University School of Medicine
New Haven, Connecticut
  Lyme Disease

Maarten Boers, MSc, MD, PhD
Professor of Clinical Epidemiology
Department of Clinical Epidemiology and Biostatistics
VU University Amsterdam Faculty of Medicine
Amsterdam, The Netherlands
Assessment of Health Outcomes

Robert Alan Bonakdar, MD
Assistant Clinical Professor, Department of Family and
  Preventive Medicine
UC San Diego School of Medicine
Director of Pain Management
Scripps Center for Integrative Medicine
La Jolla, California
*Integrative Medicine in Rheumatology:
An Evidence-Based Approach*

Dimitrios T. Boumpas, MD, FACP
Professor and Chairman, Department of Internal Medicine,
  Division of Rheumatology, Clinical Immunology, and
  Allergy
University of Crete Medical School
Chief of Medicine
Heraklion University General Hospital
Crete, Greece
*Clinical Features and Treatment of Systemic Lupus
Erythematosus*

Barry Bresnihan, MD
Professor of Rheumatology
University College Dublin School of Medicine
  and Medical Science
National University of Ireland
Consultant Rheumatologist
St. Vincent's University Hospital
Prinicipal Investigator
Conway Institute of Biomedical Research
Dublin, Ireland
Synovium

Doreen B. Brettler, MD
Professor of Medicine
University of Massachusetts Medical School
Director, New England Hemophilia Center
University of Massachusetts Memorial Healthcare
Worcester, Massachusetts
Hemophilic Arthropathy

Paul L. Briant, PhD, MS
VA Palo Alto Research & Development
Bone and Joint Research Center
Palo Alto, CA
*Joint Biomechanics: The Role of Mechanics in Joint
Pathology*

Ralph C. Budd, MD
Professor of Medicine
Director, Immunobiology Program
University of Vermont College of Medicine
Burlington, Vermont
T Lymphocytes

Leonard H. Calabrese, DO
Professor of Medicine and R.J. Fasenmyer Chair of Clinical
  Immunology
Cleveland Clinic Lerner College of Medicine
Vice Chairman, Department of Rheumatic and
  Immunologic Diseases
Cleveland Clinic Foundation
Cleveland, Ohio
*Antineutrophil Cytoplasmic Antibody–Associated
Vasculitis*

Amy C. Cannella, MD
Assistant Professor, Department of Medicine, Section of
  Rheumatology and Immunology
University of Nebraska College of Medicine
Omaha, Nebraska
*Methotrexate, Leflunomide, Sulfasalazine,
Hydroxychloroquine, and Combination Therapies*

Eugene J. Carragee, MD
Professor of Orthopaedic Surgery
Stanford University School of Medicine
Director, Spine Surgery Section
Stanford University Hospital and Clinics
Stanford, California
Low Back Pain

Steven Carsons, MD
Professor of Medicine
State University of New York at Stony Brook School
  of Medicine
Stony Brook
Chief, Division of Rheumatology, Allergy
  and Immunology
Winthrop University Hospital
Mineola, New York
Sjögren's Syndrome

James T. Cassidy, MD
Professor, Department of Child Health
University of Missouri–Columbia School of Medicine
Chief of Pediatric Rheumatology
University of Missouri Health Sciences Center
Columbia, Missouri
*Systemic Lupus Erythematosus, Juvenile
Dermatomyositis, Scleroderma, and Vasculitis*

Eliza F. Chakravarty, MD, MS
Assistant Professor, Department of Medicine, Division
  of Immunology and Rheumatology
Stanford University School of Medicine
Stanford, California
Musculoskeletal Syndromes in Malignancy

Christopher Chang, MD, PhD
Associate Clinical Professor, Department of Internal
  Medicine, Division of Rheumatology/Allergy/Clinical
  Immunology
UC Davis School of Medicine
Sacramento
Staff, UC Davis Genome and Biomedical Services
  Facility
Davis, California
Osteonecrosis

Joseph S. Cheng, MD, MS
Assistant Professor of Neurological Surgery
Vanderbilt University School of Medicine
Director, Neurosurgery Spine Program
Vanderbilt University Medical Center
Nashville, Tennessee
Neck Pain

Christopher P. Chiodo, MD
Instructor in Orthopaedic Surgery, Department
of Orthopedic Surgery
Harvard Medical School
Chief, Foot and Ankle Division
Brigham and Women's Hospital
Boston, Massachusetts
Foot and Ankle Pain

Paul P. Cook, MD
Associate Professor of Medicine
Division of Infectious Diseases
Department of Infectious Diseases
Department of Internal Medicine
Brody School of Medicine at East Carolina University
Greenville, North Carolina
Bacterial Arthritis

Joseph E. Craft, MD
Professor of Medicine and Immunobiology
Chief, Section of Rheumatology, and Director,
Investigative Medicine
Yale University School of Medicine
Chief of Rheumatology and Attending Physician
Yale–New Haven Hospital
New Haven, Connecticut
Antinuclear Antibodies

Gaye Cunnane, MD, MB, PhD, FRCPI
Senior Lecturer in Medicine
Trinity College Dublin Faculty of Health Sciences School
of Medicine
Consultant in Rheumatology and Internal Medicine
St. James' Hospital
Dublin, Ireland
Hemochromatosis

Jody A. Dantzig, BS, PhD
Medical Student
University of Pennsylvania School of Medicine
Philadelphia, Pennsylvania
Muscle: Anatomy, Physiology, and Biochemistry

John M. Davis III, MD
Assistant Professor of Medicine
Division of Rheumatology
Mayo Clinic
Rochester, Minnesota
*History and Physical Examination of the
Musculoskeletal System*

Jeroen DeGroot, MD
Operations Manager, Inflammatory and Degenerative
Diseases
BioSciences Division
TNO Quality of Life
Leiden, The Netherlands
Biologic Markers

Christopher P. Denton, PhD, FRCP
Professor of Experimental Rheumatology
Royal Free and University College Medical School
Honorary Consultant Rheumatologist, Centre for
Rheumatology
London, United Kingdom
*Systemic Sclerosis and the Scleroderma-Spectrum
Disorders*

Clinton Devin, MD
Orthopedic Surgeon, Department of Orthopaedics
and Rehabilitation
Vanderbilt Sports Medicine Center
Nashville, Tennessee
Neck Pain

Betty Diamond, MD
Professor, Department of Microbiology & Immunology
and Department of Medicine (Rheumatology)
Albert Einstein College of Medicine
Bronx
Head and Investigator, Center for Autoimmune
and Musculoskeletal Diseases
The Feinstein Institute for Medical Research
Manhasset, New York
B Cells

Federico Díaz-González, MD
Associate Professor of Rheumatology
Universidad de La Laguna Faculty of Medicine
Staff Rheumatologist
Hospital Universitario de Canarias
La Laguna, Spain
Platelets and Rheumatic Diseases

Paul E. Di Cesare, MD, FACS
Professor and Michael W. Chapman Chair, Department
of Orthopaedic Surgery
UC Davis School of Medicine
Sacramento, California
Pathogenesis of Osteoarthritis

Joost P.H. Drenth, MD, PhD
Professor of Molecular Gastroenterology and Hepatology
Department of Gastroenterology and Hepatology
Radboud University Nijmegen Medical Centre Faculty of
Medical Sciences
Nijmegen, The Netherlands
Familial Auto-inflammatory Syndromes

George F. Duna, MD, FACP
Associate Professor of Medicine
Baylor College of Medicine
Houston, Texas
*Antineutrophil Cytoplasmic Antibody–Associated
Vasculitis*

Michael L. Dustin, PhD
Irene Diamond Professor of Immunology and Associate
    Professor of Pathology
Department of Molecular Pathogenesis
The Helen L. and Martin S. Kimmel Center for Biology
    and Medicine, Skirball Institute of Biomolecular
    Medicine
New York University School of Medicine
New York, New York
    *Adaptive Immunity Including Organization of
    Lymphoid Tissues*

Hani S. El-Gabalawy, MD, FRCPC
Professor of Medicine and Immunology and Head, Division
    of Rheumatology
University of Manitoba Faculty of Medicine
Rheumatologist
Winnipeg Health Sciences Centre
Winnipeg, Manitoba, Canada
    *Synovial Fluid Analysis, Synovial Biopsy, and Synovial
    Pathology*

Keith B. Elkon, MD
Professor of Medicine and Immunology and Head, Division
    of Rheumatology
Department of Medicine
University of Washington School of Medicine
Seattle, Washington
    Cell Survival and Death in Rheumatic Diseases

Doruk Erkan, MD
Assistant Professor of Medicine
Weill Medical College of Cornell University
Associate Physician-Scientist and Assistant Attending
    Physician
Barbara Volcker Center for Women and Rheumatic
    Diseases
Hospital for Special Surgery
New York, New York
    Antiphospholipid Syndrome

Gary S. Firestein, MD
Professor of Medicine
Chief, Division of Rheumatology, Allergy,
    and Immunology
Dean, Translational Medicine
University of California, San Diego, School of Medicine
La Jolla, California
    *Etiology and Pathogenesis of Rheumatoid Arthritis;
    Clinical Features of Rheumatoid Arthritis*

Oliver FitzGerald, MD, FRCPI, FRCP(UK)
Newman Clinical Research Professor
University College Dublin School of Medicine
    and Medical Science
National University of Ireland
Consultant Rheumatologist
St. Vincent's University Hospital
Dublin, Ireland
    Psoriatic Arthritis

John P. Flaherty, MD
Professor of Medicine
Associate Chief and Director of Clinical Services, Division
    of Infectious Diseases
Northwestern University Feinberg School of Medicine
Chicago, Illinois
    *Mycobacterial Infections of Bones and Joints; Fungal
    Infections of the Bones and Joints*

Adrienne M. Flanagan, MD, PhD
Professor
Institute of Orthopaedics and Musculoskeletal Science
University College London
London
Royal National Orthopaedic Hospital
Stanmore
Department of Histopathology, University College
    Hospital
London, United Kingdom
    Synovium

Karen A. Fortner, PhD
Research Assistant Professor Immunobiology Program
Department of Medicine
University of Vermont College of Medicine
Burlington, Vermont
    T Lymphocytes

Howard A. Fuchs, MD
Associate Professor of Medicine
Division of Rheumatology
Vanderbilt University
Tennessee Valley Healthcare System
Department of Veterans Affairs Medical Center
Nashville, TN
    Polyarticular Arthritis

Steffen Gay, MD
Professor
Department of Rheumatology
University Hospital
Zurich, Switzerland
    Fibroblasts and Fibroblast-like Synoviocytes

Mark C. Genovese, MD
Professor of Medicine
Stanford University School of Medicine
Co-Chief, Division of Immunology and Rheumatology
Stanford University Medical Center
Stanford, California
    Treatment of Rheumatoid Arthritis

M. Eric Gershwin, MD
Distinguished Professor of Medicine
UC Davis School of Medicine
Sacramento, California
    Osteonecrosis

Allan Gibofsky, MD, JD, FACP, FCLM
Professor of Medicine and Public Health
Weill Medical College of Cornell University
Adjunct Professor of Law
Fordham University School of Law
Attending Rheumatologist
Hospital for Special Surgery
New York, New York
Poststreptoccocal Arthritis and Rheumatic Fever

Mark H. Ginsberg, MD
Professor, Department of Medicine, Rheumatology Section
UC San Diego School of Medicine
La Jolla, California
Platelets and Rheumatic Diseases

Joseph Golbus, MD
Associate Professor of Medicine
Northwestern University Feinberg School of Medicine
Senior Attending Physician, Division of Rheumatology
President
Evanston Northwestern Healthcare Medical Group
Chicago, Illinois
Monarticular Arthritis

Yale E. Goldman, MD, PhD
Professor, Department of Physiology
University of Pennyslvania School of Medicine
Director, Pennsylvania Muscle Institute
Philadelphia, Pennsylvania
Muscle: Anatomy, Physiology, and Biochemistry

Mary B. Goldring, PhD
Weill Medical College of Cornell University
Senior Scientist
Hospital for Special Surgery
New York, New York
Biology of the Normal Joint; Cartilage and Chondrocytes

Steven R. Goldring, MD
Weill Medical College of Cornell University
Chief Scientific Officer
Hospital for Special Surgery
New York, New York
Biology of the Normal Joint

Stuart B. Goodman, MD, PhD, FRCSC, FACS, FBSE
Robert L. and Mary Ellenburg Professor of Surgery, Department of Orthopaedic Surgery
Stanford University School of Medicine
Attending Orthopaedic Surgeon, Stanford University Medical Center
Consultant Orthopaedic Surgeon, Lucile Salter Packard Children's Hospital at Stanford
Stanford
Consultant Orthopaedic Surgeon, Palo Alto Veterans Administration Hospital
Palo Alto, California
Hip and Knee Pain

Carl S. Goodyear, PhD
Lecturer and Arthritis Research Campaign
University of Glasgow Faculty of Medicine
NCCD Fellow, Division of Clinical Neurosciences
Glasgow Biomedical Research Centre
Glasgow, United Kingdom
Rheumatoid Factors and Other Autoantibodies in Rheumatoid Arthritis

Siamon Gordon, MBChB, PhD, FRS, FMedSci
Professor Emeritus
Sir William Dunn School of Pathology
University of Oxford
Oxford, United Kingdom
Mononuclear Phagocytes in Rheumatic Diseases

Adam Greenspan, MD, FACR
Professor Emeritus of Radiology
Department of Radiology, Section of Musculoskeletal Imaging
UC Davis School of Medicine
Sacramento, California
Osteonecrosis

Peter K. Gregersen, MD
Professor of Medicine and Pathology
New York University School of Medicine
New York, New York
Genetics of Rheumatic Diseases

Christine Grimaldi, PhD
Assistant Professor, Department of Microbiology & Immunology
Albert Einstein College of Medicine
Bronx
Assistant Investigator, Center for Autoimmune and Musculoskeletal Disease
The Feinstein Institute for Medical Research
Manhasset, New York
B Cells

Bevra Hannahs Hahn, MD, FACR, MACR
Professor and Vice Chair, Department of Medicine
David Geffen School of Medicine at UCLA
Chief, Rheumatology and Arthritis
UCLA Medical Center
Los Angeles, California
Pathogenesis of Systemic Lupus Erythematosus

J. Timothy Harrington, MD
Associate Professor, Department of Medicine
University of Wisconsin School of Medicine and Public Health
Madison, Wisconsin
Mycobacterial Infections of Bones and Joints; Fungal Infections of the Bones and Joints

Edward D. Harris, Jr., MD, MACR
George DeForest Barnett Professor of Medicine, Emeritus
Stanford University School of Medicine
Academic Secretary to Stanford University, Emeritus
Stanford University
Stanford, California
Clinical Features of Rheumatoid Arthritis

David B. Hellmann, MD
Aliki Perroti Professor of Medicine
Johns Hopkins University School of Medicine
Vice Dean and Chairman, Department of Medicine
Johns Hopkins Bayview Medical Center
Baltimore, Maryland
Giant Cell Arteritis, Polymyalgia Rheumatica, and Takayasu's Arteritis

George Ho, Jr., MD
Professor of Medicine
Brody School of Medicine at East Carolina University
Greenville, North Carolina
Bacterial Arthritis

James I. Huddleston, MD
Assistant Professor, Department of Orthopaedic Surgery
Stanford University School of Medicine
Stanford, California
Hip and Knee Pain

Gene G. Hunder, MD
Professor Emeritus
Mayo Clinic College of Medical Sciences
Emeritus Member
Department of Internal Medicine, Division of Rheumatology
Mayo Clinic
Rochester, Minnesota
History and Physical Examination of the Musculoskeletal System

Johannes W.G. Jacobs, MD, PhD
Associate Professor, Department of Rheumatology and Clinical Immunology
Rheumatologist and Senior Researcher
University Medical Center Utrecht
Utrecht, The Netherlands
Glucocorticoid Therapy

Joanne M. Jordan, MD, MPH
Associate Professor of Medicine and Orthopaedics
Chief, Division of Rheumatology, Allergy, and Immunology
University of North Carolina at Chapel Hill School of Medicine
Director, Thurston Arthritis Research Center
Chapel Hill, North Carolina
Principles of Epidemiology in Rheumatic Disease

Joseph L. Jorizzo, MD
Professor and Former (Founding) Chair, Department of Dermatology
Wake Forest University School of Medicine
Winston-Salem, North Carolina
Behçet's Disease

Kenneth C. Kalunian, MD
Professor of Medicine and Director of Rheumatology, Allergy and Immunology
UC San Diego School of Medicine
La Jolla, California
Rheumatic Manifestations of Hemoglobinopathies

Arthur Kavanaugh, MD
Professor of Medicine
Center for Innovative Therapy, Division of Rheumatology, Allergy and Immunology
UC San Diego School of Medicine
La Jolla, California
Anticytokine Therapies

Alisa E. Koch, MD
Frederick G.L. Huetwell and William D. Robinson, MD Professor of Rheumatology
University of Michigan Medical School
Ann Arbor, Michigan
Cell Recruitment and Angiogenesis

Deborah Krakow, MD
Associate Professor of Obstetrics and Gynecology
David Geffen School of Medicine at UCLA
Attending Physician, Department of Obstetrics and Gynecology
Cedars-Sinai Medical Center
Los Angeles, California
Heritable Diseases of Connective Tissue

Joel M. Kremer, MD
Pfaff Family Professor of Medicine
Albany Medical College
Director of Research
The Center for Rheumatology
Albany, New York
Nutrition and Rheumatic Diseases

Hollis E. Krug, BS, MD
Associate Clinical Professor of Medicine
University of Minnesota Medical School
Staff Rheumatologist
VA Medical Center
Minneapolis, Minnesota
Management of Chronic Pain

Irving Kushner, MD
Professor of Medicine
Case Western Reserve University School of Medicine
Staff Rheumatologist
MetroHealth Medical Center
Cleveland, Ohio
Acute-Phase Reactants and the Concept of Inflammation

Robert B.M. Landewé, MD
Professor of Rheumatology, Department of Internal Medicine, Division of Rheumatology
Maastricht University Faculty of Medicine
Staff Rheumatologist
Atrium Medical Center Heerlen
Maastricht, The Netherlands
Clinical Trial Design and Analysis

Nancy E. Lane, MD
Professor of Medicine and Rheumatology
UC Davis School of Medicine
Director, Center for Healthy Aging
Sacramento, California
Metabolic Bone Disease

Daniel J. Laskin, DDS, MS
Professor and Chairman Emeritus, Department of Oral
  and Maxillofacial Surgery
School of Dentistry and School of Medicine
Virginia Commonwealth University
Richmond, Virginia
  Temporomandibular Joint Pain

David M. Lee, MD
Assistant Professor of Medicine
Harvard Medical School
Associate Physician
Brigham and Women's Hospital
Boston, Massachusetts
  Mast Cells

Lela A. Lee, MD
Professor of Dermatology and Medicine
University of Colorado School of
  Medicine
Director of Dermatology
Denver Health Medical Center
Denver, Colorado
  The Skin and Rheumatic Diseases

Marjatta Leirisalo-Repo, MD, PhD
Professor of Rheumatology, Department of Medicine,
  Division of Rheumatology
Helsinki University Faculty of Medicine
Staff Rheumatologist, Helsinki University Central
  Hospital
Helsinki, Finland
  *Undifferentiated Spondyloarthritis and Reactive
  Arthritis*

David C. Leopold, MD, DABFM
Faculty Physician and Director, Integrative Medical
  Education
Scripps Center for Integrative Medicine
La Jolla, California
  *Integrative Medicine in Rheumatology:
  An Evidence-Based Approach*

Peter E. Lipsky, MD
Chief, Autoimmunity Branch
National Institute of Arthritis and Musculoskeletal
  and Skin Diseases
National Institutes of Health
Bethesda, Maryland
  Autoimmunity

Michael D. Lockshin, MD, MACR
Professor of Medicine and Obstetrics-Gynecology
Weill Medical College of Cornell University
New York, New York
  Antiphospholipid Syndrome

Kate R. Lorig, RN, DrPH
Professor, Department of Medicine, Division of
  Immunology and Rheumatology
Stanford University School of Medicine
Director, Patient Education Research Center
Stanford, California
  Arthritis Self-Management

B. Asher Louden, MD
Resident in Dermatology
Wake Forest University Baptist Medical Center
Winston-Salem, North Carolina
  Behçet's Disease

Carlos J. Lozada, MD, FACP, FACR
Associate Professor of Medicine
University of Miami Miller School of Medicine
Director, Rheumatology Fellowship Program
  and Rheumatology Clinical Services
Jackson Memorial Hospital
Miami, Florida
  Management of Osteoarthritis

Ingrid E. Lundberg, MD, PhD
Professor of Medicine and Head, Rheumatology Unit,
  Department of Medicine
Karolinska Institute/Karolinska University Hospital
Stockholm, Sweden
  *Inflammatory Diseases of Muscle and Other
  Myopathies*

Reuven Mader, MD
Senior Clinical Lecturer
B. Rappaport Faculty of Medicine, Technion Israel
  Institute of Technology
Head, Rheumatic Diseases Unit
Ha'Emek Medical Center
Haifa, Israel
  Proliferative Bone Diseases

Rashmi M. Maganti, MD
Fellow, Division of Rheumatology and Clinical
  Immunogenetics
The University of Texas Health Science Center at Houston
Houston, Texas
  *Rheumatic Manifestations of Human
  Immunodeficiency Virus Infection*

Maren Lawson Mahowald, MD
Professor of Medicine
University of Minnesota Medical School
Rheumatology Section Chief
Minneapolis VA Medical Center
Minneapolis, Minnesota
  Management of Chronic Pain

**Walter P. Maksymowych, MBChB, FRCPC, FACP,
  FRCP(UK)**
Professor of Medicine
University of Alberta Faculty of Medicine
Senior Scientist
Alberta Heritage Foundation for Medical Research
Edmonton, Alberta, Canada
  Ankylosing Spondylitis

Scott David Martin, MD
Assistant Professor of Orthopedics
Harvard Medical School
Attending Staff Physician, Department of Orthopedics
Brigham and Women's Hospital
Boston, Massachusetts
  Shoulder Pain

Helena Marzo-Ortega, MD, MRCP
Consultant Rheumatologist and Honorary Senior Lecturer
  Academic Section of Musculoskeletal Disease
Leeds Institute of Molecular Medicine University of Leeds
  and Chapel Allerton Hospital
Leeds, United Kingdom
  *Undifferentiated Spondyloarthritis and Reactive
  Arthritis*

Dennis McGonagle, PhD, FRCPI
Professor of Investigative Rheumatology
The University of Leeds
Leeds, United Kingdom
  *Undifferentiated Spondyloarthritis and Reactive
  Arthritis*

Iain B. McInnes, PhD, FRCP
Professor of Experimental Medicine
Honorary Consultant Rheumatologist
Centre for Rheumatic Diseases, Faculty of Medicine
University of Glasgow
Glasgow, United Kingdom
  *Cytokines; Atherosclerosis in Rheumatic Disease;
  Rheumatoid Factors and Other Autoantibodies in
  Rheumatoid Arthritis*

Kevin G. Moder, MD
Consultant and Associate Professor
Division of Rheumatology and Department of Internal
  Medicine
Mayo Clinic
Rochester, Minnesota
  *History and Physical Examination of the
  Musculoskeletal System*

Eamonn S. Molloy, MD, MRCPI
Associate Staff
Department of Rheumatic and Immunologic Disease
Cleveland Clinic Foundation
Cleveland, Ohio
  *Antineutrophil Cytoplasmic Antibody–Associated
  Vasculitis*

Kanneboyina Nagaraju, PhD, DVM
Associate Professor of Pediatrics
George Washington University School of Medicine
  and Health Sciences
Director, Murine Drug Testing Facility
Center for Genetic Medicine Research
Children's Research Institute
Children's National Medical Center
Washington, DC
  *Inflammatory Diseases of Muscle and Other
  Myopathies*

Stanley J. Naides, MD
Medical Director, Immunology R&D
Quest Diagnostics Nichols Institute
San Juan Capistrano, California
  Viral Arthritis

Lee S. Newman, MD, MA
Professor, Department of Medicine, Division of Allergy
  and Clinical Immunology and Division of Pulmonary
  Sciences and Critical Care Medicine
Professor of Epidemiology, Department of Preventive
  Medicine and Biometrics
University of Colorado School of Medicine
Denver, Colorado
  Sarcoidosis

Peter A. Nigrovic, MD
Instructor in Medicine
Harvard Medical School
Staff Rheumatologist
Department of Rheumatology, Immunology, and Allergy,
  Brigham & Women's Hospital
Division of Immunology, Children's Hospital Boston
Boston, Massachusetts
  Mast Cells

Kiran Nistala, MD, MRCP, MSc
Clinical Research Fellow in Paediatric Rheumatology
Institute of Child Health
University College London
London, United Kingdome
  Juvenile Idiopathic Arthritis

James R. O'Dell, MD
Larson Professor and Vice-Chairman, Department of
  Internal Medicine
University of Nebraska College of Medicine
Chief of Rheumatology and Residency Program Director,
  Department of Internal Medicine
University of Nebraska Medical Center
Omaha, Nebraska
  *Methotrexate, Leflunomide, Sulfasalazine,
  Hydroxychloroquine, and Combination Therapies*

Peter R. Oesch, MSc, Dipl PT
Head, Department of Ergonomics and Clinical Research
Valens Rehabilitation Clinic
Valens, Switzerland
  Introduction to Physical Medicine and Rehabilitation

Yasunori Okada, MD, PhD
Professor and Chairman, Department of Pathology
Keio University School of Medicine
Tokyo, Japan
  Proteinases and Matrix Degradation

Eugenia C. Pacheco-Pinedo, MD, MSc
Postdoctoral Researcher
Department of Medicine
Molecular Cardiology Research Center
Postdoctoral Researcher
Department of Physiology
Pennsylvania Muscle Institute
Philadelphia, Pennsylvania
  Muscle: Anatomy, Physiology, and Biochemistry

Richard S. Panush, MD
Professor of Medicine
Mount Sinai School of Medicine
Chair, Department of Medicine
Saint Barnabas Medical Center
New York, New York
Occupational and Recreational Musculoskeletal Disorders

Thomas Pap, MD
Professor of Experimental Medicine
Head, Division of Molecular Medicine of Musculoskeletal Tissue
University of Münster
Institute of Experimental Musculoskeletal Medicine
Director
University Hospital Münster
Münster, Germany
Fibroblasts and Fibroblast-like Synoviocytes

Stanford L. Peng, MD, PhD
Senior Director, Translational Medicine Leader
Clinical Research and Exploratory Development
Roche Palo Alto
Palo Alto
Assistant Clinical Professor, Department of Medicine, Division of Rheumatology–Arthritis
University of California, San Francisco, School of Medicine
San Francisco, California
Antinuclear Antibodies

Harris Perlman, PhD
Associate Professor, Department of Molecular Microbiology & Immunology
Saint Louis University School of Medicine
St. Louis, Missouri
Signal Transduction

Jean-Charles Piette, MD
Department of Internal Medicine
Groupe Hospitalier Pitié-Salpêtrière
Paris, France
Relapsing Polychondritis

Michael H. Pillinger, MD
Chief of Rheumatology
New York Hospital for Joint Diseases
New York, New York
Neutrophils and Eosinophils

Robert S. Pinals, MD
Acting Chief, Division of Rheumatology & Connective Tissue Research
Professor, Department of Medicine
UMDNJ–Robert Wood Johnson Medical School
New Brunswick, New Jersey
Felty's Syndrome

Steven A. Porcelli, MD
Weinstock Professor of Microbiology & Immunology and Professor of Medicine
Albert Einstein College of Medicine
Bronx, New York
Innate Immunity

Mark D. Price, MD, PhD
Chief Resident in Orthopedic Surgery
Harvard Combined Orthopedic Surgery Program
Massachusetts General Hospital
Boston, Massachusetts
Foot and Ankle Pain

Johannes J. Rasker, MD, PhD
Professor Emeritus of Rheumatology
Faculty of Behavioral Sciences, Department of Psychology and Communication of Health and Risk
University of Twente
Enschede, The Netherlands
Fibromyalgia

John D. Reveille, MD
Professor of Internal Medicine
Director, Division of Rheumatology and Clinical Immunogenetics
Department of Internal Medicine
University of Texas Medical School at Houston
Houston, Texas
Rheumatic Manifestations of Human Immunodeficiency Virus Infection

W. Neal Roberts, Jr., MD
Rheumatology Fellowship Program Director
Chas. W. Thomas Professor of Medicine
Virginia Commonwealth University School of Medicine, Medical College of Virginia Campus
Richmond, Virginia
Psychosocial Management of Rheumatic Diseases

James T. Rosenbaum, MD
Edward E. Rosenbaum Professor of Inflammation Research and Professor of Ophthalmology, Medicine, and Cell Biology
Chair, Division of Arthritis and Rheumatic Diseases
Vice-Chair, Department of Ophthalmology
Oregon Health & Science University School of Medicine
Portland, Oregon
The Eye and Rheumatic Diseases

Andrew E. Rosenberg, MD
Associate Professor
Harvard Medical School
Director of Surgical Pathology
Massachusetts General Hospital
Boston, Massachusetts
Tumors and Tumor-like Lesions of Joints and Related Structures

Clinton T. Rubin, PhD
Distinguished Professor and Chair
Department of Biomedical Engineering
State University of New York Stony Brook University
    School of Medicine
Stony Brook, New York
    Biology, Physiology, and Morphology of Bone

Janet E. Rubin, MD
Professor of Medicine and Pharmacology
University of North Carolina at Chapel Hill School
    of Medicine
Chapel Hill, North Carolina
    Biology, Physiology, and Morphology of Bone

Holly M. Sackett, MSPH
Senior Professional Research Assistant
University of Colorado Denver
Colorado School of Public Health
Denver, Colorado
    Sarcoidosis

Jane E. Salmon, MD
Professor of Medicine
Professor of Obstetrics and Gynecology
Weill Medical College of Cornell University
Attending Physician
Hospital for Special Surgery
New York Presbyterian Hospital
New York, New York
    Antiphospholipid Syndrome

Jonathan Samuels, MD
Instructor in Medicine (Rheumatology)
NYU School of Medicine
Director, Clinical Immunulogy Laboratory
NYU Langone Medical Center
    Pathogenesis of Osteoarthritis

Naveed Sattar, MBChB, PhD, MRCPath
Professor of Metabolic Medicine
British Heart Foundation Glasgow Cardiovascular
    Research Centre
University of Glasgow
Honorary Consultant Endocrinologist
Glasgow Royal Infirmary
Glasgow, United Kingdom
    Atherosclerosis in Rheumatic Disease

John C. Scatizzi, PhD
Post-Doctoral Fellow, Division of Rheumatology, Allergy,
    & Immunology
UC San Diego School of Medicine
La Jolla, California
    Signal Transduction

Jose U. Scher, MD
Teaching Assistant
Department of Medicine, Division of Rheumatology
New York University School of Medicine
New York, New York
    Neutrophils and Eosinophils

David C. Seldin, MD, PhD
Professor of Medicine and Microbiology
Boston University School of Medicine
Director, Amyloid Treatment and Research Program
Boston Medical Center
Boston, Massachusetts
    Amyloidosis

Jérémie Sellam, MD, PhD
Assistant Professor of Rheumatology
Paris Universitas – Pierre & Marie Curie Paris VI
Assistant Professor of Rheumatology
Saint-Antoine Hospital
Paris, France
    Clinical Features of Osteoarthritis

John S. Sergent, MD, MACR
Professor of Medicine
Vice Chair for Education and Residency Program Director
Vanderbilt University School of Medicine
Nashville, Tennessee
    *Polyarticular Arthritis; Polyarteritis and Related
    Disorders; Isolated Angiitis of the Central Nervous
    System; Arthritis Accompanying Endocrine
    and Metabolic Disorders*

Richard M. Siegel, MD, PhD
Investigator, Autoimmunity Branch
National Institute of Arthritis and Musculoskeletal
    and Skin Diseases
National Institutes of Health
Bethesda, Maryland
    Autoimmunity

Karl Sillay, MD
Assistant Professor and Director, Functional Surgery,
    Department of Neurological Surgery
University of Wisconsin School of Medicine and Public
    Health
Neurosurgeon, University of Wisconsin Hospital and
    Clinics, William S. Middleton Memorial Veterans
    Hospital, St. Mary's Hospital Medical Center, and
    Meriter Hospital
Madison, Wisconsin
    Neck Pain

Anna Simon, MD, PhD
Clinical Investigator, Department of General Internal
    Medicine
Radboud University Nijmegen Medical Centre Faculty
    of Medical Sciences
Nijmegen, The Netherlands
    Familial Auto-inflammatory Syndromes

Dawd S. Siraj, MD, MPH, TM
Assistant Professor of Medicine
Brody School of Medicine at East Carolina University
Director
ECU Physicians International Travel Clinic, Section
    of Infectious Diseases
Greenville, North Carolina
    Bacterial Arthritis

Martha Skinner, MD
Professor of Medicine
Boston University School of Medicine
Boston, Massachusetts
Amyloidosis

Kathleen A. Sluka, PT, PhD
Professor of Physical Therapy
Graduate Programs in Physical Therapy and Rehabilitation
   Science, in Pain Research, and in Neuroscience
University of Iowa Carver College of Medicine
Iowa City, Iowa
Neurological Regulation of Inflammation

C. Michael Stein, MBChB, MRCP
Dan May Professor of Medicine and Professor
   of Pharmacology
Vanderbilt University School of Medicine
Nashville, Tennessee
Immunoregulatory Drugs

John H. Stone, MD, MPH
Clinical Director of Rheumatology
Massachusetts General Hospital
Boston, Massachusetts
*The Classification and Epidemiology of Systemic
Vasculitis; Immune Complex–Mediated Small Vessel
Vasculitis*

Bob Sun, MD
Instructor, Department of Medicine, Division of
   Rheumatology
Northwestern University Feinberg School of Medicine
Attending Rheumatologist
Evanston Northwestern Healthcare
Evanston, Illinois
Rheumatic Manifestations of Hemoglobinopathies

Carrie R. Swigart, MD
Assistant Professor, Department of Orthopaedics and
   Rehabilitation, Hand and Upper Extremity Section
Yale University School of Medicine
New Haven, Connecticut
Hand and Wrist Pain

Zoltán Szekanecz, MD, PhD, DSc
Professor, Department of Medicine, Division of
   Rheumatology and Immunology
Institute for Internal Medicine, Rheumatology Division
University of Debrecen Medical and Health Science
   Center
Debrecen, Hungary
Cell Recruitment and Angiogenesis

Paul P. Tak, MD, PhD
Professor of Medicine and Director, Division of Clinical
   Immunology & Rheumatology
Academic Medical Center/University of Amsterdam
Faculty of Medicine
Amsterdam, The Netherlands
Biologic Markers

Ioannis O. Tassiulas, MD
Senior Investigator, Department of Medicine, Division
   of Rheumatology
University of Crete Medical School
Heraklion, Greece
*Clinical Features and Treatment of Systemic Lupus
Erythematosus*

**H. Guy Taylor, MBChB, MRCP(UK), FRACP,
   Dipl MSM(Otago)**
Consultant Rheumatologist
Wanganui Hospital
Wanganui, New Zealand
Immunoregulatory Drugs

Peter C. Taylor, MA, PhD, FRCP
Professor of Experimental Rheumatology
Head, Clinical Trials
Kennedy Institute of Rheumatology Division
Faculty of Medicine
Imperial College London
London, United Kingdom
*Cell-Targeted Biologics and Emerging Targets:
Rituximab, Abatacept, and Other Biologics*

Robert Terkeltaub, MD
Professor of Medicine
Rheumatology Training Program Director and Associate
   Division Director for Rheumatology–Allergy/
   Immunology
UC San Diego School of Medicine
La Jolla
Section Chief, Rheumatology–Allergy
VA Medical Center San Diego
San Diego, California
*Diseases Associated with Articular Deposition of
Calcium Pyrophosphate Dihydrate and Basic Calcium
Phosphate Crystals*

Thomas S. Thornhill, MD
Professor of Orthopedics
Harvard Medical School
Chief of Orthopedics
Brigham and Women's Hospital
Boston, Massachusetts
Shoulder Pain

Helen Tighe, BSc, PhD
Associate Adjunct Professor, Department of Medicine,
   Division of Rheumatology, Allergy, and Immunology
UC San Diego School of Medicine
La Jolla, California
*Rheumatoid Factors and Other Autoantibodies in
Rheumatoid Arthritis*

Betty P. Tsao, PhD
Professor of Medicine, Department of Medicine, Division
   of Rheumatology
David Geffen School of Medicine at UCLA
Los Angeles, California
Pathogenesis of Systemic Lupus Erythematosus

Peter Tugwell, MSc, MD, FRCPC
Professor of Medicine, Department of Medicine
Ottawa Health Research Institute
University of Ottawa Faculty of Medicine
Ottawa, Ontario, Canada
Assessment of Health Outcomes

Zuhre Tutuncu, MD
Associate Professor, Department of Rheumatology, Allergy,
    and Immunology
UC San Diego School of Medicine
La Jolla, California
Anticytokine Therapies

Katherine S. Upchurch, MD
Associate Professor of Medicine
University of Massachusetts Medical School
Clinical Chief, Division of Rheumatology
UMass Memorial Medical Center
Worcester, Massachusetts
Hemophilic Arthropathy

Wim B. Van den Berg, PhD
Professor of Experimental Rheumatology, Rheumatology
    Research, and Advanced Therapeutics
Radboud University Nijmegen Medical Centre Faculty of
    Medical Sciences
Nijmegen, The Netherlands
Animal Models of Inflammatory Arthritis

Filip Van den Bosch, MD, PhD
Rheumatologist
University Hospital Gent—Department of Rheumatology
Ghent, Belgium
*Undifferentiated Spondyloarthritis and Reactive
Arthritis*

Désirée M. F. M. Van der Heijde, MD, PhD
Professor of Rheumatology, Department of
    Rheumatology
Leiden University Faculty of Medicine
Leiden, The Netherlands
*Clinical Trial Design and Analysis; Ankylosing
Spondylitis*

Sjef M. van der Linden, MD
Professor of Rheumatology, Department of Medicine
University of Maastricht Faculty of Health, Medicine,
    and Life Sciences
CAPHRI Research Institute
Head, Division of Rheumatology, Department of
    Medicine
University Hospital of Maastricht
Maastricht, The Netherlands
Ankylosing Spondylitis

Jos W.M. van der Meer, MD, PhD, FRCP
Department of General Internal Medicine
Radboud University Nijmegen Medical Centre
Nijmegen, The Netherlands
Familial Auto-inflammatory Syndromes

John Varga, MD
Hughes Distinguished Professor of Medicine
Department of Medicine, Division of Rheumatology
Northwestern University Feinberg School of Medicine
Chicago, Illinois
*Systemic Sclerosis and the Scleroderma-Spectrum
Disorders*

Philippe Vinceneux, MD
Medecine Interne 2
Hospital Pitié-Salpêtrière
Paris, France
Relapsing Polychondritis

Benjamin W.E. Wang, MD, FRCPC
Associate Professor, Department of Medicine, Division
    of Rheumatology
University of Tennessee College of Medicine
Memphis, Tennessee
Nonsteroidal Anti-inflammatory Drugs

Lucy R. Wedderburn, MD
Reader in Paediatric Rheumatology
Rheumatology Unit, Institute of Child Health–University
    College London
London, United Kingdom
Juvenile Idiopathic Arthritis

Barbara N. Weissman, MD
Professor of Radiology
Harvard Medical School
Director, Radiology Residency Program
Vice Chair, Department of Radiology
Brigham & Women's Hospital
Boston, Massachusetts
Imaging Modalities in Rheumatic Disease

Victoria P. Werth, MD
Professor of Dermatology and Medicine
University of Pennsylvania School of Medicine
Chief of Dermatology
Philadelphia VA Medical Center
Philadelphia, Pennsylvania
The Skin and Rheumatic Diseases

Karin N. Westlund-High, PhD
Professor, Department of Physiology
University of Kentucky College of Medicine
Lexington, Kentucky
Neurological Regulation of Inflammation

Michael S. Wildstein, MD
President
Wildstein Spine Center
Charleston, South Carolina
Low Back Pain

Christopher M. Wise, MD
W. Robert Irby Professor of Medicine
Department of Medicine, Division of Rheumatology,
 Allergy, and Immunology
Virginia Commonwealth University School of Medicine,
 Medical College of Virginia Campus
Richmond, Virginia
 Arthrocentesis and Injection of Joints and Soft Tissue

Frederick Wolfe, MD
Clinical Professor of Medicine
University of Kansas School of Medicine
Director, National Data Bank for Rheumatic
 Diseases
Wichita, Kansas
 Fibromyalgia

Frank A. Wollheim, MD, PhD, FRCP
Emeritus Professor, Department of Rheumatology
Lund University Faculty of Medicine/Lund University
 Hospital
Lund, Sweden
 Enteropathic Arthritis

Patricia Woo, MBBS, BSc, PhD, CBE, FRCP, FMedSci
Professor of Paediatric Rheumatology
Faculty of Medicine
University College London
London, United Kingdom
 Juvenile Idiopathic Arthritis

Anthony D. Woolf, BSc, MBBS, FRCP
Professor of Rheumatology
Peninsula College of Medicine and Dentistry, Universities
 of Exeter & Plymouth
Exeter
Consultant Rheumatologist
Duke of Cornwall Rheumatology Unit, Royal Cornwall
 Hospital
Truro, United Kingdom
 Economic Burden of Rheumatic Diseases

Robert L. Wortmann, MD
Professor of Medicine
Dartmouth-Hitchcock Medical Center
Lebanon, New Hampshire
 Gout and Hyperuricemia

David Tak Yan Yu, MD
Professor of Medicine
David Geffen School of Medicine at UCLA
Los Angeles, California
 *Undifferentiated Spondyloarthritis and Reactive
 Arthritis*

John B. Zabriskie, MD
Professor Emeritus
Rockefeller University
New York, New York
 Poststreptoccocal Arthritis and Rheumatic Fever

Robert B. Zurier, MD
Professor, Department of Medicine, Division
 of Rheumatology
University of Massachusetts Medical School
Worcester, Massachusetts
 Prostaglandins, Leukotrienes, and Related Compounds

Anne-Marie Zuurmond, PhD
Biosciences Division
TNO Quality of Life
Leiden, The Netherlands
 Biologic Markers

"Plus ça change, plus c'est la même chose" –Jean-Baptiste Alphonse Karr

As we, the editors, worked on the 8th edition of *Kelley's Textbook of Rheumatology*, we were struck by Monsieur Karr's quote from 160 years ago. This textbook continues to change and evolve. The incomparable Ted Harris, who was editor-in-chief of the 7th edition, has stepped down, leaving Gary Firestein to fill his shoes. For the first time, a European editor, Iain McInnes, joined the group and helped create a truly international edition. Full color was introduced, new chapter formats were designed to assure a consistent look and feel for each topic, and algorithms for diagnosis and treatment as well as key point boxes were included. In addition, new authors were added to the list of luminaries that already contribute to the book, and there was a major effort to provide greater availability through electronic versions of reference material and on-line access.

While change has been in the air regarding many aspects of the book, some things never vary. The book was initially designed decades ago to provide scholarly rigor to the field of rheumatology and to offer definitive reviews of scientific advances as they apply to clinical medicine. This remained the touchstone of our enterprise for the past 4 years, just as it was for the previous seven editions. The painstaking job of identifying the premier authors to present definitive information on each topic required months of work, culminating in an editors' meeting in Costa Rica to finalize the chapters (well, it wasn't *all* work!). The arduous process of guiding, reviewing, and editing the outstanding contributions of our authors was time consuming but paled compared with the efforts that the authors put into creating their chapters. The thread connecting the past to the present was also evident in the continued effort of our valued co-editors John Sergent, Ralph Budd, and Shaun Ruddy. Our trusted colleagues at Elsevier, including Cathy Carroll and Kimberly Murphy, were always available and suffered with us in Costa Rica as well.

The present looks very encouraging indeed. *Kelley's Textbook of Rheumatology*, 8th edition, is a beautiful tome that is designed to carry on the tradition of being the definitive rheumatology resource. Looking to the future, we expect that this work will continue to evolve and change. New editors, new science, new authors, and new technology will be the rule rather than the exception.

As you begin to use this edition, please know that it is truly a labor of love. We have enjoyed the experience and hope that it is as valuable to you as the previous editions.

The Editors

CONTENTS

VOLUME I

🎥 Video available on the Expert Consult Premium Edition website.
📷 Supplemental images available on the Expert Consult Premium Edition website.

◼◂ Video available on the Expert Consult Premium Edition website.
◼ Supplemental images available on the Expert Consult Premium Edition website.

📹 Video available on the Expert Consult Premium Edition website.
📷 Supplemental images available on the Expert Consult Premium Edition website.

▣◄ Video available on the Expert Consult Premium Edition website.
▣ Supplemental images available on the Expert Consult Premium Edition website.

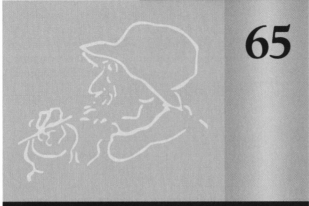

65 Etiology and Pathogenesis of Rheumatoid Arthritis

GARY S. FIRESTEIN

KEY POINTS

Rheumatoid arthritis (RA) is a complex disease involving numerous cell types, including macrophages, T cells, B cells, fibroblasts, chondrocytes, and dendritic cells.

Several genes are implicated in susceptibility to RA and severity of disease, including class II major histocompatibility complex genes, PTPN22, and peptidylarginine transferases.

Evidence of autoimmunity, including high serum levels of autoantibodies such as rheumatoid factors and anticitrullinated peptide antibodies, can be present for many years before the onset of clinical arthritis.

Adaptive and innate immune responses in the synovium have been implicated in the pathogenesis of RA.

Cytokine networks involving tumor necrosis factor, interleukin-6, and many other factors participate in disease perpetuation and can be targeted by therapeutic agents.

Bone and cartilage destruction seem to be primarily mediated by osteoclasts and fibroblast-like synoviocytes.

Rheumatoid arthritis (RA) is the most common inflammatory arthritis, affecting 0.5% to 1% of the general population worldwide. Although the prevalence is constant across the globe, regardless of geographic location and race, there are some exceptions. In China, the occurrence of RA is lower (about 0.3%), whereas it is substantially higher in other populations, such as the Pima Indians in North America (about 5%). Because of its prevalence and the ready accessibility of joint samples for laboratory investigation, RA has served as a useful model for the study of many inflammatory and immune-mediated diseases. As such, the information gleaned from these studies has provided new and unique insights into the mechanisms of normal immunity.

Although RA is properly considered a disease of the joints, abnormal immune responses can cause a variety of extra-articular manifestations. In some cases, production of rheumatoid factor (RF) with the formation of immune complexes that fix complement contributes to extra-articular findings. One of the mysteries of RA is why the synovium is the primary target.

Despite intensive work, the cause of RA remains unknown. Clues have been provided by detailed immunogenetic studies and the observation that underlying immunoreactivity antedates onset of arthritis by a decade. Progress in understanding the pathogenesis has been more robust. The roles of small molecule mediators of inflammation (e.g., arachidonic acid metabolites), autoantibodies, cytokines, growth factors, chemokines, adhesion molecules, and matrix metalloproteinases (MMPs) have been carefully defined. Synovial cells can exhibit behavior resembling a localized tumor, which invades and destroys articular cartilage, subchondral bone, tendons, and ligaments. Appreciation of these pathogenic mechanisms has increased awareness that irreversible loss of articular cartilage and bone begins soon after the onset of RA. Early interventions that suppress synovitis have a major impact on morbidity and mortality.

ROLES OF INNATE AND ADAPTIVE IMMUNITY IN ETIOLOGY AND PATHOGENESIS OF RHEUMATOID ARTHRITIS

Many mechanisms of disease are considered in this chapter. Innate immunity, which is a primitive pattern-recognition system that can lead to rapid inflammatory responses, has been implicated through the engagement of Fc receptors by immune complexes and perhaps Toll-like receptors (TLRs) by bacterial products. Antigen-driven T cell and B cell responses also may participate as a result of either xenoantigen reactivity or, more likely, responses directed at numerous autoantigens described later in the chapter. Cytokine networks participate with paracrine and autocrine loops that maintain cellular activation in the synovial intimal lining. Finally, permanent alterations in some cell types might occur during the evolution of disease that can accelerate destruction.

One potential synthesis of these data suggests that an induction phase, initiated by innate immunity, can "prepare" the joint for subsequent recruitment of inflammatory and immune cells (Fig. 65-1).[1] Cigarette smoke, bacterial products, viral components, and other environmental

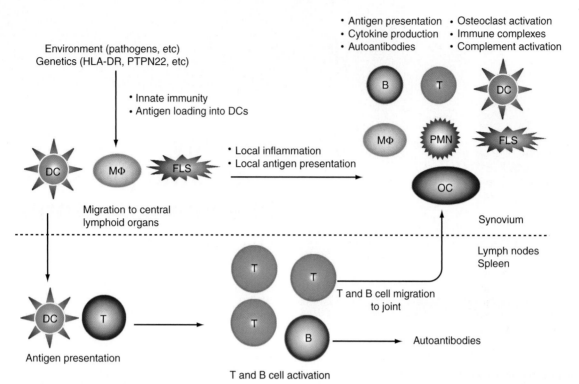

Figure 65-1 Schematic diagram of disease mechanisms that likely occur in rheumatoid arthritis. Innate immunity activates fibroblast-like synoviocytes (FLS), dendritic cells (DC), and macrophages (MΦ) in the earliest phases in individuals with underlying immune hyperreactivity as evidenced by the production of autoantibodies. The genetic makeup of an individual, including the presence of certain polymorphisms in genes that regulate immune responses, and environmental exposures are required. DC can migrate to the central lymphoid organs to present antigen and activate T cells, which can activate B cells. These lymphocytes can migrate back to the synovium and enhance adaptive immune responses in the target organ. In addition, repeated activation of innate immunity can lead directly to chronic inflammation and possibly antigen presentation in the synovium. In the latter phases of disease, many cell types activate osteoclasts (OC) through the receptor activator of nuclear factor κB (NFκB)/receptor activator of NFκB ligand (RANK/RANKL) system, although FLS and T cells likely provide the greatest stimulus. Autonomous activation of FLS also might contribute to this process.

stimuli can contribute to these responses. This process probably occurs often in normal individuals, but is self-limited. In some individuals, a predetermined propensity for immune hyperreactivity or autoreactivity might lead to a different outcome. The genome of these individuals encodes a variety of genes implicated in RA, including class II major histocompatibility complex (MHC) genes, protein tyrosine phosphatase-22 (PTPN22), cytokine promoter polymorphisms, population-specific genes (e.g., PADI4 in Japanese or Koreans), and other undefined genes. Abnormal T cell selection also could contribute by allowing autoreactive T cells to escape deletion. Immunoreactivity can be identified before clinical disease and can be manifested by the production of RFs and anticitrullinated peptide antibodies.

When cells are recruited to the synovium, or even perhaps at extrasynovial sites, antigens can be processed by dendritic cells (DCs). They can present antigen in synovial germinal centers or, more likely, migrate to central lymphoid organs, where they can activate naive T cells through interactions with the T cell receptor (TCR) and costimulatory signals. T cells can help B cells produce pathogenic antibodies or migrate to the joint where they can influence other cells through the production of cytokines such as interleukin (IL)-17 or through nonspecific cell contact mechanisms that do not require a specific antigen.

Ultimately, a destructive phase proceeds, which can be antigen dependent and independent and supported by mesenchymal elements, such as fibroblasts and synoviocytes. Bone erosions are subsequently caused by osteoclasts, whereas cartilage dissolution results from proteolytic enzymes produced by synoviocytes in the pannus or synovial fluid neutrophils. Anti-inflammatory mechanisms, such as soluble tumor necrosis factor (TNF) receptors, suppressive cytokines, cytokine binding proteins, protease inhibitors, lipoxins (LXs), antioxidants, antiangiogenic factors, and natural cytokine antagonists, are not present in sufficient concentrations to truncate the inflammatory and destructive process. The only way to suppress this response is through therapeutic interventions that either modulate pathogenic cells or neutralize the effector molecules produced by the rheumatoid process, or restore tolerance.

Although not proven, this general hypothesis takes into account many of the elements described by investigators in the field. The heterogeneity of mechanisms provides an explanation for the unpredictable response to therapeutic agents and allows clinicians to envision new therapeutic targets to prevent RA or interfere with the immunologic, inflammatory, or destructive components as separate but interrelated entities. Each of these mechanisms is discussed in detail in this chapter. Brief summaries of key points also are provided intermittently to help guide the reader through this complex maze.

ETIOLOGY OF RHEUMATOID ARTHRITIS

> ## Key Points
>
> - Genes play a key role in susceptibility to RA and disease severity.
> - Class II MHC genes, especially genes containing a specific 5-amino acid sequence in the hypervariable region of HLA-DR4, are the most prominent genetic association.
> - Newly defined genetic associations, including polymorphisms in PTPN22, PADI4, and many cytokines, suggest that the associations in RA are complex and involve many genes.

Table 65-1 Nomenclature for HLA-DR Alleles and Associations with Rheumatoid Arthritis

Old Nomenclature (HLA-DRB1* Alleles)	Current Nomenclature	Association with Rheumatoid Arthritis*
HLA-DR1	0101	+
HLA-DR4 Dw4	0401	+
HLA-DR4 Dw14	0404/0408	+
HLA-DRw14 Dw16	1402	+
HLA-DR4 Dw10	0402	−
HLA-DR2	1501, 1502, 1601, 1602	−
HLA-DR3	0301, 0302	−
HLA-DR5	1101-1104, 1201, 1202	−
HLA-DR7	0701, 0702	−
HLA-DRw8	0801, 0803	−
HLA-DR9	0901	−
HLA-DRw10	1001	−
HLA-DRw13	1301-1304	−
HLA-DRw14 Dw9	1401	−

*+, association observed; −, no association observed
From Weyand CM, Hicok KC, Conn DL, et al: The influence of HLA-DRB1 genes on disease severity in rheumatoid arthritis. Ann Intern Med 117:801, 1992.

Although the etiology of RA is unknown, many studies suggest that a blend of environmental and genetic factors is responsible; both are necessary, but are insufficient alone for full expression of the disease. The most compelling evidence for a genetic component is in monozygotic twins, in whom the concordance rate is 12% to 15% when one twin is affected compared with 1% for the general population. The risk for a fraternal twin of a patient with RA also is high (about 2% to 5%), but this is not more than the rate for other first-degree relatives. Although the immunogenetics is, at best, incompletely understood, one of the best-studied and perhaps most influential genetic risk factors is the class II MHC haplotype of an individual.

ROLE OF HLA-DR IN THE SUSCEPTIBILITY TO AND SEVERITY OF RHEUMATOID ARTHRITIS

The structure of class II MHC molecules in antigen presenting cells is associated with increased susceptibility and severity of RA and accounts for about 40% of the genetic influence. A genetic link between HLA-DR and RA was initially described in the 1970s with the observation that HLA-DR4 occurred in 70% of RA patients compared with about 30% of controls, giving a relative risk of having RA of approximately 4 to 5 to individuals with HLA-DR4.

The susceptibility to RA is associated with the third hypervariable region of DRβ-chains, from amino acids 70 through 74.[2] The epitope is glutamine-leucine-arginine-alanine-alanine (QKRAA), a sequence found in DR4 and DR14 (in which RA is more prevalent), in addition to some DR1β-chains. Current nomenclature attempts to clarify these ambiguities by including information on the specific DRβ sequences. The DR4β-chains with the greatest association with RA are referred to as DRB*0401, DRB*0404, DRB*0101, and DRB*1402 (Table 65-1). When the structure of this sequence is considered, 96% of patients with RA exhibit the appropriate HLA-DR locus in some populations.[3] In certain ethnic and racial groups, including Greeks, Pakistanis, Chileans, and African-Americans, the association with DR4 or QKRAA is not as prominent or is not associated.[4,5] The QKRAA epitope also might predict the severity of established RA, with a greater prevalence of extra-articular disease and erosions in patients with two susceptibility alleles compared with one.[6]

What is special about the shared epitope? The dose effect of the QKRAA epitope argues against a role for binding of a specific "rheumatoid antigen" because DR surface density usually does not alter T cell responses. Based on the crystal structure of HLA-DR molecules, the region associated with RA (QKRAA) primarily faces away from the antigen-binding cleft of the DR molecule that determines the specificity of peptides presented to CD4+ helper T cells. Attempts to elute peptides from the binding pocket of RA-associated alleles have not revealed a specific antigen that is either unique to or associated with RA.[7] The negative findings in RA contrast with type 1 diabetes mellitus, in which fragments of a key putative autoimmune target, glutamic acid decarboxylate 65, are bound to the diabetes-associated MHC molecules. There are several additional caveats about the role of this allele in RA, as follows:

1. Other genes must be involved because many healthy individuals carry the QKRAA motif and do not develop RA.
2. The converse hypothesis also is plausible, that is, QKRAA might have limited binding to an arthrotropic agent, preventing an appropriate T cell–mediated response.
3. The association between the shared epitope and RA might have little to do with antigen recognition and might function by shaping the T cell repertoire in the thymus (or autoantibody production, as noted with anticitrullinated peptide antibodies).
4. Specific DR sequences might alter intracellular MHC trafficking and antigen loading, indirectly affecting antigen presentation in a nonspecific fashion.
5. There is some evidence that certain DR4 epitopes are protective, such as DERAA in the same region of the molecule. Various hypotheses have attempted to explain this observation, including the possibility that the protective epitope contributes to regulatory T cell function. Although more controversial, class II associations related to the DQ region of the class II MHC locus also have been described for RA.

Another important discovery is that the shared epitope might not be an independent risk factor for RA, but instead is a marker for immunoreactivity and anticitrullinated peptide antibodies.[8] In a large series of patients with early undifferentiated inflammatory arthritis, one third of patients met criteria for RA within 1 year. Progression to RA occurred regardless of HLA-DR genotype if patients were positive for anticitrullinated peptide. When patients were stratified according to anticitrullinated peptide antibody, the shared epitope did not make an additional contribution to progression from undifferentiated arthritis to RA. These results suggest that the shared epitope contributes to immune hyperreactivity, but that anticitrullinated peptide antibodies are more closely associated with RA. In other studies, however, the presence of the shared epitope and anticitrullinated peptide antibodies together is associated with even greater disease severity.

The MHC associations can be even more complex when considering extended haplotypes in the central MHC region. The A1-B8-DR3 haplotype (also called "8.1") is linked to RA and many other autoimmune diseases independent of the HLA-DR4.[9] The locus contains more than 50 genes that could be responsible in addition to the class I and class II MHC proteins.

ADDITIONAL POLYMORPHISMS: CYTOKINES, CITRULLINATING ENZYMES, PTPN22, AND OTHERS

The clear genetic influences on RA have led to studies evaluating non-MHC genes. Single-nucleotide polymorphisms (SNPs) in promoter regions or coding regions have been extensively investigated in RA. SNPs in promoter regions could lead to altered gene regulation as a result of variable binding of transcription factors to promoters, whereas SNPs in coding regions directly change the amino acid sequence of the encoded protein. A second method for assessing genetic associations involves the evaluation of microsatellite sequences near key genes that are implicated in the disease. Microsatellites are tandem repeated sequences in the DNA that are primarily (but not exclusively) located in noncoding regions. Considerable heterogeneity exists in the length of each microsatellite, which can indirectly alter gene expression or be in linkage disequilibrium with other undefined genetic polymorphisms. Table 65-2 shows some of the SNPs and microsatellites that have been studied in RA. The relative contribution of each is still poorly defined, and variations in technique, stage of disease, and patient populations result in some disagreement among various reports.

Even some HLA associations that have been exhaustively studied remain controversial. It is easy to see why the genes with relatively weak contributions to susceptibility or severity remain uncertain. Many confounding influences can interfere with data interpretation, including remarkable differences in various racial and ethnic groups. Nevertheless, some patterns emerge. Given the importance of cytokines in RA (see later), it is not surprising that many studies have focused on these genes. The most intriguing evidence relates to TNF-α. This cytokine has been implicated in the pathogenesis of RA, and the TNF gene is located in the MHC locus on chromosome 6 in humans. Several polymorphisms of the TNF-α promoter, including two at positions −238

Table 65-2 Non–Class II Major Histocompatibility Complex Associations in Rheumatoid Arthritis

Gene	Region of Gene Studied	Associated with Rheumatoid Arthritis*
PTPN22	Coding	+
PADI4	Coding	+
STAT4	Intron	+
TRAF1-C5	Intron	+
TNF-α	Promoter	+
IL-1	Coding region; association with IL-1β strongest	+/−
IL-1Ra	Coding region	+
IL-3	Promoter	+
IL-4	Intron Promoter	+
IL-6	Promoter	−
IL-10	Promoter	−
IL-12	3′ untranslated region	−
IFN-γ	Intron microsatellite	+/−
CCR5	CCRδ32 allele	+
RANTES	Promoter	+
MIF	Promoter	+
RAGE	Ligand-binding domain	+
CTLA4	3′ untranslated region	+
TGF-β	Coding region	+
FcRγIII	Coding region	+

*+, association observed; −, no association observed; +/−, association observed in some studies, but not in others.

CCR5, chemokine receptor 5; c-5, complement 5; FcRγIII, Fc receptor γIII; IFN-γ, interferon-γ; IL, interleukin; IL-1Ra, interleukin-1 receptor antagonist; MIF, macrophage inhibitory factor; RAGE, receptor for advanced glycosylation end products; RANTES, regulated on activation, normally T cell expressed and secreted; TGF-β, transforming growth factor-β; TNF-α, tumor necrosis factor-α; TRAF1, TNF-receptor associated factor 1.

and −308, can alter gene transcription. Associations among the TNF polymorphisms and RA susceptibility and radiographic progression have been reported, although there is not uniform agreement. In addition, certain polymorphisms in cytokines, especially TNF-α or Fc receptors, have been associated with differential responses to therapy. Substitution of a T for a C at position −857 in the TNF-α promoter might confer greater responsiveness to TNF inhibitors.[10] Confirmation of such associations would require additional studies in larger patient populations and different ethnic and racial groups.

Associations with other polymorphisms or microsatellites have been identified for several other cytokines, inflammatory mediators, and chemokines, including IL-1, CCR5, and RANTES (regulated on activation, normally T cell expressed and secreted). One SNP for the T cell costimulatory molecule CTLA4 also is associated with susceptibility.[11] The contribution of each gene is relatively small compared with class II MHC, but combinations might provide an appropriate genetic background to influence the course of arthritis. No linkage has been noted with other cytokines that might play a role in RA, such as IL-6, osteopontin, and IL-12, and so far the data on IL-18 SNPs are variable.

Among the many noncytokine and non-MHC genetic linkages described for RA, the ones associated with peptidyl arginase deiminase (PADI) and PTPN22 are perhaps the most interesting. The PADI genes are responsible for the post-translational modification of arginine to citrulline. Four isoforms have been identified, known as PADI1 through PADI4. In light of the striking associations of RA with anticitrullinated peptide antibodies, several groups have investigated potential associations with these genes. The most promising is an extended haplotype in the PADI4 gene that can lead to increased levels of PADI4 protein secondary to enhanced mRNA stability.[12] In a Japanese cohort, a strong association was observed between PADI4 SNPs and susceptibility to RA. Confirmatory reports have been mixed because the association has been confirmed in other Asian populations, but not in Western Europe.[13] These studies suggest that the contribution of PADI4 to RA might be restricted, depending on the overall genetic background of the patient population.

PTPN22 associations have been discovered in large-scale screening efforts to identify SNP associations in RA.[14] Using 12,000 SNPs in the initial screens, a novel association was discovered at position 1858 in the PTPN22 gene. The allele containing thymidine leading to an amino acid substitution (R620W) was present in 8.5% of controls, but was found in nearly 15% in patients with seropositive RA. Subsequent studies have shown a similar association with systemic lupus erythematosus, type 1 diabetes, and several other autoimmune diseases. The precise function of PTPN22 is unknown, but it can regulate the phosphorylation status of several kinases important to T cell activation, including Lck and ZAP70. The R620W allele results in a gain of function that alters the threshold for TCR signaling. Because the PTPN22 allele is very rare in Japan, it is another gene (similar to PADI4) where susceptibility is specific for particular ethnic or racial populations. More recently, genetic associations linking STAT4 and the TRAF1-C5 region of the genome have been described.

GENDER

RA is one of many autoimmune diseases that is predominant in women. The ratio of female-to-male patients (2:1 to 3:1) is significant, yet not nearly as high as in Hashimoto's thyroiditis (25:1 to 50:1), systemic lupus erythematosus (9:1), or autoimmune diabetes mellitus (5:1). The gender effect also is observed in some animal models of autoimmunity, such as the NZB/NZW model of systemic lupus erythematosus in which female mice have more severe disease. The role of estrogens has been explored by various methods.[15] Auto-antibody-producing B cells exposed to estradiol are more resistant to apoptosis, suggesting that autoreactive B cell clones might escape tolerance. The effect on T lymphocytes is more difficult to reconcile with the female preponderance in RA because estrogens tend to bias T cell differentiation toward the T helper type 2 (Th2) phenotype. The cytokines produced by this subset, such as IL-4 and IL-13, usually are considered anti-inflammatory in animal models of arthritis and are present in only limited amounts in the RA synovium. The data are still controversial, however, because estradiol also can increase interferon (IFN)-γ production (typically a Th1 cytokine) by antigen-specific clones from patients with multiple sclerosis. Estrogen receptors are expressed on

fibroblast-like synoviocytes (FLS) and, when stimulated, increase production of metalloproteinases in the synovium. In macrophage cell lines, estrogen can enhance production of TNF-α. Taken together, these data suggest that the hormone milieu can have significant effects on the cells known to participate in RA. The effects are complex, however, and the specific mechanisms responsible for increased susceptibility to RA in women are uncertain.

Considerable effort also has been expended on case-controlled and retrospective studies to determine the influence of oral contraceptives. Although some suggestive data exist for a protective effect, the effect (if it exists) is probably very small and temporary (i.e., delaying rather than preventing disease). Other endocrine influences, including corticotropin-releasing hormone or estrogen synthase, have been linked with RA. Nulliparity also has been described as a risk factor, but not all studies confirm this.

Pregnancy often is associated with remission of the disease in the last trimester. More than three quarters of pregnant patients with RA improve in the first or second trimester, but 90% of these experience a flare of disease associated with an increase in RF titers in the weeks or months after delivery. The mechanism of protection is not defined, but might be due to the expression of suppressive cytokines such as IL-10 during pregnancy, production of alpha fetoprotein, or alterations in cell-mediated immunity. One intriguing finding is that fetal DNA levels in the maternal peripheral blood correlate with the propensity for improved symptoms in pregnant RA patients. It is uncertain whether the DNA itself contributes, or whether it is a marker for increased leakage of fetal cells into the maternal circulation.[16] A possible relationship between the alleviation of RA symptoms during the last trimester of pregnancy and immunogenetics may be supported by the observation that during pregnancy, alloantibodies in the maternal circulation develop against paternal HLA antigens. Maternal-fetal disparity in HLA class II phenotypes can correlate with pregnancy-induced remission. More than three fourths of pregnant women with maternal-fetal disparity of HLA-DRB1, HLA-DQA, and HLA-DQB haplotypes have significant improvement, whereas disparity is observed in only one fourth of women whose pregnancy is characterized by continuous active arthritis.[17] Suppression of maternal immune responses to paternal HLA haplotypes might be protective. This question remains unsettled because another study failed to find a correlation between the HLA disparity and clinical improvement during pregnancy.[18]

TOBACCO

Numerous environmental factors certainly contribute to RA susceptibility, although no specific exposure has been identified as a pivotal agent. Smoking is the best defined environmental risk factor for seropositive RA in certain populations. The reason for its influence on the development of synovitis is not fully defined, but could involve the activation of innate immunity and PADI in the airway. Citrullinated peptides have been detected in bronchoalveolar lavage samples of smokers, and this could provide a stimulus for generation of anticitrullinated peptide antibodies in susceptible individuals.[19] Repeated activation of innate immunity, especially in an individual with underlying genetically determined autoreactivity, potentially could contribute to autoreactivity and the initiation of RA.

RISE AND FALL OF RHEUMATOID ARTHRITIS

Any proposed etiology for RA should incorporate one additional key element: RA might be a relatively new disease in Europe and Northern Africa. Examination of ancient skeletal remains in Europe and Northern Africa fails to reveal convincing evidence of RA, even though other rheumatic diseases, such as osteoarthritis, ankylosing spondylitis, and gout, are readily discernible. In contrast, typical marginal erosions and rheumatoid lesions are present in the skeletons of Native Americans found in Tennessee, Alabama, and Central America from thousands of years ago. The first clear descriptions of RA in Europe appeared in the 17th century, and the disease was distinguished from gout and rheumatic fever by Garrod in the mid-19th century. Although still controversial, one line of thought suggests that the disease migrated from the New World to the Old World coincident with opening the trade and exploration routes. Because genetic admixture was relatively limited, an undefined environmental exposure potentially caused RA in susceptible Europeans. The most obvious explanation would be that an infectious agent is responsible. Other environmental influences, such as tobacco smoking, were introduced to the Old World at the same time, however, and could play a role.

Equally intriguing, the severity and incidence of RA seem to be decreasing (Fig. 65-2).[20] Lower severity could be related to the advent of new treatments, and decreasing incidence could be due to a "birth cohort" effect. In certain well-defined populations, including Native Americans, the incidence of RA gradually declined by 50% over the last half of the 20th century. The birth-cohort theory suggests that the earlier high incidence of disease was caused by an etiologic agent, and the exposure decreased with each succeeding generation. Changes in hygiene and other lifestyle modifications related to industrialization might contribute, and an infectious agent might be less prevalent secondary to these societal changes, as with many other infectious diseases.

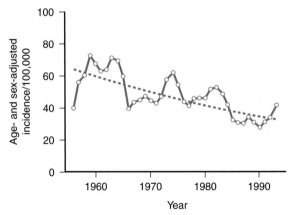

Figure 65-2 Declining incidence of rheumatoid arthritis. Population studies in Minnesota have shown a gradually decreasing incidence of rheumatoid arthritis over the last 50 years. Similar results have been observed in Native American populations. *(From Doran MF, Pond GR, Crowson CS, et al: Trends in incidence and mortality in rheumatoid arthritis in Rochester, Minnesota, over a forty-year period. Arthritis Rheum 46:635, 2002.)*

POSSIBLE CAUSES OF RHEUMATOID ARTHRITIS

Key Points

- Many pathogens have been associated with RA, including viruses, retroviruses, and *Mycoplasma*, although a precise etiologic link has not been established.
- Data suggest that a specific RA pathogen is unlikely.
- Repeated inflammatory insults, especially through specialized receptors that recognize common molecules produced by pathogens, in a genetically susceptible individual might contribute to breakdown of tolerance and subsequent autoimmunity.

Although genetic factors predispose an individual to developing RA, the environment clearly also contributes. Considerable effort has been expended to assess the role of infectious agents (Table 65-3) in addition to environmental exposures such as tobacco. The pathogen potentially could initiate disease through a variety of mechanisms, including direct infection of the synovium, activation of innate immunity by pattern-recognition receptors that bind to components of the agent, or through molecular mimicry that induces an autoreactive adaptive immune response.

INFECTIOUS AGENTS: DIRECT INFECTION AND INNATE IMMUNE RESPONSES

Toll-like Receptors and the Inflammasome in the Joint

Infectious agents could contribute to the initation or perpetuation of RA through a variety of mechanisms. Some arthrotropic microorganisms potentially could infect the synovium and cause a local inflammatory response. There is increasing awareness that the innate immune system also could directly affect the onset and course of synovitis. Pathogen-associated molecular pattern receptors, especially TLRs, are expressed by sentinel cells in the host that provide a first line of defense. These receptors recognize perserved structures in bacteria and other infectious agents and permit rapid release of inflammatory mediators, activation of antigen presenting cells, and enhancement of adaptive immune responses.

Table 65-3 Possible Infectious Causes of Rheumatoid Arthritis

Infectious Agent	Potential Pathogenic Mechanisms
Mycoplasma	Direct synovial infection; superantigens
Parvovirus B19	Direct synovial infection
Retroviruses	Direct synovial infection
Enteric bacteria	Molecular mimicry (QKRAA)
Mycobacterium	Molecular mimicry (proteoglycans, QKRAA), immunostimulatory DNA
Epstein-Barr virus	Molecular mimicry (QKRAA)
Bacterial cell walls	Macrophage activation

There are at least 11 TLRs in humans, such as TLR2 (binds peptidoglycans), TLR3 (binds double-stranded RNA), TLR4 (binds lipopolysaccharide), and TLR9 (binds bacterial DNA containing CpG motifs). When engaged, the TLRs activate signal transduction pathways such as nuclear factor κB (NFκB) and mitogen-activated protein (MAP) kinases. In some cases, such as for TLR3, additional pathways are engaged to increase expression of antiviral genes such as IFN-β.

Many of these pattern-recognition receptors are expressed by rheumatoid synovial tissue and cultured FLS, including TLR2, TLR4, and TLR9.[21-24] Exogenous TLR ligands, such as bacterial peptidoglycan and DNA, and endogenous ligands, such as heat shock proteins (HSPs), fibrinogen, and hyaluronan, are present in arthritic joints (see later). Engagement of these receptors participates in certain animal models of arthritis and can exacerbate synovial inflammation. TLR3, which recognizes viral double-stranded RNA and activates the antiviral response, also is expressed by cells in the intimal lining. Necrotic debris containing mRNA from RA synovial fluid cells activates TLR3 signaling and proinflammatory gene expression in synovitis.

As with smoking, which activates innate immunity in the lungs and leads to citrullination of peptides, current models of RA suggest that repeated engagement of this system in the synovium could help initiate the disease. This hypothesis could explain why specific pathogens have been difficult to identify in the joint. In contrast, a genetically susceptible individual potentially could break tolerance if the TLRs are repeatedly engaged.

A second mechanism that regulates innate immunity involves a novel structure called the "inflammasome." This complex includes several proteins involved in recognition of "danger signals" and pathogens, such as muramyl dipeptides and uric acid. One central component is cryopyrin, also called NALP3, which is linked to caspase 1 (IL-1 convertase) by adapter proteins. When the inflammasome is engaged, caspase 1 is activated, and IL-1 is produced. Mutations in this pathway, especially in cryopyrin, have been associated with autoinflammatory disorders such as Muckle-Wells syndrome and familial cold autoinflammatory disease. Inflammation induced by uric acid crystals or adenosine triphosphate uses this pathway and can be abrogated by IL-1 inhibitors. Cryopyrin is abundant in RA synovium and is constitutively expressed by FLS and macrophages.[25] Expression in cultured FLS is markedly increased by TNF-α. Although the role of the inflammasome in RA has not been fully defined, its ability to induce cytokine production by exposure to bacterial products and other danger signals suggests that it participates in IL-1 and IL-18 regulation.

Bacteria, Mycobacteria, Mycoplasma, and their Components

Active infection of synovial tissue by pyogenic bacteria is an unlikely cause of RA, and extensive searches for a unique or specific organism in synovial tissue or joint effusions have been negative. Antibodies to certain organisms, such as *Proteus*, are reportedly elevated in the blood of patients with RA, but this could represent an epiphenomenon or a nonspecific B cell activation.[26] Sensitive polymerase chain reaction techniques to identify the bacterial genome in synovial tissue show that a high percentage of RA and reactive arthritis

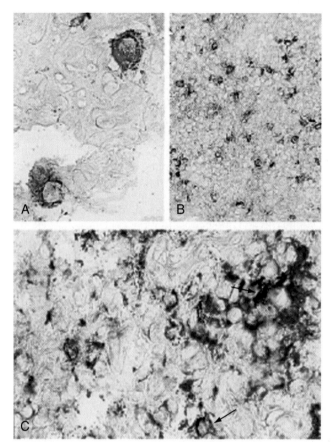

Figure 65-3 Accumulation of bacterial peptidoglycan in rheumatoid synovium. **A** and **B**, Immunohistochemistry shows synovial cells containing peptidoglycan *(red)*. **C**, Double staining studies show that bacterial peptidoglycan accumulates in synovial macrophages *(arrow)*. These bacterial products can activate Toll-like receptors and stimulate cytokine production. *(From Schrijver IA, Melief MJ, Tak PP, et al: Antigen-presenting cells containing bacterial peptidoglycan in synovial tissues of rheumatoid arthritis patients coexpress costimulatory molecules and cytokines. Arthritis Rheum 43:2160, 2000.)*

patients contain bacterial DNA sequences.[27] The bacteria identified are not unique and generally represent a cross section of skin and mucosal bacteria, including *Acinetobacter* and *Bacillus*. The synovium may function as an adjunct to the reticuloendothelial system in arthritis, allowing local macrophages to accumulate circulating bacterial products. Nucleotide sequences found in prokaryotic cells can activate TLRs and stimulate innate immune responses.

In addition to prokaryotic DNA, bacterial peptidoglycans have been detected in RA synovial tissue (Fig. 65-3).[28] Antigen presenting cells containing these products express TLRs and produce proinflammatory cytokines such as TNF-α. It is unknown whether the peptidoglycans activate cells in situ, or whether phagocytic cells from other sites or the blood engage the molecules and migrate to the joint. In either case, it is not difficult to imagine how they can contribute to synovial inflammation.

The relevance to human disease has been suggested by animal models of arthritis that depend on TLR2, TLR4, and TLR9. Rodents injected with streptococcal cell walls develop severe polyarticular arthritis. The initial phase of disease resolves and is followed by a chronic T cell–dependent phase that resembles RA. The arthritogenicity of complete

Freund's adjuvant in the rat adjuvant arthritis model largely depends on mycobacterial DNA that can bind to TLR9 and activate an adaptive immune repsonse. Endogenous TLR4 ligands also could play a role in disease perpetuation when the inflammatory response leads to local accumulation of HSPs and fibrinogen.[29]

Considerable attention has been directed toward a potential role for *Mycoplasma* and *Chlamydia* in arthritis. *Mycoplasma*-derived superantigens, such as from *Mycoplasma arthritidis*, can directly induce T cell–independent cytokine production by macrophages and can exacerbate or trigger arthritis in mice immunized with type II collagen.[30] There also is a higher prevalence of anti–*Mycoplasma pneumoniae* IgG antibodies in RA patients than matched controls. Despite this and other circumstantial evidence, most efforts to identify *Mycoplasma* and *Chlamydia* organisms or DNA in joint samples have produced negative results, and there is no direct evidence to support these organisms as etiologic agents.[31]

Epstein-Barr Virus, dnaJ Proteins, and Molecular Mimicry

Epstein-Barr virus (EBV) has been indirectly implicated in RA.[32] It is a polyclonal B lymphocyte activator that increases the production of RF, and rheumatoid macrophages and T cells have defective suppression of EBV proliferation in human B cells. Rheumatoid patients seem to have higher levels of EBV shedding in throat washings, an increased number of virus-infected B cells in the circulating blood, higher levels of antibodies to normal and citrullinated EBV antigens, and abnormal EBV-specific cytotoxic T cell responsiveness compared with controls. Patients with RA have a defect related to the control and elimination of EBV-transformed lymphocytes; this has fueled speculation that a lymphocyte defect is a triggering event in this disease.

Additional intriguing data implicating EBV in RA are derived from sequence homology between the susceptibility cassette in HLA-DR proteins and the EBV glycoprotein gp110. Similar to DRB*0401, gp110 contains the QKRAA motif, and patients with serologic evidence of a previous EBV infection have antibodies against this epitope.[33] T cell recognition of EBV epitopes in some patients with HLA-DR4, HLA-DR14, or HLA-DR1 might cause an immune response directed at innocent bystander cells through "molecular mimicry." This hypothesis could account for disease perpetuation in the absence of active infection in patients with a specific MHC genotype. Nevertheless, the data are circumstantial, and gp110 is only one of many xenoproteins that contain QKRAA. The *Escherichia coli* dnaJ protein, a bacterial HSP, contains the sequence and represents a potential link between gut bacteria and chronic arthritis. RA T cells, especially synovial fluid T cells, but not normal peripheral blood cells, have increased proliferative responses to this protein, perhaps supporting the molecular-mimicry link between a variety of QKRAA-containing proteins and arthritis.[34]

Parvovirus

Antecedent infection with parvovirus B19 has been suggested in some patients with RA based on serologic evidence.[35] Despite these cases, few rheumatoid patients have evidence of such a coincident infection, and only about 5% have evidence of recently acquired parvovirus B19 infection at the time of disease onset. Using polymerase chain reaction methods to detect B19 genes in synovial tissue, however, 75% of RA synovium samples were positive compared with about 20% of non-RA controls.[36] Immunohistochemical evidence of the B19 protein VP-1 was detected in patients with RA, but not other forms of arthritis.[37] In other studies, no evidence of the B19 genome in joint samples was detected, or the presence of B19 DNA was not specific for RA.

The mechanisms of parvovirus B19–induced synovitis, when it does occur, could be related to alterations in the function of FLS.[38] In a cell culture model of synoviocyte invasion into cartilage, infection with the parvovirus significantly increased the migration of cells into the matrix. Mice that are transgenic for the B19 protein NS1 did not develop clinical arthritis, but were more susceptible to collagen-induced arthritis even though they did not have the usual arthritis-associated genetic background. Levels of anti–type II collagen antibodies and TNF-α in the serum were similar to DBA/1 mice that had been immunized with type II collagen. These data suggest that the B19 genome might not cause arthritis, but can enhance an arthritogenic response to environmental stimuli.

Other Viruses

Because rubella virus and the rubella vaccine can cause synovitis in humans, the virus has attracted some attention as a possible triggering agent. Live rubella virus can be isolated from synovial fluid in some patients with chronic inflammatory oligoarthritis or polyarthritis in the absence of firm clinical evidence of rubella. Rubella patients do not have the classic polyarticular involvement seen so often in RA, however. Most have an oligoarthritis involving large joints. As with parvovirus B19 infection, it is possible that a subset of patients with chronic polyarthritis have disease resulting from direct infection with wild-type or attenuated rubella virus.

Studies of synovial tissue in a variety of inflammatory and noninflammatory arthropathies also have shown DNA of other viruses, such as cytomegalovirus and herpes simplex, but not adenovirus or varicella zoster.[39] As with bacterial DNA, parvovirus, and EBV, the localization of viral DNA to the inflamed joint might be related to the migration of inflammatory cells containing the viral genome or other nonspecific mechanisms, rather than an active infection. Although the hypothesis that one or more of these viral infections might serve as a triggering agent in the genetically susceptible host is appealing and intellectually satisfying, the pathogenic role of these agents is uncertain.

Retroviral infections have been suggested as a cause of RA. Extensive searches for potential agents have not been fruitful; this does not rule out the possibility that difficult-to-detect agents might be present, or even that endogenous retroviruses might play a role. Endogenous retroviruses are abundant in inflamed and normal synovium, and certain transcripts are differentially expressed in RA cells.[40] In one study, higher levels of HERV-K10 gag protein from a common endogenous retrovirus were detected by polymerase chain reaction more often in RA compared with osteoarthritis and normal peripheral blood mononuclear cells. Some indirect studies are suggestive of retroviral infection, such as the demonstration of zinc-finger transcription factors in cultured synoviocytes. In addition, the pX domain of one human retrovirus, human T-lymphotropic virus-1, causes synovitis in transgenic mice, and synoviocytes from patients infected with human T-lymphotropic virus-1 express some features of a transformed phenotype, with increased proliferation and cytokine production.[41] Other studies failed to show increased expression of human retrovirus-5 proviral DNA in rheumatoid synovium.[42] The notion that retroviruses or endogenous viruses contribute to RA is appealing, although there is no direct evidence of their involvement. Some viral products potentially could interact with receptors such as TLR3 or TLR7 to enhance production of chemokines and type I interferons.

AUTOIMMUNITY

Key Points

- Evidence of autoimmunity can be present in RA many years before the onset of clinical arthritis.
- Autoantibodies, such as RFs and anticitrullinated protein antibodies, are commonly associated with RA.
- Autoantibodies occur in RA that recognize either joint antigens, such as type II collagen, or systemic antigens, such as glucose phosphate isomerase.
- The autoantibodies potentially can contribute to synovial inflammation through several mechanisms, including local activation of complement.

The idea that aberrant immune responses are directed toward self-antigens in RA was recognized with the discovery of RF in the blood of patients with the disease. Initially described by Waaler and later by Rose, it was not until the mid-1950s that Kunkel and colleagues firmly established that RF is an autoantibody. Although understanding of autoantigens has changed over the years, and the relative contributions of cellular and humoral immunity have been debated, emphasis on the role of autoantibodies in RA has re-emerged in recent years. Autoantibody titers usually do not correlate well with disease activity. Improvement can be associated with modest decreases in levels of RFs or anticitrullinated peptide antibodies, although the changes tend to be relatively modest and are not consistent. These observations suggest that autoantibodies, although they contribute to the pathogenesis of RA, are not the primary driving factor.

Rheumatoid Factor: Evidence of Autoimmunity in Rheumatoid Arthritis

The identification and characterization of RF as a self-antibody that binds to the Fc portion of IgG was the first direct evidence that autoimmunity might play a role in RA. For many years, immune complexes comprising RF and other immunoglobulins were thought to be solely responsible for RA. Today, the presence of RF and its resultant pathogenic consequences are still considered cardinal features of RA. Longitudinal studies show that RF production often precedes the onset of RA by many years (Fig. 65-4).[43] Although some

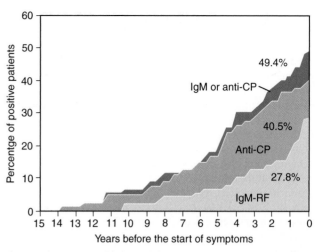

Figure 65-4 Autoantibody production in rheumatoid arthritis. Rheumatoid factors and anticitrullinated peptide (CP) antibodies are detected in the blood long before the onset of clinical arthritis in many patients. *(From Nielen MM, van Schaardenburg D, Reesink HW, et al: Specific autoantibodies precede the symptoms of rheumatoid arthritis: A study of serial measurements in blood donors. Arthritis Rheum 50:38, 2004.)*

patients are initially "seronegative" for RA and subsequently convert to "seropositive," this typically occurs during the first year of disease activity.

The role of RF in the pathogenesis of RA has been suggested by circumstantial evidence. Patients with a positive test result for RF in blood have more severe clinical disease and complications than seronegative patients. RF also is able to fix and activate complement by the classic pathway, and there is clear evidence of local complement production and consumption in the rheumatoid joint. Large quantities of IgG RF are produced by rheumatoid synovial tissue and form complexes through self-association. RF-containing immune complexes are readily detected in RA synovial tissue and the surface layers of cartilage. The latter is especially relevant because immobilized complexes can facilitate complement fixation with resultant release of chemotactic peptides. In experiments performed in patients with RA, a marked inflammatory response was elicited when RF from the patient was injected into a joint, but not when normal IgG was given.[44] B cell–targeted therapies, such as rituximab, can deplete peripheral B lymphocytes and modestly decrease titers of RF. Although this does not correlate with clinical responses, there is a suggestion that RF levels decrease in responders and increase again coincident with clinical relapses.

Three quarters of patients with RA are seropositive using standard tests for RF, although the percentage can be 90% when assayed for IgM RF with enzyme-linked immunosorbent assays. Breaking tolerance for immunoglobulin determinants recognized by RF has a genetic influence as well because first-degree relatives of seropositive patients with RA frequently are seropositive themselves. Although IgG and IgM RFs are thought to be the most abundant and pathogenic in RA, IgE RF also has been shown in some patients, especially patients with extra-articular manifestations. IgE RF potentially can complex with aggregated IgG in synovial tissue, and the subsequent complexes could degranulate synovial mast cells through activation of Fc receptors in the synovium. IgA RFs are also produced in RA, including in patients who are seronegative as determined by standard clinical tests that primarily detect IgM RF.

The RFs produced in RA patients differ from those produced in healthy individuals or from patients with paraproteins.[45] The avidity of RF for the Fc portion of IgG is several orders greater in RA than in Waldenström's macroglobulinemia or in cryoglobulins. The germline-derived RFs are produced by immature CD5-positive B cells, and many paraproteins expressed by malignant B cells (such as Waldenström's macroglobulinemia) are derived from the germline. In addition, some normal B cells in adult human tonsil tissue express and synthesize germline-encoded RFs, although they do not secrete the protein. RFs produced by RA B cells are distinct in that these proteins often are not encoded by germline genes. Instead, their sequence seems to be derived through rearrangements and somatic mutations. RF analysis in synovial membrane cultures from patients with a variety of diseases has indicated that only cells from patients with seropositive RA synthesize RF spontaneously. IgM RF represents about 7% of the total IgM produced by cells, and IgG RF represents 3% of IgG synthesized in the synovial cultures.

The expression of any particular RF idiotype is under genetic control and is related to restriction of the number of relevant or expressible variable (V) genes available in the germline.[46] RFs in RA primarily use the variable heavy 3(VH3) gene and a variety of variable light (VL) genes, whereas natural antibodies use VH1 or VH4 and the Vκ3 genes. The κ light chain repertoire expressed in RF-producing cells isolated from one patient with chronic RA was enriched for two specific Vκ genes, known as Humkv325 and Humkv328, which also are frequently associated with RF paraproteins.[47] The κ-variable domains contain many somatic mutations and non–germline-encoded nucleotides, however. Based on the extent of substitutions, the selection and production of these specific RFs were likely due to antigenic drive, rather than derived directly from the germline, as is the case with many paraproteins. Additional RFs have been identified with characteristics similar to an antigen-driven response, although some examples of germline RFs also have been isolated from RA synovium. A crystal structure of one IgM RF bound to IgG showed a key contact residue of the RF with the Fc portion of IgG containing a somatic mutation, supporting the notion that the mutations are related to affinity maturation.[48]

Autoimmunity to Citullinated Peptides

A striking recent observation related to autoantibodies is that immunoglobulins that bind to citrullinated peptides are produced by patients with RA and have significant prognostic implications. The discovery originated with reports in the 1970s that antibodies directed against keratin were detected in rheumatoid serum, and that the primary target antigen was filament-aggregating protein, filaggrin. These antibodies bind to epitopes on filaggrin that contain citrulline, which is derived from post-translational modification of arginine by PADI. Humans have four isoforms of PADI. PADI2 and PADI4 are especially abundant in synovium[49] and certain SNPs are associated with RA in Asian populations.

Induction of PADI expression and citrullination of peptides are not specific to RA and can occur in many inflammatory settings.[50] Not only are other inflammatory arthropathies marked by citrullinated proteins, but also other organs, such as the lungs in smokers, have significant PADI activity. Similarly, citrullinated peptides are present in most animal models of arthritis.[51] The specific proteins that are modified vary widely, but include many normal constituents, such as vimentin, fibrinogen and fibronectin, and xenoproteins such as EBV-derived peptides.[52] Immunohistochemistry shows citrullinated peptides in RA synovial tissue infiltrating cells (Fig. 65-5) and in extracellular deposits that often colocalize with various isoforms of PADI, especially PADI2 and PADI4.

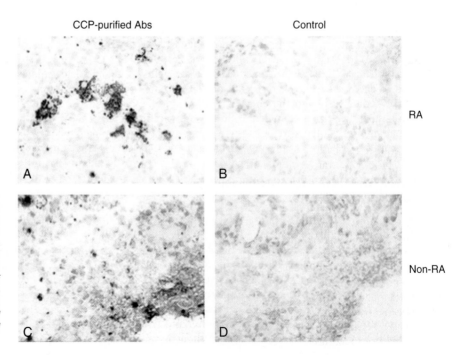

Figure 65-5 Citrullinated peptides in inflamed synovium. Rheumatoid arthritis (RA) synovium and nonrheumatoid synovium contain citrullinated peptides, detected with an anti–cyclic citrullinated peptide (CCP) antibody (*red-brown in synovium*). Control is an irrelevant antibody. Although citrullinated peptides are not specific, the production of anticitrullinated protein antibodies is more specific to RA. *(From Vossenaar ER, Smeets TJ, Kraan MC, et al: The presence of citrullinated proteins is not specific for rheumatoid synovial tissue. Arthritis Rheum 50:3485, 2004.)*

Anticitrullinated peptide antibodies have been reported in serum samples of 80% to 90% of RA patients.[53] In some studies, they are more specific for RA than RF, with specificity approaching 90%. Similar to RF, anticitrullinated peptide can appear long before the onset of clinical arthritis and could be a marker for immune hyperreactivity and subclinical inflammation leading to protein citrullination in a variety of tissues. Anticitrullinated peptide antibodies also are produced by synovial tissue B cells and can be detected in synovial fluid. The antibodies are predictors of more aggressive disease marked by bone and cartilage destruction. Some data suggest that the HLA-DR associations in RA are due to an association between the susceptibility epitope and anticitrullinated peptide antibody production.

Anticitrullinated peptide antibodies also might have pathogenic potential. Although anticitrullinated peptide antibodies have minimal effect when directly injected into mice, they enhance the arthritogenic potential of anti–type II collagen antibodies in the collagen-induced arthritis model.[54] The autoantibodies are not simply a marker of disease, but can, similar to RF, participate in the disease process. Citrullination also can increase T cell responses to arthritogenic antigens. Citrullination of rat albumin leads to the formation of antibodies that also cross-react with the unmodified protein.[55] The action of PADI on type II collagen enhances its immunogenicity, perhaps by enhancing its ability to bind to the class II MHC peptide binding groove.[56]

Autoimmunity to Cartilage-Specific Antigens

Because synovial tissue inflammation is a hallmark of RA, it is natural to assume that certain joint-specific antigens might play an etiologic or pathogenic role. The number of potential antigens is extensive, and there is no convincing evidence to date that one specific "rheumatoid" antigen exists. In contrast, the emerging picture of autoimmunity in RA tends to implicate patterns of self-directed responses, rather than a single epitope that encompasses all patients at all times during the disease. It is possible that articular autoimmunity could vary with the stage of disease, the clinical manifestations, and treatment.

Type II Collagen

The discoveries that immunization with type II collagen can cause arthritis in rats and mice, and that the disease can be passively transferred by IgG fractions containing anticollagen antibodies or by transfer of lymphocytes from affected animals have spawned extensive experiments that illustrate the antigenicity of collagen, the arthrotropic nature of the disease produced, and the dependence on class II MHC genes. It is clear that functional T cells are necessary to initiate a collagen-induced arthritis, and that a major immunogenic and arthritogenic epitope on type II collagen resides in a restricted area of the type II collagen chains.

Most data in humans suggest that RA is not caused by the development of antibodies to type II collagen, but that the inflammatory response is amplified by their production (Table 65-4). Serum samples from patients with RA contain antibody titers to denatured bovine type II collagen that are

Table 65-4 Potential Autoantigens in Rheumatoid Arthritis

Cartilage antigens
Type II collagen
gp39
Cartilage link protein
Proteoglycans
Aggrecan
Citrullinated peptides
Glucose-6-phosphoisomerase
HLA-DR (QKRAA)
Heat-shock proteins
Heavy-chain binding protein (BiP)
hnRNP-A2
Immunoglobulins (IgG)

significantly higher than the titers found in control sera[57]; however, there is no difference in antibody titers to native collagen, indicating that the denatured form generated after the breakdown of connective tissue might serve as the immunogen. Anticollagen antibodies purified from serum samples of patients with RA can activate complement, generating fragments derived from the fifth component of complement (C5a) when they bind to cartilage. This finding adds relevance to the observations that anticollagen antibodies can be eluted from rheumatoid articular cartilage. In addition, isolated synovial tissue B lymphocytes actively secrete anti–type II collagen antibodies in almost all patients with seropositive RA, whereas articular cells from non-RA patients do not.[58] Synovial fluid T cells also recognize and respond to type II collagen, and 3% to 5% of RA synovial fluid–derived T cell clones are autoreactive to the protein. T cell responses to type II collagen, especially a dominant epitope at amino acid 263-270, are much greater if the epitope is glycosylated, or if the protein is citrullinated.[59] In addition, the presence of anti–type II collagen antibodies in RA is associated with the RA-related PTPN22 polymorphism.[60]

gp39 and Other Cartilage-Specific Antigens

Several other cartilage components besides type II collagen have been implicated as potential autoantigens in RA. Among the most provocative is cartilage glycoprotein gp39. Several gp39 peptides can bind to the HLA-DR*0401 molecule and stimulate proliferation of T cells from patients with RA.[61] BALB/c mice, which are often resistant to experimental arthritis, develop polyarticular inflammatory arthritis after immunization with gp39 and complete Freund's adjuvant. Although anti-gp39 antibodies are detected in only a small percentage of patients, it seems to be reasonably specific for RA.[62] Other examples of potential cartilage autoantigens include proteoglycans, aggrecan, cartilage-link protein, and other types of collagen. T cell clones derived from RA peripheral blood can proliferate in response to aggrecan, and most of these cells have a Th1 cytokine profile, suggesting that they contribute to the Th1 bias in synovial tissue.[63] Proteomic analysis of RA serum using peptide arrays to detect multiple autoantibodies also identifies anti-gp39 antibodies in patients with early RA, and this may be associated with less aggressive disease.[64]

Autoimmunity to Nonarticular Antigens

Increasing attention has been focused on autoimmune responses that are not specific for components unique to articular structures.[65] Although their role in etiology is not always clear, at least some autoantibodies (e.g., RF and anti-citrullinated peptide) can appear before the onset of clinical disease. In other cases, the antigen-antibody system might participate in patterns of autoimmune responses that can lead to synovial inflammation.

Glucose-6-Phosphate Isomerase

A spontaneous arthritis model in K/BxN mice shows that antigen-specific immunity against a seemingly irrelevant nonarticular antigen can lead to destructive arthritis.[66] The mechanism of disease relates to the fortuitous formation of antibodies to the ubiquitous enzyme glucose-6-phosphate isomerase in the mice, and the disease can be transferred to normal mice with the serum of affected animals. The passive arthritis model is dependent on the alternate complement pathway, Fc receptors (especially FcRγIII), and mast cells, but not T cells or B cells. IL-1 seems to be more important than TNF-α, and the IL-1 knockout mice are almost completely protected from disease. This effect can be overcome by administration of a TLR ligand such as lipopolysaccharide, which shares a downstream signaling pathway with IL-1. Other cytokines, such as IL-6, and signaling pathways, such as p38 MAP kinase and upstream kinases such as MKK3, also are required for full expression of the disease.

Histochemical studies indicate that glucose-6-phosphate isomerase adheres to the surface of cartilage, permitting local antibody binding and complement fixation. Initiation of synovial inflammation in this model is complex and requires mast cells. The earliest stages also require increased vascular permeability, which provides access to the synovium and cartilage.[67] It is unclear whether the same mechanisms that start the synovial inflammatory response are required for continued arthritis. It is possible that the initial phases involving mast cell and vascular permeability are replaced by a more traditional mechanism of antibody-mediated complement fixation when serum proteins have access to cartilage with glucose-6-phosphate isomerase adherent to it.

Although the model appears at first glance to be due to a ubiquitous antigen, articular homing of the antigen suggests that it behaves similar to other arthritis models with "joint-specific" antigens. Although initial data suggested some specificity for RA, anti–glucose-6-phosphate isomerase antibodies are detected in a small percentage of RA patients and are not specific for the disease.[68] Nevertheless, glucose-6-phosphate isomerase might contribute, along with several other antibody systems, to local complement fixation and inflammation.

Heterogeneous Nuclear Ribonucleoprotein-A2 and Heavy-Chain Binding Protein

Several other autoantigens that are expressed in synovium have been characterized in RA, although they also are produced in many other locations. Antibodies directed against the heterogeneous nuclear ribonucleoprotein-A2, sometimes called RA33, occur in about one third of RA patients and patients with other systemic autoimmune diseases. There may be some specificity for RA, however, compared with osteoarthritis and seronegative spondyloarthropathies. Anti-RA33 antibodies also are produced in the TNF-α transgenic mouse model of RA, suggesting that proinflammatory cytokines can independently lead to a breakdown of tolerance for this particular protein.[69] Although not especially sensitive or specific for RA when used in isolation, an algorithm involving anti-ribonucleoprotein-A2, RF, and anticitrullinated peptide can be used to predict patients with early synovitis who will progress to erosive RA.[70] Autoantibodies that bind to stress-protein immunoglobulin heavy-chain binding protein (BiP) also have been observed.[71] About 60% of RA patients have anti-BiP antibodies, and the specificity is reportedly more than 90%. In addition to humoral responses, RA T cells can proliferate in response to this protein. Immunization of mice with BiP does not cause arthritis, but it can cross-tolerize mice and prevent collagen-induced arthritis if administered before immunization with type II collagen.[72] BiP is normally expressed in many tissues, but is markedly increased in RA synovium.

Heat Shock Proteins

The HSPs are a family of mainly medium-sized (60 to 90 kD) proteins produced in response to stress. These proteins have conserved amino acid sequences; for example, certain HSPs of *Mycobacterium tuberculosis* have considerable homology with HSPs of humans. The HSPs may facilitate intracellular folding and translocation of proteins as they protect cells from insults induced by heat, bacteria, and oxygen radicals. Immunity against HSPs contributes directly to synovitis and joint destruction in the adjuvant arthritis model in rats in which T lymphocytes recognize an epitope of mycobacterial HSP65 (amino acids 180 through 188). Some of these cells also recognize cartilage proteoglycan epitopes,[73] perhaps explaining the targeting of joints.

Some patients with RA have elevated levels of antibodies to mycobacterial HSPs, especially in synovial fluid.[74] Most T cell clones isolated from RA synovial fluid with specificity to mycobacterial components express the γδ TCR (instead of the more common αβ form) and do not display CD4 or CD8 surface antigens. Freshly isolated synovial fluid T cells from patients with RA briskly proliferate in response to the acetone-precipitable fraction of *M. tuberculosis* and recombinant 65-kD HSP.[75] Proliferation to other recall antigens, such as tetanus toxoid, is not increased, however. Synovial fluid mononuclear cells activated by 60-kD mycobacterial HSP inhibit proteoglycan production by human cartilage explants.[76] This effect depends on the generation of cytokines such as IL-1 and TNF-α by the activated cells. Human 60-kD HSP is expressed in the synovium; the amount expressed per cell seems to be similar in osteoarthritis, RA, and normal tissue.

SYNOVIAL PATHOLOGY AND BIOLOGY

The primary inflammatory site in RA is the synovium. Infiltration of synovial tissue with mononuclear cells, especially T cells and macrophages, and synovial intimal lining hyperplasia are hallmarks of the disease (Fig. 65-6). In this section, the various cell lineages and histologic patterns of rheumatoid synovium are discussed.

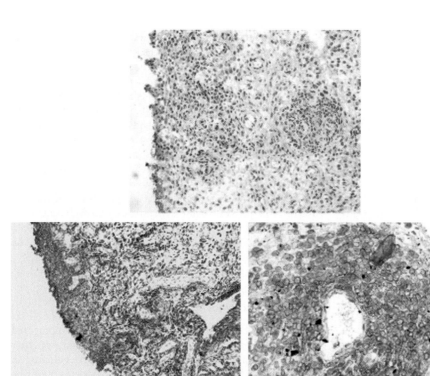

Figure 65-6 Histopathologic appearance of rheumatoid arthritis synovium. Intimal lining hyperplasia, angiogenesis, and a prominent mononuclear cell infiltrate are present. Panels show standard histology *(top)* and immunostaining for macrophages *(brown* in the intimal lining at *bottom, left)* and a perivascular T cell aggregate *(bottom right).* *(Courtesy of Dr. Paul-Peter Tak.)*

Key Points

- The synovium in RA is marked by intimal lining hyperplasia and sublining infiltration with mononuclear cells, especially CD4⁺ T cells, macrophages, and B cells.
- Synovial pathology and function of synovial cells in RA are distinctive in that:
  - Intimal lining FLS display unusually aggressive features.
  - Macrophages in the intimal lining are highly activated.
  - Lymphocytes can either diffusely infiltrate the sublining or form lymphoid aggregates with germinal centers.
  - Sublining CD4⁺ T cells mainly display the memory cell phenotype.
  - Synovial B cells and plasma cells in RA exhibit evidence of antigen-driven maturation and antibody production.
  - DCs potentially can present antigens to T cells in synovial germinal centers.
  - Mast cells produce small molecule mediators of inflammation.
  - Neutrophils are rarely present in RA synovium.

SYNOVIAL INTIMAL LINING CELLS: TYPE A AND TYPE B SYNOVIOCYTES

The synovial intimal lining is a loosely organized collection of cells that form an interface between the synovium and the synovial fluid space. The intimal lining cells lack tight junctions and a definite basement membrane. The increase in cell number in RA can be substantial. In the normal joint, the lining is only one to two cell layers deep, whereas in RA, it is often 4 to 10 cells deep. Two major cell types are found in the lining: a macrophage-like cell known as a type A synoviocyte and a fibroblast-like cell known as a type B synoviocyte. The former are derived from the bone marrow and express macrophage surface markers, such as CD68, Fc receptors, and CD14, and abundant HLA-DR, whereas the latter express little if any class II MHC antigens, are devoid of macrophage markers, and have a scant endoplasmic reticulum. The type B cells, also called FLS, express certain proteins that are unusual for mesenchymal cells, including vascular cell adhesion molecule-1 (VCAM-1), CD55 (decay accelerating factor), cadherin 11, and the proteoglycan-synthesis enzyme uridine diphosphoglucose dehydrogenase. The relative numbers of type A and type B cells are usually similar in normal synovium. There is an absolute increase in both cell types in RA, although the percentage increase in macrophage-like cells is often greater. In addition, type A synoviocytes tend to accumulate in the more superficial regions of the intimal lining.

Synovial macrophages are terminally differentiated cells that presumably do not divide in the joint, and the accumulation of cells in RA is likely from the ingress of new bone marrow–derived precursors. Mesenchymally derived type B synoviocytes can divide locally in response to the proliferative factors generated by the activated immune response. Platelet-derived growth factor (PDGF), transforming growth factor (TGF)-β, TNF-α, and IL-1 produced by many different cells combine with products of arachidonic acid metabolism to induce proliferation of these cells. In addition, pluripotential mesenchymal stem cells that arise in the bone marrow and circulate through the blood can migrate into the synovium and differentiate into type B synoviocytes.[77]

Although local proliferation of cells in the intimal lining likely occurs, rheumatoid synovium rarely shows mitotic figures, and thymidine uptake occurs in only a few synovial cells. Using a monoclonal antibody that recognizes dividing cells, an even lower rate of cell division (approximately 0.05%) is apparent.[78] A higher percentage of cells that express the cell cycle–specific antigen proliferating cell nuclear antigen are present in RA lining cells compared with osteoarthritis. This correlates with the lining cell expression of the proto-oncogene c-myc, a gene that is intimately linked with fibroblast proliferation.

The architecture of the synovial intimal lining is distinct from other lining layers in the body. In contrast to serosal surfaces, the intimal lining does not include epithelial cells, it lacks a basement membrane, and has no tight junctions. Rather than serving as a discrete barrier, it is a loose association of cells that is discontinuous in some locations. Cadherin 11, from a class of adhesion proteins that are ubiquitous in various tissues, serves as the major mediator of homotypic aggregation by FLS.[79] Immunohistochemistry shows abundant expression of this protein in the intimal lining. Its importance in the synovial architecture was confirmed in cadherin 11 knockout mice, in which the intimal lining was virtually nonexistent. Finally, cadherin 11–expressing cells self-aggregate in vitro into a structure that appears similar to a synovial lining, and this function can be blocked with a cadherin 11-Fc fusion protein. Targeting cadherin 11 with blocking antibodies suppresses arthritis in the passive K/BxN model. These data suggest that FLS, similar to T cells, B cells, and macrophages, play a crucial role in the pathogenesis of inflammatory arthritis.

After rheumatoid synovium is enzymatically dispersed in vitro, two major populations of adherent cells can be readily identified.[80] One type of cell is macrophage-like; these cells have DR antigens, Fc receptors, and monocyte lineage-differentiation antigens and are capable of phagocytosis. They have a limited life span in vitro, rarely surviving more than a few weeks even in the presence of exogenous growth factors or colony-stimulating factors (CSFs). A second type is defined by the presence of antigens expressed primarily on fibroblasts and by the absence of phagocytic capability, demonstrable DR antigens, or antigens of the monocytic lineage. When the enzymatically dispersed cells are cultured for several passages, this last cell type ultimately survives and proliferates, resulting in a relatively homogeneous population of fibroblast-like cells.

Ultrastructural studies and cell-cloning experiments of dissociated rheumatoid synovial cells have supported this classification.[81] Fibroblast-like cells grow slowly, with a doubling time of 5 to 7 days. The fibroblast-like cells grown from the dispersed cells can be passaged for several months in vitro. Their doubling rate is rapid at first, perhaps owing to the presence of cytokines produced by contaminating macrophages in the culture or a carryover effect from the synovial milieu. Over time, proliferation slows, and after 12 to 15 passages, the cells gradually become senescent and ultimately cease to grow. Although it has not been proven that these cells originate solely from the synovial intimal lining, the fact that a significant percentage of cells expresses VCAM-1 and CD55 suggests that at least some are derived from this region. Synovial fibroblasts from RA have some characteristics reminiscent of tumors or transformed cells (see following).

Experiments examining synovial tissue and FLS gene expression profiles have identified subsets of patients with specific patterns that correlated with synovial histopathology. Hierarchical clustering identified two types of FLS characterized by distinctive gene expression profiles.[82] FLS from inflammatory tissues exhibited a TGF-β gene signature that also has been described in myofibroblasts and seems to be involved in wound healing. A second pattern was reminiscent of insulin-like growth factor regulated genes and was observed in relatively noninflammatory RA tissue. Whether the pathogenic processes in the synovium imprint the synoviocytes or vice versa has not been determined. Attempts to distinguish RA and osteoarthritis FLS expression profiles from each other have offered mixed results. No consistent differences have been observed, although one study suggested that IL-32 and the chemokine CCL2 are relatively overexpressed in RA cells.

Aggressive Features of Rheumatoid Arthritis Fibroblast-like Synoviocytes

Rheumatoid FLS show some unusual properties compared with cells obtained from other synovia. Several properties reminiscent of cell transformation have been evaluated in RA and have led to the notion that synoviocytes might be permanently altered by their environment. Adherence to plastic or extracellular matrix is generally required for normal fibroblasts to proliferate and survive in culture. Although FLS typically grow and thrive under conditions that permit adherence, RA synoviocytes also can proliferate in an anchorage-independent manner.[83] In addition, cultured RA synoviocytes can exhibit defective contact inhibition and express a variety of transcription factors, such as c-Myc, which are typically abundant in tumor cells. Poorly regulated cell growth likely occurs in vivo as well; studies examining X-linked genes show oligoclonality in the synoviocyte population from RA, but not osteoarthritis, synovium.[84] This oligoclonality is especially true of cells derived from the invading pannus, which is the most aggressive region of the synovium. Increased telomerase activity, another feature of transformed tissue, also is present in RA synovium and can be observed in fibroblast growth factor (FGF)–stimulated RA synoviocytes.

In a severe combined immunodeficiency (SCID) mouse model, enzymatically dispersed FLS are coimplanted into the mice with cartilage explants. The rheumatoid cells invade the cartilage matrix, looking like destructive pannus.[85] This phenomenon occurs even if pure populations of long-term cultured RA FLS are used (Fig. 65-7).[86] Because these synoviocytes are devoid of T cells and macrophages, there is no contribution from an immune response to murine antigens. The invading cells express VCAM-1, which potentially could facilitate adhesion to cartilage or chondrocytes, and proteases that digest the cartilage matrix. Control synoviocytes from osteoarthritis patients and normal dermal fibroblasts do not invade the cartilage, indicating that the activity is unique to rheumatoid FLS. These observations form the compelling evidence that rheumatoid synoviocytes have unique characteristics that can resemble partial transformation.

Using viral vectors to introduce cytokine genes into this explanted synoviocyte, one can evaluate their respective roles in cartilage invasion. IL-1 receptor antagonist (IL-1Ra), a natural antagonist to IL-1, has no effect on

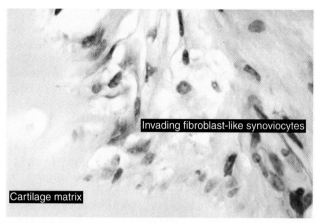

Figure 65-7 Invasion of rheumatoid arthritis synoviocytes into cartilage explants in severe combined immunodeficiency syndrome (SCID) mice. Rheumatoid arthritis fibroblast-like synoviocytes were co-implanted with normal human cartilage into the renal capsule of SCID mice. The synoviocytes attached to the cartilage and invaded the matrix. Several chondrocytes in lacunae also are present. *(Courtesy of Dr. S. Gay.)*

synoviocyte invasion, but decreases perichondrocyte matrix loss.[87] In contrast, IL-10 decreases invasion, but does not alter matrix loss. Finally, overexpression of soluble TNF receptors has no consistent effect in this model. These studies suggest that excessive production of IL-1 and underexpression of IL-10 contribute to the invasive properties of RA synoviocytes. In another study, transfecting normal synoviocytes with the human papillomavirus gene encoding E6 induced the rheumatoid phenotype.[88] The E6 protein leads to the inactivation and degradation of the p53 tumor-suppressor protein. Although this is not the sole explanation for the altered adhesion and invasion properties of RA synoviocytes, deficient p53 function potentially can contribute. The oncogenes Ras and c-Myc also contribute to synoviocytes' invasiveness in this model, and transfection of cells with dominant negative constructs decreases the aggressive phenotype of the rheumatoid cells. Antisense treatment of cells to knockdown membrane type I metalloproteinase expression also reverses the abnormality.[89]

SYNOVIAL T LYMPHOCYTES

Immunohistologic Patterns

In chronic RA, the synovium contains a collection of T lymphocytes that can lead to an organizational structure that resembles a lymph node. The distribution of lymphocytes in the tissue varies from discrete lymphoid aggregates to diffuse sheets of mononuclear cells, with the most prominent location for T cells being the perivascular region. These collections consist of small, CD4+ memory T cells (CD45RO+) with scant cytoplasm. A few scattered CD8+ T cells accumulate in the aggregates; formation of ectopic germinal centers in RA synovial tissue may depend on these cells. Peripheral to these foci is a transitional zone with a heterogeneous mixture of cells, including lymphocytes, occasional undifferentiated blast cells, plasma cells, and macrophages (see Fig. 65-6). Intercellular communication by soluble mediators and direct cell-cell contact occurs here via adhesion molecules, including the lymphocyte function-associated antigens.

Considerable heterogeneity exists in the histologic patterns within a single joint and from patient to patient. Synovial biopsy studies suggest that at least six sites must be evaluated to decrease the risk of sampling error to 10% to 20% or less.[90] In situations in which the synovia of more than one joint from an individual patient is available, the same general histopathologic patterns are usually apparent in tissue from separate sites. Although the correlation between clinical disease activity is tenuous, the presence of granulomatous lesions might be associated with extra-articular disease.

Regulation of Lymphoid Aggregate Formation

T cells often constitute 30% to 50% of cells in RA synovia, and most are CD4+. About 5% of cells are B lymphocytes or plasma cells, although in some tissues the percentage can be considerably higher. B cells are located primarily within reactive lymphoid centers, whereas plasma cells and macrophages are often found outside these centers. This arrangement is consistent with T cell–dependent B lymphocyte activation. Plasma cells, the main immunoglobulin producers, migrate away from the germinal centers after differentiation. CD4+ cells in RA synovium are in intimate contact with B lymphocytes, macrophages, and DCs. Chemokines play a key role in the organization of tissues into lymphoid structures such as aggregates and germinal centers. CXCL13 and CCL21 seem to be especially important, and their expression in rheumatoid synovium correlates with the presence of this microarchitecture.[91] CXCL13, in particular, is produced by synovial follicular DCs. Similarly, plasma cells expressing the chemokine receptor CXCR3 are present in the rheumatoid synovium. The CXCR3 ligand, Mig/CXCL9, is highly expressed in intimal lining synoviocytes and sublining cells and presumably plays a role in the recruitment and retention of plasma cells to these CD4+ T cell aggregates.[92]

The architecture of lymphoid structures in rheumatoid synovium also is regulated by members of the TNF superfamily. Lymphotoxin-α (LTα) and lymphotoxin-β (LTβ) form trimeric molecules in various combinations that can bind to distinct cell surfaces. LTα1β2 (one α chain and two β chains) binds exclusively to the LTβ receptor (LTβ-R), whereas LTα3 can bind to the TNF-R1 and TNF-R2. A third related member of the family, LIGHT, also can interact with the LTβ-R or to the herpesvirus entry mediator (HVEM). LTα, LTβ, and LIGHT regulate the function and organization of lymphoid tissues. Deletion of either LTα or LTβ seriously impairs lymphoid development, whereas lymph nodes develop normally in LIGHT-deficient mice. In the SCID mouse model using RA tissue explants, depletion of CD8+ T cells led to loss of follicular DCs, depletion of LTα1β2, and disintegration of the lymphoid follicles.[93] IL-16 production by CD8+ T cells seems to play a role in this process.

Although LTα3 is difficult to detect in RA, LTα1β2 and LIGHT are present.[94] In addition to regulating lymphoid aggregate and germinal center formation, LTα1β2 can directly stimulate FLS to produce chemokines such as CCL2 and CCL5 that attract T cells into the joint.[95] LIGHT also enhances osteoclast differentiation and induces expression of MMP9, TNF-α, IL-6, and IL-8 by macrophages.[96] When LTβ and LIGHT are inhibited in the collagen-induced arthritis model using a genetically engineered receptor, clinical arthritis is decreased.[97] The construct is not effective, however, in the passive arthritis model, in which the pathogenic antibodies are directly administered to mice. The LIGHT axis seems to play a more important role in the early phases of disease, but not in the terminal effector stages.

Synovial T Cell Phenotype

RA synovial T lymphocytes display an activated surface phenotype, with high expression of HLA-DR, CD69, and CD27. CD27+CD4+ T cells provide B cell help that potentially can increase synovial antibody production.[98] For maximal T cell responses, a second signal, in addition to antigen stimulation, is usually required. CD28 is one of these costimulatory molecules on T lymphocytes and is highly expressed by synovial T cells in RA. Its ligands, CD80 and CD86, also are displayed on antigen presenting cells in the joint, providing an excellent environment for T cell activation. The importance of the CD80/CD86-CD28 interaction is supported by the observation that an agent that blocks this interaction, abatacept, is effective in RA. One unusual phenotype of synovial T cells in RA is a population that expresses CD4 but lacks CD28. Oligoclonal expansion of CD4+CD28− T cells has been described in peripheral blood and joint samples of patients with RA.[99] The cells can be cytotoxic and can respond to autoantigens, but are inefficient B cell stimulators. This population of T cells also occurs more frequently in patients with extra-articular manifestations of RA.

CD40, another costimulatory molecule, and its ligand on T cells, CD40L, also are expressed in RA synovium.[100] CD40L, a member of the TNF superfamily, can synergize with IL-1 for the production of cytokines, such as granulocyte-macrophage colony-stimulating factor (GM-CSF), by CD40-bearing synoviocytes.[101] Synovial lymphocytes also bear adhesion molecules of the very late activation antigen (VLA) and lymphocyte function–associated antigen superfamily of integrins, which may enable the inflammatory response to localize and persist within the synovium. A high level of telomerase activity also is present in synovial lymphocytes in RA, but not in osteoarthritis or trauma patients.[102] Telomerase activity level in the synovial T cells correlates with the intimal lining hyperplasia, angiogenesis, and local lymphocyte accumulation.

T cell activation and the induction of adhesion molecules and other "activation markers" may not occur within the joint; rather, this T cell phenotype could enter the synovium and remain within the joint under the influence of locally expressed chemotactic factors and their armamentarium of adhesion molecules. The cytokine milieu of the joint induces adhesion molecules, such as intercellular adhesion molecule-1 (ICAM-1), VCAM-1, and connecting segment-1 (CS-1) fibronectin, on vascular endothelium. These, in conjunction with chemokines and other chemoattractants, call the cells to the joint based precisely on this phenotype.

Synovial T cells in RA express characteristic receptors to specific chemokines. The chemokine receptor CCR5 is the ligand for macrophage inhibitory protein (MIP)-1α and MIP-β and is highly expressed in the infiltrating RA T cells.[103] This particular receptor, along with CXCR3, is preferentially found on Th1 T cells, an observation that might explain accumulation of this phenotype in the rheumatoid synovium.

Expression of nonfunctional CCR5 alleles that protect from human immunodeficiency virus infection might diminish the risk of RA. The chemotactic factor stromal cell–derived factor-1 (SDF-1; CXCL12) also is produced by synovial tissue, and its specific receptor, CXCR4, is displayed by rheumatoid synovial T cells.[104] Other T cell phenotypes are implicated in the pathogenesis of synovitis and can be detected in RA, including Th17 cells, which produce IL-17, and CD4+CD25+ regulatory T cells (Tregs), which can suppress immune responses (see subsequent section T cell subsets).

Numerous groups have evaluated TCR gene rearrangements for clues related to antigen-specific expansion. In some patients, a pattern emerged suggesting an increased number of T cells expressing Vβ3, Vβ14, and Vβ17, especially in synovial tissue. These particular Vβ genes are structurally related and are unusually susceptible to activation by superantigens. Most studies either have not found evidence for the restricted clonality of T cells in RA synovial fluid, synovial tissue, and blood, or have not identified expansion of different Vβ or Vα genes.[105]

Overall, the data suggest that the local accumulation of T cells in the joint is not related to proliferation induced by a particular antigen. Instead, antigen-independent processes related to the expression of chemokines and adhesion molecules on vascular endothelium and circulating lymphocytes help determine the mononuclear cell infiltrate. Although local antigen-specific expansion might occur, it is probably responsible for a small component of the T cell infiltrate. The cells that encounter their appropriate antigen in the correct cytokine and antigen presenting cell environment potentially can activate other local cells through direct cell-cell contact (Fig. 65-8) or the elaboration of lymphokines. An alternative explanation is that T cell activation mainly occurs in central lymphoid organs. In this scenario, DCs that encounter antigens in the synovium or other sites migrate to lymphatic tissue and present antigen to naive T cells. When activated, these T cells enter the circulation and can home to the joint where they can produce cytokines to activate resident cells.

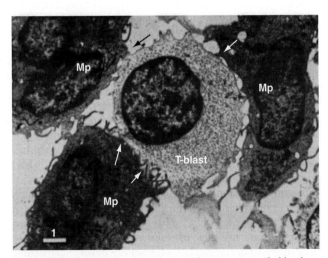

Figure 65-8 T cell in rheumatoid synovial tissue surrounded by three macrophages (Mp). *Arrows* point to probable intercellular bridging. Contact between macrophages in T cells can lead to antigen-independent activation of macrophages with production of cytokines and proteases. *(Courtesy of Dr. H. Ishikawa and Dr. M. Ziff.)*

Synovial T Cell Immune Responses

The histopathologic appearance of RA, with exuberant infiltration of the synovium with T lymphocytes, is often pointed to as evidence of a T cell–mediated disease because this is also characteristic of antigen-specific responses. The synovium can respond to inflammation in only a few ways, however. The histologic appearance of chronic arthritides that are not mediated by T cells (e.g., chronic tophaceous gout) exhibits many of the same features. Progressive destruction in RA patients despite the presence of acquired immunodeficiency syndrome suggests that non–T cell mechanisms also are important.[106] Nevertheless, efficacy of abatacept, a novel T cell–directed approach that interferes with costimulation, shows that T cell responses play a role in most patients with RA.

The microheterogeneity of the rheumatoid synovial tissue, with different numbers and proportions of cell lineages in each area, suggests that antigens presented at each location also might differ, with type II collagen presented to T cells one place, proteoglycans presented elsewhere, and responses to HSPs or viral antigens in yet another region. Although synovial T cells generally are considered activated, proliferative and cytokine responses are often less than normal peripheral blood cells or even autologous peripheral blood T cells. Spontaneous and stimulated cytokine production, including Th1 factors such as IFN-γ and IL-2, is relatively low. Responses directed toward recall antigens also are deficient, although RA synovial T cells can proliferate briskly to certain HSPs.

The mechanisms of decreased responsiveness in the synovial tissue compartment have not been studied as extensively as in synovial fluid or peripheral blood, but they likely include exposure to suppressive factors (e.g., TGF-β), abnormal redox potential that suppresses TCR signal transduction, or induction of anergy. Another contributor to local anergy is the relative lack of the costimulatory molecule CD80 on HLA-DR⁺ FLS because coculture of T cells with the synoviocytes suppresses subsequent allogeneic responses.[107]

Synovial T cells in RA functionally resemble resting peripheral blood T lymphocytes that have been activated by cytokines rather than antigen.[108] Synovial and blood T lymphocytes are able to stimulate macrophages to produce TNF-α in a cell contact–dependent manner. This process depends on NFκB and is mechanistically distinct from T cell activation via the TCR, which is independent of NFκB. The contribution of T cells to the proinflammatory cytokine milieu may be unrelated to antigen-mediated events and could result from passive activation after exposure to the cytokine environment.

Although increased immunoreactivity contributes to the etiology of RA, the search for a specific rheumatoid antigen has not been fruitful. More recent data, especially in animal models, suggest that breakdown of tolerance can be due to a combination of factors early in development. Mutations in the ZAP70 gene can lead to spontaneous T cell–dependent inflammatory arthritis in mice.[109] This protein is intimately involved with transducing TCR signals and activating T lymphocytes. An abnormal ZAP70 gene leads to defective positive and negative selection in the thymus and allows autoreactive T cells to escape. As a result, mice produce

autoantibodies (e.g., RF and anti–double-stranded DNA) and develop a severe destructive arthritis. The disease can be transferred by thymocytes or peripheral CD4⁺ T cells into syngeneic mice with a normal ZAP70 gene.

The cytokine profile of this model is much like RA, and mice with deficient TNF-α, IL-1, or IL-6 have reduced synovitis. IFN-γ deficiency has no effect, whereas IL-10 deficiency exacerbates disease. These studies show that minor changes in the TCR complex can alter T cell selection and induce T cell–dependent arthritis. Despite the clear T cell dependence of the model, the cytokines implicated are remarkably similar to autoantibody-dependent models. The cytokine profile in RA (see later) in many ways represents a final common pathway for a variety of autoimmune mechanisms.

Restoring T Cell Tolerance

Assuming that synovial T cell autoreactivity plays a key role in the pathogenesis of RA, one potential therapeutic approach is to restore tolerance. This concept has been problematic because the underlying defect has not been defined and could include abnormal thymic selection, poorly defined genetic factors that lead to immune hyperreactivity, or inadequate regulatory T cell function. The lack of a specific antigen identified as pathogenic also increases the complexity of the problem. It is clear, however, that current approaches do not "cure" RA because cessation of therapy usually leads to a recurrence of disease.

Two examples illustrate the potential for restoring homeostasis and immune tolerance. First, recent data suggest that aggressive treatment of early RA (within the year of clinical disease) with methotrexate and a TNF inhibitor could lead to long-lasting remissions.[110] In many cases, therapy was withdrawn after 1 year of treatment, and patients did not flare for at least 1 additional year. The mechanism of prolonged remission despite discontinuing therapy in early disease is not defined, but seems to differ from clinical experience in chronic RA.

Another way to induce tolerance is through mucosal immunization to enhance Th2 function. In a clinical trial, patients with RA were treated with oral administration of the dnaJP1 peptide, and T cell responses were evaluated.[111] The peptide-treated patients showed immune deviation toward a Th2 phenotype. This approach has the potential for developing individualized therapy based on specific antigens that might be pathogenic for each patient, such as QKRAA, collagen epitopes, HSPs, or many others. Additional therapies that enhance regulatory T cell function, alter costimulation, or delete only pathogenic T cells may potentially be effective in RA.

SYNOVIAL B CELLS

Synovial B cell and plasma cell hyperreactivity are viewed increasingly as key participants in the perpetuation and initiation phases of RA. This notion has been fueled by the descriptions of novel spontaneous models of arthritis in mice, such as the K/BxN model, in which loss of tolerance leads to autoantibody production, activation of innate immunity, and chronic synovitis. B cell–directed therapies, such as anti-CD20 antibody, have shown efficacy in RA.

Cytokine Regulation of Synovial B Cells

Although many rheumatoid synovial tissues exhibit a diffuse infiltration with mononuclear cells, a significant percentage also have discrete lymphoid follicles populated by B cells in the sublining region. Follicular DCs, B cells, plasma cells, and T lymphocytes collect in these aggregates. The germinal centers are highly organized structures in which affinity maturation occurs. B cells are present in the aggregates and express the maturation marker CD20 and proliferation antigens such as Ki67. The formation of these structures depends on several soluble and membrane-bound cytokines, including lymphotoxin. B cells accumulate in lymphoid aggregates in RA synovium under the influence of a variety of chemotactic factors, including CCL21 and B cell–attracting chemokine-1 (CXCL13).

A member of the TNF superfamily of cytokines known as B lymphocyte stimulator (BLyS) also has been identified as a key molecule that regulates B cell differentiation. BLyS binds to transmembrane activator and CAML interactor (TACI), which is present on B cells and T cells. If this system is blocked using recombinant TACI-Ig, the number of B cells is dramatically reduced, and antibody production is decreased. The same construct is effective as a therapeutic agent in collagen-induced arthritis, a model that depends on autoantibody production.[112]

BLyS is produced in RA synovium, especially by macrophages. Synovial lining type B synoviocytes also can release BLyS and can be induced by TNF-α and IFN-γ in vitro.[113] A related cytokine, also in the TNF superfamily, called APRIL is localized mainly to DCs in synovial germinal centers.[114] TACI-Ig, which binds BLyS and APRIL, disrupts the germinal centers and decreases immunoglobulin receptors in SCID mice implanted with rheumatoid synovium.[115] A clinical trial using an anti-BLyS antibody showed minimal benefit, however, in patients with RA. This result could be related to the fact that APRIL is still able to interact with cell surface TACI.

Synovial B Cell Maturation

B cells isolated directly from germinal centers of RA synovium show a heterogeneous pattern of V gene usage and rearrangement. Most VH genes are not mutated, suggesting that they are recent immigrants from the peripheral blood and are activated locally.[116] For RF-producing cells, shared mutations containing an identical sequence throughout the variable domain of immunoglobulins have been identified in synovial tissue.[117] Preferential use of a few VH and DH gene segments and marked preference for a DH reading frame encoding particular hydrophilic residues also have been observed, consistent with antigen-related selection and maturation. Analysis of expressed heavy-chain variable domains supports the notion that the B cell response in RA synovium is oligoclonal. Similarly, B cell clones isolated from either RA synovium or bone marrow with nurse-like cells have limited VH usage.

B cells associated with follicular DCs in the rheumatoid synovium can differentiate further and develop additional mutations, suggesting antigen-driven selection. Plasma cells in other areas of the synovium have distinct rearrangements compared with the B lymphocytes associated with DCs.

This finding raises the question of whether the plasma cells arise locally or migrate from the blood. Although plasma cell rearrangements are not similar to the B cells, groups of plasma cells used similar genes, albeit with distinct mutations. The plasma cells probably are derived from a synovial B cell clone that mutated and whose progeny proliferate and differentiate.

It is uncertain whether this process represents an ectopic lymphoid organ performing normal functions, or whether it is related to autoimmunity. The presence of abundant autoantibody-producing cells in the synovium supports the latter hypothesis, although normal immune responses also might occur in the joint. Cells that produce RFs, anti–type II collagen antibody, and anticitrulline peptide antibody populate the RA synovium. Not all B cells in the joint are activated, however. A population of CD20+CD38– B cells with impaired receptor-induced signaling as previously observed in anergic cells also infiltrates the synovium.[118] Some B cells also serve a more active role in synovial immune responses. In a SCID mouse model using synovial explants, T cell activation and cytokine production depended on B cells.[119] In the same model, treatment with TACI-Ig, which inhibits APRIL and BLyS, decreased synovial inflammation and IFN-γ production in tissues displaying germinal centers.

Maturation and survival of B cells depend on stromal cells and cells with "nurse-like cell" properties that support lymphocyte maturation in the thymus. The bone marrow and synovium of patients with RA also contain nurse-like cells, which can increase expression of CD40 and class II MHC proteins on B cells.[120] B cell survival is supported by this population of cells, whereas autoreactive clones evade deletion and produce autoantibodies. A variety of cytokines, including GM-CSF, IL-6, and IL-8, are produced by RA nurse-like cells, and direct contact with B cells is crucial for maximal proliferation and antibody production.[121] Cultured B cells spontaneously migrate beneath ordinary FLS, which permits them to survive in vitro for prolonged periods. The process depends on the interaction of the integrin α4β1 on B cells with synoviocytes expressing CD106 (VCAM-1).[122] The chemokine SDF-1 also is constitutively expressed by synoviocytes and contributes to the process. Interference with the B cell–synoviocyte interaction decreases B cell survival and is one potential mechanism by which therapeutic interventions targeted at integrins might suppress autoreactivity and inflammation in RA.

B Cell Depletion in Rheumatoid Arthritis

Although the role of T cells and cytokines attracted most of the scientific interest in recent years, clinical trials with an anti-CD20 antibody (rituximab) showing efficacy in RA refocused investigators on B cells and autoantibodies. The precise function of CD20 is not well defined; it is expressed on mature B cells, but not plasma cells. Rituximab causes a rapid and profound depletion of peripheral blood B cells. In mice, anti-CD20 antibody depletes B cells in blood, spleen, lymph nodes, and bone marrow. The few remaining B cells in the spleen were of the B1, but not B2, phenotype. Peritoneal B cells are only partially depleted, suggesting that some sites are privileged and protect B cells despite adequate drug penetration.[123] In RA, serial synovial biopsies show partial

B cell depletion after rituximab therapy despite the virtual absence of peripheral B cells. The clinical responses do not always correlate closely with the extent of synovial depletion, although some patients with the most impressive responses seem to have marked declines in the number of B cells in the post-treatment specimens.

The B cell depletion data raise many questions about the precise role of B cells in the rheumatoid synovium. Rituximab can modestly decrease autoantibody formation, but it is unclear that this is sufficient to account for the clinical responses. B cells also produce cytokines and can enhance T cell responses by serving as antigen presenting cells. Because plasma cells do not express CD20, a major source of autoantibodies is still present in the joint. The precise mechanism of anti-CD20 antibody might be complex and involve many B cell functions, rather than simply decreasing the autoantibody production and immune complex formation.

DENDRITIC CELLS

DCs are potent antigen presenting cells that populate synovial tissue and synovial effusions of patients with RA. DCs generally sample the environment, especially at mucosal and skin surfaces; process antigens; and migrate to central lymphatic sites, where they present the antigens to T cells. Rheumatoid synovium seems to function similar to lymphoid tissues in some circumstances with mature DCs expressing CD86, CD83, and DC-LAMP localized in perivascular lymphocytic infiltrates and aggregates. Ultrastructural analysis of the synovium shows the DCs in contact with lymphocytes, where they are probably presenting antigen. The presence of DCs is not unique to RA and has been identified in other inflammatory arthritides, including gout and spondyloarthropathies.

The reason that DCs reside in the synovium probably relates to the chemokine milieu in the joint.[124] DCs express the chemokine receptor CCR7, which usually permits them to home to lymphoid tissue and orchestrate organization into the appropriate germinal centers. Synoviocytes in RA express two CCR7 ligands (CCL19 and CCL21), which provide a signal for the DCs to remain in the peripheral tissue. Immature DCs and plasmacytoid DCs also have been observed scattered throughout the synovial sublining region. B cell–enriched lymphoid follicles, which are usually organized around follicular DCs, also are found in some RA joint tissues. The source of follicular DCs is not well defined, but cultured FLS can perform follicular DC functions in vitro and could contribute in vivo as well. Synoviocytes derived from RA patients can bind to germinal center B cells and suppress B cell apoptosis.[125]

Cytokines that are abundant in RA, such as GM-CSF, influence the proliferation and maturation of these antigen presenting cells. DCs can constitute 5% of synovial fluid mononuclear cells, which is almost 10-fold higher than in peripheral blood.[126] RA synovial tissue DCs can respond abnormally to certain cytokines known to be present in the rheumatoid joint. IL-10 normally suppresses DC function, partly by decreasing expression of CD86 and class II MHC molecules. RA DCs isolated from the joint are resistant to this effect, however, possibly because they express smaller amounts of the IL-10 receptor.[127] Aside from presenting

antigens, DCs also can produce cytokines that can influence T cell differentiation in the joint, including IL-12 and IL-23, which can enhance the bias toward the Th1 and Th17 (see later) phenotypes, and APRIL, which enhances B cell survival. Engineered DCs have been used in animal models to suppress disease, including cells that produce excess Th2 cytokine such as IL-4.[128]

MAST CELLS, POLYMORPHONUCLEAR LEUKOCYTES, AND NATURAL KILLER CELLS

Mast cells are present in the synovial membranes of patients with RA and, in some patients, are located at sites of cartilage erosion. Rheumatoid synovial membranes contain more than 10 times as many mast cells than do control synovial samples from patients undergoing surgery for meniscectomy. Patients with high numbers of mast cells have more intense clinical synovitis in the affected joints. Mast cells and histamine also are found in most synovial fluid specimens from inflammatory synovitis. A detailed analysis of several indicators of proliferation and the enumeration of synovial mast cells has shown strong positive correlations between the number of mast cells in synovial tissue and the degree of lymphocyte infiltration.[129] Mast cells from RA synovium express significantly greater amounts of the C5a receptor compared with osteoarthritis synovium.

Resident mast cells in synovium respond to cytokines that stimulate mast cell growth and chemotaxis. Extracts of mast cells can induce adherent rheumatoid synovial cells to increase production of prostaglandin (PG) E_2 and collagenase, and immunostaining of RA synovial mast cells shows tryptase and TNF-α. Mast cell–derived heparin has significant effects on connective tissue. In particular, it may modulate the effects of hormones on osseous cells and alter the balance of bone synthesis toward degradation.

The role of mast cells in the initiation phase of synovitis was confirmed in the passive K/BxN model, in which their absence prevented disease.[130] It is uncertain if the cells are required when synovial inflammation has been established, and other cell types, such as neutrophils, supplant the mast cells in some circumstances. The production of leukotriene (LT) B_4 in the same model requires neutrophils, but not mast cells in established disease. Treatment of synovial tissue explant cultures with a c-kit tyrosine kinase inhibitor induces mast cell apoptosis and decreased production of TNF-α.[131] These data suggest that mast cells might contribute to synovial cytokine production in established disease.

Despite the abundance of neutrophils in RA synovial effusions, only rare polymorphonuclear neutrophils (PMNs) infiltrate the synovium. Natural killer cells have been identified, however, in RA synovium.[132] Cytotoxic natural killer cells contain large amounts of granzymes, which are serine proteases. One potentially important immunoregulatory role of natural killer cells is that they can stimulate B cells to produce RFs. A subset of natural killer cells that express large amounts of CD56 is unusually abundant in RA synovial tissue and fluid.[133] These cells potentially can produce cytokines or enhance proinflammatory cytokine production by T lymphocytes and macrophages.

BONE MARROW CELLS

Although most attention has been directed at the synovium, cartilage, and cortical bone in RA, the subcortical bone and bone marrow also contribute to synovial inflammatory responses. Primitive bone marrow mesenchymal cells can traverse cortical bone through pores in murine collagen-induced arthritis before the onset of clinical disease, take up residence in the synovium, and produce mediators that enhance synovitis.[134] This process is TNF-α dependent and is abrogated in mice that lack TNF receptors. Also, CD34+ mesenchymal cells in rheumatoid bone marrow are more highly activated as judged by their NFκB status and their ability to differentiate into fibroblast-like cells that produce MMPs and proangiogenic factors.[135] The bone marrow also can contribute other relevant cells, including macrophage lineage cells that migrate to the synovium and Sertoli-like cells that support the survival of B cells. Just as the bone marrow can influence the synovium, the reverse also is true. Invasive pannus can rupture through cortical bone and invade the marrow space in some patients.[136] When this occurs, B cell aggregates are especially prominent in the marrow and occur in an environment rich in B cell chemoattractants such as CCL21 and B cell survival factors such as BLyS.

SYNOVIAL HISTOPATHOLOGY IN EARLY VERSUS LATE RHEUMATOID ARTHRITIS

Previous observations suggested that the earliest phases of RA (i.e., during the first few weeks of symptoms) exhibit distinct histopathology with a paucity of lymphocyte infiltration in the presence of endothelial cell injury, tissue edema, and neutrophil accumulation. More recent reports suggest, however, that the histologic appearance of RA is similar regardless of the duration of clinical symptoms.[137] The extent of lymphoid aggregation, T cell infiltration, and synovial lining hyperplasia can resemble chronic disease even when symptoms have been present for a short time. The cytokine patterns of these biopsy specimens as determined by immunohistochemical analysis indicated similar levels of T cell (e.g., IFN-γ) and non–T cell factors (e.g., IL-1 and TNF-α). The tumor-suppressor gene p53 also is expressed in early RA, most likely owing to intense oxidative stress in the environment.

Biopsy specimens of asymptomatic joints from patients with early or late RA also have lymphocyte infiltration, cytokine production, and p53 expression.[138] Although IFN-γ, IL-1, and TNF-α levels are increased compared with normal synovium, they are modestly lower than in clinically active joints. One difference might be the relative abundance of some cytokines, such as IL-8, and the number of macrophages, which are higher in the painful joints. Some aspects of synovial histology in early RA, such as macrophage and plasma cell infiltration, might predict more erosive or severe disease. Studies in animal models of arthritis also show increased expression of proinflammatory transcription factors, such as activator protein-1 (AP-1) and NFκB, before clinically evident arthritis.[139] These studies suggest that patients with "early" RA, as defined by the duration of symptoms, might already have chronic disease, and that evaluation of truly early disease might require assessment of patients long before the onset of symptoms (if this is even possible). The observation that autoantibodies are produced in RA patients years before the clinical arthritis also supports the notion that a preclinical phase may precede symptomatic synovitis.

SYNOVIAL FLUID

> *Key Points*
> - RA synovial effusions contain abundant neutrophils and mononuclear cells.
> - Immune complexes that contain autoantibodies such as RFs or anticitrullinated protein antibodies can fix complement, leading to the generation of chemoattractants.
> - Small molecule mediators of inflammation, such as PGs and LTs, are present in RA synovial fluid.

Synovial effusions accumulate in the joints of most patients with active RA as a result of a substantial increase in fluid influx that cannot be removed despite an increase in lymphatic flow. Components of the inflammatory and proliferative response can be evaluated in the effusions to provide clues to the proinflammatory and anti-inflammatory mechanisms that operate in RA. It has been known for many years that there is an inverse relationship between the molecular weight of proteins and their concentrations in minimally inflamed synovial fluid. High-molecular-weight serum proteins gain access more easily to synovial fluid in inflamed joints, and the relatively high concentration of IgG in RA synovial fluid is good evidence for local (synovial) synthesis of IgG. Protein traffic in human synovial effusions has been measured by determining the clearance of proteins from synovial fluid and has provided a useful measure of afferent synovial lymph flow. A markedly increased permeance of blood vessels in rheumatoid patients confirms the severity of the microvascular lesion in rheumatoid synovitis. Newer techniques evaluating the synovial fluid proteome in RA using mass spectroscopy might provide new insights into the key mediators. More than 400 proteins in RA effusions were identified as potential biomarkers of disease activity, including C-reactive protein and six members of the S100 family of calcium granule binding proteins.[140]

POLYMORPHONUCLEAR NEUTROPHILS

The presence of PMNs remains one of the most consistent indices of inflammation within a particular joint. These cells truly amplify inflammatory responses and contribute to the perpetuation of the inflammation within joints. The articular cavity serves as a depository for PMNs; they enter the synovial fluid by direct passage from postcapillary venules in the synovium. Neutrophils adhere to activated synovial microvasculature because of the action of selectins and the β2 integrins. After adherence, chemotactic agents produced by endothelium and fibroblasts may facilitate egress through the capillaries along the chemoattractant gradients of the synovium. Considering the survival time of PMNs in synovial fluid, it has been estimated that the breakdown of an average rheumatoid effusion containing 25,000/mm³ PMNs may exceed 1 billion cells each day. The ultimate fate of many of these cells is apoptosis. Neutrophil survival requires expression of the forkhead transcription factor Foxo3a.[141] Mice that are deficient in this gene are resistant to inflammatory arthritis because of the shortened PMN life span. Neutrophils lacking this factor increase expression of the apoptosis-inducing membrane protein Fas ligand after exposure to proinflammatory cytokines. Foxo3a inhibition potentially can limit the acute inflammatory response in certain diseases where neutrophils play a prominent role.

The strong attraction of chemotactic agents within the synovial fluid in RA is responsible for the large number of cells found there. Few PMNs are seen in the pannus itself and subsynovial tissue; when in the synovium, they move rapidly to the synovial fluid, drawn by the activated component of cleavage of C5a, LTB_4, platelet-activating factor, and chemokines. The CXC family of chemokines, including ENA-78 and IL-8, are especially abundant in synovial fluid and can attract neutrophils into the intra-articular space. PMNs also can release chemokines into the milieu that enhance migration of new cells into the joint space. MIP-3α mRNA is specifically produced by synovial fluid PMNs of RA patients.[142]

When in the joint, neutrophils engage immune complexes through Fc receptors and other activating signals. This engagement leads to cytoskeletal reorganization, release of granule content, generation of reactive oxygen and nitrogen species, and enhanced phagocytosis. Many of the cells contain immune complexes within phagosomes that include IgG and IgM along with complement proteins such as C1q, C3, and C4. PMNs from synovial fluid in RA release de novo synthesized proteins, including matrix proteins such as fibronectin, neutral proteinases, and IL-1. Neutrophils also secrete IL-1Ra as a major product. Although the amount of IL-1Ra each neutrophil produces is low compared with that produced by macrophages, the sheer number of PMNs allows them to produce large amounts in synovial effusions. Oncostatin M, a member of the IL-6 family, is released by synovial fluid neutrophils.[143] These cells also release numerous proteases that can adversely effect the lubricating properties of synovial fluid and the integrity of the cartilage, including elastase, trypsin, and neutrophil collagenase.

Although difficult to assess in humans, animal models show a variable role for neutrophils in the inflammatory and destructive processes. In the streptococcal cell wall model, neutrophils play a more prominent role compared with models induced by intra-articular injection with bacterial DNA. The passive K/BxN and collagen-induced arthritis models, which require systemic injection with antibodies that bind to the joint and fix complement, require neutrophils for full expression of the disease. In each case, depleting neutrophils with antibodies almost completely prevents synovial inflammation. In the K/BxN model, neutrophils initiate vascular permeability, which permits pathogenic antibodies to gain access to the joint space.

SYNOVIAL FLUID LYMPHOCYTES

The lymphocyte mix in synovial fluid differs from that of peripheral blood and synovial tissue, and analysis of synovial fluid cells is not an accurate reflection of the synovium. Although synovial effusions contain an abundance of T cells, the CD4$^+$-to-CD8$^+$ ratio is reversed compared with

that of blood or synovial tissue, with an excess of CD8$^+$ suppressor cells relative to CD4$^+$ lymphocytes. In addition, synovial tissue is nearly devoid of neutrophils, which often constitute 50% to 75% of synovial fluid cells. The synovial fluid does not contain a random distribution of cells shed from synovial tissue. The percentage of regulatory T cells (CD4$^+$CD25$^+$) also is higher in synovial fluid compared with peripheral blood.[144]

Synovial fluid contains T cells that express high levels of surface HLA-DR antigens. Other activation antigens not increased on peripheral blood cells are increased on synovial fluid lymphocytes, including VLA-1. Of CD4$^+$ cells in rheumatoid synovial fluid, most are memory cells and express CD45RO on their surface.[145] Despite the phenotypic appearance of activation, synovial fluid T cell function is deficient compared with that of peripheral blood cells. Synovial fluid lymphocyte proliferation in response to mitogens or most recall antigens, such as tetanus toxoid, is significantly less than paired blood T lymphocytes. Mycobacterial antigens and the 60-kD HSP seem to be exceptions because proliferation is greater in cells isolated from rheumatoid effusions. Cytokine production by synovial fluid T cells in vitro also is low, including mitogen-induced expression of IFN-γ and IL-1.[146]

A possible mechanism that explains defective T cell responses by synovial fluid mononuclear cells from rheumatoid patients is the presence of local inhibitors of cell activation. IL-1Ra and TGF-β are possible T cell suppressants and have been identified as components of synovial effusions that can suppress thymocyte proliferation.[147] Nonspecific components of joint effusions, such as hyaluronic acid, can be toxic to cells and can indirectly suppress T cell activation. The mechanism of diminished T cell activation could be related to abnormalities in TCR signaling. Articular T cells have diminished tyrosine phosphorylation of proteins after stimulation, especially the key signal transduction pathway p38 MAP kinase.[148] Tyrosine phosphorylation of the TCR zeta chain, an early event in TCR signaling, is low compared with peripheral blood T cells. Decreased levels of the zeta protein also are observed, suggesting that the TCR apparatus is abnormal in RA. The hyporesponsiveness of synovial fluid T cells correlates with a significant decrease in the levels of the intracellular redox-regulating agent glutathione.[149] Restoration of the intracellular glutathione enhances mitogenic-induced proliferative responses and IL-2 production in RA synovial fluid T cells. These data suggest that oxidative stress in the articular environment can suppress antigen-specific T cell responses.

IMMUNE COMPLEXES

The significance of immunoglobulin complexes circulating in blood and in synovial fluid was appreciated several decades ago. It was not until more reliable assays for immune complexes were available, however, that broad studies correlating disease activity and immune complexes could be generated. The most relevant data relate to the production of such complexes in the joint rather than the blood except in the unusual case of systemic rheumatoid vasculitis. Nevertheless, circulating IgM immune complexes are elevated in RA. In studies designed to identify the components of immune complexes in the circulation of rheumatoid patients, most studies did not find a specific antigen other than IgG complexed with RF. Using more sensitive techniques, circulating immune complexes in RA were found to contain 20 polypeptides, including albumin, immunoglobulin, complement, type II collagen, fibrinogen, and acute-phase reactants, and DNA.

Most relevant to the pathogenesis of joint destruction in RA has been the identification of immunoglobulins and complement in articular collagenous tissues from RA patients. Almost all cartilage and meniscus samples from rheumatoid patients have evidence of these components in the avascular connective tissue. Electron microscopic morphology of immunoglobulin aggregates shows that there are pathologic changes in the matrix of cartilage in the microenvironment of the aggregates themselves. Immune complexes are absent under areas of cartilage invaded actively by synovial pannus, suggesting that phagocytic cells in the invasive synovium ingest the immune complexes. This possibility lends credence to the notion that immune complexes deposited in the avascular superficial layers of cartilage in the joint may serve as chemoattractants for the pannus. Immune complexes have been extracted from cartilage of RA and osteoarthritis patients. Rheumatoid cartilage contains more than 40-fold more IgM and more than 10-fold more IgG than healthy cartilage extracts. IgM RF is found in most RA cartilage extracts, but not in osteoarthritis or healthy control extracts. In addition, more than 60% of the RA cartilage extracts are positive for native and denatured collagen type II antibody.

These observations support the hypothesis that the presence of cartilage embedded with complexes contributes to the chronicity and persistence of rheumatoid inflammation. Orthopaedic surgeons have noted for many years that joints from which all cartilage is removed do not participate in general flares of rheumatoid disease after surgery. The localization of immune complexes, as a result of either in situ formation or absorption from the synovial fluid, could be required for the full expression of RA.

ARACHIDONATE METABOLITES

Accompanying activation of PMNs is the increased mobilization of membrane phospholipids in these cells to arachidonic acid and its subsequent oxidation by cyclooxygenases (COX) to PGs and thromboxanes, or by lipoxygenases to LTs. Although the stable PGs, especially PGE_2, produce vasodilation, cause increased vascular permeability, and are involved centrally in fever production, there is increasing evidence that they have significant anti-inflammatory activities as well. Stable PG can retard the development of adjuvant arthritis, and the drug misoprostol, a PG analogue, may have significant anti-inflammatory or immunomodulatory effects. Physiologic concentrations of PGE_2 inhibit IFN-γ production by T cells, HLA-DR expression by macrophages, and T cell proliferation.

Production of PGs in RA depends on two distinct COX enzymes, COX-1 and COX-2. The former is constitutively expressed and is responsible for the normal endogenous production of PGs in the joint and in other tissues. COX-2 is an inducible enzyme responsible for increased PG synthesis in inflamed tissue. Cytokines such as IL-1 and TNF-α induce

COX-2 gene expression by cultured synoviocytes and macrophages. COX-2 mRNA and immunoreactive protein are increased in RA synovium.[150] Most nonsteroidal anti-inflammatory drugs, including indomethacin and ibuprofen, inhibit COX-1 and COX-2. Much of the anti-inflammatory activity (and analgesia) results from inhibition of the latter. Clinical experience using similar compounds in patients with osteoarthritis or RA indicates that COX-2 blockade is sufficient for the therapeutic benefit.

Although most of the emphasis has been placed on PGE, PGI_2 also can contribute to synovial inflammation. Mice lacking the PGI_2 receptor have significantly decreased arthritis severity in the collagen-induced arthritis model compared with wild-type mice even though they make similar amounts of anticollagen antibodies. Loss of PGE_2 signaling by blocking its receptors EP_2 or EP_4 was much less effective.

LTB is a potent proinflammatory product of neutrophil activation. It is chemotactic for neutrophils, eosinophils, and macrophages and promotes neutrophil aggregation and adherence to endothelium. Peripheral blood PMNs from rheumatoid patients have an enhanced capacity for the production of LTB_4 compared with similar cells from control groups.[151] In murine collagen-induced arthritis, an LTB_4 antagonist significantly decreased paw swelling and joint destruction, suggesting a pivotal role for this potent chemoattractant.[152] LTB_4 blockade in RA has been less impressive, however.

Certain arachidonic acid metabolites, such as 15-deoxy-delta(12,14)-PGJ(2), can bind to peroxisome proliferator activated receptors and inhibit cytokine production and adjuvant arthritis.[152] Cyclopentenone PGs also can inhibit NFκB by blocking IκB kinase (IKK), suppressing the NFκB-driven array of proinflammatory genes.[153] Lipoxins (LXs) represent a unique class of lipid mediators that help resolve inflammatory diseases. LXs have a trihydroxytetraene structure and are produced from arachidonic acid via the lipoxygenase pathway during cell-cell interactions. LXA_4 binds with high affinity to a G protein–coupled receptor denoted LXA_4 receptor. Activation of LXA_4 receptor inhibits recruitment of neutrophils by attenuating chemotaxis, adhesion, and transmigration into tissues, and by diminishing chemokine and cytokine production. LXA_4 significantly decreased cytokine and MMP expression in FLS through an NFκB-dependent mechanism.[154]

COMPLEMENT

The liver is the major source of complement synthesis in humans, and passive transfer of serum proteins into effusions accounts for many of the complement proteins found there. Synovial tissue also actively produces complement proteins, however.[155] Macrophages and fibroblasts produce complement proteins under the influence of cytokines such as IFN-γ, IL-1, and TNF-α. In situ hybridization shows that C2 is expressed in the synovial intimal lining, whereas C3 seems to be produced by synovial sublining macrophages. Analysis of synovial tissue shows that all complement genes from the classic pathway are expressed in RA and in healthy synovium. Despite the local production of complement components, the activities of C4, C2, and C3 and total hemolytic complement in rheumatoid synovial effusions are lower than in synovial fluids from patients with other joint diseases.[156] Although the most prominent evidence of activation implicates the classic pathway, cleavage products of the alternate pathway, including factor B and properdin, also have been documented in RA.

Using a sensitive solid-phase radioimmunoassay to quantify the activation of the classic pathway of complement by RF, IgM RF is a much more important determinant of complement activation than IgG RF in serum and synovial fluid. Combined with other data showing accelerated catabolism of C4 in RA and that the presence of C4 fragments in the plasma of rheumatoid patients correlates with titers of IgM RF, the weight of evidence indicates a role in vivo for IgM RF in complement activation.

The biologically active products of complement activation are probably the most important consequence of intraarticular complement consumption. Similar to proteases from PMNs, these inflammatory components accumulate in synovial fluid during acute inflammation. The potential for interaction between PMNs and the complement system is substantial. Neutrophil lysosomal lysates contain enzymatic activity capable of generating chemotactic activity (probably C5a) from fresh serum. C5a, in addition to being a principal chemotactic factor in inflammatory effusions, mediates lysosomal release from human PMNs; this sets up one of many amplification loops in inflammatory synovial fluid. The chemotactic anaphylatoxins C3a and C5a are often present in rheumatoid effusions, as are C5a complement components that comprise the C5b-C9 membrane attack complex. Low levels of the C5b-C9 membrane attack complex can activate synoviocytes in vitro.

Complement activation as a potential therapeutic target has received increasing attention. In rat antigen-induced arthritis, intra-articular treatment with soluble complement receptor 1 inhibits joint swelling.[157] Knockout mice lacking various complement components also provide evidence for the utility of this approach. C5-deficient mice have decreased joint inflammation in collagen-induced arthritis and the passive K/BxN model.[158] Absence of C3 or factor B also inhibits collagen-induced arthritis. In contrast to the C5 knockout mice, which had normal antibody responses, the C3-null and factor B–null animals had lower levels of anti–type II collagen antibodies.[159] The role of C3 convertase was explored in more detail using mice that were transgenic for the rodent complement regulatory protein complement receptor 1-related gene/protein y.[160] These mice have no obvious phenotype and are not more susceptible to infection. Clinical arthritis and histologic damage in collagen-induced arthritis were significantly decreased in complement receptor 1-related gene/protein y transgenic mice compared with wild-type mice.

These data suggest that classic and alternative complement pathways are implicated in inflammatory arthritis. The role of complement can be through activation of innate immune responses or classic adaptive immunity, depending on the specific model and complement components targeted. A humanized anti-C5 antibody has been evaluated in a placebo-controlled study. The antibody inhibits C5 activation and function of the C5b-C9 attack complex. Although the monoclonal antibody was well tolerated, there was only modest evidence of clinical efficacy.

PERIPHERAL BLOOD LYMPHOCYTE IMMUNE RESPONSES

Although peripheral lymphocytes are the most accessible, many investigators believe there is greater value studying cells isolated from the site of disease. Nevertheless, numerous studies show functional and phenotypic differences between RA and normal peripheral blood cells. The number of CD4$^+$ helper T cells is mildly increased in the circulation of patients with RA, with a concomitant decrease in CD8$^+$ lymphocytes (and an increased CD4$^+$-to-CD8$^+$ ratio). The surface phenotype of circulating T cells in RA suggests activation in some studies, but not in others. An increased percentage of αβ and γδ TCR-bearing cells might express HLA-DR and the adhesion protein VLA-4 (α4β1-integrin). VLA-4 plays an important role in the recruitment of cells to the synovium through interactions with VCAM-1 on endothelial cells. Other markers of activation are not elevated on RA T cells in the circulation. Peripheral blood T cells express some phenotypic characteristics of incomplete activation. It is unclear whether this process occurs in the peripheral or central lymphoid organs, or whether cells are activated in the synovium and re-enter the circulation via the synovial lymphatics.

Immunoregulatory dysfunction in RA has been described in the blood cells of some patients. An early observation was the inadequate control of EBV-infected B lymphocyte growth owing to a defect in T cell function in RA. The abnormal T cell response could be correlated with disease activity, but it also was noted that the abnormality was present in T cells of some patients with inflammatory arthropathies other than RA.[161] IFN-γ and IL-2 production can be significantly suppressed in these RA lymphocyte cultures under certain conditions.

T cell diversity and maturation are abnormal in RA. Thymic output normally decreases with age, whereas this process seems to be accelerated in RA.[162] The presence of TCR rearrangement excision circles is a measure of thymic release of mature T cells. Using this parameter, the thymic output in RA may decline prematurely. Similarly, telomere attrition suggests inappropriate "aging" of the T cells. This aging could be due to a primary defect in peripheral T cell homeostasis or due to impaired thymic function with increased T cell turnover secondary to chronic immune stimulation. This concept is supported by the observation that telomere length in RA T cells is shorter than in normal controls and more closely resembles older populations. Increased numbers of CD4$^+$CD28$^-$ T lymphocytes have been reported in the peripheral blood of RA patients.

Activated B lymphocytes also are present in the peripheral blood of patients with RA. The number of circulating B cells that spontaneously produce RF levels are significantly higher in RA patients compared with normal individuals. B cells that are enriched in autoantibody production are characterized by a surface determinant CD5.[163] This antigen is normally expressed by T cells, but it also is displayed by fetal B cells and a few immature B cells in adults. RA patients with normal circulating numbers of lymphocytes show an abnormal kappa-to-lambda-chain analysis compared with controls, implying oligoclonal B cell proliferation[164]; it is unknown whether this reflects expansion of the restricted number of clones capable of producing RF, or whether an inciting antigen is something other than IgG and related specifically to RA. Normal and RA peripheral blood B cells have equal numbers of B cells that produce IgM anti–type II collagen antibodies. The B cells that accumulate in the synovial fluid produce IgG antibodies that are more likely to be pathogenic, however.[165]

Attempts to characterize the unique gene expression profiles in the peripheral blood cells of patients with RA have met with mixed results. In some cases, RNA transcripts potentially can distinguish between RA and psoriatic arthritis and include differential expression of tumor suppressors, MAP kinases, and other proinflammatory proteins. Similar studies have been performed in animals, such as rat collagen-induced arthritis, although the ability to classify patients, stage disease, assign a diagnosis, or assess response to therapy has still eluded investigators.

ROLE OF T CELL CYTOKINES

Key Points

- Multiple subsets of T cells have been implicated in the pathogenesis of RA.
- Relatively low levels of T cell cytokines are present in RA synovium.
- The T cell cytokines that are present, such as IFN-γ and IL-17, are produced by Th1 cells or Th17 cells.
- Regulatory T cell function, which suppresses activation of other T cells, might be reduced in RA synovium.
- The contribution of T cells to synovial inflammation can be through antigen-independent mechanisms, such as direct cell-cell contact with macrophages.

Cytokines are hormone-like proteins that enable immune cells to communicate. Cytokines either can interact with cells after being released in a soluble form or can be involved with direct cell-cell communication through membrane-bound factors such as TNF-α. In addition to participating in normal immune responses, they play an integral role in the initiation and perpetuation of synovitis. The cytokine milieu in RA is not random, although early studies suggested an unrestricted abundance of cytokines. Factors produced by T lymphocytes are low in RA, whereas factors generated by macrophages and by synovial fibroblasts are markedly increased (Table 65-5).[166]

Helper T cells have been divided into cytokine-specific subsets. Th1 cells, which develop under the influence of IL-12 and perhaps IL-23, produce IFN-γ, IL-2, and IL-6, but not IL-4, IL-5, or IL-10. The cells are characterized by T-bet gene expression and use the signal transducers and activators of transcription 4 (STAT4) signaling pathway. In contrast, Th2 cells express GATA-3, use STAT6, and produce the opposite profile (IL-4$^+$, IL-5$^+$, IL-10$^+$, IL-2$^-$, IFN-γ$^-$). Some cytokines are produced by both subsets, including TNF-α, IL-3, and GM-CSF, whereas Th0 cells have an unrestricted cytokine profile. Th1 cells primarily mediate delayed-type hypersensitivity in vivo, whereas Th2 cells are more prominent regulators of isotype switching and antibody production. Some cytokines produced by Th2 cells are immunosuppressive because IL-4 and IL-10 downregulate Th1 cell differentiation and activation and delayed-type hypersensitivity.

Table 65-5 Level of Production of Synovial Cytokines in Rheumatoid Arthritis According to Cellular Source

Cellular Source	Level of Production in Rheumatoid Arthritis Synovium*
T cells	
IL-2	−
IL-3	−
IL-4	−
IL-6	±
IL-13	±
IL-17	+
IFN-γ	±
TNF-α	−
TNF-β (LTα 3)	−
RANKL	+
GM-CSF	−
Macrophages†/Fibroblasts‡	
IL-1	+++
IL-1Ra	+
IL-6	+++
IL-10	+
IL-12	+
IL-15	++
IL-16	+
IL-18	++
IL-32	+
TNF-α	++
M- CSF	+
GM-CSF	++
BLyS	++
LIGHT	++
RANKL	+
TGF-β	++
Chemokines (IL-8, MCP-1)	+++
Fibroblast growth factor	++

*−, absent or very low concentrations; +, present.
†Tissue macrophages or type A synoviocytes.
‡Tissue fibroblasts or type B synoviocytes.
BLyS, B lymphocyte stimulator; GM-CSF, granulocyte-macrophage colony-stimulating factor; IFN-γ, interferon-γ; IL, interleukin; MCP-1, monocyte chemoattractant; M-CSF, macrophage colony-stimulating factor; RANKL, receptor activator of nuclear factor κB ligand; TGF-β, transforming growth factor-β; TNF, tumor necrosis factor.

This simple system has become more complicated as new subsets have been defined. The Th3 subset that mainly produces TGF-β has been identified. The Th17 subset, which produces IL-17 but not IFN-γ and uses STAT3, seems to be especially relevant to autoimmunity and inflammatory arthritis. This phenotype can be induced when T cells are exposed to TGF-β plus IL-6 or by IL-23, all of which are present in the rheumatoid joint. Finally, a suppressive subset, Tregs, can be identified by virtue of coexpression of CD4 and CD25 on their surface. These cells are marked by Foxp3 expression and suppress the responses of other T cells through poorly defined cell contact mechanisms that involve costimulatory blockade and release of cytokines such as IL-10 and TGF-β. Defective Tregs populations have been associated with inflammatory diseases in mice, and autoimmunity can be suppressed by enhancing Tregs function.

T HELPER TYPE 1 CELL CYTOKINES

Extensive investigations into the cytokine profile of RA suggest a Th1 bias in the synovium based on cell phenotype (CXCR3 and CCR5 expression), cytokine levels in the joint (especially IFN-γ), the presence of cytokines that bias T cell differentiation toward Th1 (e.g., IL-12), and a Th1 phenotype of many T cell clones derived from RA synovial tissue. Considerable data have accumulated on the relative abundance and function of the prototypic Th1 cytokine, IFN-γ, which is the most potent inducer of MHC class II antigen on many cell types. IFN-γ also induces adhesion molecules, such as VCAM-1 and ICAM-1, on the surface of endothelial cells and can help recruit inflammatory cell accumulation at sites of injury. One of the most important functions of IFN-γ is its capacity to alter the balance of extracellular matrix synthesis and degradation by decreasing collagen synthesis and inhibiting MMP production by cytokine-stimulated cultured FLS.[167] IFN-γ knockout mice or IFN-γ receptor deficiency can exacerbate collagen-induced arthritis in mice, and this serves as a reminder that the effects of cytokines can vary depending on the model and timing of expression.

Despite the evidence for T cell activation in the rheumatoid synovium, only relatively low concentrations of IFN-γ have been detected,[168] much less than the amounts needed to induce HLA-DR expression on monocytes. The relative lack of IFN-γ in rheumatoid joints has been observed at the level of mRNA using a variety of techniques, including reverse-transcriptase polymerase chain reaction.[169] Immunohistochemical analysis shows IFN-γ in a few RA synovial T cells, although the percentage is far less than in chronically inflamed tonsils.[170]

Another Th1 cytokine, IL-2, is a T cell–derived cytokine that serves as an autocrine or paracrine T cell growth factor. Although it originally was reported to be present in synovial fluid using biologic assay, more specific immunoassays showed that IL-2 is detected in only a small percentage of RA synovial effusions and synovial tissues and, when present, is found only in low concentrations.[171] TNF-α, GM-CSF, and IL-6 can be expressed by Th1 and Th2 cells. All three are abundant in synovial fluid and produced by RA synovial tissue. The primary sources of these cytokines in the rheumatoid joint are macrophages and fibroblasts, however, rather than T cells (see later). IL-17 originally was considered a Th1 cytokine, although more recent data suggest that it is mainly produced by another distinct subset known as Th17 (see later).

T HELPER TYPE 2 CELL CYTOKINES

Although Th1 cytokines have been detected (albeit in low concentrations), Th2 cytokine levels are exceedingly low in RA. Using immunoassays, IL-4 and TNF-β generally are not detected in RA synovial fluid. In situ hybridization also shows little or no IL-4 in RA synovial tissue, although a small amount of IFN-γ is detected using the same method. When extremely sensitive nested reverse-transcriptase polymerase chain reaction techniques are used on synovial biopsy specimens, Th2 cytokines IL-4 and IL-13 are absent in RA, whereas IFN-γ and IL-12 (a cytokine that induces T cell maturation toward the Th1 phenotype) are present. In one study, IL-13 protein was detected in RA synovial effusions. IL-10, which has potent anti-inflammatory activities, is expressed in RA synovium. Macrophages rather than T cells are the major producers of IL-10 in RA, however.

T HELPER TYPE 17 CYTOKINES

The proinflammatory cytokine IL-17 exists as six isoforms (IL-17A through IL-17F). It originally was described as a Th1 cytokine, but now seems to be produced mainly by a distinct subset known as Th-17. IL-17A mimics many of the activities of IL-1 and TNF-α with respect to FLS function, including induction of collagenase and cytokine production.[172] IL-17 is present in modest, but functionally relevant, concentrations in RA synovial effusions.[173] More important, T cell–derived IL-17 in synovial tissue can synergize with IL-1 and TNF-α by activating synoviocytes to produce MMPs and other proinflammatory cytokines. Specific IL-17 receptors are expressed by synoviocytes and, when engaged, can activate the transcription factor NFκB and initiate an inflammatory cascade. In addition to its effect on mesenchymal cells, IL-17 can participate in bone erosion by enhancing osteoclast activation.[174] Bone resorption in an in vitro model using synovial explants and bone shows that blockade of IL-17, IL-1, and TNF-α is more effective than blocking the individual factors.[175]

Immunohistochemistry shows that IL-17 is mainly present in synovial sublining T cells. Because immunoreactive IL-17 can be detected near the erosive front of pannus, it also could participate in extracellular matrix destruction.[176] Animal models of arthritis show that IL-17 inhibition is anti-inflammatory and protects animals from bone and cartilage destruction.[177] It is uncertain whether Th17 cells, per se, are responsible for all IL-17 isoforms production in the joint. Either IL-23 or the combination of IL-6 and TGF-β in the joint can enhance Th17 cell differentiation. All three of these cytokines are present in RA synovium, providing an excellent milieu to encourage the generation of these cells.

REGULATORY T CELLS

The function of Tregs, defined by the CD4⁺CD25⁺ phenotype, in RA is poorly defined. Deficiency of this subset, which produces TGF-β and regulates other T cells through cell contact, might contribute to autoimmunity. Studies of RA peripheral blood show normal numbers of Tregs, although the CD4⁺CD25⁺ subset seems to accumulate in rheumatoid synovial effusions. Peripheral blood Treg responses in vitro to stimuli such as anti-CD3 and anti-CD28 antibody displayed an anergic phenotype, however, and were unable to suppress T cell or monocyte cytokine production. This abnormality might be reversed when patients are treated with TNF inhibitors.[178] These data suggest that abnormal Treg function could be secondary to cytokine imbalance in RA, rather than a primary event. Nevertheless, enhancing or restoring Treg activity as a therapeutic intervention potentially could downregulate other T cells and cytokine production. More recently, a novel phenotype defined by CD4⁺CD25⁺CD27⁺ has been identified in synovial effusions of patients with juvenile inflammatory arthritis.[179] This population expresses FoxP3 and does not produce Th1 cytokines. The suppressor function of these cells was decreased in vitro by cytokines such as IL-7 and IL-15, both of which have been identified in inflammatory synovitis.

Enhancing Treg function has been used to treat animal models of arthritis. Antigen-induced arthritis is exacerbated when CD4$^+$CD25$^+$ cells are depleted, and suppressed when the cells are passively transferred to affected animals. Treg function is reduced in some inflammation models.[180] Administration of neuropeptides, such as vasoactive intestinal peptide, seems to suppress collagen-induced arthritis by enhancing the Treg function in synovium and lymph nodes.[181]

T HELPER CELL CYTOKINE IMBALANCE IN RHEUMATOID ARTHRITIS

The relative abundance of Th1 cells and cytokines suggests that the synovium resembles a Th1-like delayed-type hypersensitivity reaction. Th2 cytokines and cellular responses that normally suppress Th1 activation are nearly absent, raising the possibility that the lack of T cell activation along the Th2 pathway in RA contributes to disease perpetuation. Addition of exogenous IL-10 or IL-4 to cultures of synovial tissue cells or synovial tissue explants suppresses synthesis of proinflammatory cytokines, such as IL-6, IL-1, TNF-α, and GM-CSF, and MMPs by cultured RA synovial tissue explants.[182] The inhibitory action of IL-4 might be mediated by decreased c-*jun* and c-*fos* expression, which is required for efficient production of MMPs and cytokines. In addition, IL-10 and IL-4 increase the release of other anti-inflammatory cytokines, such as IL-1Ra, by synovial cells. Although IL-10 protein is present in RA synovial fluid, and the gene is expressed by synovial tissue cells,[183] in vitro studies of cultured synovial cells suggest that not enough IL-10 is produced to suppress IFN-γ production.

The notion that Th1 and Th17 cytokines initiate and perpetuate arthritis, whereas Th2 cytokines are suppressive is supported by studies in animal models. IL-4 and IL-10 were administered individually or in combination in collagen-induced arthritis.[184] The cytokines had modest or no benefit when used separately, but together the effect was impressive. Clinical improvement correlated with decreased synovial IL-1, TNF-α, and cartilage destruction. Anti-IL-10 antibody therapy in collagen-induced arthritis accelerates disease. The complexity of cytokine networks in inflammatory arthritis is underscored by studies on the role of IL-12 in collagen-induced arthritis. In early arthritis, IL-12 administration increases the incidence of collagen-induced arthritis, whereas anti-IL-12 is beneficial.[185] In late disease, IL-12 administration suppresses arthritis, however, and anti-IL-12 causes an exacerbation. Although the notion that enhancing Th2 cytokines is attractive, a clinical trial using IL-10 in RA did not show significant clinical benefit or improvement in histologic evidence of synovial inflammation.[186] Combinations of Th2 cytokines might be required to coordinate a maximal effect.

ACTIVATION OF SYNOVIAL CELLS BY CELL-CELL CONTACT WITH T LYMPHOCYTES

Although T cell activation is unexpectedly modest in rheumatoid synovium, alternative mechanisms permit these cells to participate in synovial cytokine networks and matrix destruction. A second process by which T cells can activate macrophages and fibroblasts in RA is through direct cell-cell contact. Membranes prepared from activated T cells can stimulate macrophages and FLS directly to produce cytokines and MMPs.[187] The membrane constituents that regulate this process vary, depending on the particular culture conditions, but include adhesion molecules such as lymphocyte function–associated antigen-1 and membrane-bound TNF-α. A T cell displaying these proteins, even if the cell is no longer functional, potentially can contribute to macrophage and fibroblast activation in an antigen-independent fashion. One of the best-characterized consequences of this pathway is the ability of T cells to enhance synovial macrophage TNF-α production in a contact-dependent manner after exposure to macrophage-derived IL-15.[188] Cell contact–dependent activation of macrophages can be enhanced by other cytokines present in rheumatoid synovium, such as IL-7.[189]

The concept that lymphocytes can activate cells in the environment through direct contact suggests an unanticipated role for T cells in RA. The traditional paradigm assumes that T cells in the joint respond to a pathogenic stimulus and subsequently drive an antigen-specific response. Cell-cell contact influences can be antigen-independent, however, and require only colocalization of memory T cells with synoviocytes or macrophages. Because T cells with a memory phenotype accumulate in the joint owing to the release of chemoattractants, there is no requirement for a specific arthritogenic antigen to initiate the process. Instead, activation of innate immunity by nonspecific stimuli permits subsequent ingress of the correct T cell phenotype to engage resident synovial lining cells.

ROLE OF MACROPHAGE AND FIBROBLAST CYTOKINES

> ### Key Points
>
> - Macrophage and fibroblast cytokines are abundant in RA synovium.
> - Cytokine networks that involve proinflammatory cytokines, such as IL-1, TNF-α, IL-6, IL-15, IL-18, GM-CSF, and many others, can help perpetuate synovial inflammation.
> - Chemokines that recruit inflammatory cells into the joint generally are produced by macrophages and fibroblasts.
> - Anti-inflammatory cytokines, such as IL-1Ra and IL-10, are produced in rheumatoid synovium, albeit in amounts insufficient to offset proinflammatory cytokines.

Although the production of T cell cytokines is relatively low in RA, the same is not true for products of macrophages and fibroblasts. Virtually every macrophage and fibroblast proinflammatory mediator investigated in the RA synovium is abundant. This section enumerates some major cytokines and effectors produced in the joint, with an emphasis on the prevalence of macrophage and fibroblast products as driving forces during the perpetuation phase of RA. Macrophages, in particular, are the most vigorous producers of cytokines. These cells, which are present in small numbers in normal synovium, increase in number by migration from extrasynovial sites (e.g., bone marrow) after inflammation begins. Their responses include secretion of more than 100 substances and regulation of a biologic array of activity from the induction of cell growth to cell death. The role of macrophage and fibroblast cytokines in the pathogenesis of RA

Table 65-6 Effect of Cytokine Blockade in Animal Models of Arthritis and Rheumatoid Arthritis

Model	T Cell Dependence	TNF-α	IL-1	IL-6	IL-4	IL-10	IFN-γ
SKG	Yes	↓↓↓	↓↓	↓↓↓	0	↑	0
Active CIA	Yes then no	↓↓	↓↓	↓↓↓	↑	↑	↑↑
Passive CIA	No	↓↓↓	↓↓↓	0		↓	
K/BxN	Yes then no	0	↓↓↓				
Passive K/BxN	No	↓	↓↓↓	0			
SCW arthritis	No then yes	↓	↓		↑	↑	↑B
Rheumatoid arthritis	Yes	↓↓	↓	↓↓		0A	0A

↓, cytokine blockade suppresses arthritis; ↑, cytokine blockade increases arthritis; 0, minimal or no role; Aadministration of exogenous cytokine is ineffective; Badministration of exogenous IFN-γ suppresses disease.

IFN, interferon; IL, interleukin; SCW, streptococcal cell wall; TNF, tumor necrosis factor.

From Firestein GS: The T cell cometh: Interplay between adaptive immunity and cytokine networks in rheumatoid arthritis. J Clin Invest 114:471, 2004.

initially was suggested by studies involving patient samples and preclinical experiments in animal models. No animal model truly replicates RA. Table 65-6 shows the relative contribution of various cytokines to murine and rat models compared with human disease.[190] Despite dramatic differences in pathogenesis, there are remarkable similarities related to cytokine function in the various models.

PROINFLAMMATORY MACROPHAGE AND FIBROBLAST CYTOKINES

Interleukin-1 Family

The IL-1 family is a ubiquitous group of polypeptides with a wide range of biologic activity; they include IL-1α, IL-1β, IL-18, and IL-1Ra, which is a natural inhibitor of IL-1 (see the following section on suppressive cytokines and cytokine antagonists for a description of IL-1Ra). Abundant animal data indicate that IL-1 can serve as a key regulatory factor in inflammatory arthritis. Recombinant IL-1β induces the accumulation of PMNs and mononuclear leukocytes in the joint space and the loss of proteoglycan from articular cartilage when injected directly into rabbit knee joints. Transgenic mice that overexpress IL-1 also develop inflammatory arthritis, whereas mice that lack the natural IL-1 antagonist IL-1Ra have increased susceptibility to collagen-induced arthritis. In most cases, IL-1 blockade in animal models modestly decreases synovial inflammation, while markedly diminishing bone and cartilagedestruction.

Interleukin 1. Synovial macrophages are the most prolific source of IL-1 in the joint, and nearly half of all macrophages in the RA synovium express IL-1β.[191] Immunohistologic studies confirm this, with especially abundant IL-1 protein in synovial lining macrophages adjacent to type B synoviocytes and in sublining macrophages near blood vessels. The IL-1 in the lining subsequently can activate type B synoviocytes to proliferate and secrete a variety of mediators. A broad range of stimuli are capable of inducing IL-1 production by macrophages; immunoglobulin Fc fragments and, to a lesser extent, immune complexes can generate IL-1 production by rheumatoid synovial macrophages. Collagen fragments can induce IL-1 production, and type IX collagen, which has been found only in articular cartilage and localized into intersections of collagen fibrils, is a potent inducer of IL-1 by human monocytes.

Within the rheumatoid joint, IL-1 induces fibroblast proliferation; stimulates the biosynthesis of IL-6, IL-8, and GM-CSF by synovial cells; and enhances collagenase and PG production.[192] It increases glycosaminoglycan release in human synovial fibroblast cultures, although the effect of IL-1 on the production of intact proteoglycan molecules by intact articular cartilage explants can be the opposite. IL-1 induces numerous adhesion molecules on FLS and endothelial cells, including VCAM-1 and ICAM-1, and enhances bone resorption.

IL-1 has been implicated in RA, and inhibition of this mediator using IL-1Ra (anakinra) has modest anti-inflammatory activities in humans. Improvement generally has been observed in 40% to 45% of patients. IL-1Ra also has been used in combination with TNF inhibitors and provided no additional benefit even though biologic activity was shown by virtue of a decreased C-reactive protein and an increased incidence of infections.[193] The limited activity of IL-1Ra in RA was presumed to be related to its short half-life and the need for very high concentrations. The same protein is extremely effective, however, in diseases with a well-defined role for IL-1, such as Still's disease, familial cold autoinflammatory syndrome, and Muckle-Wells syndrome. Another biologic IL-1 inhibitor with high avidity for IL-1 and improved pharmacokinetics and an IL-1 convertase inhibitor had clinical responses in RA that were similar to anakinra. These data suggest that IL-1 plays a less important role in the clinical manifestations of RA than initially considered. Its contributions to cartilage and bone destruction are still uncertain.

An alternative explanation for the relatively modest benefit of IL-1 in RA relates to its signaling mechanisms. Similar to many TLRs, IL-1 activates NFκB through the kinase MyD88. Both pathways (IL-1 and TLR) converge and share a common mechanism for activating transcription of proinflammatory cytokines. When IL-1 signaling is blocked, it is possible that TLR ligands in the synovium, including exogenous ones such as peptidoglycan or endogenous ones such as HSPs, can provide the stimulus required to overcome IL-1 blockade. This concept was tested in the passive K/BxN model where mice lacking the IL-1 receptor had markedly decreased arthritis severity. When small amounts of the TLR4 ligand lipopolysaccharide were administered, robust synovitis ensued. If a similar system occurs in RA, IL-1 blockade would be unable to control synovitis as long as TLR signaling remains intact.

Interleukin-18. In addition to IL-1α and IL-1β, a homologous protein in the IL-1 family known as IL-18 has been implicated in RA. This cytokine originally was defined by its ability to bias the immune response toward the Th1 phenotype, especially in the presence of IL-12. In collagen-induced arthritis, IL-18 inhibition significantly attenuates disease.[194] The same effect was observed in IFN-γ knockout mice, indicating that other non–Th1-related activities of IL-18 might be important. Subsequent studies showed that IL-18 induces GM-CSF, nitric oxide production, and TNF-α expression by synovial macrophages.[195] Although IL-18, along with IL-12 or IL-15, can increase IFN-γ production by synovial tissue in vitro, the relative importance of this activity is uncertain compared with the IL-1-like activities of the cytokine. IL-18 is expressed by RA synovial tissue, especially by synovial fibroblasts and macrophages, and its production is markedly increased by TNF-α and IL-1β. A natural inhibitor, the IL-18 binding protein, potentially can be used as a therapeutic agent to block the proinflammatory effects and pro-Th1 effects of IL-18. One potential concern for IL-18 as a target for RA is the fact that the IL-1 convertase inhibitor had only modest benefit. IL-18, similar to IL-1β, is processed by this enzyme to produce biologically active cytokine. An effective IL-1 convertase inhibitor theoretically should block IL-1β and IL-18 release by macrophages.

Tumor Necrosis Factor Superfamily

The TNF superfamily is an extended group of related genes that play a major role in inflammation, immune responses, cell survival, and apoptosis. At least 19 members of the family have been identified, with TNF-α identified as the eponymous member. Each cytokine has its own preference for cell surface receptor, although there is some promiscuity of receptor binding and functional overlap. The TNF superfamily members exhibit conserved amino acid sequences suggesting a single ancestral gene. Many sequences include type II membrane protein characteristics and can be released from cell surfaces after proteolytic cleavage. A C-terminal conserved domain called the TNF-homology domain also is shared by several superfamily members. The active forms of the proteins are homotrimers except for LTα and LTβ, which can form either heterotrimers or homotrimers. Several members already have been discussed in the relevant sections (lymphotoxin, LIGHT, BLyS, and APRIL in Synovial Pathology and Biology; Fas ligand and TWEAK in Life and Death in the Rheumatoid Synovium; and receptor activator of NFκB ligand (RANKL) in Bone and Cartilage Destruction). In this section, one of the "founding" members of the superfamily is discussed because of its crucial role in synovial inflammation.

TNF-α is a pleiotropic cytokine that has been implicated as a key proinflammatory cytokine in RA and detected in rheumatoid synovial fluid and serum. It is produced as a membrane-bound protein that is released from the cell surface after proteolytic cleavage by TNF convertase, a membrane MMP. IL-1 and TNF-α have many similar activities, including the ability to enhance cytokine production, adhesion molecule expression, proliferation, and MMP production by cultured synoviocytes. In some systems, the effects of these two agents are synergistic. Although they share many

functions and signal transduction pathways, IL-1 and TNF use distinct surface receptors and intracellular signaling pathways. The clearly defined efficacy of TNF inhibitors in RA shows its crucial role in the disease; heterogeneity of the rheumatoid process also is apparent because only about one third of patients have a dramatic response to TNF inhibitors. Efficacy requires continuous therapy because cessation typically leads to a flare of disease. Evidence is beginning to accumulate suggesting that early aggressive therapy with anti-TNF agents can induce long-term remissions even after therapy is withdrawn. This exciting notion suggests that interventions in the earliest stages of disease could prevent the establishment of chronic synovitis.

TNF-α, similar to IL-1, stimulates collagenase and PGE_2 production by human synovial cells, induces bone resorption, inhibits bone formation in vitro, and stimulates resorption of proteoglycan and inhibits its biosynthesis in explants of cartilage.[196] In situ hybridization and immunohistochemical studies show that TNF-α is primarily produced by synovial macrophages in RA. Animal models also have supported the general role played by TNF-α in inflammatory arthritis. Overexpression of TNF-α in transgenic mice leads to an aggressive and destructive synovitis. The arthritis also spontaneously occurs in transgenic mice that express only a membrane-bound form of TNF-α on T cells.[197] TNF blockade is an effective anti-inflammatory agent in many animal models of arthritis,[198] although the effects on bone and cartilage destruction are less prominent than with IL-1 inhibitors. TNF inhibition in RA significantly decreases extracellular matrix destruction as measured by radiographic progression.[199] It is unclear why the bone-protective effects are more prominent in humans than in animal models. TNF blockade also is more effective in animal models when combined with an IL-1 inhibitor, supporting the additive or synergistic relationship between the two cytokines in animal models; this has not been observed in RA, however.

The mechanisms by which anti-TNF-α influences synovitis are distinct from the mechanisms of other biologic therapies. Individuals with an inadequate response to a TNF inhibitor are still likely to respond to either rituximab or abatacept. This likelihood supports the notion that multiple independent pathways can contribute to the pathogenesis of RA and the heterogeneous nature of the disease. Another complexity related to the role of TNF-α is that clinical responses do not always correlate with protection of the extracellular matrix. Patients with little or no clinical improvement in signs and symptoms of RA still have significant delay or arrest of joint damage. This observation supports the contention that inflammation and destruction have distinct pathogenic mechanisms.

Interleukin-6 Family

IL-6 is a protein produced by many cells including T cells, monocytes, and cultured FLS.[200] Originally defined by its B cell–stimulating properties, it induces immunoglobulin synthesis in B cell lines, is involved in the differentiation of cytotoxic T lymphocytes, and is a major factor in the regulation of acute-phase response proteins by the liver. The IL-6 receptor includes a common chain (gp130) that is shared with other cytokines and an IL-6-specific chain (IL-6R). IL-6R can be shed from cell surfaces, bind to IL-6, and deliver it to cells that lack IL-6 receptors by combining with gp130.

A striking correlation between serum IL-6 activity and serum levels of acute-phase reactants such as C-reactive protein, α_1-antitrypsin, fibrinogen, and haptoglobin occurs in patients with RA. Very high levels of IL-6 are present in RA synovial fluid, and synovial cells in culture from diverse inflammatory arthropathies produce IL-6.[200] In situ hybridization of synovial tissue also shows IL-6 mRNA in the intimal lining, and immunohistochemistry studies show IL-6 protein in the lining and sublining regions.[201] Although many synovial macrophages express the IL-6 gene, most IL-6 seems to be produced by type B synoviocytes. The pivotal role of IL-6 in RA has been shown by clinical trials using a monoclonal antibody that binds to IL-6R. The clinical responses are similar to TNF inhibitors.[202]

Cytokines with structural similarity to IL-6 and that share surface receptor subunits also have been implicated in RA. Several of these—IL-11, leukemia inhibitory factor, and oncostatin M—are expressed by rheumatoid synovium and can be detected in synovial effusions. The biologic effects of these factors are complex and can be either protective (e.g., by increasing expression of protease inhibitors, such as tissue inhibitors of metalloproteinase [TIMP]) or proinflammatory (e.g., by increasing expression of chemokines or MMPs) depending on the culture conditions or the specific model evaluated. This dichotomy among the family members is shown by the fact that IL-11 administration ameliorates collagen-induced arthritis,[203] whereas antibodies to oncostatin M are protective.[204]

Interleukin-12 Family

The IL-12 family includes a group of cytokines that play a key role in the differentiation of T cells and inflammation. IL-12 is a heterodimeric cytokine with two subunits (e.g., p35 and p40) encoded on separate genes. It is produced by antigen presenting cells and phagocytic cells. IL-23 and IL-27 have similar heterodimeric structures to IL-12, with p29/p40 and p28/EB13 components. In the context of antigen presentation, IL-12, IL-23, and IL-27 can bias T cell responses toward the Th1 phenotype. IL-23 also can play a pivotal role in the production of Th17 cells, along with IL-6 and TGF-β. The members of the IL-12 family of cytokines generally are produced by macrophages in the rheumatoid joint, but also are produced by other antigen presenting cells such as DCs. Although clinical data defining the role of these cytokines are still lacking, there are anecdotal case reports of RA patients with malignancy treated with recombinant IL-12 developing a flare of disease. Animal models, including adjuvant arthritis in rats and collagen-induced arthritis in mice, are partially ameliorated by neutralization of IL-12, IL-23, or IL-27 depending on the timing of treatment. In some situations, however, IL-27 has anti-inflammatory effects.[205,206]

Interleukin-15

IL-15 is an IL-2-like cytokine that regulates numerous immunologic functions relevant to RA, including T cell chemotaxis and proliferation, production of immunoglobulins by B cells, and the generation of natural killer cells.

The IL-15 receptor is a complex heterotrimer that includes a common chain shared with the IL-2 receptor, a common chain shared with many other cytokines, and a high-affinity specific IL-15 chain. Because it can transduce a signal directly to IL-15R-expressing cells or present the bound cytokine to stimulate neighboring cells, IL-15 can serve as an IL-2-independent mechanism for activating T cells, although its role in RA may be related to its key role in TNF-α regulation. Macrophages are the primary source of IL-15 in RA, and the cytokine is able to induce a cell-contact mechanism of macrophage TNF-α production that requires T cells. Although T lymphocytes, or at least their membranes, are required for this process, the macrophages produce the TNF-α. This network provides a potential mechanism whereby local IL-15 production in the synovium can lead to autocrine production of TNF-α in a T cell–dependent, but antigen-independent, fashion. IL-15 has been shown in RA synovial macrophages using immunohistochemical techniques.[207] Soluble IL-15 receptors can function as an IL-15 inhibitor, and when used in vivo can decrease joint inflammation in collagen-induced arthritis.[208] The mechanism of action probably includes TNF-α inhibition, although decreased IFN-γ production and immune responses to type II collagen indicate that IL-15 also regulates antigen-dependent responses.

Interleukin-32

IL-32 is a novel cytokine that activates NFκB and induces the production of several proinflammatory cytokines and chemokines, including TNF-α, IL-1, IL-6, and IL-8. It has been implicated in Crohn's disease because of its ability to enhance markedly caspase 1 activation and IL-1 production in cells that have been exposed to muramyl dipeptides. More recently, IL-32 was shown by immunohistochemistry in synovial tissues of patients with RA, especially in synovial lining macrophage-like cells.[209] The level of IL-32 expression correlated with the presence of other cytokines implicated in RA, including TNF-α, IL-1, and IL-18. Injection of IL-32 into the joints of naive mice causes a robust transient synovitis. The synovial response could be partially abrogated by anti-TNF-α antibodies, suggesting that IL-32 induces this cytokine in vivo. These data suggest that IL-32 might be upstream from several proinflammatory mediators in RA and could represent a therapeutic target.

Colony-Stimulating Factors

GM-CSF supports the differentiation of bone marrow precursor cells to mature granulocytes and macrophages. As with other major CSFs, GM-CSF also participates in normal immune responses. It is a potent macrophage activator, including the induction of HLA-DR expression, tumoricidal activity, IL-1 secretion, intracellular parasite killing, and priming for enhanced release of TNF-α and PGE$_2$. Neutrophil function also is regulated by GM-CSF, which enhances antibody-dependent cytotoxicity, phagocytosis, chemotaxis, and the production of oxygen radicals.

RA synovial fluid contains GM-CSF, which is produced by RA synovial tissue cells.[210] The major source in the synovium is macrophages, although IL-1-stimulated or TNF-α-stimulated FLS also express the GM-CSF gene.[211]

In situ hybridization studies show little or no GM-CSF mRNA in synovial T cells. The ability of GM-CSF to induce HLA-DR gene expression on macrophages might be of particular importance in RA. GM-CSF, not IFN-γ, is the major DR-inducing cytokine in RA synovial fluid and in supernatants of cultured synovial tissue cells. Collagen-induced arthritis in mice is less severe in animals that lack a functional GM-CSF gene or are treated with anti–GM-CSF antibody, which supports the hypothesis that GM-CSF is an important proinflammatory mediator.[212]

Macrophage colony-stimulating factor (M-CSF) also is expressed by RA synovium and is present in synovial effusions. Its primary pathogenic role in RA probably relates to its osteoclast-differentiating capacity. As is described later, this factor cooperates with RANKL to facilitate bone erosions.

Chemokine Families

Chemokines are a family of related chemoattractant peptides that, with the assistance of adhesion molecules, summon cells into inflammatory sites. They generally are divided into families, including C-C, C-X-C, and C-X3-C, based on the position of characteristic cysteine residues. In the C-C family, two conserved cysteines are adjacent to one another, whereas in the C-X-C family, the cysteines are separated by a nonconserved amino acid. Each individual factor has the ability to attract specific lineages of cells after interacting with specific surface receptors. Many chemokines have been identified in the rheumatoid joint. IL-8, a C-X-C chemokine that was originally characterized as a potent chemoattractant for neutrophils, along with immune complexes and other chemotactic peptides such as C5a, contributes to the large influx of PMNs into the joint. Immunohistochemical analysis of synovial tissue shows IL-8 protein in sublining perivascular macrophages and in scattered lining cells.[213] Cultured synovial tissue macrophages constitutively produce IL-8, and FLS express the gene if they are stimulated with IL-1 or TNF-α. IL-8 accounts for about 40% of the neutrophil chemoattractant activity in synovial fluid. In addition, IL-8 activates neutrophils through G protein–coupled receptors and is a potent angiogenesis factor.

Many other chemoattractant proteins are implicated in RA. MIP-1α, MIP-1β, macrophage chemoattractant protein (MCP)-1, and RANTES—members of the C-C subfamily—are produced by RA synovium.[214] CXCL16 and epithelial neutrophil-activating peptide-78 (ENA-78) are C-X-C chemokines and are abundant along with many others in that family.[215] The former, which binds to CXCR6 on T cells, can contribute to the recruitment of lymphocytes into the synovium. ENA-78 accounts for about 40% of the chemotactic activity for neutrophils in RA synovial fluid. In each case, the source of the chemokine seems to be synovial macrophages or cytokine-stimulated type B synoviocytes. The regulation of each chemokine seems to be distinct in FLS. The concentrations of chemokines are higher in RA synovial effusions compared with samples from noninflammatory arthritides, such as osteoarthritis. Although the chemokines also can be detected in the blood, the levels are considerably lower than in the joint, providing a gradient that signals cells to migrate into the synovium.

As noted earlier, lymphocyte-specific factors might contribute to the germinal center architecture of RA. The C-X-C factor B cell–activating chemokine-1 (BCA-1; CXCL13) binds to specific CXCR5 receptors on B cells. BCA-1 is expressed in the RA synovial tissues, especially by follicular DCs in germinal centers, and likely accounts for B cell migration to these regions.[216] CCL21 and several other factors participate in the anatomic organization of germinal centers, marginal zones, and other regions of lymphoid follicles. Another chemokine, SDF-1, is expressed by synoviocytes and endothelial cells and can play a major role as a chemoattractant for T cells in synovium via its receptor CXCR4.[217] In contrast to other chemokine receptors that can bind multiple members of the family, CXCR4 is highly specific for SDF-1 and is expressed by memory CD4+ lymphocytes.

Chemokine-directed approaches have garnered considerable attention as potential therapeutic targets to prevent recruitment of cells into the synovium. Numerous preclinical models support the use of chemokine blockers. Antibodies to fractalkine (CXC3L1) suppressed murine collagen-induced arthritis even though anti–type II collagen antibody production was not affected.[218] Anti-CXCL16 antibody decreased clinical arthritis in the same model. One problem is that the system is highly redundant, and several different chemotactic proteins can bind to the same receptor. No clinical improvement was observed in a study using anti-MCP-1 antibody, perhaps because the antibody also altered the kinetics of MCP-1 metabolism. Anti-IL-8 antibodies have met with limited success in psoriasis.

Alternatively, chemokines bind to G protein–coupled receptors and can be targeted to block multiple factors. A CCR1 antagonist, which blocks RANTES and MIP-1α, has been evaluated in a synovial biopsy clinical trial.[219] The compound significantly decreased synovial infiltration by CCR1-expressing cells, including macrophages and T cells. There was a trend toward clinical improvement. Chemokine receptor blockade has other levels of complexity, such as CCR2-deficient mice that develop more severe arthritis in some models. CCR2 antagonists, which block MCP-1, have not shown significant efficacy in RA clinical trials. These data suggest that the chemokine system, including the receptors, is redundant, complex, and, in some cases, perhaps protective in arthritis.

Chemokines and other chemotactic factors (e.g., C5a and LTB$_4$) can signal through a variety of mechanisms, although many pathways converge on phosphatidylinositol-3′-kinase (PI3K). Of the several PI3K isoforms, PI3Kγ is specific for chemokine signal transduction. This specificity provides an opportunity to block multiple chemokine receptors simultaneously. Proof of concept for this approach was provided by studies in PI3Kγ knockout mice, which have less synovial inflammation in passive and active collagen-induced arthritis than wild-type mice.[220] A small molecule PI3Kγ inhibitor provided similar benefit. Targeting shared intracellular pathways potentially can overcome some of the limitations presented by the complex chemoattractant system.

Platelet-Derived Growth Factor and Fibroblast Growth Factor

PDGF is a potent growth factor that is chemoattractant and mitogenic for fibroblasts and induces collagenase expression. It is the most potent stimulator of long-term growth of synovial cells in culture.[221] PDGF is expressed in vascular endothelial cells and other synovial sublining cells in rheumatoid synovium compared with healthy tissue.[222] Multiple isoforms of this molecule have been identified (PDGF A through D), all of which have been detected in RA synovial membranes. Most recently, PDGF D has been identified as an especially potent stimulator of MMP-1 expression in cultured synoviocytes. The PDGF receptor also is expressed in the same regions of RA synovium, suggesting the presence of an autocrine or paracrine system.

FGFs are a family of peptide growth factors with pleiotropic activities. In rheumatoid patients, it is likely that heparin-binding growth factor, the precursor of acidic FGF, is a major mitogen for many cell types and stimulates angiogenesis. An interaction between FGF and proteoglycans is required for biologic activity.[223] It induces capillary endothelial cells to invade a three-dimensional collagen matrix, organizing themselves to form characteristic tubules that resemble blood capillaries. Synoviocytes also can be induced to increase expression of RANKL by FGF, enhancing osteoclast activation and bone resorption. FGF is present in RA synovial fluid, and the genes are expressed by synovial cells. Synovial fibroblasts express FGF receptors and proliferate after exposure to the growth factor.

SUPPRESSIVE CYTOKINES AND CYTOKINE ANTAGONISTS

The proinflammatory cytokine network in RA is offset by a variety of suppressive and anti-inflammatory factors that attempt to re-establish homeostasis. Underproduction of these suppressive cytokines potentially can contribute to the perpetuation of the synovitis. There are many cytokine antagonists or natural immunosuppressives that represent potential therapeutic targets for the treatment of inflammatory diseases.

Interleukin-1 Receptor Antagonist

IL-1Ra is a naturally occurring IL-1 inhibitor that binds directly to type I and type II IL-1 receptors and competes with IL-1 for the ligand-binding site. Interaction of IL-1Ra with the IL-1 receptors does not result in signal transduction, and, in contrast to IL-1α or IL-1β, the receptor-ligand complex is not internalized after it binds to the IL-1 receptor. Although IL-1Ra has high affinity for the IL-1 receptor, it is a relatively weak inhibitor because IL-1 can activate cells even if only a small percentage of IL-1 receptors are occupied. Because of this, a substantial excess of the inhibitor is required to saturate the receptor and block IL-1-mediated stimulation (usually 10-fold to 100-fold excess of IL-1Ra). Recombinant IL-1Ra inhibits a variety of IL-1-mediated events in cultured cells derived from the joint, including the induction of MMP and PG production by chondrocytes and synoviocytes. It can block synovitis in rabbits induced by direct intra-articular injection of recombinant IL-1.[224]

IL-1Ra is present in rheumatoid synovial effusions; much of it is produced by neutrophils and macrophages.[225] Immunohistochemical studies of rheumatoid synovium reveal IL-1Ra protein, especially in perivascular mononuclear cells and the synovial intimal lining. The IL-1Ra protein and mRNA can be detected in synovial macrophages and, to a

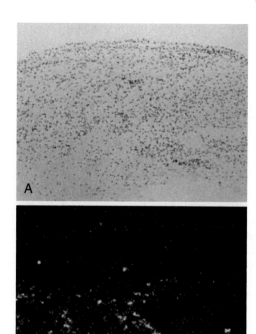

Figure 65-9 Localization of interleukin-1 receptor antagonist (IL-1Ra) messenger RNA in rheumatoid arthritis synovial tissue by in situ hybridization. The specific RNA transcript was detected in perivascular cells, especially macrophages. **A,** Bright field view. **B,** Same area using a dark field filter. Silver grains in the dark field view show the location of IL-1 Ra-positive cells.

lesser extent, in type B synoviocytes (Fig. 65-9). The presence of IL-1Ra in synovium is not specific to RA because osteoarthritis synovial tissue also contains IL-1Ra, albeit in lesser amounts; normal synovium contains little, if any, IL-1Ra protein. Despite the presence of significant amounts of IL-1Ra in synovial tissue, its importance as an IL-1 antagonist can be evaluated only in the context of the IL-1-to-IL-1Ra ratio. Studies of synovial cell culture supernatants show that the amount of IL-1Ra is insufficient to antagonize synovial IL-1.[226]

Interleukin-10

IL-10 is an immunosuppressive cytokine that was originally characterized as an inhibitor of T cell cytokine production. Its immunosuppressive actions might be important in pregnancy to suppress an immune response directed against paternal MHC antigens, and it might regulate susceptibility to some parasitic infections. As noted previously, IL-10 protein is present in RA synovial fluid, and the gene is expressed by synovial tissue macrophages. Serial synovial biopsy specimens in RA patients who were treated with recombinant IL-10 did not show any significant histologic improvement, and clinical responses were not impressive in a limited study.

Transforming Growth Factor-β

TGF-β is a key member of the TGF superfamily, which includes the bone morphogenetic proteins (BMPs) that signal through intracellular signaling molecules known as

Smads. It is widely distributed in different tissues and produced by many cells, including T cells, monocytes, and platelets. TGF-β suppresses the production of collagenase and induces the expression of TIMP. TGF-β accelerates the healing of incisional wounds and induces fibrosis and angiogenesis in experimental animal models. Substantial amounts of TGF-β are present in synovial fluid (although it is mainly present in an inactive, latent form), and mRNA can be detected in RA synovial tissue.[227] Although typically considered an immunosuppressive cytokine with wound-healing properties, the role of TGF-β in RA is complex as shown by the conflicting results of its administration in various animal models. In RA, TGF-β is one of the factors responsible for blunted responses of T cells that have been exposed to synovial fluid. TGF-β also downregulates IL-1 receptor expression on some cell types, including chondrocytes. When TGF-β is injected directly into the knees of animals, fibrosis and synovial lining hyperplasia develop.[228] In streptococcal cell wall arthritis, parenteral administration or systemic gene therapy with the TGF-β gene ameliorates the disease.[229] Intra-articular administration of anti-TGF-β antibody decreases arthritis in the injected joint, but not in the contralateral joint in the same model. Although mainly considered anti-inflammatory, TGF-β also can support the differentiation of T cells into the Th17 phenotype.

Soluble Cytokine Receptors and Binding Proteins

Soluble cytokine receptors and binding proteins can absorb free cytokines and prevent them from engaging functional receptors on cells. Although these could inhibit cytokine action, they also could act as carrier proteins that protect cytokines from proteolytic degradation or deliver them directly to cells, such as the IL-6 receptor.

TNF receptors are normally expressed as membrane-bound proteins and can be released from the cell surface after proteolytic cleavage. Soluble p55 and p75 TNF receptors have been detected in RA synovial fluid, sometimes in very high concentrations.[230] Soluble TNF receptor levels can be considerably higher than the concentration of TNF-α in blood or synovial fluid and probably explains why biologically active TNF is difficult to detect in RA synovial fluid despite the presence of immunoreactive protein. Synovial membrane mononuclear cells have increased surface expression and mRNA levels of both TNF receptors compared with osteoarthritis synovial tissue cells or peripheral blood cells.[231] Cultured FLS express TNF receptors and shed them into culture supernatants.

Many other soluble receptors and binding proteins are produced in RA, albeit in concentrations too low to suppress the exuberant proinflammatory cytokine milieu of the joint effectively. The IL-1 type II receptor is present in RA synovial fluid, along with lesser amounts of the type I receptor.[232] These soluble receptors can bind to IL-1 or IL-1Ra in synovial effusions. Soluble receptors to IL-15 and IL-17 have been characterized, and an IL-18 binding protein can inhibit cytokine activity. In some cases, a soluble receptor can protect a cytokine from degradation or transport it to the cells, as with the IL-6 receptor.

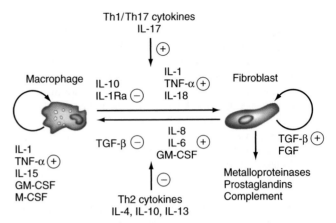

Figure 65-10 Cytokine networks in rheumatoid arthritis. Paracrine and autocrine pathways can lead to activation of fibroblast-like and macrophage-like synoviocytes in the synovial intimal lining. Positive (+) and negative (−) feedback loops are present, although in rheumatoid arthritis the former predominate. T helper type 1 (Th1) cytokines potentially can enhance the network, whereas Th2 cytokines are suppressive. FGF, fibroblast growth factor; GM-CSF, granulocyte-macrophage colony-stimulating factor; IL, interleukin; M-CSF, macrophage colony-stimulating factor; TGF, transforming growth factor; TNF, tumor necrosis factor.

PERPETUATION OF SYNOVITIS BY MACROPHAGE-FIBROBLAST CYTOKINE NETWORKS

Studies to map the cytokine profile and advances in therapy using biologic reagents to inhibit cytokines support the concept that cytokine networks play a key role in the pathogenesis of RA. Initially proposed as a potential mechanism to explain T cell–independent disease perpetuation, it is now clear that these pathways are not autonomous, and except for certain patients with early disease, discontinuation of the therapy leads to a flare. Nevertheless, paracrine and autocrine cytokine networks in the synovial intimal lining contribute largely to inflammatory arthritis in RA (Fig. 65-10).

Many cytokines that have been identified in the synovium or synovial fluid can participate in this system and might explain lining cell hyperplasia, HLA-DR and adhesion molecule induction, and synovial angiogenesis. The list of potential candidates in this highly redundant system is extensive. Several of these, including IL-1, TNF-α, and IL-6, now have well-defined roles. The first two, along with numerous other factors (e.g., IL-15, IL-18, and IL-32) are produced by synovial macrophages and stimulate synovial fibroblast proliferation and secretion of IL-6, GM-CSF, and chemokines and effector molecules such as MMPs and PGs. GM-CSF, which is produced by synovial macrophages and IL-1β-stimulated or TNF-α-stimulated synovial fibroblasts, can induce IL-1 secretion to form a positive feedback loop. GM-CSF, especially in combination with TNF-α, also increases HLA-DR expression on macrophages. Macrophage and fibroblast cytokines also can indirectly contribute to the evidence for local T cell and B cell activation, including RF production.

Cytokines also help recruit other cells into the synovium through the production of chemokines that select specific cell lineages for admission into the synovium. Many of these chemokines, including the C-X-C and C-C families, are produced by macrophages and fibroblasts and attract neutrophils, macrophages, and certain subpopulations of

T and B cells. The sublining chemokine profile helps organize these newly infiltrated cells into germinal centers in some patients. Other factors, such as IL-12 and IL-23, differentiate CD4$^+$ T cells into the Th1 phenotype to produce relatively small amounts of IFN-γ and other relevant cytokines. IL-6 and TGF-β produced mainly by the lining, along with IL-23, can support the production of Th17 cells that release the potent proinflammatory cytokine IL-17 into the local milieu. All of this occurs in the presence of inhibitor factors, soluble receptors, and binding proteins that are overwhelmed by the inflammatory drive. Other cytokines, such as RANKL and M-CSF, activate osteoclasts that remodel bone.

Although they do not cause RA per se, cytokines orchestrate the rheumatoid process. For individual patients, the pivotal cytokine or cytokines that must be blocked can be different, and even this can vary with the stage of disease. Ultimately, understanding the genetic predisposition to disease and the specific patterns of cytokine production could help determine the correct combination of cytokine inhibitors that would be effective.

SIGNAL TRANSDUCTION AND TRANSCRIPTION FACTORS

Key Points

- Complex intracellular signaling mechanisms regulate cytokine production and actions in RA synovium.
- NFκB, MAP kinases, AP-1, and several other pathways are potential therapeutic targets in RA.

Intracellular signal transduction systems transmit environmental stimuli from the cell surface to the cytoplasm or nucleus, where they subsequently are integrated at the level of transcription factor activity. The transcription factors bind to specific DNA sites in promoter regions and regulate the expression of the appropriate genes. The remarkable diversity of signaling pathways and transcription factors provides a selective mechanism for orchestrating activation and repression for appropriate arrays of genes in response to an extracellular stress. Many of the inflammatory responses observed in RA synovium, including the activation of cytokine and adhesion molecule genes, can be traced to specific transcription factors and signal transduction pathways. An extensive description of these mechanisms is beyond the scope of this chapter, and they are reviewed in Chapter 20. Considerable enthusiasm abounds for targeting signal transduction pathways. One recurrent theme is that these pathways play a role in normal cells and host defense, which raise the issues of balancing efficacy with toxicity.

NUCLEAR FACTOR κB

NFκB is a ubiquitous transcription factor that plays a key role in the expression of many genes central to RA, including IL-1β in monocytes and ICAM-1, TNF-α, IL-6, and IL-8 in rheumatoid synoviocytes. NFκB normally resides as an inactive heterodimer or homodimer in the cell cytoplasm associated with an inhibitory protein called IκB that regulates the DNA binding and subcellular localization of NFκB

proteins by masking a nuclear localization signal. Extracellular stimuli such as cytokines or TLR agonists initiate a signaling cascade leading to activation of two IKKs (IKKα and IKKβ), which phosphorylate IκB at two NH$_2$-terminal serine residues. Phosphorylated IκB is selectively ubiquitinated and degraded by the 26S proteasome. This process permits NFκB to migrate to the cell nucleus, where it binds its target genes to initiate transcription.

NFκB is abundant in rheumatoid synovium, and immunohistochemical analysis shows p50 and p65 NFκB proteins in the nuclei of cells in the synovial intimal lining.[233] Although the proteins also can be detected in osteoarthritis synovium, NFκB activation is much greater in RA because of phosphorylation and degradation of IκB in RA intimal lining cells (Fig. 65-11). Nuclear translocation of NFκB in cultured FLS occurs rapidly after stimulation by IL-1 or TNF-α through the activation of the IKK signaling complex.

The relevance of NFκB to inflammatory arthritis has been tested in several animal models. Synovial NFκB is rapidly activated, often long before clinical arthritis is evident. Adjuvant arthritis in rats is ameliorated by intra-articular gene therapy with the dominant negative IKKβ construct that blocks the IKK pathway,[234] and streptococcal cell wall arthritis is blocked by decoy oligonucleotides or a dominant negative IκB adenovirus. NFκB inhibition is associated with decreased synovial cellular infiltration and increased apoptosis. The role of this transcription factor in murine collagen-induced arthritis has been shown using selective IKKβ inhibitors, which suppress arthritis and joint destruction. The role of IKKα is less well defined in RA. It is not required for the classic IKK pathway, but an alternative signaling method through lymphotoxin specifically uses IKKα to engage NFκB. This mechanism might contribute to NFκB activation in sublining cells, especially those in lymphoid aggregates.

MITOGEN-ACTIVATED PROTEIN KINASES

MAP kinases, which are signal transduction enzymes activated in response to cellular stress, are composed of parallel protein kinase cascades that regulate cytokine and MMP gene expression. There are three different families of MAP kinases known as c-Jun N-terminal kinase (JNK), p38, and extracellular signal-regulated kinase (ERK). MAP kinases phosphorylate selected intracellular proteins, including transcription factors, which subsequently regulate the expression of various genes by transcriptional and post-transcriptional mechanisms. MAP kinases are activated by phosphorylation at conserved threonine and tyrosine residues by a cascade of dual-specificity kinases. These are activated by MAP kinase kinase kinases. The relative hierarchy of the individual MAP kinases depends on the cell type and inflammatory stimulus.

The MAP kinases are widely expressed in synovial tissue and are activated in rheumatoid synovium. Phosphorylated ERK, p38, and JNK can be detected by immunohistochemistry or Western blot analysis.[235] All three kinases are constitutively expressed by cultured FLS and can be activated within minutes after exposure to cytokines and regulate production of proinflammatory cytokines and MMPs.

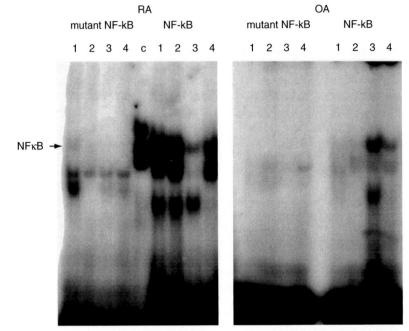

Figure 65-11 Nuclear factor κB (NFκB) activation in rheumatoid arthritis (RA) synovium. Electromobility shift assays have been performed on extracts of RA and osteoarthritis (OA) synovium. NFκB activity is significantly higher in RA synovial tissue extracts compared with extracts of OA. This is consistent with increased expression of NFκB-driven genes in RA synovium, such as proinflammatory cytokines and vascular adhesion molecules. Mutant probe is shown on the left as a negative control, and C is a positive control. *(From Han Z, Boyle DL, Manning AM, et al: AP-1 and NF-κB regulation in rheumatoid arthritis and murine collagen-induced arthritis. Autoimmunity 28:197, 1998.)*

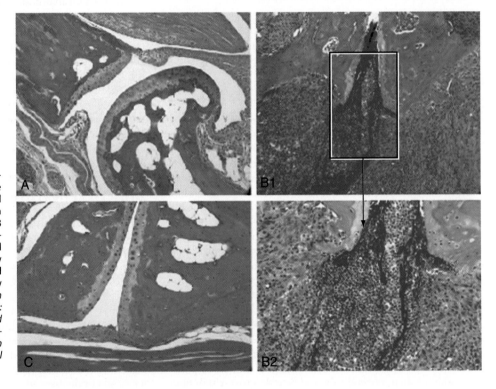

Figure 65-12 p38 mitogen-activated protein (MAP) kinase blockade suppresses murine collagen-induced arthritis. MAP kinases play a key role in cytokine regulation. Inhibitors of p38 MAP kinase suppress synovial inflammation and joint destruction in several models of arthritis. *Left panels* show near-normal joint in animal treated with p38 inhibitor. *Right panels* show control animals with arthritis. *(From Medicherla S, Ma JY, Mangadu R, et al: A selective p38α mitogen-activated protein kinase inhibitor reverses cartilage and bone destruction in mice with collagen-induced arthritis. J Pharmacol Exp Ther 318:132, 2006.)*

p38 inhibitors are effective anti-inflammatory agents in murine collagen-induced arthritis and rat adjuvant arthritis, possibly by decreasing the production of proinflammatory cytokines (Fig. 65-12).[236] Treated animals also have improved bone mineral density and decreased histologic evidence of joint inflammation. Spinal p38 also plays a major role in pain processing, and inhibitors have potential for analgesic and anti-inflammatory action. Recent studies suggest that p38 in the central nervous system can regulate peripheral inflammation because intrathecal administration

p38 blockade suppresses inflammation and joint destruction in rat adjuvant arthritis.[237] Although p38 is an attractive therapeutic target, the response rates of p38 inhibitors have been modest in RA and Crohn's disease.

JNK inhibition blocks collagenase gene expression in the cultured synoviocytes. Using a selective JNK inhibitor, marked protection of bone destruction was observed in the adjuvant arthritis model, along with decreased synovial AP-1 activation and collagenase-3 gene expression.[238] Because JNK has multiple isoforms and splice variants, some specificity possibly can be achieved by inhibiting certain forms of the enzyme to minimize potential for toxicity. This question was partially addressed in passive collagen-induced arthritis using JNK2 knockout mice and the TNF-α transgenic mice that lack JNK1. No benefit was observed in the JNK1$^{-/-}$ mice, and only modest cartilage protection was seen in the JNK2$^{-/-}$ animals.[239] However, additional studies are needed to assess the potential benefit of a selective JNK isoform inhibitor.

As an alternative to blocking MAP kinases themselves, kinases that regulate p38, JNK, and ERK also can be targeted. MKK3 and MKK6, which are upstream of p38, are activated in the rheumatoid synovial intimal lining. MKK3 knockout mice have markedly decreased joint inflammation in the passive K/BxN model.[240] These mice have nearly normal responses to lipopolysaccharide. MKK4 and MKK7 are the main kinases that modulate JNK function and are activated in the rheumatoid synovium. Small interfering RNA (siRNA) knockdown shows that only MKK7 is required for cytokine-stimulated JNK activation and MMP expression in cultured synoviocytes.[241] These studies suggest that targeting upstream kinases in RA might suppress inflammatory joint disease, while leaving other aspects of host defense or innate immunity intact.

ACTIVATOR PROTEIN-1

Similar to NFκB, AP-1 regulates many genes implicated in RA, including TNF-α and the MMPs. AP-1 activity can be induced by extracellular signals, including cytokines, growth factors, tumor promoters, and the Ras oncoprotein. AP-1 includes members of the Jun and Fos families of transcription factors, which are characterized by leucine zipper DNA-binding domains. AP-1 proteins bind to DNA and activate transcription as Jun homodimers, Jun-Jun heterodimers, or Jun-Fos heterodimers. Multiple Jun and Fos family members (c-Jun, JunB, JunD, c-Fos, FosB, Fra-1, Fra-2) are expressed in different cell types that mediate the transcription of unique and overlapping genes. AP-1-driven gene expression is greatly enhanced when one of its components, especially c-Jun, is phosphorylated. Several kinases, including JNK, ERK, p38, caseine II, and IKKε, can activate this protein complex.

AP-1 proteins and mRNA, including c-jun and c-fos, are expressed in RA synovium, especially in the nuclei of cells in the intimal lining layer.[242] c-Jun and c-Fos proteins also are expressed in the sublining inflammatory infiltrate, albeit to a lesser degree. Localization of AP-1 to the intimal lining correlates with the site where most protease and cytokine genes are overexpressed in RA. AP-1 proteins usually are not detected in normal synovium, although modest amounts also have been detected in osteoarthritis. Electromobility shift assays show high levels of AP-1-binding activity in nuclear extracts from RA synovium compared with osteoarthritis tissue.[243]

Cytokines such as IL-1 and TNF-α probably contribute to the activation of AP-1 in RA synovium. These factors are potent inducers of AP-1 nuclear binding in cultured FLS; this is accompanied by increased c-jun and c-fos mRNA and enhanced collagenase gene transcription. The specific Jun family genes that constitute AP-1 in synoviocytes have a clear effect on function. c-Jun increases the production of proinflammatory mediators, whereas JunD suppresses cytokine and

MMP production.[244] AP-1 decoy oligonucleotides suppress collagen-induced arthritis and inhibit IL-1, IL-6, TNF-α, MMP-3, and MMP-9 production by synovial tissue.[245]

SIGNAL TRANSDUCERS AND ACTIVATORS OF TRANSCRIPTION

The STATs are a family of latent cytoplasmic transcription factors that are activated in response to cytokine stimulation of cells. STAT proteins contain domains that promote docking to the appropriate tyrosine-phosphorylated cytokine receptor after activation by the Janus kinases (Jak). STATs have been implicated in the expression of many proinflammatory genes. IL-4 and IFN-α signal through STAT1, whereas IL-12 signals through STAT4. The Th2 cytokine IL-4 uses STAT6.

Active STATs have been identified in patients with RA. Using immunohistochemistry, STAT1, STAT4, and STAT6 expression was observed in rheumatoid synovium, as was a downstream target of STAT4, Jak3.[246] STAT1 expression and activation has been identified in the synovium of patients with active disease, and a STAT1 decoy oligonucleotide suppresses antigen-induced arthritis in mice.[247] STAT3 also has been detected in cells from inflamed joints and can promote survival of cultured FLS.[248] Synovial fluid from RA patients can activate STAT3, but not STAT1, in monocytes.[249] This action is independent of IFN-γ and seems to be regulated primarily by IL-6. STAT3 also is strongly phosphorylated in RA synovium and supports the hypothesis that IL-6 plays a pathogenic role in the disease. Activation of the IL-4 pathway (STAT6) also has been shown in RA tissues even though IL-4 expression is very low.[250]

Gene signature patterns using microarray technology have been evaluated in RA and correlated to histopathology. These studies can be difficult to interpret because of wide variations in the synovial cell populations, sampling error, and the statistical vagaries of managing large volumes of data. One study suggested that RA patients could be divided into two groups.[251] The first is marked by expression of proinflammatory genes, with a pattern reminiscent of regulation by the STAT1 pathway. A second pattern is dominated by genes that participate in tissue repair and remodeling, and this signature is similar to osteoarthritis tissues. With sufficient refinement, one potentially could identify subpopulations of patients that could respond to targeted therapies.

In an animal model of arthritis, treatment with the suppressor of cytokine signaling repressor (SOCS3), which blocks the activation of certain STATs, suppresses arthritis.[252] This inhibitor also is expressed in the synovium of patients with RA, although it seems to be insufficient to block STAT3 phosphorylation. These data suggest that STATs play a crucial role in cytokine signal transduction in the synovium and can be manipulated to suppress disease.

ANTIVIRAL PROTEIN REGULATION: IκB KINASE–RELATED KINASES AND INTERFERON REGULATORY FACTOR-3

The rheumatoid joint displays some characteristics that resemble an antiviral response, such as IFN-β, RANTES, IP-10, and MCP-1 expression. This group of genes can be induced by ligation of TLR3 by viruses and other TLR ligands that are present in the rheumatoid joint. The relevance of this observation to inflammatory synovitis is supported by the fact that intra-articular injection of viral double-stranded RNA induces inflammatory arthritis in mice. Synoviocytes can be activated by poly I-C (which binds to TLR3) or RNA from necrotic cells. This does not imply that RA is caused by viruses; rather, it implies that factors within the joint can activate pathways that traditionally are viewed as crucial to host defense, but also can have pathogenic results.

The antiviral response is regulated by two IKK-related kinases, known as IKKε and TANK binding kinase 1 (TBK1), which have about 30% homology to the classic IKKs. Triggered by TLR3 ligation by viral double-stranded RNA, IKKε and TBK1 phosphorylate the transcription factor interferon regulatory factor 3 (IRF3) and induce production of an array of genes that orchestrate this response, including RANTES and IFN-β. IKKε and its substrate IRF3 are expressed and highly activated in RA synovium. Using a combination of IKKε knockout mice and genetic constructs that block endogenous IKKε activity, this kinase was shown to be a key regulator of IFN-β, RANTES, and MMP expression in cultured FLS.[253]

Induction of the antiviral genes has positive and negative potential in RA. Overexpression of some IRF3-driven genes, most notably IFN-β, could have a beneficial impact on the course of inflammatory arthritis. Mice with collagen-induced arthritis injected with transduced fibroblasts expressing IFN-β have less severe disease compared with controls, including decreased bone and cartilage destruction. Despite minimal efficacy in a clinical trial of IFN-β in RA, synovial biopsy specimens in treated patients contain smaller amounts of IL-1, IL-6, MMP1, and TIMP compared with placebo controls. Ultimately, clinical interventions will be required to determine if the beneficial effects of MMP and chemokine suppression regulated by IKK-related kinases outweigh modulation of IFN-β.

LIFE AND DEATH IN THE RHEUMATOID SYNOVIUM

Key Points

- Reactive oxygen and nitrogen in RA joints contributes to a toxic environment that can damage cells and increase inflammation.
- Deficient apoptosis, or cell death, can contribute to the accumulation of cells in rheumatoid synovium.
- Abnormalities of key regulatory genes, such as the p53 tumor-suppressor gene, can enhance accumulation of cells in the joint.
- Inducing apoptosis potentially can suppress synovial inflammation and joint destruction.

Studies defining the life cycle of cells have opened a new door to understanding the pathogenesis of neoplastic and inflammatory diseases. Although most investigators previously focused on cell proliferation as a mechanism of synovial hyperplasia, increasing attention has been paid to the role of insufficient cell death in this process. In this section,

the roles of oxidative damage, programmed cell death, and permanent changes in the genome are discussed, as they can alter the natural history of RA.

REACTIVE OXYGEN AND NITROGEN

Oxidative stress in the joints of RA patients results from a confluence of several stimuli, including increased pressure in the synovial cavity, reduced capillary density, vascular changes, an increased metabolic rate of synovial tissue, and locally activated leukocytes. The generation of reactive oxygen species also can be facilitated by repetitive ischemia-reperfusion injury in the joint. Tissue injury releases iron and copper ions and heme proteins that are catalytic for free-radical reactions. Electron transport chains also are disrupted in the mitochondria and endoplasmic reticulum, leading to leakage of electrons to form superoxide.

Evidence for increased production of reactive oxygen species in RA patients includes elevated levels of lipid peroxidation products, degradation of hyaluronic acid by free radicals, decreased levels of ascorbic acid in serum and synovial fluid, and increased breath pentane excretion. The levels of thioredoxin, a marker of oxidative stress, are significantly higher in synovial fluid from RA patients compared with synovial fluid from patients with other forms of arthritis.[254] Peripheral blood lymphocyte DNA from RA patients contains significantly increased levels of the mutagenic 8-oxohydrodeoxyguanosine,[255] which is a product of oxidative damage to DNA, pointing to the genotoxic effects of oxidative stress.

Nitric oxide production also is high in rheumatoid synovial tissue.[256] Low levels of nitric oxide are constitutively produced by endothelial or neuronal synthases, and this is substantially increased by inducible nitric oxide synthase after stimulation by cytokines or bacterial products. The nitrite levels in synovial fluid are elevated in RA patients, indicating local nitric oxide production.[257] In addition, the urinary nitrate-to-creatinine ratio is increased, and inducible nitric oxide synthase is present in the synovium.

APOPTOSIS

Programmed cell death, or apoptosis, is a process by which cells can be safely eliminated in the midst of living tissue. This stereotypic response provides a mechanism for tissue development, remodeling, or cell deletion without instigating an inflammatory response. Apoptosis is a normal process that is tightly regulated and can be initiated by withdrawal of hormones and growth factors. It is evident in the elimination of autoreactive cells such as thymocytes in the thymus gland and the loss of cells after DNA damage. It also plays a crucial role in immune response by deleting activated T cells and terminating an inflammatory response by rapidly removing neutrophils.

Genes Regulating Apoptosis

The accumulation of cells in RA is typically considered as a process involving in situ cell proliferation or recruitment of cells from the bloodstream. It is equally tenable, however, that increased cell numbers could accumulate in the synovium as a result of insufficient cell deletion. T cell apoptosis in RA synovial effusions is significantly less than apoptosis of lymphocytes from crystal-induced arthropathy.[258] The RA T cells show high Fas (CD95) expression, high Bax, and low Bcl-2, which is a phenotype typically associated with increased susceptibility to apoptosis. This finding contrasts with synovial tissue cells, in which high Bcl-2 expression is found in lymphoid aggregates and protects synovial T cells from programmed cell death. Resistance to apoptosis in vitro is prolonged if the RA T cells are cocultured with FLS or IL-15. The specific adhesion molecules involved are undefined, although the integrin-binding RGD motif (arginine-glycine-asparagine) could block the protective effects of synoviocytes.

Fas and its TNF superfamily counterreceptor Fas ligand (FasL) are potent regulators of cell death for many cell types, including synovial T cells and synoviocytes. Fas is expressed by rheumatoid synovial fluid T cells, and the number of Fas+ cells in the peripheral blood of RA patients is greater than in healthy controls.[259] Anti-Fas antibody, which cross-links Fas on cell surfaces, rapidly causes apoptosis in synovial fluid B and T lymphocytes in RA, although peripheral blood T cells are more resistant. Another member of the TNF superfamily, TRAIL (TNF-related apoptosis-inducing ligand) binds to two receptors (DR4 or DR5) to induce caspase-dependent apoptosis. DR5 is expressed in RA FLS, but not osteoarthritis cells, and apoptosis can be induced by either TRAIL or agonistic anti-DR5 antibody.[260]

Studies of apoptosis in RA synovial tissue have relied on many techniques that label damaged DNA. Using the most stringent methods, only a few apoptotic nuclei have been detected in the intimal lining and the sublining.[261] Electron microscopic studies show rare cells that exhibit the typical findings of programmed cell death. Less specific techniques that detect any DNA damage show abundant cells in the intimal lining with nuclear fragmentation.[262]

There is an unexpected discrepancy between the cytologic evidence of DNA damage and the rarity of typical morphologic changes of apoptosis, even using ultrastructural criteria.[263] One explanation for synovial macrophages is that they express high levels of the caspase 8 inhibitor FLICE-like inhibitory protein, which can inhibit Fas-mediated apoptosis.[264] Despite the dearth of apoptotic cells in the lining, Bcl-2 expression (which inhibits apoptosis) is reduced in this region. The mechanisms for inducing apoptosis in FLS can involve several pathways, including induction of JNK and AP-1 activation, inhibition of the kinase Akt, or suppression of NFκB.[265] p53, which typically induces cell cycle arrest and either DNA repair or apoptosis, also is expressed in the synovial lining and sublining. One of the main effectors of p53-mediated apoptosis, PUMA (p53 upregulated modulator of apoptosis), is present in only very low concentrations, however, in the synovium and cultured synoviocytes.

Because of these unexpected findings, the regulation of apoptosis has been evaluated in cultured FLS in RA. Fas is constitutively expressed by cultured synoviocytes, and programmed cell death is initiated in a few cells (generally ≤20%) when it is cross-linked by anti-Fas antibody. Most investigators find that RA and osteoarthritis synoviocytes are equally susceptible to anti-Fas-mediated death. PUMA can induce cell death in FLS when overexpressed using genetic methods.[266] Gene transfection experiments showed,

however, that p53 directs synoviocytes to cell cycle arrest through expression of p21 instead of inducing apoptosis through PUMA. Synoviocyte apoptosis also can be initiated by oxidative stress, such as hydrogen peroxide, or by exposure to nitric oxide.

The relative paucity of apoptosis in RA also can be explained by patterns of gene expression that favor cell survival. As noted earlier, p53 preferentially induces p21 and favors survival. Sentrin-1, a ubiquitin-like protein, regulates the cell survival by modifying proteins involved in apoptosis (including p53). Sentrin-1 is expressed in RA synovium, especially at sites of cartilage invasion, and protects cells from Fas-mediated apoptosis.[267] A second protein, PTEN (phosphatase and tensine homolog on chromosome ten) originally was defined as a key factor that protects from tumorigenesis through antagonism of PI3K, Akt, and many other proliferative pathways. Underexpression of PTEN in RA has been described in rheumatoid synovial intimal lining and cultured FLS.[268]

Therapeutic Interventions That Increase Apoptosis

The potential relevance of Fas-induced death as a therapeutic modality has been shown in murine collagen-induced arthritis, in which high levels of Fas and low levels of FasL are expressed by synovial cells.[269] Mice treated with an intra-articular injection of an adenoviral vector encoding Fas ligand had decreased synovial inflammation. DNA-labeling studies showed that the construct increased synovial apoptosis. Anti-Fas antibody also induces synovial cell death in RA synovial tissue explanted in SCID mice. In the SCID mouse model using RA synovial explants, anti-DR5 antibody decreased cartilage erosion. Similarly, adenoviral transfer of TRAIL in a rabbit model of arthritis decreases synovial inflammation.[270] The importance of apoptosis as a regulator of inflammation was confirmed in murine collagen-induced arthritis, where anti-DR5 antibody or genetic DR5 deficiency exacerbated the disease.

Other targets that regulate apoptosis also have shown potential utility in animal models. NFκB blockade in streptococcal cell wall arthritis induces synovial apoptosis and suppresses arthritis. p53 gene therapy in rabbit antigen–induced arthritis induces synovial apoptosis and decreases inflammation.[271] The pleiotropic activities of p53 were shown in collagen-induced arthritis because p53 knockout mice with the disease developed increased inflammation and greater joint destruction in association with decreased apoptosis. Joint damage was mediated by increased expression of collagenase genes in the knockout mice, most likely because p53 directly suppresses MMP gene transcription.[272] p53 knockout mice with either passive collagen-induced arthritis or passive K/BxN arthritis do not manifest increased disease activity, however.[273] These data suggest that p53 mediates its protective effects through modulation of the adaptive immune response.

TUMOR-SUPPRESSOR GENES

The p53 tumor-suppressor gene is a key regulator of DNA repair and cell replication. p53 protein expression is significantly greater in the rheumatoid synovium compared with osteoarthritis and normal tissue. In long-standing disease marked by joint destruction, immunostaining localizes the protein to sublining mononuclear cells and the intimal lining.[274] p53 protein also can be detected in RA synovium from patients with very early RA and asymptomatic rheumatoid joints.[275] Its expression is much lower in other inflammatory arthropathies, however, such as reactive arthritis, which might reflect the generally greater amount of DNA damage and oxidative stress in RA.

The possibility that somatic mutations in the p53 gene might contribute to the unusual phenotype of RA synoviocytes and inadequate apoptosis in rheumatoid synovial tissue has been investigated.[276] p53 mutations have been identified in RA synovial tissue and synoviocytes, although their presence is controversial. Transition mutations, which are characteristic of damage induced by reactive oxygen or nitric oxide, account for more than 80% of the base changes. Some mutant p53 genes exhibit dominant negative characteristics and suppress the function of the wild-type allele.[277] Microdissection studies confirmed the presence of mutant islands, and the loss of p53 function in a region of RA synovium was associated with increased IL-6 gene expression in the same location.[278] The data suggest that mutations do not cause RA, but, instead, are the result of the long-standing oxidative stress. The gene alterations potentially can increase the aggressive nature of the synovium and alter the natural history of RA.

Abnormalities in other genes also have been reported in RA. Synovial T cells in RA have an increased incidence of mutations in the *hprt* gene.[279] Although not functionally important, these mutations act as a marker for oxidative damage that occurs in the synovial milieu. Some of these abnormal lymphocytes also can be detected in the peripheral blood, suggesting that articular T cells can migrate out of the joint to other parts of the body. Abnormalities of the *ras* gene, which is involved in many signal transduction pathways, also have been noted in some patients. The H-*ras* oncogene is expressed in the synovium of patients with a variety of arthritides, and mutations have been identified in RA and osteoarthritis synovium.[280] Recently, mutations in synovial vimentin have been identified that could enhance its immunogenicity.[280a] Microsatellite instability, which is marked by mutations in mononucleotide and dinucleotide repeat sequences in noncoding DNA, also is significantly greater in RA than osteoarthritis synovial tissue. Occasional mutations in a coding region microsatellite in the WISP-3 gene, which can regulate type II collagen and aggrecan expression, have been identified in RA synovium. Similar mutations were observed in osteoarthritis, suggesting that these are not specific. Mutations in mitochondrial genes also have been described in RA, most likely owing to oxidative damage.[281]

Evaluation of DNA mismatch repair genes in rheumatoid synovium suggests that the balance of two genes that protect against mutations might contribute to the pattern of DNA damage in RA, with relatively high levels of mutS homolog 3(MSH3) and low levels of MSH6 after reactive nitrogen stress.[282] The former repairs large insertions and deletions, whereas the latter repairs single base abnormalities. Because most mutations detected in RA involve single bases, the balance of mismatch repair enzymes seems to favor these limited mutations rather than more substantial ones.

BLOOD VESSELS IN ARTHRITIS

Key Points

- Angiogenesis is a dynamic process in RA that provides nutrients to expanding synovium.
- Angiogenic factors, such as IL-8 and vascular endothelial growth factor, can enhance blood vessel proliferation in the synovium.
- Microvascular endothelia in the synovium express adhesion molecules that guide circulating cells into the joint under the influence of chemoattractants.

Blood vessels previously were thought of as passive conduits through which red blood cells and leukocytes circulated while en route to an inflammatory site. This is now known to be far from the truth: The microvasculature plays an active role in such processes, not only as the means of selecting which cells should enter the tissue, but also as a determinant of tissue growth and nutrition through the proliferation of new capillaries.

ANGIOGENESIS IN RHEUMATOID ARTHRITIS: FEEDING THE STARVED SYNOVIUM

The importance of luxurious new capillary growth early in the development of synovitis has been recognized for many years. The absolute number of blood vessels is increased in RA synovium (Fig. 65-13), with a rich network of sublining capillaries and postcapillary venules in histologic sections stained with endothelium-specific antibodies. The mass of tissue outstrips angiogenesis in RA, however, as determined by the number of blood vessels per unit area and causes local tissue ischemia.[283] Synovial fluid oxygen tensions are remarkably low, lactate measurements are frequently high, and the pH can be as low as 6.8. The mean rheumatoid synovial fluid partial pressure of oxygen in samples from rheumatoid knees is approximately 30 mm Hg and occasionally less than 15 mm Hg. Another cause of diminished blood flow is increased

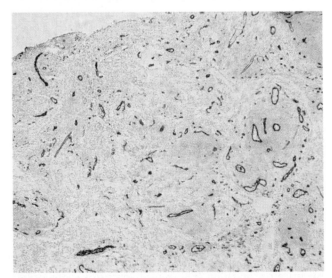

Figure 65-13 Human rheumatoid synovial membrane stained with antibody to von Willebrand factor to delineate blood vessels. Most of these blood vessels formed in response to angiogenic stimuli after the rheumatoid process had been initiated. *(Courtesy of Dr. Paul-Peter Tak.)*

positive pressure exerted by synovial effusions within the joint, a process that obliterates capillary flow, while producing ischemia-reperfusion injury in the joint. Altered vascular flow may not be the only cause of hypoxia in joints; oxygen consumption of the rheumatoid synovium (per gram of tissue) is 20 times normal.

Hypoxia is a potent stimulus for angiogenesis. One of the mechanisms by which this occurs is through the production of angiogenic factors regulated by hypoxia-inducible factor 1α (HIF-1α), such as vascular endothelial growth factor (VEGF).[284] This oxygen-sensing transcription factor regulates numerous responses to hypoxia. HIF-1α deficiency in the myeloid lineage suppresses inflammation in numerous models, including the passive K/BxN model of arthritis.[285] Low oxygen tension also leads to HIF-1α-induced transcription of VEGF, a specific endothelial cell mitogen that is present in high concentrations in rheumatoid synovial fluid and tissue. Elevated serum concentrations in early disease correlate with subsequent radiographic progress, although it is unclear if there is a causal relationship. VEGF also is able to stimulate the expression of collagenase, which can degrade the extracellular matrix to make room for the advancing vasculature and pannus.[286] VEGF expression is especially high in the synovial intimal lining, and the angiogenesis factor also is produced by cultured FLS that have been exposed to hypoxia and IL-1.[287]

VEGF can bind to two receptors with tyrosine kinase domains, VEGF-R1/Flt-1 and VEGF-R2. Genetic deletion of VEGF-R1 decreases VEGF-driven expression of IL-6 and suppresses macrophage phagocytosis. VEGF-R1$^{-/-}$ mice also are resistant to arthritis in the human T lymphotropic virus-1 pX model, which is marked by unregulated proliferation of synovial cells. Small molecule VEGF-R inhibitors also suppress acute models of inflammation, such as carrageenan paw edema, and mouse collagen-induced arthritis. Targeting this receptor with a small molecule might suppress the angiogenic and proinflammatory actions of VEGF.

In addition to the hypoxia-driven stimulus for blood vessel growth, the inflammatory cytokine milieu of the joint encourages angiogenesis. Several proinflammatory factors expressed by the rheumatoid joint, including IL-8, FGF, and TNF-α, are angiogenic. Many of these cytokines, including TNF-α, enhance angiogenesis further by increasing expression of angiopoietins (Ang-1 and Ang-2) by synoviocytes, which can then bind to their tyrosine kinase receptor, Tie-1, on RA capillary endothelial cells.[288] Additional angiogenesis factors, such as soluble E-selectin and soluble VCAM, are released by activated endothelium in RA synovium and contribute to vascular proliferation.[289] Limited quantities of some antiangiogenic mediators that inhibit capillary proliferation, such as platelet factor-4 and thrombospondin, also are produced by the joint.[290,291]

Vascular remodeling is an active process that involves the continuous creation and resorption of blood vessels. In RA, new capillaries that form under the influence of proangiogenic factors can be identified by the expression of integrins such as αvβ3. Endothelial proliferation is especially prominent in synovial tissue regions containing VEGF. Synovial blood vessel involution also can be detected as evidenced by apoptosis of the endothelium in other synovial locations. An index comparing proliferation and death of blood vessels is significantly higher in RA compared with osteoarthritis or normal synovium.

The importance of new blood vessel formation in inflammatory arthritis was elegantly shown in the collagen-induced arthritis model. The disease was markedly attenuated in animals pretreated with an angiostatic compound similar to fumagillin, which is derived from *Aspergillus*.[292] This compound is cytotoxic to proliferating, but not resting, endothelial cells. In addition, there was regression of established arthritis if treatment was initiated well into the course of the disease. Angiogenesis is essential for the establishment and progression of inflammatory arthritis because of the need for blood vessels either to recruit leukocytes or to provide nutrients and oxygen to starved tissue.

Several other antiangiogenesis approaches are effective in animal models of arthritis. Thrombospondin 1 overexpression significantly decreases blood vessel density, inflammation, and joint destruction in rat collagen-induced arthritis. Direct intra-articular administration of a cyclic RGD peptide was used in a rabbit model to block αvβ3 integrin.[293] As with RA synovium, αvβ3 is expressed by proliferating blood vessels in inflamed rabbit synovial tissue. The cyclic peptide decreased joint inflammation, increased endothelial cell apoptosis, and suppressed bone and cartilage destruction. The ability of RGD to bind selectively to proliferating blood vessels also was used to home a proapoptotic agent to synovial neovasculature in murine collagen-induced arthritis.[294] The cyclic RGD peptide was administered systemically and accumulated in inflamed synovium, but not normal joints or other organs. Apoptosis was induced in synovial blood vessels, and arthritis regressed. The potent angiogenesis inhibitor endostatin has been tested in the SCID mouse model, and it decreased synovial explant inflammatory cell infiltration and capillary density.[295] Despite the compelling rationale for antiangiogenic therapy, an anti-αv antibody showed minimal efficacy in clinical trials, perhaps because other pathways are more important in the synovium.

ADHESION MOLECULE REGULATION

The formation of new capillaries is only one aspect of blood vessel involvement in the rheumatoid process. Endothelial cells also are activated by cytokines to express adhesion molecules that bind to counterreceptors on mononuclear cells and neutrophils from the circulation and facilitate their transfer from the blood into the subsynovial tissue. There are several categories of vascular adhesion molecules. The selectins (E-selectin, L-selectin, and P-selectin) are a family of adhesion molecules whose primary ligands are carbohydrates, especially sialyl Lewis$_x$, and related oligosaccharides. A second family comprises integrins, which are heterodimers that include an α chain and a β chain. The counterreceptors depend on the specific combination of these chains and are frequently proteins in the immunoglobulin supergene family (e.g., the combination of ICAM-1 and αMβ2) or extracellular matrix proteins (e.g., the combination of fibronectin and α5β1 or vitronectin and αvβ3). Several novel peptides have been described that selectively bind to the blood vessels of human synovial explants in SCID mice.[296]

Adhesion molecule expression is increased in the RA synovium. This increased expression is almost certainly due to exposure of the vasculature to the rich cytokine milieu. Immunohistochemical techniques localize high levels of

ICAM-1 to sublining macrophages, macrophage-like synovial lining cells, and fibroblasts compared with normal tissue.[297] Significant amounts also are present on most vascular endothelial cells, although the ICAM-1 levels are quantitatively similar to those of vessels in normal endothelium. Cultured FLS also constitutively express ICAM-1, which can be markedly increased by TNF-α, IL-1, and IFN-γ.

Adhesion of α4β1-expressing mononuclear cells, such as memory T cells or monocytes, to cytokine-activated endothelial cells can be mediated by VCAM-1. VLA-4, which is predominantly expressed on lymphocytes, monocytes, and eosinophils, but not on neutrophils, serves as a receptor for VCAM-1 and an alternatively spliced region of fibronectin known as CS-1. A role for VLA-4 in arthritis has been suggested by numerous experimental observations. In adjuvant arthritis in rats, anti-α4 antibody decreases lymphocyte accumulation in the joint, but not lymph nodes, suggesting that VLA-4 is more important in recruitment to inflamed sites than to noninflamed sites.[298] In streptococcal cell wall arthritis, intravenous injection of CS-1 peptide decreases the severity of acute and chronic arthritis.[44,299] T lymphocytes isolated from the synovial fluid and synovial membrane of RA patients exhibit increased VLA-4-mediated adherence to CS-1 and VCAM-1, relative to autologous peripheral blood lymphocytes.[300] These studies also suggest that leukocytes expressing functionally activated VLA-4 are selectively recruited to inflammatory sites in RA.

Moderate amounts of VCAM-1 are expressed in RA synovial blood vessels. The intimal lining is the location of the most intense staining with anti-VCAM-1 antibodies on histologic sections. Even normal synovial tissue expresses VCAM-1 in the lining, albeit less than in RA. Cultured FLS constitutively express small amounts of VCAM-1, and the level is increased by a variety of macrophage-derived and T cell–derived cytokines. VCAM-1 also contributes to T cell adhesion to high endothelial venules in frozen sections of RA synovium.[301] The other VLA-4 counterreceptor, CS-1-containing forms of fibronectin, is restricted to inflamed RA vascular endothelium and the synovial intimal lining.[302] Normal synovial tissue contains little, if any, CS-1 fibronectin.

The integrin α4β7, which also can bind to VCAM-1, is a specific adhesion molecule involved in lymphocyte homing to Peyer's patches. Most intraepithelial and lamina propria lymphocytes express α4β7; this molecule is rarely identified in other lymphoid tissues. The expression of α4β7 on peripheral blood lymphocytes from patients with RA is low (similar to normal individuals), but a quarter of synovial fluid lymphocytes, mostly CD8+ T lymphocytes, express this adhesion molecule, which provides an interesting link between arthritis and the gut.[303]

E-selectin expression also is elevated in rheumatoid synovium, although the increase is less dramatic than for the integrins and their counterreceptors. This might be due partly to the kinetics of E-selectin expression on endothelial cells. The protein is not found on resting endothelial cells and peaks after about 3 hours of cytokine stimulation. Even in the continued presence of cytokines, however, E-selectin expression declines to near-basal levels after about 6 hours. In one study, E-selectin expression was decreased in synovial biopsy specimens after patients were treated with injectable gold and corticosteroids.[304]

The therapeutic potential for antiadhesion therapy has been studied in the SCID mouse model. Labeled human peripheral mononuclear cells were injected into engrafted mice, and migration into the tissue was examined.[305] If the mice were treated with TNF-α, ICAM-1 expression and trafficking into synovium was significantly increased. Anti-ICAM-1 antibody blocked leukocyte migration into the explant under these conditions. In another study, tonsil mononuclear cells also migrated into the RA synovial grafts in SCID mice.[306] RA clinical trials using ICAM-1 targeted therapy have been reported using anti-ICAM-1 antibody or antisense ICAM-1 oligonucleotides, although no significant clinical benefit was observed.[307] In addition, mice lacking E-selectin and P-selectin had accelerated disease in the collagen-induced arthritis model. This paradoxical result serves as a reminder of the complexity of the inflammatory process.[308]

CARTILAGE AND BONE DESTRUCTION

> ## Key Points
>
> - Distinct mechanisms and cell types regulate cartilage degradation and bone destruction in RA.
> - Several classes of proteases, including metalloproteinases, serine proteases, cathepsins, and aggrecanases, are produced by intimal lining cells in RA, especially FLS.
> - Synovial lining cells, especially FLS, can attach to and invade cartilage in RA.
> - Bone destruction is mediated by osteoclasts that are activated under the influence of RANKL and other cytokines produced by RA synovium.

CARTILAGE DESTRUCTION AND THE PANNUS-CARTILAGE JUNCTION

In RA, the cartilage is often covered by a layer of tissue composed of mesenchymal cells, which might represent the progenitor of the aggressive, mature pannus. In the established lesion, numerous areas are seen in which macrophage-like and fibroblast-like cells penetrate into cartilage matrix far from lymphocytes (Fig. 65-14).[309] Some regions show relatively acellular pannus tissue, however, suggesting that there is little, if any, enzyme-mediated tissue destruction in these areas. Invasive pannus is more commonly found in metatarsophalangeal joints compared with hip and knee joints in which a layer of resting fibroblasts seems to separate pannus from cartilage, perhaps explaining why erosions occur more often around small joints.

FLS from the intimal lining usually are considered major effectors of cartilage destruction in RA based on the prodigious amount of proteases that they produce. Rheumatoid FLS can bind to cartilage and invade into the extracellular matrix in the SCID mouse model, showing their propensity for eroding the extracellular matrix. Other cells in the joint, especially neutrophils and cells from the pannus that burrow directly into cartilage, also could be responsible for cartilage-mediated and osteoclast-mediated bone erosions. More primitive mesenchymal cells isolated directly from the cartilage-pannus junction express phenotypic and functional features of synoviocytes and chondrocytes that also have been described in the synovium.

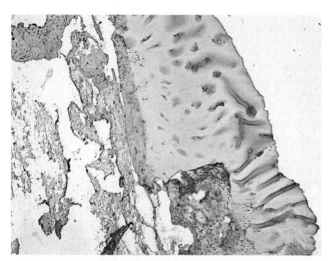

Figure 65-14 Pannus-cartilage junction. The invasive front of pannus burrows into cartilage matrix in rheumatoid arthritis joints. The pannus is primarily composed of macrophages and mesenchymal cells. Immunostaining with anti-CD68 antibody shows the distribution of macrophages in the invasive tissue. *(Courtesy of Dr. Paul-Peter Tak.)*

Cartilage is destroyed in RA by enzymatic and mechanical processes. The enzymes induced by factors such as IL-1, IL-17, TNF-α, phagocytosis of debris by synovial cells, and mechanical trauma cause the joint destruction. Early in synovitis, proteoglycans are depleted from the tissue, most likely owing to the catabolic effect of cytokines such as IL-1 on chondrocytes with the production of MMPs and aggrecanases, and this leads to mechanical weakening of cartilage. As proteoglycans are depleted, cartilage loses the ability to rebound from a deforming load and becomes susceptible to mechanical fragmentation and fibrillation. Eventually, the tissue loses functional integrity concurrent with its complete dissolution by collagenase and stromelysin. Some of the MMPs responsible for this process also are derived from the chondrocytes themselves. Multiple MMPs, especially stromelysins and collagenases, are expressed in RA cartilage, and in situ hybridization studies confirm the presence of the specific RNA transcripts within chondrocytes.[310] The cartilage is under attack from a multitude of sources: It is being bathed in protease-rich synovial fluid, it is under extrinsic attack from the invasive pannus, and the chondrocytes themselves contribute to destruction from within.

Enzymes released by PMNs in synovial fluid, including neutrophil collagenase and multiple serine proteases, also contribute to cartilage loss. Immune complexes containing RFs are embedded in the superficial layers of cartilage and can attract and activate neutrophils. Electron microscopic examinations of articular cartilage in RA reveal amorphous-appearing material and evidence of breakdown of collagen and proteoglycan consistent with superficial diffuse activity of joint fluid enzymes.[311] In a rabbit model of arthritis in which IL-1 was injected directly into the joint, the degree of cartilage damage as measured by proteoglycan levels in synovial fluid correlated best, however, with the stromelysin concentrations in synovial effusions (presumably derived from synoviocytes). Neutrophil depletion of animals did not interfere with subsequent destruction of extracellular matrix, suggesting that MMPs derived from the synovium are more important.

Most animal studies indicate that IL-1 is a key regulator of matrix degradation in arthritis[312]; this has been true across a broad range of arthritis models, including zymosan-induced arthritis, collagen-induced arthritis, antigen-induced arthritis, and streptococcal cell wall–induced arthritis. Although TNF-α blockade has clear anti-inflammatory effects, chondroprotection is less prominent. Bone and cartilage protection observed in patients receiving TNF inhibitors reminds us that animal models are imperfect predictors of RA responses. More recent data suggest that IL-17 also can contribute to joint destruction directly or by synergizing with IL-1 and TNF-α.

The rate-limiting step in cartilage loss is the cleavage of collagen because proteoglycans are degraded soon after inflammation begins. MMPs, released into the extracellular space and active at neutral pH, are probably responsible for most of the effective proteolysis of articular-cartilage proteins, but other classes of enzymes may contribute to joint destruction. Enzymes such as cathepsins B, D, G, K, L, and H may play a role within and outside cells in degrading noncollagenous matrix proteins. Serine proteinases (e.g., elastase and plasmin) and aggrecanases are doubtless involved as well.

PROTEASES—KEY MEDIATORS OF JOINT DESTRUCTION

Matrix Metalloproteinases

The MMPs are a family of enzymes that participate in extracellular matrix degradation and remodeling. MMPs usually are secreted as inactive proenzymes, and their proteolytic activity requires limited cleavage or denaturation to reveal a zinc cation at the core. Their activation can be mediated by other proteases, including trypsin, plasmin, or tryptase. The substrates for MMPs vary, but are quite specific for individual members of the family. Collagenases degrade native collagen types I, II, III, VII, and X, whereas gelatinases are able to degrade denatured or cleaved collagen. Stromelysins have broader specificity and can digest proteoglycans in addition to proteins. They also process procollagenase to the active form, serving as a positive feedback signal for matrix destruction. Some MMPs such as TNF convertase are responsible for the processing and release of cytokines from the cell surface. Many different families of proteinases are found in the joint (Table 65-7), but the MMPs are thought to play a pivotal role in joint destruction.

Regulation of Matrix Metalloproteinase Production

The cytokine milieu has the capacity to induce the biosynthesis of MMPs by synovial cells and alter the balance between extracellular matrix production and degradation. IL-1 and TNF-α, in particular, directly induce MMP gene expression by many cells, including FLS and chondrocytes. These two cytokines are additive or synergistic when used in combination. Many other cytokines implicated in rheumatoid synovitis also can induce MMP expression, including IL-17 and leukemia inhibitory factor.

MMP induction is mediated by a change in gene transcription and mRNA stabilization. Culture medium from rheumatoid synovium stimulates cartilage degradation in vitro, and this can be inhibited by an antibody against IL-1;

Table 65-7 Key Proteases and Inhibitors in Rheumatoid Arthritis Synovium

Protease	Inhibitor
Metalloproteinases Collagenase-1 Collagenase-3 Stromelysin-1 92-kD gelatinase	TIMP family; α₂-macroglobulin
Serine proteases Trypsin Chymotrypsin Tryptase	SERPINs; α₂-macroglobulin
Cathepsins Cathepsin B Cathepsin L Cathepsin K	α₂-macroglobulin

SERPIN, serine protease inhibitors; TIMP, tissue inhibitor of metalloproteinases.

these data implicate rheumatoid synovium as a source of IL-1 that activates chondrocytes to produce proteases. IL-6 does not induce MMP production by synovial cells, but instead increases the production of TIMP-1, a naturally occurring inhibitor of MMPs.[313] TGF-β inhibits collagenase synthesis in vitro and enhances the production of TIMP by fibroblasts and chondrocytes.[314] It also increases collagen production, shifting the balance to matrix repair.

Although multiple upstream regulatory sequences are involved in the regulation of MMP gene transcription, the dominant element in the promoter is AP-1. Other regulatory sites, such as an NFκB-like region, also can contribute to collagenase expression. AP-1 activity is markedly increased in FLS by proinflammatory cytokines, and its transcriptional activity is mediated by increased expression of components such as c-Jun and post-translational modification by phosphorylation. The MAP kinases are especially important for this activity, and JNK is the most efficient upstream activator. Glucocorticoid-mediated inhibition of collagenase gene expression is due to interference with the Fos-Jun complex by the glucocorticoid receptor.

Collagenases and stromelysins have the capacity to degrade virtually all of the important structural proteins in the extracellular tissues within joints. Collagenase-1 (MMP-1) cleaves through the triple-helical collagen molecule at a single glycine-isoleucine bond approximately three quarters of the distance from the NH₂ terminus. This enzyme has the capability to degrade only the interstitial helical collagens (e.g., types I, II, III, and X). It has little or no activity against types IV, V, and IX and other nonhelical collagens or denatured collagen; the degradation of the latter is primarily accomplished by the gelatinases. MMP-1 is a relatively inefficient enzyme, however, and the more recently characterized collagenase-3 (MMP-13) has more favorable kinetics. Similar to collagenase-1, collagenase-3 has an AP-1-binding site in the promoter that is an important regulator of MMP-13 gene transcription. Neutrophil collagenase, or MMP-8, is constitutively stored in neutrophil granules and is released into the milieu after degranulation. The relative importance of this enzyme in inflammatory arthritis is uncertain, and neutrophil depletion does not prevent cartilage damage in animal models. Rodents lack the collagenase-1 gene, whereas the collagenase-3 gene is preserved; this is especially important to note when evaluating effects of MMP inhibitors in animal models.

Matrix Metalloproteinase Expression in Synovium

The collagenase-1 and collagenase-3 genes are produced by RA synovial tissue, and the collagenase-3 gene is highly expressed by chondrocytes in cartilage. In situ hybridization studies show that the primary location of collagenase-1 gene expression in the synovium, similar to many other MMPs, is the intimal lining, especially in fibroblast-like cells.[315] Subchondral bone is another region in which proteinase expression occurs in RA and could participate in bone resorption. Increased MMP gene expression is an early feature of RA and occurs during the first few weeks or months of disease[316]; this underscores the need for early therapy to prevent joint destruction. High expression of collagenase-1 and gelatinases such as MMP-2 early in disease correlates with rapidly progressive erosions. Similarly, increased blood levels of the proenzymes are associated with more severe disease.

Stromelysin-1 (MMP-3) and the other members of the stromelysin family have no activity against interstitial collagen, but effectively degrade type IV collagen, fibronectin, laminin, proteoglycan core protein, and type IX collagen. Stromelysin removes the NH₂-terminal propeptides from type I procollagen and is integrally involved in the activation of procollagenase. Similar to collagenase, stromelysin gene expression is almost exclusively in the synovial intimal lining (Fig. 65-15). Prostromelysin from human synovial cells can be activated by other proteases, including cysteine proteases (the cathepsins), trypsin, chymotrypsin, plasma kallikrein, plasmin, and mast cell tryptase. Despite the putative importance of this enzyme in matrix destruction, stromelysin knockout mice are susceptible to collagen-induced arthritis and develop as much joint destruction as mice with functional stromelysin.[317]

MMP inhibitors are effective in animal models of RA and can suppress bone destruction and the inflammatory synovitis.[318] In models of osteoarthritis, deletion of MMP genes such as stromelysin does not improve outcomes. Clinical trials in RA using nonselective inhibitors have had minimal success and significant side effects, possibly related to decreased matrix turnover. Inhibitors of TNF convertase (which also can block other MMPs) appear to increase disease activity in RA for uncertain reasons. One of the most consistent side effects of MMP inhibitors is stiffness thought to result from deposition of fibrous tissue without sufficient protease activity to permit removal of matrix proteins during remodeling. This observation has been replicated in rats, which provides an opportunity to determine if highly selective MMP inhibitors would have a better risk-to-benefit ratio.[319]

Cysteine Proteases—the Cathepsins

Cathepsins are an extensive family of cysteine proteases that have broad proteolytic activity, including activity on types II, IX, and XI collagen and proteoglycans.[320] Similar to MMPs, the cathepsins are regulated by cytokines and by proto-oncogenes such as ras. IL-1 and TNF-α induce cathepsin L expression in cultured FLS.[321] In situ hybridization studies show expression of cathepsin B and L in RA synovium, especially at sites of erosion. A ribozyme that cleaves cathepsin L decreases FLS invasion and cartilage destruction in the SCID mouse model with implanted cultured synoviocytes. A novel cysteine protease called

RA synovium   Stromelysin

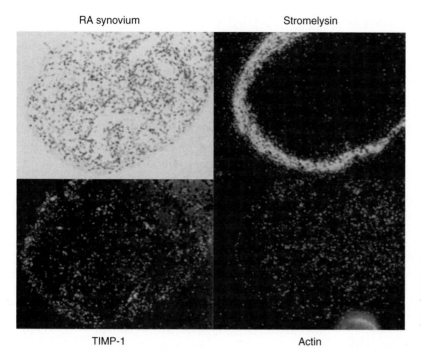

TIMP-1   Actin

Figure 65-15 Localization of stromelysin, tissue inhibitor of metalloproteinase-1 (TIMP-1), and actin mRNA in rheumatoid arthritis (RA) synovial tissue by in situ hybridization. Stromelysin is mainly expressed in the synovial intimal lining, presumably by cytokine-stimulated type B synoviocytes. Bright field and dark field views are shown. *(Courtesy of D. Boyle.)*

cathepsin K has been implicated in bone resorption by osteoclasts. It is unique among the cathepsins in its ability to degrade native type I collagen.[322] Cathepsin K is expressed in RA synovial tissue by macrophages and fibroblasts and is present in significantly higher concentrations in RA than in osteoarthritis.[323] Serum levels of cathepsin K correlate with the extent of radiographic damage. A potential role of cathepsins as mediators of bone destruction in arthritis was confirmed in studies in which a cysteine protease inhibitor significantly decreased joint damage in the rat adjuvant arthritis model.[324]

Aggrecanases

In addition to type II collagen, aggrecan is a crucial component of cartilage as one of the major proteoglycan components. Because of its large size and negative charge, aggrecan contains a considerable amount of water, which increases compressibility. Two proteolytic sites are available on aggrecan in its globular domain. One site is susceptible to MMP cleavage, whereas the other, located 32 amino acids toward the carboxy terminus, is the site for cleavage by a family of enzymes known as aggrecanases. The two sites can be identified in tissues using monoclonal antibodies after cleavage when specific neoepitopes are revealed.

Normal cartilage contains a surprising amount of aggrecanase neoepitope, suggesting continuous matrix turnover. The level of aggrecanase cleavage product increases with age. Two aggrecanase genes, aggrecanase-1 and aggrecanase-2, have been cloned and are members of the ADAMTS (a disintegrin and metalloproteinase with thrombospondin motif) family of proteins (ADAMTS-4 and ADAMTS-5).[325] These genes are expressed in osteoarthritis and RA cartilage, and their proteolytic activity can be detected in synovial fluid using bioassays. Especially high levels of the neoepitope are present in arthritic cartilage.[326] IL-1 increases aggrecanase expression in cartilage explants and cultures of chondrocytes. Aggrecanase-1 and aggrecanase-2 are constitutively expressed by RA and osteoarthritis FLS and synovial tissues.[327] Aggrecanase-1 can be induced in synoviocytes by cytokines, especially TGF-β, whereas aggrecanase-2 expression remains constant. Genetic deletion of aggrecanase-1 has no effect on a murine osteoarthritis model. Loss of aggrecanase-2 essentially prevents degenerative changes, however.[328] Although data in RA are unavailable, these studies suggest that aggrecanase-2 might be largely responsible for proteoglycan depletion from cartilage in either inflammatory or noninflammatory arthritis.

INHIBITORS OF PROTEASE ACTIVITY

α_2-Macroglobulin accounts for more than 95% of collagenase inhibitory capacity in serum. The mechanism of inhibition by α_2-macroglobulin involves hydrolysis by the proteinase of a susceptible region in one of the four polypeptide chains of α_2-macroglobulin (sometimes called the "bait"), with subsequent trapping of the proteins within the interstices of the α_2-macroglobulin. Ultimately, the protease is covalently linked to a portion of the α_2-macroglobulin molecule. The serine protease inhibitors also are abundant in synovial effusions and plasma and can serve a dual purpose of directly blocking serine protease function and indirectly decreasing MMP activity by preventing serine proteases from activating MMP proenzymes. One serine protease inhibitor, α_1-antitrypsin, has been well characterized in synovial fluid and is frequently inactivated after oxidation by reactive oxygen species.[329]

A family of proteins that specifically block MMP activity, called TIMPs, has been cloned and characterized. The TIMP proteins block proteinase activity by binding directly to MMPs in a 1:1 molar ratio. TIMP generally binds only to the active enzyme, although there are some exceptions, such as TIMP-2, which can interact with a progelatinase (MMP-2). The inhibitors bind to MMPs with extremely high avidity. Although the interaction does not result in new covalent bonds, it is essentially irreversible.

TIMP proteins are present in RA synovial fluid in excess. It is difficult to detect free active collagenase or stromelysin because these are usually complexed with the inhibitors. Most MMP is in the proenzyme form, however. Immunohistochemical and in situ hybridization studies have localized the TIMPs in hyperplastic synovial lining cells in rheumatoid synovium, but not in the cells of normal synovium. TIMP gene expression is not altered significantly by IL-1 or TNF-α, but it is increased by IL-6, oncostatin M, and TGF-β. TIMP-3 knockout mice have significantly more synovial inflammation and TNF-α production in antigen-induced arthritis, perhaps because it is unavailable to inhibit TNF convertase.[330] Similarly, TIMP-1 or TIMP-3 gene transfer limits rheumatoid FLS invasion into cartilage in a SCID mouse model. The function of these genes can extend beyond protease inhibition and can include many paracrine functions and induction of apoptosis when expressed intracellularly in cultured synoviocytes.

Given the important role of MMPs in tissue destruction, the relative balance between MMPs and TIMPs ultimately determines the fate of the extracellular matrix. The ratio in RA, with its more destructive potential, favors degradation, whereas osteoarthritis has a lower MMP-to-TIMP ratio. The levels of TIMP gene expression are similar in the two diseases and may be maximal. The higher ratio in RA results from increased MMP production. This balance between protease and inhibitor can be modified in vivo with drug therapy. Intra-articular corticosteroid injections markedly decrease synovial collagenase, stromelysin, and TIMP gene expression. In contrast, low-dose methotrexate therapy specifically decreases collagenase, but not TIMP-1 mRNA.[331] Suppressed collagenase gene expression suggests that a low collagenase-to-TIMP ratio is one mechanism of decreased tissue destruction observed in patients treated with methotrexate.

REGULATION OF BONE DESTRUCTION BY THE RECEPTOR ACTIVATOR OF NUCLEAR FACTOR κB LIGAND SYSTEM

Osteoclasts are the major cells responsible for bone degradation. RANKL, which was originally described for its role in T cell–DC interactions and lymphocyte and lymph node development, is perhaps the most important factor that modulates bone resorption.[332] Osteoclast development is complex and involves the differentiation of monocytes under the influence of cytokines such as M-CSF in combination with RANKL. Subsequent osteoclast activation can involve several pathways, most of which also depend on the presence of RANKL. Its receptor, known as RANK, is expressed by the osteoclast precursors. RANKL is produced by many cell types, including activated T cells and FLS. RANKL knockout mice have abnormally dense bones owing to a nearly complete lack of osteoclasts. When osteoclasts or their precursors are activated by soluble RANKL or by direct contact with cells displaying RANKL on their surface, bone resorption can occur through the elaboration of MMPs and cathepsin K. The RANKL-RANK system is antagonized by a soluble decoy receptor, osteoprotegerin, which binds to RANK and competes with RANKL.

Abundant evidence implicates this powerful mechanism in inflammatory arthritis. Administration of osteoprotegerin to rats with adjuvant arthritis inhibits bone destruction, but

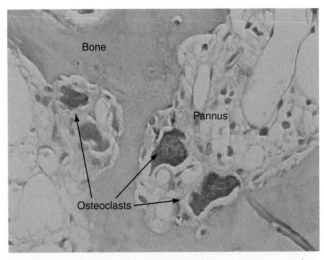

Figure 65-16 Tartrate-resistant acid phosphatase–positive osteoclasts are shown invading bone in rheumatoid arthritis (see *arrows* for examples). This process is regulated by receptor activator of nuclear factor κB ligand (RANKL) in the presence of other cytokines, such as macrophage colony-stimulating factor and tumor necrosis factor-α. *(Courtesy of Dr. Steven Goldring, Dr. Ellen Gravallese, and Dr. Allison Pettit.)*

has almost no effect on inflammation or clinical signs of arthritis.[333] RANKL knockout mice also are protected from bone erosions in the passive K/BxN model of arthritis, although cartilage destruction still occurs.[334] Animal models of arthritis point to IL-17 as a mediator of osteoclast generation. Genetic deficiency of IL-17 or anti-IL-17 antibodies has remarkable bone-sparing effects in these experiments.

RANK, RANKL, and osteoprotegerin (and M-CSF and IL-17) have been detected in the synovium and synovial fluid of patients with RA. The ratio of RANKL to osteoprotegerin is significantly higher in RA synovial effusions than in either osteoarthritis or gout, which is consistent with the more destructive nature of RA.[335] Osteoclasts expressing tartrate-resistant acid phosphatase, capable of forming resorption lacunae, can be generated from cultured RA synovial cells (Fig. 65-16).[336] This activity is blocked by the addition of exogenous osteoprotegerin. RA synoviocytes and synovial membrane T cells that display RANKL also can induce differentiation of osteoclasts from peripheral blood cells.[337]

TISSUE REPAIR

Extracellular matrix turnover in RA has been likened to wound healing owing to the crucial role of collagen production, proteases, and protease inhibitors. Remodeling the matrix by removing damaged proteins is a key element in early repair. Subsequently, the balance shifts to protease inhibition, production of cytokine inhibitors, removal of inflammatory cells through apoptosis, and release of anti-inflammatory eicosanoids such as LXs to suppress inflammation. Neutralization of oxidants via glutathione reductase or superoxide dismutase further limits tissue damage. This process permits either a return to normal architecture or scar formation. TGF-β, in particular, seems to play a key role in that it increases collagen deposition, suppresses MMP expression, and enhances production of the TIMPs. Although TGF-β levels in the joint are substantial, they are insufficient to overcome the impressive array of MMPs expressed in synovitis. The repair process seems to be inadequate in RA, perhaps because of persistent T cell activation or autonomous activation of other cell lineages. Strategies to shift from tissue damage by enhancing endogenous mechanisms not only might suppress symptoms, but also enhance appropriate remodeling of the matrix to restore homeostasis.

Because the rheumatoid synovium exhibits some properties similar to neoplastic diseases, the possibility that the tissue contains immature cells or embryonic genes that regulate repair has been explored. The embryonic growth factors from the wingless (wnt) and frizzled (fz) gene families are expressed in RA synovium.[338] Normally, these proteins participate in bone marrow progenitor differentiation and limb bud mesenchyme. Wnt5a and Fz5, in particular, are markedly elevated in RA tissues and cultured synoviocytes. When normal fibroblasts are transfected with the *wnt5a* gene, cytokine expression, such as IL-6, increases significantly. Antisense wnt-5A and dominant negative wnt-5A vectors diminish IL-6 and IL-15 expression by synoviocytes.[339] These data raise the possibility that immature mesenchymal cells populate the synovium in RA, either as a primary event or as a repair mechanism. Similar primitive mesenchymal cells circulate in the peripheral blood of RA and normal individuals, and in collagen-induced arthritis they infiltrate the synovium before clinically apparent synovial inflammation.

Restoring homeostasis and tissue repair in RA is a complex process that involves the ingress or dedifferentiation of mesenchymal cells that can remodel the matrix. In addition to TGF-β, the function of these cells is modulated by the BMPs. The BMPs are members of the TGF-β superfamily and, similar to TGF-β, signal through the Smad pathway. Several members, especially BMP-2 and BMP-7, are expressed in the joint and facilitate repair, although inappropriate release also can enhance joint damage or lead to ankylosis or enthesophyte formation.[340] BMP function also is regulated by a family of inhibitors such as Noggin, which can limit cartilage damage when overexpressed in murine antigen-induced arthritis.[341] Modulating the relative balance and timing of BMP expression ultimately could be used either to modify the destructive influence of synovitis or to regenerate damaged tissues.

SUMMARY

Understanding the etiology and pathogenesis of RA remains a complex problem, although the level of understanding has progressed considerably in recent years. T cell–dependent and T cell–independent processes contribute to disease initiation and perpetuation. It might be important to appreciate differences in disease pathogenesis at various stages of the process. These hypotheses have revealed many novel therapeutic targets and interventions that might lead to significant clinical benefit. Such was the case with the TNF inhibitors that have joined the pharmacopeia for the treatment of RA; initial observations that defined the cytokine profile in arthritis and that delineated the biology of macrophage cytokines led to this breakthrough. Similarly, understanding of apoptotic pathways, abnormalities in tumor-suppressor genes, the function of the susceptibility cassette, B cell function, or T cell differentiation might have abundant rewards.

REFERENCES

1. Firestein GS, Zvaifler NJ: How important are T cells in chronic rheumatoid synovitis? II. T cell-independent mechanisms from beginning to end. Arthritis Rheum 46:298, 2002.
2. Nepom GT, Byers P, Seyfried C, et al: HLA genes associated with rheumatoid arthritis: Identification of susceptibility alleles using specific oligonucleotide probes. Arthritis Rheum 32:15, 1989.
3. **Weyand CM, Hicok KC, Conn DL, et al: The influence of HLA-DRB1 genes on disease severity in rheumatoid arthritis. Ann Intern Med 117:801, 1992.**
4. Boki KA, Drosis AA, Tzioufas GA, et al: Examination of HLA-DR4 as a severity marker for rheumatoid arthritis in Greek patients. Ann Rheum Dis 52:517, 1993.
5. Hameed K, Bowman S, Kondeatis E, et al: The association of HLA-DRB genes and the shared epitope with rheumatoid arthritis in Pakistan. Br J Rheumatol 36:1184, 1997.
6. Calin A, Elswood J, Klouda PT: Destructive arthritis, rheumatoid factor, and HLA-DR4: Susceptibility versus severity, a case control study. Arthritis Rheum 32:1221, 1989.
7. Kirschmann DA, Duffin KL, Smith CE, et al: Naturally processed peptides from rheumatoid arthritis and non-associated HLA-DR alleles. J Immunol 155:5655, 1995.
8. van der Helm-van Mil AH, Verpoort KN, Breedveld FC, et al: The HLA-DRB1 shared epitope alleles are primarily a risk factor for anti-cyclic citrullinated peptide antibodies and are not an independent risk factor for development of rheumatoid arthritis. Arthritis Rheum 54:1117, 2006.
9. Jawaheer D, Li W, Graham RR, et al: Dissecting the genetic complexity of the association between human leukocyte antigens and rheumatoid arthritis. Am J Hum Genet 71:585, 2002.
10. Kang CP, Lee KW, Yoo DH, et al: The influence of a polymorphism at position −857 of the tumour necrosis factor alpha gene on clinical response to etanercept therapy in rheumatoid arthritis. Rheumatology (Oxf) 44:547, 2005.
11. Rodriguez MR, Nunez-Roldan A, Aguilar F, et al: Association of the CTLA4 3′untranslated region polymorphism with the susceptibility to rheumatoid arthritis. Hum Immunol 63:76, 2002.
12. Suzuki A, Yamada R, Chang X, et al: Functional haplotypes of PADI4, encoding citrullinating enzyme peptidylarginine deiminase 4, are associated with rheumatoid arthritis. Nat Genet 34:395, 2003.
13. Barton A, Bowes J, Eyre S, et al: A functional haplotype of the PADI4 gene associated with rheumatoid arthritis in a Japanese population is not associated in a United Kingdom population. Arthritis Rheum 50:1117, 2004.
14. **Begovich AB, Carlton VE, Honigberg LA, et al: A missense single-nucleotide polymorphism in a gene encoding a protein tyrosine phosphatase (PTPN22) is associated with rheumatoid arthritis. Am J Hum Genet 75:330, 2004.**
14a. Remmers EF, Plenge RM, Lee AT, et al: STAT4 and the risk of rheumatoid arthritis and systemic lupus erythematosus. N Engl J Med 357(10):977-986, 2007.
15. Lang TJ: Estrogen as an immunomodulator. Clin Immunol 113:224, 2004.
16. Yan Z, Lambert NC, Ostensen M, et al: Prospective study of fetal DNA in serum and disease activity during pregnancy in women with inflammatory arthritis. Arthritis Rheum 54:2069, 2006.
17. Nelson JL, Hughes KA, Smith AG, et al: Maternal-fetal disparity in HLA class II alloantigens and the pregnancy-induced amelioration of rheumatoid arthritis. N Engl J Med 329:466, 1993.
18. Brennan P, Barrett J, Fiddler M, et al: Maternal-fetal HLA incompatibility and the course of inflammatory arthritis during pregnancy. J Rheumatol 27:2843, 2000.
19. Linn-Rasker SP, van der Helm-van Mil AH, van Gaalen FA, et al: Smoking is a risk factor for anti-CCP antibodies only in rheumatoid arthritis patients who carry HLA-DRB1 shared epitope alleles. Ann Rheum Dis 65:366, 2006.
20. Doran MF, Pond GR, Crowson CS, et al: Trends in incidence and mortality in rheumatoid arthritis in Rochester, Minnesota, over a forty-year period. Arthritis Rheum 46:625, 2002.
21. Roelofs MF, Joosten LA, Abdollahi-Roodsaz S, et al: The expression of toll-like receptors 3 and 7 in rheumatoid arthritis synovium is increased and costimulation of toll-like receptors 3, 4, and 7/8 results in synergistic cytokine production by dendritic cells. Arthritis Rheum 52:231, 2005.

22. Radstake TR, Roelofs MF, Jenniskens YM, et al: Expression of toll-like receptors 2 and 4 in rheumatoid synovial tissue and regulation by proinflammatory cytokines interleukin-12 and interleukin-18 via interferon-gamma. Arthritis Rheum 50:3856, 2004.

23. Joosten LA, Koenders MI, Smeets RL, et al: Toll-like receptor 2 pathway drives streptococcal cell wall-induced joint inflammation: Critical role of myeloid differentiation factor 88. J Immunol 171:6145, 2003.

24. Brentano F, Kyburz D, Schorr O, et al: The role of Toll-like receptor signalling in the pathogenesis of arthritis. Cell Immunol 233:90, 2005.

25. Rosengren S, Hoffman HM, Bugbee W, et al: Expression and regulation of cryopyrin and related proteins in rheumatoid arthritis synovium. Ann Rheum Dis 64:708, 2005.

26. Rashid T, Darlington G, Kjeldsen-Kragh J, et al: Proteus IgG antibodies and C-reactive protein in English, Norwegian and Spanish patients with rheumatoid arthritis. Clin Rheumatol 18:190, 1999.

27. Gerard HC, Wang Z, Wang GF, et al: Chromosomal DNA from a variety of bacterial species is present in synovial tissue from patients with various forms of arthritis. Arthritis Rheum 44:1689, 2001.

28. Schrijver IA, Melief MJ, Tak PP, et al: Antigen-presenting cells containing bacterial peptidoglycan in synovial tissues of rheumatoid arthritis patients coexpress costimulatory molecules and cytokines. Arthritis Rheum 43:2160, 2000.

29. Choe JY, Crain B, Wu SR, et al: Interleukin 1 receptor dependence of serum transferred arthritis can be circumvented by toll-like receptor 4 signaling. J Exp Med 197:537, 2003.

30. Cole BC, Griffiths MM: Triggering and exacerbation of autoimmune arthritis by the Mycoplasma arthritidis superantigen MAM. Arthritis Rheum 36:994, 1993.

31. Hoffman RW, O'Sullivan FX, Schafermeyer KR, et al: Mycoplasma infection and rheumatoid arthritis: Analysis of their relationship using immunoblotting and an ultrasensitive polymerase chain reaction detection method. Arthritis Rheum 40:1219, 1997.

32. Blaschke S, Schwarz G, Moneke D, et al: Epstein-Barr virus infection in peripheral blood mononuclear cells, synovial fluid cells, and synovial membranes of patients with rheumatoid arthritis. J Rheumatol 27:866, 2000.

33. Roudier J, Petersen J, Rhodes GH, et al: Susceptibility to rheumatoid arthritis maps to a T-cell epitope shared by the HLA-Dw4 DR beta-1 chain and the Epstein-Barr virus glycoprotein gp 110. Proc Natl Acad Sci U S A 86:5104, 1989.

34. Albani S, Ravelli A, Mass M, et al: Immune responses to the Escherichia coli dnaJ heat shock protein in juvenile rheumatoid arthritis and their correlation with disease activity. J Pediatr 124:561, 1994.

35. Cohen BJ, Buckley MM, Clewley JP, et al: Human parvovirus infection in early rheumatoid and inflammatory arthritis. Ann Rheum Dis 45:832, 1986.

36. Saal JG, Steidle M, Einsele H, et al: Persistence of B19 parvovirus in synovial membranes of patients with rheumatoid arthritis. Rheumatol Int 12:147, 1992.

37. Takahashi Y, Murai C, Shibata S, et al: Human parvovirus B19 as a causative agent for rheumatoid arthritis. Proc Natl Acad Sci U S A 95:8227, 1998.

38. Ray NB, Nieva DR, Seftor EA, et al: Induction of an invasive phenotype by human parvovirus B19 in normal human synovial fibroblasts. Arthritis Rheum 44:1582, 2001.

39. Stahl HD, Hubner B, Seidl B, et al: Detection of multiple viral DNA species in synovial tissue and fluid of patients with early arthritis. Ann Rheum Dis 59:342, 2000.

40. Nakagawa K, Brusic V, McColl G, et al: Direct evidence for the expression of multiple endogenous retroviruses in the synovial compartment in rheumatoid arthritis. Arthritis Rheum 40:627, 1997.

41. Nakajima T, Aono H, Hasunuma T, et al: Overgrowth of human synovial cells driven by the human T cell leukemia virus type I tax gene. J Clin Invest 92:186, 1993.

42. Piper KE, Hanssen AD, Lewallen DG, et al: Lack of detection of human retrovirus-5 proviral DNA in synovial tissue and blood specimens from individuals with rheumatoid arthritis or osteoarthritis. Arthritis Rheum 55:123, 2006.

43. Nielen MM, van Schaardenburg D, Reesink HW, et al: Specific autoantibodies precede the symptoms of rheumatoid arthritis: A study of serial measurements in blood donors. Arthritis Rheum 50:38, 2004.

44. Rawson AJ, Hollander JL, Quismorio FP, et al: Experimental arthritis in man and rabbit dependent upon serum anti-immunoglobulin factors. Ann N Y Acad Sci 168:188, 1969.

45. Carson DA, Chen PP, Kipps TJ: New roles for rheumatoid factor. J Clin Invest 87:379, 1991.

46. Bouvet JP, Xin WJ, Pillot J: Restricted heterogeneity of polyclonal rheumatoid factor. Arthritis Rheum 30:998, 1987.

47. Lee SK, Bridges SL Jr, Koopman WJ, et al: The immunoglobulin kappa light chain repertoire expressed in the synovium of a patient with rheumatoid arthritis. Arthritis Rheum 35:905, 1992.

48. Sutton BJ, Corper AL, Sohi MK, et al: The structure of a human rheumatoid factor bound to IgG Fc. Adv Exp Med Biol 435:41, 1998.

49. De Rycke L, Nicholas AP, Cantaert T, et al: Synovial intracellular citrullinated proteins colocalizing with peptidyl arginine deiminase as pathophysiologically relevant antigenic determinants of rheumatoid arthritis-specific humoral autoimmunity. Arthritis Rheum 52:2323, 2005.

50. Vossenaar ER, Smeets TJ, Kraan MC, et al: The presence of citrullinated proteins is not specific for rheumatoid synovial tissue. Arthritis Rheum 50:3485, 2004.

51. Vossenaar ER, Nijenhuis S, Helsen MM, et al: Citrullination of synovial proteins in murine models of rheumatoid arthritis. Arthritis Rheum 48:2489, 2003.

52. Anzilotti C, Merlini G, Pratesi F, et al: Antibodies to viral citrullinated peptide in rheumatoid arthritis. J Rheumatol 33:647, 2006.

53. Union A, Meheus L, Humbel RL, et al: Identification of citrullinated rheumatoid arthritis-specific epitopes in natural filaggrin relevant for antifilaggrin autoantibody detection by line immunoassay. Arthritis Rheum 46:1185, 2002.

54. Kuhn KA, Kulik L, Tomooka B, et al: Antibodies against citrullinated proteins enhance tissue injury in experimental autoimmune arthritis. J Clin Invest 116:961, 2006.

55. Lundberg K, Nijenhuis S, Vossenaar ER, et al: Citrullinated proteins have increased immunogenicity and arthritogenicity and their presence in arthritic joints correlates with disease severity. Arthritis Res Ther 7:R458, 2005.

56. Burkhardt H, Sehnert B, Bockermann R, et al: Humoral immune response to citrullinated collagen type II determinants in early rheumatoid arthritis. Eur J Immunol 35:1643, 2005.

57. Watson WC, Cremer MA, Wooley PH, et al: Assessment of the potential pathogenicity of type II collagen autoantibodies in patients with rheumatoid arthritis. Arthritis Rheum 29:1316, 1986.

58. Tarkowski A, Klareskog L, Carlsten H, et al: Secretion of antibodies to types I and II collagen by synovial tissue cells in patients with rheumatoid arthritis. Arthritis Rheum 32:1087, 1989.

59. Bäcklund J, Carlsen S, Höger T, et al: Predominant selection of T cells specific for the glycosylated collagen type II epitope (263-270) in humanized transgenic mice and in rheumatoid arthritis. Proc Natl Acad Sci U S A 10:1073, 2002.

60. Burkhardt H, Huffmeier U, Spriewald B, et al: Association between protein tyrosine phosphatase 22 variant R620W in conjunction with the HLA-DRB1 shared epitope and humoral autoimmunity to an immunodominant epitope of cartilage-specific type II collagen in early rheumatoid arthritis. Arthritis Rheum 54:82, 2006.

61. Verheijden GF, Rijnders AW, Bos E, et al: Human cartilage glycoprotein-39 as a candidate autoantigen in rheumatoid arthritis. Arthritis Rheum 40:1115, 1997.

62. Sekine T, Masuko-Hongo K, Matsui T, et al: Recognition of YKL-39, a human cartilage related protein, as a target antigen in patients with rheumatoid arthritis. Ann Rheum Dis 60:49, 2001.

63. Li NL, Zhang DQ, Zhou KY, et al: Isolation and characteristics of autoreactive T cells specific to aggrecan G1 domain from rheumatoid arthritis patients. Cell Res 10:39, 2000.

64. Hueber W, Kidd BA, Tomooka BH, et al: Antigen microarray profiling of autoantibodies in rheumatoid arthritis. Arthritis Rheum 52:2645, 2005.

65. Steiner G, Smolen J: Autoantibodies in rheumatoid arthritis and their clinical significance. Arthritis Res 4:S1, 2002.

66. Kouskoff V, Korganow AS, Duchatelle V, et al: Organ-specific disease provoked by systemic autoimmunity. Cell 87:811, 1996.

67. Mandik-Nayak L, Allen PM: Initiation of an autoimmune response: Insights from a transgenic model of rheumatoid arthritis. Immunol Res 32:5, 2005.

68. Corr M, Firestein GS: Innate immunity as a hired gun: But is it rheumatoid arthritis? J Exp Med 195:F33, 2002.

69. Hayer S, Tohidast-Akrad M, Haralambous S, et al: Aberrant expression of the autoantigen heterogeneous nuclear ribonucleoprotein-A2 (RA33) and spontaneous formation of rheumatoid arthritis-associated anti-RA33 autoantibodies in TNF-alpha transgenic mice. J Immunol 175:8327, 2005.

70. Nell VP, Machold KP, Stamm TA, et al: Autoantibody profiling as early diagnostic and prognostic tool for rheumatoid arthritis. Ann Rheum Dis 64:1731, 2005.

71. Blass S, Union A, Raymackers J, et al: The stress protein BiP is overexpressed and is a major B and T cell target in rheumatoid arthritis. Arthritis Rheum 44:761, 2001.

72. Corrigall VM, Bodman-Smith MD, Fife MS, et al: The human endoplasmic reticulum molecular chaperone BiP is an autoantigen for rheumatoid arthritis and prevents the induction of experimental arthritis. J Immunol 166:1492, 2001.

73. Van Eden W, Holoshitz J, Nevo Z, et al: Arthritis induced by a T-lymphocyte clone that responds to *Mycobacterium tuberculosis* and to cartilage proteoglycans. Proc Natl Acad Sci U S A 82:5117, 1985.

74. Oda A, Miyata M, Kodama E, et al: Antibodies to 65Kd heat-shock protein were elevated in rheumatoid arthritis. Clin Rheumatol 13:261, 1994.

75. Gaston JSH, Life PF, Bailey LC, et al: In vitro responses to a 65-kilodalton mycobacterial protein by synovial T cells from inflammatory arthritis patients. J Immunol 143:2494, 1989.

76. Wilbrink B, Holewijn M, Bijlsma JW, et al: Suppression of human cartilage proteoglycan synthesis by rheumatoid synovial fluid mononuclear cells activated with mycobacterial 60-kd heat-shock protein. Arthritis Rheum 36:514, 1993.

77. Corr M, Zvaifler NJ: Mesenchymal precursor cells. Ann Rheum Dis 61:3, 2002.

78. Revell PA, Mapp PI, Lalor PA, et al: Proliferative activity of cells in the synovium as demonstrated by a monoclonal antibody, Ki67. Rheumatol Int 7:183, 1987.

79. Valencia X, Higgins JM, Kiener HP, et al: Cadherin-11 provides specific cellular adhesion between fibroblast-like synoviocytes. J Exp Med 200:1673, 2004.

80. Burmester GR, Dimitriu-Bona A, Waters SJ, et al: Identification of three major synovial lining cell populations by monoclonal antibodies directed to Ia antigens associated with monocytes/macrophages and fibroblasts. Scand J Immunol 17:69, 1983.

81. Goto M, Sasano M, Yamanaka H, et al: Spontaneous production of an interleukin 1-like factor by cloned rheumatoid synovial cells in long-term culture. J Clin Invest 80:786, 1987.

82. van der Pouw Kraan TC, van Gaalen FA, Kasperkovitz PV, et al: Rheumatoid arthritis is a heterogeneous disease: Evidence for differences in the activation of the STAT-1 pathway between rheumatoid tissues. Arthritis Rheum 48:2132, 2003.

83. Lafyatis R, Remmers EF, Roberts AB, et al: Anchorage-independent growth of synoviocytes from arthritis and normal joints: Stimulation by exogenous platelet-derived growth factor and inhibition by transforming growth factor-beta and retinoids. J Clin Invest 83:1267, 1989.

84. Imamura F, Aono H, Hasunuma T, et al: Monoclonal expansion of synoviocytes in rheumatoid arthritis. Arthritis Rheum 41:1979, 1998.

85. Geiler T, Kriegsmann J, Keyszer GM, et al: A new model for rheumatoid arthritis generated by engraftment of rheumatoid synovial tissue and normal human cartilage into SCID mice. Arthritis Rheum 37:1664, 1994.

86. **Muller-Ladner L, Kriegsmann J, Franklin BN, et al: Synovial fibroblasts of patients with rheumatoid arthritis attach to and invade normal human cartilage when engrafted into SCID mice. Am J Pathol 149:1607, 1996.**

87. Muller-Ladner U, Roberts CR, Franklin BN, et al: Human IL-1Ra gene transfer into human synovial fibroblasts is chondroprotective. J Immunol 158:3492, 1997.

88. Pap T, Aupperle KR, Gay S, et al: Invasiveness of synovial fibroblasts is regulated by p53 in the SCID mouse in vivo model of cartilage invasion. Arthritis Rheum 44:676, 2001.

89. Pap T, Nawrath M, Heinrich J, et al: Cooperation of Ras- and c-Myc-dependent pathways in regulating the growth and invasiveness of synovial fibroblasts in rheumatoid arthritis. Arthritis Rheum 50:2794, 2004.

90. Boyle DL, Rosengren S, Bugbee W, et al: Quantitative biomarker analysis of synovial gene expression by real-time PCR. Arthritis Res Ther 5:R352, 2003.

91. Manzo A, Paoletti S, Carulli M, et al: Systematic microanatomical analysis of CXCL13 and CCL21 in situ production and progressive lymphoid organization in rheumatoid synovitis. Eur J Immunol 35:1347, 2005.

92. Tsubaki T, Takegawa S, Hanamoto H, et al: Accumulation of plasma cells expressing CXCR3 in the synovial sublining regions of early rheumatoid arthritis in association with production of Mig/CXCL9 by synovial fibroblasts. Clin Exp Immunol 141:363, 2005.

93. Kang YM, Zhang X, Wagner UG, et al: CD8 T cells are required for the formation of ectopic germinal centers in rheumatoid synovitis. J Exp Med 195:1325, 2002.

94. Kim WJ, Kang YJ, Koh EM, et al: LIGHT is involved in the pathogenesis of rheumatoid arthritis by inducing the expression of pro-inflammatory cytokines and MMP-9 in macrophages. Immunology 114:272, 2005.

95. Braun A, Takemura S, Vallejo AN, et al: Lymphotoxin beta-mediated stimulation of synoviocytes in rheumatoid arthritis. Arthritis Rheum 50:2140, 2004.

96. Han S, Zhang X, Marinova E, et al: Blockade of lymphotoxin pathway exacerbates autoimmune arthritis by enhancing the Th1 response. Arthritis Rheum 52:3202, 2005.

97. Fava RA, Notidis E, Hunt J, et al: A role for the lymphotoxin/LIGHT axis in the pathogenesis of murine collagen-induced arthritis. J Immunol 171:115, 2003.

98. Ruprecht CR, Gattorno M, Ferlito F, et al: Coexpression of CD25 and CD27 identifies FoxP3+ regulatory T cells in inflamed synovia. J Exp Med 201:1793, 2005.

99. Warrington KJ, Takemura S, Goronzy JJ, et al: CD4, CD28 T cells in rheumatoid arthritis patients combine features of the innate and adaptive immune systems. Arthritis Rheum 44:13, 2001.

100. MacDonald KP, Nishioka Y, Lipsky PE, et al: Functional CD40 ligand is expressed by T cells in rheumatoid arthritis. J Clin Invest 100:2404, 1997.

101. Rissoan MC, Van Kooten C, Chomarat P, et al: The functional CD40 antigen of fibroblasts may contribute to the proliferation of rheumatoid synovium. Clin Exp Immunol 106:481, 1996.

102. Yamanishi Y, Hiyama K, Ishioka S, et al: Telomerase activity in the synovial tissues of chronic inflammatory and non-inflammatory rheumatic diseases. Int J Mol Med 4:513, 1999.

103. Patel DD, Zachariah JP, Whichard LP: CXCR3 and CCR5 ligands in rheumatoid arthritis synovium. Clin Immunol 98:39, 2001.

104. Nanki T, Hayashida K, El-Gabalawy HS, et al: Stromal cell-derived factor-1-CXC chemokine receptor 4 interactions play a central role in CD4 T cell accumulation in rheumatoid arthritis synovium. J Immunol 165:6590, 2000.

105. **Fox DA: The role of T cells in the immunopathogenesis of rheumatoid arthritis: New perspectives. Arthritis Rheum 40:598, 1997.**

106. Muller-Ladner U, Kriegsmann J, Gay RE, et al: Progressive joint destruction in a human immunodeficiency virus-infected patient with rheumatoid arthritis. Arthritis Rheum 38:1328, 1995.

107. Corrigall VM, Solau-Gervais E, Panayi GS: Lack of CD80 expression by fibroblast-like synoviocytes leading to anergy in T lymphocytes. Arthritis Rheum 43:1606, 2000.

108. Brennan FM, Hayes AL, Ciesielski CJ, et al: Evidence that rheumatoid arthritis synovial T cells are similar to cytokine-activated T cells: Involvement of phosphatidylinositol 3-kinase and nuclear factor kappaB pathways in tumor necrosis factor alpha production in rheumatoid arthritis. Arthritis Rheum 46:31, 2002.

109. Hata H, Sakaguchi N, Yoshitomi H, et al: Distinct contribution of IL-6, TNF-alpha, IL-1, and IL-10 to T cell-mediated spontaneous autoimmune arthritis in mice. J Clin Invest 114:582, 2004.

110. Quinn MA, Conaghan PG, O'Connor PJ, et al: Very early treatment with infliximab in addition to methotrexate in early, poor-prognosis rheumatoid arthritis reduces magnetic resonance imaging evidence of synovitis and damage, with sustained benefit after infliximab withdrawal: Results from a twelve-month randomized, double-blind, placebo-controlled trial. Arthritis Rheum 52:27, 2005.

111. Prakken BJ, Samodal R, Le TD, et al: Epitope-specific immunotherapy induces immune deviation of proinflammatory T cells in rheumatoid arthritis. Proc Natl Acad Sci U S A 101:4228, 2004.

112. Wang H, Marsters SA, Baker T, et al: TACI-ligand interactions are required for T cell activation and collagen-induced arthritis in mice. Nat Immunol 2:632, 2001.

113. Ohata J, Zvaifler NJ, Nishio M, et al: Fibroblast-like synoviocytes of mesenchymal origin express functional B cell-activating factor of the TNF family in response to proinflammatory cytokines. J Immunol 174:864, 2005.

114. Tan SM, Xu D, Roschke V, et al: Local production of B lymphocyte stimulator protein and APRIL in arthritic joints of patients with inflammatory arthritis. Arthritis Rheum 48:982, 2003.

115. Seyler TM, Park YW, Takemura S, et al: BLyS and APRIL in rheumatoid arthritis. J Clin Invest 115:3083, 2005.

116. Kim H-J, Berek C: B cells in rheumatoid arthritis. Arthritis Res 2:126, 2000.

117. Clausen BE, Bridges SL Jr, Lavelle JC, et al: Clonally-related immunoglobulin VH domains and nonrandom use of DH gene segments in rheumatoid arthritis synovium. Mol Med 4:240, 1998.

118. Reparon-Schuijt CC, van Esch WJ, van Kooten C, et al: Presence of a population of CD20, CD38 B lymphocytes with defective proliferative responsiveness in the synovial compartment of patients with rheumatoid arthritis. Arthritis Rheum 44:2029, 2001.

119. Takemura S, Klimiuk PA, Braun A, et al: T cell activation in rheumatoid synovium is B cell dependent. J Immunol 167:4710, 2001.

120. Shimaoka Y, Attrep JF, Hirano T, et al: Nurse-like cells from bone marrow and synovium of patients with rheumatoid arthritis promote survival and enhance function of human B cells. J Clin Invest 102:606, 1998.

121. Takeuchi E, Tomita T, Toyosaki-Maeda T, et al: Establishment and characterization of nurse cell-like stromal cell lines from synovial tissues of patients with rheumatoid arthritis. Arthritis Rheum 42: 221, 1999.

122. Burger JA, Zvaifler NJ, Tsukada N, et al: Fibroblast-like synoviocytes support B-cell pseudoemperipolesis via a stromal cell-derived factor-1- and CD106 (VCAM-1)-dependent mechanism. J Clin Invest 107:305, 2001.

123. Hamaguchi Y, Uchida J, Cain DW, et al: The peritoneal cavity provides a protective niche for B1 and conventional B lymphocytes during anti-CD20 immunotherapy in mice. J Immunol 174:4389, 2005.

124. Jongbloed SL, Lebre MC, Fraser AR, et al: Enumeration and phenotypical analysis of distinct dendritic cell subsets in psoriatic arthritis and rheumatoid arthritis. Arthritis Res Ther 8:R15, 2005.

125. Lindhout E, van Eijk M, van Pel M, et al: Fibroblast-like synoviocytes from rheumatoid arthritis patients have intrinsic properties of follicular dendritic cells. J Immunol 162:5949-5956, 1999.

126. Tsai V, Zvaifler NJ: Dendritic cell-lymphocyte clusters that form spontaneously in rheumatoid arthritis synovial effusions differ from clusters formed in human mixed leukocyte reactions. J Clin Invest 82:1731, 1988.

127. MacDonald KP, Pettit AR, Quinn C, et al: Resistance of rheumatoid synovial dendritic cells to the immunosuppressive effects of IL-10. J Immunol 163:5599, 1999.

128. Morita Y, Gupta R, Seidl KM, et al: Cytokine production by dendritic cells genetically engineered to express IL-4: Induction of Th2 responses and differential regulation of IL-12 and IL-23 synthesis. J Genet Med 7:869, 2005.

129. Malone DG, Wilder RL, Saavedra-Delgado AM, et al: Mast cell numbers in rheumatoid synovial tissues. Arthritis Rheum 30: 130, 1987.

130. Lee DM, Friend DS, Gurish MF, et al: Mast cells: A cellular link between autoantibodies and inflammatory arthritis. Science 297:1689, 2002.

131. Juurikivi A, Sandler C, Lindstedt KA, et al: Inhibition of c-kit tyrosine kinase by imatinib mesylate induces apoptosis in mast cells in rheumatoid synovia: A potential approach to the treatment of arthritis. Ann Rheum Dis 64:1126, 2005.

132. Tak PP, Kummer JA, Hack CE, et al: Granzyme-positive cytotoxic cells are specifically increased in early rheumatoid synovial tissue. Arthritis Rheum 37:1735, 1994.

133. Dalbeth N, Gundle R, Davies RJ, et al: CD56bright NK cells are enriched at inflammatory sites and can engage with monocytes in a reciprocal program of activation. J Immunol 173:6418, 2004.

134. Marinova-Mutafchieva L, Williams RO, Funa K, et al: Inflammation is preceded by tumor necrosis factor-dependent infiltration of mesenchymal cells in experimental arthritis. Arthritis Rheum 46:507, 2002.

135. Hirohata S, Miura Y, Tomita T, et al: Enhanced expression of mRNA for nuclear factor kappaB1 (p50) in CD34+ cells of the bone marrow in rheumatoid arthritis. Arthritis Res Ther 8:R54, 2006.

136. Jimenez-Boj E, Redlich K, Turk B, et al: Interaction between synovial inflammatory tissue and bone marrow in rheumatoid arthritis. J Immunol 175:2579, 2005.

137. Smeets TJ, Dolhain RJEM, Miltenburg AM, et al: Poor expression of T cell-derived cytokines and activation and proliferation markers in early rheumatoid synovial tissue. Clin Immunol Immunopathol 88:84, 1998.

138. Kraan MC, Versendaal H, Jonker M, et al: Asymptomatic synovitis precedes clinically manifested arthritis. Arthritis Rheum 41:1481, 1998.

139. Han Z, Boyle DL, Manning AM, et al: AP-1 and NF-κB regulation in rheumatoid arthritis and murine collagen-induced arthritis. Autoimmunity 28:197, 1998.

140. Liao H, Wu J, Kuhn E, et al: Use of mass spectrometry to identify protein biomarkers of disease severity in the synovial fluid and serum of patients with rheumatoid arthritis. Arthritis Rheum 50:3792, 2004.

141. Jonsson H, Allen P, Peng SL: Inflammatory arthritis requires Foxo3a to prevent Fas ligand-induced neutrophil apoptosis. Nat Med 11: 666, 2005.

142. Schlenk J, Lorenz HM, Haas JP, et al: Extravasation into synovial tissue induces CCL20 mRNA expression in polymorphonuclear neutrophils of patients with rheumatoid arthritis. J Rheumatol 32:2291, 2005.

143. Cross A, Edwards SW, Bucknall RC, et al: Secretion of oncostatin M by neutrophils in rheumatoid arthritis. Arthritis Rheum 50: 1430, 2004.

144. Mottonen M, Heikkinen J, Mustonen L, et al: CD4+ CD25+ T cells with the phenotypic and functional characteristics of regulatory T cells are enriched in the synovial fluid of patients with rheumatoid arthritis. Clin Exp Immunol 140:360, 2005.

145. Lasky HP, Bauer K, Pope RM: Increased helper inducer and decreased suppressor inducer phenotypes in the rheumatoid joint. Arthritis Rheum 31:52, 1988.

146. Nouri AME, Panayi GS: Cytokines and the chronic inflammation of rheumatic disease, III: Deficient interleukin-2 production in rheumatoid arthritis is not due to suppressor mechanisms. J Rheumatol 14:902, 1987.

147. Firestein GS, Berger AE, Tracey DE, et al: IL-1 receptor antagonist protein production and gene expression in rheumatoid arthritis and osteoarthritis synovium. J Immunol 149:1054, 1992.

148. Maurice MM, Lankester AC, Bezemer AC, et al: Defective TCR-mediated signaling in synovial T cells in rheumatoid arthritis. J Immunol 159:2973, 1997.

149. Maurice MM, Nakamura H, van der Voort EA, et al: Evidence for the role of an altered redox state in hyporesponsiveness of synovial T cells in rheumatoid arthritis. Immunology 158:1458, 1997.

150. Siegle I, Klein T, Backman JT, et al: Expression of cyclooxygenase 1 and cyclooxygenase 2 in human synovial tissue: Differential elevation of cyclooxygenase 2 in inflammatory joint diseases. Arthritis Rheum 41:122, 1998.

151. Elmgreen J, Haagen N, Ahnfelt-Ronne I: Enhanced capacity for release of leukotriene B4 by neutrophils in rheumatoid arthritis. Ann Rheum Dis 46:501, 1987.

152. Griffiths RJ, Pettipher ER, Koch K, et al: Leukotriene B4 plays a critical role in the progression of collagen-induced arthritis. Proc Natl Acad Sci U S A 92:517, 1995.

153. Rossi A, Kapahi P, Natoli G, et al: Anti-inflammatory cyclopentenone prostaglandins are direct inhibitors of IkappaB kinase. Nature 403:103, 2000.

154. Sodin-Semrl S, Spagnolo A, Barbaro B, et al: Lipoxin A4 counteracts synergistic activation of human fibroblast-like synoviocytes. Int J Immunopathol Pharmacol 17:15, 2004.

155. Neumann E, Barnum SR, Tarner IH, et al: Local production of complement proteins in rheumatoid arthritis synovium. Arthritis Rheum 46:934, 2002.

156. Pekin TJ Jr, Zvaifler NJ: Hemolytic complement in synovial fluid. J Clin Invest 43:1372, 1964.

157. Goodfellow RM, Williams AS, Levin JL, et al: Local therapy with soluble complement receptor 1 (sCR1) suppresses inflammation in rat mono-articular arthritis. Clin Exp Immunol 110:45, 1997.

158. Wang Y, Kristan J, Hao L, et al: A role for complement in antibody-mediated inflammation: C-5 deficient DBA/1 mice are resistant to collagen-induced arthritis. J Immunol 164:4340, 2000.

159. Hietala MA, Jonsson IM, Tarkowski A, et al: Complement deficiency ameliorates collagen-induced arthritis in mice. J Immunol 169: 454, 2002.

160. Banda NK, Kraus DM, Muggli M, et al: Prevention of collagen-induced arthritis in mice transgenic for the complement inhibitor complement receptor 1-related gene/protein y. J Immunol 171:2109, 2003.

161. Gaston JSH, Rickinson AB, Yao QY, et al: The abnormal cytotoxic T cell response to Epstein-Barr virus in rheumatoid arthritis is correlated with disease activity and occurs in other arthropathies. Ann Rheum Dis 45:932, 1986.

162. Goronzy JJ, Weyand CM: Thymic function and peripheral T-cell homeostasis in rheumatoid arthritis. Trends Immunol 22:251, 2001.

163. Burastero SE, Casali P, Wilder RL, et al: Monoreactive high affinity and polyreactive low affinity rheumatoid factors are produced by CD5 B cells from patients with rheumatoid arthritis. J Exp Med 168:1979, 1988.

164. Fox DA, Smith BR: Evidence for oligoclonal B cell expansion in the peripheral blood of patients with rheumatoid arthritis. Ann Rheum Dis 45:991, 1986.

165. He X, Kang AH, Stuart JM: Anti-Human type II collagen CD19 B cells are present in patients with rheumatoid arthritis and healthy individuals. J Rheumatol 28:2168, 2001.

166. Firestein GS, Zvaifler NJ: How important are T cells in chronic rheumatoid synovitis? Arthritis Rheum 33:768, 1990.

167. Unemori EN, Bair MJ, Bauer EA, et al: Stromelysin expression regulates collagenase activation in human fibroblasts: Dissociable control of two metalloproteinases by interferon-gamma. J Biol Chem 266:23, 477, 1991.

168. Firestein GS, Zvaifler NJ: Peripheral blood and synovial fluid monocyte activation in inflammatory arthritis, II: Low levels of synovial fluid and synovial tissue interferon suggest that γ-interferon is not the primary macrophage activating factor. Arthritis Rheum 30:864, 1987.

169. Chen E, Keystone EC, Fish EN: Restricted cytokine expression in rheumatoid arthritis. Arthritis Rheum 36:901, 1993.

170. Smeets TJ, Dolhain RJ, Breedveld FC, et al: Analysis of the cellular infiltrates and expression of cytokines in synovial tissue from patients with rheumatoid arthritis and reactive arthritis. J Pathol 186:75, 1998.

171. Firestein GS, Xu WD, Townsend K, et al: Cytokines in chronic inflammatory arthritis, I: Failure to detect T cell lymphokines (interleukin 2 and interleukin 3) and presence of macrophage colony-stimulating factor (CSF-1) and a novel mast cell growth factor in rheumatoid synovitis. J Exp Med 168:1573, 1988.

172. Chabaud M, Fossiez F, Taupin JL, et al: Enhancing effect of IL-17 on IL-1-induced IL-6 and leukemia inhibitory factor production by rheumatoid arthritis synoviocytes and its regulation by Th2 cytokines. J Immunol 161:409, 1998.

173. Chabaud M, Durand JM, Buchs N, et al: Human interleukin-17: a T cell-derived proinflammatory cytokine produced by the rheumatoid synovium. Arthritis Rheum 43:963, 1999.

174. Lubberts E, Joosten LA, Chabaud M, et al: IL-4 gene therapy for collagen arthritis suppresses synovial IL-17 and osteoprotegerin ligand and prevents bone erosion. J Clin Invest 105:1697, 2000.

175. Granet C, Miossec P: Combination of the pro-inflammatory cytokines IL-1, TNF-alpha and IL-17 leads to enhanced expression and additional recruitment of AP-1 family members, Egr-1 and NF-kappaB in osteoblast-like cells. Cytokine 26:169, 2004.

176. Chabaud M, Lubberts E, Joosten L, et al: IL-17 derived from juxta-articular bone and synovium contributes to joint degradation in rheumatoid arthritis. Arthritis Res 3:168, 2001.

177. Koenders MI, Lubberts E, van de Loo FA, et al: Interleukin-17 acts independently of TNF-alpha under arthritic conditions. J Immunol 176:6262, 2006.

178. Ehrenstein MR, Evans JG, Singh A, et al: Compromised function of regulatory T cells in rheumatoid arthritis and reversal by anti-TNFalpha therapy. J Exp Med 200:277, 2004.

179. Ruprecht CR, Gattorno M, Ferlito F, et al: Coexpression of CD25 and CD27 identifies FoxP3+ regulatory T cells in inflamed synovia. J Exp Med 201:1793, 2005.

180. Morgan ME, Flierman R, van Duivenvoorde LM, et al: Effective treatment of collagen-induced arthritis by adoptive transfer of CD25+ regulatory T cells. Arthritis Rheum 52:2212, 2005.

181. Gonzalez-Rey E, Fernandez-Martin A, Chorny A, et al: Vasoactive intestinal peptide induces CD4+, CD25+ T regulatory cells with therapeutic effect in collagen-induced arthritis. Arthritis Rheum 54:864, 2006.

182. Chomarat P, Banchereau J, Miossec P: Differential effects of interleukins 10 and 4 on the production of interleukin-6 by blood and synovium monocytes in rheumatoid arthritis. Arthritis Rheum 38:1046, 1995.

183. Katsikis KD, Chu CQ, Brennan FM, et al: Immunoregulatory role of interleukin 10 in rheumatoid arthritis. J Exp Med 179:1517, 1994.

184. Joosten LA, Lubberts E, Durez P, et al: Role of interleukin-4 and interleukin-10 in murine collagen-induced arthritis: Protective effect of interleukin-4 and interleukin-10 treatment on cartilage destruction. Arthritis Rheum 40:249, 1997.

185. Joosten LAB, Lubberts E, Helsen MMA, et al: Dual role of IL-12 in early and late stages of murine collagen type II arthritis. J Immunol 159:4094, 1997.

186. Smeets TJ, Kraan MC, Versendaal J, et al: Analysis of serial synovial biopsies in patients with rheumatoid arthritis: Description of a control group without clinical improvement after treatment with interleukin 10 or placebo. J Rheumatol 26:2089, 1999.

187. Burger D, Rezzonico R, Li JM, et al: Imbalance between interstitial collagenase and tissue inhibitor of metalloproteinases 1 in synoviocytes and fibroblasts upon direct contact with stimulated T lymphocytes: Involvement of membrane-associated cytokines. Arthritis Rheum 41:1748, 1998.

188. McInnes IB, Leung BP, Sturrock RD, et al: Interleukin-15 mediates T cell-dependent regulation of tumor necrosis factor-alpha production in rheumatoid arthritis. Nat Med 3:189-195, 1997.

189. van Roon JA, Verweij MC, Wijk MW, et al: Increased intraarticular interleukin-7 in rheumatoid arthritis patients stimulates cell contact-dependent activation of CD4(+) T cells and macrophages. Arthritis Rheum 52:1700, 2005.

190. Firestein GS: The T cell cometh: Interplay between adaptive immunity and cytokine networks in rheumatoid arthritis. J Clin Invest 114:471, 2004.

191. Firestein GS, Alvaro-Gracia JM, Maki R: Quantitative analysis of cytokine gene expression in rheumatoid arthritis. J Immunol 144:3347, 1990.

192. Postlethwaite AE, Lachman LB, Kang AH: Induction of fibroblast proliferation by interleukin-1 derived from human monocytic leukemia cells. Arthritis Rheum 27:995, 1984.

193. Genovese MC, Cohen S, Moreland L, et al: Combination therapy with etanercept and anakinra in the treatment of patients with rheumatoid arthritis who have been treated unsuccessfully with methotrexate. Arthritis Rheum 50:1412, 2004.

194. Joosten LA, van De Loo FA, Lubberts E, et al: An IFN-gamma-independent proinflammatory role of IL-18 in murine streptococcal cell wall arthritis. J Immunol 165:6553, 2000.

195. Gracie JA, Forsey RJ, Chan WL, et al: A proinflammatory role for IL-18 in rheumatoid arthritis. J Clin Invest 104:1393, 1999.

196. Saklatvala J: Tumour necrosis factor α stimulates resorption and inhibits synthesis of proteoglycan in cartilage. Nature 322:547, 1986.

197. Georgopoulos S, Plows D, Kollias G: Transmembrane TNF is sufficient to induce localized tissue toxicity and chronic inflammatory arthritis in transgenic mice. J Inflamm 46:86, 1996.

198. Williams RO, Mason LJ, Feldmann M, et al: Synergy between anti-CD4 and anti-tumor necrosis factor in the amelioration of established collagen-induced arthritis. Proc Natl Acad Sci U S A 91:2762, 1994.

199. Lipsky PE, van der Heijde DM, St Clair EW, et al: Infliximab and methotrexate in the treatment of rheumatoid arthritis: Anti-tumor necrosis factor trial in rheumatoid arthritis with concomitant therapy study group. N Engl J Med 343:1594, 2000.

200. Guerne PA, Zuraw BL, Vaughan JH, et al: Synovium as a source of interleukin 6 in vitro: Contribution to local and systemic manifestations of arthritis. J Clin Invest 83:585, 1989.

201. Field M, Chu C, Feldman M, et al: Interleukin-6 localisation in the synovial membrane in rheumatoid arthritis. Rheumatol Int 11: 45, 1991.

202. Nishimoto N, Yoshizaki K, Miyasaka N, et al: Treatment of rheumatoid arthritis with humanized anti-interleukin-6 receptor antibody: A multicenter, double-blind, placebo-controlled trial. Arthritis Rheum 50:1761, 2004.

203. Walmsley M, Butler DM, Marinova-Mutafchieva L, et al: An anti-inflammatory role for interleukin-11 in established murine collagen-induced arthritis. Immunology 95:31, 1998.

204. Plater-Zyberk C, Buckton J, Thompson S, et al: Amelioration of arthritis in two murine models using antibodies to oncostatin M. Arthritis Rheum 44:2697, 2001.

205. Cho ML, Kang JW, Moon YM, et al: STAT3 and NF-kappaB signal pathway is required for IL-23-mediated IL-17 production in spontaneous arthritis animal model IL-1 receptor antagonist-deficient mice. J Immunol 176:5652, 2006.

206. Villarino AV, Hunter CA: Biology of recently discovered cytokines: Discerning the pro- and anti-inflammatory properties of interleukin-27. Arthritis Res Ther 6:225, 2004.

207. Thurkow EW, van der Heijden IM, Breedveld FC, et al: Increased expression of IL-15 in the synovium of patients with rheumatoid arthritis compared with patients with *Yersinia*-induced arthritis and osteoarthritis. J Pathol 181:444, 1997.

208. Ruchatz H, Leung BP, Wei XQ, et al: Soluble IL-15 receptor alpha-chain administration prevents murine collagen-induced arthritis: A role for IL-15 in development of antigen-induced immunopathology. J Immunol 160:5654, 1998.

209. Joosten LA, Netea MG, Kim SH, et al: IL-32, a proinflammatory cytokine in rheumatoid arthritis. Proc Natl Acad Sci U S A 103:3298, 2006.

210. Xu WD, Firestein GS, Taetle R, et al: Cytokines in chronic inflammatory arthritis, II: Granulocyte-macrophage colony-stimulating factor in rheumatoid synovial effusions. J Clin Invest 83:876, 1989.

211. Alvaro-Gracia JM, Zvaifler NJ, Brown CB, et al: Cytokines in chronic inflammatory arthritis, VI: Analysis of the synovial cells involved in granulocyte-macrophage colony-stimulating factor production and gene expression in rheumatoid arthritis and its regulation by IL-1 and tumor necrosis factor-alpha. J Immunol 146:3365, 1991.

212. Cook AD, Braine EL, Campbell IK, et al: Blockade of collagen-induced arthritis post-onset by antibody to granulocyte-macrophage colony-stimulating factor (GM-CSF): Requirement for GM-CSF in the effector phase of disease. Arthritis Res 3:293, 2001.

213. Koch AE, Kunkel SL, Burrows JC, et al: Synovial tissue macrophage as a source of the chemotactic cytokine IL-8. J Immunol 147:2187, 1991.

214. Koch AE, Kunkel SL, Harlow LA, et al: Enhanced production of monocyte chemoattractant protein-1 in rheumatoid arthritis. J Clin Invest 90:772, 1992.

215. Koch AE, Kunkel SL, Harlow LA, et al: Epithelial neutrophil activating peptide-78: A novel chemotactic cytokine for neutrophils in arthritis. J Clin Invest 94:1012, 1994.

216. Schmutz C, Hulme A, Burman A, et al: Chemokine receptors in the rheumatoid synovium: Upregulation of CXCR5. Arthritis Res Ther 7:R217, 2005.

217. Blades MC, Ingegnoli F, Wheller SK, et al: Stromal cell-derived factor 1 (CXCL12) induces monocyte migration into human synovium transplanted onto SCID mice. Arthritis Rheum 46:824, 2002.

218. Nanki T, Urasaki Y, Imai T, et al: Inhibition of fractalkine ameliorates murine collagen-induced arthritis. J Immunol 173:7010, 2004.

219. Haringman JJ, Smeets TJ, Reinders-Blankert P, et al: Chemokine and chemokine receptor expression in paired peripheral blood mononuclear cells and synovial tissue of patients with rheumatoid arthritis, osteoarthritis, and reactive arthritis. Ann Rheum Dis 65:294, 2006.

220. Camps M, Ruckle T, Ji H, et al: Blockade of PI3Kgamma suppresses joint inflammation and damage in mouse models of rheumatoid arthritis. Nat Med 11:936, 2005.

221. Remmers EF, Lafyatis R, Kumkumian GK, et al: Cytokines and growth regulation of synoviocytes from patients with rheumatoid arthritis and rats with streptococcal cell wall arthritis. Growth Factors 2:179, 1990.

222. Remmers EF, Sano H, Lafyatis R, et al: Production of platelet derived growth factor B chain (PDGF-B/c-sis) mRNA and immunoreactive PDGF B-like polypeptide by rheumatoid synovium: Coexpression with heparin binding acidic fibroblast growth factor-1. J Rheumatol 18:7, 1991.

223. Yayon A, Klagsbrun M, Esko JD, et al: Cell surface, heparin-like molecules are required for binding of basic fibroblast growth factor to its high affinity receptor. Cell 64:841, 1991.

224. Henderson B, Thompson RC, Hardingham T, et al: Inhibition of interleukin-1-induced synovitis and articular cartilage proteoglycan loss in the rabbit knee by recombinant human interleukin-1 receptor antagonist. Cytokine 3:246, 1991.

225. Malyak M, Swaney RE, Arend WP: Levels of synovial fluid interleukin-1 receptor antagonist in rheumatoid arthritis and other arthropathies: Potential contribution from synovial fluid neutrophils. Arthritis Rheum 36:781, 1993.

226. Firestein GS, Boyle DL, Yu C, et al: Synovial interleukin-1 receptor antagonist and interleukin-1 balance in rheumatoid arthritis. Arthritis Rheum 37:644, 1994.

227. Fava RA, Olsen NJ, Spencer-Green G, et al: Vascular permeability factor/endothelial growth factor (VPF/VEGF): Accumulation and expression in human synovial fluids and rheumatoid synovial tissue. J Exp Med 180:34, 1994.

228. Allen JB, Manthey CL, Hand AR, et al: Rapid onset synovial inflammation and hyperplasia induced by transforming growth factor beta. J Exp Med 171:231, 1990.

229. Song XY, Gu M, Jin WW, et al: Plasmid DNA encoding transforming growth factor-beta1 suppresses chronic disease in a streptococcal cell wall-induced arthritis model. J Clin Invest 101:2615, 1998.

230. Cope AP, Aderka D, Doherty M, et al: Increased levels of soluble tumor necrosis factor receptors in the sera and synovial fluid of patients with rheumatic diseases. Arthritis Rheum 35:1160, 1992.

231. Brennan FM, Gibbons DL, Mitchell T, et al: Enhanced expression of tumor necrosis factor receptor mRNA and protein in mononuclear cells isolated from rheumatoid arthritis synovial joints. Eur J Immunol 22:1907, 1992.

232. Arend WP, Malyak M, Smith MF Jr, et al: Binding of IL-1 alpha, IL-1 beta, and IL-1 receptor antagonist by soluble IL-1 receptors and levels of soluble IL-1 receptors in synovial fluids. J Immunol 153:4766, 1994.

233. Sioud M, Mellbye O, Forre O: Analysis of the NF-kappaB p65 subunit, Fas antigen, Fas ligand and Bcl-2-related proteins in the synovium of RA and polyarticular JRA. Clin Exp Rheumatol 16:125, 1998.

234. Tak PP, Gerlag DM, Aupperle KB, et al: Inhibitor of nuclear factor kappaB kinase beta is a key regulator of synovial inflammation. Arthritis Rheum 44:1897, 2001.

235. Schett G, Tohidast-Akrad M, Smolen JS, et al: Activation, differential localization, and regulation of the stress-activated protein kinases, extracellular signal-regulated kinase, c-JUN N-terminal kinase, and p38 mitogen-activated protein kinase, in synovial tissue and cells in rheumatoid arthritis. Arthritis Rheum 43:2501, 2000.

236. Medicherla S, Ma JY, Mangadu R, et al: A selective p38α mitogen-activated protein kinase inhibitor reverses cartilage and bone destruction in mice with collagen-induced arthritis. J Pharmacol Exp Ther 318:132, 2006.

237. Boyle DL, Jones TJ, Hammaker D, et al: Modulation of peripheral inflammation by spinal p38 MAP kinase. PLoS Med 3:e338, 2006.

238. Han Z, Boyle DL, Chang L, et al: c-Jun N-terminal kinase is required for metalloproteinase expression and joint destruction in inflammatory arthritis. J Clin Invest 108:73, 2001.

239. Koller M, Hayer S, Redlich K, et al: JNK1 is not essential for TNF-mediated joint disease. Arthritis Res Ther 7:R166, 2005.

240. Inoue T, Boyle DL, Corr M, et al: Mitogen-activated protein kinase kinase 3 is a pivotal pathway regulating p38 activation in inflammatory arthritis. Proc Natl Acad Sci U S A 103:5484, 2006.

241. Inoue T, Hammaker D, Boyle DL, et al: Regulation of JNK by MKK-7 in fibroblast-like synoviocytes. Arthritis Rheum 54:2127, 2006.

242. Kinne RW, Boehm S, Iftner T, et al: Synovial fibroblast-like cells strongly express Jun-B and C-Fos proto-oncogenes in rheumatoid- and osteoarthritis. Scand J Rheumatol Suppl 101:121, 1995.

243. Han Z, Boyle DL, Manning AM, et al: AP-1 and NF-κB regulation in rheumatoid arthritis and murine collagen-induced arthritis. Autoimmunity 28:197, 1998.

244. Wakisaka S, Suzuki N, Saito N, et al: Possible correction of abnormal rheumatoid arthritis synovial cell function by jun D transfection in vitro. Arthritis Rheum 41:470, 1998.

245. Shiozawa S, Shimizu K, Tanaka K, et al: Studies on the contribution of c-fos/AP-1 to arthritic joint destruction. J Clin Invest 99:1210, 1997.

246. Walker JG, Ahern MJ, Coleman M, et al: Expression of Jak3, STAT1, STAT4, and STAT6 in inflammatory arthritis: Unique Jak3 and STAT4 expression in dendritic cells in seropositive rheumatoid arthritis. Ann Rheum Dis 65:149, 2006.

247. Huckel M, Schurigt U, Wagner AH, et al: Attenuation of murine antigen-induced arthritis by treatment with a decoy oligodeoxynucleotide inhibiting signal transducer and activator of transcription-1 (STAT-1). Arthritis Res Ther 8:R17, 2005.

248. Wang F, Sengupta TK, Zhong Z, et al: Regulation of the balance of cytokine production and the signal transducer and activator of transcription (STAT) transcription factor activity by cytokines and inflammatory synovial fluids. J Exp Med 182:1825, 1995.

249. Sengupta TK, Chen A, Zhong Z, et al: Activation of monocyte effector genes and STAT family transcription factors by inflammatory synovial fluid is independent of interferon. J Exp Med 181:1015, 1995.

250. Muller-Ladner U, Judex M, Ballhorn W, et al: Activation of the IL-4 STAT pathway in rheumatoid synovium. J Immunol 164:3894, 2000.
251. van der Pouw Kraan TC, van Gaalen FA, Kasperkovitz PV, et al: Rheumatoid arthritis is a heterogeneous disease: Evidence for differences in the activation of the STAT-1 pathway between rheumatoid tissues. Arthritis Rheum 48:2132, 2003.
252. Shouda T, Yoshida T, Hanada T, et al: Induction of the cytokine signal regulator SOCS3/CIS3 as a therapeutic strategy for treating inflammatory arthritis. J Clin Invest 108:1781, 2001.
253. Sweeney SE, Hammaker D, Boyle DL, et al: Regulation of c-Jun phosphorylation by the I kappa B kinase-epsilon complex in fibroblast-like synoviocytes. J Immunol 174:6424, 2005.
254. Maurice MM, Nakamura H, van der Voort EAM, et al: Increased expression of thioredoxin in rheumatoid arthritis. Arthritis Rheum 41:S319, 1998.
255. Bashir S, Harris G, Denman MA, et al: Oxidative DNA damage and cellular sensitivity to oxidative stress in human autoimmune diseases. Ann Rheum Dis 52:659, 1993.
256. Sakurai H, Kohsaka H, Liu MF, et al: Nitric oxide production and inducible nitric oxide synthase expression in inflammatory arthritides. J Clin Invest 96:2357, 1995.
257. Farrell AJ, Blake DR, Palmer RM, et al: Increased concentrations of nitrite in synovial fluid and serum samples suggest increased nitric oxide synthesis in rheumatic diseases. Ann Rheum Dis 51:1219, 1992.
258. Salmon M, Scheel-Toellner D, Huissoon AP, et al: Inhibition of T cell apoptosis in the rheumatoid synovium. J Clin Invest 99:439, 1997.
259. Chou CT, Yang JS, Lee MR: Apoptosis in rheumatoid arthritis: Expression of Fas, Fas-L, p53, and Bcl-2 in rheumatoid synovial tissues. J Pathol 193:110, 2001.
260. Morel J, Audo R, Hahne M, et al: Tumor necrosis factor-related apoptosis-inducing ligand (TRAIL) induces rheumatoid arthritis synovial fibroblast proliferation through mitogen-activated protein kinases and phosphatidylinositol 3-kinase/Akt. J Biol Chem 280:15709, 2005.
261. Catrina AI, Ulfgren AK, Lindblad S, et al: Low levels of apoptosis and high FLIP expression in early rheumatoid arthritis synovium. Ann Rheum Dis 61:934, 2002.
262. Firestein GS, Yeo M, Zvaifler NJ: Apoptosis in rheumatoid arthritis synovium. J Clin Invest 96:1631, 1995.
263. Matsumoto S, Muller-Ladner U, Gay RE, et al: Ultrastructural demonstration of apoptosis, Fas and Bcl-2 expression of rheumatoid synovial fibroblasts. Rheumatology 23:1345, 1996.
264. Perlman H, Pagliari LJ, Liu H, et al: Rheumatoid arthritis synovial macrophages express the Fas-associated death domain-like interleukin 1beta-converting enzyme-inhibitory protein and are refractory to Fas-mediated apoptosis. Arthritis Rheum 44:21, 2001.
265. Zhang HG, Wang Y, Xie JF, et al: Regulation of tumor necrosis factor alpha-mediated apoptosis of rheumatoid arthritis synovial fibroblasts by the protein kinase Akt. Arthritis Rheum 44:1555, 2001.
266. Cha HS, Rosengren S, Boyle DL, et al: PUMA regulation and pro-apoptotic effects in fibroblast-like synoviocytes. Arthritis Rheum 254:587, 2006.
267. Franz JK, Pap T, Hummel KM, et al: Expression of sentrin, a novel antiapoptotic molecule, at sites of synovial invasion in rheumatoid arthritis. Arthritis Rheum 43:599, 2000.
268. Pap T, Franz JK, Hummel KM, et al: Activation of synovial fibroblasts in rheumatoid arthritis: Lack of expression of the tumour suppressor PTEN at sites of invasive growth and destruction. Arthritis Res 2:59, 2000.
269. Zhang H, Yang Y, Horton JL, et al: Amelioration of collagen-induced arthritis by CD95 (Apo-1/Fas)-ligand gene transfer. J Clin Invest 100:1951, 1997.
270. Yao Q, Seol DW, Mi Z, et al: Intra-articular injection of recombinant TRAIL induces synovial apoptosis and reduces inflammation in a rabbit knee model of arthritis. Arthritis Res Ther 8:R16, 2005.
271. Yao Q, Wang S, Glorioso JC, et al: Gene transfer of p53 to arthritic joints stimulates synovial apoptosis and inhibits inflammation. Mol Ther 3:901, 2001.
272. Yamanishi Y, Boyle DL, Pinkoski MJ, et al: Regulation of joint destruction and inflammation by p53 in collagen-induced arthritis. Am J Pathol 160:123, 2002.
273. Simelyte E, Rosengren S, Boyle DL, et al: Regulation of arthritis by p53: Critical role of adaptive immunity. Arthritis Rheum 52:1876, 2005.
274. Firestein GS, Nguyen K, Aupperle K, et al: Apoptosis in rheumatoid arthritis: p53 overexpression in rheumatoid arthritis synovium. Am J Pathol 149:2143, 1996.
275. Tak PP, Smeets TJM, Boyle DL, et al: p53 overexpression in synovial tissue from patients with early and chronic rheumatoid arthritis. Arthritis Rheum 42:948, 1999.
276. Firestein GS, Echeverri F, Yeo M, et al: Somatic mutations in the p53 tumor suppressor gene in rheumatoid arthritis synovium. Proc Natl Acad Sci U S A 94:10895, 1997.
277. Han Z, Boyle DL, Shi Y, et al: Dominant negative p53 mutations in rheumatoid arthritis. Arthritis Rheum 42:1088, 1999.
278. Yamanishi Y, Boyle DL, Rosengren S, et al: Regional analysis of p53 mutations in rheumatoid arthritis synovium. Proc Natl Acad Sci U S A 99:10025, 2002.
279. Cannons JL, Karsh J, Birnboim HC, et al: HPRT mutant T cells in the peripheral blood and synovial tissue of patients with rheumatoid arthritis. Arthritis Rheum 41:1772, 1998.
280. Roivainen A, Jalava J, Pirila L, et al: H-ras oncogene point mutations in arthritic synovium. Arthritis Rheum 40:1636, 1997.
280a. Bang H, Egerer K, Gauliard A, et al: Mutation and citrullination modifies vimentin to a novel autoantigen for rheumatoid arthritis. Arthritis Rheum 56:2503-2511, 2007.
281. Da Sylva TR, Connor A, Mburu Y, et al: Somatic mutations in the mitochondria of rheumatoid arthritis synoviocytes. Arthritis Res Ther 7:R844, 2005.
282. Lee SH, Chang DK, Goel A, et al: Microsatellite instability and suppressed DNA repair enzyme expression in rheumatoid arthritis. J Immunol 170:2214, 2003.
283. Stevens CR, Blake DR, Merry P, et al: A comparative study by morphometry of the microvasculature in normal and rheumatoid synovium. Arthritis Rheum 34:1508, 1991.
284. Shweiki D, Itin A, Soffer D, et al: Vascular endothelial growth factor induced by hypoxia may mediate hypoxia-initiated angiogenesis. Nature 359:843, 1992.
285. Cramer T, Yamanishi Y, Clausen BE, et al: HIF-1alpha is essential for myeloid cell-mediated inflammation. Cell 112:645, 2003.
286. Unemori EN, Ferrara N, Bauer EA, et al: Vascular endothelial growth factor induces interstitial collagenase expression in human endothelial cells. J Cell Physiol 153:557, 1992.
287. Jackson JR, Minton JA, Ho ML, et al: Expression of vascular endothelial growth factor in synovial fibroblasts is induced by hypoxia and interleukin 1beta. Rheumatology 24:1253, 1997.
288. Scott BB, Zaratin PF, Colombo A, et al: Constitutive expression of angiopoietin-1 and -2 and modulation of their expression by inflammatory cytokines in rheumatoid arthritis synovial fibroblasts. J Rheumatol 29:230, 2002.
289. Koch AE, Halloran MM, Haskell CJ, et al: Angiogenesis mediated by soluble forms of E-selectin and vascular cell adhesion molecule-1. Nature 376:517, 1995.
290. Koch AE, Friedman J, Burrows JC, et al: Localization of the angiogenesis inhibitor thrombospondin in human synovial tissues. Pathobiology 61:1, 1993.
291. Jou IM, Shiau AL, Chen SY, et al: Thrombospondin 1 as an effective gene therapeutic strategy in collagen-induced arthritis. Arthritis Rheum 52:339, 2005.
292. Peacock DJ, Banquerigo ML, Brahn E: Angiogenesis inhibition suppresses collagen arthritis. J Exp Med 175:1135, 1992.
293. Storgard CM, Stupack DG, Jonczyk A, et al: Decreased angiogenesis and arthritis in rabbits treated with an αvβ3 antagonist. J Clin Invest 103:47, 1998.
294. Gerlag DM, Borges E, Tak PP, et al: Suppression of murine collagen-induced arthritis by targeted apoptosis of synovial neovasculature. Arthritis Res 3:357, 2001.
295. Matsuno H, Yudoh K, Uzuki M, et al: Treatment with the angiogenesis inhibitor endostatin: A novel therapy in rheumatoid arthritis. J Rheumatol 29:890, 2002.
296. Lee L, Buckley C, Blades MC, et al: Identification of synovium-specific homing peptides by in vivo phage display selection. Arthritis Rheum 46:2109, 2002.
297. Hale LP, Martin ME, McCollum DE, et al: Immunohistologic analysis of the distribution of cell adhesion molecules within the inflammatory synovial microenvironment. Arthritis Rheum 32:22, 1989.

298. Issekutz TB, Issekutz AC: T lymphocyte migration to arthritic joints and dermal inflammation in the rat: Differing migration patterns and the involvement of VLA-4. Clin Immunol Immunopathol 61:436, 1991.

299. Wahl SM, Allen JB, Hines KL, et al: Synthetic fibronectin peptides suppress arthritis in rats by interrupting leukocyte adhesion and recruitment. J Clin Invest 94:655, 1994.

300. Laffon A, Garcia-Vicuna R, Humbria A, et al: Upregulated expression and function of VLA-4 fibronectin receptors on human activated T cells in rheumatoid arthritis. J Clin Invest 88:546, 1992.

301. Van Dinther-Janssen AC, Pals ST, Scheper RJ, et al: Role of the CS1 adhesion motif of fibronectin in T cell adhesion to synovial membrane and peripheral lymph node endothelium. Ann Rheum Dis 52:672, 1993.

302. Elices MJ, Tsai V, Strahl D, et al: Expression and functional significance of alternatively spliced CS1 fibronectin in rheumatoid arthritis microvasculature. J Clin Invest 93:405, 1994.

303. Jorgensen C, Travaglio-Encinoza A, Bologna C: Human mucosal lymphocyte marker expression in synovial fluid lymphocytes of patients with rheumatoid arthritis. J Rheumatol 21:1602, 1994.

304. Corkill MM, Kirkham BW, Haskard DO, et al: Gold treatment of rheumatoid arthritis decreases synovial expression of the endothelial leukocyte adhesion receptor ELAM-1. J Rheumatol 18:1453, 1991.

305. Jorgensen C, Couret I, Canovas F, et al: Mononuclear cell retention in rheumatoid synovial tissue engrafted in severe combined immunodeficient (SCID) mice is up-regulated by tumour necrosis factor-alpha (TNF-alpha) and mediated through intercellular adhesion molecule-1 (ICAM-1). Clin Exp Immunol 106:20, 1996.

306. Jorgensen C, Couret I, Canovas F, et al: In vivo migration of tonsil lymphocytes in rheumatoid synovial tissue engrafted in SCID mice: Involvement of LFA-1. Autoimmunology 24:179, 1996.

307. Haraoui B, Strand V, Keystone E: Biologic agents in the treatment of rheumatoid arthritis. Curr Pharm Biotechnol 1:217, 2000.

308. Ruth JH, Amin MA, Woods JM, et al: Accelerated development of arthritis in mice lacking endothelial selectins. Arthritis Res Ther 7:R959, 2005.

309. Annefeld M: The potential aggressiveness of synovial tissue in rheumatoid arthritis. J Pathol 139:399, 1983.

310. Wolfe GC, MacNaul KL, Buechel FF, et al: Differential in vivo expression of collagenase messenger RNA in synovium and cartilage: Quantitative comparison with stromelysin messenger RNA levels in human rheumatoid arthritis and osteoarthritis patients and in two animal models of acute inflammatory arthritis. Arthritis Rheum 36:1540, 1993.

311. Cooke TD, Hurd ER, Jasin HE, et al: Identification of immunoglobulins and complement in rheumatoid articular collagenous tissues. Arthritis Rheum 18:541, 1975.

312. Kuiper S, Joosten LA, Bendele AM, et al: Different roles of tumour necrosis factor alpha and interleukin 1 in murine streptococcal cell wall arthritis. Cytokine 10:690, 1998.

313. Lotz M, Guerne PA: Interleukin-6 induces the synthesis of tissue inhibitor of metalloproteinases-1/erythroid potentiating activity (TIMP-1/EPA). J Biol Chem 266:2017, 1991.

314. Gunther M, Haubeck HD, van de Leur E, et al: Transforming growth factor beta 1 regulates tissue inhibitor of metalloproteinases-1 expression in differentiated human articular chondrocytes. Arthritis Rheum 37:395, 1994.

315. Firestein GS, Paine MM, Littman BH: Gene expression (collagenase, tissue inhibitor of metalloproteinases, complement, and HLA-DR) in rheumatoid arthritis and osteoarthritis synovium: Quantitative analysis and effect of intraarticular corticosteroids. Arthritis Rheum 34:1094, 1991.

316. Zvaifler NJ, Boyle D, Firestein GS: Early synovitis: Synoviocytes and mononuclear cells. Semin Arthritis Rheum 23(Suppl 2):11, 1994.

317. Mudgett JS, Hutchinson NI, Chartrain NA, et al: Susceptibility of stromelysin 1-deficient mice to collagen-induced arthritis and cartilage destruction. Arthritis Rheum 41:110, 1998.

318. Hamada T, Arima N, Shindo M, et al: Suppression of adjuvant arthritis of rats by a novel matrix metalloproteinase-inhibitor. Br J Pharmacol 131:1513, 2000.

319. Peterson JT: The importance of estimating the therapeutic index in the development of matrix metalloproteinase inhibitors. Cardiovasc Res 69:677, 2006.

320. Muller-Ladner U, Gay RE, Gay S: Cysteine proteinases in arthritis and inflammation. Perspect Drug Discovery Design 6:87, 1996.

321. Lemaire R, Huet G, Zerimech F, et al: Selective induction of the secretion of cathepsins B and L by cytokines in synovial fibroblast-like cells. Br J Rheumatol 36:735, 1997.

322. Garnero P, Borel O, Byrjalsen I, et al: The collagenolytic activity of cathepsin K is unique among mammalian proteinases. J Biol Chem 273:32347, 1998.

323. Hou WS, Li W, Keyszer G, et al: Comparison of cathepsins K and S expression within the rheumatoid and osteoarthritic synovium. Arthritis Rheum 46:663, 2002.

324. Esser RE, Angelo RA, Murphey MD, et al: Cysteine proteinase inhibitors decrease articular cartilage and bone destruction in chronic inflammatory arthritis. Arthritis Rheum 37:236, 1994.

325. Tortorella MD, Burn TC, Pratta MA, et al: Purification and cloning of aggrecanase-1: A member of the ADAMTS family of proteins. Science 284:1664, 1999.

326. Lark MW, Bayne EK, Flanagan J, et al: Aggrecan degradation in human cartilage: Evidence for both matrix metalloproteinase and aggrecanase activity in normal, osteoarthritic, and rheumatoid joints. J Clin Invest 100:93, 1997.

327. Yamanishi Y, Boyle DL, Clark M, et al: Expression and regulation of aggrecanase in arthritis: The role of TGF-beta. J Immunol 168:1405, 2002.

328. Stanton H, Rogerson FM, East CJ, et al: ADAMTS5 is the major aggrecanase in mouse cartilage in vivo and in vitro. Nature 434:648, 2005.

329. Abbink JJ, Kamp AM, Nuijens JH, et al: Proteolytic inactivation of alpha 1-antitrypsin and alpha 1-antichymotrypsin by neutrophils in arthritic joints. Arthritis Rheum 36:168, 1993.

330. Mahmoodi M, Sahebjam S, Smookler D, et al: Lack of tissue inhibitor of metalloproteinases-3 results in an enhanced inflammatory response in antigen-induced arthritis. Am J Pathol 166:1733, 2005.

331. Firestein GS, Paine MM, Boyle DL: Mechanisms of methotrexate action in rheumatoid arthritis: Selective decrease in synovial collagenase gene expression. Arthritis Rheum 37:193, 1994.

332. Goldring SR, Gravallese EM: Mechanisms of bone loss in inflammatory arthritis: Diagnosis and therapeutic implications. Arthritis Res 2:33, 2000.

333. Kong YY, Feige U, Sarosi I, et al: Activated T cells regulate bone loss and joint destruction in adjuvant arthritis through osteoprotegerin ligand. Nature 402:304, 1999.

334. Pettit AR, Ji H, von Stechow D, et al: TRANCE/RANKL knockout mice are protected from bone erosion in a serum transfer model of arthritis. Am J Pathol 159:1689, 2001.

335. Feuerherm AJ, Borset M, Seidel C, et al: Elevated levels of osteoprotegerin (OPG) and hepatocyte growth factor (HGF) in rheumatoid arthritis. Scand J Rheumatol 30:229, 2001.

336. Haynes DR, Crotti TN, Loric M, et al: Osteoprotegerin and receptor activator of nuclear factor kappaB ligand (RANKL) regulate osteoclast formation by cells in the human rheumatoid arthritis joint. Rheumatology (Oxf) 40:623, 2001.

337. Kotake S, Udagawa N, Hakoda M, et al: Activated human T cells directly induce osteoclastogenesis from human monocytes: Possible role of T cells in bone destruction in rheumatoid arthritis patients. Arthritis Rheum 44:1003, 2001.

338. Sen M, Lauterbach K, ElGabalawy H, et al: Expression and function of wingless and frizzled homologs in rheumatoid arthritis. Proc Natl Acad Sci U S A 97:2791, 2000.

339. Sen M, Chamorro M, Reifert J, et al: Blockade of Wnt-5A/frizzled 5 signaling inhibits rheumatoid synoviocyte activation. Arthritis Rheum 44:772, 2001.

340. Lories RJ, Luyten FP: Bone morphogenetic protein signaling in joint homeostasis and disease. Cytokine Growth Factor Rev 16:287, 2005.

341. Lories RJ, Daans M, Derese I, et al: Noggin haploinsufficiency differentially affects tissue responses in destructive and remodeling arthritis. Arthritis Rheum 54:1736, 2006.

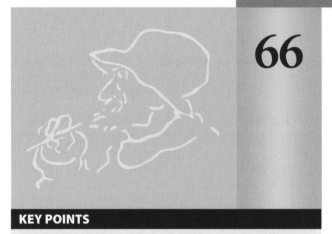

66

Clinical Features of Rheumatoid Arthritis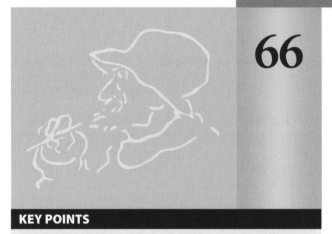

EDWARD D. HARRIS, JR. •
GARY S. FIRESTEIN

KEY POINTS

Rheumatoid arthritis is a symmetric inflammatory arthritis that mainly affects the small joints of the hands and feet.

Larger joints can be involved, usually in a symmetric fashion.

Cartilage destruction and bone erosions are common, especially in rheumatoid factor–positive or anticitrullinated protein antibody–positive patients.

Uncontrolled synovitis can lead to severe deformities, loss of function, and increased mortality.

Early aggressive therapy seems to improve long-term outcomes in rheumatoid arthritis.

Systemic manifestations include pulmonary disease, vasculitis, nodules, and eye disease.

EPIDEMIOLOGY AND THE BURDEN OF DISEASE

In past years, most investigators accepted a prevalence of rheumatoid arthritis (RA) in most populations of around 1%, with an incidence in women twice that in men. This number was based on many studies of population samples[1-3] that varied among the surveys from 0.3% to 1.5%. This figure of 1% prevalence of RA in most populations may be changing, however, as incidence rates in different decades are studied. The incidence of RA in Rochester, Minnesota, declined 50% between 1950 and 1974.[4] The differences between incidence and prevalence are enhanced by realizing that as the population ages, the prevalence of RA may increase or stay the same, even though the incidence stays the same or is decreasing, simply because individuals with RA are living longer.

The incidence of RA increases dramatically during adulthood; the exception is men in their 40s through 60s. In Olmstead County, Minnesota, this increased incidence with increasing age continues until age 85, after which the incidence declines.[5] In a 10-year extension of this study, making it a 40-year, population-based history of RA, the age-adjusted and sex-adjusted incidence per 100,000 population decreased from 62 in the decade 1955 to 1964 to 32.7 in the decade 1985 to 1994.[6] The decrease was more prominent in women than in men, and the average age at onset of the disease shifted upward. Most intriguing were the cyclic patterns of incidence within decades, suggesting the influence of environmental factors. One explanation for the decline in incidence and shift toward an older age at onset is a birth cohort effect, the greatest impact of which is early in life.[7]

Throughout the world, there are pockets of ethnic groups that have a much higher incidence of RA. Native Americans are one of these groups. In one geographic area, non–Native American populations had an RA prevalence of 1.1% to 0.9% between 1986 and 1994, whereas the prevalence in Algonquian Indians in the same region ranged from 2% to 2.1%, and the disease onset was 12 years earlier in the Native American population.[8] In Pima Indians, who bear a very high incidence of RA, a decline in incidence has been correlated with a decrease in seropositivity for rheumatoid factor (RF). The highest likelihood of seropositivity was in Pima Indians born at the turn of the 20th century, and it has decreased ever since. This is additional supportive evidence for a birth cohort effect.[9] Although newer, more effective therapy for rheumatoid patients has reduced morbidity and disability from the disease, there are still substantial dollar costs for RA. In a panel of 1156 individuals with RA in San Francisco followed for 15 years, medical care costs for RA averaged $5919 per year with an additional $2582 incurred for medical but non-RA reasons.[10] More than half of the costs were for hospitalizations, with some patients bearing costs of more than $85,000/yr, as their function declined. In another cohort of 4258 patients with RA followed for 17,085 patient-years, lifetime direct medical care costs were estimated to be $93,296.[11]

RISK FACTORS

A predisposition to RA seems to be multifactorial when one considers the following: (1) Relatively few identical twins have RA (about 15%), even though it is much more likely that there is concordance for the disease in twins than in the normal population; (2) despite the powerful influence of the "shared epitope" on HLA-DRB chains in predisposing to the severity of disease, this susceptibility cassette is not a risk factor in certain population studies; and (3) the combination of many gene polymorphisms confers a modestly increased risk of disease. A reasonable hypothesis is that the genetic predisposition to RA involves a propensity to autoimmune responses, but that repeated exposure to environmental agents is ultimately responsible for tipping the balance from subclinical autoimmunity to diseases such as RA. Many of the risk factors for RA are discussed in Chapter 65, especially genetic associations, environmental exposures, and the role of autoantibodies.

CLINICAL SYNDROMES OF EARLY RHEUMATOID ARTHRITIS

In the Northern Hemisphere, the onset of RA is more frequent in winter than in summer. In several series, the onset of RA from October to March in the Northern

Supplemental images available on the Expert Consult Premium Edition website.

Hemisphere was found to be twice as frequent as in the other 6 months.[12] Data suggest that the appearance of RF may be more likely to precede symptoms of arthritis in patients than was previously recognized. In 30 patients whose frozen serum samples were available from a time before symptoms of RA began, half had a positive latex fixation test,[13] and many more of these were men than women.

PATTERNS OF ONSET

Insidious Onset

RA has an insidious, slow onset over weeks to months in 55% to 65% of cases.[14] The initial symptoms may be systemic or articular. In some individuals, fatigue, malaise, swollen hands, and diffuse musculoskeletal pain may be the first nonspecific complaints, with joints becoming involved later. Involvement of tendon sheaths early in the process can focus attention on periarticular structures. In retrospect, the patient often can identify one joint that was involved first, quickly followed by others. Asymmetric initial presentations (often with more symmetry developing later in the course of disease) are common. The reason for the symmetry of joint involvement compared with other forms of arthritis, such as the seronegative spondyloarthropathies, is unknown.

Morning stiffness is a cardinal sign of inflammatory arthritis that can appear even before pain and may be related to the accumulation of edema fluid within inflamed tissues during sleep. The morning stiffness dissipates as edema and products of inflammation are absorbed by lymphatics and venules and returned to the circulation by motion accompanying the use of muscles and joints. To be specific for joint inflammation, morning stiffness (e.g., "difficulty moving around") should persist for at least 30 to 45 minutes before disappearing. A similar "gel" phenomenon can occur if a patient is inactive for a period during the day.

It is rare for symptoms to remit completely in one set of joints while developing in another. This quality of arthritis sets RA apart from rheumatic fever or palindromic rheumatism, in which a true migratory pattern of arthritis is common. A subtle, early change in RA is the development of muscle atrophy around affected joints. Muscle efficiency and strength become diminished. As a result, weakness develops that can be out of proportion to pain. Opening doors, climbing stairs, and doing repetitive work rapidly become more demanding. A low-grade fever without chills is rarely present. Depression and focused and nonspecific anxiety accentuate symptoms. A small but significant weight loss is common and reflects the catabolic effects of cytokines and an associated anorexia.

Acute or Intermediate Onset

Of patients, 8% to 15% have an acute onset of symptoms that peak within a few days. Rarely, a patient can pinpoint the onset of symptoms to a specific time or activity, such as opening a door or driving a golf ball. Symptoms mount, with pain developing in other joints, often in a less symmetric pattern than in patients who have an insidious

onset. Diagnosis of acute-onset RA is difficult to make, and sepsis or vasculitis must be ruled out. Fever, suggesting an infectious process, can be a prominent sign. An intermediate type of onset, in which symptoms develop over days or weeks, occurs in 15% to 20% of patients. Systemic complaints are more noticeable than in the insidious type of onset.

Joint Involvement

The joints most commonly involved first in RA are the metacarpophalangeal (MCP) joints, proximal interphalangeal (PIP) joints, metatarsophalangeal joints, and wrists (Table 66-1).[15] Larger joints generally become symptomatic after small joints. Synovitis in large joints is likely to remain asymptomatic for a longer time than in smaller ones, and a biopsy specimen of an asymptomatic knee often shows histologic evidence of synovitis. One anatomic study correlated the area, in square centimeters, of synovial membrane with that of hyaline cartilage in each joint. The joints with the highest ratio of synovium to articular cartilage correlated positively with the joints most frequently involved in the disease (see Table 66-1).[16]

EARLY SYNOVITIS: WHICH PATIENTS DEVELOP RHEUMATOID ARTHRITIS?

Distinguishing early RA from other inflammatory arthropathies can be challenging. In its earliest stages, RA might involve only a few joints and without the typical symmetric distribution. What are the diagnostic clues that can be used to determine who will progress to classic RA and who will develop an alternative inflammatory arthritis such as seronegative spondyloarthropathies or have spontaneous remission? The implications for disease management are obvious because early treatment potentially could limit or prevent joint damage and possibly permit long-term remissions or even cures. Because 30% to 40% of patients with

Table 66-1 Distribution of Joints Involved in Attacks Based on a Cumulative Experience with 227 Patients

Joint Involvement	% Patients (Mean)	% Patients (Range)
MCP, PIP	91	74-100
Wrists	78	54-82
Knees	64	41-94
Shoulders	65	33-75
Ankles	50	10-67
Feet	43	15-73
Elbows	38	13-60
Hips	17	0-40
Temporomandibular	8	0-28
Spine	4	0-11
Sternoclavicular	2	0-6
Para-articular sites	27	20-29

MCP, metacarpophalangeal; PIP, proximal interphalangeal.

Modified from Guerne P-A, Weisman MH: Palindromic rheumatism: Part of or apart from the spectrum of rheumatoid arthritis. Am J Med 16:451-460, 1992. Copyright 1992, with permission from Excerpta Medica, Inc.

Table 66-2   Evolution of Patients with Palindromic Rheumatism in Nine Series Totaling 653 Patients*

Series of Patients	No. Cases	Remission or Cure (%)	Persistent PR (%)	PR-RA (%)	Other Diseases (%)
1	34	15	85	0	0
2	140	8	52	36	4
3	179	10	47	38	5
4	39	0	56	44	0
5	70	24	34	30	12
6	38	8	66	15	11
7	43	23	23	49	5
8	50	0	46	54	0
9	60	43	21	35	2
Total or average	653	15	48	33	4

*In each series, the number of patients undergoing a remission or a cure, remaining palindromic, evolving toward rheumatoid arthritis (PR-RA), or developing another disease is expressed as a percentage

PR, palindromic rheumatism; RA, rheumatoid arthritis.

Modified from Guerne P-A, Weisman MH: Palindromic rheumatism: Part of or apart from the spectrum of rheumatoid arthritis. Am J Med 16:451-460, 1992. Copyright 1992, with permission from Excerpta Medica, Inc.

early inflammatory synovitis have spontaneous remission, accurate identification of patients with RA is essential to avoid undertreatment and overtreatment.

Some of these questions have been addressed by the Leiden Early Arthritis Clinic, which evaluates patients with less than 2 years of symptoms (most patients evaluated have symptoms for <6 months). In this cohort, only about 20% of patients met criteria for RA when initially evaluated by a rheumatologist.[17] One third of patients defied categorization and were considered to have "undifferentiated arthritis." When this group of patients was followed for 1 year, 27% ultimately developed RA, and 40% remained undifferentiated. Clinical features that were more commonly seen in the patients who developed RA included greater number of joints involved (mean of seven joints versus four joints), duration of morning stiffness (90 minutes versus 60 minutes), and the presence of autoantibodies. These features were insufficient individually to permit early diagnosis of RA, although a composite scoring system has been proposed.[18] The predictive value of this system might approach 90%.

Of the predictive features most likely to be useful in patients, serum autoantibody production might be the most powerful. Anticitrullinated protein antibodies, in particular, are strongly associated with evolution of undifferentiated arthritis into RA and progression to erosive disease. Other autoantibodies also have been used in a diagnostic algorithm for patients with very early synovitis (<3 months of symptoms), including RFs, anticitrullinated protein, and anti-RA33.[19] Using stepwise analysis of each antibody, RA could be diagnosed in 72% of patients and confirmed by subsequent clinical course.

UNUSUAL PATTERNS OR VARIANTS OF DISEASE

Palindromic Pattern of Onset

Palindromic rheumatism was described by Hench and Rosenberg in 1942.[20] Pain usually begins in one joint or in periarticular tissues; symptoms worsen for several hours to a few days and are associated with swelling and erythema. Then, in reverse sequence, symptoms resolve, leaving no residua. Table 66-2 lists joints involved in a series of 227 patients. An intercritical period, similar to that of gout, is asymptomatic. Half of patients with palindromic rheumatism go on to develop RA, particularly patients with HLA-DR4. In a compilation of 653 patients from nine series, only 15% became asymptomatic after at least 5 years with a palindromic syndrome (see Table 66-2).[21] In the remainder, multiple joints became involved, swelling did not subside completely between attacks, and tests for RF became positive. Neither the characteristics of joint fluid nor the pathologic findings of synovial biopsy specimens allow the prediction that RA will evolve from palindromic rheumatism,[22] although in the future, it may be worthwhile to measure anti–cyclic citrullinated peptide antibodies in these individuals. Individuals who do not develop RA rarely have constitutional symptoms, and the involved joints have no erosions because the synovitis does not become chronic. Of 51 patients with palindromic rheumatism, 41 experienced marked improvement in frequency and duration of attacks during treatment with antimalarials.[23]

Effect of Age on Onset

Older individuals (≥65 years old) developing RA often present with stiffness, limb girdle pain, and diffuse boggy swelling of the hands, wrists, and forearms. A clinical onset that mimics polymyalgia rheumatica or remitting seronegative synovitis with pitting edema also can occur in the elderly. Individuals with onset at age 60 years or older are less likely to have subcutaneous nodules or RF at the onset of disease, despite the high prevalence of RF in the general population in this age group. Generally, elderly individuals who develop RA tend to have a more benign course than younger patients; there is a lower frequency of positive tests for RF, but there is a strong association with HLA-DR4. The onset is slow, but the stiffness is often incapacitating.

In one study of 186 patients with RA of less than 15 months' duration, older patients had higher scores for joint space narrowing and osteophytes at baseline than patients younger than 55 years. There was no evidence, however, that the older patients had more rapid progression of damage, indicating that the osteoarthritis was responsible for a significant portion of the damage noted at the onset of disease.[24]

Rheumatoid Arthritis and Paralysis: Asymmetric Disease

Being relatively common, RA is likely to occur with many other types of chronic disease. A striking asymmetry or even unilateral involvement has been described in patients with poliomyelitis, meningioma, encephalitis, neurovascular syphilis, strokes, and cerebral palsy.[25] Joints are typically spared on the paralyzed side, and the degree of protection shows a rough correlation with the extent of paralysis. The protective effect on the affected side is less if a neurologic deficit develops in a patient who already has RA.

Arthritis Robustus

Arthritis robustus is not so much an unusual presentation of disease as an unusual reaction of patients to the disease.[26] Most patients are men; their disease is characterized by proliferative synovitis, often with deformity, that seems to cause little pain and even less disability. Patients are athletic and invariably keep working (often at physical labor). Periarticular osteopenia is unusual, whereas new bone proliferation at joint margins near significant erosions of bone and cartilage are common. Bulky subcutaneous nodules develop. Subchondral cysts also develop, presumably from the excessive pressure developed from synovial fluid within a thick joint capsule during muscular effort.

Rheumatoid Nodulosis

Whether rheumatoid nodulosis is a variant subset of RA or a different entity has not been clarified. The clinical picture is of a palindromic set of recurrent pain and swelling in different joints, radiologic subchondral bone cysts, and subcutaneous rheumatoid nodules. In one series of 16 patients followed 12 years, 6 had an aggressive course indistinguishable from classic erosive polyarticular RA. In seven patients, cholesterol crystals were found in fluid from olecranon bursae. Second-line drugs helped articular disease, but not other components of the process.[27]

COURSE AND COMPLICATIONS OF ESTABLISHED RHEUMATOID ARTHRITIS

INVOLVEMENT OF SPECIFIC JOINTS: EFFECTS OF DISEASE ON FORM AND FUNCTION

The effects of rheumatoid synovitis on joints are a complex function of the intensity of the underlying disease, its chronicity, and the stress put on individual joints by the patient. Most well-documented observations of specific joint involvement and of complications of the disease were reported in the decades before 1980. Since then, there have been refinements on these observations, but few new data.

Despite advances in understanding the pathophysiology of RA, including delineations of the cellular and enzymatic pathways that destroy joints, guidelines for the practicing physician—so that in an individual patient the probability that he or she would go on to develop erosive disease and needs aggressive treatment can be determined—are only in early stages of development. The spectrum of the clinical course of RA can range from patients who have mild pauciarticular synovitis, negative serum RF, with few radiographic changes, to patients who have unrelenting pain, synovitis, joint damage, and extra-articular manifestations.

Cervical Spine

In contrast to other nonsynovial joints, such as the manubriosternal joint or symphysis pubis, the diskovertebral joints in the cervical spine often manifest osteochondral destruction in RA and on lateral radiographs may be found to be narrowed (Fig. 66-1). There is significant pain, but passive range of motion in the absence of muscle spasm may be normal. There are at least two possible mechanisms for this process: (1) extension of the inflammatory process from adjacent neurocentral joints (the joints of Luschka), which are lined by synovium, into the diskovertebral area, and (2) chronic cervical instability initiated by apophyseal joint destruction leading to vertebral malalignment or subluxation. This process may produce microfractures of the vertebral end plates, disk herniation, and degeneration of disk cartilage. The atlantoaxial joint is prone to subluxation in several directions, as follows:

1. The atlas can move anteriorly on the axis (most common). This results from laxity of the ligaments induced by proliferative synovial tissue developing in adjacent synovial bursae or from fracture or erosion of the odontoid process.
2. The atlas can move posteriorly on the axis. This can occur only if the odontoid peg has been fractured from the axis or destroyed.
3. The atlas can sublux vertically in relation to the axis (least common). This results from destruction of the lateral atlantoaxial joints or of bone around the foramen magnum. It is apparent now that vertical (superior) migration of the odontoid can develop from unattended anterior or posterior subluxation.

The earliest and most common symptom of cervical subluxation is pain radiating up into the occiput. Two other serious, but less common, clinical patterns are as follows:

1. Slowly progressive spastic quadriparesis, frequently with painless sensory loss in the hands
2. Transient episodes of medullary dysfunction associated with vertical penetration of the dens and probable vertebral artery compression; paresthesias in the shoulders or arms may occur during movement of the head

Physical findings suggestive of atlantoaxial subluxation include a loss of occipitocervical lordosis, resistance to passive spine motion, and abnormal protrusion of the axial arch felt by the examining finger on the posterior pharyngeal wall. Radiographic views (lateral, with the neck in flexion) reveal more than 3 mm of separation between the odontoid peg and the axial arch. In symptomatic patients, the films in flexion should be taken only after radiographs (including an

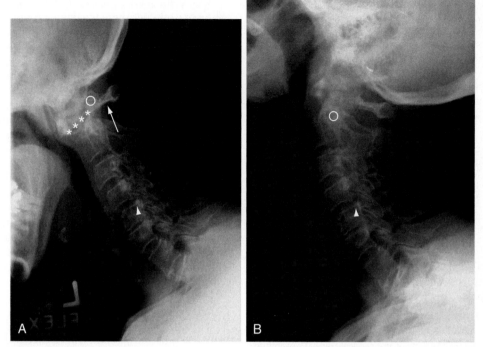

Figure 66-1   Rheumatoid arthritis of the cervical spine. **A,** Lateral radiograph in flexion shows severe anterior atlantoaxial subluxation with a wide anterior atlantodental interval *(asterisks)* and decreased posterior atlantodental interval *(arrow).* **B,** Almost complete reduction of subluxation is noted on the lateral view in extension. There also is subaxial subluxation at the level of C4-C5 *(arrowheads)* with erosive changes in various facet joints. O, odontoid. *(Courtesy of Dr. Barbara Weissman.)*

open-mouth posteroanterior view) have ruled out an odontoid fracture or severe atlantoaxial subluxation. Studies have indicated that computed tomography (CT) is useful for showing spinal cord compression by a loss of posterior subarachnoid space in patients with C1 to C2 subluxation. Magnetic resonance imaging (MRI) has proved particularly valuable in determining pathologic anatomy in this syndrome (Fig. 66-2).

Neurologic symptoms often have little relationship to the degree of subluxation and may be related to individual variations in the diameter of the spinal canal. Symptoms of spinal cord compression that demand intervention include the following:

- A sensation of the head falling forward on flexion of the cervical spine
- Altered consciousness
- Syncope
- A loss of sphincter control
- Dysphagia, vertigo, convulsions, hemiplegia, dysarthria, or nystagmus
- Peripheral paresthesias without evidence of peripheral nerve disease or compression

Some of these symptoms may be related to compression of the vertebral arteries, which must wind through foramina in the transverse processes of C1 and C2, rather than to compression of the spinal cord.

The progression of peripheral joint erosions parallels cervical spine disease in RA. The two coincide in severity and timing; the development of cervical subluxation is more likely in patients with erosion of the hands and feet. In a series of 113 patients with RA referred for hip or knee arthroplasty, 61% had radiographic evidence of cervical spine instability.[28]

Is mortality increased in patients with atlantoaxial subluxation? Neurologic signs do not inevitably develop in patients with large subluxations. When signs of cervical cord compression do appear, however, myelopathy progresses rapidly, and 50% of these patients die within 1 year.[29] These patients are at risk from small falls, whiplash injuries, and general anesthesia with intubation. Cervical collars should be prescribed for stability. Operative stabilization may be considered if symptoms are progressive.

Some data support the hypothesis that early C1-to-C2 fusion for atlantoaxial subluxation before the development of superior migration of the odontoid decreases the risk of further progression of cervical spine instability.[30] The incidence of sustained neurologic deterioration related to surgery may be 6%, however, and this emphasizes the importance of a skilled surgical team and the careful assessment of each patient. In many cases, surgical intervention in asymptomatic patients is riskier than conservative management despite the dire appearance of imaging studies.

Vertical atlantoaxial subluxation is important and may follow anterior or posterior subluxation. Symptoms associated with this collapse of the lateral support system of the atlas occur in patients with severe erosive disease. Neurologic findings include decreased sensation in the distribution of cranial nerve V, sensory loss in the C2 area, nystagmus, and pyramidal lesions.

Thoracic, Lumbar, and Sacral Spine

The thoracic, lumbar, and sacral portions of the spine are usually spared in RA. The exceptions are the apophyseal joints; rarely, synovial cysts at the apophyseal joint can

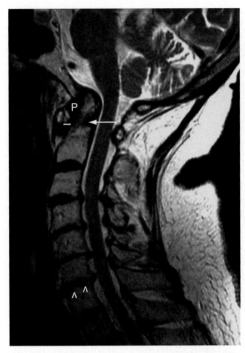

Figure 66-2 Rheumatoid arthritis of the cervical spine. T2-weighted sagittal image shows low signal periodontoid pannus (P). Odontoid process appears irregular secondary to erosions *(arrow)*. The atlantodental distance shows mild widening *(solid line)*. There also is vertical subluxation without signs of cord compression. Anterior subarachnoid space is compromised by disk protrusions at multiple levels. Erosions *(arrowheads)* are seen at the vertebral end plates at the C6-C7 level. *(Courtesy of Dr. Barbara Weissman.)*

impinge as an epidural mass on the spinal cord, causing pain, neurologic deficits, or both.

Temporomandibular Joint

The temporomandibular joint is commonly involved in RA. Histories reveal that 55% of patients have jaw symptoms at some time during the course of their disease. Radiographic examination reveals structural alterations in 78% of the joints examined. An overbite may develop as the mandibular condyle and the corresponding surface of the temporal bone, the eminentia articularis, are eroded. Physical examination of the rheumatoid patient should include palpation of the temporomandibular joint for tenderness and auscultation for crepitus. Occasionally, patients have acute pain and an inability to close the mouth, necessitating intra-articular glucocorticoid therapy to suppress the acute process.

Temporomandibular joint abnormalities are common in nonrheumatoid populations. The only specific findings for RA in the temporomandibular joint are erosions and cysts of the mandibular condyle detected by CT or MRI. There is no correlation between clinical and CT findings of the temporomandibular joint in RA.[31]

Cricoarytenoid Joints

The cricoarytenoid joints are small diarthrodial joints with an important function: They rotate with the vocal cords as the vocal cords abduct and adduct to vary the pitch and tone of the voice. Careful histories may reveal hoarseness

in 30% of rheumatoid patients. This hoarseness is not disabling in itself, but there is a danger that the cricoarytenoid joints may become inflamed and immobilized, with the vocal cords adducted to the midline, causing inspiratory stridor. Autopsy examinations have shown cricoarytenoid arthritis in almost half of the patients with RA, suggesting that much significant disease of the larynx may be asymptomatic. This suggestion is borne out by the finding that although CT scans detected laryngeal abnormalities in 54% of patients with moderately severe RA, no symptoms suggested that these abnormalities would be found.[32] In contrast, findings with indirect laryngoscopy, which detected mucosal and gross functional abnormalities (including rheumatoid nodules), were abnormal in 32% of the same patients and correlated with symptoms of sore throat and difficult inspiration. It follows that the latter examination should be obtained in symptomatic rheumatoid patients. Asymptomatic cricoarytenoid synovitis occasionally may lead to aspiration of pharyngeal contents, particularly at night.

Ossicles of the Ear

Many rheumatoid patients experience a decrease in hearing as a result of conductive hearing loss. Studies using otoadmittance measurements have been done in patients with RA in an attempt to determine whether the interossicle joints were involved.[33] The data showed that 38% of "rheumatoid ears" and only 8% of controls had a pattern characteristic of increased flaccidity of a clinically normal tympanic membrane. This finding is consistent with erosions and shortening of the ossicles produced by the erosive synovitis, not with ankylosis.

Sternoclavicular and Manubriosternal Joints

Sternoclavicular and manubriosternal joints, both possessing synovium and a large cartilaginous disk, are often involved in RA. Because of their relative immobility, there are few symptoms. Patients occasionally complain of experiencing pain in sternoclavicular joints, however, while lying on their sides in bed. When symptoms do occur, the physician must be concerned about superimposed sepsis. CT or MRI is useful for careful delineation of the sternoclavicular joint. Manubriosternal involvement is almost never clinically important, although by tomographic criteria it is common in RA.

Shoulder

RA of the shoulder not only affects synovium within the glenohumeral joint, but also involves the distal third of the clavicle, various bursae and the rotator cuff, and multiple muscles around the neck and chest wall. Severe shoulder pain is often bilateral and can lead to sleep disorders because of difficulty finding a comfortable position. Involvement of the rotator cuff in RA also has been recognized as a principal cause of morbidity. The function of the rotator cuff is to stabilize the humeral head in the glenoid. Weakness of the cuff results in superior subluxation. Rotator cuff tears or insufficiency from other causes can be shown by shoulder arthrography or MRI. In a series of 200 consecutive patients

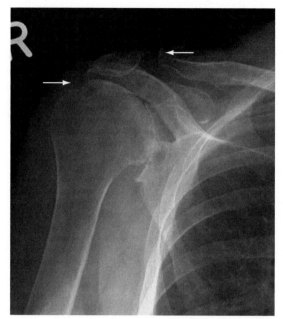

Figure 66-3 Abnormalities of the shoulder in rheumatoid arthritis. The Grashey posterior oblique view of a shoulder shows severe glenohumeral joint space narrowing with a marginal erosion and cystic change of the humeral head adjacent to the greater tuberosity *(lower arrow)*. Elevation of the humeral head with respect to the glenoid indicates chronic rotator cuff tear. There also is tapering of the distal end of the clavicle and widening of the acromioclavicular joint *(upper arrow)*. *(Courtesy of Dr. Barbara Weissman.)*

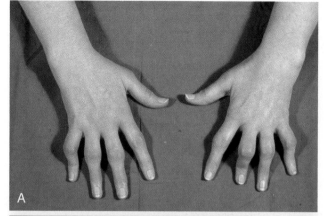

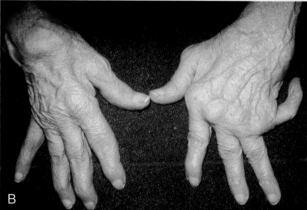

Figure 66-4 **A,** Polyarticular arthritis, especially with fusiform swelling of the proximal interphalangeal joints. Note deformity of wrists with radial deviation. **B,** Complete subluxation with marked ulnar deviation at the metacarpophalangeal joints in a patient with rheumatoid arthritis. The heads of the metacarpals are now in direct contact with the joint capsule instead of the proximal phalanges. *(Courtesy of Iain McInnes, MD.)*

with RA studied by arthrography, 21% had rotator cuff tears, and an additional 24% had evidence of frayed tendons.[34] One likely mechanism behind tears is that the rotator cuff tendon insertion into the greater tuberosity is vulnerable to erosion by the proliferative synovitis that develops there. Previous injury and aging may predispose to the development of tears. Sudden tears may be accompanied by pain and inflammation so great as to suggest sepsis.

Standard radiographic examinations of the shoulder in RA reveal erosions and superior subluxation (Fig. 66-3). Arthrograms, in addition to showing tears of the rotator cuff, can show diffuse nodular filling defects, irregular capsular attachment, bursal filling defects, adhesive capsulitis, and dilation of the biceps tendon sheath (perhaps unique to RA).[35] High-resolution CT or MRI may provide much of this information without invasive techniques.

Marked soft tissue swelling of the anterolateral aspect of the shoulders in RA may be caused by chronic subacromial bursitis rather than by glenohumeral joint effusions. In contrast to rotator cuff tears, bursal swelling is not associated with a decreased range of motion or pain. Synovial proliferation within the subdeltoid bursa may explain the resorption of the undersurface of the distal clavicle seen in this disease. Rarely, the shoulder joint may rupture, with symptoms resembling those of obstruction of venous return from the arm.

Elbow

RA rarely manifests with severe pain in the elbow, perhaps because the elbow is a stable hinge joint. Nevertheless, involvement of the elbow is common, and if lateral stability

at the elbow is lost as the disease progresses, disability can be severe.

The frequency of elbow involvement varies from 20% to 65%, depending on the severity of disease in the patient populations studied. One of the earliest findings, often unnoticed by the patient, is a loss of full extension. Because the elbow is principally a connecting joint between the hand and the trunk, the shoulder and wrists can compensate partially for the loss of elbow motion.

Hand and Wrist

The hand and wrist should be considered together because they form a functional unit. There are data linking disease of the wrist to ulnar deviation of the MCP joints.[36] The hypothesis is that weakening of the extensor carpi ulnaris muscle leads to radial deviation of the wrist as the carpal bones rotate (the proximal row in an ulnar direction and the distal ones in a radial direction). In response to this, ulnar deviation of the fingers (a "zigzag" deformity) occurs to keep the tendons to the phalanges in a normal line with the radius. Other factors, including the tendency for a power grasp to pull the fingers into an ulnar attitude and inappropriate intrinsic muscle action, are involved (Fig. 66-4). Erosion of bone or articular cartilage is

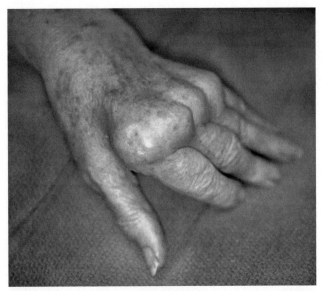

Figure 66-5 Ulnar deviation and subluxation. The hands show typical manifestations of end-stage erosive changes around the metacarpophalangeal joints, with volar dislocation and ulnar drift of the fingers. *(Copyright A.L. Ladd.)*

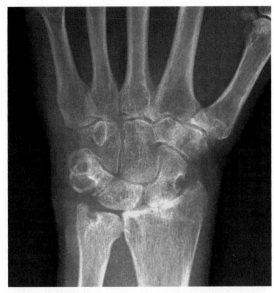

Figure 66-6 Typical sites of osseous erosion of a rheumatoid wrist shown here include triquetrum, pisiform, scaphoid, and radius. There also are erosions at the ulnar aspect of the distal radius and the distal ulnar styloid process secondary to involvement of the inferior radioulnar compartment. Diffuse cartilage loss also is evident in the radiocarpal compartment. *(Courtesy of Dr. Barbara Weissman.)*

not essential for the development of ulnar deviation (Fig. 66-5). Significant, although reducible, ulnar deviation can result from repeated synovitis or muscle weakness in the hands (e.g., in systemic lupus erythematosus [SLE] and Parkinson's disease).

Dorsal swelling on the wrist within the tendon sheaths of the extensor muscles is one of the earliest signs of disease. Typically, the extensor carpi ulnaris and extensor digitorum communis sheaths are involved. Rarely, cystic structures resembling ganglia are early findings of RA.

As the synovial proliferation develops within the wrist, pressure increases within the relatively nondistensible joint spaces. Proliferative synovium develops enzymatic machinery sufficient to destroy ligaments, tendons, and the articular disk distal to the ulnar head. Pressure and enzymes combine to produce communications among radiocarpal, radioulnar, and midcarpal joints. Integrity of the distal radioulnar joint is lost. The ulnar collateral ligament, stretched by the proliferative synovium of the radioulnar joint, finally either ruptures or is destroyed, and the ulnar head springs up into dorsal prominence, where it "floats" and is easily depressed by the examiner's fingers.

On the volar side of the wrist, synovial protrusion cysts develop; they can be palpated, and their origins can be confirmed by arthrography. The thick transverse carpal ligament provides significant resistance to decompression, however, and the hyperplastic synovium can compress the median nerve and cause carpal tunnel syndrome, often bilaterally.

Progression of disease in the wrist is characterized either by loss of joint space and bone or by ankylosis (Fig. 66-6). Disintegration of the carpus has been quantified in terms of a carpal-to-metacarpal ratio (the length of the carpus divided by the length of the third metacarpal). There is a linear decrease in the carpal-to-metacarpal ratio with progressive disease.[37] This decrease is caused by compaction of bone at the radiolunate, lunate-capitate, and capitate–

third metacarpal joints, which usually accompanies severe disease. Early detection of carpal bone involvement by RA is possible using MRI, which reveals early synovial proliferation and carpal bone erosions. Bony ankylosis is associated with the duration and the severity of disease and is found in joints that have been immobilized by pain, inflammation, treatment, or all of these.

The hand may have many joints involved in RA. A sensitive index of hand involvement is grip strength. The act of squeezing puts stress on all hand joints. Muscular contraction causes ligamentous tightening around joints, compressing inflamed synovium. The immediate result is weakness, with or without pain; the reflex inhibition of muscular contraction owing to pain may be a primary factor in this weakness. Quantitative radiographic scores for joint space narrowing, erosion, and malalignment correlate well with loss of motion, but do not correlate with joint count tenderness scores[38]; these data support the concept that inflammatory synovitis and the erosive-destructive potential of proliferative synovitis in RA are not one and the same, but rather reflect different aspects of the same disease.

The swan neck deformity is one of flexion of the distal interphalangeal (DIP) and MCP joints with hyperextension of the PIP joint. The lesion probably begins with shortening of the interosseous muscles and tendons. Shortening of the intrinsic muscles exerts tension on the dorsal tendon sheath, leading to hyperextension of the PIP joint (Fig. 66-7A).[39] Deep tendon contracture or, rarely, DIP joint involvement with RA leads to the DIP joint flexion. Marginal erosive changes in the DIP joints occur more often in patients with RA who have coexisting osteoarthritis.[40]

If, during chronic inflammation of a PIP joint, the extensor hood stretches or is avulsed, the joint may pop up in flexion, producing a boutonnière deformity (Fig. 66-7B). The DIP joint remains in hyperextension.

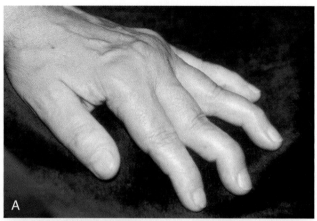
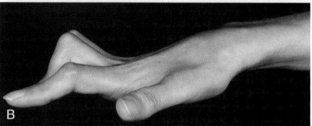

Figure 66-7 **A,** Swan neck deformity. This common deformity leads to hyperextension of the proximal interphalangeal joints and flexion of the distal interphalangeal joints. **B,** Boutonnière deformity. This deformity, which is the opposite of swan neck deformity, is marked by flexion of the proximal interphalangeal joints and extension of the distal interphalangeal joints. *(Courtesy of Iain McInnes, MD.)*

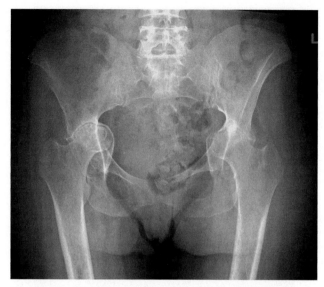

Figure 66-8 Bilateral protrusio acetabuli in rheumatoid arthritis. The medial acetabular margins protrude into the pelvis. There is severe accompanying cartilage loss. *(Courtesy of Dr. Barbara Weissman.)*

The most serious result of rheumatoid involvement of the hand is resorptive arthropathy owing to severe resorption of bone that begins at the articular cartilage and spreads along the diaphysis of the involved phalanges. Digits appear shortened, excess skin folds are present, and phalanges can be retracted (telescoped) into one another and then pulled out into abnormally long extension, often without pain. With the availability of more effective therapy for RA, resorptive arthropathy has become rare.

Three types of deformity have been described for the thumb, as follows:

Type I: MCP inflammation leads to stretching of the joint capsule and a boutonnière-like deformity.

Type II:Inflammation of the carpometacarpal joint leads to volar subluxation during contracture of the adductor hallucis.

Type III:After prolonged disease of both MCP joints, exaggerated adduction of the first metacarpus, flexion of the MCP joint, and hyperextension of the DIP joint result from the patient's need to provide a means to pinch.

One of the most common manifestations of RA in the hands is tenosynovitis in flexor tendon sheaths, and this can be a major cause of hand weakness.[41] Tenosynovitis manifests on the volar surfaces of the phalanges as diffuse swelling between joints or a palpable grating within flexor tendon sheaths in the palm and may occur in half of RA patients.

It is particularly important to diagnose de Quervain's tenosynovitis because it causes severe discomfort and yet is easily treated. de Quervain's tenosynovitis is tenosynovitis in the extensors of the thumb. Pain originating from these sheaths can be shown by Finkelstein's test—ulnar flexion at the wrist after the thumb is maximally flexed and adducted.

Frequently, rheumatoid nodules or less well-differentiated fibrin deposits develop within tendon sheaths and may "lock" the finger painfully into fixed flexion. When they are chronic and recurrent, it may be necessary to inject the tendon sheath or, if that fails, remove it surgically.

Hip

The hip is less frequently involved early in RA than in juvenile RA. Hip joint involvement must be ascertained by a careful clinical examination; symptoms of hip synovitis are pain in the lower buttock or groin. Pain on the lateral aspect of the hip is often a manifestation of trochanteric bursitis rather than synovitis.

About half of patients with well-established RA have radiographic evidence of hip disease. In contrast to osteoarthritis, in which the femoral head usually migrates superiorly, symmetric thinning of the cartilage in RA leads to axial migration. The femoral head may collapse and be resorbed, and the acetabulum is remodeled and pushed medially, leading to protrusio acetabuli (Fig. 66-8). Significant protrusion occurs in about 5% of all patients with RA.[42] Loss of internal rotation on physical examination correlates best with radiographic findings. Similar to the situation in other weight-bearing joints, the femoral head may develop cystic lesions that communicate with the joint space.

Knees

In contrast to the hips, synovial inflammation and proliferation in the knees are readily shown on physical examination. Early in knee disease, often within 1 week after the onset of symptoms, quadriceps atrophy is noticeable and leads to the application of more force than usual through the patella to the femoral surface. Another early

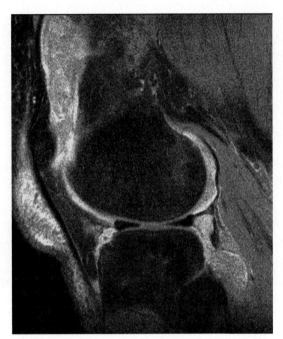

Figure 66-9 MRI of the knee in rheumatoid arthritis. Sagittal fast spin echo T2-weighted (TR 3625/TE 133) fat suppressed image allows excellent contrast. Synovial fluid is shown in white and shows a posterior fluid collection. *(Courtesy of Dr. Barbara Weissman.)*

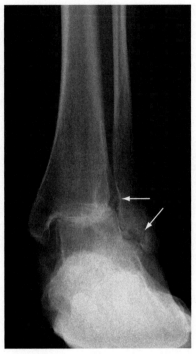

Figure 66-10 Rheumatoid arthritis of the ankle. There is diffuse loss of cartilage space with erosions of the fibula *(arrows)*. The scalloping along the medial border of the distal fibula is designated the fibular notch sign and is a characteristic finding in rheumatoid arthritis. The hindfoot is in valgus alignment.

manifestation of knee disease in RA is a loss of full extension, a functional loss that can become a fixed flexion contracture unless corrective measures are undertaken.

Some patients have a genu varum or valgus that precedes the onset of RA owing to preexisting osteoarthritis. In these individuals, the medial or lateral compartment bears the most stress from the malalignment that is first symptomatic and is likely to have radiographic evidence of erosion of bone and thinning of cartilage.

Flexion of the knee that has a moderate to large effusion markedly increases the intra-articular pressure. This increased intra-articular pressure may cause an outpouching of posterior components of the joint, producing a popliteal or Baker's cyst. Jayson and Dixon[43] have shown that fluid from the anterior compartments of the knee may enter a popliteal cyst, but does not readily return. This one-way valve may generate pressures so high in the popliteal space that it may rupture down into the calf or, less often, superiorly into the posterior thigh. Rupture occurs posteriorly between the medial head of the gastrocnemius and the tendinous insertion of the biceps. Clinically, popliteal cysts and their complications have several manifestations. An intact popliteal cyst may compress superficial venous flow to the upper part of the leg, producing dilation of superficial veins, edema, or both.[44] Rupture of the joint posteriorly with dissection of joint fluid into the calf may resemble acute thrombophlebitis with swelling and tenderness and produce systemic signs of fever with leukocytosis. One helpful sign in identifying joint rupture may be the appearance of a crescentic hematoma beneath one of the malleoli of the ankle.[45] Although arthrography clearly defines the abnormal anatomy of a Baker's cyst, this invasive procedure has been replaced by ultrasonography and, when necessary, MRI (Fig. 66-9).

Ankle and Foot

The ankle involvement is usually mild in RA, but damage can occur in severe progressive forms of the disease. Clinical evidence for ankle involvement is a cystic swelling anterior and posterior to the malleoli. Much of the stability of the ankle depends on the integrity of the ligaments holding the fibula to the tibia and these two bones to the talus. In RA, inflammatory and proliferative disease may loosen these connections by stretching and eroding the collagenous ligaments and cause erosions (Fig. 66-10). The result is incongruity, which progresses to pronation deformities and eversion of the foot.

The Achilles tendon is a major structural component and kinetic force in the foot and ankle. Rheumatoid nodules develop in this collagenous structure, and spontaneous rupture of the tendon has been reported when diffuse granulomatous inflammation is present.[46] The subtalar joint controls eversion and inversion of the foot on the talus; patients with RA invariably have more pain while walking on uneven ground, and this is related to the relatively common subtalar joint involvement in RA. Progressive eversion at the subtalar joint, combined with foot pain, leads also to a lateral subluxation beginning in the midfoot and the development of a rocker-bottom deformity. Midfoot disease leads to collapse of the arch, which contributes to difficulty walking because of pain.

More than one third of patients with RA have significant disease in the feet (Fig. 66-11). Metatarsophalangeal (MTP) joints are often involved, and gait is altered as pain develops during push-off in striding. Downward subluxation of the metatarsal heads occurs soon after the MTP joints become involved, producing "cock-up" toe deformities of

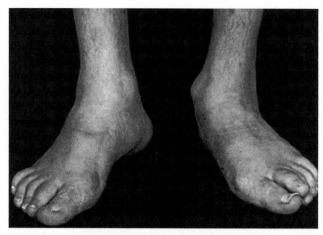

Figure 66-11 Valgus of ankle, pes planus, and forefoot varus deformity of the left foot related to painful synovitis of the ankle, forefoot, and metatarsophalangeal joint in a 24-year-old man with severe rheumatoid arthritis.

the PIP joints. Hallux valgus and bunion or callus formation occur if disease continues. Cystic collections representing outpouchings of flexor tendon sheaths often develop under the MTP joints.[47] Patients with subluxation of metatarsal heads can develop pressure necrosis of the plantar surfaces. Alternatively, patients who have subluxation of MTP joints often develop ulceration over the PIP joints that protrude dorsally (hammer toes). The net result is increased pressure on the MTPs with a sensation described as "walking on marbles" by many patients. The sequence of changes as disease progresses in the foot is as follows:[48]

1. Intermetatarsal joint ligaments stretch in response to inflammation.
2. Spread of the forefoot occurs.
3. The fibrofatty cushion on the plantar surface migrates anteriorly.
4. Subluxation of toes occurs dorsally, and extensor tendons shorten.
5. Subluxation of metatarsal heads to a subcutaneous site on the plantar surface develops.
6. Concurrently, a hallux valgus results in "stacking" of the second and third toes on top of the great toe.

DIP joints of the foot are rarely affected in RA, but a functional rigid hallux caused by muscle spasm of the great toe intrinsic muscles in an effort to relieve pressure on the lesser metatarsal heads can be extremely painful and require surgical intervention. Another cause of foot pain in rheumatoid patients is the tarsal tunnel syndrome. In a group of 30 patients with RA, erosions in the feet shown on radiographs, and foot pain, 4 (13%) were shown by electrodiagnostic techniques to have slowing of medial or lateral plantar nerve latency, or both.

Extra-articular Complications of Rheumatoid Arthritis

Generally, the number and severity of extra-articular features vary with the duration and severity of the disease. Several of these features may be related to extra-articular foci of an immune response,[49] based on evidence of independent and qualitatively different production of RF in the pleural space, pericardium, muscle, and even meninges.

These patients with systemic immune responses have true rheumatoid disease, not just RA. Other unusual proteins and protein complexes in the circulation of patients with active rheumatoid disease include antiphospholipid antibodies, circulating immune complexes, and cryoglobulins. Extra-articular manifestations of RA are associated with excess mortality.[50]

SKELETON

The skeleton has two anatomically and functionally separate components, cortical and trabecular bone, which respond differently to systemic and local diseases and to drugs. RA can be associated with generalized osteopenia and osteoporosis owing to the effects of drugs (especially corticosteroids); cytokine-induced and RANKL-induced activation of osteoclasts; and the fact that certain groups of patients with the disease, especially postmenopausal women, have other risk factors that enhance the potential for bone loss. The risk of hip fracture and vertebral compression fracture can be quite high. Bone densitometry should be performed routinely in patients with RA, and treatment with bisphosphonates should be considered as an adjunct to therapy.

Because postmenopausal women are more at risk for RA and for osteoporosis, this group should be treated aggressively. At least one study indicates that adequate management of patients with RA that addresses RA and osteoporosis can protect against bone loss.[51] Minimizing steroid use is one method to decrease the risk of osteoporosis in this group and other patients with RA. There seems to be a two-phase loss of bone induced by glucocorticoids: a rapid first phase when 12% of bone mass disappears in the first 6 to 12 months of therapy, followed by a subsequent chronic phase that has a slower rate of bone loss.[52] It is encouraging, however, that the axial bone loss in patients with RA induced early by glucocorticoids can be reversed.[53] The evaluation, biology, and management of osteoporosis is discussed in Chapter 92. Although the focus on the relationship between RA and bone is, appropriately, on osteoporosis, the diffuse loss of bone in RA, whether or not it is related to glucocorticoid therapy, leads to the high incidence of stress fractures of long bones in RA.[54] The fibula is the most common fracture site. Acute leg pain in a thin, elderly rheumatoid patient, even without a history of trauma, should generate suspicion of a stress fracture. Geodes (i.e., subchondral cysts developed by synovial penetration of the cortex or subchondral plate and subsequent proliferation) weaken bone and can predispose bone to fracture.

MUSCLE

Clinical weakness is common in RA, but is it caused by muscle involvement in the rheumatoid inflammation, or is it a reflex weakness response to pain? Most rheumatoid patients have muscle weakness, but few have muscle tenderness or elevated muscle enzymes in the blood.

In an early autopsy series, focal accumulations of lymphocytes and plasma cells with some contiguous degeneration of muscle fibers were found in all rheumatoid patients, a condition termed *nodular myositis*. More recent studies have pointed to at least five different types of muscle disease in RA, although clinically relevant active myositis is uncommon[55]:

1. Diminution of muscle bulk with atrophy of type II fibers
2. Peripheral neuromyopathy, usually due to a mononeuritis multiplex
3. Steroid myopathy
4. Active myositis and muscle necrosis with foci of endomysial mononuclear cell infiltration
5. Chronic myopathy resembling a dystrophic process, probably the end stage of inflammatory myositis

In biopsy specimens, atrophy of type II fibers is most common. Evidence of myositis and focal necrosis is found occasionally on biopsy specimens of patients with active disease, particularly in a subset with mild synovitis and a disproportionately high erythrocyte sedimentation rate (ESR). In some patients, the lymphocytes in muscle synthesize IgM RF, emphasizing the systemic nature of RA. The patchy "nodules of myositis" contain plasma cells and lymphocytes.

SKIN

The most frequently recognized skin lesion in RA is the rheumatoid nodule (discussed subsequently in a separate section), but there are several other manifestations as well. "Senile" purpura resulting from skin atrophy and capillary fragility is especially common in patients treated with glucocorticoids. Palmar erythema is common, but Raynaud's syndrome is rare. Manifestations of vasculitis range from occasional nail fold infarcts to a deep, erosive, scarring pyoderma gangrenosum. Palpable purpura in rheumatoid patients is often related to a reaction to a drug that the patient is taking, but can be primary and a direct function of the severity of articular disease. Livedo reticularis, the lacy, dusky purple, asymptomatic discoloration seen on the extremities, is believed to signify a deep dermal vasculopathy. It can be present in any or all diffuse connective tissue diseases and is associated often with antiphospholipid antibodies in the circulation.[56]

EYE

Virtually all ocular manifestations of RA can be considered complications of the disease (see Chapter 46). Keratoconjunctivitis sicca is a component of Sjögren's syndrome and is discussed in Chapter 69. More directly related to the rheumatoid process and seen in the synovium and within rheumatoid nodules are scleritis and episcleritis. The highly differentiated connective tissues in the eye make rheumatoid manifestations particularly interesting and, when they occur in aggressive form, very serious.

The episclera of the eye is highly vascular compared with the dense sclera. Scleritis, episcleritis, or both occur in less than 1% of rheumatoid patients. In episcleritis, the eye becomes red and, in contrast to conjunctivitis, results in no discharge other than tearing in response to the gritty discomfort. Loss of vision does not occur as a direct result of the episcleritis, but a keratitis or cataract developing secondarily can cause visual loss. Scleritis causes severe ocular pain and a dark red discoloration (Fig. 66-12C). No discharge is present. Depending on the intensity of the process, scleritis can be localized and superficial or generalized, with or without granulomatous resorption of the sclera down to the uveal layer; when this complication occurs, it is termed

scleromalacia perforans. In contrast to superficial eye disease, which usually can be treated conservatively with topical steroids, scleritis usually requires systemic or intraocular corticosteroid treatment. In some cases, the sclera can become thin even in the absence of overt inflammation and lead to scleromalacia (Fig. 66-12D). Rarely, perilimbic ischemic ulcers can be caused by cryoproteins (RF-IgG complexes) and if untreated can result in perforation of the anterior chamber. Patients with RA who have an associated keratoconjunctivitis sicca secondary to Sjögren's syndrome have pruritic and painful eyes, sometimes leading to chronic blepharitis.

RHEUMATOID NODULES

The mature rheumatoid nodule has a central area of necrosis rimmed by a corona of palisading fibroblasts that is surrounded in turn by a collagenous capsule with perivascular collections of chronic inflammatory cells. The earliest nodules, nests of granulation tissue, have been identified at a size of less than 4 mm. The nodules grow by accumulating cells that expand centrifugally, leaving behind central necrosis initiated by vasculopathy and compounded by protease destruction of the connective tissue matrix. Occurring in 15% to 20% of patients with definite or classic RA, nodules are found most often on extensor surfaces or pressure points, such as the olecranon process and the proximal ulna (Fig. 66-12A). They are subcutaneous and vary in consistency from a soft, amorphous, entirely mobile mass to a hard, rubbery mass attached firmly to the periosteum.

The appearance of nodules in unusual sites may lead to confusion in diagnosis, and they can sometimes appear identical to other types of nodules such as tophi. Sacral nodules may be mistaken for bedsores if the overlying skin breaks down. Occipital nodules also occur in bedridden patients. In the larynx, rheumatoid nodules on the vocal cords may cause progressive hoarseness. Nodules found in the heart and lungs are discussed later. Nodules on the sclera can produce perforation of this collagenous tissue. There have been multiple reports of rheumatoid nodule formation within the central nervous system, involving leptomeninges more than parenchyma.[57] Some patients develop rheumatoid nodules within vertebral bodies, resulting in bone destruction and signs of myelopathy.

Careful histologic study of early lesions[58] suggests that development of the nodule is mediated through affected small arterioles and resulting complement activation and terminal vasculitis. This immunologic response is linked to proliferation of resident histiocytes and fibroblasts and to an influx of macrophages from the circulation. The proliferation of cells and the supporting scaffold of connective tissue is mediated by cytokines expressed in patterns similar to those found in rheumatoid synovium. Data from studies using monoclonal antibodies against receptors for complement C3b and C3bi, monocytes, activated macrophages, and HLA-DR molecules suggest that mononuclear phagocytes are constantly being recruited into the peripheral layers and subsequently migrate into the palisade to constitute most of the cell population in this area.[59] Other studies, using cytochemical markers (nonspecific esterase and CD68—a protein associated with lysosomes—for macrophages, and prolyl hydroxylase for fibroblasts), indicate that a mixture of macrophages and nonsynoviocyte fibroblasts make up the cellular content of nodules.[60] This evidence fits with data

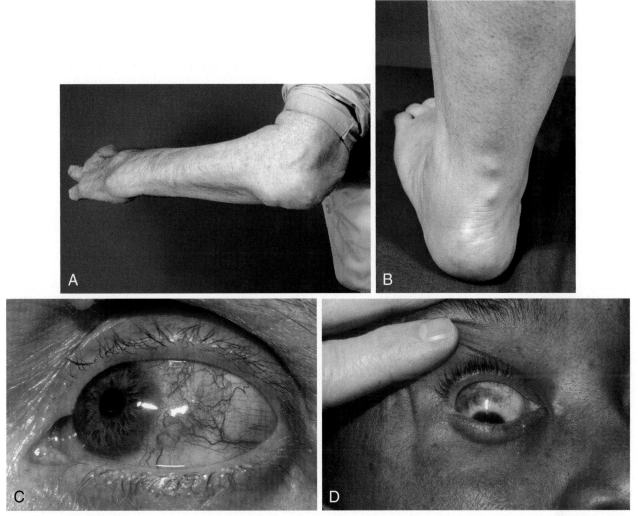

Figure 66-12 **A-D,** Manifestations of increased reactivity of mesenchymal tissue in rheumatoid arthritis include nodules on the elbow **(A)** and on the Achilles tendon **(B)**, episcleritis **(C)**, and scleromalacia **(D)**. *(Courtesy of Iain McInnes, MD.)*

from nodule tissue in organ culture; similar to synovial tissue, the cells in the palisading region have the capacity to produce collagenase and proteases in large quantity.[61]

RF is almost always found in the serum of patients with rheumatoid nodules. Rarely, such nodules are present in the absence of obvious arthritis. A condition called rheumatoid nodulosis is characterized by the presence of multiple nodules on the hands, a positive test for RF, episodes of acute intermittent synovitis, and subchondral cystic lesions of small bones of the hands and feet.[62] Many clinicians have noted that during methotrexate therapy that is successful in downregulating synovitis, existing nodules may enlarge, and new ones may develop; the pathophysiology underlying this phenomenon is unknown, although it may relate to the effects of methotrexate or adenosine (see Chapter 56). Discontinuing methotrexate in these patients usually leads to regression of some nodules. Some case reports suggest that tumor necrosis factor (TNF) inhibitors also can be associated with accelerated rheumatoid nodulosis.

The differential diagnosis of rheumatoid nodules includes the following:

1. "Benign" nodules: These usually are found in healthy children without RF or arthritis. They are nontender; appear often on the pretibial regions, feet, and scalp;

increase rapidly in size; and are histologically identical to rheumatoid nodules.
2. Granuloma annulare: These nodules are intracutaneous, but histologically identical to rheumatoid nodules. They resolve slowly and are not associated with other disease.
3. Xanthomatosis: These nodules usually have a yellow tinge, and patients have abnormally high plasma lipoprotein and cholesterol levels. There is no underlying bone involvement.
4. Tophi: These collections of monosodium urate crystals in patients with gout are associated with small, punched-out bone lesions and are found rarely in patients with a normal serum urate concentration. A search for crystals with a polarizing microscope reveals the classic needle-shaped, negatively birefringent crystals.
5. Miscellaneous nodules: The nodules of multicentric reticulohistiocytosis contain large, lipid-filled macrophages. Numerous proliferative disorders that affect cutaneous tissue, including erythema elevatum diutinum, acrodermatitis chronica atrophicans, bejel, yaws, pinta, and leprosy, can resemble rheumatoid nodules. A rheumatoid nodule, particularly when it occurs on the face, may simulate basal cell carcinoma.

FISTULA DEVELOPMENT

Cutaneous sinuses near joints develop rarely in seropositive patients with long-standing disease and positive tests for RF. These fistulas can be either sterile or septic and connect the skin surface with a joint, with a para-articular cyst in bone or soft tissues, or with a bursa. The pathogenesis of fistulas without a septic origin is particularly difficult to understand because the rheumatoid process usually is so clearly centripetal (i.e., progressing toward the center of the joint), rather than centrifugal.

INFECTION

The incidence of infections as a complication of RA has paralleled the use of glucocorticoids, biologics, and immunosuppressive agents. TNF blockers are especially noteworthy because they have been associated with reactivation of tuberculosis and other opportunistic infections such as histoplasmosis. Pulmonary infections, skin sepsis, and pyarthrosis are the most common infection in RA.[63,64] Difficulty in diagnosis is accentuated by the similarity of aggressive RA to infection, particularly in joints; a "pseudoseptic" arthritis in rheumatoid patients, associated with fever, chills, and grossly purulent synovial fluid, can be part of a severe exacerbation of RA and must be distinguished from infection.[65] A retrospective longitudinal cohort study compared the frequency of infections in a population-based incidence cohort of RA patients with that in a group of individuals without RA from the same population; this study looked at more than 7900 to 9100 person-years.[66] There were 609 RA patients and 609 non-RA patients; 73% were women, and the mean age was 58 years. Hazard ratios for RA patients versus controls after adjustment for age, sex, smoking status, leukopenia, corticosteroid use, and diabetes mellitus were as follows:

- Objectively confirmed infections = 1.7:1
- Infections requiring hospitalization = 1.83:1

Bone, joints, skin, respiratory tract, and soft tissues were the organs with highest hazard ratios. In a subsequent study in this cohort, the predictors of infection were shown to be the following:

- Increasing age
- Extra-articular manifestations of RA
- Leukopenia
- Comorbidities, such as chronic lung disease, alcoholism, diabetes mellitus, and the use of glucocorticoids

Traditional disease-modifying antirheumatic drug use generally is not associated with a major increased incidence with infection, although vigilance when using these agents, such as biologics, is essential.[67] Physicians must have a low threshold of concern for infection in rheumatoid patients.

CANCER

There is an increased risk for malignancy in RA patients, with an increased risk for lymphoma in certain patient subsets. Interstitial fibrosis may be a risk factor for lung carcinoma, particularly of the bronchoalveolar variety.[68] One exception is cancer of the gastrointestinal tract, for which there seems to be a reduced risk for RA patients.[69] It is possible that nonsteroidal anti-inflammatory drugs

(NSAIDs) lower the risk of this form of cancer, as supported by evidence that these drugs can diminish the occurrence and numbers of colonic polyps.

RA patients are at a two to three times higher risk of Hodgkin's disease, non-Hodgkin's lymphoma, and leukemia than the normal population; this is independent of immunosuppressive therapy. Of lymphomas arising in RA, about half are low grade, and half are high grade; most of these are B cell lymphomas, although there is no evidence that these originate from clonally proliferated lymphocytes associated with RA. In contrast, although the relative risk for total cancer in patients with Felty's syndrome is only 2, the relative risk for non-Hodgkin's lymphoma in this complication of RA is near 13,[70] similar to that associated with Sjögren's syndrome.

More recent data have raised the possibility that solid tumors also can be increased in patients with RA who have been treated with TNF blockers.[71] Similar data in patients with Wegener's granulomatosis suggest that the combination of etanercept and cyclophosphamide can increase the risk of cancer.[72] Several cohorts evaluating the effect of TNF inhibitors on cancer rates in RA patients suggest, however, that the oncogenic effect, if it exists, is small.

HEMATOLOGIC ABNORMALITIES

Most patients with RA have a mild normocytic normochromic anemia that correlates with ESR elevation and the activity of the disease. Anemia has mixed causes in RA. One deficiency may mask evidence of others. A useful guide is that three quarters of rheumatoid patients with anemia have the anemia of chronic disease, whereas one quarter respond to iron therapy. Patients in both groups may have superimposed vitamin B_{12} or folate deficiencies.[73] The following guidelines may be helpful in diagnosing the cause of anemia in rheumatoid patients:

1. Anemia of chronic disease is associated with significantly higher serum ferritin concentration than is found in isolated iron deficiency.
2. Folate or vitamin B_{12} deficiency or the use of methotrexate can mask iron deficiency, especially in patients taking NSAIDs with chronic gastrointestinal blood loss, by increasing the mean cell volume and mean cell hemoglobin level of erythrocytes.
3. The ESR correlates inversely with hemoglobin levels in RA, as expected in anemia of chronic disease.
4. Erythropoietin levels are higher in patients with iron deficiency anemia compared with patients with anemia of chronic disease; rheumatoid patients also have a diminished response to erythropoietin.[74]

In patients with the anemia of chronic disease, the total erythroid heme turnover is slightly reduced, and ineffective erythropoiesis accounts for a much higher than normal percentage of total heme turnover. In contrast to anemia associated with blood loss, the ineffective erythropoiesis returns to normal in RA if remission can be induced.[75] Red blood cell aplasia, immunologically mediated, is a rare finding in RA. Because erythropoiesis in animals has been shown to be dependent on T lymphocytes, however, it is logical to search for immunologic factors that can induce anemia in RA. Serum from RA patients can profoundly suppress erythroid colony formation,[76] but T lymphocytes from bone

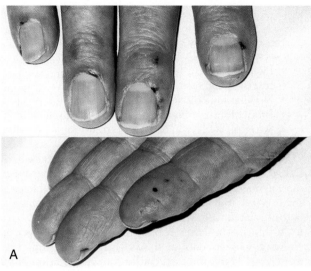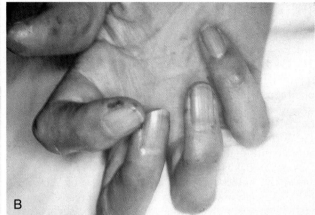

Figure 66-13 **A,** Digital vasculitis in a 65-year-old man with seropositive rheumatoid arthritis. **B,** Nail fold infarcts can occur in patients with rheumatoid arthritis, typically associated with rheumatoid factor positivity and active joint disease. *(A courtesy of Eileen Moynihan, MD.)*

marrow of rheumatoid patients have not been shown to inhibit erythroid development in vitro.

Thrombocytosis is often associated with RA. There is a significant relationship between thrombocytosis and extra-articular manifestations of rheumatoid disease and disease activity.[77] Eosinophilia (5% of total white blood cell count) also was observed in some patients.

A subset of patients with RA has increased numbers of large granular lymphocytes in the peripheral blood, bone marrow, and liver. The lymphocytes contain many azurophilic granules in the cytoplasm and may account for more than 90% of mononuclear cells in blood. They are increased in certain viral infections. The cells are Fc receptor positive, do not produce interleukin (IL)-2, respond poorly to mitogens, and have either antibody-dependent cell-mediated cytotoxicity activity (expressing CD3, CD8, and CD57) or natural killer cells (expressing CD16 and CD56).[78,79] Of previously described patients with large granular lymphocyte proliferation, almost one third have had RA.[80] Because the large granular lymphocyte syndrome in patients with RA has the same HLA-DR4 association seen in Felty's syndrome, the proposal has been made that Felty's syndrome and large granular lymphocyte syndrome represent different variants of a broader syndrome comprising RA, neutropenia, large granular lymphocyte expansions, HLA-DR4 positivity, and variable splenomegaly.[81]

Paraproteinemia, typified by monoclonal gammopathies, has a poor prognostic significance when it appears in rheumatoid patients. This evidence for monoclonal B cell proliferation carries with it a high frequency of malignant transformation to lymphoma or myeloma.[82]

VASCULITIS

The initial pathologic change in RA often includes inflammatory changes in medium and small blood vessels. It is useful, however, to use the term *vasculitis* to group extra-articular complications related not to proliferative granulomas, but rather to inflammatory vascular disease. Systemic rheumatoid vasculitis, one of the most feared complications of RA, has become increasingly uncommon in recent years. This decline in rheumatoid vasculitis likely relates to the marked improvement in therapy resulting from widespread use of methotrexate and the new biologic agents.

Variables associated with the development of rheumatoid vasculitis include the following[83]:
- Male gender
- High titers of RF in serum
- Hypocomplementemia
- Joint erosions
- Subcutaneous nodules and other extra-articular features
- Long-standing disease
- Circulating cryoglobulins

Rheumatoid vasculitis affects a subset of patients with established, often severe, RA with a prevalence of less than 5% of all cases.

Clinical vasculitis usually takes one of the following forms:
- Distal arteritis (including from splinter hemorrhage, nail fold infarcts, and gangrene) (Fig. 66-13)
- Cutaneous ulceration (including pyoderma gangrenosum)
- Peripheral neuropathy (mononeuritis multiplex)
- Arteritis of viscera, including heart, lungs, bowel, kidney, liver, spleen, pancreas, lymph nodes, and testis
- Palpable purpura

The pathologic finding in rheumatoid vasculitis is a panarteritis. All layers of the vessel wall are infiltrated with mononuclear cells. Fibrinoid necrosis is seen in active lesions. Intimal proliferation may predispose to thrombosis. Obliterative endarteritis of the finger is a common manifestation of vasculitis, and immune complex deposits have been shown in the affected vessels.[84] When larger vessels are involved, the pathologic changes resemble those of polyarteritis nodosa. In addition, a venulitis associated with RA has been described.[85] In patients with hypocomplementemia, the cellular infiltrate around the vessels contains neutrophils. In normocomplementemic patients, lymphocytes predominate.

It is unusual for vasculitis to be active in any but the sickest patients, including patients with severe deforming arthritis, extra-articular manifestations, and high RF titers[86]; this subgroup represents less than 1% of patients with RA. Although RA is more common in women than in men, vasculitis is seen more often in men than in women with RA. Supporting the hypothesis that vascular injury is mediated by deposition of circulating immune complexes are (1) depressed levels of C2 and C4; (2) hypercatabolism of C3[87]; (3) deposition of IgG, IgM, and C3 in involved arteries; and (4) the presence of large amounts of cryoimmunoglobulin in the serum of occasional patients with vasculitis.

Neurovascular disease may be the only manifestation of vasculitis. The two common clinical patterns are a mild distal sensory neuropathy and a severe sensorimotor neuropathy (mononeuritis multiplex).[88] The latter form is characterized by severe arterial damage on nerve biopsy specimens. Symptoms of the milder form may be paresthesias or "burning feet" in association with decreased touch and pin sensation distally. Patients with mononeuritis multiplex have weakness (e.g., footdrop) in addition to sensory abnormalities. Symptoms and signs are identical to those found in polyarteritis. Rheumatoid pachymeningitis is a rare complication of RA; confined to the dura and pia mater, this process may be limited to certain areas (e.g., lumbar cord or cisternae).[89] Elevated levels of IgG (including IgM and IgG RFs and low-molecular-weight IgM) and immune complexes are found in the cerebrospinal fluid.

Visceral lesions occur generally as claudication or infarction of the organ supplied by the involved arteries. Intestinal involvement with vasculitis manifests as abdominal pain, at first intermittent and progressing often to continuous pain and a tender, quiet abdomen on examination. If infarction develops, resection must be accomplished promptly. The presence of gangrene of digits and extremities, the development of intestinal lesions with bleeding or perforation, cardiac or renal involvement, and mononeuritis multiplex indicate extensive vasculitis and are associated with a poor prognosis.[90] Other entities in the differential diagnosis for rheumatoid vasculitis include diabetes mellitus, infection, atherosclerosis, and drug reactions. Current practice is to treat organ-specific vasculitis aggressively when it occurs in rheumatoid patients, similar to the treatment for patients with polyarteritis. This therapeutic approach may be responsible for the small excess mortality in rheumatoid vasculitis patients compared with "controls" with RA alone. In 61 patients with rheumatoid vasculitis, after allowance for general risk factors such as age and sex, the mortality risk was only 1.26 times that of rheumatoid patients without vasculitis.[91]

RENAL DISEASE

The kidney is rarely involved directly in RA, but often is compromised indirectly by therapy. Amyloidosis is an unusual complication of chronic RA. AA amyloidosis, along with vasculitis and sepsis, is one of the most important life-threatening complications of RA. Phenacetin abuse causes renal papillary necrosis, and salicylates and other NSAIDs may cause abnormalities as well. Membranous nephropathy is related to therapy with gold salts and penicillamine and was seen when these agents were commonly used to treat RA. Rarely, a focal necrotizing glomerulitis is seen in patients dying with RA and disseminated vasculitis.

PULMONARY DISEASE

There are at least six forms of lung disease in RA, as follows:

- Pleural disease
- Interstitial fibrosis
- Nodular lung disease
- Bronchiolitis obliterans with organizing pneumonia
- Arteritis, with pulmonary hypertension
- Small airways disease

It is not surprising that lung disease is associated with RA, considering that the drugs used to treat the disease, such as methotrexate, can cause pulmonary problems. In some cases, it may be difficult to distinguish pulmonary fibrosis related to RA from methotrexate pulmonary toxicity, although the latter is often associated with fever and eosinophilia secondary to an idiosyncratic reaction. Treatment with TNF inhibitors can lead to reactivation of pulmonary or extrapulmonary tuberculosis.

Pleural Disease

Pleuritis is commonly found on autopsy of patients with RA, but clinical disease during life is seen less frequently. In about 20% of patients, pleuritis develops concurrently with the onset of the arthritis. Pleuritic pain is not usually a major complaint. Effusions can be large enough to cause dyspnea. Characteristics of exudative rheumatoid effusions are as follows:

Glucose, 10 to 50 mg/dL
Protein, greater than 4 g/dL
Cells (mononuclear), 100 to 3500/mm^3
Lactate dehydrogenase, elevated
CH_{50}, depressed

The low glucose concentrations are of interest. Sepsis (particularly tuberculosis) is the only other condition that commonly has such a low pleural fluid glucose level. An impaired transport of glucose into the pleural space seems to be the cause of this.[92]

Interstitial Pneumonitis and Fibrosis

Pulmonary fibrosis, either slowly progressive or as a result of pulmonary inflammatory disease, can occur in RA. Similar to the findings in scleroderma, physical findings are of fine, diffuse, dry rales. Radiographs show a diffuse reticular (interstitial) or reticulonodular pattern in both lung fields; these can progress to a honeycomb appearance on plain radiographs and a characteristic lattice network seen on high-resolution CT scans. The pathologic findings are those of diffuse fibrosis in the midst of a mononuclear cell infiltrate. The principal functional defect is impairment of alveolocapillary gas exchange with decreased diffusion capacity, best measured using single-breath carbon monoxide diffusion capacities.[93] RA patients who smoke are likely to be at a higher risk for fibrotic complications in the lungs than are patients in the general population. Bronchoalveolar lavage may reveal increased numbers of lymphocytes, even in patients with only mildly abnormal chest radiographs and normal pulmonary function test results.[94] In more aggressive disease, a higher proportion of neutrophils can be found in bronchoalveolar lavage. Lymphoid interstitial pneumonitis has been described in patients with RA and Sjögren's syndrome. This is a relatively indolent disorder and is associated with elevated serum globulin levels. Bronchoalveolar lavage shows a primarily lymphocytic response.[95]

Nodular Lung Disease

Pulmonary nodules may appear singly or in clusters that coalesce. Single nodules appear as coin lesions and, when significant peripheral arthritis and nodules are present, can be diagnosed by needle biopsy without thoracotomy. Caplan's syndrome,[96] in which pneumoconiosis and RA are synergistic, producing a violent fibroblastic reaction with obliterative granulomatous fibrosis, has become a rare occurrence as the respiratory environment in mining operations has improved. Nodules may cavitate, creating a bronchopleural fistula. In several cases, solitary pulmonary nodules in RA patients have proved to be a rheumatoid nodule and a coexistent bronchogenic carcinoma,[97] a finding that suggests caution in interpreting "benign" results from fine-needle aspiration biopsy in such patients.

Bronchiolitis

An uncommon finding is an interstitial pneumonitis that progresses to alveolar involvement and bronchiolitis, respiratory insufficiency, and death. Pathologic studies show a cellular loose fibrosis and proteinaceous exudate in bronchioles and alveoli; interstitial infiltrations of lymphocytes attest to the immunogenic aspects of the disease. The course and prognosis are similar to idiopathic bronchiolitis obliterans with organizing pneumonia.

Pulmonary Hypertension

Pulmonary hypertension is more common than previously appreciated in RA. Noninvasive echocardiograms have suggested that mild pulmonary hypertension can be detected in more than 30% of patients with RA.[98] Most of these patients are asymptomatic.

Small Airways Disease

Defined by a reduced maximal midexpiratory flow rate and maximal expiratory flow rate at 50% of functional vital capacity, small airways disease was observed in 50% of 30 RA patients compared with 22% of a control population.[99] The study was adjusted for pulmonary infections, α_1-antitrypsin deficiency, penicillamine treatment, environmental pollution, and smoking. Other investigations have not found small airways dysfunction in RA and have suggested that, if present, it probably is related to factors other than RA.[100] If real, this phenomenon may be part of a generalized exocrinopathic process in the disease, expressed most flagrantly in Sjögren's syndrome.

CARDIAC COMPLICATIONS

Cardiac disease in RA can take many forms. It has become apparent that the increased risk of premature death in RA is due largely to an increased incidence of cardiovascular disease, primarily myocardial infarction and congestive heart failure. Advances in echocardiography have made the diagnosis of pericarditis and endocardial inflammation easier and more specific. Myocardial biopsy through vascular catheters has facilitated diagnosis and classification of myocarditis. In a detailed study of rheumatoid patients using echocardiography, Holter monitors, and electrocardiogram, it was reported that 70% of patients with nodular disease and 40% of patients with non-nodular RA have some cardiac involvement, including valve thickening or incompetence.[101]

Atherosclerosis

There are multiple risk factors for coronary artery disease in RA patients in addition to the risk factors that are relevant in the general population. Patients with prolonged RA have more atherosclerosis than patients of the same age with more recent disease onset.[102] Many of the same risk factors present in RA patients have been implicated in patients without rheumatic diseases, including molecules involved in the immune response, markers of inflammation, and therapeutic agents. It also is apparent that, all else being equal, tobacco smoking is an important factor in augmenting early atherosclerosis in RA patients.[103] In the large and well-studied population of rheumatoid patients at the Mayo Clinic, patients were followed until death, migration from Olmstead County, or 2001. The data showed that congestive heart failure was more important than ischemic heart disease as cause of death.[104] Even in RA patients without clinically evident cardiovascular disease, the left ventricular diastolic function and the right ventricular diastolic function are reduced.[105]

Pericarditis

Infrequently diagnosed on the basis of history and physical examination in RA, pericarditis is present in 50% of patients at autopsy. In one study, 31% of patients with RA had echocardiographic evidence of pericardial effusion. The same study revealed only rare evidence of impaired left ventricular function in prospectively studied outpatients with RA.[106] Although unusual, cardiac tamponade with constrictive pericarditis can develop in RA and may require pericardiectomy. Almost all patients have a positive test for RF, and half have nodules. The preservation of good ventricular function on echocardiography in the face of deteriorating clinical myocardial function should raise a high index of suspicion of constrictive pericarditis.

Myocarditis

Myocarditis can take the form of either granulomatous disease or interstitial myocarditis. The granulomatous process resembles subcutaneous nodules and could be considered specific for the disease. Diffuse infiltration of the myocardium by mononuclear cells may involve the entire myocardium and yet have no clinical manifestations, but it could possibly be suggested by echocardiography.

Endocardial Inflammation

Echocardiographic studies have reported evidence of previously unrecognized mitral valve disease of the anterior leaflet of the mitral valve. Although aortic valve disease and arthritis are generally associated through ankylosing spondylitis, numerous patients with granulomatous nodules on the valve have been reported.[107]

Conduction Defects

Atrioventricular block is unusual in RA, but is probably related to direct granulomatous involvement. Pathologic examination may reveal proliferative lesions or healed scars. Complete heart block has been described in more than 30 patients with RA. It generally occurs in patients with established erosive nodular disease.[108] It usually is permanent and is caused by rheumatoid granulomas in or near the atrioventricular node or bundle of His. Rarely, amyloidosis is responsible for heart block.

Coronary Arteritis

Patients with severe RA and active vasculitis who develop a myocardial infarction are likely to have coronary arteritis as a basis for the process along with accelerated atherosclerosis.

Granulomatous Aortitis or Valvular Disease

In severe rheumatoid heart disease, granulomatous disease can spread to involve even the base of the aorta. Occasionally, granulomatous disease associated with RA necessitates urgent valve replacement for aortic regurgitation.[109]

DIAGNOSIS

Criteria to establish the diagnosis of RA are based on an effective clinical history and physical examination, laboratory tests, and exclusion of other diagnoses. No single feature or laboratory test is sufficient for a definite diagnosis. The 1988 American College of Rheumatology criteria for classification usually are not used in individual cases for diagnosis; however, the requirement that objective evidence for synovitis must be present for at least 6 weeks is an important one especially because many transient forms of synovitis are observed in primary care settings (Table 66-3). A physician should not make a premature diagnosis of RA in a patient who might have a self-limited synovitis. To attempt preventing irreversible damage to joints, the diagnosis of RA should be confirmed or ruled out within 2 months after the onset of synovitis.

The characteristic patient with RA complains of pain and stiffness in multiple joints, with morning stiffness being prominent and prolonged. The joint swelling is boggy and includes soft tissue and synovial fluid. Joints are tender, especially the small joints of the hands and feet, but usually are not painful when the patient is at rest. Palmar erythema and prominent veins on the dorsum of the hand and wrist indicate increased blood flow. DIP joints are rarely involved. The temperature over the involved joints (except the hip) can be elevated, but the joints are not usually red. The range of motion is limited, and muscle strength and function around inflamed joints are diminished. Soft, poorly delineated subcutaneous nodules are often found in the extensor surface of the forearm. Findings on general physical examination are normal except for a possible low-grade fever in occasional patients (38°C) and a pulse more rapid than normal for that individual. Soft, small lymph nodes are found occasionally

in epitrochlear, axillary, and cervical areas. The history and physical examination are the most sensitive and specific tools for diagnosis of RA. Initial laboratory tests often show the results in the following list (essential tests are indicated with an asterisk (*). The other tests listed are largely of academic interest and should not be ordered routinely.

- Normal white blood cell count and differential*
- Thrombocytosis*
- Mild anemia (hemoglobin 10 g/dL), normochromic and either normocytic or microcytic*
- Normal urinalysis*
- ESR 30 mm/hr or greater and C-reactive protein level greater than 0.7 pg/mL*
- Normal renal, hepatic, and metabolic tests*
- Normal serum uric acid level
- Positive RF test (about 70% to 80% of patients; present in many normal individuals, patients with other rheumatic diseases, and individuals with chronic infections)*
- Anticitrullinated protein antibody (about 80% to 90% of patients; can be seen in other diseases, including active tuberculosis) (especially useful in early synovitis)*

Some investigators are convinced that anticitrullinated protein antibody will replace RF in the future as the autoantibody most useful in diagnosis. At this time, until it is cost-effective, it can be used to supplement RF in the presence of a strong clinical suspicion.

- Other autoantibodies (commonly found but with limited differential diagnosis utility, including antinuclear antibody, SS-A, SS-B)
- Polyclonal gammopathy as determined by serum protein electrophoresis
- Normal or elevated serum complement level
- Negative antineutrophil cytoplasmic antibody and anti–double-stranded DNA antibody tests
- "Typical" arthrocentesis, when obvious fluid is present, in RA reveals the following:
  Joint fluid is straw-colored, is slightly cloudy, and contains many flecks of fibrin 5000 to 25,000 white blood cells/mm3, and at least 50% of these are polymorphonuclear leukocytes
  No crystals
  Complement C4 and C2 levels are depressed, but C3 level can be normal
  Normal synovial fluid glucose level
  Cultures are negative

DIFFERENTIAL DIAGNOSIS

Other diseases must be excluded before the diagnosis of RA is established.[110] One of the most difficult challenges is an adult presenting with polyarthritis and fever; for this patient, a full workup may be required to define the underlying cause (Table 66-4).[111] The following sections on various diseases are listed in alphabetic order, and the illness' relative frequency is specified as common, uncommon, or rare.

Adult-Onset Still's Disease (Uncommon)

Significant fever at the onset of definite RA in adults is unusual. Later in the course, if vasculitis or serositis is present, or if there are intense exacerbations of disease, fever

Table 66-3 1988 Revised American Rheumatism Association Criteria for Classification of Rheumatoid Arthritis*

Criterion	Definition
1. Morning stiffness	Morning stiffness in and around the joints lasting at least 1 hr before maximal improvement
2. Arthritis of ≥3 joint areas	At least 3 joint areas simultaneously having soft tissue swelling or fluid (not bony overgrowth alone) observed by a physician (the 14 possible joint areas are [right or left] PIP, MCP, wrist, elbow, knee, ankle, and MTP joints)
3. Arthritis of hand joints	At least 1 joint area swollen as above in wrist, MCP, or PIP joint
4. Symmetric arthritis	Simultaneous involvement of the same joint areas (as in criterion 2) on both sides of the body (bilateral involvement of PIP, MCP, or MTP joints is acceptable without absolute symmetry)
5. Rheumatoid nodules	Subcutaneous nodules over bony prominences or extensor surfaces, or in juxta-articular regions, observed by a physician
6. Serum rheumatoid factor	Demonstration of abnormal amounts of serum rheumatoid factor by any method that has been positive
7. Radiographic changes	Changes typical of RA on posteroanterior hand and wrist radiographs, which must include erosions or unequivocal bony decalcification localized to or most marked adjacent to the involved joints (osteoarthritis changes alone do not qualify)

American College of Rheumatology Criteria	Sensitivity (%)	Specificity (%)
Morning stiffness	68	65
Arthritis of >3 areas	80	43
Arthritis of the hand joints	81	46
Symmetric arthritis	77	37
Rheumatoid nodules	3	100
Rheumatoid factor	59	93
Radiographic change	22	98

Clinical or Laboratory Variable	Persistent Nonerosive versus Self-limiting		Persistent Erosive versus Persistent Nonerosive	
	Odds Ratio	Score	Odds Ratio	Score
Symptom duration at first visit				
>6 wk, <6 mo	2.49	2	0.96	0
>6 mo	5.49	3	1.44	0
Morning stiffness >1 hr	1.96	1	1.96	1
Arthritis in ≥3 joints	1.73	1	1.73	1
Bilateral MTP compression pain	1.65	1	3.78	2
Rheumatoid factor positivity	2.99	2	2.99	2
Anticitrullinated peptide antibody positivity	4.58	3	4.58	3
Radiographic erosions (hands or feet)	2.75	2	Infinite	Infinite

*For classification purposes, a patient is said to have RA if he or she has satisfied at least four of the seven criteria. Criteria 1 through 4 must be present for at least 6 weeks. Patients with two clinical diagnoses are not excluded. Designation as classic, definite, or probable RA is not to be made.
MCP, metacarpophalangeal; MTP, metatarsophalangeal; PIP, proximal interphalangeal; RA, rheumatoid arthritis.

is more common. Adult Still's disease, in contrast, usually manifests with spiking fevers. Adult Still's disease was first described in 14 patients by Bywaters.[112] Women and men are affected equally. It usually appears during the third or fourth decade of life. Serologic studies (RF and antinuclear antibody) are negative, and patients do not have subcutaneous nodules. Most patients are febrile, and fevers can develop before arthritis. Fever patterns in these patients are often quotidian (i.e., reaching normal levels at least once each day). Occasionally, evanescent salmon-colored or pink macules appear on the trunk and extremities that become more prominent when patients are febrile. The cervical spine is involved, and loss of neck motion may be striking.

Abnormal liver function tests consistent with hepatitis and severe abdominal pain can be present and may confound attempts at diagnosis. Liver involvement is observed in most cases and was noted in more than two thirds of patients in one series[113]; hypergammaglobulinemia is present in more than 60%. Pericarditis and pleural effusions are found in less

than 25% of cases. In contrast to active SLE with nephritis, the serum complement level is normal or high. Serum ferritin levels can be enormously elevated, well beyond levels expected compared with other acute-phase reactants in the same individual.[114] Levels in serum of 30,000 ng/mL have been reported in some patients with highly active disease; when levels are greater than 10,000 ng/mL, physicians should strongly consider adult Still's disease as the diagnosis. The glycosylated form of serum ferritin, usually greater than 50% of the total, is reportedly low (mean 16%) during active phases and in remission.[115]

The diagnosis of adult-onset Still's disease still remains one of exclusion, despite the unusually elevated ferritin levels in serum. Systemic infection, malignancy (e.g., lymphoma), and diffuse vasculitis usually are entertained as diagnoses, searched for, and then discarded before a diagnosis of adult-onset Still's disease is made.

Yamaguchi and associates[116] developed criteria for establishing the diagnosis of adult Still's disease that, in

Table 66-4 Discriminating Features in Patients Presenting with Polyarthritis and Fever

Symptom or Sign	Possible Diagnoses
Temperature >40°C	Still's disease Bacterial arthritis SLE
Fever preceding arthritis	Viral arthritis Lyme disease Reactive arthritis Still's disease Bacterial endocarditis
Migratory arthritis	Rheumatic fever Gonococcemia Meningococcemia Viral arthritis SLE Acute leukemia Whipple's disease
Effusion disproportionately greater than pain	Tuberculous arthritis Bacterial endocarditis Inflammatory bowel disease Giant cell arteritis Lyme disease
Pain disproportionately greater than effusion	Rheumatic fever Familial Mediterranean fever Acute leukemia Acquired immunodeficiency syndrome
Positive test for rheumatoid factor	Rheumatoid arthritis Viral arthritis Tuberculous arthritis Bacterial endocarditis SLE Sarcoidosis Systemic vasculitis
Morning stiffness	Rheumatoid arthritis Polymyalgia rheumatica Still's disease Some viral and reactive arthritides
Symmetric small joint synovitis	Rheumatoid arthritis SLE Viral arthritis
Leukocytosis (>15,000/mm³)	Bacterial arthritis Bacterial endocarditis Still's disease Systemic vasculitis Acute leukemia
Leukopenia	SLE Viral arthritis
Episodic recurrences	Lyme disease Crystal-induced arthritis Inflammatory bowel disease Whipple's disease Mediterranean fever Still's disease SLE

SLE, systemic lupus erythematosus
From Pinals RS: Polyarthritis and fever. N Engl J Med 330:769, 1999. Copyright 1999 Massachusetts Medical Society. All rights reserved.

numerous series, have greater than 90% sensitivity (Table 66-5). After excluding other diseases, adult Still's disease should be considered if five criteria (more than two being major ones) are met. It is unknown yet whether adding hyperferritinemia would increase the specificity of diagnosis.

Table 66-5 Criteria for Diagnosis of Still's Disease

Major Criteria	Minor Criteria
Temperature >39°C for >1 wk	Sore throat
Leukocytosis >10,000/mm³ with >80% PMNs	Lymph node enlargement
Typical rash	Splenomegaly
Arthralgias >2 wk	Liver dysfunction (high AST/ALT) Negative ANA, RF

ALT, alanine transaminase; ANA, antinuclear antibody; AST, aspartate transaminase; PMNs, polymorphonuclear neutrophils; RF, rheumatoid factor.

In one series of adult-onset Still's disease, 11 patients (all of whom were white women), followed for a mean of 20.2 years after disease onset, had the following characteristics[117]:

- Ten patients had a polycyclic pattern (characterized by remissions and exacerbations).
- Patterns of exacerbations were similar to, but less severe than, the original presentations.
- Loss of wrist extension was the most common clinical abnormality, and carpal ankylosis was present in 10 patients.

In another group, 20% showed significant functional deterioration from erosive joint disease.[118] Functional class III/IV (Steinbrocker's classification) was usually related to hip disease. The overall long-term prognosis of adult-onset Still's disease is good for systemic manifestations, but less so for articular disease. The incidence of amyloidosis may be 30% within 10 years of onset of the illness, perhaps reflecting the sustained high titers of acute-phase reactants found in this disease.

Therapy must be aggressive. Full doses of NSAIDs should be prescribed soon after diagnosis. Oral glucocorticoids are often needed to control systemic symptoms. It is reasonable to prescribe weekly methotrexate to help control the inflammation and serve as a steroid-sparing drug. Because of the high likelihood that this is an example of a cytokine-driven disease, use of TNF or IL-6 blockers might be effective. Still's disease also is more likely to respond to IL-1 antagonists than is RA.[119]

Amyloidosis (Rare)

Deposits of amyloid can be found in synovial and periarticular tissues and are presumably responsible for the joint complaints of some patients. The synovial fluid in amyloid arthropathy is noninflammatory, and particulate material with apple-green fluorescence after Congo red staining may be found in the fluid. Amyloid formed of β_2-microglobulin is found in joints of patients with chronic renal failure, usually patients who are on dialysis (see Chapter 106).

Angioimmunoblastic Lymphadenopathy (Rare)

Nonerosive symmetric seronegative polyarthritis involving large joints can be an initial complaint in angioimmunoblastic lymphadenopathy.[120] Typical clinical features are lymphadenopathy, hepatosplenomegaly, rash, and hypergammaglobulinemia. It can resemble Still's disease in adults if the arthritis precedes other manifestations. Diagnosis is based on the characteristic appearance of a lymph node or skin biopsy specimen, which includes effacement of lymph node architecture, proliferation of small vessels, and a cellular infiltrate (immunoblasts, plasma cells, T lymphocytes, and histiocytes) within amorphous acidophilic interstitial material. Symptoms may be related to excessive production of IL-2 by helper T cells in this process.

Ankylosing Spondylitis, Seronegative Spondyloarthropathy, and Reactive Arthritis (Common)

Ankylosing spondylitis, psoriatic arthritis, inflammatory bowel disease–associated arthritis, and reactive arthritis are often referred to as seronegative spondyloarthropathies. These diseases are generally marked by their respective nonarticular features and the following pattern of joint disease: asymmetric, oligoarticular, lower extremities more than upper extremities, and large joints more than small joints (there are many exceptions to these general guidelines). The problem in differentiating these diseases from RA arises with a patient (particularly a woman) who has minimal back pain and definite peripheral joint involvement. The presence of low back pain and lumbar involvement also distinguish these diseases from RA.

In some unusual cases, RA and ankylosing spondylitis are present in the same patient. In one series, nine patients with RF in serum had spinal ankylosis and symmetric erosive polyarthritis; eight of the nine carried HLA-B27.[121] If these two diseases occur completely independently of each other, simultaneous appearance in the same patient should occur in 1 in 50,000 to 200,000 adults.

In distinguishing patients with Reiter's syndrome from patients with RA, a careful search for heel pain or tenderness and ocular or urethral symptoms is of great importance. Polyarthritis persists chronically in more than 80% of patients with Reiter's syndrome. The characteristics of enthesopathy in patients with Reiter's syndrome (i.e., "sausage" digits indicating periarticular soft tissue inflammation, insertional tendinitis, periostitis, and peri-insertional osteoporosis or erosions) may point to the diagnosis.

The differential diagnosis between RA with psoriasis and some forms of psoriatic arthritis may be artificial (see Chapter 47). Some patients with DIP joint involvement and severe skin involvement have a disease that is not RA. Others have a seropositive symmetric polyarthritis that appears to be RA, yet they also have psoriasis. These patients can be treated with the same disease-modifying drugs as patients with progressive RA, including TNF-α inhibitors.

A syndrome described extensively in the French literature, acne pustulosis hyperostosis osteitis,[122] may resemble psoriatic arthritis and, occasionally, when peripheral arthritis is present, RA. As the name implies, these patients variably have severe acne, palmar and plantar pustules, hyperostotic reactions (particularly in the clavicles and sternum), sacroiliitis, and peripheral inflammatory arthritis.

Inflammatory bowel disease (ulcerative colitis and Crohn's disease) is associated with arthritis in 20% of cases (see Chapter 73). Peripheral arthritis occurs more commonly than spondylitis in many series.[123] Ankles, knees, and elbows are the most typically involved peripheral joints, with PIP joints and wrists next in frequency. Simultaneous attacks of arthritis and the development of erythema nodosum are common. Only two or three joints are affected at once. Involvement is usually asymmetric, and erosions are uncommon. The occurrence of peripheral arthritis in inflammatory bowel disease is not related to HLA-B27.

Behçet's syndrome is marked by asymmetric polyarthritis in 50% to 60% of cases (see Chapter 86).[124] It is rare, with a prevalence of less than 1 in 25,000 in the United States. In more than half of cases, the attacks of arthritis are monarticular. Knees, ankles, and wrists are affected most often; synovial fluid usually contains more than 5000, but less than 30,000 white blood cells/mm^3. Joint deformity is unusual. Painful oral and genital ulcers and central nervous system involvement are characteristic. Uveal tract involvement in Behçet's syndrome must be differentiated from the scleritis characteristic of RA in patients with ocular and joint disease.

Enteric infections are complicated occasionally by inflammatory joint disease resembling RA. The joint disease associated with *Yersinia enterocolitica* infections occurs several weeks after the gastrointestinal illness. Knees and ankles are the joints most commonly involved, and most patients (even patients with peripheral arthritis and no spondylitis) have HLA-B27. Reactive arthritis also has been reported after *Salmonella*, *Shigella*, and *Campylobacter* (*Helicobacter*) *jejuni* infection.

Arthritis Associated with Oral Contraceptives (Uncommon)

A syndrome of persistent arthralgias, myalgias, and morning stiffness with occasional development of polyarticular synovitis has been described in women, usually in their 20s, who have been taking oral contraceptives (estrogens and progestins). Positive tests for antinuclear antibody are common, and patients may have circulating RF. Symptoms resolve after the oral contraceptive is discontinued.

Arthritis of Thyroid Disease (Uncommon)

In hypothyroidism (see Chapter 111), synovial effusions and synovial thickening that simulate RA have been described.[125] The ESR may be elevated because of hypergammaglobulinemia, but C-reactive protein is normal. The joint fluid is noninflammatory and may have increased viscosity. Knees, wrists, hands, and feet are involved most often, and coexisting calcium pyrophosphate dihydrate deposition disease is frequently found. This syndrome should be distinguished from arthralgias and other nonspecific musculoskeletal complaints that often accompany hyperthyroidism and hypothyroidism.

The syndrome of thyroid acropachy complicates less than 1% of cases of hyperthyroidism. This syndrome comprises periosteal new bone formation, which may be associated with a low-grade synovitis similar to hypertrophic osteoarthropathy. Patients with coexisting RA and hyperthyroidism have pain from the arthritis that, although impossible to quantify, seems to exceed the pain expected from the degree of inflammation.

Bacterial Endocarditis (Uncommon)

Arthralgias, arthritis, back pain, and myalgias occur in approximately 30% of patients with subacute bacterial endocarditis.[126] Symptoms typically occur in one or several joints, usually large, proximal ones. This synovitis is probably caused by the deposition of circulating immune complexes. Confusion with RA may arise because more than half of patients with endocarditis are seropositive for RF. Fever out of proportion to joint findings in the setting of leukocytosis should lead to a consideration of infective endocarditis as a diagnostic possibility, even in the absence of a significant heart murmur. Peripheral emboli with digital infarctions may be found, simulating palpable purpura when they occur on the lower legs. Blood cultures should be obtained in all patients with polyarthritis and significant fever. Embolic phenomena with constitutional symptoms, including arthralgias, can be presenting symptoms of atrial myxoma, but this process usually mimics systemic vasculitis or subacute bacterial endocarditis more than it does RA.

Calcium Pyrophosphate Dihydrate Deposition Disease (Common)

Calcium pyrophosphate dihydrate deposition disease is a crystal-induced synovitis that takes many forms, ranging from a syndrome of indolent osteoarthrosis to that of an acute, hot joint. About 5% of patients have a chronic polyarthritis (sometimes referred to as pseudo-RA) associated with proliferative erosions of subchondral bone. Although radiographs are helpful when chondrocalcinosis is present, calcium pyrophosphate dihydrate deposition disease may be present in the absence of calcification on radiographs.[127] Diagnosis then can be made only by arthrocentesis. A radiographic sign of calcium pyrophosphate dihydrate deposition disease that helps to differentiate it from RA is the presence of unicompartmental disease in the wrists (see Chapter 44). On physical examination, the MCPs in calcium pyrophosphate dihydrate deposition disease generally have bony enlargement rather than soft tissue swelling owing to synovial hyperplasia.

Calcific Periarthritis (Uncommon)

Although usually involving single joints, calcific periarthritis secondary to hydroxyapatite deposition can be confused with polyarthritis. The skin is red over and around the affected joints; the tissues are boggy and tender, but no joint effusion is present. Passive motion is easier than active motion. Periarticular calcification is visible on radiographs. Unless the periarthritis can be differentiated from true arthritis, the findings may mimic those of palindromic rheumatism or early monarticular RA.

Congenital Camptodactyly and Arthropathy (Rare)

Congenital camptodactyly and arthropathy is a deformity that begins in utero and produces synovial cell hypertrophy and hyperplasia without inflammatory cells.[128] Clinical manifestations include contractures of the fingers; flattening of the metacarpal heads; and short, thick femoral necks. This condition can manifest as oligoarticular seronegative RA.

Familial Mediterranean Fever (Uncommon)

The articular syndrome in familial Mediterranean fever and many other periodic fevers is an episodic monarthritis or oligoarthritis of the large joints that appears in childhood or adolescence, mimicking oligoarthritic forms of juvenile RA. The disease is caused by a genetic abnormality owing to a mutation in the pyrin gene, and 60% of reported cases have been in Sephardic Jews. Episodes of arthritis begin acutely with fever and other signs of inflammation (e.g., peritonitis or pleuritis) and can precede other manifestations of the disease. Although usually limited to days or weeks, attacks occasionally last for months and are associated with radiographic changes of periarticular osteopenia without erosions. The abdominal pain that these patients experience can be a key to diagnosis. Amyloidosis (type AA) is a late complication of this syndrome in numerous patients. Familial Mediterranean fever and related forms of periodic inflammatory syndromes are discussed fully in Chapter 113.

Fibromyalgia (Common)

In fibromyalgia, there is no evidence of synovitis. Although no specific diagnostic tests define this entity, certain nonarticular locations of pain are common to different patients. In an analysis contrasting the pain properties with those of RA,[129] the fibromyalgia patients used diverse adjectives to describe their pain, the most common being "pricking," "pressing," "shooting," "gnawing," "cramping," "splitting," and "crushing." Most patients in both groups defined the pain as aching and exhausting. Evidence is accumulating that patients with diffuse connective tissue diseases, including RA, may develop a superimposed fibromyalgia, adding to the difficulty of treating the arthritis. Rheumatoid patients have fewer psychological disturbances than patients with fibromyalgia, and RA patients who develop fibromyalgia score higher on testing scales for hypochondriasis, depression, and hysteria than patients with RA who do not have fibromyalgia (see Chapter 38).

Glucocorticoid Withdrawal Syndrome (Common)

The symptoms of glucocorticoid withdrawal are often confused with RA. Patients on glucocorticoid therapy who are being treated for nonrheumatic diseases may have diffuse polyarticular pain, particularly in the hands, if the glucocorticoid dose is tapered too rapidly.

Gout (Common)

Before a diagnosis of chronic erosive RA is made, chronic tophaceous gout must be ruled out. The reverse applies as well. Features of gouty arthritis that can mimic the features of RA include polyarthritis, symmetric involvement, fusiform swelling of joints, subcutaneous nodules, and a subacute presentation of attacks. Conversely, certain aspects of RA that suggest gouty arthritis include hyperuricemia after treatment with low doses of aspirin, periarticular nodules, and seronegative disease (particularly in men). Radiographic findings may be similar, with the appearance of the subcortical erosions of RA resembling small osseous tophi in gout. Although large asymmetric erosions with ballooning of the cortex and overhanging edges are more likely to be caused by gout than by RA, this is not always the case. Serologic test results may be misleading as well; RF has been found in 30% of patients with chronic tophaceous gout who have no clinical or radiographic signs of RA.[130] Gout occurring concomitantly with RA is extremely rare.

Hemochromatosis (Uncommon)

The characteristic articular feature of hemochromatosis that is almost diagnostic is firm bony enlargement of the MCP joints, particularly the second and third joints, with associated cystic degenerative disease and large hooklike osteophytes on radiographs and, frequently, chondrocalcinosis. Marginal erosions, juxta-articular osteoporosis, synovial proliferation, and ulnar deviation are not seen in the arthropathy of hemochromatosis, but are common in RA. Wrists, shoulders, elbows, hips, and knees are involved less often than the MCP joints. Arthritis leads the list of diagnoses provided to patients to explain their symptoms before the diagnosis of hemochromatosis.[131] In the series by McDonnell and colleagues,[131] individuals with symptoms received a diagnosis of hemochromatosis only after the symptoms had been present, on average, for an extended period (10 years) and after visiting an average of 3.5 physicians (see Chapter 108).

Hemoglobinopathies (Uncommon)

In homozygous (SS) sickle cell disease, the most common arthropathy is associated with crisis and is believed to be a result of microvascular occlusion in articular tissues. A destructive arthritis with a loss of articular cartilage that resembles severe RA has been reported in some cases, however.[132] In most patients with sickle cell disease and joint complaints, periosteal elevation, bone infarcts, fish-mouth vertebrae, and avascular necrosis can be found on radiographs. In a series of 37 patients with SS disease, from which patients with gout or avascular necrosis of the femoral head were excluded, 12 complained of a monarthritis or oligoarthritis associated with painful crises; tenderness was most marked over the epiphyses rather than the joint space, and synovial fluid was noninflammatory. Another 12 patients had arthritis of the ankle associated with a malleolar ulcer; this arthritis was chronic and resolved with improvement of the leg ulcer.[133] Episodic polyarthritis and noninflammatory synovial effusions also are found in sickle cell–β-thalassemia (see Chapter 110).

Hemophilic Arthropathy (Uncommon)

A deficiency of factor VIII or, less frequently, factor IX, sufficient to produce clinical bleeding frequently results in hemarthroses. The iron overload in the joint generates a proliferative synovitis that often leads to joint destruction. Because iron stimulates metalloproteinase production by synovial cells, when feasible, large hemarthroses should be aspirated, and the joint should be immobilized and wrapped well. The clotting abnormality is rarely overlooked, however, and it is unlikely that a diagnosis of RA would be made in the setting of hemophilia A or B (see Chapter 109).

Human Immunodeficiency Virus Infection (Common)

Several types of arthropathy have been described in association with human immunodeficiency virus (HIV) infection, including the following[134]:

1. Brief, acute arthralgias concurrent with initial HIV viremia
2. HIV-associated arthritis, lower extremity noninflammatory oligoarthritis, or a persistent polyarthritis
3. Seronegative spondyloarthropathy, resembling Reiter's syndrome, psoriatic arthritis, or reactive arthritis, often more severe than in patients without HIV infection[135]

It is crucial to rule out HIV in any patient with an acute polyarthritis and fever: HIV-positive patients have a greater risk for toxicity or opportunistic infections when using immunosuppressive drugs (see Chapter 104). HIV-positive patients also can present with syndromes of vasculitis.

Hyperlipoproteinemia (Uncommon)

Achilles tendinitis and tenosynovitis can be presenting symptoms in familial type II hyperlipoproteinemia and may be accompanied by arthritis. Synovial fluid findings may resemble the findings of mild RA, and the tendon xanthomas may be mistaken for rheumatoid nodules or gouty tophi. Conversely, bilateral pseudoxanthomatous rheumatoid nodules have been described. The treatment of hyperlipoproteinemia with statins may cause an acute or subacute muscular syndrome that resembles myositis or polymyalgia rheumatica more than RA (see Chapter 78).

Hypertrophic Osteoarthropathy (Uncommon)

Hypertrophic osteoarthropathy may present as oligoarthritis involving the knees, ankles, or wrists. The synovial inflammation accompanies periosteal new bone formation that can be seen on radiographs. Correction of the inciting factor (e.g., cure of pneumonia in a child with cystic fibrosis) is likely to alleviate the synovitis. The synovium is characterized primarily by an increased blood supply and synovial cell proliferation. Little infiltration by mononuclear cells is seen. Pain in the bones that increases when extremities are dependent is characteristic, although it is not always present. If clubbing is not present or is not noticed, this entity is easily confused with RA (see Chapter 90).

Hypercytokine Syndrome (Uncommon)

Unusual patients present to clinics and hospitals with acute or subacute wasting, often febrile diseases that have manifestations in multiple organs, but without histopathologic or clinical clues that would enable specific classification. With very high acute-phase reactants and serum ferritin levels exceedingly high, adult-onset Still's disease (without arthritis) and infection or various forms of vasculitis must be considered. These patients are inevitably given glucocorticoid therapy, and anecdotal reports have indicated successful or partially effective therapy with anti-TNF agents.

Idiopathic Hypereosinophilic Syndrome with Arthritis (Rare)

The poorly defined idiopathic hypereosinophilic syndrome often includes myalgias and arthralgias and evolves into a clinical picture of hepatomegaly with or without pericarditis, pulmonary hypertension, subcutaneous nodules, and cardiomyopathy. Synovitis, characterized by inflammatory joint fluid, is rarely erosive or deforming. The similarities between this and toxic oil syndrome and eosinophilia-myalgia syndrome, both of which are caused by the ingestion of toxic substances, suggest a basic hypersensitivity reaction.

Infectious Diseases (Including Viral Causes Such as Hepatitis C) (Common)

Bacterial sepsis may be superimposed on RA. Viral infections may manifest as arthritis, however, with many characteristics of RA. Arthritis complicates rubella more often in adults than in children and may affect the small joints of the hands. Lymphocytes predominate in synovial effusions.

Arthritis often precedes jaundice in viral hepatitis and is associated with the presence of circulating hepatitis B surface antigen and hypocomplementemia. The surface antigen has been found in synovial tissues with the use of direct immunofluorescence, and this supports the concept that this synovitis is mediated by immune complexes.[136] An acute onset of diffuse polyarthritis with small joint effusions and minimal synovial swelling, often accompanied by urticaria, should prompt the physician to obtain liver function tests in the patient with a history of exposure to hepatitis. With the onset of icterus, the arthritis usually resolves without a trace.

The increasing recognition of the RNA virus hepatitis C as a cause of joint complaints is related to the availability of specific serologic tests for this virus. About one third of individuals infected with hepatitis C virus have arthralgias or arthritis, and in a Korean series, the prevalence of cryoglobulins (mean concentration of 9.8 g/L) was 59%.[137] These individuals can present with palmar tenosynovitis, small joint synovitis, carpal tunnel syndrome, and positive tests for RF. The presence of anticitrullinated protein antibodies can be a useful feature to distinguish RA from hepatitis C–associated arthritis.[138] Other findings, including mixed cryoglobulinemia syndrome, glomerulonephritis, and cutaneous vasculitis, round out the clinical spectrum of rheumatic complaints associated with this viral infection. Because exacerbation of hepatitis can be associated with the use and the cessation of methotrexate therapy, a good case has been made for testing for hepatitis C in every patient with RA scheduled to be started on therapy with this drug.[139]

Fever, sore throat, and cervical adenopathy followed by symmetric polyarthritis are compatible with infection resulting from hepatitis B, rubella, adenovirus type 7, echovirus type 9, *Mycoplasma pneumoniae*, or Epstein-Barr virus and acute rheumatic fever or adult-onset Still's disease. In Japan, many more patients with RA have circulating antibodies against human T-lymphotropic virus 1 (HTLV-1). Multiple nodules within tendon sheaths associated with inflammation resembling rheumatoid tenosynovitis have been described in a patient with HTLV-1 arthropathy.[140]

A chronic polyarthritis resembling RA has been described after serologic proof of parvovirus infection. Usually the process is self-limited and does not progress to a destructive synovitis (see Chapter 104). Adults, often those involved in child care, present with a history of a viral-like illness, sometimes with desquamating finger involvement and a diffuse, red facial rash ("slapped cheeks") that is followed by arthralgias and synovitis.

Poststreptococcal arthritis also can resemble RA. Typically, patients have an antecedent skin or oropharynx group A streptococcal infection in the weeks preceding symptoms. Antistreptolysin O antibody titers are usually elevated. Although the same bacteria can cause glomerulonephritis, it is uncommon to see concomitant arthritis and renal disease.

Intermittent Hydrarthrosis (Common)

Intermittent hydrarthrosis is a syndrome of periodic attacks of benign synovitis in one or a few joints, usually the knee, beginning in adolescence. The difference between this and oligoarticular juvenile RA or RA is one of degree, not kind. In contrast to palindromic rheumatism, in which acute synovitis may occur in different joints during successive attacks, the same joint or joints are affected during each attack in intermittent hydrarthrosis. Joint destruction does not occur because there is no chronic, persistent, proliferative synovitis.

Lyme Disease (Common in Some Areas)

Lyme disease can closely simulate RA in adults or children because of its intermittent course with the development of chronic synovitis. A proliferative, erosive synovitis necessitating synovectomy has evolved in several cases. The histopathologic appearance of the proliferative synovium is not different from that of RA (see Chapter 100) and the Lyme synovial cells produce a similar excess of metalloproteinases. Lyme serologic tests can help distinguish this disease from RA, along with history of tick bites, characteristic skin rash, or neurologic involvement.

Malignancy (Rare)

Direct involvement by cancer of synovium usually manifests as a monarthritis. Non-Hodgkin's lymphoma can manifest as seronegative polyarthritis, however, without hepatomegaly or lymphadenopathy. Intravascular lymphoma can manifest as a symmetric polyarthritis.[141] In children, acute lymphocytic leukemia can manifest as a polyarticular arthritis. Paraneoplastic syndromes and others related to direct involvement with cancer are described in detail later.

Multicentric Reticulohistiocytosis (Rare)

Multicentric reticulohistiocytosis causes severe arthritis mutilans with an opera-glass hand (main en lorgnette).[142] Other causes of arthritis mutilans are RA, psoriatic arthritis, erosive osteoarthritis treated with glucocorticoids, and gout (after tophi are resorbed by treatment with allopurinol). The cell that causes damage to tissues is the multinucleate lipid-laden histiocyte, which apparently releases degradative enzymes sufficient to destroy connective tissue. These cells in aggregates produce multiple small nodules around joints of the hands.

Osteoarthritis (Common)

Although osteoarthritis can begin as a degenerative cartilage disease, and RA begins as synovial inflammation, the diseases can overlap as they progress (Table 66-6). In osteoarthritis, as cartilage deteriorates and joint congruence is altered and stressed, a reactive synovitis often develops.

Table 66-6 Factors Useful for Differentiating Early Rheumatoid Arthritis from Osteoarthritis

	Rheumatoid Arthritis	Osteoarthritis
Age at onset	Childhood and adults, peak incidence in 50s	Increases with age
Predisposing factors	Susceptibility epitopes (HLA-DR4, HLA-DR1) PTPN22, PADI4 polymorphisms and others Smoking	Trauma Congenital abnormalities (e.g., shallow acetabulum)
Early symptoms	Morning stiffness	Pain increases through the day and with use
Joints involved	Metacarpophalangeal joints, wrists, proximal interphalangeal joints most often; distal interphalangeal joints almost never	Distal interphalangeal joints (Heberden's nodes), weight-bearing joints (hips, knees)
Physical findings	Soft tissue swelling, warmth	Bony osteophytes, minimal soft tissue swelling early
Radiologic findings	Periarticular osteopenia, marginal erosions	Subchondral sclerosis, osteophytes
Laboratory findings	Increased C-reactive protein, rheumatoid factor, anticitrullinated peptide antibody, anemia, leukocytosis	Normal

Conversely, as the rheumatoid pannus erodes cartilage, secondary osteoarthritic changes in bone and cartilage develop. In end stages of degenerative joint disease and RA, the involved joints appear the same. To differentiate clearly between the two, the physician must delve into the early history and functional abnormalities of the disease.

Erosive osteoarthritis occurs frequently in middle-aged women (more frequently than in men) and is characterized by inflammatory changes in PIP joints with destruction and functional ankylosis of the joints. The PIP joints can be red and hot, yet there is almost no synovial proliferation or effusion; joint swelling involves hard, bony tissue and not synovium. The ESR may be slightly elevated, but RF is not found (see Chapter 90).[143]

Parkinson's Disease (Common)

Although the tremor or rigidity of Parkinson's disease is rarely confused with symptoms of RA, Parkinson's patients have a predilection for developing swan neck deformities of the hands, a phenomenon generally unappreciated by rheumatologists. This abnormality was first described in 1864,[144] and its pathogenesis is still unknown (Fig. 66-14).

Pigmented Villonodular Synovitis (Rare)

Pigmented villonodular synovitis is a nonmalignant but proliferative disease of synovial tissue that has many functional characteristics similar to those of RA and usually involves only one joint. The histopathologic appearance is characterized by proliferation of histiocytes, multinucleate giant cells, and hemosiderin and lipid-laden macrophages. Clinically, this is a painless chronic synovitis (most often of the knee) with joint effusions and greatly thickened synovium. Subchondral bone cysts and cartilage erosion may be associated with the bulky tissue. It is unclear whether this condition should be classified as an inflammation or a neoplasm of synovium (see Chapter 114).

Polychondritis (Uncommon)

Polychondritis can mimic infectious processes, vasculitis, granulomatous disease, or RA. Patients with RA and ocular inflammation (e.g., scleritis) usually have active joint

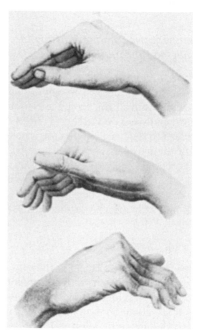

Figure 66-14 These swan neck deformities are a result of Parkinson's disease, not rheumatoid arthritis. (From Ordenstein L: Sur la Paralysie Agitante et la Sclérose en Plaques Generalisée. Paris, Imprimerie de E Martinet, 1864.)

disease before ocular problems develop; the reverse is true in polychondritis. In addition, polychondritis is not associated with RF. The joint disease is usually episodic. Nevertheless, erosions can develop that are similar to erosions of RA. In affected tissues of the external ears, nose, larynx, trachea, and costochondral areas, this disease may represent a true immune response against cartilage (see Chapter 95).

Polymyalgia Rheumatica and Giant Cell Arteritis (Common)

Although joint radionuclide imaging studies have indicated increased vascular flow in the synovium of patients with classic polymyalgia rheumatica, it is appropriate to exclude polymyalgia rheumatica as a diagnosis if significant synovitis (soft tissue proliferation or effusions) is detected. Otherwise, many patients who actually have RA would be diagnosed as having polymyalgia rheumatica and treated inappropriately with glucocorticoids. A careful history usually can differentiate shoulder or hip-girdle muscle pain from shoulder or hip joint pain. Examination of synovial biopsy specimens from patients with polymyalgia rheumatica indicates that the synovitis is usually milder than that found in RA. RA and polymyalgia rheumatica might coexist in some patients, but careful descriptions of such patients are rare.

Several patients have been described whose initial symptom of giant cell arteritis was a peripheral polyarthritis clinically indistinguishable from RA.[145] In 19 such patients in a group of 522 with biopsy-proven giant cell arteritis, however, only 3 were RF positive. The interval between the onsets of each set of symptoms was 3 years or less in 15 of the 19 patients, which also suggests a relationship between the two (see Chapter 81), and it is known that patients with giant cell arteritis often have HLA-DR4 alleles.

Relapsing Seronegative Symmetric Synovitis with Pitting Edema (Uncommon)

Relapsing seronegative symmetric synovitis with pitting edema is an uncommon syndrome marked by significant pitting edema of the hands with synovial thickening and joint tenderness. The symptoms rapidly respond to short courses of corticosteroids and can lead to residual abnormalities, including flexion contractures of the wrists and fingers. These patients are RF negative, and there has been a suggestion of increased risk of neoplastic disease. The syndrome might represent a variant of another disease, such as polymyalgia rheumatica or reflex sympathetic dystrophy, rather than a distinct entity.[146]

Rheumatic Fever (Uncommon)

Rheumatic fever is much less common than it once was, but still must be considered in adults with polyarthritis. In adults, arthritis is the most prominent clinical finding of rheumatic fever; carditis is less common than in children; and erythema marginatum, subcutaneous nodules, and chorea are rare. The presentation is often that of an additive, symmetric, large joint polyarthritis (involving lower extremities in 85% of patients), developing within 1 week and associated with a severe tenosynovitis. This extremely painful process is often dramatically responsive to salicylates. In contrast to Still's disease in adults, rheumatic fever generally has no remittent or quotidian fevers and shows evidence of antecedent streptococcal infection. It also has a less protracted course than Still's disease. There are many similarities between rheumatic fever in adults and "reactive" postinfectious synovitis developing from *Shigella*, *Salmonella*, *Brucella*, *Neisseria*, or *Yersinia* infections. As rheumatic fever becomes less common, and as penicillin prophylaxis effectively prevents recurrence of the disease, Jaccoud's arthritis (chronic post–rheumatic fever arthritis) is now quite rare. This entity, described by Bywaters in 1950,[147] results from severe and repeated bouts of rheumatic fever and synovitis, which stretches joint capsules and produces ulnar deformity of the hands without erosions. The same deformity can develop in SLE characterized by recurrent synovitis and soft tissue inflammation and in Parkinson's disease. Differentiating rheumatic fever from RA is particularly difficult when subcutaneous nodules are present with rheumatic fever.

Sarcoidosis (Uncommon)

The two most common forms of sarcoid arthritis often can be easily distinguished from RA. In the acute form with erythema nodosum and hilar adenopathy (Löfgren's syndrome), the articular complaints usually are related to periarthritis affecting large joints of the lower extremities. Differential diagnosis may be complicated because many of these patients have RF in serum. Joint erosions and proliferative synovitis do not occur in this form of sarcoidosis.

In chronic granulomatous sarcoidosis, cystlike areas of bone destruction, mottled rarefaction of bone, and a reticular pattern of bone destruction with a lacelike appearance on radiographs may simulate destructive RA. This form of sarcoidosis is often polyarticular, and biopsy of bone or synovium for diagnosis may be essential because there is often no correlation between joint disease and clinical evidence for sarcoid involvement of other organ systems. Poncet disease (tuberculous rheumatism) might actually represent granulomatous "idiopathic" arthritis (i.e., sarcoidosis) (see Chapter 105).[148]

Systemic Lupus Erythematosus (Common)

The distribution of involved joints and the deformities in SLE can be identical to RA. In contrast to RA, SLE arthritis does not usually cause cartilage destruction or bone erosions. The deformities are often reducible, sometimes leading to normal hand radiographs owing to the effect of placing the hand firmly on the film cassette. Serologies (antinuclear antibody, anti–double-stranded DNA) and major organ system involvement usually can distinguish RA from SLE.

Thiemann's Disease (Rare)

Thiemann's disease is a rare form of idiopathic vascular necrosis of the PIP joints of the hands with occasional involvement of other joints. Bony enlargement begins painlessly, and the digits (one or more may be involved) become fixed in flexion. The primary lesion is in the region of the epiphysis and generally begins before puberty, distinguishing it from erosive osteoarthritis, which it resembles radiographically. It is a heritable disease, but the genetic factors have not been defined.

Vasculitis (Common)

Patients with a variety of vasculitic syndromes can present with inflammatory arthritis, and these syndromes are readily distinguished from RA. Many small vessel vasculitides show palpable purpura and are associated with hepatitis C and cryoglobulinemia. Medium vessel forms of vasculitis, such as Wegener's granulomatosis, Churg-Strauss syndrome, or microscopic polyangiitis, include major organ system involvement (e.g., reactive airways disease, glomerulonephritis), and are usually antineutrophil cytoplasmic antibody positive. Polyarteritis nodosa usually is distinguished by renovascular hypertension and other systemic complaints. Systemic rheumatoid vasculitis can be indistinguishable from polyarteritis, necessitating a high index of suspicion.

Whipple's Disease (Common)

Since the identification of the uncultured bacillus of Whipple's disease in 1992,[149] numerous proven cases of this process that resemble adult Still's disease, in particular, have been described. Eight times as many men as women develop Whipple's disease. Many have a low-grade, intermittent fever; 80% or more have arthralgias in large joints. Diarrhea, abdominal pain, and weight loss are more common than in Still's disease, but patients with Whipple's disease do not have a characteristic skin rash.[200]

COURSE OF DISEASE

Epidemiologists have pointed out the many difficulties in attempting to establish a change in patterns of RA in different time periods or different communities. The best data suggest that the clinical manifestations of disease and the extent of disability are declining. Epidemiologic studies suggest that the disease is not changing, but that earlier, more effective treatment has diminished morbidity.

There are now well-tested criteria for clinical remission.[150] Definitions vary widely and can mean either absence of clinical and radiologic signs of disease while on treatment or a disease state with minimal or no activity after therapy is withdrawn. One composite system using the Disease Activity Score is a mathematical method that includes swollen and tender joints, ESR, and patient assessments of global health.[151] Notably, this criterion does not mean that the patient truly has complete remission without any evidence of synovitis. The American College of Rheumatology criteria require absence of joint tenderness, fatigue, joint pain, joint swelling, and morning stiffness, along with a normal ESR.

With an increased number of effective therapies available, it becomes increasingly important for physicians to be able to determine which patients would be most at risk for progressive destructive disease, and which patients would have a more benign illness that is not erosive and responsive to moderate intervention. In addition to predicting which patients may or may not develop erosions, it is equally important to identify which patients who already have erosions are more likely to progress rapidly to joint destruction. One study of an inception cohort of patients newly presenting with inflammatory polyarthritis confirmed the fact that although the initial radiographic score is, as expected, a powerful predictor of subsequent radiographic damage, a high titer of RF and anticitrullinated protein antibodies continue to be powerful predictors of deteriorating radiographic damage in subjects receiving conventional therapy.[152]

Joint erosions and deformity may not be the most important aspects of disease to the patients. It has been shown in several studies that the Health Assessment Questionnaire is an excellent predictor of work disability and mortality[153] and can be discrepant from damage measured by radiographs.

MORTALITY

In well-established RA, the median life expectancy is less than in control populations.[154,155] In one study, a 25-year prospective follow-up of 208 patients, the median life expectancy was shortened by 7 years in men and 3 years in women. Infection, renal disease, and respiratory failure traditionally have been the primary factors contributing to excess mortality in RA patients, although it has been belatedly recognized that congestive heart failure, ischemic heart disease, and peripheral atherosclerosis deserve the appellation as the prime killers of rheumatoid patients. One study published in 1990 revealed that of 100 patients with RA followed for 25 years, 63 had died—an excess mortality of approximately 40%.[156] Although it is apparent that disability develops most rapidly during the first 2 years of RA,[157] the current focus of interest is on this increased mortality.

Careful epidemiologic studies have indicated that, in addition to infection and gastrointestinal hemorrhage secondary to NSAIDs, cardiovascular mortality is increased in RA. In the Norfolk Arthritis Register, a primary care–based inception cohort, patients who were seropositive for RF died within the first 7 years of disease at an excess rate from cardiovascular causes (men 1.34, women 2.02) compared with controls.[158] This increased incidence of cardiovascular events in RA patients is independent of traditional risk factors, such as age, sex, smoking status, diabetes mellitus, hypercholesterolemia, systolic blood pressure, and body mass index.[159] The generally accepted explanation is that inflammatory cytokines that are produced in excess in RA (e.g., TNF-α, platelet-derived growth factor) have the capacity to activate endothelial and subendothelial myofibroblasts, and numerous inflammatory cells are found in atheromatous plaques. Considering that nonrheumatoid patients who have higher levels of C-reactive protein than control groups have higher incidences of coronary disease, these data are consistent with hypotheses. Ultrasonography has shown that RA patients have greater thickness of the common carotid and femoral arteries than do healthy controls, a finding that was independent of glucocorticoid therapy, but related to the duration and severity of RA.[160] Platelet-derived microparticles, the small vesicles that are released from the plasma membrane when these cells are activated, are elevated in RA in proportion to disease activity.[161] As noted earlier, the following factors and pathobiologic mechanisms could contribute to atherosclerosis in RA[162]:

- Immune complex–mediated endothelial damage
- Acute-phase reactants (C-reactive protein and serum amyloid A, both of which have proinflammatory activity)
- Inflammatory cytokines
- High expression of endothelial cell leukocyte adhesion molecules
- Medications (e.g., steroids)
- Prothrombotic factors (e.g., increased platelets, fibrinogen, and thromboxane)
- Endothelial cell dysfunction induced by inflammation

Considerations of therapy in rheumatoid patients must factor in the effects on atherogenesis. These considerations might include, in patients with an unfavorable vascular profile, supplementation with omega-3 fatty acids in the diet, early use of 3-hydroxy-3-methylglutaryl coenzyme A reductase inhibitors (statins that, in addition to lipid-lowering effects, reduce C-reactive protein), attempts to reduce elevated levels of homocysteine induced by methotrexate, avoidance of cyclosporine, and aggressive weight-loss disciplines and smoking cessation. The IL-6 receptor antibody tocilizumab suppresses several risk factors for mortality, including inflammation, elevated ESR, and elevated C-reactive protein. It also alters the lipid profile by increasing low-density lipoproteins, albeit with a concomitant increase in high density lipoproteins to maintain a similar ratio. The ultimate effects on cardiovascular risk factors and mortality are still uncertain under these circumstances.

In addition to cardiovascular causes of death associated with RA are causes of death due to the complications (articular and extra-articular) of RA and to side effects of therapy. The probability of death varies directly with the severity of complications. Potentially morbid articular complications include the various forms of atlantoaxial subluxation, cricoarytenoid synovitis, and sepsis of involved joints. Extra-articular complications directly causing a higher mortality include Felty's syndrome, Sjögren's syndrome, pulmonary complications, and diffuse vasculitis.

One of the largest and best-documented studies of survival, prognosis, and causes of death in RA was published by Mitchell and associates.[163] In this prospective study of 805 patients including 12 years of observation, 233 died during the course of the study; survivorship was only 50% of that in population controls. The increased mortality associated with RA is impressive and equals that of all patients with Hodgkin's disease, diabetes mellitus, or stroke (age adjusted). In another group of 107 patients followed for 8 years, each of whom had extra-articular disease or needed hospitalization for some aspect of the disease,[164] patients with cutaneous ulcers, vasculitic rash, neuropathy, and scleritis had a higher mortality than patients whose disease was confined to joints. Of great concern to all health care workers is the correlation of a lack of formal education with increased mortality in RA.[165]

One prediction is that tight control of inflammation might decrease the cardiovascular and cerebrovascular events and improve survival. Although the data remain preliminary, it seems that aggressive use of methotrexate can decrease mortality in patients.[166] Biologic agents such as TNF inhibitors also seem to improve survival, especially in women.[167] TNF blockade exacerbates heart disease, however, and increases mortality in individuals with preexisting congestive heart failure. Longer term studies are required to assess the impact of new agents such as rituximab and abatacept on mortality (see Chapter 59).

VARIABLES RELATED TO PROGNOSIS

In attempting to sort out the relative roles of disease manifestations, compared with nondisease factors, in generating disability in RA, investigators have generated hypothetical models of the disablement process in RA using the demographic, sociocultural, and clinical characteristics of a consecutive cohort of RA patients.[168] Although their methods were unable to explain the dynamics of disability in 41% of cases, disease-related factors explained 33%, and nondisease factors (e.g., depression and psychological status, education) accounted for 26% of the disability. Other studies have emphasized the following disease factors that correlate with a poorer prognosis and greater likelihood of joint destruction:

- Positive RF in serum[169]
- Positive anticitrullinated protein in serum
- Rheumatoid nodules[170]
- Elevated Health Assessment Questionnaire level of disability[171]
- Depression[172]
- Persistent ESR elevation (serving as a surrogate for disease control)
- Presence of the shared epitope (QKRAA) on class II major histocompatibility genes

ASSESSMENT OF THE INDIVIDUAL PATIENT

Assessment of disease activity and its progression is different from prognosis. Prognosis extrapolates from a known set of indices (as noted earlier) and the degree of measured activity of disease to a prediction of the outcome. Assessment is the accurate evaluation of disease progression over time. Although the indices listed in the previous section are useful as a way to predict the outcome from one-time measurements, having three or more assessment measures provides the physician with a graph of progression in an individual patient that he or she can try to flatten out by therapy.[173] Whatever assessment index is used, it should be used for the first time early in the patient's disease so that values before a significant loss of function are recorded.

For most patients, a self-report questionnaire based on degrees of difficulty in performing activities of daily living correlates well with the joint count, radiographic score, acute-phase reactants, grip strength, walking time, functional class estimates, and global self-assessment. One useful self-report includes only eight items from the much longer Stanford Health Assessment Questionnaire (Table 66-7).[174] The limitation of this form—failure to detect clinical improvement in patients with few impairments in activities of daily living—may be offset by its acceptability to patients within busy office practices.

In some situations, more comprehensive joint counts are needed. These include points when large changes in drug therapy are about to be instituted, and when patients are to undergo joint reconstruction by orthopaedic or hand surgeons. The Thompson index[175] uses a few joints and weights data from each joint to reflect the joint surface area, giving a better measure of the "burden of synovitis."

The choice of imaging techniques and measures is important in the assessment of the destructive lesions of RA. The inflammatory lesion in RA is reflected reasonably well by heat, pain, swelling, and tenderness. Joint destruction can occur with minimal inflammation, however. MRI and ultrasound provide ways to visualize pannus development and the loss of cartilage (see Chapter 53). It is paramount that rheumatologists and radiologists come to a consensus on cost-benefit analyses for MRI. For which patients is it appropriate to order this procedure?

In each patient, when the diagnosis of RA is reasonably certain, these measures of assessment and estimates of prognosis should be recorded. They should be major determinants of what therapies are instituted. Therapy is discussed in the following chapter.

Table 66-7 Activities of Daily Living and Visual Analog Questionnaire

A. How often is it PAINFUL for you to:	Never	Sometimes	Most of the Time	Always
Dress yourself?	_____	_____	_____	_____
Get in and out of bed?	_____	_____	_____	_____
Lift a cup or glass to your lips?	_____	_____	_____	_____
Walk outdoors on flat ground?	_____	_____	_____	_____
Wash and dry your entire body?	_____	_____	_____	_____
Bend down to pick up clothing from the floor?	_____	_____	_____	_____
Turn faucets on or off?	_____	_____	_____	_____
Get in and out of a car?	_____	_____	_____	_____

B. How much pain have you had in the PAST WEEK (mark the scale)	
No pain_____	Pain as bad as it could be
0	100

From Callahan LF, Brooks RH, Summey JA, et al: Quantitative pain assessment for routine care of rheumatoid arthritis patients, using a pain scale based on activities of daily living and a visual analog pain scale. Arthritis Rheum 30:630, 1987.

REFERENCES

1. Wolfe AM: The epidemiology of rheumatoid arthritis: A review, I: Surveys. Bull Rheum Dis 19:518-523, 1968.
2. Engel A, Roberts J, Burch TA: Rheumatoid arthritis in adults in the United States, 1960-1962. In Vital and Health Statistics, Series 11, Data from the National Health Survey, Number 17. Washington, DC, National Center for Health Statistics, 1966.
3. Mikkelsen WM, Dodge HJ, Duff IF, et al: Estimates of the prevalence of rheumatic disease in the population of Tecumseh, Michigan, 1959-1960. J Chronic Dis 20:351-369, 1967.
4. Gabriel SE, Crowson CS, O'Fallon WM: The epidemiology of rheumatoid arthritis in Rochester, Minn, 1955-1985. Arthritis Rheum 42:415-420, 1989 (abstract 1950).
5. Linos A, Worthington JW, O'Fallon WM, et al: The epidemiology of rheumatoid arthritis in Rochester, Minnesota: A study of incidence, prevalence and mortality. Am J Epidemiol 111:87-98, 1980.
6. Doran MF, Pond GR, Crowson CS, et al: Trends in incidence and mortality in rheumatoid arthritis in Rochester, Minnesota, over a forty-year period. Arthritis Rheum 46:625-631, 2002.
7. **Silman AJ: The changing face of rheumatoid arthritis: Why the decline in incidence. Arthritis Rheum 46:579-581, 2002.**
8. Peschken CA, El-Gabalawy HS, Roos LL, et al: Algonquin Indians have twice the frequency of rheumatoid arthritis with a younger age of onset. Arthritis Rheum 41(Suppl 9):558, 1998 (abstract).
9. Enzer I, Dunn G, Jacobsson L: An epidemiologic study of trends in prevalence of rheumatoid factor seropositivity in Pima Indians. Arthritis Rheum 46:1729-1734, 2002.
10. Yelin E, Wanke LA: An assessment of the annual and long-term direct costs of rheumatoid arthritis: The impact of poor function and functional decline. Arthritis Rheum 42:1209-1218, 1999.
11. Wong JB, Ramey DR, Singh G: Long-term morbidity, mortality and economics of rheumatoid arthritis. Arthritis Rheum 44:2746-2749, 2001.
12. Jacoby RK, Jayson MI, Cosh JA: Onset, early stages, and prognosis of rheumatoid arthritis: A clinical study of 100 patients with 11-year follow-up. BMJ 2:96-100, 1973.
13. Aho K, Palosuo T, Raunio V, et al: When does rheumatoid disease start? Arthritis Rheum 28:485-489, 1985.
14. Fleming A, Crown JM, Corbett M: Early rheumatoid disease, I: Onset. Ann Rheum Dis 35:357-360, 1976.
15. Fleming A, Benn RT, Corbett M, et al: Early rheumatoid disease, II: Patterns of joint involvement. Ann Rheum Dis 35:361-364, 1976.
16. Mens JM: Correlation of joint involvement in rheumatoid arthritis and in ankylosing spondylitis with the synovial:cartilaginous surface ratio of various joints. Arthritis Rheum 30:359-360, 1987 (letter).
17. van Aken J, van Dongen H, le Cessie S, et al: Comparison of long term outcome of patients with rheumatoid arthritis presenting with undifferentiated arthritis or with rheumatoid arthritis: An observational cohort study. Ann Rheum Dis 65:20-25, 2006.
18. **van der Helm-van Mil AH, Verpoort KN, le Cessie S, et al: The HLA-DRB1 shared epitope alleles differ in the interaction with smoking and predisposition to antibodies to cyclic citrullinated peptide. Arthritis Rheum 56:425-432, 2007.**
19. Nell VP, Machold KP, Stamm TA, et al: Autoantibody profiling as early diagnostic and prognostic tool for rheumatoid arthritis. Ann Rheum Dis 64:1731-1736, 2005.
20. Hench PS, Rosenberg EF: Palindromic rheumatism: New oft-recurring disease of joints (arthritis, periarthritis, para-arthritis) apparently producing no articular residues—report of 34 cases. Proc Mayo Clin 16:808, 1942.
21. Guerne P-A, Weisman MH: Palindromic rheumatism: Part of or apart from the spectrum of rheumatoid arthritis. Am J Med 93:451-460, 1992.
22. Schumacher HR: Palindromic onset of rheumatoid arthritis: Clinical, synovial fluid, and biopsy studies. Arthritis Rheum 25:361-369, 1982.
23. Youssef W, Yan A, Russell AS: Palindromic rheumatism: A response to chloroquine. J Rheumatol 18:35-37, 1991.
24. Khanna D, Ranganath VK, FitzGerald J, et al: Increased radiographic damage scores at the onset of seropositive rheumatoid arthritis in older patients are associated with osteoarthritis of the hands, but not with more rapid progression of damage. Arthritis Rheum 52:2284-2293, 2005.
25. Yoghmai I, Rooholamini SM, Faunce HF: Unilateral rheumatoid arthritis: Protective effects of neurologic deficits. AJR Am J Roentgenol 128:299-301, 1977.
26. De Haas WHD, de Boer W, Griffioen F, et al: Rheumatoid arthritis of the robust reaction type. Ann Rheum Dis 33:81-85, 1974.
27. Maldonado I, Eid H, Rodriguez GR, et al: Rheumatoid nodulosis: Is it a different subset of rheumatoid arthritis? J Clin Rheumatol 9:296-395, 2003.
28. Smith PH, Benn RT, Sharp J: Natural history of rheumatoid cervical luxations. Ann Rheum Dis 31:431-439, 1972.
29. Collins DN, Barnes CL, FitzRandolph RL: Cervical spine instability in rheumatoid patients having total hip or knee arthroplasty. Clin Orthop 272:127-135, 1991.
30. Agarwal AK, Peppelman WC, Kraus DR, et al: Recurrence of cervical spine instability in rheumatoid arthritis following previous fusion: Can disease progression be prevented by early surgery? J Rheumatol 19:1364-1370, 1992.
31. Goupille P, Fouquet B, Cotty P, et al: The temporomandibular joint in rheumatoid arthritis: Correlations between clinical and computed tomography features. J Rheumatol 17:1285-1291, 1990.
32. Lawry GV, Finerman ML, Hanafee WN, et al: Laryngeal involvement in rheumatoid arthritis: A clinical, laryngoscopic, and computerized tomographic study. Arthritis Rheum 27:873-882, 1984.
33. Moffat DA, Ramsden RT, Rosenberg JN, et al: Otoadmittance measurements in patients with rheumatoid arthritis. J Laryngol Otol 91:917-927, 1977.
34. Ennevaara K: Painful shoulder joint in rheumatoid arthritis: A clinical and radiological study of 200 cases, with special reference to arthrography of the glenohumeral joint. Acta Rheumatol Scand 11:1-116, 1967.
35. Huston KA, Nelson AM, Hunder GG: Shoulder swelling in rheumatoid arthritis secondary to subacromial bursitis. Arthritis Rheum 21:145-147, 1978.

36. Hastings DE, Evans JA: Rheumatoid wrist deformities and their relation to ulnar drift. J Bone Joint Surg Am 57:930-934, 1975.

37. Trentham DE, Masi AT: Carpometacarpal ratio: A new quantitative measure of radiologic progression of wrist involvement in rheumatoid arthritis. Arthritis Rheum 19:939-944, 1976.

38. Fuchs HA, Callahan LF, Kaye JJ, et al: Radiographic and joint count findings of the hand in rheumatoid arthritis: Related and unrelated findings. Arthritis Rheum 31:44-51, 1988.

39. Brewerton DA: Hand deformities in rheumatoid disease. Ann Rheum Dis 16:183-197, 1957.

40. Abbott GT, Bucknall RC, Whitehouse GH: Osteoarthritis associated with distal interphalangeal joint involvement in rheumatoid arthritis. Skeletal Radiol 20:495-497, 1991.

41. Gray RG, Gottlieb NL: Hand flexor tenosynovitis in rheumatoid arthritis: Prevalence, distribution, and associated rheumatic features. Arthritis Rheum 20:1003-1008, 1977.

42. Hastings DE, Parker SM: Protrusio acetabuli in rheumatoid arthritis. Clin Orthop 108:76-83, 1975.

43. Jayson MIV, Dixon A: Valvular mechanisms in juxta-articular cysts. Ann Rheum Dis 29:415-420, 1970.

44. Hench PK, Reid RT, Reames PM: Dissecting popliteal cyst stimulating thrombophlebitis. Ann Intern Med 64:1259-1264, 1966.

45. Kraag G, Thevathasan EM, Gordon DA, et al: The hemorrhagic crescent sign of acute synovial rupture. Ann Intern Med 85:477-478, 1976 (letter).

46. Rask MR: Achilles tendon rupture owing to rheumatoid disease: Case report with a nine-year follow-up. JAMA 239:435-436, 1978.

47. Bienenstock H: Rheumatoid plantar synovial cysts. Ann Rheum Dis 34:98-99, 1975.

48. Calabro JJ: A critical evaluation of the diagnostic features of the feet in rheumatoid arthritis. Arthritis Rheum 5:19-29, 1962.

49. Halla JT, Schrohenloher RE, Koopman WJ: Local immune responses in certain extra-articular manifestations of rheumatoid arthritis. Ann Rheum Dis 51:698-701, 1992.

50. **Turesson C, O'Fallon WM, Crowson CS, et al: Occurrence of extra-articular disease manifestations is associated with excess mortality in a community based cohort of patients with rheumatoid arthritis. J Rheumatol 29:62-67, 2002.**

51. Haugeberg G, Ørstavik RE, Uhlig T: Bone loss in patients with rheumatoid arthritis: Results from a population-based cohort of 366 patients followed up for two years. Arthritis Rheum 46:1720-1728, 2002.

52. Manolagas SC, Weinstein RS: Perspective: New developments in the pathogenesis and treatment of steroid-induced osteoporosis. J Bone Mineral Res 14:1061-1066, 1999.

53. Laan RF, van Riel PL, van de Putte LB, et al: Low-dose prednisone induces rapid reversible axial bone loss in patients with rheumatoid arthritis: A randomized, controlled study. Ann Intern Med 119:963-968, 1993.

54. Maddison PJ, Bacon PA: Vitamin D deficiency, spontaneous fractures and osteopenia in rheumatoid arthritis. BMJ 4:433-435, 1974.

55. Halla JT, Koopman WJ, Fallahi S, et al: Rheumatoid myositis: Clinical and histologic features and possible pathogenesis. Arthritis Rheum 27:737-743, 1984.

56. Wolf P, Gretler J, Aglas F, et al: Anticardiolipin antibodies in rheumatoid arthritis: Their relation to rheumatoid nodules and cutaneous vascular manifestations. Br J Dermatol 131:48-51, 1994.

57. Jackson CG, Chess RL, Ward JR: A case of rheumatoid nodule formation within the central nervous system and review of the literature. J Rheumatol 11:237-240, 1984.

58. Sokoloff L: The pathophysiology of peripheral blood vessels in collagen diseases. In Orbison JL, Smith DE (eds): The Peripheral Blood Vessels. Baltimore, Williams & Wilkins, 1963, p 297.

59. Palmer DG, Hogg N, Highton J, et al: Macrophage migration and maturation within rheumatoid nodules. Arthritis Rheum 30:728-736, 1987.

60. Edwards JCW, Wilkinson LS, Pitsillides AA: Palisading cells of rheumatoid nodules: Comparison with synovial intimal cells. Ann Rheum Dis 52:801-805, 1993.

61. Harris ED Jr: A collagenolytic system produced by primary cultures of rheumatoid nodule tissue. J Clin Invest 51:2973-2976, 1972.

62. Ginsberg MH, Genant HK, Yu TF, et al: Rheumatoid nodulosis: An unusual variant of rheumatoid disease. Arthritis Rheum 18:49-58, 1975.

63. Baum J: Infection in rheumatoid arthritis. Arthritis Rheum 14:135-137, 1971.

64. Huskisson EC, Hart FD: Severe, unusual and recurrent infections in rheumatoid arthritis. Ann Rheum Dis 31:118-121, 1972.

65. Singleton JD, West SG, Nordstrom DM: "Pseudoseptic" arthritis complicating rheumatoid arthritis: A report of six cases. J Rheumatol 18:1319-1322, 1991.

66. Doran MF, Crowson CS, Pond GR, et al: Frequency of infection in patients with rheumatoid arthritis compared with controls. Arthritis Rheum 46:2287-2293, 2002.

67. **Doran MF, Crowson CS, Pond GR: Predictors of infection in rheumatoid arthritis. Arthritis Rheum 46:2294-2300, 2002.**

68. Samet JM: Does idiopathic pulmonary fibrosis increase lung cancer risk? Am J Respir Crit Care Med 161:1-2, 2000.

69. Gridley G, McLaughlin JK, Ekbom A, et al: Incidence of cancer among patients with rheumatoid arthritis. J Natl Cancer Inst 85:307-311, 1993.

70. Gridley G, Klippel JH, Hoover RN, et al: Incidence of cancer among men with the Felty syndrome. Ann Intern Med 120:35-39, 1994.

71. Ongartz T, Sutton AJ, Sweeting MJ, et al: Anti-TNF antibody therapy in rheumatoid arthritis and the risk of serious infections and malignancies: Systematic review and meta-analysis of rare harmful effects in randomized controlled trials. JAMA 295:2275-2285, 2006.

72. Stone JH, Holbrook JT, Marriott MA, et al: Wegener's Granulomatosis Etanercept Trial Research Group. Solid malignancies among patients in the Wegener's Granulomatosis Etanercept Trial. Arthritis Rheum 54:1608-1618, 2006.

73. Peeters HRM, Jongen-Lavrencic M, Raja AN, et al: Course and characteristics of anaemia in patients with rheumatoid arthritis of recent onset. Ann Rheum Dis 55:162-168, 1996.

74. Vreugdenhil G, Wognum AW, van Eijk HG, et al: Anaemia in rheumatoid arthritis: The role of iron, vitamin B12, and folic acid deficiency, and erythropoietin responsiveness. Ann Rheum Dis 49:93-98, 1990.

75. Williams RA, Samson D, Tikerpae J, et al: In-vitro studies of ineffective erythropoiesis in rheumatoid arthritis. Am J Rheum Dis 41:502-507, 1982.

76. Reid CD, Prouse PJ, Baptista LC, et al: The mechanism of anaemia in rheumatoid arthritis: Effects of bone marrow adherent cells and of serum on in vivo erythropoiesis. Br J Haematol 58:607-615, 1984.

77. Farr M, Scott DL, Constable TJ, et al: Thrombocytosis of active rheumatoid disease. Ann Rheum Dis 42:545-549, 1983.

78. **Bowman SJ, Sivakumaran M, Snowden N, et al: The large granular lymphocyte syndrome with rheumatoid arthritis: Immuno-genetic evidence for a broader definition of Felty's syndrome. Arthritis Rheum 37:1326-1330, 1994.**

79. Combe B, Andary M, Caraux J, et al: Characterization of an expanded subpopulation of large granular lymphocytes in a patient with rheumatoid arthritis. Arthritis Rheum 29:672-679, 1986.

80. McEwen C, Lingg C, Kirsner JB: Arthritis accompanying ulcerative colitis. Am J Med 33:923, 1962.

81. Loughran TP Jr: Clonal diseases of large granular lymphocytes. Blood 82:1-14, 1993.

82. Kelly C, Baird G, Foster H, et al: Prognostic significance of paraproteinaemia in rheumatoid arthritis. Ann Rheum Dis 50:290-294, 1991.

83. Voskuyl AE, Zwinderman AH, Westedt ML, et al: Factors associated with the development of vasculitis in rheumatoid arthritis: Results of a case-control study. Ann Rheum Dis 55:190-192, 1996.

84. Fischer M, Mielke H, Glaefke S, et al: Generalized vasculopathy and finger blood flow abnormalities in rheumatoid arthritis. J Rheumatol 11:33-37, 1984.

85. Soter NA, Mihm MC Jr, Gigli I, et al: Two distinct cellular patterns in cutaneous necrotizing angiitis. J Invest Dermatol 66:344-350, 1976.

86. Mongan ES, Cass RM, Jacox RF, et al: A study of the relation of seronegative and seropositive rheumatoid arthritis to each other and to necrotizing vasculitis. Am J Med 47:23-25, 1969.

87. Weinstein A, Peters K, Brown D, et al: Metabolism of the third component of complement (C3) in patients with rheumatoid arthritis. Arthritis Rheum 15:49-56, 1972.

88. Conn DL, McDuffie FC, Dyck PJ: Immunopathologic study of sural nerves in rheumatoid arthritis. Arthritis Rheum 15:135-143, 1972.

89. Schmid FR, Cooper NS, Ziff M, et al: Arteritis in rheumatoid arthritis. Am J Med 30:56-83, 1961.

90. Geirsson AJ, Sturfelt G, Truedsson L: Clinical and serological features of severe vasculitis in rheumatoid arthritis: Prognostic implications. Ann Rheum Dis 46:727-733, 1987.

91. Voskkuyl AE, Zwinderman AH, Westedt ML, et al: The mortality of rheumatoid vasculitis compared with rheumatoid arthritis. Arthritis Rheum 39:266-271, 1996.

92. Dodson WH, Hollingsworth JW: Pleural effusion in rheumatoid arthritis: Impaired transport of glucose. N Engl J Med 275:1337-1342, 1966.
93. Frank ST, Weg JG, Harkleroad LE, et al: Pulmonary dysfunction in rheumatoid disease. Chest 63:27-34, 1973.
94. Tishler M, Grief J, Fireman E, et al: Bronchoalveolar lavage: A sensitive tool for early diagnosis of pulmonary involvement in rheumatoid arthritis. J Rheumatol 13:547-550, 1986.
95. Constantopoulos SH, Tsianos EV, Moutsopoulos HM: Pulmonary and gastrointestinal manifestations of Sjögren's syndrome. Rheum Dis Clin N Am 18:617-635, 1992.
96. Caplan A: Certain unusual radiographic appearances in the chest of coal miners suffering from RA. Thorax 8:29, 1953.
97. Shenberger KN, Schned AR, Taylor TH: Rheumatoid disease and bronchogenic carcinoma: case report and review of the literature. J Rheumatol 11:226-228, 1984.
98. Dawson JK, Goodson NG, Graham DR, et al: Raised pulmonary artery pressures measured with Doppler echocardiography in rheumatoid arthritis patients. Rheumatology 39:1320-1325, 2000.
99. Radoux V, Menard HA, Begin R, et al: Airways disease in rheumatoid arthritis patients: One element of a general exocrine dysfunction. Arthritis Rheum 30:249-259, 1987.
100. Sassoon CS, McAlpine SW, Tashkin DP, et al: Small airways function in non-smokers with rheumatoid arthritis. Arthritis Rheum 27:1218-1226, 1984.
101. Wislowska M, Sypula S, Kowalik I: Echocardiographic findings and 24-hour electrocardiographic Holter monitoring in patients with nodular and non-nodular rheumatoid arthritis. Rheumatol Int 18:163-169, 1999.
102. Del Rincon I, O'Leary DH, Freeman GL, et al: Acceleration of atherosclerosis during the course of rheumatoid arthritis. Atherosclerosis 195:354-360, 2006.
103. Gerli R, Sherer Y Vaudo G, et al: Early atherosclerosis in rheumatoid arthritis: Effects of smoking on thickness of the carotid artery intima media. Ann N Y Acad Sci 1051:281-290, 2005.
104. Nicola PJ, Crowson CS, Maradit-Kremers H, et al: Contribution of congestive heart failure and ischemic heart disease to excess mortality in rheumatoid arthritis. Arthritis Rheum 54:60-67, 2006.
105. Rexhepaj N, Bajraktari G, Berisha I, et al: Left and right ventricular diastolic functions in patients with rheumatoid arthritis without clinically evident cardiovascular disease. Int J Clin Pract 60:683-688, 2006.
106. MacDonald WJ Jr, Crawford MH, Klippel JH, et al: Echocardiographic assessment of cardiac structure and function in patients with rheumatoid arthritis. Am J Med 63:890-896, 1977.
107. Iveson JM, Thadani U, Ionescu M, et al: Aortic valve incompetence and replacement in rheumatoid arthritis. Ann Rheum Dis 34:312-320, 1975.
108. Ahern M, Lever JV, Cosh J: Complete heart block in rheumatoid arthritis. Ann Rheum Dis 42:389-397, 1983.
109. Camilleri JP, Douglas-Jones AG, Pritchard MH: Rapidly progressive aortic valve incompetence in a patient with rheumatoid arthritis. Br J Rheumatol 30:379-381, 1991.
110. Hoffman GS: Polyarthritis: The differential diagnosis of rheumatoid arthritis. Semin Arthritis Rheum 8:115-141, 1978.
111. Pinals RS: Polyarthritis and fever. N Engl J Med 330:769-774, 1994.
112. Bywaters EGL: Still's disease in the adult. Ann Rheum Dis 30:121-133, 1971.
113. Appenzeller S, Castro GR, Costallat LT: Adult-onset Still disease in southeast Brazil. J Clin Rheumatol 11:76-80, 2005.
114. Van Reeth C, Le Moel G, Lasne Y: Serum ferritin and isoferritins are tools for diagnosis of active adult Still's disease. J Rheumatol 21:890-895, 1994.
115. Vignes S, le Moel G, Fautrel B, et al: Percentage of glycosylated serum ferritin remains low throughout the course of adult onset Still's disease. Ann Rheum Dis 59:347-350, 2000.
116. Yamaguchi M, Ohta A, Tsunematsu T, et al: Preliminary criteria for classification of adult Still's disease. J Rheumatol 19:424-430, 1992.
117. Elkon KB, Hughes GR, Bywaters EG, et al: Adult-onset Still's disease: Twenty-year followup and further studies of patients with active disease. Arthritis Rheum 25:647-654, 1982.
118. Cush JJ, Medsger TA Jr, Christy WC, et al: Adult-onset Still's disease: Clinical course and outcome. Arthritis Rheum 30:186-194, 1987.
119. Pascual V, Allantaz F, Arce E, et al: Role of interleukin-1 (IL-1) in the pathogenesis of systemic onset juvenile idiopathic arthritis and clinical response to IL-1 blockade. J Exp Med 201:1479-1486, 2005.
120. Davies PG, Fordham JN: Arthritis and angioimmunoblastic lymphadenopathy. Ann Rheum Dis 42:516-518, 1983.
121. Fallet GH, Mason M, Berry H, et al: Rheumatoid arthritis and ankylosing spondylitis occurring together. BMJ 1:804-807, 1976.
122. Chamot AM, Benhamou CL, Kahn MF, et al: Le syndrome acne pustulose hyperostose osteite (SAPHO)—85 observations. Rev Rhum Mal Osteoartic 54:187-196, 1987.
123. McEwen C, Lingg C, Kirsner JB: Arthritis accompanying ulcerative colitis. Am J Med 33:923, 1962.
124. Zizic TM, Stevens MB: The arthropathy of Behçet's disease. Johns Hopkins Med J 136:243-250, 1975.
125. Bland JH, Frymoyer JW: Rheumatic syndromes of myxedema. N Engl J Med 282:1171-1174, 1970.
126. Churchill MD Jr, Geraci JE, Hunder GG: Musculoskeletal manifestations of bacterial endocarditis. Ann Intern Med 87:754-759, 1977.
127. Utsinger PD, Zvaifler NJ, Resnick D: Calcium pyrophosphate dihydrate deposition disease without chondrocalcinosis. J Rheumatol 2:258-264, 1975.
128. Martin JR, Huang SN, Lacson A, et al: Congenital contractural deformities of the fingers and arthropathy. Ann Rheum Dis 44:826-830, 1985.
129. Wolfe F, Cathey MA, Kleinkeksel SM, et al: Psychological status in primary fibrositis and fibrositis associated with rheumatoid arthritis. J Rheumatol 11:500-506, 1984.
130. Kozin F, McCarty DJ: Rheumatoid factor in the serum of gouty patients. Arthritis Rheum 20:1559-1560, 1977.
131. McDonnell SM, Preston BL, Jewell SA, et al: A survey of 2851 patients with hemochromatosis: Symptoms and response to treatment. Am J Med 106:619-624, 1999.
132. Schumacher HR, Dorwart BB, Bond J, et al: Chronic synovitis with early cartilage destruction in sickle cell disease. Ann Rheum Dis 36:413-419, 1977.
133. DeCeulaer K, Forbes M, Roper D, et al: Non-gouty arthritis in sickle cell disease: Report of 37 consecutive cases. Ann Rheum Dis 43:599-603, 1984.
134. Calabrese LH: Human immunodeficiency virus infection and arthritis. Rheum Dis Clin N Am 19:477-488, 1993.
135. Solomon G, Brancato L, Winchester R: An approach to the human immunodeficiency virus-positive patient with a spondyloarthropathic disease. Rheum Dis Clin N Am 17:43-58, 1991.
136. Schumacher HR, Gall EP: Arthritis in acute hepatitis and chronic active hepatitis: Pathology of the synovial membrane with evidence for the presence of Australia antigen in synovial membranes. Am J Med 57:655-664, 1974.
137. Lee YH, Ji JD, Yeon JE, et al: Cryoglobulinaemia and rheumatic manifestations in patients with hepatitis C virus infection. Ann Rheum Dis 57:728-731, 1998.
138. Wener MH, Hutchinson K, Morishima C, et al: Absence of antibodies to cyclic citrullinated peptide in sera of patients with hepatitis C virus infection and cryoglobulinemia. Arthritis Rheum 50:2305-2308, 2004.
139. Kremer JM, Alarcon GS, Lightfoot RWJ, et al: Methotrexate for rheumatoid arthritis: Suggested guidelines for monitoring liver toxicity. Arthritis Rheum 37:316-328, 1994.
140. Hasunuma T, Tadanobu M, Hoa TTM, et al: Tenosynovial nodulosis in a patient infected with human T cell lymphotropic virus I. Arthritis Rheum 40:578-582, 1997.
141. Von Kempis J, Kohler G, Herbst EW, et al: Intravascular lymphoma presenting as symmetric polyarthritis. Arthritis Rheum 41:1126-1130, 1998.
142. Gold RH, Metzger AL, Mirra JM, et al: Multicentric reticulohistiocytosis (lipoid dermato-arthritis): An erosive polyarthritis with distinctive clinical, roentgenographic and pathological features. AJR Am J Roentgenol 124:610-624, 1975.
143. Winchester RJ, Koffler D, Litwin SD, et al: Observations on the eosinophilia of certain patients with rheumatoid arthritis. Arthritis Rheum 14:650-665, 1971.
144. Ordenstein L: Sur la Paralysie Agitante et la Sclérose en Plaques Generalisée. Paris, Imprimerie de E Martinet, 1864.
145. Ginsburg WW, Cohen MD, Hall SB, et al: Seronegative polyarthritis in giant cell arteritis. Arthritis Rheum 28:1362-1366, 1985.
146. Russell EB: Remitting seronegative symmetrical synovitis with pitting edema syndrome: Followup for neoplasia. J Rheumatol 32:1760-1761, 2005.

147. Bywaters EGL: Relation between heart and joint disease including "rheumatoid heart disease" and chronic post-rheumatic arthritis (type Jaccoud). Br Heart J 12:101-131, 1950.

148. Poncet A: Address to the Congress Français de Chirurgie, 1897. Bull Acad Med Paris 46:194, 1901.

149. Relman DA, Schmidt TM, MacDermott RP, et al: Identification of the uncultured bacillus of Whipple's disease. N Engl J Med 372:293, 1992.

150. Pinals RS, Masi AT, Larsen RA: Preliminary criteria for clinical remission in rheumatoid arthritis. Arthritis Rheum 24:1308-1315, 1981.

151. van der Helm- van Mil AH, Breedveld FC, Huizinga TW: Aspects of early arthritis: Definition of disease states in early arthritis: Remission versus minimal disease activity. Arthritis Res Ther 8:21, 2006.

152. Bukhari M, Lunt M, Harrison BJ, et al: Rheumatoid factor is the major predictor of increasing severity of radiographic erosions in rheumatoid arthritis. Arthritis Rheum 46:906-912, 2002.

153. Pincus T: Why should rheumatologists collect patient self-report questionnaires in routine rheumatologic care? Rheum Dis Clin N Am 21:271-319, 1995.

154. Pinals RS: Survival in rheumatoid arthritis. Arthritis Rheum 30:473-475, 1987.

155. Vandenbroucke JP, Hazevoet HM, Cats A: Survival and cause of death in rheumatoid arthritis: A 25-year prospective followup. J Rheumatol 11:158-161, 1984.

156. Reilly PA, Cosh JA, Maddison PJ, et al: Mortality and survival in rheumatoid arthritis: A 25-year prospective study of 100 patients. Ann Rheum Dis 49:363-369, 1990.

157. Kirwan JR: The relationship between synovitis and erosions in rheumatoid arthritis. Br J Rheumatol 36:225-228, 1997.

158. Goodson NJ, Wiles NJ, Lunt M, et al: Mortality in early inflammatory polyarthritis: Cardiovascular mortality is increased in seropositive patients. Arthritis Rheum 46:2010-2019, 2002.

159. del Rincón I, Williams R, Stern MP, et al: High incidence of cardiovascular events in a rheumatoid arthritis cohort not explained by traditional cardiac risk factors. Arthritis Rheum 44:2737-2745, 2001.

160. Kumeda Y, Inaba M, Goto H, et al: Increased thickness of the arterial intima-media detected by ultrasonography in patients with rheumatoid arthritis. Arthritis Rheum 46:1489-1497, 2002.

161. Knijff-Dutmen EAJ, Koerts J, Nieuwland R, et al: Elevated levels of platelet microparticles are associated with disease activity in rheumatoid arthritis. Arthritis Rheum 46:1498-1503, 2002.

162. Van Doornum S, McColl G, Wicks IP: Accelerated atherosclerosis: An extraarticular feature of rheumatoid arthritis? Arthritis Rheum 46:862-873, 2002.

163. Mitchell DM, Spitz PW, Young DY, et al: Survival, prognosis, and causes of death in rheumatoid arthritis. Arthritis Rheum 29:706-714, 1986.

164. Erhardt CC, Mumford PA, Venables PJ, et al: Factors predicting a poor life prognosis in rheumatoid arthritis: An eight-year prospective study. Ann Rheum Dis 48:7-13, 1989.

165. Pincus T, Callahan LF, Sale WG, et al: Severe functional declines, work disability, and increased mortality in seventy-five rheumatoid arthritis patients studied over nine years. Arthritis Rheum 27:864-872, 1984.

166. Choi HK, Hernan MA, Seeger JD, et al: Methotrexate and mortality in patients with rheumatoid arthritis: A prospective study. Lancet 359:1173-1177, 2002.

167. Jacobsson LT, Turesson C, Nilsson JA, et al: Treatment with TNF-blockers and mortality risk in patients with rheumatoid arthritis. Ann Rheum Dis 66:670-675, 2007.

168. Escalante A, del Rincon I: How much disability in rheumatoid arthritis is explained by rheumatoid arthritis? Arthritis Rheum 42:1712-1721, 1999.

169. Masi AT, Maldonado-Cocco JA, Kaplan SB, et al: Prospective study of the early course of rheumatoid arthritis in young adults: Comparison of patients with and without rheumatoid factor positivity at entry and identification of variables correlating with outcome. Semin Arthritis Rheum 4:299-326, 1976.

170. Sharp JT, Calkins E, Cohen AS, et al: Observations on the clinical, chemical, and serological manifestations of rheumatoid arthritis, based on the course of 154 cases. Medicine 43:41-58, 1964.

171. **Wolfe F, Michaud K, Gefeller O, Choi HK: Predicting mortality in patients with rheumatoid arthritis. Arthritis Rheum. 48:1530-1542, 2003.**

172. Ang DC, Choi H, Kroenke K, et al: Comorbid depression is an independent risk factor for mortality in patients with rheumatoid arthritis. J Rheumatol 32:1013-1019, 2005.

173. Edworthy SM, Bloch DA, Brant RF, et al: Detecting treatment effects in patients with rheumatoid arthritis: The advantage of longitudinal data. J Rheumatol 20:40-44, 1993.

174. Pincus T, Callahan LF, Brooks RH, et al: Self-report questionnaire scores in rheumatoid arthritis compared with traditional physical, radiographic, and laboratory measures. Ann Intern Med 110:259-266, 1989.

175. Thompson PW, Silman A, Kirwan JR, et al: Articular indices of joint inflammation in rheumatoid arthritis. Arthritis Rheum 30:618-625, 1987.

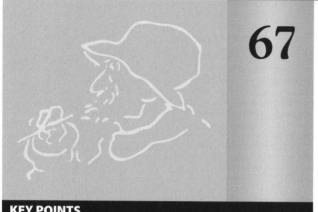

67 Treatment of Rheumatoid Arthritis

MARK C. GENOVESE

KEY POINTS

The initial approach to treatment of rheumatoid arthritis begins with a diagnosis, estimation of the patient's prognosis, and the implementation of a therapeutic plan.

The physician should employ aggressive treatment with disease-modifying antirheumatic drugs.

Combination therapies, particularly using methotrexate as the cornerstone, seem to be the most effective.

Biologic agents, particularly when used in combination with methotrexate, offer the greatest ability to slow structural damage.

Useful adjuncts to reduce pain and improve function include glucocorticoids, nonsteroidal anti-inflammatory drugs, and physical and occupational therapy.

The treatment plan should include patient education.

The patient needs to be monitored carefully for the side effects of treatment.

The ultimate goal is to induce remission; however, practical goals are to prevent structural damage, reduce the signs and symptoms of disease, and improve function.

Since the mid-1990s, there have been major changes in the treatment and management of rheumatoid arthritis (RA). Generally, approaches have been aimed at earlier identification of the disease, earlier intervention with disease-modifying antirheumatic drugs (DMARDs), aggressive dosing of existing medications, combination therapy, and the introduction of new classes of therapeutic agents such as protein-based biologic therapies. These changes have resulted in significant improvements for patients with RA, including a reduction in the symptoms and signs of disease, joint preservation and a reduction of structural progression, and an improvement in function and quality of life.

The evolution of the changes in the approach to treatment is based on the great progress investigators in many laboratories have made in understanding basic mechanisms that underlie the development of RA and its perpetuation within joints and throughout the body. In addition, sound epidemiologic studies have provided useful information on the factors that amplify disease in individuals who have it, and well-planned, double-blind, placebo-controlled clinical trials have provided the evidence-based therapy to help guide physicians.

The initial approach to treatment of RA begins with a diagnosis, estimation of the patient's prognosis, and the implementation of a therapeutic plan. It is never too early or too late to initiate treatment. This philosophy epitomizes the importance of initiating therapy at any stage of this disease. When a patient has been diagnosed with RA, or at the very least has features of inflammatory arthritis unattributed to other causes, such as infection, malignancy, or metabolic disease, therapy with DMARDs should be initiated with the goals of preventing or controlling joint damage, preventing loss of function, and decreasing pain.[1] DMARDs are the fundamental treatment for inflammatory arthritis, and all other therapeutic approaches should be considered adjuncts. Optimal therapeutic plans include more than just DMARD therapy, however. The treatment plan also should include patient education; possible consultation with physical therapists, social workers, and occupational therapists[1]; and adjunctive therapies, such as nonsteroidal anti-inflammatory drugs (NSAIDs) and glucocorticoids orally (in low dosages), intramuscularly, or intra-articularly.

DISEASE MODIFICATION THERAPY

Initiating DMARD therapy is paramount in the treatment of RA. The decision of which DMARD or DMARDs to start is less clear, however. In any given patient, any of the DMARDs can be efficacious and well tolerated, but no one DMARD is efficacious and safe in every patient. Few patients experience remission on any DMARDs, and most experience some sort of side effect from the medications prescribed to treat the disease if treated long enough. The American College of Rheumatology (ACR) treatment guidelines for the management of RA provide an important frame of reference from which to guide therapeutic decision making.[1] The ACR treatment guidelines call for a comprehensive approach to the patient with involvement of the primary care provider and the rheumatologist, and provide a general guideline for starting, changing, or adding DMARDs to the treatment of a patient with active disease (Fig. 67-1).

DMARD therapy generally begins with the initiation of therapy with the traditional small molecules, such as methotrexate (MTX), hydroxychloroquine (HCQ), or sulfasalazine (SSZ) (see Chapter 56). These agents are of proven benefit, are generally well tolerated with well-known side-effect profiles, and can be prescribed at a reasonable cost (Table 67-1). Of the three agents, MTX is the most commonly prescribed DMARD. After initiating a DMARD, patients need to be re-evaluated periodically with a goal of strict control of disease activity and monitored for potential side effects from the medications being used.

Although other small molecule treatments exist (e.g., azathioprine, gold salts, penicillamine, cyclosporine) (see Chapter 57), these agents are used infrequently and usually

ACR TREATMENT ALGORITHM

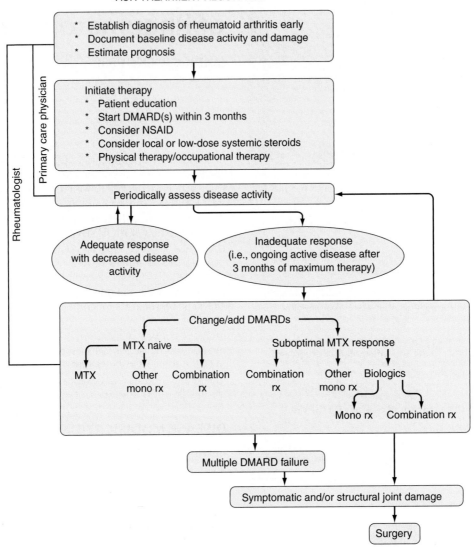

Figure 67-1 A general guide from the American College of Rheumatology (ACR) for the physician after making a diagnosis of rheumatoid arthritis. The general theme of this guideline is adding multiple drugs to basic general care until the disease has been brought under control. Although methotrexate (MTX) has become the mainstay of therapy in rheumatoid arthritis, numerous drugs can be used individually (mono rx) or more commonly added in combination (combination rx) to result in significant improvement. DMARD, disease-modifying antirheumatic drug; NSAID, nonsteroidal anti-inflammatory drug. *(From ACR: Guidelines for the management of rheumatoid arthritis: 2002 update. Arthritis Rheum 46:328-346, 2002.)*

reserved for patients refractory to other therapy or with idiosyncratic side effects with the other agents. After consideration has been given to the use of these traditional small molecule therapies, the practitioner must take stock of the growing efficacy and safety data in the support of the newer generation DMARDs such as leflunomide (see Chapter 56); the tumor necrosis factor (TNF) inhibitors adalimumab, etanercept, and infliximab (see Chapter 58); the interleukin (IL)-1 receptor antagonist anakinra (see Chapter 58); the selective costimulation modulator abatacept (see Chapter 59); and the B cell–targeted approach using rituximab (RTX) (see Chapter 59). These agents have been well studied in clinical trials showing efficacy alone or in combination with traditional therapies. The ability of these agents to slow radiographic progression of disease and restore function seems to be at least equal to, and in some cases greater than, that seen with traditional therapies.

INDIVIDUAL DISEASE-MODIFYING ANTIRHEUMATIC DRUGS

HYDROXYCHLOROQUINE

HCQ is a logical consideration as an agent in patients with mild disease, or as an adjunct to other DMARDs as part of a combination approach in patients with more aggressive disease. There are few side effects, and approximately 40% of patients receive measurable benefit. In the United States, HCQ is used more often than its cousin, chloroquine. When employing dosing schedules not exceeding 400 mg of HCQ each day, few cases of true retinopathy causing visual loss have been reported in the past,[2] providing a measure of reassurance to clinicians about its safety. It has been hypothesized that these antimalarial agents inhibit antigen processing and presentation, leading to downregulation of the CD4+ response in sites of immune damage.[3]

Table 67-1   Average Wholesale Prices of Therapy*

Medication	Cost Per Unit
Disease-Modifying Antirheumatic Drugs	
Methotrexate 2.5-mg tab	$0.30
Hydroxychloroquine 200-mg tab	$1.10
Leflunomide	
10-mg tab	$17.52
20-mg tab	$17.52
Sulfasalazine	
500-mg tablet	$0.13
500 mg EC tablet	$0.38
Biologic Agents	
Etanercept	
25-mg vial	$179.96
50-mg vial	$359.93
Adalimumab 40-mg syringe	$719.86
Infliximab 100-mg vial	$662.68
Abatacept 250-mg vial	$562.50
Rituximab	
100-mg vial	$567.99
500-mg vial	$2839.85
Anakinra 100-mg syringe	$48.16

*Based on the average wholesale price in 2006 Redbook.

It also has been shown that HCQ increases apoptosis of rheumatoid synoviocytes.[4] HCQ has been found to have equal efficacy to SSZ,[5] and as a single agent it was no less effective than the combination of SSZ and HCQ. Strong evidence supporting its utility in early and in mild disease comes from the Hydroxychloroquine in Early Rheumatoid Arthritis (HERA) trial,[6] in which patients with RA were randomly assigned to receive either HCQ or placebo over 36 weeks. At the conclusion of the study, patients who had received HCQ had improvements in joint findings, pain, and physical function superior to what was seen in the placebo group.

After 3 years of follow-up of the original cohorts, the patients who had previously been treated in the HCQ arm of the study continued to have significantly less pain and disability compared with patients who had DMARD therapy delayed for 9 months (the placebo arm). These results could not be explained based on differences in glucocorticoid, DMARD, or nonsteroidal anti-inflammatory drug (NSAID) use after the trial and were attributed to a delay in the introduction of therapy.[7] To date, there are no convincing data on the ability of HCQ to slow radiographic progression, and for patients with active, progressing disease, HCQ would be inadequate as monotherapy. Generally, the mild benefits and the lack of toxicity make HCQ a reasonable agent in early or mild disease, or as an adjunct to other DMARDs in combination therapy.

SULFASALAZINE

SSZ is another DMARD alternative in the treatment of RA (see Chapter 56). In 1942, Svartz[8] reported, in uncontrolled studies, the benefits of SSZ, which she synthesized from salicylic acid and a sulfonamide.[8] The drug was first used by gastroenterologists for treatment of inflammatory bowel disease. The drug is generally thought to be efficacious for the treatment of RA in doses of 2000 to 3000 mg/day. Although allergic reactions and rashes can occur, gastrointestinal complaints tend to be more common; these potentially can be lessened through the use of enteric-coated preparations.

Several studies have established the efficacy of SSZ in RA.[9-11] In early RA, investigators showed that SSZ was superior to placebo in reducing inflammation and clinical disease activity.[9] In a double-blind, randomized trial of 60 patients with RA who had not previously been treated with DMARDs, investigators showed that patients randomly assigned to receive SSZ had significantly less evidence of radiographic progression than did patients treated with HCQ. This difference became apparent at 24 weeks in even this small study, which suggested the possible superiority of SSZ to HCQ as a DMARD.[10]

A study comparing SSZ with leflunomide showed further the utility of SSZ in the treatment of RA.[11] In this double-blind, placebo-controlled study, patients were treated with leflunomide, SSZ, or placebo, and ACR-20 response rates were seen at 24 weeks in 49% (leflunomide), 45% (SSZ), and 29% (placebo) of patients. Leflunomide and SSZ were statistically better than placebo in reducing symptoms and signs of disease. Leflunomide and SSZ were significantly better than placebo at slowing radiographic progression of disease.

Beyond its role early in disease, or in the treatment of mild-to-moderate disease, is the potential role of SSZ in combination therapy. This therapy seems to be efficacious and well tolerated in combination with MTX and HCQ.[12-14]

METHOTREXATE

The question for rheumatologists generally is not whether to use MTX, but rather, in a given patient, whether there are any reasons not to use it. Beginning with uncontrolled trials in the 1970s, and borrowed by rheumatologists from the dermatologists, there has been a gradual increase in acceptance of MTX as the preferred DMARD in the treatment of RA (see Chapter 56). Many factors, now well documented, support this strategy, as follows:

- MTX acts quickly after being started, often within several weeks of the once-weekly dosing schedule.
- Doses can be escalated over time, from the initial levels of approximately 7.5 mg once weekly to more than 25 mg weekly (often given subcutaneously), to achieve efficacy without parallel increases in toxicity.
- MTX is inexpensive (see Table 67-1), and the monitoring necessary for toxicity is less expensive than for gold, penicillamine, other immunosuppressive agents, or cytotoxic drugs.
- MTX can suppress disease activity in a significant proportion of patients with long-standing RA in whom other traditional therapies have failed.[15]
- MTX is well tolerated with more patients likely to be taking MTX than any other nonbiologic DMARD therapy 2 to 5 years after it is first prescribed.[16]
- In addition to providing efficacy in clinical parameters, MTX slows structural damage.[17-20]
- Using MTX as a building block or the cornerstone of combination therapy has resulted in enhanced efficacy over MTX alone, without added increases in side effects.[13,14,21-26]
- There have been minimal unexpected side effects after more than 20 years of surveillance.

In early RA, after 24 months of continued use, MTX is almost as effective as etanercept.[19,20] In other studies versus biologic agents in early disease, MTX is almost as effective as adalimumab or the combination of MTX and infliximab.[25,26] For patients with disease of longer duration, MTX seemed to be equally as effective as leflunomide in head-to-head studies.[27,28]

As a practical matter, it seems that the dose of MTX can be rapidly escalated. Rapid dose escalation from 7.5 mg/wk to 20 mg/wk orally over 8 weeks has become the standard regimen for initiating therapy in early RA trials.[19,20,25,26] This rapid dose escalation is generally well tolerated and has been shown to lead to rapid and sustained benefits in patients receiving MTX.[19,20,25,26] Patients on MTX with persistent disease should have their dose titrated higher (either rapidly or in the more traditional 2.5-mg increments) until they improve, develop side effects, or reach the 20-mg to 25-mg threshold.

For patients unable to tolerate oral MTX, it is reasonable to consider changing to a subcutaneous or intramuscular injection once per week to limit some of the gastrointestinal side effects. Another alternative would be to use folic acid daily or folinic acid weekly as a means to reduce some of the side effects of the medication. Many studies, including one meta-analysis,[29] have reinforced the evidence that folic acid and folinic acid reduce the nausea and mucous membrane ulcerations that are bothersome side effects of the drug; administration of 5 mg of folic acid once weekly seems to be sufficient, although many physicians prescribe 1 mg daily. Another reason to use folic acid in MTX-treated patients is for its effectiveness in reducing plasma homocysteine levels[30]; hyperhomocysteinemia is an independent risk factor for coronary artery disease, presumably mediated by a toxic effect on the endothelium.

Concerns by rheumatologists about liver toxicity of long-term MTX therapy have gradually diminished. Although the ACR guidelines for MTX use[31] are appropriate to follow, it is generally accepted that in patients with normal liver function, minimal use of alcohol, and negative serologies for hepatitis B and C, liver function tests are necessary only once every 4 to 8 weeks. Routine biopsies of the liver, even after many years of continuous therapy, are not required as long as patients are appropriately monitored. If liver function tests suggest hepatocellular inflammation and a decreasing serum albumin despite improvement in the clinical activity of disease, biopsies should be considered if the drug is to be continued.

The other organ threatened by MTX, more in an idiosyncratic or hypersensitivity pattern than liver toxicity, has been the lungs.[32] Reasonable criteria for the diagnosis of MTX-associated pneumonitis are summarized in Chapter 56. The pathology shows interstitial pneumonitis and bronchiolitis. Initial symptoms are often vague and nonspecific—a cough, sometimes with fever and dyspnea. While anticipating such a complication, the physician also must be concerned about and rule out infection with opportunistic organisms. Patients started on MTX must be given guidance and reminded to report any upper respiratory symptoms to the physician.

It also is important to acknowledge that patients with RA are at increased risk for the development of malignancy. Although rare, lymphomas have been associated with the use of MTX, particularly in association with Epstein-Barr virus infection. This topic is discussed further in Chapter 112.

LEFLUNOMIDE

The role of leflunomide in the treatment of RA continues to evolve. It seems to be effective as a monotherapy and safe and effective as an addition to MTX in combination therapy. Leflunomide suppresses the de novo synthesis of pyrimidine (uridine and cytidine) nucleotides by inhibiting dihydroorotate dehydrogenase. T lymphocytes and B lymphocytes have low amounts of this enzyme and no salvage pathways for pyrimidine nucleotide synthesis. The action of leflunomide is specific for lymphocytes (see Chapter 56).[33]

In a trial of leflunomide versus MTX versus placebo, the number of patients achieving an ACR-20 response over the 52-week study was 52% with leflunomide, 46% with MTX, and 26% with placebo.[27] Progression of joint erosions was at a rate significantly slower for leflunomide and MTX than in the placebo group. Assays of quality of life using several instruments, such as the Health Assessment Questionnaire (HAQ),[34] were slightly better for leflunomide than MTX, and both were substantially better than placebo. Regarding adverse events, diarrhea was more common in leflunomide-treated patients, but others were the same as for MTX, including sporadic elevations of parenchymal liver enzymes.

A second multicenter phase III study compared leflunomide head to head with MTX.[28] In this study of 999 patients with RA, both agents showed substantial abilities to improve the symptoms and signs of disease. The improvements seen with MTX at 52 weeks were greater, however, than the improvements with leflunomide. Both drugs were well tolerated, and both led to inhibition of radiographic progression as assessed by radiographs. A third phase III, double-blind, randomized, multicenter trial of leflunomide, placebo, and SSZ in active RA (358 patients) showed that leflunomide was more effective than placebo in treatment, but no more effective than SSZ.[11]

Leflunomide is effective as monotherapy and has the ability to slow the radiographic progression of RA.[35] It is reasonable, however, to consider using leflunomide as an add-on to MTX for patients who have only a partial response to MTX. Starting with 10 mg of leflunomide daily after a loading dose smaller than usual (e.g., 100 mg for the first 2 days) is a reasonable strategy.[23] Based on the results of a 24-week, 263-patient multicenter study, the addition of leflunomide to MTX resulted in 46% of patients achieving an ACR-20 compared with only 24% who had placebo added to background MTX.[23] The rates of liver function test abnormalities, diarrhea, rash, and alopecia all were similar to what had been seen in the prior phase III studies.

Leflunomide has an extended plasma half-life of 15 to 18 days because it binds to plasma proteins; this has led to the recommendation that it be given as a loading dose (100 mg/day for 3 days), followed by doses of 20 mg/day. The extended plasma half-life also means, however, that if a patient has an adverse gastrointestinal event (e.g., nausea, diarrhea) during or after the loading schedule, it may take some time for the symptoms to subside. Alternative dosage schedules have evolved with time and experience with the drug, including the attenuated loading regimen and daily therapy used in the combination trial (100 mg/day for 2 days, then 10 mg/day).[23] Completely avoiding the loading dose also may decrease the likelihood of side effects in some patients, but not negatively affect the efficacy of the drug in the long-term.

In one of the first randomized, placebo-controlled (phase II) studies, leflunomide was more effective than placebo, and it was almost as effective as a 10-mg daily dose as it was as a 20-mg daily dose.[36] The higher dose had disproportionately more skin rash/allergic reactions, gastrointestinal symptoms, weight loss, and reversible alopecia than the 10-mg daily dose. It is reasonable to try the 10-mg daily dose initially, with subsequent escalation to a 20-mg daily dose after safety has been established, or after the patient has failed to achieve adequate response. Maintenance therapy of 10 mg rather than 20 mg daily, or 20 mg every other day because of the long biologic half-life, can be beneficial for some patients. It has been recommended that if serum aspartate transaminase or alanine transaminase increases to twice the upper limits of normal, or if these values are repeatedly mildly abnormal, the leflunomide dose should be reduced and discontinued if these abnormalities persist.

Generally, it is prudent to consider following the same guidelines for monitoring leflunomide that are applied to MTX,[31] including warnings for patients regarding alcohol intake and screening for preexisting hepatitis B and C. Leflunomide can be used anywhere in the treatment algorithm, but generally has been given most commonly to patients instead of MTX when the latter drug is poorly tolerated or contraindicated. It also can be used in combination with MTX in resistant active arthritis.

MINOCYCLINE AND DOXYCYCLINE

Tetracycline derivatives have a capacity to inhibit biosynthesis and activity of matrix metalloproteinases that have a principal role in degrading articular cartilage in RA. The presumed mechanism is through chelation of calcium and zinc molecules, which subsequently leads to altered molecular conformations of proenzymes sufficiently to inactive them.[37,38] Minocycline has mild but definite inhibitory effects on synovial T cell proliferation and cytokine production. Given in a dose of 100 mg daily, moderate improvement in clinical parameters of disease activity was found in patients treated with minocycline more often than in patients given placebo.[39,40]

A study of 46 patients with early RA who had not received systemic glucocorticoids or second-line drugs reported 65% of patients meeting 50% improvement in tender and swollen joints, duration of morning stiffness, and erythrocyte sedimentation rate (ESR),[41] whereas only 13% of the placebo recipients improved similarly over a 6-month period. In 2001, the results of a 2-year trial comparing minocycline with HCQ were published.[42] In this small study of patients with early RA, the patients treated with minocycline were more likely to achieve a 50% improvement than the patients treated with HCQ (60% versus 33%). This study reconfirms the potential utility of minocycline, particularly in early disease.

Although the doses used in the previously described studies do not differ from the doses for patients given

tetracyclines for acne, some bothersome side effects have been noted, including light-headed feelings, vertigo, and, rarely, liver toxicity. More worrisome have been reports of patients who are taking tetracycline derivatives who develop lupus-like syndromes, complete with autoantibodies. Minocycline-induced autoimmune syndrome is characterized by reversible polyarthralgia or arthritis, morning stiffness, fever, frequent skin involvement, occasional chronic active hepatitis, positive tests for antinuclear antibodies, and increased titers of perinuclear antineutrophil cytoplasmic antigen.[43] With proper warning to patients and careful monitoring, however, minocycline seems to be an appropriate drug for use in patients with early synovitis.

Although less studied, there is evidence supporting the use of doxycycline in the treatment of RA. In a trial of patients with early RA, doxycycline plus MTX was compared with the use of MTX alone. Investigators studied low-dose doxycycline (20 mg twice a day) and high-dose doxycycline (100 mg twice a day) in combination with MTX and found that both approaches were superior to MTX alone.[44] Despite the positive results of this study, it was small in number, and the MTX dose was escalated very slowly. It would be important to see these results replicated over time.

GOLD SALTS, PENICILLAMINE, AND AZATHIOPRINE

Three other secondary choices, some of which can be used in combinations with primary choices in active synovitis, are gold salts, penicillamine, and azathioprine. These agents generally would not be favored in early disease and have now been relegated to a role as agents used when other therapies have failed for either lack of efficacy or side effects.

There is ample published evidence that intramuscular gold therapy is beneficial for RA. Early use of gold salt injections may retard progression of joint erosions.[45] In a 48-week, placebo-controlled trial, the addition of intramuscular gold salts to patients with active disease despite the use of MTX resulted in 61% of patients achieving an ACR-20 compared with 30% of patients randomly assigned to placebo, suggesting the effectiveness of the combination of MTX and gold salts.[46] Despite the known benefits, there also is ample evidence that the two intramuscular compounds, gold sodium thiomalate and gold sodium thioglucose, are being used less by rheumatologists because of the need for meticulous monitoring for serious toxicity (e.g., cytopenias, proteinuria) and the costs of administration and monitoring.

HLA-DR3 is found in more patients who develop either thrombocytopenia or nephropathy while taking gold injections.[47] These data must be balanced against the evidence that HLA-DR3 may be associated with a better response to gold therapy.

Auranofin, the triethylphosphine gold compound taken by mouth, has been available since the mid-1980s and continues to search for its niche in treatment strategies. Several issues are clear. Auranofin has different and less severe toxicity than the intramuscular preparations. Cytopenia and proteinuria do not occur, but a bothersome mild enterocolitis that generates diarrhea leads to treatment failure in many cases. Auranofin is less efficacious than MTX, injectable gold, penicillamine, or SSZ.[48] The efficacy of auranofin, although less than the more potent drugs, has been shown,[49] and there is justification for combining it with HCQ, SSZ, or MTX in treating early stages of active synovitis.

Azathioprine, in doses of 1 to 2.5 mg/kg/day, has been used alone and in combination in RA, often as a "steroid-sparing agent." Neutropenia is the most common complication. One factor that leads to early toxicity from azathioprine is heterozygosity for mutant thiopurine methyltransferase alleles. Patients who have this defect (perhaps 10% of the population is at risk) metabolize the drug poorly and are forced to discontinue azathioprine therapy within 1 month because of hematologic side effects.[50] Although unproved, this subset of patients could be the patients who, when azathioprine was added to a stable MTX regimen, developed an acute febrile toxic reaction characterized by fever, leukocytosis, and a cutaneous leukocytoclastic vasculitis.[51]

Initially used with apparent success, penicillamine was found to cause a selective decrease in CD4[+] helper T cells. Although the "go low, go slow" sequence of starting with 125 or 250 mg/day and keeping doses no higher than 750 mg/day resulted in diminished toxicity, there have been sufficient side effects in many patients to discourage the routine use of penicillamine. Perhaps because of genetic differences among patients, the drug has been used with more apparent success and definite enthusiasm in the United Kingdom and Europe. In one study, 5 years in duration, 53% of patients remained on penicillamine, whereas only 34% remained on gold salts, 31% remained on auranofin, and 30% remained on HCQ.[52]

CYCLOSPORINE

Cyclosporine, used by transplantation immunologists for many years to reduce solid organ allograft rejection, inhibits the activation of CD4[+] helper-inducer T lymphocytes by blocking IL-2 and other T helper type 1 cytokine production,[53] and by inhibiting CD40 ligand expression in T lymphocytes.[54] The latter effect prevents T cells from delivering CD40 ligand–dependent signals to B cells. Newer microemulsion forms of cyclosporine are absorbed better and more consistently than older oil-based formulations.

Cyclosporine was first used in Europe in doses (e.g., 10 mg/kg/day) that caused unacceptable declines in renal function. Adding lower doses (2.5 to 5 mg/kg/day) to a stable dose of MTX and decreasing the cyclosporine if the patient's creatinine level increases to more than 30% of initial values have been shown to provide substantial additive benefit over MTX alone.[55] Thirty-six patients (48%) of the cyclosporine/MTX group and 12 patients (16%) of the MTX-alone group achieved 20% improvement according to the ACR criteria. No unacceptable toxicity was observed during an open label extension of the study for 1 year,[56] and similar to several of the other recommended regimens, this therapy seemed to slow radiographic progression of erosions.[57] There is little to be gained by using cyclosporine as monotherapy early in disease, but in patients with RA who have an insufficient response to MTX, cyclosporine is a reasonable alternative to be added.

TACROLIMUS

Similar to cyclosporine, tacrolimus (FK506) has specific effects limited to inhibiting CD4[+] T cell function. The adverse effects of tacrolimus are dose related and similar to cyclosporine. Tacrolimus is not absorbed as readily or consistently as is the microemulsion formulation of cyclosporine. It can be useful in patients for whom cyclosporine is inappropriate, but for whom T cell suppression is desired. It has been shown that some patients who have failed MTX treatment can respond to carefully dose-adjusted tacrolimus.[58] In a large phase III study, 464 patients with active RA were randomly assigned to receive placebo, 2 mg/day of tacrolimus, or 3 mg/day of tacrolimus. At 6 months, the results were disappointing with ACR-20 responses of 10.2%, 18.8%, and 26.8% for each of the treatment groups. Greater than 20% of patients in the tacrolimus arms experienced an increase in serum creatinine of 40% or more at some point in the trial, suggesting that careful monitoring is necessary, and that the risks may not be worth the modest benefits.[59]

TREATMENT STRATEGIES

The question of when to change or to add DMARD therapies in the treatment regimen is a difficult one, and in many cases it can be a matter of individual style. In some cases, it can be a socioeconomic decision, however, based on the costs of therapies (see Table 67-1). In some situations, use of newer DMARDs or biologic agents may be limited by third-party payers, and in most circumstances, they are allowed only after failure of one or more of the standard agents.

When initiating DMARD therapy, most patients are started on traditional small molecules, as outlined earlier, initially as monotherapy or used together in combinations. Data suggest that when given as monotherapy, these agents can be safe and effective. When an approach of careful monitoring and tight control is used, significant results can be obtained even with traditional compounds. Investigators in the United Kingdom randomly assigned patients with RA of less than 5 years' duration to receive intensive outpatient monitoring with a goal of sustained tight control of disease.[60] Patients randomly assigned to intensive control were seen monthly; their disease activity was carefully measured; and if their disease was active, they were offered joint injection with glucocorticoids, and their DMARDs were algorithmically escalated from monotherapy to combination therapy (step-up therapy). The patients in the intensive treatment group had greater improvement in most disease activity variables, including radiographic disease progression, showing that intensive outpatient monitoring with a goal of sustained tight control resulted in better outcomes than when patients are treated with routine care (Fig. 67-2).[60]

Over time, numerous different approaches to DMARD use have materialized, including sequential monotherapy, step-up combination approaches, initial combination therapy, and step-down combination approaches. Each approach has its own merits and is examined more fully subsequently. The ACR guidelines for the management of RA call for a comprehensive approach to the patient, but rely on DMARDs to result in disease modification. The traditional approach has called for sequential monotherapy, reassessment of disease, and change to an alternative DMARD if the patient has inadequate benefit or has adverse side effects. This type of approach was modified further into the "sawtooth" strategy. This approach advocated early DMARD initiation with continual serial use and careful quantitative monitoring of disability. When a patient's

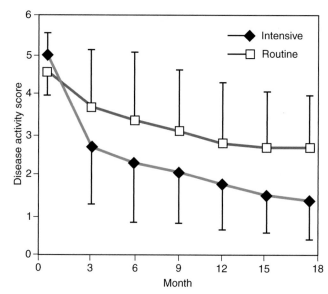

Figure 67-2 The difference in disease activity between patients treated with intensive tight control of rheumatoid arthritis versus patients treated with routine care. *(Adapted with permission from Grigor C, Capell H, Stirling A, et al: Effect of a treatment strategy of tight control for rheumatoid arthritis (the TICORA study): A single-blind randomised controlled trial. Lancet 364:263-269, 2004.)*

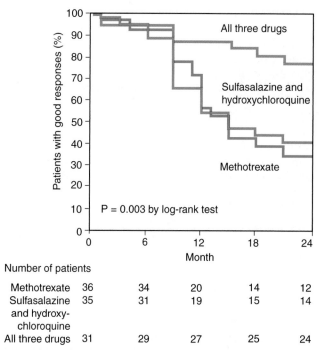

Number of patients				
Methotrexate	36	34	20	14	12
Sulfasalazine and hydroxy-chloroquine	35	31	19	15	14
All three drugs	31	29	27	25	24

Figure 67-3 The benefits of triple therapy over individual therapy with methotrexate or the combination of sulfasalazine and hydroxychloroquine. *(Adapted from O'Dell JR, Haire CE, Erikson N, et al: Treatment of rheumatoid arthritis with methotrexate alone, sulfasalazine and hydroxychloroquine, or a combination of all three medications. N Engl J Med 334: 1287, 1996.)*

disability worsens, there is a sequential change in DMARD therapy in an attempt to decrease disability to prior levels if possible.[61] This strategy has merit because it offers the potential for long-term disease modification, careful monitoring, and a reliance on DMARD approaches over that of analgesics and NSAIDs. This approach has been modified further to include combination approaches as increasing data continue to support the superiority of combinations over sequential monotherapy.

STEPPING AWAY FROM SEQUENTIAL MONOTHERAPY

Another element in the evolving optimism about treatment of RA has been the use of multiple agents in combination therapy, many of which are aimed at a different segment of the pathophysiologic processes within the synovium. Beginning with uncontrolled, but encouraging, results using combination therapy in the early 1980s,[62] it has been shown that a combination of disease-modifying drugs provides additive, perhaps synergistic, benefit to patients without increasing toxicity. Considerable data suggest that many therapies can be used in combination safely and efficaciously. In most cases, MTX has served as the building block on which combination therapy is based.[63,64] Drugs that have shown benefit when combined with MTX include HCQ, SSZ, cyclosporine, leflunomide, anakinra, adalimumab, etanercept, infliximab, abatacept, and rituximab (RTX).

As illustrated earlier, the traditional approach to the management of RA has evolved from a step-up treatment with sequential monotherapy to a step-up combination approach, where initial treatment with MTX is supplemented with a combination of DMARD interventions in patients with an inadequate response. This has become a favored approach among many rheumatologists. Other combination strategies have proved efficacious as well.

The initial use of combinations of DMARDs has significant merit and differs from the step-up approach in that combinations are used initially, rather than waiting for an inadequate response to one or more agents before adding additional agents to the regimen. Supporting this approach to combination therapy are data that "triple therapy"—MTX, SSZ, and HCQ—has been found to be more effective than MTX alone.[13] In a well-done trial, 77% of patients with active RA had a significant improvement on triple therapy compared with 33% of patients started on MTX alone over a 2-year period (Fig. 67-3).[13] A follow-up study to this one showed that the combination of all three agents was superior to MTX plus SSZ or MTX plus HCQ.[65]

The FIN-RACo trial looked further at monotherapy versus combination therapy and showed the utility, if not superiority, of the combination approach over that of monotherapy with traditional DMARD therapy.[14,66] Investigators sought to show that the combination approach with MTX, SSZ, HCQ, and prednisolone would have greater efficacy and tolerability than a single DMARD with or without prednisolone in the treatment of early RA. Ninety-seven patients were treated with combination therapy, and 98 patients were treated with a single DMARD. The primary outcome of the study was the induction of remission. At the end of 1 year, 24 of 97 patients in the combination arm met the definition of remission compared with 11 of 98 in the single DMARD arm. At 2 years, the remission rate was twice as high in the combination approach with a similar frequency of adverse events seen in both arms.

A further approach to combination therapy was first proposed by Wilske and Healey in 1989.[67] These authors proposed the "step-down bridge" approach, which advocated initial use of prednisone for the first month, a combination of DMARDs, and then an attempt to taper the multiple DMARDs to a single agent. This approach did not become more mainstream, however, until 1997 and the publication of the COBRA trial.[12] In the COBRA trial, patients were randomly assigned to receive monotherapy with SSZ or combination therapy in a step-down approach with SSZ, MTX, and high-dose glucocorticoids (Fig. 67-4). At the end of 28 weeks, there seemed to be a significant advantage for the use of the step-down combination therapy based on clinical response, and at 1 year, there also was less radiographic progression in the combination group than seen in the monotherapy group.[12] Perhaps of even greater interest is the 4-year follow-up data from this cohort. The patients who had been treated with the initial 6-month cycle of intensive combination treatment had a sustained suppression of the rate of radiographic progression independent of subsequent antirheumatic therapy. The patients initially treated with monotherapy had a change in Sharp score of 8.6 units/yr, whereas the patients on the combination regimen progressed at only 5.6 units/yr.[68] Initial combination therapy may offer longer term benefits regardless of what type of therapy or intervention is used in the future.

Perhaps the best attempt to establish the ideal algorithmic approach to the treatment of RA was done in the BeST trial.[69] In this study, patients were randomly assigned to one of four treatment strategies: monotherapy, step-up combination with traditional DMARD therapy, step-down therapy with initial combination therapy with tapered high-dose prednisone, or initial combination therapy with MTX and a TNF inhibitor (infliximab). These patients were monitored carefully with therapeutic adjustments made every 3 months. Ultimately, all the treatment approaches proved effective. Early functional benefit at 3 months was greater in the step-down (group 3) and the MTX-infliximab (group 4) arms. This finding should not be surprising given the high doses of steroids used in group 3, and this should not be a surprising result for group 4 because this group received intensive initial therapy with MTX (25 to 30 mg/wk) in addition to infliximab, which is known to have a rapid onset of action.

At 1 year, there were still functional advantages seen in groups 3 and 4, but less impressive differences seen between groups based on the ACR-20 response and the Disease Activity Score (DAS) (Fig. 67-5). Most notable were the differences seen in radiographic progression at 1 year, with median increases in radiographic scores being 2, 2.5, 1, and 0.5 in groups 1, 2, 3, and 4 (Fig. 67-6).[69] No significant differences were seen in adverse events or attrition in the different groups. Although some of the approaches may be more or less favored in different regions of the world, any of these approaches can be effective in a given patient. This study does support the conclusion, however, that initial combination therapy resulted in earlier functional improvements and less structural damage than did sequential monotherapy or step-up combination therapy. It also suggests potential advantages with the use of biologic therapy, especially combined with MTX.

BIOLOGIC DISEASE-MODIFYING ANTIRHEUMATIC DRUGS

Since the late 1990s, increasing emphasis has been placed on the use of biologic agents combined with small molecule agents such as MTX. These combinations have proved effective in the treatment of patients with severe or long-standing disease and have proved their ability to slow or prevent radiographic progression of disease.[21,22,70,71] As a class, the most effective of biologic approaches to date has been the combination of TNF antagonists (e.g., adalimumab, etanercept, and infliximab) with MTX. In refractory disease, the addition of adalimumab, etanercept, or infliximab to MTX treatment provides additional benefit to patients with persistent active disease.[21,22,24]

With all three of the available TNF inhibitors, trials have shown that more than 50% to 70% of the patients had at least a 20% response, and more than 40% of patients had a 50% improvement, as measured by the ACR criteria.[72,73] Although each of the cohorts studied in these trials was slightly different, no significant side effects were apparent in the combination arms above and beyond what was seen in the MTX-only arms of the studies, suggesting a good safety profile and strong benefit-to-risk ratio when put into perspective with the relative severity of the disease. Beyond the TNF inhibitors, there are increasing data that biologic agents such as abatacept and RTX can work effectively even in patients who have failed TNF inhibitors, continuing to provide disease control in patients with the most refractory disease.

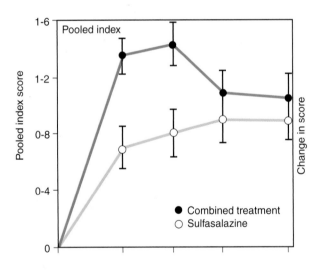
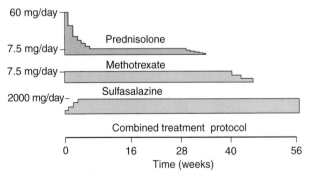

Figure 67-4 The benefits of step-down combination therapy over individual therapy with sulfasalazine. *(Adapted from Boers M, Verhoeven AC, Markusse HM, et al: Randomised comparison of combined step-down prednisolone, methotrexate and sulphasalazine with sulphasalazine alone in early rheumatoid arthritis. Lancet 350:309-318, 1997.)*

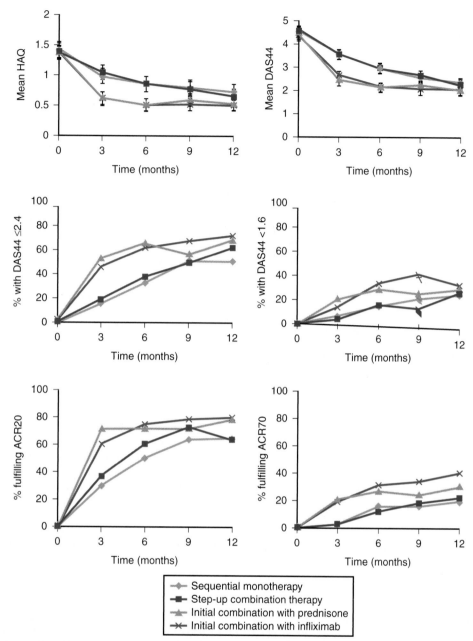

Figure 67-5 The changes in various outcome assessment tools for the four treatment strategies in rheumatoid arthritis patients over the first 12 months of treatment. *(Adapted from Goekoop-Ruiterman YP, de Vries-Bouwstra JK, Allaart CF, et al: Clinical and radiographic outcomes of four different treatment strategies in patients with early rheumatoid arthritis (the BeSt study): A randomized, controlled trial. Arthritis Rheum 52:3381-3390, 2005.)*

INHIBITION BY TUMOR NECROSIS FACTORS

The pivotal roles for TNF-α in initiation and perpetuation of the inflammatory and proliferative processes of rheumatoid synovitis are outlined in Chapter 65. As a class, the TNF inhibitors (adalimumab, etanercept, and infliximab) seem to be one of the most effective means of improving symptoms and signs of disease, increasing function, and reducing structural progression of RA.

Etanercept

Etanercept was the first TNF-α inhibitor to be approved by the U.S. Food and Drug Administration (FDA) for use in RA. It is a fusion protein of the soluble portion of the human TNF p75 chain of the receptor and the fragment crystallizable (Fc) portion of human IgG1. The receptor portion binds extracellular TNF-α, effectively neutralizing it, and the Fc moiety prolongs its circulating half-life. This drug is administered as a subcutaneous injection of 25 mg twice weekly or a single 50-mg injection once a week.

Similar to other trials of newer agents, etanercept was tested in combination with MTX (stable dose of 15 to 25 mg/wk) against MTX alone.[22] At 24 weeks, 71% of the patients receiving etanercept plus MTX and 27% of patients receiving placebo plus MTX met the ACR-20 criteria (P < .001). Particularly important were the data that 39% of the patients receiving the combination and only 3% of the patients receiving MTX alone met the ACR-50

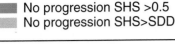

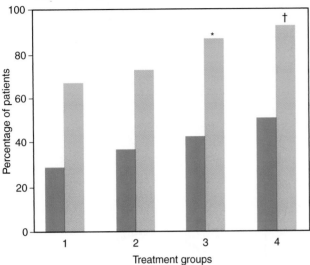

Figure 67-6 The percentage of patients without radiographic evidence of progression based on various treatment strategies in rheumatoid arthritis patients over the first 12 months of treatment. SDD, smallest detectable difference; SHS, modified Sharp–Van der Heijde score. *(Adapted from Goekoop-Ruiterman YP, de Vries-Bouwstra JK, Allaart CF, et al: Clinical and radiographic outcomes of four different treatment strategies in patients with early rheumatoid arthritis (the BeSt study): A randomized, controlled trial. Arthritis Rheum 52:3381-3390, 2005.)*

improvement criteria ($P < .001$), and 15% of the combination group met the ACR-70 criteria.[22]

A second important study evaluated etanercept as monotherapy and involved patients who had failed traditional DMARDs.[74] They were randomly assigned to etanercept or placebo, and at 6 months 59% of patients receiving 25 mg of etanercept twice weekly and 11% of the placebo group had achieved an ACR-20 criteria response.

A third important study looked at patients with early RA and compared the effects of MTX or etanercept on symptoms and signs, joint destruction, and function.[19,20] In this study, 632 patients with disease of less than 3 years' duration and who were naive to MTX and biologic agents were randomly assigned to receive either aggressively dosed MTX (20 mg/wk) or one of two different doses of etanercept (10 mg subcutaneously twice a week or 25 mg subcutaneously twice a week). Patients treated with etanercept had a more rapid response than was seen with MTX. This more rapid response led to significantly greater improvements at the ACR-20, ACR-50, and ACR-70 levels with etanercept compared with MTX for the first 4 months of the study. Although there was still a numerical trend favoring the 25-mg dose of etanercept over MTX at 1 year, the statistical significance was lost. As part of this study, radiographs also were obtained, and there was a statistically significant advantage for etanercept at 6 months, but, as with the clinical improvement, the radiographic assessments showed a trend, but no statistical significance at 1 year.[19]

At 2 years, the ACR-20 response rate was 72% in the 25-mg etanercept arm versus 59% in the MTX arm. Etanercept seemed to be better tolerated with fewer side effects than seen in the MTX cohort.[20] The most interesting result of this study was the ability of etanercept to slow radiographic

progression more than MTX. The mean change in the total Sharp score at 2 years was 1.3 in the 25-mg etanercept arm versus 3.2 in the MTX group, showing statistically meaningful differences in radiographic progression between the two arms. Patients also showed a significant improvement in function and a reduction in disability.

A fourth study, the Trial of Etanercept and Methotrexate with Radiographic Patient Outcomes (TEMPO) trial, examined the effect of monotherapy with either MTX or etanercept versus the combination of the two agents in a double-blind controlled trial. The trial randomly assigned 686 patients between the three arms. At 1 year, the results in the combination arm suggested substantially better reduction of disease activity, improvement in function, and slowing of structural damage compared with either approach as monotherapy. Similar side effects were reported in each of the three treatment arms. Possibly the most impressive finding was that the mean radiographic progression in the combination approach was a negative score.[75,76] The 2-year follow-up continued to reaffirm the superiority of the combination approach of etanercept plus MTX over either monotherapy for reducing disease activity, slowing radiographic progression, and improving function.[77]

Infliximab

Infliximab is a chimeric monoclonal antibody against TNF. It was the second anti-TNF agent approved for use by the FDA in treatment of RA and had previously been approved for use in Crohn's disease. Most of the antibody is human; however, a small portion of the Fab region is murine in origin. The antibody is given via intravenous infusions of 3 to 10 mg/kg. The recommended dosing regimen is 3 mg/kg with infusions at weeks 0, 2, and 6, and every 8 weeks thereafter. If patients fail to achieve a significant benefit, the dose can be increased, or the dosing interval can be shortened. For pharmacokinetic and pharmacoeconomic reasons, it may be more desirable to shorten the dosing interval rather than to increase the dose.[78] Concomitant administration of MTX gives more sustained benefit, may reduce the clearance of the drug, and possibly may lead to less immunogenicity, reflected by a reduction in human antichimeric antibody formation.[79,80] Whether concomitant use of other small molecules affords the same advantage is unknown, but plausible.

In the ATTRACT trial, a phase III study involving 428 patients, infliximab exhibited significant benefit in patients with long-standing and refractory RA. Patients failing to respond to MTX were randomly assigned to receive placebo, infliximab (3 mg/kg every 4 weeks or every 8 weeks), or infliximab (10 mg/kg every 4 weeks or every 8 weeks). After 54 weeks, there was a statistically significant advantage favoring all the infliximab/MTX arms compared with the placebo/MTX arm. The ACR-20 response rate seen with placebo/MTX was 17% compared with 42%, 48%, 59%, and 59% in the infliximab 3 mg/kg every 4 weeks (42%), 3 mg/kg every 8 weeks (48%), 10 mg/kg every 4 weeks (59%), and 10 mg/kg every 8 weeks (59%) groups. ACR-50 responses also were significant and exceeded 34% in the three highest dosed cohorts.[21]

Although infliximab showed marked improvement in the symptoms and signs of disease, the most impressive result of this study was the ability of infliximab to slow the radiographic progression of RA. Each of the infliximab/MTX arms showed a dramatic decrease in what would have been their predicted rate of radiographic progression and statistical superiority to the placebo/MTX arm. Commensurate with the improvement in clinical manifestations was an improvement in function and a reduction in disability measured by the HAQ and the short-form health survey (SF-36).[21]

A second large trial, the Active-Controlled Study of Patients Receiving Infliximab for the Treatment of Rheumatoid Arthritis of Early Onset (ASPIRE) study, looked at infliximab and MTX in patients with early RA. The study randomly assigned 1049 patients to receive MTX, MTX plus 3 mg/kg of infliximab, or MTX plus 6 mg/kg of infliximab. Significantly better responses were seen at 1 year in the combination MTX/infliximab arms than were seen in the MTX-only arm. This study reaffirmed that in early disease the combination of a TNF inhibitor (infliximab) plus MTX provided better clinical, radiographic, and functional improvement than seen with monotherapy with MTX alone.[26]

Adalimumab

Adalimumab is the third biologic agent directed against TNF to be approved by the FDA for the treatment of RA. Adalimumab is a fully human monoclonal antibody directed against TNF and is delivered as a subcutaneous injection once every other week, or, in patients with insufficient response, it can be given once a week. Use of background MTX with this agent also seems to increase the duration of response, possibly by slowing the clearance of the drug. As was shown with etanercept and infliximab, adalimumab showed significant benefits when combined with MTX.[24,25,70]

In the Anti-TNF Research Study Program of the Monoclonal Antibody D2E7 in Patients with Rheumatoid Arthritis (ARMADA) with adalimumab, patients with severe refractory RA were randomly assigned to receive placebo or subcutaneous adalimumab, at doses of 20 mg, 40 mg, or 80 mg every other week, in combination with MTX.[24] The efficacy of adalimumab given subcutaneously every other week in combination with MTX was significantly better than MTX plus placebo, with ACR-20, ACR-50, and ACR-70 scores of 65%, 53%, and 26% at the 40-mg every-other-week dose. In a second large study,[81] patients with active RA, after a 4-week DMARD washout period, were randomly assigned to one of five groups: 20 mg of adalimumab every other week or weekly, 40 mg of adalimumab every other week or weekly, or placebo. Patients who received 40-mg of adalimumab every other week showed substantial benefit, with an ACR-20 response of 46% compared with placebo response of 19%. The patients in the 40-mg group with weekly treatment did even better, with an ACR-20 response of 53.4%.

A 52-week, double-blind, placebo-controlled study[70] was carried out on patients with active RA who were receiving stable doses of MTX. Patients were randomly assigned to receive adalimumab, 20 mg subcutaneously once a week; adalimumab, 40 mg every other week with placebo on the alternate weeks; or placebo once a week. Substantial inhibition of radiographic progression was observed for joint space narrowing and erosions, particularly for the 40-mg every-other-week group. The authors concluded that 20 mg of adalimumab given subcutaneously weekly or 40 mg given every other week, both with concomitant MTX, significantly inhibited progression of structural joint damage and improved signs and symptoms of RA in patients who previously were incomplete responders to MTX.

Similar to the other TNF inhibitors, adalimumab also has been studied in early disease. The PREMIER study evaluated the effect of combination therapy with adalimumab and MTX versus monotherapy with either agent alone.[25] Substantial benefits were seen at 1 and 2 years in the combination arm over either of the monotherapy arms with significant advantages for the combination approach to slow structural damage, reduce disease activity, and improve function.

SAFETY OF TUMOR NECROSIS FACTOR INHIBITION

Tempering enthusiasm about the anti-TNF approaches to treatment is the reality that the beneficial effects are not permanent. Cessation of therapy is followed by a recrudescence of disease. The cytokine "rheostat" is not reset, and the as-yet-unknown forces initiating the inflammatory and proliferative process are still at work.[82] TNF inhibition does not work in all patients, and some safety concerns remain.

Serious Infections (Excluding Tuberculosis)

When TNF inhibitors were first introduced in the late 1990s, there was concern that blocking TNF might impair the host defense system. Clinicians have since been reassured that, in general, there have not been significant problems with serious bacterial infections for most patients treated with TNF inhibitors. Occasional patients taking etanercept, infliximab, or adalimumab have developed serious bacterial infections or opportunistic infection, however. Predicting which patients will develop an infection is almost impossible. A degree of vigilance and the recognition that infections can occur should be part of all treatment initiation and monitoring efforts. In addition, it is apparent that in debilitated patients (e.g., patients with infections such as skin ulcers or pneumonia or patients with other illnesses that would increase the risk of infection or diminished immune surveillance) TNF inhibition should be used with caution.

Tuberculosis

Reactivation of tuberculosis has been reported with all the TNF inhibitors. There seem to be more reports with infliximab than with etanercept or adalimumab. Researchers are unclear as to whether these differences are related to differing mechanism of action, structure, pharmacokinetics, route of administration, or the patient populations studied. Given the potential for reactivation of tuberculosis, appropriate screening should be done before the initiation of treatment with a TNF inhibitor.

Malignancies

RA conveys an increased risk for the development of lymphoproliferative disease. The development of lymphoma has been reported with each of the TNF inhibitors. It is unclear, however, whether this development is related to the medication itself or the underlying disease (see Chapter 113).

Demyelination

Rare cases of multiple sclerosis, optic neuritis, and demyelination have been reported in patients taking TNF inhibitors.[83-86] These cases have been sporadic and seem mostly to resolve when the TNF inhibitor is withdrawn. Because demyelination is a rare occurrence in the population at large, it is unclear whether these events are occurring more often than expected. It is recommended that TNF inhibition be avoided in patients with a history of demyelinating illness or who have features of unique neurologic problems.

Congestive Heart Failure

In patients with known congestive heart failure, TNF inhibitors should be used with caution because they may worsen cardiac function.

ROLE OF TUMOR NECROSIS FACTOR INHIBITION IN THE TREATMENT OF RHEUMATOID ARTHRITIS

The TNF inhibitors have exhibited a superior ability to reduce the signs and symptoms of RA, inhibit the progression of structural damage, and improve physical function in patients with this disease. Despite this, their role in the armamentarium is debated. The debate focuses on several factors, including the ability of traditional approaches to treat numerous patients effectively, particularly when used in combination; the lack of long-term safety data beyond 10 years; and the high costs of these agents (see Table 67-1).

In all of the previously mentioned studies, the combination of a TNF inhibitor plus MTX showed statistically significant benefits over MTX alone. Questions are raised, however, as to whether this numerical/statistical advantage is clinically meaningful enough to warrant the difference in cost, particularly when numerous patients on MTX alone or in combination approaches achieved substantial benefits in those studies. In the absence of truly useful biomarkers or surrogates to distinguish patients likely to respond to therapy from patients who would not respond, it is reasonable to suggest that most patients should be treated with MTX before advancing to a TNF inhibitor. Should a patient fail to achieve a significant response to MTX over a few months, however, switching the patient to a TNF inhibitor as monotherapy or adding a TNF inhibitor and treating in combination with background DMARDs should be considered.

Without head-to-head studies, the question as to which of the TNF inhibitors affords the greatest efficacy cannot be answered. There is evidence, however, that some patients may respond better to one TNF inhibitor than another. Deciding which agent to use for which patient is a difficult decision and is often influenced by a host of issues, including patient preference of injection or infusion, monotherapy or combination therapy, and, most frequently, what agent third-party payers would reimburse. Despite these factors, there continues to be an earlier adoption of TNF inhibitors in the treatment of RA.

INTERLEUKIN-1 RECEPTOR ANTAGONIST AND INTERLEUKIN-1 RECEPTOR

IL-1, similar to TNF-α, has been implicated in the pathogenesis of RA. It is produced by rheumatoid synovium and other tissues, predominantly by macrophages. There is, however, a circulating protein found in extracellular tissues, IL-1 receptor antagonist, which is a biologically important protein that functions as a naturally occurring antagonist to IL-1. A recombinant human form, anakinra, has been developed. In 2002, anakinra was approved by the FDA for the treatment of RA. It is given as a daily subcutaneous injection of 100 mg.

A 24-week, double-blind, randomized, placebo-controlled, multicenter study of 472 patients reported that of the patients who received 150 mg/day of anakinra as monotherapy, 43% met the ACR-20 criteria for improvement, although 27% of the placebo group did as well.[87] A study of combination anakinra/MTX was done in 419 patients who had failed to achieve an adequate response to MTX alone.[88] At 24 weeks, the ACR-20 response rate in the 1 mg/kg anakinra (46%) and 2 mg/kg anakinra (38%) dose groups was significantly greater than in the placebo group (19%). Anakinra also has been shown to be safe and effective with many other DMARDs, including HCQ, SSZ, and leflunomide.[89] Two separate trials looking at combination use of anakinra with etanercept showed higher rates of infections, however, and failed to show clinical benefits of the combination of these two anticytokine therapies.[90,91] In addition to the clinical benefits in signs and symptoms of disease, two studies have shown that use of anakinra can reduce radiologic progression of RA.[92,93]

Generally, anakinra has been shown to be safe and well tolerated. The most frequent side effect has been injection site reactions, which occur in more than 50% of the patients who take this medication. Although mild and self-limited, this side effect can be very uncomfortable. Anakinra is an infrequently used agent for the treatment of RA and is often reserved for patients who have failed other agents or may be inappropriate candidates for TNF inhibition. This restriction of use is partially related to its cost (see Table 67-1), the need for daily subcutaneous injections, and the perception of being less effective as a therapeutic biologic compound than are the TNF inhibitors.

PROTEIN A IMMUNOABSORPTION COLUMN

The FDA has approved a device containing staphylococcal protein A that binds IgG and IgG-antigen complexes, removing them from the circulation of patients with severe RA who are not responsive to DMARD therapy. The device has been effective in immune thrombocytopenic purpura and has been moderately more effective in RA than a "placebo" that provided sham immunoabsorption.[94] Use of this device is expensive, time-consuming for expert staff, and accompanied by side effects. The trials in RA necessitated a column treatment once a week for 12 weeks; further trials are essential to determine whether the treatment is effective in patients resistant to combinations of small molecules and biologic DMARDs. This device should be reserved as an option only for patients who have failed treatment with traditional DMARDs and the newer biologic agents.

NEW THERAPEUTIC CLASSES

New therapeutic classes also have become available with the introduction of abatacept (a selective costimulatory modulator) and RTX (a peripheral B cell–depleting agent). The addition of newer therapeutic agents generated by recombinant or monoclonal antibody biotechnology has enhanced the concept and practice of combination therapy and has effectively exploited the promise of treatments that target certain inflammatory mediators believed to play an important role in initiation and amplification of the disease process. Generally, these agents, although quite effective at various stages of disease, are most frequently reserved for patients who have developed an inadequate response to MTX and frequently have failed TNF inhibition.

Abatacept

Abatacept is a soluble, recombinant fusion protein that is composed of the extracellular domain of cytotoxic T lymphocyte–associated antigen-4 (CTLA-4) and the modified Fc portion of IgG1.[95] It seems to be effective in the treatment of RA by selectively modulating the CD80 or CD86/CD28 costimulatory signal required for full T cell activation.[96] T cells normally require two signals for full activation. The first signal is the antigen expressed in the context of the major histocompatibility complex (MHC) binding to the T cell receptor. The second signal is a costimulatory signal. One important costimulatory pathway is the engagement of CD80/CD86 on the surface of an antigen-presenting cell with CD28 on the T cell, facilitating T cell activation. In the normal sequence of events, the naturally occurring inhibitory molecule CTLA-4 is induced on the surface of the T cell downregulating the CD28-mediated T cell activation. CTLA-4 has a markedly greater affinity for CD80 or CD86 than does CD28, out-competing CD28 for CD80 or CD86 binding.[97] Abatacept, similar to CTLA-4, competes with CD28 for CD80 and CD86 binding and can be used to modulate T cell activation selectively.

Clinical trials have shown the efficacy of abatacept in the treatment of RA. In an early phase IIB trial, patients with active RA and an inadequate response to MTX were randomly assigned to MTX plus placebo, MTX plus 2 mg/kg of abatacept, or MTX plus 10 mg/kg of abatacept. Abatacept was administered as a 30-minute infusion days 1, 15, and 30, and monthly thereafter. At the 6-month end point, significantly more patients treated with 10 mg/kg of abatacept had obtained an ACR-20 response (60%) than patients on MTX alone (35%). Significantly greater ACR-50 and ACR-70 responses also were seen in the abatacept groups compared with placebo.[98] The safety profile was similar to placebo.

These results were corroborated further in a much larger phase III study looking at a similar population of patients with active RA and an inadequate response to MTX. In the AIM trial,[71] 652 patients with active RA and an inadequate response to MTX were randomly assigned to either 10 mg/kg of abatacept plus MTX or MTX alone. ACR responses (ACR-20, ACR-50, and ACR-70) at 6 and 12 months were all significantly better for the abatacept plus MTX group compared with the MTX-alone group with scores of 67% versus 39% (ACR-20), 39% versus 16% (ACR-50), and 19% versus 6% (ACR-70). At 1 year, the ACR responses

had increased in the abatacept arm. Slightly higher incidences of adverse events and serious adverse events were seen with abatacept plus MTX compared with MTX alone. An important end point of this study was structural damage assessed through radiographs taken at baseline and 12 months. Abatacept significantly slowed structural progression with an approximate 50% reduction in radiographic progression in the abatacept-treated patients.[71]

Perhaps the most important of the studies with this agent to date has been the ATTAIN trial, which was designed to assess the safety and efficacy of abatacept in anti-TNF inadequate responders with active RA who continued to receive DMARDs or anakinra.[99] In the trial, 258 patients received abatacept plus DMARD or anakinra, and 133 received placebo plus DMARD alone. Abatacept was administered as a 30-minute infusion on days 1, 15, and 29, and monthly thereafter, with a clinical end point at 6 months. At 6 months, the ACR-20, ACR-50, and ACR-70 on abatacept compared with placebo were 50% versus 19%, 20% versus 3%, and 10% versus 1%. As was true in the other studies, the abatacept arm had a significant improvement in function and reduction in pain.[99]

The largest of the phase III studies was the ASSURE trial. This randomized, double-blind, placebo-controlled trial primarily evaluated the safety of abatacept in 1441 active RA patients on traditional DMARDs and biologic DMARDs. Four groups of patients were treated for 1 year as follows: abatacept plus nonbiologic DMARD, placebo plus nonbiologic DMARD, abatacept plus biologic DMARD, or placebo plus biologic DMARD. At 1 year, there were higher rates of adverse events and serious adverse events (including serious infections) in the abatacept plus biologic DMARD group. This higher incidence led to a warning against concomitant use of abatacept with other biologic DMARDs.[100]

Rituximab

RTX is a chimeric monoclonal antibody targeting CD20+ B cells.[101] Clinical trials using RTX have shown efficacy and safety in treating RA and have provided further evidence for the role of B cells in the pathogenesis of the disease.[102,103] CD20 is a target for B cell–depleting therapy because it is uniformly expressed on B cells, but not on stem cells or plasma cells.[104] By binding CD20, RTX depletes peripheral B cells through several postulated mechanisms, including cell-mediated and complement-dependent cytotoxicity and promotion of apoptosis.[101,105,106]

In an early phase II study, 161 patients with inadequate response to MTX were treated with MTX only (n = 40), RTX only (n = 40), RTX plus cyclophosphamide (cyclophosphamide, 750 mg days 3 and 17) (n = 41), or RTX plus MTX (n = 40). All patients were treated with intravenous and oral steroids during the first 2 weeks of treatment. All RTX patients received two doses of 1000 mg, one each on days 1 and 15. At 24 weeks, all RTX treatment groups showed statistically significantly higher ACR-20 scores than MTX alone with the ACR-20 response rate of 73% in patients treated with RTX plus MTX and 38% in patients treated with MTX alone. Similarly, patients receiving RTX plus cyclophosphamide and RTX plus MTX had statistically significant ACR-50 responses over patients receiving MTX alone. A 6-month exploratory extension of treatment found

33% of patients with an ACR-20 in the RTX plus MTX group compared with 13% for RTX plus cyclophosphamide and MTX alone and 8% for RTX alone. The duration of this response, although not quite statistically significant, is impressive for a single-infusion response.[103]

A second phase II study, the DANCER trial, was designed to determine the appropriate regimen of RTX combined with MTX, with or without corticosteroids. The trial assigned 465 patients with active RA despite the use of MTX to one of nine dosing groups: placebo with no steroid, placebo with only intravenous steroids, placebo with intravenous and oral steroids, 500 mg of RTX × 2 with no steroid, 500 mg of RTX × 2 with intravenous steroids, 500 mg of RTX × 2 with intravenous and oral steroids, 1000 mg of RTX × 2 with no steroid, 1000 mg of RTX × 2 with intravenous steroids, or 1000 mg of RTX × 2 with intravenous and oral steroids. All patients were on background MTX. The RTX was given intravenously 2 weeks apart. The intravenous steroid regimen was 100 mg of methylprednisolone given on days 1 and 15. The oral steroid regimen consisted of prednisone, 60 mg/day on days 2 to 7, and prednisone, 30 mg/day on days 8 to 14.[107] The primary end point looked at only rheumatoid factor–positive patients at 24 weeks.

There was a statistically significant benefit in the RTX arms compared with the placebo arm with ACR-20 of 54%, 55%, and 28% in the 1000-mg, 500-mg, and placebo RTX regimens, respectively. The steroid regimens did not seem to affect the efficacy results at 24 weeks, but the use of intravenous steroids did reduce significantly the number of infusion reactions associated with RTX. The use of intravenous steroids before administration of RTX has become routine in an effort to limit infusion reactions. The ideal dose of RTX has become less certain given the similar results seen with the 500-mg and the 1000-mg regimens.

A more recent, and perhaps more important than the earlier trials, phase III trial studied the efficacy and safety of RTX when administered in combination with MTX in 500 patients with active RA who had an inadequate response to one or more anti-TNF-α therapies. RTX 1000 mg plus MTX or placebo plus MTX was administered by infusion on days 1 and 15. Pretreatment with intravenous methylprednisolone was followed by oral prednisone for 2 weeks after the initial RTX dosing. The primary efficacy parameter, ACR-20, was statistically significantly higher for RTX patients than for placebo patients, with 51% of patients achieving an ACR-20 compared with 18% in the placebo arm. Radiographs were obtained as part of this study, and although not achieving statistical significance at 6 months, they did show a trend toward slowing of structural progression in the RTX plus MTX arm.[72]

As with the first two studies, RTX treatment produced a rapid and sustained peripheral depletion of B cells. Additionally, immunoglobulin levels were modestly decreased, with IgM in a few patients decreasing below the lower limits of normal, but with no signs of increased infectious episodes seen during this study. Overall adverse events were reported almost equally by both treatment groups. Twenty-three percent of RTX patients developed an acute infusion reaction during or after the first infusion compared with 18% of placebo patients. Infusion-related reactions are thought to be related to cytokine release and include pruritus, fever, rash, pyrexia, rigors, sneezing, throat irritation, cough,

bronchospasm, hypotension, and hypertension. There also was a slightly higher incidence of infections and serious infections in the RTX-treated group compared with the placebo group.[72]

Overall, abatacept and RTX seem to offer significant benefits and reasonable safety profiles to date, particularly for patients who have tried and failed anti-TNF agents. Both agents improve the symptoms and signs of disease, improve function, and slow radiographic progression of disease. These agents represent a particularly noteworthy advance in the treatment of RA because they work in patients who have failed TNF inhibition, and this group represents the most refractory of RA patients. Although unique questions remain as to where each of these agents will ultimately be placed in the therapeutic armamentarium, studies with these agents have confirmed the rationale of using recombinant engineering to target crucial steps that have been identified by laboratory research in the pathogenesis of disease.

ADJUNCTIVE DRUG THERAPY

Patients with inflammatory polyarthritis have pain generated by the inflammation in their joints. The classes of compounds that treat this pain effectively are analgesics, NSAIDs, and glucocorticoids. For RA, these therapies must be considered adjuncts rather than primary therapy (disease-modifying drugs). Adjunctive therapy may be useful in the short-term, and in some cases it is sufficient for management, particularly in cases of polyarthritis that do not become chronically embedded in joints and defined as RA. The goal of RA therapy should be to make these adjunctive drugs unnecessary and redundant through control of the disease. The NSAIDs are discussed in detail in Chapter 54, and glucocorticoids are discussed in Chapter 55.

GLUCOCORTICOID THERAPY

Steroids in short courses and at low doses can result in a reduction of symptoms and signs of disease and improve patient function. Glucocorticoids are the fastest and most effective approach to immediate symptomatic improvement. It is hoped, however, that in future years their use can be minimized.

Perhaps the most common use of glucocorticoids in RA is as an adjunct in low doses as a daily therapy. Although the benefits of low-dose therapy (≤7.5 mg/day given as one dose in the morning) have been shown, data suggest that the cumulative effects on bone produce osteoporosis and other deleterious effects associated with significant morbidity. There are multiple actions of glucocorticoids on bone, including a recognized decreased production of osteoclasts and decreased production and apoptosis of osteoblasts resulting in decreased bone formation and trabecular width.[108]

The arguments supporting use of low-dose, daily prednisone are as follows. First, the rheumatoid process diminishes bone formation in patients compared with control populations.[109] Physical impairment is the major determinant of spinal and femoral bone mass deficiency in RA patients, and if the clinical activity of arthritis is factored into equations, the effect of low-dose glucocorticoid therapy on bone loss in these patients is minimal,[110] particularly if the glucocorticoid encourages more physical activity by relieving inflammation. Metabolic marker studies have indicated that generalized bone turnover is increased in RA.[111]

Second, evidence also has been presented that low-dose daily glucocorticoids reduce the rate of radiographically detected progression of disease.[112-115] This work was initially done with 128 adults with active RA of less than 2 years' duration. Patients were randomly assigned to receive 7.5 mg of prednisone per day in addition to other medications, and others received placebo. Most patients in both groups did not develop worsening radiologic scores, but the patients who did were primarily in the placebo group, and the erosions progressed more rapidly over the next 2 years.

In a more recent 2-year, double-blind, placebo-controlled trial, the benefits and risks of 10 mg of prednisone per day were evaluated. Investigators found that, particularly in the first 6 months, patients receiving prednisone had more clinical improvement, and there was significantly less radiographic progression than seen in the placebo group.[113] This finding was corroborated further in another 2-year study of patients with disease of less than 1 year's duration. Patients were randomly assigned to receive either 7.5 mg of prednisolone per day or not when they were initially started on DMARDs for the treatment of RA. After 2 years, the patients given glucocorticoids in addition to DMARDs had higher remission rates and significantly less radiographic progression than the patients treated with DMARDs alone. There was no significant difference seen in adverse events or in loss of bone between the two groups.[114] Even lower doses (5 mg of prednisolone per day) also have proved effective in substantially decreasing radiographic progression in patients with early RA with only mild increases in adverse events at 2 years.[115]

Some rheumatologists have used intramuscular injections of depot preparations of methylprednisolone intermittently in patients with active polyarthritis, although this is not a universal practice. The rationale is that this route and quantity of glucocorticoids give a sustained, gradually declining therapeutic effect that would not induce "dependence" on the drug, which often happens when even low doses are prescribed in pill form. In a 2-year randomized trial of intramuscular depot steroids in patients with RA and an incomplete response to DMARDs, the short-term and long-term (2-year) effects were assessed. In the short-term, disease activity improved faster than with placebo, but little difference remained at 6 months between the two groups. There also was a small reduction in radiographic progression in the intramuscular steroid group with fewer erosions seen. There were consequences of this approach, however, including more adverse events in the steroid arm and significant loss of bone density in the hip.[116]

Counter to efficacy data supporting glucocorticoid use are side-effect data showing that prednisone has higher cumulative toxicity over many years than nearly all other agents used to treat RA[117] and a twofold increase in standardized mortality rates.[118] Although most emphasis has been placed on osteoporosis, there is a definite association of low-dose glucocorticoid use on a daily basis with cataracts, glaucoma, impaired glucose tolerance, hirsutism, skin atrophy, and atherogenesis. Although side effects may be limited by alternate-day regimens, alternate-day administration of glucocorticoids in asthmatic patients did not produce less bone loss than daily regimens.[119]

When glucocorticoids are being used, attempts should be made to guard patients against the known side effects. The ACR task force on osteoporosis guidelines[120] has published recommendations for the following subsets of patients:

- Patients receiving long-term glucocorticoid treatment who develop a nontraumatic osteoporotic fracture
- Patients receiving long-term glucocorticoid treatment who do not have fractures
- Patients beginning long-term glucocorticoid treatment

Patients in the first group, who have developed a fracture (usually a compression fracture of the spine), are often at great risk for a higher mortality rate not only from the fracture, but also from other side effects of the glucocorticoids. These individuals not only need pharmacologic intervention, but also lifestyle changes.

Patients in the second group, who are receiving long-term glucocorticoid treatment and do not have fractures, should have baseline laboratory tests and a dual-energy x-ray absorptiometry determination of bone mineral density. Physical therapy and exercise should be started, along with calcium and vitamin D supplementation. If appropriate, additional pharmacologic therapy should be considered to prevent glucocorticoid-induced osteoporosis. Yearly measurements of bone mineral density using the same equipment in these patients would enable the physician to determine the rate of bone loss and to institute therapy appropriately.

Patients in the third group, who have RA and are beginning glucocorticoid therapy, should be evaluated carefully for associated diseases other than RA that affect bone metabolism. Women who are postmenopausal should be evaluated for the consideration of hormone replacement therapy or other antiresorptive agents. Other risk factors should be removed, when possible, and exercise, supplemental calcium, and vitamin D should be prescribed. A baseline bone mineral density determination is appropriate.

Most importantly, the potential toxicity of the glucocorticoids, if taken for long periods, must be communicated to the patient, and the patient and the physician must have as their goal to control the disease within 6 months to the point that glucocorticoids are no longer deemed necessary and can be slowly tapered. Chapter 92 contains additional discussion and therapeutic options for the treatment of osteoporosis.

Overall, the use of low-dose oral glucocorticoids for short periods as an adjunct to DMARD therapy can be justified, particularly in early disease, in a patient with refractory disease and in patients during pregnancy. Intramuscular glucocorticoid use should be considered as a short-term approach, whereas intra-articular steroids provide localized benefits particularly for patients with one or only a few active joints. Careful attention should be directed toward minimizing the potential side effects of any of these regimens.

NONSTEROIDAL ANTI-INFLAMMATORY DRUGS

More than 70 million prescriptions for NSAIDs are written each year in the United States, and more than 30 billion over-the-counter tablets are sold annually. As a class, NSAIDs are the most often used and are a very effective adjunctive therapy in RA, providing analgesic and anti-inflammatory benefits. Chapter 54 provides a comprehensive review of these compounds, with details of their molecular activity and toxicity. The introduction of the cyclooxygenase-2 (COX-2) selective agents has fueled debate further regarding safety, toxicity, and costs of NSAID therapy. Given that most patients with RA are treated with NSAID therapy, physicians must evaluate the individual patient carefully to assess chronicity of use, risk factors for NSAID toxicity, risk factors for heart disease, and the ability of the patient or the insurance plan to cover the costs of the agent prescribed. Risk factors for use of NSAIDs (including aspirin) have been identified and include the following[121]:

- Advanced age
- History of peptic ulcer (with or without a known infection with *Helicobacter pylori*)
- Concomitant use of glucocorticoids or anticoagulants
- Thrombocytopenia or platelet dysfunction
- Pregnancy
- Moderate or severe congestive heart failure, cirrhosis, or renal insufficiency
- Aspirin intolerance, asthma, and nasal polyposis

Which NSAID should be prescribed first is perhaps the most frequently encountered and possibly the most difficult question. In a young patient without any of the aforementioned risk factors, salicylates should not be excluded automatically from use. Aspirin has the advantages of being inexpensive (even in enteric-coated preparations), having an inexpensive test for blood levels, having toxicity directly related to dose, and often having a biologic manifestation of excessive blood levels (i.e., tinnitus).

Nonacetylated salicylates (e.g., salsalate, choline salicylate) also merit consideration. They are moderately effective, have a good safety profile, and are inexpensive. They have only a weak and reversible effect on COX. This finding has led to studies showing that, at concentrations below those needed to inhibit either COX-1 or COX-2, salicylates interrupt signal transduction across cell membranes in such a way that activation of inflammatory pathways in cells such as the neutrophil is inhibited.[122] If a clinician chooses to use an NSAID other than a salicylate, the only major differences, other than those afforded by the selective COX-2 inhibitors, are in frequency of dosing and in subtle differences in side-effect profiles.

The selective COX-2 inhibitors have been described in detail in Chapter 54. The fundamental difference between COX-1 and COX-2 is that COX-1 is a constitutively expressed enzyme synthesized at a constant rate by the tissues that produce it, whereas COX-2 is induced in monocytes or macrophages, endothelial cells, chondrocytes, synovial cells, and osteoblasts by cytokines and other products generated during inflammation.

The selective COX-2 inhibitors seem to be more effective than placebo in the treatment of arthritis and as effective as moderate doses of standard nonselective NSAIDs. The utility of the selective agents comes from potential safety advantages, including a lower risk of the development of gastrointestinal bleeding.[123,124] The selective agents also have no significant effects on platelets. They do not confer any advantage to the kidney, however, and risks of increasing hypertension or renal insufficiency because of their use must be recognized. Also, evidence suggests that selective COX-2 inhibition may increase risks for cardiovascular events. This controversy is discussed further in Chapter 54.

ANALGESICS

Acetaminophen is a very useful drug and can prove a useful adjunct in the treatment of arthritis. In patients without evidence of liver disease, acetaminophen can be taken in doses of 3 g or more per day without generating significant side effects. Combinations of acetaminophen with codeine or other narcotic derivatives produce a powerful but potentially addictive combination. Their use alone in polyarthritis for more than 6 weeks (i.e., the minimum period for acceptably classifying a polyarthritis as RA) should be discouraged and reserved only for patients who have severe and persistent disease despite all attempts to bring the disease under better control through the use of DMARDs and other adjuncts.

ASSESSING RESPONSE TO THERAPY

Assessing the effectiveness of a therapeutic approach is crucial to the appropriate management of an individual patient. The ACR guidelines for the management of RA call for periodic assessment of disease activity, and patients with inadequate response should have DMARDs changed or added.[1] In most clinical practices, this assessment is done by physician gestalt or global assessment after a careful history, examination, laboratory studies, and radiographs. In most situations, this approach leads to quality care; however, when intensive monitoring is applied with a goal of tighter control, better outcomes can be achieved.[60] More quantitative (but more time-consuming) approaches exist, such as the ACR response criteria, the DAS/DAS28, the HAQ, the Simplified Disease Activity Index (SDAI), and the Clinical Disease Activity Index (CDAI).

The ACR responder criteria were designed to measure improvement in disease and have been used extensively as an outcome in clinical trials.[73] The core criteria include swollen joint count, tender joint count, physician assessment of global status, patient assessment of global status, measurement of functional status (HAQ), patient assessment of pain, and a measure of inflammation such as the ESR or C-reactive protein (CRP). Although quite effective at assessing percentage improvement, such as the ACR-20, ACR-50, ACR-70, ACR responder criteria are considered a research tool and are not generally used in clinical practice.

The DAS is an effective tool to assess disease activity and measure change in activity.[125,126] It is a composite score making use of tender joint count (53 or 28), swollen joint count (44 or 28), general health assessment, and a marker of inflammation (ESR or CRP). It is a continuous measure allowing for measurement of absolute change in disease burden and percentage improvement. The DAS also has thresholds or cutoffs for low disease activity and for remission. Although a useful tool in clinical studies and in registries, the DAS is not used frequently in clinical practice; this is related partly to the need for careful joint counts, partly to the need for laboratory measures, and partly to the specific formula needed to calculate the score. DAS calculators can be found online to simplify this process for clinicians wishing to use this tool.[127]

The HAQ is a widely accepted and validated instrument for the assessment of function and disability. It is a patient self-reported questionnaire, and the HAQ disability index is frequently used in trials, registries, and many practice settings.[34] The HAQ measures eight subscales relating to physical disability and is scored between 0 and 3 (0 = no disability and 3 = completely disabled). Many variations have been made to the HAQ by other investigators, but in general they measure similar features of function and disability. Chapter 31 contains a broader discussion of health outcomes tools.

The SDAI and the CDAI are two relatively new composite scoring systems.[128,129] The SDAI is calculated using the numerical sum of the tender joint count (28 joints), the swollen joint count (28 joints), the patient's global assessment, the physician's global assessment, and the CRP (mg/dL).[128] The CDAI is similar to the SDAI, but does not use an acute-phase marker.[129] The removal of the laboratory measure makes it feasible to perform this measure directly in the office with the patient and base decisions on it without having to wait. Regardless of which tool is used, it is increasingly important to incorporate validated outcomes tools into clinical practice to assess disease activity, and to guide decision making regarding change and addition of DMARDs and expensive biologic agents.

EARLY RHEUMATOID ARTHRITIS— WINDOW OF OPPORTUNITY

For patients with a symmetric polyarthritis in three or more joint areas involving the hands, feet, or both for at least 6 weeks, and a presumptive diagnosis of RA, aggressive treatment is warranted. Patients generally are apprehensive and concerned about developing a chronic, debilitating disease. Anxiety, depression, loss of self-esteem, inability to work, and an inability to develop new coping behaviors may evolve. This "learned helplessness" must be combated by education, reassurance, counseling, and the confident attitude of the physician. Most important is the initiation of a program to downregulate activity of the synovitis with the goal of inducing a remission, or at least marked improvement, in the disease. Disease-modifying therapy is indicated at this point (see earlier), as are some adjunctive therapies. Early intervention may offer the greatest likelihood of preventing disability, and there may be a window of opportunity to have a significant impact on the trajectory of the disease over a lifetime.

The case for early intervention and for a window of opportunity has been made using several lines of evidence, as follows:

1. Functional health status declines early, with mild functional loss by 1 year and moderate-to-severe functional losses by 6 years.[130] Subsequently, work disability also occurs, especially early in disease, with work disability estimated to occur in 25% of RA patients at 6.4 years and 50% at 20.9 years after disease onset.[131]
2. Mortality rates are increased in patients with RA. Mortality rate has been shown to increase over 5 to 20 years, with 35% mortality by 20 years.[132] Morbidity and mortality rates in RA are predicted by, and are directly proportional to, clinical status. More severe and active disease has a poorer outcome.[133]
3. Radiographic changes develop early in disease.[134-136] Erosions of bone and narrowing of joint spaces develop within the first 2 years of disease in most patients and

are progressive afterward over several decades.[137] The rate of progression of radiographic scores is rapid early in disease and apparently continues along a similar trajectory for the duration of the disease if left untreated. When the proliferative synovium has begun to invade and destroy articular cartilage, joints are at risk for irreversible destruction, even when disease activity decreases.
4. In terms of economic impact, early disease activity predicts long-term costs. Data suggest that long-term medical costs and outcomes are significantly associated with early changes in disability.[138] Further data would support the fact that patients with very poor function may experience direct medical costs 2.55 to 6.97 times as high as patients with good function, with most of those costs coming from hospitalization.[139]
5. An interval of time may exist in which the introduction of DMARD therapy can result in a change in the natural course of disease—not just for a transient to short-lived time frame, but more fundamentally in the scope of the progression of the disease for a lifetime.[140] Data supporting this view have come from numerous trials looking at intervention in early RA.

In the HERA trial,[6] patients with RA were randomly assigned to receive either HCQ or placebo over 36 weeks. At the conclusion of the study, the patients who had received HCQ had improvements in joint findings, pain, and physical function superior to what was seen in the placebo group. Of more interest were the results seen after 3 years of follow-up of the original cohorts. The patients who had therapy instituted early in the disease (the HCQ arm) versus the patients who had DMARD therapy delayed for 9 months (the placebo arm) continued to have significantly less pain and disability. These results could not be explained based on differences in glucocorticoid, DMARD, or NSAID use subsequent to the trial and were attributed to the delay in the introduction of therapy.[7]

Stronger support for this line of thinking stems from data from many other trials. In the COBRA trial, patients were initially randomly assigned to receive monotherapy with SSZ or combination therapy in a step-down approach with SSZ, MTX, and high-dose glucocorticoids. At the end of 28 weeks, there seemed to be a significant advantage for the use of combination therapy based on clinical response, and at 1 year, there also was less radiographic progression in the combination group.[12] Of greatest interest is the 4-year follow-up data from this cohort. The patients who had been treated with the initial 6-month cycle of intensive combination treatment had a sustained suppression of the rate of radiographic progression independent of subsequent antirheumatic therapy. The patients initially treated with monotherapy had a change in Sharp score of 8.6 units/yr, whereas the patients on the combination regimen progressed at only 5.6 units/yr.[68]

In the FIN-RACo trial, investigators showed that combination therapy was superior to monotherapy with higher remission rates seen at 1 year and 2 years in the combination arm compared with the single DMARD arm.[14,66] Perhaps more interesting were the radiographic results at 5 years suggesting significant slowing of radiographic progression at 5 years in the patients treated with combination therapy within the first 2 years of their disease compared with the single DMARD approach.[141] Also, prompt induction of remission translated into better maintenance of work capacity at 5 years.[142] In another study, the early introduction of infliximab in addition to background MTX in patients with early RA and a poor prognosis resulted in not only a significantly better improvement in symptoms, function, and structural progression, but also an apparent ability to withdraw the infliximab and maintain the sustained benefits compared with placebo.[143]

Given the growing body of evidence, it seems that the introduction of effective therapy (particularly combination therapies) early in the course of disease can result in a profound impact on the nature of the disease years later. An interval of time may exist for intervention whereupon the outcome is a long-term change in the nature of the disease, regardless of what type of therapy or intervention is used in the future. Estimation of a patient's prognosis may assist further in choosing which patients may need the most aggressive approaches.

ESTIMATING PROGNOSIS

The challenge for the physician is to form an appreciation for the severity of a patient's disease and formulate a treatment plan accordingly. As a general guideline, the rate of progression toward joint destruction and disability in RA is proportional to the intensity of inflammatory and proliferative reactions within the joints, the degree of disability, and the persistence of this disease over time. In other words, a patient who has low-grade attacks of synovitis that are separated in time from each other would be much less likely to advance to joint deformity than a patient who has continuous, highly active synovitis.

Markers that have been identified have varied widely with individual studies, end points used, and the types of therapy implemented. An instructive study was done on 142 consecutive patients with early RA (median duration of disease was 7 months) treated actively with disease-modifying drugs and followed prospectively for an average of 6.2 years. Functional outcome and radiographic damage were the end points. The significant prognostic factors were high clinical disease activity at baseline, including morning stiffness, pain, grip strength, joint count, hemoglobin, and ESR, and a positive test for rheumatoid factor.[144] The function/disability, age, and comorbid conditions predicted 5-year mortality rate more effectively than radiographic or laboratory data.[145] The implication of this study is that functional measures may be superior to radiographs or markers of inflammatory activity in predicting outcome in RA.

In a similar cohort of 191 patients with early disease, multivariate analysis revealed that progression of joint damage was best predicted by ESR, IgM rheumatoid factor positivity, erosions at baseline, and the presence of HLA-DRB1*04 alleles.[146] Multivariate analysis of the same cohort suggested that disability at 5 years was associated with baseline HAQ scores, swollen and tender joint counts, elevated acute-phase proteins, and the presence of erosions on radiographs. Sex, age, rheumatoid factor, and the presence of HLA-DR1 alleles did not contribute to the prediction of disability at 5 years.[147] Another study of a similar cohort found that the HAQ score during the first 3 months predicted disability at 10 years with a very high odds ratio.[148]

Post-hoc analysis of clinical trials also has provided insight into factors predicting lack of clinical response to given therapies. In the ASPIRE trial,[26] patients with early disease were randomly assigned to receive MTX or MTX plus infliximab. On average, patients treated with the combination did better than patients treated with MTX alone. Certain factors predicted which of the patients treated with MTX alone might have a less than satisfactory result. Elevated acute-phase proteins, CRP or ESR, and swollen joint count were associated with greater structural damage in the MTX group, but not in the combination group, suggesting that this might be a subpopulation more likely to benefit from the combination approach early in disease.[149]

In an even larger cohort of 3500 patients, rheumatoid factor, elevated CRP, and high baseline HAQ scores all were predictors of poor outcome, and there was a strong association between the presence of HLA-DR1 alleles and the development of erosions.[150] Another indication of how function may predict outcome comes from an extensive study of the predictors for total joint replacement in 1600 patients seen during a period of observation that extended 23 years. Patients with highly abnormal values on the HAQ, global severity of disease, and ESR had a threefold to sixfold increased risk of undergoing a joint replacement.[151]

As alluded to earlier, additional markers of prognosis include genetic predispositions, such as the presence of certain genetic loci (e.g., HLA-DR alleles that are associated with RA). Although some studies have yielded conflicting results, it is generally believed that the HLA-DRB1 locus can increase the likelihood of developing RA and the severity of disease. There have already been attempts to use HLA-DRB1 typing in RA to predict responses to specific treatments.[152] In one study, the patients previously had been followed carefully in a study of combination therapy (HCQ/SSZ/MTX, HCQ/SSZ, or MTX alone).[13] Patients were classified, in simplest terms, as "successes" or "failures" in achieving 50% improvement. DR4 subtyping was detected by hybridization of the patients' DNA with allele-specific oligonucleotide probes specific for the shared epitope region. Of the patients, 74% were positive for at least one shared epitope allele, and 29% were positive for two. Although simplified, it can be concluded that patients who had one or two of the shared epitopes in their DRB1 chains were less likely to respond to MTX alone than to all three drugs, whereas the patients who had no shared epitopes in DRB1 chains did equally well on MTX alone as with all three drugs. Among patients positive for the shared epitope, 94% were "successes" if treated with triple therapy, but only 32% were "successes" if treated with MTX alone. These data are consistent with observations that patients positive for the shared epitope are at greatest risk for progressively active erosive disease and need more aggressive therapy earlier.

Further studies have suggested that the HLA-DRB1 shared epitope alleles may not be independent risk factors for the development of RA, but rather a risk factor for the development of anti–cyclic citrullinated peptide (anti-CCP) antibodies. Anti-CCP antibodies are believed to be sensitive and specific for the diagnosis of RA and may predate the development of the disease.[153] Research has continued to suggest that the presence of anti-CCP antibodies is highly specific for RA, and that anti-CCP-positive patients have more active disease and more severe radiographic evidence of destruction,[154] and that the presence of anti-CCP antibodies early in disease is a prognostic marker of erosive disease.[155,156] Data also suggest that the presence of anti-CCP is strongly associated with severe extra-articular features of RA.[157]

In the future, genetic analyses could lead to the choice of early effective therapy custom-designed for each patient. It may be possible—using relatively inexpensive microchip technology—to obtain a detailed printout that records the genetic predisposition to develop RA of each patient and the genes governing autoantibody formation and the B cell repertoire, T cell receptor sequences, cytokine and adhesion molecule production, receptor density for inflammatory ligands, and susceptibility to good and toxic effects of drugs.[158]

Refined imaging techniques can help in the staging of disease and in following effects of therapy. Magnetic resonance imaging (MRI) (see Chapter 53), although not yet justified as a cost-effective measure of synovitis, nevertheless can provide a good estimate of synovial volume within joints. In a study using gadopentetate dimeglumine–enhanced MRI,[159] it was found that the rate of erosive progression on MRI was highly correlated with the values of synovial membrane volume, but not with local or global clinical or laboratory parameters. Erosions of bone seen on MRI grew into radiographically visible erosions, but with a delay of 1 year.

Ultrasound also is proving potentially useful for diagnosing active disease at an early stage. Compared with clinical examination, MRI, three-phase bone scan, and conventional radiology in a study of 60 patients with various types of arthritis, ultrasound proved to be a sensitive tool. When looking specifically at 32 of the 60 patients without radiographic erosions, bone scan identified 58% of the joints as abnormal, ultrasound identified 54% as abnormal, and MRI showed erosions in 20% of the joints and enhancement in 41%.[160] Further radiographic studies have shown that MRI and ultrasound exhibit very high specificity and a sensitivity much higher than traditional radiographs.[161] As imaging modalities (it is hoped) decrease in cost, increase in availability, and grow in sophistication, it is possible they will have increased utility in the future for diagnostic and prognostic purposes in patients with inflammatory arthritis.

Generally, the markers discussed previously, including severe or aggressive baseline disease, poor function, the presence of rheumatoid factor and anti-CCP antibodies, and elevation of acute-phase markers, all suggest a worse prognosis. Beyond this, the presence of erosions and joint space narrowing on imaging studies early in the disease also are predictive of more destructive disease.

IMPORTANT ADJUNCTS

EDUCATION

The point has been made that a "low formal educational level is a composite/surrogate variable [that] identifies behavioral risk factors predisposing to the etiology and poor outcomes in most chronic diseases."[162] In studies of RA, morbidity and mortality rates over a 9-year period in one series were inversely proportional to the formal educational level and could not be explained by age, duration of disease,

joint count, functional measures, or medications.[163] Although the reasons behind this link of formal education to outcome are obscure, the corollary is that teaching patients about how arthritis affects people, how they can be involved in helping themselves, and what physicians use to treat arthritis leads to better outcomes.[164] Use of the Arthritis Self-Management Program has been rigorously shown to enable pain reduction, decrease visits to physicians, and save money.[165,166] Participation of spouses in educational group sessions for patients leads to additional beneficial effects.[167] Psychological counseling, a form of education, also is useful for patients with arthritis. Stress management training can be particularly effective, leading to statistically significant improvements in measures of helplessness, self-efficacy, coping, pain, and health status.[168]

Chapter 61 provides a more in-depth discussion of education and its role in arthritis; however, in general, patients need to feel they have some control over their illnesses—a capacity to do something for themselves that has a positive effect. They do not want to be bystanders, watching a contest between a disease they did nothing to bring on and physicians whose words and strategies they insufficiently understand. Education can make a big difference, enabling patients to form a therapeutic contract with their physicians and making it more likely that they will not turn, out of frustration, to alternative therapies that may do more harm than good.

PAIN CONTROL

Pain can be the factor that limits effectiveness of physical and occupational therapy, and as pointed out during a special workshop sponsored by the National Advisory Board for Arthritis and Musculoskeletal and Skin Diseases, it is frequently undertreated in patients with arthritis.[169] In addition to inhibiting function, pain is a major cause of depression in patients with polyarthritis. To maximize therapy in patients with early RA or undifferentiated polyarthritis, pain must be controlled without altering consciousness or generating addiction. Treatment strategies favoring education, rest, exercise, and disease-modifying therapies generally are favored as an approach to pain control in arthritis, and strategies that rely on narcotic derivatives alone are discouraged. In most medical centers, experts in pain management are available for consultation by rheumatologists and primary care physicians.

REST, EXERCISE, AND ACTIVITIES OF DAILY LIVING

Education and supervision of a patient by trained professionals on the importance of finding the best balance of rest and exercise for inflamed joints is essential. This component of therapy can be started well before a definitive diagnosis is made. No matter what the cause, finding this balance should ensure that a patient develops, or retains, sufficient strength to support joint function without exacerbating inflammation.

Details of physical and occupational therapy are outlined in Chapter 64. A patient with acutely and severely inflamed joints may need application of resting splints to immobilize the joint until anti-inflammatory medication takes effect. Even the most painful joints, when splinted, must be moved passively through a full range of motion each day to prevent flexion contractures, particularly in children. For moderately inflamed joints, isometric exercise with muscles contracted in a fixed position (the resting length of the muscle) provides adequate muscle tone without exacerbating joint inflammation and pain. Maximal contractions, held for 6 seconds and repeated 5 to 10 times, performed several times each day, can prevent further loss of muscle mass around arthritic joints.

Patients with inactive or well-controlled arthritis can profit from variable-resistance programs or even high-intensity strength training, which has been shown to provide significant improvements in strength, pain, and fatigue. Elderly patients with RA can benefit from progressive resistance exercises, similar to younger patients. In a study of older patients given closely regulated workouts on pneumatic resistance equipment, maximal strength of all major exercised muscle groups was increased 75% without exacerbation of clinical disease activity.[170] Not only does prescribed sustained exercise increase muscle strength, but also it helps the ability of patients to perform daily routines, improves global assessments and moods, and can decrease pain.[171]

Every patient with RA should have one or more sessions with a licensed occupational therapist to learn how to preserve joint function and alignment, while carrying out the necessary and enjoyable activities of daily living. The basic concept is to avoid excessive force applied across non–weight-bearing joints and to avoid unnecessary impact loading on weight-bearing joints. The Arthritis Society Home Service in Toronto, Canada, participated in a prospective and controlled trial showing that home therapy by occupational therapists produced a statistically significant and clinically important improvement in function in rheumatoid patients.[172]

ROLE OF THE RHEUMATOLOGIST IN MANAGEMENT

The increasing complexity of management options, combination therapies, and possible toxicities of therapy have all but necessitated that the rheumatologist be involved in the management decisions of patients with RA. Data indicate that continuing care by a rheumatologist (mean of 8.6 visits per year) results in a crude rate of progression of functional disability that is significantly less ($P = .001$) than for patients who receive only intermittent, sporadic care by a rheumatologist.[173] Analysis of the data has supported the interpretation that worsening disability was not the reason for intermittent care, but rather a consequence of it.

In another series of 561 patients with definite RA followed over 20 years, the patients seen by a rheumatologist during the first 2 years of disease improved significantly compared with others.[174] The favorable outcome could be related to an early start with aggressive therapy. It is probable that the best care is given by a team of a rheumatologist and a primary care physician working closely with each patient, plus adequate consultation from physical and occupational therapists and orthopaedic surgeons. Additional evidence

supporting this approach showed that patients who had access to a specialist (rheumatologist) had higher performance scores than patients who saw only a general practitioner. Access to primary care and specialist care resulted in significant improvements in arthritis care, comorbid illness, and health care maintenance overall beyond seeing a primary care physician alone.[175]

Among rheumatologists, there is a wide variation of frequency with which follow-up visits are scheduled, even though clinical outcome for patients varies little.[176] With the increasing restraints of managed care on medical care, all physicians must struggle to give adequate time to each patient.

COMPLEMENTARY THERAPY AND DIET

Patients with RA often want to be personally involved in attempts to control the disease. Along with direct advertising about pharmaceutical medications, patients are saturated with information about complementary therapy and diets for RA.

It is important to inform patients of the risk of taking herbal medicines that can be toxic and to let them know that there are no data to support the claims that copper bracelets, glucosamine and chondroitin sulfate, wheat germ, or tomato-free diets benefit RA. Patients interested in trying dietary modification should be informed about addition of omega-3 or omega-6 fatty acids to the diet. Eicosapentaenoic acid, in doses of 54 mg/kg/day, and docosahexaenoic acid, in doses of 36 mg/kg/day, added to the diet have been shown in double-blind, randomized, placebo-controlled studies to improve joint counts in a 30-week trial.[177] Another study proved the benefit of these fish oils over 12 months when compared with olive oil supplementation.[178]

Manipulation of the omega-6 pathway of metabolism of fatty acids has been achieved by giving 1.4 g/day of gamma-linolenic acid to RA patients in a double-blind, placebo-controlled study of 24 weeks' duration.[179] Joint tenderness improved significantly in the treated group.

Giving omega-3 fatty acids (eicosapentaenoic acid and docosahexaenoic acid) diminishes prostaglandin E_2 and leukotriene B_4 biosynthesis and increases production of prostaglandin E_3 and leukotriene B_5, both of which are less inflammatory than the usual products. Addition of gamma-linolenic acid to diets increases prostaglandin E_1 (an anti-inflammatory prostaglandin) production, and prostaglandin E_2 and leukotriene B_4 levels do not change. Data also suggest that long-term fish oil treatment may reduce cardiovascular risk factors in patients with early RA.[180]

These added oils in the diet can leave a fishy taste in the mouth and generate oily, foul-smelling stools. Some patients cannot tolerate these effects, but most can. Most important, the fish oil supplements do no apparent harm.

No other diets have been useful besides diets associated with enhancing weight loss. Excess weight is a liability for RA patients, and weight control is an important component of a good therapeutic plan. "Starvation diets," despite the fact that they may suppress the immune response, should be discouraged.

Future Directions

The growing body of data lends credence to the belief that early diagnosis and initiation of therapy in RA is appropriate and necessary to maximize the short-term and long-term benefits to the patient. It may afford a window of opportunity for substantive disease modification, which may lead to long-term protective benefits. In addition to the growing emphasis on early intervention, the rheumatology community is continually striving to improve overall response rates among current patients and to expand intervention into untreated populations. There also is a strong desire to develop therapies that work in 90% to 100% of patients, not the 60% seen today. The long-term goal of treatment intervention should be to achieve remission. Although a unique opportunity for intervention may exist early in the course of disease, it is believed that DMARDs should be introduced at all stages of disease for long-term disease modification. What also has become fundamentally clear is that even in later stages of disease, the use of DMARDs can reduce symptoms and signs, improve function, and slow structural progression.

The remarkable efficacy and safety of biologic agents has been reassuring. Monitoring for adverse events and for unforeseen occurrences must continue, however. Differences between agents also warrant considerable research. It may be that different populations and disease states would be better suited to one or another agent as monotherapy or particularly in combination with other agents. In the future, we may see improvements in combination approaches including combination biologic agents. To date, combination biologic approaches have led to increased risks of infection, however.[91,100] With the right targets or the appropriate modulations of dosages, we may be able to overcome this increased risk.

The future may see additional agents being used as adjuncts. An example would be the use of statin agents. 3-Hydroxy-3-methylglutaryl-coenzyme A (HMG-CoA) reductase inhibitors (statins) have significant benefits toward lowering cholesterol and reducing risks of cardiovascular events. The fact that patients with RA are at increased risk of cardiovascular mortality itself might be reason to consider statin use. Statins may influence other inflammatory factors, however, effecting the symptoms and signs of disease. In one study, 116 patients with RA were randomly assigned to receive placebo or 40 mg of atorvastatin in addition to their existing DMARD regimen. After 6 months, significant improvements were seen in disease activity scores and reductions in C-reactive protein and erythrocyte sedimentation rates, suggesting modest anti-inflammatory effects.[181]

In the years ahead, it will be increasingly important for rheumatologists and primary care physicians treating patients with RA to expect rigorous confirmation of efficacy and safety by double-blind, placebo-controlled studies of all new products and long-term registries to ensure the safety of these agents in the long run. Physicians must be armed with data because their patients will be armed with testimonies from the Internet and convincing ads from television, newspapers, and magazines for many diverse therapies. Another issue will be finding suitable patients to enroll in studies of the most promising medications that are ready to move into advanced phase trials. Rheumatologists must take a leading role in ensuring their patients have the chance to participate in studies of the most promising drugs and devices.

REFERENCES

1. **American College of Rheumatology: Guidelines for the management of rheumatoid arthritis: 2002 update. Arthritis Rheum 46:328-346, 2002.**
2. Bernstein HN: Ocular safety of hydroxychloroquine. Ann Ophthalmol 23:292, 1991.
3. Fox RI, Kang H: Mechanism of action of antimalarial drugs: Inhibition of antigen processing and presentation. Lupus 2(Suppl 1):S9, 1993.
4. Kim W, Yoo S, Min S, et al: Hydroxychloroquine potentiates fas-mediated apoptosis of rheumatoid synoviocytes. Clin Exp Immunol 144:503-511, 2006.
5. Faarvang KL, Egsmose C, Kryger P: Hydroxychloroquine and sulphasalazine alone and in combination in rheumatoid arthritis: A randomised double blind trial. Ann Rheum Dis 52:711, 1993.
6. A randomized trial of hydroxychloroquine in early rheumatoid arthritis. The HERA study. Am J Med 98:156-168, 1995.
7. Tsakonas E, Fitzgerald AA, Fitzcharles MA, et al: Consequences of delayed therapy with second-line agents in rheumatoid arthritis: A 3 year followup on the Hydroxychloroquine in Early Rheumatoid Arthritis (HERA) Study. J Rheumatol 27:623-629, 2000.
8. Svartz N: A new sulfanilamide preparation. Acta Med Scand 110:577, 1942.
9. Hannonen P, Mottonen T, Hakola M, et al: Sulfasalazine in early rheumatoid arthritis: A 48-week double-blind, prospective, placebo-controlled study. Arthritis Rheum 36:1501, 1993.
10. Van Der Heijde DM, Van Riel PL, Nuver-Zwart IH, et al: Effects of hydroxychloroquine and sulphasalazine on progression of joint damage in rheumatoid arthritis. Lancet 1:1036-1038, 1989.
11. Smolen JS, Kalden JR, Scott DL: Efficacy and safety of leflunomide compared with placebo and sulfasalazine in active rheumatoid arthritis: A double-blind, randomised, multicentre trial. European Leflunomide Study Group. Lancet 353:259, 1999.
12. Boers M, Verhoeven AC, Markusse HM, et al: Randomised comparison of combined step-down prednisolone, methotrexate and sulphasalazine with sulphasalazine alone in early rheumatoid arthritis. Lancet 350:309-318, 1997.
13. **O'Dell JR, Haire CE, Erikson N, et al: Treatment of rheumatoid arthritis with methotrexate alone, sulfasalazine and hydroxychloroquine, or a combination of all three medications. N Engl J Med 334:1287, 1996.**
14. Mottonen T, Hannonen P, Leirisalo-Repo M, et al: Comparison of combination therapy with single-drug therapy in early rheumatoid arthritis: A randomised trial. FIN-RACo trial group. Lancet 353:1568-1573, 1999.
15. Rau R, Schleusser B, Herborn G, et al: Long term treatment of destructive rheumatoid arthritis with methotrexate. J Rheumatol 24:1881, 1997.
16. Weinblatt ME, Maier AL: Longterm experience with low dose weekly methotrexate in rheumatoid arthritis. J Rheumatol 17(Suppl 22):33, 1990.
17. Rau R, Herborn G, Karger T, et al: Retardation of radiologic progression in rheumatoid arthritis with methotrexate therapy: A controlled study. Arthritis Rheum 34:1236, 1991.
18. Jeurissen MEC, Boerbooms AMT, van de Putte LBA, et al: Influence of methotrexate and azathioprine on radiologic progression in rheumatoid arthritis: A randomized, double-blind study. Ann Intern Med 114:999, 1991.
19. **Bathon JM, Martin RW, Fleischmann RM, et al: A comparison of etanercept and methotrexate in patients with early rheumatoid arthritis. N Engl J Med 343:1586-1593, 2000.**
20. Genovese MC, Bathon JM, Martin RW, et al: Etanercept versus methotrexate in patients with early rheumatoid arthritis: Two-year radiographic and clinical outcomes. Arthritis Rheum 46:1443-1450, 2002.
21. **Lipsky PE, van der Heijde DM, St Clair EW, et al: Infliximab and methotrexate in the treatment of rheumatoid arthritis: Anti-tumor necrosis factor trial in rheumatoid arthritis with concomitant therapy study group. N Engl J Med 343:1594-1602, 2000.**
22. Weinblatt ME, Kremer JM, Bankhurst AD, et al: A trial of etanercept, a recombinant tumor necrosis factor receptor: Fc fusion protein, in patients with rheumatoid arthritis receiving methotrexate. N Engl J Med 340:253-259, 1999.
23. Kremer JM, Genovese MC, Cannon GW, et al: Concomitant leflunomide therapy in patients with active rheumatoid arthritis despite stable doses of methotrexate: A randomized, double-blind, placebo-controlled trial. Ann Intern Med 137:726-733, 2002.

24. Weinblatt ME, Keystone EC, Furst DE, et al: Adalimumab, a fully human anti-tumor necrosis factor alpha monoclonal antibody, for the treatment of rheumatoid arthritis in patients taking concomitant methotrexate. The ARMADA trial. Arthritis Rheum 48:35-45, 2003.

25. Breedveld FC, Weisman MH, Kavanaugh AF, et al: The PREMIER study: A multicenter, randomized, double-blind clinical trial of combination therapy with adalimumab plus methotrexate versus methotrexate alone or adalimumab alone in patients with early, aggressive rheumatoid arthritis who had not had previous methotrexate treatment. Arthritis Rheum 54:26-37, 2006.

26. St Clair EW, van der Heijde DM, Smolen JS, et al: Active-controlled study of patients receiving infliximab for the treatment of rheumatoid arthritis of early onset study group: Combination of infliximab and methotrexate therapy for early rheumatoid arthritis: A randomized, controlled trial. Arthritis Rheum 50:3432-3443, 2004.

27. Strand V, Cohen S, Schiff M, et al: Treatment of active rheumatoid arthritis with leflunomide compared with placebo and methotrexate. Leflunomide Rheumatoid Arthritis Investigators Group. Arch Intern Med 159:2542-2550, 1999.

28. Emery P, Breedveld FC, Lemmel EM, et al: A comparison of the efficacy and safety of leflunomide and methotrexate for the treatment of rheumatoid arthritis. Rheumatology (Oxf) 39:655-665, 2000.

29. Ortiz Z, Shea B, Suarez-Almazoe ME, et al: The efficacy of folic acid and folinic acid in reducing methotrexate gastrointestinal toxicity in rheumatoid arthritis: A meta-analysis of randomized controlled trials. J Rheumatol 25:36, 1998.

30. Morgan SL, Baggott JE, Lee JV, et al: Folic acid supplementation prevents deficient blood folate levels and hyperhomocystinemia during long-term, low dose methotrexate therapy for rheumatoid arthritis: Implications for cardiovascular disease prevention. J Rheumatol 25:441, 1998.

31. Kremer JM, Alacron GS, Lightfoot RW, et al: Methotrexate for rheumatoid arthritis: Suggested guidelines for monitoring liver toxicity. Arthritis Rheum 37:316, 1994.

32. Barrera P, Laan RFJM, van Riel PLCM, et al: Methotrexate-related pulmonary complications in rheumatoid arthritis. Ann Rheum Dis 53:434, 1994.

33. Fox RI: Mechanisms of action of leflunomide. J Rheumatol (Suppl 53):20, 1998.

34. Bruce B, Fries JF: The Stanford Health Assessment Questionnaire: A review of its history, issues, progress, and documentation. J Rheumatol 30:167-178, 2003.

35. Sharp JT, Strand V, Leung H, et al: Treatment with leflunomide slows radiographic progression of rheumatoid arthritis: Results from three randomized controlled trials of leflunomide in patients with active rheumatoid arthritis. Leflunomide Rheumatoid Arthritis Investigators Group. Arthritis Rheum 43:495-505, 2000.

36. Mladenovic V, Domljan Z, Rozman B, et al: Safety and effectiveness of leflunomide in the treatment of patients with active rheumatoid arthritis. Arthritis Rheum 38:1595, 1995.

37. Yu LP Jr, Smith GN, Hasty KA, et al: Doxycycline inhibits type XI collagenolytic activity of extracts from human osteoarthritis cartilage and of gelatinase. J Rheumatol 18:1450, 1991.

38. Smith GN Jr, Brandt KD, Hasty KA: Activation of recombinant human neutrophil procollagenase in the presence of doxycycline results in fragmentation of the enzyme and loss of enzyme activity. Arthritis Rheum 39:235, 1996.

39. Kloppenburg M, Breedveld FC, Terwiel JP, et al: Minocycline in active rheumatoid arthritis: A double-blind, placebo-controlled trial. Arthritis Rheum 37:629, 1994.

40. Tilley B, Alarcon G, Heyse S, et al: Minocycline in rheumatoid arthritis: A 48-week, double blind, placebo-controlled trial. Ann Intern Med 122:81, 1995.

41. Odell JR, Haire CE, Palmer W, et al: Treatment of early rheumatoid arthritis with minocycline or placebo: Results of a randomized, double-blind, placebo-controlled trial. Arthritis Rheum 40:842, 1997.

42. O'Dell JR, Blakely KW, Mallek JA, et al: Treatment of early seropositive rheumatoid arthritis: A two-year, double-blind comparison of minocycline and hydroxychloroquine. Arthritis Rheum 44:2235-2241, 2001.

43. Elkayam O, Levartovsky D, Brautbar C, et al: Clinical and immunological study of 7 patients with minocycline-induced autoimmune phenomena. Am J Med 105:484, 1998.

44. O'Dell JR, Elliott JR, Mallek JA, et al: Treatment of early seropositive rheumatoid arthritis: Doxycycline plus methotrexate versus methotrexate alone. Arthritis Rheum 54:621-627, 2006.

45. Buckland-Wright JC, Clarke GS, Chikanza IC, et al: Quantitative microfocal radiography detects changes in erosion area in patients with early rheumatoid arthritis treated with Myochrysine. J Rheumatol 20:243, 1993.

46. Lehman AJ, Esdaile JM, Klinkhoff AV, et al; METGO Study Group: A 48-week, randomized double-blind, double-observer, placebo-controlled multicenter trial of combination methotrexate and intramuscular gold therapy in rheumatoid arthritis: Results of the METGO study. Arthritis Rheum 52:1360-1370, 2005.

47. Sakkas LI, Chikanza IC, Vaughn RW, et al: Gold induced nephropathy in rheumatoid arthritis and HLA class II genes. Ann Rheum Dis 52:300, 1993.

48. Felson DT, Anderson JJ, Meenan RF: The comparative efficacy and toxicity of second-line drugs in rheumatoid arthritis: Results of second-line drugs in rheumatoid arthritis. Arthritis Rheum 33:1449, 1990.

49. Borg G, Allander E, Berg E: Auranofin treatment in early rheumatoid arthritis may postpone early retirement: Results from a 2-year double blind trial. J Rheumatol 18:1015, 1991.

50. Black AJ, McLeod HL, Capell HA: Thiopurine methyltransferase genotype predicts therapy limiting severe toxicity from azathioprine. Ann Intern Med 129:716, 1998.

51. Blanco R, Martinez-Taboada VM, Gonzalez-Gay MA: Acute febrile toxic reaction in patients with refractory rheumatoid arthritis who are receiving combined therapy with methotrexate and azathioprine. Arthritis Rheum 39:1016, 1996.

52. Jessop JD, O'Sullivan MM, Lewis PA, et al: A long term five-year randomized trial of hydroxychloroquine, sodium aurothiomalate, auranofin and penicillamine in the treatment of patients with rheumatoid arthritis. Br J Rheumatol 37:992, 1998.

53. Dronke M, Leonard WJ, Depper JM, et al: Cyclosporin A inhibits T-cell growth factor gene expression at the level of mRNA transcription. Proc Natl Acad Sci U S A 81:5214, 1984.

54. Fuleihan R, Ramesh N, Horner A, et al: Cyclosporin A inhibits CD40 ligand expression in T lymphocytes. J Clin Invest 93:1315, 1994.

55. Tugwell P, Pincus T, Yocum D, et al: Combination therapy with cyclosporine and methotrexate in severe rheumatoid arthritis. N Engl J Med 333:137, 1995.

56. Stein CM, Pincus T, Yocum D, et al: Combination treatment of severe rheumatoid arthritis with cyclosporine and methotrexate for forty-eight weeks: An open-label extension study. The Methotrexate-Cyclosporine Combination Study Group. Arthritis Rheum 40:1843, 1997.

57. Tugwell P, Bombardier C, Gent M, et al: Low-dose cyclosporin versus placebo in patients with rheumatoid arthritis. Lancet 335:1051, 1990.

58. Furst DE, Saag K, Fleischmann MR, et al: Efficacy of tacrolimus in rheumatoid arthritis patients who have been treated unsuccessfully with methotrexate: A six-month, double-blind, randomized, dose-ranging study. Arthritis Rheum 46:2020-2028, 2002.

59. Yocum DE, Furst DE, Kaine JL, et al: Tacrolimus Rheumatoid Arthritis Study Group: Efficacy and safety of tacrolimus in patients with rheumatoid arthritis: A double-blind trial. Arthritis Rheum 48:3328-3337, 2003.

60. Grigor C, Capell H, Stirling A, et al: Effect of a treatment strategy of tight control for rheumatoid arthritis (the TICORA study): A single-blind randomised controlled trial. Lancet 364:263-269, 2004.

61. Fries JF: Re-evaluating the therapeutic approach to rheumatoid arthritis: The "sawtooth" strategy. J Rheumatol 22(Suppl):12-15, 1990.

62. McCarty DJ, Carrera GF: Treatment of intractable rheumatoid arthritis with combined cyclophosphamide, azathioprine and hydroxychloroquine. JAMA 255:2215, 1982.

63. Pincus T, O'Dell JR, Kremer JM: Combination therapy with multiple disease-modifying antirheumatic drugs in rheumatoid arthritis: A preventive strategy. Ann Intern Med 131:768-774, 1999.

64. Kremer JM: Rational use of new and existing disease-modifying agents in rheumatoid arthritis. Ann Intern Med 134:695-706, 2001.

65. O'Dell JR, Leff R, Paulsen G, et al: Treatment of rheumatoid arthritis with methotrexate and hydroxychloroquine, methotrexate and sulfasalazine, or a combination of the three medications: Results of a two-year, randomized, double-blind, placebo-controlled trial. Arthritis Rheum 46:1164-1170, 2002.

66. Mottonen T, Hannonen P, Korpela M, et al: Delay to institution of therapy and induction of remission using single-drug or combination-disease-modifying antirheumatic drug therapy in early rheumatoid arthritis. Arthritis Rheum 46:894-898, 2002.

67. Wilske KR, Healey LA: Remodeling the pyramid—a concept whose time has come. J Rheumatol 16:565-567, 1989.
68. Landewe RB, Boers M, Verhoeven AC, et al: COBRA combination therapy in patients with early rheumatoid arthritis: Long-term structural benefits of a brief intervention. Arthritis Rheum 46:347-356, 2002.
69. **Goekoop-Ruiterman YP, de Vries-Bouwstra JK, Allaart CF, et al: Clinical and radiographic outcomes of four different treatment strategies in patients with early rheumatoid arthritis (the BeSt study): A randomized, controlled trial. Arthritis Rheum 52:3381-3390, 2005.**
70. Keystone EC, Kavanaugh AF, Sharp JT, et al: Radiographic, clinical, and functional outcomes of treatment with adalimumab (a human anti-tumor necrosis factor monoclonal antibody) in patients with active rheumatoid arthritis receiving concomitant methotrexate therapy: A randomized, placebo-controlled, 52-week trial. Arthritis Rheum 50:1400-1411, 2004.
71. Kremer JM, Genant HK, Moreland LW, et al: Effects of abatacept in patients with methotrexate-resistant active rheumatoid arthritis: A randomized trial. Ann Intern Med 144:865-876, 2006.
72. **Cohen SB, Emery P, Greenwald MW, et al: Rituximab for rheumatoid arthritis refractory to anti-tumor necrosis factor therapy: Results of a multicenter, randomized, double-blind, placebo-controlled, phase III trial evaluating primary efficacy and safety at twenty-four weeks. Arthritis Rheum 54:2793-2806, 2006.**
73. **Felson DT, Anderson JJ, Boers M, et al: American College of Rheumatology preliminary definition of improvement in rheumatoid arthritis. Arthritis Rheum 38:727, 1995.**
74. Moreland LW, Schiff MH, Baumgartner SW, et al: Etanercept therapy in rheumatoid arthritis. Ann Intern Med 130:478, 1999.
75. Klareskog L, van der Heijde D, de Jager JP, et al: TEMPO (Trial of Etanercept and Methotrexate with Radiographic Patient Outcomes) Study Investigators: Therapeutic effect of the combination of etanercept and methotrexate compared with each treatment alone in patients with rheumatoid arthritis: Double-blind randomised controlled trial. Lancet 363:675-681, 2004.
76. van der Heijde D, Landewe R, Klareskog L, et al: Presentation and analysis of data on radiographic outcome in clinical trials: Experience from the TEMPO study. Arthritis Rheum 52:49-60, 2005.
77. van der Heijde D, Klareskog L, Rodriguez-Valverde V, et al; TEMPO Study Investigators: Comparison of etanercept and methotrexate, alone and combined, in the treatment of rheumatoid arthritis: Two-year clinical and radiographic results from the TEMPO study, a double-blind, randomized trial. Arthritis Rheum 54:1063-1074, 2006.
78. St Clair EW, Wagner CL, Fasanmade AA, et al: The relationship of serum infliximab concentrations to clinical improvement in rheumatoid arthritis: Results from ATTRACT, a multicenter, randomized, double-blind, placebo-controlled trial. Arthritis Rheum 46:1451-1459, 2002.
79. Maini RN, Breedveld FC, Kalden JR, et al: Therapeutic efficacy of multiple intravenous infusions of anti-tumor necrosis factor alpha monoclonal antibody combined with low-dose weekly methotrexate in rheumatoid arthritis. Arthritis Rheum 41:1552-1563, 1998.
80. Infliximab package insert. Malvern, Penn, Centocor, 2006.
81. van de Putte LB, Atkins C, Malaise M, et al: Efficacy and safety of adalimumab as monotherapy in patients with rheumatoid arthritis for whom previous disease modifying antirheumatic drug treatment has failed. Ann Rheum Dis 63:508-516, 2004.
82. Firestein GS, Zvaifler NJ: Anticytokine therapy in rheumatoid arthritis. N Engl J Med 337:195, 1997.
83. Robinson WH, Genovese MC, Moreland LW: Demyelinating and neurologic events reported in association with tumor necrosis factor alpha antagonism: By what mechanisms could tumor necrosis factor alpha antagonists improve rheumatoid arthritis but exacerbate multiple sclerosis? Arthritis Rheum 44:1977-1983, 2001.
84. Sicotte NL, Voskuhl RR: Onset of multiple sclerosis associated with anti-TNF therapy. Neurology 57:1885-1888, 2001.
85. van Oosten BW, Barkhof F, Truyen L, et al: Increased MRI activity and immune activation in two multiple sclerosis patients treated with the monoclonal anti-tumor necrosis factor antibody cA2. Neurology 47:1531-1534, 1996.
86. Mohan N, Edwards ET, Cupps TR, et al: Demyelination occurring during anti-tumor necrosis factor alpha therapy for inflammatory arthritides. Arthritis Rheum 44:2862-2869, 2001.
87. Bresnihan B, Alvaro-Gracia JM, Cobby M, et al: Treatment of rheumatoid arthritis with recombinant human interleukin-1 receptor antagonist. Arthritis Rheum 41:196, 1998.
88. Cohen S, Hurd E, Cush J, et al: Treatment of rheumatoid arthritis with anakinra, a recombinant human interleukin-1 receptor antagonist, in combination with methotrexate: Results of a twenty-four-week, multicenter, randomized, double-blind, placebo-controlled trial. Arthritis Rheum 46:614-624, 2002.
89. Tesser J, Fleischmann R, Dore R, et al; 990757 Study Group: Concomitant medication use in a large, international, multicenter, placebo controlled trial of anakinra, a recombinant interleukin 1 receptor antagonist, in patients with rheumatoid arthritis. J Rheumatol 31:649-654, 2004.
90. Schiff MH, Bulpitt K, Weaver AA, et al: Safety of combination therapy with anakinra and etanercept in patients with rheumatoid arthritis. Arthritis Rheum 45:157, 2001 (abstract).
91. Genovese MC, Cohen S, Moreland L, et al: Combination therapy with etanercept and anakinra in the treatment of patients with rheumatoid arthritis who have been treated unsuccessfully with methotrexate. Arthritis Rheum 50:1412-1419, 2004.
92. Jiang Y, Genant HK, Watt I, et al: A multicenter, double-blind, dose-ranging, randomized, placebo-controlled study of recombinant human interleukin-1 receptor antagonist in patients with rheumatoid arthritis: Radiologic progression and correlation of Genant and Larsen scores. Arthritis Rheum 43:1001-1009, 2000.
93. Shergy WJ, Cohen S, Greenwald M, et al: Anakinra inhibits the progression of radiographically measured joint destruction in rheumatoid arthritis. Arthritis Rheum 46:3420, 2002.
94. Wiesenhutter CW, Irish BL, Bertram JR: Treatment of patients with refractory rheumatoid arthritis with extracorporeal protein A immunoadsorption columns: A pilot trial. J Rheumatol 21:5, 1994.
95. Linsley PS, Brady W, Urnes M, et al: CTLA-4 is a second receptor for the B cell activation antigen B7. J Exp Med 174:561-569, 1991.
96. Moreland LW, Alten R, Van den Bosch F, et al: Costimulatory blockade in patients with rheumatoid arthritis: A pilot, dose-finding, double-blind, placebo-controlled clinical trial evaluating CTLA-4Ig and LEA29Y eighty-five days after the first infusion. Arthritis Rheum 46:1470-1479, 2002.
97. Collins AV, Brodie DW, Gilbert RJ, et al: The interaction properties of costimulatory molecules revisited. Immunity 17:201-210, 2002.
98. Kremer JM, Westhovens R, Leon M, et al: Treatment of rheumatoid arthritis by selective inhibition of T-cell activation with fusion protein CTLA4Ig. N Engl J Med 349:1907-1915, 2003.
99. **Genovese MC, Becker JC, Schiff M, et al: Abatacept for rheumatoid arthritis refractory to tumor necrosis factor alpha inhibition. N Engl J Med 353:1114-1123, 2005.**
100. Weinblatt M, Combe B, Covucci A, et al: Safety of the selective costimulation modulator abatacept in rheumatoid arthritis patients receiving background biologic and nonbiologic disease-modifying antirheumatic drugs: A one-year randomized, placebo-controlled study. Arthritis Rheum 54:2807-2816, 2006.
101. Reff ME, Carner K, Chambers KS, et al: Depletion of B cells in vivo by a chimeric mouse human monoclonal antibody to CD20. Blood 83:435-445, 1994.
102. Edwards JCW, Cambridge G: Sustained improvement in rheumatoid arthritis following a protocol designed to deplete B lymphocytes. Rheumatology (Oxf) 40:205, 2001.
103. Edwards JCW, Szczepanski L, Szechinski J, et al: Efficacy of B-cell-targeted therapy with rituximab in patients with rheumatoid arthritis. N Engl J Med 350:2572-2581, 2004.
104. Sell S, Max EE: All about B cells. In: Immunology, Immunopathology, and Immunity. Washington DC, ASM Press, 2001, p 101.
105. Anderson DR, Grillo-Lopez A, Varns C, et al: Targeted anti-cancer therapy using rituximab, a chimaeric anti-CD20 antibody (IDEC-C2B8) in the treatment of non-Hodgkin's B-cell lymphoma. Biochem Soc Trans 25:705-708, 1997.
106. Clynes RA, Towers TL, Presta LG, et al: Inhibitory Fc receptors modulate in vivo cytoxicity against tumor targets. Nat Med 6:443-446, 2000.
107. Emery P, Fleischmann R, Filipowicz-Sosnowska A, et al; DANCER Study Group: The efficacy and safety of rituximab in patients with active rheumatoid arthritis despite methotrexate treatment: Results of a phase IIB randomized, double-blind, placebo-controlled, dose-ranging trial. Arthritis Rheum 54:1390-1400, 2006.

108. Weinstein RS, Jilka RL, Parfitt AM, et al: Inhibition of osteoblastogenesis and promotion of apoptosis of osteoblasts and osteocytes by glucocorticoids. J Clin Invest 102:274, 1998.

109. Compton JE, Vedi S, Croucher PL, et al: Bone turnover in non-steroid treated rheumatoid arthritis. Ann Rheum Dis 53:163, 1994.

110. Kröger H, Honkanen R, Saarikoski S, et al: Decreased axial bone mineral density in perimenopausal women with rheumatoid arthritis: A population based study. Ann Rheum Dis 53:18, 1994.

111. Dequeker J, Geisems P: Osteoporosis and arthritis. Ann Rheum Dis 49:276, 1990.

112. Kirwan JR: The effect of glucocorticoids on joint destruction in rheumatoid arthritis. N Engl J Med 333:142, 1995.

113. van Everdingen AA, Jacobs JW, Siewertsz Van Reesema DR, et al: Low-dose prednisone therapy for patients with early active rheumatoid arthritis: Clinical efficacy, disease-modifying properties, and side effects: A randomized, double-blind, placebo-controlled clinical trial. Ann Intern Med 136:1-12, 2002.

114. Svensson B, Boonen A, Albertsson K, et al: Low-dose prednisolone in addition to the initial disease-modifying antirheumatic drug in patients with early active rheumatoid arthritis reduces joint destruction and increases the remission rate: A two-year randomized trial. Arthritis Rheum 52:3360-3370, 2005.

115. Wassenberg S, Rau R, Steinfeld P, et al: Very low-dose prednisolone in early rheumatoid arthritis retards radiographic progression over two years: A multicenter, double-blind, placebo-controlled trial. Arthritis Rheum 52:3371-3380, 2005.

116. Choy EH, Kingsley GH, Khoshaba B, et al; Intramuscular Methylprednisolone Study Group: A two year randomized controlled trial of intramuscular depot steroids in patients with established rheumatoid arthritis who have shown an incomplete response to disease modifying antirheumatic drugs. Ann Rheum Dis 64:1288-1293, 2005.

117. Fries JF, Williams CA, Ramsey DR, et al: The relative toxicity of disease-modifying antirheumatic drugs. Arthritis Rheum 36:297, 1993.

118. Wolfe F, Mitchell DM, Sibley JT, et al: The mortality of rheumatoid arthritis. Arthritis Rheum 37:481, 1994.

119. Ruegsegger P, Medici TC, Anliker M: Corticosteroid-induced bone loss: A longitudinal study of alternate day therapy in patients with bronchial asthma using quantitative computed tomography. Eur J Clin Pharmacol 25:615, 1994.

120. Hochberg MC, Prashker MJ, Greenwald M, et al: Recommendations for the prevention and treatment of glucocorticoid-induced osteoporosis. Am Coll Rheum 39:1791, 1996.

121. Wolfe MM, Lichtenstein DR, Singh G: Gastrointestinal toxicity of nonsteroidal antiinflammatory drugs. N Engl J Med 340:1888, 1999.

122. Abramson S, Weissmann G: The mechanisms of action of nonsteroidal anti-inflammatory drugs. Arthritis Rheum 32:1, 1989.

123. Silverstein FE, Faich G, Goldstein JL, et al: Gastrointestinal toxicity with celecoxib vs nonsteroidal anti-inflammatory drugs for osteoarthritis and rheumatoid arthritis: The CLASS (Celecoxib Long-Term Arthritis Safety Study) study: A randomized controlled trial. JAMA 284:1247-1255, 2000.

124. Bombardier C, Laine L, Reicin A, et al: Comparison of upper gastrointestinal toxicity of rofecoxib and naproxen in patients with rheumatoid arthritis. VIGOR Study Group. N Engl J Med 343:1520-1528, 2000.

125. van der Heijde DMFM, van't Hof MA, van Riel PLCM, et al: Judging disease activity in clinical practice in rheumatoid arthritis: First step in the development of a 'disease activity score.' Ann Rheum Dis 49:916-920, 1990.

126. van der Heijde DMFM, van't Hof MA, van Riel PLCM, et al: Validity of single variables and composite indices for measuring disease activity in rheumatoid arthritis. Ann Rheum Dis 51:177-181, 1992.

127. www.das-score.nl/www.das-score.nl/home.html. Accessed May 13, 2008.

128. Smolen JS, Breedveld FC, Schiff MH, et al: A simplified disease activity index for rheumatoid arthritis for use in clinical practice. Rheumatology 42:244-257, 2003.

129. Aletaha D, Smolen J: The Simplified Disease Activity Index (SDAI) and the Clinical Disease Activity Index (CDAI): A review of their usefulness and validity in rheumatoid arthritis. Clin Exp Rheumatol 23:S100-S108, 2005.

130. Wolfe F, Cathey MA: The assessment and prediction of functional disability in rheumatoid arthritis. J Rheumatol 18:1298-1306, 1999.

131. Wolfe F, Hawley DJ: The longterm outcomes of rheumatoid arthritis: Work disability: a prospective 18 year study of 823 patients. J Rheumatol 25:2108-2117, 1998.

132. Scott DL, Symmons DPM, Coulton BL, et al: Long-term outcome of treating rheumatoid arthritis: Results after 20 years. Lancet 1:1108, 1987.

133. Pincus T, Callahan LF, Sale WG, et al: Severe functional declines, work disability, and increased mortality in seventy-five rheumatoid arthritis patients studied over nine years. Arthritis Rheum 27:864, 1984.

134. Wolfe F, Sharp JT: Radiographic outcome of recent-onset rheumatoid arthritis: A 19-year study of radiographic progression. Arthritis Rheum 41:1571-1582, 1998.

135. Pincus T, Callahan LF, Fuchs HA, et al: Quantitative analysis of hand radiographs in rheumatoid arthritis: Time course of radiographic changes, relation to joint examination measures, and comparison of different scoring methods. J Rheumatol 22:1983-1989, 1995.

136. Pincus T, Fuchs HA, Callahan LF, et al: Early radiographic joint space narrowing and erosion and later malalignment in rheumatoid arthritis: A longitudinal analysis. J Rheumatol 25:636-640, 1998.

137. Fuchs HA, Kaye JJ, Callahan LF, et al: Evidence of significant radiographic damage in rheumatoid arthritis within the first two years of disease. J Rheumatol 16:585, 1989.

138. Singh G, Terry R, Ramey D, et al: Long-term medical costs and outcomes are significantly associated with early changes in disability in rheumatoid arthritis. Arthritis Rheum 39:S318, 1996.

139. Yelin E, Wanke LA: An assessment of the annual and long-term direct costs of rheumatoid arthritis: The impact of poor function and functional decline. Arthritis Rheum 42:1209-1218, 1999.

140. O'Dell JR: Treating rheumatoid arthritis early: A window of opportunity? Arthritis Rheum 46:283-285, 2002.

141. Korpela M, Laasonen L, Hannonen P, et al; FIN-RACo Trial Group: Retardation of joint damage in patients with early rheumatoid arthritis by initial aggressive treatment with disease-modifying antirheumatic drugs: Five-year experience from the FIN-RACo study. Arthritis Rheum 50:2072-2081, 2004.

142. Puolakka K, Kautiainen H, Mottonen T, et al; FIN-RACo Trial Group: Early suppression of disease activity is essential for maintenance of work capacity in patients with recent-onset rheumatoid arthritis: Five-year experiencee from the FIN-FACo trial. Arthritis Rheum 52:36-41, 2005.

143. Quinn MA, Conaghan PG, O'Connor PJ, et al: Very early treatment with infliximab in addition to methotrexate in early, poor-prognosis rheumatoid arthritis reduces magnetic resonance imaging evidence of synovitis and damage, with sustained benefit after infliximab withdrawal: Results from a twelve-month randomized double-blind, placebo-controlled trial. Arthritis Rheum 52:27-35, 2005.

144. Mottonen T, Paimela L, Leirisalo-Repo M, et al: Only high disease activity and positive rheumatoid factor indicate poor prognosis in patients with early rheumatoid arthritis treated with "sawtooth" strategy. Ann Rheum Dis 57:533, 1998.

145. Callahan LF, Pincus T, Huston JW III, et al: Measures of activity and damage in rheumatoid arthritis: Depiction of changes and prediction of mortality over five years. Arthritis Care Res 10:381, 1997.

146. Combe B, Dougados M, Goupille P, et al: Prognostic factors for radiographic damage in early rheumatoid arthritis: A multiparameter prospective study. Arthritis Rheum 44:1736-1743, 2001.

147. Combe B, Cantagrel A, Goupille P, et al: Predictive factors of 5-year health assessment questionnaire disability in early rheumatoid arthritis. J Rheumatol 30:2344-2349, 2003.

148. Lindqvist E, Saxne T, Geborek P, et al: Ten year outcome in a cohort of patients with early rheumatoid arthritis: Health status, disease process, and damage. Ann Rheum Dis 61:1055-1059, 2002.

149. Smolen JS, Van Der Heijde DM, St Clair EW, et al; Active-Controlled Study of Patients Receiving Infliximab for the Treatment of Rheumatoid Arthritis of Early Onset (ASPIRE) Study Group: Predictors of joint damage in patients with early rheumatoid arthritis treated with high-dose methotrexate with or without concomitant infliximab: Results from the ASPIRE trial. Arthritis Rheum 54:702-710, 2006.

150. Symmons DPM, Silman AJ: Aspects of early arthritis: What determines the evolution of early undifferentiated arthritis and rheumatoid arthritis? An update from the Norfolk Arthritis Register. Arthritis Res Ther 8:214, 2006.

151. Wolfe F, Zwillich SH: The long-term outcomes of rheumatoid arthritis: A 23-year prospective, longitudinal study of total joint replacement and its predictors in 1,600 patients with rheumatoid arthritis. Arthritis Rheum 41:1072, 1998.

152. O'Dell JR, Nepom BS, Haire C, et al: HLA-DRB1 typing in rheumatoid arthritis: Predicting response to specific treatments. Ann Rheum Dis 57:209, 1998.

153. van der Helm-van Mil AH, Verpoort KN, Breedveld FC, et al: The HLA-DRB1 shared epitope alleles are primarily a risk factor for anticyclic citrullinated peptide antibodies and are not an independent risk factor for development of rheumatoid arthritis. Arthritis Rheum 54:1117-1121, 2004.

154. van der Helm-van Mil AH, Verpoort KN, Breedveld FC, et al: Antibodies to citrullinated proteins and differences in clinical progression of rheumatoid arthritis. Arthritis Res Ther 7:R949-R958, 2005.

155. Vencovshy J, Machacek S, Sedova L, et al: Autoantibodies can be prognostic markers of an erosive disease in early rheumatoid arthritis. Ann Rheum Dis 62:427-430, 2003.

156. Berglin E, Johansson T, Sundin U, et al: Radiological outcome in rheumatoid arthritis is predicted by presence of antibodies against cyclic citrullinated peptide before and at disease onset, and by IgA-RF at disease onset. Ann Rheum Dis 65:453-458, 2006.

157. Turesson C, Jacobsson LT, Sturfelt G, et al: Rheumatoid factor and antibodies to cyclic citrullinated peptides are associated with severe extra-articular manifestations in rheumatoid arthritis. Ann Rheum Dis 66:59-64, 2007.

158. Weyand C, Goronzy J: Prognosis in rheumatoid arthritis: Applying new technologies to old questions. J Rheumatol 20:11, 1993.

159. Ostergaard M, Hansen M, Stoltenberg M, et al: Magnetic resonance imaging-determined synovial membrane volume as a marker of disease activity and a predictor of progressive joint destruction in the wrists of patients with rheumatoid arthritis. Arthritis Rheum 42:918, 1999.

160. Backhaus M, Kamradt T, Sandrock D, et al: Arthritis of the finger joints: A comprehensive approach comparing conventional radiography, scintigraphy, ultrasound, and contrast-enhanced magnetic resonance imaging. Arthritis Rheum 42:1232-1245, 1999.

161. Dohn UM, Ejbjerg BJ, Court-Payen M, et al: Are bone erosions detected by magnetic resonance imaging and ultrasonography true erosions? A comparison with computed tomography in rheumatoid arhritis. Arthritis Res Ther 8:R110, 2006.

162. Pincus T: Formal educational level: A marker for the importance of behavioral variables in the pathogenesis, morbidity, and mortality of most diseases? J Rheumatol 15:10, 1988.

163. Pincus T, Callahan LF: Formal education as a marker for increased mortality and morbidity in rheumatoid arthritis. J Chron Dis 311:552, 1984.

164. Lorig K, Seleznick M, Lubeck D, et al: The beneficial outcomes of the arthritis self-management course are not adequately explained by behavioral change. Arthritis Rheum 32:91, 1989.

165. Lorig KR, Mazonson PD, Holman HR: Evidence suggesting that health education for self-management in patients with chronic arthritis has sustained health benefits while reducing health care costs. Arthritis Rheum 36:439, 1993.

166. Lorig K, Ritter PL, Plant K: A disease-specific self-help program compared with a generalized chronic disease self-help program for arthritis patients. Arthritis Rheum 53:950-957, 2005.

167. Taal E, Rasker JJ, Wiegman O: Patient education and self-management in the rheumatic diseases: A self-efficacy approach. Arthritis Care Res 9:229, 1996.

168. Parker JC, Smarr KL, Buckelew SP, et al: Effects of stress management on clinical outcomes in rheumatoid arthritis. Arthritis Rheum 38:1807, 1995.

169. Bellamy N, Bradley L: Workshop on chronic pain, pain control, and patient outcomes in rheumatoid arthritis and osteoarthritis. Arthritis Rheum 39:357, 1996.

170. Rall LC, Meydani SN, Kehayias JJ, et al: The effect of progressive resistance training in rheumatoid arthritis. Arthritis Rheum 39:415, 1996.

171. Harcom TM, Lampan RM, Banwell BF, et al: Therapeutic value of graded aerobic exercise training in rheumatoid arthritis. Arthritis Rheum 28:32, 1985.

172. Helewa A, Goldsmith CH, Lee P, et al: Effects of occupational therapy home service on patients with rheumatoid arthritis. Lancet 337:1453, 1991.

173. Ward MM, Leigh JP, Fries JF: Progression of functional disability in patients with rheumatoid arthritis. Arch Intern Med 153:2229, 1993.

174. Wolfe F, Hawley DJ, Cathey MA: Clinical and health status measures over time: Prognosis and outcome assessment in rheumatoid arthritis. J Rheumatol 18:1290, 1991.

175. MacLean CH, Louie R, Leake B, et al: Quality of care for patients with rheumatoid arthritis. JAMA 284:984-992, 2000.

176. Criswell LA, Such CL, Neuhaus JM, et al: Variation among rheumatologists in clinical outcomes and frequency of office visits for rheumatoid arthritis. J Rheumatol 24:7, 1997.

177. Kremer JM, Jubiz W, Michalek A, et al: Fish-oil fatty acid supplementation in active rheumatoid arthritis: A double-blinded, controlled, crossover study. Ann Intern Med 106:497, 1987.

178. Geusens P, Wouters C, Nijs J, et al: Long-term effect of omega-3 fatty acids of active rheumatoid arthritis. Arthritis Rheum 37:824, 1994.

179. Leventhal LJ, Boyce EG, Zurier RB: Treatment of rheumatoid arthritis with gamma-linolenic acid. Ann Intern Med 119:867, 1993.

180. Cleland LG, Caughey GE, James MJ, et al: Reduction of cardiovascular risk factors with longterm fish oil treatment in early rheumatoid arthritis. J Rheumatol 33:1931-1933, 2006.

181. McCarey DW, McInnes IB, Madhok R, et al: Trial of Atorvastatin in Rheumatoid Arthritis (TARA): Double-blind, randomized placebo-controlled trial. Lancet 363:2015-2021, 2004.

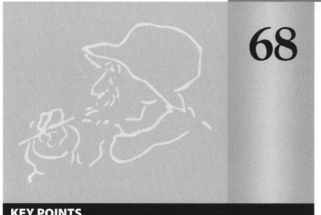

68 Felty's Syndrome

ROBERT S. PINALS

KEY POINTS

Diagnosis of Felty's syndrome requires granulocytopenia, but splenomegaly is not always present.

Felty's syndrome must be distinguished from large granular lymphocytosis.

There is a high frequency of vasculitis and other extra-articular complications.

Decreased granulocyte numbers and function lead to bacterial infections.

Treatment includes disease-modifying antirheumatic drugs and granulocyte growth factors.

Splenectomy is rarely indicated.

In 1924, Felty described the triad of chronic arthritis, splenomegaly, and granulocytopenia. Felty's syndrome represents one of many systemic complications of seropositive rheumatoid arthritis (RA) occurring in patients with unusually severe extra-articular disease and immunologic abnormalities.[1] Persistent granulocytopenia ($<2000/mm^3$) must be present, but the complete triad is not required for a diagnosis of Felty's syndrome because patients without splenomegaly resemble patients with full-blown Felty's syndrome in terms of most clinical, serologic, and immunogenetic features.[1]

EPIDEMIOLOGY

The true prevalence of Felty's syndrome is unknown, but it may be 3% in RA patients.[2] About two thirds of patients are women. HLA-DR4 is found in 95% of patients with Felty's syndrome.[1] This fact may account for the rarity of Felty's syndrome in blacks, who are known to have a low frequency of HLA-DR4. The condition usually is recognized in the fifth through seventh decades of life in patients who have had RA for 10 years or more.[2] Splenomegaly and granulocytopenia may be present before symptoms or signs of arthritis in rare instances.

GENETICS

The familial occurrence of Felty's syndrome suggests that immunogenetic factors are operative.[3] The presence of two HLA-DRB1*04 alleles encoding the shared epitope is associated with increased risk of extra-articular manifestations in RA, but only Felty's syndrome is also associated with HLA-DRB1*0401.[4]

About one third of patients with Felty's syndrome have significant clonal expansions of CD3⁺/CD8⁺ large granular

lymphocytes in their peripheral blood (Fig. 68-1). When originally described, this group of patients with RA and large granular lymphocytosis (LGL), an indolent lymphocytic leukemia, was considered to represent a separate syndrome. Immunogenetic studies have shown, however, the same HLA-DR4 associations in LGL as in other patients with Felty's syndrome.[5] Additionally, there is an absence of distinguishing clinical or serologic features, suggesting that separation on the basis of peripheral blood lymphocyte morphology may be unjustified.[5,6]

Large granular lymphocytes compose about 5% of the mononuclear cells in normal human blood. Cells with natural killer and antibody-dependent cell-mediated cytotoxic activity are found in this population. The cells usually lack surface immunoglobulin, but frequently express certain surface phenotypes, such as CD3, CD8, CD16, and CD57. Among patients with a clonal proliferation of these cells, neutropenia, splenomegaly, and susceptibility to infections are common. In some cases, there is a progressive course of malignant proliferation, but most cases are benign and require no specific therapy. About 25% of patients with LGL have inflammatory arthritis, and these patients have an immunogenetic pattern typical of Felty's syndrome. In contrast, the frequency of HLA-DR4 in patients without arthritis is not different from that in control subjects.

PATHOGENESIS

Mechanisms for the development of granulocytopenia include accelerated removal of granulocytes from the circulating pool and suppression of granulopoiesis. Ingestion and surface coating of immune complexes leads to impaired granulocyte function and facilitates their removal by the reticuloendothelial system. Specific antibodies directed against granulocyte cell surface antigens and complement activation also may be involved. Sequestration or margination of granulocytes in the spleen and venules in the lungs and elsewhere results in a diminished circulating pool.

In some patients, the marrow does not respond appropriately to granulocytopenia because of humoral or T cell suppression of myelopoiesis.[7-9] There may be different subsets of Felty's syndrome, based on humoral and cell-mediated mechanisms, and more than one mechanism may account for neutropenia in an individual patient. Autoantibodies against granulocyte colony-stimulating factor (G-CSF) may play a role in some cases.[9] Elevated levels of serum G-CSF are usually present, regardless of the presence or absence of autoantibodies, suggesting that the myeloid cells in Felty's syndrome are hyposensitive to G-CSF.

In LGL, an additional factor in the pathogenesis of neutropenia is the Fas ligand, a member of the tumor necrosis

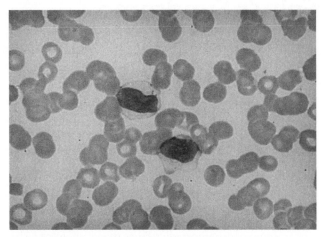

Figure 68-1 Peripheral blood smear with large granular lymphocytes.

Table 68-1 Frequency of Extra-articular Manifestations in Felty's Syndrome*

Manifestation	Frequency (%)
Rheumatoid nodules	76
Weight loss	68
Sjögren's syndrome†	56
Lymphadenopathy	34
Leg ulcers	25
Pleuritis	19
Skin pigmentation	17
Neuropathy	17
Episcleritis	8

*From a review of 10 reports since 1962.
†Determined by positive Schirmer's test.
Data from Goldberg J, Pinals RS: Felty syndrome. Semin Arthritis Rheum 10:52, 1980.

factor family.[7,10] Fas ligand is expressed on the surface of activated cytotoxic T cells, and elevated levels of soluble Fas ligand are found in sera of most patients.[11] Sera from patients with LGL have been shown to facilitate apoptosis of normal neutrophils in vitro.

The increased susceptibility to infection is probably related to several factors in addition to granulocytopenia. Granulocyte reserves are diminished, and defective function of granulocytes in phagocytosis, chemotaxis, and superoxide production has been shown.

CLINICAL FEATURES

The articular disease is usually severe, but not more so than in seropositive RA of comparable duration.[2] About one third of patients have inactive synovitis as judged by signs and symptoms, but even these patients continue to have an elevated erythrocyte sedimentation rate. In one large series, the mean erythrocyte sedimentation rate was 85 mm/hr.[12]

The spleen size varies. In 5% to 10% of patients, the spleen is not large enough to be palpable, but occasionally there is massive splenomegaly.[12] The median splenic weight in Felty's syndrome is about four times normal. There is no correlation between spleen size and the degree of granulocytopenia.[12]

Patients with Felty's syndrome tend to have more extra-articular manifestations than other patients with RA (Table 68-1). Weight loss may be striking and unexplained, often occurring for several months before the diagnosis of Felty's syndrome is made. Brown pigmentation over exposed surfaces of the extremities, especially over the tibia, may be related to stasis and to extravasation of red blood cells secondary to disease of small vessels.[12] Leg ulcers are seen frequently, but do not seem to differ from ulcers in other RA patients in terms of chronicity, recurrence, and presumed relationship to vasculitis.

COMPLICATIONS

Felty's syndrome patients have an increase in frequency of infections compared with matched RA control subjects.[1,13] The degree of granulocytopenia correlates poorly with the number and severity of infections until the granulocyte count is less than 1000/mm³. Other risk factors for infection include skin ulcers, corticosteroids, comorbid medical conditions, severity of the underlying rheumatoid process, and resulting disability.[13,14] Most infections are caused by common bacteria, such as staphylococci, streptococci, and gram-negative bacilli,[1,14] and involve common sites, particularly the skin and respiratory tract. Despite the granulocytopenia, pus may accumulate in an appropriate fashion, suggesting that the site of infection is capable of competing successfully with the spleen for available granulocytes. The response to antibiotic therapy is usually adequate.[12,14]

Mild hepatomegaly is common in Felty's syndrome, and elevations of alkaline phosphatase and the transaminases are described in about a quarter of the patients.[1,12] An unusual type of liver involvement may be associated with Felty's syndrome, but occurs rarely in other RA patients.[15] Histologically, the picture is described as nodular regenerative hyperplasia. Although there is mild portal fibrosis or infiltration with lymphocytes and plasma cells, the appearance is not characteristic of cirrhosis. Obliteration of portal venules may compromise portal blood flow, leading to atrophy and regenerative nodule formation, portal hypertension, and gastrointestinal hemorrhage. Patients with Felty's syndrome are at increased risk for the development of malignancies, particularly non-Hodgkin's lymphoma.[16]

HEMATOLOGIC AND SEROLOGIC FEATURES

The leukopenia in Felty's syndrome is relative with absolute granulocytopenia, in contrast to systemic lupus erythematosus, in which lymphopenia is a more prominent feature. There is often considerable spontaneous variation in the granulocyte count. Patients with mild lowering may return to the normal range, but this is rarely seen when depression is severe. Spontaneous remissions have been observed,[1] but are uncommon.[12] During infections or other stressful episodes, the granulocyte count often returns to the normal range, but is seldom elevated. This situation may conceal the diagnosis temporarily because blood counts may be ordered mainly in the setting of an infection or other acute illness.

The bone marrow may show no abnormality, but in most cases, there is a myeloid hyperplasia, with an excess of immature forms, often described as "maturation arrest." Although this condition might reflect an impaired myelopoietic response, early release of mature forms would result in the same appearance.[12] Rarely, in Felty's syndrome but more commonly in LGL, the marrow shows a depression in myeloid activity and increased lymphocytic infiltration.

A mild-to-moderate anemia is found in most patients, representing the anemia of chronic disease with an additional component of shortened red blood cell survival, which is corrected by splenectomy. Thrombocytopenia is seldom severe enough to cause purpura.

The alterations in immune response commonly found in RA are amplified in patients with Felty's syndrome. Rheumatoid factor is present in 98% of patients, generally in high titer[1,12]; antinuclear antibodies are found in 62% to 80%[1]; and antineutrophil cytoplasmic antibodies are found in 77%. Most of the last-mentioned are reactive against lactoferrin.[17] Immunoglobulin levels are higher than in other RA patients, and complement levels are occasionally low, although most patients have levels within the normal range.[1,12] Immune complexes have been detected by various techniques in most patients with Felty's syndrome, always in much higher frequency than in RA control subjects.[1,12]

DIFFERENTIAL DIAGNOSIS

Patients with RA also may develop superimposed illnesses that result in splenomegaly or granulocytopenia. Drug reactions, myeloproliferative disorders, reticuloendothelial malignancies, hepatic cirrhosis, amyloidosis, sarcoidosis, tuberculosis, and other chronic infections must be considered and excluded with reasonable clinical certainty before the diagnosis of Felty's syndrome is accepted.

MANAGEMENT

There have been no controlled trials of any treatment for Felty's syndrome. Specific treatment for granulocytopenia is unnecessary except in patients who have experienced bacterial infections or patients who are at high risk (granulocyte count <1000/mm^3).

Frequently, granulocytopenia may improve during treatment with disease-modifying antirheumatic drugs.[12] Gold salt injections resulted in a complete hematologic response in 60% of patients and partial response in 20% in the largest reported series, but gold salts and other older disease-modifying antirheumatic drugs have been displaced by newer drugs. Methotrexate is currently the most commonly used agent.[3,7,18] No controlled or comparative studies are available, but granulocytopenia usually improves with this treatment more rapidly than with gold salts, often within 2 months. Some patients have been followed for more than 1 year, without relapse or infection.[18] Low doses of corticosteroids do not produce consistent improvement in granulocytopenia and predispose to infection. There is limited experience with other drugs, including leflunomide and cyclosporine.[3,7] A few case reports on the use of new biologic agents have shown mixed results.[19] The mechanisms whereby second-line agents increase granulocyte counts are undetermined, as are their response rates and efficacy.

Treatment may be directed specifically at the granulocytopenia, using the granulopoietic growth factors. Several years of experience with the granulopoietic growth factors have confirmed their usefulness in increasing granulocyte counts within a short time and aiding in the resolution of infection.[20-23] Continued therapy is necessary to maintain these benefits, however, and high costs may become an issue. Prolonged use has been reported in some patients,[21-23] but it may be more reasonable to use granulopoietic growth factors for a limited period, during which disease-modifying antirheumatic drug therapy is undertaken. G-CSF seems to have fewer adverse effects than granulocyte-macrophage colony-stimulating factor. Significant adverse effects of these agents include exacerbation of arthritis, new onset of leukocytoclastic vasculitis, anemia, thrombocytopenia, and bone pain. To avoid or minimize these adverse effects, the initial use of low doses of G-CSF (3 μg/kg/day) and a short course of prednisone (20 to 30 mg/day) has been suggested.[7] A few patients are partially or completely unresponsive to G-CSF.

Because splenectomy usually reverses the hematologic abnormalities in Felty's syndrome, it has been advocated in the past as the treatment of choice.[12] The frequency of splenectomy has declined over the last 20 years, however, and currently it is reserved for patients who have not responded adequately to drug therapy. A prompt hematologic response is observed within minutes or hours after splenectomy, but granulocytopenia recurs and persists in about one quarter of these patients.[12] Continuing immune-mediated granulocyte sequestration may be responsible for these secondary failures. Recurrent or persistent infection was noted in only 26% of patients in one large series, but in 60% in four others.[12] Patients who did not experience infection before splenectomy usually continued to be free of infection afterward, whereas the patients with the most severe infections had variable and inconsistent responses to splenectomy, suggesting that functional defects in granulocytes and disease severity variables may be as important as granulocytopenia in determining susceptibility to infection.[14]

Thrombocytopenia usually improves after splenectomy, and anemia improves, to the extent that it is due to a hemolytic component. Although dramatic improvement in synovitis has been observed, it is often temporary and does not occur in most cases. Leg ulcers also may respond, even ulcers that are not significantly infected, but the variability in etiology and natural course makes these reports difficult to interpret.[12]

Remission was induced in two patients with refractory Felty's syndrome by immunoablative high-dose cyclophosphamide without stem cell rescue.[24] This approach is experimental, and long-term results are unknown.

The treatment of granulocytopenia in patients with LGL is generally similar to that in Felty's syndrome. Methotrexate[3,7,25] and G-CSF[3,20,21] have been used successfully. Cyclosporine may be indicated in refractory cases because it inhibits secretion of Fas ligand.[7] Splenectomy is less likely to be effective.[3]

PROGNOSIS

Patients with Felty's syndrome had a death rate similar to matched RA control subjects in a prospective study initiated in 1966. Despite a higher rate of infection, death as a result of sepsis (10%) was not more frequent in patients with

Felty's syndrome than in control subjects.[2] In another large series, 25% of deaths in patients with Felty's syndrome were due to sepsis.[1] There is little information on survival and prognosis in LGL, but no marked differences from Felty's syndrome have been reported.[6]

REFERENCES

1. Campion G, Maddison PJ, Goulding N, et al: The Felty syndrome: A case-matched study of clinical manifestations and outcome, serologic features, and immunogenetic association. Medicine 69:69, 1990.
2. Sibley JT, Haga M, Visram DA, et al: The clinical course of Felty's syndrome compared to matched controls. J Rheumatol 18:1163, 1991.
3. Burks EJ, Loughran TP Jr: Pathogenesis of neutropenia in large granular lymphocyte leukemia and Felty's syndrome. Blood Rev 20:245, 2006.
4. Turesson C, Schaid DJ, Weyand CM, et al: The impact of HLA-DRB1 genes on extra-articular disease manifestations in rheumatoid arthritis. Arthritis Res Ther 7:1386, 2005.
5. Bowman SJ, Corrigall V, Panayi GS, et al: Hematologic and cytofluorographic analysis of patients with Felty's syndrome: A hypothesis that a discrete event leads to large granular lymphocyte expansions in this condition. Arthritis Rheum 38:1252, 1995.
6. Starkebaum G, Loughran TP Jr, Gaur LK, et al: Immunogenetic similarities between patients with Felty's syndrome and those with clonal expansions of large granular lymphocytes in rheumatoid arthritis. Arthritis Rheum 40:62, 1997.
7. Starkebaum G: Chronic neutropenia associated with autoimmune disease. Semin Hematol 39:121, 2002.
8. Ditzel HJ, Masaki Y, Nielsen H, et al: Cloning and expression of a novel human antibody-antigen pair associated with Felty's syndrome. Proc Natl Acad Sci U S A 97:9234, 2000.
9. Hellmich B, Csernok E, Schatz H, et al: Autoantibodies against granulocyte colony-stimulating factor in Felty's syndrome and neutropenic systemic lupus erythematosus. Arthritis Rheum 46:2384, 2002.
10. Perzova R, Loughran TP: Constitutive expression of Fas ligand in large granular lymphocyte leukemia. Br J Haematol 97:123, 1997.
11. Liu JH, Wei S, Lamy T, et al: Chronic neutropenia mediated by fas ligand. Blood 95:3219, 2000.
12. Goldberg J, Pinals RS: Felty syndrome. Semin Arthritis Rheum 10:52, 1980.
13. Doran MF, Crowson CS, Pond GR, et al: Predictors of infection in rheumatoid arthritis. Arthritis Rheum 46:2294, 2002.
14. Breedveld FC, Fibbe WE, Hermans J, et al: Factors influencing the incidence of infections in Felty's syndrome. Arch Intern Med 147:915, 1987.
15. Thorne C, Urowitz MB, Wanless IR, et al: Liver disease in Felty's syndrome. Am J Med 73:35, 1982.
16. Gridley G, Klippel JH, Hoover RN, et al: Incidence of cancer among men with the Felty syndrome. Ann Intern Med 120:35, 1994.
17. Coremans IEM, Hagen EC, van der Voort EAM, et al: Autoantibodies to neutrophil cytoplasmic enzymes in Felty's syndrome. Clin Exp Rheumatol 11:255, 1993.
18. Wassenberg S, Herborn G, Rau R: Methotrexate treatment in Felty's syndrome. Br J Rheumatol 37:908, 1998.
19. Ghavami A, Genevay S, Fulpius T, et al: Etanercept in treatment of Felty's syndrome. Ann Rheum Dis 64:1090, 2005.
20. Hellmich B, Schnabel A, Gross WL: Treatment of severe neutropenia due to Felty's syndrome or systemic lupus erythematosus with granulocyte colony-stimulating factor. Semin Arthritis Rheum 29:82, 1999.
21. Stanworth SJ, Bhavnani M, Chattopadhya C, et al: Treatment of Felty's syndrome with the haemopoietic growth factor granulocyte colony-stimulating factor (G-CSF). QJM 91:49, 1998.
22. Starkebaum G: Use of colony-stimulating factors in the treatment of neutropenia associated with collagen vascular disease. Curr Opin Hematol 4:196, 1997.
23. Graham KE, Coodley GO: A prolonged use of granulocyte colony stimulating factor in Felty's syndrome. J Rheumatol 22:174, 1995.
24. Brodsky RA, Petri M, Smith BD, et al: Immunoablative high-dose cyclophosphamide without stem-cell rescue for refractory, severe autoimmune disease. Ann Intern Med 129:1031, 1998.
25. Hamidou MA, Sadr FB, Lamy T, et al: Low-dose methotrexate for the treatment of patients with large granular lymphocyte leukemia associated with rheumatoid arthritis. Am J Med 108:730, 2000.

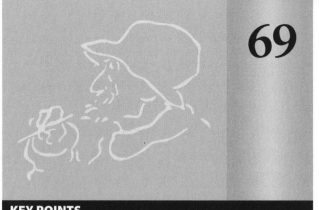

69 Sjögren's Syndrome

STEVEN CARSONS

KEY POINTS

Sicca complex consists of xerostomia, xerophthalmia, and salivary gland swelling.

Extracranial xeroses include xerotrachea, bronchitis sicca, dry skin, and vaginal dryness.

Extraglandular manifestations include neuropathy, pulmonary involvement, interstitial nephritis, cutaneous vasculitis, and lymphoproliferation.

In 1933, Sjögren[1] described the association of filamentary keratitis with arthritis. Previously, in 1882, Leber[2] had described filamentary keratitis, and in 1888, Mikulicz[3] had described a patient with bilateral lacrimal and parotid gland enlargement. Biopsy of these glands revealed extensive round cell infiltration. In 1953, Morgan and Castleman[4] noted the similarity between the glandular enlargement described by Mikulicz and the keratitis described by Sjögren. Subsequently, these disorders were considered to be variants of the same process, and the term *Sjögren's syndrome* (SS) became more widely used.[5] In 1980, Talal[6] introduced the term *autoimmune exocrinopathy*; subsequently, Skopouli and Moutsopoulos[7] introduced the term *autoimmune epitheliitis*. Both these terms emphasize the cause and systemic nature of the disease.

DEFINITIONS

The use of multiple terms to describe this condition, along with (until recently) the lack of consensus regarding classification criteria, has led to confusion. Primary SS is best defined as dry eyes and dry mouth secondary to autoimmune dysfunction of the exocrine glands. Secondary SS is the same disease in the presence of another autoimmune connective tissue disorder. Until relatively recently (1980), the terms *sicca syndrome* and *sicca complex* were used interchangeably with SS in the literature, and their routine use in clinical settings persists today. Sicca is probably best used in its most literal sense, which is "dry" (Latin). Some clinicians use the term *sicca* to describe patients with dry eyes, dry mouth, or both who do not fulfill the accepted criteria for complete SS. The term *Sjögren's syndrome* is preferred for all patients who meet the classification criteria for the disorder or who are definitively diagnosed with it.

EPIDEMIOLOGY

SS is a common autoimmune disorder. Prevalence estimates range from approximately 0.5% to 5%. The incidence rate in Olmstead County, Minnesota, was estimated to be 3.9 cases per 100,000 population.[8] Approximately half of all cases of SS are primary. Similar to most autoimmune disorders, the vast majority of cases (approximately 90%) occur in women.[8] Although the majority of cases occur in midlife, the disorder is also seen in children[9] and the elderly.[10] Remarkably little difference in clinical presentation is noted among populations that differ on the basis of age, gender, and geographic origin.[9,11-13] Prevalence rates stated in the literature vary, depending on the identifying variable chosen for study. For instance, a postmortem survey of lacrimal pathology found that 7.8% of individuals lacking a premortem diagnosis of an autoimmune disorder had moderate to severe (grade III or IV) lymphocytic infiltration.[14] Of 2500 serum samples obtained from female blood donors between the ages of 20 and 50 years, 0.44% had antibodies to SS-A.[15] Schein and colleagues[16] assessed 2481 elderly individuals residing in Salisbury, Maryland, and found the prevalence of dry eye or mouth to be 27%. In populations in which the prevalence of keratoconjunctivitis sicca (KCS) and primary SS is measured simultaneously, the prevalence of KCS always exceeds that of complete primary SS.[10,17-26] Table 69-1 describes the prevalence of primary SS in several diverse populations.

CAUSE AND PATHOGENESIS

Animal models of SS have provided some important insights regarding the immunopathogenesis of this disease: (1) SS has a strong immunogenetic component, (2) the inflammatory infiltrate is largely T cell driven, (3) autoimmune sialadenitis can be triggered by viral infection, (4) relatively specific autoantibodies are produced, and (5) genes regulating apoptosis influence the chronicity of lymphocytic infiltration and are candidates for therapeutic manipulation.

IMMUNOGENETICS

Direct clinical observation suggests a genetic component to SS, such as the presence of primary SS and autoimmune hemolytic anemia in sisters[27] and the identification of primary SS in Caucasian monozygotic twins and their mother.[28] Like many other autoimmune disorders, early human lymphocyte antigen (HLA) studies identified an association with serologically defined HLA-B8[29] and HLA-DR3.[30] Later studies demonstrated that the HLA-DR2 and -DR3 associations were secondary to linkage disequilibrium with HLA-DQ alleles.[31] Genetically defined allelic markers subsequently identified a large number of polymorphisms involving the HLA-DRB1/DQA1/DQB1 haplotype, which adds to the complexity of the genetic background of SS. These polymorphisms vary with ethnicity, clinical manifestations, and, importantly, the autoantibody response.

Table 69-1 Prevalence of Primary Sjögren's Syndrome Reported from Different Populations

Author of Study	Year of Study	Population Studied	Criteria Used	Findings	Reference
Strickland	1987	103 Caucasian females	European	PSS: 2% Probable PSS: 12%	10
Drosos	1988	62 Greek nursing home residents	Greek	PSS: 6% Probable PSS: 12%	17
Jacobsson	1989	705 Swedish adults	Copenhagen	KCS: 14.9% PSS: 2.7%	18
Zhang	1995	2166 Chinese adults	Copenhagen	PSS: 0.77%	19
Bjerrum	1997	504 Danish adults (aged 30-60 yr)	Preliminary European	KCS: 8% PSS: 0.6-2.1%	20
Dafni	1997	837 rural Greek females	Preliminary European	PSS: 0.6% Probable PSS: 2.99%	21
Thomas	1998	1000 British adults	Preliminary European	PSS: 3.3%	22
Tomsic	1999	332 Slovenian adults	Preliminary European	PSS: 0.6%	23
Bowman	2004	864 Caucasian females	AEC	PSS: <0.1-0.4%	24
Alamanos	2006	422 Greek cases	AEC	PSS: 0.92%	25
Kabasakal	2006	Turkish females	AEC	PSS: 1.56%	26

AEC, American-European consensus; KCS, keratoconjunctivitis sicca; PSS, primary Sjögren's syndrome.

In Caucasian individuals, the HLA-DRB1*0301/DQA1* 0501/DQB1*0201 haplotype has the strongest association with the production of SS-A and SS-B. Additional genes located in the major histocompatibility complex (MHC) region on chromosome 6, but not classically associated with class I or II alleles, have been linked to SS. These include transporters associated with antigen processing, genes situated between the DP and DQ regions,[32,33] and the tumor necrosis factor (TNF) alleles (particularly TNF-α)[34] located in the central MHC, telomeric to the complement synthesis genes.[31] Recently, two genes located on chromosome 1—the interleukin (IL)-10 promoter region[35] and glutathione S-transferase M1[36]—have been linked to susceptibility to SS.

IMMUNOLOGIC ALTERATIONS IN PERIPHERAL BLOOD

Similar to other autoimmune disorders, the peripheral blood of patients with SS demonstrates a relative T cell lymphopenia, normal ratios of CD4+ and CD8+ T cells, and increases in activated T cells as determined by coexpression of CD3, CD4, and CD8 antigens with HLA-DR, CD25 (IL-2R), and very late antigen-1 (CD49a).[37-39] Expression of natural killer antigens (CD16) is variable, ranging from normal to diminished.[37,40] However, killing of K562 cells by SS peripheral blood mononuclear cells is reduced compared with normal controls.[41]

In contrast to T cells, circulating B cells are increased in SS.[42] B cells from the majority of SS patients express enhanced levels of CD5 (also known as Ly-1 or B1),[43] an interesting finding in light of the role played by CD5 B cells in B cell malignancies such as chronic lymphocytic leukemia.

In addition to the presence of antibody to SS-A and SS-B in 75% and 40% of patients, respectively,[44] approximately two thirds of SS patients have serum antinuclear antibody (ANA) and rheumatoid factor (RF) activity. Many SS patients have striking polyclonal hypergammaglobulinemia. In fact, immunoglobulin (Ig) levels in SS are often higher than those seen in rheumatoid arthritis (RA), systemic lupus erythematosus (SLE), and other connective tissue disorders. Several studies point to a role for IgA in the

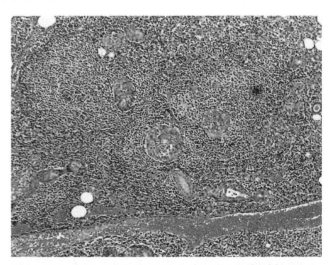

Figure 69-1 **Histopathologic section of a salivary gland from a patient with Sjögren's syndrome.** Normal glandular architecture is replaced by a sea of mononuclear cells. Remnants of acinar and ductal structures can be seen. Note the formation of a germinal center–like cluster. *(Courtesy of Dr. John Fantasia, Long Island Jewish Medical Center.)*

immunopathogenesis of this disorder, especially because it appears to be synthesized locally in inflamed glands. IgA is frequently elevated in the serum of SS patients,[45] particularly as IgA-containing RF.[46]

AUTOIMMUNE SIALADENITIS: THE IMMUNOPATHOLOGIC LESION

The hallmark of autoimmune exocrinopathy is infiltration of tissue by mononuclear cells that form distinct aggregates termed *foci*.[47] Aggregates tend to occur in periductal and periacinar locations and may become confluent, resulting in the replacement of epithelial structure (Fig. 69-1). Remnants of glands surrounded by large numbers of infiltrating mononuclear cells are known as *epimyoepithelial islands*. Plasma cells are noted within foci and at the periphery of periductal and periacinar foci. Glands with significant mononuclear infiltration may also display germinal center formation.

PHENOTYPE OF THE INFILTRATING LYMPHOCYTES

T Cell Compartment

In 1982, Fox and coworkers[48] described the classic finding of the predominance of CD4+ T cells among lymphocytes infiltrating the minor salivary gland (MSG). In this study, the CD4/CD8 ratio was 3:1. CD4+ predominance was also noted in peripheral blood. Although CD8+ T cells constitute a minority, they tend to localize around acinar epithelial cells.[49] B cells make up a minority of the lymphocyte population in tissue, and a subset of B cells present in tissue is absent in peripheral blood.[50] Infiltrating lymphocytes are activated, expressing DR, DQ, CD25, CD9, and CD10, but they are specifically distributed in the peripheral portion of the periductal foci. Bias in T cell receptor gene use has been examined as a measure of response to putative autoantigen. Most studies do not support clonal T cell restriction but rather relative expansion of certain T cell receptor genes. Studies from Japan and Europe have identified expansion of Vβ2, Vβ8, and Vβ13 T cells.[51-53]

B Cell Compartment

Plasma cells expressing IgG, IgA, and IgM are found in SS salivary glands. IgA is the predominant isotype; however, enrichment of IgM-positive cells to a level exceeding 10% appears to be specific for SS.[54] Clusters of IgA-positive cells have been localized adjacent to DR-expressing epithelium,[55] suggesting that the microenvironment of the activated glandular epithelium contributes to plasma cell differentiation and local IgA synthesis. Enhanced local synthesis of immunoglobulin is suggested by the finding of enrichment of anti–SS-B IgA in the saliva of SS patients.[56] CD20+ B cells constitute a significant and early component of periductal foci, where they eventually colocalize with distinct CD27+/CD38+ cells.[57] Germinal centers have been identified in SS glands; serum levels of membrane cofactor protein-1, interferon-γ, and B cell activating factor (BAFF) best correlate with the presence of germinal centers.[58] There is evidence that BAFF is antiapoptotic in SS, and BAFF levels are highest in SS patients with hypergammaglobulinemia.[59] Thus, BAFF may represent a new therapeutic target.

TRAFFICKING AND ADHESION OF INFLAMMATORY CELLS

The first step in inflammatory cell infiltration occurs at the glandular endothelium. Vessels in the inflamed gland express vascular cell adhesion molecule-1 (VCAM-1), intercellular adhesion molecules (ICAMs), and P- and E-selectins. Mononuclear cells surrounding blood vessels express lymphocyte function-associated antigen-1 (LFA-1), α4 and α5 integrins, and CD44.[60] Marked expression of ICAM and VCAM-1 can be observed in venules surrounded by CD4+CD45RO+ T cells.[61] High levels of the chemokine CXCL-13 has been found on endothelial cells; its counterreceptor, CXCR5, is observed on B cells organizing into germinal center–like structures.[62] Treatment of nonobese diabetic mice with antibody to VCAM-1, α4 integrin, L-selectin, or LFA-1 almost completely inhibits lymphocyte ingress into inflamed glands.[63]

Mononuclear cells use adhesion mechanisms to migrate to epithelial structures. Enhanced laminin expression is often found in the ductal epithelium of involved glands and is observed in areas not yet affected by lymphocytic infiltrate,[64] leading to speculation that laminin expression is an early event in the disease process. ICAM-1 is expressed on ductal and acinar epithelial cells together with LFA-1, which is expressed on surrounding mononuclear cells.[60] In contrast to the marked expression of CXCL-13 seen on endothelium, CXCL-12 (SDF-1) is strongly expressed on ductal epithelium, accompanied by only weak expression of CXCL-13. CXCR4, the counterreceptor for CXCL-12, localizes to periductal T cells.[62] CD8+ T cells surrounding acinar epithelium display the integrin αEβ7 and thus may use cadherin E to bind epithelial cells.[49] Importantly, acinar epithelial cells adjacent to αEβ7+ CD8+ T cells display apoptotic changes consistent with cytotoxic acinar cell destruction.

CYTOKINE PROFILE

Studies using immunohistochemical and in situ hybridization methods demonstrate the uniform presence of the proinflammatory cytokines IL-1β, TNF-α, IL-2, and IL-6 in MSG biopsies of SS patients.[65-69] These cytokines localize to mononuclear cell infiltrates and epithelium. TNF-α and TNF receptor (TNF-R) are present in the inflammatory infiltrate, vascular endothelium, and ductal epithelium, where they appear to be tightly coexpressed.[70] Acinar cells, however, do not express TNF-α or TNF-R-p75, but they do express TNF-R-p55, suggesting regional differences in susceptibility to apoptosis. Enhanced expression of STAT-1α mRNA and STAT-1α phosphorylation in SS labial salivary glands suggests a proinflammatory role for interferon-γ.[71] Interestingly, CD4+ T cell clones originating from the MSG in organ culture produce levels of IL-10 that are 15-fold higher than those produced by similar clones derived from peripheral blood. In peripheral blood, B cells and monocytes produce approximately 90% of mononuclear-derived IL-10.[72] Perhaps factors present in MSG tissue in vivo inhibit IL-10 production. BAFF levels are elevated in primary SS.

MECHANISMS OF GLANDULAR DESTRUCTION

Role of Apoptosis

Mononuclear cells infiltrating affected tissue display elevated levels of the apoptosis-related molecules Fas, FasL, and Bcl-2[73,74] and undergo apoptosis rarely (approximately 1%),[75] a phenomenon referred to as *blocked apoptosis*. Approximately 50% of infiltrating mononuclear cells express CD40 and CD40L. Bcl-2 expression colocalizes with that of CD40, suggesting that signaling through CD40 increases the expression of Bcl-2.[76] Interestingly, lymphocytes from patients with enlarged exocrine glands display reduced levels of Fas but enhanced sensitivity to steroids.[77] Despite a paucity of apoptosis in infiltrating mononuclear cells, apoptosis appears to play a role in glandular epithelial cell dysfunction. Enhanced expression of Fas and DNA strand breaks have been demonstrated on acinar epithelial cells.[73] DNA strand breaks occur even more frequently in ductal epithelium (68%) in SS, far exceeding the rate in controls (3%). This is accompanied by a significant reduction in Bcl-2 expression and enhancement of Bax expression in SS ductal epithelium.[74,78] Acinar epithelial cells adjacent to CD8⁺ T cells are apoptotic.[49]

Role of Metalloproteinases

In addition to epithelial cell death, degradation of extracellular matrix contributes to the destruction of glandular architecture. Metalloproteinase (MMP)-2, -3, and -9 are present in SS salivary glands, where they may degrade basement membrane collagen IV. Immunohistochemical studies reveal localization of MMPs to glandular cells, particularly acinar end-piece cells[79] and acinar cells adjacent to lymphocytic infiltrates.[80]

AUTOANTIGENS

The existence of a strong autoantibody response and the presence of germinal center–like structures in the salivary glands of SS patients imply that the aberrant immune response is directed against one or multiple autoantigens. Molecular characterization of B cell Ig genes has provided considerable evidence for an antigen-driven response in SS. Analysis of heavy-chain Ig rearrangements using reverse transcriptase polymerase chain reaction on tissue obtained by labial salivary gland and lymph node biopsy in SS patients revealed that 92 of 94 V(H)-D-J(H) transcripts were modified by somatic mutation.[81] Analysis of rearranged V genes from B cells obtained by microdissection of germinal center–like clusters in SS labial salivary glands revealed a mixture of polyclonality containing some somatic mutation, along with dominant B cell clones expressing hypermutated V genes.[82]

Epstein-Barr Virus

Case reports detailing the development of SS following acute mononucleosis[83,84] and the identification of salivary glands as sites of latent Epstein-Barr virus (EBV) infection have given credence to EBV's role in the pathogenesis of SS. Some studies have demonstrated elevated antibody titers to EBV antigens in SS patients,[85] whereas others have not. EBV DNA has been detected by in situ hybridization and polymerase chain reaction in SS glandular tissue, saliva, and tears.[86] These studies suggest that in certain patients, persistent glandular EBV infection may be associated with or result in immunoregulatory abnormalities, which lead to persistent inflammation and possibly lymphoma (see later).

α-Fodrin is a 120-kD constituent of the epithelial cytoskeleton that was first observed to be a target of the autoimmune response in the NFS/sld mouse model of SS.[87] Serum IgG from affected mice recognized α-fodrin in immunoblots of salivary gland homogenates. Mouse IgG and human IgG isolated from SS patients also bind to a recombinant α-fodrin fusion protein. EBV activation of lymphoid cells results in the cleavage of α-fodrin to 120-kD fragments, which occurs concomitantly with cellular apoptosis and expression of ZEBRA protein, which is a marker for activation of the lytic cycle of EBV.[88] This cleavage can be blocked by caspase inhibitors. α-Fodrin is also cleaved into a unique 155-kD fragment by enzymes present in the granules of cytotoxic lymphocytes.[89] As demonstrated by these animal and in vitro experimental models, viruses such as EBV may induce the formation of autoantigens linked to SS via intrinsic epithelial cell apoptosis and cytotoxic lymphocyte granule release,

Antimuscarinic M3 Receptor

Forty years ago, antibodies directed against salivary duct epithelium were reported[90] and were assumed to be a consequence of organ-specific autoimmunity in SS. Identification of specific glandular autoantigens was hampered by methodologic issues and perhaps by the intense interest in SS-A and SS-B, which were discovered shortly thereafter. Thirty years later, IgG present in the sera of SS patients was found to bind to and activate cholinergic receptors present on rat parotid glands.[91] Pharmacologic stimulation and inhibition studies pointed to a type M3 muscarinic receptor (M3R). Subsequently, it was demonstrated that serum and purified IgG from 11 of 15 patients with primary and secondary SS inhibited carbachol-induced contraction of isolated bladder strips, indicative of an inhibitory effect on parasympathetic neurotransmission.[92] Peptides derived from the second extracellular loop of M3R generated antibodies in rabbits that were capable of inhibiting experimental carbachol-induced colon contractions.[93] Interestingly, M3R can be cleaved in vitro by granzyme B derived from cytotoxic granules,[89] consistent with the model of autoantigen production described previously.

SS-A and SS-B

SS-A and SS-B (Ro and La) represent the dominant humoral immune target to nuclear antigen in SS. Thus, these antigens have long been speculated to be of prime diagnostic and etiologic importance, especially because the antibody response to SS-A and SS-B has characteristics of an antigen-driven response.[94] A more detailed description of these antigens is found in Chapter 20. Evidence of a local response to autoantigen is derived from studies demonstrating local antibody synthesis in salivary glands. In one study, all eight submucosal salivary gland biopsies from SS patients with circulating anti–SS-A demonstrated local production of anti–52-kD Ro.[95] In addition, the expression pattern of SS-B in acinar epithelial cells was aberrant in SS patients, demonstrating cytoplasmic and nucleoplasmic staining; in normal individuals, in contrast, staining was restricted to the nucleolus.[96]

CLINICAL MANIFESTATIONS
OCULAR

Although the most prominent ocular manifestation of SS is dry eye, patients are often unaware of dryness as a presenting symptom. Instead, they may complain of a foreign body–type sensation manifested by scratchiness, grittiness, or irritation from a "grain of sand." These symptoms may be interpreted by both the patient and the physician as atopic in nature. An early manifestation of dry eye is the inability to tolerate contact lenses. Other common symptoms of dry eye include photophobia, redness, and ocular fatigue. Thick mucous strands may cause blurring of vision, and the eyelids may be encrusted, especially on awakening. If the condition persists and is untreated, symptoms may reflect

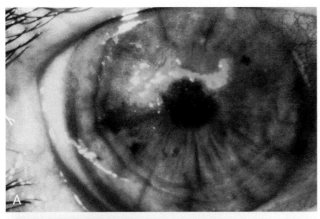

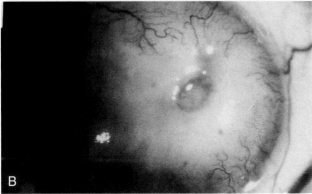

Figure 69-2 Ocular manifestations of Sjögren's syndrome. **A,** A patient with moderate dry eye, in addition to surface staining, may develop filamentary keratitis, in which the epithelium of the cornea sloughs off and becomes attached to the ocular surface, along with mucin and debris. This causes a significant foreign body sensation and discomfort. **B,** This patient with severe dry eye did not receive adequate treatment and has developed corneal scarring. (Courtesy of Dr. Reza Dana, Harvard Medical School.)

complications of xerophthalmia, including pain, intense photophobia indicative of corneal abrasion, and discharge, possibly indicative of infection (Fig. 69-2). Infections threaten sight and are most often caused by gram-positive bacteria. Previous corneal surgery, topical corticosteroid therapy, and the use of contact lenses are predisposing factors for infection.[97] Rarely, patients may present with an orbital mass, representing a swollen lacrimal gland. Examination may reveal a paucity of tears in the conjunctival sac. The conjunctivae may appear injected. Specific maneuvers such as the Schirmer test and slit-lamp examination may be able to quantitate dryness and corneal disease, respectively. Corneal examination is aided by the instillation of dye. Fluorescein stains epithelial defects, whereas rose bengal binds devitalized cells and is thus more sensitive. Small punctate defects are often first observed at the inferior corneal margin.[98] Lissamine green is thought to be equally sensitive to rose bengal but less irritating.

ORAL

In contrast to dry eye, patients often complain of a dry mouth. Physicians caring for SS patients are accustomed to seeing them carry plastic water bottles because they require a constant supply of moisture to be comfortable. The

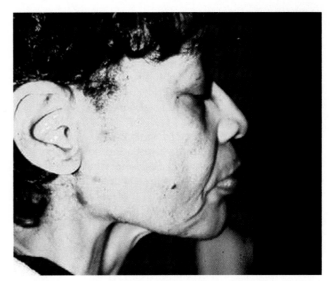

Figure 69-3 **Patient with Sjögren's syndrome and moderate parotid swelling.** In this patient, parotid enlargement fluctuates with time and is bilateral.

dry-mouth patient describes a parched feeling in the mouth, often extending to the throat. Eating is often difficult without supplemental liquids. Talal has popularized the "cracker sign," in which patients are asked whether they can chew and swallow a saltine cracker without any exogenous liquid. Dry-mouth patients often respond with visible disgust or by demonstrating a choking sign, bringing their hands up to the neck. Patients also may describe thickened saliva and may experience dysgeusia. Many of the more severe symptoms associated with dry mouth are secondary to complications of chronic dryness.

Owing to a reduction in salivary volume and the subsequent loss of the antibacterial properties of saliva, tooth decay is accelerated. In fact, unexplained rampant dental caries may be the first sign of dry mouth. Caries occurring in unusual places, such as on the incisal surfaces and at the gingival line, are common in patients with dry mouth. Enamel at the junction of fillings and crowns is particularly susceptible to decay. Fillings that fall out may also be an early sign of dry mouth. In a European Community study, 40% of SS patients experienced early dental loss. In partially or completely edentulous patients, dental loss occurred an average of 9 years before the first symptom of xerostomia.[99] For the reasons stated previously, a dry mouth is also extremely susceptible to the development of intraoral candidiasis. In one study, more than 80% of all SS subjects were culture positive for *Candida albicans*, versus none of the controls.[100] Patients report a burning mouth and tongue. During the course of their illness, the majority of SS patients will experience swelling of the salivary glands. The parotids are most commonly involved; however, the sublingual and submandibular glands may also be affected. Swelling may be bilateral or unilateral and may fluctuate with time (Fig. 69-3). In a series of patients with adult recurrent sialadenitis of the parotid glands followed prospectively, more than 50% developed SS.[101] These patients experienced parotid swelling a mean of 5 years before xerostomia. Patients may experience "glandular flares" manifested by periods of increased swelling accompanied by pain and tenderness. Thickened, inspissated saliva places SS patients at increased risk for the formation of calculi, which may be found incidentally on imaging studies. Infectious parotitis or abscess presents as erythematous, painful swelling of the gland, often accompanied by fever, chills, and malaise. The presence of a dominant hard mass should raise suspicion of lymphoma.

Examination of the oral cavity of SS patients often reveals multiple caries in the distribution noted previously. Patients with more advanced disease may be edentulous or have complete dentures. The mouth appears dry, the mucosa is thin and parchment like, and a tongue blade adheres to the tongue and buccal surfaces in a "sticky" fashion. Centers specializing in SS or dry mouth can measure the salivary flow rate quantitatively; however, by having the patient open the mouth and elevate the tongue for 1 minute, the clinician can estimate the flow rate by observing infralingual salivary pooling. Massaging the parotid yields little or no saliva from Stensen's duct. In a dry mouth, candidiasis is not manifested by thrush; rather, there is extensive erythema of the oral mucosa and loss of filiform papillae from the dorsal surface of the tongue. Small amounts of thin, whitish exudate may be found on the tongue and buccal mucosa. Bilateral angular chelitis is often observed. Examination of the parotid glands often reveals some degree of swelling, appreciated as a subtle, "grainy" enlargement. In severe cases, "chipmunk-like facies," indicative of massive bilateral glandular involvement, is seen.

OTHER XEROSES

Dry nose is common and may lead to inflammation with subsequent congestion, crusting, and epistaxis. Xerotrachea may result in a chronic dry cough. Dry skin may lead to pruritus and excoriation. Rarely, secondary infection may occur. Vaginal dryness may lead to pruritus, irritation, and dyspareunia. Although the most common cutaneous manifestation of SS is dryness, little is known about the precise cause or whether cutaneous dryness is truly part of the autoimmune exocrinopathy of SS. Sweat volume is reduced in SS patients,[102] and a skin biopsy revealed lymphocytic infiltrates surrounding eccrine glands and ducts in one patient suffering from severe anhidrosis.[103]

SYSTEMIC MANIFESTATIONS

MUSCULOSKELETAL

Patients with primary SS often experience musculoskelatal symptoms, including arthralgias and transient synovitis (Table 69-2). Prevalence estimates range from 54% to 84%.[104,105] Joint erosion is rare, but mild joint-space narrowing appears to be common.[105,106] Muscle pain is also common in SS; however, persistent and significant elevation in creatine phosphokinase is extremely uncommon.[107] Nonetheless, two studies demonstrated abnormal muscle biopsy findings in a relatively high number (72% and 73%, respectively) of primary SS patients. These abnormalities consisted of inflammatory myositis, perivascular lymphocytic infiltrates, and inclusion bodies. Despite these findings, only 11% of the combined series had clinical

Table 69-2 Systemic Manifestations Associated with Sjögren's Syndrome

Musculoskeletal
Arthralgias
Myalgias
Cutaneous
Dry skin
Hyperglobulinemic purpura
Vasculitis
Pulmonary
Xerotrachea
Pulmonary infiltrate
Micronodules
Gastrointestinal
Esophageal dysmotility
Pancreatitis
Hepatitis
Renal
Renal tubular acidosis
Interstitial nephritis
Neurologic
Peripheral neuropathy
Cranial neuropathy (especially fifth cranial nerve)
Central nervous system disease
Hematologic
Leukopenia
Anemia
Lymphoma

evidence of polymyositis.[107,108] Muscle biopsy findings did not correlate with muscle pain; 27% of patients in one series met American College of Rheumatology criteria for fibromyalgia.[107]

PULMONARY

Clinical pulmonary involvement is relatively common in primary SS. Cough reportedly occurs in 40% to 50% of patients.[109,110] It is usually a symptom of xerotrachea, which, in turn, is strongly associated with impaired mucociliary clearance.[111,112] Postmortem morphometric analysis of SS patients' lungs revealed an increase in the size of bronchial glands and goblet cells in central airways and in the mucus-occupying ratio in small airways; these changes are not dissimilar to those seen in chronic bronchitis.[113] Cough may also be secondary to bronchial hyperresponsiveness, which is found in 50% to 60% of primary SS patients studied by methacholine challenge.[114] Other pulmonary sympotms, including dyspnea and chest pain (referable to pleural and parenchymal disease, respectively), occur in 9% to 43% of patients.[115,116] When abnormalities found on pulmonary function testing are included, approximately 75% of SS patients display evidence of pulmonary involvement.[117] Abnormal findings on high-resolution computed tomography occur in 65% to 92% of SS patients and include primarily ground-glass attenuation, bronchiectasis, septal thicking, micronodules, and parenchymal cysts.[118,119] These abnormalities do not necessarily correlate with abnormal pulmonary function tests.

Despite normal chest radiographs and the absence of clinical symptoms, primary SS patients may show evidence of subclinical lung inflammation on bronchoalveolar lavage.[120] A wide range of pulmonary function test abnormalities has been reported in primary SS; however, the most common are a reduction in maximal expiratory flow, indicative of small airway disease, and reduced D_{LCO} secondary to interstitial involvement.[109,110,116] Lung biopsy reveals a spectrum of inflammatory changes, including bronchiolitis, lymphoid interstitial pneumonia, and fibrosis.[121] Recent studies have identified nonspecific interstitial pneumonitis as a common histologic subtype.[122,123] Immunohistochemical analysis demonstrates an increase in $CD4^+$ T cells in the bronchial submucosa.[124] Taken together, the predominance of small airway disease, the correlation with indicators of systemic inflammation, and $CD4^+$ T cell infiltration of bronchial submucosa imply a significant role for autoimmune exocrinopathy in SS lung disease.

RENAL

The predominant form of renal disease in primary SS is a distal renal tubular acidosis syndrome resulting from tubulointerstitial lymphocytic infiltration. On rare occasions, the first presenting symptom of SS is hypokalemic paralysis. In these cases, the sicca component was mild and previously unrecognized.[125] Overt renal disease of any form was seen in 4% of 471 patients followed for 10 years by Goules and colleagues.[126] More commonly, renal metabolic studies reveal mild disturbances in tubular function in the absence of clinical disease.[127] Proteinuria is sometimes detected in primary SS (in approximately 20% of cases) and is mainly of tubular origin (β_2-microglobulin and α_1-microglobulin), suggesting proximal tubular dysfunction. Filtration of increased amounts of proteins, such as Ig light chain and β_2-microglobulin (MHC class I–associated light chain), and local synthesis of these proteins by tubular lymphocytes may result in tubular damage. On renal biopsy, Talal and coworkers[128] noted lymphocytic infiltrates in all patients with tubular acidification defects. Similar to findings in exocrine glands, most infiltrating lymphocytes were $CD4^+$ (CD4/CD8 ratio approximately 2:1); however, lymphocytes invading tubular epithelial cells were $CD8^+$, suggesting a cytotoxic role.[129] Glomerular disease is rare but has been found in 1% to 2% of cases by clinical and biopsy studies.[126] Patients with glomerulonephritis have type II mixed cryoglobulins and low C4.[126]

GASTROINTESTINAL

Xerostomia is the most common upper alimentary abnormality in SS, and hyposalivation undoubtedly contributes to digestive abnormalities. Dysphagia has been reported in approximately 75% of patients,[130] and manometric evidence of esophageal dysmotility has been reported in at least 33%.[131] More significant dysphagia may indicate the presence of esophageal webs, which have been noted in 10% of patients.[130] Gastric symptoms have been recorded in approximately half of patients with primary SS.[132] Endoscopic examination with biopsy reveals evidence of atrophic (usually antral) gastritis in 10% to 25% and superficial gastritis in approximately 80%.[132,133] Hypopepsinogenemia has been reported in up to 67% of patients[134]; however, parietal cell antibodies have been detected in only 10%.[132] Endoscopic surveillance may be required for persistent symptoms of epigastric discomfort, fullness, and early satiety, which might indicate the presence of severe atrophic gastritis or a mucosa-associated lymphoid tissue (MALT) lymphoma (see later).

HEPATIC

Evidence of mild autoimmune hepatitis has been identified in approximaely 25% of primary SS patients,[135] with smooth muscle antibodies seen in 7% to 33%.[135,136] Antimitochondrial antibodies (AMA) have been reported in 7% to 13% of patients,[135-137] suggesting a close association between primary SS and primary biliary cirrhosis. In one series, more than 90% of AMA-positive SS patients had stage I primary biliary cirrhosis on liver biopsy.[137] Although 93% of patients with primary biliary cirrhosis display focal sialadenitis on salivary gland biopsy,[138] significant clinical evidence of SS has been reported in only 33% to 47%.[138] Some features of SS may be observed in up to 75% of patients, however.[139]

An interesting relationship has emerged between hepatitis C virus (HCV) infection and SS. As many as 57% to 77% of patients diagnosed with HCV infection exhibit clinical and histologic abnormalities suggestive of SS.[140-142] Similarly, HCV was detected in 6% to 19% of patients with SS.[143-145] Not surprisingly, patients diagnosed with SS who are HCV positive have a much higher incidence of hepatic involvement (approximately 90% versus 10%).[143,146] HCV-positive SS patients also have a higher prevalence of cryoglobulinemia, hypocomplementemia, and neurologic involvement, but they are less often SS-A or SS-B positive (10% versus 38%). Primary SS patients with cryoglobulinemia are six times more likely to have antibodies to HCV than are those without cryoglobulins.[147] Histologically, the salivary lesion in HCV-positive SS patients is similar to that in HCV-negative SS patients, except for the severity of the infiltrate. HCV-positive patients have milder lesions and lower focus scores.[141] Immunohistochemically, the lesions are also similar, displaying a preponderance of T cells with a CD4/CD8 ratio of 2:1.[148] Of interest is a report describing the onset of SS after interferon-α treatment for HCV.[149] HCV may be another viral agent that triggers autoimmune exocrinopathy given the appropriate genetic and immunologic background.

PANCREATIC

Laboratory evidence of exocrine pancreatic abnormality is not infrequent in SS. Some abnormality in pancreatic function testing has been reported in 50% to 75% of patients.[150,151] The most frequent abnormality is elevation of immunoreactive trypsin, occurring in 30% to 40%.[150] Episodes of abdominal pain and steatorrhea occur in SS but cannot always be attributed to pancreatitis, owing in part to the difficulty of interpreting serum amylase elevations. Approximately 30% of primary SS patients have elevations of P and S amylase.[152]

VASCULAR

Vasculitis has been reported in approximately 15% of SS patients. Subtypes range from hypersensitivity vasculitis to a necrotizing vasculitis resembling polyarteritis nodosa.[153] By far, the majority of cases involve the skin and manifest as recurrent crops of purpura. The lesions range from micropetechiae to large purpura and may be noninflammatory, demonstrating only extravasated red blood cells, or vasculitis. Urticarial lesions may occur. Immunopathologically, the purpura are caused by a combination of blood hyperviscosity and immune complex–mediated cutaneous vasculitis. Most biopsy specimens display immunofluorescent staining for immunoglobulin in the vessel wall.[154] Exacerbations of purpura occur secondary to increased hydrostatic pressure, such as that caused by prolonged standing and the wearing of elastic stockings. Patients with long-standing purpura often display chronic, older brawny lesions with superimposed showers of new petechiae or purpura (Fig. 69-4). In the 1980s, Alexander and colleagues[155] described the association of SS with cutaneous vasculitis, purpura, and adenopathy; 84% of their patients had antibodies to SS-A. It is important to rule out the presence of HCV in individuals presenting with cutaneous vasculitis, cryoglobulinemia, and sicca complaints. The constellation of purpura, mixed cryoglobulinemia, and hypocomplementemia (C4) has been identified as a risk for lymphoproliferation in SS patients (see later).

Raynaud's phenomenon affects 13% to 66% of SS patients.[156-159] It is often associated with nonerosive arthritis, frequently precedes the onset of xerostomia, and rarely results in digital ulceration. Nail-fold capillary microscopic changes include increased loop dilation and tortuosity and may resemble the changes seen in SLE.[160]

AUTOIMMUNE THYROID DISEASE

A strong association between SS and thyroid disease has been documented. In patients with primary SS who are examined for thyroid disease, the prevalence of thyroid abnormality ranges from 35% to 45%, and the prevalence of autoimmune thyroiditis is 18% to 24%.[161,162] Autoimmune thyroid disease occurs much more frequently in patients with SS than in those with RA.[163]

NEUROLOGIC

Neurologic disease is perhaps the most common significant extraglandular manifestation of SS. It can involve the cranial nerves, peripheral nerves, and, rarely, the central nervous system (CNS). Clinical reports suggest that half of SS patients have some form of neurologic involvement, with estimates ranging from 22% to 76%.[164-170] Peripheral neuropathy has been found in approximately 20% of SS patients[171,172]; in one study, it was symmetric in 33% of patients and was the presenting symptom in approximately 10%.[171] A predominantly sensory neuropathy may present with ataxia.[173] Sural nerve biopsy in SS patients with sensorimotor polyneuropathy reveals perivascular inflammatory infiltrates and changes suggestive or diagnostic of vasculitis in the majority.[174,175] Progressive neuropathy, especially with motor involvement (e.g., footdrop), may indicate the presence of necrotizing vasculitis, particularly in the context of palpable purpura or

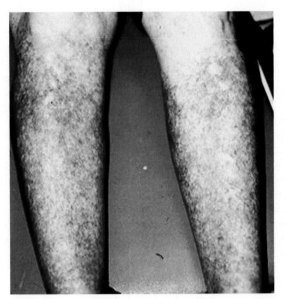

Figure 69-4 **Vascular manifestations of Sjögren's syndrome.** This patient with Sjögren's syndrome exhibits dermopathy involving the lower extremities secondary to hyperglobulinemic purpura. Recurrent showers of micropetechiae become chronic, resulting in brawny hyperpigmentation.

cutaneous ulceration. Biopsies of SS patients with pure sensory neuropathy demonstrate dorsal root ganglionitis in addition to perivascular mononuclear cell infiltrates involving cutaneous nerves.[173] Approximately one quarter of patients with peripheral neuropathy have a superimposed autonomic or cranial neuropathy.[175] Low intraepidermal nerve fiber densities indicative of small fiber neuropathy are rare.[176]

Cranial neuropathy, particularly trigeminal neuropathy, is the most distinctive type of neuropathy associated with primary SS.[166,167,177] Sensorineural hearing loss, especially involving high frequencies, is noted in approximately half of SS patients undergoing audiometric testing.[178] Disturbances in autonomic nervous system function can be demonstrated by objective testing (e.g., tilt table, digital blood flow, deep breathing) in a significant number of SS patients[179,180]; however, clinical symptoms are uncommon. Rarely, patients may develop significant postural hypotension. Adie's pupil has been described in several reports.[181,182]

The incidence of CNS disease in primary SS ranges from 0 to 30%. Interpretation of these figures is controversial owing to several issues, including lack of a uniform description of the clinical syndrome, especially when symptoms are restricted to mild cognitive or depressive features; inclusion of cases defined solely by electrophysiologic or imaging abnormalities; and the strict exclusion of SLE, primary angiitis of the CNS, antiphospholipid syndrome, or other causes, including hepatitis C. In rheumatologic practice, significant CNS disease is rare, whereas peripheral and cranial neuropathies are common. In the largest series of CNS cases reporting clinical, serologic, and pathologic characteristics, patients had an increased frequency of SS-A positivity and a strong association with peripheral inflammatory vascular disease, most commonly expressed as cutaneous vasculitis (see previous discussion); there was also an association with peripheral neuropathy and inflammatory myopathy.[183,184] Postmortem examination of primary SS patients from

Table 69-3 Risk of Lymphoproliferation in Sjögren's Syndrome

Number in Study	Region	Method	Risk (%)	Reference
110	Finland	SIR	13	202
676	Finland	SIR	8.7	203
136	USA	RR	44	201
62	France	PP	6.4	204
331	Italy	RR	33	205
55	France	PP	9	206
30	Netherlands	PP	10	207
261	Greece	IR	12.2	208
723	Greece	PP	3.9	210
138	USA	PP	6.0	211
Meta-analysis		SIR	18.8	209

IR, incidence ratio per 1000 person-years; PP, point prevalence (%); RR, relative risk; SIR, standardized incidence ratio.

another center revealed mixed inflammatory infiltrates in the leptomeninges and choroid plexus; only 5 of 11 patients had neurologic symptoms.[185]

In a study by Alexander and colleagues,[186] 75% of SS patients with active neuropsychiatric disease had abnormalities on magnetic resonance imaging (MRI), particularly in the subcortical and periventricular white matter. Twenty patients from this cohort had neurologic disease mimicking multiple sclerosis (MS).[187] Over the past several years, evidence of SS has been sought among MS outpatient populations.[188-195] Of 486 patients reported collectively, 3.3% met the criteria for SS, and 8.4% had at least one feature of SS. Of 100 consecutive patients admitted to an inpatient neurology service, 3 had SS.[196] Thus, it is likely that only a very small percentage of MS patients has undetected SS. Additionally, the existence of an SS-MS overlap syndrome cannot be excluded. Myelopathy was a prominent component of the MS-like disease reported in Alexander's series and was subsequently reported on multiple occasions, as summarized by Williams and coworkers.[197] The majority of patients demonstrate an acute or progressive transverse myelopathy. Good therapeutic outcomes have been reported with a combination of corticosteroid and cyclophosphamide. Several instances of optic neuropathy in patients with primary SS have been reported in the absence of MS.[198]

SS patients lacking clinical CNS disease may also have MRI abnormalities.[199] SS patients who displayed no evidence of neurologic abnormality except for cognitive dysfunction had abnormal single photon emission computed tomography scans but normal MRI studies.[200] Extreme caution must be used when the diagnosis of neurologic SS is entertained in patients demonstrating mild cognitive or psychiatric symptoms and minor abnormalities on sensitive imaging techniques, particularly in the absence of objective focal and serologic findings.

LYMPHOPROLIFERATIVE DISEASE

One of the major concerns of internists and rheumatologists caring for SS patients is the potential for the development of lymphoma. The original study by Kassan and colleagues[201] estimated that a primary SS patient has an approximately 40-fold enhanced risk of developing non-Hodgkin's lymphoma

(NHL) compared with age-matched controls. Subsequent studies confirmed this risk, but at a somewhat lower magnitude, which may be due in part to population differences. Table 69-3 summarizes studies examining the risk of lymphoma in primary SS.[202-212] Younger SS patients may be at somewhat higher risk than older patients.[213] A survey of 113 patients with NHL revealed that 12% had SS.[214]

SS-associated NHLs are largely B cell in origin[215] and may display a monocytoid phenotype.[216] They frequently involve MALT near the marginal zone.[217] Extranodal sites are often involved and include the salivary glands themselves (50%),[217] gastrointestinal tract (see previous discussion), lung, skin, thymus, and thyroid gland.[218-220] These NHLs are often indolent but may transform into large cell NHL.[221] Waldenström's macroglobulinemia may be heralded by the hyperviscosity syndrome, accompanied by lower extremity purpura. The clinician should be aware of signs suggestive of lymphoproliferation, including a significant increase in the size of the salivary glands, especially when accompanied by dominant masses, lymphadenopathy, splenomegaly, and pulmonary infiltrates. Longitudinal monitoring of laboratory parameters is appropriate. Development of a monoclonal protein, appearance of new-onset leukopenia and anemia, and loss of previously present specific autoantibodies (i.e., ANA, SS-A, SS-B) have all been associated with the development of lymphoma. The presence of low C3, C4, cryoglobulins, and lymphocytopenia conferred an approximate 6- to 10-fold increased risk for the development of lymphoma.[208,212] On occasion, a patient presents with significant increases in glandular swelling and lymphadenopathy suggestive of lymphoma. Tissue biopsy, however, is inconclusive, revealing lymphoid architecture that is atypical but not diagnostic of malignancy. This condition is referred to as *pseudolymphoma* and may represent an intermediate step in lymphomagenesis.[222] Molecular immunoglobulin rearrangement and immunophenotyping studies are often helpful in resolving this diagnostic issue.

SECONDARY SJÖGREN'S SYNDROME

Although secondary SS is defined as xerostomia and xerophthalmia in the presence of an autoimmune connective tissue disease, it is important to note that secondary SS is not monolithic. In other words, the characteristics of SS may vary among the different connective tissue disorders. Additionally, SS is a common accompaniment of autoimmune disorders not generally considered to be connective tissue diseases, such as thyroiditis, primary biliary cirrhosis, and MS. Thus, signs of SS should not be overlooked in these contexts.

Because of clinical, immunogenetic, and serologic overlap, many investigators and clinicians consider SS and SLE to be more intimately related than SS and other connective tissue diseases. Patients with SS-SLE overlap meet three or more criteria for both conditions and demonstrate a higher prevalence of inflammatory arthritis and renal, pulmonary, and CNS disease than those with primary SS alone.[223-225] Clinical signs suggestive of SS have been noted in 8% to 31% of patients with SLE,[226,227] whereas lymphocytic infiltration of MSGs has been reported in 50% of unselected SLE patients.[228] SLE patients who have more severe grades of lymphocytic infiltration appear to have less renal disease but more adenopathy, circulating RF, positivity to SS-A and SS-B, and erosive arthritis,[226-228] in addition to overt xerophthalmia and parotid enlargement. SLE patients with renal tubular acidosis and interstitial nephritis have been described as having concomitant primary SS.[229] In several reported series, primary SS transformed into SLE at intervals ranging from 1 to 10 years after the diagnosis of SS.[230-234]

Clinical SS affects approximately 20% of patients with RA. Thirty-one percent have positive MSG biopsies.[235] SS-A antibodies have been found in 4% to 23% of RA patients.[235-237] These patients are more likely to have severe sicca complaints and positive MSG biopsies; they are less likely to display HLA-DR4–related antigens. Interestingly, focal sialadenitis was common among an early synovitis cohort, 70% of whom were diagnosed with RA 1 year later.[238]

Between 14% and 20% of scleroderma patients have been diagnosed with SS.[239,240] On histopathologic examination, salivary glands from some patients with scleroderma display fibrosis alone, whereas others demonstrate typical lymphocytic sialadenitis and fibrosis. Despite similarities in the prevalence of SS in scleroderma and RA, individuals with scleroderma are more frequently symptomatic, perhaps due to the high prevalence of fibrosis.[239] SS is well known to complicate limited scleroderma.[241] An overlap among SS, CREST syndrome, and primary biliary cirrhosis is known to occur. Scleroderma patients meeting the criteria for SS are more likely to have limited disease.[242] Among a cohort of patients with mixed connective tissue disease, 33% had antibodies to SS-A, and 42% had sicca symptoms.[243] Approximately 15% of primary SS patients had cardiolipin antibodies.[244] When sought, β2-glycoprotein I antibodies were not detected, and clinical evidence of antiphospholipid syndrome was absent.

CLINICAL OUTCOMES

When followed over a 10-year period, approximately one third of patients with sicca complaints eventually fulfilled the criteria for SS.[245,246] Development of disease and severity of sicca symptoms correlate with the presence of autoantibodies, particularly ANA and SS-A, and the serum IgG level.[245,247] More advanced sialographic findings are seen in patients who are SS-A positive.[248] Glandular SS appears to progress very slowly. Once established,

diminished salivary flow remains relatively constant for several years, despite increases in focus score on repeat biopsy.[245,246,249] The most prevalent extraglandular manifestations developing during 9 years of follow-up were arthralgias, arthritis, Raynaud's phenomenon, dry skin, skin rash, and leukopenia.[250] The severity of extraglandular disease has been correlated to the severity of exocrine surface disease and to the presence of SS-A.[251,252] SS-A positivity has also been linked to the development of other rheumatologic diagnoses, including SLE, RA, and scleroderma.[253] Overall, there is apparently no excess mortality in patients with primary SS.[254] Recent studies from Sweden demonstrated 5- and 10-year survival rates of 96.6% and 92.8%, respectively.[255] Standardized mortality rates for the SS groups were 1.07 and 1.17 compared with the general population.[255] Excess mortality was associated only with lymphoma. Using short-form 36 (SF-36), it was found that women with primary SS had a diminished quality of life on all SF-36 scales. Although the psychological subdimension scales were similar to those of women with RA and fibromyalgia, the physical function quality of life was better in women with SS.[256] A study from the United Kingdom demonstrated that health care costs for primary SS patients were twice that of controls and approximated those for RA.[257]

DIFFERENTIAL DIAGNOSIS

Many common conditions cause dryness. Human immunodeficiency virus (HIV) causes a syndrome known as diffuse infiltrative lymphocytosis syndrome (DILS) in approximately 3% to 8% of patients.[258,259] These patients display nearly an exact replica of SS symptoms, including dry eyes, dry mouth, salivary swelling, and a propensity to develop lymphoma.[260] They are more commonly male, however, and lack specific SS-A and SS-B antibodies, although approximately 10% may exhibit ANA and RF. When it is difficult to distinguish SS from DILS, immunohistochemical study of MSGs may be useful, revealing a $CD4^+/CD8^+$ ratio of approximately 0.66 in DILS, in contrast to a ratio of more than 3.0 in SS.[258,259]

In Japan, where human T-lymphotropic virus 1 (HTLV-1) infection is endemic, a relationship between a Sjögren-like syndrome and HTLV-1 disease has been described. Clinical and serologic findings differ little between HTLV-1–positive and –negative SS patients,[261] although the former may not possess characteristic sialographic findings.[262]

Lymphocytic infiltration of salivary glands in graft-versus-host disease results in a syndrome that mimics SS[263] and appears within 12 weeks of bone marrow transplantation; infiltration peaks between 26 and 52 weeks after transplantation. Dry eye and dry mouth occur between 12 and 24 months. Symptoms may abate after 2 years.[264,265] ANA and smooth muscle antibodies are frequently positive; however, SS-A and SS-B are not.[266] Infiltrate T cell CD4/CD8 is either lower than that found in SS or inverse.[267] In these individuals, skin changes may mimic scleroderma.

Patients with sarcoidosis may present with lacrimal and salivary swelling, hypergammaglobulinemia; bone, muscle, and joint pain; and pulmonary infiltrates. In most cases, the characteristic features of sarcoidosis should pose little diagnostic difficulty. MSG biopsy reveals noncaseating granulomas.[268] Amyloid infiltration may also result in salivary gland enlargement, tongue swelling, and dry mouth, in addition to joint pain and renal insufficiency.[269]

Lymphoma may arise spontaneously in a salivary gland. The majority of tumors occur in the parotid gland and present as firm masses that are usually painless. Sicca symptoms are present in a minority (approximately 15%) of cases.[270] Other conditions causing sicca complaints are listed in Table 69-4.[271-279]

Table 69-4 Systemic Conditions Associated with Sicca Symptoms

Viral: mumps, EBV, HIV, HTLV-1
Graft-versus-host disease
Sarcoidosis
Amyloidosis
Lymphoma
Radioiodine therapy[271]
Fibromyalgia-like syndromes: chronic fatigue syndrome, dry eye and mouth syndrome[272,273]
Aging[274]
Dyslipoproteinemia[275]
Hemochromatosis[276]
Lipodystrophy[277,278]
Bulimia[279]

EBV, Epstein-Barr virus; HIV, human immunodeficiency virus; HTLV-1, human T-lymphotropic virus 1.

WORKUP

The modalities used for the workup of SS are the basis for most of the criteria proposed for the classification of SS. Thus, the evaluation of a patient with suspected SS often requires cooperation among the rheumatologist, ophthalmologist, and dental specialist. Figure 69-5 is a stepwise approach to the workup of SS based on the American-European Consensus Group modification of the European Community criteria shown in Table 69-5.[280] It is critical to ensure that the clinical conditions listed as exclusions, including medications that cause dryness, are absent. It is also important to understand the performance characteristics of the testing components used. No individual test is absolutely specific for SS, including MSG biopsy. Among ophthalmologic tests, the Schirmer test, tear breakup time, and rose bengal dye test are all sensitive; however, only the rose bengal test is specific (approximately 95%).[281,282] The Schirmer test is not very reproducible either in controls[283] or in SS patients.[284] The salivary scintigraphic time-activity pattern correlates well with salivary flow rate[285] but is diagnostically nonspecific; abnormalities could be caused by any infiltrative disorder. Sialography has the capacity to visualize the salivary ductal pattern, demonstrating abnormal arborization and ductal ectasia. Sialography appears to be as sensitive as biopsy and only slightly less specific,[286,287] but it is invasive, potentially causing flares of glandular pain and swelling. At focus scores greater than 3, scintigraphy, sialography, and biopsy display fairly good agreement.[288] Recently, parenchymal heterogeneity on ultrasonography and alterations in signal strength on

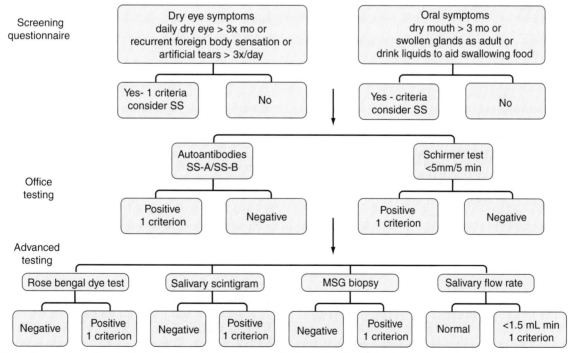

Figure 69-5 Approach to using the American-European consensus criteria for the diagnosis of Sjögren's syndrome (SS).[280] The six criteria are (1) symptoms of dry eye, (2) symptoms of dry mouth or salivary swelling, (3) evidence of dry eye by the Schirmer test or abnormal corneal staining, (4) evidence of salivary dysfunction (abnormal salivary flow, scintigram, sialogram), (5) presence of SS-A or SS-B, and (6) positive minor salivary gland (MSG) biopsy. Patients must have at least four of the six criteria, including either autoantibodies or a positive biopsy. Major exclusions include other major connective tissue disorders (for primary SS), lymphoma, sarcoidosis, amyloidosis, human immunodeficiency virus (HIV), and treatment with anticholinergic medication. The requisite four criteria may be verified by a simple office history, physical examination, and laboratory testing. If required, patients should be referred to an ophthalmologist, oral surgeon, otolaryngologist, or nuclear medicine physician to complete the workup.

Table 69-5 AEC Criteria for Sjögren's Syndrome

I. Symptoms of dry eye
  Patients must have a positive response to at least one of the following:
  Have you had daily, persistent, troublesome dry eyes for more than 3 months?
  Do you have a recurrent sensation of sand or gravel in the eyes?
  Do you use tear substitutes more than three times a day?

II. Oral symptoms
  Patients must have a positive response to at least one of the following:
  Have you had a daily feeling of dry mouth for more than 3 months?
  Have you had recurrently or persistently swollen salivary glands as an adult?
  Do you frequently drink liquids to aid in swallowing dry food?

III. Ocular signs
  Patients must have objective evidence of ocular involvement, defined as a positive result from at least one of the following two tests:
  Schirmer test performed without anesthesia (5 mm in 5 min)
  Rose bengal score or other ocular dye score (4 according to van Bijsterveld's scoring system)

IV. Histopathology
  This criterion is met if an expert histopathologist evaluates focal lymphocytic sialadenitis with a focus score of 1 in the patient's minor salivary glands (obtained through normal-appearing mucosa). The focus score is defined as the number of lymphocytic foci adjacent to normal-appearing mucous acini and containing more than 50 lymphocytes/4 mm^2 of glandular tissue.

V. Salivary gland involvement
  Patient must have objective evidence of salivary gland involvement, defined by a positive result for at least one of the following diagnostic tests:
  Unstimulated whole salivary flow (1.5 mL in 15 min)
  Parotid sialography showing the presence of diffuse sialectasis (punctate, cavitary, or destructive pattern) without evidence of obstruction in the major ducts
  Salivary scintigraphy showing delayed uptake, reduced concentration, delayed excretion of tracer, or some combination of these

VI. Autoantibodies
  Patient must have the following autoantibodies present in serum: antibodies to Ro (SS-A) or La (SS-B)

Definite Sjögren's syndrome requires the presence of four criteria, one of which must be either a positive biopsy or autoantibodies
Exclusions: prior head and neck radiation, hepatitis C infection, human immunodeficiency virus (HIV) or acquired immunodeficiency syndrome (AIDS), preexisting lymphoma, sarcoidosis, graft-versus-host disease, use of anticholinergic drugs

From Vitali C, Bombardiere S, Jonsson R, et al: Classification criteria for Sjögren's syndrome: A revised version of the European criteria proposed by the American-European Consensus Group. Ann Rheum Dis 61:554, 2002.

MRI have been shown to be relatively sensitive and specific for glandular involvement with SS.[289-291]

The MSG biopsy is often used to confirm a diagnosis of SS. It is important to verify that the biopsy is read by a pathologist experienced in interpreting salivary gland pathology. Vivino and colleagues[292] documented that the diagnosis was revised in 53% of biopsy samples reexamined at a university center. Only samples demonstrating periductal lymphocytic infiltrates in the form of foci should be regarded as being consistent with SS; biopsies revealing nonspecific scattered lymphocytic infiltrates, fibrosis, or fatty changes should not. In patients assessed specifically for

the ocular and oral components of SS, only focal sialadenitis correlates with KCS[293]; however, even biopsies with focus scores greater than 1 are not always specific for SS. Approximately 15% to 20% of specimens obtained from random postmortem samples and from healthy individuals have focus scores greater than 1.[294,295] Approximately 10% of samples from healthy elderly individuals can be interpreted as positive.[274] Focal lymphocytic sialadenitis has been found on submandibular gland biopsy, despite repeatedly negative MSG (lip) biopsies.[296] Cigarette smoking appears to lower the focus score of MSG biopsies.[297] An MSG biopsy should always be performed if the clinician cannot rule out or suspects an alternative cause of salivary swelling (e.g., lymphoma, sarcoidosis). In cases in which SS is not reasonably suspected or in which the diagnosis is readily apparent from noninvasive testing, the biopsy adds little.[298]

Serologies, particularly ANA and SS-A and SS-B, correlate with focus score on biopsy.[299] Serum IgG is the most specific predictor of a positive biopsy but has relatively low sensitivity.[300] A recent report of 41 patients tested for the presence of anti–SS-A and anti–SS-B and undergoing MSG biopsy showed a fairly high negative predictive value of anti–SS-A for MSG biopsy.[301] Anti–SS-B may be useful in identifying primary SS among patients presenting with xerostomia, xerophthalmia, and undifferentiated features of connective tissue disorder.[287] Adult classification criteria may not be applicable to children with suspected SS.[302]

TREATMENT

Therapy for SS has three phases. The first phase consists of external moisture replacement or capture. This approach can be applied to the oral cavity, eyes, nose, skin, and genital tract. The second phase consists of stimulation of endogenous secretions, which has proved effective mainly for xerostomia. This approach is currently under investigation for other xeroses, including the eyes and skin. Finally, patients with systemic manifestations, such as pulmonary disease, vasculitis, and pseudolymphoma, may require corticosteriods, cytotoxic agents, or both.

OCULAR DISEASE

Therapy of xerophthalmia begins with moisture replacement. Patients should be encouraged to use tear substitutes often. Myriad over-the-counter preparations exist. The rheumatologist should become familiar with one or two preparations from each of the following categories: (1) Standard artificial tears consist of polyvinyl alcohol or methylcellulose. (2) Preservative-free artificial tears should be used if irritation occurs with frequent use. These preparations are available as sealed, sterile, individual units that must be refrigerated or discarded after one use. (3) A subset of tear preparations has a higher viscosity by virtue of the inclusion of 0.1% dextran or 1% carboxymethylcellulose. These are useful for periods of increased symptoms but may cause some blurring. (4) Lubricating ointments and hydroxypropyl cellulose inserts are generally longer lived; however, they leave residue, may cause significant blurring, and are often reserved for nocturnal use. Vivino and Orlin[303] published an excellent compendium of these agents.

Existing tears may be retained in the eye by blocking their drainage or inhibiting their evaporation. The former can be accomplished by occluding the puncta by inserting collagen or silicone plugs (temporary) or by electrocautery (permanent). The latter can be accomplished by wearing goggles or glasses with specially constructed side chambers. These devices are not well accepted by patients but are valuable in certain environmental conditions (i.e., wind). Inflammation of the meibomian glands (blepharitis) may complicate dry eye and can be treated with warm compresses, cleansing of the lids, and a topical antibiotic when needed. Recently, data have demonstrated the efficacy of the secretagogues pilocarpine and cevimeline for xerophthalmia,[304,305] although the maximal effect may require 12 weeks of therapy.

ORAL DISEASE

Surprisingly, replacement of saliva is not as easily accomplished as tear supplementation. Artificial salivas are available,[303] but they are generally short-lived and unappetizing. A moisturizing gel (e.g., Oral Balance) is longer lived but must be applied intraorally. Patients generally find it most suitable for nighttime application. Patients should be counseled with regard to general environmental measures designed to enhance moisture, such as the use of a humidifier and the avoidance of forced hot-air heating systems and excessive air-conditioning. Emphasis should be given to fastidious dental care, including frequent examinations and office and home fluoride application. Patients should be advised not to retain sugar-containing foods in the mouth for long periods. SS patients often chew gum or candy to stimulate salivation, but only sugar-free products should be used. Some of the more severe symptoms encountered by dry-mouth patients are secondary to intraoral candidiasis.[306] Treatment should be initiated with nystatin (Mycostatin). The oral suspension (100,000 U/5 mL four times a day for 10 days) is commonly used; however, it contains significant amounts of sucrose and could, therefore, be cariogenic. Mycostatin vaginal tablets dissolved orally offer an alternative. Clotrimazole troches (10-mg troche dissolved in the mouth five times a day for 14 days) also may be used. Dentures must be removed and immersed in antifungal solutions to avoid recontamination. Oral candidiasis is recurrent and often requires retreatment. Systemic antifungals may be used, but they become ineffective as salivary flow diminishes. Interferon-α lozenges appear to increase salivary flow and reduce symptoms.[307]

SECRETORY STIMULATION

Patients whose symptoms of dryness are not optimally controlled by moisture replacement should be considered for treatment with secretory stimulants (secretagogues). Secretagogues stimulate muscarinic receptors in salivary glands and other organs, leading to enhanced secretion. Because there is a poor correlation among length of disease, biopsy findings, and response to these agents, and because M3R is upregulated in SS labial salivary gland acini,[308] a trial of secretagogue therapy should be offered. Secretagogues stimulate muscarinic activity in multiple organ systems, requiring caution in patients with asthma, narrow-angle glaucoma, acute iritis, severe cardiovascular disease, biliary

Table 69-6 Comparison of Muscarinic Stimulants for Sjögren's Syndrome

	Pilocarpine	Cevimeline
Brand name	Salagen	Evoxac
Dose form	Tablet	Capsule
Dose strength	5 mg	30 mg
Half-life	Approximately 1 hr	Approximately 5 hr
Peak onset of reaction	1 hr	1.5-2 hr
Major muscarinic side effects (%)		
Diaphoresis	40	19
Nausea	10	14
Rhinitis	9	11
Diarrhea	9	10

disease, nephrolithiasis, diarrhea, and ulcer disease. Two approved agents are available for use as secretagogues in SS: pilocarpine (Salagen) and cevimeline (Evoxac). Controlled clinical trials indicate that both drugs significantly increase the salivary flow rate in SS.[309-311] Preliminary data suggest that other xeroses may be improved as well. Pilocarpine is administered as 5-mg tablets four times a day. Cevimeline is administered as 30-mg capsules three times a day. Table 69-6 compares the properties of these agents.

Oral corticosteroids do not improve salivary flow.[312] Methotrexate and oral cyclosporine A improve subjective symptoms of dryness but not exocrine function.[313,314] Although a 14-week pilot study[315] with a subsequent 1-year follow-up[316] demonstrated a potential use for infliximab in treating the ocular, oral, and systemic inflammatory manifestations of SS, a subsequent 22-week double-blind, placebo-controlled trial revealed no advantage for infliximab-treated patients.[317] Similarly, a 12-week randomized, placebo-controlled trial revealed no benefit to etanercept treatment.[318] Additional placebo-controlled studies are required to demonstrate efficacy and safety with regard to lymphoproliferation. Recent retrospective and open-label trials suggest that anti–B cell therapy with rituximab may be useful.[319,320] B cell–directed therapies offer the potential advantages of reducing autoantibody production and interrupting B cell lymphomagenesis; however, controlled trials are required.

SYSTEMIC DISEASE

Minor musculoskeletal symptoms usually respond to non-steroidal anti-inflammatory drug therapy. Because erosive joint disease is rare, therapy with disease-modifying antirheumatic drugs is usually unnecessary; however, hydroxychloroquine at doses of 6 to 7 mg/kg per day has been used to treat fatigue, arthralgia, and myalgia in primary SS. Hydroxychloroquine does not improve dryness; however, it does reduce acute-phase proteins and elevated immunoglobulin levels in primary SS.[321] Rarely, short courses of low-dose corticosteroid (e.g., prednisolone 5 to 10 mg/day) may be necessary for very painful or disabling joint symptoms.

To combat cutaneous dryness, patients should be instructed not to dry completely after bathing; instead, they should gently blot the skin dry, leaving a slight amount of moisture, followed by application of a moisturizer. Some data suggest that secretagogues (e.g., pilocarpine) at doses of 20 to 30 mg/day ameliorate the symptoms of dry skin. Tight or constricting elastic clothing on the lower extremities may exacerbate hypergammaglobulinemic purpura; however, support hosiery may be helpful. Intermittent use of a mild corticosteroid cream may be useful to control pruritus. Mild cases of leukocytoclastic vasculitis can be treated expectantly. Severe cases manifested by necrotic or ulcerating lesions require more aggressive therapy.

Xerotrachea can be managed with humidification, secretagogues, and guaifenesin (1200 mg twice a day). Cough and dyspnea associated with pulmonary lymphocytic infiltration can be treated with a moderate-dose corticosteroid but may also require low to moderate doses of oral cyclophosphamide (50 to 150 mg/day). Frank lymphoma, when demonstrated by biopsy, requires standard chemotherapeutic intervention. Localized MALT lesions can be treated by external beam radiation or anti-CD20 monoclonal antibodies.

Treatment of mild to moderate renal tubular acidosis consists of supplementation with potassium chloride and alkalinization with potassium citrate. For cases resistant to replacement therapy or demonstrating evidence of renal insufficiency, corticosteroid therapy (0.5 to 1.0 mg/kg) should be considered.

Manifestations of gastroesophageal reflux disease are usually managed with antacids, H_2 blockers, and proton pump inhibitors. Intermittent endoscopic evaluation and intervention may be required. Sjögren's-associated hepatitis is often mild and may not require specific therapy. Persistent and progressive liver function test elevation may require therapy with prednisone and azathioprine. Standard measures for the management of acute pancreatitis or pancreatic enzyme deficiency should be used. Corticosteroid therapy has not proved useful and may itself be associated with pancreatitis; it should be avoided unless abdominal vasculitis is suspected.

Cranial and peripheral neuropathy can be treated with low-dose tricyclic antidepressants or gabapentin (300 to 1800 mg/day). Symptomatic cases resistant to the previously mentioned therapies can be treated with intravenous gammaglobulin (0.4 g/kg per day for 5 days). When demonstrated by muscle and nerve biopsy, vasculitis should be treated with moderate-dose corticosteroid (approximately 1 mg/kg per day, with subsequent tapering) and oral cyclophosphamide (50 to 150 mg/day). CNS manifestations thought to be caused by primary SS should be treated aggressively with high-dose corticosteroid orally (1 to 2 mg/kg) or by intravenous pulse (1 g/day for 3 days) and cyclophosphamide daily (50 to 150 mg/day) or monthly by intravenous pulse (0.5 to 1 g/m²).

REFERENCES

1. Sjögren H: Zur Kenntnis der keratoconjunctivitis sicca (keratitis filiformis bei hypofunktion der tranendrusen). Acta Ophthalmol (Kbh) 11(Suppl 2):1, 1933.
2. Leber: Uber die entstenhung der netzhautablosung. Klin Monatsbl Augenheilkd 20:165, 1882.
3. Mikulicz J: In discussion at Verein fur wissenschaftliche Heilkunde zu Konigsberg. Berl Klin Wochenschr 25:759, 1888.
4. Morgan WS, Castleman B: A clinicopathologic study of Mikulicz's disease. Am J Pathol 29:471, 1953.
5. Mason AM, Gumpel JM, Golding PL: Sjögren's syndrome: A clinical review. Semin Arthritis Rheum 2:301, 1973.
6. Talal N: Recent developments in the immunology of Sjögren's syndrome (autoimmune exocrinopathy). Scand J Rheumatol Suppl 61:76, 1986.
7. Skopouli FN, Moutsopoulos HM: Autoimmune epitheliitis: Sjögren's syndrome. Clin Exp Rheumatol 12(Suppl 11):S9, 1994.
8. Pillemer SR, Matteson EL, Jacobsson LT, et al: Incidence of physician-diagnosed primary Sjögren's syndrome in residents of Olmsted County, Minnesota. Mayo Clin Proc 76:593, 2001.
9. Chudwin DS, Daniels TE, Wara DW, et al: Spectrum of Sjögren's syndrome in children. J Pediatr 98:213, 1981.
10. Strickland RW, Tesar JT, Berne BH, et al: The frequency of sicca syndrome in an elderly female population. J Rheumatol 14:766, 1987.
11. Molina R, Provost TT, Arnett FC, et al: Primary Sjögren's syndrome in men: Clinical, serologic and immunogenetic features. Am J Med 80:23, 1986.
12. Brennan MT, Fox PC: Sex differences in primary Sjögren's syndrome. J Rheumatol 26:2373, 1999.
13. Cervera R, Font J, Ramos-Casals M, et al: Primary Sjögren's syndrome in men: Clinical and immunological characteristics. Lupus 9:61, 2000.
14. Nasu M, Matsubara O, Yamamoto H: Postmortem prevalence of lymphocytic infiltration of the lacrimal gland: A comparative study in autoimmune and non-autoimmune diseases. J Pathol 143:11, 1984.
15. Fritzler MJ, Pauls JD, Kinsella TD, et al: Antinuclear, anticytoplasmic, and anti-Sjögren's syndrome antigen A (SS-A/Ro) antibodies in female blood donors. Clin Immunol Immunopathol 36:120, 1985.
16. Schein OD, Hochberg MC, Munoz B, et al: Dry eye and dry mouth in the elderly: A population-based assessment. Arch Intern Med 159:1359, 1999.
17. Drosos AA, Andonopoulos AP, Costopoulos JS, et al: Prevalence of primary Sjögren's syndrome in an elderly population. Br J Rheumatol 27:123, 1988.
18. Jacobsson LT, Axell TE, Hansen BU, et al: Dry eyes or mouth: An epidemiological study in Swedish adults, with special reference to primary Sjögren's syndrome. J Autoimmun 2:521, 1989.
19. Zhang NZ, Shi CS, Yao QP, et al: Prevalence of primary Sjögren's syndrome in China. J Rheumatol 22:659, 1995.
20. Bjerrum KB: Keratoconjunctivitis sicca and primary Sjögren's syndrome in a Danish population aged 30-60 years. Acta Ophthalmol Scand 75:281, 1997.
21. Dafni UG, Tzioufas AG, Staikos P, et al: Prevalence of Sjögren's syndrome in a closed rural community. Ann Rheum Dis 56:521, 1997.
22. Thomas E, Hay EM, Hajeer A, et al: Sjögren's syndrome: A community-based study of prevalence and impact. Br J Rheumatol 37:1069, 1998.
23. Tomsic M, Logar D, Grmek M, et al: Prevalence of Sjögren's syndrome in Slovenia. Rheumatology (Oxford) 38:164, 1999.
24. Bowman SJ, Ibrahim GH, Holmes G, et al: Estimating the prevalence among Caucasian women of primary Sjögren's syndrome in two general practices in Birmingham, UK. Scand J Rheumatol 33:39, 2004.
25. Alamanos Y, Tsifetaki N, Voulgari PV, et al: Epidemiology of primary Sjögren's syndrome in north-west Greece. Rheumatology (Oxford) 45:187, 2006.
26. Kabasakal Y, Kitapcioglu G, Turk T, et al: The prevalence of Sjögren's syndrome in adult women. Scand J Rheumatol 35:379, 2006.
27. Boling EP, Wen J, Reveille JD, et al: Primary Sjögren's syndrome and autoimmune hemolytic anemia in sisters: A family study. Am J Med 74:1066, 1983.
28. Bolstad AI, Haga HJ, Wassmuth R, et al. Monozygotic twins with primary Sjögren's syndrome. J Rheumatol 27:2264, 2000.
29. Fye KH, Terasaki PI, Moutsopoulos H, et al: Association of Sjögren's syndrome with HLA-B8. Arthritis Rheum 19:883, 1976.
30. Chused TM, Kassan SS, Opelz G, et al: Sjögren's syndrome association with HLA-Dw3. N Engl J Med 296:895, 1977.
31. Arnett FC, Bias WB, Reveille JD: Genetic studies in Sjögren's syndrome and systemic lupus erythematosus. J Autoimmun 2:403, 1989.
32. Kumagai S, Kanagawa S, Morinobu A, et al: Association of a new allele of the TAP2 gene, TAP2*Bky2 (Val577), with susceptibility to Sjögren's syndrome. Arthritis Rheum 40:1685, 1997.
33. Jean S, Quelvenec E, Alizadeh M, et al: DRB1*15 and DRB1*03 extended haplotype interaction in primary Sjögren's syndrome genetic susceptibility. Clin Exp Rheumatol 16:725, 1998.
34. Guggenbuhl P, Veillard E, Quelvenec E, et al: Analysis of TNF alpha microsatellites in 35 patients with primary Sjögren's syndrome. Joint Bone Spine 67:290, 2000.

35. Hulkkonen J, Pertovaara M, Antonen J, et al: Genetic association between interleukin-10 promoter region polymorphisms and primary Sjögren's syndrome. Arthritis Rheum 44:176, 2001.

36. Morinobu A, Kanagawa S, Koshiba M, et al: Association of the glutathione S-transferase M1 homozygous null genotype with susceptibility to Sjögren's syndrome in Japanese individuals. Arthritis Rheum 42:2612, 1999.

37. Ichikawa Y, Shimizu H, Takahashi K, et al: Lymphocyte subsets of the peripheral blood in Sjögren's syndrome and rheumatoid arthritis. Clin Exp Rheumatol 7:55, 1989.

38. Ichikawa Y, Shimizu H, Yoshida M, et al: Activation antigens expressed on T cells of the peripheral blood in Sjögren's syndrome and rheumatoid arthritis. Clin Exp Rheumatol 8:243, 1990.

39. Ichikawa Y, Shimizu H, Yoshida M, et al: Activation of T cell subsets in the peripheral blood of patients with Sjögren's syndrome: Multicolor flow cytometric analysis. Arthritis Rheum 33:1674, 1990.

40. Struyf NJ, Snoeck HW, Bridts CH, et al: Natural killer cell activity in Sjögren's syndrome and systemic lupus erythematosus: Stimulation with interferons and interleukin-2 and correlation with immune complexes. Ann Rheum Dis 49:690, 1990.

41. Miyasaka N, Seaman W, Bakhshi A, et al: Natural killing activity in Sjögren's syndrome: An analysis of defective mechanisms. Arthritis Rheum 26:954, 1983.

42. Bakhshi A, Miyasaka N, Kavathas P, et al: Lymphocyte subsets in Sjögren's syndrome: A quantitative analysis using monoclonal antibodies and the fluorescence-activated cell sorter. J Clin Lab Immunol 10:63, 1983.

43. Dauphinee M, Tovar Z, Talal N: B cells expressing CD5 are increased in Sjögren's syndrome. Arthritis Rheum 31:642, 1988.

44. Carsons SE: The medical workup of Sjögren's syndrome. In Carsons SE, Harris EK (eds): The New Sjögren's Syndrome Handbook. New York, Oxford University Press, 1998, pp 29-36.

45. Basset C, Durand V, Jamin C, et al: Increased N-linked glycosylation leading to oversialylation of monomeric immunoglobulin A1 from patients with Sjögren's syndrome. Scand J Immunol 51:300, 2000.

46. Atkinson JC, Fox PC, Travis WD, et al: IgA rheumatoid factor and IgA-containing immune complexes in primary Sjögren's syndrome. J Rheumatol 16:1205, 1989.

47. Daniels TE, Aufdermonte TB, Greenspan JS: Histopathology of Sjögren's syndrome. In Talal N, Moutsopolous HM, Kassan S (eds): Sjögren's Syndrome: Clinical and Immunological Aspects. Berlin, Springer Verlag, 1987, pp 41-54.

48. Fox RI, Carstens SA, Fong S, et al: Use of monoclonal antibodies to analyze peripheral blood and salivary gland lymphocyte subsets in Sjögren's syndrome. Arthritis Rheum 25:419, 1982.

49. Fujihara T, Fujita H, Tsuoda K, et al: Preferential localization of CD8+alpha E beta 7+ T cells around acinar epithelial cells with apoptosis in patients with Sjögren's syndrome. J Immunol 163:2226, 1999.

50. Adamson TC III, Fox RI, Frisman DM, et al: Immunohistologic analysis of lymphoid infiltrates in primary Sjögren's syndrome using monoclonal antibodies. J Immunol 130:203, 1983.

51. Sumida T, Yonaha F, Maeda T, et al: T cell receptor repertoire of infiltrating T cells in lips of Sjögren's syndrome patients. J Clin Invest 89:681, 1992.

52. Smith MD, Lamour A, Boylston A, et al: Selective expression of V beta families by T cells in the blood and salivary gland infiltrate of patients with primary Sjögren's syndrome. J Rheumatol 21:1832, 1994.

53. Roncin S, Guillevin L, Beaugrand M, et al: Identification of the T cell antigen receptor V beta gene product in labial salivary glands from patients with primary Sjögren's syndrome. Ann Med Interne (Paris) 146:226, 1995.

54. Speight PM, Cruchley A, Williams DM: Quantification of plasma cells in labial salivary glands: Increased expression of IgM in Sjögren's syndrome. J Oral Pathol Med 19:126, 1990.

55. Thrane PS, Sollid LM, Haanes HR, et al: Clustering of IgA-producing immunocytes related to HLA-DR-positive ducts in normal and inflamed salivary glands. Scand J Immunol 35:43, 1992.

56. Horsfall AC, Rose LM, Maini RN: Autoantibody synthesis in salivary glands of Sjögren's syndrome patients. J Autoimmun 2:559, 1989.

57. Larsson A, Bredberg A, Henriksson G, et al: Immunohistochemistry of the B-cell component in lower lip salivary glands of Sjögren's syndrome and healthy subjects. Scand J Immunol 61:98, 2005.

58. Szodoray P, Alex P, Jonsson MV, et al: Distinct profiles of Sjögren's syndrome patients with ectopic salivary gland germinal centers revealed by serum cytokines and BAFF. Clin Immunol 117:168, 2005.

59. Szodoray P, Jellestad S, Alex P, et al: Programmed cell death of peripheral blood B cells determined by laser scanning cytometry in Sjögren's syndrome with a special emphasis on BAFF. J Clin Immunol 24:600, 2004.

60. Aziz KE, McCluskey PJ, Wakefield D: Expression of selectins (CD62 E,L,P) and cellular adhesion molecules in primary Sjögren's syndrome: Questions to immunoregulation. Clin Immunol Immunopathol 80:55, 1996.

61. Saito I, Terauchi K, Shimuta M, et al: Expression of cell adhesion molecules in the salivary and lacrimal glands of Sjögren's syndrome. J Clin Lab Anal 7:180, 1993.

62. Amft N, Curnow SJ, Scheel-Toellner D, et al: Ectopic expression of the B cell-attracting chemokine BCA-1 (CXCL13) on endothelial cells and within lymphoid follicles contributes to the establishment of germinal center-like structures in Sjögren's syndrome. Arthritis Rheum 44:2633, 2001.

63. Mikulowska-Mennis A, Xu B, Berberian JM, et al: Lymphocyte migration to inflamed lacrimal glands is mediated by vascular cell adhesion molecule-1/alpha(4)beta(1) integrin, peripheral node addressin/1-selectin, and lymphocyte function-associated antigen-1 adhesion pathways. Am J Pathol 159:671, 2001.

64. McArthur CP, Daniels PJ, Kragel P, et al: Sjögren's syndrome salivary gland immunopathology: Increased laminin expression precedes lymphocytic infiltration. J Autoimmun 10:59, 1997.

65. Oxholm P, Daniels TE, Bendtzen K: Cytokine expression in labial salivary glands from patients with primary Sjögren's syndrome. Autoimmunity 12:185, 1992.

66. Boumba D, Skopouli FN, Moutsopoulos HM: Cytokine mRNA expression in the labial salivary gland tissues from patients with primary Sjögren's syndrome. Br J Rheumatol 34:326, 1995.

67. Cauli A, Yanni G, Pitzalis C, et al: Cytokine and adhesion molecule expression in the minor salivary glands of patients with Sjögren's syndrome and chronic sialoadenitis. Ann Rheum Dis 54:209, 1995.

68. Ohyama Y, Nakamura S, Matsuzaki G, et al: Cytokine messenger RNA expression in the labial salivary glands of patients with Sjögren's syndrome. Arthritis Rheum 39:1376, 1996.

69. Sun D, Emmert-Buck MR, Fox PC: Differential cytokine mRNA expression in human labial minor salivary glands in primary Sjögren's syndrome. Autoimmunity 28:125, 1998.

70. Koski H, Janin A, Humphreys-Beher MG, et al: Tumor necrosis factor-alpha and receptors for it in labial salivary glands in Sjögren's syndrome. Clin Exp Rheumatol 19:131, 2001.

71. Wakamatsu E, Matsumoto I, Yasukochi T, et al: Overexpression of phosphorylated STAT-1alpha in the labial salivary glands of patients with Sjögren's syndrome. Arthritis Rheum 54:3476, 2006.

72. Villarreal GM, Alcocer-Varela J, Llorente L: Differential interleukin IL-10 and IL-13 gene expression in vivo in salivary glands and peripheral blood mononuclear cells from patients with primary Sjögren's syndrome. Immunol Lett 49:105, 1996.

73. Kong L, Ogawa N, Nakabayashi T, et al: Fas and Fas ligand expression in the salivary glands of patients with primary Sjögren's syndrome. Arthritis Rheum 40:87, 1997.

74. Polihronis M, Tapinos NI, Theocharis SE, et al: Modes of epithelial cell death and repair in Sjögren's syndrome (SS). Clin Exp Immunol 114:485, 1998.

75. Ohlsson M, Skarstein K, Bolstad AI, et al: Fas-induced apoptosis is a rare event in Sjögren's syndrome. Lab Invest 81:95, 2001.

76. Nakamura H, Kawakami A, Tominaga M, et al: Expression of CD40/CD40 ligand and Bcl-2 family proteins in labial salivary glands of patients with Sjögren's syndrome. Lab Invest 79:261, 1999.

77. Tsubota K, Fujita H, Tadano K, et al: Abnormal expression and function of Fas ligand of lacrimal glands and peripheral blood in Sjögren's syndrome patients with enlarged exocrine glands. Clin Exp Immunol 129:177, 2002.

78. Manganelli P, Quaini F, Andreoli AM, et al: Quantitative analysis of apoptosis and Bcl-2 in Sjögren's syndrome. J Rheumatol 24:1552, 1997.

79. Konttinen YT, Halinen S, Hanemaaijer R, et al: Matrix metalloproteinase (MMP)-9 type IV collagenase/gelatinase implicated in the pathogenesis of Sjögren's syndrome. Matrix Biol 17:335, 1998.

80. Azuma M, Motegi K, Aota K, et al: Role of cytokines in the destruction of acinar structure in Sjögren's syndrome salivary glands. Lab Invest 77:269, 1997.
81. Gellrich S, Rutz S, Borkowski A, et al: Analysis of V(H)-D-J(H) gene transcripts in B cells infiltrating the salivary glands and lymph node tissues of patients with Sjögren's syndrome. Arthritis Rheum 42:240, 1999.
82. Stott DI, Hiepe F, Hummel M, et al: Antigen-driven proliferation of B cells within the target tissue of an autoimmune disease: The salivary glands of patients with Sjögren's syndrome. J Clin Invest 102:938, 1998.
83. Whittingham S, McNeilage J, Mackay IR: Primary Sjögren's syndrome after infectious mononucleosis. Ann Intern Med 102:490, 1985.
84. Gaston JS, Rowe M, Bacon P: Sjögren's syndrome after infection by Epstein-Barr virus. J Rheumatol 17:558, 1990.
85. Inoue N, Harada S, Miyasaka N, et al: Analysis of antibody titers to Epstein-Barr virus nuclear antigen in sera of patients with Sjögren's syndrome and with rheumatoid arthritis. J Infect Dis 164:22, 1991.
86. Fox RI, Pearson G, Vaughan JH: Detection of Epstein-Barr virus-associated antigens and DNA in salivary gland biopsies from patients with Sjögren's syndrome. J Immunol 137:3162, 1986.
87. Haneji N, Nakamura T, Takio K, et al: Identification of alpha-fodrin as a candidate autoantigen in primary Sjögren's syndrome. Science 276:604, 1997.
88. Inoue H, Tsubota K, Ono M, et al: Possible involvement of EBV-mediated alpha fodrin cleavage for organ-specific autoantigen in Sjögren's syndrome. J Immunol 166:5801, 2001.
89. Nagaraju K, Cox A, Casciola-Rosen L, et al: Novel fragments of the Sjögren's syndrome autoantigens alpha-fodrin and type 3 muscarinic acetylcholine receptor generated during cytotoxic lymphocyte granule-induced cell death. Arthritis Rheum 44:2376, 2001.
90. MacSween RN, Goudie RB, Anderson JR, et al: Occurrence of antibody to salivary duct epithelium in Sjögren's disease, rheumatoid arthritis, and other arthritides: A clinical and laboratory study. Ann Rheum Dis 26:402, 1967.
91. Bacman S, Sterin-Borda L, Camusso JJ, et al: Circulating antibodies against rat parotid gland M3 muscarinic receptors in primary Sjögren's syndrome. Clin Exp Immunol 104:454, 1996.
92. Waterman SA, Gordon TP, Rischmueller M: Inhibitory effects of muscarinic receptor autoantibodies on parasympathetic neurotransmission in Sjögren's syndrome. Arthritis Rheum 43:1647, 2000.
93. Cavill D, Waterman SA, Gordon TP: Antibodies raised against the second extracellular loop of the human muscarinic M3 receptor mimic functional autoantibodies in Sjögren's syndrome. Scand J Immunol 59:261, 2004.
94. Lindstrom FD, Eriksson P, Tejle K, et al: IgG subclasses of anti-SS-A/Ro in patients with primary Sjögren's syndrome. Clin Immunol Immunopathol 73:358, 1994.
95. Tengner P, Halse AK, Haga HJ, et al: Detection of anti-Ro/SSA and anti-La/SSB autoantibody-producing cells in salivary glands from patients with Sjögren's syndrome. Arthritis Rheum 41:2238, 1998.
96. de Wilde PC, Kater L, Bodeutsch C, et al: Aberrant expression pattern of the SS-B/La antigen in the labial salivary glands of patients with Sjögren's syndrome. Arthritis Rheum 39:783, 1996.
97. Ormerod LD, Fong LP, Foster CS: Corneal infection in mucosal scarring disorders and Sjögren's syndrome. Am J Ophthalmol 105:512, 1988.
98. Friedlaender MH: Ocular manifestations of Sjögren's syndrome: Keratoconjunctivitis sicca. Rheum Dis Clin North Am 18:591, 1992.
99. Baudet-Pommel M, Albuisson E, Kemeny JL, et al: Early dental loss in Sjögren's syndrome: Histologic correlates. European Community Study Group on Diagnostic Criteria for Sjögren's Syndrome (EEC COMAC). Oral Surg Oral Med Oral Pathol 78:181, 1994.
100. Rhodus NL, Bloomquist C, Liljemark W, et al: Prevalence, density and manifestations of oral Candida albicans in patients with Sjögren's syndrome. J Otolaryngol 26:300, 1997.
101. Wang SL, Zou ZJ, Yu SF, et al: Recurrent swelling of parotid glands and Sjögren's syndrome. Int J Oral Maxillofac Surg 22:362, 1993.
102. Katayama I, Yokozeki H, Nishioka K: Impaired sweating as an exocrine manifestation in Sjögren's syndrome. Br J Dermatol 133:716, 1995.
103. Mitchell J, Greenspan J, Daniels T, et al: Anhidrosis (hypohidrosis) in Sjögren's syndrome. J Am Acad Dermatol 16:233, 1987.
104. Castro-Poltronieri A, Alarcon-Segovia D: Articular manifestations of primary Sjögren's syndrome. J Rheumatol 10:485, 1983.
105. Pease CT, Shattles W, Barrett NK, et al: The arthopathy of Sjögren's syndrome. Br J Rheumatol 32:609, 1993.
106. Tsampoulas CG, Skopouli FN, Sartoris DJ, et al: Hand radiographic changes in patients with primary and secondary Sjögren's syndrome. Scand J Rheumatol 15:333, 1986.
107. Lindvall B, Bengtsson A, Ernerudh J, et al: Subclinical myositis is common in primary Sjögren's syndrome and is not related to muscle pain. J Rheumatol 29:717, 2002.
108. Vrethem M, Lindvall B, Holmgren H, et al: Neuropathy and myopathy in primary Sjögren's syndrome: Neurophysiological, immunological and muscle biopsy results. Acta Neurol Scand 82:126, 1990.
109. Papiris SA, Maniata M, Constantopoulos SH, et al: Lung involvement in primary Sjögren's syndrome is mainly related to the small airway disease. Ann Rheum Dis 58:61, 1999.
110. Mialon P, Barthelemy L, Sebert P, et al: A longitudinal study of lung impairment in patients with primary Sjögren's syndrome. Clin Exp Rheumatol 15:349, 1997.
111. Fairfax AJ, Haslam PL, Pavia D, et al: Pulmonary disorders associated with Sjögren's syndrome. Q J Med 50:279, 1981.
112. Mathieu A, Cauli A, Pala R, et al: Tracheobronchial mucociliary clearance in patients with primary and secondary Sjögren's syndrome. Scand J Rheumatol 24:300, 1995.
113. Andoh Y, Shimura S, Sawai T, et al: Morphometric analysis of airways in Sjögren's syndrome. Am Rev Respir Dis 148:1358, 1993.
114. La Corte R, Potena A, Bajocchi G, et al: Increased bronchial responsiveness in primary Sjögren's syndrome: A sign of tracheobronchial involvement. Clin Exp Rheumatol 9:125, 1991.
115. Strimlan CV, Rosenow EC III, Divertie MB, et al: Pulmonary manifestations of Sjögren's syndrome. Chest 70:354, 1976.
116. Kelly C, Gardiner P, Pal B, et al: Lung function in primary Sjögren's syndrome: A cross sectional and longitudinal study. Thorax 46:180, 1991.
117. Constantopoulos SH, Papadimitriou CS, Moutsopoulos HM: Respiratory manifestations in primary Sjögren's syndrome: A clinical, functional, and histologic study. Chest 88:226, 1985.
118. Uffmann M, Kiener HP, Bankier AA, et al: Lung manifestation in asymptomatic patients with primary Sjögren's syndrome: Assessment with high resolution CT and pulmonary function tests. J Thorac Imaging 16:282, 2001.
119. Koyama M, Johkoh T, Honda O, et al: Pulmonary involvement in primary Sjögren's syndrome: Spectrum of pulmonary abnormalities and computed tomography findings in 60 patients. J Thorac Imaging 16:290, 2001.
120. Hatron PY, Wallaert B, Gosset D, et al: Subclinical lung inflammation in primary Sjögren's syndrome: Relationship between bronchoalveolar lavage cellular analysis findings and characteristics of the disease. Arthritis Rheum 30:1226, 1987.
121. Deheinzelin D, Capelozzi VL, Kairalla RA, et al: Interstitial lung disease in primary Sjögren's syndrome: Clinical pathological evaluation and response to treatment. Am J Respir Crit Care Med 154:794, 1996.
122. Ito I, Nagai S, Kitaichi M, et al: Pulmonary manifestations of primary Sjögren's syndrome: A clinical, radiologic and pathological study. Am J Respir Crit Care Med 171:632, 2005.
123. Parambil JG, Myers JL, Lindell RM, et al: Interstitial lung disease in primary Sjögren's syndrome. Chest 130:1489, 2006.
124. Papiris SA, Saetta M, Turato G, et al: CD-4 positive T-lymphocytes infiltrate the bronchial mucosa of patients with Sjögren's syndrome. Am J Respir Crit Care Med 156:637, 1997.
125. Raskin RJ, Tesar JT, Lawless OJ: Hypokalemic periodic paralysis in Sjögren's syndrome. Arch Intern Med 141:1671, 1981.
126. Goules A, Masouridi S, Tzioufas AG, et al: Clinically significant and biopsy-documented renal involvement in primary Sjögren's syndrome. Medicine 79:241, 2000.
127. Shiozawa S, Shiozawa K, Shimizu S, et al: Clinical studies of renal disease in Sjögren's syndrome. Ann Rheum Dis 46:768, 1987.
128. Talal N, Zisman E, Schur PH: Renal tubular acidosis, glomerulonephritis and immunologic factors in Sjögren's syndrome. Arthritis Rheum 11:774, 1968.
129. Matsumura R, Kondo Y, Sugiyama T, et al: Immunohistochemical identification of infiltrating mononuclear cells in tubulointerstitial nephritis associated with Sjögren's syndrome. Clin Nephrol 30:335, 1988.

130. Kjellen G, Fransson SG, Lindstrom F, et al: Esophageal function, radiography, and dysphagia in Sjögren's syndrome. Dig Dis Sci 31:225, 1986.
131. Tsianos EB, Chiras CD, Drosos AA, et al: Oesophageal dysfunction in patients with primary Sjögren's syndrome. Ann Rheum Dis 44:610, 1985.
132. Ostuni PA, Germana B, DiMario F, et al: Gastric involvement in primary Sjögren's syndrome. Clin Exp Rheumatol 11:21, 1993.
133. Pokorny G, Karacsony G, Lonovics J, et al: Types of atrophic gastritis in patients with primary Sjögren's syndrome. Ann Rheum Dis 50:97, 1991.
134. Maury CP, Tornroth T, Teppo AM: Atrophic gastritis in Sjögren's syndrome: Morphologic, biochemical and immunologic findings. Arthritis Rheum 28:388, 1985.
135. Lindgren S, Manthorpe R, Eriksson S: Autoimmune liver disease in patients with primary Sjögren's syndrome. J Hepatol 20:354, 1994.
136. Manthorpe R, Permin H, Tage-Jensen U: Autoantibodies in Sjögren's syndrome, with special reference to liver-cell membrane antibody (LMA). Scand J Rheumatol 8:168, 1979.
137. Skopouli FN, Barbatis C, Moutsopoulos HM: Liver involvement in primary Sjögren's syndrome. Br J Rheumatol 33:745, 1994.
138. Hansen BU, Lindgren S, Eriksson S, et al: Clinical and immunological features of Sjögren's syndrome in patients with primary biliary cirrhosis with emphasis on focal sialadenitis. Acta Med Scand 224:611, 1988.
139. Uddenfeldt P, Danielsson A, Forssell A, et al: Features of Sjögren's syndrome in patients with primary biliary cirrhosis. J Intern Med 230:443, 1991.
140. Haddad J, Deny P, Munz-Gotheil C, et al: Lymphocyte sialadenitis of Sjögren's syndrome associated with chronic hepatitis C virus liver disease. Lancet 339:321, 1992.
141. Pirisi M, Scott C, Fabris C, et al: Mild sialoadenitis: A common finding in patients with hepatitis C virus infection. Scand J Gastroenterol 29:940, 1994.
142. Verbaan H, Carlson J, Eriksson S, et al: Extrahepatic manifestations of chronic hepatitis C infection and the interrelationship between primary Sjögren's syndrome and hepatitis C in Swedish patients. J Intern Med 245:127, 1999.
143. Jorgensen C, Legouffe MC, Perney P, et al: Sicca syndrome associated with hepatitis C virus infection. Arthritis Rheum 39:1166, 1996.
144. Garcia-Carrasco M, Ramos M, Cervera R, et al: Hepatitis C virus infection in primary Sjögren's syndrome: Prevalence and clinical significance in a series of 90 patients. Ann Rheum Dis 56:173, 1997.
145. Szodoray P, Csepregi A, Hejjas M, et al: Study of hepatitis C virus infection in 213 Hungarian patients with Sjögren's syndrome. Rheumatol Int 21:6, 2001.
146. **Ramos-Casals M, Garcia-Carrasco M, Cervera R, et al: Hepatitis C virus infection mimicking primary Sjögren's syndrome: A clinical and immunologic description of 35 cases. Medicine 80:1, 2001.**
147. Ramos-Casals M, Cervera R, Yague J, et al: Cryoglobulinemia in primary Sjögren's syndrome: Prevalence and clinical characteristics in a series of 115 patients. Semin Arthritis Rheum 28:200, 1998.
148. Coll J, Gambus G, Corominas J, et al: Immunohistochemistry of minor salivary gland biopsy specimen from patients with Sjögren's syndrome with and without hepatitis C virus infection. Ann Rheum Dis 56:390, 1997.
149. Unoki H, Moriyama A, Tabaru A, et al: Development of Sjögren's syndrome during treatment with recombinant human interferon-alpha-2b for chronic hepatitis C. J Gastroenterol 31:723, 1996.
150. Coll J, Navarro S, Tomas R, et al: Exocrine pancreatic function in Sjögren's syndrome. Arch Intern Med 149:848, 1989.
151. Nishimori I, Morita M, Kino J, et al: Pancreatic involvement in patients with Sjögren's syndrome and primary biliary cirrhosis. Int J Pancreatol 17:47, 1995.
152. Tsianos EB, Tzioufas AG, Kita MD, et al: Serum isoamylases in patients with autoimmune rheumatic diseases. Clin Exp Rheumatol 2:235, 1984.
153. **Tsokos M, Lazarou SA, Moutsopoulos HM: Vasculitis in primary Sjögren's syndrome: Histologic classification and clinical presentation. Am J Clin Pathol 88:26, 1987.**
154. Sugai S, Shimizu S, Tachibana S, et al: Hypergammaglobulinemic purpura in patients with Sjögren's syndrome: A report of nine cases and a review of the Japanese literature. Jpn J Med 28:148, 1989.
155. Alexander EL, Arnett FC, Provost TT, et al: Sjögren's syndrome: Association of anti-Ro(SS-A) antibodies with vasculitis, hematologic abnormalities, and serologic hyperreactivity. Ann Intern Med 98:155, 1983.
156. Youinou P, Pennec YL, Katsikis P, et al: Raynaud's phenomenon in primary Sjögren's syndrome. Br J Rheumatol 29:205, 1990.
157. Skopouli FN, Talal A, Galanopoulou V, et al: Raynaud's phenomenon in primary Sjögren's syndrome. J Rheumatol 17:618, 1990.
158. Kraus A, Caballero-Uribe C, Jakez J, et al: Raynaud's phenomenon in primary Sjögren's syndrome: Association with other extraglandular manifestations. J Rheumatol 19:1572, 1992.
159. Garcia-Carrasco M, Siso A, Ramos-Casals M, et al: Raynaud's phenomenon in primary Sjögren's syndrome: Prevalence and clinical characteristics in a series of 320 patients. J Rheumatol 29:726, 2002.
160. Ohtsuka T: Nailfold capillary abnormalities in patients with Sjögren's syndrome and systemic lupus erythematosus. Br J Rheumatol 136:94, 1997.
161. Ramos-Casals M, Garcia-Carrasco M, Cervera R, et al: Thyroid disease in primary Sjögren's syndrome: Study in a series of 160 patients. Medicine (Baltimore) 79:103, 2000.
162. Perez B, Kraus A, Lopez G, et al: Autoimmune thyroid disease in primary Sjögren's syndrome. Am J Med 99:480, 1995.
163. Youinou P, Mangold W, Jouquan J, et al: Organ-specific autoantibodies in non-organ-specific autoimmune diseases with special reference to rheumatoid arthritis. Rheumatol Int 7:123, 1987.
164. Andonopoulos AP, Lagos G, Drosos AA, et al: The spectrum of neurologic involvement in Sjögren's syndrome. Br J Rheumatol 29:21, 1990.
165. Hietaharju A, Yli-Kerttula U, Hakkinen V, et al: Nervous system manifestations in Sjögren's syndrome. Acta Neurol Scand 81:144, 1990.
166. Mauch E, Volk C, Kratzsch G, et al: Neurological and neuropsychiatric dysfunction in primary Sjögren's syndrome. Acta Neurol Scand 89:31, 1994.
167. Tajima Y, Mito Y, Owada Y, et al: Neurological manifestations of primary Sjögren's syndrome in Japanese patients. Intern Med 36:690, 1997.
168. Govoni M, Bajocchi G, Rizzo N, et al: Neurological involvement in primary Sjögren's syndrome: Clinical and instrumental evaluation in a cohort of Italian patients. Clin Rheumatol 18:299, 1999.
169. **Lafitte C, Amoura Z, Cacoub P, et al: Neurological complications of primary Sjögren's syndrome. J Neurol 248:577, 2001.**
170. Terenzi TJ, Dennis KA, Carsons SE: Primary Sjögren's with systemic manifestations: Effects of classification utilizing the new European-American consensus criteria and the ACR criteria for SLE. Arthritis Rheum 46:S367, 2002.
171. Gemignani F, Marbini A, Pavesi G, et al: Peripheral neuropathy associated with primary Sjögren's syndrome. J Neurol Neurosurg Psychiatry 57:983, 1994.
172. Barendregt PJ, van den Bent MJ, van Raaij-van den Aarssen VJ, et al: Involvement of the peripheral nervous system in primary Sjögren's syndrome. Ann Rheum Dis 60:876, 2001.
173. Griffin JW, Cornblath DR, Alexander E, et al: Ataxic sensory neuropathy and dorsal root ganglionitis associated with Sjögren's syndrome. Ann Neurol 27:304, 1990.
174. Malinow K, Yannakakis GD, Glusman SM, et al: Subacute sensory neuronopathy secondary to dorsal root ganglionitis in primary Sjögren's syndrome. Ann Neurol 20:535, 1986.
175. Mellgren SI, Conn DL, Stevens JC, et al: Peripheral neuropathy in primary Sjögren's syndrome. Neurology 39:390, 1989.
176. Goransson LG, Herigstad A, Tjensvoll AB, et al: Peripheral neuropathy in primary Sjögren's syndrome: A population-based study. Arch Neurol 63:1612, 2006.
177. Kaltreider HB, Talal N: The neuropathy of Sjögren's syndrome: Trigeminal nerve involvement. Ann Intern Med 70:751, 1969.
178. Tumiati B, Casoli P, Parmeggiani A: Hearing loss in Sjögren's syndrome. Ann Intern Med 126:450, 1997.
179. Mandl T, Jacobsson L, Lilja B, et al: Disturbances of autonomic nervous function in primary Sjögren's syndrome. Scand J Rheumatol 26:401, 1997.
180. Andonopoulos AP, Christodoulou J, Ballas C, et al: Autonomic cardiovascular neuropathy in Sjögren's syndrome: A controlled study. J Rheumatol 25:2385, 1998.
181. Vetrugno R, Liguori R, Cevoli S, et al: Adie's tonic pupil as a manifestation of Sjögren's syndrome. Ital J Neurol Sci 18:293, 1997.
182. Bachmeyer C, Zuber M, Dupont S, et al: Adie syndrome as the initial sign of primary Sjögren's syndrome. Am J Ophthalmol 123:691, 1997.

183. Molina R, Provost TT, Alexander EL: Peripheral inflammatory vascular disease in Sjögren's syndrome: Association with nervous system complications. Arthritis Rheum 28:1341, 1985.
184. Alexander EL, Ranzenbach MR, Kumar AJ, et al: Anti-Ro(SS-A) autoantibodies in central nervous system disease associated with Sjögren's syndrome (CNS-SS): Clinical, neuroimaging, and angiographic correlates. Neurology 44:899, 1994.
185. de la Monte SM, Hutchins GM, Gupta PK: Polymorphous meningitis with atypical mononuclear cells in Sjögren's syndrome. Ann Neurol 14:455, 1983.
186. Alexander EL, Beall SS, Gordon B, et al: Magnetic resonance imaging of cerebral lesions in patients with Sjögren's syndrome. Ann Intern Med 108:815, 1988.
187. Alexander EL, Malinow K, Lejewski JE, et al: Primary Sjögren's syndrome with central nervous system disease mimicking multiple sclerosis. Ann Intern Med 104:323, 1986.
188. Noseworthy JH, Bass BH, Vandervoort MK, et al: The prevalence of primary Sjögren's syndrome in a multiple sclerosis population. Ann Neurol 25:95, 1989.
189. Montecucco C, Franciotta DM, Caporali R, et al: Sicca syndrome and anti-SSA/Ro antibodies in patients with suspected or definite multiple sclerosis. Scand J Rheumatol 18:407, 1989.
190. Metz LM, Seland TP, Fritzler MJ: An analysis of the frequency of Sjögren's syndrome in a population of multiple sclerosis patients. J Clin Lab Immunol 30:121, 1989.
191. Miro J, Pena-Sagredo JL, Berciano J, et al: Prevalence of primary Sjögren's syndrome in patients with multiple sclerosis. Ann Neurol 27:582, 1990.
192. Ellemann K, Krogh E, Arlien-Soeborg P, et al: Sjögren's syndrome in patients with multiple sclerosis. Acta Neurol Scand 84:68, 1991.
193. Sandberg-Wollheim M, Axell T, Hansen BU, et al: Primary Sjögren's syndrome in patients with multiple sclerosis. Neurology 42:845, 1992.
194. de Andres C, Guillem A, Rodriguez-Mahou M, et al: Frequency and significance of anti-Ro(SS-A) antibodies in multiple sclerosis patients. Acta Neurol Scand 104:83, 2001.
195. de Seze J, Devos D, Castelnovo G, et al: The prevalence of Sjögren's syndrome in patients with primary progressive multiple sclerosis. Neurology 57:1359, 2001.
196. Olsen ML, O'Connor S, Arnett FC, et al: Autoantibodies and rheumatic disorders in a neurology inpatient population: A prospective study. Am J Med 90:479, 1991.
197. Williams CS, Butler E, Roman GC: Treatment of myelopathy in Sjögren's syndrome with a combination of prednisone and cyclophosphamide. Arch Neurol 58:815, 2001.
198. Wise CM, Agudelo CA: Optic neuropathy as an initial manifestation of Sjögren's syndrome. J Rheumatol 15:799, 1988.
199. Pierot L, Suave C, Leger JM, et al: Asymptomatic cerebral involvement in Sjögren's syndrome: MRI findings of 15 cases. Neuroradiology 35:378, 1993.
200. Belin C, Moroni C, Caillat-Vigneron N, et al: Central nervous system involvement in Sjögren's syndrome: Evidence from neuropsychological testing and HMPAO-SPECT. Ann Med Interne (Paris) 150:598, 1999.
201. **Kassan SS, Thomas TL, Moutsopoulos HM, et al: Increased risk of lymphoma in sicca syndrome. Ann Intern Med 89:888, 1978.**
202. Pertovaara M, Pukkala E, Laippala P, et al: A longitudinal cohort study of Finnish patients with primary Sjögren's syndrome: Clinical, immunological, and epidemiologic aspects. Ann Rheum Dis 60:467, 2001.
203. Kauppi M, Pukkala E, Isomaki H: Elevated incidence of hematologic malignancies in patients with Sjögren's syndrome compared with patients with rheumatoid arthritis (Finland). Cancer Causes Control 8:201, 1997.
204. Pariente D, Anaya JM, Combe B, et al: Non Hodgkin's lymphoma associated with primary Sjögren's syndrome. Eur J Med 1:337, 1992.
205. Valesini G, Priori R, Bavoillot D, et al: Differential risk of non-Hodgkin's lymphoma in Italian patients with primary Sjögren's syndrome. J Rheumatol 24:2376, 1997.
206. Zufferey P, Meyer OC, Grossin M, et al: Primary Sjögren's syndrome (SS) and malignant lymphoma: A retrospective cohort study of 55 patients with SS. Scand J Rheumatol 24:342, 1995.
207. Kruize AA, Hene RJ, van der Heide A, et al: Long-term follow-up of patients with Sjögren's symdrome. Arthritis Rheum 39:297, 1996.

208. **Skopouli FN, Dafni U, Ioannidis JP, et al: Clinical evolution, and morbidity and mortality of primary Sjögren's syndrome. Semin Arthritis Rheum 29:296, 2000.**
209. Zintzaras E, Voulgarelis M, Moutsopoulos HM: The risk of lymphoma development in autoimmune diseases: A meta-analysis. Arch Intern Med 165:2337, 2005.
210. Ioannidis JP, Vassikiou VA, Moutsopoulos HM: Long-term risk of mortality and lymphoproliferative disease and predictive classification of primary Sjögren's syndrome. Arthritis Rheum 46:741, 2002.
211. McCurley T, Collins RD, Ball E, et al: Nodal and extranodal lymphoproliferative disorders in Sjögren's syndrome: A clinical and immunopathologic study. Hum Pathol 21:482, 1990.
212. Theander E, Henriksson G, Ljungberg O, et al: Lymphoma and other malignancies in primary Sjögren's syndrome: A cohort study on cancer incidence and lymphoma predictors. Ann Rheum Dis 65:796, 2006.
213. Ramos-Casals M, Cervera R, Font J, et al: Young onset of primary Sjögren's syndrome: Clinical and immunological characteristics. Lupus 7:202, 1998.
214. Janin A, Morel P, Quiquandon I, et al: Non-Hodgkin's lymphoma and Sjögren's syndrome: An immunopathological study of 113 patients. Clin Exp Rheumatol 10:565, 1992.
215. Zulman J, Jaffe R, Talal N: Evidence that the malignant lymphoma of Sjögren's syndrome is a monoclonal B-cell neoplasm. N Engl J Med 299:1215, 1978.
216. Sheibani K, Burke JS, Swartz WG, et al: Monocytoid B-cell lymphoma: Clinicopathological study of 21 cases of a unique type of low-grade lymphoma. Cancer 62:1531, 1988.
217. Voulgarelis M, Dafni UG, Isenberg DA, et al: Malignant lymphoma in primary Sjögren's syndrome: A multicenter, retrospective, clinical study by the European Concerted Action on Sjögren's Syndrome. Arthritis Rheum 42:1765, 1999.
218. Isaacson P, Wright DH: Extranodal malignant lymphoma arising from mucosa-associated lymphoid tissue. Cancer 53:2515, 1984.
219. Hansen LA, Prakash UB, Colby TV: Pulmonary lymphoma in Sjögren's syndrome. Mayo Clin Proc 64:920, 1989.
220. Royer B, Cazals-Hatem D, Sibilia J, et al: Lymphomas in patients with Sjögren's syndrome are marginal zone B cell neoplasms, arise in diverse extranodal and nodal sites and are not associated with viruses. Blood 90:766, 1997.
221. Biasi D, Caramaschi P, Ambrosetti A, et al: Mucosa-associated lymphoid tissue lymphoma of the salivary glands occurring in patients affected by Sjögren's syndrome: Report of 6 cases. Acta Haematol 105:83, 2001.
222. Talal N, Aufdemorte TB, Kincaid WL, et al: Two patients illustrating lymphoma transition and response to therapy in Sjögren's syndrome. J Autoimmun 1:171, 1988.
223. Ramos-Casals M, Brito-Zeron P, Font J: The overlap of Sjögren's syndrome with other systemic autoimmune diseases. Semin Arthritis Rheum 36:246, 2007.
224. Szanto A, Szodoray P, Kiss E, et al: Clinical, serologic and genetic profiles of patients with associated Sjögren's syndrome and systemic lupus erythematosus. Hum Immunol 67:924, 2006.
225. Manoussakis MN, Georgopoulou C, Zintzaras E, et al: Sjögren's syndrome associated with systemic lupus erythematosus: Clinical and laboratory profiles and comparison with primary Sjögren's syndrome. Arthritis Rheum 50:882, 2004.
226. Andonopoulos AP, Skopouli FN, Dimou GS, et al: Sjögren's syndrome in systemic lupus erythematosus. J Rheumatol 17:201, 1990.
227. Grennan DM, Ferguson M, Williamson J, et al: Sjögren's syndrome in SLE. Part 1. The frequency of the clinical and subclinical features of Sjögren's syndrome in patients with SLE. N Z Med J 86:374, 1977.
228. Skopouli F, Siouna-Fatourou H, Dimou GS, et al: Histologic lesion in labial salivary glands of patients with systemic lupus erythematosus. Oral Surg Oral Med Oral Pathol 72:208, 1991.
229. Graninger WB, Steinberg AD, Meron G, et al: Interstitial nephritis in patients with systemic lupus erythematosus: A manifestation of concomitant Sjögren's syndrome? Clin Exp Rheumatol 9:41, 1991.
230. Romero RW, Nesbitt LT Jr, Ichinose H: Mikulicz disease and subsequent lupus erythematosus development. JAMA 237:2507, 1977.
231. Provost TT, Talal N, Harley JB, et al: The relationship between anti-Ro(SS-A) antibody-positive Sjögren's syndrome and anti-Ro (SS-A) antibody-positive lupus erythematosus. Arch Dermatol 124:63, 1988.

232. Chevalier X, de Bandt M, Bourgeois P, et al: Primary Sjögren's syndrome preceding the presentation of systemic lupus erythematosus as a benign intracranial hypertension syndrome. Ann Rheum Dis 51:808, 1992.
233. Zufferey P, Meyer OC, Bourgeois P, et al: Primary systemic Sjögren's syndrome (SS) preceding systemic lupus erythematosus: A retrospective study of 4 cases in a cohort of 55 SS patients. Lupus 4:23, 1995.
234. Satoh M, Yamagata H, Watanabe F, et al: Development of anti-Sm and anti-DNA antibodies followed by clinical manifestation of systemic lupus erythematosus in an elderly woman with long-standing Sjögren's syndrome. Lupus 4:63, 1995.
235. Andonopoulos AP, Drosos AA, Skopouli FN, et al: Secondary Sjögren's syndrome in rheumatoid arthritis. J Rheumatol 14:1098, 1987.
236. Skopouli FN, Andonopoulos AP, Moutsopoulos HM: Clinical implications of the presence of anti-Ro(SSA) antibodies in patients with rheumatoid arthritis. J Autoimmun 1:381, 1988.
237. Boire G, Menard HA, Gendron M, et al: Rheumatoid arthritis: Anti-Ro antibodies define a non-HLA-DR associated clinicoserological cluster. J Rheumatol 20:1654, 1993.
238. Brennan MT, Pillemer SR, Goldbach-Mansky R, et al: Focal sialadenitis in patients with early synovitis. Clin Exp Rheumatol 19:444, 2001.
239. Cipoletti JF, Buckingham RB, Barnes EL, et al: Sjögren's syndrome in progressive systemic sclerosis. Ann Intern Med 87:535, 1977.
240. Andonopoulos AP, Drosos AA, Skopouli FN, et al: Sjögren's syndrome in rheumatoid arthritis and progressive systemic sclerosis: A comparative study. Clin Exp Rheumatol 7:203, 1989.
241. Frayha RA, Tabbara KF, Geha RS: Familial CREST syndrome with sicca complex. J Rheumatol 4:53, 1977.
242. Avouac J, Sordet C, Depinay C, et al: Systemic sclerosis-associated Sjögren's syndrome and relationship to the limited cutaneous subtype: Results of a prospective study of sicca syndrome in 133 consecutive patients. Arthritis Rheum 54:2243, 2006.
243. Setty YN, Pittman CB, Mahale AS, et al: Sicca symptoms and anti-SSA/Ro antibodies are common in mixed connective tissue disease. J Rheumatol 29:487, 2002.
244. Jedryka-Goral A, Jagiello P, D'Cruz DP, et al: Isotype profile and clinical relevance of anticardiolipin antibodies in Sjögren's syndrome. Ann Rheum Dis 51:889, 1992.
245. Pertovaara M, Korpela M, Uusitalo H, et al: Clinical follow-up study of 87 patients with sicca symptoms (dryness of eyes or mouth, or both). Ann Rheum Dis 58:423, 1999.
246. Kruize AA, van Bijsterveld OP, Hene RJ, et al: Long-term course of tear gland function in patients with keratoconjunctivitis sicca and Sjögren's syndrome. Br J Ophthalmol 81:435, 1997.
247. Haga HJ: Clinical and immunological factors associated with low lacrimal and salivary flow rate in patients with primary Sjögren's syndrome. J Rheumatol 29:305, 2002.
248. Miyachi K, Naito M, Maeno Y, et al: Sialographic study in patients with and without antibodies to Sjögren's syndrome A (Ro). J Rheumatol 10:387, 1983.
249. Jonsson R, Kroneld U, Backman K, et al: Progression of sialadenitis in Sjögren's syndrome. Br J Rheumatol 32:578, 1993.
250. Markusse HM, Oudkerk M, Vroom TM, et al: Primary Sjögren's syndrome: Clinical spectrum and mode of presentation based on an analysis of 50 patients selected from a department of rheumatology. Neth J Med 40:125, 1992.
251. Asmussen K, Andersen V, Bendixen G, et al: Quantitative assessment of clinical disease status in primary Sjögren's syndrome: A cross-sectional study using a new classification model. Scand J Rheumatol 26:197, 1997.
252. Kelly CA, Foster H, Pal B, et al: Primary Sjögren's syndrome in northeast England: A longitudinal study. Br J Rheumatol 30:437, 1991.
253. Davidson BK, Kelly CA, Griffiths ID: Primary Sjögren's syndrome in the northeast of England: A long-term follow-up study. Rheumatology (Oxford) 38:245, 1999.
254. Martins PB, Pillemer SR, Jacobsson LT, et al: Survivorship in a population based cohort of patients with Sjögren's syndrome, 1976-1992. J Rheumatol 26:1296, 1999.
255. Theander E, Manthorpe R, Jacobsson LT: Mortality and causes of death in primary Sjögren's syndrome: A prospective cohort study. Arthritis Rheum 50:1262, 2004.
256. Strombeck B, Ekdahl C, Manthorpe R, et al: Health-related quality of life in primary Sjögren's syndrome, rheumatoid arthritis and fibromyalgia compared to normal population data using SF-36. Scand J Rheumatol 29:20, 2000.
257. Callaghan R, Prabu A, Allan RB, et al: Direct healthcare costs and predictors of costs in patients with primary Sjögren's syndrome. Rheumatology (Oxford) 46:105, 2007.
258. Williams FM, Cohen PR, Jumshyd J, et al: Prevalence of the diffuse infiltrative lymphocytosis syndrome among human immunodeficiency virus-type 1-positive outpatients. Arthritis Rheum 41:863, 1998.
259. Kordossis T, Paikos S, Aroni K, et al: Prevalence of Sjögren's-like syndrome in a cohort of HIV-1-positive patients: Descriptive pathology and immunopathology. Br J Rheumatol 37:691, 1998.
260. Ulirsch RC, Jaffe ES: Sjögren's syndrome-like illness associated with the acquired immunodeficiency syndrome-related complex. Hum Pathol 18:1063, 1987.
261. Nakamura H, Kawakami A, Tominaga M, et al: Relationship between Sjögren's syndrome and human T-lymphotropic virus type 1 infection: Follow-up study of 83 patients. J Lab Clin Med 135:139, 2000.
262. Izumi M, Nakamura H, Nakamura T, et al: Sjögren's syndrome (SS) in patients with human T cell leukemia virus 1 associated myelopathy: Paradoxical features of the major salivary glands compared to classical SS. J Rheumatol 26:2609, 1999.
263. Gratwhol AA, Moutsopoulos HM, Chused TM, et al: Sjögren-type syndrome after allogeneic bone marrow transplantation. Ann Intern Med 87:703, 1977.
264. Lindahl G, Lonnquist B, Hedfors E: Lymphocytic infiltration of lip salivary glands in bone marrow recipients: A model for the development of the histopathological changes in Sjögren's syndrome?. J Autoimmun 2:579, 1989.
265. Janin-Mercier A, Devergie A, Arrago JP, et al: Systemic evaluation of Sjögren-like syndrome after bone marrow transplantation in man. Transplantation 43:677, 1987.
266. Rouquette-Gally AM, Boyeldieu D, Gluckman E, et al: Auto-immunity in 28 patients after allogeneic bone marrow transplantation: Comparison with Sjögren's syndrome and scleroderma. Br J Haematol 66:45, 1987.
267. Hiroki A, Nakamura S, Shinohara M, et al: A comparison of glandular involvement between chronic graft-versus-host disease and Sjögren's syndrome. Int J Oral Maxillofac Surg 25:298, 1996.
268. Drosos AA, Constantopoulos SH, Psychos D, et al: The forgotten cause of sicca complex: Sarcoidosis. J Rheumatol 16:1548, 1989.
269. Gogel HK, Searles RP, Volpicelli NA, et al: Primary amyloidosis presenting as Sjögren's syndrome. Arch Intern Med 143:2325, 1983.
270. Nime FA, Cooper HS, Eggleston JC: Primary malignant lymphomas of the salivary glands. Cancer 37:906, 1976.
271. Solans R, Bosch JA, Galofre P, et al: Salivary and lacrimal gland dysfunciton (sicca syndrome) after radioiodine therapy. J Nucl Med 42:738, 2001.
272. Sirois DA, Natelson B: Clinicopathological findings consistent with primary Sjögren's syndrome in a subset of patients diagnosed with chronic fatigue syndrome: Preliminary observations. J Rheumatol 28:126, 2001.
273. Price EJ, Venables PJ: Dry eyes and mouth syndrome: A subgroup of patients presenting with sicca symptoms. Rheumatology (Oxford) 41:416, 2002.
274. De Wilde PC, Baak JP, van Houwelingen JC, et al: Morphometric study of histological changes in sublabial salivary glands due to aging process. J Clin Pathol 39:406, 1986.
275. Goldman JA, Julian EH: Pseudo-Sjögren's syndrome with hyperlipoproteinemia. JAMA 237:1582, 1977.
276. Takeda Y, Ohya T: Sicca symptom in a patient with hemochromatosis: Minor salivary gland biopsy for differential diagnosis. Int J Oral Maxillofac Surg 16:745, 1987.
277. Alarcon-Segovia D: Ramos-Niembro F: Association of partial lipodystrophy and Sjögren's syndrome. Lett Ann Intern Med 85:474, 1976.
278. Ipp MM, Howard NJ, Tervo RC, et al: Sicca syndrome and total lipodystrophy. Ann Intern Med 85:443, 1976.
279. Levin PA, Falko JM, Dixon K, et al: Benign parotid enlargement in bulimia. Ann Intern Med 93:827, 1980.
280. Vitali C, Bombardiere S, Jonsson R, et al: Classification criteria for Sjögren's syndrome: A revised version of the European criteria proposed by the American-European Consensus Group. Ann Rheum Dis 61:554, 2002.
281. Paschides CA, Kitsios G, Karakostas KX, et al: Evaluation of tear break-up time, Schirmer's-1 test and rose bengal staining as confirmatory tests for keratoconjunctivitis sicca. Clin Exp Rheumatol 7:155, 1989.

282. Kalk WW, Mansour K, Vissink A, et al: Oral and ocular manifestations in Sjögren's syndrome. J Rheumatol 29:924, 2002.

283. Clinch TE, Benedetto DA, Felberg NT, et al: Schirmer's test. Arch Ophthalmol 101:1383, 1983.

284. Haga HJ, Hulten B, Bolstad AI, et al: Reliability and sensitivity of the diagnostic tests for primary Sjögren's syndrome. J Rheumatol 26:604, 1999.

285. Saito T, Fukuda H, Horikawa M, et al: Salivary gland scintigraphy with 99mTc-pertechnetate in Sjögren's syndrome: Relationship to clinicopathologic features of salivary and lacrimal glands. J Oral Pathol Med 26:46, 1997.

286. Vitali C, Tavoni A, Simi U, et al: Parotid sialography and minor salivary gland biopsy in the diagnosis of Sjögren's syndrome: A comparative study of 84 patients. J Rheumatol 15:262, 1988.

287. Vitali C, Monti P, Giuiggioli C, et al: Parotid sialography and lip biopsy in the evaluation of oral component in Sjögren's syndrome. Clin Exp Rheumatol 7:131, 1989.

288. Lindvall AM, Jonsson R: The salivary gland component of Sjögren's syndrome: An evaluation of diagnostic methods. Oral Surg Oral Med Oral Pathol 62:32, 1986.

289. Niemela RK, Paakko E, Suramo I, et al: Magnetic resonance imaging and magnetic resonance sialography of parotid glands in primary Sjögren's syndrome. Arthritis Rheum 45:512, 2001.

290. Izumi M, Eguchi K, Ohki M, et al: MR imaging of the parotid gland in Sjögren's syndrome: A proposal for new diagnostic criteria. AJR Am J Roentgenol 166:1483, 1996.

291. Niemela RK, Takalo R, Paakko E, et al: Ultrasonography of salivary glands in primary Sjögren's syndrome: A comparison with magnetic resonance imaging and magnetic resonance sialography of parotid glands. Rheumatology (Oxford) 43:875, 2004.

292. Vivino FB, Gala I, Hermann GA: Change in final diagnosis on second evaluation of labial minor salivary gland biopsies. J Rheumatol 29:938, 2002.

293. Daniels TE, Whitcher JP: Association of patterns of labial salivary gland inflammation with keratoconjunctivitis sicca: Analysis of 618 patients with suspected Sjögren's syndrome. Arthritis Rheum 37:869, 1994.

294. Segerberg-Konttinen M: A postmortem study of focal adenitis in salivary and lacrimal glands. J Autoimmun 2:553, 1989.

295. Radfar L, Kleiner DE, Fox PC, et al: Prevalence and clinical significance of lymphocytic foci in minor salivary glands of healthy volunteers. Arthritis Rheum 47:520, 2002.

296. Katz J, Yamase H, Parke A: A case of Sjögren's syndrome with repeatedly negative findings on lip biopsy. Arthritis Rheum 34:1325, 1991.

297. Manthorpe R, Benoni C, Jacobsson L, et al: Lower frequency of focal lip sialadenitis (focus score) in smoking patients: Can tobacco diminish the salivary gland involvement as judged by histological examination and anti-SSA/Ro and anti-SSB/La antibodies in Sjögren's syndrome? Ann Rheum Dis 59:54, 2000.

298. Lee M, Rutka JA, Slomovic AR, et al: Establishing guidelines for the role of minor salivary gland biopsy in clinical practice for Sjögren's syndrome. J Rheumatol 25:247, 1998.

299. Shah F, Rapini RP, Arnett FC, et al: Association of labial salivary gland histopathology with clinical and serologic features of connective tissue diseases. Arthritis Rheum 33:1682, 1990.

300. Brennan MT, Sankar V, Leakan RA, et al: Risk factors for positive minor salivary gland biopsy findings in Sjögren's syndrome and dry mouth patients. Arthritis Rheum 47:189, 2002.

301. Kessel A, Toubi E, Rozenbaum M, et al: Sjögren's syndrome in the community: Can serology replace salivary gland biopsy? Rheumatol Int 26:337, 2006.

302. Houghton K, Malleson P, Cabral D, et al: Primary Sjögren's syndrome in children and adolescents: Are proposed diagnostic criteria applicable? J Rheumatol 32:2225, 2005.

303. Vivino FB, Orlin SE: Sjögren's syndrome: Giving dry mouth and dry eye the full treatment. J Musculoskel Med 17:350, 2000.

304. Papas AS, Sherrer YS, Charney M, et al: Successful treatment of dry mouth and dry eye symptoms in Sjögren's syndrome patients with oral pilocarpine: A randomized, placebo-controlled, dose-adjustment study. J Clin Rheumatol 10:169, 2004.

305. Ono M, Takamura E, Shinozaki K, et al: Therapeutic effect of cevimeline on dry eye in patients with Sjögren's syndrome: A randomized, double-blind clinical study. Am J Ophthalmol 138:6, 2004.

306. Hernandez YL, Daniels TE: Oral candidiasis in Sjögren's syndrome: Prevalence, clinical correlations, and treatment. Oral Surg Oral Med Oral Pathol 68:324, 1989.

307. Shiozawa S, Tanaka Y, Shiozawa K: Single-blinded controlled trial of low-dose oral IFN-alpha for the treatment of xerostomia in patients with Sjögren's syndrome. J Interferon Cytokine Res 18:255, 1998.

308. Beroukas D, Goodfellow R, Hiscock J, et al: Up-regulation of M3-muscarinic receptors in labial salivary gland acini in primary Sjögren's syndrome. Lab Invest 82:203, 2002.

309. Fox PC, Atkinson JC, Macynski AA, et al: Pilocarpine treatment of salivary gland hypofunction and dry mouth (xerostomia). Arch Intern Med 151:1149, 1991.

310. Vivino FB, Al-Hashimi I, Khan Z, et al: Pilocarpine tablets for the treatment of dry mouth and dry eye symptoms in patients with Sjögren's syndrome: A randomized, placebo-controlled, fixed-dose, multicenter trial: P92-01 Study Group. Arch Intern Med 159:174, 1999.

311. Fife RS, Chase WF, Dore RK, et al: Cevimeline for the treatment of xerostomia in patients with Sjögren's syndrome: A randomized trial. Arch Intern Med 162:1293, 2002.

312. Fox PC, Datiles M, Atkinson JC, et al: Prednisone and piroxicam for treatment of primary Sjögren's syndrome. Clin Exp Rheumatol 11:149, 1993.

313. Skopouli FN, Jagiello P, Tsifetaki N, et al: Methotrexate in primary Sjögren's syndrome. Clin Exp Rheumatol 14:555, 1996.

314. Drosos AA, Skopouli FN, Costopoulos JS, et al: Cyclosporin A (CyA) in primary Sjögren's syndrome: A double-blind study. Ann Rheum Dis 45:732, 1986.

315. Steinfeld SD, Demols P, Salmon I, et al: Infliximab in patients with primary Sjögren's syndrome: A pilot study. Arthritis Rheum 44:2371, 2001.

316. Steinfeld SD, Demols P, Appelboom T: Infliximab in primary Sjögren's syndrome: One year follow-up. Arthritis Rheum 46:3301, 2002.

317. Mariette X, Ravaud P, Steinfeld S, et al: Inefficacy of infliximab in primary Sjögren's syndrome: Results of the randomized, controlled trial of Remicade in primary Sjögren's syndrome. Arthritis Rheum 50:1270, 2004.

318. Sankar V, Brennan MT, Kok MR, et al: Etanercept in Sjögren's syndrome: A twelve-week randomized, double-blind, placebo-controlled pilot clinical trial. Arthritis Rheum 50:2240, 2004.

319. Pijpe J, van Imhoff GW, Spijkervet FK, et al: Rituximab treatment in patients with primary Sjögren's syndrome: An open-label phase II study. Arthritis Rheum 52:2740, 2005.

320. Seror R, Sordet C, Guillevin L, et al: Tolerance and efficacy of rituximab and changes in serum B cell biomarkers in patients with systemic complications of primary Sjögren's syndrome. Ann Rheum Dis 66:351, 2007.

321. Fox RI, Chan E, Benton L, et al: Treatment of primary Sjögren's syndrome with hydroxychloroquine. Am J Med 85:62, 1988.

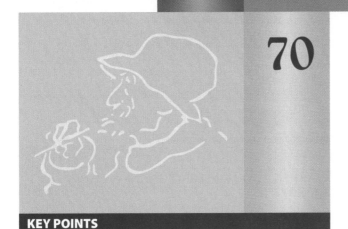

70   Ankylosing Spondylitis 📹

SJEF M. VAN DER LINDEN •
DÉSIRÉE VAN DER HEIJDE •
WALTER P. MAKSYMOWYCH

KEY POINTS

In early stages of ankylosing spondylitis (AS), radiographic evidence of sacroiliitis may be absent.

Magnetic resonance imaging may be helpful in cases of suspected AS.

The modified New York criteria are useful primarily to classify groups of patients (e.g., for clinical or epidemiologic studies). They are not well suited to establish the diagnosis of AS in individual patients.

Radiographic sacroiliitis is a usual but by no means obligatory sign of AS.

Observer variation in reading pelvic radiographs for the presence or absence of sacroiliitis is considerable.

Inflammatory back pain is the usual clue to the early diagnosis of AS.

A positive family history of AS or other manifestations of spondyloarthritis increases the likelihood of AS if an individual's symptoms suggest that disease.

Among patients with chronic inflammatory back pain, HLA-B27 typing may aid in establishing the diagnosis AS.

Physiotherapy and spa exercise therapy are important components of disease management.

Group physiotherapy is more effective than exercises performed at home by the patient.

If treatment with nonsteroidal anti-inflammatory drugs (NSAIDs) fails, biologics should be considered.

For AS patients with active disease, the response to treatment with tumor necrosis factor (TNF) blockers is usually quick, impressive, and sustained.

Most AS patients have a normal or marginally elevated erythrocyte sedimentation rate and C-reactive protein level. Patients with normal levels of acute-phase reactants tend to have a somewhat lower response to anti-TNF agents.

AS patients who have full ankylosis of the spine may still respond to TNF blockers if they have inflammatory back pain.

The Bath ankylosing spondylitis disease activity index (BAS-DAI) is the most frequently used instrument to assess patient-reported disease activity.

Expert's opinion and BASDAI greater than 4 (scale 0 to 10) are important in considering TNF blocking agents if conservative treatment with NSAIDs and physiotherapy fails.

In many populations, AS occurs in 1% to 3% of HLA-B27–positive individuals. The disease is more common (about 10%) among first-degree relatives of HLA-B27–positive AS patients.

Ankylosing spondylitis (AS) is a chronic inflammatory disease of unknown cause associated with human leukocyte antigen (HLA)-B27. It usually affects the sacroiliac joints at early stages and may involve the axial skeleton at later stages of the disease. Peripheral joint involvement may also be an important feature. The disease can be accompanied by extraskeletal manifestations such as acute anterior uveitis, aortic incompetence, cardiac conduction defects, fibrosis of the upper lobes of the lungs, neurologic involvement, or renal (secondary) amyloidosis. AS causes significant pain, disability, and social burden around the world. Favorable results of treating AS with anti–tumor necrosis factor (TNF) agents have largely redefined the entire therapeutic approach to this disease. AS belongs to the group of diseases known as the spondyloarthropathies or spondyloarthritides. This group of disorders constitutes a family of related but heterogeneous conditions rather than a single disease with different clinical manifestations[1] (Tables 70-1 and 70-2).

HISTORICAL ASPECTS

It is controversial whether the skeletal abnormalities described in many Egyptian pharaohs, including Rameses II, were due to AS, diffuse skeletal hyperostosis, or spondylosis deformans.[2] In 1850, Brodie described the clinical features of a 31-year-old man with an ankylosed spine who "occasionally suffer[ed] severe inflammation of the eye." In 1884, Struempell from Leipzig, Germany, described two patients with complete ankylosis of the spine and hip joints.[3] This report was soon followed by descriptions of the disease by von Bechterew from St. Petersburg, Russia, and Marie from Paris, France.[4,5] Although Roentgen had developed his radiographic technique by 1896,

Table 70-1 Spondyloarthropathies

Ankylosing spondylitis

Reiter's syndrome or reactive arthritis

Arthropathy of inflammatory bowel disease (Crohn's disease, ulcerative colitis)

Psoriatic arthritis

Undifferentiated spondyloarthropathies

Juvenile chronic arthritis and juvenile-onset ankylosing spondylitis

Table 70-2 Clinical Characteristics of Spondyloarthropathies

Typical pattern of peripheral arthritis—predominantly of lower limb, asymmetric

Tendency toward radiographic sacroiliitis

Absence of rheumatoid factor

Absence of subcutaneous nodules and other extra-articular features of rheumatoid arthritis

Overlapping extra-articular features characteristic of the group (e.g., anterior uveitis)

Significant familial aggregation

Association with HLA-B27

it was not until 1930 that sacroiliac disease, now considered the radiographic hallmark of AS, was fully recognized.

NOMENCLATURE

The term *ankylosing spondylitis* is derived from the Greek roots *ankylos,* or "bent" (although it now usually implies fusion or adhesions), and *spondylos,* or "vertebral disk." Because ankylosis of the spine tends to appear in late stages of the disease and does not occur in many patients with mild disease, it has been suggested that it would be better to rename the disease spondylitis or spondylitic disease.[6]

CLASSIFICATION

CLASSIFICATION CRITERIA FOR SPONDYLOARTHROPATHIES

The spectrum of spondyloarthropathies is wider than the disorders listed in Table 70-1. To encompass patients with seronegative oligoarthritis, dactylitis, or polyarthritis of the lower extremities; heel pain due to enthesitis; and other undifferentiated spondyloarthropathies, classification criteria for the whole group of spondyloarthropathies were developed[1] (Table 70-3). The European Spondyloarthropathy Study Group (ESSG) criteria resulted in a sensitivity of 86% and a specificity of 87%. In the subgroup of early cases (i.e., those in whom signs and symptoms had developed within the last year), the sensitivity declined to 68%, although the specificity increased to 93%. These criteria, though clearly not intended for diagnostic purposes, might be useful to identify atypical and undifferentiated forms of spondyloarthropathies. This set of criteria performed quite well in patients with different sociocultural and geographic characteristics.[7]

Table 70-3 European Spondyloarthropathy Study Group Classification Criteria

Inflammatory spinal pain
OR
Synovitis (asymmetric, predominantly in lower limbs)
AND
Any one of the following (sensitivity, 77%; specificity, 89%):
    Positive family history
    Psoriasis
    Inflammatory bowel disease
    Alternate buttock pain
    Enthesopathy
Adding sacroiliitis (sensitivity, 86%; specificity, 87%)

From Dougados M, van der Linden S, Juhlin R, et al: The European Spondyloarthropathy Study Group preliminary criteria for the classification of spondyloarthropathy. Arthritis Rheum 34:1218-1227, 1991.

CLASSIFICATION CRITERIA FOR ANKYLOSING SPONDYLITIS

The diagnosis of AS is based on clinical features. The disease is "primary" or "idiopathic" if no associated disorder is present; it is "secondary" if the disease is associated with psoriasis or chronic inflammatory bowel disease.

In daily practice, a presumptive clinical diagnosis of AS is usually supported by radiographic evidence of sacroiliitis; indeed, many think of AS as symptomatic sacroiliitis. The presence of sacroiliitis does not necessarily indicate the presence of AS, however. Moreover, although radiographic sacroiliitis is frequent in AS, it is by no means an early or obligate manifestation of the disease.[8] Lack of either sensitivity or specificity in previous classifications led to a modification of the New York criteria for AS[9] (Table 70-4). Two criteria—limitation of lumbar spine motion and limitation of chest expansion—appear to reflect disease duration; they are usually not present in early disease.[10] It should be stressed that classification criteria are usually not useful for early diagnosis owing to a lack of sensitivity. In particular, in the early phase of AS, conventional sacroiliac radiographs may be normal. An approach based on pretest probabilities and likelihood ratios has been proposed to diagnose the disease with predominantly axial manifestations before the presence of radiographic sacroiliitis.[11]

EPIDEMIOLOGY

PREVALENCE

The prevalence of AS closely parallels the frequency of HLA-B27. This holds true for those B27 subtypes that are associated with the disease, but it is not true for populations in which certain subtypes that lack an association with AS occur rather frequently, such as the Indonesian population.[12-14]

Among whites, the estimated prevalence rate of AS as defined by the modified New York criteria ranges from 68 per 100,000 population older than 20 years in the Netherlands to 197 per 100,000 in the United States.[15,16] The prevalence of clinical AS in France is 150 per 100,000 adults, whereas in Norway it is 210 per 100,000 adults.[17,18] The prevalence of the disease in Finland is similar, with a figure of 150 per 100,000 people.[19]

Higher prevalence rates have been reported in central Europe. An epidemiologic study from Berlin reported a prevalence figure of 0.86%.[20] In the general population, AS

Table 70-4 Criteria for Ankylosing Spondylitis

Rome, 1961

Clinical Criteria

1. Low back pain and stiffness for more than 3 months, not relieved by rest
2. Pain and stiffness in thoracic region
3. Limited motion in lumbar spine
4. Limited chest expansion
5. History or evidence of iritis or its sequelae

Radiographic Criterion

6. Radiograph showing bilateral sacroiliac changes characteristic of ankylosing spondylitis (this excludes bilateral osteoarthritis of sacroiliac joints)

Definite Ankylosing Spondylitis

Grade 3 or 4 bilateral sacroiliitis with at least one clinical criterion
OR
At least four clinical criteria

New York, 1966

Diagnostic Criteria

1. Limitation of lumbar spine motion in all three planes: anterior flexion, lateral flexion, extension
2. Pain at dorsolumbar junction or in lumbar spine
3. Limitation of chest expansion to 2.5 cm or less measured at level of fourth intercostal space

Grading of Radiographs

Normal, 0; suspicious, 1; minimal sacroiliitis, 2; moderate sacroiliitis, 3; ankylosis, 4

Definite Ankylosing Spondylitis

Grade 3 or 4 bilateral sacroiliitis with at least one diagnostic criterion
OR
Grade 3 or 4 unilateral or grade 2 bilateral sacroiliitis with diagnostic criterion 1 or with criteria 2 and 3

Probable Ankylosing Spondylitis

Grade 3 or 4 bilateral sacroiliitis with no diagnostic criteria

Modified New York, 1984

Criteria

1. Low back pain of at least 3 months' duration improved by exercise and not relieved by rest
2. Limitation of lumbar spine in sagittal and frontal planes
3. Chest expansion decreased relative to normal values for age and sex
4. Bilateral sacroiliitis grade 2 to 4
5. Unilateral sacroiliitis grade 3 or 4

Definite Ankylosing Spondylitis

Unilateral grade 3 or 4, or bilateral grade 2 to 4 sacroiliitis and any clinical criterion

Data from van der Linden SM, Valkenburg HA, Cats A: Evaluation of diagnostic criteria for ankylosing spondylitis: A proposal for modification of the New York criteria. Arthritis Rheum 27:361-368, 1984.

Table 70-5 HLA-B27 Prevalence in White Populations

Population Subgroup	HLA-B27 Phenotype Frequency (%)
Urgo Finnish	12-18
Northern Scandinavian	10-16
Slavic	7-14
Western European	6-9
Southern European	2-6
Basque	9-14
Gypsy (Spain)	16-18
Arab, Jew, Armenian, Iranian	3-5
Pakistani	6-8
Indian	2-6

INCIDENCE

There is no adequate evidence that the incidence of AS has changed in the last few decades. Clinical features, age of onset, and survival time have remained stable.[22] One study revealed an overall age and gender-adjusted incidence of 7.3 per 100,000 person-years. This U.S. figure compares quite well with the Finnish study, which revealed a stable incidence of 8.7 (95% confidence interval [CI] 6.4 to 11.0) per 100,000 people aged 16 or older.[17]

RACIAL DISTRIBUTION

AS occurs in all parts of the world, but there are race-related differences in prevalence. This might reflect differences in the distribution of HLA-B27 among races (Table 70-5). Approximately 90% of white patients with AS possess HLA-B27, whereas AS and HLA-B27 are nearly absent (prevalence of B27 < 1%) in African blacks and Japanese. In African Americans, owing to racial admixture with whites, 2% possess B27, but only about 50% of black patients with AS possess B27. Correspondingly, African Americans are affected far less frequently than American whites.

BURDEN OF DISEASE

AS is associated with a considerable burden to the patient and society. Apart from the axial and articular manifestations, extra-articular manifestations, such as enthesitis and acute anterior uveitis, and comorbidities, such as inflammatory bowel disease and psoriasis, contribute to the burden of disease. In addition, a large proportion of patients has spinal osteoporosis, leading to vertebral fractures and thoracic kyphosis. All these features result in a decreased quality of life. Disease status scores for physical functioning and disease activity correlate clearly with psychological scores for anxiety and depression.[23] The impact of AS also can be seen in various aspects of employment, ranging from requiring assistance at work to withdrawal from the workforce.[24] Apart from the impact on labor force participation, AS patients have an important impact on health care and non–health care resource utilization, resulting in mean total costs (direct and productivity) of about $6700 to $9500 per year per patient when applying the human capital approach to calculate productivity costs.[25-27]

is likely to develop in about 1% to 2% of HLA-B27–positive adults who have a disease-associated B27 subtype, although there may be regional or geographic differences. For example, in northern Norway, AS may develop in 6.7% of HLA-B27–positive people.[21]

The disease is much more common among HLA-B27–positive first-degree relatives of HLA-B27–positive AS patients; roughly 10% to 30% of them have signs or symptoms of AS.[15] In fact, a positive family history of AS is a strong risk factor for the disease.

Table 70-6 Components of Disease Duration

Onset of axial AS manifestations (inflammatory back pain)
Onset of extra-axial AS manifestations (peripheral arthritis, enthesitis)
Onset of associated spondyloarthropathic diseases (acute anterior uveitis, inflammatory bowel disease, psoriasis)
Time since diagnosis of AS by health care provider

AS, ankylosing spondylitis.
From Davis, JC, Dougados M, Braun J, et al: Definition of disease duration in ankylosing spondylitis: Reassessing the concept. Ann Rheum Dis 65: 1518-1520, 2006.

The burden of illness increases with duration of disease. Important components of the definition of disease duration are provided in Table 70-6.[28] Because the burden reduces quality of life, and because all types of costs associated with AS result from loss of function and disease activity, early diagnosis and treatment are necessary to prevent or reduce functional decline and improve patient outcome.[29]

CAUSE AND GENETICS

The precise cause of AS is still unclear, although several dominant themes have emerged. First, there is a major genetic contribution. Although it is now well established that HLA-B27 is directly involved in the pathogenesis of disease, its precise pathophysiologic role is unclear, and additional non–major histocompatibility complex (MHC) genes contribute to the risk for disease. Second, cartilage appears to be the primary target tissue for the abnormal immune response. Third, cytokine dysregulation, with overexpression of TNF-α, and intestinal inflammation are prominent features of disease. Fourth, emerging evidence implicates bone morphogenetic proteins in the pathogenesis of ankylosis.

The dominant role of genetic factors is highlighted by data demonstrating disease concordance in 75% of monozygotic twins compared with 13% of nonidentical twins,[30] familial aggregation,[31] and population data demonstrating associations with B27.[32] Genetic data also suggest that 97% of the population variance can be explained by additive genetic effects, the environmental trigger is ubiquitous, three to nine genes are involved in addition to B27, and genes influence disease severity and phenotype.[33]

HLA-B27

Despite the near-pervasive nature of this association, it has been estimated that B27 contributes only 16% of the total genetic risk. The association with B27 is also less evident in other populations, such as native Indonesians, Lebanese, Thais, and West African blacks. It is present in only 60% to 80% of those with concomitant psoriasis and inflammatory bowel disease. Forty-five subtypes have been assigned on the basis of nucleotide sequence homology that encodes more than 20 different products. The most common subtype in Caucasians is B*2705, followed by B*2702; both are associated with disease. The most common subtype in Chinese and Japanese is B*2704, which is associated with disease. B*2706 is the most common subtype in other Asians, but it is neutral or only weakly associated with disease.[13] B*2709 is observed primarily in southern Italy and is not associated with axial disease, although peripheral arthritis has been

reported.[34] There are insufficient epidemiologic data on other subtypes to evaluate disease associations.

The main function of HLA class I molecules such as B27 is to present peptides to CD8+ T cells. Crystallographic analysis of B*2705 shows a peptide-binding groove with pockets (A to F) that accommodate the side chains and amino and carboxyl termini of the bound peptide.[35] The B pocket is conserved among B27 subtypes but differs from most other B molecules. It has a glutamine amino acid at its apex at amino acid position 45 that interacts with arginine at position 2 of B27-bound peptides; this pocket conveys specificity for the type of peptide bound to B27. In addition, both B*2706 and B*2709 differ from B*2705 at a single amino acid position in the F pocket that binds the peptide C terminal amino acid. This influences the type of peptide bound to disease-associated and nonassociated B27 subtypes and thereby recognition by CD8+ T cells.

NON-B27 GENES

It has been estimated that the entire HLA region contributes about half the total genetic risk for disease, implicating additional HLA genes beyond B27. Population and family studies have implicated HLA-B60 in B27-positive Caucasians but not in non-Caucasians.[36] Several B alleles (B60, B61, B7, B13, B22, B39, B40, B41, B42) have been implicated in B27-negative AS. Some alleles, such as B39, have a peptide-binding groove that shares similarities with B27. Several case-control studies have now reported associations with HLA-DRB1*01, 07, and 08 that are independent of B27.[37]

Two observations clearly suggest a role for non-HLA genes. First, there is an increased risk for disease in B27-positive first-degree relatives of AS probands (10% to 20%) compared with B27-positive individuals in the general population (2% to 5%).[15] Second, disease concordance is 75% in identical twins versus 27% in HLA-B27 concordant dizygotic twins.[30] The contribution of non-HLA genes is comparable to the entire genetic contribution to insulin-dependent diabetes. Case-control studies in Caucasian and Taiwanese populations support an association with the cytochrome P-450 CYP2D6 gene on chromosome 22, which is involved in the metabolism of drugs.[38] An association has also been described with the CARD15 gene in AS patients with concomitant intestinal inflammation.[39] CARD15 binds bacterial cell wall components and is a regulator of the proinflammatory transcriptional factor nuclear factor κB (NFκB).

Several gene consortia have used linkage approaches and microsatellite markers to identify regions of the genome demonstrating nonrandom inheritance in AS families. Relatively weak linkage has been demonstrated with regions on chromosomes 1p, 6q, 9q, 10q, 11q, 16q, and 19q; there has been little agreement among studies, however, likely reflecting the weak contributions of individual loci and the small sample size of each study.[40-42] Several case-control and family-based association studies have now reported associations with the interleukin (IL)-1 gene cluster on chromosome 2.[43-45] This cluster includes genes for IL-1A, IL-1B, IL-1RN, and six genes demonstrating structural homology to these genes, namely, IL-1F5 to F10. A meta-analysis of these studies suggests that the primary association is with a locus at or close to IL-1A.[46] Additional reports show that despite a male predominance, there is no association with loci on the X chromosome, and non-HLA genes may influence disease severity.[47] Recently, genome-wide association studies have identified two new genes definitely involved in the pathogenesis of the disease, IL23R and ARTS1.[47a]

HYPOTHESES

The primary hypotheses address the pathophysiologic role of B27 and focus either on some aspect of its principal function, which is to present peptides to CD8+ T cells, or on less conventional properties of B27, such as its propensity to misfold and its expression as heavy-chain dimers on the cell surface. The former hypothesis proposes that CD8+ T cell autoreactivity to self-peptide from joint tissue is induced by cross-reactivity with bacterial peptide that demonstrates molecular mimicry with this self peptide; both peptides are therefore presented by B27 in the course of T cell–mediated defense to bacterial infection. This arthritogenic peptide hypothesis is supported by epidemiologic data demonstrating differential disease associations with B27 subtypes that vary in their ability to bind and present peptides. The relevance to human disease has been reinforced in crystallographic studies showing that although B*2709 binds a self-peptide—vasoactive intestinal peptide receptor 1—in a single conformation that does not elicit CD8 T cell reactivity, B*2705 binds the same peptide in a dual conformation that does elicit CD8 T cell reactivity.[48] There are, however, no in vivo studies of patients showing CD8 T cell cross-reactivity to bacterial peptides demonstrating molecular mimicry with joint tissue–derived self-peptides presented by B27.

An alternative hypothesis is based on the finding that B27 is more likely to misfold than are other class I HLA molecules, which may be due to its weaker binding of peptides in the endoplasmic reticulum. This property appears to be dependent on the unique structural properties of the B27 peptide-binding pocket.[49] The accumulation of misfolded B27 within the cell activates the unfolded protein response, which includes activation of a variety of proinflammatory transcriptional factors (e.g., NFκB) and cytokines (e.g., IL-1, TNF-α). Evidence of this unfolded protein response has been obtained from synovial fluid cells from AS patients. This hypothesis does not address the differential B27 subtype associations with disease, but this property of B27 may be important in expanding and perpetuating the inflammatory response.

A third hypothesis proposes that B27 forms heavy-chain homodimers on the cell surface through the formation of a disulfide bond linking the cysteine residues at position 67.[50] The likelihood of dimer formation appears to be linked to B27's propensity to misfold. These structures have been detected in patients with AS, and their formation has been shown to stimulate the release of TNF-α, but B27 is not the only class I molecule that can form such dimers.

ANIMAL MODELS

Our understanding of the direct role of B27 in the pathogenesis of disease was advanced with the first report of a B27 transgenic rat model of arthritis. HLA-B27 is overexpressed in these animals, which develop chronic intestinal inflammation similar to Crohn's disease at 16 weeks of age, followed by peripheral arthritis in 70% of animals by 20 weeks and occasional spondylitis of tail vertebrae.[51] Disease is more common in males and is related to the degree of overexpression of B27. The presence of T cells and B27 expression on a bone marrow–derived cell are required. Moreover, animals maintained in a germ-free environment do not develop either colitis or arthritis until they are introduced into the normal laboratory environment.[52] The lack of spondylitis in this model, however, raises questions about its relevance to human disease. In a more recent B27 transgenic rat model, B27 is overexpressed together with human β2-microglobulin. These animals show a much higher incidence of spondylitis, despite the absence of concomitant colitis.[53] This model more closely resembles human disease.

Several animal models of AS have also been developed, based on the induction of autoimmunity to antigens present in cartilage and fibrous tissue, such as aggrecan and versican.[54,55] The importance of TNF-α to the pathogenesis of AS is highlighted in the phenotype of a transgenic mouse model that overexpresses TNF-α. These animals develop sacroiliitis characterized by the formation of osteoclasts and granulation tissue.[56]

HUMAN STUDIES

Pathologic studies show a disease predilection for sites rich in cartilage, particularly fibrocartilage. These include articular sites such as the sacroiliac joints, intervertebral disks, and facet joints, but also certain entheses, such as the Achilles tendon, where the presence of fibrocartilage allows dissipation of compressive forces against bone. Immunohistochemical studies have shown an abundance of aggrecan and type II collagen at the fibrocartilaginous insertions of entheses.[57] The presence of fibrocartilage extends to extraskeletal sites such as the anterior uvea and the root and wall of the aorta. This strongly implies that cartilage may be the primary target for an immune response as the initiating event in this disease. Cellular immunity to the G1 domain of aggrecan has been observed in AS as well as in other inflammatory joint disorders, implying a nonspecific response to joint damage.[58] However, a specific HLA-B27–restricted CD8+ T cell response to a cartilage antigen derived from type VI collagen has now been identified in the peripheral blood and synovial fluid of AS patients.[59] The pathogenetic significance of these T cells requires further study.

ROLE OF BACTERIA

B27 transgenic rats do not develop arthritis if maintained in a germ-free environment. Exposure of these animals to bacteria, especially *Bacteroides* species, triggers the onset of both intestinal and joint inflammation. In humans, evidence of intestinal inflammation is present in up to 60% of AS patients; its presence in juvenile patients with only peripheral joint inflammation increases the likelihood of the development axial disease.[60] Oligoclonal T cell expansions have been reported in both the colonic mucosa and synovial fluid of patients with enterogenic AS, suggesting a common antigenic stimulus.[61] Examination of peripheral blood and colonic lamina propria T cells from patients with AS demonstrated impaired production of interferon-γ, TNF-α, and IL-2 compared with healthy B27-positive controls.[62] This, together with evidence of increased intestinal permeability, might account for impaired immune responses to bacteria. Elevated immunoglobulin (Ig) A antibodies to several bacteria have been observed, such as *Klebsiella pneumoniae* and *Escherichia coli*, but bacterial products have not been detected in sacroiliac joint biopsies.[63] Another mechanism that implicates intestinal bacteria focuses on the finding of antigen presenting cells in both intestinal mucosa and synovium that express the CD163 scavenger receptor and possess the capacity to secrete TNF-α and IL-1 in response to bacterial lipopolysaccharide.[64] This subset of macrophages is increased in AS compared with rheumatoid arthritis (RA) synovium.

ANKYLOSIS

The development of ankylosis may be a sequela of prior inflammation, but this remains to be proved. An animal model of ankylosing enthesitis showed evidence of the uncoupling of inflammation and ankylosis, the latter being regulated by bone morphogenetic proteins; these members of the transforming growth factor-ß superfamily control a wide array of cellular processes, such as proliferation, differentiation, and motility.[65] Expression of bone morphogenetic protein has also been documented in the entheses of AS patients.

PATHOLOGY

Characteristic pathologic features of AS include inflammation in axial joints, large peripheral joints, and entheses associated with inflammation in subchondral bone marrow. Reparation is also characteristic in terms of the development of chondroid metaplasia, followed by calcification of cartilage and formation of bone, particularly in the axial joints.

SACROILIAC JOINT

Disease typically originates in the sacroiliac joints, where magnetic resonance imaging (MRI) reveals inflammation in the posteroinferior capsular region and subchondral bone of the synovial portion of the joint.[66] Detailed histopathologic studies in early disease are limited owing to the inaccessibility of biopsy material. A controlled study of sacroiliac biopsies from AS patients at various stages of disease and controls showed cellular infiltration with lymphocytes, macrophages, and plasma cells in the synovium and subchondral marrow as the earliest features of disease.[67] Later features include the development of pannus extending from both synovium and subchondral bone marrow, with erosion of articular cartilage and its replacement by granulation tissue. Osteoclast formation and erosion of subchondral bone account for the typical widening of the joint space seen on plain radiography. Enthesitis is also evident in later stages of disease at the insertion of the posterior capsule. Reparative changes include cartilage metaplasia at sites of active inflammation, followed by its calcification and then replacement by endochondral bone, leading to obliteration of the joint space by ankylosis. Para-articular changes include bone sclerosis and fat replacement of bone marrow. Immunohistologic studies show the presence of dense cellular infiltrates of T lymphocytes and macrophages expressing TNF-α.[68] Transforming growth factor is evident at sites of new bone formation.

SPINE

Several regions of the spine are affected, although histopathologic reports that clearly document the findings in early disease are confined to single case studies. Inflammation typically ascends the spine but may involve the cervical region first and may skip vertebral segments. Chronic inflammation with lymphocytes, plasma cells, and macrophages is first observed in the outer annulus fibrosus, particularly at its insertion into the rim of the vertebral end plate. This leads to resorption of bone, followed by reparative changes in adjacent trabecular bone and bone apposition on the waist of the vertebral body during postinflammatory remodeling, accounting for the squaring and shining corner appearance on plain radiography. Cartilage metaplasia of granulation tissue is followed by its calcification and then replacement by bone at the vertebral margin and in the outer annulus. This extends across the vertical length of the disk, eventually leading to complete bony fusion of adjacent vertebrae and the appearance of a syndesmophyte on plain radiography. Extensive involvement of the entire spine results in the "bamboo spine" appearance on plain radiography. The process of inflammation may also involve the central portion of the disk, which is best seen on MRI as spondylodiscitis. Involvement of the atlantoaxial structures, particularly the insertion of the transverse ligament into the arch of the atlas and the capsular insertion of the lateral atlantoaxial joint, may lead to atlantoaxial dislocation and cord compression.

Chronic inflammation is also seen at the capsular insertion of apophyseal joints. The characteristic sequence of pannus formation, subchondral inflammation, erosion of articular cartilage and bone at the capsular insertion, cartilage metaplasia, and ossification of subsynovium and fibrous capsule at its insertion is observed. This leads first to marginal and then complete bony ankylosis of the joint. There is evidence that ankylosis of the apophyseal joint precedes and is a factor in the development of ankylosis in the adjacent intervertebral disk.[69] Immunohistologic analysis shows subchondral lymphocyte infiltrates with CD4+ and CD8+ T cells, together with hypervascularization and foci of CD68+ osteoclastic cells.[70]

Pathologic involvement of costotransverse and costovertebral joints follows the same pattern described earlier, and MRI indicates that involvement of these joints is common.[71] Enthesitis with bone erosion and then ossification may affect the insertions of the supraspinous and intraspinous ligaments. Osteoporosis with kyphosis is a typical feature of late stages of disease.

EXTRASPINAL LESIONS

Extraspinal lesions can be broadly divided into articular and nonarticular inflammatory lesions. The former include synchondrotic joints such as the manubriosternal joint and symphysis pubis, large synovial joints such as the hips and knees, and entheses. The pathologic sequence of changes in synchondrotic joints is typical of those observed in the spine. Involvement of the hips is characterized by subchondral granulation tissue and osteoclast formation in the femoral heads and acetabulum that is associated with degradation of overlying articular cartilage.[72] Knee assessment has been conducted in patients representing a broad category of spondyloarthritis, with limited information specific to AS. The appearance of synovitis appears to be similar to that observed in RA, although with more pronounced vascularity and differential expression of integrins.[73] Entheseal involvement most frequently occurs at sites rich in fibrocartilage, such as the Achilles tendon. Inflammation and chronic cellular infiltration of soft tissues are relatively sparse but may be extensive within the adjacent subchondral bone, particularly in B27-positive individuals.[74] A comparative study of the subchondral marrow from knee and hip joint entheses showed that AS patients clearly differ from those with RA and osteoarthritis with respect to the frequency of marrow inflammation, infiltration with CD8+ T cells, and presence of hyperosteoclastic erosive lesions.

Inflammation in nonarticular sites may involve the anterior uvea and ciliary body. Elsewhere, granulation tissue forms, with an accumulation of lymphocytes and plasma cells around the small blood vessels in the adventitia of the ascending aorta, followed by fibrosis extending below the base of the aortic valve to form a characteristic subvalvular ridge. Apical fibrosis of the lungs also occurs.

CLINICAL MANIFESTATIONS

SKELETAL MANIFESTATIONS

Low Back Pain and Stiffness

Back pain is an extremely common symptom, occurring in up to 80% of the general population. Therefore, it is important to note that back pain in AS has special features that differentiate it from mechanical back pain[75,76] (Table 70-7).

The pain is initially felt primarily deep in the gluteal region, is dull in character, is difficult to localize, and is insidious in onset. The pain can be severe at this early phase of the disease; it localizes in the sacroiliac joints but is occasionally referred toward the iliac crest or greater trochanteric region or down the dorsal thigh. Radiation of buttock pain may suggest root compression of the ischiadic nerve. The buttock pain typically alternates from side to side. Coughing, sneezing, or other maneuvers that cause a sudden twist of the back may accentuate pain. Although the pain is often unilateral or intermittent at first, within a few months it usually becomes persistent and bilateral, and the lower lumbar area becomes stiff and painful. The pain is associated with a feeling of low back stiffness that is worse in the morning and may awaken the patient from sleep, particularly during the second half of the night. Many patients do not differentiate between low back pain and stiffness. The morning stiffness may last up to 3 hours. Both the stiffness and the pain tend to be eased by a hot shower, an exercise program, or physical activity; they do not improve with rest. Fatigue as a result of chronic back pain and stiffness may be an important problem and can be accentuated by sleep disturbances due to these symptoms.

Chest Pain

With subsequent involvement of the thoracic spine (including costovertebral and costotransverse joints) and the occurrence of enthesopathy at the costosternal and manubriosternal joints, patients may experience chest pain

Table 70-7 Diagnostic Features of Ankylosing Spondylitis

Inflammatory spinal pain
    Onset before age 40 yr
    Insidious onset
    Persistence for at least 3 mo
    Morning stiffness of at least 30 min duration
    Improvement with exercise but not with rest

Awakening because of back pain during second half of night
Chest pain
Alternate buttock pain
Acute anterior uveitis
Synovitis (predominantly of lower limbs, asymmetric)
Enthesitis (heel, plantar)
Radiographic sacroiliitis

Positive family history of
    Ankylosing spondylitis
    Chronic inflammatory bowel disease
    Psoriasis

accentuated by coughing or sneezing, which is sometimes characterized as "pleuritic." The chest pain is often associated with tenderness over the sternocostal or costosternal junctions. Mild to moderate reduction of chest expansion is often detectable in an early stage of AS. Chest pain occurs relatively often in HLA-B27–positive relatives, even in the absence of radiographic evidence of sacroiliitis.[77]

Tenderness

Extra-articular tenderness at certain loci is a prominent complaint in some patients. These lesions are due to enthesitis. Common tender sites are the costosternal junctions, spinous processes, iliac crests, greater trochanters, ischial tuberosities, tibial tubercles, and heels (Achilles tendinitis or plantar fasciitis). Radiographically, bone spurs may develop at these sites.

Joints

The girdle or "root" joints (hips and shoulders) are the most frequently involved extra-axial joints in AS, and pain in these areas is the presenting symptom in up to 15% of patients. Shoulder involvement, but especially hip involvement, may cause considerable physical disability. Coexisting disease in the lumbar spine often contributes significantly to disability of the lower extremities. Hips and shoulders are involved at some stage of disease in up to 35% of patients. Hip disease is more common in Algeria, India, and Mexico. It is relatively more common as a presenting manifestation if the disease starts in childhood (juvenile AS). In boys 8 to 10 years of age, hip disease as a manifestation of juvenile AS is the most frequent type of chronic arthritis. These children with hip disease are mostly HLA-B27 positive, and they are serologically negative for antinuclear antibodies.

The knee joint may also be affected in AS, often as an intermittent effusion. The temporomandibular joint is involved in about 10% of patients.

EXTRASKELETAL MANIFESTATIONS

Constitutional symptoms, such as fatigue, weight loss, and low-grade fever, occur frequently. Other extraskeletal manifestations are more localized.

Eye Disease

Acute anterior uveitis or iridocyclitis is the most common extra-articular manifestation of AS, occurring in 25% to 30% of patients at some time during the course of the disease. There is no clear relationship between activity of the articular disease and this extra-articular manifestation. The onset of eye inflammation is usually acute and typically unilateral, but the attacks may alternate. The eye is red and painful, with visual impairment. Photophobia and increased lacrimation may be present. If the eye remains untreated or if treatment is delayed, posterior synechiae and glaucoma may develop. Most attacks subside in 4 to 8 weeks without sequelae if early treatment is provided. Acute anterior uveitis is more common in B27-positive than B27-negative patients with AS.[78] Relatives who have acute anterior uveitis seem to be at higher risk for AS themselves. The calculated incidence of acute anterior uveitis in a Swiss family study was 89 attacks per 1000 patient-years for AS patients, but only 8 per 1000 person-years among healthy B27-positive relatives.[79]

Cardiovascular Disease

Cardiac involvement may be clinically silent or may cause considerable problems. Manifestations of cardiac involvement include ascending aortitis, aortic valve incompetence, conduction abnormalities, cardiomegaly, and pericarditis. In rare situations, aortitis may precede other features of AS. Aortic incompetence was noted in 3.5% of patients who had the disease for 15 years and in 10% after 30 years.[80] Inflammation and dilation of the aorta are the main cause of aortic valve incompetence. Cardiac conduction disturbances are seen with increasing frequency with the passage of time, occurring in 2.7% of those with disease of 15 years' duration and in 8.5% after 30 years.[80] Both aortic incompetence and cardiac conduction defects occur twice as often in patients with peripheral joint involvement.

Pulmonary Disease

Lung involvement is a rare and late manifestation of AS. It is characterized by slowly progressive fibrosis of the upper lobes of the lungs, appearing, on average, 2 decades after the onset of AS. Patients may complain of cough, dyspnea, and sometimes hemoptysis.[81]

High-resolution computed tomography (CT) may be helpful in detecting interstitial lung disease in patients with respiratory symptoms whose chest radiographs are normal.[82] This imaging technique reveals a high prevalence of lung changes even among AS patients with early disease and without respiratory symptoms. The clinical significance of these findings is unknown. Long-term prospective studies need to be performed.[83]

Pulmonary ventilation is usually well maintained; an increased diaphragmatic contribution helps compensate for chest wall rigidity, which is due to involvement of the thoracic joints in the inflammatory process. Vital capacity and total lung capacity may be moderately reduced as a consequence of the restricted chest wall movement, whereas residual volume and functional residual capacity are usually increased.

Neurologic Involvement

Neurologic complications of AS can be caused by fracture, instability, compression, or inflammation. Traffic accidents or minor trauma can cause spinal fractures. The C5-C6 or C6-C7 level is the most commonly involved site.

As in RA, atlantoaxial joint subluxation, atlanto-occipital subluxation, and upward subluxation of the axis may occur in AS as a consequence of instability resulting from the inflammatory process. Spontaneous anterior atlantoaxial subluxation is a well-recognized complication in about 2% of patients and manifests with or without signs of spinal cord compression. It is observed more commonly in patients with spondylitis and peripheral arthritis than in those with exclusively axial involvement.[84]

Causes of neurologic complications due to compression include ossification of the posterior longitudinal ligament (which may lead to compressive myelopathy), destructive intervertebral disk lesions, and spinal stenosis.

The cauda equina syndrome is a rare but serious complication of long-standing AS. The syndrome affects lumbosacral nerve roots. This gives rise to pain and sensory loss, but frequently there are also urinary and bowel symptoms. There is a gradual onset of urinary and fecal incontinence, impotence, saddle anesthesia, and occasionally loss of ankle jerks. Motor symptoms, if present, are usually mild. Newer imaging techniques, such as CT and MRI, allow the accurate noninvasive diagnosis of this complication of AS.[85] There are no compressive lesions. Arachnoiditis and arachnoid adhesions may be important in the pathogenesis.

Renal Involvement

IgA nephropathy has been reported in many patients with AS. These patients often have an elevated IgA level (93%) and renal impairment (27%) at presentation.[86] Microscopic hematuria and proteinuria may occur in up to 35% of patients. The significance of these findings in terms of subsequent deterioration of renal function is unclear.[87] Amyloidosis (secondary type) is a rare complication. Amyloid deposits detected through abdominal subcutaneous fat aspiration are not invariably associated with a poor renal prognosis.[88]

Osteoporosis

Osteopenia is seen in the early stages of AS.[89] In patients with this disease, osteoporotic deformities of the thoracic spine contribute significantly to abnormal posture, particularly fixed hyperkyphosis.[90] Radiographic damage to the cervical and lumbar spine, thoracic wedging, and disease activity are determinants of hyperkyphosis in AS.[91] An increased occiput-to-wall distance is associated with vertebral fractures. The prevalence of symptomatic osteoporotic spinal fractures is increased in AS.[92] Neurologic complications occur rather frequently, even after minor trauma.[93] Proper assessment of bone density in the spine is difficult in the presence of syndesmophytes, because they may give rise to falsely high values. This measurement error can be avoided by using quantitative CT. Further research is needed to determine the true fracture risk and complication rate in early and late disease and the relation to disease activity. Currently, it is unclear whether any specific therapy to prevent osteoporotic spinal fractures is effective.

PHYSICAL FINDINGS

SPINAL MOBILITY

To arrive at an early diagnosis, the physician must perform a thorough physical examination. On examination of the spine, there may be some limitation of motion of the lumbar spine as elicited by forward flexion, hyperextension, or lateral flexion. Early loss of the normal lumbar lordosis is often the first sign and is easily assessed on inspection.

The Schober test (or its modifications) is useful to detect any limitation of forward flexion of the lumbar spine, although it is typically normal in early disease. As the patient stands erect, one mark is placed with a pen on the skin overlying the fifth lumbar spinous process (usually at the level of the posterosuperior iliac spine or the "dimple of Venus"), and another mark is placed 10 cm above in the midline. The patient is then asked to bend forward maximally without bending the knees. In healthy people, the distance between the two marks on the skin should increase as the skin stretches. If the distance between both marks does not reach 15 cm, this indicates reduced lumbar spine mobility. Lateral flexion may also be diminished, and spinal rotation may cause pain.

CHEST EXPANSION

Mild to moderate reduction of chest expansion is often detectable in early stages of AS. Normal values are age and sex dependent, and there is considerable overlap between normal values and those obtained from AS patients. Reduction below 5 cm in young persons with an insidious onset of chronic, inflammatory low back pain strongly suggests AS. Chest expansion should be measured on maximal inspiration after forced maximal expiration at the level of the fourth intercostal space in males and just below the breasts at the xiphisternal level in females.

ENTHESITIS

Examination of the ischial tuberosities, greater trochanters, spinous processes, costochondral and manubriosternal junctions, supraspinatus insertion, and iliac crests can determine the presence of enthesitis. Heel pain, especially when getting out of bed, is a characteristic manifestation of Achilles and plantar fasciitis enthesitis.

SACROILIITIS

Direct pressure over the sacroiliac joints may elicit pain, as may special testing maneuvers, although the latter lack specificity and sensitivity. These signs may also be negative in early disease or may become negative in late stages as inflammation is replaced by fibrosis or bony ankylosis.

POSTURE

Over the course of the disease, the patient may lose normal posture. Involvement of the cervical spine is manifested by pain and limitation of neck movement. A forward slope of the neck can be detected by having the patient stand against a wall and try to position his or her occiput against it.

After many years of progression in patients with severe disease, the entire spine may become increasingly stiff, with loss of normal posture from gradual loss of lumbar lordosis and the development of thoracic kyphosis. The abdomen becomes protuberant; breathing is primarily by diaphragmatic action. These typical deformities usually evolve after a disease duration of 10 years or more.

LABORATORY TESTS

Generally, routine blood tests are not helpful. A normal erythrocyte sedimentation rate (ESR) or normal C-reactive protein (CRP) level does not exclude active disease. An elevated ESR or CRP is reported in up to 75% of patients, but it may not correlate with clinical disease activity.[94] In an unselected patient population, an elevated ESR and CRP was present in 45% and 38%, respectively, of patients with spinal disease only, compared with 62% and 61%, respectively, of patients with peripheral arthritis with or without inflammatory bowel disease. Neither ESR nor CRP is superior in assessing disease activity.[95] A mild normochromic anemia may be present in 15% of patients. Elevation of serum alkaline phosphatase (derived primarily from bone) is seen in some patients but is unrelated to disease activity or duration. Some elevation of serum IgA is frequent in AS. Its level correlates with acute-phase reactants. Active disease is associated with decreased lipid levels, particularly high-density lipoprotein cholesterol, resulting in a more atherogenic lipid profile.[96]

IMAGING STUDIES

CONVENTIONAL RADIOGRAPHY

The typical radiographic changes of AS are seen primarily in the axial skeleton, especially in the sacroiliac, discovertebral, apophyseal, costovertebral, and costotransverse joints. They evolve over many years, with the earliest, most consistent, and most characteristic findings seen in the sacroiliac joints. However, otherwise typical AS has been described in the absence of radiographic evidence of sacroiliitis.[15] The radiographic findings of sacroiliitis are usually symmetric and consist of blurring of the subchondral bone plate, followed by erosions and sclerosis of the adjacent bone. The changes in the synovial portion of the joint (i.e., the lower two thirds of the joint) result from inflammatory synovitis and osteitis of the adjacent subchondral bone.[97] The cartilage covering the iliac side of the joint is much thinner than that covering the sacral side. Therefore, the erosions and subchondral sclerosis are typically seen first and tend to be more prominent on the iliac side.

Table 70-8 Grading of Sacroiliitis: New York Criteria

Grade 0, normal
Grade 1, suspicious
Grade 2, minimal sacroiliitis
Grade 3, moderate sacroiliitis
Grade 4, ankylosis

In the upper one third of the sacroiliac joint, where strong intra-articular ligaments hold the bones together, the inflammatory process may lead to similar radiographic abnormalities. Progression of the subchondral bone erosions can lead to pseudowidening of the sacroiliac joint space. Over time, gradual fibrosis, calcification, interosseous bridging, and ossification occur. Erosions become less obvious, but the subchondral sclerosis persists, becoming the most prominent radiographic feature.

Ultimately, usually after several years, there may be complete bony ankylosis of the sacroiliac joints, with resolution of bony sclerosis. It is practical to grade radiographic sacroiliitis according to the New York criteria (Table 70-8).

Bony erosions and osteitis ("whiskering") at sites of osseous attachment of tendons and ligaments are frequently seen, particularly at the calcaneus, ischial tuberosities, iliac crest, femoral trochanters, supraspinatus insertion, and spinous processes of the vertebrae. In the early stages of the evolution of syndesmophytes, there is inflammation of the superficial layers of the annulus fibrosus, with subsequent reactive sclerosis and erosions of the adjacent corners of the vertebral bodies. This combination of destructive osteitis and repair leads to "squaring" of the vertebral bodies. This squaring is associated with gradual ossification of the annulus fibrosus and eventual "bridging" between vertebrae by syndesmophytes.[98] There are often concomitant inflammatory changes, ankylosis in the apophyseal joints, and ossification of the adjacent ligaments. In a number of patients, this may ultimately result in a virtually complete fusion of the vertebral column ("bamboo spine").

Hip involvement may lead to symmetric, concentric joint space narrowing, irregularity of the subchondral bone with subchondral sclerosis, osteophyte formation at the outer margin of the articular surface, and, ultimately, bony ankylosis of these joints.

There are several validated scoring methods available to quantify structural damage in AS: the Bath AS radiology index (BASRI), the stoke AS spondylitis score (SASSS), and the modified SASSS.[99-101] The BASRI includes scores for the cervical and lumbar spine as well as the sacroiliac joints. A similar score for the hips is also available. The SASSS evaluates the lumbar spine only; the modified SASSS assesses the cervical and lumbar spine. These scoring methods are most suited for use in clinical trials and observational studies.

COMPUTED TOMOGRAPHY AND MAGNETIC RESONANCE IMAGING

The conventional plain pelvic radiograph is still the initial tool for the evaluation of sacroiliac joints in patients with inflammatory low back pain. This technique, however, lacks

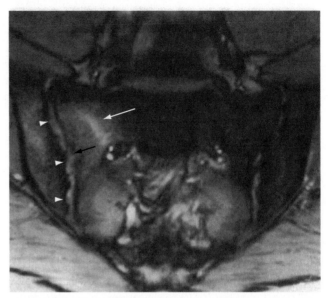

Figure 70-1 T1-weighted, opposed-phase, gradient echo magnetic resonance image 3 minutes after the intravenous injection of gadolinium-DTPA in a 23-year-old man with ankylosing spondylitis and severe inflammatory back pain localized mainly to the right side, of 3 years' duration. Acute sacroiliitis is demonstrated by the strong contrast enhancement of the right sacroiliac joint (*arrowheads*), with impressive bone marrow edema (*white arrow*) and erosions (*black arrow*). (Enhancement factor 150%, graded 3B right, 1× left.)

sensitivity in the early stages of sacroiliac inflammation. In such cases, dynamic MRI with a T1-weighted sequence after the intravenous injection of gadolinium diethylenetriaminepentaacetic acid (Gd-DTPA) is able to demonstrate early stages of sacroiliitis[102,103] (Fig. 70-1). Fat-saturating techniques such as short tau inversion recovery (STIR) sequences are very sensitive in the detection of bone marrow edema, which is a frequent finding in AS-related inflammation of the musculoskeletal system.[104] STIR imaging is cheaper than Gd-DTPA sequences and almost as good. Thus, active, early sacroiliitis can best be searched for by STIR or contrast-based sequences.

Similarly, spinal involvement is first assessed by conventional radiography. Square vertebrae, shiny corners (the Romanus lesion), spondylodiscitis (the Anderson lesion), and syndesmophytes with partial and complete fusion are typical radiographic features of AS. Spinal inflammation cannot be assessed by conventional radiography but can be visualized by MRI,[20] where it is typically seen in the vertebrae, at both anterior and posterior sites as well as around the intervertebral disk. Posterior elements such as the facet joints, pedicles, and transverse processes can show inflammatory lesions as well. MRI and ultrasonography can be very useful to assess enthesitic problems such as Achilles tendinitis and heel pain.

To quantify spinal inflammation, mainly for use in clinical trials, several scoring methods exist. Currently, one cannot prioritize among these methods. The relation between clinical symptoms and structural damage needs to be explored further.[105]

For the detection of bone changes, such as erosions and ankylosis, CT is usually considered superior to MRI, but MRI is better in the imaging of cartilage and provides the possibility of dynamic measurements.[102,106,107] CT is definitely not indicated in the routine evaluation of the sacroiliac joint. CT scanning may be useful in the diagnosis of spinal fractures, spinal stenosis, or thecal diverticula. A major difference between CT and MRI is the radiation exposure associated with the former but not with the latter.

DIAGNOSIS

Clinical manifestations of AS usually begin in late adolescence or early adulthood; only rarely do they begin after age 40 years.[15] The diagnosis of AS at an early stage of disease depends primarily on a careful history and physical examination. Two features of the history are critical: the presence of inflammatory low back pain and stiffness, and a positive family history for AS.

Low back pain is very common in the general population and is frequently due to noninflammatory, nonspecific mechanical causes. However, the low back pain in AS has typical "inflammatory" features (see Table 70-7). A history of inflammatory low back pain can be used as a diagnostic tool. A reassessment of the clinical history for diagnostic purposes among young to middle-aged adults (younger than 50 years) with chronic back pain and an established diagnosis of either AS or mechanical back pain revealed a sensitivity of 37% (95% CI 28 to 46), a specificity of 84% (95% CI 76 to 90), a positive likelihood ratio of 2.3 (95% CI 1.4 to 3.7), and a post-test probability of AS of 11% (given a pre-test probability of 5%) if two of the four parameters listed in Table 70-9 were present. If three or four of these items were present, the sensitivity was 34% (95% CI 25 to 43), the specificity was 97% (95% CI 92 to 99), the positive likelihood ratio was 12.4 (95% CI 4.0 to 40), and the post-test probability of AS was 39%.[76] Because the prevalence of AS in many white populations is as low as approximately 0.1% to 0.3%, applying the clinical history as a test for the disease in such low-probability settings provides rather low post-test probability values. However, a positive family history increases the pretest probability of AS from 0.1% for a person belonging to the general population to about 10% for any first-degree relative of an AS proband.[15] The probability of having AS for a first-degree relative with a positive family history of AS increases from 10% to nearly 50% if this relative has inflammatory low back pain. In contrast, the likelihood of having AS increases from 0.1% to only 1% for a person who has inflammatory back pain (without any other inflammatory indications listed in Table 70-9) but has a negative family history for AS.

A definite diagnosis of AS is usually established by radiographic evidence of bilateral sacroiliitis. The plain anteroposterior view of the pelvis is usually adequate for diagnostic purposes. There is, however, considerable intra- and interobserver variation in the radiographic diagnosis of sacroiliitis for both conventional pelvic films and CT of the sacroiliac joints. Training in reading these films has limited value. Improvement in sensitivity tends to be associated with a decrease in specificity.[108]

In most adult patients, AS can be diagnosed clinically without the HLA-B27 test. This assessment has no additional value in established disease or as a pure screening tool.[109] However, in young patients with inflammatory chronic back pain, a positive HLA-B27 test increases the likelihood of having AS, particularly if imaging of the

Table 70-9 Proposed Criteria for Inflammatory Back Pain in Young to Middle-aged Adults* with Chronic Back Pain

Morning stiffness of at least 30 min duration
Improvement of back pain with exercise but not with rest
Awakening because of back pain during second half of night only
Alternating buttock pain

*Younger than 50 yr.

From Rudwaleit M, Metter A, Listing J, et al: Inflammatory back pain in ankylosing spondylitis: A reassessment of the clinical history for application as classification and diagnostic criteria. Arthritis Rheum 65:569-578, 2006.

sacroiliac joints does not provide conclusive results. Usually, however, the contribution of MRI and HLA-B27 typing to purely clinical factors in diagnosing axial manifestations of AS among patients with inflammatory back pain of short duration is rather limited.[110]

Physicians are reluctant to make the diagnosis of AS when radiographic evidence of sacroiliitis is not present. In particular, relatives of AS patients may have signs and symptoms of AS, including inflammatory back pain, but sometimes do not show radiographic sacroiliitis even after lengthy follow-up. Radiographic sacroiliitis is frequent in AS but is by no means an early or obligate manifestation of the disease. In patients with a clinical diagnosis of possible AS, radiographic sacroiliitis may become manifest only after appropriate follow-up. Therefore, diagnosing the disease early, before (conventional) radiographic evidence of sacroiliitis is manifest, constitutes a challenge to the clinician. This is especially true as more effective treatments become increasingly available. In this context, the term *preaxial* AS is often used. An approach based on pretest probabilities and likelihood ratios has been proposed to diagnose early disease with predominantly axial manifestations before convincing evidence of radiographic sacroiliitis is present.[76]

AS rarely develops after age 40; however, late-onset AS does occur. In this case, there may be little or no clinical involvement of the axial skeleton initially, but patients may show moderate oligoarthritis with low cell counts in the synovial fluid and pitting edema of the lower limbs.[111]

At the other end of the age scale, juvenile-onset AS is not uncommon among patients with spondyloarthropathies. Such patients tend to have enthesopathy and peripheral arthritis that may be severe and disabling.

GENDER ISSUES

Clinically, AS is more common in males, with a reported male-female ratio of about 2:1 to 3:1. However, extrapolation of studies employing the genetic marker HLA-B27 suggests that, based on radiographs of the sacroiliac joints, prevalence rates are about equal in both sexes.[15]

Disease expression is thought to be different in males and females. A case-control study comparing 35 female patients to 70 male patients as controls showed no differences in spinal symptoms, chest expansion, peripheral arthritis, extra-articular manifestations, or functional outcome. The males with AS more often had radiographic spinal changes and hip joint involvement than their female counterparts. There is still some controversy, but overall, there are no significant clinical or radiographic differences between women and men with AS. However, on average, the disease seems to be more severe in men.[112,113]

Fertility among female patients with AS is normal.[114] Most patients (50% to 60%) do not experience major changes in disease activity during pregnancy, but an increase in morning stiffness and low back pain, particularly at night, may occur at about the 20th week of gestation and last for a few days to weeks.[115] In about 50% of patients, an exacerbation of symptoms is seen within the first half year after delivery. Sacroiliitis, including complete ankylosis of the sacroiliac joints, does not constitute a contraindication for vaginal delivery. Epidural anesthesia is usually possible, because most patients have a rather short duration of disease and do not have extensive spinal syndesmophytes. The fetal outcome is not impaired in patients with AS. Every pregnancy in patients with this disease should be considered high risk, however, and such pregnancies require close collaboration between rheumatologists and obstetricians.

PROGNOSIS

The course of AS is highly variable, characterized by spontaneous remissions and exacerbations. Its prognosis has generally been considered rather favorable. The disease may run a relatively mild or self-limited course. However, the disease may also remain active over many years. Life expectancy is somewhat reduced, particularly after 10 years of disease.[116] A study from Finland indicates that the risk of dying for patients with AS is increased by 50% compared with controls matched for age and gender. Causes of death include complications of the disease such as amyloidosis and spinal fractures, as well as cardiovascular, gastrointestinal, and renal disease.[117] There is no convincing evidence that the natural history of the disease has essentially changed over the last few decades.[118,119] No differences exist between familial and sporadic AS in terms of age at onset, age at diagnosis, or prevalence of peripheral arthritis and acute anterior uveitis.[120]

Functional limitations increase with disease duration. Although structural damage seen on radiographs is clearly associated with physical function and spinal mobility at the group level, individual patients with normal radiographs might exhibit a major reduction in spinal mobility, whereas those with severe radiographic abnormalities might function quite well in everyday tasks.[121]

Recent data show that the functional prognosis of AS is less favorable than was previously thought. Withdrawal from work in those with paid jobs varies from 10% after 20 years of disease duration to 30% after 10 years, depending on the characteristics of the patients included and the social security system considered[122-125] (Table 70-10). The age- and sex-adjusted withdrawal rate from labor-force participation was 3.1 times higher among Dutch patients compared with the general population.[125] Older age at disease onset, manual work, lower educational level, and coping strategies characterized by the limitation and pacing of activities were associated with a higher risk for work disability.[123-125] Vocational counseling, job training, easy access to the workplace, and support of colleagues and management may reduce the probability of withdrawal from work.[122,126] Sick leave in those

Table 70-10 Withdrawal from Workforce Due to Disability among Patients with Ankylosing Spondylitis

Country	Withdrawal Rate	Comments
Mexico (103 patients)	3%/yr	
France (182 patients)	36% after 20 yr	
Netherlands (529 patients)	30% after 20 yr	RR compared to general population: 3.1 (95% CI: 2.5 to 3.7)
USA (234 patients)	10% after 20 and 30 yr	Highly educated patients; IBD excluded

CI, confidence interval; IBD, inflammatory bowel disease; RR, relative risk.

with paid jobs was linked to disease activity and presence of extraspinal disease manifestations.[122,125,127] Patients with peripheral joint involvement are more likely to take sick leave than are AS patients with axial manifestations only.

Overall, the first 10 years of disease are particularly important with respect to subsequent outcome. Most of the loss of function among patients with AS occurs within this period and is associated with the presence of peripheral arthritis, spinal radiographic changes, and development of a so-called bamboo spine.[128] In a retrospective study of patients with spondyloarthropathies, including AS, of at least 10 years' duration, seven variables were associated with disease severity if these factors occurred within the first 2 years of follow-up. These factors, expressed as an odds ratio together with its 95% CI, are as follows: arthritis of hip joints (22.9; 4.4 to 118), ESR more than 30 mm/hr (7; 4.8 to 9.5), poor efficacy of nonsteroidal anti-inflammatory drugs (NSAIDs) (8.3; 2.6 to 27.1), limitation of lumbar spine (7; 2 to 25), sausage-like digits (8.5; 1.5 to 9.0), oligoarthritis (4.3; 1.4 to 13.1), and onset before age 16 years (3.5; 1.1 to 12.8).[129] However, the only factor consistently associated with a severe course is involvement of the hip.

The long-term results of total hip replacement in AS are satisfactory. The outcome of 138 total hip replacements and 12 revisions was good or very good in 86%, and 63% of patients had no pain. Mobility was good or very good in 44%. The mean follow-up was 7.5 years (range, 1 to 34 years). Altogether, 69% of the male hip recipients younger than 60 years were at work at the time of the survey.[130]

ASSESSMENT AND MONITORING

Signs and symptoms such as spinal pain and limitation of motion might be due to current disease activity or to damage. A plethora of tools is available to assess these dimensions. For example, there are many ways to measure limitation of motion of the lumbar spine. New instruments have been developed to assess various aspects of the disease, including the Bath and Edmonton AS metrology indexes, Bath AS global index, BASRI, Bath AS disease activity index, and Dougados functional index.[131-134] However, standardization and validation of many of these instruments are lacking or incomplete. An international Assessment in Ankylosing Spondylitis (ASAS) working group was formed with the aim of selecting, proposing, and testing core sets of measures for different settings.[135] It was thought that a certain set of variables should be targeted to a specific task. For example, when assessing the efficacy of

Table 70-11 World Health Organization–International League of Associations for Rheumatology Core Sets for Ankylosing Spondylitis

Domain	Instrument
1. Function	BASFI or Functional Index Dougados
2. Pain	VAS: last week, spine pain at night due to AS VAS: last week, spine pain due to AS
3. Spinal mobility	Chest expansion and modified Schober and occiput to wall distance (lateral spinal flexion or BASMI)
4. Patient global assessment	VAS: last week
5. Stiffness	Duration of morning spine stiffness, last week
6. Peripheral joints and entheses	Number of swollen joints (44 joint count); validated enthesis index
7. Acute-phase reactants	Erythrocyte sedimentation rate
8. Spine radiographs	Lateral view of lumbar spine and lateral view of cervical spine
9. Hip radiographs	Pelvic radiograph including sacroiliac joints and hips
10. Fatigue	VAS on fatigue from BASDAI

Disease-controlling antirheumatic therapy domains: 1-10; symptom-modifying antirheumatic drug domains: 1-5, 10; physical therapy domains: 1-5, 10; clinical record-keeping domains: 1-7.

AS, ankylosing spondylitis; BASDAI, Bath ankylosing spondylitis disease activity index; BASFI, Bath ankylosing spondylitis functional index; BASMI, Bath ankylosing spondylitis metrology index; VAS, visual analog scale.

From van der Heijde D, Calin A, Dougados M, et al: Selection of instruments in the core set for DC-ART, SMARD, physical therapy, and clinical record keeping in ankylosing spondylitis: Progress report of ASAS Working Group—assessments in ankylosing spondylitis. J Rheumatol 26:951-954, 1999.

Table 70-12 Assessment in Ankylosing Spondylitis (ASAS) International Working Group Improvement Criteria and Partial Remission Criteria

ASAS-20 Improvement Criteria
At least 20% improvement and 10 units improvement in three of the four following domains, without 20% or more worsening and 10 units worsening in the remaining domain: BASFI Morning stiffness Patient global assessment Pain
ASAS-40 Improvement Criteria
At least 40% improvement and 20 units improvement in three of the four following domains, without any worsening in the remaining domain: BASFI Morning stiffness Patient global assessment Pain
ASAS-5/6 Improvement Criteria
At least 20% improvement in five of the six following domains: BASFI Morning stiffness Patient global assessment Pain Acute-phase reactants Spinal mobility
ASAS Partial Remission Criteria
A value below 20 units in all four domains of the ASAS-20 improvement criteria

Data from Anderson et al[136] and Brandt et al[137]
BASFI, Bath ankylosing spondylitis functional index.

physical therapy, it would not be realistic to include measures of radiographic changes of the spine. Clearly, the set of measures for a drug's disease-modifying capabilities will differ from a set that measures analgesic effectiveness only. Four settings have been defined: disease-controlling antirheumatic therapy; symptom-modifying antirheumatic drugs, such as NSAIDs; physical therapy; and clinical record keeping in daily practice (Table 70-11).[135] Also, criteria to assess the response of individual patients have been developed and validated. These ASAS-20 improvement criteria are frequently used in clinical trials.[136] In addition, more stringent improvement criteria—ASAS-40 and ASAS-5/6—have been proposed,[137] as well as criteria to define partial remission. The three sets of improvement criteria and the partial remission criteria are presented in Table 70-12.[136,137]

A needs-based quality of life instrument specific for AS has been developed. It is well accepted and easy to perform and, in terms of assessing the impact of interventions, has shown good scaling and psychometric properties and sensitivity to change.[138,139]

MANAGEMENT

A recent systematic review of the literature on the management of AS culminated in a series of treatment propositions developed by ASAS/European League Against Rheumatism (EULAR) that emphasize the key evidence-based

components of disease management (Table 70-13; Fig. 70-2).[140,141] For most patients, AS is a relatively mild disease with a good functional prognosis. Most do not experience significant extraskeletal manifestations except for acute anterior uveitis, which occurs in about 30% of patients. Usually, this eye disease can be well managed with eye drops containing corticosteroids to reduce inflammation and with pupil-dilating, atropine-like agents to prevent or diminish synechiae. At the outset, patients should be warned that acute anterior uveitis may occur at any time during the course of the disease.

The treatment objectives in AS are to relieve pain, stiffness, and fatigue and to maintain good posture and good physical and psychosocial functioning.[142] No drug is currently available that significantly influences the course of spinal disease and retards the process of ossification in particular. Similarly, evidence is lacking that any of the conventional disease-modifying antirheumatic drugs, including sulfasalazine and methotrexate, alter or inhibit the inflammation seen in the spine and entheses in AS.

A full explanation of the disease, its course, possible complications (e.g., acute anterior uveitis), and its prognosis is essential to achieve compliance by the patient. Self-help groups provide important information and social support. In addition, patient organizations often provide access to hydrotherapy and group physiotherapy. Exercises are the mainstay of treatment. Preferably, they should be started after a hot shower or a hot bath. Swimming and extension-promoting exercises or sporting activities such as volleyball or cross-country skiing are appropriate. These

Table 70-13 Treatment Recommendations

1. Treatment of AS should be tailored according to:
   Current manifestations of disease (axial, peripheral, entheseal, extra-articular symptoms and signs)
   Level of current symptoms, clinical findings, and prognostic indicators
   Disease activity, inflammation
   Pain
   Function, disability, handicap
   Structural damage, hip involvement, spinal deformities
   General clinical status (age, sex, comorbidity, concomitant drugs)
   Patient's wishes and expectations

2. Disease monitoring of patients with AS should include patient history (e.g., questionnaires), clinical parameters, laboratory tests, and imaging, all based on clinical presentation and ASAS core set. Monitoring frequency is individualized, based on symptoms, severity, and drug treatment.

3. Optimal management of AS requires a combination of non-pharmacologic and pharmacologic treatments.

4. Nonpharmacologic treatment of AS should include patient education and regular exercise. Individual and group physical therapy should be considered. Patient associations and self-help groups may be useful

5. NSAIDs are recommended as first-line drug treatment for patients with pain and stiffness. In those with increased GI risk, nonselective NSAIDs plus a gastroprotective agent or a selective COX-2 inhibitor could be used.

6. Analgesics, such as paracetamol and opioids, might be considered for pain control in patients in whom NSAIDs are insufficient, contraindicated, or poorly tolerated.

7. Corticosteroid injections directed to the local site of musculoskeletal inflammation may be considered. The use of systemic corticosteroids for axial disease is not supported by evidence.

8. There is no evidence of the efficacy of DMARDs, including sulfasalazine and methotrexate, for the treatment of axial disease. Sulfasalazine may be considered in patients with peripheral arthritis.

9. Anti-TNF treatment should be given to patients with persistently high disease activity despite conventional treatments, according to ASAS recommendations. There is no evidence to support the obligatory use of DMARDs before or concomitant with anti-TNF treatment in patients with axial disease.

10. Total hip arthroplasty should be considered in patients with refractory pain or disability and radiographic evidence of structural damage, independent of age. Spinal surgery—for example, corrective osteotomy and stabilization procedures—may be of value in selected patients.

AS, ankylosing spondylitis; ASAS, Assessment in Ankylosing Spondylitis; COX, cyclooxygenase; DMARDs, disease-modifying antirheumatic drugs; GI, gastrointestinal; NSAIDs, nonsteroidal anti-inflammatory drugs; TNF, tumor necrosis factor.
From Zochling J, van der Heijde D, Burgos-Vargas R, et al: ASAS/EULAR recommendations for the management of ankylosing spondylitis. Ann Rheum Dis 65:444-452, 2006.

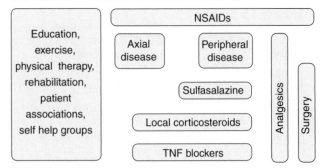

Figure 70-2 Recommended management of ankylosing spondylitis (AS), based on clinical expertise and research evidence. The disease progression with time moves vertically from top to bottom. ASAS/EULAR, Assessment in Ankylosing Spondylitis European League Against Rheumatism; NSAIDs, nonsteroidal anti-inflammatory drugs; TNF, tumor necrosis factor.

PHYSIOTHERAPY

There is now ample evidence that physiotherapy in the form of exercises is effective, at least in the short term (up to 1 year), and particularly in groups of patients with AS (level A evidence). Scientific evidence of long-term effectiveness is not yet available.[143-145]

In a randomized, controlled trial, a program of supervised physiotherapy in groups was found to be superior to individualized programs in improving thoracolumbar mobility and fitness. The program, which consisted of hydrotherapy, exercises, and sporting activities twice weekly for 3 hours per session, resulted in improved overall health and less stiffness, as reported by the patient.[144] An intensive 3-week spa exercise therapy program resulted in marked improvement in both subjective and objective assessments that lasted for up to 9 months. Health resource utilization, in particular NSAID use and sick leave, was significantly reduced during this 9-month follow-up period. The clinical benefits of such treatments can be achieved at acceptable costs.[146,147] Level A evidence from a recent Cochrane review on the efficacy of physiotherapeutic interventions, including exercises, is summarized in Table 70-14.[148]

Lying prone for 15 to 30 minutes once or several times a day is useful to reverse the tendency toward kyphosis, which is aggravated by pain and fatigue, and flexion contractures of the hip joints. Patients should sleep fully supine on a firm mattress with only a small neck-support pillow.

MEDICATION

Nonsteroidal Anti-inflammatory Drugs

The efficacy and effectiveness of NSAID therapy for the alleviation of symptoms have been well established (level A evidence). When given for prolonged periods of up to a year, there may be improvement in spinal mobility and acute-phase reactants.[149] Many NSAIDs are effective in patients with AS, and no NSAID has documented superiority in terms of efficacy. Selective cyclooxygenase-2 (COX-2) inhibitors have similar efficacy to conventional NSAIDs (level A evidence).[150] A nonselective NSAID is appropriate for most patients with AS, who tend to be relatively young

activities counteract the kyphotic effects of pain and fatigue on posture and reduce stiffness. Patients should avoid vigorous or contact sports if the spine has become fused or osteoporotic, because such a spine is susceptible to fracture.

Appliances such as driving mirrors may improve comfort and safety, especially if there is considerable involvement of the cervical spine. In that case, appropriate neck support is also required to reduce the risk of fracturing the vulnerable osteoporotic cervical spine as a consequence of traffic accidents. For the same reason, automobile air bags are strongly recommended.

Table 70-14 Cochrane Review of Physiotherapeutic Interventions and Spa Therapy for Patients with Ankylosing Spondylitis: Conclusions

Home exercise programs are better than no intervention
Supervised group physiotherapy is better than home exercise
Combined inpatient spa and exercise therapy followed by supervised outpatient weekly group physiotherapy is better than weekly group physiotherapy alone

From Dagfinrud H, Kvien TK, Hagen KB: Physiotherapy interventions for ankylosing spondylitis. Cochrane Database of Systematic Reviews 4, art. no.CD002822.pub2.DOI, 2004.

and without comorbidity. A COX-2 selective agent may be used in the presence of risk factors for peptic ulceration, although both categories of NSAIDs may exacerbate inflammatory bowel disease. Once-daily drug regimens may improve patient compliance. Up to 2 weeks may be required to demonstrate maximal symptomatic benefit from an NSAID. If symptomatic relief is inadequate, a switch to another NSAID may be worthwhile; failure of two NSAIDs should prompt an exploration of other management strategies.

Given the gastrointestinal and cardiovascular risks of taking NSAIDs or coxibs, one must address whether this treatment should be on a daily or an "on-demand" basis. A 2-year randomized, prospective, controlled trial in AS patients compared the efficacy of continuous NSAID therapy to that of intermittent on-demand use. The results suggest that continuous therapy retards radiographic disease progression.[151] This study is in line with an older study that also suggested a possible disease-controlling effect of continuous therapy.[152] However, these findings are controversial.[153]

Second-Line Drugs

Borrowing well-established concepts in the treatment of RA, disease-controlling therapy for AS has been defined as an agent that decreases inflammatory manifestations of disease, sustains or improves function, and prevents or decreases the rate of progression of structural damage. Although most of the second-line agents developed primarily for RA have been studied in AS, none can be considered disease controlling in AS. The greatest amount of data is available for sulfasalazine, which was first proposed as a therapy for AS in 1984, based on the common association between inflammatory bowel disease and spondyloarthropathies, the description of inflammatory lesions in the ileum of patients with spondyloarthropathies, and its success in the treatment of intestinal inflammation.[154] A total of 11 double-blind, placebo-controlled trials have been published, as well as two meta-analyses. The results of the two largest trials were consistent, demonstrating no significant benefit for sulfasalazine in AS, although subgroup analysis showed that patients with (peripheral) polyarthritis—mostly those with psoriatic arthritis, but also AS patients with peripheral joint involvement—had a significant but modest response.[155,156] An important limitation in most of these studies was the long disease duration (> 10 years) of recruited patients, and it has been suggested that early disease may be more responsive to therapy. However, a 24-week placebo-controlled trial that recruited 230 patients meeting ESSG criteria for spondyloarthropathies and with symptom duration of less than 5 years confirmed that sulfasalazine was ineffective.[157] The most recent meta-analysis, based on 11 trials, concluded that this agent has a significant impact only on the ESR and the severity of spinal stiffness (level A evidence).[158] The primary indication for the use of sulfasalazine in routine practice is a patient who has concomitant peripheral arthritis and has had an inadequate response to NSAIDs and physical modalities.

The evaluation of methotrexate in AS has been limited to case reports and open analyses, mostly reported in abstract form. These studies have included limited numbers of patients for periods of 6 months to 3 years, at doses from 7.5 to 15 mg weekly. The results have been mixed, with some benefit noted in patients with concomitant peripheral arthritis. Two small placebo-controlled trials assessed methotrexate in doses of 10 and 7.5 mg weekly for 24 weeks, with contradictory findings.[159,160] A meta-analysis concluded that there was no evidence of efficacy and that higher-quality trials, larger sample sizes, longer durations of treatment, and higher dosages of methotrexate were necessary before any definitive conclusions could be drawn (level B evidence).[161]

Corticosteroids may be effective for local intra-articular treatment in AS, including the sacroiliac joints, if given under fluoroscopic guidance (level B evidence). Systemic steroids are of unproven benefit and are thought to be less effective than in RA (level C evidence). Leflunomide has been studied in AS, and although an open-label study suggested a benefit in patients with peripheral arthritis, a small placebo-controlled study reported no benefit (level B evidence).[162,163] A controlled dose-response (60 mg versus 10 mg) evaluation of a bisphosphonate, pamidronate, given intravenously on a monthly basis for 6 months showed evidence of symptomatic efficacy, primarily in patients with only axial disease (level B evidence).[164] However, this finding needs to be confirmed.

Thalidomide has been used in two open-label studies in AS because it enhances the degradation of TNF-α messenger RNA. In a Chinese study, improvement was reported in 80% of patients, with deterioration 3 months after treatment discontinuation. Frequent side effects are drowsiness, constipation, and dizziness (level B evidence).[165]

BIOLOGIC THERAPIES

A milestone in the treatment of AS is the development of anti–TNF-α therapies. The rationale is based on the finding of TNF-α expression in sacroiliac joint biopsies of AS patients, the observation that overexpression of TNF-α leads to sacroiliitis in animal models, and earlier clinical trial data demonstrating the efficacy of one anti–TNF-α agent, infliximab, in Crohn's disease. Three anti–TNF-α agents are of proven benefit in AS according to pivotal phase III trials (level A evidence): infliximab, etanercept, and adalimumab. Infliximab is an IgG1 chimeric monoclonal antibody with the Fab portion derived from the mouse. It is given in a dose of 3 to 5 mg/kg every 6 to 8 weeks after loading at 0, 2, and 6 weeks. Etanercept is a recombinant 75-kD TNF receptor IgG1 fusion protein that is self-administered by subcutaneous injection either once (50 mg) or twice (25 mg) weekly. Adalimumab is a human monoclonal antibody that is self-administered by subcutaneous injection on alternate weeks (40 mg). None requires concomitant therapy with methotrexate.

Table 70-15 Assessment in Ankylosing Spondylitis (ASAS) Recommendations for the Initiation of Treatment with Biologics

Patient Selection
Diagnosis

Patients normally fulfilling modified New York criteria for definitive AS
Modified New York criteria 1984:
    Radiological criterion: sacroiliitis, grade ≥ II bilaterally or grade III to IV unilaterally
    Clinical criteria (two of three): low back pain and stiffness for >3 mo that improves with exercise but is not relieved by rest; limitation of motion
        of lumbar spine in both sagittal and frontal planes; limitation of chest expansion relative to normal values correlated for age and sex

Active Disease
Active disease for ≥ 4 wk BASDAI ≥ 4 (scale, 0–10) and an expert* opinion†
Treatment Failure

All patients should have had adequate therapeutic trials of at least two NSAIDs. An adequate therapeutic trial is defined as:
    Treatment for at least 3 mo at maximum recommended or tolerated anti-inflammatory dose unless contraindicated
    Treatment for <3 mo if treatment was withdrawn because of intolerance, toxicity, or contraindications
Patients with pure axial manifestations do not have to take DMARDs before anti-TNF treatment can be started
Patients with symptomatic peripheral arthritis should have an insufficient response to at least one local corticosteroid injection, if appropriate
Patients with persistent peripheral arthritis must have had a therapeutic trial of sulfasalazine‡
Patients with symptomatic enthesitis must have failed appropriate local treatment

Contraindications

Women who are pregnant or breastfeeding; effective contraception must be practiced
Active infection
Patients at high risk of infection, including those with:
    Chronic leg ulcer
    Previous tuberculosis (follow local recommendations for prevention or treatment)
    Septic arthritis of a native joint within the past 12 mo
    Sepsis of a prosthetic joint within the past 12 mo, or indefinitely if the joint remains in situ
    Persistent or recurrent chest infections
    Indwelling urinary catheter
History of lupus or multiple sclerosis
Malignancy or premalignancy states, excluding:
    Basal cell carcinoma
    Malignancies diagnosed and treated more than 10 yr previously (and the probability of total cure is very high)

Assessment of Disease
ASAS Core Set for Daily Practice
Physical function (BASFI or Dougados functional index) Pain (VAS for spine at night from AS in the past week and VAS for spine from AS in the past week) Spinal mobility (chest expansion, modified Schober and occiput to wall distance, and lateral lumbar flexion) Patient's global assessment (VAS for the past week) Stiffness (duration of morning spine stiffness in the past week) Peripheral joints and entheses (number of swollen joints [44 total], enthesitis score such as developed in Maastricht, Berlin, or San Francisco) Acute-phase reactants (ESR or CRP) Fatigue (VAS)
BASDAI
VAS for overall level of fatigue or tiredness in the past week VAS for overall level of AS neck, back, or hip pain in the past week VAS for overall level of pain or swelling in joints other than neck, back, or hips in the past week VAS for overall discomfort from any areas tender to touch or pressure in the past week VAS for overall level of morning stiffness from time of awakening in the past week Duration and intensity (VAS) of morning stiffness from time of awakening (up to 120 min)
Assessment of Response
Responder criteria: BASDAI—50% relative change or absolute change of 20 mm (scale between 0 and 100) and expert opinion in favor of   continuation Time of evaluation: 6 to 12 wk

*The expert is a physician, usually a rheumatologist, with expertise in inflammatory back pain and the use of biologic agents. *Expert* should be locally defined.

†The expert should consider clinical features (history and examination), serum acute-phase reactant levels, or imaging results, such as radiographs demonstrating rapid progression or magnetic resonance images indicating ongoing inflammation.

‡Sulfasalazine treatment for at least 4 mo at standard target dose or maximally tolerated dose unless contraindicated or not tolerated. Treatment for less than 4 mo if treatment was withdrawn because of intolerance or toxicity or contraindicated.

AS, ankylosing spondylitis; BASDAI, Bath ankylosing spondylitis disease activity index; BASFI, Bath ankylosing spondylitis functional index; CRP, C-reactive protein; DMARD, disease-modifying antirheumatic drug; ESR, erythrocyte sedimentation rate; NSAID, nonsteroidal anti-inflammatory drug; TNF, tumor necrosis factor; VAS, visual analog scale (all VASs can be replaced by a numerical rating scale).

From Braun J, Davis J, Dougados M, et al: ASAS Working Group: First update of the international ASAS consensus statement for the use of anti-TNF agents in patients with ankylosing spondylitis. Ann Rheum Dis 65:316-320, 2006. See also http://www.ASAS-group.org.

All three agents demonstrate ASAS-20 response rates of 55% to 60% and ASAS-40 response rates of 45% to 50% in phase III trials.[166-168] Improvement is evident by 2 to 4 weeks and is sustained as long as the patient remains on treatment; virtually all patients relapse by 4 months after discontinuation of treatment.[169] Significant improvement is also observed in function, spinal mobility, peripheral synovitis, enthesitis score, and quality of life. Sick leave and work disability are reduced. The number of patients who must be treated to achieve one patient who experiences at least 50% improvement in disease activity is just two (95% CI 1 to 6). Objective parameters of disease activity that show improvement include acute-phase reactants, synovial histopathology, and MRI features of inflammation in the spine and sacroiliac joints.[170] There is as yet no evidence that these agents are disease controlling with respect to the prevention of structural damage on plain radiography. Response to treatment appears to be increased in those with high disease activity and worse in those with a long disease duration, impaired function, and no discernible evidence of inflammation on MRI.[171] However, patients with complete spinal ankylosis may benefit from these treatments.[168] Adverse events in AS patients are no different from those reported in RA, and infusion reactions in patients receiving infliximab have been no more frequent than in RA patients on concomitant methotrexate.

Recommendations for the use of anti–TNF-α therapies have been developed (Table 70-15).[172-174] These new therapeutic modalities identify important clinical questions to be answered by further research. All the anti–TNF-α agents examined to date have disease-modifying properties, but their long-term safety and disease-controlling effects in terms of preventing structural damage have yet to be demonstrated.

SURGERY

Involvement of the hip joint may cause serious disability. Ectopic bone formation may occur, but the outcome of total hip replacement is generally favorable.[130]

Vertebral osteotomy may be required in selected cases to correct marked flexion deformity when forward vision is severely impaired. Diaphragmatic herniation may result from the procedure.

SUMMARY

Although our understanding of the genetics of AS has improved greatly, our knowledge about its cause and pathogenesis is far from complete. A lot has been accomplished in terms of classification and assessment of the disease. Treatment with biologics such as anti–TNF-α is very effective and may be the first therapy that actually controls the disease. The challenge now is to determine how to predict and improve outcomes at the level of individual patients.

Future Directions

Diagnostic criteria must be defined for individual patients with AS at an early stage of the disease.

The long interval (on average) between the first symptoms of AS and the clinical diagnosis must be shortened.

Research into factors that accurately predict final outcome at the time of diagnosis is essential.

Study of which factors predict response to biologic therapy for individual AS patients is highly desirable. In addition, the long-term effects of treatment with biologics are not yet known.

Evidence of the effectiveness of preventing damage in terms of the development of syndesmophytes is contradictory. It is largely unknown what triggers the process of ankylosing.

A few studies suggest that continuous (versus intermittent) use of NSAIDs or coxibs may slow the progression of axial radiographic manifestations of AS. These findings, however, are controversial.

REFERENCES

1. Dougados M, van der Linden S, Juhlin R, et al: The European Spondylarthropathy Study Group: Preliminary criteria for the classification of spondylarthropathy. Arthritis Rheum 34:1218-1227, 1991.
2. Chhem RK, Schmit P, Faure C: Did Ramesses II really have ankylosing spondylitis? A reappraisal. Can Assoc Radiol J 55:211-217, 2004.
3. Struempell A: Lehrbuch der speziellen Pathologie und Therapie der inneren Krankheiten. Leipzig, Vogel, 1884, Band 2, Teil 2 pp152-153.
4. Von Bechterew W: Steifheit der Wirbelsaeule und ihre Verkruemmung als besondere Erkrankungsform. Neurol Zentralbl 12:426, 1893.
5. Marie P: Sur la spondylose rhizomélique. Rev Med 18:285, 1889.
6. Arnett F: Seronegative spondylarthropathies. Bull Rheum Dis 37:1-12, 1987.
7. Cury SE, Vilar MJP, Ciconelli RM, et al: Evaluation of the European Spondyloarthropathy Study Group (ESSG) preliminary classification criteria in Brazilian patients. Clin Exp Rheumatol 15:79-82, 1997.
8. Khan MA, van der Linden SM, Kushner I, et al: Spondylitic disease without radiologic evidence of sacroiliitis in relatives of HLA-B27 positive ankylosing spondylitis patients. Arthritis Rheum 28:40-43, 1985.
9. **Van der Linden SM, Valkenburg HA, Cats A: Evaluation of diagnostic criteria for ankylosing spondylitis: A proposal for modification of the New York criteria. Arthritis Rheum 27:361-368, 1984.**
10. Goethé HS, Steven MM, van der Linden S, et al: Evaluation of diagnostic criteria for ankylosing spondylitis: A comparison of the Rome, New York and modified New York criteria in patients with a positive clinical history screening test for ankylosing spondylitis. Br J Rheumatol 24:242-249, 1985.
11. Rudwaleit M, van der Heijde D, Khan MA, et al: How to diagnose axial spondyloarthritis early. Ann Rheum Dis 63:535-543, 2004.
12. D'Amato M, Fiorillo MT, Carcassi C, et al: Relevance of residue 116 of HLA-B27 in determining susceptibility to ankylosing spondylitis. Eur J Immunol 25:3199-3201, 1995.
13. Lopez-Larrea C, Sujirachato K, Mehra NK, et al: HLA-B27 subtypes in Asian patients with ankylosing spondylitis. Tissue Antigens 45:169-176, 1995.

14. Nasution AR, Marjuadi A, Kunmartini S, et al: HLA-B27 subtypes positively and negatively associated with spondylarthropathy. J Rheumatol 24:1111-1114, 1997.

15. Van der Linden SM, Valkenburg HA, de Jongh BM, et al: The risk of developing ankylosing spondylitis in HLA-B27 positive individuals: A comparison of relatives of spondylitis patients with the general population. Arthritis Rheum 27:241-249, 1984.

16. Ahearn JM, Hochberg MC: Epidemiology and genetics of ankylosing spondylitis. J Rheumatol 16(Suppl):22-28, 1988.

17. Bakland G, Nossent HC, Gran JT: Incidence and prevalence of ankylosing spondylitis in Northern Norway. Arthritis Rheum 53:850-855, 2005.

18. Saraux A, Guillemin F, Guggenbuhl F, et al. Prevalence of spondyloarthropathies in France: 2001. Ann Rheum Dis 64:1431-1435, 2005.

19. Kaipiainen-Seppanen O, Aho K, Heliovaara M: Incidence and prevalence of ankylosing spondylitis in Finland. J Rheumatol 24:496-499, 1997.

20. Braun J, Bollow M, Remlinger G, et al: Prevalence of spondyloarthropathies in HLA-B27 positive and negative blood donors. Arthritis Rheum 41:58-67, 1998.

21. Gran JT, Husby G: Ankylosing spondylitis: A comparative study of patients in an epidemiological survey, and those admitted to a department of rheumatology. J Rheumatol 11:788-793, 1984.

22. Carbone LD, Cooper C, Michet CJ, et al: Ankylosing spondylitis in Rochester, Minnesota, 1935-1989. Arthritis Rheum 35:1476-1482, 1992.

23. Martindale J, Smith J, Sutton CJ, et al: Disease and psychological status in ankylosing spondylitis. Rheumatology 45:1288-1293, 2006.

24. Boonen A, Chorus A, Miedema H, et al: Employment, work disability, and work days lost in patients with ankylosing spondylitis: A cross sectional study of Dutch patients. Ann Rheum Dis 60:353-358, 2001.

25. Boonen A, van der Heijde D, Landewe R, et al: Work status and productivity costs due to ankylosing spondylitis: Comparison of three European countries. Ann Rheum Dis 61:429-437, 2002.

26. Boonen A, van der Heijde D, Landewé R, et al: Direct costs of ankylosing spondylitis and its determinants: An analysis among three European countries. Ann Rheum Dis 62:732-740, 2003.

27. Ward MM: Functional disability predicts total costs in patients with ankylosing spondylitis. Arthritis Rheum 46:223-231, 2002.

28. Davis JC, Dougados M, Braun J, et al: Definition of disease duration in ankylosing spondylitis: Reassessing the concept. Ann Rheum Dis 65:1518-1520, 2006.

29. Kobelt G, Andlin-Sobocki P, Maksymowych WP: Costs and quality of life of patients with ankylosing spondylitis in Canada. J Rheumatol 33:289-295, 2006.

30. Brown MA, Kennedy LG, MacGregor AJ, et al: Susceptibility to ankylosing spondylitis in twins: The role of genes, HLA, and the environment. Arthritis Rheum 40:1823-1828, 1997.

31. Brown MA, Laval SH, Brophy S, Calin A: Recurrence risk modeling of the genetic susceptibility to ankylosing spondylitis. Ann Rheum Dis 59:268-270, 2000.

32. Gonzalez-Roces S, Alvarez MV, Gonzalez S, et al: HLA-B27 and worldwide susceptibility to ankylosing spondylitis. Tissue Antigens 49:116-123, 1997.

33. Hamersma J, Cardon LR, Bradbury L, et al: Is disease severity in ankylosing spondylitis genetically determined? Arthritis Rheum 44:1396-1400, 2001.

34. D'Amato M, Fiorillo MT, Carcassi C, et al: Relevance of residue 116 of HLA-B27 in determining susceptibility to ankylosing spondylitis. Eur J Immunol 25:3199-3201, 1995.

35. Jardetzky TS, Lane WS, Robinson RA, et al: Identification of self peptides bound to purified HLA-B27. Nature 353:326-329, 1991.

36. Robinson WP, van der Linden S, Khan MA, et al: HLA-Bw60 increases susceptibility to ankylosing spondylitis in HLA-B27+ patients. Arthritis Rheum 32:1135-1141, 1989.

37. Brown MA, Kennedy LG, Darke C, et al: The effect of HLA-DR genes on susceptibility to and severity of ankylosing spondylitis. Arthritis Rheum 52:460-465, 1998.

38. Brown MA, Edwards S, Hoyle E, et al: Polymorphisms of the CYP2D6 gene increase susceptibility to ankylosing spondylitis. Hum Mol Genet 9:1563-1566, 2000.

39. Laukens D, Peeters H, Marichal D, et al: CARD15 gene polymorphisms in patients with spondyloarthropathies identify a specific phenotype previously related to Crohn's disease. Ann Rheum Dis 64:930-935, 2005.

40. Zhang G, Luo J, Bruckel J, et al: Genetic studies in familial ankylosing spondylitis susceptibility. Arthritis Rheum 50:2246-2254, 2004.

41. Laval SH, Timms A, Edwards S, et al: Whole-genome screening in ankylosing spondylitis: Evidence of non-MHC genetic-susceptibility loci. Am J Hum Genet 68:918-926, 2001.

42. Miceli-Richard C, Zouali H, Said-Nahal R, et al: Groupe Francais d'Etude Genetique des Spondylarthropathies. Significant linkage to spondyloarthropathy on 9q31-34. Hum Mol Genet 13:1641-1648, 2004.

43. Maksymowych WP, Reeve JP, Reveille JD, et al: High-throughput single nucleotide polymorphism (SNP) analysis of the interleukin-1 receptor antagonist (IL1RN) locus in patients with ankylosing spondylitis (AS) by mass ARRAY matrix assisted laser desorption ionization time of flight mass spectroscopy. Arthritis Rheum 48; 2011-2018, 2003.

44. Maksymowych WP, Rahman P, Reeve J, et al: The interleukin-1 locus is associated with susceptibility to ankylosing spondylitis: A Spondyloarthritis Research Consortium of Canada (SPARCC) analysis of 3 Canadian populations. Arthritis Rheum 54:974-985, 2006.

45. Timms AE, Crane AM, Sims AM, et al: The interleukin 1 gene cluster contains a major susceptibility locus for ankylosing spondylitis. Am J Hum Genet 75:587-595, 2004.

46. Sims A-M, Timms AE, Pointon J, et al: IL-1 gene family members are associated with ankylosing spondylitis in both Caucasian and Asian populations. Clin Exp Rheumatol 24:463, 2006.

47. Hoyle E, Laval SH, Calin A, et al: The X-chromosome and susceptibi lity to ankylosing spondylitis. Arthritis Rheum 43:1353-1355, 2000.

47a. Brown MA: Breakthroughs in genetic studies of ankylosing spondylitis. Rheumatology 47:132-137, 2008.

48. Hülsmeyer M, Fiorillo MT, Bettosini F, et al: Dual, HLA-B27 subtype-dependent conformation of a self-peptide. J Exp Med 199:271-281, 2004.

49. Mear JP, Schreiber KL, Munz C, et al: Misfolding of HLA-B27 as a result of its B pocket suggests a novel mechanism for its role in susceptibility to spondyloarthropathies. J Immunol 163:6665-6670, 1999.

50. Kollnberger S, Bird L, Sun MY, et al: Cell-surface expression and immune receptor recognition of HLA-B27 homodimers. Arthritis Rheum 46:2972-2982, 2002.

51. Hammer RE, Maika SD, Richardson JA, et al: Spontaneous inflammatory disease in transgenic rats expressing HLA-B27 and human beta 2m: An animal model of HLA-B27-associated human disorders. Cell 63:1099-1112, 1990.

52. Taurog JD, Richardson JA, Croft JT, et al: The germfree state prevents development of gut and joint inflammatory disease in HLA-B27 transgenic rats. J Exp Med 180:2359-2364, 1994.

53. Tran TM, Dorris ML, Satumtira N, et al: Additional human beta-2 microglobulin curbs HLA-B27 misfolding and promotes arthritis and spondylitis without colitis in male HLA-B27-transgenicrats. Arthritis Rheum 54:1317-1327, 2006.

54. Glant T, Mikecz K, Arzoumanian A, et al: Proteoglycan-induced arthritis in Balb/c mice. Arthritis Rheum 30:201-212, 1987.

55. Shi S, Ciurli C, Cartman A, et al: Experimental immunity to the G1 domain of the proteoglycan versican induces spondylitis and sacroiliitis, of a kind seen in human spondyloarthropathies. Arthritis Rheum 48:2903-2915, 2003.

56. Redlich K, Gortz B, Hayer S, et al: Overexpression of tumor necrosis factor causes bilateral sacroiliitis. Arthritis Rheum 50:1001-1005, 2004.

57. Benjamin M, McGonagle D: The anatomical basis for disease localisation in seronegative spondyloarthropathy at entheses and related sites. J Anat 199:503-526, 2001.

58. Zou J, Zhang Y, Thiel A, et al: Predominant cellular immune response to the cartilage autoantigenic G1 aggrecan in ankylosing spondylitis and rheumatoid arthritis. Rheumatology 42:846-855, 2003.

59. Atagunduz P, Appel H, Kuon W, et al: HLA-B27-restricted CD8+ T cell response to cartilage-derived self peptides in ankylosing spondylitis. Arthritis Rheum 52:892-901, 2005.

60. Mielants H, Veys EM, Goemaere S, et al: Gut inflammation in the spondyloarthropathies: Clinical, radiologic, biologic and genetic features in relation to the type of histology. A prospective study. J Rheumatol 18:1542-1551, 1991.

61. Van Damme N, Elewaut D, Baeten D, et al: Gut mucosal T cell lines from ankylosing spondylitis patients are enriched with alphaEbeta7 integrin. Clin Exp Rheumatol 19:681-687, 2001.

62. Van Damme N, De Vos M, Baeten D, et al: Flow cytometric analysis of gut mucosal lymphocytes supports an impaired Th1 cytokine profile in spondyloarthropathy. Ann Rheum Dis 60:495-499, 2001.

63. Braun J, Tuszewski M, Ehlers S, et al: Nested polymerase chain reaction strategy simultaneously targeting DNA sequences of multiple bacterial species in inflammatory joint diseases. II. Examination of sacroiliac and knee joint biopsies of patients with spondyloarthropathies and other arthritides. J Rheumatol 24:1101-1105, 1997.

64. Baeten D, Demetter P, Cuvelier CA, et al: Macrophages expressing the scavenger receptor CD163: A link between immune alterations of the gut and synovial inflammation in spondyloarthropathy. J Pathol 196:343-350, 2002.

65. Lories RJU, Derese I, Luyten FP: Modulation of bone morphogenetic protein signaling inhibits the onset and progression of ankylosing enthesitis. J Clin Invest 115:1571-1579, 2005.

66. Muche B, Bollow M, Francois RJ, et al: Anatomic structures involved in early- and late-stage sacroiliitis in spondyloarthritis. Arthritis Rheum 48:1374-1384, 2003.

67. Francois RJ, Gardner DL, Degrave EJ, Bywaters EGL: Histopathologic evidence that sacroiliitis in ankylosing spondylitis is not merely enthesitis. Arthritis Rheum 43:2011-2024, 2000.

68. Braun J, Bollow M, Neure L, et al: Use of immunohistologic and in situ hybridization techniques in the examination of sacroiliac joint biopsy specimens from patients with ankylosing spondylitis. Arthritis Rheum 38:499-505, 1995.

69. de Vlam K, Mielants H, Veys EM: Involvement of the zygapophyseal joint in ankylosing spondylitis: Relation to the bridging syndesmophyte. J Rheumatol 26:1738-1745, 1999.

70. Appel H, Kuhne M, Spiekermann S, et al: Immunohistologic analysis of zygapophyseal joints in patients with ankylosing spondylitis. Arthritis Rheum 54:2845-2851, 2006.

71. Maksymowych WP, Rennie WJ, Dhillon SS, et al: Is the costovertebral joint the primary site of inflammation in the thoracic spine of patients with ankylosing spondylitis? A systematic evaluation by MRI. Clin Exp Rheumatol 24:465, 2006.

72. Appel H, Kuhne M, Spiekermann S, et al: Immunohistochemical analysis of hip arthritis in ankylosing spondylitis: Evaluation of the bone-cartilage interface and subchondral bone marrow. Arthritis Rheum 54:1805-1813, 2006.

73. Baeten D, Kruithof E, De Rycke L, et al: Diagnostic classification of spondyloarthropathy and rheumatoid arthritis by synovial histopathology: A prospective study in 154 consecutive patients. Arthritis Rheum 50:2931-2941, 2004.

74. McGonagle D, Marzo-Ortega H, O'Connor P, et al: Histological assessment of the early enthesitis lesion in spondyloarthropathy. Ann Rheum Dis 61:534-537, 2002.

75. Calin A, Porta J, Fries JF, Schurman DJ: Clinical history as a screening test for ankylosing spondylitis. JAMA 237:2613-2614, 1977.

76. Rudwaleit M, Metter A, Listing J, et al: Inflammatory back pain in ankylosing spondylitis: A reassessment of the clinical history for application as classification and diagnostic criteria. Arthritis Rheum 65:569-578, 2006.

77. Van der Linden S, Khan MA, Rentsch HU, et al: Chest pain without radiographic sacroiliitis in relatives of patients with ankylosing spondylitis. J Rheumatol 15:836-839, 1988.

78. Khan MA, Kushner I, Braun WE: Comparison of clinical features in HLA-B27 positive and negative patients with ankylosing spondylitis. Arthritis Rheum 20:909-912, 1977.

79. Van der Linden S, Rentsch HU, Gerber N, et al: The association between ankylosing spondylitis, acute anterior uveitis and HLA-B27: The results of a Swiss family study. Br J Rheumatol 27(Suppl 2):39-41, 1988.

80. Graham DC, Smythe HA: The carditis and aortitis of ankylosing spondylitis. Bull Rheum Dis 9:171-174, 1958.

81. Strobel ES, Fritschka E: Case report and review of the literature: Fatal pulmonary complications in ankylosing spondylitis. Clin Rheumatol 16:617-622, 1997.

82. Casserly IP, Fenlon HM, Breatnach E, et al: Lung findings on high-resolution computed tomography in idiopathic ankylosing spondylitis: Correlation with clinical findings, pulmonary function testing and plain radiography. Br J Rheumatol 36:677-682, 1997.

83. Quismorio F Jr: Pulmonary involvement in ankylosing spondylitis. Curr Opin Pulm Med 2:342-345, 2006.

84. Ramos-Remus C, Gomez-Vargas A, Hernandez-Chavez A, et al: Two year follow-up of anterior and vertical atlantoaxial subluxation in ankylosing spondylitis. J Rheumatol 24:507-510, 1997.

85. Tyrrell PNM, Davies AM, Evans N: Neurological disturbances in ankylosing spondylitis. Ann Rheum Dis 53:714-717, 1994.

86. Lai KN, Li PKT, Hawkins B, et al: IgA nephropathy associated with ankylosing spondylitis: Occurrence in women as well as in men. Ann Rheum Dis 48:435-437, 1989.

87. Vilar MJ, Cury SE, Ferraz MB, et al: Renal abnormalities in ankylosing spondylitis. Scand J Rheumatol 26:19-23, 1997.

88. Gratacos J, Orellana C, Sanmarti R, et al: Secondary amyloidosis in ankylosing spondylitis: A systematic review of 137 patients using abdominal fat aspiration. J Rheumatol 24:912-915, 1997.

89. Lee YSL, Schlotzhauer T, Ott SM, et al: Skeletal status of men with early and late ankylosing spondylitis. Am J Med 103:233-241, 1997.

90. Geusens P, Vosse D, van der Heijde D, et al: High prevalence of thoracic vertebral deformities and discal wedging in ankylosing spondylitis patients with hyperkyphosis. J Rheumatol 28:1856-1861, 2001.

91. Vosse D, van der Heijde D, Landewe R, et al: Determinants of hyperkyphosis in patients with ankylosing spondylitis. Ann Rheum Dis 65:770-774, 2006.

92. Cooper C, Carbone L, Michet CJ, et al: Fracture risk in patients with ankylosing spondylitis: A population based study. J Rheumatol 21:1877-1882, 1994.

93. Graham B, van Peteghem PK: Fractures of the spine in ankylosing spondylitis: Diagnosis, treatment, and complications. Spine 14:803-807, 1989.

94. Khan MA, Kushner I: Diagnosis of ankylosing spondylitis. In Cohen AS (ed): Progress in Clinical Rheumatology, Vol 1, Orlando, Grune & Stratton, 1984, pp 145-178.

95. Spoorenberg A, van der Heijde D, de Klerk E, et al: Relative value of erythrocyte sedimentation rate and C-reactive protein in assessment of disease activity in ankylosing spondylitis. J Rheumatol 26:980-984, 1999.

96. van Halm VP, van Denderen JC, Peters MJL, et al: Increased disease activity is associated with a deteriorated lipid profile in patients with ankylosing spondylitis. Ann Rheum Dis 65:1473-1477, 2006.

97. Schichikawa K, Tsujimoto M, Nishioka J, et al: Histopathology of early sacroiliitis and enthesitis in ankylosing spondylitis. In Ziff M, Cohen SB (eds): The Spondyloarthropathies: Advances in Inflammation Research, Vol 9. New York, Raven Press, 1985.

98. Aufdermaur M: Pathogenesis of square bodies in ankylosing spondylitis. Ann Rheum Dis 48:628-631, 1989.

99. Calin A, Mackay K, Santos H, Brophy S: A new dimension to outcome: Application of the Bath ankylosing spondylitis radiology index. J Rheumatol 26:988-992, 1999.

100. Dawes PT: Stoke ankylosing spondylitis spine score. J Rheumatol 26:993-996, 1999.

101. Creemers MC, Franssen MJ, van't Hof MA, et al: Assessment of outcome in ankylosing spondylitis: An extended radiographic scoring system. Ann Rheum Dis 64:127-129, 2005.

102. Braun J, Bollow M, Eggens U, et al: Use of dynamic magnetic resonance imaging with fast imaging in the detection of early and advanced sacroiliitis in spondylarthropathy patients. Arthritis Rheum 37:1039-1045, 1994.

103. Braun J, Bollow M, Remlinger G, et al: Prevalence of spondyloarthropathies in HLA-B27 positive and negative blood donors. Arthritis Rheum 41:58-67, 1998.

104. McGonagle D, Gibbon W, O'Connor P, et al: Characteristic magnetic resonance imaging entheseal changes of knee synovitis in spondyloarthropathy. Arthritis Rheum 41:694-700, 1998.

105. Lukas C, Braun J, van der Heijde D, et al: Scoring inflammatory activity of the spine by magnetic resonance imaging in ankylosing spondylitis. A multi-reader experiment. J Rheumatol (in press).

106. Wittram C, Whitehouse GH, Williams JW, et al: A comparison of MR and CT in suspected sacroiliitis. J Comput Assist Tomogr 20:68-72, 1996.

107. Geijer M, Sihlbom H, Gothlin JH, et al: The role of CT in the diagnosis of sacroiliitis. Acta Radiol 39:265-268, 1998.

108. van Tubergen A, Heuft-Dorenbosch L, Schulpen G, et al: Radiographic assessment of sacroiliitis by radiologists and rheumatologists: Does training improve quality? Ann Rheum Dis 62:519-525, 2003.

109. Khan MA, Khan MK: Diagnostic value of HLA-B27 testing in ankylosing spondylitis and Reiter's syndrome. Ann Intern Med 96:70-76, 1982.

110. Heuft-Dorenbosch L, Landewe R, Weijers R, et al: Performance of various criteria sets in patients with inflammatory back pain of short duration: The Maastricht Early Spondyloarthritis Clinic. Ann Rheum Dis 66:92-98, 2007.

111. Dubost JJ, Sauvezie B: Late onset peripheral spondyloarthropathy. J Rheumatol 16:1214-1217, 1989.

112. Kidd B, Mullee M, Frank A, et al: Disease expression of ankylosing spondylitis in males and females. J Rheumatol 15:1407-1409, 1988.

113. Jimenez-Balderas FJ, Mintz G: AS: Clinical course in women and men. J Rheumatol 20:2069-2072, 1993.

114. Østensen M, Østensen H: Ankylosing spondylitis—the female aspect. J Rheumatol 25:120-124, 1998.

115. Østensen M, Fuhrer L, Mathieu R, et al: A prospective study of pregnant patients with rheumatoid arthritis and ankylosing spondylitis using validated clinical instruments. Ann Rheum Dis 63:1212-1217, 2004.

116. Khan MA, Khan MK, Kushner I: Survival among patients with ankylosing spondylitis: A lifetable analysis. J Rheumatol 8:86-90, 1981.

117. Lehtinen K: Mortality and causes of death in 398 patients admitted to hospital with ankylosing spondylitis. Ann Rheum Dis 52:174-176, 1993.

118. Calin A, Elswood J, Rigg S, et al: Ankylosing spondylitis: An analytical review of 1500 patients—the changing pattern of disease. J Rheumatol 15:1234-1238, 1988.

119. Fries JF, Singh G, Bloch DA, et al: The natural history of ankylosing spondylitis: Is the disease really changing? J Rheumatol 16:860-863, 1989.

120. Van der Paardt M, Dijkmans B, Giltay E, van de Horst-Bruinsma I: Dutch patients with familial and sporadic ankylosing spondylitis do not differ in disease phenotype. J Rheumatol 29:2583-2584, 2002.

121. Wanders A, Landewe R, Dougados M, et al: Association between radiographic damage of the spine and spinal mobility for individual patients with ankylosing spondylitis: Can assessment of spinal mobility be a proxy for radiographic evaluation? Ann Rheum Dis 64:988-994, 2005.

122. Guillemin F, Briancon S, Pourel J, Gaucher A: Long-term disability and prolonged sick leaves as outcome measurements in ankylosing spondylitis: Possible predictive factors. Arthritis Rheum 33:1001-1006, 1990.

123. Ramos-Remus C, Prieto-Parra RE, Michel-Diaz J, et al: A five-year cumulative analysis of labor-status and lost working days in patients with ankylosing spondylitis (AS). Arthritis Rheum 41(Suppl):1136, 1998.

124. Ward M, Kuzis S: Risk factors for work disability in patients with ankylosing spondylitis. J Rheumatol 28:315-321, 2001.

125. Boonen A, Chorus A, Miedema H, et al: Withdrawal from labour force due to work disability in patients with ankylosing spondylitis. Ann Rheum Dis 60:1033-1039, 2001.

126. Chorus AMJ, Boonen A, Miedema HS, van der Linden S: Employment perspectives of patients with ankylosing spondylitis. Ann Rheum Dis 61:693-699, 2002.

127. Boonen A, Chorus A, Miedema H, et al: Employment, work disability, and work days lost in patients with ankylosing spondylitis: A cross sectional study of Dutch patients. Ann Rheum Dis 60:353-358, 2001.

128. Gran JT, Skomsvolly JF: The outcome of ankylosing spondylitis: A study of 100 patients. Br J Rheumatol 36:766-771, 1997.

129. Amor B, Silva-Santos R, Nahal R, et al: Predictive factors for the long-term outcome of spondyloarthropathies. J Rheumatol 21:1883-1887, 1994.

130. Calin A, Elswood J: The outcome of 138 total hip replacements and 12 revisions in ankylosing spondylitis: High success rate after a mean followup of 7.5 years. J Rheumatol 16:955-958, 1989.

131. Calin A, Garrett S, Whitelock H, et al: A new approach to defining functional ability in ankylosing spondylitis: The development of the Bath ankylosing spondylitis functional index (BASFI). J Rheumatol 21:2281-2285, 1994.

132. Dougados M, Gueguen A, Nakache JP, et al: Evaluation of a functional index and an articular index in ankylosing spondylitis. J Rheumatol 15:302-307, 1988.

133. Garrett S, Jenkinson T, Whitelock H, et al: A new approach to defining disease status in AS: The Bath ankylosing spondylitis disease activity index (BASDAI). J Rheumatol 21:2286-2291, 1994.

134. Jenkinson TR, Mallorie PA, Whitelock H, et al: Defining spinal mobility in ankylosing spondylitis (AS): The Bath AS metrology index (BASMI). J Rheumatol 21:1694-1698, 1994.

135. **Van der Heijde D, Calin A, Dougados M, et al: Selection of specific instruments for each domain in core set for DC-ART, SM-ARD, physical therapy and clinical record keeping in ankylosing spondylitis: Progress report of ASAS working group. J Rheumatol 26: 951-954, 1999.**

136. Anderson JJ, Baron G, van der Heijde D, et al: Ankylosing spondylitis assessment group preliminary definition of short-term improvement in ankylosing spondylitis. Arthritis Rheum 44:1876-1886, 2001.

137. Brandt J, Listing J, Sieper J, et al: Development and preselection of criteria for short term improvement after anti-TNFα treatment in ankylosing spondylitis. Ann Rheum Dis 63:1438-1444, 2004.

138. Doward LC, Spoorenberg A, Cook SA, et al: Development of the ASQoL: A quality of life instrument specific to ankylosing spondylitis. Ann Rheum Dis 62:20-26, 2003.

139. Davis J, Revicki D, van der Heijde D, et al: Health-related quality of life outcomes in patients with active ankylosing spondylitis treated with adalimumab: Results from a randomized controlled study. Arthritis Rheum (in press).

140. **Zochling J, van der Heijde D, Dougados M, et al: Current evidence for the management of ankylosing spondylitis: A systematic literature review for the ASAS/EULAR management recommendations in ankylosing spondylitis. Ann Rheum Dis 65:423-432, 2006.**

141. **Zochling J, van der Heijde D, Burgos-Vargas R, et al: ASAS/EULAR recommendations for the management of ankylosing spondylitis. Ann Rheum Dis 65:444-452, 2006.**

142. Khan MA, Skosey JL: Ankylosing spondylitis and related spondyloarthropathies. In Samter M (ed): Immunological Diseases. Boston, Little, Brown, 1988, pp 1509-1538.

143. Band DA, Jones SD, Kennedy LG, et al: Which patients with ankylosing spondylitis derive most benefit from inpatient management program? J Rheumatol 24:2381-2384, 1997.

144. Hidding A, van der Linden S, Boers M, et al: Is group physical therapy superior to individualized therapy in ankylosing spondylitis? A randomized controlled trial. Arthritis Care Res 6:117-125, 1993.

145. Dagfinder H, Hagen K: Physiotherapy interventions for ankylosing spondylitis (Cochrane review). Oxford, Cochrane Library, 2001.

146. van Tubergen A, Landewé R, van der Heijde D, et al: Combined spa-exercise therapy is effective in patients with ankylosing spondylitis: A randomized controlled trial. Arthritis Rheum 45:430-438, 2001.

147. van Tubergen A, Boonen A, Landewé R, et al: Cost-effectiveness of combined spa-exercise therapy in ankylosing spondylitis: A randomized controlled trial. Arthritis Rheum 47:459-467, 2002.

148. **Dagfnrud H, Kvien TK, Hagen KB: Physiotherapy interventions for ankylosing spondylitis. Cochrane Database of Systematic Reviews 4, art. no.CD002822.pub2.DOI, 2004.**

149. Dougados M, Gueguen A, Nakache JP, et al: Ankylosing spondylitis: What is the optimum duration of a clinical study? A one year versus 6 weeks non-steroidal anti-inflammatory drug trial. Rheumatology 38:235-244, 1999.

150. Dougados M, Behier JM, Jolchine I, et al: Efficacy of celecoxib, a cyclooxygenase 2-specific inhibitor, in the treatment of ankylosing spondylitis: A six week controlled study with comparison against placebo and against a conventional nonsteroidal anti-inflammatory drug. Arthritis Rheum 44:180-185, 2001.

151. Wanders A, van der Heijde D, Landewe R, et al: Nonsteroidal anti-inflammatory drugs reduce radiographic progression in patients with ankylosing spondylitis: A randomized controlled trial. Arthritis Rheum 52:1756-1765, 2005.

152. Boersma JW: Retardation of ossification of the lumbar vertebral column in ankylosing spondylitis by means of phenylbutazone. Scand J Rheumatol 5:60-64, 1976.

153. Akkoc N, van der Linden S, Khan MA: Ankylosing spondylitis and symptom-modifying vs disease-modifying therapy. Clin Rheumatol 20:539-557, 2006.

154. Amor B, Kahan A, Dougados M, Delrieu F: Sulphasalazine in ankylosing spondylitis. Ann Intern Med 101:878, 1984.

155. Dougados M, van der Linden S, Leirisalo-Repo M, et al: Sulfasalazine in the treatment of spondyloarthropathy. Arthritis Rheum 38:618-627, 1995.

156. Clegg DO, Reda DJ, Weisman MH, et al: Comparison of sulfasalazine and placebo in the treatment of ankylosing spondylitis. Arthritis Rheum 39:2004-2012, 1996.

157. Braun J, Zochling J, Baraliakos X, et al: Efficacy of sulfasalazine in patients with inflammatory back pain due to undifferentiated spondyloarthritis and early ankylosing spondylitis: A multicentre randomised controlled trial. Ann Rheum Dis 65:1147-1153, 2006.

158. **Chen J, Liu C: Is sulfasalazine effective in ankylosing spondylitis? A systematic review of randomized controlled trials. J Rheumatol 33:722-731, 2006.**

159. Roychowdhury B, Bintley-Bagot S, Hunt J, Tunn EJ: Methotrexate in severe ankylosing spondylitis: A randomised placebo controlled, double-blind observer study. Rheumatology 40(Suppl 1):43, 2001.

160. Gonzalez-Lopez L, Garcia-Gonzalez A, Vazquez-del-Mercado M, et al: Efficacy of methotrexate in ankylosing spondylitis: A randomized, double-blind, placebo-controlled trial. J Rheumatol 31:1568-1574, 2004.

161. **Chen J, Liu C: Methotrexate for ankylosing spondylitis. Cochrane Database of Systematic Reviews 3, art. no. CD004524.pub2, 2003.**

162. Haibel H, Rudwaleit M, Braun J, et al: Six month open label trial of leflunomide in ankylosing spondylitis. Ann Rheum Dis 64:124-126, 2005.

163. Van Denderen JC, Van der Paardt M, Nurmohamed MT, et al: Double-blind study of leflunomide in the treatment of active ankylosing spondylitis. Ann Rheum Dis 63(Suppl 1):SAT0033, 2004.

164. Maksymowych WP, Jhangri GS, Fitzgerald AA, et al: A six-month randomized, controlled, double-blind, dose response comparison of intravenous pamidronate (60 mg versus 10 mg) in the treatment of nonsteroidal antiinflammatory drug-refractory ankylosing spondylitis. Arthritis Rheum 46:766-773, 2002.

165. Huang F, Gu J, Zhao W, et al: One-year open-label trial of thalidomide in ankylosing spondylitis. Arthritis Rheum 47:249-254, 2002.

166. Van der Heijde D, Dijkmans B, Geusens P, et al: Efficacy and safety of infliximab in patients with ankylosing spondylitis: Results of a randomized placebo-controlled trial (ASSERT). Arthritis Rheum 52:582-591, 2005.

167. Davis JC Jr, van der Heijde D, Braun J, et al: Recombinant human tumor necrosis factor receptor (etanercept) for treating ankylosing spondylitis. Arthritis Rheum 48:3230-3236, 2003.

168. Van der Heijde D, Kivitz A, Schiff MH, et al: Efficacy and safety of adalimumab in patients with ankylosing spondylitis: Results of a multicenter, randomized, double-blind, placebo-controlled trial. Arthritis Rheum 54:2136-2146, 2006.

169. Baraliakos X, Listing J, Brandt J, et al: Clinical response to discontinuation of anti-TNF therapy in patients with ankylosing spondylitis after 3 years of continuous treatment with infliximab. Arthritis Res Ther 7:439-444, 2005.

170. Braun J, Landewe R, Hermann KG, et al: Major reduction in spinal inflammation in patients with ankylosing spondylitis after treatment with infliximab: Results of a multicenter, randomized, double-blind, placebo-controlled magnetic resonance imaging study. Arthritis Rheum 54:1646-1652, 2006.

171. Rudwaleit M, Listing J, Brandt J, et al: Prediction of a major clinical response (BASDAI 50) to tumour necrosis factor α blockers in ankylosing spondylitis. Ann Rheum Dis 63:665-670, 2004.

172. Maksymowych WP, Inman RD, Gladman D, et al: Canadian Rheumatology Association consensus on the use of anti-TNFα-directed therapies in the treatment of spondyloarthritis. J Rheumatol 30:1356-1363, 2003.

173. **Braun J, Pham T, Sieper J, et al: International ASAS consensus statement for the use of anti-tumour necrosis factor agents in patients with ankylosing spondylitis. Ann Rheum Dis 62:817-824, 2003.**

174. **Braun J, Davis J, Dougados M, et al: ASAS Working Group: First update of the international ASAS consensus statement for the use of anti-TNF agents in patients with ankylosing spondylitis. Ann Rheum Dis 65:316-320, 2006.**

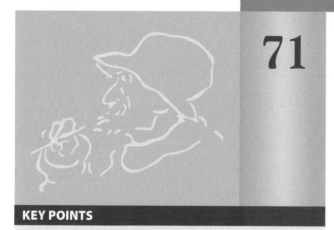

71

Undifferentiated Spondyloarthritis and Reactive Arthritis

DAVID TAK YAN YU •
DENNIS McGONAGLE •
HELENA MARZO-ORTEGA •
FILIP VAN DEN BOSCH •
MARJATTA LEIRISALO-REPO

KEY POINTS

Undifferentiated spondyloarthritis and reactive arthritis are members of the spondyloarthritis family.

Spondyloarthritis is characterized by inflammatory spinal pain or asymmetric oligoarthritis predominantly of the lower extremities.

Undifferentiated spondyloarthritis is distinguished by an absence of ankylosing spondylitis, preceding infection, psoriasis, ulcerative colitis, or Crohn's disease.

Reactive arthritis is characterized by the presence of a triggering infection.

No prospectively validated diagnostic criteria or algorithms exist for undifferentiated spondyloarthritis or reactive arthritis.

Enthesitis is an underlying feature unifying the spondyloarthritis family.

The course of undifferentiaed spondyloarthritis and reactive arthritis varies from individual to individual.

Nonsteroidal anti-inflammatory drugs are the first line of treatment.

The only effective disease-modifying antirheumatic drug is sulfasalazine.

There is a high probability that biologics that block tumor necrosis factor-α are very effective.

The spondyloarthritis family consists of ankylosing spondylitis (AS), undifferentiated spondyloarthritis, some forms of psoriatic arthritis, reactive arthritis, Reiter's syndrome, and arthritis associated with inflammatory bowel disease. The first two are the most common. AS is the best defined, using a series of classification criteria; the most recent are the 1984 modified New York criteria (see Chapter 70). Until recently, this family was known as the spondyloarthropathies. In 2002, however, the Assessment in Ankylosing Spondylitis (ASAS) international working group replaced *spondyloarthropathy* with *spondyloarthritis* to stress that these are inflammatory diseases.[1]

There has also been some confusion over the definition of Reiter's syndrome. Initially, based on a 1916 report of a single patient, the syndrome consisted of the triad of arthritis, urethritis, and conjunctivitis. Eventually, by convention, the term was applied to patients who did not have all three features, as well as being used interchangeably with the term *reactive arthritis*. At this time, the term *Reiter's syndrome* is probably of historical value only.

UNDIFFERENTIATED SPONDYLOARTHRITIS

Because undifferentiated spondyloarthritis is a member of the spondyloarthritis family, strictly speaking, one must define *spondyloarthritis* before one can define *undifferentiated spondyloarthritis*. Spondyloarthritis is caused by multiple genetic and environmental factors, each contributing to various degrees in individual patients. Thus, as in most rheumatic diseases caused by multiple factors, diagnosis ultimately relies on what is termed *expert opinion*. In other words, when an expert in the field, after weighing all the available clinical, laboratory, and imaging information, diagnoses a particular patient as having spondyloarthritis, that patient is regarded as having spondyloarthritis. Although this approach can be effective in clinical practice, if used in research, it would lead to chaos. For purposes of comparing data among different studies, a unified classification definition of spondyloarthritis is needed.

CLASSIFICATION CRITERIA FOR SPONDYLOARTHRITIS

To generate classification criteria for spondyloarthritis, investigators first use the expert-opinion approach to generate two groups of patients: one with spondyloarthritis, and one with other rheumatic diseases. A predetermined set of clinical, laboratory, and radiographic data is collected from these two groups of patients and then submitted to statistical analysis to arrive at a distinguishing set of parameters. Unfortunately, in the case of spondyloarthritis, no single parameter has sufficient discriminating power. To distinguish between the spondyloarthritis group and the control group, investigators must resort to either an algorithm or a combination of parameters. Using these strategies, two sets of classification criteria have been generated by two groups of investigators.

In 1990, a group of French investigators devised a point system, assigning values of 1 to 3 points to each of 12 parameters.[2] A patient is regarded as having spondyloarthritis if the sum of the points is greater than 6. This set is known as the Amor criteria (Table 71-1). Independent of this French study, in 1991, a task force of 11 spondyloarthritis specialists from five different European countries (the European Spondyloarthropathy Study Group [ESSG]) also compared a group of spondyloarthritis patients with a control group of patients with other rheumatic diseases.[3] Again, no single parameter had the power to discriminate between the two groups. This study group selected two parameters as "entry criteria" with moderate discriminative power

Supplemental images available on the Expert Consult Premium Edition website.

1191

Table 71-1   Amor Multiple Entry Criteria for Diagnosing Spondyloarthropathies

A. Clinical Symptoms or Past History

1. Lumbar or dorsal pain at night, or morning stiffness of lumbar or dorsal spine..............................1
2. Asymmetric oligoarthritis..2
3. Buttock pain...1
   If affecting the right and left buttock alternately..2
4. Sausage-like toe or digit..2
5. Heel pain...2
6. Iritis..2
7. Nongonococcal urethritis or cervicitis accompanying, or within 1 mo before, the onset of arthritis.....................1
8. Acute diarrhea accompanying, or within 1 mo before, the onset of arthritis...................................1
9. Presence or history of psoriasis, balanitis, or inflammatory bowel disease (ulcerative colitis or Crohn's disease)... ...2

B. Radiographic Finding

10. Sacroiliitis (grade ≥2 if bilateral; grade ≥3 if unilateral)...3

C. Genetic Background

11. Presence of HLA-B27 or family history of ankylosing spondylitis, Reiter's syndrome, uveitis, psoriasis, or chronic
    enterocolopathies..2

D. Response to Treatment

12. Clear-cut improvement of rheumatic complaints with nonsteroidal anti-inflammatory drugs (NSAIDs) in less than
    48 hr or relapse of pain in less than 48 hr if NSAIDs discontinued...2
A patient is considered to be suffering from a spondyloarthropathy if the sum of the applicable criteria is at least 6.

and minimum overlap: inflammatory low back pain or asymmetric oligoarthritis, preferably of the lower extremities (Table 71-2). Any patient with one of these entry criteria is classified as having spondyloarthritis if he or she satisfies one additional ESSG parameter. This classification system also divides spondyloarthritis patients into two overlapping groups—one with predominantly axial involvement and the other with peripheral involvement. The axial type is mostly likely forme fruste or early AS (see Chapter 70).

Using the ESSG criteria, about half of spondyloarthritis patients can be classified as having AS, reactive arthritis, or arthritis associated with psoriasis or with Crohn's disease or ulcerative colitis. For those patients who cannot be classified into these categories, the term *undifferentiated spondyloarthritis* is used.

DIAGNOSTIC ALGORITHMS

The ESSG classification criteria are not very useful in clinical practice because they do not assign to individual patients a degree of probability of having spondyloarthritis. In clinical practice, a considerable number of patients are diagnosed as having "probable" spondyloarthritis, based on expert opinion, but they might not satisfy the classification criteria. For example, data from the ESSG indicate that inflammatory spinal pain is pivotal in axial spondyloarthritis, but it is not sufficient for a diagnosis.

Rudwaleit and colleagues[4] extracted data from more than 25 publications on patients with axial spondyloarthritis and arrived at a diagnostic algorithm. The probability, expressed as likelihood ratio, of an individual patient having spondyloarthritis can be calculated according to the number of positive parameters. A patient has a greater than 90% probability of having spondyloarthritis if he of she has inflammatory spinal pain plus three to four other features of the disease. This algorithm is called the Berlin criteria for spondyloarthritis.

Table 71-2   European Spondyloarthropathy Study Group Criteria for Spondyloarthropathy

A patient might have a spondyloarthropathy if he or she has at least one of the two following entry criteria:
1. Inflammatory spinal pain: This is defined as a history or present symptoms of spinal pain in the back, dorsal, or cervical region, with at least 4 of the following: (a) onset before age 45 yr, (b) insidious onset, (c) improved by exercise, (d) associated with morning stiffness, (e) at least 3 mo duration.
2. Synovitis: This is defined as past or present asymmetric arthritis or arthritis predominantly in the lower limbs.

A patient who satisfies at least one of the entry criteria is classified as having a spondyloarthropathy if he or she also has one or more of the following parameters:
Positive family history—presence in first-degree or second-degree relatives of any of the following: (a) ankylosing spondylitis, (b) psoriasis, (c) acute uveitis, (d) reactive arthritis, (e) inflammatory bowel disease
Psoriasis—past or present, diagnosed by a physician
Inflammatory bowel disease—past or present Crohn's disease or ulcerative colitis diagnosed by a physician and confirmed by radiographic examination or endoscopy
Urethritis, cervicitis, or acute diarrhea within 1 mo before arthritis—nongonococcal
Buttock pain alternating between right and left gluteal areas—past or present
Enthesopathy—past or present spontaneous pain or tenderness at sites of insertion of the Achilles tendon or plantar fascia
Sacroiliitis—bilateral grade 2 to 4 or unilateral grade 3 or 4, according to the following radiographic grading system: 0 = normal, 1 = possible, 2 = minimal, 3 = moderate, 4 = ankylosis

Most of the studies that have generated the various spondyloarthritis criteria have been based on patients with a disease duration of several years. To address early diagnosis, and to compare the various sets of criteria, a Dutch group examined 68 patients with inflammatory back pain of less than 2 years' duration.[5] Their analysis showed that only 6% of these patients did not fulfill any of the sets of criteria. As many as 53% of patients fulfilled all three sets of criteria for spondyloarthritis. The most sensitive set was the ESSG criteria.

Thus, at this point, we have a plethora of clinical criteria and algorithms for the classification and diagnosis of spondyloarthritis. It is clear that large-scale prospective studies are necessary to arrive at even more useful diagnostic criteria. It is also clear that additional parameters are required to provide a higher degree of predictive power. The most promising involves magnetic resonance imaging (MRI).

SIGNS, SYMPTOMS, AND COURSE OF SPONDYLOARTHRITIS

No large-scale multinational studies have reported on the signs and symptoms of undifferentiated spondyloarthritis. Because it is defined by the exclusion of traditionally well-recognized arthritides, patients determined to have undifferentiated spondyloarthritis probably exhibit a mixture of diverse signs and symptoms, one of which is either inflammatory low back pain or asymmetric oligoarthritis.

No large-scale longitudinal studies are available concerning the course and prognosis of undifferentiated spondyloarthritis. Some studies show that after several years of follow-up, some patients go into remission, some develop AS, and others continue to have undifferentiated spondyloarthritis.[1] A considerable number of patients were initially misdiagnosed with spondyloarthritis, and their actual diagnoses, such as rheumatoid arthritis (RA) or gout, did not become clear until several years later. Clearly, a diagnostic method based on something other than expert opinion or classification criteria is needed. Most useful would be parameters that can predict whether a patient will progress rapidly into AS, because these patients might benefit from early, aggressive therapy. In addition, a unifying hypothesis regarding the basic underlying concept of spondyloarthritis would be helpful.

ENTHESITIS

Both spondyloarthritis and rheumatoid arthritis (RA) are inflammatory rheumatic diseases that attack multiple joints. At one time, spondyloarthritis was considered a form of RA. It was Ball[6] who first reported that inflammation at insertions is the important anatomic difference between RA and spondyloarthritis. Inflammation at these areas is termed *enthesitis*. Currently, enthesitis is recognized as one of the three cardinal anatomic lesions in spondyloarthritis; the other two are osteitis and synovitis. Enthesitis has been proposed as the unifying lesion among the diverse inflammatory abnormalities seen in spondyloarthritis.[7]

Anatomy

The enthesis is the site of insertion of a ligament, tendon, fascia, or joint capsule to bone. There are two types of entheses: fibrocartilaginous and fibrous. Fibrocartilaginous entheses are much more numerous than fibrous entheses, and they are usually situated close to the articular margin of the joints. Fibrous entheses are situated at a considerable distance from the joint; the most typical example is the deltoid insertion. Fibrocartilaginous entheses are composed of four regions: tendon, ligament, or joint capsule; fibrocartilage; calcified fibrocartilage; and underlying bone. Hence, the enthesis is

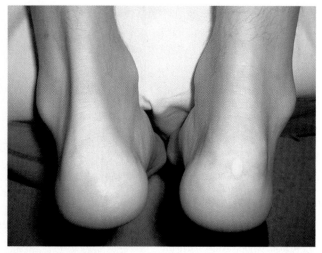

Figure 71-1 Swelling of the right Achilles tendon in a 26-year-old man with spondyloarthritis.

an *organ*, defined as a group of tissues working collectively to carry out a shared function.[8] The enthesis organ functions to aid movement and to limit damage from joint locomotion. The function of fibrocartilage is to dissipate stress and prevent the breakdown of protective mechanisms. Because of the complexity of the entheses and the weight bearing that takes place, there are myriad forces acting at these sites. Insertions are in fact highly prone to microdamage, which includes disruption of the bone cortex, altered vascularity, and tissue repair responses. Therefore, it appears that even healthy, normal insertions have constant tissue turnover and repair and probably microinflammation.[9] These factors are likely important for the localization of inflammatory responses in spondyloarthritis patients.

From the clinical perspective, enthesitis is recognized at characteristic sites, including the Achilles tendon, plantar fascia, patellar tendon, and others (Fig. 71-1). Because of clinical inaccessibility, it has not been well understood until recently that enthesitis is very common at virtually all sites of disease in spondyloarthritis, including the spine and synovial joints.

Histology

Because of the inaccessibility of the enthesis in comparison to the synovium, there is a paucity of data on acute entheseal lesions. However, studies from the sacroiliac joint and peripheral sites confirm the presence of an inflammatory cell infiltrate as well as cytokines, such as tumor necrosis factor-α (TNF-α), at these sites.[10-12]

Historically, enthesitis and osteitis were viewed as separate processes. However, it is now clear that the underlying trabecular bone network plays an integral role in enthesitis. Indeed, the bone cortex and insertions may be focally absent, and the enthesis insertions appear to be linked directly to trabecular bone. This allows for a smooth transition between the soft tissue and the enthesis component and the hard tissue from the adjacent bone component. This close relationship between the entheses and the underlying bone is clinically relevant and is often the basis for recognizing enthesis-related pathology on MRI, where it translates into bone marrow edema or osteitis.[13]

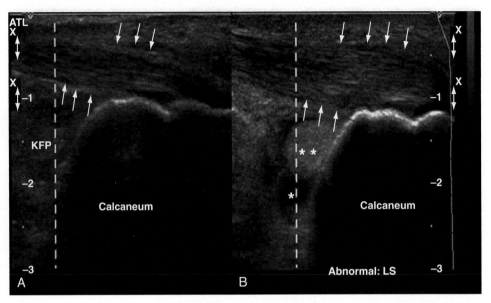

Figure 71-2 Ultrasound (US) images for the patient in Figure 71-1. Images were taken with an HDI 5000 using a linear 12.5-MHz transducer. Both images are longitudinal sections. **A,** Left Achilles tendon (AT), which was normal on both clinical and US examination. The short *white arrows* point to the edges of the tendon, and the *white dotted line (with arrows)* indicates the depth of the tendon. **B,** Abnormal right side, with thickening and hypoechogenicity of the Achilles tendon extending to the insertion. There is also a distended retrocalcaneal bursa. KFP, Kager's fat pad; *, fluid; **, fat pad or synovium.

Imaging

Conventional plain radiography shows enthesitis only at skeletal sites, such as the Achilles tendon or the plantar fascia. However, on MRI or ultrasonography, enthesitis is commonly found at all sites of disease, including the spine and synovial joints.[14] The ultrasound appearance of enthesitis is that of hypoechoic thickening and edema, with erosion, new bone formation, or changes in entheseal vascularity on power Doppler ultrasonography (Fig. 71-2). On MRI, enthesitis can be visualized as perientheseal inflammation with adjacent bone edema in fat-suppressed T2-weighted sequences (Fig. 71-3). Although both MRI and ultrasonography are useful, they are not perfect. Many entheseal sites are inaccessible to the ultrasound probe. In the case of MRI, the intrinsic low water content of insertions makes it difficult to appreciate changes at attachments, especially in small joints.

Clinical Assessment

Only a few entheses are accessible enough for accurate physical examination. The majority of spinal entheses, a common target for spondyloarthritis, are inaccessible. The same is true for entheses around peripheral joints such as the knee, where only 5 or 6 of the more than 30 insertions are accessible to clinical examination. Further, when synovial joints are inflamed and distended, it may be clinically impossible to differentiate among bursitis, synovitis, and enthesitis. For plantar fasciitis, physical examination cannot distinguish between inflammatory and degenerative enthesitis, so the clinician must rely on other features. Also, conditions such as fibromyalgia must be considered, because entheseal sites are commonly affected in this disease.

Notwithstanding these limitations, investigators have developed clinical schemes for scoring enthesitis. These have proved to be of some benefit as disease outcome measures during drug trials.[15]

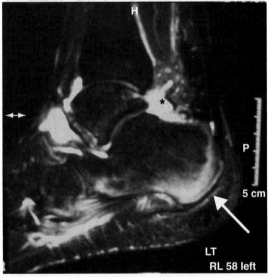

Figure 71-3 Fat-suppressed magnetic resonance image of the foot of a young patient with ankylosing spondylitis. The high signal is consistent with marrow edema, reflecting acute plantar fasciitis *(white arrow)*. In addition, there is retrocalcaneal bursitis *(asterisk)*.

Therapy and Future Directions

There is a misconception that treatment for enthesitis in spondyloarthritis is restricted to isolated lesions, such as those at the Achilles tendon or the plantar fascia. It must be recognized that spondyloarthritis is an inflammatory disease of multiple entheses and associated osteitis. Global treatment of spondyloarthritis is discussed in the next section; however, we have noted that up to 60% of enthesitis or osteitis inflammatory lesions regress almost completely after treatment with a TNF-α blocker.[16] The concept of a functional enthesis as a joint-specific factor, perhaps playing as great a role as the HLA-B27 gene in spondyloarthritis, opens up novel avenues for research into the pathogenesis of spondyloarthritis.

TREATMENT

There are no studies focusing specifically on the pharmacologic approach to undifferentiated spondyloarthritis. Consequently, undifferentiated spondyloarthritis is treated with drugs that are effective for AS: nonsteroidal anti-inflammatory drugs (NSAIDs), conventional disease-modifying antirheumatic drugs (DMARDs), and drugs that block TNF-α.

Nonsteroidal Anti-inflammatory Drugs

The efficacy of NSAIDs in AS and, more generally, in spondyloarthritis is so well accepted that a clear-cut improvement in pain and morning stiffness within 48 hours after starting NSAID therapy, or a rapid relapse of pain after discontinuation of the agent, is one of the Amor spondyloarthritis classification criteria (see Table 71-1). In a multicenter study specifically addressing the effect of NSAIDs in spondyloarthritis,[17] 741 of the 2228 patients suffered from back pain, with spondyloarthritis in 69 and mechanical disorders in 672. Treatment with NSAIDs was considered effective by 53 spondyloarthritis patients (77%), in contrast to only 102 mechanical disorder patients (15%). No data exist on the superiority of one particular NSAID over another, whether NSAIDs should be used continually or on demand, or whether NSAIDs by themselves modify the course of undifferentiated spondyloarthritis. The dosage should be individualized to obtain a good clinical response with minimal side effects. In a substantial number of cases, NSAIDs have to be given at the maximal tolerable dosage.

Disease-Modifying Antirheumatic Drugs

Sulfasalazine at a dose of 2 g/day is the only DMARD that has been tested specifically in undifferentiated spondyloarthritis in a placebo-controlled study.[18] The entry criteria for that 230-patient study were inflammatory low back pain for less than 5 years and classification of spondyloarthritis according to the ESSG criteria (see Table 71-2). None of the patients had radiographic spinal ankylosis, but more than half of them also had peripheral arthritis or enthesitis. After 6 months of therapy, there was no difference between the sulfasalazine group and the placebo group in the primary outcome, which was the Bath ankylosing spondylitis disease activity index (BASDAI). In the subgroup of patients with back pain but no peripheral arthritis, there was significant improvement with sulfasalazine in BASDAI, spinal pain, and morning stiffness. Efficacy in the subgroup without peripheral arthritis contradicted the findings of an earlier study of 619 patients with AS, psoriatic arthritis, and reactive arthritis.[19] There, sulfasalazine was effective only in the subgroup of patients with peripheral arthritis and not the subgroup with predominantly axial disease. Because the entry criteria and primary outcome measures in the two studies were different, it is difficult to determine why the outcomes were different.

At this time, it is reasonable for practicing physicians to provide undifferentiated spondyloarthritis patients a limited trial of sulfasalazine. There are no data that use of sulfasalazine beyond 6 months is useful even in those with a positive response. Although other conventional DMARDs, such as methotrexate, leflunomide, or cyclosporine, are regularly used in psoriatic arthritis, there is no evidence of a beneficial effect in undifferentiated spondyloarthritis.

Antibiotics

Three studies have addressed the usefulness of antimicrobial drugs in patients with undifferentiated spondyloarthritis. In two of the studies, a 3-month course of ciprofloxacin or doxycycline did not produce favorable results in comparison to placebo.[20,21] The third study compared doxycycline alone with a combination of doxycycline and rifampin in 30 undifferentiated spondyloarthritis subjects over a 9-month period.[22] The combination was more effective in treating pain and morning stiffness and in reducing the swollen and tender joint count; however, there was no placebo control.

Tumor Necrosis Factor-α Blockers

As a consequence of the dramatic improvements observed with TNF-α blocking agents in AS and psoriatic arthritis, this cytokine has also been regarded as a prime therapy in other spondyloarthritides. However, it must be stressed that the only evidence in undifferentiated spondyloarthritis comes from case reports or small open-label studies. Brandt and coworkers[23] published their experience in six patients with severe undifferentiated spondyloarthritis treated with 3 or 5 mg/kg infliximab at weeks 0, 2, and 6. The authors reported a significant improvement on day 1 after the first infusion, which lasted until week 12 in five of six patients. Improvement of 50% or greater in disease activity, function, pain, and swollen joint scores was observed in the patients taking 5 mg/kg. The same investigators treated 10 undifferentiated spondyloarthritis patients with etanercept 25 mg twice weekly for 12 weeks and reported a similar 50% or greater regression of disease activity in 60% of patients.[24] After cessation of anti–TNF-α therapy, four of eight patients relapsed after 3 to 6 weeks; two patients went into long-standing remission.

Future Directions in Spondyloarthritis

Even though the prevalence of undifferentiated spondyloarthritis is comparable to that of AS, there is no category I evidence-based recommendation for treatment, with the exception of sulfasalazine; even with that drug, the results of studies are conflicting. There is a high likelihood that TNF-α blockers can be highly effective in many patients. Given the fact that undifferentiated spondyloarthritis is the second most frequent spondyloarthritis subset and that almost 60% of these patients go on to develop AS within 10 years, it is imperative to identify those patients at high risk for functional disability or evolution to more specified diseases. Whether TNF-α therapies can arrest disease progression in this subgroup of patients needs to be studied.

REACTIVE ARTHRITIS

DEFINITION AND CAUSE

The term *reactive arthritis* was defined in 1969 as an arthritis that develops soon after or during an extra-articular infection but in which the microorganism does not enter the joint.[25] Since then, there have been several attempts to generate a validated set of classification and diagnostic criteria; however, at this time, universal agreement has not been reached.[26,27] In 1999, during the Fourth International Workshop on Reactive Arthritis in Berlin, a consensus was reached to use the term *reactive arthritis* only if the clinical picture and the triggering pathogens are "typical."[26] The typical pathogen and most common cause of genital infections is *Chlamydia trachomatis*; 4% of infected patients develop reactive arthritis.[28] The typical microbes in the gastrointestinal tract include *Yersinia*, *Salmonella*, *Shigella*, *Campylobacter*, and, less frequently, *Clostridium difficile*. Besides these classic pathogens, there is a growing list of other alleged candidates (Table 71-3).

GENETICS AND PATHOGENESIS

In hospital-based series, about 60% to 80% of patients are human leukocyte antigen (HLA)-B27 positive. The presence of HLA-B27 is associated with more severe arthritis and extra-articular features and predicts a prolonged disease. In studies of individual outbreaks or in epidemiologic surveys at the population level, there is only a slight or no increased frequency of HLA-B27.[29,30]

The classic reactive arthritis–triggering pathogens are gram-negative obligate or facultative intracellular aerobic bacteria with a lipopolysaccharide-containing outer membrane. They are invasive, and in reactive arthritis, bacterial antigens seem to disseminate from the mucosa to the joints. *Chlamydia*, *Yersinia*, *Salmonella*, and *Shigella* antigens as well as nucleotides have been detected

Table 71-3 Microbial Infections Associated with Reactive Arthritis

Enteric Bacteria
Salmonella: various serovars
Shigella
S. flexneri
S. dysenteriae
S. sonnei
Yersinia
Y. enterocolitica (especially O:3 and O:9)
Y. pseudotuberculosis
Campylobacter
C. jejuni
C. coli
Clostridium difficile
Bacteria Causing Urethritis
Chlamydia trachomatis
*Mycoplasma genitalium**
*Ureaplasma urealyticum**
Bacteria Causing Upper Respiratory Infection
Beta-hemolytic streptococcus*
Chlamydia pneumoniae

*Not well accepted as triggers for reactive arthritis.

in the synovial compartment. The significance of these findings is not clear because bacterial macromolecules and nucleotides have also been found in other types of arthritis and, in the case of *Chlamydia*, in some asymptomatic controls.[31-33]

A recent and more comprehensive hypothesis is one proposed by Gaston and Lillicrap.[34] After invasion via a mucosal route, the microbes persist either in the epithelium or within associated lymphoid tissues, liver, and spleen. The viable organisms or bacterial antigens are disseminated to the joint, causing a local inflammatory response there. A CD4+ T cell response to the invading microorganism drives the arthritic process, most likely supported by a CD8+ T cell response. A deviating or poor T helper type 2 cytokine response may favor the persistence of the microbes or the microbial antigens and contribute to poor elimination of the antigens in the host. Although HLA-B27 is not required for the development of reactive arthritis, its presence contributes to the chronicity of the disease. The favorite hypothesis involves a cross-reaction between microbial structures and HLA-B27 or that HLA-B27 itself might be a target of the immune response.

EPIDEMIOLOGY

There are a few population-based studies on the annual incidence of reactive arthritis, most from Scandinavia. The total incidence has been estimated at 10 to 30 per 100,000.[35-38] Two community-based epidemiologic studies found that *C. trachomatis* and Enterobacteriae play an equal causative role.[38] Single-source epidemics have been observed in association with *Yersinia enterocolitica*, *Yersinia pseudotuberculosis*, *Campylobacter jejuni*, *Shigella flexneri*, and *Salmonella enterica*. The results show that the frequency of reactive arthritis varies greatly among outbreaks, from 0% to 21%.

CLINICAL FEATURES

There is usually a lag of 1 to 4 weeks from the start of infection to the onset of musculoskeletal symptoms. The triggering infection can also be asymptomatic. The patients are usually young adults; reactive arthritis is uncommon in children.[39] Male and female patients have a similar risk of developing reactive arthritis induced by gastrointestinal infection, whereas reactive arthritis triggered by *C. trachomatis* is more frequent in males.

The clinical features of reactive arthritis are summarized in Table 71-4. The typical clinical picture is asymmetric oligoarthritis, often in the large joints of the lower extremities; however, about 50% of patients have arthritis in the upper limbs as well. A mild polyarticular form of arthritis in the small joints has been observed when reactive arthritis is being studied at the population level. Patients can also have dactylitis (Fig. 71-4). About 30% of patients have acute low back pain, typically worse at night, that radiates to the buttocks.

Extra-articular inflammatory symptoms and signs are frequent (see Table 71-4). Enthesitis or bursitis can occur, either in association with arthritis or as the only reactive complication. Other extra-articular features (common

Table 71-4 Clinical Features of Reactive Arthritis in Hospital-Based Studies

	Triggering infection					
	Yersinia	Salmonella	Shigella	Campylobacter	Clostridium difficile	Chlamydia/ Urethritis
Number of joints, mean (range)	6 (1-22)	6 (0-22)	4 (2-11)	3 (1-10)	NA	7 (1-24)
Low back pain (%), mean (range)	30 (16-45)	37 (18-67)	3 (2-50)	24	NA	47
Radiographic sacroiliitis (%), mean (range)	19 (11-20)	11	NA	NA	NA	
Urethritis (%), mean (range)	15 (4-23)	14	69 (50-69)	NA	NA	93
Conjunctivitis (%), mean (range)	6 (6-7)	13 (6-18)	72 (17-78)	NA	NA	41
Iritis (%), mean (range)	7 (6-17)	3	4 (3-17)	NA	NA	
Skin lesions (%), mean (range)	5 (4-7)	2 (2-6)	17	NA	NA	14
Duration of arthritis (mo), mean (range)	3 (1-13)	5 (0-30)	1	0	NA	5 (1-16)
Chronic (>12 mo) course (%), mean (range)	4 (1-24)	19 (0-30)	1	0	NA	14
HLA-B27 positive (%), mean (range)	71 (56-72)	77 (0-94)	83 (83-85)	59	NA	81

NA, not available.

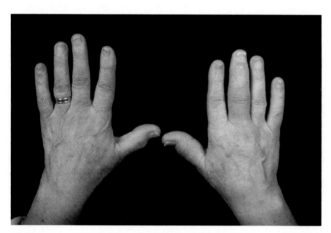

Figure 71-4 Dactylitis (sausage digit) of the right third finger. *(Courtesy of Filip De Keyser.)*

to the other spondyloarthritides as well) include eye symptoms such as conjunctivitis (usual) or acute anterior uveitis (less frequent), various skin rashes, and, in prolonged or chronic cases, nail changes resembling those seen in psoriasis.

LABORATORY TESTS

The only reactive arthritis–specific laboratory tests are those aimed at identifying the triggering pathogens. The most specific tests involve the isolation of microbes from patient samples. Most chlamydial infections are asymptomatic, but for diagnosis, a search for *Chlamydia* in the first portion of the morning urine by ligase reaction is the test of choice. During the acute phase of enteric infections, isolation is usually possible from the stools. However, by the time arthritic complications appear, patients may have recovered from the gastroenteritis, and the microbes may not be detectable in the feces. *Salmonella* and *Yersinia* infections are usually associated with a strong antibody response; consequently, the laboratory diagnosis of reactive arthritis is often dependent on the detection of specific antibodies in the serum.[40] The problem is that there are no international standards for the constellation of serologic tests. Therefore, the usefulness of a test must be validated in each community before it can be applicable to the diagnosis of reactive arthritis. In only about 60% of clinically diagnosed cases of reactive arthritis is evidence of previous infection detected either by serology or by cultures from urogenital or stool samples.

If the clinical picture is typical of reactive arthritis, a positive serologic finding of *Chlamydia*, *Yersinia*, or *Salmonella* has a sensitivity of 73% to 90% and a specificity of 78% to 90%; if *Chlamydia* is detected in the urogenital tract, the sensitivity is 50% and the specificity is 96%. If the clinical picture is not compatible with reactive arthritis, the post-test probability of diagnosing reactive arthritis is much lower.[41] Hence, the clinical picture is pivotal in the diagnosis.

Routine laboratory tests such as acute-phase reactants and synovial fluid analysis are not specific for reactive arthritis. HLA-B27 is not a useful diagnostic tool.

NATURAL HISTORY

Following the acute episode, residual episodic or continuous mild joint or enthesopathy pain is common. Also, one third of patients have occasional attacks of low back pain. Among patients with previous postenteric reactive arthritis, signs and symptoms of chronic spondyloarthritis may occur in 14%. Duration of arthritis for longer than 6 months is arbitrarily regarded as a sign of chronicity. A prolonged (>1 year) extension of acute arthritis has been described in about 4% of *Yersinia*, 19% of *Salmonella*, 19% of *Shigella*, and 17% of *Chlamydia* arthritis patients.[29,30,42] Depending on the triggering infection and the duration of follow-up, chronic arthritis is observed in 2% to 18%, sacroiliitis in 14% to 49%, and AS in 12% to 26% (Table 71-5).

Factors determining the progression of acute reactive arthritis to chronic spondyloarthritis are not clear, but they include the species of the triggering pathogen, the presence of HLA-B27, a positive family history for spondyloarthritis, and the presence of chronic gut inflammation. Patients with Reiter's syndrome triggered by urogenital infection seem to

Table 71-5 Long-Term Prognosis of Enteric Reactive Arthritis

	Salmonella		Yersinia enterocolitica		Shigella
Follow-up time (yr)	5	11	4-5	10	20
No. of patients	27	50	58	107	100
Males (%)	NA	57	39	49	93
HLA-B27 positive (%)	22	88	NA	78	NA
Recovered (%)	33	40	19	49	20
Arthralgia (%)	NA	20	32	19	NA
Low back pain (%)	30	44	NA	37	NA
Recurrent arthritis (%)	37	22	NA	5	18
Iritis during follow-up (%)	NA	NA	NA	14	7
Chronic arthritis (%)	52	16	16	2	18
Ankylosing spondylitis (%)	NA	12	9	16	14
Radiographic sacroiliitis (%)	NA	12	9	30	32
Patients with radiographic erosions in peripheral joints (%)	15	NA	3	0	12

Each column represents results from a single study.
NA, not available.

Table 71-6 Randomized, Double-Blind, Placebo-Controlled Studies of Antimicrobial Chemotherapy for Reactive Arthritis

Reference	Cause	Number of Patients	Duration of Therapy (mo)	Treatment	Result Compared with Placebo
45	Chlamydia	21	3	Lymecycline	Lymecycline effective
	Enteric infections	19	3	Lymecycline	No difference
46	Yersinia	36	3	Ciprofloxacin	No difference
20	Various triggers	55	3	Ciprofloxacin	No difference
47	Various triggers	71	3	Ciprofloxacin	No difference
44	Clinical suspicion of reactive arthritis	152	3	Azithromycin	No difference

be more vulnerable to recurrent urethritides and recurrent episodes of arthritides. In a genetically predisposed subject, it is still uncertain to what extent reactive arthritis contributes to the cause of sacroiliitis or AS. It is possible that sacroiliac changes would have occurred anyway, even in the absence of preceding reactive arthritis.

TREATMENT

Treatment of the Triggering Infection

All patients with acute C. trachomatis infection, as well as their partners, should receive the standard treatment for chlamydial infections. At this time, uncomplicated enteritis preceding reactive arthritis is not an indication for treatment with antimicrobials.

Treatment of Arthritis

The use of NSAIDs, often at the full dose, is usually of major benefit for acute arthritis and spinal pain. Local glucocorticoid injections are also beneficial in patients with mon- or oligoarthritis. Enthesitis responds to local corticosteroid injections as well. Systemic corticosteroids are used if the

patient is bedridden due to severe polyarthritis, is febrile, or has carditis or an atrioventricular conduction disturbance. Reactive arthritis patients seem to need higher doses of systemic prednisone or prednisolone, such as 20 to 40 mg/day, compared with RA patients.

Antibiotics

The effect of short-term and long-term antibiotic therapy to treat reactive arthritis has been a focus of research during the last 20 years. Although no controlled studies exist, some evidence speaks in favor of antibiotics during the infectious phase, even before the arthritis has had time to develop.[43] Once arthritis has developed, however, the introduction of antibiotics does not modify the course of the disease[20, 44-47] (Table 71-6).

Disease-Modifying Antirheumatic Drugs

Because about 50% of patients recover from reactive arthritis within the first 6 months, use of DMARDs is often not considered. There is only limited information on the efficacy of such drugs. Patients with acute reactive arthritis who started sulfasalazine treatment during the first 3 months reached clinical remission more rapidly compared with those in the placebo arm.[48] Sulfasalazine is also effective in chronic reactive arthritis.[49] However, if the drug is ineffective, it should not be continued for more than 6 months. TNF-α blockers are effective in chronic HLA-B27–associated AS, but their use has been reported in only a few cases of reactive arthritis. There appears to be a benefit, and these agents do not cause a relapse of the triggering infection.[50]

REFERENCES

1. Zochling J, Brandt J, Braun J: The current concept of spondyloarthritis with special emphasis on undifferentiated spondyloarthritis. Rheumatology (Oxford) 44:1483-1491, 2005.
2. Amor B, Dougados M, Mijiyawa M: Criteria of the classification of spondylarthropathies. Rev Rhum Mal Osteoartic 57:85-89, 1990.
3. Dougados M, van der Linden S, Juhlin R, et al: The European Spondylarthropathy Study Group preliminary criteria for the classification of spondylarthropathy. Arthritis Rheum 34:1218-1227, 1991.
4. Rudwaleit M, van der Heijde D, Khan MA, et al: How to diagnose axial spondyloarthritis early. Ann Rheum Dis 63:535-543, 2004.
5. Heuft-Dorenbosch L, Landewe R, Weijers R, et al: Performance of various criteria sets in patients with inflammatory back pain of short duration: The Maastricht early spondyloarthritis clinic. Ann Rheum Dis 2006. Available at http://www.ncbi.nlm.nih.gov/entrez/query.fcgi?cmd=Retrieve&db=PubMed&dopt=Citation&list_uids=16868021 (accessed July 25, 2006).
6. Ball J: Enthesopathy of rheumatoid and ankylosing spondylitis. Ann Rheum Dis 30:213-223, 1971.
7. McGonagle D, Gibbon W, Emery P: Classification of inflammatory arthritis by enthesitis. Lancet 352:1137-1140, 1998.
8. Benjamin M, Moriggl B, Brenner E, et al: The "enthesis organ" concept: Why enthesopathies may not present as focal insertional disorders. Arthritis Rheum 50:3306-3313, 2004.
9. Benjamin M, Toumi H, Suzuki D, et al: Microdamage and altered vascularity at the enthesis bone interface provides an anatomical explanation for bone involvement in the HLA-B27 associated spondyloarthropathies and allied disorders. Arthritis Rheum.56:224-233, 2007.
10. Braun J, Bollow M, Neure L, et al: Use of immunohistologic and in situ hybridization techniques in the examination of sacroiliac joint biopsy specimens from patients with ankylosing spondylitis. Arthritis Rheum 38:499-505, 1995.
11. Laloux L, Voisin MC, Allain J, et al: Immunohistological study of entheses in spondyloarthropathies: Comparison in rheumatoid arthritis and osteoarthritis. Ann Rheum Dis 60:316-321, 2001.
12. McGonagle D, Marzo-Ortega H, O'Connor P, et al: Histological assessment of the early enthesitis lesion in spondyloarthropathy. Ann Rheum Dis 61:534-537, 2002.
13. McGonagle D, Marzo-Ortega H, Benjamin M, et al: Report on the Second International Enthesitis Workshop. Arthritis Rheum 48:896-905, 2003.
14. Balint PV, Kane D, Wilson H, et al: Ultrasonography of entheseal insertions in the lower limb in spondyloarthropathy. Ann Rheum Dis 61:905-910, 2002.
15. Mander M, Simpson JM, McLellan A, et al: Studies with an enthesis index as a method of clinical assessment in ankylosing spondylitis. Ann Rheum Dis 46:197-202, 1987.
16. Marzo-Ortega H, McGonagle D, O'Connor P, et al: Efficacy of etanercept in the treatment of the entheseal pathology in resistant spondylarthropathy: A clinical and magnetic resonance imaging study. Arthritis Rheum 44:2112-2117, 2001.
17. Amor B, Dougados M, Listrat V, et al: Evaluation of the Amor criteria for spondylarthropathies and European Spondylarthropathy Study Group (ESSG): A cross-sectional analysis of 2228 patients. Ann Med Interne (Paris) 142:85-89, 1991.
18. **Braun J, Zochling J, Baraliakos X, et al: Efficacy of sulfasalazine in patients with inflammatory back pain due to undifferentiated spondyloarthritis and early ankylosing spondylitis: A multicentre randomised controlled trial. Ann Rheum Dis 65:1147-1153, 2006.**
19. **Clegg DO, Reda DJ, Abdellatif M: Comparison of sulfasalazine and placebo for the treatment of axial and peripheral articular manifestations of the seronegative spondylarthropathies: A Department of Veterans Affairs cooperative study. Arthritis Rheum 42:2325-2329, 1999.**
20. **Sieper J, Fendler C, Laitko S, et al: No benefit of long-term ciprofloxacin treatment in patients with reactive arthritis and undifferentiated oligoarthritis: A three-month, multicenter, double-blind, randomized, placebo-controlled study. Arthritis Rheum 42:1386-1396, 1999.**
21. **Smieja M, MacPherson DW, Kean W, et al: Randomised, blinded, placebo controlled trial of doxycycline for chronic seronegative arthritis. Ann Rheum Dis 60:1088-1094, 2001.**
22. Carter JD, Valeriano J, Vasey FB: Doxycycline versus doxycycline and rifampin in undifferentiated spondyloarthropathy, with special reference to chlamydia-induced arthritis: A prospective, randomized 9-month comparison. J Rheumatol 31:1973-1980, 2004.
23. Brandt J, Haibel H, Reddig J, et al: Successful short term treatment of severe undifferentiated spondyloarthropathy with the anti-tumor necrosis factor-alpha monoclonal antibody infliximab. J Rheumatol 29:118-122, 2002.
24. Brandt J, Khariouzov A, Listing J, et al: Successful short term treatment of patients with severe undifferentiated spondyloarthritis with the anti-tumor necrosis factor-alpha fusion receptor protein etanercept. J Rheumatol 31:531-538, 2004.
25. Ahvonen P, Sievers K, Aho K: Arthritis associated with *Yersinia enterocolitica* infection. Acta Rheumatol Scand 15:232-253, 1969.
26. Kingsley G, Sieper J: Third International Workshop on Reactive Arthritis. 23-26 September 1995, Berlin, Germany: Report and abstracts. Ann Rheum Dis 55:564-584, 1996.
27. Pacheco-Tena C, Burgos-Vargas R, Vazquez-Mellado J, et al: A proposal for the classification criteria for clinical and experimental studies on reactive arthritis. J Rheumatol 26:1338-1346, 1999.
28. Rich E, Hook EW 3rd, Alarcon GS, et al: Reactive arthritis in patients attending an urban sexually transmitted diseases clinic. Arthritis Rheum 39:1172-1177, 1996.
29. Leirisalo-Repo M, Helenius P, Hannu T, et al: Long-term prognosis of reactive salmonella arthritis. Ann Rheum Dis 56:516-520, 1997.
30. Leirisalo-Repo M, Suoranta H: Ten-year follow-up study of patients with *Yersinia* arthritis. Arthritis Rheum 31:533-537, 1988.
31. Cox CJ, Kempsell KE, Gaston JS: Investigation of infectious agents associated with arthritis by reverse transcription PCR of bacterial rRNA. Arthritis Res Ther 5:R1-8, 2003.
32. Schumacher HR Jr, Arayssi T, Crane M, et al: *Chlamydia trachomatis* nucleic acids can be found in the synovium of some asymptomatic subjects. Arthritis Rheum 42:1281-1284, 1999.
33. Wilkinson NZ, Kingsley GH, Jones HW, et al: The detection of DNA from a range of bacterial species in the joints of patients with a variety of arthritides using a nested, broad-range polymerase chain reaction. Rheumatology (Oxford) 38:260-266, 1999.
34. Hill Gaston JS, Lillicrap MS: Arthritis associated with enteric infection. Best Pract Res Clin Rheumatol 17:219-239, 2003.
35. Isomaki H, Raunio J, von Essen R, et al: Incidence of inflammatory rheumatic diseases in Finland. Scand J Rheumatol 7:188-192, 1978.
36. Kvien TK, Glennas A, Melby K, et al: Reactive arthritis: Incidence, triggering agents and clinical presentation. J Rheumatol 21:115-122, 1994.
37. Savolainen E, Kaipiainen-Seppanen O, Kroger L, et al: Total incidence and distribution of inflammatory joint diseases in a defined population: Results from the Kuopio 2000 arthritis survey. J Rheumatol 30:2460-2468, 2003.
38. Soderlin MK, Kautiainen H, Puolakkainen M, et al: Infections preceding early arthritis in southern Sweden: A prospective population-based study. J Rheumatol 30:459-464, 2003.
39. Rudwaleit M, Richter S, Braun J, et al: Low incidence of reactive arthritis in children following a salmonella outbreak. Ann Rheum Dis 60:1055-1057, 2001.
40. Granfors K, Viljanen M, Tiilikainen A, et al: Persistence of IgM, IgG, and IgA antibodies to *Yersinia* in *Yersinia* arthritis. J Infect Dis 141:424-429, 1980.
41. Sieper J, Rudwaleit M, Braun J, et al: Diagnosing reactive arthritis: Role of clinical setting in the value of serologic and microbiologic assays. Arthritis Rheum 46:319-327, 2002.
42. Sairanen E, Paronen I, Mahonen H: Reiter's syndrome: A follow-up study. Acta Med Scand 185:57-63, 1969.
43. Bardin T, Enel C, Cornelis F, et al: Antibiotic treatment of venereal disease and Reiter's syndrome in a Greenland population. Arthritis Rheum 35:190-194, 1992.
44. **Kvien TK, Gaston JS, Bardin T, et al: Three month treatment of reactive arthritis with azithromycin: A EULAR double blind, placebo controlled study. Ann Rheum Dis 63:1113-1119, 2004.**

45. Lauhio A, Leirisalo-Repo M, Lahdevirta J, et al: Double-blind, placebo-controlled study of three-month treatment with lymecycline in reactive arthritis, with special reference to Chlamydia arthritis. Arthritis Rheum 34:6-14, 1991.

46. Toivanen A, Yli-Kerttula T, Luukkainen R, et al: Effect of antimicrobial treatment on chronic reactive arthritis. Clin Exp Rheumatol 11:301-307, 1993.

47. Yli-Kerttula T, Luukkainen R, Yli-Kerttula U, et al: Effect of a three month course of ciprofloxacin on the outcome of reactive arthritis. Ann Rheum Dis 59:565-570, 2000.

48. Egsmose C, Hansen TM, Andersen LS, et al: Limited effect of sulphasalazine treatment in reactive arthritis: A randomised double blind placebo controlled trial. Ann Rheum Dis 56:32-36, 1997.

49. Clegg DO, Reda DJ, Weisman MH, et al: Comparison of sulfasalazine and placebo in the treatment of reactive arthritis (Reiter's syndrome): A Department of Veterans Affairs cooperative study. Arthritis Rheum 39:2021-2027, 1996.

50. Flagg SD, Meador R, Hsia E, et al: Decreased pain and synovial inflammation after etanercept therapy in patients with reactive and undifferentiated arthritis: An open-label trial. Arthritis Rheum 53:613-617, 2005.

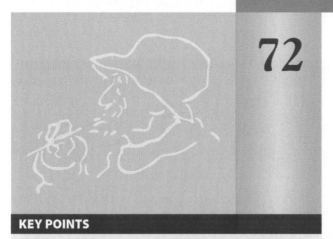

72 Psoriatic Arthritis 📷 🎥

OLIVER FITZGERALD

KEY POINTS

Psoriatic arthritis should be suspected in a patient with an asymmetric joint distribution pattern who may have additional clinical features, such as dactylitis, enthesitis, or inflammatory-type back pain, and who is negative for rheumatoid factor. In such patients, a careful search for psoriasis is warranted.

New classification criteria, the Classification of Psoriatic Arthritis (CASPAR) criteria, have been published more recently.

Psoriatic arthritis is a progressive disease, with 47% of patients developing erosions within 2 years of diagnosis. Polyarticular disease and an elevated erythrocyte sedimentation rate are markers of poor outcome.

An essential core set of domains and instruments is now agreed as being necessary for inclusion in clinical trials.

Studies of synovial tissue have highlighted an increase in vascularity and the presence of neutrophils as helping to distinguish spondyloarthropathy from rheumatoid arthritis.

Prominent entheseal involvement with bone marrow edema at entheseal insertions on magnetic resonance imaging has prompted the hypothesis that psoriatic arthritis may originate at the enthesis.

A role for CD8+ T cells and the innate immune response has been proposed.

Although there is a paucity of evidence for efficacy of disease-modifying antirheumatic drugs in psoriatic arthritis, tumor necrosis factor inhibitors have proved effective for skin and joint disease.

Psoriatic arthritis is a member of the spondyloarthropathy family and may be defined as an inflammatory arthropathy associated with psoriasis and usually negative for rheumatoid factor. Until the 1950s, an inflammatory arthritis occurring in the presence of psoriasis was thought to represent rheumatoid arthritis (RA) occurring coincidentally with psoriasis. Based primarily on clinical and radiologic grounds and using the rheumatoid factor, the distinction between RA and psoriatic arthritis became gradually accepted. Wright described the classic clinical features in 1959 and together with his colleague Moll, he published his classification criteria in 1973.[1,2] These criteria have remained until more recently the simplest and the most frequently used in clinical studies. The American Association of Rheumatism included psoriatic arthritis as a distinct clinical entity in the classification of rheumatic diseases for the first time in 1964.[3]

EPIDEMIOLOGY

Epidemiologic studies have supported the concept that psoriatic arthritis is a unique disease entity separate from RA. The prevalence of inflammatory arthritis is increased among patients with psoriasis, ranging from 7% to 25% compared with a general population estimate of 2% to 3%. The prevalence of psoriasis subjects with arthritis also is increased at 2.6% to 7% compared with a general population estimate of 0.1% to 2.8%.[4]

Psoriasis affects about 2% of the population. The prevalence varies, with 5% to 10% of Russians and Norwegians affected and only 0% to 0.3% of West Africans or Native Americans affected.[5] Onset of psoriasis may be at any age, but most frequently peaks in the 20s. Although there is no gender predilection, there is a genetic predisposition.

Of patients with psoriasis, 7% to 42% develop arthritis. This figure varies so widely partly because of a lack of widely accepted diagnostic criteria, but also depending on what population is being studied. The exact prevalence and incidence of psoriatic arthritis are unknown. The reported prevalence of psoriatic arthritis varied from 0.056% to 0.28% in a large population-based study in the United States.[6] Cases were defined as patients who reported a "physician diagnosis" of psoriasis and psoriatic arthritis. The prevalence was calculated at 0.25% (95% confidence interval, 0.18% to 0.31%). Kay and colleagues[7] did a prevalence study in northeast England evaluating records from six general practices; 81 of 772 psoriasis subjects had an inflammatory arthritis with a prevalence of 0.28%. The reported incidence of psoriatic arthritis has varied from 3 to 23 per 100,000. Data from Rochester, New York, have shown an incidence rate of 6.59 per 100,000, whereas in Finland, 16 new cases of psoriatic arthritis were identified in a population of 87,000, giving a mean incidence rate of 23 per 100,000.[8,9]

CLINICAL FEATURES

Plaque psoriasis or psoriasis vulgaris is the most common skin phenotype in patients with psoriatic arthritis. Other patterns of skin involvement may be seen (Fig. 72-1). Although the arthritis usually develops in a setting of an established diagnosis of psoriasis, some patients may be unaware that they have psoriasis, or psoriasis may develop after the onset of arthritis in approximately 15% of cases.[10] If a patient presents with the classic articular manifestations of psoriatic arthritis, but does not volunteer psoriasis or the presence of a rash, it is incumbent on the physician to examine the patient's skin carefully, including the scalp and nails because psoriasis frequently lurks in such areas. Examples of nail dystrophic changes are shown in Figure 72-2.

📷 Supplemental images available on the Expert Consult Premium Edition website.
🎥 Video available on the Expert Consult Premium Edition website.

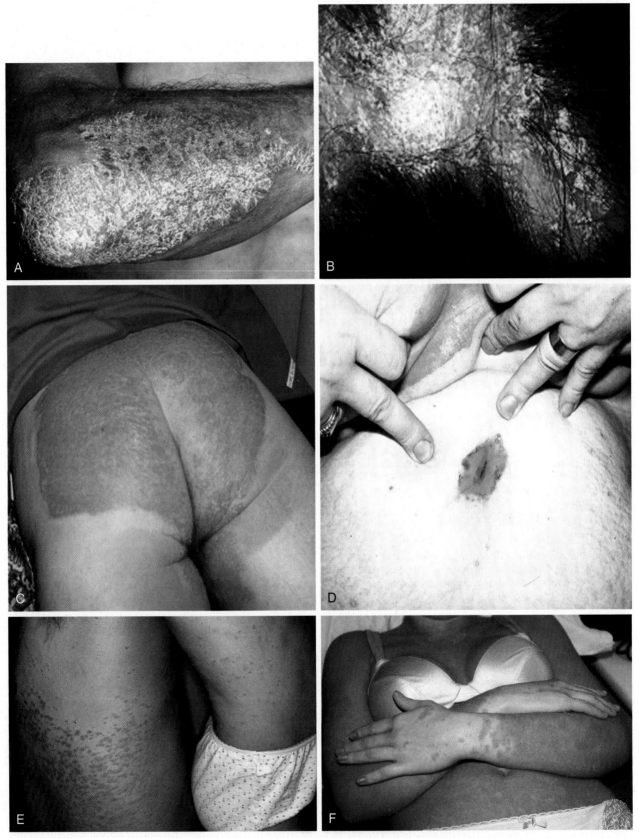

Figure 72-1 Clinical phenotypes in psoriasis; **A** to **H,** Plaque psoriasis (psoriasis vulgaris). **A,** At extensor surface of elbow and on scalp (**B**); genital psoriasis (**C**); inframammary and umbilical flexural psoriasis (**D**); guttate psoriasis in a father and child (**E**); erythrodermic psoriasis on the trunk and upper limbs (**F**).

Continued

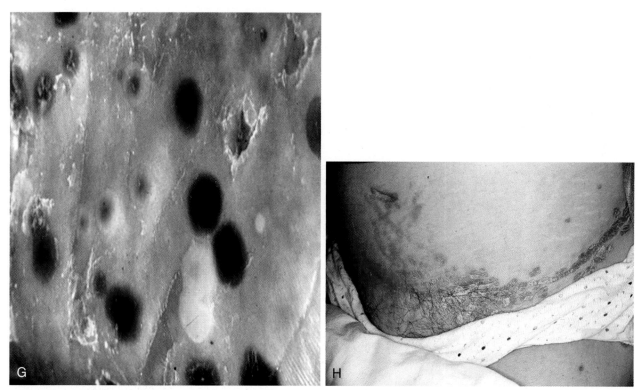

Figure 72-1, cont'd **G,** Pustular psoriasis on the foot; and the Koebner phenomenon on a surgical abdominal wound (**H**).

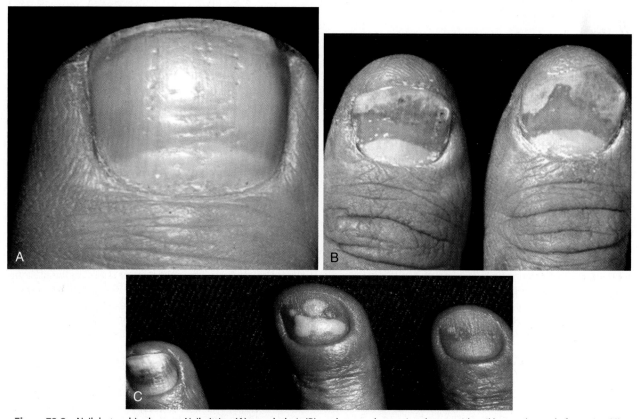

Figure 72-2 Nail dystrophic changes. Nail pitting (**A**); onycholysis (**B**), and severe destructive change with nail loss and pustule formation (**C**).

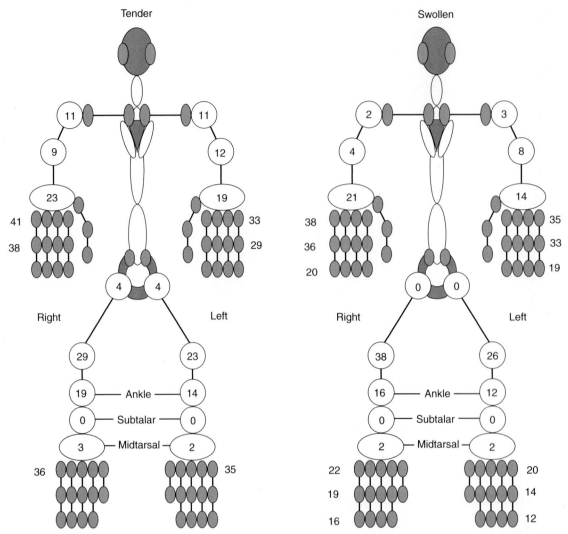

Figure 72-3 Frequency (%) of peripheral limb joint involvement in 129 patients with early psoriatic arthritis as assessed by joint tenderness and swelling (distal interphalangeal joints of hand and proximal and distal interphalangeal joints of feet not assessed for tenderness as part of Ritchie Articular Index).

Although a more recent U.S. study suggests that the prevalence of psoriatic arthritis among psoriasis patients increases with psoriasis severity,[6] in clinical practice, there seems to be little relationship between severity of skin involvement and severity of arthritis. In one prospective study, only 35% of patients reported that their skin and joint components flared at the same time.[10]

Patients with psoriatic arthritis present with symptoms and signs of joint, entheseal, or spinal inflammation. The joints involved at presentation in 129 early psoriatic arthritis patients are shown in Figure 72-3. In one of their seminal papers on psoriatic arthritis, Wright and Moll[11] described five clinical patterns of psoriatic arthritis (Fig. 72-4):

1. Asymmetric oligoarthritis
2. Symmetric polyarthritis
3. Predominant distal interphalangeal (DIP) joint involvement
4. Predominant spondyloarthritis
5. Destructive (mutilans) arthritis

These classification criteria are the most commonly quoted, although many alternative criteria have been proposed. Variability in the definition of terms has led to

differences in the reported frequency of psoriatic arthritis subsets among the different studies. The pattern of joint involvement is not fixed; the patient's disease may fluctuate and may be influenced by treatment. In a study of 129 patients with early psoriatic arthritis, 53 of 77 initially classified as polyarticular were reassessed at 2 years; 26 of 53 (49%) patients were subsequently classified as oligoarticular, 19 of 53 (36%) remained classified as polyarticular, and 12 of 53 (23%) were in remission.[12]

The Classification of Psoriatic Arthritis (CASPAR) study has included in the analysis a breakdown of disease pattern subtypes.[13] This multicenter study included data on 588 psoriatic arthritis cases and 536 controls. In contrast to the original Moll and Wright paper, but similar to many subsequent publications, approximately 63% of patients had polyarticular joint involvement compared with 13% with oligoarticular disease. The other patterns of joint involvement described by Moll and Wright occurred much less commonly. Predominant DIP disease was found in less than 5%, but DIP involvement can occur in any of the subtypes. Predominant spondyloarthritis also is uncommon, although spinal involvement may be found in 40% to 70% of psoriatic

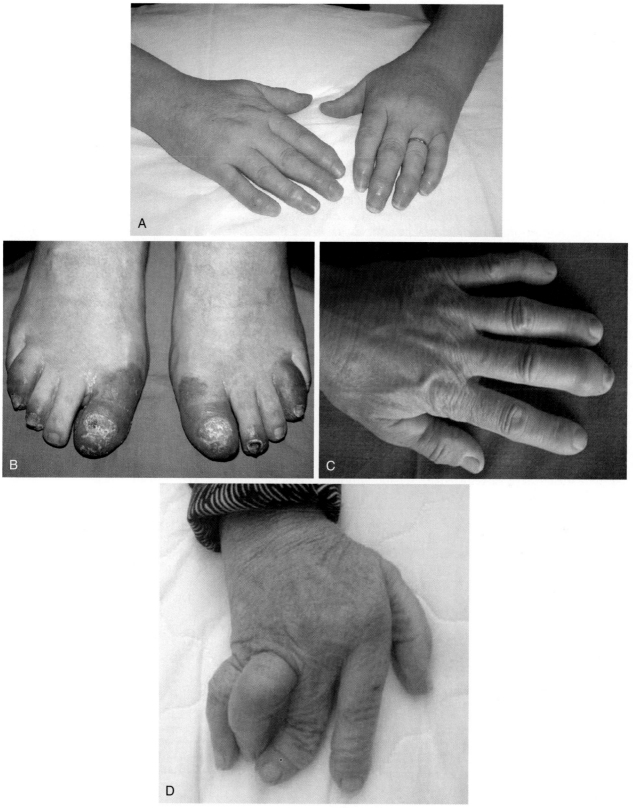

Figure 72-4 Patterns of peripheral joint disease. **A-D,** Asymmetric polyarticular disease. **A,** Distal interphalangeal joint involvement and forearm lymphedema; toe dactylitis with skin and nail change **(B)**; predominant distal interphalangeal joint involvement **(C)**; and arthritis mutilans **(D)**.

arthritis cases depending on whether or not radiographs are taken.[14] Finally, arthritis mutilans, a destructive form of arthritis associated with flail joints, is rare, although more patients may develop this form of joint involvement with time if their disease is not properly controlled.

Features that are typical of psoriatic arthritis are helpful in diagnosis, including dactylitis and enthesitis. Dactylitis, in which there is a sausage-shaped swelling of the fingers or toes (see Fig. 72-4B), may be found in 29% to 33.5% of psoriatic arthritis patients at first presentation, and 48% may have an episode of dactylitis during follow-up.[12,15] Ultrasound and magnetic resonance imaging (MRI) studies have shown that joint and tenosynovial inflammation are prominent in involved digits.[16,17] Enthesitis, inflammation at tendon or ligament insertion into bone, is a feature of all of the spondyloarthropathies and may be a presenting feature in psoriatic arthritis. Overall, enthesitis is found in 38% of patients at presentation.[12] The most common entheseal sites involved are the Achilles and plantar fascia insertions. Other sites include the insertions of the quadriceps and patellar tendons, the iliac crest, the rotator cuff, and the epicondyles at the elbow. Patients complain of pain at these sites with tenderness and sometimes swelling found on examination. Entheseal involvement may be asymptomatic, with ultrasound being more sensitive than clinical palpation. Often spurs are detected on x-ray, although spurs are not always associated with symptoms.

With the obvious exception of psoriasis and nail dystrophic change, extra-articular disease is less common in psoriatic arthritis compared with RA. Iritis or uveitis occurs in 7% to 18%, more bilateral than in ankylosing spondylitis, but usually found in patients with spinal involvement.[10,18] Numerous studies have suggested that psoriatic arthritis patients have a higher prevalence of inflammatory bowel disease, sometimes asymptomatic and detected only on biopsy specimen.[19,20] Whether this inflammatory bowel disease is coincidental or possibly related to medication effects remains to be clarified. Distal limb edema or lymphedema may occur more commonly in psoriatic arthritis; one case-control study found it in 21% of psoriatic arthritis patients compared with 4.9% of controls (see Fig. 72-4A).[21] Finally, amyloid is rare, but is described in psoriatic arthritis.

DIFFERENTIAL DIAGNOSIS

Certain articular features if present are useful in distinguishing psoriatic arthritis from RA, including dactylitis, DIP involvement, and inflammation at entheseal sites (Table 72-1; see Fig. 72-4). In addition, inflammatory-type back pain or sacroiliitis on plain-x-ray or MRI should raise the suspicion of psoriatic arthritis because spinal involvement is uncommon in RA. The absence of rheumatoid nodules or other systemic features common to RA can be another useful differentiating feature.

Distinguishing psoriatic arthritis from other spondyloarthropathies also is important. Dactylitis may be a feature in reactive arthritis where a palmoplantar pustular rash (keratoderma blennorrhagicum) may be clinically and histologically indistinguishable from pustular psoriasis (see Fig. 72-1G). In relation to spinal involvement, sacroiliitis may be unilateral more frequently, and the spinal changes

Table 72-1 Clinical Features That Best Distinguish Psoriatic Arthritis from Rheumatoid Arthritis

	Psoriatic Arthritis	Rheumatoid Arthritis
Psoriasis	+	−
Symmetric	+	++
Asymmetric	++	+
Enthesopathy	+	−
Dactylitis	+	−
Nail dystrophy	+	−
HIV association	+	−

HIV, human immunodeficiency virus.

on plain radiography may be more asymmetric in psoriatic arthritis compared with classic ankylosing spondylitis. Finally, crystal-associated arthropathies occasionally can confuse, especially with monarticular disease, and are best distinguished by synovial fluid crystal analysis. Serum urate levels may be increased in patients with psoriatic arthritis adding to the confusion.

LABORATORY FEATURES

There is no diagnostic laboratory test for psoriatic arthritis. Although the absence of rheumatoid factor is considered an important distinguishing feature from RA, low levels of rheumatoid factor may be found in patients (5% to 16%) with typical psoriatic arthritis features. Until there is a more definitive diagnostic test, it is difficult to be categorical about diagnosis in these patients. Cyclic citrullinated peptide antibodies were initially thought to be specific to RA, but it is now recognized that cyclic citrullinated peptide antibodies are found in approximately 5% of psoriatic arthritis patients as well.[22] Acute-phase markers, such as erythrocyte sedimentation rate, C-reactive protein, or serum amyloid A, all may be elevated in psoriatic arthritis patients, but less commonly and to a lesser degree than in RA patients. These markers are elevated in particular in patients with polyarticular disease and act as a marker of poor prognosis.[23] Finally, as mentioned previously, hyperuricemia may be found in association with metabolic abnormalities in psoriatic arthritis patients and not reflecting the extent of skin involvement.

RADIOGRAPHIC FEATURES

Although there have been substantial advances in the application, in particular, of musculoskeletal ultrasound (MSUS) and of MRI in patients with arthritis, including psoriatic arthritis, plain radiographic imaging remains the "gold standard" for assessing bony changes in peripheral joints in psoriatic arthritis.

PLAIN RADIOGRAPHY

Sixty-seven percent of patients with established psoriatic arthritis have radiographic abnormalities,[10] and 47% of patients with recent-onset psoriatic arthritis will have developed erosions within 2 years of disease onset.[12] Distinctive radiographic features reflect in some cases the clinical

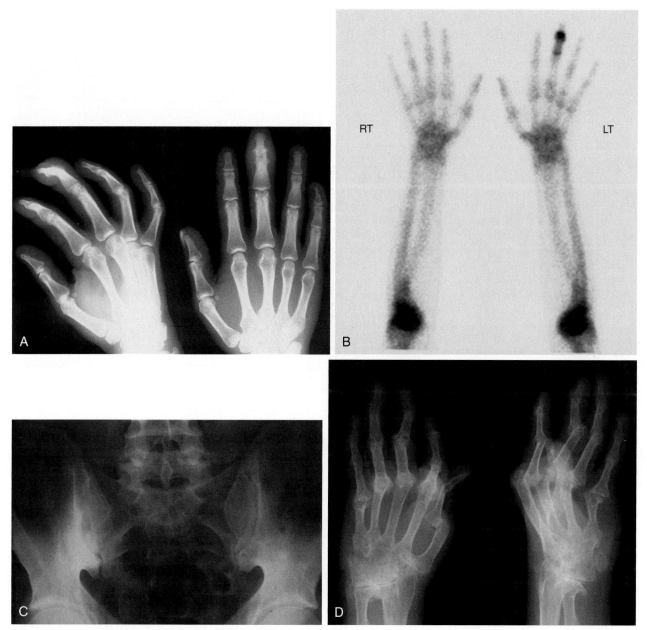

Figure 72-5 Radiologic features in psoriatic arthritis. **A,** Third left distal interphalangeal joint monarthritis with prominent new bone formation. **B,** Bone scan from same patient as in **A. C,** Asymmetric right-sided sacroiliitis. **D,** Severe destructive changes (arthritis mutilans) with multiple erosions and "pencil-in-cup" deformities. *(Courtesy of Dr. Robin Gibney.)*

phenotype (Fig. 72-5). These features include asymmetric joint involvement; involvement of the interphalangeal joints of the fingers and toes, with features of bony erosion and resorption sometimes seen together and resulting in the classic "pencil-in-cup" deformity; joint space narrowing or involvement of entheseal sites, often with bony spurs developing or periostitis; and spinal involvement, frequently less severe and asymmetric compared with classic ankylosing spondylitis.

Radiographic progression in psoriatic arthritis is slow in early psoriatic arthritis with the mean modified Sharp (to include DIP joints in the hands) erosion score at presentation increasing from 1.2 to 3 at 2 years.[12] The Larson and the Sharp scoring systems have been used in psoriatic arthritis, but neither the Larson nor the Sharp score has been developed

specifically for psoriatic arthritis or has been extensively validated.

MUSCULOSKELETAL ULTRASOUND

There are many MSUS applications in psoriatic arthritis, and the applications are likely to develop further as the technology, in particular power Doppler to allow identification of blood flow, develops further (Fig. 72-6). Already it has been shown that MSUS is more sensitive than clinical examination in detecting knee synovitis in patients with various arthritides, including psoriatic arthritis.[24] One study has suggested further that this increased sensitivity may result in reclassification of some patients as polyarticular when they were previously diagnosed as oligoarticular on clinical grounds.[25] This

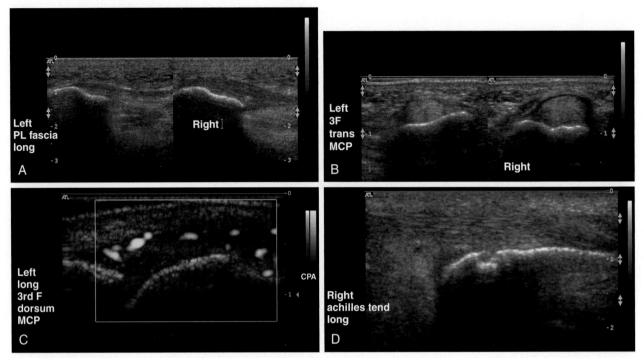

Figure 72-6 Musculoskeletal ultrasound features in psoriatic arthritis. **A,** Right plantar fascia thickening compared with the left. **B,** Transverse section through left third finger at the metacarpophalangeal joint showing right tenosynovitis. **C,** Power Doppler ultrasound through left third finger at the metacarpophalangeal joint confirming increased vascularity (synovitis). **D,** Right Achilles tendinitis with calcaneal erosion. *(Courtesy of Dr. Robin Gibney.)*

reclassification may result in significant changes in prognosis and therapy. Finally, MSUS has been used in the objective monitoring of response of synovitis to therapy.[26]

The MSUS features at the enthesis include entheseal thickening, hypoechoic change, increased vascularity as shown on power Doppler, tenosynovitis, and bony erosions or enthesophyte formation.[27,28] MSUS has been shown to be more sensitive than clinical examination in detecting lower limb enthesopathy.[28,29] MSUS has been used in studies of dactylitic digits. Together with MRI, MSUS has shown dactylitis to be due to a combination of synovial and tenosynovial inflammation.[16,17] Finally, MSUS guidance for small joint or entheseal aspiration or injection may have particular application in patients with psoriatic arthritis.

MAGNETIC RESONANCE IMAGING

MRI studies have been particularly useful in offering new insights into disease pathogenesis in psoriatic arthritis. Based on the prominent entheseal-related bone marrow edema seen on MRI, McGonagle and colleagues[30] have proposed that psoriatic arthritis, in contrast to RA, is an entheseal-based disease. MRI can be used to study all aspects of joint involvement including the enthesis, but the use of MRI as a routine clinical tool in psoriatic arthritis is not yet clarified. The application of MRI to the spine or sacroiliac joints in psoriatic arthritis may prove especially helpful as has been shown in ankylosing spondylitis, but studies in psoriatic arthritis patients are awaited. Preliminary studies have suggested that MRI can be useful as an outcome measure in the detection of synovitis or of vascularity in patients with psoriatic arthritis undergoing biologic therapies (Fig. 72-7). More detailed studies are required.

OTHER IMAGING MODALITIES

The use of other imaging modalities, such as computed tomography (CT) or scintigraphy, has largely been superseded by MRI. CT is now mainly reserved for patients in whom MRI is contraindicated or for whom MRI is unavailable. Positron emission tomography has been found to be comparable to MSUS and MRI in RA knees; this work needs to be extended to psoriatic arthritis.

DIAGNOSIS

A diagnostic test for psoriatic arthritis is currently unavailable. Nevertheless, in its simplest form, psoriatic arthritis can be considered as an arthritis occurring in the presence of psoriasis, but in the absence of rheumatoid factor. Most psoriatic arthritis patients meet this simple definition. The arthritis can be predominantly spinal, it may involve only entheseal sites, psoriasis may present after the arthritis in 15%, and low-titer positive rheumatoid factor may be found. Recognizing these difficulties, the CASPAR group have published new classification criteria based on an analysis of 588 psoriatic arthritis cases and 536 controls (Table 72-2).[31] These criteria have yet to be validated in other large patient cohorts, and they should not be used in individual patient diagnosis. In the setting of clinical research, the CASPAR criteria have a specificity of 0.987 and a sensitivity of 0.914. For the individual patient, an algorithm for diagnosis is suggested in Figure 72-8.

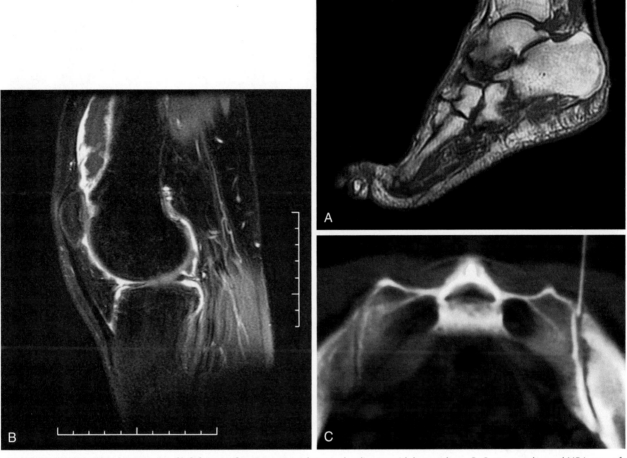

Figure 72-7 **A,** T1-weighted MR image of left foot confirming severe talonavicular disease with bone edema. **B,** Contrast-enhanced MR image of an inflamed knee joint in psoriatic arthritis showing synovial enhancement and large suprapatellar effusion. **C,** CT scan of sacroiliac joint showing sclerosis, erosion, and needle in place just before corticosteroid injection. *(Courtesy of Dr. Robin Gibney.)*

CLINICAL COURSE AND OUTCOME

Five early psoriatic arthritis cohorts have been studied.[12,32-35] The mean disease duration in these cohorts was 6 to 12 months, the median age at onset of psoriasis was 27 to 31 years, and the median age at onset of arthritis was 38 to 52 years. Overall, there was little relationship between skin disease severity and psoriatic arthritis onset; the small joints of hands and feet were the most common joints involved; the DIP joints were involved in one third of patients, usually associated with nail disease, which was present in two thirds; dactylitis and enthesitis were present in one third; and spinal involvement only was found in 2% to 4%, but was present in 20% overall. In follow-up, disease continued to progress in most patients with 47% developing erosive disease within 2 years.[12] Markers for progression included polyarticular disease and an elevated erythrocyte sedimentation rate. Long-term follow-up studies have shown significant morbidity and increased mortality in psoriatic arthritis: 17% have five or more deformed joints, 40% to 57% have a deforming arthritis, 20% to 40% have spinal involvement, 11% to 19% are disabled, and mortality is increased compared with the general population.[10,36,37] In a more recent study, carotid intimal medial thickness was increased in psoriatic arthritis patients compared with controls, but significantly reduced compared with an RA cohort of similar disease duration (unpublished observations).

OUTCOME DOMAINS AND INSTRUMENTS

Measuring response to treatment of psoriatic arthritis in clinical trials has been the subject of much interest for members of the Group for Research and Assessment of Psoriasis and Psoriatic Arthritis (GRAPPA) and Outcome Measures in Rheumatoid Arthritis Clinical Trials (OMERACT). Much of the data that have been used to date in clinical trials have been adapted from RA and have not been validated. Controversial issues have included the number of joints to count, the usefulness of the acute-phase response in psoriatic arthritis, and how important is it to include a measure of function or quality of life. An essential core set of domains that must be included in clinical trials has now been agreed on with other domains necessary but not mandatory, and yet others requiring considerably more research (Fig. 72-9). Instruments for many of these domains have yet to be developed and validated, and some instruments, such as the Psoriasis Assessment Severity Index (PASI), have acknowledged limitations. Table 72-3 lists the currently available instruments for the core domains.

Table 72-2 CASPAR Classification Criteria for Psoriatic Arthritis

Inflammatory articular disease (joint, spine, or entheseal) with ≥3 points from the following:

1. Evidence of psoriasis (one of a, b, c)
   a. Current psoriasis*—psoriatic skin or scalp disease present today as judged by a rheumatologist or dermatologist
   b. Personal history of psoriasis—history of psoriasis that may be obtained from patient, family physician, dermatologist, rheumatologist, or other qualified health care provider
   c. Family history of psoriasis—history of psoriasis in a first-degree or second-degree relative according to patient report
2. Psoriatic nail dystrophy—typical psoriatic nail dystrophy, including onycholysis, pitting, and hyperkeratosis observed on current physical examination
3. Negative test for rheumatoid factor—by any method except latex, but preferably by ELISA or nephelometry, according to the local laboratory reference range
4. Dactylitis (one of a, b)
   a. Current swelling of an entire digit
   b. History—history of dactylitis recorded by a rheumatologist
5. Radiologic evidence of juxta-articular new bone formation—ill-defined ossification near joint margins (but excluding osteophyte formation) on plain x-rays of hand or foot

Specificity 0.987, sensitivity 0.914.
   *Current psoriasis scores 2, whereas all other items score 1.
   CASPAR, Classification of Psoriatic Arthritis; ELISA, enzyme-linked immunosorbent assay.

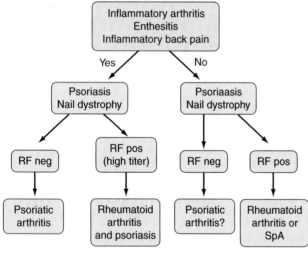

Figure 72-8 Algorithm to be used in diagnosis of individual patients presenting with possible psoriatic arthritis. Some patients may present with typical articular manifestations of psoriatic arthritis, but in the absence of skin or nail disease. They can be diagnosed as definite psoriatic arthritis only when psoriasis subsequently develops. RF, rheumatoid factor; SpA, spondyloarthropathy.

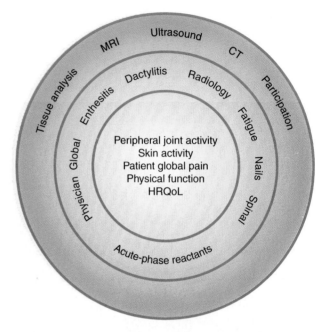

Figure 72-9 Outcome domains in psoriatic arthritis. The central core domains are considered essential for inclusion in clinical trials. The middle circle contains domains that are considered important, but not essential. The outer circle contains domains that all require further research and validation. HRQoL, health-related quality of life.

Table 72-3 Core Set Instruments Proposed for Use in Clinical Trials

Domain	Instrument
Peripheral joint inflammation	Tender/swollen joint count 68/66
Patient global assessment	Instrument under study
Skin assessment	PASI (if BSA ≥3%) Lesion score (erythema, induration, scale) BSA
Pain	Visual analogue scale or numerical rating scale
Physical function	HAQ/SF-36 physical function composite
Health-related quality of life	Generic Disease specific (e.g., DLQI or PsAQoL)

BSA, body surface area; DLQI, Dermatology Life Quality Index; HAQ, health assessment questionnaire; PASI, Psoriasis Assessment Severity Index; PsAQoL psoriatic arthritis quality of life; SF-36, short-form health survey.

In the setting of clinical trials, numerous composite scores (e.g., American College of Rheumatology [ACR]-20, ACR-50, ACR-70; European League Against Rheumatism (EULAR) Disease Activity Score [DAS] response criteria) have been used in psoriatic arthritis, most again adapted from RA and not extensively validated in psoriatic arthritis. One scoring system was developed for psoriatic arthritis, the PsARC, and although it has been used in numerous studies, it too has not been extensively validated and is considered perhaps less responsive and discriminant.[38] Much work is required to develop a validated and responsive composite instrument in psoriatic arthritis.

PATHOGENESIS

Many more recent studies have explored key components of disease pathogenesis, including the contribution of genetic factors, the role of infection or trauma, studies of animal models or involved sites of disease, and the importance of components of the immune system such as cytokines.

GENETIC FACTORS

Familial clustering of psoriasis and psoriatic arthritis is well described. Twin studies in psoriasis also have shown a high rate of concordance in monozygotic twins.[39] The genetic basis for this clustering has been the subject of extensive investigations in psoriasis, but has been much less well studied in psoriatic arthritis. Studies of psoriatic arthritis have often included patients as a subset of larger psoriasis cohorts, and there has been little recognition of the diversity of clinical phenotypes.

It has long been recognized that there is a strong association between psoriasis and the HLA-C region of the major histocompatibility complex (MHC). Whether this was HLA-Cw6 itself, found in approximately 60% of psoriasis cohorts, or a region telomeric to this has been the subject of much controversy. More recently, Elder[40] has definitively shown that the HLA susceptibility region for psoriasis is HLA-Cw6, often in linkage disequilibrium with other HLA-B alleles—HLA-B57, HLA-B37, and HLA-B13. The presence of HLA-Cw6 is associated with an earlier age of onset of psoriasis (type 1 disease, <40 years old) and with more extensive and severe disease. In individuals with psoriatic arthritis, the association with HLA-Cw6 is slightly weaker, whereas additional associations have been found with HLA-B27, chiefly in patients with predominant spinal disease, and with HLA-B38 and HLA-B39.[41]

These findings have been interpreted to suggest that the MHC association with psoriasis lies close to the HLA-C region, whereas the association with the articular manifestations more likely lies in or close to the HLA-B region. A study of a large cohort of psoriatic arthritis patients in the United Kingdom has found HLA-Cw6 to be in linkage disequilibrium with HLA-DRBI*07, and that possession of both alleles were associated with fewer involved or damaged joints (Pauline Ho, et al: personal communication, 2007).

Other genes within the MHC region have been explored in psoriasis and psoriatic arthritis. Tumor necrosis factor (TNF)-α promoter polymorphisms or a gene in linkage disequilibrium with TNF-α may predispose the patient to or increase susceptibility to psoriasis and to psoriatic arthritis. One study has found further an association between the TNF-308A allele and disease progression in early psoriatic arthritis.[42] Whole-genome scans in psoriasis also have identified additional non-MHC susceptibility regions, known as the PSORS regions on chromosomes 4, 6, and 17. To date, no candidate genes have been identified.

Increasing evidence suggests that an additional or distinct genetic contribution is responsible for the development of psoriatic arthritis. More recent work has pointed to an MHC class I chain-related A (MICA)-A9 polymorphism, which confers additional relative risk in particular for polyarticular disease in psoriasis patients who carry Cw*0602.[43] MICA-A9 polymorphism was found in linkage disequilibrium with HLA-B alleles (B*5701, B*3801). These results suggest that the MICA gene or other nearby genes may be involved in the development of psoriatic arthritis. Additionally, a genome scan identified a paternally influenced locus on chromosome 16, a region not known to be implicated in psoriasis susceptibility.[44]

ENVIRONMENTAL FACTORS

The role of environmental factors in triggering either skin or joint disease in patients with psoriasis or psoriatic arthritis has been supported largely by clinical observations, although the mechanism is poorly understood. It has long been recognized that there is a strong association between guttate psoriasis and preceding streptococcal infections in children.[45] That this association might be related to a streptococcal superantigen has been proposed. Some authors also have found bacterial antigens in synovial tissue samples from psoriatic arthritis patients, but this may be no different from noninflammatory control subjects.[46]

The Koebner phenomenon (see Fig. 72-1H) has been reported to occur in 52% of patients with psoriasis. The Koebner phenomenon is the development of psoriasis along the site of skin trauma. It has been proposed that trauma also may play a role in triggering episodes of joint inflammation, and the term *deep Koebner phenomenon* has been coined. Although the role of trauma has not been proved, in one study, 24.6% of patients reported a traumatic event before the onset of arthritis.[47]

Finally, a link between stress and exacerbation of psoriasis has been proposed, supported largely by clinical observational studies. A similar association may exist in psoriatic arthritis, but this has not been systematically examined.

ANIMAL MODELS

Although spondyloarthropathy has been detected in a variety of primates, more recent rodent models have proved helpful in deciphering pathogenic pathways. In rodents transgenic for HLA-B27 class I molecules, skin, nail, and joint features have been described that mimic some of the features of the human phenotype.[48] When HLA-B27 transgenic rats were raised in a germ-free environment, they seemed to be protected from joint disease. Mice genetically lacking MHC class II also have developed skin and joint disease, but confined to the distal phalanges with skin and nail disease also on the affected digits.[49] Involvement of the distal phalanges and nails also was reported in aging male DBA/1 mice from different litters that were caged together from 12 weeks.[50] In these animals, dactylitis, periostitis, and ankylosing enthesitis were observed.

Finally, in a more recent study, JunB protein was shown to be expressed in normal and in clinically uninvolved psoriatic skin, but expression was considerably reduced in involved psoriatic lesions.[51] Epidermal deletion of JunB and c-Jun in a mouse model resulted in skin and joint disease with 100% penetrance and a clinical and histologic phenotype highly consistent with human psoriasis and psoriatic arthritis. In further experiments, the same authors showed that the joint disease, but not the skin disease, required T and B cells and intact TNF receptor 1 signaling.

IMMUNOPATHOLOGY

The key pathologic events in psoriatic arthritis occur in the skin, synovium, entheseal sites, and cartilage and bone. The pathobiologic features in the skin and synovium have been well described, but only a few studies have focused on the enthesis. In relation to cartilage and bone, more recent studies have shown the presence of osteoclasts at the cartilage-pannus junction and high numbers of circulating osteoclast precursors in the circulation of psoriatic arthritis patients. Detailed studies similar to those done in RA on the synovial-cartilage-bone interface possibly could yield valuable information regarding joint destruction in psoriatic arthritis.

Psoriasis Skin

Involved psoriasis skin is characterized by epidermal hyperplasia, mononuclear leukocytes in the papillary dermis, neutrophils in the stratum corneum, and an increase in various subsets of dendritic cells.[52] CD8[+] T cells are the predominant T cell subset chiefly found in the epidermis, whereas dermal T cells contain a mixture of CD4[+] and CD8[+]. Most T cells in skin lesions express the addressin, cutaneous lymphocyte antigen, in contrast to circulating T cells and T cells found in the inflamed synovium in psoriatic arthritis.[53] Finally, vascular changes also are prominent in psoriasis with an impressive growth and dilation of superficial blood vessels.

Psoriatic Synovium

Many early studies of synovial pathology in psoriatic arthritis highlighted the presence of prominent and striking vascular changes. In the first study that compared psoriatic arthritis and RA synovial tissue, quantitative immunopathologic analysis confirmed these prominent vascular changes and found that vessel number was significantly increased in psoriatic arthritis.[54] Lining layer hyperplasia was less marked in psoriatic arthritis, and fewer macrophages were seen trafficking into the synovium and out to the lining layer. The number of T lymphocytes and their subsets and the number of B cells were similar to the frequency found in RA. Although neutrophil infiltration was not assessed, this study examined adhesion molecule expression further in the two patient subgroups and found E-selectin expression to be considerably reduced in psoriatic arthritis. Many of these observations have been confirmed by other authors.

In a more recent study by Kruithof and coworkers,[55] the synovial immunopathologic features in patients with spondyloarthropathy, including psoriatic arthritis, were compared with the features seen in RA.[55] Using a semiquantitative scoring system, the authors identified many features characteristic of the spondyloarthropathy group as a whole and in the psoriatic arthritis subgroup alone. Increased vascularity, higher neutrophil numbers (also seen in involved psoriasis skin), and a higher number of infiltrating CD163[+] macrophages, a marker of mature tissue macrophages, reliably distinguished spondyloarthropathy from RA. No significant differences were seen between oligoarticular versus polyarticular psoriatic arthritis.

The important role of the vasculature in psoriatic arthritis pathogenesis is perhaps most elegantly shown by the large numbers of tortuous and dilated blood vessels observed through an arthroscopic view of psoriatic joints.[56] An interaction of key growth factors is thought to regulate closely the new vessel formation or angiogenic process. Growth factors, including TNF-α, transforming growth factor (TGF)-β, platelet-derived growth factor (PDGF), angiopoietins (ANG-1, ANG-2), and vascular endothelial growth factor (VEGF), have been described in skin and synovial tissue.[57,58] Because this expression is found at an early stage of inflammation, it may represent a primary event in psoriatic arthritis as opposed to a reaction or response to hypoxia. One possibility is that there is a genetic predisposition to endothelial activation, which results in new vessel formation and increased cellular trafficking.

Entheseal Sites

Laloux and associates[59] described the immunopathologic features of the enthesis in patients undergoing joint replacement surgery with spondyloarthropathy, including psoriatic arthritis, and compared with RA. Numbers of patients were small in this study, but there was a consistent increase in CD8[+] T cell expression at the enthesis in patients with psoriatic arthritis compared with RA patients. Ultrasound-guided biopsy of five sites of acute enthesitis in early spondyloarthropathy also confirmed an inflammatory response with increased vascularity and cellular, predominantly macrophage, infiltration.[60] These findings are consistent with the well-described association of psoriatic arthritis with HLA class I antigens. They also are consistent with the previously described dominance of activated and mature CD8[+] T cells in psoriatic arthritis synovial fluid samples compared with RA.[61] It is attractive to suggest that entheseal-derived antigens might trigger an immune response in the adjacent synovial tissue. To date, evidence for this hypothesis has not been found, although it is clearly an area for future study. A search for candidate antigens common to the enthesis and the skin might be informative.

CYTOKINES

Synovial explant tissues obtained from psoriatic arthritis joints have been shown to produce higher levels of the T helper type 1 cytokines interleukin (IL)-2 and interferon-γ protein than explants similarly cultured from osteoarthritis and RA patients.[62] This T helper type 1 lymphocyte profile also has been observed in psoriasis plaques.[63] The cytokines IL-1β and TNF-α also were released by psoriasis synovial explants in high concentrations. In contrast, IL-4 and IL-5 were not identified, but IL-10 was highly expressed in psoriatic synovium, although not in skin. A similar pattern of cytokine production in psoriatic arthritis synovium was shown using immunohistochemical and gene expression techniques.[64,65] Other innate cytokines, such as IL-18 and IL-15, also are present in psoriatic arthritis synovial tissue and are downregulated by methotrexate therapy.

TNF-α levels are elevated in psoriatic skin, synovium, and joint fluid of patients with psoriatic arthritis.[62,66] Several lines of evidence support the concept that TNF-α is an important cytokine in the psoriatic joint. TNF-α transgenic mice exhibit extensive bone destruction similar to that observed in some psoriatic arthritis patients. In a study of 129 patients with early psoriatic arthritis, patients with erosions were significantly more likely to have the TNF-α-308 A allele, an allele associated with high TNF-α production.[42] As mentioned earlier, immunohistochemical and gene expression studies have shown marked upregulation of TNF-α in the psoriatic synovial membrane. Histopathologic analysis of synovial specimens from eight spondyloarthropathy patients, four of whom had psoriatic arthritis, treated with the anti-TNF-α monoclonal antibody infliximab revealed decreased vascularity, synovial lining thickness, and mononuclear cell infiltration after therapy.[67,68] In another study, a significant reduction in the quantity of infiltrating macrophages, the CD31+ vascular area, αvβ3-positive neovessels/*Ulex europaeus* agglutinin–positive vessels, VEGF and its receptor KDR/flk-1 (VEGFR-2), and SDF-1-positive vessels in psoriatic arthritis synovium was noted after 8 weeks (three infusions) of infliximab treatment.[69]

MATRIX METALLOPROTEINASES AND CARTILAGE DESTRUCTION

Radiographs of psoriatic joints often reveal cartilage loss manifested as joint space narrowing. Similar to RA, matrix metalloproteinases (MMPs) and tissue inhibitors of MMPs (TIMPs) were identified in psoriatic arthritis synovial lining and sublining layers.[70,71] In particular, immunohistochemical studies revealed that MMP-9 localized to blood vessel walls, whereas MMP-1, MMP-2, MMP-3, TIMP-1, and TIMP-2 showed a cellular and interstitial staining pattern in the synovial lining. Serum levels of MMP-3 exhibited a marked and rapid decrease after successful anti-TNF-α therapy raising the possibility that this molecule may serve as a biomarker. In another study, similar levels of MMP-1 and MMP-3 mRNA were detected in RA and psoriatic arthritis synovial tissue despite the fact that the RA patients exhibited more erosions on plain radiographs.[72] The elevated ratio of MMPs to TIMP-1 in the synovial tissue favored cartilage degradation, although the expression of MMPs was not significantly elevated at the cartilage-pannus junction compared with other sites. These reports indicate that MMPs are upregulated in psoriatic arthritis synovium, but their precise functions remain to be defined.

BONE REMODELING

Radiographs of psoriatic arthritis joints also can reveal markedly altered bone remodeling in the form of bone resorption (tuft resorption or osteolysis, large eccentric erosions, and pencil-in-cup deformities) and new bone formation (periostitis, spur or enthesophyte formation, bony ankylosis). Important in bone resorption, psoriatic joint biopsy specimens show large multinucleated osteoclasts in deep resorption pits at the bone-pannus junction.[73] Osteoclastogenesis (differentiation of monocytes into osteoclasts) is a contact-dependent process directed by osteoblasts and stromal cells in the bone marrow. These cells release signals necessary for differentiation of an osteoclast precursor derived from the CD14+ monocyte population into an osteoclast.

One of these signals is the receptor activator of nuclear factor κB ligand (RANKL), a member of the TNF superfamily that binds to RANK on the surface of osteoclast precursors and osteoclasts. This ligand-receptor interaction stimulates proliferation and differentiation of osteoclast precursors and activation of osteoclasts. It has been proposed that the relative expression of RANKL and of its natural antagonist osteoprotegerin ultimately controls osteoclastogenesis.

In psoriatic arthritis synovial tissues, marked upregulation of RANKL protein and low expression of osteoprotegerin were detected in the adjacent synovial lining.[73] Osteoclasts also were noted in cutting cones traversing the subchondral bone supporting a bidirectional attack on the bone in psoriatic joints. In addition, osteoclast precursors, derived from circulating CD14+ monocytes, were markedly elevated in the peripheral blood of patients with psoriatic arthritis compared with healthy controls. Treatment of patients with psoriatic arthritis with anti-TNF-α agents significantly decreased the level of circulating osteoclast precursor, supporting a central role for TNF-α in the generation of this precursor population.

The mechanisms responsible for new bone formation in the psoriatic joint are poorly understood. TGF-β and VEGF may be pivotal in this process given that TGF-β is strongly expressed in synovial tissues isolated from patients with ankylosing spondylitis and synergizes with VEGF to induce bone formation in animal models.[74] De Klerck and colleagues[75] showed that the bone morphogenetic proteins (BMPs) BMP-2 and BMP-7 are upregulated in regions of pathologic new bone formation. The same investigators showed that the expression of phosphorylated Smad-1 and Smad-5, important signaling molecules downstream of BMP, was markedly increased in regions of new bone formation taken from the calcaneus in a patient with Achilles tendinitis and periostitis. These studies provide evidence that potential mediators of ankylosis and periostitis in the psoriatic enthesis and joint include BMP molecules and possibly VEGF and TGF-β.

SUMMARY

In considering a model for disease pathogenesis in psoriatic arthritis, we have to try to take into account the genetic susceptibility; the role of the environment; cellular immunologic mechanisms; and secreted cytokines, chemokines, and other proteins. For some time, the primary hypothesis has been that psoriatic arthritis is an HLA class I–restricted, antigen-driven immune process (Fig. 72-10). Considerable evidence has been presented to support this hypothesis; however, despite careful analysis of T cell receptor phenotype, no antigen-driven process other than that driven by Epstein-Barr virus has been identified.[75a] The potential role of components of the innate immune response, such as Toll-like receptors or cells bearing natural killer receptors, is currently under active investigation. It is possible that the interaction of environmental factors, such as those derived from pathogens or expressed after trauma, with Toll-like receptors in a genetically susceptible individual may set in train intracellular signaling events leading to cytokine release, immune activation, and release of destructive enzymes such as MMPs (Fig. 72-11).

TREATMENT

In considering treatment strategies for psoriatic arthritis, the diverse nature of the clinical phenotype (peripheral arthritis, skin and nail disease, axial disease, dactylitis and enthesitis) may complicate therapeutic decisions because not all treatments are effective for all of the features, and patients often display a mixture of all of the features

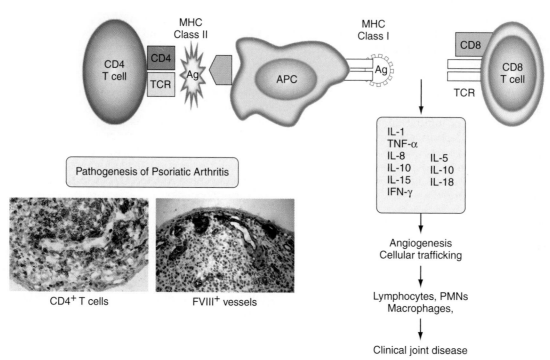

Pathogenesis of Psoriatic Arthritis

CD4+ T cells

FVIII+ vessels

Figure 72-10 Traditional disease pathogenesis model in psoriatic arthritis. APC, antigen-presenting cell; IFN, interferon; IL, interleukin; PMNs, polymorphonuclear neutrophils; TCR, T cell receptor; TNF, tumor necrosis factor.

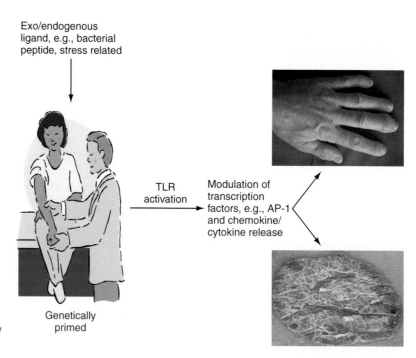

Figure 72-11 Alternative model incorporating new disease pathogenesis concepts. TLR, Toll-like receptor.

simultaneously. GRAPPA published a systematic review of the evidence for treatment strategies in psoriatic arthritis, and this review provides treatment guidelines that are currently being devised. The reader is referred to this GRAPPA publication for a detailed review of the evidence; Figure 72-12 is a proposed preliminary algorithm for treatment choices.[76] Treatment choices may be driven by the disease feature considered most severe at the time of the evaluation. Finally, in reviewing the evidence for therapeutic effect presented next, the recommendations from the Agency for

Health Care Policy Research were used where interventions are scored by categories of evidence (level 1 through 4) and strength of recommendation (grade A through D).[77]

TRADITIONAL AGENTS

Although there is little published evidence of a favorable therapeutic effect in psoriatic arthritis, nonsteroidal anti-inflammatory drugs are most often the agents first used in psoriatic arthritis whatever the clinical phenotype (level 1b,

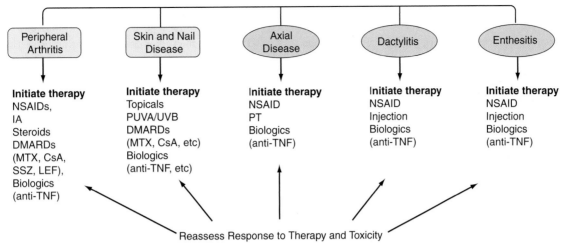

Figure 72-12 Preliminary treatment algorithm for the various clinical manifestations in psoriatic arthritis. *(From Kavanaugh AF, Ritchlin CT: Systematic review of treatments for psoriatic arthritis: An evidence based approach and basis for treatment guidelines. J Rheumatol 33:1417-1421, 2006.)*

grade A).[78] Expert opinion supports use of nonsteroidal anti-inflammatory drugs, although occasional exacerbations of psoriasis have been reported. The use of systemic corticosteroids is not evidence-based (level 4, grade D), although 24% of patients in one study were taking prednisolone.[79] There are concerns that exacerbations of psoriasis may follow corticosteroid withdrawal. There have been no randomized controlled trials of intra-articular steroids in psoriatic arthritis or of local entheseal or dactylitis injections. Expert opinion indicates that intra-articular steroids can be quite effective, especially in oligoarticular disease or where there is localized entheseal involvement, such as in plantar fasciitis (level 4, grade D). Mild skin disease (PASI <10) is usually controlled with topical steroids or vitamin D derivatives, with the latter best used for maintenance therapy.[80]

Systemic therapy is considered in patients with three or more inflamed joints despite conventional therapy as described previously; persistent or treatment-resistant axial, entheseal, or dactylitic disease especially where multiple sites are involved; or moderate or severe psoriasis (PASI >10). Randomized controlled trials of disease-modifying antirheumatic drugs (DMARDs) are few and limited by size. Based on evidence and expert opinion, nearly all DMARDs may have small-to-moderate beneficial effects on peripheral joints, enthesitis, and dactylitis.[78,81,82] Axial features and nail disease do not seem to respond.[83] Good or moderate improvements in skin disease have been reported with some of the older systemic agents, such as methotrexate, cyclosporine, sulfasalazine, leflunomide, and acetretin (all level 1b, grade A).[80]

The best evidence for DMARD use comes from studies of peripheral joint disease and of psoriasis. There have been six randomized controlled trials of sulfasalazine in psoriatic arthritis (level 1a, grade A), the largest including 221 patients. Fifty-nine percent of patients achieved a therapeutic response (PsARC), but in keeping with other studies a high therapeutic response (42.7%) also was noted in placebo-treated patients.[38]

Methotrexate remains for many rheumatologists the DMARD of first choice for patients with psoriatic arthritis, but evidence for its use is limited (level 3, grade B). A small,

prospective randomized controlled trial concluded that methotrexate was as effective as cyclosporine, and a more recent study of 72 patients with active psoriatic arthritis and an incomplete response to methotrexate, in which cyclosporine was added in, showed significant differences only in synovitis as detected by MSUS and PASI score in favor of the combination therapy.[26,84] Although evidence for methotrexate is lacking, an open study reported significant reductions in synovial cellular infiltration and in cytokine gene expression after 3 months of therapy.[65] Although there is evidence that cyclosporine may be as effective as methotrexate, its use is limited because its toxicity profile is considered to be high (level 1b, grade B).[85]

Perhaps the best randomized controlled trial in psoriatic arthritis of a DMARD is with leflunomide (level 1b, grade A).[86] This trial included 190 patients who received either leflunomide or placebo for 24 weeks. Fifty-nine percent of patients treated with leflunomide compared with 30% of patients given placebo met the primary response criteria (PsARC) with significant, although small improvements in other individual parameters, including joint scores, health assessment questionnaire, PASI, and Dermatology Life Quality Index. Regarding some older DMARDs, such as gold salts and antimalarials, there is no evidence of treatment benefit; exacerbation of psoriasis is reported, and they cannot be recommended. One small randomized controlled trial with azathioprine suggested benefit with a reduction in Ritchie score (level 2b, grade B). Finally, apart from the cyclosporine/methotrexate study referred to earlier, there is little or no evidence that DMARD combination therapy is either beneficial or safe in psoriatic arthritis.

With the exception of psoriasis, there is a paucity of evidence that DMARDs are beneficial for the other features of psoriatic arthritis, including dactylitis, axial disease, or enthesitis. The absence of evidence does not mean the absence of an effect, however. Further randomized controlled trials specifically examining these features in psoriatic arthritis are required. In psoriasis, methotrexate and cyclosporine have been shown to be highly and probably equally effective (level 1b, grade A).[80] Adverse effects, in particular with cyclosporine, may limit usage in some patients.

BIOLOGICS

The approach to treatment in psoriatic arthritis has changed considerably with the introduction of biologic therapies. As a result of numerous large, well-conducted, randomized controlled trials, there is now accumulating evidence that anti-TNF treatments are effective in controlling peripheral arthritis symptoms and signs, improving quality of life, and preventing radiologic progression (overall level 1b, grade A).[78] Patients receiving 25 mg subcutaneously twice weekly of etanercept had significant improvements in ACR-20 responses (59% versus 15%) at 12 weeks compared with placebo.[87] At 12 months, radiographic disease progression (modified total Sharp score) was inhibited in the etanercept group (−0.03 unit) compared with worsening of +1.00 unit in the placebo group.

Although the anti-TNF therapies have not been compared in any study, the effect on peripheral arthritis seems to be similar. There also is evidence that anti-TNF therapies are effective for other disease features, such as nail disease, enthesitis, and dactylitis.[81,82,88] These studies are limited by the absence of a validated instrument to measure these features. With psoriasis, the effects of anti-TNF therapies can be quite dramatic.[89] In particular with the antibody therapy, highly significant improvements in PASI scores were achieved (e.g., PASI = 75 in 59% of adalimumab-treated patients versus 1% of placebo-treated patients after 24 weeks, and PASI = 90 in 50%).[90]

Alefacept is a fusion protein of soluble lymphocyte function antigen 3 with Fc fragments of IgG1. Alefacept was the first biologic agent approved for moderate-to-severe psoriasis (level 1b, grade A). Efficacy was dose dependent and slow, but PASI = 75 was achieved in 33% of patients at some point.[91] More recently, alefacept in combination with methotrexate was evaluated in 185 patients with active psoriatic arthritis.[92] At 6 months, 54% of alefacept-treated patients versus 23% of placebo-treated patients achieved an ACR-20 response. Finally, efalizumab, a humanized monoclonal antibody targeting the CD11a component of lymphocyte function antigen 1, also has been approved for

psoriasis with PASI = 75 achieved in 22% to 39% in randomized controlled trials.[89] To date, there is no evidence for beneficial effect of efalizumab in other psoriatic arthritis disease manifestations.

Future Directions

The surge of interest in new therapies for psoriatic arthritis is most welcome, in particular for patients with poor prognostic features (polyarticular disease, elevated erythrocyte sedimentation rate, dactylitis, and progressive change on radiograph) who fail to respond to standard treatment approaches. Much additional research on currently available agents and on new treatments is required. New instruments to measure key outcome domains, such as enthesitis, need to be developed and validated, and comparisons of newer agents with standard DMARDs, such as methotrexate, are required to inform treatment decisions. GRAPPA is currently developing treatment guidelines based on current evidence, but there are many gaps in our knowledge, and expert opinion is the best available guide in many situations. It is hoped, however, that guidelines or recommendations can be agreed on that would help inform the physician when treating psoriatic arthritis and its diverse clinical manifestations.

REFERENCES

1. Wright V: Rheumatism and psoriasis: A re-evaluation. Am J Med 27:454-462, 1959.
2. Moll JMH, Wright V: Psoriatic arthritis. Semin Arthritis Rheum 3:55-78, 1973.
3. Blumberg BS, Bunim JJ, Calkins E, et al: ARA nomenclature and classification of arthritis and rheumatism (tentative). Arthritis Rheum 7:93-97, 1964.
4. Gladman DD, Antoni C, Mease P, et al: Psoriatic arthritis: Epidemiology, clinical features, course, and outcome. Ann Rheum Dis 64(Suppl 2):ii-14-ii-17, 2005.
5. Krueger G, Ellis CN: Psoriasis—recent advances in understanding its pathogenesis and treatment. J Am Acad Dermatol 53(Suppl 1):S94-S100, 2005.
6. Gelfand JM, Gladman DD, Mease PJ, et al: Epidemiology of psoriatic arthritis in the population of the United States. J Am Acad Dermatol 53:573, 2005.
7. Kay L, Perry-James J, Walker D: The prevalence and impact of psoriasis in the primary care population in northeast England. Arthritis Rheum 42:S299, 1999.
8. Shbeeb M, Uramoto KM, Gibson LE, et al: The epidemiology of psoriatic arthritis in Olmsted County, Minnesota, USA, 1982-1991. J Rheumatol 27:1247-1250, 2000.
9. Savolainen E, Kaipiainen-Seppanen O, Kroger L, et al: Total incidence and distribution of inflammatory joint diseases in a defined population: Results from the Kuopio 2000 arthritis survey. J Rheumatol 30:2460-2468, 2003.
10. Gladman DD, Shuckett R, Russell ML, et al: Psoriatic arthritis (PSA)—an analysis of 220 patients. QJM 62:127-141, 1987.
11. **Moll JMH, Wright V: Familial occurrence of psoriatic arthritis. Ann Rheum Dis 22:181-195, 1973.**
12. **Kane D, Stafford L, Bresnihan B, et al: A prospective, clinical and radiological study of early psoriatic arthritis: An early synovitis clinic experience. Rheumatology (Oxf) 42:1460-1468, 2003.**
13. Helliwell PS, Porter G, Taylor WJ: Polyarticular psoriatic arthritis is more like oligoarticular psoriatic arthritis, than rheumatoid arthritis. Ann Rheum Dis 66:113-117, 2007.
14. Battistone MJ, Manaster BJ, Reda DJ, et al: The prevalence of sacroiliitis in psoriatic arthritis: New perspectives from a large, multicenter cohort. A Department of Veterans Affairs Cooperative Study. Skeletal Radiol 28:196-201, 1999.
15. Brockbank JE, Stein M, Schentag CT, et al: Dactylitis in psoriatic arthritis: A marker for disease severity? Ann Rheum Dis 64:188-190, 2005.
16. Kane D, Greaney T, Bresnihan B, et al: Ultrasonography in the diagnosis and management of psoriatic dactylitis. J Rheumatol 26:1746-1751, 1999.
17. Olivieri I, Barozzi L, Pierro A, et al: Toe dactylitis in patients with spondyloarthropathy: Assessment by magnetic resonance imaging. J Rheumatol 24:926-930, 1997.
18. Queiro R, Torre JC, Belzunegui J, et al: Clinical features and predictive factors in psoriatic arthritis-related uveitis. Semin Arthritis Rheum 31:264-270, 2002.
19. Schatteman L, Mielants H, Veys EM, et al: Gut inflammation in psoriatic arthritis: A prospective ileocolonoscopic study. J Rheumatol 22:680-683, 1995.
20. Williamson L, Dockerty JL, Dalbeth N, et al: Gastrointestinal disease and psoriatic arthritis. J Rheumatol 31:1469-1470, 2004.
21. Cantini F, Salvarani C, Olivieri I, et al: Distal extremity swelling with pitting edema in psoriatic arthritis: A case-control study. Clin Exp Rheumatol 19:291-296, 2001.
22. Korendowych E, Owen P, Ravindran J, et al: The clinical and genetic associations of anti-cyclic citrullinated peptide antibodies in psoriatic arthritis. Rheumatology (Oxf) 44:1056-1060, 2005.
23. **Gladman DD, Farewell VT, Nadeau C: Clinical indicators of progression in psoriatic arthritis: Multivariate relative risk model. J Rheumatol 22:675-679, 1995.**

24. Karim Z, Wakefield RJ, Quinn M, et al: Validation and reproducibility of ultrasonography in the detection of synovitis in the knee: A comparison with arthroscopy and clinical examination. Arthritis Rheum 50:387-394, 2004.

25. Wakefield RJ, Green MJ, Marzo-Ortega H, et al: Should oligoarthritis be reclassified? Ultrasound reveals a high prevalence of subclinical disease. Ann Rheum Dis 63:382-385, 2004.

26. Fraser AD, van Kuijk AW, Westhovens R, et al: A randomised, double blind, placebo controlled, multicentre trial of combination therapy with methotrexate plus cyclosporine in patients with active psoriatic arthritis. Ann Rheum Dis 64:859-864, 2005.

27. Balint PV, Sturrock RD: Inflamed retrocalcaneal bursa and Achilles tendonitis in psoriatic arthritis demonstrated by ultrasonography. Ann Rheum Dis 59:931-933, 2000.

28. D'Agostino MA, Said-Nahal R, Hacquard-Bouder C, et al: Assessment of peripheral enthesitis in the spondylarthropathies by ultrasonography combined with power Doppler: A cross-sectional study. Arthritis Rheum 48:523-533, 2003.

29. Balint PV, Kane D, Wilson H, et al: Ultrasonography of entheseal insertions in the lower limb in spondyloarthropathy. Ann Rheum Dis 61:905-910, 2002.

30. **McGonagle D, Conaghan PG, Emery P: Psoriatic arthritis: A unified concept twenty years on. Arthritis Rheum 42:1080-1086, 1999.**

31. **Taylor W, Gladman D, Helliwell P, et al: Classification criteria for psoriatic arthritis: Development of new criteria from a large international study. Arthritis Rheum 54:2665-2673, 2006.**

32. Harrison BJ, Silman AJ, Barrett EM, et al: Presence of psoriasis does not influence the presentation or short-term outcome of patients with early inflammatory polyarthritis. J Rheumatol 24:1744-1749, 1997.

33. Jones SM, Armas JB, Cohen MG, et al: Psoriatic arthritis: Outcome of disease subsets and relationship of joint disease to nail and skin disease. Br J Rheumatol 33:834-839, 1994.

34. Punzi L, Pianon M, Rossini P, et al: Clinical and laboratory manifestations of elderly onset psoriatic arthritis: A comparison with younger onset disease. Ann Rheum Dis 58:226-229, 1999.

35. Khan M, Schentag C, Gladman DD: Clinical and radiological changes during psoriatic arthritis disease progression. J Rheumatol 30:1022-1026, 2003.

36. Torre Alonso JC, Rodriguez Perez A, Arribas Castrillo JM, et al: Psoriatic arthritis (PA): A clinical, immunological and radiological study of 180 patients. Br J Rheumatol 30:245-250, 1991.

37. Hanly JG, Russell ML, Gladman DD: Psoriatic spondyloarthropathy: A long term prospective study. Ann Rheum Dis 47:386-393, 1988.

38. Clegg DO, Reda DJ, Mejias E, et al: Comparison of sulfasalazine and placebo in the treatment of psoriatic arthritis. A Department of Veterans Affairs Cooperative Study. Arthritis Rheum 39:2013-2020, 1996.

39. Eastmond CJ: Psoriatic arthritis: Genetics and HLA antigens. Baillieres Clin Rheumatol 8:263-276, 1994.

40. Elder JT: PSORS1: Linking genetics and immunology. J Invest Dermatol 126:1205-1206, 2006.

41. Gladman DD, Farewell VT: The role of HLA antigens as indicators of disease progression in psoriatic arthritis: Multivariate relative risk model. Arthritis Rheum 38:845-850, 1995.

42. Balding J, Kane D, Livingstone W, et al: Cytokine gene polymorphisms: Association with psoriatic arthritis susceptibility and severity. Arthritis Rheum 48:1408-1413, 2003.

43. Gonzalez S, Martinez-Borra J, Lopez-Vazquez A, et al: MICA rather than MICB, TNFA, or HLA-DRB1 is associated with susceptibility to psoriatic arthritis. J Rheumatol 29:973-978, 2002.

44. Karason A, Gudjonsson JE, Upmanyu R, et al: A susceptibility gene for psoriatic arthritis maps to chromosome 16q: Evidence for imprinting. Am J Hum Genet 72:125-131, 2003.

45. Rasmussen JE: The relationship between infection with group A beta hemolytic streptococci and the development of psoriasis. Pediatr Infect Dis J 19:153-154, 2000.

46. Wilbrink B, van der Heijden IM, Schouls LM, et al: Detection of bacterial DNA in joint samples from patients with undifferentiated arthritis and reactive arthritis, using polymerase chain reaction with universal 16S ribosomal RNA primers. Arthritis Rheum 41:535-543, 1998.

47. Langevitz P, Buskila D, Gladman DD: Psoriatic arthritis precipitated by physical trauma. J Rheumatol 17:695-697, 1990.

48. Yanagisawa H, Richardson JA, Taurog JD, et al: Characterization of psoriasiform and alopecic skin lesions in HLA-B27 transgenic rats. Am J Pathol 147:955-964, 1995.

49. Bardos T, Zhang J, Mikecz K, et al: Mice lacking endogenous major histocompatibility complex class II develop arthritis resembling psoriatic arthritis at an advanced age. Arthritis Rheum 46:2465-2475, 2002.

50. Lories RJ, Matthys P, de Vlam K, et al: Ankylosing enthesitis, dactylitis, and onychoperiostitis in male DBA/1 mice: A model of psoriatic arthritis. Ann Rheum Dis 63:595-598, 2004.

51. Zenz R, Eferl R, Kenner L, et al: Psoriasis-like skin disease and arthritis caused by inducible epidermal deletion of Jun proteins. Nature 437:369-375, 2005.

52. Bos JD, de Rie MA, Teunissen MB, et al: Psoriasis: Dysregulation of innate immunity. Br J Dermatol 152:1098-1107, 2005.

53. Pitzalis C, Cauli A, Pipitone N, et al: Cutaneous lymphocyte antigen-positive T lymphocytes preferentially migrate to the skin but not to the joint in psoriatic arthritis. Arthritis Rheum 39:137-145, 1996.

54. **Veale D, Yanni G, Rogers S, et al: Reduced synovial membrane macrophage numbers, ELAM-1 expression, and lining layer hyperplasia in psoriatic arthritis as compared with rheumatoid arthritis. Arthritis Rheum 36:893-900, 1993.**

55. Kruithof E, Baeten D, De Rycke L, et al: Synovial histopathology of psoriatic arthritis, both oligo- and polyarticular, resembles spondyloarthropathy more than it does rheumatoid arthritis. Arthritis Res Ther 7:R569-R580, 2005.

56. Reece RJ, Canete JD, Parsons WJ, et al: Distinct vascular patterns of early synovitis in psoriatic, reactive, and rheumatoid arthritis. Arthritis Rheum 42:1481-1484, 1999.

57. Fearon U, Griosios K, Fraser A, et al: Angiopoietins, growth factors, and vascular morphology in early arthritis. J Rheumatol 30:260-268, 2003.

58. Leong TT, Fearon U, Veale DJ: Angiogenesis in psoriasis and psoriatic arthritis: Clues to disease pathogenesis. Curr Rheumatol Rep 7:325-329, 2005.

59. Laloux L, Voisin MC, Allain J, et al: Immunohistological study of entheses in spondyloarthropathies: Comparison in rheumatoid arthritis and osteoarthritis. Ann Rheum Dis 60:316-321, 2001.

60. McGonagle D, Marzo-Ortega H, O'Connor P, et al: Histological assessment of the early enthesitis lesion in spondyloarthropathy. Ann Rheum Dis 61:534-537, 2002.

61. Costello P, Bresnihan B, O'Farrelly C, et al: Predominance of CD8+ T lymphocytes in psoriatic arthritis. J Rheumatol 26:1117-1124, 1999.

62. Ritchlin C, Haas-Smith SA, Hicks D, et al: Patterns of cytokine production in psoriatic synovium. J Rheumatol 25:1544-1552, 1998.

63. Austin LM, Ozawa M, Kikuchi T, et al: The majority of epidermal T cells in psoriasis vulgaris lesions can produce type 1 cytokines, interferon-gamma, interleukin-2, and tumor necrosis factor-alpha, defining TC1 (cytotoxic T lymphocyte) and TH1 effector populations: A type 1 differentiation bias is also measured in circulating blood T cells in psoriatic patients. J Invest Dermatol 113:752-759, 1999.

64. Danning CL, Illei GG, Hitchon C, et al: Macrophage-derived cytokine and nuclear factor kappaB p65 expression in synovial membrane and skin of patients with psoriatic arthritis. Arthritis Rheum 43:1244-1256, 2000.

65. Kane D, Gogarty M, O'Leary J, et al: Reduction of synovial sublining layer inflammation and proinflammatory cytokine expression in psoriatic arthritis treated with methotrexate. Arthritis Rheum 50:3286-3295, 2004.

66. Partsch G, Steiner G, Leeb BF, et al: Highly increased levels of tumor necrosis factor-alpha and other proinflammatory cytokines in psoriatic arthritis synovial fluid. J Rheumatol 24:518-523, 1997.

67. Baeten D, Kruithof E, Van den Bosch F, et al: Immunomodulatory effects of anti-tumor necrosis factor alpha therapy on synovium in spondylarthropathy: Histologic findings in eight patients from an open-label pilot study. Arthritis Rheum 44:186-195, 2001.

68. Kruithof E, De Rycke L, Roth J, et al: Immunomodulatory effects of etanercept on peripheral joint synovitis in the spondylarthropathies. Arthritis Rheum 52:3898-3909, 2005.

69. Canete JD, Pablos JL, Sanmarti R, et al: Antiangiogenic effects of anti-tumor necrosis factor alpha therapy with infliximab in psoriatic arthritis. Arthritis Rheum 50:1636-1641, 2004.

70. Ribbens C, Martin y Porras M, et al: Increased matrix metalloproteinase-3 serum levels in rheumatic diseases: Relationship with synovitis and steroid treatment. Ann Rheum Dis 61:161-166, 2002.

71. Vandooren B, Kruithof E, Yu DT, et al: Involvement of matrix metalloproteinases and their inhibitors in peripheral synovitis and down-regulation by tumor necrosis factor alpha blockade in spondylarthropathy. Arthritis Rheum 50:2942-2953, 2004.

72. Kane D, Jensen LE, Grehan S, et al: Quantitation of metalloproteinase gene expression in rheumatoid and psoriatic arthritis synovial tissue distal and proximal to the cartilage-pannus junction. J Rheumatol 31:1274-1280, 2004.
73. **Ritchlin CT, Haas-Smith SA, Li P, et al: Mechanisms of TNF-alpha- and RANKL-mediated osteoclastogenesis and bone resorption in psoriatic arthritis. J Clin Invest 111:821-831, 2003.**
74. Peng H, Wright V, Usas A, et al: Synergistic enhancement of bone formation and healing by stem cell-expressed VEGF and bone morphogenetic protein-4. J Clin Invest 110:751-759, 2002.
75. De Klerck B, Carpentier I, Lories RJ, et al: Enhanced osteoclast development in collagen-induced arthritis in interferon-gamma receptor knock-out mice as related to increased splenic CD11b+ myelopoiesis. Arthritis Res Ther 6:R220-R231, 2004.
75a. Curran SA, Fitzgerald OM, Costello PJ, et al: Nucleotide sequencing of psoriatic arthritis tissue before and during methotrexate administration reveals a complex inflammatory T cell infiltrate with very few clones exhibiting features that suggest they drive the inflammatory process by recognizing autoantigens. J Immunol 172:1935-1944, 2004.
76. **Kavanaugh AF, Ritchlin CT: Systematic review of treatments for psoriatic arthritis: An evidence based approach and basis for treatment guidelines. J Rheumatol 33:1417-1421, 2006.**
77. Shiffman RN, Shekelle P, Overhage JM, et al: Standardized reporting of clinical practice guidelines: A proposal from the Conference on Guideline Standardization. Ann Intern Med 139:493-498, 2003.
78. Soriano ER, McHugh NJ: Therapies for peripheral joint disease in psoriatic arthritis: A systematic review. J Rheumatol 33:1422-1430, 2006.
79. Grassi W, De Angelis R, Cervini C: Corticosteroid prescribing in rheumatoid arthritis and psoriatic arthritis. Clin Rheumatol 17:223-226, 1998.
80. Strober BE, Siu K, Menon K: Conventional systemic agents for psoriasis: A systematic review. J Rheumatol 33:1442-1446, 2006.
81. Ritchlin CT: Therapies for psoriatic enthesopathy: A systematic review. J Rheumatol 33:1435-1438, 2006.
82. Helliwell PS: Therapies for dactylitis in psoriatic arthritis: A systematic review. J Rheumatol 33:1439-1441, 2006.
83. Nash P: Therapies for axial disease in psoriatic arthritis: A systematic review. J Rheumatol 33:1431-1434, 2006.
84. Spadaro A, Riccieri V, Sili-Scavalli A, et al: Comparison of cyclosporin A and methotrexate in the treatment of psoriatic arthritis: A one-year prospective study. Clin Exp Rheumatol 13:589-593, 1995.
85. Mihatsch MJ, Wolff K: Consensus conference on cyclosporin A for psoriasis, February 1992. Br J Dermatol 126:621-623, 1992.
86. Kaltwasser JP, Nash P, Gladman D, et al: Efficacy and safety of leflunomide in the treatment of psoriatic arthritis and psoriasis: A multinational, double-blind, randomized, placebo-controlled clinical trial. Arthritis Rheum 50:1939-1950, 2004.
87. **Mease P.J., Kivitz A.J., Burch F.X., et al: Etanercept treatment of psoriatic arthritis: Safety, efficacy, and effect on disease progression. Arthritis Rheum 50:2264-2272, 2004.**
88. Cassell S, Kavanaugh AF: Therapies for psoriatic nail disease: A systematic review. J Rheumatol 33:1452-1456, 2006.
89. Boehncke WH, Prinz J, Gottlieb AB: Biologic therapies for psoriasis: A systematic review. J Rheumatol 33:1447-1451, 2006.
90. Mease PJ, Gladman DD, Ritchlin CT, et al: Adalimumab for the treatment of patients with moderately to severely active psoriatic arthritis: Results of a double-blind, randomized, placebo-controlled trial. Arthritis Rheum 52:3279-3289, 2005.
91. Lebwohl M, Christophers E, Langley R, et al: An international, randomized, double-blind, placebo-controlled phase 3 trial of intramuscular alefacept in patients with chronic plaque psoriasis. Arch Dermatol 139:719-727, 2003.
92. Mease PJ, Gladman DD, Keystone EC: Alefacept in combination with methotrexate for the treatment of psoriatic arthritis: Results of a randomized, double-blind, placebo-controlled study. Arthritis Rheum 54:1638-1645, 2006.

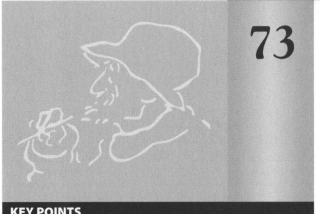

73 Enteropathic Arthritis 📷

FRANK A. WOLLHEIM

KEY POINTS

The gut microflora (biota) is essential for early childhood development and maintenance of adult health. Loss of normal tolerance causes diseases such as asthma and inflammatory bowel disease (IBD).

The gut-associated lymphoid tissue is the largest immune organ in the body, disseminating cells to other organs, including the joints. These lymphocytes produce protective secretory immunoglobulin (Ig) A and IgM but also leak complement-binding IgG, mediating both local protection and inflammation.

Genetic polymorphism causes impaired defense to microbes in Crohn's disease.

Peripheral and central joint disease in IBD is determined by different genes on several chromosomes.

HLA-B27 contributes to the pathogenesis of enteric reactive arthritis by molecular mechanisms that involve misfolding and are unrelated to antigen recognition. Aggressive antibiotic therapy is of no benefit.

Celiac disease has been underdiagnosed in adults and is associated with arthritis in 25% of patients.

Whipple's disease induces a reduced T helper type 1 response against the agent. Joint complaints are the presenting symptom in two thirds of patients.

Microscopic colitis is an underdiagnosed entity in elderly women, and chronic arthritides are overrepresented in collagenous colitis.

Enteropathic arthritis is the name given to several different conditions in which pathology in the gut and the musculoskeletal system dominates. It was realized centuries ago that dysentery was sometimes followed by arthritis, a condition now known as reactive arthritis. Inflammatory bowel disease (IBD) and reactive arthritis are the dominant entities discussed in this chapter.

The gut has three major biologic functions: it is a barrier against hostile factors in the environment, it has an obvious role in nutrition and in the excretion of waste, and it has major trophic functions in the host. The gut is constantly exposed to living and dead antigenic material, and 25% of it consists of lymphoid tissue. The gut is a privileged tissue, in that it is tolerant of food constituents and most microbes. Tolerance, however, is not a passive process; it involves active host immune responses.[1] Disturbances in these responses result in signs and symptoms, such as food allergy or IBD (Fig. 73-1). The generation of arthritis is at the core of this chapter, and different mechanisms are operative, many of which are still elusive.

GUT BIOLOGY

PHYSIOLOGY

The gut has an estimated surface area of 300 to 400 m², which is 200 times the body's skin surface area. Molecules smaller than 5000 daltons can pass through the epithelial membranes of the microvilli, whereas larger molecules can enter Peyer's patches by endocytosis. Altered gut permeability can be observed in several diseases; the causes are genetic in part but are triggered by exogenous factors such as drugs and microorganisms.[3] Oral feeding of lactalbumin, lactoglobulin, polyethylene glycol particles, ^{51}Cr-labeled EDTA, and sugars such as lactulose and mannitol, followed by urinalysis, is used to quantify pathologic changes, including changes in permeability and absorptive mechanisms. In addition, intestinal permeability and function can be studied by regional perfusion with the help of endoscopic techniques that close off segments of the gut with inflatable balloons.[4] A recent study applying enzyme-linked immunosorbent assays to fluid collected by this technique showed marked local immunity to a number of food-related antigens in patients with rheumatoid arthritis.[5] Ethnic differences in gut permeability have also been described.[6]

The healthy gut harbors a mixture of native bacteria acquired at birth or shortly thereafter that retains a relatively constant composition; it also has a smaller population of transient bacteria of varying composition. The former are essential for health and live in symbiosis; the latter contain potential pathogens. Whereas the stomach and duodenum normally contain less than 10³ mucosa-adhering bacteria, the number of bacteria increases to 10⁴ in the jejunum and 10⁷ in the ileum. Most of this last group are gram-negative aerobic species. In the colon, the bacterial density is 10¹² or more, consisting mostly of anaerobic bacteria. Transit time is fast in the upper gut and slow in the distal gut, but the immunologic impact of the microflora is higher in the proximal parts of the gut.[7]

The trophic functions of the gut require this microflora, as demonstrated by host defects in germ-free animals. Bacteria digest food carbohydrates into short-chain fatty acids, which facilitates the absorption of Ca^{2+}, Mg^{2+}, and Fe^{2+} ions, and they synthesize amino acids and vitamins and secrete antibacterial protective substances. Commensal bacteria also produce immunomodulatory saccharides that regulate the T helper type 1 (Th1)–T helper type 2 (Th2) balance. Some 300 to 500 different species are represented, and the composition is unique for each individual. Some of the common colonic species and their functions are shown in Figure 73-2.[7]

📷 Supplemental images available on the Expert Consult Premium Edition website.

1219

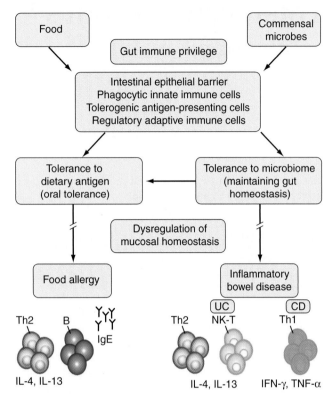

Figure 73-1 Immune privilege in the gut. CD, Crohn's disease; IFN, interferon; IL, interleukin; UC, ulcerative colitis. (*From Iweala OI, Nagler CR: Immune privilege in the gut: The establishment and maintenance of nonresponsiveness to dietary antigens and commensal flora. Immunol Rev 213:82-100, 2006.*)

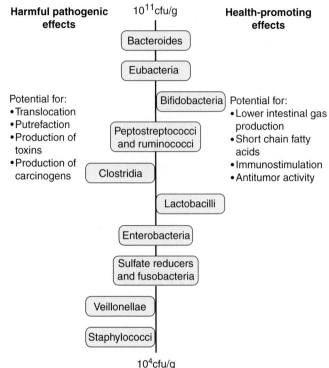

Figure 73-2 Physiologic roles of the intestinal microflora. (*From Guarner F: Enteric flora in health and disease. Digestion 73(Suppl 1):5-12, 2006.*)

GUT-ASSOCIATED LYMPHOID TISSUE

Gut-associated lymphoid tissue (GALT) is the largest lymphoid organ of the body, constituting 25% of the mucosal mass. GALT components are found in Peyer's plaques, gut lymphoid follicles, lamina propria, and intraepithelial T cells. The epithelial glycoprotein called secretory component or polymeric immunoglobulin receptor is a 100-kD transmembrane receptor for polymeric immunoglobulin, that is, J chain–containing immunoglobulin (Ig) A and IgM. It is abundantly present in Peyer's patches in the distal ileum. It forms complexes—secretory IgA and, to some extent, secretory IgM—that are secreted into the lumen and constitute a noninflammatory, non–complement-binding first line of defense. It is estimated that a healthy adult secretes 3 to 5 g of secretory IgA into the gut daily (Fig. 73-3). Breastfeeding provides the newborn with secretory IgA and IgM, which confers passive protection and also regulates much of the child's immune system (Fig. 73-4).

From the Peyer's patches, primed B lymphocytes disseminate throughout the body's mucous membranes, notably to other parts of the alimentary tract. Primed T lymphocytes also disseminate into the circulation and lymph nodes and home into target organs, such as salivary glands (in Sjögren's disease), lungs, and synovium.[8] Vascular adhesion protein-1 (VAP-1) expressed on synovial epithelial cells is involved in lymphocyte homing, and P-selectin is a part of macrophage recruitment. VAP-1 is a bifunctional glycoprotein with both adhesive and oxidative properties.[9] The inhibition of this molecule may become a target in the treatment of enteropathic arthritis. Most T lymphocytes in the mucosal lamina propria are CD4[+], whereas intraepithelial T cells are mostly CD8[+]. Gut-associated lymphocytes preferentially express the integrins α4β7 and αEβ7 and the integrin receptor CCR9 upon stimulation by intestinal dendritic cells.[9]

A chain of events in the pathogenesis of enteropathic arthritis can begin with gastrointestinal infection with the appropriate microorganism in a genetically predisposed patient. This causes local inflammation in the gut mucosa, formation of secretory IgA, increased permeability, absorption of foreign material, and triggering of T lymphocytes. Circulating immune complexes and memory T cells localize to joints and cause synovitis (Fig. 73-5).

SPONDYLOARTHROPATHIES

Seronegative spondyloarthropathy is the designation for a group of diseases exhibiting some common characteristics and with overlapping genetic and clinical features. Included in this group, among other conditions, are arthritis with IBD, reactive arthritis, and a syndrome termed undifferentiated spondyloarthritis. The gut is a putative or proven port of entry for microbial agents, and the joint disease is characterized by sacroiliitis, spinal involvement, enthesopathy, or peripheral oligoarthritis with dominant localization to the lower extremities. Systemic manifestations involving the eyes, skin, heart, and urogenital tract are also common.

INFLAMMATORY BOWEL DISEASE

EPIDEMIOLOGY

The prevalence of Crohn's disease and ulcerative colitis is about equal, and in the United States, there are between 50 and 100 cases per 100,000 population.[3] In recent years,

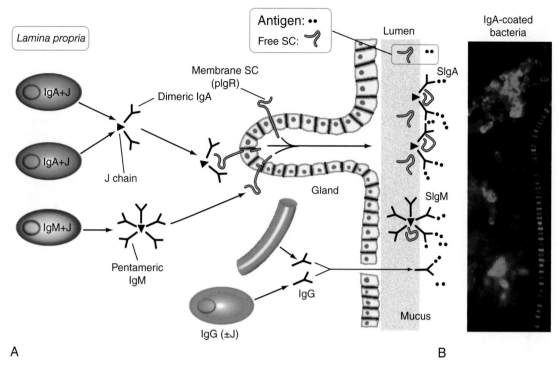

A   B

Figure 73-3   Mucosal immunoglobulin defense system. IgA and IgM are coupled to secretory component (SC), whereas IgG passes into the lumen unattached and is still complement binding. *(From Brandtzaeg P, Johansen FE: Mucosal B cells: Phenotypic characteristics, transcriptional regulation, and homing properties. Immunol Rev 206:32-63, 2005.)*

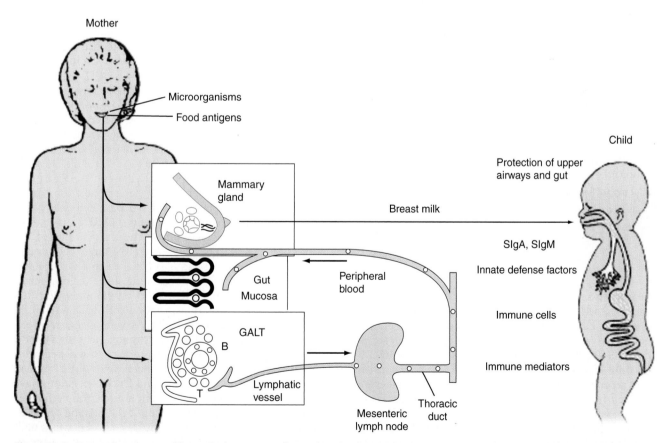

Figure 73-4   Integration of mucosal immunity between mother and newborn. Primed B (and probably T) cells from Peyer's patch migrate via lymph and peripheral blood to the lactating mammary gland, resulting in the presence in breast milk of secretory antibodies (SIgA and SIgM) specific for enteric antigens. *(From Brandtzaeg P: Mucosal immunity: Integration between mother and the breast-fed infant. Vaccine 21:3382-3388, 2003.)*

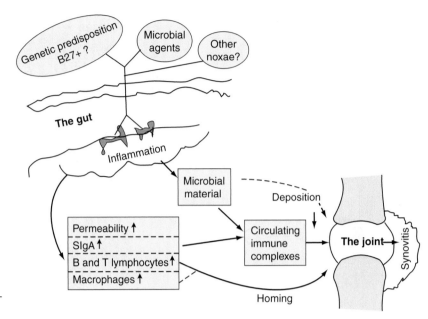

Figure 73-5 Immune pathogenesis of enteropathic arthritis.

Table 73-1 Extraintestinal Manifestations of Inflammatory Bowel Disease

Feature or Disease	Crohn's	Ulcerative Colitis
Peripheral arthritis	≈15%	≈10%
Axial or sacroiliac arthritis	≈15%-20%	≈10%-15%
Septic arthritis	Rare	Not reported
Skin		
Erythema nodosum	Up to 15%	<15%
Erythema multiforme	Rare	?
Pyoderma gangrenosum	0.5%-2%	0.3%-0.4% in severe disease
Aphthous ulcers	Rare	1%-8%
Nephrolithiasis (oxalate)	<15%	?
Amyloidosis	Very rare	Not reported
Liver disease	3%-5%	7%
Uveitis	13%	4%
Vasculitis	Takayasu's	<5%
Clubbing of fingers	Yes	1%-5%
Increased prevalence of asthma	Yes	Yes
Increased prevalence of multiple sclerosis	No	Yes

the incidence of ulcerative colitis has decreased in Western countries, whereas the previously low incidence of IBD in eastern Europe, South America, and the Pacific have increased.[10] This may be due in part to better reporting. The overall concordance in monozygotic twins is 36%, but it is only 16% in ulcerative colitis.[11] Joint involvement has been reported in up to 25% of patients.[4] Lower figures were reported from a large population-based Canadian study,[12] but it excluded peripheral arthritis, which may explain why less than 10% of patients had "arthritis." Interestingly, asthma and multiple sclerosis were overrepresented in two recent studies of extraintestinal autoimmune manifestations of IBD (Table 73-1).[13]

CAUSE

Intestinal microflora remain a major suspect in the cause of IBD, but final proof is lacking. Experimental models require gut bacteria. Postoperative therapy with metronidazole has prolonged the time to relapse.[14] Genome-wide screening has identified a region on chromosome 16 with polymorphisms that in 2001 were linked to CARD15 (caspase-activating recruitment domain 15), also known as NOD2 (nuclear oligomerization domain 2). This region, named IBD1, shows mutations in up to 80% of patients with Crohn's disease. A number of putative susceptibility loci (IBD1 to 9), seven of which have been confirmed in independent studies, are present on different genes[15] (Fig. 73-6). CARD15 and CARD4 are cytosolic sensors for the bacterial peptidoglycan muramide dipeptide and trigger the synthesis of antibacterial α-defensins.[16,17] Reduced mucosal expression of these defensins is found in patients with Crohn's disease.[18] Whereas CARD15 mutations were present in 43% of patients in the initial French study,[19] later population studies found a much lower prevalence in northern European populations and no correlation in Asians. CARD15 mutations are not related to susceptibility in the United States. High expression of CARD15 messenger RNA has been found in the small intestine, and it is believed to be a regulator of nuclear factor κB (NFκB) signaling after the engagement of Toll-like receptors (TLRs). IBD3 on chromosome 6 has shown the most constant association with IBD, and HLA-DRB1*0103 has been linked to severe ulcerative colitis in several studies.[9] Further, a tumor necrosis factor-α (TNF-α) microsatellite gene factor was associated with Crohn's disease but not with ulcerative colitis. Human leukocyte antigen (HLA)-DR2 and DR3 associations have been linked to ulcerative colitis but not to Crohn's disease.

Mutations of the detoxifying ATP-binding cassette, subfamily B, member 1 gene (ABCB1), also known as multidrug resistance 1 gene (MDR1), are strongly downregulated in unaffected colonic tissue of both Crohn's disease and ulcerative colitis patients. TLR4 and TLR5 associations

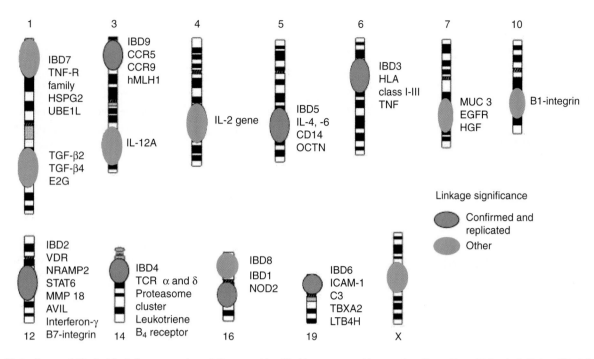

Figure 73-6 Susceptibility loci for inflammatory bowel disease as identified by genome-wide scanning. *(From Ahmad T, Tamboli CP, Jewell D, Colombel JF: Clinical relevance of advances in genetics and pharmacogenetics of IBD. Gastroenterology 126:1533-1549, 2004.)*

have been identified in several populations; this may be of special interest, because they act in synergy with CARD15 and CARD4 in the induction of proinflammatory cytokines. TLR inhibitors are being investigated for therapeutic efficacy. The relation of these new genetic factors to the occurrence of joint or other extraintestinal manifestations has not been studied in detail. Recently, several new susceptibility loci for IBD have been confirmed using genome-wide screening. These involve IL23R and other factors influencing the barrier function of the gut and innate immunity.[19a] IL23 and its receptor deserve special attention since gene-manipulated mice are resistant to colitis and since IL23 is upregulated in patients with CD.[19b]

PATHOGENESIS

Crohn's disease and ulcerative colitis are clinically distinct entities with a different pathogenesis, but new genetic evidence also shows some common features. Both are familial, but hereditary factors are more important in Crohn's disease, according to twin studies.

Whereas the entire gut wall is involved in a patchy way in Crohn's disease, diffuse mucosal pathology is typical of ulcerative colitis. T lymphocyte proliferation and cytokine generation are also different. In Crohn's disease, a Th1 response dominates,[20] but no such dominance has been documented for ulcerative colitis. Increased amounts of proinflammatory cytokines, TNF-α, interleukin (IL)-1β, IL-6, and IL-8, are released locally in both diseases (see Fig. 73-1).[21]

The interplay between the intestinal microflora and genetic host factors is disturbed in IBD. The microbial contribution is still largely unclear, and animal work indicates that parts of the normal gut flora may be involved. In addition, pathogenic organisms, such as *Clostridium difficile*, have been linked to exacerbations of IBD.[22] As discussed earlier, genetic factors related to innate immunity are involved in susceptibility to IBD. Experimental work with transgenic animals

transfected with human HLA-B27 and β$_2$-microglobulin has shown that certain strains of conventional mice and rats develop spondyloarthropathies, whereas identical animals in a germ-free environment are protected.[23,24] In human disease, HLA-B27 is clearly one predisposing factor, but only in the minority of cases with spinal joint involvement. Jejunal fluid from patients with ankylosing spondylitis (AS) and rheumatoid arthritis collected with the closed-segment endoscopic technique contained antibodies against *Klebsiella pneumoniae*, *Escherichia coli*, and *Proteus mirabilis*.[3] A disturbed and augmented local immune response in parts of the gut against a variety of microorganisms is emerging as a prevalent feature of several chronic joint diseases, but it has not been examined in IBD with this endoscopic technique.

Gene manipulation in mice indicates that IL-2, IL-10, and transforming growth factor-β may be protective factors and that HLA-B27 may influence cytokine expression.[25] Altered cytokine balance in the gut mucosa may be an important contributing pathogenic factor.

Increased gut permeability has already been alluded to as an important factor in pathogenesis.[4] Bacteria recovered from the gut lumen in IBD are covered by immunoglobulin, part of which is circulatory IgG.[26] Increased leakage of tissue fluid from the inflamed mucosa allows the egress of complement-binding IgG, which may contribute to inflammation and further augment permeability. The altered immune response to bacteria differs between Crohn's disease and ulcerative colitis.[27] Increased gut permeability in IBD is under genetic influence. Basal permeability was normal in a study of relatives of patients with Crohn's disease, but it became abnormally increased after the ingestion of acetylsalicylic acid.[28] Environmental influences on permeability may be partly mediated by bacterial endotoxin. An in vitro perfusion study on rat gut showed that serosal rather than mucosal application of endotoxin impairs the barrier.[29] Absorbed bacterial material could therefore add to an already damaged barrier.

Table 73-2 Distinct Features of Inflammatory Bowel Disease

Feature	Crohn's	Ulcerative Colitis
Genetic base	Strong, recessive	Weaker, dominant
Concordance in monozygotic twins	36%	19%
Non-HLA genes	Yes	Yes
Gut permeability sensitive to ASA on genetic base	Yes	?
T lymphocyte response in gut	Th1 (IFN-γ↑)	No Th1-Th2 imbalance
Fas ligand expression	No	Yes
Effect of smoking	None (?)	Protective
Correlation of gut activity to arthritis symptoms	No	Yes
ICAM-1 antisense therapy	Beneficial	No response (?)
Response to anti-TNF therapy	Well established	Probably effective

ASA, acetylsalicylic acid; HLA, human leukocyte antigen; ICAM, intercellular adhesion molecule; IFN, interferon; Th1, T helper type 1; Th2, T helper type 2; TNF, tumor necrosis factor.

CLINICAL FEATURES

Although Crohn's disease and ulcerative colitis are clinically distinct entities, they share many features (Table 73-2). Spinal involvement occurs in 10% to 20% of cases. The back symptoms are often silent, so their prevalence is underestimated; they may precede the onset of IBD or appear later.[4] In contrast to AS, there is an equal sex distribution. In general, the involvement is similar to or identical with that in classic AS, although small differences have been found.[30] Changes in enteropathic disease tended to be milder, squaring was more prevalent, and Romanus lesions were not found. The majority of radiographic features were similar. As noted, spinal involvement is often asymptomatic, but when symptoms are present, they do not correlate with intestinal symptoms. The issue is complicated by the association of AS with silent Crohn's disease, as diagnosed by biopsy.[31] Isolated sacroiliitis is not strongly associated with HLA-B27. In full-blown IBD-related AS, the prevalence of B27 is between 50% and 70%.[4]

Between 5% and 15% of patients in most studies develop peripheral arthritis, slightly more often in Crohn's disease than in ulcerative colitis (Table 73-3). It is often nondestructive and reversible, but erosive changes may also occur. Limited histopathologic evidence indicates the presence of granulomas in Crohn's disease and nonspecific synovitis in ulcerative colitis.[4] In Crohn's patients, rapidly destructive septic arthritis has been reported in the hip. Joint symptoms tend to coincide with gut activity in ulcerative colitis but not in Crohn's disease. Total colectomy is associated with remission of arthritis in half the patients with ulcerative colitis, but paradoxically, arthritis may also begin after surgery.[32] This may represent a form of bypass arthritis related to altered gut microbiology.

Based on the examination of about 1500 patients with IBD, a distinction was made between two forms of peripheral arthritis[33] (Fig. 73-7). Oligoarthritis, or type 1, affects less than five joints, while polyarthritis, or type 2, involves more than five joints. The highest prevalence was found in metacarpophalangeal, proximal interphalangeal, knee, and

Table 73-3 Peripheral Joint Disease in Inflammatory Bowel Disease

Feature	Type 2 (>5 Joints)	Type 1 (< 5 Joints)
Ulcerative colitis	3; 3%	2; 5%
Crohn's disease	6; 0%	4; 6%
Clinical course	Self-limited arthritis	Persistent arthritis
Course of IBD	Relapsing in <85%	Relapsing in 30%-40%
MHC association	HLA-B27, B35, DRB1*0103	HLA-B44

HLA, human leukocyte antigen; IBD, inflammatory bowel disease; MHC, major histocompatibility complex.

ankle joints. Shoulder involvement was more common in ulcerative colitis, but joint involvement was otherwise strikingly similar. It is important that the majority of type 1 cases were acute and resolved within 6 weeks, whereas the type 2 cases persisted.[34] Type 1 arthritis was 12 times more prevalent in carriers of the rare HLA-DRB1*0103 allele. This is an example of genetic influence on disease phenotype and may be a clue to pathogenesis.

Clubbing of fingers, uveitis, and skin manifestations are other extraintestinal manifestations of IBD, with a higher frequency in Crohn's disease. Erythema nodosum, which is usually self-limited, is most frequent in young female patients with ulcerative colitis. Pyoderma gangrenosum is a more severe, painful, ulcerating skin reaction that is frequently associated with systemic disease[35] (Fig. 73-8). In a series of 86 patients with pyoderma gangrenosum seen at the Mayo Clinic between 1970 and 1983, 31 had IBD.[4] Erythema nodosum, uveitis, and peripheral arthritis commonly occur together in IBD and have been linked to HLA-DRB1*0103 and TNF-α gene polymorphism.[36] Uveitis is also a feature of other spondyloarthropathies, such as AS and reactive arthritis. In IBD, however, uveitis is more often bilateral, and the tendency toward chronicity is more pronounced.[37,38]

DIAGNOSIS

A careful history and clinical examination, supplemented by imaging, are the principal diagnostic tools. As mentioned, genetic mapping has shown interesting clinical correlates, but genotyping is not part of the routine clinical workup at present, except perhaps for HLA-B27. Stool cultures should be performed when infection with special pathogens is suspected.

TREATMENT

Joint manifestations are considered secondary to active IBD. Current dogma states that treating the latter will benefit the former, but there is no rigorous proof that this is so. Placebo effects account for perhaps 20% of the treatment response in IBD; therefore, only placebo-controlled evidence can be trusted. Sulfasalazine and its derivative 5-ASA inhibit the function of NFκB, and several studies have shown the efficacy of these drugs compared with placebo in ulcerative colitis but not in Crohn's disease.[3] Glucocorticoids are effective in both forms of IBD, although the response of uveitis to topical therapy with glucocorticoids may be less prompt than in uveitis of other causes.[4]

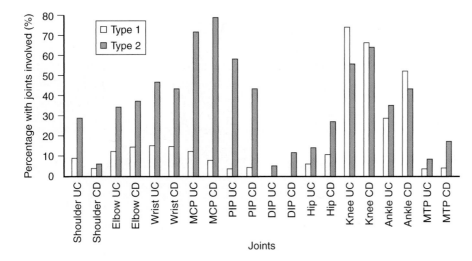

Figure 73-7 Articular distribution of peripheral arthropathies in inflammatory bowel disease. See also Table 73-3. CD, Crohn's disease; DIP, distal interphalangeal joint; MCP, metacarpophalangeal joint; MTP, metatarsophalangeal joint; PIP, proximal interphalangeal joint.; UC, ulcerative colitis. *(From Orchard TR, Wordsworth BP, Jewell DP: Peripheral arthropathies in inflammatory bowel disease: Their articular distribution and natural history. Gut 42:387, 1998.)*

tested in controlled studies, but there is no convincing evidence that they are better than placebo, and they are usually inferior to glucocorticoids.[45]

OUTCOME

There are no prospective studies addressing the outcome of arthritis complicating IBD.

ENTERIC REACTIVE ARTHRITIS

Enteric reactive arthritis is a common postinfectious condition related to uroarthritis but triggered from the gut. The French physician Broussais founded the so-called physiologic medicine, claiming that all human disease was caused by gastrointestinal infections; he was familiar with postdysenteric arthritis. Various eponyms have been attached to reactive arthritis, perhaps the best being Fiessinger-Leroy syndrome.[46] *Yersinia* was identified by Winblad and coworkers[47] in Sweden as a human pathogen causing enteritis. Ahvonen and colleagues[48] in Finland confirmed it as a trigger for reactive arthritis in 1969.

EPIDEMIOLOGY

The occurrence of enteric reactive arthritis is determined by the prevalence of exposure to triggering agents and the susceptibility of infected individuals. Therefore, incidence and prevalence figures vary among populations and over time. A population-based study from Oslo over 2 years estimated that the minimum annual incidence of enteric reactive arthritis among individuals aged 18 to 60 years was 5 per 100,000.[49] The risk of developing enteric reactive arthritis in exposed individuals varies from very low to 20% in different outbreaks[3]; it may be lower in children.[50] The prevalence of *Yersinia* infections has diminished in recent years, probably as a consequence of improved slaughterhouse hygiene. *Salmonella* and *Campylobacter* are presently the two dominant causes of enteric reactive arthritis in most countries.[50]

CAUSE

The triggering agents are usually gram-negative obligate or facultative intracellular organisms. Table 73-4 shows the agents most commonly implicated as triggers. In most series,

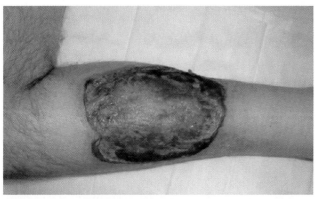

Figure 73-8 Pyoderma gangrenosum in a case of Crohn's disease. *(From Rothfuss KS, Stange EF, Herrlinger KR: Extraintestinal manifestations and complications in inflammatory bowel diseases. World J Gastroenterol 12:4819-4831, 2006.)*

Azathioprine has been widely used to maintain remission in IBD. It has proven long-term efficacy in both ulcerative colitis and Crohn's disease, according to a large European study.[39] It should not be combined with 5-ASA owing to a pharmacokinetic interaction.[40]

TNF inhibition with infliximab (but not with etanercept) results in remission of gastrointestinal manifestations in close to 60% of patients with Crohn's disease, as confirmed in several placebo-controlled studies.[41] More recently, infliximab was found to be superior to placebo in ulcerative colitis patients resistant to conventional drug therapy, although the evidence is less robust if compared to glucocorticoid therapy.[42] Anecdotal evidence supports the efficacy of infliximab in the treatment of pyoderma gangrenosum. Natalizumab, an antibody against α4 integrin, has shown promising effects in both multiple sclerosis and Crohn's disease. However, enthusiasm was reduced after the occurrence of three cases of the severe form of leukoencephalitis; two of the patients died.[43] The drug is still in limited use.

Pain control with nonsteroidal anti-inflammatory drugs is a potential problem owing to their potential induction of flares. However, they are widely used and often well tolerated. Probiotics, though widely promoted, have not been effective in IBD.[44] Metronidazole, ciprofloxacin, and other poorly absorbed broad-spectrum antibiotics have been widely

Table 73-4 Causative Agents in Postenteric Reactive Arthritis

Common	Less Common
Shigella flexneri	Shigella sonnei
Salmonella typhimurium	Shigella dysenteriae
Salmonella enteritidis	Salmonella paratyphi B
Yersinia enterocolitica O3	Salmonella paratyphi C
Yersinia enterocolitica O9	Yersinia enterocolitica O8
Yersinia pseudotuberculosis	Giardia lamblia (septic?)
Campylobacter jejuni	Group A streptococci

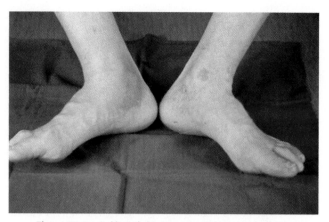

Figure 73-9 Ankle arthritis in a man with *Yersinia* arthritis.

no organism can be identified in one quarter of patients.[4,49,50] The list of confirmed triggering organisms remains remarkably short. Group A streptococcus is a relatively new trigger of reactive arthritis. In one pediatric center in Florida, 25 children with this trigger were identified,[4] but the majority of cases have been published by one group in Canada.[51] These reports have not been followed up by more recent studies. *Giardia lamblia* has been implicated in occasional cases.[1] Although other triggers may still be identified, clearly only a small number of microorganisms have the potency to trigger reactive arthritis. It is not clear which features determine arthritogenicity.[4] *Brucella* infection is also frequently associated with arthritis, which is an important differential diagnosis in endemic areas (see later).

PATHOGENESIS

In enteric reactive arthritis, a triggering gut pathogen starts an inflammatory reaction in the gut; immune cells and antigenic material then disseminate into the joint. By definition, no living organisms are present in the joint after the outbreak of arthritis. Several steps in the pathogenesis remain elusive. The humoral immune response to the trigger involves secretory IgA and IgM and also IgG, and it is prolonged in comparison to patients who do not develop enteric reactive arthritis. This indicates a surviving reservoir of the trigger, perhaps only in the form of antigenic material, somewhere in the body.[52,53] Living pathogens are not considered instrumental in enteric reactive arthritis.

The role of HLA-B27 has been studied intensely for decades. Some evidence indicates that it enhances the activation of NFκB and the expression of proinflammatory signals, resulting in a glutamic acid located in the B pocket.[54] In vitro experiments have shown normal cellular uptake of bacteria but delayed elimination.[53] Ex vivo studies have identified antigenic material, in part in the form of processed lipopolysaccharid, and DNA in the joints.[52,53] It is not known how this material gets into the joints. Bacterial lipopolysaccharide and heat shock protein can be found in joint tissue up to 4 years after the acute episode.[48] Carriage of HLA-B27 does not influence the duration of bacterial presence in feces in salmonellosis, and joint involvement does not correlate with carriage. However, transfection of human HLA-B27 into monocytes and macrophages did prolong the intracellular persistence of *Salmonella* in comparison to untransfected cells and cells transfected with HLA-A2.[53] For many years, molecular mimicry was suspected to play a part, but this has never been confirmed.[4] New insights implicate mechanisms unrelated to antigen presentation. The discovery of a propensity toward misfolding

of the HLA-B27 B pocket, leading to impaired elimination, opens new vistas to explain the enhanced lipopolysaccharide-stimulated formation of TNF-α.[55]

CLINICAL FEATURES

Reactive arthritis is characterized by the acute onset of asymmetric oligoarthritis, with dominant localization to the lower extremities and often affecting the large joints (Fig. 73-9). Aseptic urethritis is a common feature, and the presence of circinate balanitis is almost pathognomonic. Enthesopathy, manifested by heel pain, is very common. Erythema nodosum is rather unusual. Unequivocal signs of synovitis are often accompanied by less distinct arthralgias, which may outlast synovitis by several months. The enteritis is typically mild and may escape recognition, suggesting that a vigorous inflammatory response in the gut may provide protection against arthritis. Fever and acute-phase reactants may be low grade or intense. Self-limited glomerulonephritis, myocarditis, and conjunctivitis are other clinical features.

Streptococcus-triggered enteric reactive arthritis develops, on average, 3 weeks after throat infection, at which time high-titer antistreptococcal antibodies are found, most often against nonhemolytic atypical streptococci. The arthritis is not migratory, in contrast to that seen in rheumatic fever. Symptoms last an average of 60 days, and there is an equal sex distribution . HLA-B27 is not prevalent.[47]

DIAGNOSIS

Asymmetric, nondestructive oligoarthritis starting some weeks after mild gastroenteritis in a previously healthy individual should raise the suspicion of enteric reactive arthritis. The presence of balanitis blennorrhagica in males is almost pathognomonic. Rheumatoid factor and anticyclic citrullinated peptide antibody (anti-CCP) should be negative. A triggering agent may be cultured from the stools or traced serologically in the blood. However, even a systematic search reveals a trigger in only 60% of cases. Conversely, it is not unusual to find triggers in patients without previous symptomatic disease.[49]

TREATMENT

Importantly, enteric reactive arthritis cannot be prevented with aggressive antibiotic therapy, even when started early.[4,56] Symptomatic analgesic treatment is usually sufficient but may be supplemented by short periods of systemic glucocorticoids or antimalarials. Short-term antibiotic therapy is usually administered if a triggering agent can be identified. The rationale for the use of antibiotics is to eradicate remaining microorganisms (e.g., *Salmonella*) in carriers and to prevent recurrence. However, there is no evidence that antibiotics influence the outcome. One small, controlled Finnish study showed no effect after 12 months but claimed that after 5 years, chronic symptoms were more common in patients who had not received antibiotics during the initial episode of enteric reactive arthritis. This study may not be valid owing to incomplete data and unbalanced patient groups.[57]

OUTCOME

Full recovery from the acute joint episode is the rule, but this may take 3 to 18 months or longer. When *Salmonella* is the trigger, the duration is often long. Enteric reactive arthritis was once considered less likely to result in chronic or recurrent disease than uroarthritis.[3] However, several follow-up studies have documented arthralgias, tendinitis, or even frank spondyloarthropathy in two thirds of patients.[4,52,57,58] Spinal disease eventually develops in approximately 20% of patients.[3]

BRUCELLA ARTHRITIS

EPIDEMIOLOGY

Brucellosis has been eradicated in western Europe and North America but is still a major zoonosis in areas of South America, the Middle East, India, and other places where goat and sheep farming is practiced and poverty is prevalent. With increased global travel, sporadic cases can be expected in Europe and the United States. In endemic areas, the reported incidence is between 1 and 200 cases per 100,000.[58]

CAUSE AND PATHOGENESIS

Brucella are small gram-negative bacteria that infect macrophages and are harbored in the liver, spleen, and bone marrow; from there, they can spread to joints. The four species causing human disease are *Brucella melitensis*, *Brucella abortus*, *Brucella suis*, and *Brucella canis*. *Brucella* arthritis is thought to be reactive, based on the failure to grow microorganisms from joint fluid and the poor response to antibiotic therapy, but this has never been proved.[4]

CLINICAL FEATURES AND DIAGNOSIS

Brucellosis causes arthritis in about one third of cases. The main locations are the spine in adults and the peripheral joints in children and adolescents. Knees, hips, and ankles are the dominant peripheral locations. Sacroiliitis can be extremely acute and painful. Rising titers of serum antibodies and a confirmatory culture solidify the diagnosis.

TREATMENT AND OUTCOME

Rifampicin 600 to 900 mg and doxycycline 200 mg daily for at least 6 weeks are recommended by the World Health Organization, but other combinations have been tried.[58]

The arthritis can become destructive unless treated early. Spinal stenosis may be a complication.

BYPASS ARTHRITIS-DERMATITIS SYNDROME

EPIDEMIOLOGY

Improved surgical techniques for overweight treatment have eliminated a major cause of bypass arthritis-dermatitis syndrome. It may occur as a rare complication in gastrointestinal diseases with defective peristalsis, systemic sclerosis, and IBD, particularly after colorectal surgery.[4]

CAUSE AND PATHOGENESIS

Bacterial overgrowth in a blind loop is the likely cause. The formation and absorption of complement-binding immune complexes with increased gut permeability are contributing factors in pathogenesis.

CLINICAL FEATURES AND DIAGNOSIS

The main features seen in patients in the 1970s were an intensely painful oligoarthritis of the large and small joints and the spine, without structural changes, and a recurrent papulopustular rash (Fig. 73-10). Today, gastrointestinal dysfunction in combination with painful, nondestructive oligoarthritis and intermittent papular skin rash is seen.

TREATMENT AND OUTCOME

Correction of gastrointestinal function, nonresorbed antibiotics such as neomycin, and symptomatic pain relief are the principal therapeutic options. Prolonged complaints have been reported, but cure is the rule.

CELIAC DISEASE

EPIDEMIOLOGY

Celiac disease is a common condition with a global distribution. It used to be considered most prevalent in children, but new evidence shows that it is even more common in adults. Intestinal symptoms are often minimal or absent; consequently, published prevalence figures of 1% may be too low.[4,59]

CAUSE AND PATHOGENESIS

Celiac disease is caused by an immune reaction to partly digested wheat gluten by T lymphocytes in the gut of genetically HLA-DQ2–positive or HLA-DQ8–positive individuals.

It was shown in 2002 that dietary gluten is partly digested by gastric enzymes to generate a stable 33–amino acid peptide that is deamidated by tissue transglutaminase.[60] The peptide is then presented in the context of HLA-DQ2 or HLA-DQ8 to CD4+ T cells, resulting in interferon-γ release and inflammation, altered gut permeability, and eventually villus atrophy. Autoantibodies against tissue transglutaminase are also formed.[59]

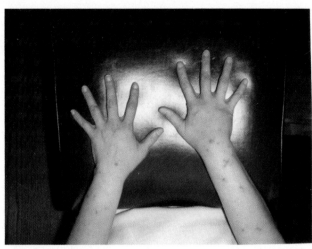

Figure 73-10   Relapsing pustulosis in a woman with bypass arthritis-dermatitis syndrome.

CLINICAL FEATURES AND DIAGNOSIS

Only two thirds of patients present with diarrhea or irritated bowel symptoms. Celiac disease is a systemic disease that can involve type 1 diabetes, anemia, osteoporosis, neuropathies, and joint symptoms in up to 25% of patients.[61] This can be an asymmetric oligoarthritis or polyarthritis, and axial involvement is common. Arthritis may be the presenting symptom of the disease.[62]

In addition to small-bowel biopsy, the diagnosis can be established by assay of anti–tissue glutaminase antibodies of the IgA type.[59]

TREATMENT AND OUTCOME

Elimination of gluten from the diet is the rational therapy and is often the only one required. In addition, various experimental approaches have been discussed but are not yet supported by data. These include the administration of IL-10 to boost regulatory T cells, the induction of tolerance by nasal application of gluten peptides, and gene therapy. No specific therapy has been established for the joint problems.

Children with verified celiac disease still have abnormal mucosa in adulthood and must continue the dietary restriction. There are no outcome reports dealing with joint involvement.

WHIPPLE'S DISEASE

EPIDEMIOLOGY

Whipple's disease is a rare condition. Incidence and prevalence figures are unknown. A retrospective French study identified 52 patients, 73% of whom were men.[4]

CAUSE AND PATHOGENESIS

Whipple's disease, or intestinal lipodystrophy, as it was initially called in 1907,[4] is an intestinal infection with a unique microorganism called *Tropheryma whippelii*, belonging to the Actinomycetes family. The organism has been found in sewage, but the source of infection in humans is not known. Six different genotypes have been confirmed in culture from diseased tissue.[63]

The organism lives in macrophages, and these elicit a skewed lymphocyte response, with suppressed Th1 dominating Th2 cells. Expression of the cytokine IL-16 stimulates growth of the pathogen.[64] Altered gut permeability may be implicated in joint involvement.

CLINICAL FEATURES

The disease can have many faces and may remain undiagnosed for many years. Recurrent fever; malaise; hematologic, pulmonary, and cardiac disturbances; and neurologic and ophthalmic symptoms are sometimes present and misinterpreted. Articular symptoms, however, are the presenting feature in 67% of cases, compared with intestinal symptoms in only 15%. Eventually, 83% of patients develop diarrhea, abdominal pain, and malnutrition. Arthralgias and arthritis are most commonly seen in knee joints but can localize in any peripheral joint, as well as in spinal joints and disks. Sacroiliitis has been described.

DIAGNOSIS

The diagnosis rests on immune histology, with the occurrence of periodic acid–Schiff–positive material, an abundance of CD68+ macrophages, and staining with antisera specific for *T. whippelii*. It is now also possible to grow the organism in culture, which takes an average of 30 days. In one study, only 2 of 10 small-bowel specimens were growth positive; the yield is higher using sterile cardiac or nerve tissue.[63] Culture therefore remains a research tool.

TREATMENT

There are no randomized, controlled studies available. Initial treatment should be ceftriaxone for 2 weeks to ensure entrance into the central nervous system. Then oral trimethoprim-sulfamethoxazole is administered for a prolonged or indefinite period. In case of intolerance or lack of efficacy, tetracycline can be used. Use of penicillin, streptomycin, and chloramphenicol has been abandoned.[65]

OUTCOME

Without treatment, Whipple's disease is chronic or relapsing, usually progressive, and ultimately fatal. With adequate antibiotic therapy, clinical remission is usually complete or near complete. However, immune histology still shows some evidence of remaining pathology, indicating that therapy should not be interrupted.[65]

MICROSCOPIC COLITIS

Chronic diarrhea is common, and its prevalence increases in the elderly.[66] Microscopic colitis includes two diseases presenting with diarrhea—collagenous colitis and lymphocytic colitis, described in 1976 and 1989, respectively—and associated with rheumatologic conditions.[67]

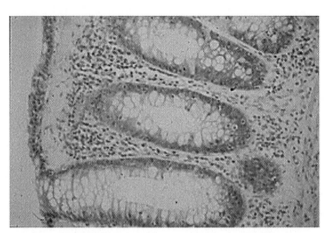

Figure 73-11   Collagenous colitis. Note the intact epithelium and massive subepithelial collagen layer. *(Courtesy of Dr. Claes Lindström.)*

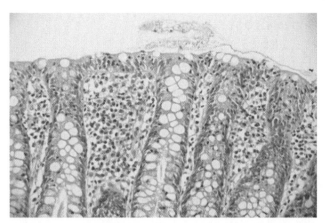

Figure 73-12   Lymphocytic colitis. Note the epithelial lesions with intraepithelial lymphocytosis and inflammation of the lamina propria. *(From Wollheim FA: Collagenous colitis and rheumatology. Curr Rheumatol Rep 2:183-184, 2000.)*

EPIDEMIOLOGY

Microscopic colitis is the recognized cause in 10% to 20% of patients investigated for nonbloody diarrhea in Europe and North America. The annual incidence for collagenous and lymphocytic colitis is 4 to 12 per 100,000 each in population-based studies from Sweden and Minnesota, and the figures are rising.[67] The female-male ratio is 7:1 in collagenous colitis and 2:1 in lymphocytic colitis. The peak incidence is among those 60 to 80 years old.

CAUSE

The cause is unknown. No genetic factors have been identified. Exposure to antirheumatic therapy has been suspected in patients with rheumatoid arthritis, based on the observation that arthritis usually precedes the onset of collagenous colitis. Reaction against some luminal factor is deduced from the observation that histology is normalized when ileostomy is performed but recurs after closure. Drugs that are prime suspects include NSAIDs and acetylsalicylic acid, lansoprazole, ranitidine, sertraline, and ticlopidine.[67]

PATHOGENESIS

Infection is suspected, but no agent has been identified. Luminal factors are strongly suggested by almost complete histologic normalization after performing ileostomy and recurrence of pathology and symptoms after its closure.

CLINICAL FEATURES

The intestinal symptoms consist of chronic, intermittent (or sometimes chronic, persistent) painful watery stools; weight loss; and fatigue. There is no difference between collagenous and lymphocytic colitis. The course is acute or chronic but usually benign.

Collagenous colitis is associated with a variety of joint syndromes in at least 20% of cases. These include Sjögren's syndrome, nondestructive oligoarthritis, migratory arthralgias, sacroiliitis, and rheumatoid arthritis. A survey of 63 consecutive cases in one Swedish center identified 8 cases of rheumatoid arthritis and 3 cases of AS, clearly suggesting a correlation between colitis and chronic joint disease.[66] The prevalence of rheumatologic conditions in lymphocytic colitis is probably lower, but no study has been published.

DIAGNOSIS

The diagnosis can be made only by histology obtained at colonoscopy. The barium radiograph is essentially normal, and laboratory tests are unhelpful. Lindström found a characteristic thickening of the collagen layer under the gut epithelium. This layer is normally 3 μm, but in collagenous colitis, it is more than 10 μm and may reach 50 to 100 μm (Fig. 73-11). In addition, one can see inflammation and an increased number of lymphocytes. The histology of lymphocytic colitis shows an abundance of epithelial lymphocytes (Fig. 73-12). In both conditions, the gut epithelium remains intact, although colonic mucosal tears are occasionally present.

TREATMENT AND OUTCOME

Seven randomized, placebo-controlled studies of collagenous colitis have been published, but none on lymphocytic colitis. Budesonide resulted in clinical and histologic improvement in three studies. Bismuth subsalicylate, probiotics, *Boswellia serrata* extract, and various antibiotics have been tried in a few patients but did not prove effective and cannot be recommended.[67] Most patients recover after an illness of variable length.

PONCET'S DISEASE AND BACILLE CALMETTE-GUÉRIN–INDUCED ARTHRITIS

Tuberculous arthritis, or Poncet's disease, is a rare aseptic form of insidious fever, weakness, and arthritis described mostly in young adults suffering from extrapulmonary tuberculosis.[14] It responds slowly to antituberculous therapy, and in the absence of pulmonary changes, the intestine is assumed to be the port of entry. The attenuated *Mycobacterium* strain bacille Calmette-Guérin (BCG) is used intradermally as an adjuvant in cancer therapy to stimulate T cell–mediated immunity; it is also instilled into the urinary bladder to treat superficial cancer.

EPIDEMIOLOGY

No epidemiologic data are available. A recent review identified 50 bona fide cases of Poncet's disease.[68] Aseptic arthritis occurs in 0.4% to 0.8% of patients treated with the instillation of BCG for bladder malignancy,[4] and anecdotal evidence indicates an increased prevalence of HLA-B27 among them.[51] This finding was associated with sacroiliitis in 20% and oligoarthritis with predominant localization to the lower limbs; it occurred more often in men. In cases of reactive arthritis occurring after the intradermal administration of BCG, 6 of 10 patients were women, and symmetric hand arthritis dominated.

CAUSE AND PATHOGENESIS

An aseptic complication of active tuberculosis or the administration of BCG precipitates the process. By definition, it is a reactive arthritis, which means that the infectious agent triggers an immune reaction; however, the enteropathic nature is not firmly established. HLA-B27 may be a susceptibility factor in post-BCG arthritis.[4]

Mycobacterium heat shock protein 65 has been incriminated in both these sterile forms of arthritis, as well as in others.[52] Mycobacterial and human heat shock proteins are 50% homologous, and one hypothesis is that both the therapeutic efficacy and the arthritis are caused by cross-reactive T lymphocytes. Heat shock protein also has homologies with proteoglycan and HLA-DR. The pathogenesis of arthritis after intravesical instillation of BCG might be different and related to antigen persistence, setting the stage for a kind of reactive arthritis.

CLINICAL FEATURES AND DIAGNOSIS

Insidious fever, weakness, and arthritis are described mostly in young adults suffering from extrapulmonary tuberculosis.[4] The arthritis consists of oligo- or polyarthritis of large or small joints, or both. The onset is not as acute as in regular enteric reactive arthritis. Most peripheral joints can be affected.[4]

Arthritis developing in the presence of active tuberculosis or after recent exposure to BCG and proven to be aseptic is sufficient for diagnosis.

TREATMENT AND OUTCOME

There is no established treatment. Post-BCG cases usually heal within 3 months.

REFERENCES

1. Iweala OI, Nagler CR: Immune privilege in the gut: The establishment and maintenance of non-responsiveness to dietary antigens and commensal flora. Immunol Rev 213:82-100, 2006.
2. Wollheim FA: Enteropathic arthritis: How do the joints talk with the gut? Curr Opin Rheumatol 13:305-309, 2001.
3. Wollheim FA: Enteropathic arthritis. In Kelley WN, Harris ED Jr, Ruddy S, Sledge CB (eds): Textbook of Rheumatology, 5th ed. Philadelphia, WB Saunders, 1997, p 1006.
4. Wollheim FA: Enteropathic arthritis. In Kelley WN, Harris ED Jr, Ruddy S, Sledge CB (eds): Textbook of Rheumatology, 7th ed. Philadelphia, WB Saunders, 2005, p 1165.
5. Hvatum M, Kanerud L, Hallgren R, Brandtzaeg P: The gut-joint axis: Cross reactive food antibodies in rheumatoid arthritis. Gut 55:1240-1247, 2006.
6. Iqbal TH, Lewis KO, Gearty JC, Cooper BT: Small intestinal permeability to mannitol and lactulose in the three ethnic groups resident in west Birmingham. Gut 39:199, 1996.
7. **Guarner F: Enteric flora in health and disease. Digestion 73(Suppl 1): 5-12, 2006.**
8. Brandtzaeg P: Mucosal immunity: Integration between mother and the breast-fed infant. Vaccine 21:3382-3388, 2003.
9. Marttila-Ichihara F, Smith DJ, Stolen C, et al: Vascular amine oxidases are needed for leukocyte extravasation into inflamed joints in vivo. Arthritis Rheum 54:2852-2862, 2006.
10. Lakatos PL: Recent trends in the epidemiology of inflammatory bowel diseases: Up or down? World J Gastroenterol 12:6102-6108, 2006.
11. **Tysk C, Lindberg E, Jarnerot G, Floderus-Myrhed B: Ulcerative colitis and Crohn's disease in an unselected population of monozygotic and dizygotic twins: A study of heritability and the influence of smoking. Gut 29:990, 1988.**
12. **Bernstein CN, Wajda A, Blanchard JF: The clustering of other chronic inflammatory diseases in inflammatory bowel disease: A population-based study. Gastroenterology 129:827-836, 2005.**
13. Loftus EV Jr: Inflammatory bowel disease extending its reach. Gastroenterology 129:1117-1120, 2005.
14. Perencevich M, Burakoff R: Use of antibiotics in the treatment of inflammatory bowel disease. Inflamm Bowel Dis 12:651-664, 2006.
15. Gaya DR, Russell RK, Nimmo ER, Satsangi J: New genes in inflammatory bowel disease: Lessons for complex diseases? Lancet 367:1271-1284, 2006.
16. Vermeire S: Review article: Genetic susceptibility and application of genetic testing in clinical management of inflammatory bowel disease. Aliment Pharmacol Ther 24(Suppl 3):2-10, 2006.
17. Voss E, Wehkamp J, Wehkamp K, et al: NOD2/CARD15 mediates induction of the antimicrobial peptide human beta-defensin-2. J Biol Chem 281:2005-2011, 2006.
18. Hugot JP, Laurent-Puig P, Gower-Rousseau C, et al: Mapping of a susceptibility locus for Crohn's disease on chromosome 16. Nature 379:821-823, 1996.
19. Fuss IJ, Neurath M, Boirivant M, et al: Disparate CD4⁺ lamina propria (LP) lymphokine secretion profiles in inflammatory bowel disease: Crohn's disease LP cells manifest increased secretion of IFN-γ, whereas ulcerative colitis LP cells manifest increased secretion of IL-5. J Immunol 157:1261, 1996.
19a. Xavier RJ, Podolsky DK: Unravelling the pathogenesis of inflammatory bowel disease. Nature 448:427-434, 2007.
19b. Neurath M: IL-23: A master regulator in Crohn disease. Nature Med 13:26-28, 2007.
20. Camoglio L, Te Velde AA, Tigges AJ, et al: Altered expression of interferon-γ and interleukin-4 in inflammatory bowel disease. Inflamm Bowel Dis 4:285, 1998.
21. Guimbaud R, Bertrand V, Chauvelot-Moachon L, et al: Network of inflammatory cytokines and correlation with disease activity in ulcerative colitis. Am J Gastroenterol 93:2397, 1998.
22. Mylonaki M, Langmead L, Pantes A, et al: Enteric infection in relapse of inflammatory bowel disease: Importance of microbiological examination of stool. Eur J Gastroenterol Hepatol 16:775-778, 2004.
23. Hammer RE, Maika SD, Richardson JA, et al: Spontaneous inflammatory disease in transgenic rats expressing HLA-B27 and human β₂m: An animal model of HLA-B27-associated human disorders. Cell 63:1099, 1990.
24. **Taurog JD, Richardson JA, Croft JT, et al: The germfree state prevents development of gut and joint inflammatory disease in HLA-B27 transgenic rats. J Exp Med 180:2359, 1994.**
25. Rath HC, Herfarth HH, Ikeda JS, et al: Normal luminal bacteria, especially *Bacteroides* species, mediate chronic colitis, gastritis, and arthritis in HLA-B27/human β₂-microglobulin transgenic rats. J Clin Invest 98:945, 1996.
26. van der Waaij LA, Kroese FG, Visser A, et al: Immunoglobulin coating of faecal bacteria in inflammatory bowel disease. Eur J Gastroenterol Hepatol 16:669-674, 2004.
27. Macpherson A, Khoo UY, Forgacs I, et al: Mucosal antibodies in inflammatory bowel disease are directed against intestinal bacteria. Gut 38:365, 1996.
28. Söderholm JD, Olaison G, Lindberg E, et al: Different intestinal permeability patterns in relatives and spouses of patients with Crohn's disease: An inherited defect in mucosal defence? Gut 44:96, 1999.
29. Osman NE, Wäström B, Karlsson B: Serosal but not mucosal endotoxin exposure increases intestinal permeability in vitro in the rat. Scand J Gastroenterol 33:1170, 1998.

30. Helliwell PS, Hickling P, Wright V: Do the radiological changes of classical ankylosing spondylitis differ from the changes found in the spondylitis associated with inflammatory bowel disease, psoriasis, and reactive arthritis? Ann Rheum Dis 57:135, 1998.

31. Mielants H, Veys EM, Goemaere S, et al: A prospective study of patients with spondylarthropathy with special reference to HLA-B27 and to gut histology. J Rheumatol 20:1353, 1993.

32. Andreyev HJ, Kamm MA, Forbes A, Nicholls RJ: Joint symptoms after restorative proctocolectomy in ulcerative colitis and familial polyposis coli. J Clin Gastroenterol 23:35, 1996.

33. **Orchard TR, Wordsworth BP, Jewell DP: Peripheral arthropathies in inflammatory bowel disease: Their articular distribution and natural history. Gut 42:387, 1998.**

34. Orchard TR, Thiyagaraja S, Welsh KI, et al: Clinical phenotype is related to HLA genotype in the peripheral arthropathies of inflammatory bowel disease. Gastroenterology 118:274, 2000.

35. Rothfuss KS, Stange EF, Herrlinger KR: Extraintestinal manifestations and complications in inflammatory bowel diseases. World J Gastroenterol 12:4819-4831, 2006.

36. von den Driesch P: Pyoderma gangrenosum: A report of 44 cases with follow-up. Br J Dermatol 137:1000, 1997.

37. Orchard TR, Chua CN, Ahmad T, et al: Uveitis and erythema nodosum in inflammatory bowel disease: Clinical features and the role of HLA genes. Gastroenterology 123:714, 2002.

38. Banares A, Hernandez-Garcia C, Fernandez-Guitierrez B, Jover JA: Eye involvement in the spondyloarthropathies. Rheum Dis Clin North Am 24:771, 1998.

39. Holtmann MH, Krummenauer F, Claas C, et al: Long-term effectiveness of azathioprine in IBD beyond 4 years: A European multicenter study in 1176 patients. Dig Dis Sci 51:1516-1524, 2006.

40. Hande S, Wilson-Rich N, Bousvaros A, et al: 5-Aminosalicylate therapy is associated with higher 6-thioguanine levels in adults and children with inflammatory bowel disease in remission on 6-mercaptopurine or azathioprine. Inflamm Bowel Dis 12:251-257, 2006.

41. Akobeng AK, Zachos M: Tumor necrosis factor-alpha antibody for induction of remission in Crohn's disease. Cochrane Database Syst Rev 1:CD003574, 2004.

42. Lawson MM, Thomas AG, Akobeng AK: Tumour necrosis factor alpha blocking agents for induction of remission in ulcerative colitis. Cochrane Database Syst Rev 3:CD005112, 2006.

43. Berger JR: Natalizumab and progressive multifocal leucoencephalopathy. Ann Rheum Dis 65(Suppl 3):iii48-iii53, 2006.

44. Rolfe V, Fortun P, Hawkey C, Bath-Hextall F: Probiotics for maintenance of remission in Crohn's disease. Cochrane Database Syst Rev 4:CD004826, 2006.

45. Perencevich M, Burakoff R: Use of antibiotics in the treatment of inflammatory bowel disease. Inflamm Bowel Dis 12:651-664, 2006.

46. Wallace DJ, Weisman M: Should a war criminal be rewarded with eponymous distinction? The double life of Hans Reiter (1881-1969). J Clin Rheumatol 6:49, 2000.

47. Winblad S, Nilehn B, Jonsson M: Two further cases, bacteriologically verified, of human infection with "Pasteurella X" (syn. Yersinia enterocolitica). Acta Pathol Microbiol Scand 67:537-541, 1966.

48. **Ahvonen P, Sievers K, Aho K: Arthritis associated with Yersinia enterocolitica infection. Acta Rheumatol Scand 15:232-253, 1969.**

49. Kvien TK, Glennas A, Melby K, et al: Reactive arthritis: Incidence, triggering agents and clinical presentation. J Rheumatol 21:115-122, 1994.

50. Rudwaleit M, Richter S, Braun J, Sieper J: Low incidence of reactive arthritis in children following a salmonella outbreak. Ann Rheum Dis 60:1055-1057, 2001.

51. Jansen TL, Janssen M, Traksel R, de Jong AJ: A clinical and serological comparison of group A versus non-group A streptococcal reactive arthritis and throat culture negative cases of post-streptococcal reactive arthritis. Ann Rheum Dis 58:410-414, 1999.

52. **Gaston JS, Lillicrap MS: Arthritis associated with enteric infection. Best Pract Res Clin Rheumatol 17:219-239, 2003.**

53. Hannu T, Inman R, Granfors K, Leirisalo-Repo M: Reactive arthritis or post-infectious arthritis? Best Pract Res Clin Rheumatol 20: 419-433, 2006.

54. **Penttinen MA, Heiskanen KM, Mohapatra R, et al: Enhanced intracellular replication of Salmonella enteritidis in HLA-B27-expressing human monocytic cells: Dependency on glutamic acid at position 45 in the B pocket of HLA-B27. Arthritis Rheum 50:2255-2263, 2004.**

55. **Turner MJ, Sowders DP, DeLay ML, et al: HLA-B27 misfolding in transgenic rats is associated with activation of the unfolded protein response. J Immunol 175:2438-2448, 2005.**

56. Kvien TK, Gaston JS, Bardin T, et al: Three month treatment of reactive arthritis with azithromycin: A EULAR double blind, placebo controlled study. Ann Rheum Dis 63:1113-1119, 2004.

57. Yli-Kerttula T, Luukkainen R, Yli-Kerttula U, et al: Effect of a three month course of ciprofloxacin on the late prognosis of reactive arthritis. Ann Rheum Dis 62:880-884, 2003.

58. McGill PE: Geographically specific infections and arthritis, including rheumatic syndromes associated with certain fungi and parasites, Brucella species and Mycobacterium leprae. Best Pract Res Clin Rheumatol 17:289-307, 2003.

59. Lee SK, Green PH: Celiac sprue (the great modern-day imposter). Curr Opin Rheumatol 18:101-107, 2006.

60. Shan L, Molberg O, Parrot I, et al: Structural basis for gluten intolerance in celiac sprue. Science 297:2275-2279, 2002.

61. Lubrano E, Ciacci C, Ames PR, et al: The arthritis of coeliac disease: Prevalence and pattern in 200 adult patients. Br J Rheumatol 35:1314, 1996.

62. **Slot O, Locht H: Arthritis as presenting symptom in adult coeliac disease: Two cases and review of the literature. Scand J Rheumatol 29:260, 2000.**

63. Fenollar F, Birg ML, Gauduchon V, Raoult D: Culture of Tropheryma whippelii from human samples: A 3-year experience (1999 to 2002). J Clin Microbiol 41:3816-3822, 2003.

64. Moos V, Kunkel D, Marth T, et al: Reduced peripheral and mucosal Tropheryma whippelii-specific Th1 response in patients with Whipple's disease. J Immunol 177:2015-2022, 2006.

65. Mahnel R, Marth T: Progress, problems, and perspectives in diagnosis and treatment of Whipple's disease. Clin Exp Med 4:39-43, 2004.

66. Nyhlin N, Bohr J, Eriksson S, Tysk C: Systematic review: Microscopic colitis. Aliment Pharmacol Ther 23:1525-1534, 2006.

67. **Wollheim FA: Collagenous colitis and rheumatology. Curr Rheumatol Rep 2:183-184, 2000.**

68. Kroot EJ, Hazes JM, Colin EM, Dolhain RJ: Poncet's disease: Reactive arthritis accompanying tuberculosis. Two case reports and a review of the literature. Rheumatology (Oxford) 46:484-489, 2007.

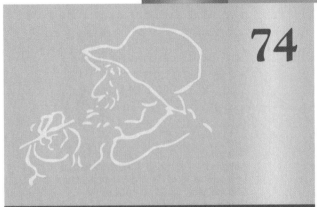

74

Pathogenesis of Systemic Lupus Erythematosus

BEVRA HANNAHS HAHN •
BETTY P. TSAO

KEY POINTS

Systemic lupus erythematosus (SLE) results from failure to regulate production of pathogenic autoantibodies, which appear years before the first clinical symptom of disease.

Pathogenic autoantibodies are subsets of antibodies to various antigens, including nucleosome, double-stranded DNA, Ro, NR2, band 3 on erythrocytes, and phospholipids—usually IgG and complement-fixing.

Antigens that stimulate production of antibodies are derived from blebs on apoptotic cells (nucleosomes, Ro, La, ribonucleoprotein [RNP], phospholipids), bacterial CpG DNA and viral RNA (both of which stimulate the innate immune system), and membranes of activated cells.

Abnormalities of regulation of the immune responses include decreased ability to clear immune complexes and apoptotic cells, intrinsic hyperactivation of B lymphocytes and T lymphocytes, skewed cytokine production favoring immunity and inflammation (including increases in interferon [IFN]-α, IFN-γ, interleukin [IL]-6, and IL-10, and decreases in IL-2 and transforming growth factor [TGF]-β), and defective numbers/function of regulatory CD4+CD25+Foxp3+ and CD8+ inhibitory T cells.

Genetic predisposition to SLE involves multiple genes, with homozygous deficiencies of complement components (which are uncommon) accounting for the highest risk. HLA-D (especially DR2 and DR3) and HLA class III haplotypes increase risk, as do genes in several non-HLA regions on other chromosomes.

Gene variants predisposing to SLE may influence clearance of immune complexes or apoptotic bodies (FCGR2A, C1q), activation of B cells or T cells (IL-10 promoter, protein tyrosine phosphatase 22 (PTPN22), programmed cell death 1 [PDCD1]), and inflammation related to dendritic cell activation (interferon regulatory factor 5 [IRF5]).

Studies of pedigrees stratified by clinical manifestations of SLE have identified linkages with "SLE loci" for hemolytic anemia, neuropsychiatric disease, and renal disease.

Environmental/microenvironmental factors that predispose to or activate SLE include ultraviolet B light, infection with Epstein-Barr virus, female gender, and exposure to estrogen-containing medications or "lupus-inducing" medications.

The pathogenesis of systemic lupus erythematosus (SLE) is complex, as shown in Figure 74-1.[1] Target tissue damage is caused primarily by pathogenic autoantibodies and immune complexes. The abnormal immune response that permits persistence of pathogenic B cells and T cells has multiple components, including activation of the innate immune system by DNA-containing and RNA-containing antigens (probably from infectious agents), processing of increased quantities of self-antigens by antigen presenting cells (APCs), hyperactivation of T cells and B cells, and failure of multiple regulatory networks to interrupt this process. The immunologic abnormalities occur in a framework of interactions between multiple susceptibility genes (and insufficient protective genes)[2,3]; gender influences; and environmental stimuli, at least one of which (ultraviolet [UV] light) can induce apoptosis in dermal cells that results in presentation of RNA protein, DNA protein, and phospholipid self-antigens to the immune system.[4]

EFFECTORS OF SYSTEMIC LUPUS ERYTHEMATOSUS

PATHOGENIC AUTOANTIBODIES

All individuals produce numerous antibodies that react with self-molecules. Characteristics of the normal background antiself repertoire include the following: most of the antibodies are IgM, they have weak avidity for self-antigens, and they are widely cross-reactive with multiple antigens. Pathogenic autoantibodies are different (Table 74-1). They are usually IgG, have high avidity for self-antigens, and have restricted specificity.[5,6] High-avidity antiself antibodies can be constructed from many different immunoglobulin genes, but they tend to derive from a few "preferred" families of genes, suggesting derivation from initial, antigen-activated "mother" B cells.[7,8] Pathogenic immunoglobulin molecules are often highly mutated, particularly in the hypervariable (complementarity determining) regions of their heavy and light chains.[5-10]

Several features of autoantibodies influence their pathogenic potential, including what antigens they bind, avidity for those antigens, the net charge of the immunoglobulin

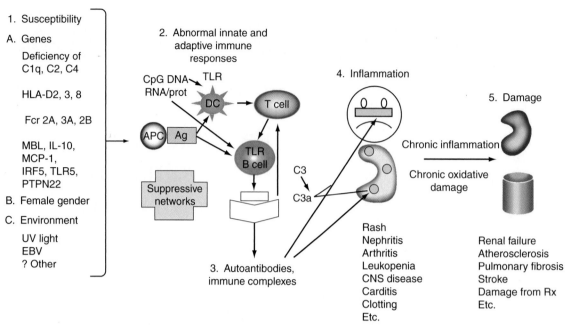

Figure 74-1   Overview of the stages and pathogenesis of systemic lupus erythematosus (SLE). The immune abnormalities that characterize SLE are pictured in five phases. In phase 1, an individual is susceptible to SLE because of genetics, gender, and the external environment that influences antigen presentation and other immune responses. In an individual with adequate numbers of predisposing factors, stage 2 develops, consisting of abnormal persistence of antigens, including hypomethylated DNA (CpG DNA) in DNA/anti-DNA complexes, and other DNA/protein and RNA/protein self-antigens. These antigens activate cells of innate (dendritic cells [DC]) and adaptive (B cells) immune systems via Toll-like receptors (TLR); the activated cells then activate T lymphocytes. The adaptive system is working at the same time, where antigen presenting cells (APC) present self-antigens to T lymphocytes and B lymphocytes; the B cells mature to plasma cells and secrete autoantibodies. At the same time, suppressive networks (regulatory and inhibitory T cells, phagocytic cells, idiotypic networks) are in place to dampen the harmful immune responses. Phase 3 begins with a clinically healthy individual having positive tests for autoantibodies in the serum. Immune complexes form. Phase 4, following phase 3 by a mean of 3 years, is clinical disease. The result of complement activation and other proinflammatory responses from tissue attacked by autoantibodies and immune complexes causes symptoms and signs of disease, which can include the features listed in the figure. Phase 5 occurs after months and years of chronic inflammation and chronic oxidative damage, which promote scarring of tissue such as kidney and lung, plaque deposition in arteries, and clotting. Irreversible tissue damage occurs. It is likely that at each of these phases, some individuals progress to the next phase, and others do not. CNS, central nervous system; EBV, Epstein-Barr virus; UV, ultraviolet.

molecule and the immune complex it forms with antigen, the presence in the immunoglobulin molecule of charged amino acids that interact with opposite charges on cell membranes or DNA, presence in the immunoglobulin molecules of sequences recognized by helper T cells, and ability to fix and activate complement.[9] Although we understand many of these principles, it is difficult to predict that a given monoclonal antiself antibody will be a pathogen. Two high-avidity, IgG2a, complement-fixing murine monoclonal anti-DNA antibodies were transferred to normal mice—one caused nephritis, whereas the other did not.[11] Among monoclonal human antibodies to DNA, some caused proteinuria on transfer to severe combined immunodeficiency mice, whereas others did not.[12]

In terms of antigens bound, it is convenient to think of the autoantibodies of SLE as belonging to one of several groups directed against DNA/protein complexes, RNA/protein complexes, cell membrane structures, and intracellular molecules that reach cell surfaces during cell activation. The antibodies considered to be the hallmark of SLE are IgG antibodies to double-stranded (ds) DNA. These antibodies probably develop from antibodies to histone proteins on nucleosomes (antinucleosomal antibodies). Nucleosomes are presented to the immune system in surface membrane blebs of cells undergoing apoptosis and are released from cells undergoing programmed cell death.[4,13]

Studies in mice suggest that the initial antibodies to DNA/protein are directed against nucleosomes.[13] As the antibodies mature and gain somatic mutations, some daughter cells bind single-stranded (ss) DNA, and then ultimately anti-ssDNA and anti-dsDNA. In support of this "antinucleosome-to-anti-dsDNA" hypothesis are observations that mice and humans with SLE have T cells activated by nucleosomes and nucleosomal peptides; such cells can help B cell synthesis of IgG anti-dsDNA.[14-16] In addition, CpG regions of DNA from bacteria, viruses, or mammalian self (rare in human DNA, but increased in SLE patients) can activate B cells and dendritic cells directly via Toll-like receptor 9 (TLR9), using the innate immune system that protects against pathogens to initiate an immune response to self.[17-19]

Similarly, dsRNA and ssRNA from viruses and self-antigens can activate innate immunity via TLR7 (dsRNA) and TLR3 (ssRNA).[20,21] It is likely that at least some pathogenic anti-DNA antibodies bind directly or in complexes to DNA deposited in basement membranes and to other renal structures, including heparan sulfate, histone, laminin, α-actinin, and collagen in glomerular basement membranes.[22-24] Sera from patients with lupus nephritis contain antibodies that bind to glomeruli; some bind DNA, and others do not. More recent data suggest that most antibodies binding to human glomeruli recognize nucleosomes,[24]

Table 74-1 Characteristics of Pathogenic Autoantibodies

Most are immunoglobulin isotypes that fix complement—primarily IgG (and some IgM)

Most are T cell–dependent antibodies derived from B cells reacting to specific autoantigens

High quantities are more likely to be associated with clinical disease and active disease than low quantities

Many different V-region, D-region, and J-region genes of the immunoglobulin heavy chain and V-region and J-region genes of the light chain used to assemble protective antibodies against external antigens also can be used to assemble pathogenic autoantibodies

There is probably some restriction in the immunoglobulin genes used to assemble autoantibodies because they tend to be derived from a few families, suggesting that many cells are daughters of cells initially activated by antigen

Many pathogenic autoantibodies are mutated in variable regions (and often in framework regions), suggesting modification by specific antigenic stimulation

General characteristics that favor ability of an autoantibody to be pathogenic:
   Ability to bind directly to target tissues, such as erythrocyte, lymphocyte, and platelet membranes, or to glomerular antigens
   Ability to activate complement
   Cationic charge favoring adherence to polyanionic regions of membranes
   High avidity for the autoantigens present in target tissue*

*Presence of amino acids in antigen-contacting region of the immunoglobulin molecule that favor charge-charge or hydrogen-bonding interactions with molecules in the antigen; this contributes to high avidity for antigen.

confirming a major role of antinucleosome/DNA in lupus nephritis. Non–DNA-binding autoantibodies that probably can cause nephritis include antibodies to C1q[25,26] and Ro/SS-A.[27]

A subset of autoantibodies has been discovered within the anti-DNA repertoire that bind the glutamate receptor on neurons (N-methyl-D-aspartate receptor subunits NR2a and NR2b).[28] These antiglutamate receptors have been found in cerebrospinal fluid of a patient with SLE central nervous system disease. In vitro, they cause apoptosis of neurons; transferred to mice, they fix primarily to the hippocampus or lateral amygdala, depending on the method used to open the blood-brain barrier.[29] In patients with SLE, antibodies to NR2 are associated with depression, rather than with cognitive defects.[30]

Another autoantibody highly specific for SLE is anti-Smith (anti-Sm). High-affinity anti-Sm antibodies have a prevalence of 5% to 25% in SLE patients. They are usually of IgG subclass, suggesting T cell dependence. T cell immunity against Sm peptides has been described in peripheral blood mononuclear cells and lymphoid tissues of SLE patients and mice.[31] Sm-reactive T cells show highly restricted T cell receptor (TCR) usage, which is characteristic of an antigen-driven response. SmD1 seems to be the most frequently recognized peptide in the molecule. It is remarkably conserved and bears a 99% homology with the mouse D1 protein. The epitope $SmD1_{83-119}$ seems to be recognized with remarkable sensitivity and specificity by human SLE sera (70% in SLE patients versus 8.3% in healthy controls and patients with other autoimmune diseases), possibly owing to its highly positive charge and its conformation.[32,33] In murine systems, $SmD1_{83-119}$ is effective as an immunogen (accelerating disease) and as a tolerogen (preventing or delaying disease) in lupus-prone mice.[31,33]

Other autoantibodies that directly cause disease include autoantibodies that coat platelets or erythrocytes. Antibodies that cause hemolysis in SLE are primarily warm-reactive IgG non-Rhesus, often reactive with oligomerized band 3, an anion transporter protein on erythrocyte membranes. Such erythrocytes usually have deficient surface expression of CD55 or CD59 or both, which are glycoprotein-anchored molecules that control complement activation. Hemolysis probably requires antibody plus C3b deposition on membranes, with subsequent phagocytosis after interaction with CR1 (complement) receptors or fragment crystallizable (Fc) receptors or both on phagocytes.[34]

Antibodies against platelets in SLE patients with thrombocytopenia recognize a wider variety of antigens than do antibodies in patients with idiopathic thrombocytopenic purpura. In both diseases, antibodies are directed against surface glycoprotein II and glycoprotein III antigens on intact platelets, but in SLE there are additional antibodies against cytoplasmic antigens, which come to the surface of activated platelets, and against phospholipids, suggesting that activated, damaged cells and cells undergoing apoptosis (in which antigenic portions of phospholipids in cell membranes are directed outward rather than inward) are important in stimulating pathogenic responses in SLE.[35]

Antibodies against proteins associated with the Ro/La particle are probably also direct pathogens, particularly in congenital heart block.[36-40] IgG anti-Ro crosses the placenta, can bind to certain areas of the fetal heart conduction system tissue, can alter myosin-actin function, and probably can cause heart block. The syndrome has been essentially reproduced in fetal mice; infusion of IgG anti-Ro from mothers with fetuses with congenital heart block induces electrocardiographic abnormalities in the fetal mouse heart compatible with heart block.[37] When a woman has produced a fetus with congenital heart block, the chances of subsequent fetuses having the same problem are greatly increased. Most infants with congenital heart block have mothers with anti-Ro (or rarely anti-ribonucleoprotein [RNP] or anti-La). Many of these mothers are healthy at the time of this occurrence, but some develop SLE or lupus-like syndromes later.[36]

Antibodies against phospholipids (either anticardiolipin or the lupus anticoagulant) increase the risk for venous or arterial thrombosis, for fetal loss, and for thrombocytopenia. They are likely to be involved directly in induction or maintenance of blood clots.[41] Their ability to cause fetal loss has been confirmed by transfer of human antiphospholipid to pregnant mice. Fetal death was increased and depended on activation of complement by the antibodies.[42,43] Antibodies to ribosomal P have been associated with depression and psychosis in SLE patients in some studies and with hepatitis and nephritis in others.[44-46] The mechanism by which they cause disease is unclear, but may be related to the fact that they, similar to some antibodies to DNA and RNP, can penetrate membranes of living cells, bind cytoplasmic or nuclear structures, and alter cell function.[47]

Table 74-2 Factors Favoring Tissue Deposition and Pathogenicity of Immune Complexes

Excessive quantities of immune complexes, which overwhelm clearance mechanisms
"Correct" size (large complexes are bound by the mononuclear phagocytic system and cleared rapidly; small complexes are excreted in urine; intermediate-size complexes are most likely to escape these mechanisms and to be tissue bound)
Tissue tropism of immune complexes (cationic charge of complexes allows binding to anions in tissue; antibody in complex may recognize components of tissues such as actinin in glomeruli)
Decreased immune complex and apoptotic bodies clearance and catabolism (relates to acquired and genetically determined low levels of surface complement receptors, genetic acquisition of fragment crystallizable [Fcγ] receptors that are inefficient binders of immunoglobulin in immune complexes, decreased solubilization of immune complexes by complement as complement levels fall or are genetically low, delayed phagocytosis of apoptotic bodies)
CpG regions in DNA of DNA/anti-DNA complexes (binds TLR9 in dendritic cells and B cells)

PATHOGENIC IMMUNE COMPLEXES

Similar to autoreactive antibodies, some immune complexes are pathogenic, and others are not. The characteristics of pathogenic immune complexes are summarized in Table 74-2 and reviewed elsewhere.[48] The size of the immune complex is important. Large immune complexes are cleared by the mononuclear phagocytic cell system on their first pass through the circulation, whereas small immune complexes are more likely to deposit in tissue. Excessive quantities of immune complexes overwhelm the mechanisms used to clear them, as discussed earlier. Finally, some immune complexes are "tissue tropic" and prone to bind to tissues because they have a net cationic charge or because the antibodies they contain are directed against tissue components. It is well accepted that immune complexes that fix complement are responsible for much of the tissue damage that characterizes SLE. In mammals, immune complexes are transported bound to complement receptor 1 (CR1), predominantly on erythrocytes. If surface CR1 molecule numbers are low, either because of genetic factors or because they have been stripped from the cell surfaces by an overload of activated complement, pathogenic immune complexes may persist long enough to cause tissue damage.[49,50]

GENETICS OF SYSTEMIC LUPUS ERYTHEMATOSUS

As with other autoimmune diseases, susceptibility to SLE depends on multiple genes.[3,51,52] Susceptibility genes are defined as genes that increase the relative risk for a disease, even though most individuals with that gene are healthy. The number of genes an individual must inherit to develop clinical SLE is unknown. It is likely to be several, with full gene effect depending partly on other modifying or protective genes in the same individual, gender, and the strength of environmental stimuli that can trigger disease (e.g., a severe sunburn in an individual with susceptibility genes).

Evidence for genetic predisposition in humans includes the following:

1. An approximately 10-fold increase in clinical disease in monozygotic compared with dizygotic twins[53-55]
2. A 5-fold to 29-fold relative risk for SLE in first-degree relatives, with approximately 10% of patients with SLE having an affected first-degree, second-degree, or third-degree relative[56]
3. Eight established and confirmed chromosomal regions linked to SLE, and five such genomic segments linked to disease subsets[3,52]
4. Many established and confirmed associations of SLE with particular gene variants and haplotypes[1,3,52]
5. Functional demonstration of a few SLE-associated gene polymorphisms[1,3,52]

Because the highest reported concordance rate in monozygotic twins is 57%,[53] it is likely that environmental factors and epigenetic factors also are required. The evidence for genetic control of disease is even more compelling in mice. Several strains are predisposed to SLE, with almost all individuals (gender dependent in some strains) developing the disease as they age. Major histocompatibility complex (MHC) class II genes on chromosome 17 (similar to HLA-D on chromosome 6) and regions on several other chromosomes contribute to susceptibility in these strains.[57,58] Some locations on mouse chromosomes have potential homologues in the human genome. Mice predisposed to SLE that also inherit the lpr or gld genes have accelerated disease based on mutations in the genes encoding Fas (in lpr) and Fas ligand (in gld) that impair apoptosis and permit autoreactive T cells and B cells to persist for abnormally long periods.[59] Abnormalities of the human Fas or Fas ligand genes are responsible for the hereditary autoimmune lymphoproliferative syndrome, a disease characterized by lymphoid hyperplasia and hematologic autoimmunity (Online Mendelian Inheritance in Man #601859).

B6 × satin beige (BXSB) male mice spontaneously develop severe systemic autoimmunity owing to the presence of the yaa gene in the Y chromosome, which is the duplicated Tlr7 gene usually located on the X chromosome, but in the BXSB strain it is translocated to the Y chromosome.[60] Compared with normal mice, male mice carrying the yaa gene have increased expression levels of TLR7 in B cells, which activates B cells to produce autoantibodies to RNA-containing nucleolar antigens and accelerates a lupus-like disease mediated by interactions with several genes in the BXSB genome.[60,61]

HUMAN GENETIC STUDIES

Multiple ethnic populations have been analyzed for susceptibility genes. The following four principles have emerged:

1. Some of the susceptibility gene variants differ between ethnic/racial populations.
2. There are individual gene variants that predispose to disease across multiple ethnic groups.
3. There are individual gene variants that predispose to multiple autoimmune diseases.
4. Genetic predisposition may be linked to autoantibody repertoires and to clinical subsets of disease.

The currently known genes and gene regions associated with murine and human SLE are shown in Table 74-3.

Table 74-3 Genetic Basis of Systemic Lupus Erythematosus (SLE)

Genes Involved in Murine Lupus

MHC (chromosome 17)—H2z of NZW mouse permits production of pathogenic IgG antibodies to DNA

Ipr (chromosome 19)—contains mutation in Fas that accelerates SLE on permissive genetic backgrounds, such as MRL/Ipr

gld (chromosome 1)—contains mutation in Fas ligand that accelerates SLE on permissive genetic backgrounds

yaa (chromosome Y)—accelerates SLE in males of genetically predisposed strains (BXSB)

Multiple regions on different chromosomes protect NZW mice from developing SLE, although they possess several predisposing genes

In mice with combined New Zealand Black (NZB) and New Zealand White (NZW) backgrounds

Chromosome 1—contains at least two regions that predispose to SLE

Nba2—associated with break in tolerance to DNA-containing molecules; a candidate susceptibility gene for the Nba2 locus has been identified—Ifi202 (chromosome 1)—a NZB-derived interferon-inducible gene

Sle1—promotes loss of tolerance to nucleosomes and permits development of histone-specific T cells; ANA develops along with minimal nephritis; this chromosomal region contains four separate susceptibility loci—Sle1a, Sle1b, Sle1c, and Sle1d—the NZM2410/NZW-derived complement receptor 2 gene, Cr2, has been implicated as a candidate susceptibility gene for the Sle1c locus

Chromosome 4—Sle2 permits hyperactivation of B cells with high levels of IgM, no nephritis

Chromosome 7—Sle3 permits hyperactivation of T cells, increased numbers of CD4+ T cells with delayed apoptosis, increased IgG antibodies to nucleosomal antigens, moderate nephritis

Combination of Sle1 and Sle3 permits severe SLE with IgG antibodies to DNA and lethal, early nephritis

Sle1 suppressor in MHC regimen reduces percentage of mice with lethal nephritis in Sle1 + Sle2 + Sle1s

Genes Involved in Human Lupus

Histocompatibilty (HLA) Genes

Extended haplotypes predispose to lupus in some ethnic groups:
HLA-B8/DRB1*0301/DQB1*0201/C4AQO (anti-Ro)
HLA-DRB1*1501/DQB1*0602 (nephritis, low levels of tumor necrosis factor-α)
HLA-DRB1*0801/DQB1*0402
HLA-A10/B18/C4A4/C4B2/BFS (associated with C2 deficiency)
DR2 (increases relative risk twofold to threefold)
DR3 (increases relative risk twofold to threefold)
DR2/DQw1 (anti-Ro)
DR3/DQw2 (anti-Ro plus anti-La)
DR2 or DR3 with DQB1*0201, DQB1*0602, DQB1*0302 (anti-DNA)
DR4 with DQw5, DQw8, and others (anti-U1 RNP)
DR2 with DQw6 or DQw7 and others (anti-Sm)
DR4, DR7 with DQw7, DQw8, DQw6, and others (lupus anticoagulant)
Homozygous deficiencies of early complement components (C2, C4)

Nonhistocompatibility Genes

Protein tyrosine phosphatase 22 (PTPN22) polymorphism c chromosome 1
C1q (chromosome 1)
FcγRIIA receptor allele (chromosome 1)
FcγRIIIA receptor allele (chromosome 1)
Promoter polymorphisms of interleukin-10 (chromosome 1)
PDCD1 polymorphisms (chromosome 2)
Interferon regulating factor 5 polymorphisms

Table 74-4 Putative Susceptibility Loci Significantly Linked to Systemic Lupus Erythematosus by Genome Scanning

Locus	LOD Scores	Candidate Genes	Syntenic Murine Susceptibility Loci
1q22-24	3.4	FCGR2A, FCGR3A	Sle1a, Sle1b
1q31	3.79		
1q41-43	3.3, 3.5		Sle1d, Bxs3
2q35-37	4.2	PDCD1	
4p16-15	3.8		
6p11-22	4.2	DR, DQ	Lbw1, Sle1s
12q24	4.0		
16q12-13	3.8		

LOD scores, logarithm of the odds that the two loci are linked; PDCD1, programmed cell death 1 gene.

chromosomes contain susceptibility genes, with general agreement that those linked to SLE include two regions on chromosome 1, and chromosomes 2, 4, and 16.[62-66]

Extended haplotypes predispose to disease in certain ethnic groups. As shown in Table 74-3, several investigators have reported an association between HLA class I-B8 and SLE in whites of Western and Northern European ancestry.[3,67-71] There is linkage disequilibrium between class I-B8 and class II-DR3. DR3 and DR2 are linked to SLE in different haplotypes and predispose to different clinical subsets of disease.[67,69,70,72-85] HLA-B8/DR3/DQw2/C4AQO is a haplotype associated with a deletion of class III genes—C4A and a neighboring CYP21A gene[72,76,78,80,81]—and predisposes to SLE in whites.

Abnormalities in C4, particularly C4A gene expression, are common in SLE patients from multiple ethnic/race groups (including northern and central Europeans, Anglo-Saxons, U.S. whites, African-Americans, Asian Chinese, Koreans, and Japanese), and various molecular mechanisms result in C4AQ0 (the null allele of C4).[86] The significant association between C4AQ0 and SLE in the context of multiple MHC haplotypes, ethnic/racial groups, and molecular mechanisms strongly supports the notion that no or low expression level of C4A protein predisposes to SLE susceptibility. The extended haplotype HLA-A10/B18/C4A4/C4B2/BFS is in disequilibrium with class III complement C2 deficiency[2]; homozygous deficiency for C2 occurs in 1 in 10,000 individuals,[87-90] many of whom have SLE or similar disease. The SLE is clinically distinct; patients have primarily joint and skin disease and are often antinuclear antibody (ANA) negative.

A more recent study using a large cohort (334 families containing 576 SLE patients) identified three distinct SLE-associated haplotypes containing DRB1*1501/DQB1*0602, DRB1*0801/DQB1*0402, and DRB1*0301/DQB1*0201 alleles.[91] By defining ancestral recombinants, the DRB1*1501 (formerly known as DR2) risk haplotype contains the DRB1 and DQB1 genes, but excludes the class I and class III regions including tumor necrosis factor (TNF)-α. The DRB1*0301 haplotype corresponds to the HLA A1-B8-DR3 haplotype of the Northern European origin that has been associated with several other autoimmune diseases, including type 1 diabetes, Graves' disease, and myasthenia gravis.[92] The extensive linkage disequilibrium of the DRB1*0301 haplotype makes

Table 74-4 shows the putative susceptibility loci significantly linked to SLE by genome scanning. Some genes associated with SLE in humans are located on chromosome 6, in the region that encodes HLA genes, especially class II (DR, DQ, DP) and class III (C2, C4).[2,3,62] Other ancestral recombinants within this region rare and difficult to narrow the SLE-associated region beyond the 1-Mb interval containing most class III and class II genes.[91] The DRB1*0801 (DR8) haplotype is less common in this cohort, and ancestral recombinants narrow the risk region to approximately 500 kb containing the DRB1 and DQB1 genes.[91]

These three SLE class II risk haplotypes are highly enriched in white families; among the 254 families carrying at least one risk haplotype, 229 (90%) were white or had known white admixture. Analysis of haplotype frequencies in 280 female SLE cases from the family collection and 174 female white controls revealed an approximately twofold increase in frequencies of risk haplotypes of SLE patients compared with controls and a doubling of risk for homozygotes compared with heterozygotes.[91] The disease-associated HLA genotypes seem to be not-as-strong contributors for risks to develop SLE compared with other autoimmune diseases, such as ankylosing spondylitis, type 1 diabetes, or rheumatoid arthritis.

INDIVIDUAL HUMAN LEUKOCYTE ANTIGEN GENES PREDISPOSING TO SYSTEMIC LUPUS ERYTHEMATOSUS

High risk for SLE is conferred by homozygous deficiencies of early complement components or their inhibitors, including C2 and C4 within the HLA gene complex and non-HLA C1q, C1r, and C1-INH.[87-90] Individuals with nearly total absence of these proteins are rare and account for less than 5% of patients with SLE. Most individuals with homozygous deficiencies have SLE or SLE-like diseases, however. Although null alleles for C4 are genes predisposing to SLE in multiple ethnic groups (see Table 74-3), complete deficiency of C4 is rare because four alleles (two at C4A and two at C4B) contribute to synthesis of the protein. In affected populations, about 50% of SLE patients have a C4 gene abnormality compared with 15% or less in healthy, ethnically matched control subjects.

DR3 and DR2 are individual genes that predispose to SLE in multiple ethnic groups, but the relative risk conferred by those genes alone is 2 to 3.[2,67,69,79,84-93] As described previously, DR3 is a part of an extended HLA haplotype in linkage disequilibrium with the promoter polymorphism of the TNF-α gene (−308A TNFA).[94] The −308A TNFA allele has been shown to confer higher transcriptional activity than the −308G TNFA allele.[95] The high-activity allele has been associated with SLE in multiple studies and may be an independent risk factor or a part of the HLA risk haplotype.[96-100] Neither the disease association nor the elevated activity has been consistently shown in similar studies, however.[101]

GENES ASSOCIATED WITH AUTOANTIBODY PRODUCTION

Familial aggregation of autoantibody profiles (including ANA; rheumatoid factor; IgM antiphospholipid antibodies; and antibodies to dsDNA, Sm, Ro/SSA, La/SSB, or RNP) has been established in 1506 individuals from 229 SLE multiplex families.[102] In this study, genome-wide linkage analyses have identified several non-HLA chromosomal regions that may contain gene variants that predispose to the generation of specific autoantibody. Major autoantigens in SLE

are nuclear complexes containing either RNA or DNA, which may serve as ligands to particular TLRs on B cells or dendritic cells, or both, leading to the initiation and perpetuation of autoantibody production (also known as Toll hypothesis).[103]

In murine lupus, TLR7 (a receptor for ssRNA) and TLR9 (a receptor for CpG-containing dsDNA) control the generation of autoantibodies to RNA-containing antigens (including Sm antigen) and DNA-containing antigens (such as anti-dsDNA and antinucleosome antibodies).[104] TLR8 also may be important in the recognition of autoantigens containing RNA in humans.[105] Members in the TLR7/TLR8/TLR9 activation pathways are candidate genes for increased risk of the generation of autoantibodies to nuclear complexes that are frequently found in SLE patients. TLR9 gene variants have not been associated, however, with the production of autoantibodies (Sm, RNP, Ro, and La) and SLE susceptibility in Asians,[106] or with SLE/lupus nephritis in whites.[107] Other TLRs may play a role in the pathogenesis of SLE. TLR4 (innate receptor for bacterial liposaccharide) and commensal flora are required for the production of anti-dsDNA and the development of immune complex–mediated glomerulonephritis in a mouse model.[58] A TLR5 stop codon has been associated with protection from the development of SLE susceptibility in whites, particularly in anti-dsDNA seronegative subsets, suggesting a role for flagellated bacteria triggering TLR5 activation in the pathogenesis of SLE.[108]

Associations between HLA genes and autoantibodies have been reported for anti-DNA,[109] anti-U1 RNP,[110] the 70-kD polypeptide of U1 RNP,[110,111] the lupus anticoagulant,[112] and autoantibodies to nucleosomes.[65] A strong association exists between certain HLA genes, particularly amino acid sequences in the DR and DQα and DQβ regions, and the ability to make certain autoantibodies.[3,109-114] Anti-Ro/SS-A and La/SS-B are examples.[113,114] They are genetically linked antibodies specific for proteins associated with small nuclear RNP; they are associated clinically with sicca complex, neonatal lupus, and subacute cutaneous lupus. Anti-Ro without anti-La is associated with DR2/DQw1; anti-Ro plus anti-La is associated with DR3/DQw2 and exhibits a gene-dose effect. That is, patients heterozygous for DQw1/DQw2 have high quantities of anti-Ro,[113] which strengthens the evidence linking the genes and the autoantibodies. Most patients who have anti-Ro plus anti-La have three or four of the relevant DR/DQ alleles, and none has less than two.[3]

All of the DQα alleles associated with anti-Ro share a Glu in position 34; all the DQβ alleles have Leu in position 26. These amino acids are found in those positions in the I-A molecules of MRL/lpr mice, the only murine lupus model that makes large quantities of anti-Ro and anti-La.[3,114] Many of these autoantibodies are associated with certain clinical manifestations of SLE. The genetic background may control the autoantibody pattern, which helps determine the clinical subset.

NONLEUKOCYTE ANTIGEN GENES PREDISPOSING TO SYSTEMIC LUPUS ERYTHEMATOSUS IN HUMANS

Non-HLA gene/genomic regions linked to or associated with SLE are listed in Table 74-3. A strong association between the rare disorder of complement C1q deficiency and SLE reveals the importance of C1q in preventing the development of SLE. Of approximately 40 individuals of European or Asian ethnic origin identified to have homozygous deficiency of C1q, more than 90% (30 individuals) developed SLE.[115,116] Mice lacking C1q are defective in removal of apoptotic bodies, and many develop lupus-like glomerulonephritis on a permissive genetic background.[117] Structurally similar to C1q, mannose-binding ligand (MBL) activates classic and alternative pathways of the complement cascade and opsonizes bacteria. Polymorphisms in the MBL promoter and exon 1, which result in lower levels of MBL, are more prevalent in SLE patients than in ethnically matched white, Asian, and African-American controls.[118-121]

C-reactive protein (CRP), a pendraxin similar to C1q and MBL, assists in complement binding to foreign and damaged cells and is involved in clearance of immune complexes and apoptotic cells. The CRP gene is located on chromosome 1q23 within an interval linked to SLE in multiple populations. CRP variants that result in defective clearance of apoptotic products may provide autoantigens in SLE. Two CRP single-nucleotide polymorphisms (SNPs) have been associated with decreased levels (rs1800947, rs1205), ANA production (rs1800947), and risk for SLE (rs1800947) in a British family-based association study.[122] An intronic GT repeat of CRP has been associated with plasma levels of CRP, and the GT^{20} allele is associated with high basal CRP in normal populations.

The CRP GT^{20} allele occurs more frequently in African-American and Hispanic SLE patients than in white SLE patients, and SLE patients carrying this allele are at risk for vascular arterial events.[123] Administration of a single dose of CRP reverses lupus nephritis and nephrotoxic nephritis in mice, which suggests that CRP may reduce tissue inflammation and damage as the acute-phase reactant.[124] Genetic effects of CRP may be modulated by FCGR2A variants. FcγRIIa receptor is the major receptor for CRP, and the R131 FCGR2a allele confers higher binding than the H131 allele.[125] Current results of genetic studies are promising, and future investigation of this gene not only would allow better understanding of the genetic influence of CRP, but also its role in the pathogenesis of SLE manifestations.

The Fc gene cluster located on chromosome 1q23 contains a set of structurally similar genes derived from gene duplications evolutionally. Human leukocytes express surface receptors that bind the Fc portions of IgG in immune complexes, which mediate immune clearance. Missense polymorphisms in the genes encoding FcγIIA or FcγIIIA receptors (H131R FCGR2A or V176F FCGR3A) result in differential affinity to IgG-containing immune complexes. The low binding alleles (the R131 allele of FCGR2A for IgG2 and the 176F allele of FCGR3A for IgG1/IgG3) are risk factors for susceptibility to SLE in multiple ethnic populations[125-127] probably by virtue of decreased capacity in clearance of circulating immune complexes, which may result in tissue deposition and inflammation.

In contrast, the V176 FCGR3A high binding allele may be a risk factor for progression of renal disease to end-stage renal disease among SLE patients.[128] It is possible that when renal disease is initiated, the high binding allele may cause more tissue deposition of immune complexes and severe local damage. The risk allele of these two activating receptor genes are often coinherited as a risk haplotype for SLE.[129] Of the two gene effects, V176 FCGR3A is associated with SLE more consistently and is associated with other autoimmune diseases, such as rheumatoid arthritis.[130,131] Another member of Fc receptor genes, FCGR3B, has copy number variations that are associated with susceptibility to lupus nephritis.[132] The gene copy number varies from zero to four, causing a dose effect of expression levels of FcγRIIIb.[132] SLE patients with low FCGR3B copy number have reduced expression on surfaces of neutrophils, which may reduce glomerular clearance of immune complexes and increase risk for glomerulonephritis.

FCRL3 encodes Fc receptor–like 3, which is structurally similar to FcγRs. A Japanese case-control study revealed the association of a functional SNP −C169T in the promoter region of FCRL3 with multiple autoimmune diseases, including SLE.[133] This association with SLE was not confirmed in a Spanish study, however.[134] FCGR2B is an inhibitory receptor that can downmodulate B cell receptor (BCR) signaling and decrease antibody-mediated phagocytosis in macrophages.[135] The I232T allele affects the inclusion of the FcγIIb in membrane lipid rafts, in resting stage and in coligation with BCR, and the SLE-associated T232 allele is less potent in inhibition of B cell activation.[136] The T232 FCGR2B is associated with SLE in multiple Asian populations, but this allele is rare in whites. Promoter polymorphisms of FCGR2B associated with SLE identified in two white cohorts are not found in Asians, supporting the notion of ethnic variations in FCGR2B variants predisposing to SLE.[136]

Interleukin (IL)-10, an immunoregulatory cytokine, can inhibit monocyte and dendritic cell function, but it stimulates B cell activation, proliferation, differentiation, and immunoglobulin secretion.[137] Increased serum levels of IL-10 in SLE patients compared with normals have been shown consistently.[137] The molecular basis of high IL-10 levels in SLE has been associated with several promoter polymorphisms (including two CA-repeat microsatellites and 10 SNPs). One microsatellite, IL-10.G, has been associated with susceptibility to SLE in Scottish, Mexican-American, and Italian populations, but not in Mexican, Swedish, or Taiwanese populations.[138-143] Although no association between the three SNP haplotypes (−1082 G/A, −819 C/T, and −592 C/A) and SLE has been established in five studies, significant association with various SLE manifestations has been reported.[144-148] The remaining seven promoter SNPs were identified more recently and led to the definition of eight SNP haplotypes.[149] These haplotypes correlated with IL-10 production in normals and were significantly associated with SLE in African-Americans.[149] These genetic studies suggested a molecular basis for elevated levels of IL-10 contributing to the pathogenesis of SLE.

Polymorphisms of cytotoxic T lymphocyte antigen 4 (CTLA4), programmed cell death 1 (PDCD1), and protein tyrosine phosphatase PTPN22 may be a shared genetic factor for multiple autoimmune diseases in humans. CTLA4, a structural homologue of CD28 that competes with CD28 for the binding of B7 on APCs, can transduce inhibitory signals by activation of serine/threonine phosphatases, downregulate T cell function, and prevent autoimmune diseases by promoting anergy. The CT60A/G in the 3′UTR of CTLA4 decreased the production of a spliced variant with inhibitory activity and has been associated with multiple autoimmune diseases, including type 1 diabetes, autoimmune hypothyroidism, and Graves' disease.[150] Association between CTLA4 and SLE has yielded inconsistent results. Polymorphisms within the *CTLA4* promoter (−1722T/C, −1661A/G, −319C/T) and exon 1 (+49G/A) have been associated with SLE in multiple ethnic groups.[151]

PDCD1 (also known as PD-1), a member of the CD28/CTLA4/ICOS costimulatory receptor family containing an inhibitory immunoreceptor tyrosine-based motif, is expressed on activated T cell and B cell surfaces to regulate their peripheral tolerance.[152] An intronic *PDCD1* SNP (PD1.3A; the minor A allele of 7146 G/A) was associated with SLE in Europeans and Mexicans,[153] with type 1 diabetes,[154] and with rheumatoid arthritis subsets.[155] This allele subsequently was associated with renal manifestations in SLE patients from Northern Sweden, but not with overall SLE susceptibility.[156] Functionally, this SNP affects the binding of runt-related transcription factor 1 (RUNX1) in the intronic enhancer, which may influence hyperactivity of lymphocytes in SLE.

The R620W polymorphism of PTPN22 disrupts the interaction of its protein product and Src tyrosine kinase (Csk), and alters negative regulation of T cell signaling.[157] The 620W PTPN22 polymorphism was first identified as a candidate gene for type 1 diabetes[158] and was subsequently associated with rheumatoid arthritis, SLE, autoimmune thyroid disease, and other autoimmune disorders in whites.[159] Association of 620W PTPN22 with SLE has been variable—not consistently shown in sporadic SLE, but more likely to be found in SLE patients who have another overlapping autoimmune disease, family history of SLE, or other autoimmune diseases.[160-163] The 620W is twice as active as R620 in suppressing TCR signaling, which presumably permits autoreactive T cells to escape from deletion during thymic development.[159] Variants of CTLA4, PDCD1, and PTPN22 that affect either expression levels or functions have been associated with multiple autoimmune diseases, but their cellular pathways leading to disease onset await further investigation.

A link between type 1 interferon (IFN) and the pathogenesis of SLE in humans and mice has been established by a series of studies.[164] Genetic factors that cause increased production of type 1 IFN or stimulation of the IFN pathway or both may predispose to SLE. An initial screen of 13 genes in the type 1 IFN pathway identified association between SLE and variants in tyrosine kinase 2 (TYK2) and interferon regulatory factor 5 (IRF5) in a Scandinavian population.[165] Tyk2 binds to type 1 IFN receptor α subunit, and its catalytic activity promotes ligand-induced downmodulation of receptor expression and negatively regulates cellular signaling.[166] IRF5 is important for transactivation of type 1 IFN and IFN-responsive genes and for the production of proinflammatory cytokines (IL-6, IL-12, and TNF-α) after TLR signaling.[167]

Functions of these two gene products provide potential mechanisms to predispose to the development of SLE. Allelic association of IRF5 SNP (the T allele of rs2004640, 2 bp downstream from exon 1B) with SLE has been convincingly replicated using case-control and family-based cohorts in which the SLE-associated allele introduces an alternative splice site and expression of several unique IRF5 isoforms

with different coding and noncoding sequences.[168] This allele together with an independent variant (rs2280714 T allele, approximately 5 kb downstream of IRF5, previously associated with elevated expression of IRF5 transcripts) forms a common haplotype that is strongly associated with increased risk for SLE.[168] This IRF5 haplotype may cause increased production of various IRF5 isoforms with different activation properties, affinity to transcription cofactors, or stability, predisposing to the development of SLE.

Linkage analysis in complex diseases (e.g., SLE) usually leads to the identification of large genomic intervals of approximately 20 centimorgans (approximately 20 million bp) that are likely to contain disease-susceptibility genes. This method uses DNA samples from families with multiple affected members to assess cosegregation of the test genetic marker allele with a phenotype of interest (e.g., SLE). As shown in Table 74-4, genome scanning of genetic markers from several groups using different collections of multiplex pedigree materials shows significant linkage of the 1q22-24,[63] 1q31,[169] 1q41-42,[63,66,170] 2q37,[171] 4p16-15,[172] 6p21-11,[62,173] 12q24,[174] and 16q12-13[62,173] chromosomal regions to SLE (the threshold for significant linkage is defined as a logarithm of odds [LOD] scores = 3.3 or 3.6 depending on linkage methods).[175] Confirmation of significant linkage in an independent cohort has been established for all eight loci, providing strong evidence for the presence of SLE susceptibility genes in each putative locus.[64,170,172-174,176-178]

Because linkage analysis identifies large genomic intervals that are likely to harbor disease-susceptibility genes, efforts to fine-map and assess positional candidate genes (candidate genes mapped within the linked region) are in progress. To this end, a positional candidate gene for the 2q37 locus,[171,179] PDCD1, has been associated with SLE.[153] PDCD1 is a strong candidate because mice deficient in PDCD1 are defective in peripheral tolerance of T cells and B cells and develop lupus-like arthritis and glomerulonephritis.[150,180,181] An intronic SNP in PDCD1 is associated with susceptibility to SLE in Europeans and Mexicans with relative risks of 2.6 and 3.5.[153] This SLE-associated SNP located in an intronic enhancer abolishes binding to the RUNX1 transcription factor, which could lead to aberrant regulation of PDCD1 contributing to breakdown of immune tolerance and development of SLE.

The 1q41-42 linked region contains poly(adenosine diphosphate–ribose) polymerase, an enzyme that participates in DNA repair triggered by apoptosis, and that has been associated with SLE by one group of investigators,[66] but not confirmed by others.[182-184] The 1q22-24-linked region contains FCGR2A and FCGR3A, which have been associated with SLE susceptibility in many studies as described previously. These two genes may be in linkage disequilibrium because of their physical proximity, which complicates the assessment of the relative role of each gene in susceptibility to SLE. A more recent study provides strong genetic evidence (linkage and family-based and population-based association) to support a role of FCGR3A in susceptibility to SLE.[185]

No positional candidate genes within the 4p16-15 region have been associated so far with SLE. The 6p21-11-linked region contains the approximately 3.6-Mb HLA region that contains several class II risk haplotypes of SLE. CARD15/NOD2, encoding a protein involved in bacterial recognition by monocytes, is the positional candidate gene within the 16q12-13 region linked to SLE. The functional role of CARD15 in innate immunity makes its genetic variants candidates for predisposition to autoimmune diseases. Multiple polymorphisms of CARD15 have been shown to contribute to susceptibility to Crohn's disease.[186-188] The three most common polymorphisms associated with Crohn's disease are not associated with SLE in a Spanish population,[189] but the 908R CARD15 allele is associated with SLE in a larger study of European whites.[190] Interaction between genetic risk factors may affect susceptibility; data supporting linkage and genetic interaction of 1q23 and 16q12 have been observed in a multiethnic cohort containing 145 SLE-affected sibling pairs.[176]

The highly heterogeneous nature of manifestations among SLE patients may represent genetic heterogeneity that confounds the identification of lupus-susceptibility genes. One approach to reduce heterogeneity is to stratify pedigrees for the presence of a single manifestation and to re-evaluate the genome-wide scanning data for linkage evidence for the particular manifestation-associated SLE locus. This strategy has led to the identification of (1) a vitiligo-related SLE locus, SLEV1, at chromosome 17p13,[191] which has been confirmed by an independent study[192]; (2) an SLE susceptibility locus, SLEH1, at 11q14 in African-American SLE pedigrees stratified by hemolytic anemia (maximum LOD = 4.5 at D11S2002)[193] and a nucleolar antibody pattern (maximum LOD = 5.62 at D11S2002)[194]; (3) an SLEB3 locus at 4p16 in 23 European-American SLE pedigrees stratified by neuropsychiatric manifestations (maximum LOD = 5.19 at D4S2366)[195]; (4) an SLED1 locus at 19p13.2 (maximum LOD = 4.93 at D19S714) and another SLED2 at 18q21.1 (maximum LOD = 3.40 at D18S858) in 37 European-American and 29 African-American pedigrees, containing at least one affected case with a positive anti-dsDNA[196]; and (5) SLEN1 at 10q22.3 (maximum LOD = 3.16 at D10S2470) and SLEN2 at 2q34-35 (maximum LOD = 2.15 at D2S2972) in 31 European-American pedigrees and SLEN3 at 11p15.6 (maximum LOD = 3.34 at D11S1984) stratified by renal disease in 20 African-American pedigrees with two or more patients with SLE and renal disease,[197] in which SLEN1 and SLEN2 have been confirmed.[198]

The advantage of this approach is the improved evidence for linkage revealed by pedigree stratification based on select clinical manifestations compared with the disease status of SLE. These results from testing each manifestation separately increase the possibility of false-positive results using a smaller subset of family materials, however, which highlights the importance of replications in independent samples.

MURINE LUPUS GENETIC STUDIES

Several inbred mouse strains are genetically "programmed" to develop SLE.[199,200] New Zealand Bielchowsky/Black (NZB/Bl) mice develop IgG1 antibodies to erythrocytes, IgM antibodies to ssDNA, and mild lymphoproliferation; most die of hemolytic anemia, with disease earlier in females than in males. NZB/NZW and NZB/SWR F1 hybrids develop IgG2a and IgG2b anti-dsDNA; females die of glomerulonephritis mediated primarily by anti-DNA, and males develop slowly progressive disease at a later age.

NZB/NZW F1 hybrid brother-sister matings have generated substrains of mice designated NZM mice that vary widely in prevalence and severity of nephritis, serum levels of IgG and IgM, and antibodies to nucleosomes and DNA.

Linkage studies of the entire mouse genome of the New Zealand genetic background have identified specific chromosomal regions that harbor lupus susceptibility genes, including genes located on chromosomes 1, 4, 7, and 17 (containing the MHC region). The importance of these chromosomal regions has been elucidated by detailed phenotypic characterization and successive backcrosses into another normal mouse strain (C57BL/6 or B6) to analyze the locations and component phenotypes of individual susceptibility genes. Heterozygosity at the H2 locus on chromosome 17 (particularly containing H2z from NZW) has been identified as important in conferring certain autoantibodies and nephritis.[201-204] The regions of interest on chromosomes 1 and 4 contain DNA contributed by NZB and NZW parents.

One NZB-derived locus on chromosome 1, Nba2, may contribute to loss of tolerance to DNA-containing self-antigens.[200,202,203] The Nba2 lupus susceptibility locus was characterized further by developing congenic mice via repeatedly backcrossing mice containing the NZB chromosome 1 interval into the normal B6 genetic background and then intercrossing siblings to generate B6.Nba2 congenic mice homozygous for the Nba2 locus. Comparisons of 11,000 gene microarrays revealed only two differentially expressed genes of spleen cells from B6.Nba2 and B6 mice: IFN-inducible Ifi202 and Ifi203.[205] Ifi202 has been implicated as a candidate susceptibility gene supported by studies of strain distribution of expression, promoter polymorphisms, and effects on cell proliferation and apoptosis.

A similar approach has produced multiple congenic strains of mice, each carrying a single susceptibility locus from the NZM2410 genome.[206] The region designated Sle1 on chromosome 1 (close to Nba2), when expressed in B cells and T cells of a normal B6 background (B6.NZMc1), promotes development of IgG antibodies to nucleosome and generates histone-specific T cells.[207-210] Although the mice lose tolerance to nucleosome and develop ANAs induced by the exposed portion of chromatin (H2A/H2B/DNA)—antibodies thought to precede pathogenic anti-DNA—these antibodies do not evolve, and animals develop minimal nephritis. Subsequent studies reveal that the potent autoimmunity conferred by the genomic interval of Sle1 reflects the combined effects of a cluster of four independent, but functionally related, susceptibility genes: *Sle1a, Sle1b, Sle1c,* and *Sle1d.*[211]

Congenic strains for each of these four subintervals have been generated, in which *Sle1b* is the strongest contributor of the observed Sle1 phenotype and has been isolated to a small genomic segment containing the SLAM family of lymphocyte adhesion receptors. The lupus-susceptible allele results in alternative splicing of messenger RNA of one SLAM family member, Ly108, which reduces the ability of self-reactive BCR to signal clonal anergy and receptor editing, resulting in accumulation of self-reactive B cells in the spleen and lymph nodes.[212] The congenic interval of *Sle1c* results in the production of autoreactive B cells and T cells mediated through three genes.[213] One of these genes, *Cr2*, which encodes complement receptors 1 and 2 by alternative splicing of a common transcript, has been implicated as a lupus susceptibility gene.[214] An SNP of the NZM2410/ NZW Cr2, creating a novel glycosylation site within the C3d binding domain, may interfere with receptor dimerization, reduce receptor-mediated signaling, and consequently lower the threshold for negative selection of autoreactive B cells.[214]

Mice congenic for the region on chromosome 4 (B6. NZMc4 expressing the Sle2 region) show hyperactivation of B cells with hypersecretion of IgM, but develop no nephritis.[210] Mice congenic for the chromosome 7 region (B6.NZMc7 containing the Sle3 region) have hyperactivation of T cells, increased numbers of CD4+ helper T cells, reduced apoptosis, and increased levels of IgG antibodies to multiple nucleosomal antigens; they develop moderate nephritis.[210] When mice are bred to express Sle1 and Sle3, they develop severe disease, with IgG antibodies to DNA and other self-antigens, and lethal, early glomerulonephritis—confirming the hypothesis that multiple genes conferring multiple abnormalities in immune tolerance and B cell and T cell function are required for an individual to develop severe SLE.[210]

Finally, studies of this type have shown that several chromosome regions in NZW mice (a strain that inherits multiple susceptibility genes, including H2z, Sle1, and Sle3) are linked to protection from disease.[210] One of these, Sle1 suppressor (*Sle1s*), when bred into mice with Sle1 plus Sle3, reduces the incidence of severe nephritis by half.[215] *Sle1s* has been narrowed to a 956-kb genomic interval that definitely excludes TNFA, but includes many functionally important candidates, including MHC class II genes, the complement genes proximal to TNF-α, and others.[215] Modifying and protective genes are crucial in determining exactly how "predisposed" an individual is to this autoimmune disease.

ENVIRONMENTAL FACTORS, GENDER, AND APOPTOSIS AS SOURCES OF AUTOANTIGENS

As mentioned in the discussion of genetics, the fact that most monozygotic twins are discordant for clinical SLE suggests that environmental factors play a role in disease pathogenesis (Table 74-5).[53-55,216] Two environmental factors are clearly important: UV light and gender. There also is increasing evidence for a role for Epstein-Barr virus (EBV) infection. Seventy percent of SLE patients experience disease flares after exposure to UV light[217]; the B spectrum may be more important than the A spectrum in activating disease in humans. Although patients might be wise to avoid intense exposure to UVA and UVB spectra, some data suggest that exposure to UVA might benefit SLE.[218]

Several experiments have suggested mechanisms by which exposure to UV light might accelerate disease. Exposure of DNA to UV light increases thymine dimers, which renders the DNA more immunogenic.[219] It has been observed that exposure of keratinocytes to UV light induces apoptosis.[4,220] During apoptosis, three events occur that probably expose self-molecules to the immune system or render them immunogenic, or both: (1) movement of nuclear and cytoplasmic DNA-protein and RNA-protein antigens to the surface of cells in membrane-encased blebs (e.g., nucleosomes, Ro/SS-A, and U1 RNP antigens),[4,220]

(2) flipping of the membrane inside-out so that antigenic portions of membrane phospholipids are exposed on the cell surface, and (3) modification of intracellular proteins that might render them antigenic.[221] Each of these changes presents nucleoprotein and cytoplasmic and phospholipid self-antigens to the immune system; this might be the major stimulus that allows the few lymphocytes that escape self-tolerance mechanisms to become self-reactive. More recent evidence indicates that apoptotic lymphocytes also release lipid microparticles, which have proinflammatory and anti-inflammatory effects and can induce apoptosis in monocytes/macrophages, contributing to the defective clearance of apoptotic cells and immune complexes characteristic of SLE.[222]

The potential role of EBV in inducing or flaring SLE, originally suggested by James and colleagues in 1997,[223] has been confirmed in more recent work. Because EBV lives chronically in B cells, and B cell activation is a feature of SLE, it is difficult to say whether EBV infection initiates B cell hyperactivity, autoantibody formation, and disease, or whether the upregulation of EBV in B cells results from other activating stimuli. It may not matter which is true because the appearance of the response is likely to initiate much broader autoimmunity in susceptible individuals.

Patients with SLE have abnormally high frequencies of EBV-infected cells in their blood, and in one study high copy numbers were associated with disease flares.[224] EBV latency membrane proteins also are expressed, and these

Table 74-5 Environmental Factors That May Play a Role in the Pathogenesis of Systemic Lupus Erythematosus (SLE)

Definite
UVB light
EBV
Probable
Estrogen and prolactin—in humans, female-to-male ratio is 9:1 between menarche and menopause, 3:1 in young and old
Lupus-inducing medications*
Hydralazine
Procainamide
Isoniazid
Hydantoins
Chlorpromazine
Methyldopa
Penicillamine
Minocycline
Tumor necrosis factor-α inhibitors
Interferon-α
Possible
Dietary factors
Alfalfa sprouts and related sprouting foods containing Canavanine
Pristane and similar substances
Infectious agents other than EBV
Bacterial DNA
Human retroviruses
Endotoxins, bacterial lipopolysaccharides

*Although each of the drugs listed, and many others, can induce lupus-like symptoms in predisposed individuals, there is little evidence that they can induce true SLE or even activate disease in individuals with spontaneous, established SLE. If the clinical care of a patient with SLE would benefit from use of one of these drugs, the drug should not be withheld.
EBV, Epstein-Barr virus; UVB, ultraviolet B.

proteins can heighten activation of TLR, a mechanism that could allow autoreactive B cells to avoid tolerance.[225] In another study,[226] EBV viral loads measured by multiple methods showed a 40-fold increase in SLE patients compared with controls and a greater frequency of EBV-specific CD69[+]CD4[+] T cells producing IFN-γ. EBV viral loads were inversely correlated, however, with the frequency of EBV-specific CD69[+]CD4[+] IFN-γ-producing cells, and with lower levels of HLA-A2 tetramer-positive CD8[+] T cells.

Whether EBV infection triggers SLE or is stimulated by it, T cell control of the viral production is inadequate, and the response persists too long; this fits with the general principle that immunoregulation of autoantibody production is defective. Children with SLE are 50 times more likely to have been infected with EBV than children from the same clinics who do not have SLE (discussed subsequently).[223] Even in adults with SLE, the odds ratio for infection with EBV is 8.[227] Infection with EBV results in production of the viral protein EBV nuclear antigen-1 (EBNA-1). Antibodies against EBNA-1 are found in all infected individuals, but in SLE the antibodies diversify more than in normals, developing cross-reactivity with Ro, Sm B/B′, and SmD1—all antibodies characteristic of SLE. In the permissive genetic background, the single common infection with EBV can lead to unusually extensive epitopic spreading, generating multiple autoantibodies.[228,229] IgA and IgG antibodies to EBV were associated with SLE in African-Americans and in older whites with the disease. There was an additional association between an allelic variant of the CTLA4 gene promoter and the anti-EBV response.[230]

It is likely that EBV (but not other herpesviruses tested or cytomegalovirus) can push a predisposed individual from nonautoimmunity to autoantibody production, starting the cycle that may lead to disease. In addition, cycles of disease worsening could relate to B cell activation with increased EBV antigens stimulating production of other autoantibodies. Breakthroughs in understanding of the role of the innate immune system in predisposing to SLE are likely to lead to discovery of other inciting infectious agents. Administration of bacterial lipopolysaccharides to mice with SLE accelerates disease.[231] One study[232] detected antibodies to the retroviral gag protein p24 from human immunodeficiency virus type 1 in one third of SLE patients compared with 1 of 120 control subjects. Type C coronavirus has been implicated in the nephritis of NZB/Bl mice and related strains.[233] One group found persistent BK polyomavirus more frequently in patients with SLE than in control subjects.[234] To date, only the EBV explanation has consistent support from multiple laboratories.

Gender is of great importance in susceptibility to SLE, which is predominantly a disease of women, particularly during the reproductive years.[216,235] The basis of this sex predisposition is not fully understood. It seems unlikely that gene polymorphisms on the X chromosome are involved because the disease does not follow a sex-linked genetic pattern. More recent work shows, however, that regulatory regions controlling expression of CD40L on T cells, located on the inactive X chromosome in women with SLE, are demethylated (compared with healthy women), resulting in increased CD40L expression, which should provide increased activation signals between T and B cells.[236]

Epigenetic changes in methylation of DNA also can be induced by environmental exposure to drugs[237] and may play a role in drug-induced lupus. In lupus-prone mice (BXSB) strain, a lupus-accelerating gene (Yaa) has been mapped to the Y chromosome; Yaa results from increased copy numbers of TLR7 after translocation of the TLR7 gene from X to Y. This translocation probably leads to increased immunoreactivity to RNA-containing antigens.[61] It is unknown whether increased copy numbers of TLR7 predispose to SLE in humans.

Another idea is that women who have been pregnant have fetal cells that persist for decades in their circulation or tissues; the fetal cells induce chronic graft-versus-host disease, which resembles SLE.[238] Similarly, maternal cells persist in offspring for many years. Abnormalities in sex hormone metabolism might contribute to gender differences in susceptibility to SLE. Men and women with SLE have accelerated metabolism of testosterone.[235,239,240] Estrone is preferentially hydroxylated at the C-16 position in men and women with SLE and in their first-degree relatives, resulting in the accumulation of 16-hydroxylated metabolites, which have sustained high estrogenic activity. Men and women with SLE might have too much estrogenic and too little androgenic hormone, shifting their immune system toward increased responses.

Among menopausal nurses (N = approximately 70,000), those treated with hormone replacement therapy had an increased risk for development of SLE compared with nurses who did not receive hormone replacement therapy (age-adjusted relative risk 2.1 to 2.5),[241] and women in this cohort exposed to estrogen-containing oral contraceptives also had slightly increased risk for SLE (relative risk 1.4 to 1.9).[242] The increased risk conferred by prior use of oral contraceptives was not confirmed in a subsequent study of a smaller population (N = 240) of women who already had SLE.[243]

A lupus-enhancing effect of estrogen was confirmed in a study in which treatment of women with 1 year of hormone replacement therapy containing estradiol and progesterone significantly increased the rate of mild and moderate disease flares, although not severe flares.[244] In contrast, treatment with oral contraceptives for 1 year was not associated with increased flare rates.[245,246] Prolactin levels are elevated in some individuals with SLE and may increase disease activity.[247]

Finally, there is evidence that T cells (from humans) and B cells (from mice), when exposed to estradiol, develop resistance to tolerance. In a transgenic mouse model of anti-DNA expression, B cells that bind DNA with high avidity are deleted in the bone marrow and do not reach peripheral tissues. Treatment of the mice with estradiol (or prolactin) rescues those cells, however; they survive to enter either marginal zones (T cell–independent responses) or follicular regions (T cell–dependent antibody responses) of peripheral lymphoid tissues.[248] In the estradiol group, Bcl-2 is upregulated (probably protecting from apoptosis),[249] and calcium signaling and tyrosine protein kinase phosphorylation are diminished.

The presence of female sex hormones is a factor that allows autoreactive B cells to survive tolerance and persist in peripheral tissues, where they can increase autoantibody production if the correct activating signals are provided.

In SLE, some B cells fail to be appropriately deleted when exposed to self-antigen. There is substantial evidence in mice and humans that lymphocytes resistant to apoptosis lead to lymphoid compartment expansion and autoimmunity (e.g., the *lpr* and *gld* mutations that permit mice with susceptible genetic backgrounds to develop full-blown SLE). With regard to T cells, in vitro exposure of human SLE T cells to estradiol upregulates surface CD40L expression and production of calcineurin, along with reducing apoptosis in those cells.[250,251] The general theme here is that estradiol is likely to prolong the life of autoreactive B cells and T cells, providing another permissive factor for development of disease.

An additional factor that may promote development of disease in genetically predisposed individuals is diet. Some macaque monkeys fed alfalfa sprouts developed SLE; sprouting vegetables contain an aromatic amino acid, canavanine, that is immunostimulatory.[252] Mice with SLE are protected from disease if they have severely restricted calorie intake, restricted fat intake, or high intake of omega-3 unsaturated fat such as eicosapentaenoic acid (fish oil).[253-255] A study in human SLE suggested that 20 g of fish oil daily may be steroid sparing.[256] The role of these dietary observations in human disease is uncertain, but we recommend that patients with SLE minimize their dietary intake of sprouts, excessive calories, and saturated fat. Reports suggesting that exposure of women to hair dye, permanent-wave solutions, and lipstick increased their risk for SLE were not confirmed in subsequent studies.[257,258]

Drugs appear on the list of environmental exposures that might induce SLE-like disease. The drugs listed in Table 74-5 are frequently implicated in drug-induced SLE.[259] This disease is probably different from spontaneous SLE. The clinical manifestations of drug-induced SLE are predominantly arthritis, serositis, fatigue, malaise, and low-grade fever; nephritis and central nervous system disease are rare. These manifestations disappear in most patients within a few weeks of discontinuation of the offending drug, never to reappear unless re-exposure occurs. Although ANAs appear in all patients, it is unusual for high titers of anti-dsDNA or profound hypocomplementemia to develop.

Antibodies to histones are common with some of the inducing drugs; these antibodies also are found in SLE. In drug-induced SLE and spontaneous SLE, the response is probably directed primarily against chromatin nucleosomes, with different histones dominating the response in the two diseases.[259] Antibodies to lymphocytes, platelets, erythrocytes, and phospholipids occur in drug-induced SLE and spontaneous SLE.

It is possible that an individual predisposed to SLE might have the disease triggered by exposure to one of these drugs. Experience has suggested that such an event is rare, however. If a patient with spontaneous SLE needs one of these drugs (e.g., hydantoin or isoniazid), the drug should not be withheld. If one drug has probably induced SLE, the patient should not be rechallenged with that agent. Specificity of autoantibodies to DNA-protein or RNA-protein complexes may spread over time to involve other self-antigens in individuals with the correct permissive genes. Of note to rheumatologists is the more recent implication of therapies with minocycline,[260] statins, and TNF inhibitors[261,262] as potential inducers of SLE-like reactions.

What are the antigens that induce SLE? Are the stimulating antigens foreign (cross-reacting or mimicking "self," such as EBV, which contains a sequence found in proteins associated with Ro), or are they normal or altered self-molecules (e.g., apoptotic bodies) that induce responses that overwhelm tolerance? The role of DNA has been a particular mystery because mammalian DNA (in contrast to bacterial DNA) is weakly immunogenic,[263,264] and yet the IgG anti-dsDNA response correlates with disease activity and nephritis in some patients with SLE, and antibodies to DNA cause nephritis in mice.[11] Immunogenic DNA could originate from certain bacteria after infection,[265] but it is likely that mammalian DNA-protein complexes, particularly those in nucleosomes, are the initial stimulators of this response.[266,267]

Early responses in mice are directed against nucleosomes and "spread" to involve ssDNA and dsDNA over time.[267] Helper T cells that support anti-DNA production are activated by nucleosomes,[266] and some nephritogenic monoclonal antibodies to DNA bind DNA-histone complexes; the anti-DNA/DNA-histone complex can bind to heparan sulfate in glomerular basement membranes.[11] Some antibodies of this type can penetrate cells and bind to cytoplasmic and nuclear structures, probably altering cell function and contributing to disease by mechanisms other than classic complement-mediated tissue injury.[47,268]

The stimulatory role of the Ro molecules is probably similar in that RNA-protein globular complexes induce an immune response in B cells that spreads to include reactivity to other antigens.[269] Cells undergoing apoptosis are capable of presenting nucleosomes, Ro, U1 RNP, and antigenic portions of membrane phospholipids to immune systems and may be crucial in inducing autoreactivity or permitting it to persist.[270,271] It is likely that apoptosis must be precisely balanced to avoid autoimmunity. In humans, defects in Fas (Fas is required for normal apoptosis) are associated with lymphoproliferative disease and autoimmunity, particularly hemolytic anemia and thrombocytopenia—the Canale-Smith syndrome.[270]

Apoptosis that is too rapid might allow quantitative increases in presentation of self-antigens. Apoptosis in some patients with SLE is defective; levels of the Bcl-2 protein that protects from apoptosis are high in human SLE T cells,[271] but levels of Fas ligand (which promotes apoptosis) also are high, and in vitro apoptosis of lymphocytes is increased.[270,272] Another potential mechanism promoting SLE through altered apoptosis involves deficiencies of C1q. It is likely that C1q is involved in clearance of cells undergoing apoptosis[273]; perhaps failure to clear such cells is important in individuals with homozygous deficiencies of C1q, almost all of whom develop SLE.[88,89] Mice homozygous for C1q deficiency also are predisposed to lupus nephritis.[274]

There are likely to be four major sources of nucleosome-like antigens that stimulate antinucleosomal immunity so central to SLE: (1) CpG DNA in bacteria and in DNA/anti-DNA complexes that bind to TLR in dendritic cells and B cells, (2) viral RNA that binds TLR and other receptors in dendritic cells and B cells, (3) apoptotic bodies, and (4) debris from dying cells. In addition to the available sources, normal clearance mechanisms for immune complexes (e.g., nucleosome/antinucleosome) and for apoptotic cells are defective.

ABNORMAL IMMUNE RESPONSES CHARACTERISTIC OF SYSTEMIC LUPUS ERYTHEMATOSUS

The result of interactions between susceptibility genes and triggering environmental factors is development of the pathogenic autoantibodies and immune complexes that characterize SLE. This development requires hyperactivity of B cells and T cells and failure of multiple immunoregulatory circuits to downregulate those responses. The most prominent of these abnormalities are listed in Tables 74-6, 74-7, and 74-8.

CHARACTERISTICS OF LUPUS B CELLS

Abnormalities of B cells are summarized in Table 74-6. B cells play a central role in SLE. Along with their traditional functions as precursors of antibody-producing plasma cells, B cells are efficient APCs and regulate T cell functions, produce cytokines, and express receptor-ligand pairs (i.e., CD154-CD40) previously thought to be restricted to other cell types.[275] B cells develop in bone marrow from stem cells to progenitor B cells to pro-B cells to pre-B cells (pre-B cells are the earliest cells that express surface CD20), then to immature B cells that circulate in the peripheral blood and populate lymphoid tissues. In the periphery, B cells become mature. There are several transitional stages between immaturity and maturity, and at each of these points are mechanisms designed to eliminate highly autoreactive cells.

In the presence of a new antigen, mature B cells recognizing it become activated, then die from activation-induced death; form blast cells, which become antibody-secreting plasma cells; or become memory B cells stored in peripheral compartments. During periods of clinically active SLE in humans, numbers of plasma cells increase, numbers of naive mature B cells decline, and the proportion of memory B cells increases.[276] Long-lived plasma cells (which express little, if any, CD20) are resistant to most of the treatments currently used in SLE, and their persistence might account for flares.[276,277]

In the periphery, at least three types of B cells participate in autoimmunity: (1) the B-1 B cell (about 20% of circulating B cells in adults), which has limited antigen reactivity, secretes IgM, and is primarily self-renewing; (2) the marginal zone B cell in peripheral lymphoid tissue, which is largely responsible for T cell–independent antibody production; and (3) the follicular B cell, which exists in peripheral lymphoid tissue in close approximation to T cells and matures into cells that make T cell–dependent antibodies. All of these B cells can make anti-DNA, but the large quantities of IgG subsets that are major pathogens probably derive primarily from follicular B cells.

Table 74-6 Characteristics of B Cells in the Abnormal Immune Response in Patients with Systemic Lupus Erythematosus (SLE)

Numbers	Surface/Cytoplasm Markers	Functions
Increased immunoglobulin-synthesizing plasma cells	Increased surface CD40L (enhances activation)	Activation via BCR produces increased intracellular Ca^{2+}
Increased mature B cells	Increased surface CD80 and CD86 (enhances activation)	
Decreased naive B cells	Decreased surface CR2 (decreased binding C′, interferon-α)	
Increased memory B cells	Increased BlyS in serum drives maturation, immunoglobulin secretion Mature B express RAG1 and RAG2 (ready for immunoglobulin secretion)	
Expression of VH4.34 H chain	Increased germinal center phenotype (exposed to T cells)	Genetic variants that reduce activity of inhibitory pathways (lyn, FcγRIIB1) predispose to SLE Increased production of IL-6 and IL-10 supports B cell maturation and proliferation

BCR, B cell receptor; IL, interleukin.

Table 74-7 Abnormalities in T Cells in Systemic Lupus Erythematosus

Numbers	Functions	Responses to T Cell Receptor Stimulation
Decreased CD4$^+$ T cells	Abnormal rates of apoptosis lead to imbalance	Autoantigens stimulate T cell help
Decreased CD8$^+$ T cells	Hyperreaction to signaling through TCR	TCR recognizes peptides from immunoglobulin VH, histone in nucleosomes, Sm, RNP, Ro
Increased double negative T cells	Activation results in reduced IL-2 production with increased intracellular Ca^{2+}, increased phosphorylation of tyrosine kinases, increased CREM	T cells of many phenotypes provide help
Decreased iNK T cells	Respond to interferon-α from dendritic cells Mitochondrial abnormalities	Defective regulation of T cell help by CD4$^+$CD25$^+$ regulatory T cells and CD8$^+$ T cells Increased release of sIL-2R, TNFR, sCD40L Increased secretion of IL-10, interferon-γ

IL, interleukin; TCR, T cell receptor.

Table 74-8 Abnormalities in Immunoregulation in Systemic Lupus Erythematosus

B Cells	T Cells	Dendritic Cells (and Monocytes)
Deletion of cells with high affinity for self is defective	Deletion of cells with high affinity for self is defective, delayed, or accelerated	Helper dendritic cells are activated and express surface MHC class II, CD80, CD40, FasL (poised to activate B and T)
Resistant to apoptosis		
BCR receptor editing may be defective	Inadequate generation of regulatory T cells and inhibitory/cytotoxic T cells	Defects in maturity arrest necessary for tolerizing T cells, or in IL-10 production
Antibody idiotypic networks fail to suppress B cells	T cell–activating determinants fail to activate CD4+CD25+ regulatory T cells and CD8+CD28− suppressive T cells Cytokine shift favors activation of T cell help, rather than regulation	Phagocytic cells fail to remove immune complexes and apoptotic cells adequately

BCR, B cell receptor; IL, interleukin.

The following abnormalities of SLE B cells have been described in human and murine lupus:

1. Aberrant survival of autoreactive autoantibody-producing cells in the periphery
2. Enhanced B cell activation resulting from increased signaling responses after ligation of surface receptors, and diminished activity of inhibitory signaling pathways[278]
3. Enhanced production of and response to several cytokines and other growth factors
4. Secretion of high-affinity IgG antibodies to self-antigens

The descriptions that follow apply to B cells identified after the diagnosis of SLE, and by that time, many factors have influenced the B cells. B cell–B cell interactions mediated by CD154-CD40 are essential for differentiation of germinal center B cells into memory cells and for the formation of secondary germinal center structures that allow reactivated memory B cells to differentiate into plasma cells secreting high-affinity antibodies.[275,279] IL-21 also drives naive and memory B cells to mature into plasma cells, particularly cells activated by the costimulatory CD154-CD40 interaction.[280] Autoantibody-producing B cells may be redirected into T cell–dependent germinal center regions, leading to differentiation into plasma cells secreting pathogenic autoantibodies.[275]

Evidence from studies in MRL/lpr and (NZB/NZW) F1 mice suggests that autoreactive B cells are able to form or enter splenic follicles where they contact T cells, whereas in normal mice, autoreactive B cells are retained outside follicles.[281,282] Freshly isolated B cells from the periphery of patients with active SLE are poised to be easily activated and to escape regulation. Their surfaces constitutively express CD154; they are enriched in cells that express a germinal center phenotype or TLR9 or both,[275,276,283] and they have downregulated the complement-inhibitory proteins CD55 and CD59.[284] In addition, they are pushed to activation and survival by a microenvironment rich in B cell growth factors, such as B cell activating factor (BAFF), or BlyS, and IL-10.[285] In addition, SLE memory B cells have decreased expression of the downregulating Fc receptor, FcIIB, in contrast to cells from normal healthy controls.[286]

When B cells from SLE patients are activated, aberrant cell signaling occurs.[278,287-290] This occurrence is characterized by recruitment of a low-molecular-weight isoform of CD45 to lipid rafts on cell membranes, with resultant reduced recruitment of Lyn, a protein tyrosine kinase, which alters signal transduction. There is increased intracellular calcium flux and abnormal phosphorylation of multiple proteins; these changes are independent of disease activity[287] and are indicative of intrinsic abnormalities in SLE B cells. As further evidence of intrinsic B cell defects, in the MRL/lpr mouse model of SLE, mice unable to generate T cell help because they are TCR−/− still develop anti-DNA and nephritis,[291] and mice with B cells expressing surface BCR, but unable to secrete immunoglobulin, still develop nephritis, although in lower frequency than the wild-type MRL/lpr mice.[292]

Although these abnormal B cells might be accounted for by delayed apoptosis with the lpr (mutated Fas) background, there also is evidence for intrinsic B cell abnormalities in the Fas-intact (NZB × NZW)F1 mice, where adoptive transfer of pre-B cells from embryonic liver into severe combined immunodeficiency mice resulted in production of anti-DNA and nephritis.[293] Finally, expression of the antiapoptotic molecule, Bcl-2, is increased in SLE B cells of some mouse models and of some patients, probably contributing to prolonged survival.[271,294]

Defects in the induction or regulation of B cell apoptosis have been well characterized in human and murine systems of SLE and can be summarized as follows:

1. Autoantigens that drive B cells are readily available.
2. Altered homeostasis of apoptosis favors either antigen presentation (acclerated apoptosis) or persistence of autoreactive B cells (delayed apoptosis).
   a. Mutations of Fas or Fas ligand genes are associated with delayed apoptosis in lymphocytes, including B cells, of lpr and gld mice, resulting in lymphoproliferation and systemic autoimmunity. Sporadic cases of humans with Fas and Fas ligand mutations have been reported who also develop lymphoproliferative diseases with some lupus-like features.[295] Increased expression of Fas ligand on anti-DNA–secreting B cells in patients with SLE may increase killing of Fas-expressing immunoregulatory T cells, facilitating escape of autoreactive B cells from the immune tolerance system.[296]
   b. Mice congenitally deficient for the proapoptotic protein Bim[297] or transgenic for the antiapoptotic protein Bcl-2[294] develop a lupus-like disorder.

c. Bcl-2 expression is increased in peripheral lymphocytes and sera of some SLE patients, but not all.[298-300]

3. B cell growth factors play a role in promoting B cell maturation and immunoglobulin secretion in individuals with predisposing genetic or environmental factors. Mice transgenic for BlyS (a member of the TNF superfamily, also called BAFF or TALL-1) develop lymphoproliferation and a lupus-like disorder associated with inhibition of B cell apoptosis mediated by Bcl-2 upregulation.[301,302] BlyS is important for driving immature B cells to mature B cells.[303] Some SLE patients exhibit elevated serum levels, lymphocyte levels, and target tissue levels of this protein.[304]

4. Estradiol and prolactin sex hormones influence the location and activation of B cells. Altered selection of naive B cells and their rescue from tolerance induction, with subsequent persistence in the periphery, as a result of hormonal treatment with estradiol or prolactin,[247-249,300] is associated with an upregulation of Bcl-2 expression and impaired apoptosis in these cells.

The antigens recognized by B cells are important in stimulating pathogenic autoantibody production by the hyperactivatable cells. In lupus mice, polyclonal activation of B cells precedes the high-avidity, single autoantigen–specific B cell activation that characterizes well-developed disease. This fact suggests that B cells in SLE are subject to increased polyclonal activation and antigen-specific activation before disease appears.[305,306] Either type of stimulation induces altered intracellular events that result in increased B cell function and delayed apoptosis. Because patients have autoantibody repertoires that differ among individuals (e.g., almost all have ANAs, but only some have anti-dsDNA, anti-Ro, anti-RNP, or antiplatelet antibodies), it is likely that many B cells are activated by specific antigens.

After autoantibody responses are initiated, B cells and helper T cells develop that recognize additional antigens—a process known as epitope spreading. A lupus-predisposed individual may make an antibody to immunogenic portions of nucleosome, Sm peptides, or immunoglobulin-derived peptides, and a few months later, B cells can be detected that make antinucleosome or anti-Sm, anti-dsDNA, and ANAs.[306-308] Whether spreading is more common in SLE than in normal individuals may depend on intrinsic abnormalities of B cells and T cells, failure to regulate the initial response, the presence of an antigen that mimics these DNA-protein or RNA-protein complexes (especially on their surface), or engagement of dendritic cells via DNA-protein and RNA-protein complexes, or all four.[307-309]

Another possible reason for hyperactivity of B cells in SLE is abnormalities in the CR2 pathway.[310] CR2 is a polymeric surface complex containing CD21, CD19, and CD81; it binds EBV, C3b, C3dg, C3d, and IFN-α, and possibly DNA in immune complexes. When BCR and CR2 are cross-linked, the activating signal for B cells is greatly magnified. In SLE patients, CR2 expression is decreased during active disease. Although one might predict that low CR2 would result in less B cell activity, full expression of CR2 may be required for enough activation to induce apoptosis. Low CR2 might result in defective B cell tolerance. In addition, inhibitory signaling pathways may be impaired in SLE B cells. The coreceptors that negatively regulate surface immunoglobulin signaling, CD22 and CD45, and a

downstream signal transduction molecule (SH2-containing phosphatase 1) all have been shown to be downregulated in SLE B cells.[311-313]

An additional abnormality of SLE B cells is enhanced production and response to cytokines, such as IL-6 and IL-10. SLE B cells are more easily driven to differentiate by IL-6 than are normal B cells.[314] SLE patients have increased numbers of IL-6-secreting cells, and SLE B cells constitutively express surface receptors for IL-6, in contrast to B cells from normal controls.[314,315] IL-6 increases in vitro production by B cells of IgG and anti-DNA-IgG, whereas addition of anti-IL-6 inhibits those effects.[315] Administration of IL-6 to mice accelerates lupus.[316] IL-10 has immunostimulatory and immunosuppressive effects. SLE patients display increased serum concentrations of IL-10 and increased numbers of IL-10-secreting cells during active disease.[317,318]

Administration of anti-IL-10 to SLE-predisposed mice is effective in preventing disease, probably by permitting transforming growth factor (TGF)-β–mediated suppression of T cell and B cell functions.[319] In patients with SLE, anti-IL-10 monoclonal antibody suppressed the in vitro production of autoantibody from B cells, whereas recombinant IL-10 promoted it.[317] An immunoprotective role of IL-10 was found in lupus-prone MRL/lpr mice; mice made deficient in IL-10 developed severe lupus with earlier skin lesions, increased lymphadenopathy, and more severe glomerulonephritis than IL-10-sufficient mice. The protective effect of IL-10 was mediated through downregulation of pathogenic T helper type 1 (Th1) responses.[320] A hypothesis reconciling the previous contrasting observations is that during the initial phase of SLE, in which IFN-γ (which stimulates helper T cells) and its induced IgG2a autoantibody production promote disease, IL-10 is needed to suppress the pathogenic Th1 responses. By contrast, at later phases of disease, excessive IL-10 production may lead to enhanced autoantibody production and subsequent formation of pathogenic immune complexes.

CHARACTERISTICS OF LUPUS T CELLS

Abnormalities in T cell function are reviewed in Table 74-7. These abnormalities play a major role in murine and human SLE. In all the strains of lupus mice that have been tested, elimination or inactivation of CD4+ helper T cells protects from disease,[321,322] and athymic mice do not develop SLE.[323] Quantitative variations in T cells and their subsets may be important. In human SLE, the total number of T cells is usually reduced, probably as a result of the effects of antilymphocyte antibodies.[324,325] Decreased CD4+ T cell numbers correlate well with antilymphocyte antibodies specifically reactive against CD4+, and there is strong correlation among high antilymphocyte antibody titers, lymphopenia, and disease activity.[326,327]

Data vary as to which T cell subset is most frequently reduced, and the characteristics of cells in peripheral blood may not be as important as cells in target organs. Although CD4+ and CD8+ T cells are often decreased in blood of SLE patients, numbers of double-negative T cells are increased.[328,329] Double-negative natural killer T cells respond to glycolipid antigens presented by nonpolymorphic MHC molecules such as CD1 and can provide help for autoantibody production in SLE.[329-331] In addition, certain subsets of double-negative cells possess potent suppressive activity. Such a subset (bearing the invariant Va24JaQ TCR) was decreased in peripheral blood of Japanese SLE patients.[332] Generally, many T cell subsets of human SLE peripheral blood T cells (CD4+CD8−, CD4−CD8+, and CD4−CD8−) can provide help for autoantibody production, whereas only CD4+CD8− cells have this capacity in healthy individuals.

Several functional abnormalities have been reported in SLE T cells in terms of proliferation, activation, expression of costimulatory or effector surface molecules, intracellular signaling pathways, helper or cytolytic activity, and ability to synthesize IL-2 after TCR activation. Accessory cell–dependent TCR/CD3-mediated proliferation in unfractionated peripheral blood mononuclear cell cultures from SLE patients is significantly decreased compared with normal controls,[333] whereas CD3/TCR-mediated proliferation of purified SLE T cells ranges from low to normal to enhanced.[334] Decreased proliferative responses have been reported in some patients in response to mitogenic lectins (PHA, ConA, PWM), anti-CD2, and allogeneic and autologous mixed lymphocyte reactions.[324,335] There is considerable evidence for the presence of in vivo polyclonal T cell activation in SLE. Increased numbers of circulating T cells show spontaneous proliferation[336] and express proliferating cell nuclear antigen.[337] There is increased expression of MHC class II molecules[336] on T cell surfaces and increased release of soluble IL-2 receptors,[338] TNF receptors,[339] and soluble CD40L into the serum.[340]

A pan–T cell dysfunction seems to exist in SLE, which is characterized by exaggerated helper and diminished regulatory/suppressor CD4+CD25+ and CD8+ T cell activities.[341] Natural killer cell functions are defective.[342] Partly as a result of loss of effective CD8+ T and natural killer cell negative feedback on B cells,[343] autoreactive B cell clones produce autoantibodies against an array of intracellular and extracellular autoantigens (see the preceding section for discussion of intrinsic abnormalities in SLE B cells). The ability of T cells to help antibody production and their inability to suppress it are probably the T cell functions most pertinent to clinical SLE. Because many of the pathogenic autoantibodies in patients with SLE are IgG, T cell help plays a major role in their production and maintenance.

As mentioned previously, in human SLE, T cells with many different surface phenotypes give help for autoantibody production,[331,344] including classic helper cells (CD4+CD8− α/β TCR), CD4+CD8− γ/δ TCR cells, CD4−CD8+ α/β TCR cells, and CD1-restricted double-negative natural killer T cells.[345] This unusual situation of cells of many phenotypes providing help to B cells may represent intrinsic defects in the T cells and B cells, failure of regulatory CD4+CD25+ or suppressive CD8+ T cells to mature or function to regulate their targets, or absence of other downregulating networks.

CD8 T cell function is impaired in peripheral blood T cells from patients with SLE.[346,347] Impaired generation of CD8 cytolytic T cells against allogeneic targets[348] and cytolytic activity induced by anti-CD3 stimulation have been reported.[347,349] CD8 cells from some SLE patients sustain, rather than suppress, spontaneous polyclonal IgG production; they synergize with CD4 T cells to support autoantibody synthesis.[344,350] CD8 suppressive activity for autoantibody production also is defective in several murine

models of SLE, and becomes increasingly apparent as the mice age.[351]

Inquiries into the mechanisms causing T cell dysfunctions have led to identification of several defects of signal transduction. In contrast to T cells from the peripheral blood of normal individuals or patients with nonlupus rheumatic diseases, peripheral blood T cells from SLE patients show diminished TCR ζ chain expression.[352,353] An enhanced and prolonged increase in intracellular Ca^2 concentration ($[Ca^2]$) following TCR-mediated cell activation has been identified in human primary SLE T cells, T cell lines, and antigen-specific T cell clones,[278] which is unrelated to disease activity. Ca^2 as a second messenger mediates calcineurin-catalyzed dephosphorylation of nuclear factor of activated T cell and its nuclear translocation, and overexpression of CD154, Fas ligand, and c-myc in SLE T cells.[352-354] There are reports of defective cyclic adenosine monophosphate (cAMP)–dependent protein phosphorylation in peripheral blood T cells from SLE patients. This defect may be attributed to deficient activities of type I and type II isoenzymes of protein kinase A.[355-357] Among SLE patients, the prevalences of deficient type I and type II protein kinase A activities are approximately 80% and 40%. These deficiencies are persistent over time and are independent of clinical disease activity.

Regulation of apoptosis in human and murine lupus T cells is impaired. Although mutations in the apoptosis-mediating Fas receptor or the Fas ligand in the *lpr* and *gld* mouse backgrounds are associated with impaired lymphocyte apoptosis or lupus-like disease, the Fas-mediated signaling pathway seems to be normal in human SLE.[358] SLE T cells in many patients show defective activation-induced cell death, however; this could be due to abnormalities in a second major pathway leading to activation-induced cell death, which involves signaling between members of the TNF-α surface receptor family and their ligands. T cells from peripheral blood of some SLE patients show decreased intracellular synthesis of TNF-α, which could result in undesirable survival of autoreactive cells.[359]

In contrast, increased spontaneous apoptosis also has been observed in SLE.[360] This accelerated apoptosis is likely to provide more autoantigens to stimulate the immune system. Apoptosis must be in perfect balance for avoidance of autoreactivity—if autoreactive lymphocytes persist too long, as in MRL/lpr mice, or are increased in quantity with cell survival too brief, as in some patients with active SLE, autoimmunity results. Disruption of the mitochondrial transmembrane potential with mitochondrial hyperpolarization has been proposed as the point of no return in apoptotic signaling. This phenomenon precedes caspase activation and phosphatidylserine externalization in the early phase of Fas-induced, p53-induced, and hydrogen peroxide–induced apoptosis.[361-363] Deviations in key mitochondrial checkpoints associated with abnormal T cell apoptosis in SLE have been identified:[363] (1) deficient elevation of transmembrane potential, (2) diminished CD3/CD28-induced reactive oxygen intermediates and hydrogen peroxide production, and (3) reduced hydrogen peroxide–induced apoptosis.

One of the cardinal biochemical abnormalities in SLE T cells is a global decrease in genomic deoxymethylcytosine content.[364] Because methylation of deoxycytosine in regulatory sequences can suppress transcription of the associated gene,[365] abnormal hypomethylation could contribute to overexpression of some genes in SLE T cells. More importantly, T cells treated with methylation inhibitors, including procainamide and hydralazine, become autoreactive as a result of surface lymphocyte function antigen-1 (CD11a) overexpression, leading to a lupus-like disease in murine models.[366] Lymphocyte function antigen-1 overexpression lowers the threshold for T cell activation, allowing the cells to respond to self-class II MHC molecules presenting inappropriate antigens.[367]

In particular, lymphocyte function antigen-1 overexpression seems to overstabilize the normally low-affinity interaction between the TCR and class II MHC molecules lacking the relevant antigenic peptide, allowing the signaling apparatus to assemble and transmit its signal.[368] Defective signaling via the extracellular regulating kinase pathway in active SLE T cells has been associated with DNA hypomethylation. More recently, hypomethylation of the "silenced" X chromosome in women with SLE has been shown and associated with increased expression of CD40L on T cell surfaces, another example of hypomethylation in regulatory sequences permitting upregulation of the protein-encoding gene.[57]

More recent work has shown that peripheral blood T cells from SLE patients on TCR stimulation with anti-CD8 and anti-CD28 produce abnormally low levels of IL-2.[357,369] Such a deficiency could lead to failure of autoreactive T cells to undergo apoptosis after strong activation signals and to defective generation of regulatory and suppressor T cells. The basis of this defect is multifactorial, with (1) reduced generation of p65 (required for activation of NF-κB on the IL-2 promoter), (2) elevation of CREM/CREB ratios (CREM is cAMP-responsive element modulator—a transcriptional repressor that binds to cAMP response elements and downregulates the expression of genes having this binding site), and (3) increased CREM binding of the c-fos promoter (which decreases transcription of c-fos, reducing AP-1 binding of the IL-2 promoter), all of which lead to (4) inadequate IL-2 production.

Increased expression of Ca^{2+}/calmodulin-dependent kinase IV and of protein phosphatase 2A may contribute to increased production of CREM. To summarize this work, several molecules required for full activation of the IL-2 promoter are altered in SLE T cells, possibly centering on increased expression of CREM, with the end result being reduced production of IL-2, an essential growth cytokine for T cells.[357,370-372]

Altered cytokine homeostasis characterizes T cells, B cells, and dendritic cells in active SLE. Increased levels of IL-10 in the serum and increased numbers of IL-10-secreting cells are observed. IL-10 inhibits some T cell functions and can lead to downregulation of IL-2, TNF-α, and IFN-γ,[373] each of which plays a cardinal role in the generation of cytotoxic and suppressive T cells. Secretion of IL-2 by SLE T cells is often low as discussed in the preceding paragraphs, whereas secretion of IFN-γ may be high.[374] Murine lupus seems to depend strongly on increased levels of IFN-γ, however, because mice that are congenitally deficient for the IFN-γ receptor are partially protected from developing SLE,[375] and treatment with soluble IFN-γ receptor prevents disease.[376] Perhaps the cells isolated from patients with active disease are exhausted, and the cytokine profile they produce does not reflect the initiation of disease or flares.

Several investigators have found dramatic elevations in expression of genes that are IFN-inducible (particularly by IFN-α) during periods of SLE activity.[377-382] A major source of this cytokine is plasmacytoid dendritic cells, rather than lymphocytes, but many cells can secrete IFN-α. IFN-α activates immature dendritic cells, providing APCs that drive innate and adaptive autoimmunity. The upregulation of IFN-inducible genes is associated with disease activity, but is much more common in SLE than in other chronic inflammatory diseases. The presence of a granulopoiesis signature in gene expression by peripheral blood cells from SLE patients also is notable, and we expect to understand the importance of these cells in SLE over the next few years.

Autoantigens that activate T cells are crucial in SLE. These are derived from nucleosomes, RNA/protein antigens such as RNP and Sm, and the autoantibodies themselves. Autoantibodies can activate their own T cell help; B cells process their surface immunoglobulin and present immunoglobulin-derived peptides in their surface MHC class II molecules to nearby helper T cells, which are activated to help the synthesis of additional autoantibody.[383-387] This may be an important mechanism for sustaining the production of pathogenic autoantibodies in SLE.

In human and murine lupus, the V regions of anti-DNA antibodies contain peptide determinants that activate T cells and can accelerate the disease process.[374,383] Peripheral blood T cells from many patients with SLE recognize V_H determinants of human anti-DNA.[374] Used as a tolerogen, an artificial V_H peptide (pCONSENSUS), based on V_H peptides, inhibits responses to nucleosomes and other autoantigens, but it leaves the murine immune system intact and able to generate responses to external antigens.[384] Similar observations have been made with a peptide from the V_H region of another monoclonal antibody anti-DNA; that product (Edratide) is in clinical trials in patients with SLE.[388,389]

Similarly, patients with SLE have circulating T cells that recognize peptides from nucleosomes, and it is likely that these cells also upregulate anti-DNA antibody production.[390,391] These peptides also can be used as tolerogens.[385-389] It is the authors' opinion that the main mechanism by which these tolerizing peptides suppress SLE-like autoimmunity is by induction of regulatory $CD4^+CD25^+$ cells and of suppressive $CD8^+$ T cells.[386,387,389,391]

The role of T cells in directly causing tissue damage in SLE has not been emphasized, but it is probably important. Because 50% of individuals with subacute cutaneous lupus and anti-Ro/SS-A do not have immunoglobulin and complement deposited at the dermal-epidermal junction, dermatitis in those individuals may be caused by T cells sensitized to Ro.[392] Finally, although the classic explanation for vasculitis is deposition of immune complexes in vessel walls, some T cells, probably sensitized to endothelial cell antigens, can cause vasculitis.[393] Kidney-infiltrating T cells in SLE patients show a relatively restricted TCR Vβ repertoire. TCR Vβ8 and Vβ20 were preferentially expressed in 50% and 40% of kidney biopsy specimens in one study,[394] and junctional sequences of complementary DNA encoding the TCR Vβ8 and Vβ20 genes in intrarenal T cells showed oligoclonal expansion, indicating antigen-driven stimulation.

Where are the suppressor/regulatory T cells that should eliminate these pathogenic, hyperactive T cells and B cells?

More recent work has suggested abnormalities in interactions between CD4 T cells that are required for maturation of CD4+CD25+ regulatory T cells and cytotoxic CD8 cells. These abnormalities might result from the inability of natural killer cells from SLE patients to secrete adequate quantities of activated TGF-β.[395] It is likely that CD4 T cells stimulate natural killer cells to secrete active TGF-β under normal circumstances, but not when SLE is active. In the chronic graft-versus-host mouse model of lupus-like disease, autoantibody formation and nephritis are delayed by administration of T cells preincubated with TGF-β, suggesting that this cytokine may partially restore suppression/regulation in individuals with autoimmunity.[395]

T lymphocytes are quantitatively and qualitatively abnormal in human lupus and in murine models of the disease. Qualitative abnormalities include increased responsiveness to surface activating signals, which results in increased calcium flux that may depend on defects in protein kinase A type I and II isoenzymes. The end result is decreased synthesis of IL-2. Hypomethylation of DNA may be another outcome. For unknown reasons, T cells with many different surface phenotypes promote help of autoantibody production without appropriate suppression. Quantitative abnormalities in several cytokines, such as IL-2 (low), IFN-γ (high), IL-10 (high), and TGF-β (low), are important in aberrant cell function. There are several adverse outcomes of all these abnormalities, including resistance to apoptosis in some autoreactive T cells, accelerated apoptosis in other T lymphocytes that release autoantigens, and defective regulation of the skewing of many different subsets to provide help. Finally, defects in regulatory, cytotoxic, and suppressive T cells are important in allowing autoantibody production.

ABNORMALITIES IN IMMUNOREGULATION

The ability to make pathogenic subsets of autoantibodies and immune complexes must be accompanied by inability to downregulate them if disease is to be sustained. In murine lupus, when autoantibodies appear, they increase steadily until organ damage occurs, and death follows. In humans, autoantibodies of SLE appear years before the first clinical manifestation of disease, and after disease onset the levels of many autoantibodies fluctuate, sometimes increasing with clinical exacerbations and decreasing during periods of improvement (e.g., ANA, anti-DNA, anti-SmD peptide). Autoantibodies including ANA, anti-DNA, anti-phospholipids, anti-Sm, and anti-RNP appear years before the first symptom of disease in most patients, suggesting that for many months regulatory mechanisms are effective in preventing disease. Nevertheless, when the diagnosis of SLE has been made, virtually every mechanism of regulating antibodies that has been studied is abnormal.

IMMUNE TOLERANCE

Highly autoreactive B lymphocytes and T lymphocytes are deleted, inactivated, or suppressed in healthy individuals by immune tolerance. Mechanisms of tolerance include deletion (B cells and T cells), anergy (B cells and T cells), BCR editing (B cells), cytokine shifts (T cells), and induction of regulatory cells (suppressing B cells and T cells). Tolerance steps occur at several points along cell development, beginning with immature or naive cells in the thymus (T cells) or bone marrow (B cells) and extending to peripheral lymphoid organs (B cells and T cells).[396-402]

For T cells, strong interaction between autoantigen-recognizing TCRs and MHC class I and class II molecules on thymic epithelial cells (containing autoantigens) may deliver one or two signals to the cells: (1) cross-linking of antigen receptors, followed by (2) engagement of second surface receptors after activation of T cell help (especially CD28 and its B7 ligands, CD80 and CD86). If two signals are received, apoptosis results; the cells are deleted. A few that "leak" into the periphery can be deleted there. Cells that receive only one activation signal are anergized; they are difficult to activate when they reach the periphery, and they may eventually undergo apoptosis. B cells undergo the same processes, with the bone marrow and peripheral lymphoid organs as sites of deleting and anergizing signals. In addition, B cells can undergo receptor editing—a process in which an autoreactive surface immunoglobulin molecule is changed by different combinations of heavy and light chains within each cell. The resultant surface immunoglobulin molecule (BCR) is no longer highly autoreactive; the edited "safe" B cells are selected for expansion.[396-399]

Dendritic cells also influence tolerance, particularly in T cells. One paradigm is that immature dendritic cells educate T cells to be tolerant (i.e., anergic or regulatory), whereas mature dendritic cells activate T cells. More recent data suggest that dendritic cells are tolerogenic or activating not because of their maturity, but because of the cytokines they secrete, with IL-10, TGF-β, granulocyte colony-stimulating factor, and hepatic growth factor all playing roles in induction of tolerance.[402]

In murine and human B cells, there are several points in cell development during which deletion of autoreactive cells can occur.[398,399] The first is the step between an immature cell in the bone marrow and the transitional T1 cell in peripheral lymphoid tissue, the second is between the T1 and more mature T2/3 stage, and the third is between the Tr/3 and mature B cell. The mature B cells that can make pathogenic autoantibodies include marginal zone B2 cells, B1 self-renewing B cells, and follicular, germinal center B2 cells (which are the cells best poised to receive T cell help and to generate long-lived memory B cells and plasma cells). Autoreactive B cells from SLE patients can enter germinal centers in greater numbers than cells from healthy individuals, suggesting increased exposure to T cell stimulation.[403]

These intrinsic checkpoints in B cell development are influenced by sex hormones; second signals (especially CD40/CD40L, both of which are overexpressed in SLE B cells and T cells); BAFF, which is elevated in some SLE patients; and cytokines that are B cell growth factors, such as IL-6 and IL-10 (both increased in some SLE patients). Ability of this intrinsic B cell tolerance to proceed in an orderly fashion is altered by the external factors listed, and by genetic background and the tolerogenic or activated states of APCs, including dendritic cells.[212,404] In addition, B cells can be activated independent of BCR via TLR9 receptors.[21]

T cell functions can be altered by shifts in the cytokines they release; deviation from Th1 to Th2 patterns protects from some T cell–induced autoimmune diseases in animals, such as experimental allergic encephalitis and diabetes.[347] Finally, T cells and dendritic cells can be generated that suppress effector T cells or B cells or both; most authorities consider this a form of tolerance.[402,405]

In patients with SLE, immune tolerance is presumably defective with enhanced numbers and survival of autoreactive T cells and B cells. Many of the abnormalities that could account for this finding are discussed under the previous B lymphocyte and T lymphocyte sections and listed in Table 74-8.

INADEQUATE CLEARING OF IMMUNE COMPLEXES

Several defects contribute to inadequate clearing of soluble and insoluble immune complexes.[48] Immune complexes are transported by complement receptors, primarily on erythrocytes in humans. The numbers of complement receptors (CR1 and CR2) on cell surfaces are reduced in patients with active SLE[90,406] so that immune complexes are not transported adequately to the mononuclear phagocytic cell system that clears them, leaving the immune complexes to deposit in tissues. In some individuals, the low numbers of complement receptors may be genetically determined; in most, they are probably low because they have been stripped away by large quantities of immune complex.[90,406] CR2 is of additional importance because it is a receptor for EBV and IFN-α, each of which has been implicated in the pathogenesis of SLE.[310]

Phagocytosis of immune complexes occurs after binding to Fcγ receptors of several types on monocytes, macrophages, and neutrophils. Binding and internalization of immunoglobulin in immune complexes may be less than normal in some SLE patients with certain alleles of Fcγ RIIA and FcγRIIIA.[125-129,134,135,407] In many SLE patients, immune complexes are not phagocytosed properly, and this permits persistence of harmful immune complexes in the circulation.[48,207] In an earlier section, we discussed impaired clearing of apoptotic bodies in patients with SLE[59,270,271]; persistence of these bodies probably permits sustained exposure of the immune system to autoantigens contained in them and contributes to autoantibody production.

INADEQUATE DOWNREGULATION BY T CELLS

Autoimmune disease is prevented by mechanisms of central and peripheral immune tolerance, among which a cardinal role is played by regulatory/inhibitory cells.[386,387,408-410] These cells belong to the CD4, CD8, or natural killer T cell compartments and exert an array of complex functions on diverse cell subsets. Several functional abnormalities have been described for each of these T cell subsets in human and murine lupus.

In the CD8+ compartment, at least two distinct subsets of suppressor cells have been identified in mice and humans that share the CD8+CD28− surface phenotype, are not cytotoxic, and do not induce apoptosis. The first CD8+ suppressor subset induces antigen-specific immunosuppression through cell-to-cell contact with APC presenting antigen.[411] The second subset mediates an antigen-nonspecific suppression of T cell proliferation via soluble factors, such as IFN-α, IL-10,

and TGF-β.[386,412] This subset is functionally impaired in SLE,[346,347] suggesting involvement in disease pathogenesis. In human SLE, there is impaired generation of CD8 cytolytic T cells against allogeneic targets[348] and depressed anti-CD3–dependent cytolytic activity.[349] CD8 lymphocytes from lupus patients sustain, rather than suppress, spontaneous polyclonal IgG production; they synergize with CD4 T cells to support autoantibody synthesis.[350]

In addition to loss of function, numbers of CD8+ T cells also may decline as autoimmune disease appears. Studies in mice and dogs have shown that CD8 cells decline in number or do not expand at the rapid rate occurring in CD4+ T cells and B cells as the animals develop SLE.[351] In patients with SLE, there is considerable variation in numbers of CD8+ cells[413]; in some individuals, they are lower than normal.[414,415] How do suppressor T cells evolve? In mice and humans, interactions between CD4 and CD8 cell subsets are required to induce suppression of immunoglobulin production in antigen, PWM, or autologous mixed lymphocyte response systems.[416,417] Similarly, differentiation of cytotoxic CD8 precursors into cytotoxic CD8+ effectors requires the presence of CD4 cells, possibly as a source of IL-2. In some systems, TGF-β may be an additional requirement; its major source in humans is the natural killer cell.[343,348,351,417]

In combination with IL-2, TGF-β can induce peripheral CD8+ T cells to become inhibitory and naive CD4+ T cells to become CD4+CD25+ regulatory T cells.[343] Such cells, either CD4+ or CD8+, suppress antibody production.[345,387,418,419] Unmanipulated adult BWF1 mice and SLE patients cannot generate CD8+ inhibitory/cytotoxic T cells capable of suppressing autoantibody production.[346,351] That could result from defects in generation of inhibitory/cytotoxic T cells, inadequate functional capacities of inhibitory/cytotoxic T cells, antibodies to inhibitory/cytotoxic T cells or to their CD4+ precursor cells, or defective CD4+ precursor cells (e.g., making inadequate quantities of IL-2). There is evidence for all of these hypotheses.[347-349,357,363,368,420] CD4+ T cells, dendritic cells, and possibly other APCs participate in generation of inhibitory/cytotoxic T cells. Generation of cytotoxic CD8+ cells requires help from a CD4 helper cell through CD40-CD40L interactions, usually with the surface of a dendritic cell.[421-423] Other studies have reported, however, that if CD8 cytotoxic precursor frequencies are high, priming of CD8 T cell responses may not require CD4 T cell help.[424]

When generated, the CD8 suppressor/effector can subsequently act directly on the CD4 T helper cell and abrogate its ability to provide help. Alternatively, it can act on an APC via cell-to-cell contact and render it tolerogenic through induction of surface expression of inhibitory receptors, such as ILT-3 and ILT-4, and downregulation of surface expression of CD80 and CD86.[425] Such a "tolerogenic" APC, on subsequent contact with a CD4 T helper or CD8+CD28− suppressor, would render it anergic. Based on this model, failure to generate CD8 inhibitory/cytotoxic T cells in patients with SLE or lupus-prone mice could result from abnormalities in dendritic cells or in CD4 T cell suppressor/inducers. It also is possible that the inhibitory/cytotoxic T cells are generated, but cannot function well enough to oppose activated T helper cells and B cells.

The multiple defects described in the CD8 T cells can be overcome. More recent evidence suggests that, in the BWF1 model of lupus, CD8 inhibitory cells still may be present and may be induced to protect against the development of systemic autoimmunity in young BWF1 mice. Vaccination of BWF1 mice with plasmid DNA vectors encoding immunoglobulin V_H-derived MHC class I–binding epitopes activates cytotoxic T cells that ablate autoantibody-producing B cells and inhibit the development of lupus nephritis.[419] Similarly, injection of tolerogenic doses of peptides from anti-DNA or from the histone of nucleosomes can activate CD4[+] regulatory T cells and CD8[+] inhibitory T cells.[387,391] In human SLE, functional CD8[+] inhibitory/cytotoxic T cells seem to be restored during periods of clinical improvement.[346] Novel therapies that aim to restore suppressive capacity to CD8[+] inhibitory/cytotoxic T cells are an attractive option.

Natural killer T cells, which are double negative (which is CD4[−]CD8[−]TCR[+]CD56[+]), possess potent suppressive activity. Such a subset (bearing the invariant Va24JaQ TCR; iNKT) was reported to be decreased in peripheral blood of two groups of SLE patients.[332,426] The role of natural killer and iNKT cells in various models of lupus has varied, and the authors are reluctant to state a general principle about the role of these cells in pathogenesis. Studies of these cells are in progress.

Another important subset of regulatory cells is a thymus-derived CD4 subset constitutively expressing the IL-2 receptor β chain (CD25); these cells protect the host from spontaneous organ-specific autoimmune disease. CD4[+]CD25[+] T cells have been called "professional" suppressor cells and have a contact-dependent mechanism of action in vitro.[427] In mice, CD4[+]CD25[+] T cells appear in the peripheral immune system on day 3 of life. CD4[+]CD25[−] T cells in the absence of CD4[+]CD25[+] T cells cause severe and progressive organ-specific autoimmune disease. In human SLE, some groups have reported reduced numbers of presumptive regulatory T cells (CD4[+]CD25[High] cells) in adults or children with active SLE, and that the numbers of those cells correlated inversely with clinical disease activity.[428,429] Induction of CD4[+]CD25[+] regulatory T cells by tolerization with selected peptides protects lupus mice from developing disease.[387,389,391]

Several sets of regulatory/suppressor T cells, including CD8[+]CD28[−] inhibitory/cytotoxic T cells, CD4[+]CD25[+] regulatory T cells, and natural killer T cells, protect from autoimmunity in normal mice, and probably in healthy humans. It is likely that abnormalities affecting any of these subsets contribute to the imbalance between autoantibody synthesis and regulation that is characteristic of SLE.

INADEQUATE IDIOTYPIC CIRCUITS CONTROLLING PATHOGENIC B CELLS AND T CELLS

In human and murine SLE, a substantial proportion of autoantibodies express a restricted number of public idiotypes (Ids).[430-432] Ids are sequences within the heavy and light chains of immunoglobulin molecules that are themselves antigenic; they induce anti-Id responses. Normally, anti-Ids can suppress Ids and downregulate production of Id[+] antibodies. Some Ids (e.g., 16/6, O-81, and IdGN2) dominate tissue lesions in human SLE.[430] In murine lupus, treating mice with anti-Ids directed against the public Ids dominating their anti-dsDNA antibodies can prevent or

suppress disease, at least temporarily.[430] T cells have a similar idiotypic regulatory system; the Ids reside in the TCR molecules, and the anti-Ids reside on TCRs of regulatory T cells that are expected to suppress the Id[+] T cells. It is unclear why this idiotypic B cell and T cell process is not operating normally to suppress disease in either human or murine lupus.

SUMMARY

As shown in Table 74-9, many of the clinical manifestations of SLE are probably caused by or are associated with the pathogenic autoantibodies, immune complexes, and B cell and T cell abnormalities that have been described. Certain immune complexes, selected antibodies to DNA or Ro/SS-A, and antibodies that bind glomerular structures can cause nephritis. Antibodies that bind to the fetal conduction system or cell membranes (lymphocytes, erythrocytes, platelets, neurons) or enter cells and alter cell functions also have the potential to cause disease. Immune complexes, antibodies to endothelial cells, antineutrophil cytoplasmic antibodies, and T cells may participate in vasculitis and in endothelial cell damage that promotes accelerated atherosclerosis—onto which may be added the prothrombotic effects of antibodies to phospholipids.

An individual's ability to manufacture pathogenic immunoglobulin and sustain its production depends on intrinsic abnormalities of immune complex and apoptotic cell clearance and of B lymphocytes and T lymphocytes, and these abnormalities depend on inheriting an appropriate

Table 74-9 Correlation among Clinical Manifestations of Systemic Lupus Erythematosus and Autoantibodies, Immune Complexes, and T Cells

Manifestation	Autoantibodies	Immune Complexes	T Cells
Nephritis	Anti-dsDNA Anti-Ro Anti-C1q Ids 16/6, 3l and GN2	+	+
Arthritis	?	+	+
Dermatitis	Anti-Ro Anti-dsDNA Id 16/6		+
Vasculitis	Anti-Ro	+	+
Central nervous system	Anti-ribosomal P Antineuronal Anti-NR2	+	
Hematologic Lymphopenia Hemolysis Thrombocytopenia Clotting	Antilymphocyte Antierythrocyte Antiplatelet Antiphospholipid	+	
Fetal loss	Antiphospholipid		
Neonatal lupus	Anti-Ro		
Sicca syndrome	Anti-Ro		+
Mild disease	Anti-RNP without other autoantibody except ANA		

ANA, antinuclear antibody; anti-dsDNA, anti–double-stranded DNA.

number of susceptibility genes, lacking protective genes, and encountering an environmental stimulus such as EBV infection that sets the whole process into action. Even after an individual has detectable autoantibodies, years pass before the first clinical symptom of disease appears, suggesting that immunoregulation is effective for a while in most individuals, and then becomes exhausted. Understanding this complex process is evolving rapidly, making the study of the pathogenesis of SLE a fascinating area in modern medicine.

REFERENCES

1. Croker JA, Kimberly RP: SLE: Challenges and candidates in human disease. Trends Immunol 26:580-586, 2005.
2. Forabosco P, Gorman JD, Cleveland C, et al: Meta-analysis of genome-wide linkage studies of systemic lupus erythematosus. Genes Immun 7:609-614, 2006.
3. Harley JB, Kelly JA, Kaufman KM: Unraveling the genetics of systemic lupus erythematosus. Springer Semin Immunopathol 28:119-130, 2006.
4. Casciola-Rosen L, Rosen A: Ultraviolet light-induced keratinocyte apoptosis: A potential mechanism for the induction of skin lesions and autoantibody production in LE. Lupus 6:175-180, 1997.
5. Katz JB, Limpanasithikul W, Diamond B: Mutational analysis of an autoantibody: Differential binding and pathogenicity. J Exp Med 180:925-932, 1994.
6. **Frenchi G, Putterman C, Diamond B: The structure and derivation of antibodies and autoantibodies. In Wallace DR, Hahn BH (eds): Dubois' Lupus Erythematosus, 7th ed. Philadelphia, Lippincott Williams & Wilkins, 2007, pp 408-431.**
7. Shlomchik M, Mascelli M, Shan H, et al: Anti-DNA antibodies from autoimmune mice arise by clonal expansion and somatic mutation. J Exp Med 171:265-292, 1990.
8. Tillman DM, Jou NT, Hill RJ, et al: Both IgM and IgG anti-DNA antibodies are the products of clonally selective B cell stimulation in (NZB x NZW)F1 mice. J Exp Med 176:761-779, 1992.
9. Hahn BH: Antibodies to DNA. N Engl J Med 338:1359-1368, 1998.
10. van Es JH, Gmelig Meyling FH, van de Akker WR, et al: Somatic mutations in the variable regions of a human IgG anti-double-stranded DNA autoantibody suggest a role for antigen in the induction of systemic lupus erythematosus. J Exp Med 173:461-470, 1991.
11. Ohnishi K, Ebling FM, Mitchell B, et al: Comparison of pathogenic and non-pathogenic murine antibodies to DNA: Antigen binding and structural characteristics. Int Immunol 6:817-830, 1994.
12. Ehrenstein MR, Katz DR, Griffiths MH, et al: Human IgG anti-DNA antibodies deposit in kidneys and induce proteinuria in SCID mice. Kidney Int 48:705-711, 1995.
13. Burlingame RW, Rubin RL: Autoantibody to the nucleosome subunit (H2A-H2B)-DNA is an early and ubiquitous feature of lupus-like conditions. Mol Biol Rep 23(3-4):159-166, 1996.
14. Bruns A, Blass S, Hausdorf G, et al: Nucleosomes are major T and B cell autoantigens in systemic lupus erythematosus. Arthritis Rheum 43:2307-2315, 2000.
15. Kaliyaperumal A, Michaels MA, Datta SK: Naturally processed chromatin peptides reveal a major autoepitope that primes pathogenic T and B cells of lupus. J Immunol 168:2530-2537, 2002.
16. Lu L, Kaliyaperumal A, Boumpas DT, et al: Major peptide autoepitopes for nucleosome-specific T cells of human lupus. J Clin Invest 104:345-355, 1999.
17. Viglianti GA, Lau CM, Hanley TM, et al: Activation of autoreactive B cells by CpG dsDNA. Immunity 19:837-847, 2003.
18. Christensen SR, Kashgarian M, Alexopoulou L, et al: Toll-like receptor 9 controls anti-DNA autoantibody production in murine lupus. J Exp Med 202:321-331, 2005.
19. Boule MW, Broughton C, Mackay F, et al: Toll-like receptor 9-dependent and -independent dendritic cell activation by chromatin-immunoglobulin G complexes. J Exp Med 199:1631-1640, 2004.
20. Lau CM, Broughton C, Tabor AS, et al: RNA-associated autoantigens activate B cells by combined B cell antigen receptor/Toll-like receptor 7 engagement. J Exp Med 202:1171-1177, 2005.
21. **Marshak-Rothstein A: Toll-like receptors in systemic autoimmune disease. Nat Rev Immunol 6:823-835, 2006.**
22. Chan TM, Leung JK, Ho SK, et al: Mesangial cell-binding anti-DNA antibodies in patients with systemic lupus erythematosus. J Am Soc Nephrol 13:1219-1229, 2002.
23. Deocharan B, Qing X, Lichauco J, et al: Alpha-actinin is a cross-reactive renal target for pathogenic anti-DNA antibodies. J Immunol 168:3072-3078, 2002.
24. Li QZ, Xie C, Wu T, et al: Identification of autoantibody clusters that best predict lupus disease activity using glomerular proteome arrays. J Clin Invest 115:3428-3439, 2005.
25. Horvath L, Czirjak L, Fekete B, et al: High levels of antibodies against C1q are associated with disease activity and nephritis but not with other organ manifestations in SLE patients. Clin Exp Rheumatol 19:667-672, 2001.
26. Siegert CE, Daha MR, Tseng CM, et al: Predictive value of IgG autoantibodies against C1q for nephritis in systemic lupus erythematosus. Ann Rheum Dis 52:851-856, 1993.
27. Maddison PJ, Reichlin M: Deposition of antibodies to a soluble cytoplasmic antigen in the kidneys of patients with systemic lupus erythematosus. Arthritis Rheum 22:858-863, 1979.
28. DeGiorgio LA, Konstantinov KN, Lee SC, et al: A subset of lupus anti-DNA antibodies cross-reacts with the NR2 glutamate receptor in systemic lupus erythematosus. Nat Med 7:1189-1193, 2001.
29. Huerta PT, Kowal C, DeGiorgio LA, et al: Immunity and behavior: Antibodies alter emotion. Proc Natl Acad Sci U S A 103:678-683, 2006.
30. Lapteva L, Nowak M, Yarboro CH, et al: Anti-N-methyl-D-aspartate receptor antibodies, cognitive dysfunction, and depression in systemic lupus erythematosus. Arthritis Rheum 54:2505-2514, 2006.
31. Riemekasten G, Kawald A, Weiss C, et al: Strong acceleration of murine lupus by injection of the SmD1(83-119) peptide. Arthritis Rheum 44:2435-2445, 2001.
32. Riemekasten G, Weiss C, Schneider S, et al: T cell reactivity against the SmD1(83-119) C terminal peptide in patients with systemic lupus erythematosus. Ann Rheum Dis 61:779-785, 2002.
33. Riemekasten G, Langnickel D, Ebling FM, et al: Identification and characterization of SmD183-119-reactive T cells that provide T cell help for pathogenic anti-double-stranded DNA antibodies. Arthritis Rheum 48:475-485, 2003.
34. Giannouli S, Voulgarelis M, Ziakas PD, et al: Anaemia in systemic lupus erythematosus: From pathophysiology to clinical assessment. Ann Rheum Dis 65:144-148, 2006.
35. Rioux JD, Zdarsky E, Newkirk MM, et al: Anti-DNA and anti-platelet specificities of SLE-derived autoantibodies: Evidence for CDR2H mutations and CDR3H motifs. Mol Immunol 32:683-696, 1995.
36. Buyon JP, Clancy RM: Neonatal lupus: Basic research and clinical perspectives. Rheum Dis Clin N Am 31:299-313, vii, 2005.
37. Mazel JA, El-Sherif N, Buyon J, et al: Electrocardiographic abnormalities in a murine model injected with IgG from mothers of children with congenital heart block. Circulation 99:1914-1918, 1999.
38. Reichlin M, Brucato A, Frank MB, et al: Concentration of autoantibodies to native 60-kd Ro/SS-A and denatured 52-kd Ro/SS-A in eluates from the heart of a child who died with congenital complete heart block. Arthritis Rheum 37:1698-1703, 1994.
39. Salomonsson S, Dorner T, Theander E, et al: A serologic marker for fetal risk of congenital heart block. Arthritis Rheum 46:1233-1241, 2002.
40. Tran HB, Ohlsson M, Beroukas D, et al: Subcellular redistribution of la/SSB autoantigen during physiologic apoptosis in the fetal mouse heart and conduction system: A clue to the pathogenesis of congenital heart block. Arthritis Rheum 46:202-208, 2002.
41. Pierangeli SS, Chen PP, Gonzalez EB: Antiphospholipid antibodies and the antiphospholipid syndrome: An update on treatment and pathogenic mechanisms. Curr Opin Hematol 13:366-375, 2006.
42. Girardi G, Redecha P, Salmon JE: Heparin prevents antiphospholipid antibody-induced fetal loss by inhibiting complement activation. Nat Med 10:1222-1226, 2004.
43. Holers VM, Girardi G, Mo L, et al: Complement C3 activation is required for antiphospholipid antibody-induced fetal loss. J Exp Med 195:211-220, 2002.
44. Bonfa E, Golombek SJ, Kaufman LD, et al: Association between lupus psychosis and anti-ribosomal P protein antibodies. N Engl J Med 317:265-271, 1987.

45. Hulsey M, Goldstein R, Scully L, et al: Anti-ribosomal P antibodies in systemic lupus erythematosus: A case-control study correlating hepatic and renal disease. Clin Immunol Immunopathol 74:252-256, 1995.

46. Schneebaum AB, Singleton JD, West SG, et al: Association of psychiatric manifestations with antibodies to ribosomal P proteins in systemic lupus erythematosus. Am J Med 90:54-62, 1991.

47. Reichlin MN: Autoantibodies to intracellular antigens in SLE that bind and penetrate cells. In Kammer GM, Tsokos GC (eds): Molecular and Cellular Pathogenesis. Totowa, NJ, Humana Press, 1999.

48. **Salmon JE: Abnormalities in immune complex clearance and Fcgamma receptor function. In Wallace DJ, Hahn BH (eds): Dubois' Lupus Erythematosus, 7th ed. Philadelphia, Lippincott Williams & Wilkins, 2007, pp 191-213.**

49. Carroll MC: The role of complement in B cell activation and tolerance. Adv Immunol 74:61-88, 2000.

50. Cook HT, Botto M: Mechanisms of disease: The complement system and the pathogenesis of systemic lupus erythematosus. Nat Clin Pract Rheumatol 2:330-337, 2006.

51. Croker BP, Gilkeson G, Morel L: Genetic interactions between susceptibility loci reveal epistatic pathogenic networks in murine lupus. Genes Immun 4:575-585, 2003.

52. Wong M, Tsao BP: Current topics in human SLE genetics. Springer Semin Immunopathol 28:97-107, 2006.

53. Block SR, Winfield JB, Lockshin MD, et al: Studies of twins with SLE: A review of the literature and presentation of 12 additional sets. Am J Med 59:533-552, 1979.

54. Deapen D, Escalante A, Weinrib L, et al: A revised estimate of twin concordance in SLE. Arthritis Rheum 35:311, 1992.

55. Jarvinen P, Kaprio J, Makitalo R, et al: Systemic lupus erythematosus and related systemic diseases in a nationwide twin cohort: An increased prevalence of disease in MZ twins and concordance of disease features. J Intern Med 231:67-72, 1992.

56. Alarcon-Segovia D, Alarcon-Riquelme ME, Cardiel MH, et al: Familial aggregation of systemic lupus erythematosus, rheumatoid arthritis, and other autoimmune diseases in 1,177 lupus patients from the GLADEL cohort. Arthritis Rheum 52:1138-1147, 2005.

57. Kono DH, Theofilopoulos AN: Genetics of SLE in mice. Springer Semin Immunopathol 28:83-96, 2006.

58. Liu K, Mohan C: What do mouse models teach us about human SLE? Clin Immunol 119:123-130, 2006.

59. Cohen PL: Apoptotic cell death and lupus. Springer Semin Immunopathol 28:145-152, 2006.

60. Pisitkun P, Deane JA, Difilippantonio MJ, et al: Autoreactive B cell responses to RNA-related antigens due to TLR7 gene duplication. Science 312:1669-1672, 2006.

61. Subramanian S, Tus K, Li QZ, et al: A Tlr7 translocation accelerates systemic autoimmunity in murine lupus. Proc Natl Acad Sci U S A 103:9970-9975, 2006.

62. Gaffney PM, Kearns GM, Shark KB, et al: A genome-wide search for susceptibility genes in human systemic lupus erythematosus sib-pair families. Proc Natl Acad Sci U S A 95:14875-14879, 1998.

63. Moser KL, Neas BR, Salmon JE, et al: Genome scan of human systemic lupus erythematosus: Evidence for linkage on chromosome 1q in African-American pedigrees. Proc Natl Acad Sci U S A 95: 14869-14874, 1998.

64. Shai R, Quismorio FP Jr, Li L, et al: Genome-wide screen for systemic lupus erythematosus susceptibility genes in multiplex families. Hum Mol Genet 8:639-644, 1999.

65. Tsao BP, Cantor RM, Kalunian KC, et al: Evidence for linkage of a candidate chromosome 1 region to human systemic lupus erythematosus. J Clin Invest 99:725-731, 1997.

66. Tsao BP, Cantor RM, Grossman JM, et al: PARP alleles within the linked chromosomal region are associated with systemic lupus erythematosus. J Clin Invest 103:1135-1140, 1999.

67. Bell DA, Rigby R, Stiller CR, et al: HLA antigens in systemic lupus erythematosus: Relationship to disease severity, age at onset, and sex. J Rheumatol 11:475-479, 1984.

68. Gibofsky A, Winchester RJ, Patarroyo M, et al: Disease associations of the Ia-like human alloantigens: Contrasting patterns in rheumatoid arthritis and systemic lupus erythematosus. J Exp Med 148: 1728-1732, 1978.

69. Schur PH, Marcus-Bagley D, Awdeh Z, et al: The effect of ethnicity on major histocompatibility complex complement allotypes and extended haplotypes in patients with systemic lupus erythematosus. Arthritis Rheum 33:985-992, 1990.

70. So AK, Fielder AH, Warner CA, et al: DNA polymorphism of major histocompatibility complex class II and class III genes in systemic lupus erythematosus. Tissue Antigens 35:144-147, 1990.

71. Stastny P: HLA-D and Ia antigens in rheumatoid arthritis and systemic lupus erythematosus. Arthritis Rheum 21(5 suppl):S139-S143, 1978.

72. Carroll MC, Palsdottir A, Belt KT, et al: Deletion of complement C4 and steroid 21-hydroxylase genes in the HLA class III region. EMBO J 4:2547-2552, 1985.

73. Christiansen FT, Zhang WJ, Griffiths M, et al: Major histocompatibility complex (MHC) complement deficiency, ancestral haplotypes and systemic lupus erythematosus (SLE): C4 deficiency explains some but not all of the influence of the MHC. J Rheumatol 18:1350-1358, 1991.

74. De JD, Martin-Villa JM, Gomez-Reino JJ, et al: Differential contribution of C4 and HLA-DQ genes to systemic lupus erythematosus susceptibility. Hum Genet 91:579-584, 1993.

75. Dunckley H, Gatenby PA, Hawkins B, et al: Deficiency of C4A is a genetic determinant of systemic lupus erythematosus in three ethnic groups. J Immunogenet 14(4-5):209-218, 1987.

76. Fielder AH, Walport MJ, Batchelor JR, et al: Family study of the major histocompatibility complex in patients with systemic lupus erythematosus: Importance of null alleles of C4A and C4B in determining disease susceptibility. BMJ (Clin Res Ed) 286:425-428, 1983.

77. Hawkins BR, Wong KL, Wong RW, et al: Strong association between the major histocompatibility complex and systemic lupus erythematosus in southern Chinese. J Rheumatol 14:1128-1131, 1987.

78. Howard PF, Hochberg MC, Bias WB, et al: Relationship between C4 null genes, HLA-D region antigens, and genetic susceptibility to systemic lupus erythematosus in Caucasian and black Americans. Am J Med 81:187-193, 1986.

79. Kachru RB, Sequeira W, Mittal KK, et al: A significant increase of HLA-DR3 and DR2 in systemic lupus erythematosus among blacks. J Rheumatol 11:471-474, 1984.

80. Kemp ME, Atkinson JP, Skanes VM, et al: Deletion of C4A genes in patients with systemic lupus erythematosus. Arthritis Rheum 30:1015-1022, 1987.

81. Sturfelt G, Truedsson L, Johansen P, et al: Homozygous C4A deficiency in systemic lupus erythematosus: Analysis of patients from a defined population. Clin Genet 38:427-433, 1990.

82. Tokunaga K, Omoto K, Akaza T, et al: Haplotype study on C4 polymorphism in Japanese: Associations with MHC alleles, complotypes, and HLA-complement haplotypes. Immunogenetics 22:359-365, 1985.

83. Wilson WA, Perez MC, Armatis PE: Partial C4A deficiency is associated with susceptibility to systemic lupus erythematosus in black Americans. Arthritis Rheum 31:1171-1175, 1988.

84. Gladman DD, Terasaki PI, Park MS, et al: Increased frequency of HLA-DRW2 in SLE. Lancet 2:902, 1979.

85. Reveille JD, Schrohenloher RE, Acton RT, et al: DNA analysis of HLA-DR and DQ genes in American blacks with systemic lupus erythematosus. Arthritis Rheum 32:1243-1251, 1989.

86. Yang Y, Chung EK, Zhou B, et al: The intricate role of complement component C4 in human systemic lupus erythematosus. Curr Dir Autoimmun 7:98-132, 2004.

87. Agnello V: Lupus diseases associated with hereditary and acquired deficiencies of complement. Springer Semin Immunopathol 9(2-3): 161-178, 1986.

88. Bowness P, Davies KA, Norsworthy PJ, et al: Hereditary C1q deficiency and systemic lupus erythematosus. QJM 87:455-464, 1994.

89. Walport MJ, Davies KA, Morley BJ, et al: Complement deficiency and autoimmunity. Ann N Y Acad Sci 815:267-281, 1997.

90. Atkinson JP, Schifferli JA: Complement system and systemic lupus erythematosus. In Kammer GM, Tsokos GC (eds): Lupus: Molecular and Cellular Pathogenesis. Totowa, NJ, Humana Press, 1999.

91. Graham RR, Ortmann WA, Langefeld CD, et al: Visualizing human leukocyte antigen class II risk haplotypes in human systemic lupus erythematosus. Am J Hum Genet 71:543-553, 2002.

92. Erlich HA, Nepom GT, Tyan DB: Autoimmunity: Genetics and immunological mechanisms. In Rimoin DL, Connor JM, Pyeritz RE, et al (eds): Emery and Rimoin's Principles and Practice of Medical Genetics, 5th ed. London, Harcourt Publisher Ltd, 2006.

93. Hochberg MC, Boyd RE, Ahearn JM, et al: Systemic lupus erythematosus: A review of clinico-laboratory features and immunogenetic markers in 150 patients with emphasis on demographic subsets. Medicine (Balt) 64:285-295, 1985.

94. Wilson AG, de Vries N, Pociot F, et al: An allelic polymorphism within the human tumor necrosis factor alpha promoter region is strongly associated with HLA A1, B8, and DR3 alleles. J Exp Med 177:557-560, 1993.
95. Wilson AG, Symons JA, McDowell TL, et al: Effects of a polymorphism in the human tumor necrosis factor alpha promoter on transcriptional activation. Proc Natl Acad Sci U S A 94:3195-3199, 1997.
96. Lu LY, Ding WZ, Fici D, et al: Molecular analysis of major histocompatibility complex allelic associations with systemic lupus erythematosus in Taiwan. Arthritis Rheum 40:1138-1145, 1997.
97. Rood MJ, van Krugten MV, Zanelli E, et al: TNF-308A and HLA-DR3 alleles contribute independently to susceptibility to systemic lupus erythematosus. Arthritis Rheum 43:129-134, 2000.
98. Rudwaleit M, Tikly M, Khamashta M, et al: Interethnic differences in the association of tumor necrosis factor promoter polymorphisms with systemic lupus erythematosus. J Rheumatol 23:1725-1728, 1996.
99. Sullivan KE, Wooten C, Schmeckpeper BJ, et al: A promoter polymorphism of tumor necrosis factor alpha associated with systemic lupus erythematosus in African-Americans. Arthritis Rheum 40:2207-2211, 1997.
100. Wilson AG, Gordon C, di Giovine FS, et al: A genetic association between systemic lupus erythematosus and tumor necrosis factor alpha. Eur J Immunol 24:191-195, 1994.
101. Bidwell J, Keen L, Gallagher G, et al: Cytokine gene polymorphism in human disease: On-line databases, supplement 1. Genes Immun 2:61-70, 2001.
102. Ramos PS, Kelly JA, Gray-McGuire C, et al: Familial aggregation and linkage analysis of autoantibody traits in pedigrees multiplex for systemic lupus erythematosus. Genes Immun 7:417-432, 2006.
103. Martin DA, Elkon KB: Autoantibodies make a U-turn: The toll hypothesis for autoantibody specificity. J Exp Med 202:1465-1469, 2005.
104. Christensen SR, Shupe J, Nickerson K, et al: Toll-like receptor 7 and TLR9 dictate autoantibody specificity and have opposing inflammatory and regulatory roles in a murine model of lupus. Immunity 25:417-428, 2006.
105. Vollmer J, Tluk S, Schmitz C, et al: Immune stimulation mediated by autoantigen binding sites within small nuclear RNAs involves Toll-like receptors 7 and 8. J Exp Med 202:1575-1585, 2005.
106. Hur JW, Shin HD, Park BL, et al: Association study of Toll-like receptor 9 gene polymorphism in Korean patients with systemic lupus erythematosus. Tissue Antigens 65:266-270, 2005.
107. De Jager PL, Richardson A, Vyse TJ, et al: Genetic variation in toll-like receptor 9 and susceptibility to systemic lupus erythematosus. Arthritis Rheum 54:1279-1282, 2006.
108. Hawn TR, Wu H, Grossman JM, et al: A stop codon polymorphism of Toll-like receptor 5 is associated with resistance to systemic lupus erythematosus. Proc Natl Acad Sci U S A 102:10593-10597, 2005.
109. Fronek Z, Timmerman LA, Alper CA, et al: Major histocompatibility complex genes and susceptibility to systemic lupus erythematosus. Arthritis Rheum 33:1542-1553, 1990.
110. Hoffman RW, Rettenmaier LJ, Takeda Y, et al: Human autoantibodies against the 70-kd polypeptide of U1 small nuclear RNP are associated with HLA-DR4 among connective tissue disease patients. Arthritis Rheum 33:666-673, 1990.
111. Kaneoka H, Hsu KC, Takeda Y, et al: Molecular genetic analysis of HLA-DR and HLA-DQ genes among anti-U1-70-kd autoantibody positive connective tissue disease patients. Arthritis Rheum 35:83-94, 1992.
112. Arnett FC, Olsen ML, Anderson KL, et al: Molecular analysis of major histocompatibility complex alleles associated with the lupus anticoagulant. J Clin Invest 87:1490-1495, 1991.
113. Hamilton RG, Harley JB, Bias WB, et al: Two Ro (SS-A) autoantibody responses in systemic lupus erythematosus: Correlation of HLA-DR/DQ specificities with quantitative expression of Ro (SS-A) autoantibody. Arthritis Rheum 31:496-505, 1988.
114. Reveille JD, Macleod MJ, Whittington K, et al: Specific amino acid residues in the second hypervariable region of HLA-DQA1 and DQB1 chain genes promote the Ro (SS-A)/La (SS-B) autoantibody responses. J Immunol 146:3871-3876, 1991.
115. Pickering MC, Botto M, Taylor PR, et al: Systemic lupus erythematosus, complement deficiency, and apoptosis. Adv Immunol 76:227-324, 2000.
116. Slingsby JH, Norsworthy P, Pearce G, et al: Homozgous hereditary C1q deficiency and systemic lupus erythematosus: A new family and the molecular basis of C1q deficiency in three families. Arthritis Rheum 39:663-670, 1995.
117. Botto M, Dell'Agnola C, Bygrave AE, et al: Homozygous C1q deficiency causes glomerulonephritis associated with multiple apoptotic bodies. Nat Genet 19:56-59, 1998.
118. Davies EJ, Snowden N, Hillarby MC, et al: Mannose-binding protein gene polymorphism in systemic lupus erythematosus. Arthritis Rheum 38:110-114, 1995.
119. Ip WK, Chan SY, Lau CS, et al: Association of systemic lupus erythematosus with promoter polymorphisms of the mannose-binding lectin gene. Arthritis Rheum 41:1663-1668, 1998.
120. Lee YH, Witte T, Momot T, et al: The mannose-binding lectin gene polymorphisms and systemic lupus erythematosus: Two case-control studies and a meta-analysis. Arthritis Rheum 52:3966-3974, 2005.
121. Sullivan KE, Wooten C, Goldman D, et al: Mannose-binding protein genetic polymorphisms in black patients with systemic lupus erythematosus. Arthritis Rheum 39:2046-2051, 1996.
122. Russell AI, Cunninghame Graham DS, Shepherd C, et al: Polymorphism at the C-reactive protein locus influences gene expression and predisposes to systemic lupus erythematosus. Hum Mol Genet 13:137-147, 2004.
123. Szalai AJ, Alarcon GS, Calvo-Alen J, et al: Systemic lupus erythematosus in a multiethnic US Cohort (LUMINA), XXX: Association between C-reactive protein (CRP) gene polymorphisms and vascular events. Rheumatology (Oxf) 44:864-868, 2005.
124. Rodriguez W, Mold C, Kataranovski M, et al: Reversal of ongoing proteinuria in autoimmune mice by treatment with C-reactive protein. Arthritis Rheum 52:642-650, 2005.
125. Salmon JE, Pricop L: Human receptors for immunoglobulin G: Key elements in the pathogenesis of rheumatic disease. Arthritis Rheum 44:739-750, 2001.
126. Karassa FB, Trikalinos TA, Ioannidis JP: Role of the Fcgamma receptor IIa polymorphism in susceptibility to systemic lupus erythematosus and lupus nephritis: A meta-analysis. Arthritis Rheum 46:1563-1571, 2002.
127. Karassa FB, Trikalinos TA, Ioannidis JP: The Fc gamma RIIIA-F158 allele is a risk factor for the development of lupus nephritis: a meta-analysis. Kidney Int 63:1475-1482, 2003.
128. Alarcon GS, McGwin G, Petri M, et al: Time to renal disease and end-stage renal disease in PROFILE: A multiethnic lupus cohort. PLoS Med 3:e396, 2006.
129. Magnusson V, Johanneson B, Lima G, et al: Both risk alleles for FcgammaRIIA and FcgammaRIIIA are susceptibility factors for SLE: A unifying hypothesis. Genes Immun 5:130-137, 2004.
130. Morgan AW, Barrett JH, Griffiths B, et al: Analysis of Fcgamma receptor haplotypes in rheumatoid arthritis: FCGR3A remains a major susceptibility gene at this locus, with an additional contribution from FCGR3B. Arthritis Res Ther 8:R5, 2005.
131. Kyogoku C, Tsuchiya N, Matsuta K, et al: Studies on the association of Fc gamma receptor IIA, IIB, IIIA and IIIB polymorphisms with rheumatoid arthritis in the Japanese: Evidence for a genetic interaction between HLA-DRB1 and FCGR3A. Genes Immun 3:488-493, 2002.
132. Aitman TJ, Dong R, Vyse TJ, et al: Copy number polymorphism in Fcgr3 predisposes to glomerulonephritis in rats and humans. Nature 439:851-855, 2006.
133. Kochi Y, Yamada R, Suzuki A, et al: A functional variant in FCRL3, encoding Fc receptor-like 3, is associated with rheumatoid arthritis and several autoimmunities. Nat Genet 37:478-485, 2005.
134. Sanchez E, Callejas JL, Sabio JM, et al: Polymorphisms of the FCRL3 gene in a Spanish population of systemic lupus erythematosus patients. Rheumatology (Oxf) 45:1044-1046, 2006.
135. Daeron M: Fc receptor biology. Annu Rev Immunol 15:203-234, 1997.
136. Tsuchiya N, Honda Z, Tokunaga K: Role of B cell inhibitory receptor polymorphisms in systemic lupus erythematosus: A negative times a negative makes a positive. J Hum Genet 51:741-750, 2006.
137. Beebe AM, Cua DJ, de Waal MR: The role of interleukin-10 in autoimmune disease: Systemic lupus erythematosus (SLE) and multiple sclerosis (MS). Cytokine Growth Factor Rev 13(4-5):403-412, 2002.
138. D'Alfonso S, Rampi M, Bocchio D, et al: Systemic lupus erythematosus candidate genes in the Italian population: Evidence for a significant association with interleukin-10. Arthritis Rheum 43:120-128, 2000.

139. Eskdale J, Wordsworth P, Bowman S, et al: Association between polymorphisms at the human IL-10 locus and systemic lupus erythematosus. Tissue Antigens 49:635-639, 1997.

140. Mehrian R, Quismorio FP Jr, Strassmann G, et al: Synergistic effect between IL-10 and bcl-2 genotypes in determining susceptibility to systemic lupus erythematosus. Arthritis Rheum 41:596-602, 1998.

141. Alarcon-Riquelme ME, Lindqvist AK, Jonasson I, et al: Genetic analysis of the contribution of IL-10 to systemic lupus erythematosus. J Rheumatol 26:2148-2152, 1999.

142. Johansson C, Castillejo-Lopez C, Johanneson B, et al: Association analysis with microsatellite and SNP markers does not support the involvement of BCL-2 in systemic lupus erythematosus in Mexican and Swedish patients and their families. Genes Immun 1:380-385, 2000.

143. Ou TT, Tsai WC, Chen CJ, et al: Genetic analysis of interleukin-10 promoter region in patients with systemic lupus erythematosus in Taiwan. Kaohsiung J Med Sci 14:599-606, 1998.

144. Rood MJ, Keijsers V, Van der Linden MW, et al: Neuropsychiatric systemic lupus erythematosus is associated with imbalance in interleukin 10 promoter haplotypes. Ann Rheum Dis 58:85-89, 1999.

145. Crawley E, Woo P, Isenberg DA: Single nucleotide polymorphic haplotypes of the interleukin-10 5′ flanking region are not associated with renal disease or serology in Caucasian patients with systemic lupus erythematosus. Arthritis Rheum 42:2017-2018, 1999.

146. Lazarus M, Hajeer AH, Turner D, et al: Genetic variation in the interleukin-10 gene promoter and systemic lupus erythematosus. J Rheumatol 24:2314-2317, 1997.

147. Mok CC, Lanchbury JS, Chan DW, et al: Interleukin-10 promoter polymorphisms in Southern Chinese patients with systemic lupus erythematosus. Arthritis Rheum 41:1090-1095, 1998.

148. van der Linden MW, Westendorp RG, Sturk A, et al: High interleukin-10 production in first-degree relatives of patients with generalized but not cutaneous lupus erythematosus. J Invest Med 48:327-334, 2000.

149. Gibson AW, Edberg JC, Wu J, et al: Novel single nucleotide polymorphisms in the distal IL-10 promoter affect IL-10 production and enhance the risk of systemic lupus erythematosus. J Immunol 166:3915-3922, 2001.

150. Ueda H, Howson JM, Esposito L, et al: Association of the T-cell regulatory gene CTLA4 with susceptibility to autoimmune disease. Nature 423:506-511, 2003.

151. Krishnan S, Chowdhury B, Tsokos GC: Autoimmunity in systemic lupus erythematosus: Integrating genes and biology. Semin Immunol 18:230-243, 2006.

152. Nishimura H, Honjo T: PD-1: An inhibitory immunoreceptor involved in peripheral tolerance. Trends Immunol 22:265-268, 2001.

153. Prokunina L, Castillejo-Lopez C, Oberg F, et al: A regulatory polymorphism in PDCD1 is associated with susceptibility to systemic lupus erythematosus in humans. Nat Genet 32:666-669, 2002.

154. Nielsen C, Hansen D, Husby S, et al: Association of a putative regulatory polymorphism in the PD-1 gene with susceptibility to type 1 diabetes. Tissue Antigens 62:492-497, 2003.

155. Prokunina L, Padyukov L, Bennet A, et al: Association of the PD-1.3A allele of the PDCD1 gene in patients with rheumatoid arthritis negative for rheumatoid factor and the shared epitope. Arthritis Rheum 50:1770-1773, 2004.

156. Johansson M, Arlestig L, Moller B, et al: Association of a PDCD1 polymorphism with renal manifestations in systemic lupus erythematosus. Arthritis Rheum 52:1665-1669, 2005.

157. Vang T, Congia M, Macis MD, et al: Autoimmune-associated lymphoid tyrosine phosphatase is a gain-of-function variant. Nat Genet 37:1317-1319, 2005.

158. Bottini N, Musumeci L, Alonso A, et al: A functional variant of lymphoid tyrosine phosphatase is associated with type I diabetes. Nat Genet 36:337-338, 2004.

159. Bottini N, Vang T, Cucca F, et al: Role of PTPN22 in type 1 diabetes and other autoimmune diseases. Semin Immunol 18:207-213, 2006.

160. Criswell LA, Pfeiffer KA, Lum RF, et al: Analysis of families in the Multiple Autoimmune Disease Genetics Consortium (MADGC) collection: The PTPN22 620W allele associates with multiple autoimmune phenotypes. Am J Hum Genet 76:561-571, 2005.

161. Kyogoku C, Langefeld CD, Ortmann WA, et al: Genetic association of the R620W polymorphism of protein tyrosine phosphatase PTPN22 with human SLE. Am J Hum Genet 75:504-507, 2004.

162. Wu H, Cantor RM, Graham DS, et al: Association analysis of the R620W polymorphism of protein tyrosine phosphatase PTPN22 in systemic lupus erythematosus families: Increased t allele frequency in systemic lupus erythematosus patients with autoimmune thyroid disease. Arthritis Rheum 52:2396-2402, 2005.

163. Kaufman KM, Kelly JA, Herring BJ, et al: Evaluation of the genetic association of the PTPN22 R620W polymorphism in familial and sporadic systemic lupus erythematosus. Arthritis Rheum 54:2533-2540, 2006.

164. **Bancereau J, Pascual V: Type I interferon in systemic lupus erythematosus and other autoimmune diseases. Immunity 25:383-392, 2006.**

165. Sigurdsson S, Nordmark G, Goring HH, et al: Polymorphisms in the tyrosine kinase 2 and interferon regulatory factor 5 genes are associated with systemic lupus erythematosus. Am J Hum Genet 76:528-537, 2005.

166. Marijanovic Z, Ragimbeau J, Kumar KG, et al: TYK2 activity promotes ligand-induced IFNAR1 proteolysis. Biochem J 397:31-38, 2006.

167. Takaoka A, Yanai H, Kondo S, et al: Integral role of IRF-5 in the gene induction programme activated by Toll-like receptors. Nature 434:243-249, 2005.

168. Graham RR, Kozyrev SV, Baechler EC, et al: A common haplotype of interferon regulatory factor 5 (IRF5) regulates splicing and expression and is associated with increased risk of systemic lupus erythematosus. Nat Genet 38:550-555, 2006.

169. Johanneson B, Lima G, Von Salome J, et al: A major susceptibility locus for systemic lupus erythematosus maps to chromosome 1q31. Am J Hum Genet 71:1060-1071, 2002.

170. Graham RR, Langefeld CD, Gaffney PM, et al: Genetic linkage and transmission disequilibrium of marker haplotypes at chromosome 1q41 in human systemic lupus erythematosus. Arthritis Res 3:299-305, 2001.

171. Lindqvist AK, Steinsson K, Johanneson B, et al: A susceptibility locus for human systemic lupus erythematosus (hSLE1) on chromosome 2q. J Autoimmun 14:169-178, 2000.

172. Gray-McGuire C, Moser KL, Gaffney PM, et al: Genome scan of human systemic lupus erythematosus by regression modeling: Evidence of linkage and epistasis at 4p16-15.2. Am J Hum Genet 67:1460-1469, 2000.

173. Gaffney PM, Ortmann WA, Selby SA, et al: Genome screening in human systemic lupus erythematosus: Results from a second Minnesota cohort and combined analyses of 187 sib-pair families. Am J Hum Genet 66:547-556, 2000.

174. Nath SK, Quintero-Del-Rio AI, Kilpatrick J, et al: Linkage at 12q24 with systemic lupus erythematosus (SLE) is established and confirmed in Hispanic and European American families. Am J Hum Genet 74:73-82, 2004.

175. Lander E, Kruglyak L: Genetic dissection of complex traits: Guidelines for interpreting and reporting linkage results. Nat Genet 11:241-247, 1995.

176. Tsao BP, Cantor RM, Grossman JM, et al: Linkage and interaction of loci on 1q23 and 16q12 may contribute to susceptibility to systemic lupus erythematosus. Arthritis Rheum 46:2928-2936, 2002.

177. Johansson CM, Zunec R, Garcia MA, et al: Chromosome 17p12-q11 harbors susceptibility loci for systemic lupus erythematosus. Hum Genet 115:230-238, 2004.

178. Moser KL, Gray-McGuire C, Kelly J, et al: Confirmation of genetic linkage between human systemic lupus erythematosus and chromosome 1q41. Arthritis Rheum 42:1902-1907, 1999.

179. Magnusson V, Lindqvist AK, Castillejo-Lopez C, et al: Fine mapping of the SLEB2 locus involved in susceptibility to systemic lupus erythematosus. Genomics 70:307-314, 2000.

180. Nishimura H, Honjo T: PD-1: An inhibitory immunoreceptor involved in peripheral tolerance. Trends Immunol 22:265-268, 2001.

181. Nishimura H, Nose M, Hiai H, et al: Development of lupus-like autoimmune diseases by disruption of the PD-1 gene encoding an ITIM motif-carrying immunoreceptor. Immunity 11:141-151, 1999.

182. Boorboor P, Drescher BE, Hartung K, et al: Poly(ADP-ribose) polymerase polymorphisms are not a genetic risk factor for systemic lupus erythematosus in German Caucasians. J Rheumatol 27:2061, 2000.

183. Criswell LA, Moser KL, Gaffney PM, et al: PARP alleles and SLE: Failure to confirm association with disease susceptibility. J Clin Invest 105:1501-1502, 2000.

184. Delrieu O, Michel M, Frances C, et al: Poly(ADP-ribose) polymerase alleles in French Caucasians are associated neither with lupus nor with primary antiphospholipid syndrome. GRAID Research Group. Group for Research on Auto-Immune Disorders. Arthritis Rheum 42:2194-2197, 1999.

185. Edberg JC, Langefeld CD, Wu J, et al: Genetic linkage and association of Fcgamma receptor IIIA (CD16A) on chromosome 1q23 with human systemic lupus erythematosus. Arthritis Rheum 46:2132-2140, 2002.

186. Hugot JP, Chamaillard M, Zouali H, et al: Association of NOD2 leucine-rich repeat variants with susceptibility to Crohn's disease. Nature 411:599-603, 2001.

187. Lesage S, Zouali H, Cezard JP, et al: CARD15/NOD2 mutational analysis and genotype-phenotype correlation in 612 patients with inflammatory bowel disease. Am J Hum Genet 70:845-857, 2002.

188. Ogura Y, Bonen DK, Inohara N, et al: A frameshift mutation in NOD2 associated with susceptibility to Crohn's disease. Nature 411:603-606, 2001.

189. Ferreiros-Vidal I, Garcia-Meijide J, Carreira P, et al: The three most common CARD15 mutations associated with Crohn's disease and the chromosome 16 susceptibility locus for systemic lupus erythematosus. Rheumatology (Oxf) 42:570-574, 2003.

190. De Jager PL, Graham R, Farwell L, et al: The role of inflammatory bowel disease susceptibility loci in multiple sclerosis and systemic lupus erythematosus. Genes Immun 7:327-334, 2006.

191. Nath SK, Kelly JA, Namjou B, et al: Evidence for a susceptibility gene, SLEV1, on chromosome 17p13 in families with vitiligo-related systemic lupus erythematosus. Am J Hum Genet 69:1401-1406, 2001.

192. Spritz RA, Gowan K, Bennett DC, et al: Novel vitiligo susceptibility loci on chromosomes 7 (AIS2) and 8 (AIS3), confirmation of SLEV1 on chromosome 17, and their roles in an autoimmune diathesis. Am J Hum Genet 74:188-191, 2004.

193. Kelly JA, Thompson K, Kilpatrick J, et al: Evidence for a susceptibility gene (SLEH1) on chromosome 11q14 for systemic lupus erythematosus (SLE) families with hemolytic anemia. Proc Natl Acad Sci U S A 99:11766-11771, 2002.

194. Sawalha AH, Namjou B, Nath SK, et al: Genetic linkage of systemic lupus erythematosus with chromosome 11q14 (SLEH1) in African-American families stratified by a nucleolar antinuclear antibody pattern. Genes Immun 3(Suppl 1):S31-S34, 2002.

195. Nath SK, Kelly JA, Reid J, et al: SLEB3 in systemic lupus erythematosus (SLE) is strongly related to SLE families ascertained through neuropsychiatric manifestations. Hum Genet 111:54-58, 2002.

196. Namjou B, Nath SK, Kilpatrick J, et al: Genome scan stratified by the presence of anti-double-stranded DNA (dsDNA) autoantibody in pedigrees multiplex for systemic lupus erythematosus (SLE) establishes linkages at 19p13.2 (SLED1) and 18q21.1 (SLED2). Genes Immun 3(Suppl 1):S35-S41, 2002.

197. Quintero-Del-Rio AI, Kelly JA, Kilpatrick J, et al: The genetics of systemic lupus erythematosus stratified by renal disease: Linkage at 10q22.3 (SLEN1), 2q34-35 (SLEN2), and 11p15.6 (SLEN3). Genes Immun 3(Suppl 1):S57-S62, 2002.

198. Quintero-Del-Rio AI, Kelly JA, Garriott CP, et al: SLEN2 (2q34-35) and SLEN1 (10q22.3) replication in systemic lupus erythematosus stratified by nephritis. Am J Hum Genet 75:346-348, 2004.

199. Andrews BS, Eisenberg RA, Theofilopoulos AN, et al: Spontaneous murine lupus-like syndromes: Clinical and immunopathological manifestations in several strains. J Exp Med 148:1198-1215, 1978.

200. Hahn BH, Singh RR: Animal models of systemic lupus erythematosus. In Wallace DJ, Hahn BH (eds): Dubois' Lupus Erythematosus, 7th ed. Philadelphia, Lippincott Williams & Wilkins, 2007, pp 299-355.

201. Morel L, Tian XH, Croker BP, et al: Epistatic modifiers of autoimmunity in a murine model of lupus nephritis. Immunity 11:131-139, 1999.

202. Vyse TJ, Rozzo SJ, Drake CG, et al: Contributions of Ea(z) and Eb(z) MHC genes to lupus susceptibility in New Zealand mice. J Immunol 160:2757-2766, 1998.

203. Vyse TJ, Rozzo SJ, Drake CG, et al: Control of multiple autoantibodies linked with a lupus nephritis susceptibility locus in New Zealand black mice. J Immunol 158:5566-5574, 1997.

204. Rozzo SJ, Vyse TJ, David CS, et al: Analysis of MHC class II genes in the susceptibility to lupus in New Zealand mice. J Immunol 162:2623-2630, 1999.

205. Rozzo SJ, Allard JD, Choubey D, et al: Evidence for an interferon-inducible gene, Ifi202, in the susceptibility to systemic lupus. Immunity 15:435-443, 2001.

206. Morel L, Yu Y, Blenman KR, et al: Production of congenic mouse strains carrying genomic intervals containing SLE-susceptibility genes derived from the SLE-prone NZM2410 strain. Mamm Genome 7:335-339, 1996.

207. Sobel ES, Satoh M, Chen Y, et al: The major murine systemic lupus erythematosus susceptibility locus Sle1 results in abnormal functions of both B and T cells. J Immunol 169:2694-2700, 2002.

208. Sobel ES, Mohan C, Morel L, et al: Genetic dissection of SLE pathogenesis: Adoptive transfer of Sle1 mediates the loss of tolerance by bone marrow-derived B cells. J Immunol 162:2415-2421, 1999.

209. Mohan C, Alas E, Morel L, et al: Genetic dissection of SLE pathogenesis: Sle1 on murine chromosome 1 leads to a selective loss of tolerance to H2A/H2B/DNA subnucleosomes. J Clin Invest 101:1362-1372, 1998.

210. Mohan C, Morel L, Wakeland EK: Genetic insights into murine lupus. In Kammer GM, Tsokos GC (eds): Lupus: Molecular and Cellular Pathogenesis. Totowa, NJ, Humana Press, 1999.

211. Morel L, Blenman KR, Croker BP, et al: The major murine systemic lupus erythematosus susceptibility locus, Sle1, is a cluster of functionally related genes. Proc Natl Acad Sci U S A 98:1787-1792, 2001.

212. Kumar KR, Li L, Yan M, et al: Regulation of B cell tolerance by the lupus susceptibility gene Ly108. Science 312:1665-1669, 2006.

213. Chen Y, Perry D, Boackle SA, et al: Several genes contribute to the production of autoreactive B and T cells in the murine lupus susceptibility locus Sle1c. J Immunol 175:1080-1089, 2005.

214. Boackle SA, Holers VM, Chen X, et al: Cr2, a candidate gene in the murine Sle1c lupus susceptibility locus, encodes a dysfunctional protein. Immunity 15:775-785, 2001.

215. Subramanian S, Yim YS, Liu K, et al: Epistatic suppression of systemic lupus erythematosus: Fine mapping of Sles1 to less than 1 mb. J Immunol 175:1062-1072, 2005.

216. Cooper GS, Dooley MA, Treadwell EL, et al: Hormonal, environmental, and infectious risk factors for developing systemic lupus erythematosus. Arthritis Rheum 41:1714-1724, 1998.

217. Wysenbeek AJ, Block DA, Fries JF: Prevalence and expression of photosensitivity in systemic lupus erythematosus. Ann Rheum Dis 48:461-463, 1989.

218. McGrath H Jr: Ultraviolet-A1 irradiation decreases clinical disease activity and autoantibodies in patients with systemic lupus erythematosus. Clin Exp Rheumatol 12:129-135, 1994.

219. Natali PG, Tan EM: Experimental skin lesions in mice resembling systemic lupus erythematosus. Arthritis Rheum 16:579-589, 1973.

220. Casciola-Rosen LA, Anhalt G, Rosen A: Autoantigens targeted in systemic lupus erythematosus are clustered in two populations of surface structures on apoptotic keratinocytes. J Exp Med 179:1317-1330, 1994.

221. Casiano CA, Ochs RL, Tan EM: Distinct cleavage products of nuclear proteins in apoptosis and necrosis revealed by autoantibody probes. Cell Death Differ 5:183-190, 1998.

222. Distler JH, Huber LC, Gay S, et al: Microparticles as mediators of cellular cross-talk in inflammatory disease. Autoimmunity 39:683-690, 2006.

223. James JA, Kaufman KM, Farris AD, et al: An increased prevalence of Epstein-Barr virus infection in young patients suggests a possible etiology for systemic lupus erythematosus. J Clin Invest 100:3019-3026, 1997.

224. Gross AJ, Hochberg D, Rand WM, et al: EBV and systemic lupus erythematosus: A new perspective. J Immunol 174:6599-6607, 2005.

225. Wang H, Nicholas MW, Conway KL, et al: EBV latent membrane protein 2A induces autoreactive B cell activation and TLR hypersensitivity. J Immunol 177:2793-2802, 2006.

226. Kang I, Quan T, Nolasco H, et al: Defective control of latent Epstein-Barr virus infection in systemic lupus erythematosus. J Immunol 172:1287-1294, 2004.

227. James JA, Neas BR, Moser KL, et al: Systemic lupus erythematosus in adults is associated with previous Epstein-Barr virus exposure. Arthritis Rheum 44:1122-1126, 2001.

228. McClain MT, Poole BD, Bruner BF, et al: An altered immune response to Epstein-Barr nuclear antigen 1 in pediatric systemic lupus erythematosus. Arthritis Rheum 54:360-368, 2006.

229. Poole BD, Scofield RH, Harley JB, et al: Epstein-Barr virus and molecular mimicry in systemic lupus erythematosus. Autoimmunity 39:63-70, 2006.

230. Parks CG, Cooper GS, Hudson LL, et al: Association of Epstein-Barr virus with systemic lupus erythematosus: Effect modification by race, age, and cytotoxic T lymphocyte-associated antigen 4 genotype. Arthritis Rheum 52:1148-1159, 2005.

231. Cavallo T, Granholm NA: Bacterial lipopolysaccharide transforms mesangial into proliferative lupus nephritis without interfering with processing of pathogenic immune complexes in NZB/W mice. Am J Pathol 137:971-978, 1990.

232. Talal N, Garry RF, Schur PH, et al: A conserved idiotype and antibodies to retroviral proteins in systemic lupus erythematosus. J Clin Invest 85:1866-1871, 1990.

233. Erausquin C, Merino R, Izui S, et al: Therapeutic effect of early thymic irradiation in (NZB x NZW)F1 mice, associated with a selective decrease in the levels of IgG3 and gp70-anti-gp70 immune complexes. Cell Immunol 161:207-212, 1995.

234. Sundsfjord A, Osei A, Rosenqvist H, et al: BK and JC viruses in patients with systemic lupus erythematosus: Prevalent and persistent BK viruria, sequence stability of the viral regulatory regions, and non-detectable viremia. J Infect Dis 180:1-9, 1999.

235. Lahita RG: Sex hormones and systemic lupus erythematosus. Rheum Dis Clin N Am 26:951-968, 2000.

236. Lu Q, Tresmer L, Wu A, et al: Women and lupus: The inactive X awakens. Arthritis Rheum 54:S775, 2006.

237. Ballestar E, Esteller M, Richardson BC: The epigenetic face of systemic lupus erythematosus. J Immunol 176:7143-7147, 2006.

238. Nelson JL: Microchimerism and autoimmune disease. N Engl J Med 338:1224-1225, 1998.

239. Lahita RG, Kunkel HG, Bradlow HL: Increased oxidation of testosterone in systemic lupus erythematosus. Arthritis Rheum 26:1517-1521, 1983.

240. Lahita RG, Bradlow L, Fishman J, et al: Estrogen metabolism in systemic lupus erythematosus: Patients and family members. Arthritis Rheum 25:843-846, 1982.

241. Sanchez-Guerrero J, Liang MH, Karlson EW, et al: Postmenopausal estrogen therapy and the risk for developing systemic lupus erythematosus. Ann Intern Med 122:430-433, 1995.

242. Sanchez-Guerrero J, Karlson EW, Liang MH, et al: Past use of oral contraceptives and the risk of developing systemic lupus erythematosus. Arthritis Rheum 40:804-808, 1997.

243. Cooper GS, Dooley MA, Treadwell EL, et al: Hormonal and reproductive risk factors for development of systemic lupus erythematosus: Results of a population-based, case-control study. Arthritis Rheum 46:1830-1839, 2002.

244. Buyon JP, Petri MA, Kim MY, et al: The effect of combined estrogen and progesterone hormone replacement therapy on disease activity in systemic lupus erythematosus: A randomized trial. Ann Intern Med 142(12 Pt 1):953-962, 2005.

245. Petri M, Kim MY, Kalunian KC, et al: Combined oral contraceptives in women with systemic lupus erythematosus. N Engl J Med 353:2550-2558, 2005.

246. Sanchez-Guerrero J, Uribe AG, Jimenez-Santana L, et al: A trial of contraceptive methods in women with systemic lupus erythematosus. N Engl J Med 353:2539-2549, 2005.

247. Walker SE, McMurray RW, Houri JM, et al: Effects of prolactin in stimulating disease activity in systemic lupus erythematosus. Ann N Y Acad Sci 840:762-772, 1998.

248. Venkatesh J, Peeva E, Xu X, et al: Cutting edge: Hormonal milieu, not antigenic specificity, determines the mature phenotype of autoreactive B cells. J Immunol 176:3311-3314, 2006.

249. Bynoe MS, Grimaldi CM, Diamond B: Estrogen up-regulates Bcl-2 and blocks tolerance induction of naive B cells. Proc Natl Acad Sci U S A 97:2703-2708, 2000.

250. Evans MJ, MacLaughlin S, Marvin RD, et al: Estrogen decreases in vitro apoptosis of peripheral blood mononuclear cells from women with normal menstrual cycles and decreases TNF-alpha production in SLE but not in normal cultures. Clin Immunol Immunopathol 82:258-262, 1997.

251. Rider V, Li X, Peterson G, et al: Differential expression of estrogen receptors in women with systemic lupus erythematosus. J Rheumatol 33:1093-1101, 2006.

252. Malinow MR, Bardana EJ Jr, Pirofsky B, et al: Systemic lupus erythematosus-like syndrome in monkeys fed alfalfa sprouts: Role of a nonprotein amino acid. Science 216:415-417, 1982.

253. Jolly CA, Muthukumar A, Avula CP, et al: Life span is prolonged in food-restricted autoimmune-prone (NZB x NZW)F(1) mice fed a diet enriched with (n-3) fatty acids. J Nutr 131:2753-2760, 2001.

254. Jolly CA, Muthukumar A, Reddy Avula CP, et al: Maintenance of NF-kappaB activation in T-lymphocytes and a naive T-cell population in autoimmune-prone (NZB/NZW)F(1) mice by feeding a food-restricted diet enriched with n-3 fatty acids. Cell Immunol 213:122-133, 2001.

255. Kelley VE, Ferretti A, Izui S, et al: A fish oil diet rich in eicosapentaenoic acid reduces cyclooxygenase metabolites, and suppresses lupus in MRL-lpr mice. J Immunol 134:1914-1919, 1985.

256. Walton AJ, Snaith ML, Locniskar M, et al: Dietary fish oil and the severity of symptoms in patients with systemic lupus erythematosus. Ann Rheum Dis 50:463-466, 1991.

257. Freni-Titulaer LW, Kelley DB, Grow AG, et al: Connective tissue disease in southeastern Georgia: A case-control study of etiologic factors. Am J Epidemiol 130:404-409, 1989.

258. Sanchez-Guerrero J, Karlson EW, Colditz GA, et al: Hair dye use and the risk of developing systemic lupus erythematosus. Arthritis Rheum 39:657-662, 1996.

259. Rubin RL: Drug-induced lupus. In Wallace DJ, Hahn BH (eds): Dubois' Lupus Erythematosus, 7th ed. Philadelphia, Lippincott Williams & Wilkins, 2007, pp 870-900.

260. Elkayam O, Yaron M, Caspi D: Minocycline-induced autoimmune syndromes: An overview. Semin Arthritis Rheum 28:392-397, 1999.

261. Sandborn WJ, Hanauer SB: Antitumor necrosis factor therapy for inflammatory bowel disease: A review of agents, pharmacology, clinical results, and safety. Inflamm Bowel Dis 5:119-133, 1999.

262. Schiff MH, Burmester GR, Kent JD, et al: Safety analyses of adalimumab (HUMIRA) in global clinical trials and US postmarketing surveillance of patients with rheumatoid arthritis. Ann Rheum Dis 65:889-894, 2006.

263. Gilkeson GS, Grudier JP, Karounos DG, et al: Induction of anti-double stranded DNA antibodies in normal mice by immunization with bacterial DNA. J Immunol 142:1482-1486, 1989.

264. Schwartz RS, Stollar BD: Origins of anti-DNA autoantibodies. J Clin Invest 75:321-327, 1985.

265. Neujahr DC, Reich CF, Pisetsky DS: Immunostimulatory properties of genomic DNA from different bacterial species. Immunobiology 200:106-119, 1999.

266. Datta SK, Kaliyaperumal A: Nucleosome-driven autoimmune response in lupus: Pathogenic T helper cell epitopes and costimulatory signals. Ann N Y Acad Sci 815:155-170, 1997.

267. Burlingame RW, Boey ML, Starkebaum G, et al: The central role of chromatin in autoimmune responses to histones and DNA in systemic lupus erythematosus. J Clin Invest 94:184-192, 1994.

268. Reichlin M: Cellular dysfunction induced by penetration of autoantibodies into living cells: Cellular damage and dysfunction mediated by antibodies to dsDNA and ribosomal P proteins. J Autoimmun 11:557-561, 1998.

269. McCluskey J, Farris AD, Keech CL, et al: Determinant spreading: Lessons from animal models and human disease. Immunol Rev 164:209-229, 1998.

270. Vaishnaw AK, McNally JD, Elkon KB: Apoptosis in the rheumatic diseases. Arthritis Rheum 40:1917-1927, 1997.

271. Lorenz HM, Grunke M, Hieronymus T, et al: In vitro apoptosis and expression of apoptosis-related molecules in lymphocytes from patients with systemic lupus erythematosus and other autoimmune diseases. Arthritis Rheum 40:306-317, 1997.

272. Georgescu L, Vakkalanka RK, Elkon KB, et al: Interleukin-10 promotes activation-induced cell death of SLE lymphocytes mediated by Fas ligand. J Clin Invest 100:2622-2633, 1997.

273. Korb LC, Ahearn JM: C1q binds directly and specifically to surface blebs of apoptotic human keratinocytes: Complement deficiency and systemic lupus erythematosus revisited. J Immunol 158:4525-4528, 1997.

274. Mitchell DA, Taylor PR, Cook HT, et al: Cutting edge: C1q protects against the development of glomerulonephritis independently of C3 activation. J Immunol 162:5676-5679, 1999.

275. Grammer AC, Lipsky PE: CD154-CD40 interactions mediate differentiation to plasma cells in healthy individuals and persons with systemic lupus erythematosus. Arthritis Rheum 46:1417-1429, 2002.

276. Grammer AC, Lipsky PE: B cell abnormalities in systemic lupus erythematosus. Arthritis Res Ther 5(Suppl 4):S22-S27, 2003.

277. Hoyer BF, Manz RA, Radbruch A, et al: Long-lived plasma cells and their contribution to autoimmunity. Ann N Y Acad Sci 1050: 124-133, 2005.
278. Tsokos GC, Wong HK, Enyedy EJ, et al: Immune cell signaling in lupus. Curr Opin Rheumatol 12:355-363, 2000.
279. Shakhov AN, Nedospasov SA: Expression profiling in knockout mice: Lymphotoxin versus tumor necrosis factor in the maintenance of splenic microarchitecture. Cytokine Growth Factor Rev 12: 107-119, 2001.
280. Ettinger R, Sims GP, Fairhurst AM, et al: IL-21 induces differentiation of human naive and memory B cells into antibody-secreting plasma cells. J Immunol 175:7867-7879, 2005.
281. Wellmann U, Werner A, Winkler TH: Altered selection processes of B lymphocytes in autoimmune NZB/W mice, despite intact central tolerance against DNA. Eur J Immunol 31:2800-2810, 2001.
282. Jacobson BA, Rothstein TL, Marshak-Rothstein A: Unique site of IgG2a and rheumatoid factor production in MRL/lpr mice. Immunol Rev 156:103-110, 1997.
283. Papadimitraki ED, Choulaki C, Koutala E, et al: Expansion of toll-like receptor 9-expressing B cells in active systemic lupus erythematosus: Implications for the induction and maintenance of the autoimmune process. Arthritis Rheum 54:3601-3611, 2006.
284. Garcia-Valladares I, Tisha-Fregoso Y, Richaud-Patin Y, et al: Diminished expression of complement regulatory proteins (CD55 and CD59) in lymphocytes from systemic lupus erythematosus patients with lymphopenia. Lupus 15:600-605, 2006.
285. Stohl W, Metyas S, Tan SM, et al: B lymphocyte stimulator overexpression in patients with systemic lupus erythematosus: Longitudinal observations. Arthritis Rheum 48:3475-3486, 2003.
286. Mackay M, Stanevsky A, Wang T, et al: Selective dysregulation of the FcgammaIIB receptor on memory B cells in SLE. J Exp Med 203:2157-2164, 2006.
287. Flores-Borja F, Kabouridis PS, Jury EC, et al: Altered lipid raft-associated proximal signaling and translocation of CD45 tyrosine phosphatase in B lymphocytes from patients with systemic lupus erythematosus. Arthritis Rheum 56:291-302, 2006.
288. **Kyttaris VC, Krishnan S, Tsokos GC: Systems biology in systemic lupus erythematosus: Integrating genes, biology and immune function. Autoimmunity 39:705-709, 2006.**
289. Pugh-Bernard AE, Cambier JC: B cell receptor signaling in human systemic lupus erythematosus. Curr Opin Rheumatol 18:451-455, 2006.
290. Liossis SN, Kovacs B, Dennis G, et al: B cells from patients with systemic lupus erythematosus display abnormal antigen receptor-mediated early signal transduction events. J Clin Invest 98:2549-2557, 1996.
291. Peng SL, Madaio MP, Hughes DP, et al: Murine lupus in the absence of alpha beta T cells. J Immunol 156:4041-4049, 1996.
292. Chan OT, Hannum LG, Haberman AM, et al: A novel mouse with B cells but lacking serum antibody reveals an antibody-independent role for B cells in murine lupus. J Exp Med 189:1639-1648, 1999.
293. Reininger L, Radaszkiewicz T, Kosco M, et al: Development of autoimmune disease in SCID mice populated with long-term "in vitro" proliferating (NZB x NZW)F1 pre-B cells. J Exp Med 176:1343-1353, 1992.
294. Strasser A, Whittingham S, Vaux DL, et al: Enforced BCL2 expression in B-lymphoid cells prolongs antibody responses and elicits autoimmune disease. Proc Natl Acad Sci U S A 88:8661-8665, 1991.
295. Vaishnaw AK, Toubi E, Ohsako S, et al: The spectrum of apoptotic defects and clinical manifestations, including systemic lupus erythematosus, in humans with CD95 (Fas/APO-1) mutations. Arthritis Rheum 42:1833-1842, 1999.
296. Nagafuchi H, Wakisaka S, Takeba Y, et al: Aberrant expression of Fas ligand on anti-DNA autoantibody secreting B lymphocytes in patients with systemic lupus erythematosus: "Immune privilege"-like state of the autoreactive B cells. Clin Exp Rheumatol 20:625-631, 2002.
297. Bouillet P, Metcalf D, Huang DC, et al: Proapoptotic Bcl-2 relative Bim required for certain apoptotic responses, leukocyte homeostasis, and to preclude autoimmunity. Science 286:1735-1738, 1999.
298. Miret C, Font J, Molina R, et al: Relationship of oncogenes (sFas, Bcl-2) and cytokines (IL-10, alfa-TNF) with the activity of systemic lupus erythematosus. Anticancer Res 21:3053-3059, 2001.
299. Rose LM, Latchman DS, Isenberg DA: Bcl-2 expression is unaltered in unfractioned peripheral blood mononuclear cells in patients with systemic lupus erythematosus. Br J Rheumatol 34:316-320, 1995.
300. Fathi NA, Hussein MR, Hassan HI, et al: Glomerular expression and elevated serum Bcl-2 and Fas proteins in lupus nephritis: Preliminary findings. Clin Exp Immunol 146:339-343, 2006.
301. Khare SD, Sarosi I, Xia XZ, et al: Severe B cell hyperplasia and autoimmune disease in TALL-1 transgenic mice. Proc Natl Acad Sci U S A 97:3370-3375, 2000.
302. Gross JA, Johnston J, Mudri S, et al: TACI and BCMA are receptors for a TNF homologue implicated in B-cell autoimmune disease. Nature 404:995-999, 2000.
303. Baker KP: BLyS—an essential survival factor for B cells: Basic biology, link to pathology and therapeutic target. Autoimmun Rev 3: 368-375, 2004.
304. Cheema GS, Roschke V, Hilbert DM, et al: Elevated serum B lymphocyte stimulator levels in patients with systemic immune-based rheumatic diseases. Arthritis Rheum 44:1313-1319, 2001.
305. Dziarski R: Autoimmunity: Polyclonal activation or antigen induction? Immunol Today 9:340-342, 1988.
306. Stamatis N, Liossis C, Tsokos GC: B cells in systemic lupus erythematosus. In Wallace DJ, Hahn BH (eds): Dubois' Lupus Erythematosus, 7th ed. Philadelphia, Lippincott Williams & Wilkins, 2007, pp 176-190.
307. Craft J, Fatenejad S: Self antigens and epitope spreading in systemic autoimmunity. Arthritis Rheum 40:1374-1382, 1997.
308. James JA, Harley JB: B-cell epitope spreading in autoimmunity. Immunol Rev 164:185-200, 1998.
309. Singh RR, Hahn BH, Tsao BP, et al: Evidence for multiple mechanisms of polyclonal T cell activation in murine lupus. J Clin Invest 102:1841-1849, 1998.
310. Asokan R, Hua J, Young KA, et al: Characterization of human complement receptor type 2 (CR2/CD21) as a receptor for IFN-alpha: A potential role in systemic lupus erythematosus. J Immunol 177: 383-394, 2006.
311. Huck S, Le CR, Youinou P, et al: Expression of B cell receptor-associated signaling molecules in human lupus. Autoimmunity 33:213-224, 2001.
312. Majeti R, Xu Z, Parslow TG, et al: An inactivating point mutation in the inhibitory wedge of CD45 causes lymphoproliferation and autoimmunity. Cell 103:1059-1070, 2000.
313. Mary C, Laporte C, Parzy D, et al: Dysregulated expression of the Cd22 gene as a result of a short interspersed nucleotide element insertion in Cd22a lupus-prone mice. J Immunol 165:2987-2996, 2000.
314. Honda M, Linker-Israeli M: Cytokine gene expression in human systemic lupus erythematosus. In Kammer GM, Tsokos GC (eds): Lupus: Molecular and Cellular Pathogenesis. Totowa, NJ, Humana Press, 1999.
315. Nagafuchi H, Suzuki N, Mizushima Y, et al: Constitutive expression of IL-6 receptors and their role in the excessive B cell function in patients with systemic lupus erythematosus. J Immunol 151: 6525-6534, 1993.
316. Finck BK, Chan B, Wofsy D: Interleukin 6 promotes murine lupus in NZB/NZW F1 mice. J Clin Invest 94:585-591, 1994.
317. Llorente L, Zou W, Levy Y, et al: Role of interleukin 10 in the B lymphocyte hyperactivity and autoantibody production of human systemic lupus erythematosus. J Exp Med 181:839-844, 1995.
318. Hagiwara E, Gourley MF, Lee S, et al: Disease severity in patients with systemic lupus erythematosus correlates with an increased ratio of interleukin-10:interferon-gamma-secreting cells in the peripheral blood. Arthritis Rheum 39:379-385, 1996.
319. Ishida H, Muchamuel T, Sakaguchi S, et al: Continuous administration of anti-interleukin 10 antibodies delays onset of autoimmunity in NZB/W F1 mice. J Exp Med 179:305-310, 1994.
320. Yin Z, Bahtiyar G, Zhang N, et al: IL-10 regulates murine lupus. J Immunol 169:2148-2155, 2002.
321. Wofsy D, Seaman WE: Successful treatment of autoimmunity in NZB/NZW F1 mice with monoclonal antibody to L3T4. J Exp Med 161:378-391, 1985.
322. Wofsy D: Administration of monoclonal anti-T cell antibodies retards murine lupus in BXSB mice. J Immunol 136:4554-4560, 1986.
323. Mihara M, Ohsugi Y, Saito K, et al: Immunologic abnormality in NZB/NZW F1 mice: Thymus-independent occurrence of B cell abnormality and requirement for T cells in the development of autoimmune disease, as evidenced by an analysis of the athymic nude individuals. J Immunol 141:85-90, 1988.

324. Horwitz D, Gray D: The interaction of T cells with cells of the innate immune system and B cells in the pathogenesis of SLE. In Wallace DJ, Hahn BH (eds): Dubois' Lupus Erythematosus, 7th ed. Philadelphia, Lippincott Williams & Wilkins, 2007, pp 133-160.

325. Winfield JB: Antilymphocyte autoantibodies. In Wallace DJ, Hahn BH (eds): Dubois' Lupus Erythematosus, 5th ed. Baltimore, Williams & Wilkins, 1997.

326. Butler WT, Sharp JT, Rossen RD, et al: Relationship of the clinical course of systemic lupus erythematosus to the presence of circulating lymphocytotoxic antibodies. Arthritis Rheum 15:251-258, 1972.

327. Yamada A, Winfield JB: Inhibition of soluble antigen-induced T cell proliferation by warm-reactive antibodies to activated T cells in systemic lupus erythematosus. J Clin Invest 74:1948-1960, 1984.

328. Devi BS, Van NS, Krausz T, et al: Peripheral blood lymphocytes in SLE—hyperexpression of CD154 on T and B lymphocytes and increased number of double negative T cells. J Autoimmun 11:471-475, 1998.

329. Sieling PA, Porcelli SA, Duong BT, et al: Human double-negative T cells in systemic lupus erythematosus provide help for IgG and are restricted by CD1c. J Immunol 165:5338-5344, 2000.

330. Rajagopalan S, Zordan T, Tsokos GC, et al: Pathogenic anti-DNA autoantibody-inducing T helper cell lines from patients with active lupus nephritis: Isolation of CD4-8− T helper cell lines that express the gamma delta T-cell antigen receptor. Proc Natl Acad Sci U S A 87:7020-7024, 1990.

331. Shivakumar S, Tsokos GC, Datta SK: T cell receptor alpha/beta expressing double-negative (CD4−/CD8−) and CD4+ helper cells in humans augment the production of pathogenic anti-DNA autoantibodies associated with lupus nephritis. J Immunol 143:103-112, 1989.

332. Oishi Y, Sumida T, Sakamoto A, et al: Selective reduction and recovery of invariant Valpha24JalphaQ T cell receptor T cells in correlation with disease activity in patients with systemic lupus erythematosus. J Rheumatol 28:275-283, 2001.

333. Kaneoka H, Morito F, Yamaguchi M: Low responsiveness to the anti-Leu 4 antibody by T cells from patients with active systemic lupus erythematosus. J Clin Lab Immunol 28:15-26, 1989.

334. Stohl W: Impaired generation of polyclonal T cell-mediated cytolytic activity despite normal polyclonal T cell proliferation in systemic lupus erythematosus. Clin Immunol Immunopathol 63:163-172, 1992.

335. Tsokos GC, Liossis SN: Lymphocytes, cytokines, inflammation, and immune trafficking. Curr Opin Rheumatol 10:417-425, 1998.

336. Raziuddin S, Nur MA, al-Wabel AA: Increased circulating HLA-DR+ CD4+ T cells in systemic lupus erythematosus: Alterations associated with prednisolone therapy. Scand J Immunol 31:139-145, 1990.

337. Horwitz DA, Stastny P, Ziff M: Circulating deoxyribonucleic acid-synthesizing mononuclear leukocytes, I: Increased numbers of proliferating mononuclear leukocytes in inflammatory disease. J Lab Clin Med 76:391-402, 1970.

338. Manoussakis MN, Papadopoulos GK, Drosos AA, et al: Soluble interleukin 2 receptor molecules in the serum of patients with autoimmune diseases. Clin Immunol Immunopathol 50:321-332, 1989.

339. Davas EM, Tsirogianni A, Kappou I, et al: Serum IL-6, TNFalpha, p55 srTNFalpha, p75srTNFalpha, srIL-2alpha levels and disease activity in systemic lupus erythematosus. Clin Rheumatol 18:17-22, 1999.

340. Kato K, Santana-Sahagun E, Rassenti LZ, et al: The soluble CD40 ligand sCD154 in systemic lupus erythematosus. J Clin Invest 104:947-955, 1999.

341. Hahn BH, Ebling F, Singh RR, et al: Cellular and molecular mechanisms of regulation of autoantibody production in lupus. Ann N Y Acad Sci 1051:433-441, 2005.

342. Stohl W, Elliott JE, Hamilton AS, et al: Impaired recovery and cytolytic function of CD56+ T and non-T cells in systemic lupus erythematosus following in vitro polyclonal T cell stimulation: Studies in unselected patients and monozygotic disease-discordant twins. Arthritis Rheum 39:1840-1851, 1996.

343. Horwitz DA: Transforming growth factor beta: taking control of T cells' life and death. Immunity 25:399-401, 2006.

344. Datta SK, Patel H, Berry D: Induction of a cationic shift in IgG anti-DNA autoantibodies: Role of T helper cells with classical and novel phenotypes in three murine models of lupus nephritis. J Exp Med 165:1252-1268, 1987.

345. Zeng D, Dick M, Cheng L, et al: Subsets of transgenic T cells that recognize CD1 induce or prevent murine lupus: Role of cytokines. J Exp Med 187:525-536, 1998.

346. Filaci G, Bacilieri S, Fravega M, et al: Impairment of CD8+ T suppressor cell function in patients with active systemic lupus erythematosus. J Immunol 166:6452-6457, 2001.

347. Filaci G, Rizzi M, Setti M, et al: Non-antigen-specific CD8+ T suppressor lymphocytes in diseases characterized by chronic immune responses and inflammation. Ann N Y Acad Sci 1050:115-123, 2005.

348. Tsokos GC, Smith PL, Christian CB, et al: Interleukin-2 restores the depressed allogeneic cell-mediated lympholysis and natural killer cell activity in patients with systemic lupus erythematosus. Clin Immunol Immunopathol 34:379-386, 1985.

349. Stohl W: Impaired polyclonal T cell cytolytic activity: A possible risk factor for systemic lupus erythematosus. Arthritis Rheum 38:506-516, 1995.

350. Linker-Israeli M, Quismorio FP Jr, Horwitz DA: CD8+ lymphocytes from patients with systemic lupus erythematosus sustain, rather than suppress, spontaneous polyclonal IgG production and synergize with CD4+ cells to support autoantibody synthesis. Arthritis Rheum 33:1216-1225, 1990.

351. Karpouzas GA, La CA, Ebling FM, et al: Differences between CD8+ T cells in lupus-prone (NZB x NZW) F1 mice and healthy (BALB/c x NZW) F1 mice may influence autoimmunity in the lupus model. Eur J Immunol 34:2489-2499, 2004.

352. Liossis SN, Ding XZ, Dennis GJ, et al: Altered pattern of TCR/CD3-mediated protein-tyrosyl phosphorylation in T cells from patients with systemic lupus erythematosus: Deficient expression of the T cell receptor zeta chain. J Clin Invest 101:1448-1457, 1998.

353. Koshy M, Berger D, Crow MK: Increased expression of CD40 ligand on systemic lupus erythematosus lymphocytes. J Clin Invest 98:826-837, 1996.

354. Kovacs B, Liossis SN, Dennis GJ, et al: Increased expression of functional Fas-ligand in activated T cells from patients with systemic lupus erythematosus. Autoimmunity 25:213-221, 1997.

355. Kammer GM, Khan IU, Malemud CJ: Deficient type I protein kinase A isozyme activity in systemic lupus erythematosus T lymphocytes. J Clin Invest 94:422-430, 1994.

356. Mishra N, Khan IU, Tsokos GC, et al: Association of deficient type II protein kinase A activity with aberrant nuclear translocation of the RII beta subunit in systemic lupus erythematosus T lymphocytes. J Immunol 165:2830-2840, 2000.

357. Kammer GM: Altered regulation of IL-2 production in systemic lupus erythematosus: An evolving paradigm. J Clin Invest 2005;115:836-840, 2005.

358. Mysler E, Bini P, Drappa J, et al: The apoptosis-1/Fas protein in human systemic lupus erythematosus. J Clin Invest 93:1029-1034, 1994.

359. Kovacs B, Vassilopoulos D, Vogelgesang SA, et al: Defective CD3-mediated cell death in activated T cells from patients with systemic lupus erythematosus: Role of decreased intracellular TNF-alpha. Clin Immunol Immunopathol 81:293-302, 1996.

360. Emlen W, Niebur J, Kadera R: Accelerated in vitro apoptosis of lymphocytes from patients with systemic lupus erythematosus. J Immunol 152:3685-3692, 1994.

361. Banki K, Hutter E, Gonchoroff NJ, et al: Elevation of mitochondrial transmembrane potential and reactive oxygen intermediate levels are early events and occur independently from activation of caspases in Fas signaling. J Immunol 162:1466-1479, 1999.

362. Li PF, Dietz R, von Harsdorf R: p53 regulates mitochondrial membrane potential through reactive oxygen species and induces cytochrome c-independent apoptosis blocked by Bcl-2. EMBO J 18:6027-6036, 1999.

363. Gergely P Jr, Grossman C, Niland B, et al: Mitochondrial hyperpolarization and ATP depletion in patients with systemic lupus erythematosus. Arthritis Rheum 46:175-190, 2002.

364. Richardson B, Scheinbart L, Strahler J, et al: Evidence for impaired T cell DNA methylation in systemic lupus erythematosus and rheumatoid arthritis. Arthritis Rheum 33:1665-1673, 1990.

365. Bird AP, Wolffe AP: Methylation-induced repression—belts, braces, and chromatin. Cell 99:451-454, 1999.

366. Yung R, Powers D, Johnson K, et al: Mechanisms of drug-induced lupus, II: T cells overexpressing lymphocyte function-associated antigen 1 become autoreactive and cause a lupuslike disease in syngeneic mice. J Clin Invest 97:2866-2871, 1996.

367. Kaplan MJ, Beretta L, Yung RL, et al: LFA-1 overexpression and T cell autoreactivity: Mechanisms. Immunol Invest 29:427-442, 2000.

368. Katsiari CG, Tsokos GC: Transcriptional repression of interleukin-2 in human systemic lupus erythematosus. Autoimmun Rev 5:118-121, 2006.

369. Kammer GM, Perl A, Richardson BC, et al: Abnormal T cell signal transduction in systemic lupus erythematosus. Arthritis Rheum 46:1139-1154, 2002.

370. Sassone-Corsi P: Coupling gene expression to cAMP signalling: Role of CREB and CREM. Int J Biochem Cell Biol 30:27-38, 1998.

371. Wong HK, Kammer GM, Dennis G, et al: Abnormal NF-kappa B activity in T lymphocytes from patients with systemic lupus erythematosus is associated with decreased p65-RelA protein expression. J Immunol 163:1682-1689, 1999.

372. Powell JD, Lerner CG, Ewoldt GR, et al: The −180 site of the IL-2 promoter is the target of CREB/CREM binding in T cell anergy. J Immunol 163:6631-6639, 1999.

373. Mosmann TR: Properties and functions of interleukin-10. Adv Immunol 56:1-26, 1994.

374. Kalsi JK, Grossman J, Kim J, et al: Peptides from antibodies to DNA elicit cytokine release from peripheral blood mononuclear cells of patients with systemic lupus erythematosus: Relation of cytokine pattern to disease duration. Lupus 13:490-500, 2004.

375. Schwarting A, Wada T, Kinoshita K, et al: IFN-gamma receptor signaling is essential for the initiation, acceleration, and destruction of autoimmune kidney disease in MRL-Fas(lpr) mice. J Immunol 161:494-503, 1998.

376. Ozmen L, Roman D, Fountoulakis M, et al: Experimental therapy of systemic lupus erythematosus: The treatment of NZB/W mice with mouse soluble interferon-gamma receptor inhibits the onset of glomerulonephritis. Eur J Immunol 25:6-12, 1995.

377. Bennett L, Palucka AK, Arce E, et al: Interferon and granulopoiesis signatures in systemic lupus erythematosus blood. J Exp Med 197:681-685, 2003.

378. Baechler EC, Batliwalla FM, Karypis G, et al: Interferon-inducible gene expression signature in peripheral blood cell of patients with severe lupus. Proc Natl Acad Sci U S A 100:2610-2615, 2003.

379. Kirou KA, Lee C, George S, et al: Activation of the interferon-alpha pathway identifies a subgroup of systemic lupus erythematosus patients with distinct serologic features and active disease. Arthritis Rheum 52:1491-1503, 2005.

380. Feng X, Wu H, Grossman JM, et al: Association of increased interferon-inducible gene expression with disease activity and lupus nephritis in patients with systemic lupus erythematosus. Arthritis Rheum 54:2951-2962, 2006.

381. Banchereau J, Pascual V: Type I interferon in systemic lupus erythematosus and other autoimmune diseases. Immunity 25:383-392, 2006.

382. Bauer JW, Baechler EC, Petri M, et al: Elevated serum levels of interferon-regulated chemokines are biomarkers for active human systemic lupus erythematosus. PLoS Med 19:e491, 2006.

383. Singh RR, Kumar V, Ebling FM, et al: T cell determinants from autoantibodies to DNA can upregulate autoimmunity in murine systemic lupus erythematosus. J Exp Med 181:2017-2027, 1995.

384. Singh RR, Ebling FM, Sercarz EE, et al: Immune tolerance to autoantibody-derived peptides delays development of autoimmunity in murine lupus. J Clin Invest 96:2990-2996, 1995.

385. Hahn BH, Singh RR, Wong WK, et al: Treatment with a consensus peptide based on amino acid sequences in autoantibodies prevents T cell activation by autoantigens and delays disease onset in murine lupus. Arthritis Rheum 44:432-441, 2001.

386. Hahn BH, Singh RP, La Cava A, et al: Tolerogenic treatment of lupus mice with consensus peptide induces Foxp3-expressing, apoptosis-resistant, TGFbeta-secreting CD8+ T cell suppressors. J Immunol 175:7728-7737, 2005.

387. LaCava Ebling FM, Hahn BH: Ig-reactive CD4+CD25+ T cells from tolerized (New Zealand Black x New Zealand White)F1 mice suppress in vitro production of antibodies to DNA. J Immunol 173:3542-3548, 2004.

388. Mauermann N, Stoeger Z, Zinger H, et al: Amelioration of lupus manifestations by a peptide based on the complementarity determining region 1 of an autoantibody in severe combined immunodeficient (SCID) mice engrafted with peripheral blood lymphocytes of systemic lupus erythematosus (SLE) patients. Clin Exp Immunol 137:513-520, 2004.

389. Sela U, Dayan M, Hershkoviz R, et al: The negative regulators Foxj1 and Foxo3 are up-regulated by a peptide that inhibits systemic lupus erythematosus-associated T cell responses. Eur J Immunol 36:2971-2980, 2006.

390. Kaliyaperumal A, Mohan C, Wu W, et al: Nucleosomal peptide epitopes for nephritis-inducing T helper cells of murine lupus. J Exp Med 183:2459-2469, 1996.

391. Kang HK, Michaels MA, Berner BR, et al: Very low-dose tolerance with nucleosomal peptides controls lupus and induces potent regulatory T cell subsets. J Immunol 174:3247-3255, 2005.

392. Werth VP, Dutz JP, Sontheimer RD: Pathogenetic mechanisms and treatment of cutaneous lupus erythematosus. Curr Opin Rheumatol 9:400-409, 1997.

393. Danning CL, Illei GG, Boumpas DT: Vasculitis associated with primary rheumatologic diseases. Curr Opin Rheumatol 10:58-65, 1998.

394. Murata H, Matsumura R, Koyama A, et al: T cell receptor repertoire of T cells in the kidneys of patients with lupus nephritis. Arthritis Rheum 46:2141-2147, 2002.

395. Horwitz DA, Gray JD, Zheng SG: The potential of human regulatory T cells generated ex vivo as a treatment for lupus and other chronic inflammatory diseases. Arthritis Res 4:241-246, 2002.

396. Chen C, Radic MZ, Erikson J, et al: Deletion and editing of B cells that express antibodies to DNA. J Immunol 152:1970-1982, 1994.

397. Tiegs SL, Russell DM, Nemazee D: Receptor editing in self-reactive bone marrow B cells. J Exp Med 177:1009-1020, 1993.

398. Jacobi AM, Diamond B: Balancing diversity and tolerance: Lessons from patients with systemic lupus erythematosus. J Exp Med 202:341-344, 2005.

399. Yurasov S, Hammersen J, Tiller T, et al: B-cell tolerance checkpoints in healthy humans and patients with systemic lupus erythematosus. Ann N Y Acad Sci 1062:165-174, 2005.

400. Kang HK, Datta SK: Regulatory T cells in lupus. Int Rev Immunol 25(1-2):5-25, 2006.

401. Allen PM: Defining yourself: Tolerance development in the immune system. J Immunol 177:1369-1372, 2006.

402. Rutella S, Danese S, Leone G: Tolerogenic dendritic cells: Cytokine modulation comes of age. Blood 198:1435-1440, 2006.

403. Cappione A III, Anolik JH, Pugh-Bernard A, et al: Germinal center exclusion of autoreactive B cells is defective in human systemic lupus erythematosus. J Clin Invest 115:3205-3216, 2005.

404. Zhu J, Liu X, Xie C, et al: T cell hyperactivity in lupus as a consequence of hyperstimulatory antigen-presenting cells. J Clin Invest 115:1869-1878, 2005.

405. Palucka AK, Laupeze B, Aspord C, et al: Immunotherapy via dendritic cells. Adv Exp Med Biol 560:105-114, 2005.

406. Holers VM: Complement receptors and the shaping of the natural antibody repertoire. Springer Semin Immunopathol 26:405-423, 2005.

407. Munoz LE, Gaipl US, Franz S, et al: SLE—a disease of clearance deficiency? Rheumatology (Oxf) 44:1101-1107, 2005.

408. Mason D: T-cell-mediated control of autoimmunity. Arthritis Res 3:133-135, 2001.

409. Sakaguchi S, Sakaguchi N, Shimizu J, et al: Immunologic tolerance maintained by CD25+ CD4+ regulatory T cells: Their common role in controlling autoimmunity, tumor immunity, and transplantation tolerance. Immunol Rev 182:18-32, 2001.

410. Shevach EM: Regulatory T cells in autoimmmunity. Annu Rev Immunol 18:423-449, 2000.

411. Liu Z, Tugulea S, Cortesini R, et al: Specific suppression of T helper alloreactivity by allo-MHC class I-restricted CD8+. Int Immunol 10:775-783, 1998.

412. Balashov KE, Khoury SJ, Hafler DA, et al: Inhibition of T cell responses by activated human CD8+ T cells is mediated by interferon-gamma and is defective in chronic progressive multiple sclerosis. J Clin Invest 95:2711-2719, 1995.

413. Koide J, Takano M, Takeuchi T, et al: Direct demonstration of immunoregulatory T-cell defects in patients with systemic lupus erythematosus. Scand J Immunol 23:449-459, 1986.

414. Morimoto C, Reinherz EL, Schlossman SF, et al: Alterations in immunoregulatory T cell subsets in active systemic lupus erythematosus. J Clin Invest 66:1171-1174, 1980.

415. Tsokos GC, Balow JE: Phenotypes of T lymphocytes in systemic lupus erythematosus: Decreased cytotoxic/suppressor subpopulation is associated with deficient allogeneic cytotoxic responses rather than with concanavalin A-induced suppressor cells. Clin Immunol Immunopathol 26:267-276, 1983.

416. Morimoto C, Distaso JA, Borel Y, et al: Communicative interactions between subpopulations of human T lymphocytes required for generation of suppressor effector function in a primary antibody response. J Immunol 128:1645-1650, 1982.
417. Gatenby PA, Kotzin BL, Kansas GS, et al: Immunoglobulin secretion in the human autologous mixed leukocyte reaction: Definition of a suppressor-amplifier circuit using monoclonal antibodies. J Exp Med 156:55-67, 1982.
418. Feinberg MB, Silvestri G: T(S) cells and immune tolerance induction: A regulatory renaissance? Nat Immunol 3:215-217, 2002.
419. Fan GC, Singh RR: Vaccination with minigenes encoding V(H)-derived major histocompatibility complex class I-binding epitopes activates cytotoxic T cells that ablate autoantibody-producing B cells and inhibit lupus. J Exp Med 196:731-741, 2002.
420. Tanaka S, Matsuyama T, Steinberg AD, et al: Antilymphocyte antibodies against CD4+2H4+ cell populations in patients with systemic lupus erythematosus. Arthritis Rheum 32:398-405, 1989.
421. Bennett SR, Carbone FR, Karamalis F, et al: Help for cytotoxic-T-cell responses is mediated by CD40 signalling. Nature 393:478-480, 1998.
422. Ridge JP, Di RF, Matzinger P: A conditioned dendritic cell can be a temporal bridge between a CD4+ T-helper and a T-killer cell. Nature 393:474-478, 1998.
423. Schoenberger SP, Toes RE, van der Voort EI, et al: T-cell help for cytotoxic T lymphocytes is mediated by CD40-CD40L interactions. Nature 393:480-483, 1998.
424. Mintern JD, Davey GM, Belz GT, et al: Cutting edge: Precursor frequency affects the helper dependence of cytotoxic T cells. J Immunol 168:977-980, 2002.
425. Chang CC, Ciubotariu R, Manavalan JS, et al: Tolerization of dendritic cells by T(S) cells: The crucial role of inhibitory receptors ILT3 and ILT4. Nat Immunol 3:237-243, 2002.
426. Green MR, Kennell AS, Larche MJ, et al: Natural killer cell activity in families of patients with systemic lupus erythematosus: Demonstration of a killing defect in patients. Clin Exp Immunol 141:165-173, 2005.
427. Shevach EM: Certified professionals: CD4(+)CD25(+) suppressor T cells. J Exp Med 193:F41-F46, 2001.
428. Lee JH, Wang LC, Lin YT, et al: Inverse correlation between CD4+ regulatory T-cell population and autoantibody levels in paediatric patients with systemic lupus erythematosus. Immunology 117:280-286, 2006.
429. Liu MF, Wang CR, Fung LL, et al: Decreased CD4+CD25+ T cells in peripheral blood of patients with systemic lupus erythematosus. Scand J Immunol 59:198-202, 2004.
430. Hahn BH: Idiotypes and idiotype networks. In Wallace DJ, Hahn BH (eds): Dubois' Lupus Erythematosus, 7th ed. Philadelphia, Lippincott Williams & Wilkins, 2007, pp 255-272.
431. Shoenfeld Y, Mozes E: Pathogenic idiotypes of autoantiodies in autoimmunity: Lessons from new experimental models of SLE. FASEB J 4:2646-2651, 1990.
432. Kalunian KC, Panosian-Sahakian N, Ebling FM, et al: Idiotypic characteristics of immunoglobulins associated with systemic lupus erythematosus: Studies of antibodies deposited in glomeruli of humans. Arthritis Rheum 32:513-522, 1989.

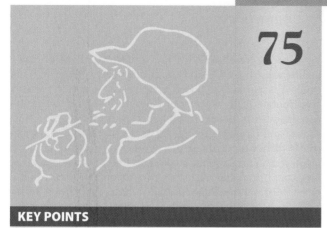

75

Clinical Features and Treatment of Systemic Lupus Erythematosus

IOANNIS O. TASSIULAS •
DIMITRIOS T. BOUMPAS

KEY POINTS

The diagnosis of systemic lupus erythematosus (SLE) remains largely clinical.

Undifferentiated connective tissue disease and incomplete lupus represent 10% to 20% of patients referred to rheumatologists.

Antiphospholipid antibody–mediated morbidity is an important part of the natural history of SLE.

SLE patients are at increased risk for certain comorbidities secondary to the disease or its treatment or both.

Evidence-based recommendations for the management of SLE have been developed.

Systemic lupus erythematosus (SLE) is the prototypic autoimmune disease characterized by the production of autoantibodies to components of the cell nucleus in association with diverse clinical manifestations encompassing almost all organ systems. SLE is a complex disease with variable presentations, course, and prognosis characterized by remissions and flares. The extreme heterogeneity of the disease has led some investigators to propose that SLE represents a syndrome rather than a single disease.

This chapter discusses clinical aspects of SLE, including diagnosis and treatment. Important aspects of the disease are highlighted, and practical information that could be used by readers with various backgrounds and expertise is presented. SLE is an intensively studied disease with abundant data. Where possible, evidence-based recommendations are presented based on a systematic review of the literature.[1] Where data are scarce, a critical overview of expert-based opinions is presented.

HISTORICAL BACKGROUND

The term *lupus* (Latin for "wolf") was first used during the Middle Ages to describe erosive skin lesions that were evocative of a wolf's bite. The "classical" period of lupus starts in 1846 with the Viennese physician von Hebra (1816-1880), who introduced the butterfly metaphor to describe the malar rash. Von Hebra also used the term *lupus erythematosus* and published the first illustrations in his *Atlas of Skin Diseases* in 1856. The "neoclassical" period of lupus starts with the recognition of lupus as a systemic disease with visceral manifestations. Kaposi (1837-1902) first recognized the systemic nature of the disease. The existence of a systemic form was

firmly established by Osler in Baltimore and Jadassohn in Vienna. Other important milestones in this period include the description of the false-positive test for syphilis in SLE by Reinhart and Hauck from Germany (1909); the description of the typical endocarditis lesions in SLE by Libman and Sacks in New York (1923); the description of the typical glomerular changes by Baehr (1935); and finally the use of the term *diffuse connective tissue disease* by Klemperer, Pollack, and Baehr (1941).

The major serologic breakthrough in the diagnosis of SLE was the discovery of the LE cell by Hargraves, Richmond, and Morton at the Mayo Clinic in 1948; this marks the beginning of the modern era in SLE. Major advances in understanding of the pathology and immunology of SLE include the identification of antibodies to DNA and other extractable nuclear antigens; the development of animal models of SLE and the recognition of the role of genetic predisposition to the development of SLE; and the contribution of the major histocompatibility complex loci, various cytokines, cellular components of the innate and adaptive immune system, mechanisms of central and peripheral immune tolerance, and apoptotic cell death. Intensive study of the immune system abnormalities and the genetics in SLE has identified new therapeutic targets for this complex disease.

EPIDEMIOLOGY AND CLASSIFICATION

EPIDEMIOLOGY

Prevalence rates in SLE are estimated to be 51 per 100,000 in the United States.[2] The incidence of SLE has nearly tripled in the last 40 years, mainly as a result of improved diagnosis of mild disease.[3] Estimated incidence rates in North America, South America, and Europe range from 2 to 8 per 100,000 per year.[4,5] Women are affected nine times more frequently than men, and African-Americans and Hispanics are affected much more frequently than whites and have a higher disease morbidity.[6-9] The disease seems to be more common in urban than rural areas. Of patients with SLE, 65% have disease onset between ages 16 and 55, 20% present before age 16, and 15% present after the age of 55.[10] Men with SLE tend to have less photosensitivity, more serositis, an older age at diagnosis, and a higher 1-year mortality compared with women.[11,12] SLE tends to be milder in the elderly with a lower incidence of malar rash, photosensitivity, purpura, alopecia, Raynaud's phenomenon, renal system involvement, and central nervous system (CNS) involvement, but a greater prevalence of serositis, pulmonary involvement, sicca symptoms, and musculoskeletal manifestations.[13]

CLASSIFICATION CRITERIA

Many autoimmune rheumatic diseases are characterized by overlapping organ system involvement and lack a pathognomonic test. Criteria for disease classification were developed in 1971, revised in 1982, and revised again in 1997 (Table 75-1).[14] Classification criteria help to distinguish patients with the disease in question from individuals without the disease. The American College of Rheumatology (ACR) classification criteria for SLE were developed for clinical studies to ensure that SLE patients reported in the literature actually have the disease. In addition to the wide variety of manifestations, SLE runs an unpredictable course. The dynamic nature of the disease makes its diagnosis challenging in some cases. Often a prolonged period of observation is required before making a definitive diagnosis.

USE OF CLASSIFICATION CRITERIA FOR DIAGNOSTIC PURPOSES

Although the classification criteria also may be used as diagnostic aids, there are several caveats for their use for diagnostic purposes. These criteria were developed and validated for the classification of patients with long-standing established disease and may exclude patients with early disease or disease limited to a few organs. Despite excellent sensitivity (>85%) and specificity (>95%) for patients with established disease, the sensitivity of the criteria for patients early in the disease may be significantly lower. Some systems are overrepresented; the mucocutaneous manifestations of lupus are represented with four criteria (photosensitivity, malar rash, discoid lesions, and oral ulcers). At the same time, all features included in the classification criteria contribute equally without any weight based on sensitivity and specificity for each individual criterion. Studies have shown and experience supports that criteria such as objective evidence of renal disease (significant proteinuria, active urine sediment, or renal biopsy specimen with evidence of lupus nephritis), discoid rash, and cytopenias are more useful in establishing the diagnosis of SLE than the other criteria.

Because SLE is a disease whose course is typified by periodic involvement of one organ system after another, it is apparent that patients must have the disease for years before they fulfill the classification criteria; medical literature may overestimate the diagnostic utility of some tests or features of the disease because they are usually analyzed among patients with an uncertain cause of symptoms, as is common in practice. Data from tertiary care centers among patients referred for SLE suggest that two thirds of patients fulfill ACR criteria for SLE; approximately 10% have clinical SLE, but do not fulfill criteria; and 25% have fibromyalgia-like symptoms and positive antinuclear antibody (ANA), but never develop SLE.[15]

ACTIVITY AND DAMAGE INDICES

SLE has a chronic course that is often complicated by exacerbations and flares of varying severity. Assessing disease activity in a patient with SLE is crucial to the physician because it forms the basis of most treatment decisions. Disease activity in chronic diseases such as SLE needs to be

Table 75-1 American College of Rheumatology Revised Classification Criteria for Systemic Lupus Erythematosus

Criteria	Definition
Malar rash	Fixed erythema, flat or raised, over the malar eminences, tending to spare the nasolabial folds
Discoid rash	Erythematous raised patches with adherent keratotic scaling and follicular plugging; atrophic scarring occurs in older lesions
Photosensitivity	Skin rash as a result of unusual reaction to sunlight, by patient history or physician observation
Oral ulcers	Oral or nasopharyngeal ulceration, usually painless, observed by a physician
Arthritis	Nonerosive arthritis involving two or more peripheral joints, characterized by tenderness, swelling, or effusion
Serositis	a. Pleuritis—convincing history of pleuritic pain or rub heard by a physician or evidence of pleural effusion *or* b. Pericarditis—documented by ECG or rub or evidence of pericardial effusion
Renal disorder	a. Persistent proteinuria >0.5 g/day >3+ if quantitation is not performed *or* b. Cellular casts—may be red blood cell, hemoglobin, granular tubular, or mixed
Neurologic disorder	a. Seizures—in the absence of offending drugs or known metabolic derangements (e.g., uremia, acidosis, or electrolyte imbalance) *or* b. Psychosis—in the absence of offending drugs or known metabolic derangements (e.g., uremia, acidosis, or electrolyte imbalance)
Hematologic disorder	a. Hemolytic anemia with reticulocytosis, *or* b. Leukopenia—<4000/mm^3, *or* c. Lymphopenia—<1500/mm^3, *or* d. Thrombocytopenia—<100,000/mm^3 in the absence of offending drugs
Immunologic disorder	a. Anti-DNA—antibody to native DNA in abnormal titer, *or* b. Anti-Sm—presence of antibody to Sm nuclear antigen, *or* c. Positive finding of antiphospholipid antibodies based on (1) abnormal serum concentration of IgG or IgM anticardiolipin antibodies, (2) positive test result for lupus anticoagulant using a standard method, or (3) false-positive serologic test for syphilis known to be positive for at least 6 mo and confirmed by *Treponema pallidum* immobilization or fluorescent treponemal antibody absorption test
ANA	Abnormal titer of ANA by immunofluorescence or equivalent assay at any point in time and in the absence of drugs known to be associated with drug-induced lupus syndrome

ANA, antinuclear antibody; ECG, electrocardiogram.
Adapted from Hochberg MC: Updating the American College of Rheumatology revised criteria for the classification of systemic lupus erythematosus. Arthritis Rheum 40:1725, 1997.

Table 75-2   Systemic Lupus Erythematosus Disease Activity Index

Descriptor	Definition	Weighted Score
Seizure	Recent onset; exclude metabolic, infectious, or drug-related causes	8
Psychosis	Altered ability to function in normal activity owing to severe disturbance in the perception of reality; includes hallucinations, incoherence marked by loose associations, impoverished thought content, marked illogical thinking, and bizarre disorganized or catatonic behavior; exclude the presence of uremia and offending drugs	8
Organic brain syndrome	Altered mental function with impaired orientation or impaired memory or other intellectual function, with rapid onset and fluctuating clinical features; includes clouding of consciousness with reduced capacity to focus and inability to sustain attention on environment, and at least two of the following—perceptual disturbance, incoherent speech, insomnia or daytime drowsiness, and increased or decreased psychomotor activity; exclude metabolic infectious and drug-related causes	8
Visual	Retinal changes from systemic lupus erythematosus cytoid bodies, retinal hemorrhages, serous exudate or hemorrhage in choroid, optic neuritis (not due to hypertension, drugs, or infection)	8
Cranial nerve	New onset of sensory or motor neuropathy involving a cranial nerve	8
Lupus headache	Severe, persistent headache; may be migrainous, unresponsive to narcotic analgesia	8
Cerebrovascular accident	New syndrome; exclude arteriosclerosis	8
Vasculitis	Ulceration, gangrene, tender finger nodules, periungual infarction, splinter hemorrhages; vasculitis confirmed by biopsy or angiogram	8
Arthritis	More than two joints with pain and signs of inflammation (tenderness, swelling, or effusions)	4
Myositis	Proximal muscle aching or weakness associated with elevated creatine phosphokinase/aldolase levels, electromyographic changes, or biopsy specimen showing myositis	4
Casts	Heme, granular, or erythrocyte	4
Hematuria	>5 erythrocytes per high-power field; exclude other causes (stone, infection)	4
Proteinuria	>0.5 g of urinary protein excreted per 24 hr; new onset or recent increase of >0.5 g/24 hr	4
Pyuria	>5 leukocytes per high-power field; exclude infection	4
New malar rash	New onset or recurrence of inflammatory type of rash	4
Alopecia	New or recurrent; patch of abnormal, diffuse hair loss	4
Mucous membrane	New onset or recurrence of oral or nasal ulceration	4
Pleurisy	Pleuritic chest pain with pleural rub or effusion, or pleural thickening	4
Pericarditis	Pericardial pain with at least one rub or effusion; confirmation by ECG or echocardiography	4
Low complement	Decrease in CH50, C3, or C4 levels (to less than the lower limit of the laboratory-determined normal range)	2
Increased DNA binding	>25% binding by Farr assay (to more than the upper limit of the laboratory-determined normal range, e.g., 25%)	2
Fever	>38°C after exclusion of infection	1
Thrombocytopenia	<100,000 platelets	1
Leukopenia	Leukocyte count <3000/mm^3 (not due to drugs)	1

ECG, electrocardiogram.

distinguished from damage. This distinction has important implications for the long-term prognosis and the appropriate treatment in individual patients. A detailed history and physical examination should be done in every SLE patient. Appropriate laboratory evaluation, including pulmonary function tests, magnetic resonance imaging (MRI), high-resolution computed tomography (CT), magnetic resonance arteriography, and conventional arteriography, should be used to help differentiate active from chronic lesions where applicable.

Several validated global and organ-specific activity indices are widely used in the evaluation of SLE patients.[16,17] These include British Isles Lupus Assessment Group Scale, European Consensus Lupus Activity Measure (ECLAM), Lupus Activity Index, National Institutes of Health SLE Index Score, Systemic Lupus Activity Measure, and Systemic Lupus Erythematosus Disease Activity Index (SLEDAI).

These indices have been developed in the context of long-term observational studies and have been shown to be strong predictors of damage and mortality, and to reflect change in disease activity. They have been validated against each other.

We recommend the use of at least one of these indices for monitoring of disease activity. In our experience, the ECLAM and the SLEDAI (Table 75-2) are more convenient for use in daily practice. Computerized clinical charts that compute several disease activity indices simultaneously have been developed.[18] The Systemic Lupus International Collaborating Clinics/ACR damage index is a validated instrument specifically designed to ascertain damage in SLE.[19] The damage in SLE may be due to SLE itself or to drug therapy. The index records damage in 12 organs or systems (Table 75-3). There is no index to measure damage caused by drugs in SLE at present. The change must have been present for at least

Table 75-3   Systemic Lupus International Collaborating Clinics/American College of Rheumatology Damage Index for Systemic Lupus Erythematosus

Item	Score
Ocular (either eye by clinical assessment)	
Any cataract ever	0, 1
Retinal change or optic atrophy	0, 1
Neuropsychiatric	
Cognitive impairment (e.g., memory deficit, difficulty with calculation, poor concentration, difficulty in spoken or written language, impaired performance level) or major psychosis	0, 1
Seizures requiring therapy for 6 mo	0, 1
Cerebrovascular accident ever (score 2 if >1)	0, 1, 2
Cranial or peripheral neuropathy (excluding optic)	0, 1
Transverse myelitis	0, 1
Renal	
Estimated or measured glomerular filtration rate <50%	0, 1
Proteinuria >3.5 g/24 hr	0, 1
or End-stage renal disease (regardless of dialysis or transplantation)	*or* 3
Pulmonary	
Pulmonary hypertension (right ventricular prominence, or loud P_2)	0, 1
Pulmonary fibrosis (physical and radiographic)	0, 1
Shrinking lung (radiograph)	0, 1
Pleural fibrosis (radiograph)	0, 1
Pulmonary infarction (radiograph)	0, 1
Cardiovascular	
Angina or coronary artery bypass	0, 1
Myocardial infarction ever (score 2 if >1)	0, 1, 2
Cardiomyopathy (ventricular dysfunction)	0, 1
Valvular disease (diastolic murmur, or systolic murmur >3/6)	0, 1
Pericarditis for 6 mo or pericardiectomy	0, 1
Peripheral vascular	
Claudication for 6 mo	0, 1
Minor tissue loss (pulp space)	0, 1
Significant tissue loss ever (e.g., loss of digit or limb) (score 2 if >1 site)	0, 1, 2
Venous thrombosis with swelling, ulceration, or venous stasis	0, 1
Gastrointestinal	
Infarction or resection of bowel below duodenum, spleen, liver or gallbladder ever, for any cause (score 2 if >1 site)	0, 1, 2
Mesenteric insufficiency	0, 1
Chronic peritonitis	0, 1
Stricture or upper gastrointestinal tract surgery ever	0, 1
Chronic pancreatitis	0, 1
Musculoskeletal	
Muscle atrophy or weakness	0, 1
Deforming or erosive arthritis (including reversible deformities, excluding avascular necrosis)	0, 1
Osteoporosis with fracture or vertebral collapse (excluding avascular necrosis)	0, 1
Avascular necrosis (score 2 if >1)	0, 1, 2
Osteomyelitis	0, 1
Tendon rupture	0, 1
Skin	
Scarring chronic alopecia	0, 1
Extensive scarring of panniculus other than scalp and pulp space	0, 1
Skin ulceration (excluding thrombosis for >6 mo)	0, 1
Premature gonadal failure	0, 1
Diabetes (regardless of treatment)	0, 1
Malignancy (exclude dysplasia) (score 2 if >1 site)	0, 1

6 months and is ascertained clinically or by simple investigations. Several independent studies have shown that the early acquisition of damage is a poor prognostic sign.[20,21]

CLINICAL FEATURES

MUCOCUTANEOUS INVOLVEMENT

Mucocutaneous involvement is almost universal in SLE. Cutaneous lesions in SLE can be classified as lupus specific and nonspecific (Table 75-4). The lupus-specific lesions

can be subclassified further as acute, subacute, and chronic lesions.[22,23]

Acute Rashes—Malar Rash

The classic lupus butterfly rash manifests acutely as an erythematous, elevated lesion, pruritic or painful, in a malar distribution, commonly precipitated by exposure to sunlight (Fig. 75-1). The rash may last days to weeks and is commonly accompanied by other inflammatory manifestations of the disease. The acute butterfly rash should be

Table 75-4 Classification of Lupus Erythematosus–
Associated Skin Lesions

LE-Specific Skin Lesions
Acute cutaneous LE
Localized
Generalized
Subacute cutaneous LE
Annular
Papulosquamous (psoriasiform)
Chronic cutaneous LE
"Classic" DLE
Localized
Generalized
Hypertrophic (verrucous) DLE
Lupus panniculitis (profundus)
Mucosal LE
Tumid lupus
Chilblain lupus

LE-Nonspecific Skin Lesions
Cutaneous vascular disease
Vasculitis
Leukocytoclastic
Palpable purpura
Urticarial vasculitis
Polyarteritis nodosa–like
Papulonodular mucinosis
Degos disease–like
Atrophie blanche–like
Livedo reticularis
Thrombophlebitis
Raynaud's phenomenon
Erythromelalgia
LE-nonspecific bullous lesions
Acquired epidermolysis bullosa
Dermatitis herpetiformis–like bullous LE
Pemphigus erythematosus
Porphyria cutanea tarda
Urticaria
Vasculopathy
Anetoderma/cutis laxa
Acanthosis nigricans (type B insulin resistance)
Periungal telangiectasia
Erythema multiforme
Leg ulcers
Lichen planus
Alopecia (nonscarring)
"Lupus hair"
Telogen effluvium
Alopecia areata
Sclerodactyly
Rheumatoid nodules
Calcinosis cutis

DLE, discoid lupus erythematosus; LE, lupus erythematosus.
Modified from Sontheimer RD, Provost TT: Cutaneous Manifestations of
Rheumatic Diseases. Baltimore, Williams & Wilkins, 1996.

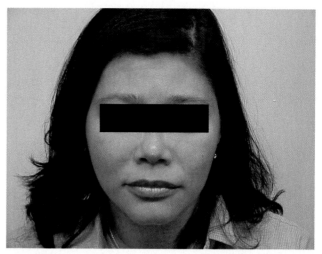

Figure 75-1 Localized acute cutaneous lupus erythematosus (malar rash). These lesions are abrupt in onset, frequently appear after exposure to the sun, and are characterized by erythema and edema. The sparing of the nasolabial folds and the absence of discrete papules and pustules help to differentiate this condition from acne rosacea (including glucocorticoid-induced rosacea).

present with annular or psoriasiform skin lesions, and this is strongly associated with anti-Ro (SS-A) and anti-La (SS-B) antibodies. Patients with SCLE have a high incidence of photosensitivity and rarely can present with erythema multiforme–like lesions (Rowell's syndrome).[26] SCLE lesions begin as small, erythematous, slightly scaly papules that evolve into either a psoriasiform (papulosquamous) or annular form. The latter lesions often coalesce to form polycyclic or figurative patterns (Fig. 75-2). The lesions typically have erythematous, and sometimes crusted, margins. The most frequently affected areas in SCLE are the shoulders, forearms, neck, and upper torso. The face is usually spared.

Chronic Rashes

Discoid lupus erythematosus (DLE) lesions develop in 25% of patients with SLE, but also may occur in the absence of any other clinical features of SLE.[27] Patients with DLE have approximately a 5% to 10% risk of developing SLE, which tends to be mild. Patients with numerous and widespread lesions seem to be more likely to develop SLE. Discoid lesions are characterized by discrete, erythematous, slightly infiltrated plaques covered by a well-formed adherent scale that extends into dilated hair follicles (follicular plugging) (Fig. 75-3). Discoid lesions are most often seen on the face, neck, and scalp, but also occur on the ears and infrequently on the upper torso. They tend to expand slowly with active inflammation at the periphery, and then to heal, leaving depressed central scars, atrophy, telangiectasias, and dyspigmentation (hyperpigmentation or hypopigmentation). The differential diagnosis of discoid lesions includes hypertrophic lichen planus, eczema, and actinic keratosis; some early and scaly discoid lesions also must be differentiated from psoriasis.

Other Rashes

Additional SLE-specific skin lesions include lupus profundus, presenting as a firm nodular lesion with or without an overlying cutaneous lesion. The nodules are often painful and consist of

differentiated from other causes of facial erythema, such as rosacea; seborrheic, atopic, and contact dermatitis; glucocorticoid-induced dermal atrophy; and flushing. Other acute cutaneous lesions include generalized erythema and bullous lesions. The rash of acute cutaneous lupus erythematosus can be transient and heal without scarring.[22,23]

Subacute Rashes

Subacute cutaneous lupus erythematosus (SCLE) is not uniformly associated with SLE.[24] Approximately 50% of affected patients have SLE, and about 10% of patients with SLE have this type of skin lesion.[25] Patients with SCLE may

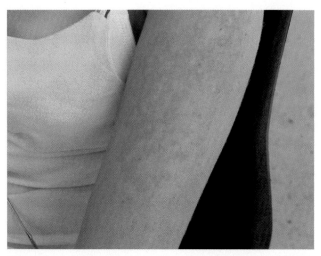

Figure 75-2 Subacute cutaneous lupus lesions. Typical features include symmetric, widespread, superficial, and nonscarring lesions. Involvement of the neck, shoulders, upper chest, upper back, and extensor surface of the hand is common. These lesions begin as small photosensitive, erythematous, scaly papules or plaques that evolve into a papulosquamous (psoriasiform) or annular polycyclic form as in this patient. Subacute cutaneous lupus erythematosus has been associated with the presence of anti-Ro/SS-A antibodies, genetic deficiencies of complement C2 and C4, and certain medications, such as hydrochlorothiazide.

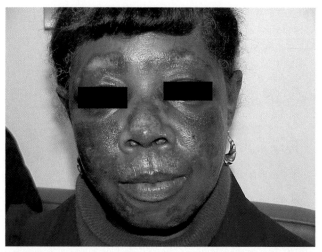

Figure 75-3 Discoid lupus erythematosus. Refractory to treatment, facial discoid lupus erythematosus lesions produce large areas of disfigurement on confluence. Note the erythema (indicating disease activity), keratin-plugged follicles, and dermal atrophy. The characteristic pattern of hyperpigmentation at the active border and hypopigmentation at the inactive center is especially evident in black patients. Discoid lesions are usually found on the face, scalp, ears, or neck. Facial involvement of this sort can produce extreme psychosocial disability.

perivascular infiltrates of mononuclear cells plus panniculitis, manifested as hyaline fat necrosis with mononuclear cell infiltration and lymphocytic vasculitis. The nodules usually appear on the scalp, face, arms, chest, back, thighs, and buttocks; ulcerations are uncommon, and they usually resolve leaving a depressed area. Some patients with lupus profundus exhibit no other manifestations of SLE. Tumid lupus, a rare variant, is characterized by photodistributed lesions with chronic pink-to-violaceous papules, nonscarring plaques, and nodules.

Alopecia

Hair loss occurs in most patients with lupus and in some cases can precede other manifestations of SLE.[28] Lupus alopecia may involve the scalp, eyebrows, eyelashes, beard, and body hair. Scarring alopecia is a complication of DLE that typically affects the scalp. Lupus hair is characterized by thin hair that easily fractures, usually occurs along the frontal hairline, is associated with disease activity, and grows back normally as the disease subsides.

Photosensitivity

Photosensitivity refers to the development of a rash after exposure to ultraviolet B (UVB) radiation found in sunlight or fluorescent lights. It occurs in 60% to 100% of patients with SLE. Some patients also are sensitive to UVA radiation (emitted from photocopiers) and rarely may even be sensitive to the visible light spectrum. Not all photosensitive individuals have SLE, and the two disorders are not causally linked in every patient with SLE. Acute, subacute, and DLE lesions and some bullous and urticarial lesions are photosensitive. The severity of cutaneous reaction depends on the intensity of the UV source and the duration of exposure. Although the exact mechanism by which UV radiation causes skin lesions is unknown, it may be related to

the enhanced apoptosis of keratinocytes that leads to the exposure of autoantigens and the production of proinflammatory cytokines and other immune mediators by keratinocytes and Langerhans cells.[29,30]

Differential Diagnosis

Several dermatologic entities can simulate the appearance of lupus-specific lesions and should be considered in patients with atypical features or refractoriness to standard therapy or both. Acne rosasea can result in a red face and is often confused with acute cutaneous lupus erythematosus. Photosensitive psoriasis can simulate papulosquamous SCLE, whereas occasionally erythema multiforme may be confused with annular SCLE. Finally, other common dermatoses that are not related to SLE may be found in SLE patients, such as contact dermatitis, eczema, and seborrheic dermatitis.

Mucous Membranes

Involvement of the mucous membranes occurs in 25% to 45% of patients with SLE.[31] The most common manifestations include irregularly shaped, raised, white plaques; areas of erythema; silvery white scarred lesions; and ulcers with surrounding erythema on the soft or hard palate or buccal mucosa.[32] These lesions should be distinguished clinically from lichen planus, candidiasis, aphthous stomatitis, intraoral herpes, Behçet syndrome (also known as Adamantiades-Behçet syndrome), bite marks, leukoplakia, and malignancy. The oral ulcers in SLE are usually painless, and sometimes there is no apparent association between their presence and systemic disease activity. Oral lesions may be the first signs of SLE. Characteristic discoid lesions with erythema, atrophy, and depigmentation can occur on the lips. Nasal ulcers have been noted in patients with SLE. They usually are found in the lower nasal septum, tend to be bilateral, and are associated with active disease. Nasal septum perforation has been reported in 4% of SLE patients and is secondary to vasculitis.[33] Involvement of the upper airway mucosa also can occur and cause hoarseness.

Pathology

Biopsy specimens of skin lesions from patients with DLE and SLE contain the membrane attack complex, which comprises C5b through C9, and immune complexes at the dermal-epidermal junction.[34] The basilar epithelium in these areas is vacuolated and edematous, and the dermis contains an inflammatory infiltrate. In contrast, 19 of 29 specimens of normal-appearing skin from patients with DLE or SLE showed only immune complexes at the dermal-epidermal junction, without the membrane attack complex. The other 10 specimens, all from patients without cutaneous involvement, showed neither immune complexes nor membrane attack complexes. These data suggest that immune complexes within skin lesions selectively generate the assembly of the membrane attack complex, which mediates membrane injury. A synergistic interaction of immune complexes and cofactors may be required to activate complement in areas of skin that are predisposed to tissue injury.[34]

The search for immunoreactant deposition in nonlesional skin of SLE patients has been referred to as the "lupus band test." The diagnostic and prognostic significance of the nonlesional lupus band test is controversial. The following issues should be taken into account when interpreting a nonlesional lupus band test: The biopsy specimen should be taken from a non–sun-exposed area because a lupus band test is positive in 20% of sun-exposed areas of normal individuals[35]; the diagnostic specificity for SLE is very high when three or more immunoglobulin or complement components are identified.[36] Under these conditions, a positive nonlesional LBT can serve as a useful piece of information in cases with atypical clinical and laboratory manifestations of SLE.

MUSCULOSKELETAL INVOLVEMENT

The musculoskeletal system is the most commonly involved system in SLE, affecting 53% to 95% of patients.

Arthritis and Arthropathy

Joint involvement in SLE is classically described as nonerosive, nondeforming arthralgias and arthritis in a distribution similar to that of rheumatoid arthritis, primarily affecting the small joints of the hands, wrists, and knees (Fig. 75-4). It may be the presenting symptom of SLE or accompany other manifestations during a flare of the disease. A study of hand arthritis in SLE found deforming arthritis in only 17 of 176 patients. The authors described three patterns of deforming arthritis in SLE: a deforming and typically nonerosive arthropathy known as Jaccoud's arthritis (8 of 17), an erosive arthropathy (3 of 17), and a mild deforming arthropathy (6 of 17).[37]

Patients' symptoms (pain and stiffness) are usually out of proportion to the degree of synovitis present on physical examination, and synovitis may be transient (resolving within a few days in some patients), migratory, and reversible.[38] At the other extreme are a few patients with an impressive synovitis indistinguishable from rheumatoid

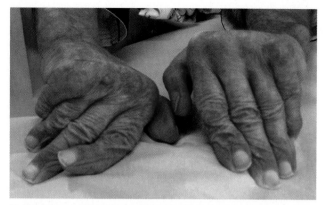

Figure 75-4 Jacoud-type arthropathy. Deformities in the hands, such as ulnar drift at the metacarpophalangeal joints, swan-neck and boutonnière deformities, and hyperextension at the interphalangeal joint of the thumb, closely resemble the deformities seen in rheumatoid arthritis. The absence of erosions on radiographs and their reducibility distinguish this condition from the deforming arthritis of rheumatoid arthritis. *(Courtesy of Dr. D. Vassilopoulos.)*

arthritis, for whom the term "rhupus" has been coined.[39] Radiologic features in lupus hand arthritis include scapholunate dissociation, joint space narrowing, cystic change, and palmar/ulnar subluxation in the wrist. In the fingers, metacarpophalangeal hook erosions, metacarpophalangeal subluxation, and cystic changes are the most common features, but marginal erosions are rare. With the use of more sensitive imaging techniques, such as high-resolution ultrasound combined with power Doppler, wrist synovial hypertrophy and effusion were detected in 16 (94%) of 17 patients with SLE hand arthritis. Eight patients (47%) had erosions at the second and third metacarpophalangeal joints, which were not detectable by simple x-rays in three of them. Eleven patients (65%) had evidence of tenosynovitis, with detectable power Doppler signal in half of them.[40]

Tenosynovitis is an early manifestation of SLE, and tendon rupture syndromes have been reported in many different sites in the body, including the patellar tendons, the Achilles tendon, the long head of the biceps, the triceps, and the extensor tendons of the hands.[41,42] Tendon rupture has been associated with male gender, trauma, oral and intra-articular steroid use, and long disease duration.[43] Flexure tendon contractures of the elbow also have been reported.[44] Synovitis can induce the carpal tunnel syndrome, which may be the initial manifestation of SLE or drug-induced lupus (DIL).[45] Although septic arthritis is uncommon in SLE, it should be suspected when one joint is inflamed out of proportion to all others. Aspiration and culture of the synovial fluid are essential to rule out infection in this case. Subcutaneous nodules along the flexor tendons of the hand can be found in SLE. The histologic appearance is similar to that of rheumatoid nodules.[46] Periarticular calcification has been reported in the small joints of the hand, whereas soft tissue calcification is rarely seen in SLE.[47,48]

Myositis

Generalized myalgia and muscle tenderness are common, especially during disease exacerbations. Inflammatory myositis involving the proximal muscles has been reported to occur in 5% to 11% of patients and may develop at any time during the course of the disease.[49,50] The differential diagnosis of proximal muscle weakness in SLE includes a drug-related myopathy secondary to corticosteroid, antimalarial, or statin medications use. Concurrent hypothyroidsm also can cause an increase in creatine phosphokinase and proximal myopathy. Muscle biopsy, electromyographic studies, and elevation of the serum creatine phosphokinase or aldolase levels help to differentiate between inflammatory and drug-related myopathy.

The histologic features of myositis in SLE may be less striking than in idiopathic polymyositis. Histologic features include muscle atrophy, microtubular inclusions, and a mononuclear cell infiltrate. Fiber necrosis is an uncommon finding, but immunoglobulin deposition is almost always present despite the rarity of concurrent inflammation.[51-53] A low serum creatine phosphokinase value can be found in patients with connective tissue disease including SLE; a normal creatine phosphokinase value in the presence of symptoms and signs of myositis should not dissuade the physician from a diagnosis of myopathy. The skin lesions of dermatomyositis also can appear in patients with SLE. Chest pain or discomfort secondary to costochondritis has been reported in SLE, and other conditions, such as angina pectoris, pericarditis, and esophageal spasm, must be ruled out first. Relapsing polychondritis also has been described in patients with SLE and in most cases responds to low-dose corticosteroid treatment.[54,55]

Avascular Bone Necrosis

Avascular necrosis of bone is a major cause of significant morbidity and disability in patients with SLE. Symptomatic avascular necrosis occurs in 5% to 12% of SLE patients. Higher prevalences have been reported in series that used MRI for its detection.[56] Acute joint pain manifesting late in the course of SLE and localized to a very few areas, especially shoulders, hips, and knees, may indicate the development of avascular necrosis. The initial pathologic lesion that leads to osteonecrosis begins by interruption of the blood supply to the bone followed by reactive hyperemia of the adjacent bone resulting in demineralization, trabecular thinning, and finally collapse if stressed. In SLE, factors that can induce ischemia leading to bone necrosis include Raynaud's phenomenon, vasculitis, fat emboli, corticosteroids, and antiphospholipid antibody syndrome (APS). A large study of 744 patients followed for an average of 25 years found that only the presence of arthritis and the use of corticosteroids or cytotoxic medications or both are independent risk factors for development of avascular necrosis in patients with SLE.[57] Osteonecrosis often develops a short time after the onset of corticosteroid therapy, within 1 month in some patients who receive high doses.[58-61]

RENAL INVOLVEMENT

Renal involvement is a major cause of morbidity and hospital admissions in SLE patients and occurs in 40% to 70% of all patients. Generally, renal involvement tends to occur within the first 2 years of SLE with its frequency decreasing significantly after the first 5 years of disease. The disease displays a remarkable clinical and histologic heterogeneity (see later). Almost half of patients present with asymptomatic urine abnormalities, such as hematuria and proteinuria. Nephrotic or nephritic syndrome or both also may be observed in 30% of patients. Rarely (<5%), patients may present with chronic renal insufficiency, rapidly progressive glomerulonephritis, or a pulmonary-renal vasculitis syndrome.

Immunopathology

Immune complex formation and deposition in the kidney results in intraglomerular inflammation with recruitment of leukocytes and activation and proliferation of resident renal cells.[62] A plethora of humoral and cellular elements contributes to glomerular injury. Intense inflammation may destroy resident renal cells by necrosis or apoptosis, resulting in fibrinoid necrosis. In a few patients, intense capillary inflammation results in rupture of the capillary wall and the capsule itself with epithelial cells, mononuclear cells, fibrin basement membrane material, and collagen accumulating in the urinary space of the glomerulus (crescentic glomerulonephritis). When injury is less intense, endocapillary cells respond by proliferating and producing extracellular matrix (proliferative lesions). Extreme injury or protracted inflammation activates a final common pathway of all types of glomerular injury, resulting in atrophy and scarring.

In lupus nephritis, the location of immune complex deposition and formation is closely linked to histopathology and the intensity of the inflammatory response. Deposition of immune complexes in the mesangium is characteristic of mesangial lupus nephritis. Immune complex deposition in the subendothelial area of the capillary loops results in proliferative lupus nephritis (focal or diffuse) with exuberant glomerular hypercellularity. This hypercellularity is due to proliferation of mesangial and endothelial cells and leukocytic infiltrates, resulting in compromised capillary flow and renal function. Epimembranous (subepithelial) deposits along peripheral glomerular capillary loops that are diffusely thickened and the lack of inflammatory infiltrate are characteristic of membranous nephropathy.

The standard 1982 World Health Organization classification has been revised to provide a clearer and unequivocal description of various lesions and classes of lupus nephritis (Table 75-5).[63] In several studies of lupus nephritis, type IV nephritis is the most common (approximately 40%), whereas type III and type V follow with an approximate frequency of 25% and 15%. Transformation from one class to another can occur, spontaneously and as a result of treatment. Prognosis is worse when membranous and proliferative changes coexist.[62]

Laboratory Findings

Proteinuria of various levels is the dominant feature of lupus nephritis and is usually accompanied by glomerular hematuria.[64] Nephritic syndrome accounts for an additional 30% to 40% of patients; rapidly progressive glomerulonephritis is rare and accounts for less than 10% of the initial presentations. Generally, untreated patients with mesangial nephritis have small amounts of proteinuria (<1 g/day) with hematuria, but typically no cellular casts. Patients with membranous glomerulopathy have proteinuria often at nephrotic range, but otherwise unremarkable urine sediments.

Table 75-5 Histologic Classification of Lupus Nephritis According to the International Society of Nephrology/Renal Pathology Society, 2003

WHO Type	
Class I	*Minimal mesangial lupus nephritis* Normal glomeruli by light microscopy, but mesangial immune deposits by immunofluorescence
Class II	*Mesangial proliferative nephritis* Purely mesangial hypercellularity of any degree or mesangial matrix expansion by light microscopy, with mesangial immune deposits Few isolated subepithelial or subendothelial deposits may be visible by immunofluorescence or electron microscopy, but not by light microscopy
Class III	*Focal lupus nephritis* Active or inactive focal, segmental, or global endocapillary or extracapillary glomerulonephritis involving <50% of all glomeruli, typically with focal subendothelial immune deposits, with or without mesangial alterations
Class IV	*Diffuse lupus nephritis* Active or inactive diffuse, segmental, or global endocapillary or extracapillary glomerulonephritis involving ≥50% of all glomeruli, typically with diffuse subendothelial immune deposits, with or without mesangial alterations. This class is subdivided into *diffuse segmental (IV-S)* lupus nephritis when ≥50% of the involved glomeruli have segmental lesions, and *diffuse global (IV-G)* lupus nephritis when ≥50% of the involved glomeruli have global lesions. Segmental is defined as a glomerular lesion that involves less than half of the glomerular tuft. This class includes cases with diffuse wire loop deposits, but with little or no glomerular proliferation
Class V	*Membranous lupus nephritis* Global or segmental subepithelial immune deposits or their morphologic sequelae by light microscopy and by immunofluorescence or electron microscopy, with or without mesangial alterations Class V nephritis may occur in combination with class III or class IV, in which case both are diagnosed Class V nephritis may show advanced sclerotic lesions
Class VI	*Advanced sclerotic lupus nephritis* ≥90% of glomeruli globally sclerosed without residual activity

WHO, World Health Organization.
Adapted from Weening JJ, et al: The classification of glomerulonephritis in systemic lupus erythematosus revisited. J Am Soc Nephrol 15:241, 2004.

C3 tends to be normal, and anti-DNA antibodies when present are usually found in low titers. In contrast, patients with proliferative nephritis have hypertension, a nephritic urine sediment with various degrees of proteinuria (often at nephrotic range), low C3, and typically high titers of anti-DNA antibodies. The clinical presentation does not always predict the underlying histologic class of nephritis. In patients who have been previously treated with steroids, the findings in the urinalysis may be more subtle than previously, creating a sense of false security. In these cases, a high index of suspicion is crucial.

Urinalysis

Urinalysis is the most important and effective method to detect and monitor disease activity in lupus nephritis.[64] To ensure quality, several steps have to be taken, including expeditious examination of a fresh, early morning, midstream, clean-catch, nonrefrigerated specimen and flagging of specimens from patients at substantial risk to develop nephritis to ensure careful examination at central laboratories. Hematuria (usually microscopic, rarely macroscopic) indicates inflammatory glomerular or tubulointerstitial disease. Erythrocytes are fragmented or misshapen (dysmorphic). Granular and fatty casts reflect proteinuric states, whereas red blood cell, white blood cell, and mixed cellular casts reflect nephritic states (Fig. 75-5). Broad and waxy casts reflect chronic renal failure. In severe proliferative disease, urine sediment containing the full range of cells and casts can be found ("telescopic urine sediment") as a result of severe glomerular and tubular ongoing disease superimposed on chronic renal damage.

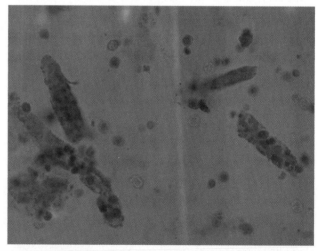

Figure 75-5 Urinary specimen in active lupus nephritis. Urinalysis is the most useful test to monitor for renal involvement and relapses after remission in lupus patients. Dysmorphic urinary red blood cells (RBCs) are seen in the urine of a patient with active glomerulonephritis and an active urine sediment. Note the fragmented RBCs and the abnormal sizes and shapes of most of them. The proteinacious matrix of this cellular cast in the middle of the figure contains RBCs. (*Courtesy of Dr. D. Vassilopoulos.*)

Renal Biopsy

Indications. Renal biopsy rarely helps in the diagnosis of SLE, but is the best way of documenting the renal pathology. In the absence of renal abnormalities, renal biopsy has nothing to offer and should not be done. Standard indications for renal biopsy before treatment include (1) nephritic urine sediment (glomerular hematuria and cellular casts); (2) glomerular hematuria with proteinuria greater than 0.5 to 1 g/day; (3) glomerular hematuria with proteinuria less than 0.3 to 0.5 g/day, and low C3 or positive anti–double-stranded DNA (dsDNA); and (4) proteinuria greater than 1 to 2 g/day (especially if C3 is low or anti-dsDNA antibodies are present or both).

Selected patients with clinical and laboratory evidence of severe lupus nephritis, nephritic or nephrotic syndrome, azotemia, and hypertension may not require a renal biopsy before treatment with cytotoxic drugs. Patients with concomitant serologic abnormalities (i.e., low C3, positive anti-dsDNA) or patients who had previous immunosuppressive treatment may be candidates for renal biopsy even with more subtle findings. Studies have suggested (and experience supports) that patients and physicians are more willing to decide on aggressive therapies when faced with a renal biopsy specimen indicating severe renal involvement; this translates into earlier institution of cytotoxic therapy and better renal outcomes.[65] The decision for repeat biopsy is more complex and should be considered in cases of (1) unexplained worsening proteinuria (e.g., >2 g/day increase if non-nephrotic at baseline or >50% increase if nephrotic), (2) unexplained worsening of renal function (e.g., reproducible 30% increase in serum creatinine), (3) persistent glomerular hematuria with proteinuria greater than 2 g/day or proteinuria greater than 3 g/day (especially if C3 is decreased), and (4) nephritic or nephrotic flare.

Evaluation and Interpretation of Renal Biopsy Specimen. Evaluation of the renal biopsy specimen is of paramount importance and typically includes light microscopy, immunofluorescence, and electron microscopy (Figs. 75-6 and 75-7).[62] Evaluation of specimens with less than 10 glomeruli is suboptimal. Light microscopy stains commonly used include hematoxylin and eosin (best to identify inflammatory cells), Masson trichrome (best for interstitial fibrosis and glomerulosclerosis), and periodic acid–Schiff (best

for basement membrane abnormalities). Immunofluorescence studies do not help if the diagnosis of SLE is established. In SLE, the "pan-house" staining is usually observed with numerous deposits of immunoglobulins and complement. Electron microscopy helps to define distribution (i.e., subendothelial, epithelial, membranous deposits) of immune complexes and may be useful in the recognition of early proliferative changes when the light microscopy findings may be more subtle. In such cases, the presence of subendothelial deposits—even if scarce—may help guide treatment, especially in the presence of other features of proliferative nephritis (nephritic sediment, low C3, anti-DNA antibodies).

Activity and chronicity indices are useful in the renal biopsy report as a complement to the World Health Organization classification. In the activity index, a variety of lesions are scored 0 to 3+ with a maximum score of 24 points. This index includes features suggesting active inflammation such as proliferative changes, necrosis/karyorrhexis, cellular crescents, leukocyte infiltration, hyaline thrombi, and interstitial inflammation. In the chronicity index, lesions are scored 0 to 3+ with a maximum score of 12 points. This index includes chronic, irreversible features such as sclerotic glomeruli, fibrous crescents, tubular atrophy, and interstitial fibrosis.

In our experience, the most important elements to recognize and consider in a renal biopsy specimen are (1) the presence of crescents, fibrinoid necrosis, or a high activity index (e.g., >9) and (2) interstitial fibrosis, tubular atrophy, glomerular sclerosis, or moderate-to-high chronicity scores (e.g., >3). Their presence denotes severe disease with an ominous prognosis unless treated aggressively (Fig. 75-7).

Monitoring of Lupus Nephritis

Renal Function. Serum creatinine is a practical, but insensitive, early indicator of abnormalities in glomerular filtration rate. Its absolute level is affected by muscle mass and age in addition to glomerular filtration rate. In clinical practice,

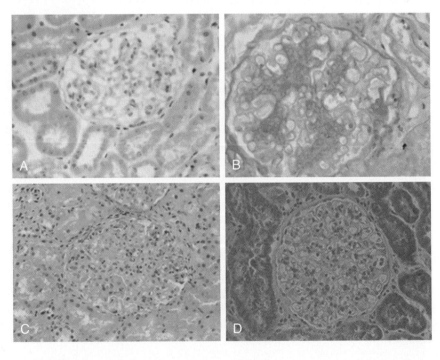

Figure 75-6 World Health Organization types of lupus nephritis (see Table 75-5 for a detailed description of histologic findings). **A,** Normal glomerulus (type I). **B,** Mesangial disease (type II). Note mesangial hypercellularity and expansion of the mesangial matrix, which does not compromise the capillary loops. **C,** Proliferative nephritis. Dramatic increase in mesangial and endocapillary cellularity produce a lobular appearance of the glomerular tufts and compromise the patency of most capillary loops. When less than 50% of glomeruli are involved, nephritis is denoted as focal (type III). When more than 50% of glomeruli are involved, nephritis is denoted as diffuse (type IV). **D,** Membranous nephropathy (type V). In membranous lupus nephropathy, the capillary walls of the glomerular tuft are prominent and widely patent, resembling "stiff" structures with decreased compliance.

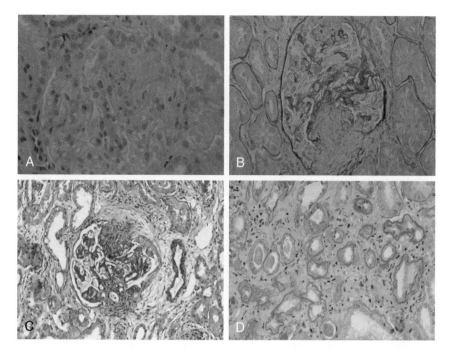

Figure 75-7 High-risk histologic features suggesting severe nephritis. **A,** Fibrinoid necrosis with karyorrhexis in a patient with focal proliferative glomerulonephritis. **B** and **C,** Cellular crescents with layers of proliferative endothelial cells and monocytes lining Bowman's capsule along with a predominantly mononuclear interstitial infiltrate. **D,** Severe interstitial fibrosis and tubular atrophy. Note the thickening of the tubular basement membranes and tubular epithelial degeneration with separation of residual tubules owing to deposition of collagenous connective tissue among tubules.

detecting changes in renal function is more important than the absolute level. Creatinine clearance has several shortcomings in estimating changes in function, the most important of which is overestimation of true glomerular filtration rate with declining renal function. Serum creatinine is a more practical approach for detecting changes in the glomerular filtration rate and is the examination of choice. Significant reproducible changes in serum creatinine (e.g., 20% to 30% increase) are of concern—even if they fall within the normal range—because they indicate significant loss of renal function.[64] Serum cystatin C may be a more sensitive and specific biomarker for renal function and glomerular filtration rate, but its role in monitoring patients with lupus nephritis has not been studied.

Urine Collection. Two or three timed collections of urine to determine 24-hour protein excretion and baseline creatinine clearance is the "gold standard." We obtain urine samples before therapy and periodically thereafter before decisions regarding assessing response and changes in therapy. Urine samples containing creatinine concentrations that deviate significantly from population averages for men (20 mg/kg/day) or women (15 mg/kg/day) should raise suspicions about the adequacy of the urine collection. Spot urine protein/creatinine is a simpler method to estimate the severity of proteinuria and could be used in between 24-hour collections to provide (together with serum albumin and cholesterol levels) rough estimates of the response of proteinuria to therapy. The numeric ratio generally approaches the number of grams per day of proteinuria. If the ratio is 3.4, the 24-hour protein excretion is approximately 3.4 g/day.[64]

Urinalysis. Resolution of active urine sediment is a feature of renal remission, but to be clinically meaningful, it has to be sustained for several months. Reappearance of cellular casts with significant proteinuria is an early and reliable

predictor of renal relapse and in most patients usually precedes increases in anti-DNA titers or decreases in C3 by several weeks.[66]

Serology. Anti-DNA antibodies and C3 and C4 complement components are useful in monitoring activity of lupus nephritis and in guiding treatment. Generally, changes in anti-DNA titers are more valuable than their absolute values. Patients with rising titers of anti-DNA antibodies warrant close monitoring for evidence of lupus activity. Because C4 deficiency is common in patients with lupus nephritis and C3 levels correlate best with renal histology on repeat renal biopsy specimens, C3 is the preferred choice for monitoring disease activity.

Assessment of Prognosis and Risk Stratification

Prognosis varies greatly among the many clinical and pathologic forms of lupus nephritis and has important implications for treatment decisions. Numerous demographic and clinical variables can affect prognosis, and individual patients have unique combinations of such risk factors. Although individual risk factors are extremely heterogeneous and vary in their overall impact, patients with the largest number of risk factors carry a worse prognosis, are less likely to respond to therapy, tend to respond more slowly, and need more aggressive treatment.

Patient characteristics associated with bad outcomes include African-American race, azotemia, anemia, APS, failure to respond to initial immunosuppressive therapy, and flares with worsening in renal function.[67-70] Combinations of severe active (crescents and fibrinoid necrosis) with marked chronic changes (moderate-to-severe tubulointerstitial fibrosis and tubular atrophy, e.g., chronicity index >3) are particularly ominous. The impact of race in determining severity of disease, response to treatment, and final outcome is becoming increasingly apparent. Significant differences in

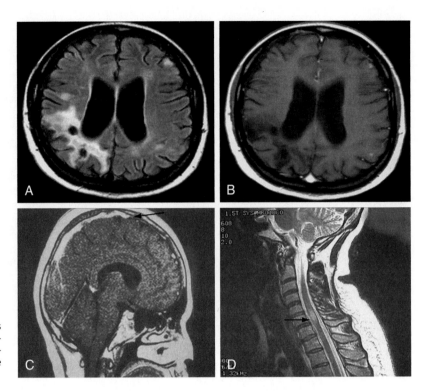

Figure 75-8 Severe neuropsychiatric systemic lupus erythematosus. **A-D,** MRI showing cerebrovascular disease (**A** and **B**), thrombosis in the sagittal sinus in a patient with antiphospholipid antibodies (**C**), and acute transverse myelitis (**D**).

these risk factors may explain the marked heterogeneity in course, prognosis, and treatment responses in randomized controlled studies around the world.

NERVOUS SYSTEM INVOLVEMENT

SLE affects the CNS and the peripheral nervous system. Nervous system involvement in SLE is a major cause of morbidity and mortality. Nervous system involvement in SLE is the least understood manifestation of the disease and remains a complex diagnostic entity as a result of its multiple clinical presentations (Fig. 75-8). The ACR described case definitions and classification criteria for 19 CNS and peripheral nervous system syndromes that have been observed in patients with SLE, which collectively are referred to as neuropsychiatric systemic lupus erythematosus (NPSLE) syndromes (Table 75-6).[71] Approximately 40% of the NPSLE manifestations develop before the onset of SLE or at the time of diagnosis, and 63% develop within the first year after the diagnosis.[72] Table 75-7 shows an approach to the management of neuropsychiatric symptoms and findings in SLE.

The prevalence of specific NPSLE syndromes varied widely in the literature before the introduction of the ACR criteria for NPSLE, with estimates of the overall prevalence ranging from 14% to 75%.[73] The plethora of neuropsychiatric manifestations reported in SLE points to multiple pathogenic mechanisms. Neuropsychiatric events in SLE may be caused by a primary manifestation of the disease; secondary complications of the disease or therapy, such as hypertension, infection, or drug-induced aseptic meningitis, especially with nonsteroidal anti-inflammatory drugs (NSAIDs); or a coincidental problem unrelated to SLE. Vascular abnormalities, autoantibodies, and inflammatory mediators have been reported to play significant pathogenic roles in the development of NPSLE. A bland non-inflammatory vasculopathy involving small vessels was the

Table 75-6   Neuropsychiatric Syndromes in Systemic Lupus Erythematosus

Central Nervous System
Aseptic meningitis
Cerebrovascular disease
Demyelinating syndrome
Headache (including migraine and benign intracranial hypertension)
Movement disorder (chorea)
Myelopathy
Seizure disorder
Acute confusional state
Anxiety disorder
Cognitive dysfunction
Mood disorder
Psychosis

Peripheral Nervous System
Acute inflammatory demyelinating polyradiculoneuropathy (Guillain-Barré syndrome)
Autonomic disorder
Mononeuropathy, single/multiplex
Myasthenia gravis
Neuropathy, cranial
Plexopathy
Polyneuropathy

Adapted from The American College of Rheumatology nomenclature and case definitions for neuropsychiatric lupus syndrome. Arthritis Rheum 42:599, 1999.

predominant finding in neuropathologic autopsy studies.[74] In the same study, vasculitis of small and large vessels was rare, and brain microinfarcts occurred in association with microangiopathy.

A variety of autoantibodies has been associated with the pathogenesis of different manifestations of NPSLE. Autoantibodies include, among others, antineuronal antibodies,[75] antiganglioside antibodies,[76,77] anti-NR2 glutamate receptor antibodies,[78] anti-DNA antibodies,[79] antiribosomal (P) antibodies,[80,81] anti-β_2-glycoprotein I antibodies, antiprothrombin antibodies,[82] and lupus anticoagulants.[83] Increased intracranial and intrathecal levels of cytokines, such as interleukin-6, interferon-α, interleukin-10, interleukin-8, and tumor necrosis factor-α, have been associated with seizures and psychosis.[84-87]

Cognitive dysfunction has been reported in 80% of SLE patients.[88] The association between SLE and headache is controversial. Psychosis is reported in 8% of SLE patients and is characterized by the presence of either delusions or hallucinations.[88-92] The latter are most frequently auditory.

Table 75-7 Approach to the Management of Neuropsychiatric Symptoms in Systemic Lupus Erythematosus

Diffuse or focal process? Classify symptoms (see Table 75-6)
Primary or secondary?
Evidence for generalized lupus activity? If yes, probably related to lupus
Exclude nonlupus-related causes (e.g., infections, drugs, electrolyte abnormalities, hypoxia)
Recent evolving or old, inactive process?
Thrombotic or inflammatory process?
Inflammatory
Generalized lupus activity (clinical or serologic)
High-grade abnormalities in lumbar puncture (i.e., protein, cells)
MRI findings suggestive of cerebritis or myelitis
Thrombotic
Antiphospholipid antibodies or stigmata for APS
MRI findings suggestive of thrombosis
Severe inflammatory disease?
Myelitis, cerebritis, coma, status epilepticus, large (or multiple) cerebrovascular accident, mononeuritis multiplex, severe psychosis, catatonia
Consider cytotoxic therapy

APS, antiphospholipid antibody syndrome; MRI, magnetic resonance imaging.

When psychosis is present, it must be distinguished from other causes, including drug abuse, schizophrenia, and depression. Generalized and focal seizures are reported in 6% to 51% of patients and may occur either in the setting of active generalized multisystem SLE or as isolated neurologic events. Seizures frequently are associated with the presence of antiphospholipid antibodies, which are associated with microangiopathy, arterial thrombosis, and subsequent cerebral infarction. Demyelination, transverse myelopathy, and chorea are rare manifestations of NPSLE and occur in 1% to 3% of patients. Clinical and neuroimaging evidence of demyelination may be indistinguishable from multiple sclerosis.[93] Transverse myelopathy and chorea manifest acutely and often are associated with the presence of antiphospholipid antibodies (see Fig. 75-8).[94,95] A peripheral sensorimotor neuropathy has been reported in 28% of SLE patients and may occur independently of other disease characteristics.[96]

CARDIOVASCULAR INVOLVEMENT

A variety of cardiac manifestations can be seen in SLE, with pericarditis being the most common and found in approximately one quarter of the patients. Pericardial effusions may be asymptomatic and are usually mild to moderate. Tamponade is rare, but can occur. Myocardial involvement is rare (<5% of patients) and typically occurs in the presence of generalized SLE activity. Clinical features of left ventricular dysfunction, nonspecific ST/T wave changes, segmental wall motion abnormalities, and decreased ejection fraction are found in greater than 80% of patients. MRI has been used to detect clinical and subclinical myocardial involvement in SLE (Fig. 75-9). Patients may present with fever, dyspnea, tachycardia, and congestive heart failure. Patients with SLE have substantially increased morbidity

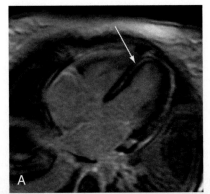

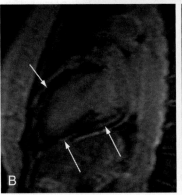
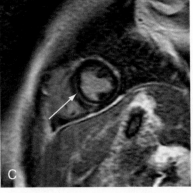

Figure 75-9 Lupus myocarditis. MRI shows enhancement of the myocardium, which spares the endocardium. **A-C,** Contrast-enhanced inversion recovery technique with late imaging after contrast administration in horizontal long-axis plane (**A**), vertical long-axis plane (**B**), and short-axis plane (**C**). Strong enhancement is found in the midwall of the ventricular septum (**A** and **C**), in the apex (**A**), and in the mid-anterior and posterior wall (**B**).

and mortality from cardiovascular disease.[97-99] Morbidity includes accelerated, premature atherosclerosis and valvular heart disease.

Cardiovascular disease and atherosclerosis are a common cause of morbidity and mortality in various SLE cohorts. Autopsy studies from the early 1980s showed severe atherosclerosis in 40% of SLE patients compared with 2% of control subjects, matched for age at the time of death.[100] Analysis of the Swedish Hospital Discharge Register followed by linkage to the Cause of Death Register during the period 1964 to 1995 showed that SLE patients were at increased risk for death as a result of coronary heart disease or stroke (standardized mortality ratio 2.97, 95% confidence interval 2.78 to 3.16).[101] The risk was substantially higher in the younger group of patients (20 to 39 years old; standardized mortality ratio 16, 95% confidence interval 10.4 to 23.6).

Other studies have shown that SLE patients carry an increased risk for myocardial infarction or stroke compared with the healthy population. This risk cannot be fully explained by the traditional cardiovascular disease risk factors.[98,102-104] Atherosclerosis—defined by coronary artery calcification or carotid plaque size—also is more common in SLE patients than in healthy controls (e.g., 31% versus 9%, in subjects with an average age of 40; relative risk 9.8, 95% confidence interval 2.5 to 39), even after adjustment for possible confounding factors, and it correlates with disease activity and damage scores.[105,106]

Valvular Heart Disease

Valvular heart disease is common in patients with SLE. In a prospective study evaluating 69 SLE patients and 56 healthy controls with transesophageal echocardiograms over 2 years, the prevalence of valvular heart disease was 61% in SLE patients compared with 9% of the controls.[107] The most common abnormality was diffuse thickening of the mitral and aortic valves followed by vegetations, valvular regurgitation, and stenosis in decreasing order of frequency. Valvular abnormalities frequently resolved, appeared for the first time, or persisted but changed in appearance or size between the two studies. Mild or moderate valvular regurgitation did not progress to become severe, and new stenoses did not develop. Neither the presence of valvular disease nor changes in the echocardiographic findings were temporally related to the duration, activity, or severity of SLE or to its treatment.

The combined incidence of stroke, peripheral embolism, heart failure, infective endocarditis, and the need for valve replacement was 22% in patients with valvular disease and 8% in patients without valvular disease. Several pathologic studies of SLE patients have shown active and healed valvulitis and active Libman-Sacks vegetations with acute thrombus, healed vegetations with or without hyalinized thrombus, or active and healed vegetations, in the same or different valves. Thrombotic vegetations secondary to a hypercoagulable state also have been shown in patients with lupus.[108-111] These vegetations cannot be clearly differentiated from Libman-Sacks vegetations on echocardiography.[112,113] Valvular vegetations can embolize, which may result in a change in their appearance or resolution.[109,110,114,115] Acute and subacute bacterial endocarditis may occur on previously involved valves (see later).

Pleura and Lungs

The most common pleuropulmonary manifestation of SLE is pleuritis (Table 75-8). Pleuritic pain is present in 45% to 60% of patients and may occur with or without a pleural effusion.[116,117] Clinically apparent pleural effusions have been reported in 50% of patients with SLE and may be found in 93% of cases at autopsy. Effusions are usually bilateral, but may be unilateral, equally distributed between the left and the right hemithoraces. Pleural effusions in SLE are invariably exudative, but with higher glucose and lower lactate dehydrogenase levels than those found in rheumatoid arthritis.[118] Pleural biopsy findings are nonspecific and include lymphocytic and plasma cell infiltration, fibrosis, and fibrinous pleuritis. Thoracoscopy has revealed nodules on the visceral pleura, and immunofluorescence of biopsy samples of these nodules revealed immunoglobulin deposits.[119]

Clinically significant interstitial lung disease complicates SLE in 3% to 13% of patients, but is rarely severe.[116,120] Asymptomatic involvement is more common, and abnormalities in pulmonary function tests have been reported in two

Table 75-8 Pleuropulmonary Manifestations of Systemic Lupus Erythematosus

Pleuropulmonary Manifestation	Common
Pleuritic chest pain or pleurisy	Common, with or without effusion or friction rub
Pleural effusion	Exudate; unilateral or bilateral
Acute pneumonitis	Not common; presentation includes fever, nonproductive cough, infiltrates, hypoxia; high mortality rates
Interstitial lung disease	Insidious onset of dyspnea on exertion, nonproductive cough, pleuritic chest pain
Bronchiolitis obliterans with organizing pneumonia	Can be difficult to diagnose; requires biopsy; responds to corticosteroids
Pulmonary capillaritis or diffuse alveolar hemorrhage	Rare, associated with antiphospholipid antibodies; poor prognosis
Shrinking-lung syndrome	Occurs in patients with long-standing SLE; diaphragmatic weakness possible cause
Pulmonary embolism or infarction	Common in patients with antiphospholipid antibodies
Pulmonary hypertension	Insidious onset of dyspnea on exertion, chronic fatigue, weakness, palpitations, edema
Lymphadenopathy	Massive mediastinal lymphadenopathy uncommon in patients with SLE alone; cervical and auxillary lymphadenopathy common, correlates with disease activity
Infection	Typical and atypical pathogens; caused by immune dysfunction and immunosuppressive medications
Malignant tumor	Lung cancer; lymphoma more common in SLE

SLE, systemic lupus erythematosus.

thirds of patients with SLE in some studies.[116] Abnormalities in high-resolution CT have been reported in 70% of patients with SLE.[121] Symptomatic interstitial lung disease is rarely an early or dominant feature of SLE, and severe pulmonary fibrosis is extremely rare. Histologic features of interstitial lung disease complicating SLE are nonspecific and include varying degrees of chronic inflammatory cell infiltrates, peribronchial lymphoid hyperplasia, interstitial fibrosis, and hyperplasia of type II pneumocytes.[116] The presence of Raynaud's phenomenon, swollen fingers, sclerodactyly, telangiectasia, and nail-fold capillary abnormalities among patients with SLE was associated with a higher prevalence of restrictive defects and decreased diffusing capacity.[122]

Acute lupus pneumonitis manifesting as cough, dyspnea, pleuritic pain, hypoxemia, and fever occurs in 1% to 4% of patients with SLE. Chest radiographs reveal infiltrates, which may be unilateral or bilateral. Histologic features are nonspecific and include alveolar wall damage and necrosis, inflammatory cell infiltration, edema, hemorrhage, and hyaline membranes. A microangiitis involving capillaries, with fibrin thrombi and infiltration with necrotic neutrophils, may be present.[123]

Pulmonary hemorrhage is a rare but potentially catastrophic complication of SLE. Mortality has been reported to be 50% to 90%.[124] Clinical features are nonspecific, but diffuse alveolar infiltrates, hypoxemia, dyspnea, and anemia are characteristic. Alveolar hemorrhage usually occurs in patients with a known history of SLE, high titers of anti-DNA antibodies, and active extrapulmonary disease. Fiberoptic bronchoscopy with bronchoalveolar lavage and transbronchial lung biopsy is usually adequate to substantiate the diagnosis in patients with suspected alveolar hemorrhage. Lung biopsy specimens show extensive hemorrhage within alveolar spaces and capillaritis. Deposits of IgG, C3, or immune complexes have been found in 50% of patients with alveolar hemorrhage complicating SLE.[123]

The "shrinking lung syndrome" is characterized by progressive dyspnea and small lung volumes on chest radiographs and is thought to be secondary to diaphragmatic dysfunction.[125] It can be difficult to differentiate from respiratory muscle weakness, primary parenchymal disease, or pleural causes of low lung volumes without the use of invasive studies.

LYMPH NODE AND SPLEEN INVOLVEMENT

Lymphadenopathy occurs in approximately 40% of patients usually at the onset of disease or during disease flares. The nodes are typically soft, nontender, and discrete, and usually are detected in the cervical, axillary, and inguinal area. Biopsy specimens reveal areas of follicular hyperplasia and necrosis.[126] The appearance of hematoxylin bodies is highly suggestive of SLE, but is uncommon. Clinically significant lymphadenopathy that raises diagnostic issues is less common. Generally, patients with lymphadenopathy are more likely to have nonspecific symptoms, such as fever and malaise. A lymph node biopsy may be warranted when the degree of lymphadenopathy is out of proportion to the activity of the lupus.

Splenomegaly occurs in 10% to 45% of patients, particularly during active disease, and is not associated with cytopenias. Periarterial fibrosis, or "onionskin" lesions, in the spleen has been considered pathognomonic of SLE and is thought to represent healed vasculitis. Splenic atrophy and functional hyposplenism also have been reported in SLE and may predispose to severe septic complications.[127,128]

HEMATOLOGIC INVOLVEMENT

Hematologic abnormalities are common and can be the presenting symptom in SLE. Major clinical manifestations include anemia, leukopenia, thrombocytopenia, and APS.

Anemia

Anemia is common and affects most SLE patients at some time during the course of their disease. The mechanisms of anemia in SLE vary and include anemia of chronic disease, hemolysis (immune or microangiopathic), blood loss, renal insufficiency, medications, infection, hypersplenism, myelodysplasia, myelofibrosis, and aplastic anemia.[129-133] A frequent cause of anemia in SLE is suppressed erythropoiesis from chronic inflammation. The mechanism is multifactorial and includes suppression of hematopoiesis by inflammatory cytokines via apoptosis of progenitor cells or other mechanisms and antibodies against red blood cell growth factors or progenitor cells.[129] Overt autoimmune hemolytic anemia has been reported in 10% of patients with SLE.[133] SLE patients may have a positive Coombs test without overt hemolysis. Blood loss, either from the gastrointestinal tract, usually secondary to medications (NSAIDs), or as a result of excessive menstrual bleeding may cause iron deficiency anemia. A rare cause of iron deficiency anemia in SLE may be low-grade pulmonary hemorrhage without actual hemoptysis.

A microangiopathic hemolytic anemia with or without the other features (e.g., fever, thrombocytopenia, kidney involvement, and neurologic symptoms) of thrombotic thrombocytopenic purpura has been rarely described in SLE.[134] The presence of schistocytes in the peripheral blood smear and increased lactate dehydrogenase levels are the hallmarks of this disorder. When this disorder occurs in the setting of generalized lupus activity, we prefer to call it thrombotic thrombocytopenic purpura–like syndrome and use immunosuppressive therapy when it is severe. In the absence of generalized lupus activity, we view this disorder as bona fide thrombotic thrombocytopenic purpura. Autoantibodies against a metalloprotease that is responsible for cleaving the high-molecular-weight von Willebrand factor have been implicated in the pathogenesis of this disorder.[135] A similar syndrome can occur in the presence of antiphospholipid antibodies.[136] Red blood cell aplasia resulting from antibodies against erythrocyte progenitors has been rarely reported in SLE patients.[131,132] Bone marrow suppression also can be induced by medications, including immunosuppressive drugs and antimalarials.

Leukopenia

Leukopenia is common in SLE; it can be the presenting symptom and usually is associated with disease activity. A white blood cell count of less than 4500/μL has been reported in approximately 50% of patients, especially patients with active disease.[133] Severe leukopenia (neutrophil count <500/μL) is rare, however. Lymphocytopenia (lymphocyte count <1500/μL) occurs in approximately 20% of SLE patients.[137] Cytotoxic lymphocyte antibodies have been detected in the serum of SLE patients, and their titers have been correlated with the degree of lymphocytopenia.[138] Another potential mechanism of lymphopenia is increased apoptosis secondary to increased Fas antigen expression on the peripheral T cells in patients with SLE.[139] Neutropenia in SLE patients can result from immune mechanisms, medications, bone marrow suppression, or hypersplenism.[140] Decreased eosinophil and basophil counts are usually secondary to corticosteroid use in lupus. Leukocytosis in lupus can occur and usually reflects an infection or the use of high-dose corticosteroids.[141]

Thrombocytopenia

Mild thrombocytopenia (platelet counts 100,000 to 150,000/μL) has been reported in 25% to 50% of patients; counts less than 50,000/μL occur in only 10%.[133,140] The most common cause of thrombocytopenia in SLE is immune-mediated platelet destruction, but increased platelet consumption also may occur as a result of microangiopathic hemolytic anemia or hypersplenism. Impaired platelet production as a result of bone marrow suppression secondary to medications is another potential contributing factor (Table 75-9). The major mechanism is immunoglobulin binding to platelets followed by destruction in the spleen, as in idiopathic thrombocytopenic purpura.[142] Antibodies against thrombopoietin have been reported in the serum of SLE patients and correlated with thrombocytopenia.[143] Idiopathic thrombocytopenic purpura may be the first sign of SLE, followed by other symptoms even many years later. In such cases, the presence of high-titer ANAs or the presence of extractable nuclear antigens raises the possibility of underlying SLE. A careful history and physical examination in many of these cases may reveal additional features of SLE.

LIVER AND GASTROINTESTINAL TRACT INVOLVEMENT

Gastrointestinal manifestations have been reported in 25% to 40% of patients with SLE and reflect either lupus of the gastrointestinal tract or the effects of medications.[144,145] Esophageal involvement has been reported in less than 5% of SLE patients. Dysphagia caused by esophageal dysmotility and aperistalsis is the most usual symptom, tends to be episodic, and is associated with Raynaud's phenomenon and the presence of antiribonucleoprotein antibodies.[146] The esophageal dysmotility may be caused by an inflammatory reaction in the esophageal muscles, by ischemia, or by vasculitic changes in Auerbach's plexus. Other causes of dysphagia in lupus include gastroesophageal reflux disease resulting in esophagitis, esophageal spasm, and esophageal strictures; esophageal candidiasis, especially in patients treated with corticosteroids or immunosuppressive agents or both; and esophageal ulcers.

Dyspepsia has been reported in 11% to 50% of patients with SLE, and peptic ulcers (usually gastric) have been reported in 4% to 21%. These complications are more common in patients treated with NSAIDs. It also has been suggested that SLE itself predisposes to ulcer formation.[147] Bleeding

Table 75-9 Management of Thrombocytopenia in Systemic Lupus Erythematosus

Lupus related?
Rule out drug effects. Ask about over-the-counter drugs such as quinine for leg cramps, vitamins, supplements, or herbal medicines
Discontinue all but absolutely essential drugs
Discontinue agents that may interfere with platelet function (e.g., aspirin, NSAIDs)
Confirm autoimmune etiology by examining peripheral smear. Rule out platelet clumping that can cause false thrombocytopenia and abnormalities of the white or red blood cells
Consider bone marrow examination, especially in older patients, to rule out occult myelodysplasia
Tests for antiplatelet antibodies are not helpful
Rule out thrombotic thrombocytopenic purpura or antiphospholipid-related microangiopathic hemolytic anemia (anemia with pronounced reticulocytosis and fragmented erythrocytes in the peripheral smear), antiphospholipid antibodies, or antiphospholipid antibody syndrome
Look for evidence of lupus activity in other organs (especially major organs)
Determine severity
Severe: platelets $<20 \times 10^3/\mu L$
Moderate-to-severe: platelets $20-50 \times 10^3/\mu L$
Treat. Goal is not a normal platelet count, but a safe platelet count $(30-50 \times 10^3/\mu L)$

NSAIDs, nonsteroidal anti-inflammatory drugs.

from peptic ulcer disease in SLE is uncommon, and perforation is rare.

Abdominal pain accompanied by nausea and vomiting occurs in 30% of patients with SLE.[144,148] Special consideration should be given to conditions associated with SLE, such as peritonitis, mesenteric vasculitis with intestinal infarction, pancreatitis, and inflammatory bowel disease. Mesenteric vasculitis with infarction is a serious and potentially life-threatening manifestation. Risk factors for the development of mesenteric vasculitis include peripheral vasculitis and CNS lupus.[149] The clinical presentation is usually with insidious symptoms that may be intermittent for months before the development of an acute abdomen with nausea, vomiting, diarrhea, gastrointestinal bleeding, and fever.[144,149] Patients with mesenteric vasculitis occasionally have an acute presentation with mesenteric thrombosis and infarction, often in association with antiphospholipid antibodies.

The diagnosis of mesenteric vasculitis may be difficult to establish. Plain radiographic studies may reveal segmental bowel dilation, air-fluid levels, "thumbprinting" or narrowing of the lumen, and pseudo-obstruction. Abdominal CT scan findings compatible with mesenteric vasculitis include prominence of mesenteric vessels with a comblike appearance supplying dilated bowel loops, small bowel thickening, and ascites.[150] Arteriography may reveal evidence of vasculitis or ischemia of the small intestine or colon. Vasculitis generally involves small arteries, which can lead to a negative arteriogram. Pancreatitis associated with SLE may result from vasculitis or thrombosis and occurs in 2% to 8% of patients.[151] Elevated levels of serum amylase have been described in patients with SLE without pancreatitis and should be interpreted in light of the overall clinical examination. The role of azathioprine and corticosteroids as a cause of acute pancreatitis in patients with SLE is controversial.[152]

Hepatic disease may be more common in SLE than previously thought. Clinically significant hepatic disease is generally unusual in SLE. The incidence of hepatomegaly is 12% to 55% depending on the series.[153,154] Pathologically, a wide variety of lesions may be seen. Excessive fatty infiltration (steatosis) is a common finding and may occur as part of the disease process or may be secondary to corticosteroid treatment.[155] Liver chemistries (e.g., aspartate aminotransferase, alanine aminotransferase, lactate dehydrogenase, alkaline phosphatase) may be abnormal in patients with active SLE or in patients receiving NSAIDs.

The term *lupoid hepatitis* was formerly used to describe autoimmune hepatitis because of clinical and serologic similarities to SLE. Autoantibodies may help to distinguish between autoimmune hepatitis and liver disease associated with SLE. ANAs can be seen in both disorders, but anti–smooth muscle and antimitochondrial antibodies are uncommon in SLE (<30%) and usually when found are in low titers. Histology in lupus-associated hepatitis rarely shows the periportal (interface) hepatitis with piecemeal necrosis characteristic of autoimmune hepatitis, and liver-associated chemistries tend to be lower in SLE with only mild (usually three to four times normal) elevations. The absence of these antibodies and the presence of anti–ribosomal P protein antibodies suggest lupus hepatitis.[153]

Ascites is uncommon in SLE, and when detected, infectious causes or perforation or both must be excluded by paracentesis. Congestive heart failure and hypoalbuminemia secondary to nephrotic syndrome or protein-losing enteropathy represent other possible causes of ascites in patients with SLE. Protein-losing enteropathy has been described in some patients with SLE and can be the first manifestation of the disease. It usually occurs in young women and is characterized by the onset of profound edema and hypoalbuminemia.[145]

OPHTHALMIC INVOLVEMENT

Eight percent of patients with SLE develop inflammation of the retinal artery during the course of their disease. An equal number of patients have infarction of the retinal vasculature secondary to the presence of antiphospholipid antibodies. Both conditions can lead to the presence of cotton-wool spots in the retina visible on ophthalmoscopy or fluorescein angiography (where perivascular exudates and patches of dye leakage along the vessels are seen). Cotton-wool spots result from focal ischemia and are not pathognomonic for SLE. The presence of retinal vasculitis is usually associated with generalized active systemic disease, and retinal vasculitis occurs early in the disease process.[156] Corneal and conjunctival involvement is usually part of secondary Sjögren's syndrome; uveitis and scleritis are extremely rare manifestations in SLE.

DIAGNOSIS

DIAGNOSTIC TESTS

Antinuclear Antibodies

ANA testing is usually the first step in the immunologic diagnosis of SLE and other systemic autoimmune diseases. A retrospective study has shown that autoantibodies are typically present and accumulate progressively many years before the clinical diagnosis of SLE.[157] Immunofluorescence is the standard approach for detecting ANAs, and the staining patterns (i.e., homogeneous or diffuse, speckled, rim, nucleolar, or centromere) depend on the location of the target antigen. These patterns correspond to the presence of autoantibodies against different nuclear antigens. The ANA assay is an ideal screening test because of its sensitivity (95% when using human cultured cells as the substrate) and simplicity.[158] The entity of "ANA-negative lupus" described in previous years is usually associated with the presence of other cytoplasmic autoantibodies, such as anti-Ro (SS-A) and anti-ribosomal P protein.

The specificity of ANAs for SLE is low because multiple other conditions are associated with a positive ANA (i.e., scleroderma, polymyositis, dermatomyositis, rheumatoid arthritis, autoimmune thyroiditis, autoimmune hepatitis, infections, neoplasms, and many drugs). Also, some healthy individuals test positive for ANAs.[159] The formation of ANAs is age-dependent; it is estimated that 10% to 35% of individuals older than 65 years have ANAs. The titers are generally lower (<1:40), however, than the titers in systemic autoimmune diseases. In contrast to the low positive predictive value of ANA testing, a patient with a negative test has less than a 3% chance of having SLE; a negative ANA test is useful for excluding the diagnosis of SLE. In the presence of typical features of SLE, a negative ANA test does not exclude the diagnosis.

Antibodies to Extractable Nuclear Antigens

The nucleosome, a complex of DNA and histones, was the first lupus autoantigen to be identified. Autoantibodies to single-stranded DNA (ssDNA) and individual histones are commonly detected in SLE and in DIL and are nonspecific. Antibodies to dsDNA are found in 70% of SLE patients at some point during the course of their disease and are 95% specific for SLE, making them a valuable disease marker.

A subset of anti-dsDNA antibodies has been shown to be nephritogenic, and their titer usually correlates with the activity of kidney disease.[160] Anti-Sm (Smith) antibodies are detected in 10% to 30% of SLE patients, and their presence is pathognomonic for SLE. Anti–nuclear ribonucleoprotein antibodies are associated with anti-Sm, but are not disease specific. Their role in diagnosis or prognosis of the disease is limited. Anti-Ro (SS-A) and anti-La (SS-B) antibodies are detected in 10% to 50% and 10% to 20% of SLE patients, but are not disease specific. Their presence has been associated with the development of secondary Sjögren's syndrome, photosensitivity, CNS disease, neonatal lupus, and development of congenital heart block in the children of mothers who carry these antibodies.

Antiribosomal antibodies are highly specific for the diagnosis of SLE, but less sensitive than anti-dsDNA or anti-Sm antibodies. Anti–ribosomal P antibodies have been linked retrospectively with neuropsychiatric manifestations of SLE, especially lupus psychosis. It is unclear why some autoantibodies are specific for SLE and some are not. There is experimental and clinical evidence that some of these autoantibodies may play a role in the pathogenesis of the disease (e.g., anti-dsDNA and renal disease). Alternatively, autoantibodies may reflect disease-specific immune mechanisms, but not be pathogenetic by themselves.

TYPICAL AND ATYPICAL PRESENTATIONS

As in other systemic rheumatic diseases, the diagnosis of SLE requires an integration of the patient's symptoms, physical examination findings, and results of diagnostic tests. Table 75-10 shows the frequency of various manifestations of SLE at disease onset and during the disease course. The presence of one or more of these features or the involvement of at least two different organs in young women should always raise the possibility of SLE. Many of these features are not unique to SLE, however, and could be seen in other infectious, metabolic, and malignant diseases and in other systemic rheumatic diseases.

The recognition that systemic rheumatic diseases have several common features, which makes a specific diagnosis difficult, has led to the concept of the undifferentiated connective tissue syndrome. These patients account for 10% to 20% of patients referred to tertiary care centers. Among patients presenting with symptoms suggestive of a connective tissue disease, only 10% to 15% fulfill classification criteria for SLE 5 years later. Prognostic factors for SLE were young age, alopecia, serositis, DLE, positive Coombs test, and positive anti-Sm and anti-DNA antibodies.[161] Latent or incomplete lupus describes patients who present with a constellation of symptoms suggestive of SLE, but do not qualify by clinical intuition or classification criteria as having classic SLE.[162,163] These patients usually present with one or two of the ACR criteria and other features not included in the classification criteria. Most of these patients do not develop SLE, or if they do, it is usually mild and rarely involves major organs.

Table 75-10 Frequency of Various Manifestations of Systemic Lupus Erythematosus at Disease Onset and during the Disease

Manifestation	Onset (%)	During (%)
Arthralgia	77	85
Constitutional	53	77
Skin	53	78
Arthritis	44	63
Renal	38	74
Raynaud's phenomenon	33	60
Central nervous system	24	54
Vasculitis	23	56
Mucous membranes	21	52
Gastrointestinal	18	45
Lymphadenopathy	16	32
Pleurisy	16	30
Pericarditis	13	23
Lung	7	14
Nephrotic syndrome	5	11
Azotemia	3	8
Myositis	3	3
Thrombophlebitis	2	6
Myocarditis	1	3
Pancreatitis	1	2

Modified from Gladman DD, Urowitz MB: Systemic lupus erythematosus. In Klippel JH, Weyend CM, Wortmann RL: Primer on the Rheumatic Diseases, 11th ed. Atlanta, Arthritis Foundation, 1997.

Patients presenting with unusual manifestations of SLE without accompanying features that help establish the diagnosis constitute a small but challenging group of patients. Case reports and case series suggest that SLE may manifest with high fever and lymphadenopathy simulating lymphoid or hematologic malignancy, neurologic events (e.g., chorea, cerebrovascular accident, myelitis), unusual skin rashes such as chronic urticaria or panniculitis, abdominal vasculitis, pneumonitis and pulmonary hemorrhage, pulmonary hypertension, isolated serositis, myocarditis, aplastic anemia, and isolated cytopenias. In such cases, a careful history for manifestations of SLE in the past and a careful physical examination together with serology may help to recognize the disease early.

In our experience with such cases, nonrheumatologists may fail to recognize subtle evidence for the disease, such as a faint or transient malar rash, transient arthritis, or oral and nasal ulcers. Nonrheumatologists also may fail to elicit a history of photosensitivity or Raynaud's phenomenon or other features of SLE that are not present at the time of the evaluation. The latter are typically not volunteered by the patient unless specifically asked for. In some cases, this information may have been retrieved but not integrated into the diagnostic thinking.

SLE remains largely a clinical diagnosis. The diagnosis of mild SLE at the early stages of the disease may present considerable challenges. Strict adherence to the classification criteria may miss many patients. In cases of patients with typical features of SLE with low-titer or, rarely, a negative ANA, the diligent clinician should not hesitate to establish the diagnosis after excluding other diseases. At the same time, knowledge of the epidemiology of the disease in the age or sex group of the patient helps; autoimmune thyroid disease is more common in young women than SLE, and young girls with positive ANA and arthralgias are more likely to have autoimmune thyroid disease. Patients may manifest numerous features suggestive of SLE, yet never develop the disease. In such cases, use of the term "possible or probable lupus" with longer follow-up is recommended. These patients should be reassured that their prognosis is excellent.

DIFFERENTIAL DIAGNOSIS

Because of the pleiotropic manifestations of SLE, the differential diagnosis is large depending on the specific manifestations in each patient. Differential diagnosis from other polyarticular diseases affecting young women, such as rheumatoid arthritis or Still disease, may not be easy in the initial stages. Many other diseases also may be confused with early SLE, including undifferentiated connective tissue disease, primary Sjögren's syndrome, primary APS, fibromyalgia with positive ANA, idiopathic thrombocytopenic purpura, DIL, and autoimmune thyroid disease.

The differential in patients presenting with fever or splenomegaly and lymphadenopathy must include infectious diseases or lymphoma. In febrile patients with known SLE, leukocytosis, neutrophilia, shaking chills, and normal levels of anti-DNA antibodies favor infection.[164] SLE may manifest with localized or generalized lymphadenopathy or splenomegaly, but the size of lymph nodes is rarely more than 2 cm, and splenomegaly is mild to moderate. Patients with known or suspected SLE with prominent lymphadenopathy, massive splenomegaly, or expansion of a monoclonal CD19$^+$/CD22$^+$ B cell population should raise the suspicion of non-Hodgkin's lymphoma.[165] In patients presenting with neurologic symptoms, infections, cerebrovascular accidents, or immune-mediated neurologic diseases (e.g., multiple sclerosis, Guillain-Barré disease) must be considered. Finally, in patients presenting with a pulmonary renal syndrome, the disease must be differentiated from Goodpasture syndrome and antineutrophilic cytoplasmic antibody–associated vasculitis. In patients presenting with glomerulonephritis, the differential diagnosis includes postinfectious glomerulonephritis (streptococcal, staphylococcal, subacute bacterial endocarditis, or hepatitis C virus), membranoproliferative glomerulonephritis, or renal vasculitis (antineutrophilic cytoplasmic antibody or anti–glomerular basement membrane associated).

TREATMENT

GENERAL PRINCIPLES OF MANAGEMENT

The management of SLE requires a comprehensive assessment of disease activity and damage from the disease and careful tailoring of the treatment according to the organ involved and its severity. Patient education and multidisciplinary interventions, particularly in newly diagnosed patients, are an important aspect of the management of SLE. Generally, the management of the disease is divided between the management of disease with nonmajor organ (or nonvisceral) involvement and disease with major organ (or visceral) involvement. In the first case, the agents that are used have fewer side effects, whereas the management in the second case involves agents that suppress the immune system (immunosuppressive/cytotoxic agents). Because of their significant side effects, cytotoxic agents in SLE are reserved only for patients with moderate-to-severe disease.

MANAGEMENT OF MILD SYSTEMIC LUPUS ERYTHEMATOSUS WITHOUT MAJOR ORGAN INVOLVEMENT

NSAIDs, antimalarials, glucocorticoids, and, in severe, refractory cases, immunosuppressive agents (azathioprine, mycophenolate mofetil, methotrexate) are used in the treatment of SLE patients without major organ involvement. Despite their widespread use, there are few randomized controlled trials showing their efficacy in uncomplicated SLE. Although most studies have shown improvement, it is not apparent whether patients were left with residual disease activity or its extent.

NSAIDs are believed to be effective in the treatment of musculoskeletal disorders and complaints in SLE patients, based mostly on experience with musculoskeletal complaints in other conditions. In view of their gastrointestinal toxicity together with concerns about the cardiovascular safety of NSAIDs, we recommend judicious use of NSAIDs for limited periods for patients at low risk for gastrointestinal, renal, and cardiovascular toxicity. Dehydroepiandrosterone, an adrenal hormone with androgenic properties, has shown efficacy in mild lupus in several controlled trials, but its use is limited in SLE.

Antimalarials—mainly hydroxychloroquine—are widely used for musculoskeletal and cutaneous manifestations of lupus. The drug has a long-term effect in preventing major flares in SLE.[166,167] Additional nonrandomized studies have shown favorable effects of hydroxychloroquine on disease activity, damage accrual, and serum total cholesterol. Several studies indicate beneficial effects of methotrexate on disease activity and articular and cutaneous manifestations in SLE. In SLE patients without CNS or renal involvement, azathioprine therapy has been associated with fewer hospitalizations (0.02/patient-year versus 0.17/patient-year; $P < .05$), but no decrease in prednisone maintenance requirement. Mycophenolate mofetil also has been used in the treatment of SLE without major organ involvement in a few uncontrolled case studies.

TREATMENT OF MODERATE-TO-SEVERE SYSTEMIC LUPUS ERYTHEMATOSUS

Table 75-11 presents a working, albeit arbitrary, definition of moderate-to-severe SLE. To date, most experts agree that the treatment of moderate-to-severe SLE consists of a period of intensive immunosuppressive therapy (induction therapy) followed by a longer period of less intensive maintenance therapy.[70] The primary objective of the induction therapy is to halt injury, recover function, and induce remission by controlling immunologic activity. Maintenance therapy is used to consolidate remission and prevent flares with agents (or schedules) that are associated with a lower risk for complications and are more convenient to the patient. Table 75-12 summarizes randomized controlled trials for the treatment of moderate-to-severe SLE.

Immunosuppressive, Cytotoxic, and Biologic Agents

Corticosteroids. For patients with moderate-to-severe disease, corticosteroids are used either as single or as background

Table 75-11 Indications for Cytotoxic Drug Use in Systemic Lupus Erythematosus

General
Involvement of major organs or extensive involvement of nonmajor organs (i.e., skin) refractory to first-line agents
Failure to respond to or inability to taper corticosteroids to acceptable doses for long-term use
Specific Organ Involvement
Renal
Proliferative or membranous nephritis (nephritic or nephritic syndrome)
Hematologic
Severe thrombocytopenia (platelets $<20 \times 10^3/\mu L$)
Thrombotic thrombocytopenic purpura–like syndrome
Severe hemolytic or aplastic anemia, or immune neutropenia not responding to corticosteroids
Pulmonary
Lupus pneumonitis or alveolar hemorrhage
Cardiac
Myocarditis with depressed left ventricular function, pericarditis with impending tamponade
Gastrointestinal
Abdominal vasculitis
Nervous system
Transverse myelitis, cerebritis, psychosis refractory to corticosteroids, mononeuritis multiplex, severe peripheral neuropathy

Table 75-12 Randomized Controlled Trials for Moderate-to-Severe Systemic Lupus Erythematosus

Author, Year	Main Findings and Comments
Austin et al, 1986	Renal function was better preserved in patients who received IV-CY plus low-dose prednisone compared with high-dose prednisone alone; long-term study with approximately 10 yr of follow-up; significant differences among groups emerged only after the first 5 yr
Lewis et al, 1992	Treatment with plasmapheresis plus a standard regimen of prednisone and cyclophosphamide therapy does not improve the clinical outcome in patients with lupus nephritis
Boumpas et al, 1992	Extended course of pulse cyclophosphamide (15 pulses) is more effective than 6 mo of pulse methylprednisolone in preserving renal function in patients with severe lupus nephritis; addition of a quarterly maintenance regimen to monthly pulse cyclophosphamide reduces the rate of exacerbations
Gourley et al, 1996	In patients with lupus nephritis, monthly bolus therapy with methylprednisolone was less effective than monthly bolus therapy with cyclophosphamide; a trend toward greater efficacy with combination therapy also was noted; cyclophosphamide therapy was accompanied by increased risk for adverse effects (amenorrhea, cervical dysplasia, infections)
Illei et al, 2001	With extended follow-up (median 11 yr), pulse cyclophosphamide continued to show superior efficacy over pulse methylprednisolone alone for treatment of lupus nephritis; the combination of pulse cyclophosphamide and methylprednisolone provided additional benefit over pulse cyclophosphamide alone without conferring additional risk for adverse events
Illei et al, 2002	Nephritic flares are common (observed in approximately one third of patients) in subjects with proliferative lupus nephritis, even in those with a complete response to therapy, but flares do not result in loss of renal function if treated with additional immunosuppressive agents; renal flares are an important feature of the natural history of lupus nephritis
Chan et al, 2000	For treatment of diffuse proliferative lupus nephritis, the combination of MMF and prednisolone is as effective as a regimen of daily oral cyclophosphamide (≤6 mo) and prednisolone followed by azathioprine and prednisolone; short-term study (2-yr follow-up) involving Chinese patients with most patients with nephritis of <6 mo duration
Chan et al, 2005	With longer follow-up, flares in the MMF group were twice as many compared with the cyclophosphamide group and were observed on discontinuation of MMF; for this reason, during the extension period of this study, MMF was continued as a maintenance therapy at lower doses (from 2 g/day initially, reduced to 1.5 g/day and then 1 g/day in 6-mo intervals); rates of doubling of baseline creatinine and relapse-free survival were similar in the MMF group (MMF as induction and maintenance) compared with those of cyclophosphamide as induction with azathioprine as maintenance; MMF treatment was associated with fewer infections and fewer infections that required hospitalization; azathioprine is a reasonable option for maintenance therapy in lupus nephritis after induction with IV-CY; medium-term study with 5 yr of follow-up
Houssiau et al, 2002	In European SLE patients with proliferative lupus nephritis, a remission-inducing regimen of low-dose intravenous cyclophosphamide (cumulative dose 3 g) followed by azathioprine achieves clinical results comparable to those obtained with a high-dose intravenous cyclophosphamide regimen (a course of 8 pulses of IV-CY); patients had milder nephritis compared with NIH studies (Austin, Boumpas, Gourley, Illei)
Houssiau et al, 2004	Extended follow-up (median 73 mo) of previous trial with similar results; early response (6 mo) to therapy (defined as a decrease in serum creatinine level and proteinuria <1 g/24 hr) is predictive of good long-term renal outcome
Contreras et al, 2004	After induction therapy with monthly and maintenance with quarterly IV-CY, MMF (0.5-3 g/day), or azathioprine, rates of event-free survival (composite end point including death or renal failure) and relapse-free survival better with MMF; no significant differences between MMF and azathioprine; efficacy and dose of IV-CY significantly lower than in other randomized controlled studies; 95% of patients were Hispanic or African-American
Ginzler et al, 2005	Short-term induction therapy with evaluation at 24 mo and approximately 2 yr follow-up; more remissions with MMF compared with monthly pulses of IV-CY; most patients in both groups did not achieve remission; patients with no improvement at 12 wk were crossed to the other group; this was more common with IV-CY, resulting in a smaller number of patients in the IV-CY available for comparison; 56% of patients were African-American (approximately 20% in the NIH studies)
Barile-Fabris et al, 2005	32 Mexican SLE patients presenting with severe neuropsychiatric SLE manifestations (peripheral/cranial neuropathy, optic neuritis, transverse myelitis, brainstem disease, or coma) were treated with induction therapy with 3 pulses of IV-MP, followed by monthly cyclophosphamide (IV-CY) versus IV-MP bimonthly every 4 mo for 1 year, and then by IV-CY or IV-MP every 3 mo for another year; IV-CY was more effective than IV-MP, resulting in significant improvement in clinical, laboratory, or specific neurologic testing variables

IV-CY, intravenous pulse cyclophosphamide; IV-MP, intravenous methylprednisolone; MMF, mycophenolate mofetil; NIH, National Institutes of Health; SLE, systemic lupus erythematosus.

therapy in combination with immunosuppressive agents at prednisone doses ranging from 0.5 to 1 mg/kg/day in a single dose, usually in the morning. When corticosteroids are combined with immunosuppressive agents, we rarely use more than 0.5 to 0.6 mg/kg of prednisone because of concerns for infections, including opportunistic infections (see later). Corticosteroid toxicity is a major problem in SLE, and tapering of the dosage is a primary concern. Generally, tapering

starts after the first 4 to 6 weeks of therapy. The goal is a dose of 0.25 mg/kg every other day at 2 to 3 months, which is an acceptable dosage for long-term use. The concomitant use of other immunosuppressive agents facilitates tapering and decreases toxicity. In cases of doses greater than 0.6 mg/kg/day or in rapidly progressing severe disease, we use bolus therapy (1 to 3 daily pulses of methylprednisolone at a dose of 1000 mg/day followed by 0.5 mg/kg/day of prednisone).

Protection from osteoporosis is of paramount importance and should be initiated as soon as use of these agents is anticipated. In patients with severe or life-threatening disease, the use of a low dose of prednisone for several years after remission is widely accepted.

Azathioprine. The starting dose of azathioprine is 1 mg/kg/day with the usual maintenance dose being 2 to 3 mg/kg/day in one to three doses taken with food. The role of screening patients in advance for thiopurine methyltransferase activity is controversial, but is recommended by many authors to detect the roughly 1 in 300 individuals with very low levels. These patients are susceptible to abrupt and prolonged marrow aplasia at the usual doses of azathioprine. When the drug is instituted, monitoring includes complete blood count with platelets, creatinine, and aspartate aminotransferase or alanine aminotransferase. Liver enzyme activity should be measured every 3 to 4 months (see Table 75-2). Azathioprine should be used cautiously in patients with renal or liver disease and in patients who use allopurinol. Randomized controlled trials in lupus nephritis have not shown superiority for azathioprine compared with high-dose corticosteroids, and the drug is used as a corticosteroid-sparing agent in various manifestations of SLE (see later).

In moderate-to-severe SLE, azathioprine has been used as a maintenance therapy at doses ranging from 1 to 3 mg/kg/day, especially in women of reproductive age because of its acceptable safety profile during pregnancy (see later). Although discontinuation of the drug because of side effects is common, in SLE, more often the drug is discontinued for lack of efficacy.

Mycophenolate Mofetil. After its introduction in transplantation, mycophenolate mofetil was used to treat SLE patients refractory to corticosteroids or cytotoxic agents in small case series. It subsequently was studied in randomized controlled trials in lupus nephritis where it was compared (in doses of 1 to 3 g/day for 6 to 24 months) with either oral or pulse cyclophosphamide for the induction and maintenance of remission.[168-171] In these studies, mycophenolate mofetil showed comparable efficacy and fewer side effects than cyclophosphamide. In the absence of long-term data and harder outcomes (e.g., doubling of serum creatinine or end-stage renal disease), claims of superiority in terms of efficacy to cyclophosphamide cannot be adequately substantiated at present. This is especially true for the most severe cases, where cyclophosphamide has a track record of efficacy, something that it is hoped will also be shown for mycophenolate mofetil. In these patients, the combination of pulse intravenous cyclophosphamide with intravenous methylprednisolone is the treatment of choice (see later).

Mycophenolate mofetil has been used for the treatment of a variety of other manifestations of SLE in addition to proliferative nephritis, including membranous nephropathy, skin disease, refractory thrombocytopenia, and pulmonary hemorrhage.[52-56] Further controlled trials are needed, however, to establish the role of this agent for other disease manifestations.

Cyclophosphamide. Although some centers still employ daily oral cyclophosphamide regimens for short periods (2 mg/kg/day every morning in a single dose for 3 to 12 months

until remission), the National Institutes of Health protocol has become the protocol of choice for most physicians (Table 75-13). With the notable exception of NPSLE, randomized controlled trials are available only for lupus nephritis; recommendations for other indications are based on extrapolation from those data.

Randomized controlled trials with long-term follow-up have shown that intermittent pulse cyclophosphamide therapy (intravenous cyclophosphamide) is effective for moderate-to-severe proliferative lupus nephritis with a better toxicity profile than daily oral cyclophosphamide.[172] After induction therapy, a maintenance regimen is essential to decrease the risk of flares.[173] Subsequent studies from the National Institutes of Health have shown that combination pulse therapy with cyclophosphamide and methylprednisolone (intravenous methylprednisolone) improves renal outcomes without increasing toxicity.[174,175] Based on these studies, we propose 7 monthly pulses of intravenous cyclophosphamide (0.5 to 1 g/m^2) followed by quarterly pulses for at least 1 year beyond remission (Table 75-14). For patients with moderate-to-severe disease, monthly pulses of intravenous methylprednisolone are added during the induction period.[174,175] Ovarian toxicity (found to be age-related and dose-related),[176] infections (especially herpes zoster), flares (observed in approximately one third of patients), incomplete response, and, in rare cases, refractoriness to treatment have emerged from these studies as significant limitations of current cytotoxic therapy.

Because of concerns about the toxicity, together with the appreciation that lupus nephritis may be less severe in whites, European investigators sought alternative protocols to administer cyclophosphamide (Euro-Lupus Nephritis Trial). In studies involving mostly patients with milder forms of disease, less intensive regimens of cyclophosphamide (6 semiweekly pulses at a fixed dose of 500 mg each in combination with three daily doses of 750 mg of intravenous methylprednisolone) followed with azathioprine as maintenance had comparable efficacy—but less toxicity—than a short course of high-dose intravenous cyclophosphamide (8 pulses).[177] By multivariate analysis, early response to therapy at 6 months (defined as a decrease in serum creatinine level and proteinuria <1 g/24 hr) was the best predictor of good long-term renal outcome.[178] In addition to showing that in patients with milder forms of lupus nephritis less intensive regimens of intravenous cyclophosphamide may be used, this study showed that sequential therapy with a short course of intravenous cyclophosphamide followed by azathioprine is a valid approach in lupus.

In addition to proliferative and membranous lupus nephritis, case reports, case series, and uncontrolled clinical studies support the efficacy of intravenous cyclophosphamide in severe thrombocytopenia, neurologic disease (myelitis, encephalitis, psychosis, mononeuritis multiplex, and polyneuropathy), abdominal vasculitis, acute pneumonitis and alveolar hemorrhage, dermatologic disease, and other severe manifestations of SLE. A randomized controlled trial in NPSLE has confirmed its efficacy in severe NPSLE.[179] Reversible alopecia and nausea are the most commonly observed side effects of cyclophosphamide; myelotoxicity, gonadal toxicity, and malignancy are less frequent, although much more serious adverse effects. A variety of different infections can occur, including bacterial infections

Table 75-13 Recommended Monitoring of Cytotoxic Drug Therapy in Systemic Lupus Erythematosus

Drug	Dosage	Toxicities Requiring Monitoring	Baseline Evaluation	Laboratory Monitoring
Azathioprine (FDA pregnancy category D*)	50-100 mg/day in 1-3 doses with food	Myelosuppression, hepatotoxicity, lymphoproliferative diseases	CBC, platelets, creatinine, AST or ALT	CBC and platelets every 2 wk, with changes in dosage; baseline tests every 1-3 mo
Mycophenolate mofetil (FDA pregnancy category C)	1-3 g/day in 2 divided doses with food	Myelosuppression, hepatotoxicity, infection	CBC, platelet, creatinine, AST or ALT	CBCs and platelets every 1-2 wk with changes in dosage; baseline tests every 1-3 mo
Cyclophosphamide (FDA pregnancy category D)	50-150 mg/day in a single dose with breakfast; lots of fluids, empty bladder before bedtime	Myelosuppression, hemorrhagic cystitis, myeloproliferative disease, malignancies	CBC, platelet, creatinine, AST or ALT, urinalysis	CBC with differential every 1-2 wk, with changes in dosage and then every 1-3 mo; keep WBC >4000/mm^3 with dosage adjustment; urinalysis and AST or ALT every 3 mo; urinalysis every 6-12 mo after cessation
Methotrexate (FDA pregnancy category X)	7.5-15 mg/wk in 1-3 doses with food or milk/water	Myelosuppression, hepatic fibrosis, pneumonitis	Chest x-ray, hepatitis B and C serology in high-risk patients, AST or ALT, albumin, alkaline phosphatase and creatinine	CBC with platelet, AST, albumin, creatinine every 1-3 mo
Cyclosporine (FDA pregnancy category C)	100-400 mg/day in 2 doses at the same time every day with meal or between meals	Renal insufficiency, anemia, hypertension	CBC, creatinine, uric acid, LFTs, blood pressure	Creatinine every 2 wk until dose is stable, then monthly; CBC, potassium, and LFTs every 1-3 mo; cyclosporine levels only with high doses

*Azathioprine may be used during pregnancy if needed.
ALT, alanine transaminase; AST, aspartate transaminase; CBC, complete blood count; FDA, Food and Drug Administration; LFTs, liver function tests; WBC, white blood cell count.
Modified from ACR Ad Hoc committee on clinical guidelines for monitoring drug therapy in rheumatoid arthritis. Arthritis Rheum 39:723-731, 1996.

and opportunistic infections, such as *Pneumocystitis jiroveci* (*carinii*), fungal infections, and *Nocardia*, and reactivation of latent infections, including herpes zoster, tuberculosis, and human papillomavirus.

More recent studies have shown by multivariate analysis that the dosage of corticosteroids is the overriding independent determinant of the risk of infection among patients with SLE receiving cyclophosphamide with concomitant high doses of corticosteroids. The risk of developing premature ovarian failure depends on the age of the patient at the initiation of treatment and the cumulative dose of the drug, as we first reported in 1993. In our study, the rates of sustained amenorrhea after a short course (≤7 pulses) of cyclophosphamide were 0% for patients younger than 25 years old, 12% for patients 26 to 30 years old, and 25% for patients older than 30 years. A long course (≥15 pulses) of cyclophosphamide induced sustained amenorrhea in 17% of patients younger than 25 years old, 43% of patients of 26 to 30 years old, and 100% of patients older than 30 years. In men, gonadal toxicity may be observed with 7 g cumulative dose, corresponding to approximately 2 months of daily oral therapy.

To reduce morbidity from cyclophosphamide treatment, gonadal protection and less intensive regimens of cyclophosphamide have been advocated. Preliminary data suggest that gonadal protection from cyclophosphamide may be feasible, a finding requiring further confirmation. In a nonrandomized trial, the use of depot leuprolide acetate, a synthetic gonadotropin-releasing hormone analogue, significantly decreased rates of gonadal failure (30% versus 5%)

in young women with severe SLE treated with cyclophosphamide (n = 20 in both groups).[180] For white patients with proliferative disease, sequential therapy with a short course of intravenous cyclophosphamide followed by azathioprine has been found to be effective and to decrease the cumulative dose of cyclophosphamide. Other strategies for preserving fertility, such as cryopreservation of unfertilized ova and ovarian tissue germ cell transplantation, are currently under investigation and should be considered experimental at present. In male patients receiving cyclophosphamide for malignancies, the frequency of azoospermia ranges from 50% to 90%. The administration of testosterone 100 mg intramuscularly and sperm banking represent valid strategies for testicular function preservation.[181]

The use of intermittent pulse cyclophosphamide, together with adequate hydration, has practically eliminated the cases of bladder carcinoma, although hemorrhagic cystitis may be seen in patients who are unable to empty the bladder (e.g., neurogenic bladder) or in cases where the practice of adequate hydration and frequent emptying of the bladder are not followed meticulously. We routinely give mesna—an agent that has been advocated to reduce the concentration of acrolein and probably other toxic metabolites in the bladder—although controlled studies showing its efficacy in SLE are unavailable.

Rituximab. Rituximab is an anti-CD20 chimeric murine/human monoclonal antibody that depletes B cells—but not plasma cells—resulting in a dramatic and predictable

Table 75-14 National Institutes of Health Protocol for Administration and Monitoring of Pulse Cyclophosphamide Therapy

Estimate creatinine clearance by standard methods
Calculate body surface area (m²): BSA = √height (cm) × weight (kg)/3600
CY dosing and administration Initial dose CY 0.75g/m² (0.5g/m² of CY if creatinine clearance rate is less than one third of expected normal) Administer CY in 150 mL normal saline intravenously over 30-60 min (alternative: equivalent dose of pulse CY may be taken orally in highly motivated and compliant patients)
WBC at days 10 and 14 after each CY treatment (patient should delay prednisone until after blood tests are drawn to avoid transient corticosteroid-induced leukocytosis)
Adjust subsequent doses of CY to maximum dose of 1 g/m² to keep nadir WBC >1500/μL. If WBC nadir becomes <1500/μL, decrease next dose by 25%
Repeat CY doses monthly (every 3 wk in patients with extremely aggressive disease) for 6 mo (7 pulses), then quarterly for 1 yr after remission is achieved (inactive urine sediment, proteinuria <1 g/day, normalization of complement [and ideally anti-DNA], and minimal or no extrarenal lupus activity). Alternative maintenance therapy: azathioprine or MMF for 1-2 yr
Protect bladder against CY-induced hemorrhagic cystitis Diuresis with 5% dextrose and 0.45% saline (e.g., 2 L at 250 mL/hr). With frequent voiding, continue high-dose oral fluids for 24 hr. Patients should return to clinic if they cannot sustain inadequate fluid intake Consider mesna (each dose 20% of total CY dose) intravenously or orally at 0, 2, 4, and 6 hr after CY dosing. Mesna is especially important to use when sustained diuresis may be difficult to achieve, or if pulse CY is administered in outpatient setting If anticipated difficulty with sustaining diuresis (e.g., severe nephrotic syndrome) or with voiding (e.g., neurogenic bladder), insert a three-way urinary catheter with continuous bladder flushing with standard antibiotic irrigating solution (e.g., 3 L) or normal saline for 24 hr to minimize risk of hemorrhagic cystitis
Antiemetics (usually administered orally) Dexamethasone 10 mg single dose *plus* Serotonin receptor antagonists: granisetron (Kytril) 1 mg with CY dose (usually repeat dose in 12 hr); ondansetron (Zofran) 8 mg 3 times a day for 1-2 days
Monitor fluid balance during hydration. Use diuresis if patient develops progressive fluid accumulation
Complications of pulse CY *Expected*: nausea and vomiting (central effect of CY) mostly controlled by serotonin receptor antagonists; transient hair thinning (rarely severe at CY doses ≤1 g/m²) *Common*: significant infection diathesis only if leukopenia not carefully controlled; modest increase in herpes zoster (very low risk of dissemination); infertility (male and female); amenorrhea proportional to age of patient during treatment and to the cumulative dose of CY. In women at high risk for persistent amenorrhea, consider using leuprolide 3.75 mg subcutaneously 2 wk before each dose of CY. In men, use testosterone 100 mg intramuscularly every 2 wk

CY, Cyclophosphamide (Cytoxan); MMF, mycophenolate mofetil; WBC, white blood cell count.

peripheral blood B cell lymphopenia in most patients that lasts for at least 4 to 12 months after therapy. Response to therapy does not consistently correlate with B cell depletion. To date, experience comes from uncontrolled trials in various manifestations of SLE refractory to conventional therapy (renal, CNS, cytopenias, serositis, APS). Treatment protocols range from the usual regimen of 375 mg/m² × 4 weeks to shorter schemes (500 to 1000 mg × 2 weeks). In a case series involving severe refractory pemphigus vulgaris, a different scheme using rituximab as induction (3 weekly pulses) and maintenance (4 monthly pulses of 375 mg/m²) was used.[182] Most, but not all, patients were on concurrent intravenous cyclophosphamide, corticosteroids, or mycophenolate mofetil. No opportunistic infections have been reported so far, but allergic reactions, usually mild to moderate, may occur.

Response (partial or complete) has been seen in half of the patients, but follow-up is short. In some patients, the disease relapses after 6 to 12 months, and they have been successfully retreated.[183] Open questions with rituximab concern (1) optimal treatment regimen (i.e., frequency, use of concomitant immunosuppressive agents), (2) better documentation of potential for retreatment after relapse without developing neutralizing antibodies, and (3) randomized controlled trials versus intravenous cyclophosphamide. Although the drug potentially could be used for induction and maintenance, at present we view it more as a remission-inducing agent in patients with severe SLE who have failed intravenous cyclophosphamide combined with intravenous methylprednisolone.

Immunosuppressive Therapy in Systemic Lupus Erythematosus: Which Agent and for Whom?

Table 75-15 provides cytotoxic therapy recommendations for SLE patients based on severity of disease. Although azathioprine is considered by many authors to be superior to corticosteroids, in randomized controlled trials, the superiority of azathioprine is marginal at best, and its primary use is as induction therapy in mild cases of SLE or as maintenance therapy in patients with various degrees of severity. Although azathioprine and mycophenolate mofetil have not been formally tested "head-to-head" as induction therapy, published and anecdotal experience suggests that some patients with disease refractory to intravenous cyclophosphamide (which usually does not respond to azathioprine) may respond to mycophenolate mofetil, an observation that underscores the potential superiority of mycophenolate mofetil to azathioprine as induction treatment. The initial data so far in the Contreras study[169] have failed to show superiority of mycophenolate mofetil as maintenance treatment, however. Because of the significant difference in the cost between the two drugs, comparison studies are needed.

Mycophenolate mofetil is less toxic than cyclophosphamide, does not cause ovarian failure, and is more acceptable to patients than cyclophosphamide. Taking all these facts together, at present we view mycophenolate mofetil as an agent for moderate cases of SLE where in the past intravenous cyclophosphamide may have been used. This is especially the case in patients for whom ovarian toxicity is an important consideration (see Table 75-5). Although there are uncertainties regarding the optimal administration and its long-term safety and efficacy, the more recent follow-up study by Chan and coworkers[170] has resolved several of these issues.

For severe cases or cases where the disease does not remit after the first 4 to 6 months of therapy with mycophenolate mofetil (or does not improve substantially after the first 3 months of therapy), the combination of pulses of

Table 75-15 Recommended Cytotoxic Therapy for Major Organ Involvement in Systemic Lupus Erythematosus

Disease Severity	Induction Therapy	Maintenance Therapy
Mild	High-dose corticosteroids (i.e., 0.5-1 mg/kg/day prednisone for 4-6 wk with gradual tapering to 0.125 mg/kg every other day within 3 mo) alone or in combination with azathioprine (1-2 mg/kg/day)	Low-dose corticosteroids (i.e., prednisone ≤0.125 mg/kg on alternate days) alone or with azathioprine (1-2 mg/kg/day)
	If no remission within 3 mo, treat as moderately severe	Consider further gradual tapering at the end of each year of remission
Moderate	MMF (2 g/day) (or azathioprine) with corticosteroids as above; if no remission after the first 6-12 mo, advance to next therapy or	If remission after first 6-12 mo, MMF may be tapered to 1.5 g/day twice a day for 6-12 mo and then to 1 g/day; consider further tapering at the end of each year in remission or
	Pulse cyclophosphamide alone or in combination with pulse corticosteroids for the first 6 mo (background corticosteroids 0.5 mg/kg/day for 4 wk, then taper) for 7 pulses	Quarterly pulses of cyclophosphamide or
		Azathioprine (1-2 mg/kg/day)
Severe	Monthly pulses of cyclophosphamide combined with pulse corticosteroids for 6-12 mo	Quarterly pulses of cyclophosphamide for at least 1 yr beyond remission
	If no response, consider adding rituximab or switch to MMF	Azathioprine (1-2 mg/kg/day)
		MMF (1-2 g/day)

MMF, mycophenolate mofetil.

intravenous cyclophosphamide and intravenous methylprednisolone until remission remains the treatment of choice (see Table 75-5). Initial data and anecdotal experience suggest that individual patients may respond unpredictably to one treatment or the other, and that it may be necessary to switch therapy if response is inadequate within the first few months of disease. For patients who enter into remission within 6 months, maintenance therapy with mycophenolate mofetil for the initial 1 to 2 years of remission may be preferable to azathioprine, although the efficacy of this approach has not been tested in patients with severe disease, in contrast to the quarterly pulses of intravenous cyclophosphamide.

Figure 75-10 is an algorithm for the treatment of lupus nephritis. Regardless of the agent used, early effective cytotoxic therapy is of paramount importance as first show in lupus nephritis by Esdaile and colleagues.[184] Whether physicians, in view of the better toxicity profile of mycophenolate mofetil, would be more likely to use this drug earlier in the course of the disease remains to be seen.

OTHER AGENTS

Methotrexate

Although there has been substantial evidence supporting the effectiveness of methotrexate in rheumatoid arthritis, there are scarce data on its use in SLE. Current recommendations suggest its use as a steroid-sparing agent for articular and cutaneous manifestations of the disease. A randomized double-blind, placebo-controlled trial of methotrexate in SLE patients showed that a weekly dose of 15 to 20 mg for 6 months effectively controlled disease activity and allowed for corticosteroid reduction.[185]

Cyclosporine

Cyclosporine is most commonly used for membranous lupus nephropathy at doses of 1 to 2 mg/kg. Small case series also suggest a clinical benefit in other manifestations of SLE, such as skin rashes, thrombocytopenia, and aplastic anemia. More recently, cyclosporine has shown comparable efficacy to azathioprine in preventing flares in patients with proliferative lupus nephritis after induction of remission with oral cyclophosphamide. Despite this evidence, and with the notable exception of membranous nephropathy, use of cyclosporine in SLE is limited.

Intravenous Gamma Gobulin

Intravenous gamma globulin has been used for the treatment of a variety of severe SLE manifestations. Proposed mechanisms of action include Fcγ receptor blockade, downregulation of the immune response by anti-idiotype antibodies, a decrease in T suppressor cells, accelerated immunoglobulin catabolism, and neutralization of C3a and C5a, all of which have been advocated to contribute to its therapeutic effect in SLE. Intravenous gamma globulin is administered in doses of 400 mg/kg/day for 5 consecutive days and is most commonly used for the treatment of severe, refractory thrombocytopenia, usually achieving a rapid increase in the number of platelets within hours of administration. Nephritis, arthritis, fever, rashes, and immunologic parameters improve with intravenous gamma globulin.[186] Side effects of intravenous gamma globulin include fever, myalgia, headache, arthralgia, and, rarely, aseptic meningitis. The drug is contraindicated in cases of known IgA deficiency.

GENERAL ISSUES

CYTOTOXIC DRUGS IN SEVERE, LIFE-THREATENING DISEASE

Controlled trials and clinical experience suggest that intravenous cyclophosphamide in combination with intravenous methylprednisolone is the treatment of choice for most patients. For refractory patients, based on initial experience,

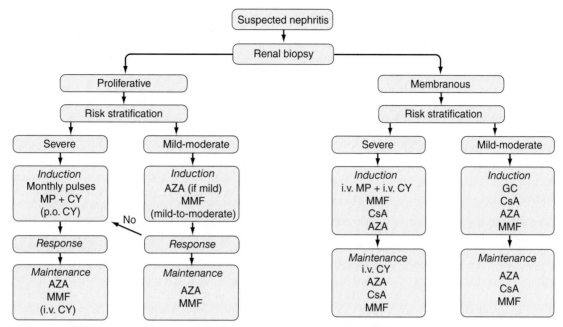

Figure 75-10 Algorithm for the treatment of lupus nephritis. All regimens include a background of glucocorticosteroids (0.5 to 0.8 mg/kg for the first 4 weeks of induction, 0.25 mg/kg every other day for maintenance). AZA, azathioprine; CsA, cyclosporine; CY, cyclophosphamide; GC, glucocorticosteroids; MMF, mycophenolate mofetil; MP, methylprednisolone.

availability, and potential side effects, combinations of intravenous cyclophosphamide with rituximab may be an acceptable strategy. Mycophenolate mofetil may rescue a few refractory patients, but its efficacy in critically ill patients requires further documentation. For selected patients (e.g., patients with neurologic disease, antiphospholipid antibody syndrome, thrombocytopenia), intravenous gamma globulin may be considered as an adjunctive therapy. In critically ill patients, plasmapheresis may offer some benefit to selected patients.

Cyclophosphamide may be administered either orally or as pulse therapy in the intensive care unit. The major concern is bladder protection and respiratory and intravenous line infections. Bladder irrigation through a three-way catheter in case of urine output less than 100 mL/hr is essential along with diligent care of the lines and tapering of corticosteroids. An aggressive search for infection is essential before and after therapy. Until infection is ruled out, we usually use high-dose corticosteroids. An aggressive tapering of corticosteroids when the patient improves is essential to minimize the risk of infectious and other complications. The importance of a multidisciplinary approach involving several medical subspecialties cannot be overemphasized.

PREVENTION AND MANAGEMENT OF INFECTION AND IMMUNIZATIONS

Infections attributed predominantly to corticosteroids and cytotoxic drugs are an important cause of hospital admissions and account for approximately one quarter of all deaths. In one of the earliest studies from the National Institutes of Health, 60% of the febrile episodes were ascribed to active SLE alone and 23% to infections. Leukocytosis, neutrophilia, shaking chills, and normal levels of anti-DNA

antibodies were associated with infection in febrile patients with SLE.[164] Judicious use of corticosteroids and immunizations may decrease the frequency of infections. Strategies to decrease the impact of infections include (1) simple hygienic measures and education aimed at patients and physicians; (2) antimicrobial prophylaxis in cohorts of patients with increased prevalence of certain infections, patients who receive heavy doses of immunosuppressive agents, or patients who undergo procedures associated with temporary bacteremia; and (3) immunizations similar to those available to the general population.

Bacterial Endocarditis

Clinical or subclinical valvular abnormalities are common in patients with moderate-to-severe SLE and may predispose to bacterial endocarditis. Patients with known valvular abnormalities should receive endocarditis prophylaxis before invasive dental, intestinal, or genitourinary procedures according to the standard regimens of the American Heart Association. For patients without known valvular abnormalities, some investigators also have advocated the use of prophylactic antibiotic prophylaxis. In our opinion, this is a reasonable suggestion, especially when patients receive high-intensity immunosuppressive therapy, but firm data to support this suggestion are lacking at present.

Tuberculosis and Pneumocystis jiroveci

Widely applicable guidelines for tuberculosis prophylaxis in SLE do not exist. Purified protein derivative testing may be considered in areas with a high prevalence of tuberculosis for patients who may receive long-term prednisone equal to or greater than the equivalent of 15 mg/day of prednisone. In such cases, a 5-mm tuberculin reaction represents a realistic cutoff. For patients living in low-prevalence countries, current data do not support the routine use of purified protein derivative testing before cytotoxic therapy. In contrast to patients with systemic vasculitis, we do not routinely employ prophylaxis for *Pneumocystis jiroveci* in patients with SLE. Some authors recommend prophylaxis, however, for patients on high-dose corticosteroids alone or in combination with cytotoxic drugs if the CD4 count is less than 300 cells/μL (1 double-strength tablet of trimethoprim-sulfamethoxazole three times a week or dapsone 100 mg/day if allergic to sulfamethoxazole).

Immunizations

Although vaccination theoretically may induce polyclonal activation in SLE and induce a flare, it is believed to be safe. More specifically, the influenza vaccine has been shown to be safe and effective; the pneumococcal vaccine also is safe, but the resultant antibody titers may be decreased in patients with SLE compared with controls. The use of corticosteroids may contribute to the blunted antibody response. A protective immune response can be achieved safely in patients with SLE with tetanus toxoid and *Haemophilus influenzae* type B in addition to pneumococcus. Immunization with live vaccines (e.g., measles, mumps, rubella, polio, varicella, varicella-zoster virus) is contraindicated in patients on corticosteroids at doses equivalent to 20 mg/day of prednisone for more than 2 weeks and in patients on cytotoxic drugs. The efficacy and safety of hepatitis B vaccination in SLE patients requires further documentation. Rheumatic syndromes temporally related to vaccination have been described, but a causal relationship has not been established.

PULMONARY INFILTRATES

Pulmonary complications are a major cause of morbidity and mortality in SLE patients receiving cytotoxic drugs. The differential diagnosis in this setting is broad and includes infectious and noninfectious processes. The radiographic findings are rarely specific for one disease, and most potential etiologies have overlapping clinical and radiographic appearances. An aggressive approach to identifying a specific etiology is of paramount importance; this includes bronchoscopy and early use of CT.

SCREENING FOR MALIGNANCY

Certain cancers occur more frequently in SLE compared with the general population, as more recent data substantiate, and may be due partly to cytotoxic/immunosuppressive drugs. The risk seems to be most heightened for lymphoma.[187] Cooperative efforts to evaluate this risk have been undertaken by several groups. An increased frequency of abnormal cervical Papanicolaou (Pap) smears in women with SLE has been reported by several groups.[188,189] In one study, the risk factors for the development of an abnormal Pap smear include a history of sexually transmitted diseases, the use of oral contraceptives, and the use of immunosuppressive drugs, especially cyclophosphamide.[189] Vigilance in cancer preventive strategies similar to that of the general population is essential. This vigilance is particularly important in view of more recent data suggesting that appropriate cancer screening may be overlooked in patients with SLE.[190]

USE OF CYTOTOXIC DRUGS IN PREGNANCY

Pregnant patients with active SLE and mild disease generally are managed with corticosteroids. In moderate-to-severe disease, corticosteroids, azathioprine, cyclosporine, and intravenous gamma globulin may be acceptable for the fetus. In life-threatening disease, cyclophosphamide may be used only if there are no alternative therapies. Cyclophosphamide and methotrexate are contraindicated (U.S. Food and Drug Administration category D—positive evidence for risk), whereas adequate information is lacking for mycophenolate mofetil (category C—risk cannot be ruled out). Because azathioprine may be excreted in breast milk, breastfeeding is not recommended. The American Academy of Pediatrics recommends that nursing is permissible for women receiving corticosteroids, but the interval between dose and nursing should be at least 4 hours if the prednisone dose is more than 20 mg/day. The American Academy of Pediatrics recommendations also indicate that hydroxychloroquine is compatible with breastfeeding. Although low concentrations of this drug are found in breast milk, because of the slow elimination rate and potential for accumulation of toxic amounts in the infant, breastfeeding during daily therapy should be undertaken cautiously.

ADJUNCT THERAPY

Photoprotection may be beneficial in patients with skin manifestations and is commonly used throughout the year. Lifestyle modifications (e.g., smoking cessation, weight control, exercise) are likely to be beneficial for outcomes in SLE and should be encouraged. Depending on the individual medication and the clinical situation, other agents (e.g., low-dose aspirin, calcium/vitamin D, bisphosphonates, statins, antihypertensives including angiotensin-converting enzyme inhibitors) are commonly used. The efficacy and safety of oral estrogen contraceptives in SLE patients has been assessed in two randomized controlled trials, which concluded that they do not increase the risk for flare in stable disease.[191,192] These results may not be generalized to patients with increased risk for thrombo-occlusive events, and accompanying risks should be assessed before estrogen therapy is prescribed.

SPECIAL CONSIDERATIONS

PREGNANCY: THE MOTHER AND FETUS IN SYSTEMIC LUPUS ERYTHEMATOSUS

SLE affects predominantly women of childbearing age. Sterility and fertility rates for women with SLE are comparable to healthy control groups. Secondary amenorrhea is associated with increased disease activity. Menstrual irregularities have been reported in women taking high doses of corticosteroids, and premature ovarian failure occurs in women receiving cyclophosphamide. SLE patients also are at risk for various adverse pregnancy outcomes, including miscarriage, stillbirth, and premature delivery (relative risk 2.2 to 5.8).[193] This risk is even higher for patients with antiphospholipid antibodies, as suggested by several prospective and retrospective studies, with relative risks ranging from 1.4 to 12.3 depending on the adverse outcome studied.[194-199]

The management of a pregnant SLE patient has always been a challenge for the practicing physician because SLE may affect pregnancy and vice versa (Table 75-16). There is not enough evidence to support a deleterious effect of SLE on fertility.[200-202] An increased frequency of SLE has been reported in endometriosis patients, which may have an impact on fertility.[203] A meta-analysis of epidemiologic studies that were published during 1980 to 1992[204] and subsequent controlled[196,205-211] and uncontrolled studies[193,197,198,212,213] have indicated that pregnancy may increase SLE disease activity and cause flares (reported frequency of flares 13% to 74%), but these flares are usually (33% to 88%) mild to moderate, involving mostly skin, joints, and blood.

SLE may affect the outcome of pregnancy. Lupus nephritis has been identified as risk factor for hypertensive complications and preeclampsia.[206,210,214-216] In a prospective study of SLE pregnancies, patients with preexisting lupus nephritis developed hypertension more frequently (50% versus 12%) than patients without nephritis.[206] The presence of antiphospholipid antibodies also is associated with increased risk for preeclampsia during pregnancy,[217,218] and the relative risk was estimated to be 16.8 (95% confidence interval 1.3 to 2.58) in a study of Chinese patients.[219] Patients with active nephritis also carry increased risk for adverse pregnancy outcomes, although the evidence comes from fewer studies.[211,220] In a retrospective analysis of 70 pregnancies in 48 women with lupus nephritis, the prevalence of fetal loss was 52% in active nephritis compared with 11% in cases of complete remission.[221] A single retrospective study in African-American women with SLE showed that anti-Ro positivity is associated with fetal wastage (71% versus 18%).[222]

SLE pregnancies are accompanied by increased rates (12% to 35%) of intrauterine growth restriction, with a relative risk of 8.6 (95% confidence interval 3 to 24.3) determined in a retrospective case-control study.[223] Antiphospholipid antibodies and nephritis also are associated with low birth weight and intrauterine growth restriction.[224-226]

Women with SLE have higher rates of spontaneous abortion, intrauterine fetal death, and premature birth compared with healthy women. Pregnancy outcome is optimal when the disease is in clinical remission for 6 to 12 months, and the patient's renal function is stable and normal or near-normal. Contraception and family planning are important.[193]

Proteinuria may increase during pregnancy in women with underlying kidney disease. Differentiation of preeclampsia from lupus activity in the kidneys is not difficult in most cases. Very low serum complement, active urine sediment, and evidence of generalized lupus activity favor lupus nephritis. Other features, such as hypertension, thrombocytopenia, an increase in serum uric acid levels, and proteinuria, may be observed in both conditions. Low-grade activation of the classic complement pathway may be attributable to pregnancy alone. Lupus placentae are small in size, and they exhibit ischemic-hypoxic changes, decidual vasculopathy and thrombi, chronic villitis, and perivillous fibrin.

Fetal growth and development in SLE may be affected by disease activity, by abnormality of maternal kidney function,

Table 75-16 Approach to the Management of Pregnancy in Systemic Lupus Erythematosus

Planning of pregnancy
　Ensure that lupus is inactive for at least 6 mo. Reassure patient (small risk for major flare)
　Discourage pregnancy if creatinine is >2 mg/dL

Check for antiphospholipid antibodies and other antibodies that may be relevant during pregnancy (e.g., anti-SSA, anti-SSB)

Check baseline laboratory tests (serology, serum chemistry including creatinine, albumin, uric acid, anti-dsDNA, C3, C4)

Be aware of the small risk for CHB, especially in women with anti-SSA and anti-SSB antibodies or with a prior episode of CHB. In such cases, monitor for CHB between 16 and 24 wk of gestation

Monitor blood pressure and proteinuria closely. Should this develop, differentiate between active nephritis and preeclampsia. The presence of generalized lupus activity and active urine sediment, and significantly low serum complement suggests lupus nephritis

For patients with APS, consider combined heparin and aspirin to reduce risk for pregnancy loss and thrombosis. For patients with antiphospholipid antibodies, consider aspirin, although there are no adequate data to support its use

APS, antiphospholipid antibody syndrome; CHB, congenital heart block.

by antiphospholipid antibody, and by SS-A/Ro and SS-B/La antibodies. Elevation of maternal alpha fetoprotein levels occurs in patients with SLE and is associated with preterm delivery, high corticosteroid dosage, and the presence of antiphospholipid antibody.[227] False elevation in human chorionic gonadotropin also has been reported.[228] Maternal IgG-mediated thrombocytopenia may be transmitted to the fetus; however, most infants born of thrombocytopenic mothers with SLE have normal platelet counts. IgG Coombs hemolytic antibody may be transmitted and cause hemolysis in the fetus and newborn. Anti-DNA antibodies have no pathologic effect on the fetus. Antiphospholipid antibodies cause placental insufficiency, intrauterine growth restriction, and fetal death. They do not usually cause abnormalities in the infant.

Neonatal lupus is a passively transferred autoimmune disease that occurs in some infants born to mothers with anti-SS-A/Ro or anti-SS-B/La antibodies or both. The most serious complication in the neonate is complete heart block, which occurs in 2% of such pregnancies.[229,230] Isolated skin rash occurs in a similar percentage. When a woman has given birth to an infant with congenital heart block, the risk in future pregnancies is about 15%. Ovarian induction and fertilization can be successful in SLE patients, but rates of fetal and maternal complications may be higher.

There is only a little evidence regarding therapy of SLE during pregnancy. Prednisolone, other nonfluorinated glucocorticoids, and azathioprine may be used in SLE pregnancy, but their efficacy and safety have not been shown in randomized trials.[198,211,215,231,232] Low-dose aspirin has been used in SLE pregnancy.[233] Evidence is stronger for hydroxychloroquine, and its efficacy and safety have been evaluated in one randomized controlled trial,[234] three nonrandomized studies (one prospective, two retrospective),[220,235,236] and several case series.[215,237,238] These recommendations differ from those of the Food and Drug Administration (see Table 75-12). There is no evidence to support the use of mycophenolate mofetil, cyclophosphamide, or methotrexate, and these agents must be avoided during pregnancy.[239-241] Although cyclosporine has been used in pregnancy, its safety has not been established.[242,243]

ANTIPHOSPHOLIPID ANTIBODY SYNDROME

Antiphospholipid antibodies (see Chapter 76) are commonly encountered in SLE patients and are associated with increased risk for thrombo-occlusive incidents. In such patients, primary or secondary prevention of thrombosis is warranted, but the clinical decision is often hampered by accompanying risks for treatment-related adverse effects (i.e., major bleeding). Despite the lack of evidence for primary prevention of thrombosis and pregnancy loss, some experts recommend the use of low-dose aspirin in SLE patients with antiphospholipid antibodies, especially when other risk factors for thrombosis coexist.

The effectiveness of oral anticoagulation over aspirin alone in secondary prevention of thrombosis in (non-pregnant) SLE patients with a history of antiphospholipid antibodies and thrombosis has been established in several retrospective controlled studies[244-248] and randomized controlled trials with mixed APS populations (i.e., primary and SLE-related).[249,250] The intensity of anticoagulation has been a matter of debate, however. The two randomized controlled trials of 114 and 109 patients have shown no superiority of high-intensity warfarin (target international normalized ratio [INR] 3.1 to 4.0) over moderate-intensity warfarin (target INR 2.0 to 3.0) for secondary prevention, and there was an increased risk for minor bleeding incidents in the high-intensity arm (hazard ratio 2.92, 95% confidence interval 1.13 to 7.52). In these studies, most patients (>70%) had a history of venous, rather than arterial, thrombosis, and patients who had already had recurrent events on oral anticoagulation were excluded.

Retrospective studies including more patients with previous arterial thrombosis or stroke have concluded that high-intensity warfarin is more efficacious in secondary prevention of thrombosis, and it carries a risk for major bleeding that is similar to that of lower intensity anticoagulation. Based on these findings, it is recommended that in patients with APS and a first event of venous thrombosis, oral anticoagulation should target INR 2.0 to 3.0. In the case of arterial or recurrent thrombosis, high-intensity anticoagulation (target INR 3.0 to 4.0) is warranted.

As for pregnant SLE patients with APS, a Cochrane Database Review concluded that combined unfractionated heparin and aspirin may reduce the risk for pregnancy loss (relative risk 0.46, 95% confidence interval 0.29 to 0.71).[251] The combination of low-molecular-weight heparin and aspirin also seems to be effective, although the results did not reach statistical significance (relative risk 0.78, 95% confidence interval 0.39 to 1.57). These results are based on findings from randomized controlled trials[252-254] and prospective[232,255,256] and retrospective controlled studies[247,257-259] in SLE pregnancies complicated by antiphospholipid antibodies or APS and previous history of pregnancy loss or thrombosis. No randomized trials have assessed the usefulness of anticoagulation in prevention of recurrent thrombosis during pregnancy. We recommend the use of aspirin and anticoagulation for the prevention of APS-related thrombosis during pregancy.

SYSTEMIC LUPUS ERYTHEMATOSUS IN CHILDHOOD AND ADOLESCENCE

Approximately 15% to 20% of all cases of SLE are diagnosed in childhood. Pediatric SLE may differ from adult SLE in regard to disease expression and physiologic, developmental, and psychosocial issues. Because of a paucity of data in pediatric SLE, little is known about its epidemiology, long-term outcome, and optimal management. Generally, the same principles are applied in the management of pediatric SLE; however, the special needs of this population have to be taken into consideration.

DRUG-INDUCED LUPUS

DIL represents a paradigm of an environmental agent triggering lupus in a genetically predisposed individual. It is well established that certain drugs induce autoantibodies in numerous patients, most of whom do not develop signs of an autoantibody-associated disease.[260] More than 100 drugs have been reported to cause DIL, including many of the newer biologics and antiviral therapeutics.

The incidence of DIL in the United States has been estimated to be 15,000 to 20,000 new cases per year. The frequency of DIL is probably underreported; many cases are mild and self-limited when the offending drug is removed. DIL should be suspected in patients who do not have a diagnosis or history of SLE, who develop a positive ANA and at least one clinical feature of SLE after an appropriate duration of drug exposure, and whose symptoms resolve after discontinuation of the drug. The clinical features of DIL include fever, myalgias, rash, arthritis, and serositis. Hematologic abnormalities, kidney disease, and CNS lupus are rare, although they have been reported. Antihistone antibodies are present in more than 95% of cases, whereas hypocomplementemia and anti-DNA antibodies are rare (with the exception of disease associated with use of interferon-α and anti–tumor necrosis factor therapies). A variety of drugs have been identified as being definite, probable, or possible causes of lupus (Table 75-17).

Although the pathogenesis of DIL is not well understood, a genetic predisposition may play a role in the case of certain drugs, particularly agents that are metabolized by acetylation, such as procainamide and hydralazine. The disease is more likely to develop in patients who are slow acetylators.[261] Data also suggest that these drugs may alter gene expression by inhibiting T cell DNA methylation.[262] Pharmacologic levels of these drugs induce overexpression of leukocyte function–associated 1 antigen by this mechanism, causing autoreactivity in CD4$^+$ T cells.

DIALYSIS AND RENAL TRANSPLANTATION

End-Stage Renal Disease and Dialysis

Approximately 10% to 20% of patients with SLE develop end-stage renal disease. Progression of lupus nephritis to the point of dialysis does not indicate end-stage renal disease. Approximately 5% to 10% of SLE patients requiring dialysis recover sufficient function to interrupt dialysis temporarily or for long periods. Patients with rapid deterioration of renal function are more likely to have a reversible physiologic

Table 75-17 Drugs Reported to Induce Lupus-like Disease and Associated Autoantibodies

Agent	Risk
Antiarrhythmics	
Procainamide	High
Quinidine	Moderate
Disopyramide	Very low
Propafenone	Very low
Antihypertensives	
Hydralazine	High
Methyldopa	Low
Captopril	Low
Enalapril	Low
Acebutolol	Low
Labetalol	Very low
Pindolol	Very low
Clonidine	Very low
Minoxidil	Very low
Prazosin	Very low
Antipsychotics	
Chlorpromazine	Low
Perphenazine	Very low
Phenelzine	Very low
Lithium carbonate	Very low
Anticonvulsants	
Carbamazepine	Low
Phenytoin	Very low
Trimethadione	Very low
Primidone	Very low
Ethosuximide	Very low
Antibiotics	
Isoniazid	Low
Minocycline	Very low
Nitrofurantoin	Very low
Anti-inflammatories	
Penicillamine	Low
Sulfasalazine	Low
Phenylbutazone	Very low
Zafirlukast	Very low
Mesalamine	Low
Diuretics	
Chlorthalidone	Very low
Hydrochlorothiazide	Very low
Antihyperlipidemics	
Lovastatin	Very low
Simvastatin	Very low
Miscellaneous	
Propylthiouracil	Low
Levodopa	Very low
Aminoglutethimide	Very low
Timolol eye drops	Very low
Biologic Agents	
Tumor necrosis factor-α blockers	High
Interferon-α	Low

Discontinuation of immunosuppressive therapy is an emotional issue for patients and physicians. We generally consider discontinuing therapy in patients with steadily increasing creatinine to 3.5 mg/dL with inactive urine sediment, renal biopsy specimen showing exclusively scarring and atrophy, or contracted renal size. Peritoneal dialysis is a reasonable option for SLE patients and offers greater independence. Most SLE patients with advancing renal disease experience a significant decline in lupus activity. Half of patients on maintenance hemodialysis continue to experience lupus activity, however, which often is difficult to distinguish from the complication of uremia.[263] Lupus activity is more likely to persist on dialysis when renal failure develops rapidly.

Uremia is a major predisposing factor for infections, and judicious use of corticosteroids and immunosuppressive drug therapy is essential to minimize the high risk of septic death in SLE patients with end-stage renal disease. Cardiovascular and cerebrovascular mortality and morbidity are increased in SLE patients with end-stage renal disease compared with SLE patients without end-stage renal disease.[264] Data from the United States Renal Data System (USRDS) suggest that, similar to other primary renal diseases, the incidence of end-stage renal disease secondary to lupus nephritis increased steadily over the period 1982 to 1995, despite the introduction of efficacious new treatment regimens; this may be related to the limited or delayed use of these modalities.[265]

Renal Transplantation

There are no firm rules for the optimal timing of renal transplantation in lupus nephritis patients. Although some patients with living related donors proceed directly to transplantation without prior dialysis, a period of at least 3 months on dialysis may allow some patients to recover adequate function for significant periods. A study in 8481 patients with a variety of renal diseases has suggested that avoiding long-term dialysis improves allograft survival of renal transplants from living donors. Improved immune function after dialysis may have contributed to this effect.[266]

Kidney transplantation is a viable alternative for SLE patients. Data from the USRDS and a European center suggest that graft and patient survival are similar between patients with end-stage renal disease caused by SLE and controls.[267,268] Recurrence of lupus nephritis in the renal allograft is a rare event (approximately 2% of transplants) and not an important cause of graft loss. The importance of antiphospholipid antibodies in vascular thrombosis in transplant recipients that was suggested by previous studies[263] was confirmed in a retrospective multicenter study.[269] In this study, all seven of the patients with APS not treated with anticoagulation therapy lost their allografts within 1 week as a result of renal thrombosis. In contrast, three out of four transplant patients with APS treated with anticoagulation therapy maintained their allografts for more than 2 years. The authors concluded that patients with APS are at high risk of post-transplant renal thrombosis and recommended anticoagulation therapy. The risk for thrombotic complications in antiphospholipid-positive SLE patients was confirmed more recently from a single-center European study.[267] In a subsequent pediatric study involving 100 renal transplants performed in 94 young SLE patients, comparable

(e.g., acute tubular necrosis) or pathologic (e.g., crescentic glomerulonephritis) component accounting for their renal failure. In these patients, immunosuppressive therapy (pulse of methylprednisolone with pulses of cyclophosphamide, 0.4 to 0.5 g/m², administered 8 to 10 hours before dialysis) may continue during dialysis.

CRITICAL ILLNESS

Life-threatening illness can develop in patients with SLE from any of the following causes: (1) exacerbation of preexisting manifestations of SLE; (2) development of new life-threatening manifestations of SLE; (3) infections resulting from immunosuppression; (4) adverse effects of drugs used to treat SLE; (5) malignancy resulting from prolonged use of cytotoxic drugs; and (6) acute serious illnesses that are unrelated to SLE, but whose manifestations are altered or exaggerated by it. Infection is the most common form of pulmonary involvement in patients with SLE.[271]

Infections in patients with SLE can be confused with exacerbation of the underlying disease process, and empiric therapy with broad-spectrum antibiotics is warranted until infection is conclusively ruled out. Bronchoscopy or open lung biopsy may be needed in addition to routine cultures to exclude an infectious origin. A diagnosis of acute lupus pneumonitis can be made after rigorously excluding infections in patients presenting with features resembling infectious pneumonia. Unilateral or bilateral alveolar infiltrates are seen on the chest radiograph, hypoxemia and respiratory alkalosis may be seen on arterial blood gases, and ventilatory assistance may be required in severe cases.[272,273] Mortality in patients with lupus pneumonitis may be 50%. A high index of suspicion should be maintained for a young female patient presenting with unexplained pulmonary infiltrates.

Alveolar hemorrhage is a serious but rare complication of SLE with high morbidity and mortality. The severity of alveolar hemorrhage in SLE may range from an uncommon mild and chronic form to massive bleeding resulting in death. The classic triad of hemoptysis, falling hematocrit, and pulmonary infiltrates is not uniformly present in all patients.[124,274] Bilateral diffuse alveolar infiltrates are seen on chest radiograph, but may be patchy, with lower lobe predominance. Respiratory failure may occur, and more than half of affected patients in most series required mechanical ventilation. Patients with alveolar hemorrhage usually have lupus nephritis as a preexisting condition.[275,276] Early bronchoscopy with bronchoalveolar lavage is recommended to show alveolar hemorrhage and to collect specimens for culture. Mortality in patients with alveolar hemorrhage is 40% to 90%.[124,273,277-279]

Cardiovascular disease secondary to premature accelerated atherosclerosis is increasingly recognized among SLE patients.[105,106,280] Although patients with SLE are often concerned about vasculitis, most coronary occlusive disease in SLE results from atherosclerosis or thrombosis.[281] Cases of left ventricular free wall rupture, acute mitral regurgitation after rupture of chordae tendinae, and aortic dissection have been described in patients with SLE. Cerebrovascular accidents manifesting acutely with hemiplegia, aphasia, cerebral dysfunction, cortical blindness, or other deficits of cerebral function can be caused by intracranial hemorrhage from ruptured aneurysms, thrombotic strokes from vasculitis or vasculopathy secondary to antiphospholipid antibodies, or embolic strokes from cardiac emboli.[114,282]

Spinal cord myelopathy is a devastating manifestation of SLE. Patients present with weakness or paralysis, bilateral sensory deficits, and impaired sphincter control. Symptoms usually evolve in a matter of hours or days. MRI of the spinal cord may show characteristic abnormalities of cord edema if obtained early. Because of the poor prognosis, early diagnosis and aggressive therapy are important.[94,283]

Patients with SLE presenting with an acute abdomen are challenging. The clinical syndrome may be secondary to mesenteric arterial thrombosis; ischemic bowel; ruptured hepatic aneurysms; cholecystitis; pancreatitis; or perforation of a viscus including a peptic ulcer, the appendix, the cecum, or the colon.[284,285] Patients with active SLE presenting with an acute abdomen and a high SLEDAI score are more likely to have active intra-abdominal vasculitis than patients with active lupus, but low SLEDAI scores. The former group, in view of the high mortality, should be considered for early laparotomy.[286]

Recommended Assessment and Monitoring and Referral Guidelines

Because of the low prevalence of moderate-to-severe SLE, most general internists do not have experience in its management. The role of the general internist in the early diagnosis, monitoring of patients with mild, stable diseases, and referral of patients with unstable or moderate-to-severe disease is essential, however.[287] Table 75-18 presents guidelines for the initial assessment and frequency of monitoring for general use.

Table 75-18 Recommended Initial Assessment and Monitoring of Systemic Lupus Erythematosus

History and review of systems
  Joint pain and swelling, Raynaud's phenomenon
  Photosensitivity, rash, hair loss
  Shortness of breath, pleuritic chest pain
  General symptoms (depression, fatigue, fever, weight change)

Physical examination
  Rashes (acute, subacute, chronic, nonspecific, others), alopecia, oral or nasal ulcers
  Lymphadenopathy, splenomegaly, pericardial or pleural effusions
  Funduscopic examination, edema
  Other features as suggested by history and symptoms

Imaging and laboratory tests
  Hematology*
  Chemistry*
  PT/PTT, antiphospholipid antibodies
  Urinalysis*
  Serology (ANA, ENA including anti-dsDNA,† complement†)
  Chest x-ray
  ECG
  Other tests as suggested by history and symptoms

Disease activity index (at each visit or at major changes in therapy)

Side effects of therapy

Damage index (SLICC) (every 1-2 yr)

*Every 3-6 months, if stable.
†Every 3-6 months in patients with active renal disease.
ANA, antinuclear antibody; ECG, electrocardiogram; ENA, extractable nuclear antigen; PT/PTT, prothrombin time/partial thromboplastin time; SLICC, Systemic Lupus International Collaborating Clinics.

Prognosis, Morbidity, and Mortality

A bimodal mortality pattern in SLE was first described in 1974 showing that early mortality in SLE is associated with SLE disease activity and infection, whereas late mortality is associated with atherosclerotic complications.[288] Although current treatment of SLE has improved survival, prolonged and complete remission—defined as 5 years without clinical and laboratory evidence of active disease and on no treatment—has remained elusive, occurring in 1.7% of patients.[289,290] In the Hopkins Lupus Cohort, hemolytic anemia was significantly associated with mortality risk in adjusted analyses, regardless of whether it was present at diagnosis or at a later time.[291] Other factors associated with decreased survival in the same cohort were lower socioeconomic status, age older than 50 years at the time of diagnosis, male gender, and low complement level at diagnosis. Renal disease was less strongly associated with survival, as had been reported in previous studies.[97,292]

Many patients (20% to 40% in various studies) do not respond adequately to current immunosuppressive therapies. Half (50%) of these patients reach end-stage renal disease. A relapsing remitting, or "flare," pattern is the classic pattern of SLE activity. Flares are common in SLE patients. The incidence of flare has been estimated to be 0.65 per patient-year of follow-up.[209] In patients with moderate-to-severe lupus nephritis participating in a randomized controlled trial, renal flares were seen in 20% to 40% of patients. The mean time for flare is 3 years—hence long follow-up is important. Of patients who flare, one third reach end-stage renal disease despite therapy.[293]

In SLE, treatment-related morbidity may not be easily separable from disease-related morbidity. The incidence of hospital admissions for patients with SLE is 0.69 admissions per patient-year. Infections, coronary artery disease, and orthopaedic management of osteonecrosis were prominent reasons for hospitalization.[294]

EVIDENCE-BASED RECOMMENDATIONS FOR THE MANAGEMENT OF SYSTEMIC LUPUS ERYTHEMATOSUS

SLE is a complex disease with variable presentations, course, and prognosis. Because of the systemic nature of the disease, multiple medical subspecialties are involved in the care of patients dictating an integrated approach to its care. To this end, the European League Against Rheumatism task force on SLE has developed recommendations covering the most important aspects in the management.[1] These recommendations, developed not only for specialists, but for all internists, were based on a combined research-based evidence approach and expert opinion consensus. The recommendations for the management of SLE are shown in Table 75-19.

Acknowledgments

The authors thank Drs. P. Sidiropoulos, G. Bertsias, and Eva Padimitraki for critical review of the manuscript; Dr. D. Vassilopoulos for sharing of patient and laboratory pictures; and Dr. K. Pagonidis for his help with the imaging studies.

Table 75-19 Summary of Statements and Recommendations on the Management of Systemic Lupus Erythematosus Based on Evidence and Expert Opinion*

General Management
Prognosis
In patients with SLE, new clinical signs (rashes (B), arthritis (B), serositis (B), neurologic manifestations [seizures/psychosis] (B)), routine laboratory (CBC (B), serum creatinine (B), proteinuria (B), and urinary sediment (B)), and immunologic tests (serum C3 (B), anti-dsDNA (B), anti-Ro/SSA (B), anti-La/SSB (C), antiphospholipid antibody (B), anti-RNP (B)) may provide prognostic information for the outcome in general and involvement of major organs, and should be considered in the evaluation of patients. Confirmation by imaging (brain MRI (B)) and pathology (renal biopsy (B)) may add prognostic information and should be considered in selected patients
Monitoring
New clinical manifestations, such as number and type of skin lesions (C) or arthritis (D), serositis (D), and neurologic manifestations (seizures/psychosis) (D); laboratory tests (CBC) (B); immunologic tests (serum C3/C4 (B), anti-C1q (B), anti-dsDNA (B)); and validated global activity indices (D) have diagnostic ability for monitoring for lupus activity and flares, and may be used in the monitoring of lupus patients
Comorbidities
SLE patients are at increased risk for certain comorbidities secondary to the disease or its treatment or both. These comorbidities include infections (urinary tract infections (B), other infections (C)), atherosclerosis (B), hypertension (B), dyslipidemias (B), diabetes (C), osteoporosis (C), avascular necrosis (C), and malignancies (especially non-Hodgkin's lymphoma) (B). Minimization of risk factors together with a high index of suspicion, prompt evaluation, and diligent follow-up of these patients is recommended
Treatment
In the treatment of SLE without major organ manifestations, antimalarials (A) or glucocorticoids (A) or both are beneficial and may be used. NSAIDs may be used judiciously for limited periods in patients at low risk for their complications (D). In nonresponsive patients or patients in whom steroids cannot be reduced below doses acceptable for long-term use, immunosuppressive agents such as azathioprine (B), mycophenolate mofetil (D), and methotrexate (A) also should be considered

*The strength of each statement (**A-D**) is given in parentheses, in bold. **A**=Evidence from randomized controlled trials or meta-analyses of randomized controlled trials without concerns for the validity. **B**=As in **A**, but with concerns about the validity of the evidence, or evidence from meta-analyses of epidemiologic studies or prospective controlled studies without concerns about the validity of the evidence. **C**=Evidence from nonprospective controlled (retrospective cohort, case-control, or cross-sectional) or uncontrolled studies without concerns about the validity. **D**=Based on evidence from meta-analyses from epidemiologic studies, nonrandomized controlled studies (prospective or nonprospective), or uncontrolled studies with major concerns about the validity of the evidence; or no data (expert opinion).

APS, antiphospholipid antibody syndrome; CBC, complete blood count; MRI, magnetic resonance imaging; NSAIDs, nonsteroidal anti-inflammatory drugs; RNP, ribonucleoprotein; SLE, systemic lupus erythematosus.

Continued

Table 75-19 Summary of Statements and Recommendations on the Management of Systemic Lupus Erythematosus Based on Evidence and Expert Opinion—cont'd

Adjunct Therapy

Photoprotection may be beneficial in patients with skin manifestations and should be considered (**B**). Lifestyle modifications (smoking cessation, weight control, exercise) (**D**) are likely to be beneficial for lupus outcomes and should be encouraged. Depending on the individual medication and the clinical situation, other agents (low-dose aspirin (**D**), calcium/vitamin D (**D**), bisphosphonates (**A**), statins (**D**), antihypertensives [including angiotensin-converting enzyme inhibitors] (**D**)) should be considered. Estrogens (oral contraceptives (**A**), hormonal replacement therapy (**A**)) may be used, but accompanying risks should be assessed

Neuropsychiatric Lupus

Diagnosis

In SLE patients, the diagnostic workup (clinical (**A-C**), laboratory (**B**), neuropsychologic (**C**), and imaging tests (**B-C**)) of neuropsychiatric manifestations should be similar to that in the general population presenting with the same neuropsychiatric manifestations

Treatment

SLE patients with major neuropsychiatric manifestations considered to be of inflammatory origin (optic neuritis, acute confusional state/coma, cranial or peripheral neuropathy, psychosis, and transverse myelitis/myelopathy) may benefit from immunosuppressive therapy (**A**)

Pregnancy in Lupus

Pregnancy affects mothers with SLE and their offspring in several ways
Mother: There is no significant difference in fertility in lupus patients (**C**). Pregnancy may increase lupus disease activity, but these flares are usually mild (**B**). Patients with lupus nephritis and antiphospholipid antibodies are more at risk of developing preeclampsia and should be monitored more closely (**B**)
Fetus: SLE may affect the fetus in several ways, especially if the mother has a history of lupus nephritis or antiphospholipid, anti-Ro, or anti-La antibodies. These conditions are associated with an increase of the risk of miscarriage (**B**), stillbirth (**B**), premature delivery (**B**), intrauterine growth restriction (**C**), and fetal heart block (**B**). Prednisolone (**D**), azathioprine (**D**), hydroxychloroquine (**A**), and low-dose aspirin (**D**) may be used in lupus pregnancies. Current evidence suggests that mycophenolate mofetil, cyclophosphamide, and methotrexate must be avoided (**D**)

APS

In patients with SLE and antiphospholipid antibodies, low-dose aspirin may be considered for primary prevention of thrombosis and pregnancy loss (**D**). Other risk factors for thrombosis also should be assessed. Estrogen-containing drugs increase the risk for thrombosis (**D**). In nonpregnant patients with SLE and APS-associated thrombosis, long-term anticoagulation with oral anticoagulants is effective for secondary prevention of thrombosis (**A**). In pregnant patients with SLE and APS combined, unfractionated or low-molecular-weight heparin and aspirin reduce pregnancy loss and thrombosis and should be considered (**A**)

Lupus Nephritis

Monitoring

Renal biopsy (**B**), urine sediment analysis (**B**), proteinuria (**B**), and kidney function (**B**) may have independent predictive ability for clinical outcome in therapy of lupus nephritis, but need to be interpreted in conjunction. Changes in immunologic tests (anti-dsDNA, serum C3) (**B**) have limited ability to predict the response to treatment and may be used only as supplemental information

Treatment

In patients with proliferative lupus nephritis, glucocorticoids combined with immunosuppressive agents are effective against progression to end-stage renal disease (**A**). In short-term and medium-term trials, mycophenolate mofetil has shown at least similar efficacy compared with pulse cyclophosphamide and a more favorable toxicity profile (**A**); failure to respond by 6 mo should lead to discussions for intensification of therapy. Long-term efficacy has been shown only for cyclophosphamide-based regimens, which are associated with considerable adverse effects (**A**). Flares after remission are common and require diligent follow-up

End-Stage Renal Disease

Dialysis (**B**) and transplantation (**B**) in SLE have comparable rates for long-term patient and graft survivals as those observed in nondiabetic, non-SLE patients, with transplantation being the method of choice (**C**)

APS, antiphospholipid antibody syndrome; CBC, complete blood count; MRI, magnetic resonance imaging; NSAIDs, nonsteroidal anti-inflammatory drugs; RNP, ribonucleoprotein; SLE, systemic lupus erythematosus.

REFERENCES

1. Bertsias G, et al: EULAR recommendations for the management of systemic lupus erythematosus. Report of a Task Force of the European Standing Committee for International Clinical Studies Including Therapeutics (ESCISIT). Ann Rheum Dis 65(Suppl II):194, 2006.
2. Lawrence RC, Helmick CG, Arnett FC, et al: Estimates of the prevalence of arthritis and selected musculoskeletal disorders in the United States. Arthritis Rheum 41:778-799, 1998.
3. Uramoto KM, Michet CJ Jr, Thumboo J, et al: Trends in the incidence and mortality of systemic lupus erythematosus, 1950-1992. Arthritis Rheum 42:46-50, 1999.
4. Vilar MJ, Sato EI: Estimating the incidence of systemic lupus erythematosus in a tropical region (Natal, Brazil). Lupus 11:528-532, 2002.
5. Jimenez S, Cervera R, Font J, et al: The epidemiology of systemic lupus erythematosus. Clin Rev Allergy Immunol 25:3-12, 2003.
6. Bresnihan B: Outcome and survival in systemic lupus erythematosus. Ann Rheum Dis 48:443-445, 1989.
7. Rivest C, Lew RA, Welsing PM, et al: Association between clinical factors, socioeconomic status, and organ damage in recent onset systemic lupus erythematosus. J Rheumatol 27:680-684, 2000.
8. Alarcon GS, Friedman AW, Straaton KV, et al: Systemic lupus erythematosus in three ethnic groups, III: A comparison of characteristics early in the natural history of the LUMINA cohort. LUpus in MInority populations: NAture vs. Nurture. Lupus 8:197-209, 1999.
9. Alarcon GS, Roseman J, Bartolucci AA, et al: Systemic lupus erythematosus in three ethnic groups, II: Features predictive of disease activity early in its course. LUMINA Study Group. LUpus in MInority populations: NAture vs. Nurture. Arthritis Rheum 41:1173-1180, 1998.

10. Ballou SP, Khan MA, Kushner I: Clinical features of systemic lupus erythematosus: Differences related to race and age of onset. Arthritis Rheum 25:55-60, 1982.
11. **Cervera R, Khamashta MA, Font J, et al: Systemic lupus erythematosus: Clinical and immunologic patterns of disease expression in a cohort of 1,000 patients. The European Working Party on Systemic Lupus Erythematosus. Medicine (Balt) 72:113-124, 1993.**
12. Miller MH, Urowitz MB, Gladman DD, et al: Systemic lupus erythematosus in males. Medicine (Balt) 62:327-334, 1983.
13. Boddaert J, Huong DL, Amoura Z, et al: Late-onset systemic lupus erythematosus: A personal series of 47 patients and pooled analysis of 714 cases in the literature. Medicine (Balt) 83:348-359, 2004.
14. Hochberg MC: Updating the American College of Rheumatology revised criteria for the classification of systemic lupus erythematosus. Arthritis Rheum 40:1725, 1997.
15. Calvo-Alen J, Bastian HM, Straaton KV, et al: Identification of patient subsets among those presumptively diagnosed with, referred, and/or followed up for systemic lupus erythematosus at a large tertiary care center. Arthritis Rheum 38:1475-1484, 1995.
16. Griffiths B, Mosca M, Gordon C: Assessment of patients with systemic lupus erythematosus and the use of lupus disease activity indices. Best Pract Res Clin Rheumatol 19:685-708, 2005.
17. Urowitz MB, Gladman DD: Measures of disease activity and damage in SLE. Baillieres Clin Rheumatol 12:405-413, 1998.
18. Vitali C, Bencivelli W, Mosca M, et al: Development of a clinical chart to compute different disease activity indices for systemic lupus erythematosus. J Rheumatol 26:498-501, 1999.
19. Gladman D, Ginzler E, Goldsmith C, et al: The development and initial validation of the Systemic Lupus International Collaborating Clinics/American College of Rheumatology damage index for systemic lupus erythematosus. Arthritis Rheum 39:363-369, 1996.
20. Stoll T, Seifert B, Isenberg DA: SLICC/ACR Damage Index is valid, and renal and pulmonary organ scores are predictors of severe outcome in patients with systemic lupus erythematosus. Br J Rheumatol 35:248-254, 1996.
21. Rahman P, Gladman DD, Urowitz MB, et al: Early damage as measured by the SLICC/ACR damage index is a predictor of mortality in systemic lupus erythematosus. Lupus 10:93-96, 2001.
22. Patel P, Werth V: Cutaneous lupus erythematosus: a review. Dermatol Clin 20:373-385, v, 2002.
23. Gilliam JN, Sontheimer RD: Skin manifestations of SLE. Clin Rheum Dis 8:207-218, 1982.
24. Gilliam JN, Sontheimer RD: Subacute cutaneous lupus erythematosus. Clin Rheum Dis 8:343-352, 1982.
25. Wollina U, Barta U, Uhlemann C, et al: Lupus erythematosus-associated red lunula. J Am Acad Dermatol 41:419-421, 1999.
26. Rowell NR, Beck JS, Anderson JR: Lupus erythematosus and erythema multiforme-like lesions: A syndrome with characteristic immunological abnormalities. Arch Dermatol 88:176-180, 1963.
27. Pistiner M, Wallace DJ, Nessim S, et al: Lupus erythematosus in the 1980s: A survey of 570 patients. Semin Arthritis Rheum 21:55-64, 1991.
28. Wysenbeek AJ, Leibovici L, Amit M, et al: Alopecia in systemic lupus erythematosus: Relation to disease manifestations. J Rheumatol 18:1185-1186, 1991.
29. Casciola-Rosen LA, Anhalt G, Rosen A: Autoantigens targeted in systemic lupus erythematosus are clustered in two populations of surface structures on apoptotic keratinocytes. J Exp Med 179:1317-1330, 1994.
30. Hruza LL, Pentland AP: Mechanisms of UV-induced inflammation. J Invest Dermatol 100:35S-41S, 1993.
31. Urman JD, Lowenstein MB, Abeles M, et al: Oral mucosal ulceration in systemic lupus erythematosus. Arthritis Rheum 21:58-61, 1978.
32. Jonsson R, Heyden G, Westberg NG, et al: Oral mucosal lesions in systemic lupus erythematosus—a clinical, histopathological and immunopathological study. J Rheumatol 11:38-42, 1984.
33. Rahman P, Gladman DD, Urowitz MB: Nasal-septal perforation in systemic lupus erythematosus—time for a closer look. J Rheumatol 26:1854-1855, 1999.
34. Biesecker G, Lavin L, Ziskind M, et al: Cutaneous localization of the membrane attack complex in discoid and systemic lupus erythematosus. N Engl J Med 306:264-270, 1982.
35. Fabre VC, Lear S, Reichlin M, et al: Twenty percent of biopsy specimens from sun-exposed skin of normal young adults demonstrate positive immunofluorescence. Arch Dermatol 127:1006-1011, 1991.
36. Velthuis PJ, Kater L, van der Tweel I, et al: Immunofluorescence microscopy of healthy skin from patients with systemic lupus erythematosus: More than just the lupus band. Ann Rheum Dis 51:720-725, 1992.
37. van Vugt RM, Derksen RH, Kater L, et al: Deforming arthropathy or lupus and rhupus hands in systemic lupus erythematosus. Ann Rheum Dis 57:540-544, 1998.
38. Reilly PA, Evison G, McHugh NJ, et al: Arthropathy of hands and feet in systemic lupus erythematosus. J Rheumatol 17:777-784, 1990.
39. Panush RS, Edwards NL, Longley S, et al: 'Rhupus' syndrome. Arch Intern Med 148:1633-1636, 1988.
40. Wright S, Filippucci E, Grassi W, et al: Hand arthritis in systemic lupus erythematosus: An ultrasound pictorial essay. Lupus 15:501-506, 2006.
41. Furie RA, Chartash EK: Tendon rupture in systemic lupus erythematosus. Semin Arthritis Rheum 18:127-133, 1988.
42. Pritchard CH, Berney S: Patellar tendon rupture in systemic lupus erythematosus. J Rheumatol 16:786-788, 1989.
43. Petri M: Clinical features of systemic lupus erythematosus. Curr Opin Rheumatol 7:395-401, 1995.
44. Grigor R, Edmonds J, Lewkonia R, et al: Systemic lupus erythematosus: A prospective analysis. Ann Rheum Dis 37:121-128, 1978.
45. Sidiq M, Kirsner AB, Sheon RP: Carpal tunnel syndrome: First manifestation of systemic lupus erythematosus. JAMA 222:1416-1417, 1972.
46. Hahn BH, Yardley JH, Stevens MB: "Rheumatoid" nodules in systemic lupus erythematosus. Ann Intern Med 72:49-58, 1970.
47. Sugimoto H, Hyodoh K, Kikuno M, et al: Periarticular calcification in systemic lupus erythematosus. J Rheumatol 26:574-579, 1999.
48. Carette S, Urowitz MB: Systemic lupus erythematosus and diffuse soft tissue calcifications. Int J Dermatol 22:416-418, 1983.
49. Isenber DA, Snaith ML: Muscle disease in systemic lupus erythematosus: A study of its nature, frequency and cause. J Rheumatol 8:917-924, 1981.
50. Tsokos GC, Moutsopoulos HM, Steinberg AD: Muscle involvement in systemic lupus erythematosus. JAMA 246:766-768, 1981.
51. Russell ML, Hanna WM: Ultrastructural pathology of skeletal muscle in various rheumatic diseases. J Rheumatol 15:445-453, 1988.
52. Cronin ME: Musculoskeletal manifestations of systemic lupus erythematosus. Rheum Dis Clin N Am 14:99-116, 1988.
53. Finol HJ, Montagnani S, Marquez A, et al: Ultrastructural pathology of skeletal muscle in systemic lupus erythematosus. J Rheumatol 17:210-219, 1990.
54. Kitridou RC, Wittmann AL, Quismorio Jr FP: 1987. Chondritis in systemic lupus erythematosus: Clinical and immunopathologic studies. Clin Exp Rheumatol 5:349-353, 1987.
55. Harisdangkul V, Johnson WW: Association between relapsing polychondritis and systemic lupus erythematosus. South Med J 87:753-757, 1994.
56. Halland AM, Klemp P, Botes D, et al: Avascular necrosis of the hip in systemic lupus erythematosus: The role of magnetic resonance imaging. Br J Rheumatol 32:972-976, 1993.
57. Gladman DD, Urowitz MB, Chaudhry-Ahluwalia V, et al: Predictive factors for symptomatic osteonecrosis in patients with systemic lupus erythematosus. J Rheumatol 28:761-765, 2001.
58. Abeles M, Urman JD, Rothfield NF: Aseptic necrosis of bone in systemic lupus erythematosus: Relationship to corticosteroid therapy. Arch Intern Med 138:750-754, 1978.
59. Weiner ES, Abeles M: Aseptic necrosis and glucocorticosteroids in systemic lupus erythematosus: A reevaluation. J Rheumatol 16:604-608, 1989.
60. Massardo L, Jacobelli S, Leissner M, et al: High-dose intravenous methylprednisolone therapy associated with osteonecrosis in patients with systemic lupus erythematosus. Lupus 1:401-405, 1992.
61. Oinuma K, Harada Y, Nawata Y, et al: Osteonecrosis in patients with systemic lupus erythematosus develops very early after starting high dose corticosteroid treatment. Ann Rheum Dis 60:1145-1148, 2001.
62. Grande JP, Balow JE: Renal biopsy in lupus nephritis. Lupus 7:611-617, 1998.
63. Weening JJ, D'Agati VD, Schwartz MM, et al: The classification of glomerulonephritis in systemic lupus erythematosus revisited. Kidney Int 65:521-530, 2004.
64. Austin HA: Clinical evaluation and monitoring of lupus kidney disease. Lupus 7:618-621, 1998.

65. Esdaile JM, Joseph L, MacKenzie T, et al: The benefit of early treatment with immunosuppressive drugs in lupus nephritis. J Rheumatol 22:1211, 1995.

66. Hebert LA, Dillon JJ, Middendorf DF, et al: Relationship between appearance of urinary red blood cell/white blood cell casts and the onset of renal relapse in systemic lupus erythematosus. Am J Kidney Dis 26:432-438, 1995.

67. Austin HA 3rd, Boumpas DT, Vaughan EM, et al: High-risk features of lupus nephritis: Importance of race and clinical and histological factors in 166 patients. Nephrol Dial Transplant 10:1620-1628, 1995.

68. Tektonidou MG, Sotsiou F, Nakopoulou L, et al: Antiphospholipid syndrome nephropathy in patients with systemic lupus erythematosus and antiphospholipid antibodies: Prevalence, clinical associations, and long-term outcome. Arthritis Rheum 50:2569-2579, 2004.

69. Moroni G, Ventura D, Riva P, et al: Antiphospholipid antibodies are associated with an increased risk for chronic renal insufficiency in patients with lupus nephritis. Am J Kidney Dis 43:28-36, 2004.

70. Boumpas DT, Sidiropoulos P, Bertsias G: Optimum therapeutic approaches for lupus nephritis: What therapy and for whom? Nat Clin Pract Rheumatol 1:22-30, 2005.

71. American College of Rheumatology nomenclature and case definitions for neuropsychiatric lupus syndromes. Arthritis Rheum 42:599-608, 1999.

72. De Marcaida JA, Reik Jr L: Disorders that mimic central nervous system infections. Neurol Clin 17:901-941, 1999.

73. Sibbitt WL Jr, Sibbitt RR, Brooks WM: Neuroimaging in neuropsychiatric systemic lupus erythematosus. Arthritis Rheum 42:2026-2038, 1999.

74. Hanly JG, Walsh NM, Sangalang V: Brain pathology in systemic lupus erythematosus. J Rheumatol 19:732-741, 1992.

75. Hanson VG, Horowitz M, Rosenbluth D, et al: Systemic lupus erythematosus patients with central nervous system involvement show autoantibodies to a 50-kD neuronal membrane protein. J Exp Med 176:565-573, 1992.

76. Galeazzi M, Annunziata P, Sebastiani GD, et al: Anti-ganglioside antibodies in a large cohort of European patients with systemic lupus erythematosus: clinical, serological, and HLA class II gene associations. European Concerted Action on the Immunogenetics of SLE. J Rheumatol 27:135-141, 2000.

77. Pereira RM, Yoshinari NH, De Oliveira RM, et al: Antiganglioside antibodies in patients with neuropsychiatric systemic lupus erythematosus. Lupus 1:175-179, 1992.

78. DeGiorgio LA, Konstantinov KN, Lee SC, et al: A subset of lupus anti-DNA antibodies cross-reacts with the NR2 glutamate receptor in systemic lupus erythematosus. Nat Med 7:1189-1193, 2001.

79. Williamson RA, Burgoon MP, Owens GP, et al: Anti-DNA antibodies are a major component of the intrathecal B cell response in multiple sclerosis. Proc Natl Acad Sci U S A 98:1793-1798, 2001.

80. Teh LS, Isenberg DA: Antiribosomal P protein antibodies in systemic lupus erythematosus: A reappraisal. Arthritis Rheum 37:307-315, 1994.

81. Bonfa E, Golombek SJ, Kaufman LD, et al: Association between lupus psychosis and anti-ribosomal P protein antibodies. N Engl J Med 317:265-271, 1987.

82. Hanly JG: Antiphospholipid syndrome: An overview. Can Med Assoc J 168:1675-1682, 2003.

83. Love PE, Santoro SA: Antiphospholipid antibodies: Anticardiolipin and the lupus anticoagulant in systemic lupus erythematosus (SLE) and in non-SLE disorders: Prevalence and clinical significance. Ann Intern Med 112:682-698, 1990.

84. Hirohata S, Miyamoto T: Elevated levels of interleukin-6 in cerebrospinal fluid from patients with systemic lupus erythematosus and central nervous system involvement. Arthritis Rheum 33:644-649, 1990.

85. Shiozawa S, Kuroki Y, Kim M, et al: Interferon-alpha in lupus psychosis. Arthritis Rheum 35:417-422, 1992.

86. Trysberg E, Carlsten H, Tarkowski A: Intrathecal cytokines in systemic lupus erythematosus with central nervous system involvement. Lupus 9:498-503, 2000.

87. Jonsen A, Bengtsson AA, Nived O, et al: The heterogeneity of neuropsychiatric systemic lupus erythematosus is reflected in lack of association with cerebrospinal fluid cytokine profiles. Lupus 12:846-850, 2003.

88. Ainiala H, Hietaharju A, Loukkola J, et al: Validity of the new American College of Rheumatology criteria for neuropsychiatric lupus syndromes: A population-based evaluation. Arthritis Rheum 45:419-423, 2001.

89. Brey RL, Holliday SL, Saklad AR, et al: Neuropsychiatric syndromes in lupus: Prevalence using standardized definitions. Neurology 58:1214-1220, 2002.

90. Hanly JG, McCurdy G, Fougere L, et al: Neuropsychiatric events in systemic lupus erythematosus: Attribution and clinical significance. J Rheumatol 31:2156-2162, 2004.

91. Sanna G, Bertolaccini ML, Cuadrado MJ, et al: Neuropsychiatric manifestations in systemic lupus erythematosus: Prevalence and association with antiphospholipid antibodies. J Rheumatol 30:985-992, 2003.

92. Sibbitt WL Jr, Brandt JR, Johnson CR, et al: The incidence and prevalence of neuropsychiatric syndromes in pediatric onset systemic lupus erythematosus. J Rheumatol 29:1536-1542, 2002.

93. Graham JW, Jan W: MRI and the brain in systemic lupus erythematosus. Lupus 12:891-896, 2003.

94. Kovacs B, Lafferty TL, Brent LH, et al: Transverse myelopathy in systemic lupus erythematosus: An analysis of 14 cases and review of the literature. Ann Rheum Dis 59:120-124, 2000.

95. Cervera R, Asherson RA, Font J, et al: Chorea in the antiphospholipid syndrome: Clinical, radiologic, and immunologic characteristics of 50 patients from our clinics and the recent literature. Medicine (Balt) 76:203-212, 1997.

96. Omdal R, Loseth S, Torbergsen T, et al: Peripheral neuropathy in systemic lupus erythematosus—a longitudinal study. Acta Neurol Scand 103:386-391, 2001.

97. Abu-Shakra M, Urowitz MB, Gladman DD, et al: Mortality studies in systemic lupus erythematosus: Results from a single center, I: Causes of death. J Rheumatol 22:1259-1264, 1995.

98. Ward MM: Premature morbidity from cardiovascular and cerebrovascular diseases in women with systemic lupus erythematosus. Arthritis Rheum 42:338-346, 1999.

99. Rubin LA, Urowitz MB, Gladman DD: Mortality in systemic lupus erythematosus: The bimodal pattern revisited. QJM 55:87-98, 1985.

100. Haider YS, Roberts WC: Coronary arterial disease in systemic lupus erythematosus: Quantification of degrees of narrowing in 22 necropsy patients (21 women) aged 16 to 37 years. Am J Med 70:775-781, 1981.

101. Bjornadal L, Yin L, Granath F, et al: Cardiovascular disease a hazard despite improved prognosis in patients with systemic lupus erythematosus: Results from a Swedish population based study 1964-95. J Rheumatol 31:713-719, 2004.

102. Manzi S, Meilahn EN, Rairie JE, et al: Age-specific incidence rates of myocardial infarction and angina in women with systemic lupus erythematosus: Comparison with the Framingham Study. Am J Epidemiol 145:408-415, 1997.

103. Fischer LM, Schlienger RG, Matter C, et al: Effect of rheumatoid arthritis or systemic lupus erythematosus on the risk of first-time acute myocardial infarction. Am J Cardiol 93:198-200, 2004.

104. Bessant R, Hingorani A, Patel L, et al: Risk of coronary heart disease and stroke in a large British cohort of patients with systemic lupus erythematosus. Rheumatology (Oxf) 43:924-929, 2004.

105. Roman MJ, Shanker BA, Davis A, et al: Prevalence and correlates of accelerated atherosclerosis in systemic lupus erythematosus. N Engl J Med 349:2399-2406, 2003.

106. Asanuma Y, Oeser A, Shintani AK, et al: Premature coronary-artery atherosclerosis in systemic lupus erythematosus. N Engl J Med 349:2407-2415, 2003.

107. Roldan CA, Shively BK, Crawford MH: An echocardiographic study of valvular heart disease associated with systemic lupus erythematosus. N Engl J Med 335:1424-1430, 1996.

108. Deppisch LM, Fayemi AO: Non-bacterial thrombotic endocarditis: Clinicopathologic correlations. Am Heart J 92:723-729, 1976.

109. Gorelick PB, Rusinowitz MS, Tiku M, et al: Embolic stroke complicating systemic lupus erythematosus. Arch Neurol 42:813-815, 1985.

110. Devinsky O, Petito CK, Alonso DR: Clinical and neuropathological findings in systemic lupus erythematosus: The role of vasculitis, heart emboli, and thrombotic thrombocytopenic purpura. Ann Neurol 23:380-384, 1988.

111. Bidani AK, Roberts JL, Schwartz MM, et al: Immunopathology of cardiac lesions in fatal systemic lupus erythematosus. Am J Med 69:849-858, 1980.

112. Blanchard DG, Ross RS, Dittrich HC: Nonbacterial thrombotic endocarditis: Assessment by transesophageal echocardiography. Chest 102:954-956, 1992.

113. Lopez JA, Fishbein MC, Siegel RJ: Echocardiographic features of nonbacterial thrombotic endocarditis. Am J Cardiol 59:478-480, 1987.
114. Futrell N, Millikan C: Frequency, etiology, and prevention of stroke in patients with systemic lupus erythematosus. Stroke 20:583-591, 1989.
115. Sturfelt G, Eskilsson J, Nived O, et al: Cardiovascular disease in systemic lupus erythematosus: A study of 75 patients form a defined population. Medicine (Balt) 71:216-223, 1992.
116. Orens JB, Martinez FJ, Lynch 3rd JP: Pleuropulmonary manifestations of systemic lupus erythematosus. Rheum Dis Clin N Am 20:159-193, 1994.
117. Fishback N, Koss MN: Pulmonary involvement in systemic lupus erythematosus. Curr Opin Pulm Med 1:368-375, 1995.
118. Sahn SA: The pathophysiology of pleural effusions. Annu Rev Med 41:7-13, 1990.
119. Mathlouthi A, Ben M'rad S, Merai S, et al: Massive pleural effusion in systemic lupus erythematosus: Thoracoscopic and immunohistological findings. Monaldi Arch Chest Dis 53:34-36, 1998.
120. Haupt HM, Moore GW, Hutchins GM: The lung in systemic lupus erythematosus: Analysis of the pathologic changes in 120 patients. Am J Med 71:791-798, 1981.
121. Fenlon HM, Doran M, Sant SM, et al: High-resolution chest CT in systemic lupus erythematosus. AJR Am J Roentgenol 166:301-307, 1996.
122. Groen H, ter Borg EJ, Postma DS, et al: Pulmonary function in systemic lupus erythematosus is related to distinct clinical, serologic, and nailfold capillary patterns. Am J Med 93:619-627, 1992.
123. Myers JL, Katzenstein AA: Microangiitis in lupus-induced pulmonary hemorrhage. Am J Clin Pathol 85:552-556, 1986.
124. Zamora MR, Warner ML, Tuder R, et al: Diffuse alveolar hemorrhage and systemic lupus erythematosus: Clinical presentation, histology, survival, and outcome. Medicine (Balt) 76:192-202, 1997.
125. Thompson PJ, Dhillon DP, Ledingham J, et al: Shrinking lungs, diaphragmatic dysfunction, and systemic lupus erythematosus. Am Rev Respir Dis 132:926-928, 1985.
126. Kojima M, Nakamura S, Morishita Y, et al: Reactive follicular hyperplasia in the lymph node lesions from systemic lupus erythematosus patients: A clinicopathological and immunohistological study of 21 cases. Pathol Int 50:304-312, 2000.
127. Dillon AM, Stein HB, English RA: Splenic atrophy in systemic lupus erythematosus. Ann Intern Med 96:40-43, 1982.
128. Piliero P, Furie R: Functional asplenia in systemic lupus erythematosus. Semin Arthritis Rheum 20:185-189, 1990.
129. Giannouli S, Voulgarelis M, Ziakas PD, et al: Anaemia in systemic lupus erythematosus: From pathophysiology to clinical assessment. Ann Rheum Dis 65:144-148, 2006.
130. Voulgarelis M, Kokori SI, Ioannidis JP, et al: Anaemia in systemic lupus erythematosus: Aetiological profile and the role of erythropoietin. Ann Rheum Dis 59:217-222, 2000.
131. Habib GS, Saliba WR, Froom P: Pure red cell aplasia and lupus. Semin Arthritis Rheum 31:279-283, 2002.
132. Liu H, Ozaki K, Matsuzaki Y, et al: Suppression of haematopoiesis by IgG autoantibodies from patients with systemic lupus erythematosus (SLE). Clin Exp Immunol 100:480-485, 1995.
133. Keeling DM, Isenberg DA: Haematological manifestations of systemic lupus erythematosus. Blood Rev 7:199-207, 1993.
134. Nesher G, Hanna VE, Moore TL, et al: Thrombotic microangiographic hemolytic anemia in systemic lupus erythematosus. Semin Arthritis Rheum 24:165-172, 1994.
135. Niewold TB, Alpert D, Scanzello CR, et al: Rituximab treatment of thrombotic thrombocytopenic purpura in the setting of connective tissue disease. J Rheumatol 33:1194-1196, 2006.
136. Sultan SM, Begum S, Isenberg DA: Prevalence, patterns of disease and outcome in patients with systemic lupus erythematosus who develop severe haematological problems. Rheumatology (Oxf) 42:230-234, 2003.
137. Rivero SJ, Diaz-Jouanen E, Alarcon-Segovia D: Lymphopenia in systemic lupus erythematosus: Clinical, diagnostic, and prognostic significance. Arthritis Rheum 21:295-305, 1978.
138. Winfield JB, Winchester RJ, Kunkel HG: Association of cold-reactive antilymphocyte antibodies with lymphopenia in systemic lupus erythematosus. Arthritis Rheum 18:587-594, 1975.
139. Amasaki Y, Kobayashi S, Takeda T, et al: Up-regulated expression of Fas antigen (CD95) by peripheral naive and memory T cell subsets in patients with systemic lupus erythematosus (SLE): A possible mechanism for lymphopenia. Clin Exp Immunol 99:245-250, 1995.
140. Budman DR, Steinberg AD: Hematologic aspects of systemic lupus erythematosus: Current concepts. Ann Intern Med 86:220-229, 1977.
141. Boumpas DT, Chrousos GP, Wilder RL, et al: Glucocorticoid therapy for immune-mediated diseases: Basic and clinical correlates. Ann Intern Med 119:1198-1208, 1993.
142. Pujol M, Ribera A, Vilardell M, et al: High prevalence of platelet autoantibodies in patients with systemic lupus erythematosus. Br J Haematol 89:137-141, 1995.
143. Fureder W, Firbas U, Nichol JL, et al: Serum thrombopoietin levels and anti-thrombopoietin antibodies in systemic lupus erythematosus. Lupus 11:221-226, 2002.
144. Hoffman BI, Katz WA: The gastrointestinal manifestations of systemic lupus erythematosus: A review of the literature. Semin Arthritis Rheum 9:237-247, 1980.
145. Sultan SM, Ioannou Y, Isenberg DA: A review of gastrointestinal manifestations of systemic lupus erythematosus. Rheumatology (Oxf) 38:917-932, 1999.
146. Gutierrez F, Valenzuela JE, Ehresmann GR, et al: Esophageal dysfunction in patients with mixed connective tissue diseases and systemic lupus erythematosus. Dig Dis Sci 27:592-597, 1982.
147. Ginzler EM, Aranow C: Prevention and treatment of adverse effects of corticosteroids in systemic lupus erythematosus. Baillieres Clin Rheumatol 12:495-510, 1998.
148. Jovaisas A, Kraag G: Acute gastrointestinal manifestations of systemic lupus erythematosus. Can J Surg 30:185-188, 1987.
149. Zizic TM., Classen JN, Stevens MB: Acute abdominal complications of systemic lupus erythematosus and polyarteritis nodosa. Am J Med 73:525-531, 1982.
150. Ko SF, Lee TY, Cheng TT, et al: CT findings at lupus mesenteric vasculitis. Acta Radiol 38:115-120, 1997.
151. Pascual-Ramos V, Duarte-Rojo A, Villa AR, et al: Systemic lupus erythematosus as a cause and prognostic factor of acute pancreatitis. J Rheumatol 31:707-712, 2004.
152. Breuer GS, Baer A, Dahan D, et al: Lupus-associated pancreatitis. Autoimmun Rev 5:314-318, 2006.
153. Runyon BA, LaBrecque DR, Anuras S: The spectrum of liver disease in systemic lupus erythematosus: Report of 33 histologically-proved cases and review of the literature. Am J Med 69:187-194, 1980.
154. Miller MH, Urowitz MB, Gladman DD, et al: The liver in systemic lupus erythematosus. QJM 53:401-409, 1984.
155. Abraham S, Begum S, Isenberg D: Hepatic manifestations of autoimmune rheumatic diseases. Ann Rheum Dis 63:123-129, 2004.
156. Ushiyama O, Ushiyama K, Koarada S, et al: Retinal disease in patients with systemic lupus erythematosus. Ann Rheum Dis 59:705-708, 2000.
157. Arbuckle MR, McClain MT, Rubertone MV, et al: Development of autoantibodies before the clinical onset of systemic lupus erythematosus. N Engl J Med 349:1526-1533, 2003.
158. Emlen W, O'Neill L: Clinical significance of antinuclear antibodies: Comparison of detection with immunofluorescence and enzyme-linked immunosorbent assays. Arthritis Rheum 40:1612-1618, 1997.
159. Tan EM, Feltkamp TE, Smolen JS, et al: Range of antinuclear antibodies in "healthy" individuals. Arthritis Rheum 40:1601-1611, 1997.
160. Lefkowith JB, Gilkeson GS: Nephritogenic autoantibodies in lupus: Current concepts and continuing controversies. Arthritis Rheum 39:894-903, 1996.
161. Calvo-Alen J, Alarcon GS, Burgard SL, et al: Systemic lupus erythematosus: Predictors of its occurrence among a cohort of patients with early undifferentiated connective tissue disease: Multivariate analyses and identification of risk factors. J Rheumatol 23:469-475, 1996.
162. Swaak AJ, van de Brink H, Smeenk RJ, et al: Incomplete lupus erythematosus: Results of a multicentre study under the supervision of the EULAR Standing Committee on International Clinical Studies Including Therapeutic Trials (ESCISIT). Rheumatology (Oxf) 40:89-94, 2001.
163. Ganczarczyk L, Urowitz MB, Gladman DD: "Latent lupus." J Rheumatol 16:475-478, 1989.

164. Stahl NI, Klippel JH, Decker JL: Fever in systemic lupus erythematosus. Am J Med 67:935-940, 1979.
165. Papadaki HA, Xylouri I, Katrinakis G, et al: Non-Hodgkin's lymphoma in patients with systemic lupus erythematosus. Leuk Lymphoma 44:275-279, 2003.
166. Tsakonas E, Joseph L, Esdaile JM, et al: A long-term study of hydroxychloroquine withdrawal on exacerbations in systemic lupus erythematosus. The Canadian Hydroxychloroquine Study Group. Lupus 7:80-85, 1998.
167. A randomized study of the effect of withdrawing hydroxychloroquine sulfate in systemic lupus erythematosus. The Canadian Hydroxychloroquine Study Group. N Engl J Med 324:150-154, 1991.
168. **Ginzler EM, Dooley MA, Aranow C, et al: Mycophenolate mofetil or intravenous cyclophosphamide for lupus nephritis. N Engl J Med 353:2219-2228, 2005.**
169. **Contreras G, Pardo V, Leclercq B, et al: Sequential therapies for proliferative lupus nephritis. N Engl J Med 350:971-980, 2004.**
170. Chan TM, Tse KC, Tang CS, et al: Long-term study of mycophenolate mofetil as continuous induction and maintenance treatment for diffuse proliferative lupus nephritis. J Am Soc Nephrol 16:1076-1084, 2005.
171. Chan TM, Li FK, Tang CS, et al: Efficacy of mycophenolate mofetil in patients with diffuse proliferative lupus nephritis. Hong Kong-Guangzhou Nephrology Study Group. N Engl J Med 343:1156-1162, 2000.
172. **Austin HA 3rd, Klippel JH, Balow JE, et al: Therapy of lupus nephritis: Controlled trial of prednisone and cytotoxic drugs. N Engl J Med 314:614-619, 1986.**
173. **Boumpas DT, Austin HA 3rd, Vaughn EM, et al: Controlled trial of pulse methylprednisolone versus two regimens of pulse cyclophosphamide in severe lupus nephritis. Lancet 340:741-745, 1992.**
174. Illei GG, Austin HA, Crane M, et al: Combination therapy with pulse cyclophosphamide plus pulse methylprednisolone improves long-term renal outcome without adding toxicity in patients with lupus nephritis. Ann Intern Med 135:248-257, 2001.
175. Gourley MF, Austin HA 3rd, Scott D, et al: Methylprednisolone and cyclophosphamide, alone or in combination, in patients with lupus nephritis: A randomized, controlled trial. Ann Intern Med 125:549-557, 1996.
176. Boumpas DT, Austin HA 3rd, Vaughan EM, et al: Risk for sustained amenorrhea in patients with systemic lupus erythematosus receiving intermittent pulse cyclophosphamide therapy. Ann Intern Med 119:366-369, 1993.
177. Houssiau FA, Vasconcelos C, D'Cruz D, et al: Immunosuppressive therapy in lupus nephritis: The Euro-Lupus Nephritis Trial, a randomized trial of low-dose versus high-dose intravenous cyclophosphamide. Arthritis Rheum 46:2121-2131, 2002.
178. Houssiau FA, Vasconcelos C, D'Cruz D, et al: Early response to immunosuppressive therapy predicts good renal outcome in lupus nephritis: Lessons from long-term followup of patients in the Euro-Lupus Nephritis Trial. Arthritis Rheum 50:3934-3940, 2004.
179. Barile-Fabris L, Ariza-Andraca R, Olguin-Ortega L, et al: Controlled clinical trial of IV cyclophosphamide versus IV methylprednisolone in severe neurological manifestations in systemic lupus erythematosus. Ann Rheum Dis 64:620-625, 2005.
180. Somers EC, Marder W, Christman GM, et al: Use of a gonadotropin-releasing hormone analog for protection against premature ovarian failure during cyclophosphamide therapy in women with severe lupus. Arthritis Rheum 52:2761-2767, 2005.
181. Masala A, Faedda R, Alagna S, et al: Use of testosterone to prevent cyclophosphamide-induced azoospermia. Ann Intern Med 126:292-295, 1997.
182. Ahmed AR, Spigelman Z, Cavacini LA, et al: Treatment of pemphigus vulgaris with rituximab and intravenous immune globulin. N Engl J Med 355:1772-1779, 2006.
183. **Smith KG, Jones RB, Burns SM, et al: Long-term comparison of rituximab treatment for refractory systemic lupus erythematosus and vasculitis: Remission, relapse, and re-treatment. Arthritis Rheum 54:2970-2982, 2006.**
184. Esdaile JM, Joseph L, MacKenzie T, et al: The benefit of early treatment with immunosuppressive agents in lupus nephritis. J Rheumatol 21:2046-2051, 1994.
185. Carneiro JR, Sato EI: Double blind, randomized, placebo controlled clinical trial of methotrexate in systemic lupus erythematosus. J Rheumatol 26:1275-1279, 1999.
186. Boletis JN, Ioannidis JP, Boki KA, et al: Intravenous immunoglobulin compared with cyclophosphamide for proliferative lupus nephritis. Lancet 354:569-570, 1999.
187. Bernatsky S, Boivin JF, Joseph L, et al: An international cohort study of cancer in systemic lupus erythematosus. Arthritis Rheum 52:1481-1490, 2005.
188. Ognenovski VM, Marder W, Somers EC, et al: Increased incidence of cervical intraepithelial neoplasia in women with systemic lupus erythematosus treated with intravenous cyclophosphamide. J Rheumatol 31:1763-1767, 2004.
189. Bernatsky S, Ramsey-Goldman R, Gordon C, et al: Factors associated with abnormal Pap results in systemic lupus erythematosus. Rheumatology (Oxf) 43:1386-1389, 2004.
190. Bernatsky SR, Cooper GS, Mill C, et al: Cancer screening in patients with systemic lupus erythematosus. J Rheumatol 33:45-49, 2006.
191. Sanchez-Guerrero J, Uribe AG, Jimenez-Santana L, et al: A trial of contraceptive methods in women with systemic lupus erythematosus. N Engl J Med 353:2539-2549, 2005.
192. Petri M, Kim MY, Kalunian KC, et al: Combined oral contraceptives in women with systemic lupus erythematosus. N Engl J Med 353:2550-2558, 2005.
193. Mintz G, Niz J, Gutierrez G, et al: Prospective study of pregnancy in systemic lupus erythematosus: Results of a multidisciplinary approach. J Rheumatol 13:732-739, 1986.
194. Derksen RH, Bouma BN, Kater L: The prevalence and clinical associations of the lupus anticoagulant in systemic lupus erythematosus. Scand J Rheumatol 16:185-192, 1987.
195. Ishii Y, Nagasawa K, Mayumi T, et al: Clinical importance of persistence of anticardiolipin antibodies in systemic lupus erythematosus. Ann Rheum Dis 49:387-390, 1990.
196. Cortes-Hernandez J, Ordi-Ros J, Paredes F, et al: Clinical predictors of fetal and maternal outcome in systemic lupus erythematosus: A prospective study of 103 pregnancies. Rheumatology (Oxf) 41:643-650, 2002.
197. Kiss E, Bhattoa HP, Bettembuk P, et al: Pregnancy in women with systemic lupus erythematosus. Eur J Obstet Gynecol Reprod Biol 101:129-134, 2002.
198. Lima F, Buchanan NM, Khamashta MA, et al: Obstetric outcome in systemic lupus erythematosus. Semin Arthritis Rheum 25:184-192, 1995.
199. Lynch A, Marlar R, Murphy J, et al: Antiphospholipid antibodies in predicting adverse pregnancy outcome: A prospective study. Ann Intern Med 120:470-475, 1994.
200. Silva CA, Leal MM, Leone C, et al: Gonadal function in adolescents and young women with juvenile systemic lupus erythematosus. Lupus 11:419-425, 2002.
201. Geva E, Lerner-Geva L, Burke M, et al: Undiagnosed systemic lupus erythematosus in a cohort of infertile women. Am J Reprod Immunol 51:336-340, 2004.
202. Balasch J, Creus M, Fabregues F, et al: Antiphospholipid antibodies and human reproductive failure. Hum Reprod 11:2310-2315, 1996.
203. Sinaii N, Cleary SD, Ballweg ML, et al: High rates of autoimmune and endocrine disorders, fibromyalgia, chronic fatigue syndrome and atopic diseases among women with endometriosis: A survey analysis. Hum Reprod 17:2715-2724, 2002.
204. Hayslett JP: The effect of systemic lupus erythematosus on pregnancy and pregnancy outcome. Am J Reprod Immunol 28:199-204, 1992.
205. Tandon A, Ibanez D, Gladman DD, et al: The effect of pregnancy on lupus nephritis. Arthritis Rheum 50:3941-3946, 2004.
206. Carmona F, Font J, Cervera R, et al: Obstetrical outcome of pregnancy in patients with systemic lupus erythematosus: A study of 60 cases. Eur J Obstet Gynecol Reprod Biol 83:137-142, 1999.
207. Ruiz-Irastorza G, Lima F, Alves J, et al: Increased rate of lupus flare during pregnancy and the puerperium: A prospective study of 78 pregnancies. Br J Rheumatol 35:133-138, 1996.
208. **Petri M, Howard D, Repke J: Frequency of lupus flare in pregnancy. The Hopkins Lupus Pregnancy Center experience. Arthritis Rheum 34:1538-1545, 1991.**
209. Petri M, Genovese M, Engle E, et al: Definition, incidence, and clinical description of flare in systemic lupus erythematosus: A prospective cohort study. Arthritis Rheum 34:937-944, 1991.
210. Nossent HC, Swaak TJ: Systemic lupus erythematosus, VI: Analysis of the interrelationship with pregnancy. J Rheumatol 17:771-776, 1990.
211. Georgiou PE, Politi EN, Katsimbri PV, et al: Outcome of lupus pregnancy: A controlled study. Rheumatology (Oxf) 39:1014-1019, 2000.

212. Lockshin MD: Pregnancy does not cause systemic lupus erythematosus to worsen. Arthritis Rheum 32:665-670, 1989.
213. Le Thi Huong D, Wechsler B, Piette JC, et al: Pregnancy and its outcome in systemic lupus erythematosus. QJM 87:721-729, 1994.
214. Soubassi L, Haidopoulos D, Sindos M, et al: Pregnancy outcome in women with pre-existing lupus nephritis. J Obstet Gynaecol 24: 630-634, 2004.
215. Huong DL, Wechsler B, Vauthier-Brouzes D, et al: Pregnancy in past or present lupus nephritis: A study of 32 pregnancies from a single centre. Ann Rheum Dis 60:599-604, 2001.
216. Julkunen H, Kaaja R, Palosuo T, et al: Pregnancy in lupus nephropathy. Acta Obstet Gynecol Scand 72:258-263, 1993.
217. Faden D, Tincani A, Tanzi P, et al: Anti-beta 2 glycoprotein I antibodies in a general obstetric population: Preliminary results on the prevalence and correlation with pregnancy outcome: Anti-beta2 glycoprotein I antibodies are associated with some obstetrical complications, mainly preeclampsia-eclampsia. Eur J Obstet Gynecol Reprod Biol 73:37-42, 1997.
218. Branch DW, Andres R, Digre KB, et al: The association of antiphospholipid antibodies with severe preeclampsia. Obstet Gynecol 73:541-545, 1989.
219. Mok MY, Chan EY, Fong DY, et al: Antiphospholipid antibody profiles and their clinical associations in Chinese patients with systemic lupus erythematosus. J Rheumatol 32:622-628, 2005.
220. Moroni G, Quaglini S, Banfi G, et al: Pregnancy in lupus nephritis. Am J Kidney Dis 40:713-720, 2002.
221. Moroni G, Ponticelli C: The risk of pregnancy in patients with lupus nephritis. J Nephrol 16:161-167, 2003.
222. Watson RM, Braunstein BL, Watson AJ, et al: Fetal wastage in women with anti-Ro(SSA) antibody. J Rheumatol 13:90-94, 1986.
223. Julkunen H, Jouhikainen T, Kaaja R, et al: Fetal outcome in lupus pregnancy: A retrospective case-control study of 242 pregnancies in 112 patients. Lupus 2:125-131, 1993.
224. Lockwood CJ, Romero R, Feinberg RF, Clyne LP, et al: The prevalence and biologic significance of lupus anticoagulant and anticardiolipin antibodies in a general obstetric population. Am J Obstet Gynecol 161:369-373, 1989.
225. Polzin WJ, Kopelman JN, Robinson RD, et al: The association of antiphospholipid antibodies with pregnancies complicated by fetal growth restriction. Obstet Gynecol 78:1108-1111, 1991.
226. Rubbert A, Pirner K, Wildt L, et al: Pregnancy course and complications in patients with systemic lupus erythematosus. Am J Reprod Immunol 28:205-207, 1992.
227. Petri M, Ho AC, Patel J, et al: Elevation of maternal alpha-fetoprotein in systemic lupus erythematosus: A controlled study. J Rheumatol 22:1365-1368, 1995.
228. Clark F, Dickinson JE, Walters BN, et al: Elevated mid-trimester hCG and maternal lupus anticoagulant. Prenat Diagn 15:1035-1039, 1995.
229. Buyon JP, Hiebert R, Copel J, et al: Autoimmune-associated congenital heart block: Demographics, mortality, morbidity and recurrence rates obtained from a national neonatal lupus registry. J Am Coll Cardiol 31:1658-1666, 1998.
230. Lockshin MD, Bonfa E, Elkon K, et al: Neonatal lupus risk to newborns of mothers with systemic lupus erythematosus. Arthritis Rheum 31:697-701, 1988.
231. Clowse ME, Magder LS, Witter F, et al: The impact of increased lupus activity on obstetric outcomes. Arthritis Rheum 52:514-521, 2005.
232. Buchanan NM, Khamashta MA, Morton KE, et al: A study of 100 high risk lupus pregnancies. Am J Reprod Immunol 28:192-194, 1992.
233. Tincani A, Faden D, Tarantini M, et al: Systemic lupus erythematosus and pregnancy: A prospective study. Clin Exp Rheumatol 10: 439-446, 1992.
234. Levy RA, Vilela VS, Cataldo MJ, et al: Hydroxychloroquine (HCQ) in lupus pregnancy: Double-blind and placebo-controlled study. Lupus 10:401-404, 2001.
235. Costedoat-Chalumeau N, Amoura Z, Duhaut P, et al: Safety of hydroxychloroquine in pregnant patients with connective tissue diseases: A study of one hundred thirty-three cases compared with a control group. Arthritis Rheum 48:3207-3211, 2003.
236. Buchanan NM, Toubi E, Khamashta MA, et al: Hydroxychloroquine and lupus pregnancy: Review of a series of 36 cases. Ann Rheum Dis 55:486-488, 1996.
237. Parke A, West B: Hydroxychloroquine in pregnant patients with systemic lupus erythematosus. J Rheumatol 23:1715-1718, 1996.
238. Al-Herz A, Schulzer M, Esdaile JM: Survey of antimalarial use in lupus pregnancy and lactation. J Rheumatol 29:700-706, 2002.
239. Armenti VT, Radomski JS, Moritz MJ, et al: Report from the National Transplantation Pregnancy Registry (NTPR): Outcomes of pregnancy after transplantation. Clin Transpl 121-130, 2002.
240. Ramsey-Goldman R, Schilling E: Immunosuppressive drug use during pregnancy. Rheum Dis Clin N Am 23:149-167, 1997.
241. Ramsey-Goldman R, Mientus JM, Kutzer JE, et al: Pregnancy outcome in women with systemic lupus erythematosus treated with immunosuppressive drugs. J Rheumatol 20:1152-1157, 1993.
242. Doria A, Di Lenardo L, Vario S, et al: Cyclosporin A in a pregnant patient affected with systemic lupus erythematosus. Rheumatol Int 12:77-78, 1992.
243. Hussein MM, Mooij JM, Roujouleh H: Cyclosporine in the treatment of lupus nephritis including two patients treated during pregnancy. Clin Nephrol 40:160-163, 1993.
244. Ruiz-Irastorza G, Khamashta MA, Hunt BJ, et al: Bleeding and recurrent thrombosis in definite antiphospholipid syndrome: Analysis of a series of 66 patients treated with oral anticoagulation to a target international normalized ratio of 3.5. Arch Intern Med 162: 1164-1169, 2002.
245. Rosove MH, Brewer PM: Antiphospholipid thrombosis: Clinical course after the first thrombotic event in 70 patients. Ann Intern Med 117:303-308, 1992.
246. Rivier G, Herranz MT, Khamashta MA, et al: Thrombosis and antiphospholipid syndrome: A preliminary assessment of three antithrombotic treatments. Lupus 3:85-90, 1994.
247. Munoz-Rodriguez FJ, Font J, Cervera R, et al: Clinical study and follow-up of 100 patients with the antiphospholipid syndrome. Semin Arthritis Rheum 29:182-190, 1999.
248. Khamashta MA, Cuadrado MJ, Mujic F, et al: The management of thrombosis in the antiphospholipid-antibody syndrome. N Engl J Med 332:993-997, 1995.
249. Finazzi G, Marchioli R, Brancaccio V, et al: A randomized clinical trial of high-intensity warfarin vs. conventional antithrombotic therapy for the prevention of recurrent thrombosis in patients with the antiphospholipid syndrome (WAPS). J Thromb Haemost 3:848-853, 2005.
250. Crowther MA, Ginsberg JS, Julian J, et al: A comparison of two intensities of warfarin for the prevention of recurrent thrombosis in patients with the antiphospholipid antibody syndrome. N Engl J Med 349:1133-1138, 2003.
251. Empson M, Lassere M, Craig J, et al: Prevention of recurrent miscarriage for women with antiphospholipid antibody or lupus anticoagulant. Cochrane Database Syst Rev CD002859, 2005.
252. Triolo G, Ferrante A, Ciccia F, et al: Randomized study of subcutaneous low molecular weight heparin plus aspirin versus intravenous immunoglobulin in the treatment of recurrent fetal loss associated with antiphospholipid antibodies. Arthritis Rheum 48:728-731, 2003.
253. Farquharson RG, Quenby S, Greaves M: Antiphospholipid syndrome in pregnancy: A randomized, controlled trial of treatment. Obstet Gynecol 100:408-413, 2002.
254. Rai R, Cohen H, Dave M, et al: Randomised controlled trial of aspirin and aspirin plus heparin in pregnant women with recurrent miscarriage associated with phospholipid antibodies (or antiphospholipid antibodies). BMJ 314:253-257, 1997.
255. Franklin RD, Kutteh WH: Antiphospholipid antibodies (APA) and recurrent pregnancy loss: Treating a unique APA positive population. Hum Reprod 17:2981-2985, 2002.
256. Balasch J, Carmona F, Lopez-Soto A, et al: Low-dose aspirin for prevention of pregnancy losses in women with primary antiphospholipid syndrome. Hum Reprod 8:2234-2239, 1993.
257. Pauzner R, Dulitzki M, Langevitz P, et al: Low molecular weight heparin and warfarin in the treatment of patients with antiphospholipid syndrome during pregnancy. Thromb Haemost 86:1379-1384, 2001.
258. Many A, Pauzner R, Carp H, et al: Treatment of patients with antiphospholipid antibodies during pregnancy. Am J Reprod Immunol 28:216-218, 1992.
259. Carmona F, Font J, Azulay M, et al: Risk factors associated with fetal losses in treated antiphospholipid syndrome pregnancies: A multivariate analysis. Am J Reprod Immunol 46:274-279, 2001.

260. Olsen NJ: Drug-induced autoimmunity. Best Pract Res Clin Rheumatol 18:677-688, 2004.

261. Reidenberg MM, Drayer DE, Lorenzo B, et al: Acetylation phenotypes and environmental chemical exposure of people with idiopathic systemic lupus erythematosus. Arthritis Rheum 36:971-973, 1993.

262. Kretz-Rommel A, Rubin RL: Disruption of positive selection of thymocytes causes autoimmunity. Nat Med 6:298-305, 2000.

263. Stone JH: End-stage renal disease in lupus: Disease activity, dialysis, and the outcome of transplantation. Lupus 7:654-659, 1998.

264. Ward MM: Cardiovascular and cerebrovascular morbidity and mortality among women with end-stage renal disease attributable to lupus nephritis. Am J Kidney Dis 36:516-525, 2000.

265. Ward MM: Changes in the incidence of end-stage renal disease due to lupus nephritis, 1982-1995. Arch Intern Med 160:3136-3140, 2000.

266. Mange KC, Joffe MM, Feldman HI: Effect of the use or nonuse of long-term dialysis on the subsequent survival of renal transplants from living donors. N Engl J Med 344:726-731, 2001.

267. Moroni G, Tantardini F, Gallelli B, et al: The long-term prognosis of renal transplantation in patients with lupus nephritis. Am J Kidney Dis 45:903-911, 2005.

268. Ward MM: Outcomes of renal transplantation among patients with end-stage renal disease caused by lupus nephritis. Kidney Int 57:2136-2143, 2000.

269. Vaidya S, Sellers R, Kimball P, et al: Frequency, potential risk and therapeutic intervention in end-stage renal disease patients with antiphospholipid antibody syndrome: A multicenter study. Transplantation 69:1348-1352, 2000.

270. Bartosh SM, Fine RN, Sullivan EK: Outcome after transplantation of young patients with systemic lupus erythematosus: A report of the North American pediatric renal transplant cooperative study. Transplantation 72:973-978, 2001.

271. Murin S, Wiedemann HP, Matthay RA: Pulmonary manifestations of systemic lupus erythematosus. Clin Chest Med 19:641-665, viii, 1998.

272. Matthay RA, Schwarz MI, Petty TL, et al: Pulmonary manifestations of systemic lupus erythematosus: Review of twelve cases of acute lupus pneumonitis. Medicine (Balt) 54:397-409, 1975.

273. Carette S, Macher AM, Nussbaum A, et al: Severe, acute pulmonary disease in patients with systemic lupus erythematosus: Ten years of experience at the National Institutes of Health. Semin Arthritis Rheum 14:52-59, 1984.

274. Santos-Ocampo AS, Mandell BF, Fessler BJ: Alveolar hemorrhage in systemic lupus erythematosus: Presentation and management. Chest 118:1083-1090, 2000.

275. Liu MF, Lee JH, Weng TH, et al: Clinical experience of 13 cases with severe pulmonary hemorrhage in systemic lupus erythematosus with active nephritis. Scand J Rheumatol 27:291-295, 1998.

276. Lee JG, Joo KW, Chung WK, et al: Diffuse alveolar hemorrhage in lupus nephritis. Clin Nephrol 55:282-288, 2001.

277. Mintz G, Galindo LF, Fernandez-Diez J, et al: Acute massive pulmonary hemorrhage in systemic lupus erythematosus. J Rheumatol 5:39-50, 1978.

278. Eagen JW, Memoli VA, Roberts JL, et al: Pulmonary hemorrhage in systemic lupus erythematosus. Medicine (Balt) 57:545-560, 1978.

279. Marino CT, Pertschuk LP: Pulmonary hemorrhage in systemic lupus erythematosus. Arch Intern Med 141:201-203, 1981.

280. Bruce IN, Gladman DD, Urowitz MB: Premature atherosclerosis in systemic lupus erythematosus. Rheum Dis Clin N Am 26:257-278, 2000.

281. Karrar A, Sequeira W, Block JA: Coronary artery disease in systemic lupus erythematosus: A review of the literature. Semin Arthritis Rheum 30:436-443, 2001.

282. Kitagawa Y, Gotoh F, Koto A, et al: Stroke in systemic lupus erythematosus. Stroke 21:1533-1539, 1990.

283. Boumpas DT, Patronas NJ, Dalakas MC, et al: Acute transverse myelitis in systemic lupus erythematosus: Magnetic resonance imaging and review of the literature. J Rheumatol 17:89-92, 1990.

284. Kojima E, Naito K, Iwai M, et al: Antiphospholipid syndrome complicated by thrombosis of the superior mesenteric artery, co-existence of smooth muscle hyperplasia. Intern Med 36:528-531, 1997.

285. McCollum CN, Sloan ME, Davison AM, et al: Ruptured hepatic aneurysm in systemic lupus erythematosus. Ann Rheum Dis 38:396-398, 1979.

286. Medina F, Ayala A, Jara LJ, et al: Acute abdomen in systemic lupus erythematosus: The importance of early laparotomy. Am J Med 103:100-105, 1997.

287. Guidelines for referral and management of systemic lupus erythematosus in adults. American College of Rheumatology Ad Hoc Committee on Systemic Lupus Erythematosus Guidelines. Arthritis Rheum 42:1785-1796, 1999.

288. Urowitz MB, Bookman AA, Koehler BE, et al: The bimodal mortality pattern of systemic lupus erythematosus. Am J Med 60:221-225, 1976.

289. Tozman EC, Urowitz MB, Gladman DD: Prolonged complete remission in previously severe SLE. Ann Rheum Dis 41:39-40, 1982.

290. Urowitz MB, Feletar M, Bruce IN, et al: Prolonged remission in systemic lupus erythematosus. J Rheumatol 32:1467-1472, 2005.

291. Kasitanon N, Magder LS, Petri M: Predictors of survival in systemic lupus erythematosus. Medicine (Balt) 85:147-156, 2006.

292. Mok CC, Lee KW, Ho CT, et al: A prospective study of survival and prognostic indicators of systemic lupus erythematosus in a southern Chinese population. Rheumatology (Oxf) 39:399-406, 2000.

293. Illei GG, Takada K, Parkin D, et al: Renal flares are common in patients with severe proliferative lupus nephritis treated with pulse immunosuppressive therapy: Long-term followup of a cohort of 145 patients participating in randomized controlled studies. Arthritis Rheum 46:995-1002, 2002.

294. Petri M, Genovese M: Incidence of and risk factors for hospitalizations in systemic lupus erythematosus: A prospective study of the Hopkins Lupus Cohort. J Rheumatol 19:1559-1565, 1992.

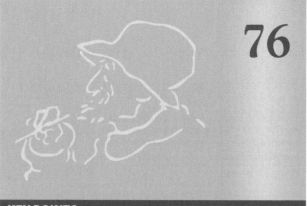

76

Antiphospholipid Syndrome 📷

DORUK ERKAN •
JANE E. SALMON •
MICHAEL D. LOCKSHIN

KEY POINTS

Antiphospholipid antibodies (aPLs) are a family of autoantibodies directed against phospholipid-binding plasma proteins, most commonly ß$_2$-glycoprotein I.

The origin of aPLs is unknown but is hypothesized to be an incidental exposure to infectious agents that induce autoantibodies in susceptible individuals.

The clinical manifestations of aPLs range from asymptomatic to catastrophic antiphospholipid syndrome (APS); thus, patients should not be evaluated and managed as if they had a single disease.

Stroke is the most common presentation of arterial thrombosis; deep vein thrombosis is the most common venous manifestation of APS. Pregnancy losses in patients with aPLs typically occur after 10 weeks' gestation (fetal loss), but earlier losses also occur.

Catastrophic APS is a rare, abrupt, life-threatening complication that consists of multiple thromboses of medium and small arteries occurring over days.

The diagnosis of APS should be made in the presence of characteristic clinical manifestations and *persistently* positive aPLs (measured at least 12 weeks apart).

The prevention of secondary thrombosis in persistently aPL-positive individuals lacks a risk-stratified approach; the effectiveness of high-intensity anticoagulation in APS patients with vascular events is not supported by prospective controlled studies.

A common strategy to prevent fetal loss in aPL-positive patients with a history of pregnancy morbidities is low-dose aspirin and heparin; if patients fail this regimen, the next step is to add intravenous immunoglobulin (IVIG), although this approach is not supported by controlled studies.

Prevention of primary thrombosis in persistently aPL-positive individuals lacks an evidence-based approach; elimination of reversible thrombosis risk factors and prophylaxis during high-risk periods (e.g., surgical procedures) are crucial.

Currently, there is no evidence that anticoagulation is effective for nonthrombotic manifestations of aPLs, such as livedo reticularis, thrombocytopenia, hemolytic anemia, or heart valve disease.

Catastrophic APS patients usually receive a combination of anticoagulation, corticosteroids, IVIG, and plasma exchange.

DEFINITION

Diagnosis of the antiphospholipid syndrome (APS) requires that a patient have both a clinical event (thrombosis or pregnancy morbidity) and the persistent presence of antiphospholipid antibody (aPL), documented by a solid-phase serum assay (anticardiolipin or anti–ß$_2$-glycoprotein I [anti-ß$_2$GPI] immunoglobulin [Ig] G or M), a coagulation assay (inhibitor of phospholipid-dependent clotting—the lupus anticoagulant test), or both. Preliminary (Sapporo) classification criteria for APS,[1] revised in 2004,[2] are listed in Table 76-1.

Certain factors are not included as criteria but may be helpful in the diagnosis of individual patients. These include IgA anticardiolipin or anti-ß$_2$GPI, valvular heart disease, thrombocytopenia, early preeclampsia, and livedo reticularis (Table 76-2). These factors are rare, nonstandardized, or nonspecific phenomena that are too unreliable for use in clinical studies but occur in a sufficient number of patients to support a suspected diagnosis. A false-positive test for syphilis does not fulfill the laboratory criterion.

APS can occur as an isolated diagnosis, or it can be associated with systemic lupus erythematosus (SLE) or another rheumatic disease. Antiphospholipid antibodies, but probably not the syndrome, can be induced by drugs and infections.[3]

EPIDEMIOLOGY

Low-titer, usually transient, anticardiolipin occurs in up to 10% of normal blood donors,[4,5] and moderate- to high-titer anticardiolipin or a positive lupus anticoagulant test occurs in less than 1%. The prevalence of positive aPL tests increases with age. Ten percent to 40% of SLE patients[5] and approximately 20% of rheumatoid arthritis patients[6] have positive aPL tests.

Based on a limited number of uncontrolled and non–risk-stratified studies, asymptomatic (no history of vascular or pregnancy events) aPL-positive patients have a 0% to 4% annual risk of thrombosis; patients with other autoimmune diseases such as SLE are at the higher end of the range.[7,8] The aPL profile (low versus high risk for thrombosis) and patients' clinical characteristics (presence or absence of other acquired or genetic thrombosis risk factors) influence the individual risk of thrombosis.[9] Ten percent of first-stroke victims have aPLs,[10] especially those who are young (up to 29%),[5,11] as do up to 20% of women who have suffered three or more consecutive fetal losses.[12] Fourteen percent of patients with recurrent venous thromboembolic disease have aPLs.[13]

CAUSE

The main antigen to which aPLs bind is not a phospholipid but rather a phospholipid-binding plasma protein—namely, ß$_2$GPI (apolipoprotein H). ß$_2$GPI is normally present at a

📷 Supplemental images available on the Expert Consult Premium Edition website.

1301

Table 76-1   Revised Sapporo Classification Criteria for Antiphospholipid Syndrome

Clinical Criteria
1. Vascular thrombosis*
One or more clinical episodes[†] of arterial, venous, or small vessel thrombosis[‡] in any tissue or organ.
2. Pregnancy morbidity
(a) One or more unexplained deaths of a morphologically normal fetus at or beyond the 10th week of gestation, or
(b) One or more premature births of a morphologically normal neonate before the 34th week of gestation because of eclampsia, severe preeclampsia, or recognized features of placental insufficiency[§], or
(c) Three or more unexplained consecutive spontaneous abortions before the 10th week of gestation, with maternal anatomic or hormonal abnormalities and paternal and maternal chromosomal causes excluded.

Laboratory Criteria[ǁ]
1. Lupus anticoagulant present in plasma on two or more occasions at least 12 weeks apart, detected according to the guidelines of the International Society on Thrombosis and Hemostasis
2. Anticardiolipin antibody of immunoglobulin (Ig) G or IgM isotype in serum or plasma, present in medium or high titer (>40 GPL or MPL, or >99th percentile), on two or more occasions at least 12 weeks apart, measured by a standardized enzyme-linked immunosorbent assay (ELISA).
3. Anti–β_2-glycoprotein I antibody of IgG or IgM isotype in serum or plasma (in titer >99th percentile) present on two or more occasions at least 12 weeks apart, measured by a standardized ELISA.
Definite antiphospholipid syndrome (APS) is present if at least one of the clinical criteria and one of the laboratory criteria are met. Classification of APS should be avoided if less than 12 weeks or more than 5 years separate the positive antiphospholipid antibody test and the clinical manifestation. In studies of populations of patients who have more than one type of pregnancy morbidity, investigators are strongly encouraged to stratify groups of subjects according to a, b, or c above.

*Coexisting inherited or acquired factors for thrombosis are not reasons to exclude patients from APS trials. However, two subgroups of APS patients should be recognized, based on the presence and absence of additional risk factors for thrombosis. Indicative (but not exhaustive) cases include age (>55 yr in men and >65 yr in women) and the presence of any of the established risk factors for cardiovascular disease (hypertension, diabetes mellitus, elevated low-density lipoprotein or low high-density lipoprotein cholesterol, cigarette smoking, family history of premature cardiovascular disease, body mass index >30 kg/m², microalbuminuria, estimated glomerular filtration rate <60 mL/min), inherited thrombophilias, oral contraceptive use, nephritic syndrome, malignancy, immobilization, and surgery. Thus, patients who fulfill criteria should be stratified according to contributing causes of thrombosis.

[†]A thrombotic episode in the past can be considered a clinical criterion, provided that thrombosis is proved by appropriate diagnostic means and that no alternative diagnosis or cause of thrombosis is found.

[‡]Superficial venous thrombosis is not included in the clinical criteria.

[§]Generally accepted features of placental insufficiency include an abnormal or nonreassuring fetal surveillance test (e.g., nonreactive nonstress test) suggestive of fetal hypoxemia, an abnormal Doppler flow velocimetry waveform analysis suggestive of fetal hypoxemia (e.g., absent end-diastolic flow in the umbilical artery), oligohydramnios (e.g., amniotic fluid index ≤5 cm), or a postnatal birth weight less than the 10th percentile for gestational age.

[ǁ]Investigators are strongly advised to classify APS patients participating in studies into one of the following categories: I, more than one laboratory criteria present (any combination); IIa, only lupus anticoagulant present; IIb, only anticardiolipin antibody present; IIc, only anti-β_2-glycoprotein I antibody present.

From Miyakis S, Lockshin MD, Atsumi T, et al: International consensus statement on an update of the classification criteria for definite antiphospholipid syndrome. J Thromb Haemost 4:295-306, 2006.

Table 76-2   Other Features Suggesting the Presence of Antiphospholipid Antibodies

Clinical
Livedo reticularis
Thrombocytopenia (usually 50,000-100,000 platelets/mm³)
Autoimmune hemolytic anemia
Cardiac valve disease (vegetations or thickening)
Multiple sclerosis–like syndrome, chorea, or other myelopathy

Laboratory
Immunoglobulin A anticardiolipin antibody
Immunoglobulin A anti–β_2-glycoprotein I

concentration of 200 mg/mL, is a member of the complement control protein family, and has five repeating domains and several alleles. An octapeptide in the fifth domain and critical cysteine bonds are necessary for both phospholipid binding and antigenicity[14]; a first-domain site activates platelets.[15,16] In vivo, β_2GPI binds to phosphatidylserine on activated or apoptotic cell membranes, including those of trophoblasts, platelets, and endothelial cells. Under physiologic conditions, β_2GPI may function in the elimination of apoptotic cells[17] and as a natural anticoagulant.[18]

Other, less relevant antigens targeted by aPLs are prothrombin, annexin V, protein C, protein S, high- and low-molecular-weight kininogens, tissue plasminogen activator, factor VII, factor XI, factor XII, complement component C4, and complement factor H.[19]

In experimental animal models, passive or active immunization with viral peptides,[20] bacterial peptides,[21] and heterologous β_2GPI[22] induces polyclonal aPLs and clinical events associated with APS. These data suggest that pathologic autoimmune aPL is induced in susceptible humans by infections via molecular mimicry.

However, infection-induced aPLs (syphilitic and non-syphilitic *Treponema*, *Borrelia burgdorferi*, human immunodeficiency virus, *Leptospira*, or parasites) are usually β_2GPI independent and bind phospholipids directly.[23] Drugs (chlorpromazine, procainamide, quinidine, and phenytoin) and malignancies (lymphoproliferative disorders) can also induce β_2GPI-independent aPLs. Conversely, autoimmune aPLs bind β_2GPI or other phospholipid-binding plasma proteins, which in turn bind negatively charged phospholipids such as cardiolipin (β_2GPI-dependent aPLs).

Low levels of aPLs may be present normally; one of the functions of normal aPLs may be to participate in the physiologic removal of oxidized lipids.

PATHOGENESIS

Antiphospholipid antibody is most likely related to thrombosis through multiple mechanisms; a proposed pathogenesis is illustrated in Figure 76-1. The process begins with activation or apoptosis of platelets, endothelial cells, or trophoblasts, during which phosphatidylserine (a negatively charged phospholipid) migrates from the inner to the normally electrically neutral outer cell membrane. Circulating β_2GPI binds to phosphatidylserine, and then aPL binds to a β_2GPI dimer.[24]

Antiphospholipid antibody–β_2GPI dimer binding activates the complement cascade extracellularly; initiates an

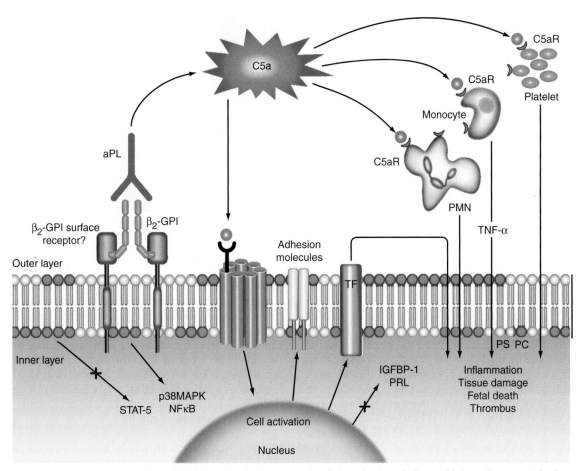

Figure 76-1 **Proposed mechanism of antiphospholipid antibody (aPL)–related thrombosis and placental injury.** The negatively charged phospholipid phosphatidylserine (PS, *yellow circles*) migrates from the inner to the outer cell membrane during activation or apoptosis of platelets and endothelial cells, and it is normally present on trophoblasts. The neutral phospholipid phosphatidylcholine (PC, *red circles*) is the major constituent of the outer layer of unactivated cells. Dimeric ß$_2$-glycoprotein I (ß$_2$GPI) then binds to PS (probably via ß$_2$GPI surface receptors such as apoER2′, annexin A2, or a Toll-like receptor), and aPL binds to ß$_2$GPI, activating the classic complement pathway and leading to the generation of C5a, which induces (a) expression of adhesion molecules (e.g., intracellular adhesion molecule [ICAM]-1 and tissue factor [TF]) and (b) activation of monocytes, polymorphonuclear (PMN) cells, and platelets, resulting in the release of proinflammatory mediators (e.g., tumor necrosis factor [TNF]-α, vascular endothelial growth factor receptor-1 [VEGFR1]) and the prothrombotic stage. Both nuclear factor κB (NFκB) and p38 mitogen-activated protein kinase (p38MAPK) may play a role in the intracellular signaling cascade. Antiphospholipid antibodies also downregulate the expression of trophoblast signal transducer and activator of transcription 5 (STAT-5), reducing the endometrial stromal cell production of prolactin (PRL) and insulin growth factor binding protein-1 (IGFBP-1).

intracellular signaling cascade, probably through the C5a and ß$_2$GPI surface receptors; and recruits and activates inflammatory effector cells, including monocytes, neutrophils, and platelets, leading to the release of proinflammatory products (e.g., tumor necrosis factor [TNF]-α, oxidants, proteases) and the induction of a prothrombotic phenotype.[25-27] The putative receptor of ß$_2$GPI binding protein that transduces signals from the cell membrane to the nucleus is not yet identified and may vary among cells. The following candidates have been suggested: apoER2′ (a member of the low-density lipoprotein receptor superfamily), annexin A2, and a Toll-like receptor.[28,29] Both nuclear factor κB and p38 mitogen-activated protein kinase may play a role in the intracellular signaling cascade[30,31]

In addition, through downregulation of the signal transducer and activator of transcription 5 (Stat5), aPLs inhibit the production of placental prolactin and insulin growth factor binding protein-1,[32] and they adversely affect the formation of a trophoblast syncytium, placental apoptosis, and trophoblast invasion—all processes that are required for the normal establishment of placental function.

Other possible contributory mechanisms of aPL-mediated thrombosis include inhibition of coagulation cascade reactions catalyzed by phospholipids (e.g., activation of circulating procoagulant proteins or inhibition of protein C and S activation), induction of tissue factor (a physiologic initiator of coagulation) expression on monocytes, reduction of fibrinolysis, and interaction with the annexin V anticoagulant shield in the placenta.[29]

In experimental animal models, aPLs cause fetal resorption and increase the size and duration of trauma-induced venous and arterial thrombi.[33,34] Inhibiting complement activation prevents experimental aPL-induced fetal death, and C5 knockout mice carry pregnancies normally despite aPL,[35] implying that a complement-mediated effector mechanism is an absolute requirement for fetal death to occur. Complement activation is also required for experimental thrombosis.[36]

Because high-level aPLs may persist for years in asymptomatic persons, it is likely that vascular injury, endothelial cell activation, or both immediately precede the occurrence of thrombosis in those bearing the antibody (second-hit hypothesis). Of note, at least 50% of APS patients with vascular factors possess other acquired thrombosis risk factors at the time of their events.[37,38]

Both persons congenitally lacking β_2GPI[39] and β_2GPI knockout mice appear normal.[40] β_2GPI polymorphisms influence the generation of aPLs in individuals, but they have only a weak relationship to the occurrence of APS.[41] A cluster of 50 upregulated genes may have an effect on the occurrence of thrombosis in aPL-positive individuals.[42]

CLINICAL FEATURES

The clinical manifestations range from asymptomatic aPL positivity (no history of vascular or pregnancy events) to catastrophic APS (multiple thromboses occurring over days). Thus, patients should not be evaluated and managed as if they have a single disease.

VASCULAR OCCLUSION

APS affects all organ systems. Its principal manifestations are venous or arterial thromboses and pregnancy loss (see Table 76-1). Except for their severity, the youth of affected patients, and the unusual anatomic locations (Budd-Chiari syndrome; sagittal sinus and upper extremity thromboses), venous thromboses in APS do not differ clinically from thromboses attributable to other causes. Similarly, arterial thromboses differ from non–aPL-associated thromboses only by their recurrent nature, unusual locations, and occurrence in young patients. Deep vein thrombosis and stroke are the most common clinical manifestations of APS. Renal thrombotic microangiopathy, glomerular capillary endothelial cell injury, and thrombosis of renal vessels cause proteinuria without celluria or hypocomplementemia and may lead to severe hypertension, renal failure, or both.[43]

PREGNANCY MORBIDITY

Pregnancy losses in patients with aPLs typically occur after 10 weeks' gestation (fetal loss), although earlier losses also occur. However, these pre-embryonic or embryonic pregnancy losses (<10 weeks' gestation) are more commonly due to chromosomal and other genetic defects. Pregnancy in those with APS is often normal until the second trimester, when fetal growth slows and amniotic fluid volume decreases. APS patients may develop severe, early preeclampsia or HELLP (hemolysis, elevated liver enzymes, low platelets) syndrome. Placental infarction is a cause of fetal growth restriction or death; nonthrombotic mechanisms of placental dysfunction also occur.[44] Prior late pregnancy losses predict future losses, independent of the aPL profile.

MISCELLANEOUS MANIFESTATIONS

Many patients have livedo reticularis (Fig. 76-2), although this is not specific for APS. Cardiac valve disease (vegetations, thickening, or both), a late manifestation, may necessitate valve replacement. Its pathogenesis in APS is unknown. Recent studies suggest that APS does not add to the risk of atherosclerosis imparted by SLE.[45] Pulmonary hypertension may develop due to recurrent pulmonary

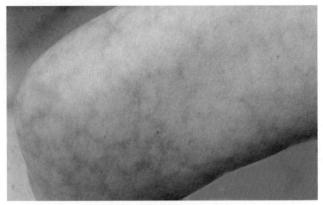

Figure 76-2 Livedo reticularis in antiphospholipid syndrome.

embolism or small vessel thrombosis; rarely, aPL-positive patients may present with diffuse pulmonary hemorrhage. Some patients develop nonfocal neurologic symptoms such as lack of concentration, forgetfulness, and dizzy spells. Multiple small, hyperintense lesions seen on magnetic resonance imaging (MRI), primarily in the periventricular white matter, do not correlate well with clinical symptoms. Rarely, high-affinity antiprothrombin antibodies may cause hemorrhage by depleting prothrombin (lupus anticoagulant hypoprothrombinemia syndrome).[46]

CATASTROPHIC ANTIPHOSPHOLIPID SYNDROME

Catastrophic APS is a rare, abrupt, life-threatening complication. It consists of multiple thromboses of medium and small arteries occurring (despite apparently adequate anticoagulation) over a period of days and causing stroke; cardiac, hepatic, adrenal, renal, and intestinal infarction; and peripheral gangrene.[4,47] In a review of 220 patients with catastrophic APS, the main clinical manifestations included renal involvement in 154 patients (70%), pulmonary in 146 (66%), cerebral in 133 (60%), cardiac in 115 (52%), and cutaneous in 104 (47%).[48] Acute adrenal failure may be the initial clinical event. Proposed formal criteria for this syndrome are shown in Table 76-3.[49] Patients often have moderate thrombocytopenia; erythrocytes are less fragmented than in the hemolytic uremic syndrome or thrombotic thrombocytopenic purpura, and fibrin split products are not strikingly elevated. Renal failure and pulmonary hemorrhage may occur. Tissue biopsies show noninflammatory vascular occlusion.

DIAGNOSIS AND DIAGNOSTIC TESTS

LABORATORY STUDIES

The diagnosis of APS requires a positive lupus anticoagulant test or a moderate- to high-titer anticardiolipin IgG or IgM test in patients with characteristic clinical manifestations. Patients with negative lupus anticoagulant and anticardiolipin tests should be tested for IgA anticardiolipin and IgG, IgM, or IgA anti-β_2GPI when there is a high suspicion for APS. Positive aPL results require a repeat test after 12 or more weeks to exclude a transient, clinically unimportant

Table 76-3 Preliminary Criteria for the Classification of Catastrophic Antiphospholipid Syndrome (APS)

1. Evidence of involvement of three or more organs, systems, or tissues*
2. Development of manifestations simultaneously or in less than 1 wk
3. Confirmation by histopathology of small vessel occlusion in at least one organ or tissue†
4. Laboratory confirmation of the presence of antiphospholipid antibody (lupus anticoagulant or anticardiolipin or anti–β_2-glycoprotein I antibodies)‡
Definite Catastrophic APS
All 4 criteria
Probable Catastrophic APS
Criteria 2 through 4 and two organs, systems, or tissues involved
Criteria 1 through 3, except no confirmation 6 wk apart due to early death of patient not tested before catastrophic episode
Criteria 1, 2, and 4
Criteria 1, 3, and 4 and development of a third event more than 1 wk but less than 1 mo after the first, despite anticoagulation

*Usually, clinical evidence of vessel occlusions, confirmed by imaging techniques when appropriate. Renal involvement is defined by a 50% rise in serum creatinine, severe systemic hypertension, proteinuria, or some combination of these.

†For histopathologic confirmation, significant evidence of thrombosis must be present, although vasculitis may coexist occasionally.

‡If the patient had not previously been diagnosed with APS, laboratory confirmation requires that the presence of antiphospholipid antibody be detected on two or more occasions at least 6 weeks apart (not necessarily at the time of the event), according to the proposed preliminary criteria for the classification of APS.

From Asherson RA, Cervera R, de Groot PG, et al: Catastrophic antiphospholipid syndrome: International consensus statement on classification criteria and treatment guidelines. Lupus 12:530-534, 2003.

antibody. The diagnosis of APS should be questioned if less than 12 weeks or more than 5 years separate the positive aPL test from the clinical manifestation.[2]

The lupus anticoagulant test is a more specific but less sensitive predictor of thromboses than is anticardiolipin; it correlates better with aPL-related clinical events.[50] Documentation of a lupus anticoagulant requires a four-step process: (1) demonstration of a prolonged phospholipid-dependent coagulation screening test, such as activated partial thromboplastin time or dilute Russell viper venom time (however, low-level abnormalities are not clearly linked to APS); (2) failure to correct the prolonged screening test by mixing the patient's plasma with normal platelet-poor plasma, demonstrating the presence of an inhibitor; (3) shortening or correction of the prolonged screening test by the addition of excess phospholipid, demonstrating phospholipid dependency; and (4) exclusion of other inhibitors.[51] Approximately 80% of patients with lupus anticoagulant have anticardiolipin, and 20% of patients positive for anticardiolipin have lupus anticoagulant.[52]

The anticardiolipin enzyme-linked immunosorbent assay (ELISA) is sensitive but not specific for the diagnosis of APS.[53] Although the widely available ELISA test for IgG and IgM anticardiolipin is standardized, considerable variability exists among commercial laboratories that perform the test, especially for the IgA isotype.[54] Low-titer anticardiolipin or anti-ß$_2$GPI, transient aPLs, and antibody to noncardiolipin phospholipids (phosphatidylserine, phosphatidylethanolamine) have no proven relationship to APS. The ELISA tests other than anticardiolipin and anti-ß$_2$GPI are neither standardized nor widely accepted as predictors of clinical illness.

Whether to test persons with venous occlusive disease or recurrent fetal loss simultaneously for protein C, protein S, and antithrombin III deficiency or for the factor V Leiden and prothrombin mutations is a matter of economics and clinical likelihood; such testing is advisable when feasible. It is useful to test persons with arterial occlusive disease for hyperhomocysteinemia.

Antinuclear and anti-DNA antibodies occur in approximately 45% of patients clinically diagnosed as having primary APS without an accompanying illness[55]; these antibodies do not mandate the additional diagnosis of SLE if the patient has no clinical indicators of SLE. Thrombocytopenia in APS is usually modest ($>50,000/mm^3$); proteinuria and renal insufficiency occur in patients with thrombotic microangiopathy. Pathologic examination demonstrates small artery and glomerular thrombi and recanalization (Fig. 76-3). Hypocomplementemia, erythrocyte casts, and pyuria are not characteristic of thrombotic microangiopathy and, when present, imply lupus glomerulonephritis. Erythrocyte sedimentation rate, hemoglobin, and leukocyte count are usually normal in patients with uncomplicated primary APS, except during acute thrombosis. Prothrombin fragment 1 + 2 and other markers of coagulation activation do not predict impending thrombosis.

IMAGING STUDIES

MRI shows vascular occlusion and infarction consistent with clinical symptoms, with no special characteristics (other than multiple, otherwise unexplained cerebral infarctions in a young person). Multiple small, hyperintense white-matter lesions are common and do not unequivocally imply brain infarction. Occlusions usually occur in vessels below the resolution limits of angiography; hence, angiography or magnetic resonance angiography is not indicated unless clinical findings suggest medium- or large-vessel disease. Echocardiography or cardiac MRI may show severe Libman-Sacks endocarditis and intracardiac thrombi.[56]

PATHOLOGY

Skin, renal, and other tissues show noninflammatory occlusion of all caliber arteries and veins, acute and chronic endothelial injury and its sequelae, and recanalization in late lesions. Uteroplacental insufficiency was once thought to be due to thrombosis or spiral artery vasculopathy (atherosis, intimal thickening, fibrinoid necrosis, and absence of physiologic changes in the spiral arteries).[57] Consistent with the importance of inflammation in murine models of APS, recent findings demonstrate inflammatory infiltrates, particularly macrophages, and suggest that inflammation contributes to placental injury in patients.[58] The finding of necrotizing vasculitis suggests concomitant lupus or other connective tissue disease. There are no other diagnostic immunofluorescence or electron microscopic findings.

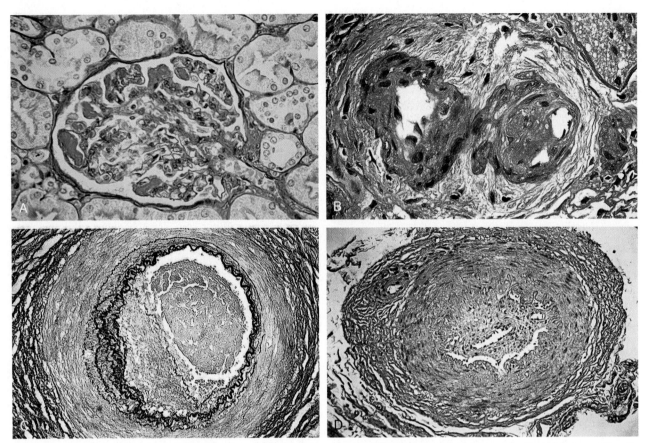

Figure 76-3 Renal thrombotic microangiopathy in antiphospholipid syndrome (APS). **A,** Kidney biopsy from a 35-year-old woman with primary APS, microhematuria, and non-nephrotic proteinuria. The glomerulus contains microthrombi, occluding capillary lumina, and there is endothelial swelling. **B,** The same patient's small renal artery contains organized thrombus, with recanalization and arteriosclerosis (periodic acid–Schiff, ×100). **C,** Autopsy specimen from a 45-year-old man with primary APS. Note the thrombus in various stages of organization, intact elastic lamina with focal reduplication, and medial thickening (elastic Verhoeff stain, ×100). **D,** The same patient's medium-sized peripheral artery. Note the organized thrombus with recanalization, severe fibrointimal thickening, medial hypertrophy, and extreme stenosis of lumen (hematoxylin and eosin, ×75). *(Courtesy of Dr. Surya V. Seshan.)*

DIFFERENTIAL DIAGNOSIS

Infection-induced anticardiolipin is usually transient and is more commonly IgM than IgG.[59] Transient aPLs or low-titer anticardiolipin is inconclusive for diagnosis. Research laboratories can distinguish autoimmune from infection-induced aPLs by determining the antibody's β_2GPI dependence. In a patient who has lupus or lupus-like disease, livedo reticularis, or long-standing thrombocytopenia and who has a persistently positive aPL test, it is usually unnecessary to exclude other diagnoses.

Because the prevalence of aPL-positive ELISA tests increases with age, and because the differential diagnosis of vascular occlusion is broader than it is in young adults, particular care is necessary in diagnosing APS in patients older than 60 years. Sustained high-titer anticardiolipin IgG, livedo reticularis, thrombocytopenia, coexisting rheumatic disease, and absence of other causes support a diagnosis of APS.

Five percent to 21% of women with recurrent pregnancy losses, and 0.5% to 2% of normal pregnant women, have aPLs. Heritable deficiency of protein C, protein S, and anti-thrombin III and the presence of the factor V Leiden (A506G), prothrombin (G20210A), and methylene tetrahydrofolate reductase (MTHFR, C677T) mutations are less

common causes of fetal loss.[60] Attribution of pregnancy loss to APS is most certain when there is no coexisting plausible explanation, when the loss occurs after the demonstration of a fetal heartbeat (10 weeks), when a significant aPL profile is repeatedly positive before and after pregnancy, and when the placenta shows vasculopathy and infarction. A single pregnancy loss before 10 weeks' gestation in a patient with a low-positive anticardiolipin test is more likely to be attributable to fetal chromosomal abnormalities, infection, or maternal hormonal or anatomic abnormalities.

Independent coagulopathies may further increase the thrombotic risk in patients with aPLs. These and other acquired thrombotic risk factors (hypertension, diabetes, nephrotic syndrome, venous insufficiency, immobility) are alternative causes of thromboembolic disease. Arterial occlusion occurs in patients with thrombotic thrombocytopenic purpura, infected or sterile emboli of cardiac or vascular origin, septicemia, hyperhomocysteinemia, myxoma, Takayasu's arteritis, polyarteritis nodosa, and severe Raynaud's disease. The relationship of Sneddon's syndrome (stroke and livedo reticularis, with or without aPLs) to APS is uncertain.

Catastrophic APS has few mimics. Among them are sepsis, disseminated intravascular coagulation, thrombotic thrombocytopenic purpura, hemolytic uremic syndrome, polyarteritis nodosa, and disseminated embolization from myxoma, atrial thrombus, or atherosclerotic plaque. Small vessel occlusions occurring in rapid succession suggest disseminated intravascular coagulation. Severe cerebral and renal disease suggests thrombotic thrombocytopenic purpura; renal failure and hemolysis suggest hemolytic uremic syndrome. Antiphospholipid antibodies are rarely present in patients with the alternative diagnoses. Acute adrenal insufficiency is characteristic of APS and Waterhouse-Friderichsen syndrome.

TREATMENT

THROMBOSIS

Treatment recommendations are summarized in Table 76-4. Anticoagulation with heparin is the treatment for acute thrombosis in APS patients. Warfarin, occasionally in association with low-dose aspirin, is used for secondary thrombosis prophylaxis. Two randomized, controlled trials demonstrated that moderate warfarin (international normalized ratio [INR] 2 to 3) and high-intensity warfarin (INR 3 to 4) are equally protective against recurrence in APS patients after the first thrombosis.[61,62] The intensity of anticoagulation for aPL-related arterial thrombosis is still a matter for debate, because in both studies, patients with arterial events constituted less than half the study population. Although APS patients with arterial thrombosis who are at high risk for recurrence may require high-intensity anticoagulation, in the absence of risk-stratified studies, *high risk* has no consensus definition and is currently based solely on clinical judgment.

Aspirin is the standard of care after an ischemic stroke or transient ischemic attack to prevent a recurrence in aPL-negative patients. Although most aPL-positive patients with ischemic strokes receive warfarin, the Antiphospholipid Antibody in Stroke Study (APASS) concluded that for selected aPL-positive patients who do not have atrial fibrillation or high-grade stenosis, aspirin and warfarin (target INR 2.2) are equivalent in terms of both efficacy and major bleeding complications.[63] The APASS results probably do not apply to conventionally defined APS, because the average age of study participants was much higher than that of the average APS population; in addition, the aPL determination was performed only once at study entry, and the titer cutoff for assigning a patient to the positive anticardiolipin group was very low. However, aspirin is an option for older aPL-positive patients who have a single low-titer anticardiolipin test and whose presentation is one stroke.

Some patients require larger than expected doses of both heparin and warfarin to achieve therapeutic anticoagulation. Uncommonly, positive lupus anticoagulant tests cause the INR to be unreliable.[64] Such patients may be treated with high-dose warfarin or unfractionated or low-molecular-weight heparin, monitored by the measurement of anti–factor Xa activity or other appropriate assay.

For well-anticoagulated patients who continue to have thromboses, aspirin (81 to 325 mg/day), hydroxychloroquine, a statin drug, intravenous immunoglobulin (IVIG), and plasmapheresis have theoretical bases for efficacy, and all have been used.[65] Corticosteroids have no established role in the treatment of APS but are used for rheumatic

Table 76-4 Treatment Recommendations for Persistently Antiphospholipid Antibody–Positive Individuals

Clinical Circumstance	Recommendation
Asymptomatic	No treatment*
Venous thrombosis	Warfarin INR 2.5 indefinitely
Arterial thrombosis	Warfarin INR 2.5 indefinitely
Recurrent thrombosis	Warfarin INR 3 to 4 + low-dose aspirin
Pregnancy	
First pregnancy	No treatment*
Single pregnancy loss at <10 wk	No treatment*
≥1 Fetal or ≥3 (pre) embryonic loss, no thrombosis	Prophylactic heparin† + low-dose aspirin throughout pregnancy, discontinue 6-12 wk post partum
Thrombosis regardless of pregnancy history	Therapeutic heparin‡ or low-dose aspirin throughout pregnancy, warfarin post partum
Valve nodules or deformity	No known effective treatment; full anticoagulation if emboli or intracardiac thrombi demonstrated
Thrombocytopenia >50,000/mm³	No treatment
Thrombocytopenia <50,000/mm³	Prednisone, IVIG
Catastrophic APS	Anticoagulation + corticosteroids + IVIG or plasmapheresis

*Aspirin (81 mg/day) may be given.
†Enoxaparin 0.5 mg/kg subcutaneously once daily.
‡Enoxaparin 1 mg/kg subcutaneously twice daily or 1.5 mg/kg subcutaneously once daily.
APS, antiphospholipid syndrome; INR, international normalized ratio; IVIG, intravenous immunoglobulin.

symptoms in patients with accompanying systemic autoimmune illness. However, high doses of corticosteroids are usually given empirically to patients with severe thrombocytopenia, hemolytic anemia, and catastrophic APS.

No controlled studies in APS patients have been published for clopidogrel, pentoxifylline, aspirin-dipyridamole, argatroban, hirudin, and other new anticoagulant agents. Neither hirudin nor fondaparinux inactivates complement, and neither drug protects mice with experimental APS against pregnancy loss, so they may be ineffective in human disease. Clinical experience suggests that thrombolytic agents for acute thrombosis are unhelpful, because reocclusion occurs rapidly.

Currently available data, although retrospective and not risk-stratified, indicate that lifelong anticoagulation of APS patients with vascular events is appropriate.[66] However, the recent recognition that some patients have full remission of antibody and that most thrombotic events have recognizable triggers raises the possibility of discontinuing anticoagulation in highly selected patients when the triggers are eliminated.

PREGNANCY MORBIDITY

Heparin anticoagulation is indicated at the diagnosis of pregnancy in an aPL-positive woman who has had prior pregnancy losses attributable to APS. Because warfarin is teratogenic, only unfractionated or low-molecular-weight heparin is used for the treatment of affected pregnancies in the United States; in other countries, converting to warfarin after the first trimester may be considered acceptable.[67] Most physicians with a special interest in this field now use low-molecular-weight heparin owing to the decreased risk of thrombocytopenia and osteoporosis.

Patients with prior fetal losses later than 10 gestational weeks should be treated with prophylactic heparin (enoxaparin 30 to 40 mg subcutaneously once daily), together with low-dose aspirin; this regimen increases the fetal survival rate from 50% (untreated) to 80%.[68,69] Women who have had prior thromboses must be fully anticoagulated (enoxaparin 1 mg/kg subcutaneously twice daily or 1.5 mg/kg subcutaneously once daily) throughout pregnancy, because the risk of new thrombosis markedly increases both during pregnancy and post partum. Even with treatment, prematurity and fetal growth restriction still occur. Clopidogrel and newer antithrombotic agents are not cleared for use in pregnancy, but together with IVIG and hydroxychloroquine, they may be considered in patients who are unable to use heparin or who fail heparin treatment.

In aPL-positive women with prior thrombosis, warfarin is changed to heparin or low-molecular-weight heparin before conception, if possible, or at the first missed menstrual period. In aPL-positive women without prior thrombosis, heparin treatment begins after confirmation of pregnancy, continues until 48 hours before anticipated delivery (to allow epidural anesthesia), and resumes for 8 to 12 weeks post partum. Some physicians recommend the initiation of heparin before conception; no clinical trial supports this recommendation, however, and the risk of longer-duration heparin therapy is considerable. Patients in most published series received low-dose aspirin as well as heparin, but the benefit of adding aspirin is unknown.

Because of the risk of postpartum thrombosis, it is prudent to continue anticoagulation for 8 to 12 weeks post partum and then discontinue it by tapering the doses. If desired, conversion from heparin to warfarin may be accomplished after the first or second postpartum week. Breastfeeding is permissible with both heparin and warfarin.

No studies unequivocally justify the treatment of women with aPLs during a first pregnancy, women with only very early losses, or women whose aPL titers are low or transient. Nonetheless, it is common to offer such patients low-dose aspirin.

ASYMPTOMATIC ANTIPHOSPHOLIPID ANTIBODY–POSITIVE INDIVIDUALS

Persistence of aPLs for decades without clinical events is well documented. The probability that an asymptomatic person incidentally found to have aPLs will eventually develop the syndrome is likely low.[7] Anticoagulation is not indicated for the prophylactic treatment of asymptomatic aPL-positive individuals. For those with moderate- to high-titer anticardiolipin and persistent aPLs, education about the meaning of abnormal tests is appropriate, as is a discussion of warning signs to report. Elimination of reversible thrombosis risk factors and prophylaxis during high-risk periods, such as surgical procedures, are crucial. Ongoing prospective clinical trials will determine whether asymptomatic persons with high-titer aPLs should be treated prophylactically.

Although drugs that induce lupus (hydralazine, phenytoin) may also induce aPLs, if no alternatives are available, they may be prescribed for patients with aPLs. Drugs that promote thrombosis (estrogen and estrogen-containing oral contraceptives) are not currently deemed safe, even for asymptomatic women serendipitously known to have high-titer antibodies. This advice does not translate to a recommendation to test all normal women before the prescription of such medications, but it does suggest that special attention and further evaluation be provided to those with family histories or clinical suggestions of rheumatic disease, livedo reticularis, biologic false-positive tests for syphilis, or borderline thrombocytopenia. There is no reliable information regarding the safety of progestin-only contraception, "morning after" contraception, or the use of raloxifene, bromocriptine, or leuprolide in APS patients. A small retrospective review of women undergoing artificial reproductive technology (in vitro fertilization) procedures demonstrated no thrombotic events.[70]

ANTIPHOSPHOLIPID ANTIBODY–POSITIVE INDIVIDUALS WITH AMBIGUOUS EVENTS

Some patients with positive aPL tests have clinical events of ambiguous meaning (dizzy or confusional episodes, nonspecific visual disturbance, very early pregnancy loss). There is no consensus for the treatment of such persons. Because full anticoagulation carries high risk, many physicians prescribe low-dose (81 mg) aspirin, hydroxychloroquine, or both daily. No published data support or repudiate this recommendation.

Based on the presumed pathogenesis, some physicians prescribe anticoagulation for patients with livedo reticularis, thrombocytopenia, leg ulcers, thrombotic microangiopathy, or valvulopathy. The efficacy of anticoagulation is unknown in these conditions. One small, descriptive, cross-sectional study provides evidence that B cell depletion with rituximab is well tolerated and can be effective for refractory thrombocytopenia and skin ulcers in aPL-positive patients.[71]

CATASTROPHIC ANTIPHOSPHOLIPID SYNDROME

The onset of catastrophic APS is usually sudden and immediately life threatening. Early diagnosis can be a challenge, but it is critical because, in contrast to other causes of multiple organ dysfunction syndrome, appropriate therapy includes anticoagulation and corticosteroids in combination with repeated plasma exchange, IVIG, and, in desperate situations, other modalities such as cyclophosphamide or rituximab. However, mortality remains as high as 48% despite all attempts at effective therapy.[72] There are no systematic studies of the treatment of catastrophic APS owing to the rarity of the condition.

ANTIPHOSPHOLIPID ANTIBODY–NEGATIVE INDIVIDUALS WITH A CLINICAL EVENT

In patients clinically suspected of having APS but with normal anticardiolipin, lupus anticoagulant, and anti-ß₂GPI tests, alternative causes of clotting must be sought. Even among patients with concomitant rheumatic disease, APS may not be the cause of recurrent thromboembolism or pregnancy loss. Patients with SLE develop emboli from

SLE-related cardiac valvular disease, vasculitis, or atheroma. Other patients have factor V Leiden or some other procoagulant mutation. Recurrent pregnancy losses may be caused by chromosomal abnormalities, uterine infection, diabetes, hypertension, or non-aPL coagulopathy. The concept of "seronegative" APS is not recognized.

PROGNOSIS

Pulmonary hypertension, neurologic involvement, myocardial ischemia, nephropathy, gangrene of extremities, and catastrophic APS are associated with a worse prognosis. During long-term follow-up, serious morbidity and disability occur in an unpredictable proportion of primary APS patients who experience major vascular events and in those who have delays in diagnosis and treatment. Thus, the long-term functional outcome of primary APS patients is poor; at 10 years, one third of patients develop permanent organ damage, and one fifth are unable to perform everyday activities.[73]

In a retrospective study of obstetric APS patients without thrombosis, 35% developed aPL-related clinical events during 8 years of follow-up. The studied populations were highly selected referral populations that may have been biased toward severe disease, but follow-up studies of obstetric patients with autoantibodies show similar results.[74]

Long-term outcomes of children born of APS pregnancies are not known. In many patients with long-standing APS, the development of severe cardiac valvular disease necessitates valve replacement, and rare patients develop renal failure due to thrombotic microangiopathy. Immediate thrombosis may cause loss of a transplanted kidney or other organ; aPL positivity correlates with poor graft survival after renal transplantation in SLE patients.[75]

Serious perioperative complications may occur despite prophylaxis in aPL-positive patients, because they are at additional risk for thrombosis when undergoing surgical procedures. Thus, perioperative strategies should be clearly identified before any surgical procedure, pharmacologic and physical antithrombosis interventions should be vigorously employed, periods without anticoagulation should be kept to an absolute minimum, intravascular manipulation for access and monitoring should be minimized, and any deviation from a normal course should be considered a potential disease-related event.[76]

REFERENCES

1. Wilson WA, Gharavi AE, Koike T, et al: International consensus statement on preliminary classification criteria for antiphospholipid syndrome: Report of an international workshop. Arthritis Rheum 42:1309-1311, 1999.
2. **Miyakis S, Lockshin MD, Atsumi T, et al: International consensus statement on an update of the classification criteria for definite antiphospholipid syndrome. J Thromb Haemost 4:295-306, 2006.**
3. Gharavi AE, Sammaritano LR, Wen J, et al: Characteristics of human immunodeficiency virus and chlorpromazine-induced antiphospholipid antibodies: Effect of beta 2 glycoprotein I on binding to phospholipid. J Rheumatol 21:94-99, 1994.
4. Vila P, Hernandez MC, Lopez-Fernandez MF, et al: Prevalence, follow-up and clinical significance of the aCL in normal subjects. Thromb Haemost 72:209-213, 1994.
5. Petri M: Epidemiology of the antiphospholipid antibody syndrome. J Autoimmun 15:145-151, 2000.
6. Olech E, Merrill JT: The prevalence and clinical significance of antiphospholipid antibodies in rheumatoid arthritis. Curr Rheumatol Rep 8:100-108, 2006.
7. Giron-Gonzalez JA, Garcia del Rio E, Rodriguez C, et al: Antiphospholipid syndrome and asymptomatic carriers of antiphospholipid antibody: Prospective analysis of 404 individuals. J Rheumatol 31:1560-1567, 2004.
8. Somers E, Magder LS, Petri ML: Antiphospholipid antibodies and incidence of venous thrombosis in a cohort of patients with systemic lupus erythematosus. J Rheumatol 29:2531-2536, 2002.
9. Erkan D, Harrison MJ, Levy R, et al: APLASA—a randomized double-blind placebo-controlled primary thrombosis prevention trial in asymptomatic persistently antiphospholipid antibody (APL)-positive individuals with aspirin (ASA) [abstract]. Clin Exp Rheumatol 25:14, 2007.
10. The Antiphospholipid Antibody Stroke Study (APASS) Group: Anticardiolipin antibodies are an independent risk factor for first ischemic stroke. Neurology 43:2069-2073, 1993.
11. Levine SR, Brey RL, Sawaya KL, et al: Recurrent stroke and thromboocclusive events in the antiphospholipid syndrome. Ann Neurol 38:119-124, 1995.
12. Stephenson MD: Frequency of factors associated with habitual abortion in 197 couples. Fertil Steril 66:24-29, 1996.
13. Ginsberg JS, Wells PS, Brill-Edwards P, et al: Antiphospholipid antibodies and venous thromboembolism. Blood 86:3685-3691, 1995.
14. Koike T, Ichikawa K, Kasahara H: Epitopes on beta2-GPI recognized by anticardiolipin antibodies. Lupus 7(Suppl 2):S14, 1998.
15. Shi T, Giannakopoulos B, Yan X, et al: Anti-beta2-glycoprotein I antibodies in complex with beta2-glycoprotein I can activate platelets in a dysregulated manner via glycoprotein Ib-IX-V. Arthritis Rheum 54:2558-2567, 2006.
16. Reddel SW, Wang YX, Sheng YH, et al: Epitope studies with anti-beta 2-glycoprotein I antibodies from autoantibody and immunized sources. J Autoimmun 15:91-96, 2000.
17. Casciola-Rosen L, Rosen A, Petri M, et al: Surface blebs on apoptotic cells are sites of enhanced procoagulant activity: Implications for coagulation events and antigenic spread in systemic lupus erythematosus. Proc Natl Acad Sci U S A 93:1624-1629, 1996.
18. Mori T, Takeya H, Nishioka J, et al: Beta 2-glycoprotein I modulates the anticoagulant activity of activated protein C on the phospholipid surface. Thromb Haemost 75:49-55, 1996.
19. Bertolaccini ML, Hughes GR: Antiphospholipid antibody testing: Which are most useful for diagnosis? Rheum Dis Clin North Am 32:455-463, 2006.
20. Gharavi AE, Pierangeli SS, Harris EN: Origin of antiphospholipid antibodies. Rheum Dis Clin North Am 27:551-563, 2001.
21. **Blank M, Krause I, Fridkin M, et al: Bacterial induction of autoantibodies to beta2-glycoprotein-I accounts for the infectious etiology of antiphospholipid syndrome. J Clin Invest 109:797-804, 2002.**
22. Gharavi AE, Sammaritano LR, Wen J, et al: Induction of antiphospholipid antibodies by immunization with beta 2 glycoprotein I (apolipoprotein H). J Clin Invest 90:1105-1109, 1992.
23. Arvieux J, Renaudineau Y, Mane I, et al: Distinguishing features of anti-beta2 glycoprotein I antibodies between patients with leprosy and the antiphospholipid syndrome. Thromb Haemost 87:599-605, 2002.
24. Lutters BC, Derksen RH, Tekelenburg WL, et al: Dimers of beta 2-glycoprotein 1 increase platelet deposition to collagen via interaction with phospholipids and the apolipoprotein E receptor 2'. J Biol Chem 278:33831-33838, 2003.
25. Bordron A, Dueymes MY, Levy Y, et al: Anti-endothelial cell antibody binding makes negatively charged phospholipids accessible to antiphospholipid antibodies. Arthritis Rheum 41:1738-1747, 1998.
26. Simantov R, LaSala J, Lo SK, et al: Activation of cultured vascular endothelial cells by antiphospholipid antibodies. J Clin Invest 96:2211-2219, 1996.
27. Font J, Espinosa G, Tassies D, et al: Effects of β2-glycoprotein I and monoclonal anticardiolipin antibodies in platelet interaction with subendothelium under flow conditions. Arthritis Rheum 46:3283-3289, 2002.
28. van Lummel M, Pennings MT, Derksen RH, et al: The binding site in β2-glycoprotein I for ApoER2' on platelets is located in domain V. J Biol Chem 280:36729-36736, 2005.
29. Erkan D, Lockshin MD: What is antiphospholipid syndrome? Curr Rheumatol Rep 6:451-457, 2004.
30. Dunoyer-Geindre S, de Moerloose P, Galve-de Rochemonteix B, et al: NFkappaB is an essential intermediate in the activation of endothelial cells by anti-beta2-glycoprotein 1 antibodies. Thromb Haemost 88:851-857, 2002.

31. Pierangeli SS, Vega-Ostertag M, Harris EN: Intracellular signaling triggered by antiphospholipid antibodies in platelets and endothelial cells: A pathway to targeted therapies. Thromb Res 114:467-476, 2004.

32. Mak IYH, Brosens JJ, Christian M, et al: Regulated expression of signal transducer and activator of transcription, Stat5, and its enhancement of PRL expression in human endometrial stromal cells in vitro. J Clin Endocrinol Metab 87:2581-2587, 2002.

33. Pierangeli SS, Liu XW, Barker JH, et al: Induction of thrombosis in a mouse model by IgG, IgM, and IgA immunoglobulins from patients with the antiphospholipid syndrome. Thromb Haemost 74:1361-1367, 1995.

34. Jankowski M, Vreys I, Wittevrongel C, et al: Thrombogenicity of β2-glycoprotein I-dependent antiphospholipid antibodies in a photochemically-induced thrombosis model in the hamster. Blood 101:157-162, 2003.

35. **Girardi G, Bulla R, Salmon JE, et al: The complement system in the pathophysiology of pregnancy. Mol Immunol 43:68-77, 2006.**

36. Fleming SD, Egan RP, Chai C, et al: Anti-phospholipid antibodies restore mesenteric ischemia/reperfusion-induced injury in complement receptor 2/complement receptor 1-deficient mice. J Immunol 173:7055-7061, 2004.

37. Kaul M, Erkan D, Sammaritano L, et al: Assessment of the 2006 revised antiphospholipid syndrome (APS) classification criteria [abstract]. Arthritis Rheum 54:S796, 2006.

38. Erkan D, Yazici Y, Peterson MG, et al: A cross-sectional study of clinical thrombotic risk factors and preventive treatments in antiphospholipid syndrome. Rheumatology (Oxford) 41:924-929, 2002.

39. Bancsi LF, van der Linden IK, Bertina RM: Beta 2-glycoprotein I deficiency and the risk of thrombosis. Thromb Haemost 67:649-653, 1992.

40. Sheng Y, Reddel SW, Herzog H, et al: Impaired thrombin generation in beta 2-glycoprotein I null mice. J Biol Chem 276:13817-13821, 2001.

41. Kamboh MI, Manzi S, Mehdi H, et al: Genetic variation in apolipoprotein H (beta2-glycoprotein I) affects the occurrence of antiphospholipid antibodies and apolipoprotein H concentrations in systemic lupus erythematosus. Lupus 8:742-750, 1999.

42. Potti A, Bild A, Dressman HK, et al: Gene-expression patterns predict phenotypes of immune-mediated thrombosis. Blood 107:1391-1396, 2006.

43. Bhandari S, Harnden P, Brownjohn AM, et al: Association of anticardiolipin antibodies with intraglomerular thrombi and renal dysfunction in lupus nephritis. QJM 91:401-409, 1998.

44. Rand JH, Wu X, Andree HAM, et al: Pregnancy loss in the antiphospholipid-antibody syndrome: A possible thrombogenic mechanism. N Engl J Med 337:154-160, 1997.

45. Roman MJ, Shanker BA, Davis A, et al: Prevalence and correlates of accelerated atherosclerosis in systemic lupus erythematosus. N Engl J Med 349:2399-2406, 2003.

46. Erkan D, Bateman H, Lockshin MD: Lupus-anticoagulant-hypoprothrombinemia syndrome associated with systemic lupus erythematosus: Report of 2 cases and review of literature. Lupus 8:560-564, 1999.

47. Erkan D, Cervera R, Asherson RA: Catastrophic antiphospholipid syndrome: Where do we stand? Arthritis Rheum 48:3320-3327, 2003.

48. Cervera R, Font J, Gomez-Puerta JA, et al: Validation of the preliminary criteria for the classification of catastrophic antiphospholipid syndrome. Ann Rheum Dis 64:1205-1209, 2005.

49. **Asherson RA, Cervera R, de Groot PG, et al: Catastrophic antiphospholipid syndrome: International consensus statement on classification criteria and treatment guidelines. Lupus 12:530-534, 2003.**

50. **Galli M, Luciani D, Bertolini G, et al: Lupus anticoagulants are stronger risk factors for thrombosis than anticardiolipin antibodies in the antiphospholipid syndrome: A systematic review of the literature. Blood 101:1827-1832, 2003.**

51. Brandt JT, Triplett DA, Alving B, et al: Criteria for the diagnosis of lupus anticoagulants: An update. Thromb Haemost 74:1185-1190, 1995.

52. Cervera R, Piette JC, Font J, et al: Antiphospholipid syndrome: Clinical and immunologic manifestations and patterns of disease expression in a cohort of 1000 patients. Arthritis Rheum 46:1019-1027, 2002.

53. Day HM, Thiagarajan P, Ahn C, et al: Autoantibodies to β2-glycoprotein I in systemic lupus erythematosus and primary antiphospholipid syndrome: Clinical correlations in comparison with other antiphospholipid antibody tests. J Rheumatol 25:667-674, 1998.

54. Erkan D, Derksen WJ, Kaplan V, et al: Real world experience with antiphospholipid antibody tests: How stable are results over time? Ann Rheum Dis 64:1321-1325, 2005.

55. Lockshin MD, Sammaritano LR, Schwartzman S: Brief report: Validation of the Sapporo criteria for antiphospholipid antibody syndrome. Arthritis Rheum 43:440-443, 2000.

56. Erel H, Erkan D, Lehman TJ, et al: Diagnostic usefulness of 3 dimensional gadolinium enhanced magnetic resonance venography in antiphospholipid syndrome. J Rheumatol 29:1338-1339, 2002.

57. Khong TY, De Wolf F, Robertson WB, et al: Inadequate maternal vascular response to placentation in pregnancies complicated by preeclampsia and by small-for-gestational-age infants. Br J Obstet Gynaecol 93:1049-1059, 1986.

58. Stone S, Pijnenborg R, Vercruysse L, et al: The placental bed in pregnancies complicated by primary antiphospholipid syndrome. Placenta 27:457-467, 2006.

59. Levy RA, Gharavi AE, Sammaritano LR, et al: Characteristics of IgG antiphospholipid antibodies in patients with systemic lupus erythematosus and syphilis. J Rheumatol 17:1036-1041, 1990.

60. Kupferminc MJ, Eldo A, Steinman N, et al: Increased frequency of genetic thrombophilia in women with complications of pregnancy. N Engl J Med 340:9-13, 1999.

61. **Crowther MA, Ginsberg JS, Julian J, et al: Comparison of two intensities of warfarin for the prevention of recurrent thrombosis in patients with the antiphospholipid antibody syndrome. N Engl J Med 349:1133-1138, 2003.**

62. **Finazzi G, Marchioli R, Brancaccio V, et al: A randomized clinical trial of high-intensity warfarin vs conventional antithrombotic therapy for the prevention of recurrent thrombosis in patients with the antiphospholipid syndrome (WAPS). J Thromb Haemost 3:848-853, 2005.**

63. Levine SR, Brey RL, Tilley BC, et al: Antiphospholipid antibodies and subsequent thrombo-occlusive events in patients with ischemic stroke. JAMA 291:576-584, 2004.

64. Ortel TL, Moll S: Monitoring warfarin therapy in patients with lupus anticoagulants. Ann Intern Med 127:177-185, 1997.

65. Erkan D, Lockshin MD: New treatments for antiphospholipid syndrome. Rheum Dis Clin North Am 32:129-148, 2006.

66. Brunner HI, Chan WS, Ginsberg JS, et al: Long term anticoagulation is preferable for patients with antiphospholipid antibody syndrome: Result of a decision analysis. J Rheumatol 29:490-501, 2002.

67. Vilela VS, de Jesus NR, Levy RA: Prevention of thrombosis during pregnancy. Isr Med Assoc J 4:794-797, 2002.

68. **Kutteh WH: Antiphospholipid antibody-associated recurrent pregnancy loss: Treatment with heparin and low-dose aspirin is superior to low-dose aspirin alone. Am J Obstet Gynecol 174:1584-1589, 1996.**

69. **Rai R, Cohen H, Dave M, et al: Randomised controlled trial of aspirin and aspirin plus heparin in pregnant women with recurrent miscarriage associated with phospholipid antibodies (or antiphospholipid antibodies). BMJ 314:253-257, 1997.**

70. Guballa N, Sammaritano L, Schwartzman S, et al: Ovulation induction and in vitro fertilization in systemic lupus erythematosus and antiphospholipid syndrome. Arthritis Rheum 43:550-556, 2000.

71. Tenedios F, Erkan D, Lockshin MD: Rituximab in the primary antiphospholipid syndrome (PAPS) [abstract]. Arthritis Rheum 52:4078, 2005.

72. Vero S, Asherson RA, Erkan D: Critical care review: Catastrophic antiphospholipid syndrome. J Intensive Care Med 21:144-159, 2006.

73. Erkan D, Yazici Y, Sobel R, et al: Primary antiphospholipid syndrome: Functional outcome after 10 years. J Rheumatol 27:2817-2821, 2000.

74. Erkan D, Merrill JT, Yazici Y, et al: High thrombosis rate after fetal loss in antiphospholipid syndrome: Effective prophylaxis with aspirin. Arthritis Rheum 44:1466-1467, 2001.

75. Raklyar I, DeMarco PJ, Wu J, et al: Anticardiolipin antibody correlates with poor graft survival in renal transplantation for systemic lupus erythematosus. Arthritis Rheum 52:S384, 2005.

76. **Erkan D, Leibowitz E, Berman J, Lockshin MD: Perioperative medical management of antiphospholipid syndrome: Hospital for Special Surgery experience, review of the literature and recommendations. J Rheumatol 29:843-849, 2002.**

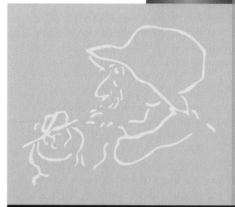

77

Systemic Sclerosis and the Scleroderma-Spectrum Disorders

JOHN VARGA • CHRISTOPHER P. DENTON

KEY POINTS

Systemic sclerosis (SSc) is a multisystem connective tissue disease of unknown etiology that occurs more commonly in women, follows a chronic course, and is associated with substantial morbidity and mortality.

SSc has a complex pathogenesis and protean clinical manifestations that reflect the underlying autoimmunity, vasculopathy, and fibrosis.

The hallmark of SSc is induration of the skin (scleroderma), whereas leading causes of death are pulmonary arterial hypertension; pulmonary fibrosis; and complications of cardiac, renal, and gastrointestinal tract involvement.

Scleroderma may occur in localized forms and in a distinct group of scleroderma-spectrum disorders

Systemic sclerosis (SSc) is a multisystem connective tissue disease of unknown etiology. Similar to other connective tissue diseases, SSc follows a chronic course, occurs more commonly in women, and is highly heterogeneous in its protean clinical manifestations. The hallmarks of SSc are autoimmunity and inflammation, functional and structural abnormalities in small blood vessels in multiple vascular beds, and progressive interstitial and vascular fibrosis in the skin and internal organs. This constellation of seemingly disparate pathophysiologic and clinical features occurs in most patients, and helps to differentiate SSc from other connective tissue diseases. Although the outcome of SSc has improved considerably during the past 2 decades, the disease carries the highest case fatality among the connective tissue diseases and is still considered incurable.

CLASSIFICATION OF SCLERODERMA-SPECTRUM DISORDERS

The hallmark of SSc is induration and thickening of the skin (scleroderma). The scleroderma spectrum of disorders encompasses, in addition to SSc, numerous disparate conditions that exhibit common clinical and pathologic features (Table 77-1). In SSc, the skin involvement ranges from widespread thickening (diffuse cutaneous SSc) to thickening limited to the face and distal extremities (limited cutaneous SSc), and may be altogether absent in some cases (SSc sine scleroderma). Localized scleroderma is a family of disorders that includes morphea, linear scleroderma, and coup de sabre. These disorders are more common in childhood, and in marked contrast to SSc are almost never associated with significant systemic involvement. Related disorders include hemifacial atrophy and inflammatory fibrosing conditions affecting the subcutaneous tissue, such as eosinophilic fasciitis and eosinophilia-myalgia syndrome, which are associated with chronic scleroderma-like skin changes.

Differentiation of the major subset of SSc into limited or diffuse cutaneous forms is based on the maximum extent of skin involvement.[1] In diffuse cutaneous SSc, there is widespread involvement of the skin with thickening proximal to the elbows or knees and often involving the chest or abdominal wall (Fig. 77-1). In limited cutaneous SSc, skin involvement is limited to the distal extremities or face, or may involve only the fingers (sclerodactyly) (Fig. 77-2). Another subgroup of SSc includes patients who manifest features of another autoimmune rheumatic disease (overlap syndrome). Some patients with characteristic vascular and internal organ manifestations and serologic findings of SSc lack typical skin sclerosis. This subset, called SSc sine scleroderma, comprises only approximately 1% of cases, but presents a particular diagnostic challenge.[2] Some patients with unexplained pulmonary fibrosis or pulmonary arterial hypertension (PAH) likely fall into this category. Clues to this diagnosis include the presence of Raynaud's phenomenon, nail-fold capillary changes of SSc, and hallmark SSc-associated autoantibodies. Some patients with isolated Raynaud's phenomenon eventually develop SSc or another full-blown connective tissue disease.

There is no single test that is diagnostic for SSc. For the purposes of distinguishing SSc from other autoimmune connective tissue diseases, preliminary criteria were developed.[3,4] These criteria had a high sensitivity and specificity for the diffuse cutaneous form, but not the limited cutaneous form, of SSc. In addition, the criteria do not take into account the hallmark autoantibodies now recognized in SSc. Key clinical features of the major subsets of SSc are summarized

Table 77-1 Scleroderma-Spectrum Disorders

Skin Sclerosis
Systemic sclerosis
Limited cutaneous
Diffuse cutaneous
Localized scleroderma
Infiltrative disorders
Amyloidosis
Scleromyxedema
Sclerodema of Buschke
Lichen sclerosis et atrophicus
Inflammatory
Overlap connective tissue diseases
Eosinophilic fasciitis
Chronic graft-versus-host disease
Sarcoidosis
Metabolic disorders
Myxedema
Porphyria cutanea tarda
Congenital porphyrias
Acromegaly
Digital Vascular Insufficiency
Raynaud's phenomenon
Primary Raynaud's phenomenon
Associated Raynaud's phenomenon
Other autoimmune rheumatic disorders (e.g., SLE, polymyositis, undifferentiataed connective tissue disease, overlap [mixed] connective tissue disease)
Other vascular disease
Hematologic
Cryoglobulinaemia
Cold agglutinin disease
Hyperviscosity syndrome
Systemic vasculitis
Buerger disease (thromboangiitis obliterans)
Macrovascular disease (e.g., thrombotic, embolic, atherosclerotic)

SLE, systemic lupus erythematosus.

in Table 77-2. Beyond classification of SSc by subset, it is important to consider the stage of disease. Diffuse cutaneous SSc tends to have a more abrupt onset and progressive course, with organ failure often developing within 5 years of the first symptoms. In limited cutaneous SSc, major visceral complications generally occur later.

Placing SSc patients into subsets of diffuse and limited cutaneous forms represents a clinically useful approach to risk stratification. In the early stage of diffuse cutaneous SSc, there is progressive extension of skin sclerosis and new onset of internal organ complications. In many cases, skin involvement peaks within 12 to 18 months of onset, often followed by declining extent and severity.[5] In contrast, patients with limited cutaneous SSc generally have insidious progression of skin involvement. Localized forms of scleroderma generally do not affect the internal organs and are not associated with Raynaud's phenomenon. Plaque morphea is the most common form of localized scleroderma in adults (Fig. 77-3), whereas linear scleroderma predominates in childhood.

EPIDEMIOLOGY

SSc is a sporadic disease that has a worldwide distribution and occurs in every ethnic group. No seasonal or geographic clustering of cases has been convincingly documented. The epidemiology of SSc has proven difficult to establish, reflecting the clinical diversity of the disease, the absence of widely accepted criteria for diagnosis or classification, and the methodologic challenges associated with population-based case ascertainment. Incidence estimates range from 9 to 19 cases/1 million/yr, with prevalence rates ranging from 28 to 253 cases/1 million/yr in the United States,[6,7] and 120 cases/1 million/yr in the United Kingdom.[8,9] Based on incidence and survival rates, it is estimated that there are 75,000 to 100,000 cases of SSc in the United States. The only community-based survey of SSc yielded a prevalence of 286 cases/1 million population.[10] This study also suggested that SSc is frequently misdiagnosed, implying that its true prevalence may be higher than previously estimated.

Similar to other connective tissue diseases, SSc is more frequent in women than men, with the most common age of disease onset in the 30 to 50 years range. The incidence of SSc is higher and disease onset occurs at an earlier age among African-Americans compared with whites. African-Americans with SSc are more likely to have diffuse skin involvement and pulmonary fibrosis and to have a worse prognosis.[11]

ETIOLOGY

GENETIC FACTORS

The genetics of SSc are complex, and the disease is not inherited in a straightforward mendelian fashion. Twins show a low rate of disease concordance (<5%).[12] This rate is similar between monozygotic and dizygotic twin pairs. Other studies have shown that SSc occurs significantly more frequently in families with SSc (1.6%) than in the general population (0.026%).[13] Although the absolute risk of SSc for each family member is low, a positive family history represents the strongest risk factor yet identified for SSc, indicating an important role for heredity in disease susceptibility. First-degree relatives of SSc patients also are more likely to have a positive antinuclear antibody than controls.[14]

In contrast to other connective tissue diseases, HLA linkages are generally weak in SSc. Particular HLA haplotypes do show associations with distinct serologically defined SSc subsets, however. A cluster of SSc cases had been described among Choctaw Native Americans living in Oklahoma, with affected individuals sharing a unique American Indian HLA haplotype.[15] Current investigations in SSc genetics focus primarily on polymorphisms in candidate genes. Associations of specific single nucleotide polymorphisms have been reported in genes involved in immunity and inflammation, vascular function, and connective tissue homeostasis.[16]

VIRUSES

The etiology of SSc is unknown. Along with exposure to certain environmental and occupational agents and drugs, infection with human cytomegalovirus (CMV) and other viruses has been implicated as a potential trigger.[17] Several reports have described the presence of antibodies directed against human CMV in the serum of patients with SSc. These antibodies recognized the UL83 and UL94 protein epitopes on human CMV.[18-20] Anti–topoisomerase I antibodies in some SSc patients show cross-reactivity with human CMV–derived proteins, providing evidence for molecular mimicry as a potential mechanistic link between

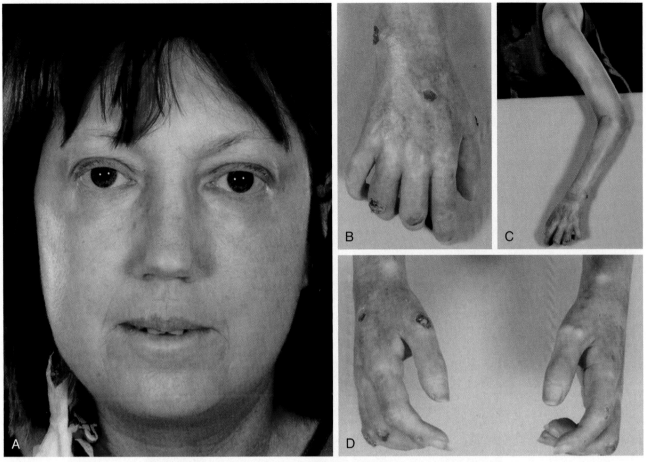

Figure 77-1 Diffuse cutaneous systemic sclerosis. Characteristic features of diffuse cutaneous systemic sclerosis are illustrated. **A,** Skin over the face is tightened; there is reduced opening of the mouth, owing in part to diminished oral aperture, but also to contractural changes in the soft tissues around the face and jaw. **B-D,** Hands exhibit reduced flexion and extension and fixed contractures at the interphalangeal joints. Ulceration occurs at sites of pressure or trauma, distinct from the ischemic digital lesions of limited cutaneous systemic sclerosis. Skin changes proximal to the knees or elbows on the limb, or involving the chest or abdominal wall, define the diffuse cutaneous subset.

human CMV infection and SSc.[21] Antibodies to UL94 can induce endothelial cell apoptosis and fibroblast activation in cell culture assays, suggesting a direct role for antiviral antibodies in tissue damage.[22,23] CMV infection is implicated in allograft vasculopathy, a complication of organ transplantation characterized by vascular neointima formation and smooth muscle cell proliferation reminiscent of the obliterative proliferative vasculopathy seen in SSc. In human dermal fibroblasts, CMV can directly induce the synthesis of the profibrotic growth factor connective tissue growth factor (CTGF), or CCN2, in vitro.[24] Evidence of infection with human parvovirus B19 also has been described in patients with SSc.[25,26]

ENVIRONMENTAL EXPOSURES, DRUGS, AND RADIATION

Although reports of putative geographic clustering of SSc cases suggest shared environmental exposures, careful investigations have generally failed to substantiate apparent clusters. Well-documented epidemic outbreaks of SSc-like multisystemic illnesses with acute onset and chronic persistence have been reported. One such illness, called the toxic oil syndrome, was linked to the ingestion of contaminated rapeseed cooking oils in Spain.[27] In the United

States, dietary supplements of tryptophan were implicated in an outbreak of the eosinophilia-myalgia syndrome epidemic in 1989.[28-30] Although scleroderma-like chronic skin lesions, multisystem involvement, and evidence of autoimmunity were prominent features of these apparently novel toxicoepidemic syndromes, associated clinical, histopathologic, and laboratory features clearly distinguished them from SSc.[31,28]

The frequency of SSc seems to be increased among men with occupational exposure to silica dust. Other occupational exposures linked with SSc include polyvinyl chloride, trichloroethylene, and organic solvents.[32,33] Anecdotal reports also have alleged an association between SSc and environmental exposures to pesticides, hair dyes, and industrial fumes.[32,34-36] No well-controlled studies have shown a causative association between cigarette smoking and SSc, in contrast to rheumatoid arthritis, in which smoking is the most definitive environmental risk factor.

Drugs implicated as potentially causative for SSc-like illnesses include bleomycin, pentazocine, and cocaine. The use of fenfluramine appetite suppressants has been linked to the development of PAH. The occurrence of SSc in women who had undergone cosmetic breast augmentation with silicone implants raised concern regarding a possible association.[28] Subsequent large-scale epidemiologic surveys

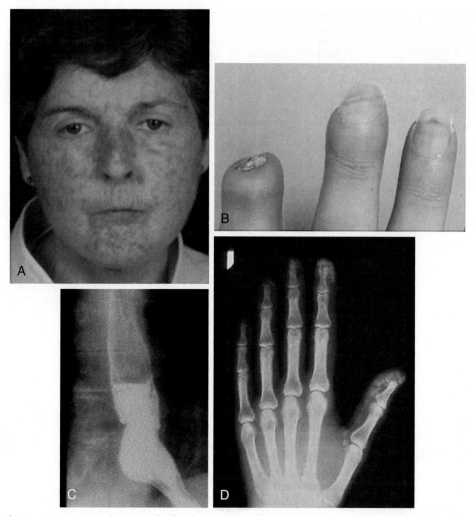

Figure 77-2 Limited cutaneous systemic sclerosis. **A,** The facial appearance of limited cutaneous systemic sclerosis contrasts markedly with diffuse cutaneous systemic sclerosis. There is marked perioral furrowing and much less skin induration. Telangiectasias are common and often widespread. **B-D,** Raynaud's phenomenon and digital ischemia may be severe and may lead to autoamputation. Subcutaneous calcinosis occurs. Esophageal involvement is common.

did not indicate an increased risk of SSc, however, or of other well-defined connective tissue diseases among women with silicone breast implants.[37-39] Radiation treatment for malignant neoplasms has been linked with the onset of de novo SSc and exacerbation of tissue fibrosis in patients with preexisting SSc.[40,41] Table 77-3 lists some environmental agents and drugs that have been linked with the development of SSc.

PATHOLOGY

GENERAL FEATURES

The characteristic pathologic findings in SSc are a noninflammatory proliferative/obliterative vasculopathy affecting small arteries and arterioles in multiple vascular beds, in combination with interstitial and vascular fibrosis in the skin, lungs, and multiple other internal organs.[42] Although in long-standing SSc these lesions generally occur in the absence of inflammation, in early-stage disease, inflammatory cell infiltrates are prominent in many organs. In the skin, the infiltrates are located predominantly around

Table 77-2 Classification of Systemic Sclerosis (SSc)*

Limited cutaneous SSc	Skin thickening restricted to sites distal to elbows and knees, but may involve face and neck
CREST syndrome	Subset of limited cutaneous SSc with prominent calcinosis, Raynaud's phenomenon, esophageal dysmotility, sclerodactyly, and telangiectasia
Diffuse cutaneous SSc	Skin thickening on the trunk and proximal extremities in addition to distal extremities and face
Overlap SSc	Skin changes and other characteristic features of SSc coexisting with features of another connective tissue disease, including SLE, myositis, or rheumatoid arthritis
SSc sine scleroderma	Raynaud's phenomenon, characteristic internal organ complications, and serologic abnormalities of SSc, but no apparent skin involvement

*Limited SSc has been suggested as a classification to define patients with Raynaud's phenomenon and capillaroscopic changes and serologies characteristic of SSc.

SLE, systemic lupus erythematosus.

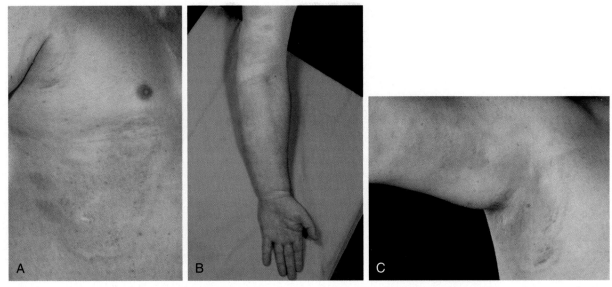

Figure 77-3 Localized scleroderma. **A-C,** Localized forms of scleroderma include morphea and linear scleroderma. When extensive, morphea can be a substantial problem. Clinical activity is suggested by pain, aching, or itching of affected areas of skin; enlargement of an existing plaque; or development of new lesions. Although localized scleroderma may occur in patients with systemic sclerosis, evolution to systemic disease has not been described.

Table 77-3 Environmental Agents and Drugs Implicated in Scleroderma-like Syndromes

Chemicals
Silica
Heavy metals
Mercury
Organic chemicals
Vinyl chloride
Benzene
Toluene
Trichloroethylene

Drugs
Bleomycin
Pentazocine
Paclitaxel
Cocaine
Dietary supplement/appetite suppressants
Tryptophan (contamination)
Mazindol
Fenfluramine
Diethylpropion

blood vessels and in the reticular dermis and are composed primarily of CD4$^+$ T lymphocytes and monocytes, whereas in the lungs, cellular infiltrates consist predominantly of CD8$^+$ T lymphocytes (Fig. 77-4).

VASCULAR PATHOLOGY

Vascular injury and activation are the earliest and possibly primary events in the pathogenesis of SSc. Histopathologic evidence of vascular damage is present before fibrosis and can be detected in involved and uninvolved skin, indicating a generalized process.[43] Manifestations of vascular involvement, such as Raynaud's phenomenon, generally precede other disease manifestations. Additional clinical signs of SSc vasculopathy include cutaneous telangiectasia, nail-fold capillary alterations, PAH, digital pit formation,

gastric antral vascular ectasia (also called watermelon stomach), and scleroderma renal crisis.

In patients with established SSc, the most characteristic vascular finding is bland intimal proliferation in the small and medium-sized arteries (Fig. 77-5). Expansion of the intimal layer, a striking finding that SSc shares with chronic allograft arteriopathy, is thought to be due to increased proliferation and migration of myointimal cells and local accumulation of collagen.[44] The vascular basement membranes are thickened and reduplicated. The blood vessels of the heart, lungs, kidneys, and intestinal tract are prominently affected. Impaired fibrinolysis, increased levels of von Willebrand factor, and ongoing platelet aggregation are noted.[45] Endothelial cell injury results in further platelet aggregation, release of platelet-derived growth factor (PDGF) and endothelin-1 (ET-1), and endothelial cell apoptosis.[45,46] Vasculitic lesions and immune complex deposition in the vessel walls are uncommon.

In late stages of the disease, extensive fibrin deposition and perivascular fibrosis cause progressive luminal occlusion, and there is striking paucity of small blood vessels in lesional tissue.[47] Loss of vascular supply leads to chronic tissue hypoxia. Widespread proliferative/obliterative vasculopathy of small and medium-sized arteries in multiple vascular beds is the pathologic hallmark of all forms of SSc.

TISSUE FIBROSIS

Fibrosis is characterized by accumulation of excessive amounts of type I collagen and other fibrillar collagens, fibronectin, elastin, proteoglycans, and other connective tissue molecules in the extracellular matrix (ECM). The process causes disruption of tissue architecture. In SSc, interstitial and vascular fibrosis in the skin and parenchymal organs contributes directly to their progressive dysfunction and eventual failure. Most prominently affected are the lungs, gastrointestinal tract, heart, tendon sheath, and perifascicular tissue surrounding skeletal muscle. Histopathologic

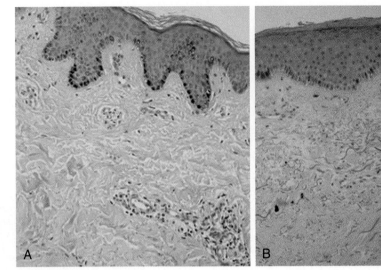

Figure 77-4 Histology of skin in diffuse cutaneous systemic sclerosis. **A,** There is perivascular infiltration in the dermis with inflammatory cells of multiple lineages. Microvascular endothelial cell activation and increased extracellular matrix deposition also are seen. **B,** Later, there is regression of the inflammatory features. Secondary structures within the skin, such as hair follicles and sweat glands, are reduced, and rete pegs are flattened. (Hematoxylin and eosin stain, original magnification ×40.)

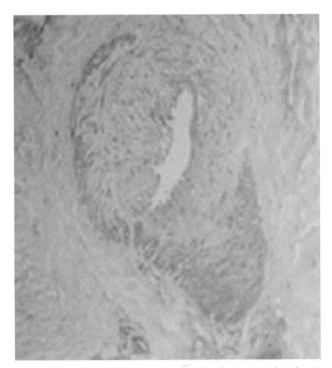

Figure 77-5 Histologic appearance of scleroderma vasculopathy. In the finger, changes in the digital artery may narrow the lumen and reduce response to vasodilators. Pulmonary arterial changes may lead to pulmonary arterial hypertension. The histologic appearance is reminiscent of idiopathic pulmonary arterial hypertension (previously termed primary pulmonary hypertension).

examination of these organs indicates accumulation of homogeneous and acellular connective tissue with thick hyalinized collagen bundles.

ORGAN-SPECIFIC PATHOLOGIC FINDINGS

Skin

Fibrosis of the skin, the hallmark of SSc, causes marked expansion of the dermis. The process obliterates the hair follicles, sweat glands, and other skin appendages. Collagen fiber accumulation is most prominent in the reticular (deep) dermis, and gradually invades the subjacent adipose layer with entrapment of fat cells. Skin biopsy in early stages of SSc may reveal deep dermal perivascular infiltrates composed of T lymphocytes and monocytes. Less commonly, mast cells[48] and eosinophils[46,49,50] may be detected. The proportion of alpha smooth muscle actin–positive myofibroblasts, a mesenchymal cell that is intermediate between fibroblasts and contractile smooth muscle cells and plays a major role in fibrogenesis, is increased in the lesional skin.[51]

With disease progression, the skin undergoes atrophy with thinning of the epidermis and effacement of the rete pegs (see Fig. 77-4). The fibrotic dermis is largely acellular and contains dense accumulation of compact hyalinized collagen bundles, fibronectin, and other structural matrix proteins. Paucity of dermal capillaries is associated with chronic tissue hypoxia that induces vascular endothelial growth factor (VEGF) and other angiogenic factors. Evidence of tissue hypoxia can be found in clinically uninvolved, apparently "normal" skin.[52]

Biochemically, the collagens in the fibrotic dermis are normal, and relative proportions of the main fibrillar collagens (type I and type III) are comparable to those of normal skin. In contrast, the minor nonfibrillar type VII collagen, normally restricted to the dermal-epidermal basement membrane zone, is abundant throughout the lesional dermis.[53] The levels of enzymes mediating post-translational collagen modification, such as lysyl hydroxylase (PLOD2), are elevated, resulting in an increase in aldehyde-derived collagen cross-links, which may account for the dense sclerotic nature of the fibrotic dermis.[54] Studies using DNA microarray technology have defined better the sequence of activation events that underlie the development of irreversible fibrosis. The results reveal strikingly altered patterns of gene expression in skin from SSc patients compared with healthy controls. Clinically involved skin and uninvolved skin seem to be indistinguishable in terms of their gene expression profiles. The expression of many genes involved in ECM homeostasis, and in transforming growth factor (TGF)-β, CCN2, and Wnt signaling pathways, is elevated.[55,56]

Lungs

In early SSc, patchy infiltration of the alveolar walls with lymphocytes, plasma cells, macrophages, and eosinophils is seen (Fig. 77-6). At this stage, elevated proportions of inflammatory leukocytes can be found in alveolar lavage fluid. With progression, interstitial lung fibrosis and vascular damage predominate, often coexisting within the same lesions. Intimal thickening of the pulmonary arteries, best seen with elastin stain, underlies PAH, and at autopsy is often associated with multiple pulmonary emboli and myocardial fibrosis.

Fibrosis in the lungs is characterized by expansion of the alveolar interstitium, owing to accumulation of collagens and other connective tissue proteins. The typical histologic pattern seen on lung biopsy specimen is nonspecific interstitial pneumonitis, a form of interstitial lung disease characterized by mild-to-moderate interstitial inflammation, type II pneumocyte hyperplasia, and uniform distribution of fibrosis. Less commonly, SSc is associated with the usual interstitial pneumonia pattern, which is characterized by scattered fibroblastic foci and patchy distribution of fibrosis and has a worse prognosis.[57,58] Progressive thickening of the alveolar septa ultimately results in obliteration of the airspaces and honeycombing, and consequent loss of pulmonary blood vessels. This process impairs gas exchange and contributes to worsening of PAH. Extensive pulmonary fibrosis may predispose to primary lung carcinoma.[47]

Gastrointestinal Tract

Prominent pathologic changes can occur at any level from the mouth to the rectum. The esophagus is virtually always affected, with fibrosis in the lamina propria, submucosa, and muscular layers, and characteristic vascular lesions.[42,59] Replacement of the normal intestinal architecture results in disordered peristaltic activity, gastroesophageal reflux and small bowel dysmotility, pseudo-obstruction, and bacterial overgrowth. Chronic gastroesophageal reflux is complicated by esophageal inflammation, ulcerations, and stricture formation. One third of SSc patients with severe gastroesophageal reflux develop Barrett's esophagus, characterized by metaplasia of the normal squamous lining of the esophagus into columnar epithelium.[60,61] Because it is a premalignant lesion associated with a greater than 30-fold increased risk of adenocarcinoma, patients with Barrett's metaplasia need monitoring for the development of dysplasia and adenocarcinoma.

Kidneys

In the kidneys, vascular lesions predominate, and glomerulonephritis is rare except in overlap syndromes. Chronic renal ischemia is associated with shrunken glomeruli and other ischemic changes. Patients with acute scleroderma renal crisis show dramatic histopathologic changes that are indistinguishable from the changes observed in other forms of malignant hypertension.[62] Vascular changes in SSc kidneys are most prominent in the small interlobular and arcuate renal arteries, which show reduplication of elastic lamina, marked intimal proliferation, and accumulation of

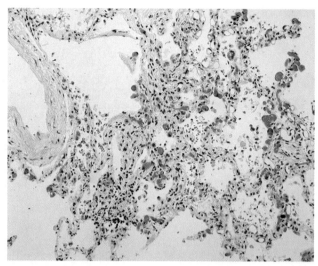

Figure 77-6 Histologic appearance of the lung. Evidence of interstitial lung disease is common in systemic sclerosis. Although there is substantial variation in the appearance of lung histology, consistent features include reduction in airspaces and thickening of alveolar walls with increased extracellular matrix deposition. Inflammatory cell infiltrates may be prominent. Lung biopsy is rarely required for diagnosis of interstitial lung disease in SSc.

ground substance.[63] These changes also can be found in SSc patients who do not have renal crisis.[64]

Fibrinoid necrosis of the arteriolar walls may be seen. Intimal thickening leads to severe narrowing and total obliteration of the lumen, often with microangiopathic hemolysis. Tubular changes occur secondary to vascular insufficiency and include flattening and degeneration of tubular cells. The clinical picture may resemble thrombotic thrombocytopenic purpura, especially in severe cases of scleroderma renal crisis. The reported association of thrombotic thrombocytopenic purpura with low levels of activity of the enzyme plasma von Willebrand factor cleaving protease (ADAMTS13) has not been reported in SSc renal crisis, however. Nonspecific immunoglobulin and complement C3 deposition may be found, but inflammatory infiltrates are uncommon. Histologic features of scleroderma renal crisis are shown in Figure 77-7.

Heart

At autopsy, evidence of cardiac involvement is found in 80% of patients with SSc.[42,65] Modest pericardial effusions are common; occasionally, fibrosis and constrictive pericarditis may occur. A characteristic pathologic finding is myocardial contraction band necrosis, which is thought to reflect repeated ischemia-reperfusion injury and may be a manifestation of "myocardial Raynaud's phenomenon."[65] Significant interstitial and perivascular fibrosis may occur in the absence of clinically evident heart involvement.[66,67] Skeletal muscle myositis in SSc may be accompanied by acute myocarditis.[65,68,69]

PATHOLOGIC FINDINGS IN OTHER ORGANS

The major patterns of organ-based disease in SSc are summarized in Table 77-4. Many other systems can be affected by the disease, however. Fibrosis of the thyroid glands is

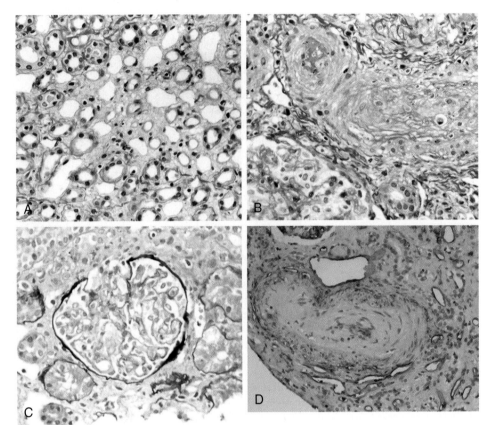

Figure 77-7 Histologic appearance of scleroderma renal crisis. **A** and **B**, Typical histologic features are present, including interstitial fibrosis (**A**), occlusion of intrarenal arteries with neointima formation, fibrinoid necrosis of the vessel wall, and reduplication of the internal elastic lamina (**B**). **C**, The glomeruli are shrunken and lack inflammatory cells or proliferative changes. **D**, In severe cases, there is evidence of intravascular thrombosis resembling the changes of thrombotic thrombocytopenic purpura.

Table 77-4 Prevalence of Major Internal Organ–Based Complications in Systemic Sclerosis (SSc)

Organ Involved	Approximate Frequency (%)	
	Limited Cutaneous SSc	Diffuse Cutaneous SSc
Raynaud's phenomenon	99	98
Gastrointestinal tract	74	60
Kidney (scleroderma renal crisis)	1	15
Heart	9	12
Lungs	50	65
Pulmonary hypertension	25	20
Interstitial lung disease	25	40
Skeletal myopathy	10	25
Thyroid	15	10

common.[70,71] Broad bands of fibrous tissue are seen in the thyroid gland, with atrophy and obliteration of the follicles, in the absence of inflammation.[72] Patients with SSc frequently have abnormal thyroid function tests and antithyroid antibodies.[73,74] Erectile dysfunction is common in men with SSc and may be a presenting manifestation of the disease. Pathologic examination shows extensive proliferative/obliterative changes in the penile blood vessels.[75] Fibrosis of the salivary and lacrimal glands in the absence of inflammation can occur and may be associated with Sjögren's syndrome. Synovial biopsy specimens show fibrosis and characteristic vascular changes in the small arterioles.[76]

ANIMAL MODELS OF SCLERODERMA

Animal models of human disease can be valuable for investigating complex pathogenesis, for identifying the genetic underpinnings and cellular and molecular components of the process and their interactions, and for developing novel treatment strategies and evaluating their efficacy. A variety of animal models have been investigated as potential models for SSc. Although none reproduce all three cardinal features of the disease (obliterative/proliferative vasculopathy, autoimmunity, and fibrosis), some models do recapitulate selected characteristics.[77] Mouse models of scleroderma can be divided into three types: (1) naturally occurring, where spontaneous mutations are associated with a genetically transmitted scleroderma-like phenotype, such as tight skin (Tsk1/+ mouse); (2) induced models, where the scleroderma phenotype is elicited by chemical exposures or manipulation of the immune system (bleomycin-induced skin and lung fibrosis); and (3) transplantation of HLA-mismatched bone marrow cells resulting in chronic sclerodermatous graft-versus-host disease and genetic manipulations giving rise to mouse strains with heritable scleroderma-like traits (Table 77-5).

HERITABLE ANIMAL MODELS OF SCLERODERMA

The tight skin mouse (Tsk1/+) is characterized by diffuse thickening and tethering of the skin. Although mice homozygous for the Tsk1 mutation die in utero at 8 to 10 days of gestation, heterozygous mice (Tsk1/+) survive and develop tight skin that is firmly bound to the underlying

Table 77-5 Mouse Models of Scleroderma

Model	Aspects of Pathogenesis				Key Features
	Vasculopathy, Vascular Activation	Inflammation	Autoimmunity	Fibrosis	
Naturally Occurring					
Tsk-1	−	−	+	+	Duplication mutation in fibrillin-1 gene
Tsk-2	−	+	+	+	Unknown genetic defect; early cutaneous inflammatory cell infiltrate
Induced					
Bleomycin (subcutaneous injection)	−	+	−	+	Production of reactive oxygen species, monocytic inflammation, skin and lung fibrosis
GVHD (B10.D2 versus Balb/C)	+	+	−	+	Transfer of spleen cells from B10.D2 mice into irradiated Balb/C mice results in chronic GVHD and fibrosis
GVHD (B10.D2 versus Rag-2$^{-/-}$)	+	+	+	+	Transfer of spleen cells into RAG-2 null mice results in systemic fibrosis, inflammation, and autoantibodies
Transgenic					
TGFβRII DN	−	+	−	+	Mice expressing a dominant negative TFGβRII develop systemic tissue fibrosis
MRL/lpr/IFNγR$^{-/-}$	−	+	+	+	MRL/lpr mouse strain lacking IFN-γ receptors spontaneously develop systemic fibrosis
Conditional TGFβRI	+	+	−	+	Conditional expression of constitutively active TGF-β receptor in fibroblasts causes tissue fibrosis and inflammation

GVHD, graft-versus-host disease; IFN, interferon; TGF, transforming growth factor.

subcutaneous tissue. In contrast to human SSc, Tsk1/+ mice have subcutaneous hyperplasia, with unremarkable dermis.[78] Tsk1/+ mice develop emphysematous changes in the lungs rather than fibrosis, and vasculopathy does not occur. Although skin inflammation is uncommon, Tsk1/+ mice do mount an autoimmune response with serum antibodies directed against topoisomerase I.

The Tsk1 mutation has been localized to mouse chromosome 2, and subsequently identified as an intragenic tandem duplication in the gene encoding fibrillin-1.[79] Fibrillin-1 is a large structural protein that is widely distributed in connective tissue microfibrils and is involved in the regulation of the latency and activation of TGF-β.[80] Mutations in the fibrillin-1 gene are responsible for Marfan syndrome, characterized by activation of TGF-β in multiple tissues. The Tsk1/+ fibrillin-1 duplication mutation gives rise to an abnormally large 450-kD protein.[79] No corresponding mutations in the fibrillin-1 gene have been shown in patients with SSc.

As mentioned previously, the skin lesions in Tsk1/+ are due to tethering and thickening of the hypodermal tissue, rather than the dermal fibrosis characteristic of SSc, raising some doubt regarding the relevance of the Tsk1/+ mouse as a bona fide model for the human disease.[78,81] Although it has been hypothesized that accumulation of abnormally large mutant fibrillin-1 in Tsk1/+ mice destabilizes the ECM,[82,81] or perturbs the homeostatic control of TGF-β latency, the precise mechanisms linking the Tsk1/+ mutation in fibrillin-1 to the development of cutaneous hyperplasia are unknown.[77]

Another potential animal model of scleroderma is the Tsk2 mouse. Heterozygous Tsk2 mice spontaneously develop scleroderma-like skin changes by age 3 to 4 weeks.[83] The dermis is fibrotic and, in contrast to Tsk1/+ mice, shows extensive infiltration with mononuclear inflammatory cells. Tsk2/+ mice have evidence of autoimmunity.[84] The Tsk2 mutation, originally induced by exposure of normal mice to ethyl nitrosurea, is located on mouse chromosome 1 and is inherited as an autosomal dominant trait, although the underlying molecular defect has not yet been identified.[77]

INDUCIBLE ANIMAL MODELS OF SCLERODERMA

Chronic skin and lung fibrosis can be induced in normal BALB/c or C57 mice by subcutaneous bleomycin injections.[85] The sequence of histopathologic changes in the lesional skin closely resembles that seen in SSc: early and self-limited mononuclear cell infiltration and upregulation of cytokines such as TGF-β and monocyte chemotactic protein (MCP)-1, followed by development of dermal fibrosis with excessive collagen deposition and accumulation of alpha smooth muscle actin–positive myofibroblasts.[86,87] In contrast to SSc, bleomycin-induced scleroderma in the mouse is not associated with either vascular changes or autoantibodies, and skin fibrosis is limited in its extent and duration. Nevertheless, in light of its reproducibility, relative strain independence, and ease of induction, this mouse model of scleroderma is now widely used for investigating the pathogenic roles of specific gene products in fibrosis.[87,88]

Subcutaneous injection of TGF-β in newborn mice causes granulation tissue formation and transient fibrosis. Simultaneous injection of CTGF with TGF-β causes persistent fibrosis, suggesting that CTGF is required for sustaining the fibrotic response.[89] Transplantation of HLA-mismatched bone marrow or spleen cells into sublethally irradiated recipient mice results in sclerodermatous graft-versus-host disease, characterized by chronic fibrosis of the skin and lung, perivascular fibrosis, and autoimmunity.[90,91] In this model, skin fibrosis is preceded by mononuclear cell infiltration and elevation of TGF-β and chemokines.

GENETIC MANIPULATIONS IN MICE GIVING RISE TO SYSTEMIC SCLEROSIS PHENOTYPES

Various mouse strains with genetic modifications resulting in spontaneous development of scleroderma-like phenotypes have been created (see Table 77-5). These transgenic and knockout mice are currently undergoing intensive study and provide robust novel experimental tools in scleroderma research.[92,93,88] Mouse strains with constitutive or inducible upregulation of TGF-β signaling in fibroblasts recapitulate key clinical, histologic, and biochemical features of SSc and provide support for the likely role of perturbed TGF-β signaling in pathogenesis.[94,92]

PATHOGENESIS

INTEGRATED OVERVIEW

The pathogenesis of SSc is complex and incompletely understood. Animal models reproduce only some of the diverse pathologic and clinical attributes of the disease. A holistic view of pathogenesis must integrate the three cardinal features of SSc: vascular injury and damage, activation of the innate and adaptive arms of the immune system autoimmunity, and generalized interstitial and vascular fibrosis.[71,95] Although each of these processes occurs in each patient, their relative contribution to the disease varies from one patient to another. The clinical heterogeneity of SSc is likely to be a reflection of the variable contributions of these pathogenetic processes. As illustrated in Figure 77-8, complex and dynamic interplay between these distinct processes is thought to be responsible for initiating, amplifying, and sustaining tissue damage in SSc.[70]

VASCULOPATHY

Vascular Injury and Activation

Vascular injury and activation are likely to be the initiating events in SSc. Evidence of vascular involvement is early and widespread, and is associated with significant

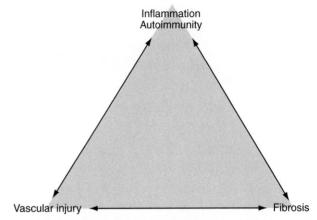

Figure 77-8 Pathogenetic triad of systemic sclerosis. Patients with systemic sclerosis display evidence of autoimmunity and inflammation, vasculopathy, and fibrosis. Autoimmunity and vasculopathy apparently precede the onset, and contribute to the development and progression, of fibrosis. Vascular injury and fibrosis may contribute to chronic autoimmunity and inflammation.

clinical sequelae. The initial vascular insult apparently is endothelial cell injury, possibly triggered by unidentified serum cytotoxic factors or T cell–derived proteolytic granzymes.[96] Other potential causes include endothelial cell–directed autoantibodies, vasculotropic viruses, inflammatory cytokines, and environmental stress. Vascular injury causes endothelial cell activation and dysfunction, with increased expression of vascular endothelial cell adhesion molecule-1 and endothelial leukocyte adhesion molecule-1, altered secretion of vasoactive mediators, and activation of platelets and fibrinolytic pathways.[97,98] Activated platelets release thromboxane A$_2$, PDGF, and TGF-β, which potentiate vasoconstriction, and contribute to fibroblast activation and myofibroblast transdifferentiation. Pericytes, which are smooth muscle–like structural cells normally found in the walls of small blood vessels, show marked hyperplasia in lesional skin from patients with early-stage SSc, and express the surface marker Thy-1 (CD90) and receptors for PDGF.[99-101]

Production of and responsiveness to endothelium-derived vasodilatory factors (nitric oxide, calcitonin gene–related peptide, and prostacyclin) are defective in SSc endothelium, and the altered vasodilator/vasoconstrictor balance results in impaired blood flow responses and episodes of ischemia-reperfusion with oxidative stress that amplifies vascular injury. Microvessels show increased permeability and enhanced transendothelial leukocyte migration. Fibrinolytic cascades are activated, and platelets are exposed to subendothelial structures, with resultant platelet activation and aggregation culminating in thrombosis.

Activated endothelial cells release ET-1, the most potent potent vasoconstrictor known (Fig. 77-9). In addition, ET-1 promotes leukocyte adhesion and vascular smooth muscle cell proliferation, and induces fibroblast activation. The levels of ET-1 are elevated in the blood and in bronchoalveolar lavage fluids from patients with SSc.[102-104] Expression of allograft inflammatory protein (AIF)-1, a macrophage-derived protein important in the immune response and proliferative vasculopathy that occur during chronic allograft rejection (allograft vasculopathy), is elevated in blood

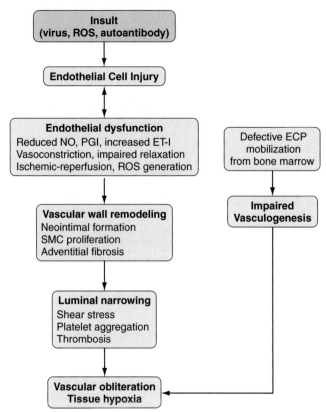

Figure 77-9 Pathogenesis of vasculopathy. Initial endothelial insult results in endothelial cell activation, with reversible functional changes, increased expression of adhesion molecules, and enhanced leukocyte diapedesis resulting in perivascular inflammation. Damaged endothelial cells have impaired production of vasodilators, such as nitric oxide, and increased production of vasoconstrictors, such as endothelin-1. Consequent vasoconstriction and defective vasodilation aggravate vascular damage, leading to irreversible and progressive vascular wall remodeling, luminal occlusion, platelet aggregation, in situ thrombosis, and tissue ischemia. Loss of blood vessels may be compounded further by insufficient vasculogenesis.

and in affected vessels in lesional skin and lungs of patients with SSc.[104a] Because AIF-1 stimulates vascular smooth muscle cell proliferation, its increased expression and induction by TGF-β are likely to contribute to the vasculopathy of SSc.

Vascular Damage and Defective Vasculogenesis in Systemic Sclerosis

Hypertrophy of the intimal and medial layers of small blood vessels in combination with adventitial fibrosis causes progressive luminal narrowing. Together with endothelial cell apoptosis, the process culminates in obliterative vasculopathy and vascular rarefaction, with the characteristic striking decrease of blood vessels seen on angiograms of SSc patients with late-stage disease.[104b] Loss of microvasculature leads to chronic tissue hypoxia, which induces hypoxia-inducible factor-1–dependent genes such as VEGF and its receptors. Plasma levels of the angiogenesis inhibitor endostatin, a degradation product of type XVIII collagen, were reported to be increased in SSc (Fig. 77-10).[105] Other studies found elevated levels of angiogenic factors VEGF, fibroblast growth factor, and PDGF. The expression of VEGF and its receptors were elevated in lesional tissue.[52,106,107]

An apparent paradox is why, in the face of tissue hypoxia and ongoing angiogenic drive, is SSc associated with progressive loss of blood vessels. More recent studies implicate failure of vasculogenesis, owing to a reduction in the number of circulating endothelial progenitor cells and their impaired differentiation into mature endothelial cells.[108-110] Because bone marrow–derived CD34+ circulating endothelial progenitor cells are essential for physiologic vasculogenesis in ischemic tissues, their defective mobilization or function compromises the vascular repair process. Whether the reduction in circulating endothelial progenitor cells noted in SSc patients is due to "exhaustion" of the bone marrow, or destruction in the peripheral circulation, remains unresolved.

INFLAMMATION AND AUTOIMMUNITY

T Cell Activation in Systemic Sclerosis

The innate and the adaptive arms of the immune system seem to be activated in early SSc, and autoimmunity is prominent; however, the role of cellular and humoral autoimmune effector pathways in the pathogenesis is uncertain. Activation of T cells is evident in lesional tissues and in peripheral blood, and seems to play a direct role in tissue injury. In early stages of the disease, activated CD4 and CD8 T lymphocytes and monocytes/macrophages, and less commonly B cells, eosinophils, mast cells, and natural killer cells, are observed in perivascular regions in the lesional skin, lungs, and other affected organs; these inflammatory cell infiltrates are detectable before the appearance of fibrosis.[43,111,112] Studies using in situ hybridization of skin biopsy specimens from patients with early SSc show that procollagen gene expression is higher in fibroblasts that are adjacent to inflammatory cells, suggesting a role for the inflammatory cells or their soluble products in inducing fibroblast activation.[113] The extent of lymphocytic tissue infiltration correlates with the severity and progression of skin fibrosis.[111]

Tissue-infiltrating mononuclear cells are predominantly CD3+ and CD4+; express activation markers CD45, HLA-DR, and the interleukin (IL)-2 receptor; and display restricted T cell receptor signatures indicative of oligoclonal T cell expansion in specific response to antigen.[114,115] In the lungs, a predominance of CD8+ cells and γ/δ T cells is observed.[115] It is unknown whether T cells in lesional tissue are activated nonspecifically (by cytokines or chemokines) or specifically in response to an (unknown) antigen.[116]

Evidence of T cell activation in SSc also is detected in the peripheral blood. Serum levels of IL-2 are elevated, and circulating T cells show spontaneous cytokine secretion and increased expression of the IL-2 receptor. The mechanisms responsible for the migration and homing of activated mononuclear cells from the peripheral blood to target tissues, and their retention and accumulation there, are not well understood. Increased expression of lymphocyte function–associated antigen-1 and other adhesion molecules on SSc T lymphocytes may enable them to adhere directly to fibroblasts.[117] Circulating CD4+ T cells in SSc cells also express elevated chemokine receptors and α1 integrin adhesion molecules, accounting for their enhanced binding ability to endothelium and to fibroblasts.[118] Vascular endothelial cells express intracellular adhesion molecule-1,

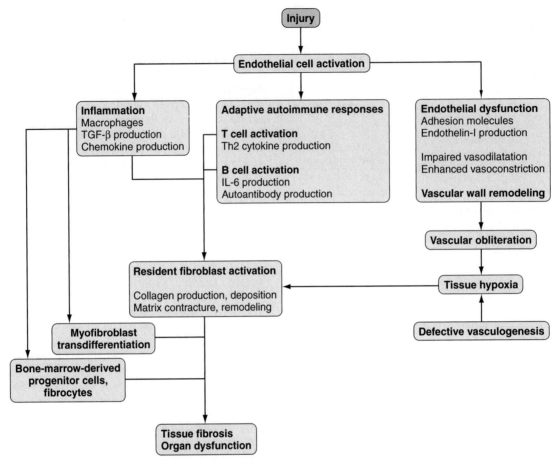

Figure 77-10 Pathogenesis of fibrosis in systemic sclerosis. Fibrosis is the end result of chronic inflammation and autoimmunity and vascular damage and hypoxia. Injury results in vascular damage and perivascular inflammation, with local secretion and activation of fibrogenic cytokines and chemokines, inducing fibroblast activation and myofibroblast accumulation. Circulating mesenchymal progenitor cells traffic to and accumulate within the lesional tissue and transdifferentiate into fibrotic fibroblasts, accelerating matrix accumulation. Tissue hypoxia, matrix remodeling, and contraction contribute further to the fibrotic process, which disrupts tissue architecture and interferes with organ function.

E-selectin, and other adhesion molecules that facilitate leukocyte diapedesis. Studies employing DNA microarray analysis indicate that peripheral blood leukocytes from patients with SSc show increased expression of interferon (IFN)-regulated genes[119] and genes encoding AIF-1, and selectins and integrins mediating leukocyte adhesion to the endothelium.[120]

T Helper Type 1/T Helper Type 2 Cytokine Balance and T Helper Type 2 Polarized Immune Responses in Systemic Sclerosis

An emerging hypothesis for the pathogenesis of fibrotic disorders implicates an altered balance between T helper type 1 (Th1) and T helper type 2 (Th2) cytokines in aberrant response to tissue injury. T cells polarized to a Th2 pattern secrete abundant IL-4, IL-5, and IL-13, with a paucity of the hallmark Th1 cytokine IFN-γ. The Th2 cytokines are profibrogenic because they can directly stimulate collagen synthesis and myofibroblast transdifferentiation, and induce TGF-β, a powerful modulator of immunoregulation and ECM accumulation. In contrast, the Th1 cytokine IFN-γ blocks these responses and exerts antifibrotic effects. Skewing of the immune response toward a Th2 pattern contributes to a more profibrotic environment.

Animal studies have provided support for the significance of a Th2-polarized immune response in the pathogenesis of fibrosis. Cells that have been polarized in vitro to a Th2 pattern induce fibrosis when passively transferred in vivo.[121] Mice lacking the transcription factor T-bet, which directs differentiation of T cells toward a Th1-predominant phenotype, spontaneously show a Th2-polarized immune response and develop exaggerated skin fibrosis in response to injection of bleomycin.[122,123] Patients with SSc display a relative shift in the Th1/Th2 cytokine balance toward a Th2 predominance. The serum levels of IFN-γ, and its in vitro production by peripheral blood monocytes, are reduced.[124,125] Peripheral blood leukocytes from SSc patients show elevated expression of the gene for the transcription factor GATA3, which drives Th2 polarization.[126] Clones of CD4+ T cells generated from SSc skin biopsy specimens show a Th2 cytokine profile, with in vitro secretion of IL-4, but not IFN-γ.[127] Alveolar CD8+ T cells from SSc patients show elevated Th2 cytokine production, and the Th2 predominance predicts accelerated decline in lung function.[128,129] Proteomic analysis also showed a predominance of Th2 cytokines in SSc bronchoalveolar lavage fluids.[130] Using DNA microarray technology, bronchoalveolar lavage fluid CD8+ cells from patients with SSc were shown to have an activated Th2 pattern of gene expression with increased levels of IL-4 and IL-13, and reduced production of IFN-γ.[129] A longitudinal study of 26 patients with diffuse cutaneous SSc showed that improvement in skin involvement over time was associated with a decline in serum Th2 cytokines and a concomitant increase in IL-12, a Th1-inducing cytokine.[131] The specific roles of the regulatory T cell and T helper type 3 T cell subsets in SSc have not yet been characterized.

Monocytes and Macrophages

Phagocytic monocytes and macrophages have central roles in host defense, innate immunity, and tissue repair. Monocytes are a major source of regulatory cytokines and chemokines, including IL-1, tumor necrosis factor (TNF)-α, MCP-1, PDGF, and TGF-β, all of which are important in regulating immune, inflammatory, and fibroproliferative responses. In addition, monocytes produce collagenases and other matrix metalloproteinase enzymes that mediate tissue remodeling. Macrophages are prominent among the mononuclear cells infiltrating the lesional skin in early SSc.[132] In addition, evidence of local mast cell and eosinophil activation and degranulation are seen in lesional skin. In SSc patients with active lung disease, alveolar macrophages obtained by bronchoalveolar lavage have an alternatively activated phenotype, characterized by secretion of the profibrotic mediators TGF-β, PDGF, and IL-13.[133]

Autoantibodies and Humoral Autoimmunity in Systemic Sclerosis

Circulating autoantibodies with multiple antigenic specificities can be detected in virtually all patients with SSc, but a direct role of humoral autoimmunity in the pathogenesis of tissue damage has not been conclusively established. Autoantibodies in SSc tend to be highly specific and mutually exclusive (see later), and show strong associations with individual disease phenotypes. Serum levels of autoantibodies, in particular anti–topoisomerase I, may correlate with the extent of skin and lung fibrosis and show fluctuations with disease activity.[134]

Various hypotheses have been proposed to explain the generation of autoantibodies in SSc. According to one hypothesis involving the altered processing of self-antigens, patients with SSc-specific self-antigens, such as topoisomerase I, undergo fragmentation owing to proteolytic cleavage by reactive oxygen species. This fragmentation results in exposure of normally cryptic epitopes, and a break in immune tolerance with recognition of the peptide as immunogenic.[135] Other mechanisms invoked to explain the generation of specific autoantibodies in SSc include molecular mimicry as a consequence of viral infection, chronic B cell hyperreactivity resulting from intrinsic abnormalities in B cell signaling, and increased expression or altered subcellular localization of potential autoantigenic peptides.[136]

Although SSc-associated autoantibodies have validated clinical utility as diagnostic markers, their contribution to disease manifestations is uncertain. More recent studies highlight the occurrence and potential biologic activities of autoantibodies directed against ECM components, fibroblasts, and endothelial cells or the PDGF receptor in some patients with SSc. The antibodies can induce target

Table 77-6 Autoantibody Associations in Systemic Sclerosis

Antibody	Prevalence (%)*	Clinical Association
Antinuclear antibody	>95	Limited and diffuse skin subsets
Anti–topoisomerase 1 (Scl-70)	15-20	Diffuse skin, tendon rubs, pulmonary fibrosis, increased mortality
Anticentromere	15-20	Limited skin (CREST), severe Raynaud's phenomenon, digital ischemia, pulmonary hypertension
Nucleolar antibodies RNA polymerases	4-20	Diffuse skin, tendon friction rubs, scleroderma renal crisis, increased mortality
Fibrillarin (U3-RNP)	8	Diffuse skin, African-American, male
Th	5	Limited skin, isolated pulmonary hypertension
PM/Scl	1	Limited skin, myositis

*Estimated prevalence in North American patients.
CREST, calcinosis, Raynaud's phenomenon, esophageal dysmotility, sclerodactyly, and telangiectasia.

cell activation or apoptosis in vitro.[15,137-139] It is unknown whether these autoantibodies precede, or are a consequence of, fibrosis, and their direct pathogenetic role in SSc remains to be established. Target specificities and clinical associations of key autoantibodies in SSc are summarized in Table 77-6.

B Cell Activation and Function in Systemic Sclerosis

More recent studies provide evidence for a potential direct role for B lymphocytes in the pathogenesis of SSc. B cells have multiple immunoregulatory functions in addition to the generation of antibodies, including antigen presentation, cytokine production, lymphoid organogenesis, and T cell differentiation. Although B cells are not generally prominent in lesional tissue, an activated B cell "signature" with increased expression of immunoglobulin genes was shown by DNA microarray analysis in SSc skin.[55] Patients with SSc display intrinsic abnormalities of B cells.[140] The number of naive B cells is elevated in the circulation, whereas plasma cells are markedly decreased. Memory B cells are chronically activated and display increased CD95, CD86, and CD19, a cell surface signaling receptor that regulates intrinsic and antigen receptor–induced B cell responses.[140]

Upregulation of CD19 seems to be specific for SSc and was not seen in other autoimmune diseases. Mice transgenic for CD19 develop spontaneous autoimmunity with production of high titers of anti–topoisomerase I antibodies.[141] Altered B cell function and chronic activation in SSc may account not only for autoantibody production, but also fibrosis because activated B cells secrete IL-6, which directly stimulates fibroblast activation and the synthesis of collagen. Patients with SSc also have elevated levels of the potent

B cell survival factor B cell activating factor belonging to the TNF family (BAFF) in the serum and in lesional skin, and B cells express increased levels of the BAFF receptor.[131]

FIBROSIS

Overview: Molecular and Cellular Determinants of the Extracellular Matrix

Interstitial and vascular fibrosis, the most characteristic and prominent pathologic manifestation of SSc, is characterized by replacement of normal tissue architecture with dense connective tissue. The ECM consists of a cellular compartment of resident and infiltrating cells, and connective tissue composed of collagens, proteoglycans, fibrillins, and adhesion molecules. The ECM also serves as a reservoir for growth factors and matricellular proteins that, together with the connective tissue compartment, control the differentiation, function, and survival of fibroblasts. Excessive connective tissue accumulation results from overproduction by fibroblasts and related mesenchymal cells that are activated by soluble factors in an autocrine/paracrine manner, by the surrounding ECM, or via cell-cell interactions. Impaired matrix degradation and turnover, and expansion of the pool of mesenchymal cells contributing to ECM synthesis also play a role.

Regulation of Collagen Synthesis

The collagens, the most abundant proteins of the ECM, constitute a family of more than two dozen structural proteins with critical roles in organ development, growth, and differentiation. Collagens can be classified as fibrillar and nonfibrillar. The ECM of the skin, bones, and tendons is composed largely of type I collagen, with smaller amounts of associated type III collagen. Type II collagen is found mainly in articular cartilage. The fibrillar collagens consist of three α chains wound into a characteristic triple helix, a structure made possible by the presence of a glycine at every third residue of repeating Gly-X-Y sequence, where X is frequently a proline, and Y is frequently a hydroxyproline. During their biosynthesis, fibrillar collagens undergo extensive enzymatic modifications inside the cell, and additional processing after their secretion. Covalent cross-linking stabilizes the collagen fiber network in the extracellular space.

In normal fibroblasts, type I collagen synthesis can be regulated by cytokines and other soluble extracellular factors, and cell-cell and cell-matrix contact and tissue hypoxia (Table 77-7). These environmental cues allow fibroblast to respond to dynamic tissue requirements during development and tissue repair.[71] The genes encoding the various collagens harbor cis-acting regulatory elements with conserved nucleotide sequences that are specifically recognized by DNA-binding transcription factors, including Sp1, Ets1, Smad2 and Smad3, Egr-1, and CCAAT-binding factor, which stimulate transcription, and Sp3, C/EBP, YB1, c-Krox, and Fli1, which suppress transcription.[141] These transcription factors interact with one another and with non–DNA-binding cofactors, scaffold proteins, and chromatin-modifying enzymes such as p300/CREB binding protein (p300/CBP), PCAF, and histone deacetylases.

Table 77-7 Signaling Molecules Implicated in the Pathogenesis of Fibrosis in Systemic Sclerosis

Molecule	Cellular Source	Elevated in Systemic Sclerosis
Transforming growth factor-β	Inflammatory cells, platelets, fibroblasts, macrophages	+
Platelet-derived growth factor	Platelets, macrophages, fibroblasts, endothelial cells	+
CTGF/CCN2	Fibroblasts	+
Insulin-like growth factor-I	Fibroblasts	+
IL-4, IL-13	T helper type 2 lymphocytes, mast cells	+
IL-6	Macrophages, B cells, T cells, fibroblasts	+
Chemokines (MCP-1, MCP-3)	Neutrophils, epithelial cells, endothelial cells, fibroblasts	+
Fibroblast growth factor	Fibroblasts	+
Endothelin-1	Endothelial cells	+
Serotonin	Platelets	+

The activities and interactions of transcription factors and cofactors are controlled by extracellular cues. Because enzymes that modify chromatin structure at target gene promoters enhance the availability of DNA-binding factors to their corresponding cis-acting regulatory sequences and induce transcription, the histone acetyltransferase p300/CBP and related chromatin-modifying enzymes are important components of the transcriptional regulatory network.[142,157] Alterations in the expression levels, activities, or interactions among the various transcription factors and cofactors contribute to persistent fibroblast activation in SSc.[143]

Cellular Determinants of Fibrosis

Fibroblasts. Fibroblasts are capable of synthesis and degradation of ECM and are key effectors of the process of fibrosis. Under the influence of appropriate extracellular signals, these cells or their progenitors synthesize collagens and other ECM macromolecules; adhere to and contract connective tissue; secrete growth factors, cytokines, and chemokines or express surface receptors for them; and undergo transdifferentiation into myofibroblasts. Together, these biosynthetic, proinflammatory, contractile, and adhesive functions enable fibroblasts to mediate effective wound healing. Although under physiologic conditions the fibroblast repair program is self-limited, pathologic fibrosis is characterized by sustained and amplified fibroblast activation, resulting in exaggerated ECM accumulation and remodeling. Inappropriate fibroblast activation is the fundamental pathogenetic alteration underlying fibrosis in SSc.[70]

Fibroblasts are spindle-shaped cells that are responsible for connective tissue synthesis and turnover, and they play essential roles in organ development, tissue repair, and ECM homeostasis. Studies with DNA microarrays revealed that fibroblasts from different anatomic locations differ markedly in their pattern of gene expression, suggesting that fibroblasts in different sites in the body could be considered distinct differentiated cell types.[144,145] The apparent "positional memory" of fibroblasts is governed by genetic imprinting by the HOX family transcription factors.

Myofibroblasts, Pericytes, and Mesenchymal Cell Plasticity. In fibrosis, the pool of activated mesenchymal cells contributing to ECM accumulation and remodeling in a tissue is expanded not only by proliferation of resident fibroblasts, but also by local transdifferentiation of other cell types, and the influx of mesenchymal progenitor cells from the circulation. Myofibroblasts are specialized cells that develop from fibroblasts in response to mechanical tension and TGF-β and express the cytoskeletal protein alpha–smooth muscle actin.[146] Myofibroblasts synthesize collagens, tissue inhibitors of metalloproteinase (TIMP), and other ECM components, and are a major source of activated TGF-β during the fibrotic response.[147] Their primary physiologic role is contraction of early granulation tissue. Contracting matrix, in turn, provides mechanical tension that promotes further myofibroblast differentiation.[147a] During normal wound healing, myofibroblasts are detected transiently and disappear; their removal from the lesion by apoptosis is a crucial step in wound resolution. In pathologic fibrogenesis, myofibroblasts persist, resulting in excessively contracted ECM characteristic of chronic scar. The presence of alpha–smooth muscle actin–positive myofibroblasts expressing Thy-1 is strongly associated with fibrotic disoders and SSc, but is absent from normal skin.[51,101]

Pericytes are mesenchymal cells that normally reside in the walls of microvessels in intimate contact with the underlying endothelium; they regulate vascular homeostasis. The microvascular pericyte compartment in SSc shows marked hyperplasia and increased expression of PDGF receptors.[101] Activated pericytes can transdifferentiate into collagen-producing fibroblasts and myofibroblasts, linking microvascular injury and fibrosis.[101] Under certain conditions, epithelial cells also can undergo transformation to fibroblasts. The process of epithelial-mesenchymal transition plays a vital role during vertebrate embryonic development. Epithelial-mesenchymal transition is induced by TGF-β and suppressed by bone morphogenetic protein-7. Pathologic epithelial-mesenchymal transition occurs in cancer, renal fibrosis, and idiopathic pulmonary fibrosis.[148] To date, the role of epithelial cells and epithelial-mesenchymal transition in the pathogenesis of SSc has not been examined.

Mesenchymal Progenitor Cells in the Circulation. Fibrocytes are CD34+ mesenchymal cells normally present in small numbers in the peripheral blood that can synthesize collagen and present antigen.[149] These bone marrow–derived cells express CD14+ (a monocyte marker) and chemokine receptors (CCR3, CCR5, and CXCR4), which allows them to traffic into and accumulate in specific tissues. The role for circulating fibrocytes and their trafficking into lesional tissue in the pathogenesis of fibrosis was established in animal models using neutralizing antibodies, and in mice genetically deficient in CXCR4.[150] It has been suggested that fibrocytes originating from bone marrow–derived monocyte precursor cells traffic into fibrotic lesional tissue, where they undergo specialization into fibroblasts and myofibroblasts, losing the CD14 and CD34 markers in the process, and contribute to the progression of fibrosis.[151] Other studies have identified

multipotent monocyte-derived mesenchymal progenitor cells in peripheral blood.[108] The role of pericytes, fibrocytes, and other monocyte-derived fibroblast progenitor cells in tissue damage in SSc remains speculative, however.[152]

MOLECULAR DETERMINANTS OF FIBROSIS: TRANSFORMING GROWTH FACTOR-β

The expression of ECM genes is normally tightly regulated by paracrine/autocrine mediators, cell-cell contact, hypoxia, and contact with the surrounding ECM. Of the multiple cytokines implicated in SSc (see Table 77-7), TGF-β is considered to be the master regulator of physiologic fibrogenesis (wound healing and tissue repair) and pathologic fibrosis.[153] TGF-β is highly pleiotropic and plays essential roles in normal tissue repair, angiogenesis, immunoregulation, and cell proliferation and differentiation, but it also is implicated in cancer, fibrosis, and autoimmunity.[154] It is likely that a dynamic interplay between TGF-β and many other cytokines and growth factors contributes to fibrosis in SSc. Most cell types secrete TGF-β as a latent, inactive complex that is sequestered within the ECM. Under appropriate conditions, latent TGF-β is converted to its biologically active form capable of inducing responses through specific TGF-β receptors expressed on the surface of target cells. The activation of latent TGF-β is mediated by integrins, thrombospondins, and proteolytic enzymes.

Cellular Signaling by Transforming Growth Factor-β

A member of a large cytokine superfamily that also includes activin and bone morphogenetic proteins, TGF-β is secreted by platelets, monocytes/macrophages, T cells, and fibroblasts. Most cell types express specific surface receptors for TGF-β. The responses elicited by TGF-β are specific for target cell lineage and are highly context-dependent. In mesenchymal cells, TGF-β acts as a potent inducer of fibrillar collagen synthesis; stimulates fibroblast proliferation, migration, adhesion, and transdifferentiation into myofibroblasts; and suppresses the production of matrix-degrading metalloproteinases (Table 77-8).

Most cells generate TGF-β as a biologically inactive precursor molecule that resides as a latent complex in the ECM reservoir and is unable to interact with the TGF-β receptors. The conversion of latent TGF-β to its active form capable of binding its cell surface receptors is a complex process mediated by thrombospondin-1, integrins αvβ6 and αvβs, and various proteases, and is under tight regulation. On its activation, TGF-β binds to the type II TGF-β receptor, triggering an intracellular signal transduction cascade that leads to the induction of target genes.[155]

The evolutionarily conserved canonical TGF-β signal transduction pathway involves phosphorylation of the type I TGF-β receptor activin-like kinase 5, a transmembrane serine-threonine kinase that phosphorylates a group of intracellular signaling proteins called Smads. Ligand-induced phosphorylation of Smad2/3 allows them to form heterocomplexes with Smad4 and translocate from the cytoplasm into the nucleus. Within the nucleus, the activated Smad complex specifically recognizes and binds to a *cis*-acting DNA sequence (CAGAC) that defines the consensus Smad-binding element. On binding to the Smad-binding

Table 77-8 Fibrogenic Activities of Transforming Growth Factor-β

Recruits monocytes
Stimulates synthesis of collagens, fibronectin, proteoglycans, elastin, TIMP; inhibits matrix metalloproteinases
Stimulates fibroblast proliferation, chemotaxis
Induces fibrogenic cytokine production (CTGF), autoinduction; blocks synthesis and activity of interferon-γ
Stimulates production of endothelin-1
Stimulates expression of surface receptors for TGF-β, PDGF
Induces fibroblast mitogenic responses to PDGF-AA
Promotes fibroblast-myofibroblast differentiation, monocyte-fibrocyte differentiation
Promotes epithelial-mesenchymal transition
Inhibits fibroblast apoptosis

CTGF, connective tissue growth factor; PDGF, platelet-derived growth factor; TGF, transforming growth factor; TIMP, tissue inhibitor of metalloproteinases.

element, activated Smads recruit transcriptional cofactors to the DNA, resulting in induction of gene transcription. The conserved Smad-binding element is found in the promoters of many TGF-β-inducible genes, including type I collagens, plasminogen activator inhibitor 1, alpha–smooth muscle actin, and CTGF. Ligand-induced signal transduction through the Smad pathway is tightly controlled by endogenous inhibitors such as Smad7.

Although the Smad pathway is the central mediator of signals from the TGF-β receptors, more recent evidence indicates the existence of alternative non-Smad pathways that also participate in TGF-β signaling.[156] Non-Smad signaling molecules activated by TGF-β include protein kinases (mitogen-activated protein kinases p38 and JNK, focal adhesion kinase FAK, and TGF-β activated kinase TAK1), lipid kinases such as PI3 kinase and its downstream target Akt, the calcium-dependent phosphatase calcineurin, and the tyrosine kinase c-Abl. These non-Smad pathways interact with one another and with Smads, creating complex signaling networks. Their importance and role in physiologic and pathologic fibrogenic responses remain to be established.[157]

MOLECULAR EFFECTORS OF FIBROSIS: CYTOKINES, GROWTH FACTORS, CHEMOKINES, AND LIPID MEDIATORS

Multiple cytokines, growth factors, chemokines, and eicosanoids regulate ECM accumulation and mesenchymal cell function, and have been found to be elevated in SSc. These soluble mediators—most prominently CTGF, PDGF, IL-4, IL-6, and IL-13—contribute to the pathogenesis of fibrosis, and represent potential targets for antifibrotic therapy.

Connective Tissue Growth Factor (CCN2)

CTGF, a cysteine-rich 40-kD member of the CCN early-response gene family, is a matricellular growth factor implicated in angiogenesis, wound healing, and development. Tissue expression of CTGF is undetectable in normal adults, but is markedly elevated in SSc and other fibrotic

conditions. In SSc, the serum levels of CTGF correlate with the extent of skin and pulmonary fibrosis.[140,158] In normal fibroblasts, CTGF expression can be induced by TGF-β, IL-4, and VEGF, whereas TNF-α and iloprost block stimulation.[159] In vivo, CTGF induces a transient fibrotic response in mice and markedly enhances the TGF-β response.[160] In vitro, CTGF stimulates fibroblast proliferation, chemotaxis, and synthesis of collagen and fibronectin. Because many CTGF effects closely parallel the effects induced by TGF-β, it has been suggested that TGF-β responses are mediated through endogenous CTGF. The fibroblast receptors for CTGF and the mechanism of action underlying CTGF profibrotic responses are still incompletely characterized.

Platelet-Derived Growth Factor and Other Fibrogenic Cytokines

PDGFs are disulfide-bonded heterodimeric proteins consisting of an A and a B chain that act mainly on stromal cells and regulate the wound healing process. Originally isolated from platelets, PDGF isoforms also are produced by macrophages, endothelial cells, and fibroblasts. PDGF is a potent fibroblast mitogen and chemoattractant for fibroblasts; induces the synthesis of collagen, fibronectin, and proteoglycans; and stimulates the secretion of TGF-β1, MCP-1, and IL-6. Fibroblasts from patients with SSc show elevated expression of PDGF and PDGF-β receptor,[161] and PDGF levels are increased in bronchoalveolar lavage fluid.[162] Serum antibodies to the PDGF receptor from patients with SSc induce fibroblast activation in vitro[138]; however, stimulatory antibodies to the PDGF receptor are not specific for SSc and have been detected in the sera of patients with graft-versus-host disease as well.

The immunomodulatory cytokine IL-4 plays a major role in Th2 diseases. In normal fibroblasts, IL-4 stimulates proliferation, chemotaxis, collagen synthesis, and production of TGF-β, CTGF, and TIMP.[152] Serum levels of IL-4 are elevated in patients with SSc,[163] and the number of IL-4-producing T lymphocytes is increased in peripheral blood.[114,164] Expression of IL-4 and its mRNA is markedly elevated in SSc lesional skin and cultured fibroblasts. IL-6, produced by monocytes, T lymphocytes, fibroblasts, and endothelial cells, stimulates collagen and TIMP-1 synthesis, and promotes a Th2-polarized immune response. The biologic activities of IL-6 are mediated via the Jak-Stat intracellular signaling pathway shared with other cytokines. Serum levels of IL-6 are elevated in patients with SSc and correlated with the severity of skin involvement.[165] IL-13 is implicated in asthma and other fibrotic conditions. The profibrotic effects of IL-13 involve indirect mechanisms secondary to stimulation of TGF-β production by macrophages and direct stimulation of fibroblast proliferation and collagen synthesis.[166-168] Serum levels of IL-13 are elevated in patients with SSc.

Chemokines represent a superfamily of more than 40 low-molecular-weight soluble mediators originally characterized by their chemotactic effects on leukocytes, but now recognized to have a broad range of cellular targets and biologic activities, and to play important roles in angiogenesis, wound healing, and fibrosis.[169] The CC chemokine MCP-1 stimulates collagen production directly and through induction of endogenous TGF-β production. Serum levels of

MCP-1, macrophage inflammatory protein (MIP)-1α, IL-8, CXCL8, and CCL18 are elevated in SSc and correlate with the severity of skin fibrosis.[85,163,170,171] Mononuclear cells and dermal fibroblasts from SSc patients spontaneously produce these chemokines, and lesional SSc fibroblasts show constitutive upregulation of the MCP-1 receptor CCR2.[172]

Because MCP-1 is capable of polarizing the immune response to a Th2 predominance, the MCP-1-CCR2 axis is thought to play a major role in the pathogenesis of SSc by amplifying collagen stimulation and promoting Th2 cytokine polarization. Significantly, mice defective for MCP-1 are resistant to the development of fibrosis induced by bleomycin injection.[88] Strong expression of MCP-1 and MCP-3 was noted in lesional skin in SSc, particularly in early disease.[173] These chemokines promote mononuclear leukocyte migration across the endothelial layer in vitro.[92] The levels of MIP-1α, CXCL8, and CCL18 also are elevated in SSc bronchoalveolar lavage fluid. One study showed that elevated CCL18 levels identified SSc patients who had pulmonary fibrosis, and changes in CCL18 serum levels showed a strong negative correlation with changes in lung function in this cohort. Additional chemokines that have been shown to be overexpressed in lesional tissue or serum in patients with SSc or in animal models of scleroderma include the CC chemokines RANTES and PARC, and the CXC chemokines IL-8, MIP-2, and fractalkine.

Insulin-like growth factor binding protein-1 (IGFBP-1) stimulates collagen synthesis and fibroblast proliferation and induces TGF-β.[174,175] Patients with SSc have elevated levels of IGF-1 in bronchoalveolar lavage fluids.[175] Expression of IGFBP-3 is markedly elevated in SSc fibroblasts.[12] Adenovirally mediated overexpression of IGFBP-5 resulted in the induction of chronic scleroderma-like fibrosis in mice.[176]

Intrinsic Negative Regulation of Extracellular Matrix Accumulation

To prevent excessive matrix accumulation and scarring in response to injury, redundant biologic mechanisms have evolved for suppressing ECM synthesis and fibroblast proliferation and differentiation. Fibroblasts are equipped with endogenous molecules that repress ECM gene expression and TGF-β stimulation. Smad7 is an inhibitory member of the Smad family that blocks Smad-mediated TGF-β signal transduction by accelerating ubiquitin-mediated TGF-β receptor degradation. Functional impairment of Smad7 was shown in SSc fibroblasts.[177,178] Other cell-intrinsic endogenous repressors of collagen synthesis include the transcription factors Sp3, Fli-1, p53, and Ras, the corepressor Nab2, and the nuclear hormone receptor peroxisome proliferator-activated receptor (PPAR)-γ.[142,157,179] In SSc, diminished expression, induction, or function of these endogenous inhibitors, or their impaired responsiveness to extracellular ligands, may be responsible for failure to extinguish fibroblast activation, contributing to ECM upregulation in fibrosis.

Interferon-γ

IFN-γ, produced primarily by Th1 lymphocytes, is a major negative regulator of collagen gene expression and fibroblast activation. IFN-γ represses collagen gene expression[71,180,181] and abrogates stimulation induced by TGF-β.[157] IFN-γ also

is a potent inhibitor of fibroblast proliferation, fibroblast-mediated matrix contraction, and myofibroblast transdifferentiation. Significantly, some studies have shown that fibroblasts from patients with SSc are resistant to the inhibitory effects of IFN-γ.[182] Clinical trials of IFN-γ in SSc have shown a modest and inconsistent improvement in skin fibrosis.[183-185]

SCLERODERMA FIBROBLAST

Fibroblasts explanted from lesional skin or fibrotic lungs of patients with SSc display an abnormal activated phenotype that persists during their serial passage in vitro, indicating autonomous alteration in cell function.[143] The "SSc phenotype" is characterized by the following: enhanced ECM synthesis, secretion of profibrotic cytokines and chemokines and increased expression of their cell surface receptors, and resistance to IFN-γ and other inhibitory signals. SSc fibroblasts show features of myofibroblast transdifferentiation, partly as a result of constitutive activation of the focal adhesion kinase FAK.[186] It is not established whether the activated phenotype of SSc fibroblasts represents an abnormality intrinsic to these cells, or reflects their activation in responses to exogenous stimuli.

Numerous molecules involved in intracellular signal transduction and transcriptional regulation are elevated or activated in SSc fibroblasts, including protein kinase C, Smad3, Egr-1, p300, and c-Abl. Elevated expression of the prosurvival factors Bcl-2 and Akt in SSc fibroblasts may play a role in their resistance to apoptosis.[187] Because most of the SSc fibroblast characteristics can be induced in normal fibroblasts by treatment with TGF-β, it has been suggested that the SSc phenotype is due to autocrine TGF-β signaling. The levels of TGF-β receptors are elevated on SSc fibroblasts, enabling these cells to mount a robust response to endogenously produced TGF-β or to low levels of environmental TGF-β.[143,188-190]

SSc fibroblasts have elevated levels of thrombospondin, αvβ5 and αvβ3 integrins, which mediate latent TGF-β activation at the cell surface.[191] Consistent with the autocrine TGF-β hypothesis, SSc fibroblasts show constitutive activation of intracellular TGF-β signaling, with elevated expression and nuclear accumulation of activated Smad3,[31,167,177] and constitutive interaction with the transcriptional coactivator and histone acetyltranferase p300/CBP.[193,194] Other studies show defective expression or function of endogenous suppressors of TGF-β signaling and ECM production, suggesting that failure to terminate fibroblast activation may represent a fundamental defect in SSc.

Endogenous molecules that negatively regulate fibroblast activation include Fli-1, PPAR-γ, Nab2, and Smad7.[195,196] Autocrine TGF-β activation of fibroblasts cannot fully account for all of the phenotypic hallmarks of SSc fibroblasts, such as constitutive CTGF production, indicating that Smad-independent TGF-β signaling mechanisms and non–TGF-β-mediated activation events are involved in the induction or maintenance of the SSc phenotype. The autonomous SSc phenotype also could result from abnormal integrin-mediated signaling from the surrounding ECM. More recent evidence indicates that epigenetic alterations in SSc fibroblasts are associated with persistent and heritable fibroblast dysfunction. Silencing the

Fli-1 gene, an important endogenous negative regulator of collagen gene expression, by DNA methylation or chromatin histone deacetylation, suppresses its expression in fibroblasts from lesional skin, with resultant increase in collagen synthesis.[196]

CLINICAL FEATURES

The clinical manifestations of SSc are protean, reflecting its complex underlying pathology. The frequency of various clinical features differs according to the stage and subset of disease. In addition, the severity and activity of each complication needs to be considered in making treatment decisions. Fatigue and lethargy are common throughout the illness, although usually more pronounced in its early phases. Fever is uncommon; if fever is present, other causes, such as infection or underlying malignancy, should be excluded. Reactive depression is a frequent accompaniment to this often relentless and disfiguring disorder. Patients often feel isolated or depressed, and support groups can provide an invaluable service to them.

SKIN MANIFESTATIONS

Skin thickening and hardening are the hallmarks of SSc. In patients with limited cutaneous SSc, skin changes generally are restricted to the hands and face, with some extension to the neck and forearms, and are generally preceded by Raynaud's phenomenon. Different patterns of skin involvement can develop. In some cases, there is puffiness and swelling of the skin, especially over the digits. In other cases, the skin changes are more atrophic with tightened fingers and loss of subcutaneous tissue. Complications of digital ischemia including pitting scars and ulceration occur (see later).

The skin changes in diffuse cutaneous SSc are more consistent. Typically, the first manifestation is soft tissue edema affecting the hands, wrists, and lower limbs, followed by inflammation of the skin with intense pruritus that might persist for the first 12 to 18 months of disease. Skin thickening with dermal fibrosis and sclerosis follows. The sclerosis typically moves proximally, and at this stage of diffuse cutaneous SSc an advancing edge of involved skin can be identified. Simultaneously, involvement of truncal skin and in more severe cases upper arms and thighs may occur. Proximal skin involvement defines the diffuse cutaneous SSc subset, but may be absent in early stages of disease.

The changes in the skin usually proceed through three phases: early, established, and late. The early stage can be difficult to diagnose, and a high level of suspicion is needed when the only feature may b e puffiness of the hands and feet, most marked in the mornings. Nonpitting dependent edema may occur and lead to symptoms of neural compression, including carpal tunnel syndrome. The subsequent, often sudden, development of firm, taut, hidebound skin proximal to the metacarpophalangeal joints, adherent to deeper structures such as tendons and joints and limiting their movement, permits a definitive diagnosis of SSc. The skin may be coarse, pigmented, and dry at this stage. The epidermis thins, hair growth ceases, sweating is impaired, and skin creases disappear. Later,

as secondary epithelial structures recover, hair growth and sweating may return before there is softening of the affected skin.

Careful assessment of the extent of skin involvement is the best clinical technique for detecting the patient at risk for life-threatening internal organ involvement. Numerous scoring systems to quantify skin sclerosis have been developed. The most widely applied system consists of a 0-to-3 grading at 17 skin sites (maximum score 51). In this grading, normal skin scores 0, mild (or equivocal) thickening scores 1, established (or definite) thickening without fixation to deeper tissues scores 2, and severe thickening with fixation to deep tissues (hidebound) scores 3. Overall within-patient variability in scoring (derived from multiple examinations) is about 5 skin-thickness units.[196a] Controlled trials of penicillamine and recombinant relaxin have provided insight into the natural history of skin involvement in SSc, emphasizing that after 2 to 3 years there is often plateauing or improvement of skin score even without effective treatment. Novel assessment tools for skin involvement, such as high-frequency ultrasound,[196b] skin deformity,[197] or durometry,[198] are under investigation.

Ischemic Ulceration

Ischemic ulceration is a common complication in limited and diffuse cutaneous forms of SSc. Ulcers may occur on the fingertips, in the finger creases, over extensor surfaces of joints, and in association with calcinosis cutis, and cause pain and functional impairment. Several pathologic mechanisms operate to cause digital ulceration and critical ischemia. The latter describes the context in which there is inadequate tissue nutrition affecting a digit, but without ulceration. It is frequently painful and generally is taken as a sign of impending ischemic ulceration. Local trauma, such as cuts or abrasions, may be an initiating event, which, in concert with impaired healing owing to poor vascular flow, dermal fibrosis, and epidermal atrophy, leads to chronic, poorly healing skin ulcerations.

Management of digital ulceration requires a multifaceted approach (Fig. 77-11). Treatment of vasospasm, use of skin emollients, and treatment of secondary infection all are important. Prostacyclin infusions have been shown to improve healing of ischemic digital ulcers and may reduce recurrent ulcer formation. Endothelin receptor blockers have been shown to reduce the formation of new digital ulcers, but have no effect on healing of established ulcers.[199]

Cutaneous Telangiectasia

Cutaneous telangiectasia, dilations of dermal blood vessels, occur in limited cutaneous SSc and diffuse cutaneous SSc, but are more extensive in limited cutaneous SSc, particularly the subgroup previously designated as CREST (calcinosis, Raynaud's phenomenon, esophageal involvement, sclerodactyly, and telangiectasia) syndrome. Telangiectasias are often prominent on the palms and lips, have a typical oval appearance, and tend to increase in number over time, possibly indicating progression of the vascular manifestations at other sites.[200] Although previously considered a hallmark of limited cutaneous SSc, it seems that late-stage diffuse cutaneous SSc also is associated with extensive cutaneous and

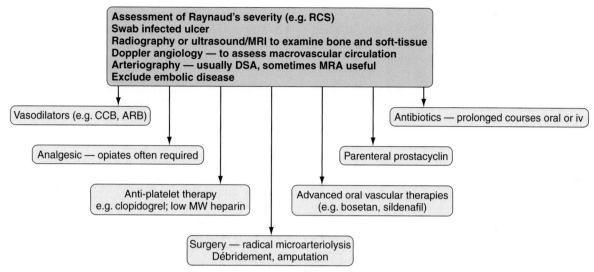

Figure 77-11 Algorithm summarizing the management of digital vasculopathy in systemic sclerosis. Manifestations of vasculopathy include Raynaud's phenomenon, ischemic digital ulceration, and critical digital ischemia—fixed ischemia with threatened tissue viability, ischemic pain, and refractory digital infection. Treatment includes local measures to maximize tissue viability and quantify any large vessel pathology or source for emboli. Pain control, treatment of infection, and optimization of blood supply to ischemic territories are paramount. Modern treatments that have been effective in treatment of pulmonary arterial hypertension, such as endothelin receptor antagonists or phosphodiesterase type 5 inhibitors, have been evaluated. Prostacyclin analogues are widely used for acute management. RCS, Raynaud clinical severity.

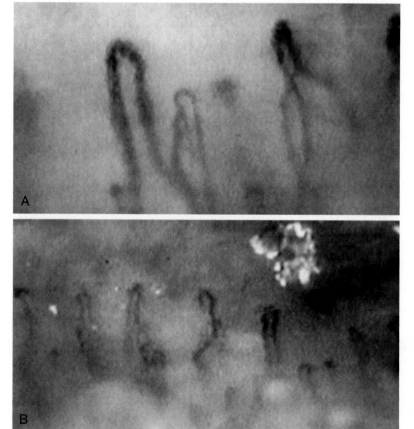

Figure 77-12 Nail-fold capillaroscopy. Digital nail-fold capillaroscopy can identify microvascular abnormalities in patients with Raynaud's phenomenon. In systemic sclerosis, small vessel density, diameter, and tortuosity are abnormal. **A,** The most prominent feature is capillary dropout. **B,** Even capillary distribution with tortuosity at upper limit of normal, a pattern consistent with primary Raynaud's phenomenon.

mucosal vascular lesions. The nail-fold capillaries are almost always abnormal in SSc (Fig. 77-12). Dropout of capillary loops is the cardinal abnormality, with later changes including dilation of loops and evidence of neovascularization. Systematic examination suggests that capillary dropout is a hallmark of progression in SSc.[201]

VASCULAR FEATURES

Raynaud's Phenomenon

Episodic vasospasm induced by cold or emotional stress is common in the general population, affecting a substantial number of otherwise healthy individuals. The overall prevalence of Raynaud's phenomenon is 3% to 10% of adults worldwide, although it may affect 20% of young women. The prevalence varies depending on climate, skin color, ethnic background, and occupational exposure to vibrating machines.[202] The clinical classification of Raynaud's phenomenon and related disorders is summarized in Table 77-9.

Although Raynaud's phenomenon may occur in most connective tissue and rheumatic diseases, it is a near-universal accompaniment of SSc. Raynaud's phenomenon can predate the development of other features of SSc by several years, particularly in patients with the limited cutaneous

Table 77-9 Classification of Raynaud's Phenomenon

Isolated Raynaud's phenomenon
Occupational Raynaud's phenomenon
Cold injury
Vibrating tools
Polyvinyl chloride exposure
Secondary Raynaud's phenomenon
Systemic sclerosis
Mixed connective tissue disease
Sjögren's syndrome
SLE
Polymyositis/dermatomyositis
Rheumatoid arthritis
Arteritis
Antiphospholipid antibody syndrome
Primary biliary cirrhosis
Carpal tunnel syndrome
Cryoglobulinemia
Vasospastic disorders (migraine, Prinzmetal angina)
Infection
Hepatitis C
Cytomegalovirus (?)
Obstructive vascular disease
Atherosclerosis
Thromboangiitis obliterans
Thoracic outlet syndrome (cervical rib)
Metabolic syndrome
Hypothyroid
Carcinoid syndrome
Drug-induced
Antimigraine
β-blocker
Bleomycin
Interferons
Ergotamine derivatives

SLE, systemic lupus erythematosus.

form. Key features that distinguish Raynaud's phenomenon evolving into SSc include the presence of significant structural change in the nail-fold capillaries, the presence of trophic changes and pitting scars or keratin plugs on the pulp surface of digits (Fig. 77-13), and the presence of antinuclear autoantibodies. Complications of severe Raynaud's phenomenon include critical digital ischemia and ulceration.

The clinical syndrome, first described by Maurice Raynaud in 1862 as episodic digital ischemia provoked by cold and emotion, is classically manifest by intermittent pallor of the digits followed by cyanosis, suffusion, or pain and tingling. Blanching reflects digital arterial vasospasm, cyanosis reflects the deoxygenation of static venous blood, and redness reflects reactive hyperemia after the return of blood flow. Continuous blanching, blueness, or pain is not Raynaud's phenomenon. Important clues to secondary Raynaud's phenomenon include onset in children or adults older than 45 years; severe symptoms occurring all year round; digital ulcerations, which rarely, if ever, occur in primary Raynaud's phenomenon; and asymmetric symptoms.

The most distal parts of the skin and its appendages receive their nutrient blood supply from capillary loops that arise from and return to a vascular plexus deeper in the skin. These capillary loops can be visualized in the skin fold of the fingernail just proximal to the cuticle, where the capillary is visible over its long axis.[203] The characteristic changes seen in individuals destined to develop connective tissue disease are enlargement of capillary loops and loss of capillaries, either diffusely or adjacent to enlarged capillaries. Small hemorrhages around disordered capillaries also may be seen.

Tests for autoantibodies and nail-fold capillaroscopy together detect more than 90% of patients destined to develop SSc.[204] Of the population with Raynaud's phenomenon, 15% are positive for one or both findings. Conversely, these tests are even stronger as negative predictors of progression; individuals with isolated Raynaud's phenomenon, normal nail-fold capillaroscopy, and no antinuclear antibodies almost never develop connective tissue disease.[205] There is little evidence that symptomatic treatment of Raynaud's phenomenon influences the evolution of SSc. Some individuals with little skin involvement have typical capillaroscopic and serologic features of SSc and additional features such as esophageal reflux. These patients have previously been designated as "autoimmune Raynaud's," but the term *limited* SSc might be more appropriate.[206]

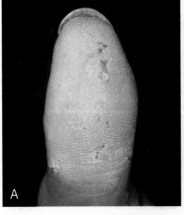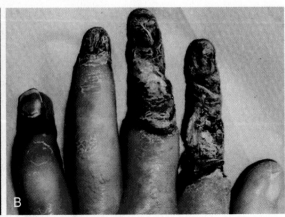

Figure 77-13 Spectrum of ischemic tissue secondary to Raynaud's phenomenon. In a mild form, digital ischemia contributes to the development of small hyperkeratotic plugs of ischemic scar tissue over the finger pulp. **A,** In patients with systemic sclerosis, these plugs evolve to form digital pitting scars. **B,** More severe ischemia leads to digital ulceration, digital infarction, gangrene, and mummification.

Critical Digital Ischemia

Critical digital ischemia and digital gangrene represent medical emergencies that require intensive treatment. Although Raynaud's phenomenon undoubtedly contributes to these complications, critical ischemia develops only in the setting of fixed structural vascular disease. Amputation specimens show occlusive vasculopathic changes resembling those observed in other vascular beds. Occlusive vasculopathy affects medium-sized arteries, especially the ulnar artery.[207] Management of critical digital ischemia includes optimal treatment for Raynaud's phenomenon, together with antiplatelet agents such as aspirin or clopidogrel. Parenteral prostacyclin and selective phosphodiesterase inhibitors may be helpful.[208,209]

Involvement of Large Vessels

Similar to other autoimmune rheumatic diseases, including systemic lupus erythematosus and rheumatoid arthritis, macrovascular disease can occur in SSc, although its frequency is unknown. Large vessel involvement has important implications for organ-based complications, such as renal disease, peripheral ischemia, and bowel involvement. Noninvasive studies have shown blood flow abnormalities in the large vessels in the cerebral and renal circulation in patients with SSc,[210] and symptomatic and asymptomatic macrovascular disease are increased.[211,212] A more recent study of macrovascular involvement showed a predilection for the ulnar artery.[207] Postmortem studies have reported that cerebrovascular disease, especially with vascular calcification, may be disproportionately severe in patients with limited cutaneous SSc compared with macrovascular disease at other sites.[212a]

GASTROINTESTINAL TRACT MANIFESTATIONS

The gastrointestinal tract is the most commonly involved internal organ system in diffuse and limited cutaneous subsets of SSc, and almost any part may be affected. Gastrointestinal tract involvement results in substantial morbidity. The earliest lesion is neural dysfunction, possibly resulting from arteriolar changes in the vasa nervorum[42,213] or compression of nerve fibers by fibrous tissue.[214] The burden of gastrointestinal complications is outlined in Table 77-10.

The oral aperture becomes diminished, and there is a reduction in bulk of the lips. These changes result in compromised dental care, dental and gum disease, and dry mouth. The cosmetic effect can be substantial.[215] Esophageal involvement is frequent with dysmotility and lower esophageal sphincter dysfunction, and consequent gastroesophageal reflux is almost universal in SSc.[216] The earliest clinical symptoms may be subtle, or patients may experience retrosternal discomfort or even overt pain, which can be nocturnal. Over time, chronic gastroesophageal reflux disease and its complications develop. In patients with frank dysphagia, esophagoscopy may be required to identify structural changes, such as hiatal hernia, esophageal strictures, or Barrett's metaplasia.[60,217] The stomach is frequently involved, with delayed gastric emptying that can lead to postprandial bloating and vomiting.

Table 77-10 Gastrointestinal Manifestations of Systemic Sclerosis

Site	Manifestation
Mouth	Perioral tight skin Reduced oral aperture Dental caries; xerostomia
Esophagus	Dysmotility, reflux Stricture, Barrett's metaplasia
Stomach	Gastroparesis
Small bowel	Hypomotility, stasis Bacterial overgrowth Pseudo-obstruction Intestinal pneumatosis
Large bowel	Hypomotility, pseudo-obstruction Colonic pseudodiverticula
Anorectum	Sphincter incompetence

Severe involvement of the small intestine typically occurs in patients with established SSc and can be a major cause of morbidity and mortality. In its most severe form, small intestinal involvement leads to recurrent episodes of intestinal pseudo-obstruction secondary to ileus with dilated small bowel loops. Although clinical suspicion is raised by features of pseudo-obstruction, there also are characteristic abnormalities on diagnostic imaging. Contrast studies may show the "stack of coins" sign, owing to close apposition of the valvulae conniventes. Small bowel bacterial overgrowth complicating hypomotility results in recurrent diarrhea and bloating, and in more severe cases leads to malabsorption, weight loss, malnutrition, and cachexia. The classic symptoms are change in bowel pattern, with frequent loose, floating, foul-smelling stools, and abdominal distention.

Management of advanced bowel disease includes rotating antibiotics, stimulation of intestinal motility with prokinetic agents such as erythromycin or domperidone, and supplemental alimentation. In the short-term, nocturnal feeding to maintain nutrition and a nasogastric or nasojejunal feeding tube may be effective. Longer term nutritional supplementation requires percutaneous jejunostomy, or gastroscopy if stomach emptying is not delayed. When malnutrition is the major problem, intermittent parenteral hyperalimentation may be required.[218]

Large bowel involvement is commonly manifested by constipation, which may be complicated by sigmoid volvulus. Anorectal incontinence is a frequent manifestation. Investigations include anal manometry and imaging to assess the integrity of the internal and external anal sphincter. Atony and hypomotility of the rectum and sigmoid colon is a frequent and early manifestation of SSc that may be missed because patients are reluctant to discuss these symptoms. Constipation is initially managed conservatively with dietary manipulation and stool volume expanders. Codeine can cause constipation and should be avoided. Surgery in the gastrointestinal tract must be viewed with caution. Manometric and radiographic localization of affected segments of stomach, small intestine, and colon may allow judicious surgical resection or venting procedures, but these are not risk-free and are not always successful.[219]

Vascular Abnormalities within the Gastrointestinal Tract

Vascular lesions of the intestinal mucosa, a cause of chronic anemia in SSc due to intermittent bleeding, may be scattered throughout the gut (Fig. 77-14), or take the form of vascular ectasia around the cardia of the stomach. This lesion, previously called "watermelon stomach" (owing to its characteristic endoscopic appearance) is now termed *gastric antral vascular ectasia*.[220] Vascular lesions in the intestinal tract can be treated by laser or argon plasma photocoagulation.[221,222]

Liver and Pancreas

The liver is generally spared in SSc. The exception is primary biliary cirrhosis, which may rarely occur in patients with SSc, especially the limited cutaneous form, and has a better prognosis than isolated primary biliary cirrhosis.[223] Pancreatic exocrine insufficiency can contribute to malabsorption and diarrhea. Formal pancreatic function testing indicates that pancreatic exocrine function is frequently reduced, but rarely to an extent that is clinically important.[224]

MUSCULOSKELETAL INVOLVEMENT

Joints

The fibrotic process of SSc commonly affects the tendons (causing tendon friction rubs), ligaments, and joint capsules, restricting movement. In addition, fibrosis is found in the synovium, but frank arthritis and joint destruction are uncommon. Management of soft tissue and joint problems in SSc is closely linked to skin care and to overall skeletal mobility. Resorption of the distal tufts of the digits (acro-osteolysis) is frequent in late-stage disease and is due to inadequate vascular supply required for viable bone. Other sites of bone resorption include the mandible and the ribs. Contraction of the fingers is a hallmark of SSc, may develop rapidly, and has a significant impact on hand function. Less commonly, contractures can affect large joints. Tendon friction rubs, most common in patients with early-stage diffuse cutaneous SSc,

are correlated with rapidly progressive skin involvement and increased risk of scleroderma renal crisis.[225] Tendinitis may cause severe inflammatory pain in SSc and contributes to the development of tendon contractures. Swelling of the tendons and soft tissues in the wrist often leads to median nerve compression with carpal tunnel syndrome.

Arthralgia is common, especially in the early stage of the diffuse cutaneous form of SSc. The presence of arthralgia often causes diagnostic uncertainty, particularly in patients with early disease who have not yet developed other cardinal features of SSc, such as Raynaud's phenomenon or esophagitis. Frank arthritis may rarely occur as a complication, or as part of an overlap syndrome; this is important to recognize because arthritis may be quite responsive to therapy, and because the combination of joint pain and reduced mobility in the context of active skin involvement in SSc often leads to particularly severe hand deformity. Symmetric polyarthritis, usually seronegative, anodular, and nonerosive, may be the presenting feature in rare patients destined to develop SSc.[226]

Skeletal Muscle Involvement

Some degree of skeletal muscular involvement is common in SSc. Although muscle weakness and atrophy may result from disuse secondary to joint contractures or chronic disease, about 20% of SSc patients develop a true myopathy characterized by mild chronic weakness and atrophy, minimal elevation of creatine phosphokinase, subtle abnormalities on electromyography, and modest noninflammatory histologic alterations with focal replacement of myofibrils with collagen and perimysial and epimysial fibrosis. This form of myopathy is generally unresponsive to anti-inflammatory medication.[227] Some patients develop inflammatory myositis indistinguishable from polymyositis. Caution must be observed with patients who develop myositis in the context of early diffuse cutaneous SSc, when treatment with high-dose corticosteroids might precipitate renal crisis. An atypical inflammatory myositis that requires special histochemical stains to show the differences in fiber size and composition has been reported in association with myocarditis

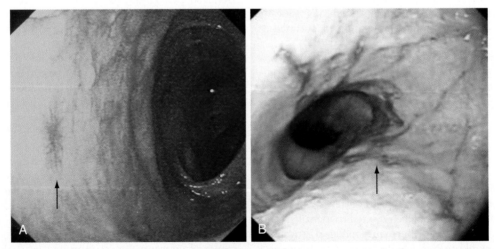

Figure 77-14 Mucosal vascular lesions in systemic sclerosis. Telangiectatic lesions can occur on mucosal surfaces and contribute to gastrointestinal blood loss. **A,** Typical lesion on the colonic mucosa is shown. **B,** Florid vascular dilation *(arrow)* can develop in the gastric antrum and lead to the development of gastric antral venous ectasia ("watermelon stomach"), with upper gastrointestinal hemorrhage.

in some patients with diffuse cutaneous SSc. In practice, it is important to distinguish between inflammatory myositis (true SSc-myositis overlap) and a chronic low-grade, predominantly fibrotic, myopathy.

CARDIAC INVOLVEMENT

The frequency of significant cardiac involvement in SSc has been difficult to ascertain, although it is believed to be frequent and can have a major impact on survival.[66,231,242-244] A potential consequence of myocardial involvement is reduction in the ability to cope well with intercurrent hemodynamics of cardiac stress such as that due to electrolyte disturbance, fluid shift, or acidosis. The pericardium and the myocardium are frequently affected. In contrast to myocardial involvement, abnormalities of the pericardium are easy to detect by virtue of the formation of a pericardial effusion. Thirty-five percent of SSc patients are found to have hemodynamically insignificant effusions. Larger effusions are less frequent.[232] Pericardial effusions in SSc are often associated with complications such as PAH and scleroderma renal crisis, where they may precede the onset of renal failure.

Numerous cardiac manifestations may develop in SSc, reflecting the disparate pathologic processes that can affect the myocardium. Clinically, it is useful to distinguish abnormalities of cardiac rate and rhythm that reflect inflammation or fibrosis from diffuse myocardial involvement leading to altered hemodynamics. Current approaches to investigation and treatment of cardiac involvement in SSc are summarized in Figure 77-15.

Cardiac involvement in SSc may be due to ischemic damage, myocarditis, replacement fibrosis, systemic hypertension, and PAH. Evidence of diastolic dysfunction, suggesting abnormal ventricle wall stiffness or defective ventricular relaxation or both, is found in most patients.[233-236,248] The abnormalities predominantly affect the longitudinal (endocardial) fibers, which fits well with the histologic findings of diffuse patchy fibrosis found in more than 40% of autopsies. It has been suggested that this lesion results from intermittent vasospastic ischemia, and that therapy directed at relieving ischemia may improve outcome.[238] Ambulatory monitoring shows reduced heart rate variability, suggestive of widespread autonomic dysfunction, in most patients with SSc.[239]

Myocardial involvement may be due to myocardial ischemia, fibrosis, and myocarditis. Potential mechanisms for ischemic damage include coronary arterial vasospasm, small vessel disease, and occlusive coronary artery disease. Histologic examination of the coronary arteries in SSc has not

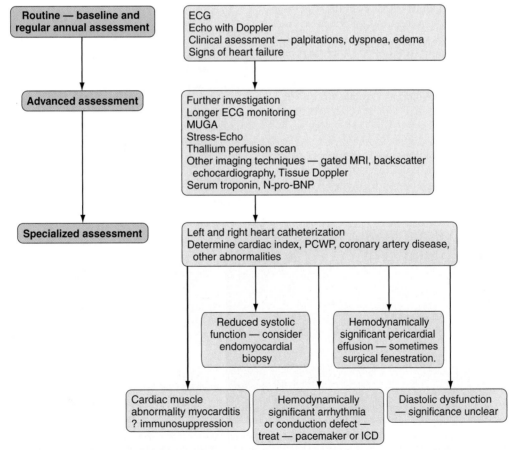

Figure 77-15 Evaluation and management of cardiac complications of systemic sclerosis. All patients with systemic sclerosis should undergo cardiac assessment, including clinical evaluation, chest radiograph, electrocardiogram (ECG), and Doppler echocardiography at baseline and on an annual basis. Determination of serum markers such as NT-proBNP and troponin may be useful. Long-term monitoring is required to assess intermittent arrhythmias; generally, only hemodynamically significant cardiac manifestations are treated. When inflammatory myocarditis is suspected, steroids and immunosuppression may be appropriate. Coincidental viral myocarditis should be considered in the differential diagnosis.

shown excess fibromuscular hypertrophy, however. The frequency of angiographically proven coronary artery disease does not seem to be increased.[240] An association between cardiac mortality and myositis has been shown in SSc, raising the possibility of associated myocarditis. Myocarditis may explain the frequent occurrence of exudative pericardial effusions in SSc, endocardial lesions found on histology, and ECG evidence of conducting tissue damage.

Although at present there are few published data suggesting low-grade myocarditis leading to diastolic dysfunction and the other cardiac abnormalities in SSc, we have described excess of troponin T release.[241] An attractive hypothesis is that low-grade intermittent myocardial inflammation causes subtle myocardial damage in the first few years when the disease process is most active, leading to mild fibrosis with diastolic dysfunction in later stages. Gated magnetic resonance imaging (MRI) is a novel tool potentially useful for detecting myocardial fibrosis and for quantitation of abnormal contraction or relaxation.[241a] Sudden death in young and middle-aged patients with SSc has been reported and is believed to be caused by ischemic damage to the cardiac conduction system.

PULMONARY INVOLVEMENT

Although interstitial lung disease has long been recognized as a common and significant complication of SSc, PAH has been less well appreciated until more recently. Although these two major pulmonary complications of SSc are considered separately, subsequently, they commonly occur together. Additional pulmonary complications of SSc include aspiration pneumonia, pleural disease, spontaneous pneumothorax, drug-induced pneumonitis, pneumoconiosis, and cancer. Table 77-11 summarizes the respiratory complications of SSc.

Pulmonary Fibrosis

The most common forms of interstitial lung disease in SSc are histologically classified as usual interstitial pneumonia and nonspecific interstitial pneumonitis. Investigation and assessment of interstitial lung disease in SSc focuses on early detection, assessment of severity, and determination of progression and is best performed by regular pulmonary function tests. High-resolution computed tomography (CT) remains the most valuable tool for detection of early lung fibrosis (Fig. 77-16).[242]

Interstitial lung disease develops insidiously and generally progresses to fibrosis. Because lung fibrosis is irreversible, early diagnosis is vital. The most common initial symptoms are breathlessness, especially on exertion, and a dry cough. Chest pain is infrequent, and hemoptysis is rare; the presence of either one indicates additional pathology. On physical examination, the most frequent finding is bilateral inspiratory crackles at the lung bases. Radiographic features consist of reticulonodular shadowing, usually symmetric and most marked at the lung bases. Because the chest radiograph is an insensitive indicator of alveolitis or early pulmonary fibrosis, however, it should be used only as an initial screen or to exclude infection or aspiration.

Mildly symptomatic SSc patients often have normal chest radiographs despite interstitial lung disease, and pulmonary function tests are more discriminatory. The single-breath diffusion capacity of lung for carbon monoxide is abnormal in more than 70% of patients with diffuse cutaneous SSc, including asymptomatic patients with no complaints and an unremarkable chest radiograph.[243] A reduction in diffusion capacity is the earliest detected abnormality in SSc patients who go on to develop interstitial lung disease. The

Table 77-11 Pulmonary Manifestations of Systemic Sclerosis

Pulmonary fibrosis, alveolitis

Pulmonary hypertension
    Primary (PAH)
    Secondary to pulmonary fibrosis, loss of vascular beds

Aspiration pneumonitis
Pleural effusions, pleuritis
Bronchiectasis
Lung cancer

PAH, pulmonary arterial hypertension.

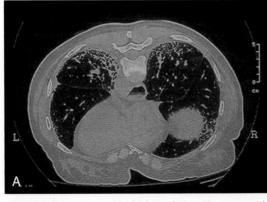 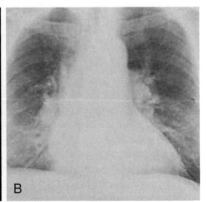

Figure 77-16 Computerized chest imaging. The high-resolution CT scan provides the most sensitive method of detecting lung fibrosis in systemic sclerosis. **A,** The earliest CT feature of lung fibrosis is increase in interstitial opacity. Amorphous change in the absence of traction bronchiectasis may suggest alveolitis, but similar changes may be caused by fine fibrosis. Later more reticular change develops, sometimes with associated cysts. Chest CT also may identify severe esophageal involvement with air in the esophagus, and enlargement of the proximal pulmonary vascular tree in advanced pulmonary arterial hypertension. **B,** In contrast, chest radiography detects only more advanced fibrotic change, but can exclude other pathology. In this example, severe lung fibrosis is associated with pulmonary arterial hypertension causing increased vascular markings in the hilar region with attenuation of vascular markings peripherally.

combination of normal lung volumes but reduced gas transfer in the face of normal chest imaging suggests pulmonary vascular disease.[244]

The application of high-resolution CT has been of immense value for definition and assessment of diffuse lung diseases and has revealed the character and distribution of fine structural abnormalities not visible on chest radiographs.[245] The earliest detectable high-resolution CT abnormality is a narrow, often ill-defined, subpleural crescent of increased density in the posterior segments of the lower lobes.[175] When more extensive, the shadowing takes on a characteristic reticulonodular appearance and becomes associated with fine, honeycomb airspaces and ultimately large cystic airspaces, an appearance that mirrors the macroscopic picture. Pleural disease and mediastinal lymphadenopathy also may be identified by high-resolution CT. It is important to perform high-resolution CT in prone and supine positions, particularly in patients with early SSc, to exclude the contribution of gravity to the radiographic appearances from vascular and interstitial pooling in the dependent areas. In addition to identifying early disease, high-resolution CT can be used to quantify the extent and delineate the pattern of lung abnormality.

Management of Interstitial Lung Disease

The mainstay of therapy for SSc-associated interstitial lung disease has long been corticosteroids or cyclophosphamide or both, given orally or as intermittent intravenous bolus. Two randomized controlled trials completed more recently showed a modest benefit for cyclophosphamide over placebo.[246,247] Reports of treatment with mycophenolate mofetil have been encouraging.[248,249] The place of immunosuppressive strategies remains uncertain, however, and requires randomized controlled trials. In idiopathic pulmonary fibrosis, more recent clinical trials of pirfenidone, etanercept, IFN-γ, and acetylcysteine (Mucodyne) have shown some efficacy, and these agents are currently undergoing further evaluation. The management of lung fibrosis in SSc is likely to be informed by the results from idiopathic pulmonary fibrosis studies.[250] For selected SSc patients with advanced pulmonary involvement, lung transplantation may be an option. Single lung transplant is now considered to be the most successful transplantation approach for interstitial lung disease and for PAH.[251]

Pulmonary Arterial Hypertension

PAH, defined as an elevation in the mean pulmonary artery pressure greater than 25 mm Hg at rest, occurs in limited and diffuse cutaneous forms of SSc and is a leading cause of mortality. The outcome in SSc-associated PAH is considerably worse than that of idiopathic PAH.[252] This worse outcome may reflect comorbidity or differences in under lying pathogenetic mechanisms. In SSc, PAH resulting from intrinsic fibroproliferative abnormalities in the pulmonary vasculature, pathologically indistinguishable from idiopathic PAH, is most common, with a prevalence of approximately 10% to 15%. The second pattern of PAH occurs in association with pulmonary interstitial fibrosis and is driven by hypoxia and the destruction of the pulmonary vascular bed. PAH in SSc also occurs in the context of pulmonary fibrosis,

and typical histologic appearance of PAH can be found in lung biopsy specimens from SSc patients with lung fibrosis. It has been suggested that coexistent vasculopathy determines outcome and survival in many cases of SSc-associated pulmonary fibrosis.[253]

PAH may remain asymptomatic until quite advanced. The initial symptoms include exertional breathlessness, and less often chest pain or syncope. In patients with SSc, PAH typically is discovered during regular monitoring with pulmonary function tests, Doppler echocardiography, and electrocardiography. An isolated reduction in diffusion capacity with preservation of lung volumes suggests PAH.[254] Definitive diagnosis requires exclusion of thromboembolic disease by ventilation-perfusion lung scan, spiral CT scan or pulmonary angiography, and hemodynamic demonstration of a mean pulmonary artery pressure greater than 25 mm Hg at rest or greater than 30 mm Hg with exercise. There is a correlation between peak pulmonary artery pressure estimated by Doppler echocardiography and direct measurements at right heart catheterization except when pulmonary artery pressures are in the 30 to 50 mm Hg range.[241]

Cardiac catheterization is essential for the workup because it allows the recognition of pulmonary venous hypertension and the precise determination of pulmonary vascular resistance, cardiac output (cardiac index), and pulmonary artery pressures. Serum levels of the N-terminal pro-brain natriuretic peptide (N-pro-BNP) may be helpful for screening and monitoring PAH. The levels correlate with survival in patients with SSc-associated PAH.[255]

Although historically PAH was associated with a grave prognosis, substantial progress in its management has been achieved recently. Figure 77-17 is an algorithm for detection and assessment of PAH. The current focus in the evaluation is on early identification and determination of severity. The World Health Organization/New York Heart Association functional classification is useful for assessing the severity of PAH and for treatment decisions. Exercise capacity, typically assessed by the distance walked in 6 minutes under standard conditions, has prognostic implications and is used for risk stratification.[256]

Current approaches to the treatment of PAH in SSc are summarized in Figure 77-18. Oral anticoagulation, spironolactone, and oxygen supplementation, when appropriate, may be used as supportive therapy. Specific treatments for PAH are initiated only for advanced disease (functional class III or IV); earlier intervention may be advantageous and is under investigation.[257] Treatment options for class III PAH include oral ET-1 receptor blockade[258] and phosphodiesterase inhibition.[259] Alternative therapies include inhaled and subcutaneous prostacyclin analogues.[260] Intravenous agents generally are reserved for patients with severe or advancing PAH.

Despite more recent progress, the management of PAH remains a major challenge; this is a result of the poor outcome of SSc-associated PAH compared with idiopathic PAH, and the lack of high-quality evidence addressing issues such as combination therapy and the benefits of early intervention. Our approach to the management of PAH in patients with SSc is summarized in Figure 77-18. When the diagnosis of PAH is confirmed, the contribution of associated interstitial lung disease is considered. Patients with significant hypoxemia benefit from supplemental oxygen. It is possible that lung fibrosis treatments such as immunosuppression may be

```
┌──────────────────────┐        ┌──────────────────────┐
│ Clinical suspicion   │        │ Regular screening    │
│ Breathlessness       │────────│ Annual assessment    │
│ Syncope              │        │   in all SSc patients│
│ Chest pain           │        │                      │
└──────────────────────┘        └──────────────────────┘
                           │
                           ▼
        ┌──────────────────────────────────────┐
        │ Differential diagnosis               │
        │ Ascertain pulmonary fibrosis         │
        │ Exclude thromboembolic disease       │
        │ Exclude pulmonary venous hypertension│
        │ Other causes: HIV, portal HT, anorexigen,│
        │   CTEPH, PVOD                        │
        └──────────────────────────────────────┘
                           │
                           ▼
        ┌──────────────────────────────────────┐
        │ Diagnosis                            │
        │ ECG, CXR                             │
        │ Doppler-echocardiography             │
        │ Pulmonary function tests             │
        │ Right heart catheter                 │
        └──────────────────────────────────────┘
                           │
                           ▼
 ┌──────────────────────────────────────────┐
 │ Risk stratification                      │
 │ WHO functional class*, Dyspnea index     │      ┌──────────┐
 │ Submaximal exercise test (e.g. six minute walk)│─│ Therapy  │
 │ Cardiodynamic assessment: peak and       │      └──────────┘
 │   mean PA pressure, cardiac index,       │
 │   pulmonary vascular resistance          │
 └──────────────────────────────────────────┘
```

Figure 77-17 Evaluation of pulmonary arterial hypertension (PAH) in systemic sclerosis. All patients with systemic sclerosis should have routine screening for evidence of PAH. An echocardiogram, pulmonary function test, and clinical review are recommended on at least a yearly basis. Patients who have evidence or suspicion of PAH should undergo further assessment as indicated. Diagnosis must be made by right heart catheterization. Diastolic dysfunction is common and leads to elevated pulmonary capillary wedge pressure. Other forms of PAH may require alternative therapies, such as CTEPH. The New York Heart Association/World Health Organization functional class is important in determining optimal therapy and outcome.* CTEPH, chronic thromboembolic pulmonary hypertension; PVOD, peripheral vascular occlusive disease.

appropriate (see later). In the absence of contraindication, supportive therapy with diuretics, oral anticoagulation, and in some cases digoxin is considered. Patients with functional class III disease are eligible for advanced therapy.

Our practice is to begin treatment with an oral ET-1 receptor antagonist when functional class III is reached; lack of response prompts switching to a phosphodiesterase inhibitor, whereas partial response or transient response generally results in addition of a phosphodiesterase inhibitor. Further deterioration can be managed by adding inhaled

iloprost or parenteral prostacyclin. Although surgical intervention may be useful for symptom control (septostomy) or long-term benefit (single lung transplant), these approaches are feasible in only a small number of SSc patients.[251]

RENAL MANIFESTATIONS

The kidney is the internal organ that most clearly and acutely shows the consequences of blood vessel spasm and arterial damage in SSc. In contrast to PAH, which is characterized

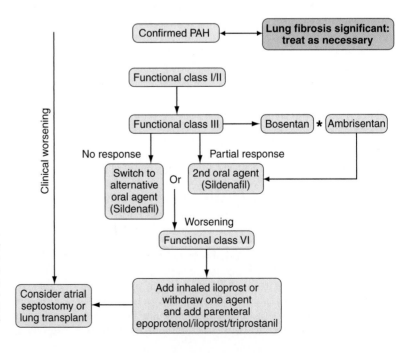

Figure 77-18 Management of pulmonary arterial hypertension (PAH). Patients with PAH in functional class II, III, or IV are candidates for therapy, generally an oral endothelin receptor antagonist as a single agent. Partial response prompts combination therapy with a 5′ phosphodiesterase (PDE5) inhibitor, whereas lack of response leads to switching to a PDE5 inhibitor. Adding inhaled iloprost or switching to subcutaneous triprostanil or intravenous prostacyclin is considered for patients who fail to respond.

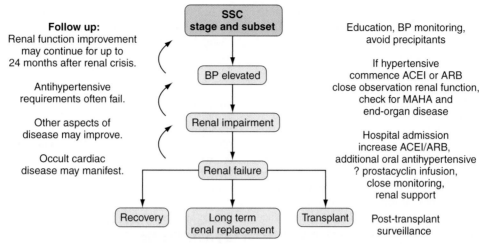

Figure 77-19   Management of scleroderma renal crisis. The overriding principle in management is vigilance and monitoring. Patients should be educated about the risk of renal crisis. Precipitating factors, such as corticosteroids, and potentially nephrotoxic agents, such as nonsteroidal anti-inflammatory drugs or high-dose diuretics, should be minimized. Hypertension must be treated promptly with an angiotensin-converting enzyme inhibitor (ACEI). Evidence of renal crisis, such as microangiopathic hemolytic anemia, declining renal function, or hypertensive retinopathy, mandates inpatient management. In addition to maximizing angiotensin-converting enzyme inhibition, additional antihypertensive agents may be required, and some centers introduce prostacyclin infusion in light of its effects on renal perfusion. Renal function may recover, and dialysis can be discontinued for 2 years after renal crisis. ACEI, angiotensin converting enzyme inhibitor; ARB, angiotensin receptor blocker.

by slowly progressive vasculopathy evolving over a long time, the vascular changes in renal scleroderma may develop rapidly, perhaps owing to the much higher levels of systemic blood pressure compared with the pulmonary circulation. In both cases, it seems likely that an abnormal response to vascular injury underlies the pathology. In scleroderma renal crisis, intrinsic systemic vasospasm leads to accelerated hypertension.

Scleroderma Renal Crisis

Scleroderma renal crisis, first reported in 1863,[260] typically causes accelerated hypertension and acute renal failure. Until the advent of angiotensin-converting enzyme (ACE) inhibitors, scleroderma renal crisis was associated with a very high mortality. In recent decades, mortality at 1 year declined from 85% to 24%.[261] Other patterns of renal involvement in SSc include chronic vasculopathy with reduced glomerular filtration rate. Patients with overlap SSc may develop inflammatory glomerular disease including glomerulonephritis, characteristically associated with serologic features.

Scleroderma renal crisis occurs in 10% to 15% of patients with diffuse cutaneous SSc and only vary rarely (1% to 2%) in limited cutaneous SSc.[262] Most cases occur within the first 12 months of disease, and in a quarter of patients with scleroderma renal crisis, the diagnosis of SSc is made at the time of the renal presentation.[5] Typically, patients present with accelerated hypertension and progressive renal impairment. End-organ damage can result in encephalopathy with generalized seizures or flash pulmonary edema. Microangiopathic hemolytic anemia is common, and disseminated intravascular coagulation may develop. Thrombocytopenia may be present. Approximately two thirds of cases of scleroderma renal crisis require renal replacement therapy.[262] Of these, half eventually recover sufficiently to discontinue dialysis; this can occur for 24 months, and decisions about renal transplantation should be postponed until that time. The possi-

bility for delayed renal recovery distinguishes scleroderma renal crisis from other causes of end-stage renal failure.

Improved outcomes are achieved with early use of ACE inhibitors as routine therapy for renal crisis. The efficacy of ACE inhibitors precludes future placebo-controlled studies in treating established scleroderma renal crisis. It is unclear whether related drugs, such as angiotensin receptor blockers, are effective in preventing or abrogating scleroderma renal crisis. Corticosteroids, along with cyclosporine, have been implicated as precipitants of scleroderma renal crisis.[225,263]

The management of scleroderma renal crisis is summarized schematically in Figure 77-19. Currently, our approach is to hospitalize patients at diagnosis (based on new-onset accelerated hypertension with evidence of renal impairment, microangiopathic hemolysis, or significant end-organ damage in the context of SSc) and treat with a full-dose ACE inhibitor. The dose should be increased daily to achieve a blood pressure reduction of 10 to 20 mm Hg systolic per 24 hours, even if there is continued deterioration in renal function, which can be followed by daily creatinine clearance or calculated glomerular filtration rate. In Europe, patients may be given continuous low-dose prostacyclin, which may help control blood pressure and has potentially beneficial effects on renal blood flow,[264] endothelial cell function, and production of proinflammatory or profibrotic factors. Additional antihypertensive agents may be useful, including combinations of angiotensin receptor blocker or ACE inhibitor drugs or calcium channel blockers, nitrates, or other vasodilator agents such as doxazosin. Care must be taken to monitor cardiac function closely because vasodilation may be associated with relative hypovolemia.

The outcome of scleroderma renal crisis is poor, with early mortality approaching 10%, and half of patients needing dialysis.[265] The dialysis may be temporary, and many patients requiring renal replacement therapy eventually come off dialysis 6 to 24 months after the renal crisis. For this reason, even though transplantation is no less successful in SSc than in systemic lupus erythematosus, final decisions should not be made until at least 2 years after the renal crisis.[266] Renal biopsy may provide prognostic information and confirms the diagnosis. Cases of SSc with inflammatory glomerular pathology have been identified, and they require potentially very different treatment compared with classic scleroderma renal crisis.

Rarely, patients have apparently primary accelerated or severe hypertension as an initial presentation of SSc.[267] It is important to examine such cases carefully for the presence of this disease, and follow up clinical suspicion with appropriate investigations. The diagnosis of early SSc has been facilitated by nail-fold capillaroscopy, together with autoimmune serology, including hallmark SSc-associated autoantibodies. Not only do these investigations often confirm the clinical diagnosis of SSc, but they also can help identify patients with isolated Raynaud's phenomenon who are at high risk of developing a connective tissue disorder.

Other Forms of Renal Involvement

Other acute renal complications may occur, especially in overlap syndromes with lupus nephritis. There may be serologic clues that a patient is evolving within the connective tissue disease spectrum that anticipate clinical changes, such as the development of a rise in titer of an associated anti–double-stranded DNA antibody. It has been suggested that anti–neutrophil cytoplasmic antibody reactivity may predict unusual renal complications of SSc, such as glomerulonephritis and renal vasculitis.[268] Some of these changes occur in SSc patients treated with penicillamine.[269] Indolent chronic renal involvement, characterized by a slow reduction in glomerular filtration rate accompanied by proteinuria, has been described in SSc.[270]

Renal Transplantation in Systemic Sclerosis

Considerable recovery of renal function may occur after acute scleroderma renal crisis, sometimes allowing discontinuation of dialysis. Because improvement of renal function may continue for 2 years, decisions regarding renal transplantation should be deferred. The survival of renal allografts in SSc is comparable to that seen in other autoimmune rheumatic diseases, including systemic lupus erythematosus.[266] It is possible that post-transplant immunosuppressive regimens have beneficial effects on underlying disease that diminish involvement in the grafted kidney. Nonrenal manifestations of SSc also may improve after renal transplantation.[271] Nevertheless, recurrent scleroderma renal disease in grafted organs has been described.[272]

OTHER MANIFESTATIONS
Neurologic Manifestations

In early-stage diffuse cutaneous SSc, patients commonly report symptoms of median nerve compression, and many patients undergo surgical treatment for carpal tunnel syndrome before the diagnosis of SSc is established. As the inflammatory phase of SSc passes, these symptoms often improve without specific therapies. Isolated, or occasionally multiple, involvement of the cranial nerves can

occur, sometimes in association with specific autoantibody profiles, such as anti-U1-RNP.[270] As in other connective tissue diseases, a symmetric peripheral neuropathy is sometimes identified and may occur in the setting of overlap vasculitis.

Sicca Symptoms

In addition to overlap SSc that fulfills classification criteria for Sjögren's syndrome,[273] sicca symptoms are common. These symptoms probably reflect the loss of minor exocrine glandular structures, together with the atrophic changes of associated tissues.

DIAGNOSIS AND DIAGNOSTIC EVALUATION

The differential diagnosis for scleroderma-spectrum disorders is extensive (see Table 77-1). The list includes conditions in which skin induration is due to deposition of abnormal protein within the dermis, as in amyloidosis or scleromyxedema, or to inflammation and secondary scarring in metabolic disorders such as porphyria. The most important differential diagnoses for SSc are the scleroderma-spectrum disorders. Features such as Raynaud's phenomenon provide an important clinical clue of systemic involvement. The hallmark SSc autoantibodies do not occur in scleroderma-like diseases resulting from metabolic abnormalities or infiltration. The diagnosis of SSc usually is made on clinical grounds and is supported by laboratory investigations. Classification criteria were developed to discriminate SSc from other connective tissue diseases in clinical research, rather than for diagnostic purposes; patients with mild SSc or with early disease frequently fail to fulfill these criteria.

DISEASE ASSESSMENT

Assessment starts with diagnosis and classification. In a patient with features of a scleroderma-spectrum disorder, the first consideration is to determine if the condition is localized disease or SSc. The simplest discriminators are the presence of Raynaud's phenomenon and internal organ manifestations, of which the earliest is often reflux esophagitis, although Raynaud's phenomenon and gastroesophageal reflux are common in otherwise healthy individuals. The distribution of skin involvement provides crucial information about SSc subset and classification. Acral involvement is almost universal in SSc, whereas asymmetric skin induration and acral sparing suggest localized scleroderma.

Autoantibody testing is the most useful laboratory investigation (see later). Nail-fold capillary microscopy is an additional clinical investigation that helps to discriminate primary Raynaud's phenomenon from early SSc because the latter is associated with classic changes, including capillary dropout and dilation. In localized scleroderma, capillaroscopy is entirely normal. In contrast to other connective tissue diseases, such as systemic lupus erythematosus or inflammatory arthritis, characterized by a relapsing-remitting clinical course, in SSc damage tends to occur gradually and to progress over time. It is more useful to evaluate severity and cumulative damage than disease activity. Preliminary indices for evaluating disease activity[274,275] and severity[275a] have been proposed.

Because these tools remain to be validated, they are more relevant to research than clinical practice.

AUTOANTIBODIES IN ASSESSMENT

Most patients with SSc have serum antinuclear autoantibodies, including hallmark autoantibodies specifically associated with SSc (see Table 77-6). The most common immunofluorescence pattern with Hep2 cell substrates is speckled; in contrast, PM-Scl, anti-fibrillarin Th/T$_o$, and anti–RNA polymerase antibodies generate a nucleolar pattern of staining. These different staining patterns are valuable in practice when patients present with an undifferentiated connective tissue disease because a scleroderma pattern of immunoreactivity can be a useful first sign of the disease. The major SSc-associated autoantibodies are anticentromere, anti–topoisomerase I, anti–RNA polymerase I/III, and antifibrillarin. These autoantibodies are almost always mutually exclusive, reflecting their immunogenetic basis linked to the MHC class II associations.[276] The strongest association between an SSc autoantibody and a specific clinical pattern is between lung fibrosis and anti–topoisomerase I antibodies, most frequently in patients with diffuse cutaneous SSc. Anti–RNA polymerase I/III reactivity is associated with scleroderma renal crisis.[277] Other autoantibodies can predict coexisting disease, such as thyroiditis, primary biliary cirrhosis,[223] and overlap syndromes.

TREATMENT OF SYSTEMIC SCLEROSIS

There have been major advances in the treatment of organ-specific complications of SSc. In particular, the management and outcome of scleroderma renal crisis has been transformed by the judicious use of ACE inhibitors. Morbidity from Raynaud's phenomenon and esophagitis has been markedly reduced. Progress also has been made in treating PAH, and more recent reports indicate that immunosuppression using cyclophosphamide may slow the progression of interstitial lung disease complicating SSc.

Despite these positive developments, no SSc therapy to date has been proved to be effective in altering the natural history of the disease. The choice and evaluation of any treatment regimen for SSc is challenging because the disease is complex, and its pathogenesis is poorly understood; it is heterogeneous in its extent, severity, and rate of progression. Treatment typically includes a combination of agents targeting the immune, vascular, and fibrotic processes underlying the pathogenesis of SSc. Therapy must be tailored to the individual patient, however, carefully taking into consideration disease subset and duration, rate of progression, and pattern and severity of internal organ involvement. Careful baseline assessment of organ-based complications and long-term follow-up are essential.

IMMUNOMODULATORY THERAPY

Immunosuppressive strategies in SSc are most likely to be effective in early-stage disease when inflammatory features are prominent. Numerous immunosuppressive drugs have been used, but with the exception of cyclophosphamide, none have been shown to be effective in randomized clinical trials (Table 77-12). Adding to a substantial body of uncontrolled

Table 77-12 Immunomodulatory and Immunosuppressive Interventions Used in Systemic Sclerosis

Methotrexate
Cyclosporine
Cyclophosphamide*
Azathioprine
Mycophenolate mofetil
Thalidomide
Antithymocyte globulin
Intravenous immunoglobulin
Extracorporeal photopheresis
Immunoablation with autologous stem cell rescue (transplantation)

*Found to be effective in a randomized, clinical trial.

or retrospective studies suggesting benefit for cyclophosphamide in SSc-associated interstitial lung disease, two more recent randomized double-blind, placebo-controlled trials have shown a modest benefit. Intensive immunosuppression with autologous hematopoietic stem cell rescue is a promising novel form of intervention. Uncontrolled studies show the feasibility of stem cell therapy,[278] and several randomized clinical trials comparing stem cell therapy with other forms of immunosuppression are currently under way. Because of its substantial cost and potential treatment-related complications, including death, stem cell therapy may be best suited for diffuse cutaneous SSc patients with severe disease.

Other approaches to immunosuppression include use of antithymocyte globulin[279] or anti-CD25 monoclonal antibody.[280] Mycophenolate mofetil is increasingly used in diffuse cutaneous SSc, and results from pilot studies suggest that it is well tolerated and may be beneficial in SSc-associated lung fibrosis.[248,281] It is possible that immunosuppressive or antimetabolic agents also modulate nonimmune processes contributing to pathogenesis of SSc such as fibroblast activation or vasculopathy, and that drugs whose primary mode of action is believed to be antifibrotic also modulate immune cell function; examples include IFN-γ and penicillamine.[95]

Low-dose corticosteroids (≤5 mg prednisone/day) are useful for controlling inflammatory symptoms that are frequent in early-stage SSc and are commonly used in combination with immunosuppressive agents for the treatment of lung fibrosis and of myositis. Long-term corticosteroids should be avoided, however, because they may precipitate scleroderma renal crisis (see earlier). Steroid use is ideally restricted to patients with myositis, symptomatic serositis, the early edematous phase of the skin disease, refractory arthritis, and tenosynovitis. The lowest possible therapeutically effective dose should be used in cases of SSc that require corticosteroid administration. We advise daily monitoring of blood pressure in patients at high risk.

ANTIFIBROTIC AGENTS

Although many current treatment strategies are immunomodulatory, in patients with established SSc, the most effective agents are likely to be those with antifibrotic activity. To date, no drug has been proven to be effective as an antifibrotic, and many drugs used in the past for this indication have been shown to be ineffective in controlled trials.

Table 77-13 Therapeutic Approaches to Management of Raynaud's Phenomenon

Class of Drug	Example
Calcium channel blockers	Nifedipine
Angiotensin II receptor antagonists	Losartan
α-adrenergic blockade	Prazosin
Prostacyclin	Iloprost (parenteral)
Endothelin receptor blockers	Bosentan
Phosphodiesterase inhibitors	Sildenafil
Surgery	Sympathectomy

A pilot study of a human monoclonal antibody directed against TGF-β1 showed no efficacy compared with placebo.[252] The antibiotic minocycline has been suggested as a potential antifibrotic agent, but a prospective controlled trial showed a lack of benefit in diffuse cutaneous SSc.[282] Because oxidant stress may play a role in the pathogenesis of SSc, antioxidant agents have been considered as potential therapies. In theory, such an approach might influence the vascular, fibrotic, and immunologic processes of the disease.

VASCULAR THERAPIES

Vasculopathy affecting small blood vessels is a universal feature of all forms of SSc and accounts for substantial morbidity. Many vasodilator drugs have been used as treatment for Raynaud's phenomenon (Table 77-13). The primary goal of such treatments is to reduce vasospasm or promote vasodilation. Some agents may have broader effects on endothelial cell function or vascular remodeling, and it has been suggested that some drugs for Raynaud's phenomenon also might have beneficial effects on other aspects of SSc.[199] Oral therapy may be insufficient, and in these cases parenteral prostacyclin analogues are often used. In some cases, surgical intervention with digital sympathectomy is valuable, especially if there is a single ischemic digit or refractory ischemic digital ulceration (see Fig. 77-11).

Because widespread vascular damage commonly occurs in SSc, drugs that protect injured endothelial cells and prevent platelet aggregation and subsequent release of platelet-derived mediators could be helpful. None of the drugs that have been evaluated, including ketanserin, a serotonin antagonist, dipyridamole, and aspirin, were clinically effective in altering vascular damage in randomized clinical trials. The ACE inhibitor captopril has been used for the primary and possibly prophylactic treatment of vascular disease.[283] However, a randomized, prospective clinical trial failed to show any long-term clinical benefit of prophylactic ACE inhibitor therapy in SSc.[283a]

As in other autoimmune rheumatic diseases, therapy with statin drugs potentially may be beneficial for vascular disease in SSc beyond their lipid-lowering effects. There have been no controlled clinical trials, but small studies suggest that statins have possible beneficial effects on markers of endothelial cell injury.[284] A recent report suggested that atorvastatin might favorably modulate the number of circulating endothelial cell precursors in patients with SSc and vascular complications.[109]

Although specific management approaches are considered elsewhere in this chapter, general principles apply to damage

occurring across numerous vascular beds; this is because of the similarity between histopathologic abnormalities within medium-sized arterial vessels in the lung, kidney, and digital circulation. Vasospasm is especially prominent in the digital circulation, but structural changes with mural fibrosis and lumen narrowing are more important in late-stage disease. With this in mind, treatment goals are to induce vasodilation or prevent vasoconstriction, and to remodel damaged blood vessels.

Prevention of thrombosis is logical, but results of clinical studies with antithrombotic agents have been equivocal. Prostacyclin analogues given by intravenous infusion have been used in Europe for digital vasculopathy and Raynaud's phenomenon.[285] Antioxidants may reduce vascular damage, and some patients choose to take high-dose antioxidant vitamin supplements. Calcium channel blockers are of proven effectiveness in Raynaud's phenomenon and are widely used.[286] Losartan was superior to nifedipine in a small clinical trial.[287] Serotonin reuptake inhibitors, such as fluoxetine, may be beneficial in SSc-associated Raynaud's phenomenon.[288] In contrast, the benefit of long-term ACE inhibitor therapy in Raynaud's phenomenon is unproven.

MANAGEMENT PRINCIPLES

The first principle of management is accurate diagnosis. The differential diagnosis of scleroderma-like conditions is considered in Table 77-1. Historically, SSc has been perceived as a grievous disease, and widely approached with a degree of therapeutic nihilism. In the current era, such an attitude serves the patient with SSc poorly. Instead, we prefer to view SSc as a chronic, treatable disease similar to diabetes mellitus. Ample evidence shows improved survival of patients with SSc and improved outcomes from major organ-based complications, including renal, pulmonary vascular, and interstitial lung disease. Certain aspects of the disease continue to defy effective management—most notably cardiac and lower gastrointestinal tract involvement.

Education

There is often considerable confusion among patients and health care professionals regarding the nature, clinical manifestations, and natural history of SSc, and its evaluation, monitoring, and long-term management. Education is an important component of the management.[289] We find that patients who have a good understanding of their disease become active partners in its management, and cope better with its burdens over time.

Screening for Organ-based Disease

A mainstay of management of established SSc is regular screening for the development of new complications and for progression of abnormalities noted at baseline. Currently, we recommend that in SSc patients with early disease (i.e., the first 2 to 4 years), careful assessment for renal, cardiac, and respiratory function be performed on a yearly basis, recognizing that more than half of patients develop at least one significant complication during follow-up, and reflecting a growing body of evidence supporting effectiveness of therapies.[5] The challenge of reversing established organ damage leads to the hypothesis that earlier detection of major complications could allow treatment at an earlier stage and improve outcome. Although this is a compelling strategy and forms the basis for active management, trials of effective therapies are needed to confirm the validity of this construct, and to determine how various treatments, often potentially toxic and expensive, should be used.

Disease Modification versus Organ-specific Strategies

Therapeutic progress in SSc has largely come from the application of interventions that are valuable in related conditions. Use of these agents in SSc often requires adjustments to standard protocols, and outcomes may be different. Examples include the use of ACE inhibitors in scleroderma renal crisis, proton-pump inhibitors for gastroesophageal reflux disease, cytotoxic agents for interstitial lung disease, broad-spectrum antibiotics and enteral or parenteral nutritional supplementation for midgut disease, and novel therapies for PAH.

OUTCOME AND PROGNOSIS

The long-term outcome of SSc is a major concern at the time of diagnosis. The heterogeneity of the disease and its major subsets necessitates careful assessment. Ideally, patients should be stratified according to the likelihood of developing major organ-based complications or of progression of already existing complications.

The past 25 years have witnessed substantial improvement in the mortality of SSc, and more recent analysis indicates greater than 80% 5-year survival.[5] Certain subsets of SSc have a worse outcome, however. Advanced PAH is associated with a less than 50% 2-year survival.[255] Historically, the highest mortality is seen in patients with scleroderma renal crisis, with 1-year survival less than 15%.[228] Major improvements followed the introduction and widespread early use of ACE inhibitors; more recent case-control analysis suggests greater than 85% 1-year survival. Longer term outcome remains poor, with high mortality at 3 years from multiple causes. The outcome of patients with SSc-associated PAH is worse than the outcome of patients with idiopathic PAH. More recent studies have indicated improved survival in SSc-associated PAH with greater than 70% 2-year survival.[255] Although SSc remains a grievous disease with life-threatening complications, subsets without significant internal organ involvement and limited skin involvement have normal survival,[228] and it is likely that prognosis will continue to improve.

LOCALIZED SCLERODERMA

Localized forms of scleroderma are distinguished from SSc not only by the absence of vasospasm, structural vascular damage, and involvement of internal organs, but also by the distribution of the skin lesions.[292] The three main varieties of localized scleroderma are morphea, linear scleroderma, and coup de sabre. These conditions are characterized by localized inflammation and fibrosis of the skin and underlying tissue. Patches of abnormality, termed *plaque morphea*, develop as single or multiple lesions. In linear scleroderma, lesions

develop along the limbs, or less commonly, on the trunk in a linear fashion, sometimes in association with plaques of morphea as a mixed pattern. Linear scleroderma on the forehead or scalp is called coup de sabre.[293]

Early localized scleroderma lesions are associated with inflammatory changes in the dermis and violaceous discoloration, and are often accompanied by localized itching or discomfort. With time, the lesions become indurated and sclerotic, and in late stages there may be a pale waxy central area with an erythematous border. Eventually, the skin texture softens, although pigmentary abnormalities often persist. In morphea profunda, the lesions occur in the deeper dermis, and overlying skin features are less apparent.

In adults with localized scleroderma, the main concerns generally relate to discomfort and cosmetic changes; however, in children, the disease is more serious. Linear scleroderma can be associated with growth failure that may be profound; on the face, this leads to hemifacial atrophy, also known as Parry-Romberg syndrome. Occasionally, localized scleroderma is associated with extensive skin changes affecting the trunk (pansclerotic morphea) that can resemble diffuse cutaneous SSc. The absence of Raynaud's phenomenon and normal nail-fold capillaroscopy are useful diagnostic features distinguishing all forms of localized scleroderma from SSc. Autoantibody testing is less robust for this purpose because localized scleroderma may be associated with antinuclear antibody, anti–single-stranded DNA, and other autoantibodies. Although progression of localized scleroderma to SSc almost never occurs, some patients with SSc develop plaques of morphea or areas of linear localized scleroderma.

The etiology of localized scleroderma is unclear. Local triggers, such as trauma, are implicated, and association with infection, including *Borrelia burgdorferi*, has been described.[294] Management of patients with localized scleroderma must be individualized. Adults with mild disease often do not require treatment or may be treated locally with topical immunosuppressant agents, such as tacrolimus[295] or calcipotriene (a form of vitamin D_3), or with phototherapy. In severe or progressive localized scleroderma, systemic therapy with corticosteroids and immunosuppressants may be appropriate. Methotrexate, penicillamine, mycophenolate mofetil, azathioprine, hydroxychloroquine sulfate, and cyclosporine have been used with variable success. In rapidly progressive disease, initial treatment may include intravenous pulses of methylprednisolone. Treatment also must include physiotherapy to minimize growth asymmetry and to maximize function. Table 77-14 summarizes approaches to evaluation and management for the major types of localized scleroderma.

MORPHEA

Morphea may occur in a circumscribed or a generalized form. In circumscribed morphea, there may be just one or two lesions with no generalized spread. The changes often begin with small, violaceous or erythematous skin lesions, which enlarge and progress to firm hidebound skin with variable degrees of hypopigmentation or hyperpigmentation. These lesions eventually assume a waxy, pale appearance with subsequent atrophy. Pruritus is often a problem with the early lesion. Lesions vary in diameter from 10 mm to 10 cm.

Table 77-14 Management of Localized Scleroderma in Adults and Children

Pattern of Disease	Clinical Features	Treatment	Prognosis
Plaque morphea	One or a few circumscribed sclerotic plaques with hypopigmentation or hyperpigmentation and an inflamed violaceous border	Often unnecessary. Topical steroids, immunosuppression (e.g., tacrolimus) or phototherapy may be considered. Serial measurement to assess progress	Good prognosis. Lesions less active within 3 yr, but pigmentary changes often persist
Generalized morphea	Widespread pruritic lesions, often symmetric and following distribution of superficial veins	Suppress inflammatory component using corticosteroids: in children oral doses 15 mg/day have been used. Intravenous infusions often effective. Methotrexate, immunosuppressive maintenance therapy often used, although benefit not proven in controlled trials. Vitamin D–containing creams may be useful. Topical corticosteroids rarely helpful. PUVA has been used	Internal organ pathology or Raynaud's phenomenon rare. Generally improves within 5 yr of onset, although textural and pigmentary changes may persist
Linear scleroderma	Sclerotic areas in linear distribution on limbs, asymmetric; in childhood can lead to growth defect. Serial measurements of limb length and girth essential to monitor progression	Suppress inflammatory component using corticosteroids: in children oral doses 15 mg/day have been used. Intravenous infusion has been used. Methotrexate, other immunosuppressive maintenance therapy often used, although benefit not proven in controlled trials. Vitamin D–containing creams may be useful. Physiotherapy and appropriate regular exercise important to minimize growth defect in childhood disease. Surgical correction of limb defects may be considered when disease is inactive	Long-term effects of childhood-onset form are minimized by effective suppression of the inflammatory process and by good physiotherapy. Tends to resolve, but can remain active for years
Coup de sabre	Linear scleroderma affecting the face or scalp, often involving the underlying subcutaneous tissues, muscles, periosteum, and bone. Cerebral abnormalties also reported, including intracranial calcification	Therapeutic options as for linear scleroderma; systemic treatment only for active inflammatory lesions	Scarring, growth defects, and alopecia persist, but the inflammatory component usually resolves

PUVA, psoralens and ultraviolet A.

The condition often resolves within 3 to 5 years, although patches may persist for more than 25 years.[292]

In some patients, morphea is widespread and generalized. Fingers and toes usually are spared, but the trunk and legs are generally involved. Generalized morphea can be disfiguring and may continue to extend, resulting in joint contractures, disability, and troublesome ulceration. In guttate morphea, there are multiple hypopigmented and pigmented papules 2 to 10 mm in diameter, with minimal sclerosis. These lesions are commonly localized to the neck, shoulders, and anterior chest wall, and resemble those of lichen sclerosus et atrophicus.

LINEAR SCLERODERMA

Linear scleroderma occurs most frequently in childhood, but also may develop in adults.[296,297] In this very rare process, sclerotic areas have a linear, bandlike pattern and often follow a dermatomal distribution. Lesions generally predominate on one side of the body, although some degree of contralateral involvement may be present at later stages, suggesting that there may be a systemic process. When linear scleroderma lesions cross joint lines, they can be associated with atrophy of the soft tissue, muscle, periosteum, bone, and occasionally synovium. In some cases, the lesions cause extensive growth defects in a limb or a part thereof, which can be extremely disfiguring. Fixed valgus deformities occur, and scoliotic changes in the spine can develop as a

result of limb-length inequality. When the toes or fingers are affected, hammer toes or claw hand may develop. These changes are more noticeable in a growing child.[298] It is common for patients to present with morphea and later develop linear lesions. This evolution should be anticipated carefully because the linear lesions tend to have much greater morbidity than the circumscribed patches of morphea.

Because the linear lesions may be insidiously progressive, lengthy follow-up of these patients is important. Laboratory investigation generally reveals normal erythrocyte sedimentation rate and rheumatoid factor, but autoantibodies are often present. Some children with morphea or linear lesions or both develop synovitis, with an elevated erythrocyte sedimentation rate, rheumatoid factor, and circulating autoantibodies, and accelerated development of contractures. At the time of presentation, there may be only a small area of localized or linear scleroderma, distant from the joint symptoms.

The evaluation of localized forms of scleroderma is challenging. Although charting of the involved areas is cumbersome and imprecise, the lesions should be carefully recorded; leg length, limb circumferences, and posture should be monitored; and muscle function and neurologic status should be assessed on a regular basis. Charting of new lesions also is essential. Thermography has been used to assess the activity of localized disease,[299] and high-frequency ultrasound or MRI may help to determine the depth of localized scleroderma lesions.[300]

COUP DE SABRE

Linear scleroderma occurring on the face or scalp may assume a depressed, ivory appearance. The lesion was considered reminiscent of the scar from a sabre wound and termed *coup de sabre*. The linear lesion often is associated with ipsilateral facial hemiatrophy. It also may be associated with vascular abnormalities of the brain and distant morphea lesions. There is overlap between this form of linear scleroderma and specific localized growth defects, such as idiopathic hemifacial atrophy (Parry-Romberg syndrome). In the latter, the overlying skin may be texturally normal, however.[293]

PSEUDOSCLERODERMA SYNDROMES

SCLEREDEMA AND SCLEROMYXEDEMA

Scleredema and scleromyxedema are distinct idiopathic connective tissue disorders that must be distinguished from SSc and from localized scleroderma.[31] Approximately half of cases of scleredema have diabetes mellitus, typically long-standing and insulin-dependent. The histopathologic hallmark is an increase in mucin-rich ECM in involved skin, although this may diminish as the disease becomes more long-standing.[301] In scleromyxedema, there is a more florid epidermal abnormality, often with papule formation. Both conditions can be associated with an initial inflammatory cell infiltrate, but this diminishes over time.[302] Histologic similarities between scleredema, scleromyxedema, and nephrogenic systemic fibrosis (see later) are striking, and suggest that similar pathogenic mechanisms may be involved.[303]

Scleredema and scleromyxedema may be associated with paraproteinemia and with a plasma cell dyscrasia, and less commonly with multiple myeloma.[304] There have been no randomized clinical trials for evaluating treatments for scleredema and scleromyxedema. Interventions that have been reported to be effective in individual cases include immunoglobulin infusions often given together with immunosuppression, such as methotrexate or mycophenolate mofetil.[305] In severe cases, immunoablation and autologous stem cell transplantation have been used.[306] There have been some reports of successful treatment with plasmapheresis, although long-term outcomes have been disappointing.[307]

EOSINOPHILIC FASCIITIS

Eosinophilic fasciitis (alternatively called "diffuse fasciitis with eosinophilia") is an uncommon disorder characterized by the development of indurated subcutaneous connective tissue. The lesions most commonly occur on the lower limbs and forearms. The affected areas have a characteristic "woody" consistency on palpation. Elevation of involved territories reveals the "groove sign" as veins within indurated subcutaneous tissue empty (Fig. 77-20). This sign can be seen for superficial veins in other scleroderma spectrum disorders and is not specific for eosinophilic fasciitis.

Eosinophilic fasciitis is associated with peripheral blood eosinophilia, which is often transient. In the early stage, histologically affected tissue shows thickening and inflammation in the subcutaneous fascia. The fascial infiltrate

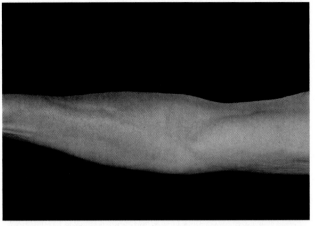

Figure 77-20 The arm of a patient with eosinophilic fasciitis. Eosinophilic fasciitis is associated histologically with inflammation and fibrosis in the subcutaneous tissues, yielding the characteristic woody texture of distal limbs. Loss of perivascular fat tissue accounts for the groove sign when the arm is elevated. There may be contractural changes owing to shortening of the flexor tendons and tissue fibrosis. Absence of Raynaud's phenomenon and sparing of the digits distinguish fasciitis from systemic sclerosis. Peripheral blood eosinophilia and eosinophilic infiltrates in the affected tissue are common, but may be transient. Full-thickness skin biopsy including deep fascia is required for histologic confirmation of the diagnosis.

typically, but not always, includes eosinophils.[308] With progression, fascial inflammation is replaced by thickening and fibrosis that may extend deeper into the perimuscular tissue. Because the lesion may extend superficially to the dermis, it can clinically resemble scleroderma. Contractures at large joints and limitation of the range of movement can develop. Constitutional symptoms may occur in the early stages of the disease.[40]

Corticosteroids have been commonly used in the treatment of acute eosinophilic fasciitis. Other immunosuppressive agents include methotrexate, but there have been no randomized clinical trials evaluating the efficacy of any therapy. The etiology of eosinophilic fasciitis is uncertain. Some individuals develop the disorder after episodes of unaccustomed vigorous exercise. MRI has been found to be useful in confirmation of the inflammatory changes in the subcutaneous tissues, and determination of ongoing activity at later stages. Occasionally, there is evidence of other complications of eosinophilia, including myocarditis, and there are reports of paraneoplastic cases. The most common association has been with T cell lymphoma[309] or with myeloma.[310] Other hematologic associations include aplastic or hemolytic anemia.[311] There are distinct clinical and pathologic differences between eosinophilic fasciitis and the eosinophilia-myalgia syndrome that was associated with consumption of contaminated tryptophan dietary supplement.[40]

NEPHROGENIC SYSTEMIC FIBROSIS OR NEPHROGENIC FIBROSING DERMOPATHY

Nephrogenic fibrosing dermatopathy, first described in 1997 and now recognized as an emerging problem in patients with chronic renal failure, shares histopathologic and clinical features with other scleroderma-spectrum disorders, notably fasciitis and scleromyxedema. Although most patients are on long-term dialysis, no association with a particular route or type of renal replacement therapy could be shown, and 10% of cases occur in patients who have never received dialysis.[312] Histologic hallmarks include cutaneous and sub-cutaneous fibrosis with accumulation of spindle-shaped cells, including numerous CD34+ cells.[303] There is an increase in acid mucin accumulation in lesional skin at early stages, drawing parallels with other forms of fibromucinosis (see earlier). Serum from patients with nephrogenic fibrosing dermatopathy can stimulate fibroblast proteoglycan secretion in vitro.[313] Because visceral fibrosis and skeletal muscle involvement have been described in some patients with nephrogenic fibrosing dermopathy, the term *dialysis-associated systemic fibrosis* has been proposed as an alternative.[314]

Clinical features include loss of subcutaneous fat, thickening and tightness of skin over the limbs, and contracture formation at large joints.[315] The subdermal tissues become hard or "woody," resembling established fasciitis, and there can be waxy plaques of morphea-like skin over affected areas. Raynaud's phenomenon and hallmark SSc autoantibodies do not occur. The similarity between nephrogenic fibrosing dermatopathy and other scleroderma-spectrum disorders and environmentally induced forms of cutaneous fibrosis, such as toxic oil syndrome[316] or eosinophilia-myalgia syndrome,[317] is noteworthy. The development of a new syndrome suggests that a change in practice or novel environmental trigger may be responsible. Risk factors for the development of nephrogenic fibrosing dermatopathy include exposure to gadolinium-containing MRI contrast agents[318] and possibly high-dose erythropoietin.[319,320] Some patients with nephrogenic fibrosing dermatopathy improve with adjustment to renal replacement therapy, and others respond to renal transplantation. Agents that may be helpful in scleromyxedema or scleroderma also have been used.

Future Directions

DISEASE-MODIFYING THERAPY

Although there is now a much better understanding of the pathogenesis in SSc and the potential links between the key pathologic processes, there is still little that can be offered as effective disease-modifying therapy. Effective therapies likely would target key mediators, pathways, or intercellular interactions. At present, a combination of vascular, immunomodulatory, and antifibrotic strategies is envisaged, although it is possible that if vascular or immune-directed treatments were given at an early stage, some of the fibrotic consequences of SSc could be prevented. Evidence from studies of skin sclerosis suggests, however, that even in early disease, the profibrotic processes are well established.

RISK STRATIFICATION

The clinical heterogeneity of SSc is one of the most challenging aspects of the disease because it is difficult to determine at presentation whether and when major internal organ disease will occur. Serologic markers are of some use, and it is likely that in the future there may be genetic markers. Within each organ system, investigation is usually multifaceted, and assessments of probability have been made to try to determine the likelihood of a particular complication, such as PAH. Studies of the

hallmark serum autoantibodies in SSc have highlighted clinical associations with particular reactivities. Limited cutaneous disease and PAH are associated with anticentromere reactivity, lung fibrosis with antitopoisomerase reactivity, renal involvement, and diffuse skin disease with antibodies to RNA polymerases I and III.[290,291]

INDIVIDUALIZED THERAPY

For most cases of SSc, therapy is individualized. Some generic aspects can be considered, such as management of Raynaud's phenomenon and esophagitis, skin care, and disease education. The use of major potential disease-modifying therapy is considered on a case-specific basis, however. Sometimes treatment directed to one system, such as lung fibrosis or PAH, may be of more general benefit.

Early Intervention—Prevention Paradigm for Internal Organ Disease

Although some patients with SSc present with clinically significant internal organ disease, such as scleroderma renal crisis or PAH, this is uncommon. Even in such patients, the history often reveals preexisting clinical features of SSc. In most cases, symptoms of Raynaud's phenomenon or skin involvement precede major organ-based complications. There is often the potential for early detection and clinical intervention, especially for respiratory and gastrointestinal tract involvement. Cardiac or renal involvement may be more difficult to detect early, but clinical markers that suggest risk for these manifestations may be present (see earlier).

Our recommendation is that all patients should have careful screening at diagnosis, and a program of regular follow-up should be instituted. This program must be combined with diligent patient education so that relevant symptoms are heeded, and appropriate advice is sought. The clinical heterogeneity of SSc represents a substantial challenge to the practicing rheumatologist, and precludes generalizable treatment protocols. This heterogeneity also confounds clinical trials. Nevertheless, it is assumed that outcomes could be improved and severe internal organ disease prevented, if complications are detected earlier. It is possible, although not yet formally shown, that treatments that have been shown to work in advanced disease may be beneficial at an earlier stage.

REFERENCES

1. LeRoy EC, Black C, Fleischmajer R, et al: Scleroderma (systemic sclerosis): Classification, subsets and pathogenesis. J Rheumatol 15:202-205, 1988.
2. Poormoghim H, Lucas M, Fertig N, et al: Systemic sclerosis sine scleroderma: Demographic, clinical, and serologic features and survival in forty-eight patients. Arthritis Rheum 43:444-451, 2000.
3. Anonymous: Preliminary criteria for the classification of systemic sclerosis (scleroderma). Subcommittee for scleroderma criteria of the American Rheumatism Association Diagnostic and Therapeutic Criteria Committee. Arthritis Rheum 23:581-590, 1980.
4. Pope JE, Bellamy N: Outcome measurements in scleroderma clinical trials. Semin Arthritis Rheum 23:22-33, 1993.
5. Shand L, Lunt M, Nihtyanova S, et al: Relationship between change in skin score and disease outcome in diffuse cutaneous systemic sclerosis: Application of a latent linear trajectory model. Arthritis Rheum 56:2422-2431, 2007.
6. Steen VD, Oddis CV, Conte CG, et al: Incidence of systemic sclerosis in Allegheny County, Pennsylvania: A twenty-year study of hospital-diagnosed cases, 1963-1982. Arthritis Rheum 40:441-445, 1997.

7. **Mayes MD, Lacey JV Jr, Beebe-Dimmer J, et al: Prevalence, incidence, survival, and disease characteristics of systemic sclerosis in a large US population. Arthritis Rheum 48:2246-2255, 2003.**

8. Hopkinson N: Prevalence of scleroderma in South East England. Rheumatology S64, 2000 (abstract).

9. Allcock RJ, Forrest I, Corris PA, et al: A study of the prevalence of systemic sclerosis in northeast England. Rheumatology (Oxf) 43: 596-602, 2004.

10. Maricq HR, Weinrich MC, Keil JE, et al: Prevalence of scleroderma spectrum disorders in the general population of South Carolina. Arthritis Rheum 32:998-1006, 1989.

11. Nietert PJ, Mitchell HC, Bolster MB, et al: Racial variation in clinical and immunological manifestations of systemic sclerosis. J Rheumatol 33:263-268, 2006.

12. Feghali-Bostwick C, Medsger TA Jr, Wright TM: Analysis of systemic sclerosis in twins reveals low concordance for disease and high concordance for the presence of antinuclear antibodies. Arthritis Rheum 48:1956-1963, 2003.

13. Arnett FC, Cho M, Chatterjee S, et al: Familial occurrence frequencies and relative risks for systemic sclerosis (scleroderma) in three United States cohorts. Arthritis Rheum 44:1359-1362, 2001.

14. Maddison PJ, Skinner RP, Pereira RS, et al: Antinuclear antibodies in the relatives and spouses of patients with systemic sclerosis. Ann Rheum Dis 45:793-799, 1986.

15. Arnett FC, Howard RF, Tan F, et al: Increased prevalence of systemic sclerosis in a Native American tribe in Oklahoma. Arthritis Rheum 39:1362-1370, 1996.

16. Ahmed SS, Tan FK: Identification of novel targets in scleroderma: Update on population studies, cDNA arrays, SNP analysis, and mutations. Curr Opin Rheumatol 15:766-771, 2003.

17. Pandey JP, LeRoy EC: Human cytomegalovirus and the vasculopathies of autoimmune diseases (especially scleroderma), allograft rejection, and coronary restenosis. Arthritis Rheum 41:10-15, 1998.

18. Neidhart M, Kuchen S, Distler O, et al: Increased serum levels of antibodies against human cytomegalovirus and prevalence of autoantibodies in systemic sclerosis. Arthritis Rheum 42:389-392, 1999.

19. Namboodiri AM, Rocca KM, Kuwana M, et al: Antibodies to human cytomegalovirus protein UL83 in systemic sclerosis. Clin Exp Rheumatol 24:176-178, 2006.

20. Namboodiri AM, Rocca KM, Pandey JP: IgG antibodies to human cytomegalovirus late protein UL94 in patients with systemic sclerosis. Autoimmunity 37:241-244, 2004.

21. Muryoi T, Kasturi KN, Kafina MJ, et al: Antitopoisomerase I monoclonal autoantibodies from scleroderma patients and tight skin mouse interact with similar epitopes. J Exp Med 175:1103-1109, 1992.

22. Lunardi C, Dolcino M, Peterlana D, et al: Antibodies against human cytomegalovirus in the pathogenesis of systemic sclerosis: A gene array approach. PLoS Med 3:e2, 2006.

23. Lunardi C, Bason C, Navone R, et al: Systemic sclerosis immunoglobulin G autoantibodies bind the human cytomegalovirus late protein UL94 and induce apoptosis in human endothelial cells. Nat Med 6:1183-1186, 2000.

24. Markiewicz M, Smith EA, Rubinchik S, et al: The 72-kilodalton IE-1 protein of human cytomegalovirus (HCMV) is a potent inducer of connective tissue growth factor (CTGF) in human dermal fibroblasts. Clin Exp Rheumatol 22(3 Suppl 33):S31-S34, 2004.

25. Ferri C, Zakrzewska K, Longombardo G, et al: Parvovirus B19 infection of bone marrow in systemic sclerosis patients. Clin Exp Rheumatol 17:718-720, 1999.

26. Ghinoi A, Mascia MT, Giuggioli D, et al: Coexistence of non-specific and usual interstitial pneumonia in a patient with severe cystic scleroderma lung involvement and parvovirus B19 infection. Clin Exp Rheumatol 23:431-433, 2005.

27. Tabuenca JM: Toxic-allergic syndrome caused by ingestion of rapeseed oil denatured with aniline. Lancet 2:567-568, 1981.

28. Varga J, Schumacher HR, Jimenez SA: Systemic sclerosis after augmentation mammaplasty with silicone implants. Ann Intern Med 111:377-383, 1989.

29. Hertzman PA, Blevins WL, Mayer J, et al: Association of the eosinophilia-myalgia syndrome with the ingestion of tryptophan. N Engl J Med 322:869-873, 1990.

30. Silver RM, Heyes MP, Maize JC, et al: Scleroderma, fasciitis, and eosinophilia associated with the ingestion of tryptophan. N Engl J Med 322:874-881, 1990.

31. Mori Y, Kahari VM, Varga J: Scleroderma-like cutaneous syndromes. Curr Rheumatol Rep 4:113-122, 2002.

32. Nietert PJ, Sutherland SE, Silver RM, et al: Is occupational organic solvent exposure a risk factor for scleroderma? Arthritis Rheum 41:1111-1118, 1998.

33. Diot E, Lesire V, Guilmot JL, et al: Systemic sclerosis and occupational risk factors: A case-control study. Occup Environ Med 59: 545-549, 2002.

34. Garabrant DH, Lacey JV Jr, Laing TJ, et al: Scleroderma and solvent exposure among women. Am J Epidemiol 157:493-500, 2003.

35. Maitre A, Hours M, Bonneterre V, et al: Systemic sclerosis and occupational risk factors: Role of solvents and cleaning products. J Rheumatol 31:2395-2401, 2004.

36. Bovenzi M, Barbone F, Pisa FE, et al: A case-control study of occupational exposures and systemic sclerosis. Int Arch Occup Environ Health 77:10-16, 2004.

37. Janowsky EC, Kupper LL, Hulka BS: Meta-analyses of the relation between silicone breast implants and the risk of connective-tissue diseases. N Engl J Med 342:781-790, 2000.

38. Hochberg MC, Perlmutter DL, Medsger TA Jr, et al: Lack of association between augmentation mammoplasty and systemic sclerosis (scleroderma). Arthritis Rheum 39:1125-1131, 1996.

39. Burns CJ, Laing TJ, Gillespie BW, et al: The epidemiology of scleroderma among women: Assessment of risk from exposure to silicone and silica. J Rheumatol 23:1904-1911, 1996.

40. Varga J, Haustein UF, Creech RH, et al: Exaggerated radiation-induced fibrosis in patients with systemic sclerosis. JAMA 265: 3292-3295, 1991.

41. Darras-Joly C, Wechsler B, Bletry O, et al: De novo systemic sclerosis after radiotherapy: A report of 3 cases. J Rheumatol 26:2265-2267, 1999.

42. **D'Angelo WA, Fries JF, Masi AT, et al: Pathologic observations in systemic sclerosis (scleroderma): A study of fifty-eight autopsy cases and fifty-eight matched controls. Am J Med 46:428-440, 1969.**

43. Freemont AJ, Hoyland J, Fielding P, et al: Studies of the microvascular endothelium in uninvolved skin of patients with systemic sclerosis: Direct evidence for a generalized microangiopathy. Br J Dermatol 126:561-568, 1992.

44. Prescott RJ, Freemont AJ, Jones CJ, et al: Sequential dermal microvascular and perivascular changes in the development of scleroderma. J Pathol 166:255-263, 1992.

45. Kahaleh MB: Endothelin, an endothelial-dependent vasoconstrictor in scleroderma: Enhanced production and profibrotic action. Arthritis Rheum 34:978-983, 1991.

46. Varga J, Heiman-Patterson TD, Emery DL, et al: Clinical spectrum of the systemic manifestations of the eosinophilia-myalgia syndrome. Semin Arthritis Rheum 19:313-328, 1990.

47. Yousem SA: The pulmonary pathologic manifestations of the CREST syndrome. Hum Pathol 21:467-474, 1990.

48. Hawkins RA, Claman HN, Clark RA, et al: Increased dermal mast cell populations in progressive systemic sclerosis: A link in chronic fibrosis? Ann Intern Med 102:182-186, 1985.

49. Cox D, Earle L, Jimenez SA, et al: Elevated levels of eosinophil major basic protein in the sera of patients with systemic sclerosis. Arthritis Rheum 38:939-945, 1995.

50. Varga J, Bashey RI: Regulation of connective tissue synthesis in systemic sclerosis. Int Rev Immunol 12(2-4):187-199, 1995.

51. Jelaska A, Korn JH: Role of apoptosis and transforming growth factor beta1 in fibroblast selection and activation in systemic sclerosis. Arthritis Rheum 43:2230-2239, 2000.

52. Davies CA, Jeziorska M, Freemont AJ, et al: The differential expression of VEGF, VEGFR-2, and GLUT-1 proteins in disease subtypes of systemic sclerosis. Hum Pathol 37:190-197, 2006.

53. Rudnicka L, Varga J, Christiano AM, et al: Elevated expression of type VII collagen in the skin of patients with systemic sclerosis: Regulation by TGF-β. J Clin Invest 93:1709-1715, 1994.

54. van der Slot AJ, Zuurmond AM, Bardoel AF, et al: Identification of PLOD2 as telopeptide lysyl hydroxylase, an important enzyme in fibrosis. J Biol Chem 278:40967-40972, 2003.

55. **Whitfield ML, Finlay DR, Murray JI, et al: Systemic and cell type-specific gene expression patterns in scleroderma skin. Proc Natl Acad Sci U S A 100:12319-12324, 2003.**

56. Gardner H, Shearstone JR, Bandaru R, et al: Gene profiling of scleroderma skin reveals robust signatures of disease that are imperfectly reflected in the transcript profiles of explanted fibroblasts. Arthritis Rheum 54:1961-1973, 2006.

57. Kim DS, Yoo B, Lee JS, et al: The major histopathologic pattern of pulmonary fibrosis in scleroderma is nonspecific interstitial pneumonia. Sarcoidosis Vasc Diffuse Lung Dis 19:121-127, 2002.

58. Bouros D, Wells AU, Nicholson AG, et al: Histopathologic subsets of fibrosing alveolitis in patients with systemic sclerosis and their relationship to outcome. Am J Respir Crit Care Med 165:1581-1586, 2002.

59. Roberts CG, Hummers LK, Ravich WJ, et al: A case-controlled study of the pathology of oesophageal disease in systemic sclerosis (scleroderma). Gut 55:1697-1703, 2006.

60. Wipff J, Allanore Y, Soussi F, et al: Prevalence of Barrett's esophagus in systemic sclerosis. Arthritis Rheum 52:2882-2888, 2005.

61. Katzka DA, Reynolds JC, Saul SH, et al: Barrett's metaplasia and adenocarcinoma of the esophagus in scleroderma. Am J Med 82:46-52, 1987.

62. Fisher ER, Rodnan GP: Pathologic observations concerning the kidney in progressive systemic sclerosis. AMA Arch Pathol 65:29-39, 1958.

63. Trostle DC, Bedetti CD, Steen VD, et al: Renal vascular histology and morphometry in systemic sclerosis: A case-control autopsy study. Arthritis Rheum 31:393-400, 1988.

64. Kovalchik MT, Guggenheim SJ, Silverman MH, et al: The kidney in progressive systemic sclerosis: A prospective study. Ann Intern Med 89:881-887, 1978.

65. Follansbee WP, Zerbe TR: Medsger TA Jr: Cardiac and skeletal muscle disease in systemic sclerosis (scleroderma): A high risk association. Am Heart J 125:194-203, 1993.

66. Fernandes F, Ramires FJ, Arteaga E, et al: Cardiac remodeling in patients with systemic sclerosis with no signs or symptoms of heart failure: An endomyocardial biopsy study. J Card Fail 9:311-317, 2003.

67. Murata I, Takenaka K, Shinohara S, et al: Diversity of myocardial involvement in systemic sclerosis: An 8-year study of 95 Japanese patients. Am Heart J 135(6 Pt 1):960-969, 1998.

68. Kerr LD, Spiera H: Myocarditis as a complication in scleroderma patients with myositis. Clin Cardiol 16:895-899, 1993.

69. Clemson BS, Miller WR, Luck JC, et al: Acute myocarditis in fulminant systemic sclerosis. Chest 101:872-874, 1992.

70. Varga J, Abraham DJ: Systemic sclerosis: Paradigm multisystem fibrosing disorder. J Clin Invest 117:557-567, 2007.

71. Jimenez SA, Derk CT: Following the molecular pathways toward an understanding of the pathogenesis of systemic sclerosis. Ann Intern Med 140:37-50, 2004.

72. Gordon MB, Klein I, Dekker A, et al: Thyroid disease in progressive systemic sclerosis: Increased frequency of glandular fibrosis and hypothyroidism. Ann Intern Med 95:431-435, 1981.

73. De Keyser L, Narhi DC, Furst DE, et al: Thyroid dysfunction in a prospectively followed series of patients with progressive systemic sclerosis. J Endocrinol Invest 13:161-169, 1990.

74. Kahl LE, Medsger TA Jr, Klein I: Prospective evaluation of thyroid function in patients with systemic sclerosis (scleroderma). J Rheumatol 13:103-107, 1986.

75. Nehra A, Hall SJ, Basile G, et al: Systemic sclerosis and impotence: A clinicopathological correlation. J Urol 153:1140-1146, 1995.

76. Schumacher HR Jr: Joint involvement in progressive systemic sclerosis (scleroderma): A light and electron microscopic study of synovial membrane and fluid. Am J Clin Pathol 60:593-600, 1973.

77. Clark SH: Animal models in scleroderma. Curr Rheumatol Rep 7:150-155, 2005.

78. Baxter RM, Crowell TP, McCrann ME, et al: Analysis of the tight skin (Tsk1/+) mouse as a model for testing antifibrotic agents. Lab Invest 85:1199, 2005.

79. Siracusa LD, McGrath R, Ma Q, et al: A tandem duplication within the fibrillin 1 gene is associated with the mouse tight skin mutation. Genome Res 6:300-313, 1996.

80. Neptune ER, Frischmeyer PA, Arking DE, et al: Dysregulation of TGF-beta activation contributes to pathogenesis in Marfan syndrome. Nat Genet 33:407-411, 2003.

81. Lemaire R, Farina G, Kissin E, et al: Mutant fibrillin 1 from tight skin mice increases extracellular matrix incorporation of microfibril-associated glycoprotein 2 and type I collagen. Arthritis Rheum 50:915-926, 2004.

82. Wallis DD, Tan FK, Kielty CM, et al: Abnormalities in fibrillin 1-containing microfibrils in dermal fibroblast cultures from patients with systemic sclerosis. Arthritis Rheum 44:1855-1864, 2001.

83. Christner PJ, Peters J, Hawkins D, et al: The tight skin 2 mouse: An animal model of scleroderma displaying cutaneous fibrosis and mononuclear cell infiltration. Arthritis Rheum 38:1791-1798, 1995.

84. Gentiletti J, McCloskey LJ, Artlett CM, et al: Demonstration of autoimmunity in the tight skin-2 mouse: A model for scleroderma. J Immunol 175:2418-2426, 2005.

85. Yamamoto T, Takagawa S, Katayama I, et al: Animal model of sclerotic skin, I: Local injections of bleomycin induce sclerotic skin mimicking scleroderma. J Invest Dermatol 112:456-462, 1999.

86. Takagawa S, Lakos G, Mori Y, et al: Sustained activation of fibroblast transforming growth factor-beta/Smad signaling in a murine model of SSc. J Invest Dermatol 121:41-50, 2003.

87. Lakos G, Takagawa S, Chen SJ, et al: Targeted disruption of TGF-beta/Smad3 signaling modulates skin fibrosis in a mouse model of scleroderma. Am J Pathol 165:203-217, 2004.

88. Ferreira AM, Takagawa S, Fresco R, et al: Diminished induction of skin fibrosis in mice with MCP-1 deficiency. J Invest Dermatol 126:1900-1908, 2006.

89. Chujo S, Shirasaki F, Kawara S, et al: Connective tissue growth factor causes persistent proalpha2(I) collagen gene expression induced by transforming growth factor-beta in a mouse fibrosis model. J Cell Physiol 203:447-456, 2005.

90. Zhang Y, McCormick LL, Desai SR, et al: Murine sclerodermatous graft-versus-host disease, a model for human scleroderma: cutaneous cytokines, chemokines, and immune cell activation. J Immunol 168:3088-3098, 2002.

91. Ruzek MC, Jha S, Ledbetter S, et al: A modified model of graft-versus-host-induced systemic sclerosis (scleroderma) exhibits all major aspects of the human disease. Arthritis Rheum 50:1319-1331, 2004.

92. Denton CP, Lindahl GE, Khan K, et al: Activation of key profibrotic mechanisms in transgenic fibroblasts expressing kinase-deficient type II Transforming growth factor-β receptor (TβRIIδk). J Biol Chem 280:16053-16065, 2005.

93. Samuel CS, Zhao C, Yang Q, et al: The relaxin gene knockout mouse: A model of progressive scleroderma. J Invest Dermatol 125:692-699, 2005.

94. Sonnylal S, Denton CP, Zheng B, et al: Postnatal induction of transforming growth factor beta signaling in fibroblasts of mice recapitulates clinical, histologic, and biochemical features of scleroderma. Arthritis Rheum 56:334-344, 2007.

95. Charles C, Clements P, Furst DE: Systemic sclerosis: Hypothesis-driven treatment strategies. Lancet 367:1683-1691, 2006.

96. Kahaleh MB, Sherer GK, LeRoy EC: Endothelial injury in scleroderma. J Exp Med 149:1326-1335, 1979.

97. Cerinic MM, Valentini G, Sorano GG, et al: Blood coagulation, fibrinolysis, and markers of endothelial dysfunction in systemic sclerosis. Semin Arthritis Rheum 32:285-295, 2003.

98. Hummers LK: Microvascular damage in systemic sclerosis: Detection and monitoring with biomarkers. Curr Rheumatol Rep 8:131-137, 2006.

99. Helmbold P, Nayak RC, Marsch WC, et al: Isolation and in vitro characterization of human dermal microvascular pericytes. Microvasc Res 61:160-165, 2001.

100. Rajkumar VS, Sundberg C, Abraham DJ, et al: Activation of microvascular pericytes in autoimmune Raynaud's phenomenon and systemic sclerosis. Arthritis Rheum 42:930-941, 1999.

101. Rajkumar VS, Howell K, Csiszar K, et al: Shared expression of phenotypic markers in systemic sclerosis indicates a convergence of pericytes and fibroblasts to a myofibroblast lineage in fibrosis. Arthritis Res Ther 7:R1113-R1123, 2005.

102. Vancheeswaran R, Azam A, Black C, et al: Localization of endothelin-1 and its binding sites in scleroderma skin. J Rheumatol 21:1268-1276, 1994.

103. Cambrey AD, Harrison NK, Dawes KE, et al: Increased levels of endothelin-1 in bronchoalveolar lavage fluid from patients with systemic sclerosis contribute to fibroblast mitogenic activity in vitro. Am J Respir Cell Mol Biol 11:439-445, 1994.

104. Yamane K, Miyauchi T, Suzuki N, et al: Significance of plasma endothelin-1 levels in patients with systemic sclerosis. J Rheumatol 19:1566-1571, 1992.

104a. Del Galdo F, Maul GG, Jiménez SA, Artlett CM. Expression of allograft inflammatory factor 1 in tissues from patients with systemic sclerosis and in vitro differential expression of its isoforms in response to transforming growth factor beta. Arthritis Rheum 54:2616-2625, 2006.

104b. Fleming JN, Nash RA, McLeod DO, et al: Capillary regeneration in scleroderma: Stem cell therapy reverses phenotype? PLoS ONE. Jan 16; 3:e1452, 2008.

105. Hebbar M, Peyrat JP, Hornez L, et al: Increased concentrations of the circulating angiogenesis inhibitor endostatin in patients with systemic sclerosis. Arthritis Rheum 43:889-893, 2000.

106. Distler O, Distler JH, Scheid A, et al: Uncontrolled expression of vascular endothelial growth factor and its receptors leads to insufficient skin angiogenesis in patients with systemic sclerosis. Circ Res 95:109-116, 2004.

107. Distler O, Del Rosso A, Giacomelli R, et al: Angiogenic and angiostatic factors in systemic sclerosis: Increased levels of vascular endothelial growth factor are a feature of the earliest disease stages and are associated with the absence of fingertip ulcers. Arthritis Res 4:R11, 2002.

108. Kuwana M, Okazaki Y, Yasuoka H, et al: Defective vasculogenesis in systemic sclerosis. Lancet 364:603-610, 2004.

109. Kuwana M, Kaburaki J, Okazaki Y, et al: Increase in circulating endothelial precursors by atorvastatin in patients with systemic sclerosis. Arthritis Rheum 54:1946-1951, 2006.

110. Del Papa ND, Quirici N, Soligo D, et al: Bone marrow endothelial progenitors are defective in systemic sclerosis. Arthritis Rheum 54:2605-2615, 2006.

111. Roumm AD, Whiteside TL, Medsger TA Jr, et al: Lymphocytes in the skin of patients with progressive systemic sclerosis: Quantification, subtyping, and clinical correlations. Arthritis Rheum 27:645-653, 1984.

112. Kalogerou A, Gelou E, Mountantonakis S, et al: Early T cell activation in the skin from patients with systemic sclerosis. Ann Rheum Dis 64:1233-1235, 2005.

113. Kahari VM, Sandberg M, Kalimo H, et al: Identification of fibroblasts responsible for increased collagen production in localized scleroderma by in situ hybridization. J Invest Dermatol 90:664-670, 1988.

114. Sakkas LI, Xu B, Artlett CM, et al: Oligoclonal T cell expansion in the skin of patients with systemic sclerosis. J Immunol 168:3649-3659, 2002.

115. Yurovsky VV, Wigley FM, Wise RA, et al: Skewing of the CD8+ T-cell repertoire in the lungs of patients with systemic sclerosis. Hum Immunol 48(1-2):84-97, 1996.

116. Sakkas LI, Platsoucas CD: Is systemic sclerosis an antigen-driven T cell disease? Arthritis Rheum 50:1721-1733, 2004.

117. Piela TH, Korn JH: Lymphocyte-fibroblast adhesion induced by interferon-gamma. Cell Immunol 114:149-160, 1988.

118. Rudnicka L, Majewski S, Blaszczyk M, et al: Adhesion of peripheral blood mononuclear cells to vascular endothelium in patients with systemic sclerosis (scleroderma). Arthritis Rheum 35:771-775, 1992.

119. York MR, Nagai T, Mangini AJ, et al: A macrophage marker, siglec-1, is increased on circulating monocytes in patients with systemic sclerosis and induced by type I interferons and Toll-like receptor agonists. Arthritis Rheum 56:1010-1020, 2007.

120. Tan FK, Zhou X, Mayes MD, et al: Signatures of differentially regulated interferon gene expression and vasculotrophism in the peripheral blood cells of systemic sclerosis patients. Rheumatology (Oxf) 45:694-702, 2006.

121. Wangoo A, Sparer T, Brown IN, et al: Contribution of Th1 and Th2 cells to protection and pathology in experimental models of granulomatous lung disease. J Immunol 166:3432-3439, 2001.

122. Lakos G, Melichian D, Wu M, et al: Increased bleomycin-induced skin fibrosis in mice lacking the Th1-specific transcription factor T-bet. Pathobiology 73:224-237, 2006.

123. Aliprantis AO, Wang J, Fathman JW, et al: Transcription factor T-bet regulates skin sclerosis through its function in innate immunity and via IL-13. Proc Natl Acad Sci U S A 104:2827-2830, 2007.

124. Kantor TV, Friberg D, Medsger TA Jr, et al: Cytokine production and serum levels in systemic sclerosis. Clin Immunol Immunopathol 65:278-285, 1992.

125. Prior C, Haslam PL: In vivo levels and in vitro production of interferon-gamma in fibrosing interstitial lung diseases. Clin Exp Immunol 88:280-287, 1992.

126. Tan FK, Stivers DN, Arnett FC, et al: HLA haplotypes and microsatellite polymorphisms in and around the major histocompatibility complex region in a Native American population with a high preva-

lence of scleroderma (systemic sclerosis). Tissue Antigens 53:74-80, 1999.

127. Mavalia C, Scaletti C, Romagnani P, et al: Type 2 helper T-cell predominance and high CD30 expression in systemic sclerosis. Am J Pathol 151:1751-1758, 1997.

128. Atamas SP, Yurovsky VV, Wise R, et al: Production of type 2 cytokines by CD8+ lung cells is associated with greater decline in pulmonary function in patients with systemic sclerosis. Arthritis Rheum 42:1168-1178, 1999.

129. Luzina IG, Atamas SP, Wise R, et al: Occurrence of an activated, profibrotic pattern of gene expression in lung CD8+ T cells from SSc patients. Arthritis Rheum 48:2262-2274, 2003.

130. Rottoli P, Magi B, Perari MG, et al: Cytokine profile and proteome analysis in bronchoalveolar lavage of patients with sarcoidosis, pulmonary fibrosis associated with systemic sclerosis and idiopathic pulmonary fibrosis. Proteomics 5:1423-1430, 2005.

131. Matsushita T, Hasegawa M, Yanaba K, et al: Elevated serum BAFF levels in patients with systemic sclerosis: Enhanced BAFF signaling in systemic sclerosis B lymphocytes. Arthritis Rheum 54:192-201, 2006.

132. Kraling BM, Maul GG, Jimenez SA: Mononuclear cellular infiltrates in clinically involved skin from patients with systemic sclerosis of recent onset predominantly consist of monocytes/macrophages. Pathobiology 63:48-56, 1995.

133. Hamilton RF Jr, Parsley E, Holian A: Alveolar macrophages from systemic sclerosis patients: Evidence for IL-4-mediated phenotype changes. Am J Physiol Lung Cell Mol Physiol 286:L1202-L1209, 2004.

134. Hu PQ, Fertig N, Medsger TA Jr, et al: Correlation of serum anti-DNA topoisomerase I antibody levels with disease severity and activity in systemic sclerosis. Arthritis Rheum 48:1363-1373, 2003.

135. Casciola-Rosen L, Wigley F, Rosen A: Scleroderma autoantigens are uniquely fragmented by metal-catalyzed oxidation reactions: Implications for pathogenesis. J Exp Med 185:71-79, 1997.

136. Harris ML, Rosen A: Autoimmunity in scleroderma: The origin, pathogenetic role, and clinical significance of autoantibodies. Curr Opin Rheumatol 15:778-784, 2003.

137. Carvalho D, Savage CO, Black CM, et al: IgG antiendothelial cell autoantibodies from scleroderma patients induce leukocyte adhesion to human vascular endothelial cells in vitro: Induction of adhesion molecule expression and involvement of endothelium-derived cytokines. J Clin Invest 97:111-119, 1996.

138. Baroni SS, Santillo M, Bevilacqua F, et al: Stimulatory autoantibodies to the PDGF receptor in systemic sclerosis. N Engl J Med 354:2667-2676, 2006.

139. Henault J, Robitaille G, Senecal JL, et al: DNA topoisomerase I binding to fibroblasts induces monocyte adhesion and activation in the presence of anti-topoisomerase I autoantibodies from systemic sclerosis patients. Arthritis Rheum 54:963-973, 2006.

140. Sato S, Hasegawa M, Fujimoto M, et al: Quantitative genetic variation in CD19 expression correlates with autoimmunity. J Immunol 165:6635-6643, 2000.

141. Ramirez F, Tanaka S, Bou-Gharios G: Transcriptional regulation of the human alpha 2(I) collagen gene (COL1A2), an informative model system to study fibrotic diseases. Matrix Biol 25:365-372, 2006.

142. Ghosh AK, Varga J: Transcriptional coactivators p300/CBP and Type I collagen gene expression. Curr Sci 85:155-161, 2003.

143. Pannu J, Trojanowska M: Recent advances in fibroblast signaling and biology in scleroderma. Curr Opin Rheumatol 16:739-745, 2004.

144. Chang HY, Chi JT, Dudoit S, et al: Diversity, topographic differentiation, and positional memory in human fibroblasts. Proc Natl Acad Sci U S A 99:12877-12882, 2002.

145. Rinn JL, Bondre C, Gladstone HB, et al: Anatomic demarcation by positional variation in fibroblast gene expression programs. PLoS Genet 2:e119, 2006.

146. Tomasek JJ, Gabbiani G, Hinz B, et al: Myofibroblasts and mechanoregulation of connective tissue remodelling. Nat Rev Mol Cell Biol 3:349-363, 2002.

147. Kirk TZ, Mark ME, Chua CC, et al: Myofibroblasts from scleroderma skin synthesize elevated levels of collagen and tissue inhibitor of metalloproteinase (TIMP-1) with two forms of TIMP-1. J Biol Chem 270:3423-3428, 1995.

147a. Wipff PJ, Rifkin DB, Meister JJ, Hinz B: Myofibroblast contraction activates latent TGF-beta1 from the extracellular matrix. J Cell Biol 179:1311-1323, 2007.

148. Kalluri R, Neilson EG: Epithelial-mesenchymal transition and its implications for fibrosis. J Clin Invest 112:1776-1784, 2003.

149. Abe R, Donnelly SC, Peng T, et al: Peripheral blood fibrocytes: Differentiation pathway and migration to wound sites. J Immunol 166:7556-7562, 2001.

150. Phillips RJ, Burdick MD, Hong K, et al: Circulating fibrocytes traffic to the lungs in response to CXCL12 and mediate fibrosis. J Clin Invest 114:438-446, 2004.

151. Quan TE, Cowper SE, Bucala R: The role of circulating fibrocytes in fibrosis. Curr Rheumatol Rep 8:145-150, 2006.

152. Postlethwaite AE, Shigemitsu H, Kanangat S: Cellular origins of fibroblasts: Possible implications for organ fibrosis in systemic sclerosis. Curr Opin Rheumatol 16:733-738, 2004.

153. Denton CP, Abraham DJ: Transforming growth factor-beta and connective tissue growth factor: Key cytokines in scleroderma pathogenesis. Curr Opin Rheumatol 13:505-511, 2001.

154. Mauviel A: Transforming growth factor-beta: A key mediator of fibrosis. Methods Mol Med 117:69-80, 2005.

155. Massague J, Seoane J, Wotton D: Smad transcription factors. Genes Dev 19:2783-2810, 2005.

156. Moustakas A, Heldin CH: Non-Smad TGF-beta signals. J Cell Sci 118:3573-3584, 2005.

157. Varga J: SSc and Smads: Dysfunctional Smad family dynamics culminating in fibrosis. Arthritis Rheum 46:1703-1713, 2002.

158. Igarashi A, Nashiro K, Kikuchi K, et al: Connective tissue growth factor gene expression in tissue sections from localized scleroderma, keloid, and other fibrotic skin disorders. J Invest Dermatol 106:729-733, 1996.

159. Leask A, Abraham DJ: The role of connective tissue growth factor, a multifunctional matricellular protein, in fibroblast biology. Biochem Cell Biol 81:355-363, 2003.

160. Chujo S, Shirasaki F, Kawara S, et al: Connective tissue growth factor causes persistent proalpha2(I) collagen gene expression induced by transforming growth factor-beta in a mouse fibrosis model. J Cell Physiol 203:447-456, 2005.

161. Klareskog L, Gustafsson R, Scheynius A, et al: Increased expression of platelet-derived growth factor type B receptors in the skin of patients with systemic sclerosis. Arthritis Rheum 33:1534-1541, 1990.

162. Ludwicka A, Ohba T, Trojanowska M, et al: Elevated levels of platelet derived growth factor and transforming growth factor-beta 1 in bronchoalveolar lavage fluid from patients with scleroderma. J Rheumatol 22:1876-1883, 1995.

163. Hasegawa M, Fujimoto M, Kikuchi K, et al: Elevated serum levels of interleukin 4 (IL-4), IL-10, and IL-13 in patients with systemic sclerosis. J Rheumatol 24:328-332, 1997.

164. Tsuji-Yamada J, Nakazawa M, Minami M, et al: Increased frequency of interleukin 4 producing CD4+ and CD8+ cells in peripheral blood from patients with systemic sclerosis. J Rheumatol 28:1252-1273, 2001.

165. Sato S, Hasegawa M, Takehara K: Serum levels of interleukin-6 and interleukin-10 correlate with total skin thickness score in patients with systemic sclerosis. J Dermatol Sci 27:140-146, 2001.

166. Fichtner-Feigl S, Fuss IJ, Young CA, et al: Induction of IL-13 triggers TGF-beta1-dependent tissue fibrosis in chronic 2,4,6-trinitrobenzene sulfonic acid colitis. J Immunol 178:5859-5870, 2007.

167. Jinnin M, Ihn H, Yamane K, et al: Interleukin-13 stimulates the transcription of the human alpha2(I) collagen gene in human dermal fibroblasts. J Biol Chem 279:41783-41791, 2004.

168. Kaviratne M, Hesse M, Leusink M, et al: IL-13 activates a mechanism of tissue fibrosis that is completely TGF-beta independent. J Immunol 173:4020-4029, 2004.

169. Chizzolini C: Update on pathophysiology of scleroderma with special reference to immuno-inflammatory events. Ann Med 39:42-53, 2007.

170. Galindo M, Santiago B, Rivero M, et al: Chemokine expression by systemic sclerosis fibroblasts: Abnormal regulation of monocyte chemoattractant protein 1 expression. Arthritis Rheum 44:1382-1386, 2001.

171. Kodera M, Hasegawa M, Komura K, et al: Serum pulmonary and activation-regulated chemokine/CCL18 levels in patients with systemic sclerosis: A sensitive indicator of active pulmonary fibrosis. Arthritis Rheum 52:2889-2896, 2005.

172. Carulli MT, Ong VH, Ponticos M, et al: Chemokine receptor CCR2 expression by systemic sclerosis fibroblasts: Evidence for autocrine regulation of myofibroblast differentiation. Arthritis Rheum 52:3772-3782, 2005.

173. Ong VH, Evans LA, Shiwen X, et al: Monocyte chemoattractant protein 3 as a mediator of fibrosis: Overexpression in systemic sclerosis and the type 1 tight-skin mouse. Arthritis Rheum 48:1979-1991, 2003.

174. Ghahary A, Shen Q, Shen YJ, et al: Induction of transforming growth factor beta 1 by insulin-like growth factor-1 in dermal fibroblasts. J Cell Physiol 174:301-309, 1998.

175. Harrison NK, Glanville AR, Strickland B, et al: Pulmonary involvement in systemic sclerosis: The detection of early changes by thin section CT scan, bronchoalveolar lavage and 99mTc-DTPA clearance. Respir Med 83:403-414, 1989.

176. Yasuoka H, Jukic DM, Zhou Z, et al: Insulin-like growth factor binding protein 5 induces skin fibrosis: A novel murine model for dermal fibrosis. Arthritis Rheum 54:3001-3010, 2006.

177. Asano Y, Ihn H, Yamane K, et al: Involvement of alphavbeta5 integrin-mediated activation of latent transforming growth factor beta1 in autocrine TGF beta signaling in systemic sclerosis fibroblasts. Arthritis Rheum 52:2897-2905, 2005.

178. Dong C, Zhu S, Wang T, et al: Deficient Smad7 expression: A putative molecular defect in scleroderma. Proc Natl Acad Sci U S A 99:3908-3913, 2002.

179. Czuwara-Ladykowska J, Shirasaki F, Jackers P, et al: Fli-1 inhibits collagen type I production in dermal fibroblasts via an Sp1-dependent pathway. J Biol Chem 276:20839-20848, 2001.

180. Yuan W, Yufit T, Li L, et al: Negative modulation of alpha1(I) procollagen gene expression in human skin fibroblasts: Transcriptional inhibition by interferon-gamma. J Cell Physiol 179:97-108, 1999.

181. Higashi K, Inagaki Y, Suzuki N, et al: Y-box binding protein YB-1 mediates transcriptional repression of human alpha 2(I) collagen gene expression by interferon-gamma. J Biol Chem 278:5156-5162, 2003. [Erratum in 278:12598, 2003].

182. Chizzolini C, Rezzonico R, Ribbens C, et al: Inhibition of type I collagen production by dermal fibroblasts upon contact with activated T cells: Different sensitivity to inhibition between systemic sclerosis and control fibroblasts. Arthritis Rheum 41:2039-2047, 1998.

183. Hunzelmann N, Anders S, Fierlbeck G, et al: Systemic scleroderma: Multicenter trial of 1 year of treatment with recombinant interferon gamma. Arch Dermatol 133:609-613, 1997.

184. Polisson RP, Gilkeson GS, Pyun EH, et al: A multicenter trial of recombinant human interferon gamma in patients with systemic sclerosis: Effects on cutaneous fibrosis and interleukin 2 receptor levels. J Rheumatol 23:654-658, 1996.

185. Freundlich B, Jimenez SA, Steen VD, et al: Treatment of systemic sclerosis with recombinant interferon-gamma: A phase I/II clinical trial. Arthritis Rheum 35:1134-1142, 1992.

186. Mimura Y, Ihn H, Jinnin M, et al: Constitutive phosphorylation of focal adhesion kinase is involved in the myofibroblast differentiation of SSc fibroblasts. J Invest Dermatol 124:886-892, 2005.

187. Santiago B, Galindo M, Rivero M, et al: Decreased susceptibility to Fas-induced apoptosis of systemic sclerosis dermal fibroblasts. Arthritis Rheum 44:1667-1676, 2001.

188. Kawakami T, Ihn H, Xu W, et al: Increased expression of TGF-beta receptors by scleroderma fibroblasts: Evidence for contribution of autocrine TGF-beta signaling to scleroderma phenotype. J Invest Dermatol 110:47-51, 1998.

189. Yamane K, Ihn H, Kubo M, et al: Increased transcriptional activities of transforming growth factor beta receptors in scleroderma fibroblasts. Arthritis Rheum 46:2421-2428, 2002.

190. Pannu J, Gardner H, Shearstone JR, et al: Increased levels of transforming growth factor beta receptor type I and up-regulation of matrix gene program: A model of scleroderma. Arthritis Rheum 54:3011-3021, 2006.

191. Mimura Y, Ihn H, Jinnin M, et al: Constitutive thrombospondin-1 overexpression contributes to autocrine TGF-beta signaling in cultured scleroderma fibroblasts. Am J Pathol 166:1451-1463, 2005.

192. Yamane K, Miyauchi T, Suzuki N, et al: Significance of plasma endothelin-1 levels in patients with systemic sclerosis. J Rheumatol 19:1566-1571, 1992.

193. Bhattacharyya S, Ghosh AK, Pannu J, et al: Fibroblast expression of the coactivator p300 governs the intensity of profibrotic response to transforming growth factor beta. Arthritis Rheum 52:1248-1258, 2005.

194. Ihn H, Yamane K, Asano Y, et al: Constitutively phosphorylated Smad3 interacts with Sp1 and p300 in scleroderma fibroblasts. Rheumatology (Oxf) 45:157-165, 2006.

195. Kubo M, Czuwara-Ladykowska J, Moussa O, et al: Persistent down-regulation of Fli1, a suppressor of collagen transcription, in fibrotic scleroderma skin. Am J Pathol 163:571-581, 2003.

196. Wang Y, Fan PS, Kahaleh B: Association between enhanced type I collagen expression and epigenetic repression of the FLI1 gene in scleroderma fibroblasts. Arthritis Rheum 54:2271-2279, 2006.

196a. Clements PJ, Lachenbruch PA, Ng SC, et al: Skin score: A semiquantitative measure of cutaneous involvement that improves prediction of prognosis in systemic sclerosis. Arthritis Rheum 33:1256-1263, 1990.

196b. Moore TL, Lunt M, McManus B, et al: Seventeen-point dermal ultrasound scoring system—a reliable measure of skin thickness in patients with sclerosis. Rheumatology (Oxf), 42:1559-1563, 2003.

197. Balbir-Gurman A, Denton CP, Nichols B, et al: Non-invasive measurement of biomechanical skin properties in systemic sclerosis. Ann Rheum Dis 61:237-241, 2002.

198. Kissin EY, Schiller AM, Gelbard RB, et al: Durometry for the assessment of skin disease in systemic sclerosis. Arthritis Rheum 55:603-609, 2006.

199. Korn JH, Mayes M, Matucci Cerinic M, et al: Digital ulcers in systemic sclerosis: Prevention by treatment with bosentan, an oral endothelin receptor antagonist. Arthritis Rheum 50:3985-3993, 2004.

200. Walker JG, Stirling J, Beroukas D, et al: Histopathological and ultrastructural features of dermal telangiectasias in systemic sclerosis. Pathology 37:220-225, 2005.

201. Anderson ME, Allen PD, Moore T, et al: Computerized nailfold video capillaroscopy—a new tool for assessment of Raynaud's phenomenon. J Rheumatol 32:841-848, 2005.

202. Herrick AL: Pathogenesis of Raynaud's phenomenon. Rheumatology (Oxf) 44:587-596, 2005.

203. Carpentier PH, Satger B, Poensin D, et al: Incidence and natural history of Raynaud phenomenon: A long-term follow-up (14 years) of a random sample from the general population. J Vasc Surg 44:1023-1028, 2006.

204. Cutolo M, Pizzorni C, Sulli A: Capillaroscopy. Best Pract Res Clin Rheumatol 19:437-452, 2005.

205. Spencer-Green G: Outcomes in primary Raynaud phenomenon: A meta-analysis of the frequency, rates, and predictors of transition to secondary diseases. Arch Intern Med 158:595-600, 1998.

206. LeRoy EC, Medsger TA Jr: Criteria for the classification of early systemic sclerosis. J Rheumatol 28:1573-1576, 2001.

207. Taylor MH, McFadden JA, Bolster MB, et al: Ulnar artery involvement in systemic sclerosis (scleroderma). J Rheumatol 29:102-106, 2002.

208. Fries R, Shariat K, von Wilmowsky H, et al: Sildenafil in the treatment of Raynaud's phenomenon resistant to vasodilatory therapy. Circulation 112:2980-2985, 2005.

209. Gore J, Silver R: Oral sildenafil for the treatment of Raynaud's phenomenon and digital ulcers secondary to systemic sclerosis. Ann Rheum Dis 64:1387, 2005.

210. Cheng KS, Tiwari A, Boutin A, et al: Carotid and femoral arterial wall mechanics in scleroderma. Rheumatology (Oxf) 42:1299-1305, 2003.

211. Youssef P, Englert H, Bertouch J: Large vessel occlusive disease associated with CREST syndrome and scleroderma. Ann Rheum Dis 52:564-569, 1993.

212. Ho M, Veale D, Eastmond C, et al: Macrovascular disease and systemic sclerosis. Ann Rheum Dis 59:39-43, 2000.

212a. Héron E, Fornes P, Rance A, et al: Brain involvement in scleroderma: Two autopsy cases. Stroke 29:719-721, 1998.

213. Greydanus MP, Camilleri M: Abnormal post-cibal gastric and small bowel motility due to neuropathy or myopathy in systemic sclerosis. Gastroenterology 96:110-115, 1989.

214. Dessein PH, Joffe BI, Metz RM, et al: Autonomic dysfunction in systemic sclerosis: Sympathetic overactivity and instability. Am J Med 93:143-150, 1992.

215. Spackman GK: Scleroderma: What the general dentist should know. Gen Dent 47:576-579, 1999.

216. Yarze JC, Varga J, Stampfl D, et al: Esophageal function in systemic sclerosis: A prospective evaluation of motility and acid reflux in 36 patients. Am J Gastroenterol 88:870-876, 1993.

217. Bonino JA, Sharma P: Barrett's esophagus. Curr Opin Gastroenterol 22:406-411, 2006.

218. Sallam H, McNearney TA, Chen JD: Systematic review: Pathophysiology and management of gastrointestinal dysmotility in systemic sclerosis (scleroderma). Aliment Pharmacol Ther 23:691-712, 2006.

219. Sjogren RW: Gastrointestinal motility disorders in scleroderma. Arthritis Rheum 37:1265-1282, 1994.

220. Watson M, Hally RJ, McCue PA, et al: Gastric antral vascular ectasia (watermelon stomach) in patients with systemic sclerosis. Arthritis Rheum 39:341-346, 1996.

221. Yusoff I, Brennan F, Ormonde D, et al: Argon plasma coagulation for treatment of watermelon stomach. Endoscopy 34:407-410, 2002.

222. Calamia KT, Scolapio JS, Viggiano TR: Endoscopic YAG laser treatment of watermelon stomach (gastric antral vascular ectasia) in patients with systemic sclerosis. Clin Exp Rheumatol 18:605-608, 2000.

223. Rigamonti C, Shand LM, Feudjo M, et al: Clinical features and prognosis of primary biliary cirrhosis associated with systemic sclerosis. Gut 55:388-394, 2006.

224. Shawis TN, Chaloner C, Herrick AL, et al: Pancreatic function in systemic sclerosis. Br J Rheumatol 35:298-299, 1996.

225. Steen VD, Medsger TA Jr: The palpable tendon friction rub: An important physical examination finding in patients with systemic sclerosis. Arthritis Rheum 40:1146-1151, 1997.

226. Doran M, Wordsworth P, Bresnihan B, et al: A distinct syndrome including features of systemic sclerosis, erosive rheumatoid arthritis, anti-topoisomerase antibody, and rheumatoid factor. J Rheumatol 28:921-922, 2001.

227. Akesson A, Fiori G, Krieg T, et al: Assessment of skin, joint, tendon and muscle involvement. Clin Exp Rheumatol 21(3 Suppl 29):S5-S8, 2003.

228. Steen VD: Medsger TA Jr: Long-term outcomes of scleroderma renal crisis. Ann Intern Med 133:600-603, 2000.

229. Abbott KC, Trespalacios FC, Welch PG, et al: Scleroderma at end stage renal disease in the United States: Patient characteristics and survival. J Nephrol 15:236-240, 2002.

230. Bulpitt KJ, Clements PJ, Lachenbruch PA, et al: Early undifferentiated connective tissue disease, III: Outcome and prognostic indicators in early scleroderma (systemic sclerosis). Ann Intern Med 118:602-609, 1993.

231. Lee P, Langevitz P, Alderdice CA, et al: Mortality in systemic sclerosis (scleroderma). QJM 82:139-148, 1992.

232. Satoh M, Tokuhira M, Hama N, et al: Massive pericardial effusion in scleroderma: A review of five cases. Br J Rheumatol 34:564-567, 1995.

233. Plazak W, Zabinska-Plazak E, Wojas-Pelc A, et al: Heart structure and function in systemic sclerosis. Eur J Dermatol 12:257-262, 2002.

234. Candell-Riera J, Armadans-Gil L, Simeon CP, et al: Comprehensive noninvasive assessment of cardiac involvement in limited systemic sclerosis. Arthritis Rheum 39:1138-1145, 1996.

235. Armstrong GP, Whalley GA, Doughty RN, et al: Left ventricular function in scleroderma. Br J Rheumatol 35:983-988, 1996.

236. Di Bello V, Ferri C, Giorgi D, et al: Ultrasonic videodensitometric analysis in scleroderma heart disease. Coron Artery Dis 10:103, 1999.

237. Nakajima K, Taki J, Kawano M, et al: Diastolic dysfunction in patients with systemic sclerosis detected by gated myocardial perfusion SPECT: An early sign of cardiac involvement. J Nucl Med 42:183-188, 2001.

238. Alexander EL, Firestein GS, Weiss JL, et al: Reversible cold-induced abnormalities in myocardial perfusion and function in systemic sclerosis. Ann Intern Med 105:661-668, 1986.

239. Morelli S, Piccirillo G, Fimognari F, et al: Twenty-four hour heart period variability in systemic sclerosis. J Rheumatol 23:643-645, 1996.

240. Akram MR, Handler CE, Williams M, et al: Angiographically proven coronary artery disease in scleroderma. Rheumatology (Oxf) 45:1395-1398, 2006.

241. Mukerjee D, St George D, Coleiro B, et al: Prevalence and outcome in systemic sclerosis associated pulmonary arterial hypertension: Application of a registry approach. Ann Rheum Dis 62:1088-1093, 2003.

241a. Karwatowski SP, Chronos NA, Sinclaire H, et al: Effect of systemic sclerosis on left ventricular long-axis motion and left ventricular mass assessed by magnetic resonance. J Cardiovasc Magn Reson 2:109-117, 2000.

242. Latsi PI, Wells AU: Evaluation and management of alveolitis and interstitial lung disease in scleroderma. Curr Opin Rheumatol 15:748-755, 2003.

243. Wells AU, Hansell DM, Rubens MB, et al: Fibrosing alveolitis in systemic sclerosis: Indices of lung function in relation to extent of disease on computed tomography. Arthritis Rheum 40:1229-1236, 1997.

244. Robertson L, Pignone A, Kowal-Bielecka O, et al: Pulmonary arterial hypertension in systemic sclerosis: Diagnostic pathway and therapeutic approach. Ann Rheum Dis 64:804-807, 2005.

245. Desai SR, Veeraraghavan S, Hansell DM, et al: CT features of lung disease in patients with systemic sclerosis: Comparison with idiopathic pulmonary fibrosis and nonspecific interstitial pneumonia. Radiology 232:560-567, 2004.

246. **Tashkin DP, Elashoff R, Clements PJ, et al; Scleroderma Lung Study Research Group: Cyclophosphamide versus placebo in scleroderma lung disease. N Engl J Med 354:2655-2666, 2006.**

247. Hoyles RK, Ellis RW, Wellsbury J, et al: A multicenter, prospective, randomized, double-blind, placebo-controlled trial of corticosteroids and intravenous cyclophosphamide followed by oral azathioprine for the treatment of pulmonary fibrosis in scleroderma. Arthritis Rheum 54:3962-3970, 2006.

248. Nihtyanova SI, Brough GM, Black CM, et al: Mycophenolate mofetil in diffuse cutaneous systemic sclerosis—a retrospective analysis. Rheumatology (Oxf) 46:442-445, 2007.

249. Gerbino AJ, Goss CH, Molitor JA: Effect of mycophenolate mofetil on pulmonary function in scleroderma-associated interstitial lung disease. Chest 133:455-460, 2008.

250. Walter N, Collard HR, King TE Jr: Current perspectives on the treatment of idiopathic pulmonary fibrosis. Proc Am Thorac Soc 3:330-338, 2006.

251. Schachna L, Medsger TA Jr, Dauber JH, et al: Lung transplantation in scleroderma compared with idiopathic pulmonary fibrosis and idiopathic pulmonary arterial hypertension. Arthritis Rheum 54:3954-3961, 2006.

252. Denton CP, Humbert M, Rubin L, et al: Bosentan treatment for pulmonary arterial hypertension related to connective tissue disease: A subgroup analysis of the pivotal clinical trials and their open-label extensions. Ann Rheum Dis 65:1336-1340, 2006.

253. Steen V: Predictors of end stage lung disease in systemic sclerosis. Ann Rheum Dis 62:97-99, 2003.

254. **Steen V, Medsger TA Jr: Predictors of isolated pulmonary hypertension in patients with systemic sclerosis and limited cutaneous involvement. Arthritis Rheum 48:516-522, 2003.**

255. Williams MH, Handler CE, Akram R, et al: Role of N-terminal brain natriuretic peptide (N-TproBNP) in scleroderma-associated pulmonary arterial hypertension. Eur Heart J 27:1485-1494, 2006.

256. Villalba WO, Sampaio-Barros PD, Pereira MC, et al: Six-minute walk test for the evaluation of pulmonary disease severity in scleroderma patients. Chest 131:217-222, 2007.

257. Hachulla E, Gressin V, Guillevin L, et al: Early detection of pulmonary arterial hypertension in systemic sclerosis: A French nationwide prospective multicenter study. Arthritis Rheum 52:3792-3800, 2005.

258. Barst RJ, Langleben D, Frost A, et al: STRIDE-1 Study Group: Sitaxsentan therapy for pulmonary arterial hypertension. Am J Respir Crit Care Med 169:441-447, 2004.

259. Galie N, Ghofrani HA, Torbicki A, et al: Sildenafil Use in Pulmonary Arterial Hypertension (SUPER) Study Group: Sildenafil citrate therapy for pulmonary arterial hypertension. N Engl J Med 353:2148-2157, 2005.

260. Rodnan GP, Benedek TG: An historical account of the study of progressive systemic sclerosis (diffuse scleroderma). Ann Intern Med 57:305-319, 1962.

261. Steen VD, Constantino JP, Shapiro AP, et al: Outcome of renal crisis in systemic sclerosis: Relation to the availability of converting enzyme inhibitors (ACE). Ann Intern Med 113:352-357, 1990.

262. Penn H, Howie A, Kingdon EJ, et al: Scleroderma renal crisis: Patient characteristics and long-term outcomes. Q J Med 100:485-494, 2007.

263. DeMarco PJ, Weisman MH, Seibold JR, et al: Predictors and outcomes of scleroderma renal crisis: The high-dose versus low-dose D-penicillamine in early diffuse systemic sclerosis trial. Arthritis Rheum 46:2983-2989, 2002.

264. Della Bella S, Molteni M, Mocellin C, et al: Novel mode of action of iloprost: In vitro down-regulation of endothelial cell adhesion molecules. Prostaglandins 65(2-3):73-83, 2001.

265. Walker JG, Ahern MJ, Smith MD, et al: Scleroderma renal crisis: Poor outcome despite aggressive antihypertensive treatment. Intern Med J 33(5-6):216-220, 2003.

266. Chang YJ, Spiera H: Renal transplantation in scleroderma. Medicine (Balt) 78:382-385, 1999.

267. Lally EV, Jimenez SA, Kaplan SR: Progressive systemic sclerosis: Mode of presentation, rapidly progressive disease course, and mortality based on an analysis of 91 patients. Semin Arthritis Rheum 18:1-13, 1988.

268. Locke IC, Worrall JG, Leaker B, et al: Autoantibodies to myeloperoxidase in systemic sclerosis. J Rheumatol 24:86-89, 1997.

269. Hillis GS, Khan IH, Simpson JG, et al: Scleroderma, D-penicillamine treatment, and progressive renal failure associated with positive antimyeloperoxidase antineutrophil cytoplasmic antibodies. Am J Kidney Dis 30:279-281, 1997.

270. Hietarinta M, Lassila O, Hietaharju A: Association of anti-U1RNP- and anti-Scl-70-antibodies with neurological manifestations in systemic sclerosis. Scand J Rheumatol 23:64-67, 1994.

271. Gibney EM, Parikh CR, Jani A, et al: Kidney transplantation for systemic sclerosis improves survival and may modulate disease activity. Am J Transplant 4:2027-2031, 2004.

272. Pham PT, Pham PC, Danovitch GM, et al: Predictors and risk factors for recurrent scleroderma renal crisis in the kidney allograft: Case report and review of the literature. Am J Transplant 5:2565-2569, 2005.

273. Coll J, Rives A, Grino MC, et al: Prevalence of Sjogren's syndrome in autoimmune diseases. Ann Rheum Dis 46:286-289, 1987.

274. Valentini G, Bencivelli W, Bombardieri S, et al: European Scleroderma Study Group to define disease activity criteria for systemic sclerosis, III: Assessment of the construct validity of the preliminary activity criteria. Ann Rheum Dis 62:901-903, 2003.

275. Merkel PA, Herlyn K, Martin RW, et al: Scleroderma Clinical Trials Consortium: Measuring disease activity and functional status in patients with scleroderma and Raynaud's phenomenon. Arthritis Rheum 46:2410-2420, 2002.

275a. Medsger TA, Silman AJ, Steen VD, et al: A disease severity scale for systemic sclerosis: developing and testing. J Rheumatol 26(10):2159-2167, 1999.

276. Kuwana M, Inoko H, Kameda H, et al: Association of human leukocyte antigen class II genes with autoantibody profiles, but not with disease susceptibility in Japanese patients with systemic sclerosis. Intern Med 38:336-344, 1999.

277. Bunn CC, Denton CP, Shi-Wen X, et al: Anti-RNA polymerases and other autoantibody specificities in systemic sclerosis. Br J Rheumatol 37:15-20, 1998.

278. Farge D, Passweg J, van Laar JM, et al: EBMT/EULAR Registry: Autologous stem cell transplantation in the treatment of systemic sclerosis: Report from the EBMT/EULAR Registry. Ann Rheum Dis 63:974-981, 2004.

279. Stratton RJ, Wilson H, Black CM: Pilot study of anti-thymocyte globulin plus mycophenolate mofetil in recent-onset diffuse scleroderma. Rheumatology (Oxf) 40:84-88, 2001.

280. Scherer HU, Burmester GR, Riemekasten G: Targeting activated T cells: Successful use of anti-CD25 monoclonal antibody basiliximab in a patient with systemic sclerosis. Ann Rheum Dis 65:1245-1247, 2006.

281. Liossis SN, Bounas A, Andonopoulos AP: Mycophenolate mofetil as first-line treatment improves clinically evident early scleroderma lung disease. Rheumatology 45:1005-1008, 2006.

282. Mayes MD, O'Donnell D, Rothfield NF, et al: Minocycline is not effective in systemic sclerosis: Results of an open-label multicenter trial. Arthritis Rheum 50:553-557, 2004.

283. Maddison P: Prevention of vascular damage in scleroderma with angiotensin-converting enzyme (ACE) inhibition. Rheumatology 41:965-971, 2002.

283a. Gliddon AE, Doré CJ, Black CM, et al: Prevention of vascular damage in scleroderma and autoimmune Raynaud's phenomenon: A multicenter, randomized, double-blind, placebo-controlled trial of the angiotensin-converting enzyme inhibitor quinapril. Arthritis Rheum 56:3837-3846, 2007.

284. Furukawa S, Yasuda S, Amengual O, et al: Protective effect of pravastatin on vascular endothelium in patients with systemic sclerosis: A pilot study. Ann Rheum Dis 65:1118-1120, 2006.

285. Milio G, Corrado E, Genova C, et al: Iloprost treatment in patients with Raynaud's phenomenon secondary to systemic sclerosis and the

quality of life: A new therapeutic protocol. Rheumatology (Oxf) 45:999-1004, 2006.

286. Thompson AE, Pope JE: Calcium channel blockers for primary Raynaud's phenomenon: A meta-analysis. Rheumatology (Oxf) 44:145-150, 2005.

287. Dziadzio M, Denton CP, Smith R, et al: Losartan therapy for Raynaud's phenomenon and scleroderma: Clinical and biochemical findings in a fifteen-week, randomized, parallel-group, controlled trial. Arthritis Rheum 42:2646-2655, 1999.

288. Coleiro B, Marshall SE, Denton CP, et al: Treatment of Raynaud's phenomenon with the selective serotonin reuptake inhibitor fluoxetine. Rheumatology (Oxf) 40:1038-1043, 2001.

289. Samuelson UK, Ahlmen EM: Development and evaluation of a patient education program for persons with systemic sclerosis (scleroderma). Arthritis Care Res 13:141-148, 2000.

290. Bunn CC, Black CM: Systemic sclerosis: An autoantibody mosaic. Clin Exp Immunol 117:207-208, 1999.

291. Reveille JD, Solomon DH: American College of Rheumatology Ad Hoc Committee of Immunologic Testing Guidelines: Evidence-based guidelines for the use of immunologic tests: Anticentromere, Scl-70, and nucleolar antibodies. Arthritis Rheum 49:399-412, 2003.

292. Laxer RM, Zulian F: Localized scleroderma. Curr Opin Rheumatol 18:606-613, 2006.

293. Tollefson MM, Witman PM: En coup de sabre morphea and Parry-Romberg syndrome: A retrospective review of 54 patients. J Am Acad Dermatol 56:257-263, 2007.

294. Weide B, Walz T, Garbe C: Is morphoea caused by *Borrelia burgdorferi*? Br J Dermatol 142:636-644, 2000.

295. Mancuso G, Berdondini RM: Topical tacrolimus in the treatment of localized scleroderma. Eur J Dermatol 13:590-592, 2003.

296. Marzano AV, Menni S, Parodi A, et al: Localized scleroderma in adults and children: Clinical and laboratory investigations on 239 cases. Eur J Dermatol 13:171-176, 2003.

297. Vancheeswaran R, Black CM, David J, et al: Childhood-onset scleroderma: Is it different from adult-onset disease. Arthritis Rheum 39:1041-1049, 1996.

298. Zulian F, Athreya BH, Laxer R, et al: Juvenile Scleroderma Working Group of the Pediatric Rheumatology European Society (PRES): Juvenile localized scleroderma: Clinical and epidemiological features in 750 children: An international study. Rheumatology (Oxf) 45:614-620, 2006.

299. Birdi N, Shore A, Rush P, et al: Childhood linear scleroderma: A possible role of thermography for evaluation. J Rheumatol 19:968-973, 1992.

300. Cosnes A, Anglade MC, Revuz J, et al: Thirteen-megahertz ultrasound probe: Its role in diagnosing localized scleroderma. Br J Dermatol 148:724-729, 2003.

301. Tate BJ, Kelly JW, Rotstein H: Scleredema of Buschke: A report of seven cases. Australas J Dermatol 37:139-142, 1996.

302. Cokonis Georgakis CD, Falasca G, Georgakis A, et al: Scleromyxedema. Clin Dermatol 24:493-497, 2006.

303. Kucher C, Xu X, Pasha T, et al: Histopathologic comparison of nephrogenic fibrosing dermopathy and scleromyxedema. J Cutan Pathol 32:484-490, 2005.

304. Dziadzio M, Denton CP, Smith R, et al: Losartan therapy for Raynaud's phenomenon and scleroderma: Clinical and biochemical findings in a fifteen-week, randomized, parallel-group, controlled trial. Arthritis Rheum 42:2646-2655, 1999.

305. Lister RK, Jolles S, Whittaker S, et al: Scleromyxedema: Response to high-dose intravenous immunoglobulin (hdIVIg). J Am Acad Dermatol 43(2 Pt 2):403-408, 2000.

306. Donato ML, Feasel AM, Weber DM, et al: Scleromyxedema: Role of high-dose melphalan with autologous stem cell transplantation. Blood 107:463-466, 2006.

307. Keong CH, Asaka Y, Fukuro S, et al: Successful treatment of scleromyxedema with plasmapheresis and immunosuppression. J Am Acad Dermatol 22(5 Pt 1):842-844, 1990.

308. Barnes L, Rodnan GP, Medsger TA, et al: Eosinophilic fasciitis: A pathologic study of twenty cases. Am J Pathol 96:493-517, 1979.

309. Eklund KK, Anttila P, Leirisalo-Repo M: Eosinophilic fasciitis, myositis and arthritis as early manifestations of peripheral T-cell lymphoma. Scand J Rheumatol 32:376-377, 2003.

310. Khanna D, Verity A, Grossman JM: Eosinophilic fasciitis with multiple myeloma: A new haematological association. Ann Rheum Dis 61:1111-1112, 2002.

311. Garcia VP, de Quiros JF, Caminal L: Autoimmune hemolytic anemia associated with eosinophilic fasciitis. J Rheumatol 25:1864-1865, 1998.

312. Cassis TB, Jackson JM, Sonnier GB, et al: Nephrogenic fibrosing dermopathy in a patient with acute renal failure never requiring dialysis. Int J Dermatol 45:56-59, 2006.

313. Edward M, Fitzgerald L, Thind C, et al: Cutaneous mucinosis associated with dermatomyositis and nephrogenic fibrosing dermopathy: Fibroblast hyaluronan synthesis and the effect of patient serum. Br J Dermatol 156:473-479, 2007.

314. Mendoza FA, Artlett CM, Sandorfi N, et al: Description of 12 cases of nephrogenic fibrosing dermopathy and review of the literature. Semin Arthritis Rheum 35:238-249, 2006.

315. Mackay-Wiggan JM, Cohen DJ, Hardy MA, et al: Nephrogenic fibrosing dermopathy (scleromyxedema-like illness of renal disease). J Am Acad Dermatol 48:55-60, 2003.

316. Posada de la Paz M, Philen RM, Borda AI: Toxic oil syndrome: The perspective after 20 years. Epidemiol Rev 23:231-247, 2001.

317. Bolster MB, Silver RM: Eosinophilia-myalgia syndrome, toxic-oil syndrome, and diffuse fasciitis with eosinophilia. Curr Opin Rheumatol 6(6):642-649, 1994.

318. Swaminathan S, Ahmed I, McCarthy JT, et al: Nephrogenic fibrosing dermopathy and high-dose erythropoietin therapy. Ann Intern Med 145:234-235, 2006.

319. Grobner T: Gadolinium—a specific trigger for the development of nephrogenic fibrosing dermopathy and nephrogenic systemic fibrosis? Nephrol Dial Transplant 21:1104-1108, 2006.

320. Antic M, Lautenschlager S, Itin PH: Eosinophilic fasciitis 30 years after—what do we really know? Report of 11 patients and review of the literature. Dermatology 213:93-101, 2006.

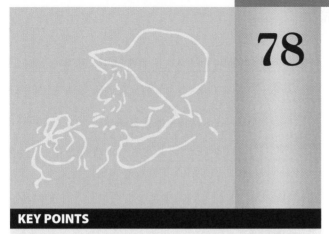

78 Inflammatory Diseases of Muscle and Other Myopathies

KANNEBOYINA NAGARAJU •
INGRID E. LUNDBERG

This heterogeneous group of muscle diseases is characterized by symmetric proximal muscle weakness and frequent involvement of other organs.

Myopathies are often accompanied by elevated levels of serum muscle enzymes and abnormal electromyograms.

Histology shows varying degrees of inflammation and muscle fiber degeneration and regeneration.

Some patients have autoantibodies to molecules involved in protein synthesis, and these antibodies are often associated with distinct clinical phenotypes.

Corticosteroids and cytotoxic drugs are common therapies.

HISTORY OF INFLAMMATORY MUSCLE DISEASES

Inflammatory muscle diseases are a heterogeneous group of systemic autoimmune rheumatic disorders characterized by chronic muscle weakness, muscle fatigue, and mononuclear cell infiltration into skeletal muscle. These disorders were described in the literature more than a century ago as generalized muscle disorders affecting principally the trunk and proximal limb muscles, with or without skin involvement.[1-5] It was also recognized that these diseases can range from acute and even fatal to slow, progressive, chronic, insidious conditions, with patterns of relapse and remission. Steiner's[6] summary of myositis cases in 1903 made a clear distinction between idiopathic polymyositis and other forms of myositis caused by bacteria and parasites,[6] and Stertz[7] in 1916 first reported an association between dermatomyositis and internal malignancy.[7] At about the same time, Batten[8] described the first case of dermatomyositis with classic histologic features in a child.

Since the1940s, it has been recognized that polymyositis may occur in the absence of cutaneous lesions, muscle pain, or constitutional symptoms, and it may present in an acute, subacute, or chronic insidious form, with some fraction of cases showing systemic features or involvement of organs and tissues.[9] The differential diagnosis has been described independently by several investigators, and the most chronic form was differentiated from an adult variety of muscular dystrophy.[10-12] Banker and Victor[13] noted that dermatomyositis in children was different and involved a greater degree of vascular inflammation and thrombosis (systemic angiopathy). The first, and still widely used, classification scheme and set of diagnostic criteria for myositis were proposed by Bohan

and Peter in 1975.[14,15] These include polymyositis and dermatomyositis but not the later-described subset known as inclusion body myositis (IBM). IBM was later defined by the presence of distinct histopathologic changes, including vacuoles and nuclear and cytoplasmic inclusions, as well as by distinct clinical features, including resistance to glucocorticoids.[16,17] Debate continues whether IBM should be considered an idiopathic inflammatory myopathy (IIM). We have chosen to include information on IBM in this chapter because it is clinically relevant to the differential diagnosis of polymyositis.

EPIDEMIOLOGY

The actual annual incidence of inflammatory myopathy is currently unknown. Because these diseases are so rare, no large-scale epidemiologic studies have been reported; however, several retrospective studies have reported an annual incidence of fewer than 10 per million individuals[18-22] (Table 78-1). This may be an overestimate, given that the Peter and Bohan diagnostic criteria used in these studies did not distinguish IBM as a separate disease entity. The prevalence of IBM has been estimated to be 10.7 per million in the United States, 9.3 per million in Australia, and 4.9 per million in the Netherlands.[23-25] The age-adjusted prevalence of IBM for those older than 50 years was reported as 16 to 35 per million.[24,25] In some geographic areas, IBM appears to be the most common acquired progressive myopathy, representing 16% to 28% of all inflammatory myopathies.[25] There may be referral biases in these studies. The incidence-prevalence studies need to be interpreted cautiously, given that most have not reported confidence intervals for their rates.

The incidence of the various myopathies varies according to ethnicity, age, and gender. Some studies have reported that the incidence of polymyositis is higher in black patients than in white patients.[18] IIMs can occur in any age group, from early childhood to late in adult life. The onset of polymyositis is usually in the late teens or older, with the mean age at onset being 50 to 60 years; dermatomyositis shows two peaks—5 to 15 years and 45 to 65 years. IBM is commonly seen in individuals older than 50 years and is rare in younger adults. Some studies have reported gender-specific incidence rates. For example, in the case of polymyositis and dermatomyositis, females are more commonly affected than males (ratio >2:1), whereas in IBM, the converse is true (again, >2:1 ratio).

Inflammatory myopathies can occur in association with other autoimmune connective tissue diseases, such as scleroderma, systemic lupus erythematosus (SLE), rheumatoid arthritis, Sjögren's syndrome, polyarthritis nodosa, and

Table 78-1 Incidence of Inflammatory Myopathies by Country

Country	Study Dates	Incidence (million/yr)	Reference
USA	1963-1982	5.5	18
USA	1947-1968	5.0	20
Australia	1989-1991	7.4	21
Sweden	1984-1993	7.6	22
Israel	1960-1976	2.1	178

sarcoidosis. Significant proportions of all myositis patients (11% to 40%) have an associated connective tissue disease.[23,26,27] Several studies have also confirmed an association between malignancies and inflammatory myopathies. The frequency of malignancies varies widely (4% to 42%) in different studies,[19,28] but in general, the incidence of malignancy is higher in dermatomyositis patients than in IBM or polymyositis patients.[29] It is difficult to determine the relative risks for a particular malignancy because a variety of malignancies are associated with myositis, and only small numbers of individual malignancies have been reported in any one study.

CAUSE

GENETIC RISK FACTORS

An association with immune response genes and occasional reports of familial clustering of myositis support the role of genetic factors in these diseases.[30-35] Polymorphisms in human leukocyte antigen (HLA) class I and II genes are known genetic risk factors for several autoimmune diseases, including myositis, but the mechanisms for these associations remain unclear. One possibility is that because the gene products influence T cell repertoire development, tolerance, and immune responses to foreign agents, certain polymorphisms may be selected based on environmental triggers. It appears that haplotypes HLA-DRB1*0301 and HLA-DQA1*0501 are the strongest known genetic risk factors for all forms of myositis in Caucasians; however, different phenotypes have additional HLA risk and protective factors.[35,36] The HLA-B8/DR3/DR52/DQ2 haplotype is found in a significant proportion of IBM patients.[37] The risk and protection conferred by HLA associations differ significantly among different ethnic and serologic groups. For example, in some populations (e.g., Koreans and Mesoamericans), there is no association with HLA genes.[33] Further, HLA-DRB1*0301, which is a risk factor in Caucasians, is a protective factor in the Japanese population.[38] The HLA-DRB1*0301, HLA-DQA1*0501, and HLA-DQB1*0201 alleles are strongly associated with myositis-specific antibodies in polymyositis patients.[39] Mechanistic data supporting the role of HLA molecules in disease pathogenesis are, unfortunately, lacking at present. Some studies have reported that maternally derived chimeric cells are present in the peripheral blood and muscle tissues of juvenile dermatomyositis patients, suggesting that HLA alleles control the occurrence of chimerism and explain the HLA association found in these disorders.[40,41] Like other autoimmune disease conditions, myositis is a complex multigenic disorder involving other

Table 78-2 Possible Environmental Risk Factors

Infectious Agents
Viruses
Picornavirus family, enteroviruses
Polio, coxsackievirus types A and B, echoviruses
Retroviruses
HIV-1, HTLV-1
Parvovirus B19
Hepatitis C virus
Hepatitis B virus
Bacteria
Staphylococci
Clostridia
Mycobacteria
Parasites
Toxoplasma gondii
Trypanosoma cruzi
Borrelia burgdorferi

Noninfectious Agents
Drugs
D-penicillamine
Corticosteroids
Chloroquine
Statins (atorvastatin, lovastatin, pravastatin, simvastatin)
Lipid-lowering fibrates (bezafibrate, clofibrate, gemfibrozil)
L-tryptophan
Biologic agents (e.g., growth hormone, interferon-α, interleukin-2)
Vaccination for tetanus, BCG, diphtheria, hepatitis B, hepatitis A
Miscellaneous drugs (e.g., local anesthesia, hydroxyurea, leuprolide acetate)
Ultraviolet radiation exposure
Miscellaneous agents (e.g., silicone breast implants, chronic graft-versus-host disease associated with bone marrow transplantation, collagen injection, silica exposure)

BCG, bacille Calmette-Guérin; HIV, human immunodeficiency virus; HTLV-1, human T-lymphotropic virus 1.

non-HLA immune response genes (e.g., cytokines and receptors, including tumor necrosis factor-α [TNF-α], interleukin [IL]-1, and tumor necrosis factor receptor [TNFR]-1), complement components (e.g., C4, C2), immunoglobulin heavy-chain allotypes, and T cell receptors.[42] The exact contribution of the genetic component in these disorders is currently unknown, in part because of their rarity, the small number of subjects in any single cohort, and the heterogeneity in disease phenotype. International collaborative efforts are currently under way to address these issues and to identify potential genetic and environmental risk factors in myositis.

ENVIRONMENTAL RISK FACTORS

The temporal association of myositis onset and environmental agents in certain individuals suggests that specific exposures in the context of certain genetic backgrounds can initiate muscle inflammation. Common environmental agents implicated in myositis include infectious organisms, such as viruses and bacteria, and noninfectious agents, such as drugs and food supplements (Table 78-2). For example, enteroviruses (influenza, coxsackievirus, echoviruses) and retroviruses (human T-lymphotrophic virus-1) are known to induce muscle inflammation. The myositis associated with enteroviruses usually occurs in children and is generally self-limited. A viral cause is strengthened by the presence of high-titer antiviral antibodies and viral particles in patients' serum and tissue samples,[43,44] as well as the induction of muscle inflammation by enteroviruses in animal models. Attempts to identify virus in the tissues of IIM patients by sensitive techniques such as polymerase chain reaction have failed, leading to doubts about the viral cause of these diseases[45] and ruling out continual viral infection as a cause of the ongoing muscle inflammation in these patients. However, it is possible that viruses initially trigger the disease process before being eliminated by the host's immune response, thus explaining the absence of viral genomes in the myositis muscle tissue. Similarly, some microorganisms, such as staphylococci, clostridia, and mycobacteria, are known to affect skeletal muscle and cause acute muscle inflammation, but there is no evidence that these organisms actually cause chronic, self-sustaining muscle inflammation.

Parasites such as *Toxoplasma gondii*, *Trypanosoma cruzi*, and *Borrelia burgdorferi* have been implicated in the triggering of IIMs. The evidence in support of a parasitic cause include the recovery of parasites from some myositis patients and their serologic response to the parasites; improvement in myositis symptoms after treatment with antiparasitic drugs; a histologic picture of inflammation, including infiltration of macrophages and CD4 T cells; and induction of myositis after parasitic infection in animal models.[46-51a] Despite these observations, it is difficult to establish a direct link between any parasitic infections and myositis in human patients, because there is often no history of antecedent parasitic infection.

Ultraviolet (UV) light irradiation is likely to be a risk factor for the development of dermatomyositis, because epidemiologic data that have demonstrated a latitude gradient of polymyositis and dermatomyositis, with the latter being more frequent closer to the equator and the former being more frequent in northern countries. The ratio between polymyositis and dermatomyositis is associated with a latitude gradient and is directly correlated with UV light irradiation. This observed correlation is particularly strong in a subset of dermatomyositis patients with anti–Mi-2 autoantibodies, indicating that UV light may be an environmental risk factor for its development. The association between UV light exposure and subtype of myositis suggests that UV light is an exogenous modifier that can influence the clinical phenotype in polymyositis and dermatomyositis.[52]

It appears that malignancy is an additional risk factor for the development of myositis, and there is a strong association between dermatomyositis and malignancies. This early clinical observation has been confirmed in epidemiologic studies.[28,53] With regard to polymyositis and IBM, the association with malignancy is less convincing. The increased risk of malignancy associated with dermatomyositis has been established both at the time of dermatomyositis diagnosis and more than 10 years after diagnosis. The pathophysiologic mechanism for the association between malignancy and dermatomyositis has not been clarified, but there could be several explanations. The strong association between malignancy and the onset of dermatomyositis indicates that the latter could be a paramalignant phenomenon; that is, the development of myositis is a consequence of the malignancy (related to autoantigens), or the malignancy and dermatomyositis share disease mechanisms. Thus, the molecular mechanisms underlying this unique association are currently unclear. However, there is circumstantial evidence that removal of a tumor sometimes results in amelioration of muscle weakness, and tumor reappearance sometimes coincides with muscle weakness, suggesting that these two are linked. A recent report has shed some light on this connection by showing that myositis-specific antigens are highly expressed in cancer tissues as well as in regenerating muscle cells of myositis patients.[54,55] The authors propose that in cancer-associated myositis, an autoimmune response directed against cancer cross-reacts with regenerating muscle cells, enabling a feed-forward loop of tissue damage and antigen selection.[56] This association must be explored further, because cancer-associated myositis patients almost never develop myositis-specific autoantibodies, which are protective for the development of cancer. For malignancies that develop during established disease, the potential explanations include the presence of chronic inflammation or prolonged immunosuppressive treatment, which could contribute to the development of malignancy.

MIMICS OF MYOSITIS

A variety of insults induce the clinical and pathologic spectrum that mimics myositis in some individuals (see Table 78-2). A number of drugs are known to cause a myopathy that closely mimics myositis. For example, D-penicillamine causes clinically and histologically indistinguishable IIM.[57] Likewise, commonly used lipid-lowering drugs such as statins (e.g., atorvastatin, lovastatin) can cause a myopathy that resembles inflammatory myositis. These agents inhibit 3-hydroxy-3-methylglutaryl-coenzyme A (HMG-CoA) reductase, a rate-limiting enzyme involved in the conversion of HMG-CoA to mevalonic acid, thereby preventing the synthesis of bioactive sterol and nonsterol metabolic intermediates in the cholesterol synthetic pathway. The mechanism by which these drugs cause myopathy is not known.[58-60] Other drugs such as hydroxyurea can cause skin rashes that resemble dermatomyositis.[61] Recent reports implicate the vaccine adjuvant aluminum hydroxide as a cause of macrophagic myofasciitis. The histology shows infiltration by macrophages and some CD8 T cells into the endomysium, perimysium, and epimysium, together with clinically elevated creatine kinase (CK) levels, muscle weakness, myalgias, fatigue, and arthralgias.[62] Despite some reports of vaccine-induced myositis, systematic investigation has failed to link any vaccine to myositis.[63]

PATHOGENESIS

Significant advances have been made in our understanding of the pathogenesis of the human inflammatory myopathies.[64-69] It is generally thought that IIMs are autoimmune in origin because they are frequently associated with other autoimmune diseases (e.g., Hashimoto's thyroiditis) and collagen vascular diseases (e.g., scleroderma); many patients exhibit an autoantibody response, including the presence of myositis-specific autoantibodies; some studies provide evidence for lymphocyte-mediated muscle fiber injury; and a favorable response to immunosuppressive therapies in some patients supports an autoimmune cause of these disorders.

HUMORAL IMMUNE RESPONSE

More than 50% of all IIM patients have uniquely defined auto-antibodies—some of which are specific to myositis, and some of which are merely associated with myositis. These are generally referred to as myositis-specific autoantibodies (MSAs) and myositis-associated autoantibodies (MAAs), respectively. MAAs includes autoantibodies to various nuclear and cyto-plasmic antigens. Antinuclear antibodies (ANAs) present in myositis are not particularly associated with any disease sub-group, whereas MSAs that are directed against antigens of the protein synthesis pathway (e.g., aminoacyl–transfer RNA [tRNA] synthetases and signal recognition particles) and nuclear components (e.g., nuclear helicase [Mi-2]) are often associated with distinct clinical disease groups and subgroups (e.g., tRNA synthetases with interstitial lung disease, and Mi-2 with dermatomyositis) (Table 78-3).

Anti–histidyl tRNA synthetase antibodies are the most frequent and are present in about 16% to 20% of myositis patients.[70-72] Antibodies against other aminoacyl-tRNA synthetases, such as threonyl-tRNA synthetase (PL-7), alanyl-tRNA synthetase (PL-12), isoleucyl-tRNA synthetase (OJ), glycyl-tRNA synthetase (EJ), and asparaginyl-tRNA synthetase (KS), are found less frequently (1% to 3%). Anti–Mi-2 antibodies are strongly associated with derma-tomyositis,[73,74] with prominent features such as Gottron's papules, heliotrope rash, the V sign, and the shawl sign. An individual usually has only one MSA, because they are often mutually exclusive. The MSAs are most common in patients with other autoimmune diseases and are infrequent or absent in IBM patients and those with malignancies, mus-cular dystrophies, or other myopathies. These antibodies are sometimes present before the onset of clinical disease.[75]

MAAs such as PM-Scl are frequently associated with a characteristic overlap syndrome that includes features of scleroderma[76,77] This syndrome is characterized by mild muscle disease, prominent arthritis, and limited skin involve-ment; it frequently responds to therapy.[78] Some myositis patients also have other MAAs, such as anti-snRNP, anti-Ro/SSA, anti-Ku, and anti-PMS1. Antibodies recognizing an uncharacterized 56-kD large nuclear ribonucleoprotein have been found in a majority of myositis patients (86%), and the antibody titer appears to vary with disease activity, suggesting its importance in our understanding of disease pathogenesis and its potential usefulness as a clinical disease marker.[79] Some of the MSAs show strong immunogenetic associations; for example, antibodies against aminoacyl-tRNA synthetases are associated with HLA-DQA1*0501, anti-SRP with DR5, anti–Mi-2 with DR7, and anti–PM-Scl with DR3.[35] Neither the molecular mechanisms that initiate and perpetuate the autoimmune response nor the precise role of these autoantibodies in the pathogenesis of myosi-tis is currently known. It is likely that these autoantibod-ies are not the primary pathogenic event leading to muscle fiber damage because they are present in only a fraction of all myositis patients; they are directed not against muscle-specific antigens but against ubiquitously expressed cellular proteins; and they are usually specific for intracellular target antigens that are not easily accessible to antibodies. How-ever, these antibodies serve as excellent clinical markers and can help diagnose and categorize these heterogeneous disorders into homogeneous subgroups.

Table 78-3 Myositis-Specific Antibodies

Autoantibodies	Clinical Disease/Features
Antisynthetase autoantibodies*	More common in polymyositis than dermatomyositis; inter-stitial lung disease, arthritis, Raynaud's phenomenon, fevers, mechanic's hands
Signal recognition particle (SRP)†	Polymyositis; possible severe dis-ease and cardiac involvement
Chromodomain helicase DNA binding proteins 3 and 4 (Mi-2α and β)‡	Dermatomyositis

*Common antisynthetase antibodies found in myositis are targeted to histidyl-tRNA synthetase (Jo-1), threonyl-tRNA synthetase (PL-7), alanyl-tRNA synthetase (PL-12), isoleucyl-tRNA synthetase (OJ), glycyl-tRNA synthetase (EJ), and asparaginyl-tRNA synthetase (KS).

†Autoantibodies commonly bind to a 54-kD SRP protein in the U.S. patient population and 72-, 54-, and 9-kD proteins in the Japanese population

‡Targets a 240-kD helicase protein that is part of the nucleosome remodeling deacetylase complex.

CELL-MEDIATED IMMUNE RESPONSE

At the cellular level, there are distinct differences in the distribution and location of the various lymphocyte subsets in the muscle tissues in different IIMs. Two major patterns of inflammatory cell infiltrates are seen in muscle tissue. The first has a predominantly perivascular distribution (Fig. 78-1A), often in perimysial areas (Fig. 78-1C), and is largely made up of CD4+ T cells, macrophages, and dendritic cells. In occasional patients, B cells are present. This pattern in seen mainly in dermatomyositis patients with skin rash, but occasionally in patients without a rash. The second pattern has a predominantly endomysial distribution (Fig. 78-1B), with mononuclear inflammatory cells often surrounding and sometimes invading non-necrotic muscle fibers. These inflammatory cellular infiltrates are made up primarily of CD8+ T cells and macrophages, but CD4+ T cells and dendritic cells are also present. This pattern is generally seen in patients without skin rash and often in those clas-sified as having polymyositis or IBM. In some patients, the two patterns of inflammation are seen in the same biopsy. The two distinct locations and the varying compositions of the inflammatory cell populations in the two areas suggest two different pathogenic mechanisms—one that targets the blood vessels, and one that targets the muscle fibers. Notable inflammation is also seen in other organs.

The vascular involvement in patients with dermatomyo-sitis is also manifested in the skin and can be seen clini-cally in the form of nail-fold changes and changes in the gastrointestinal (GI) tract. The capillaries show clear hyper-plasia, vacuolization, and necrosis, contributing to an ischemia that could cause fiber damage.[80,81] One of the earli-est events in the pathogenesis of dermatomyositis appears to be activation of the complement cascade. This leads to the subsequent deposition of complement components, which in turn results in the deposition of lytic membrane attack complexes in the endothelial cells and the eventual loss of capillaries due to complement-mediated damage. The capil-laries are abnormally thickened and enlarged and look like high endothelial venules, which are characteristics of ves-sels that facilitate lymphocyte trafficking (Fig. 78-2). The

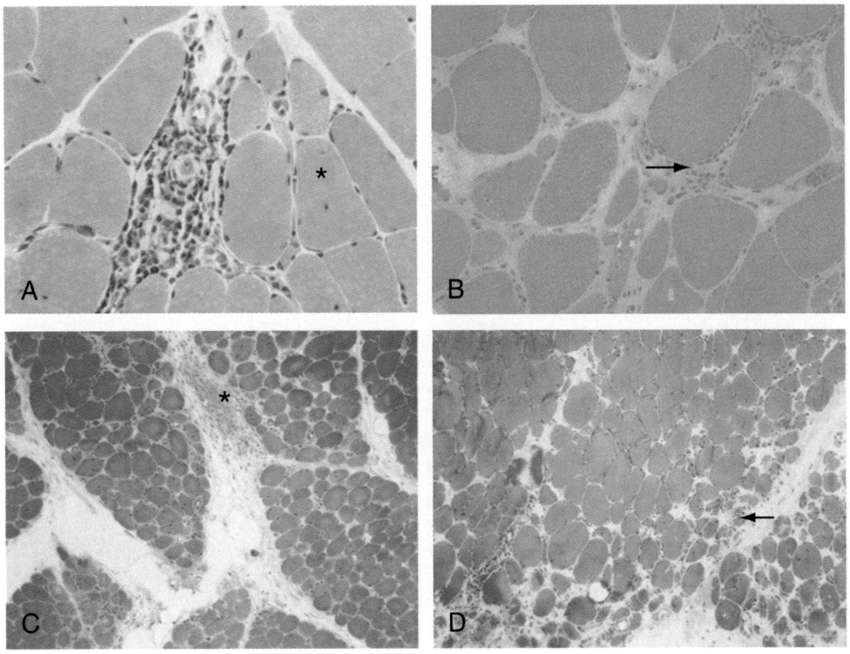

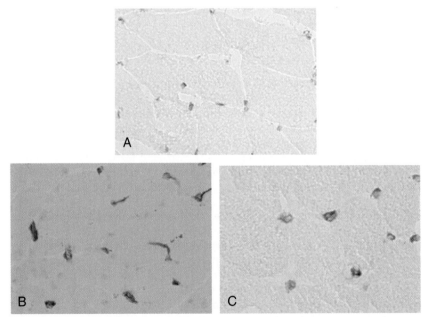

Figure 78-1 Hematoxylin and eosin staining of muscle biopsy showing perivascular inflammation. A, Variation in fiber size and central nucleation *(star)*. **B,** Endomysial inflammation and increased fibrosis. **C,** Perimysial inflammation *(star)*. **D,** Perifascicular atrophy *(arrow)*. *(B, Courtesy of Dr. Inger Nemmesmo. D, Courtesy of Dr. Paul Plotz.)*

Figure 78-2 Muscle biopsy staining with CD146 (Mel-CAM), an endothelial cell marker. Results are shown in normal **(A)**, dermatomyositis **(B)**, and polymyositis **(C)** subjects. Note the abnormal capillary size in both dermatomyositis and polymyositis.

capillaries also show signs of neovascularization.[82] This loss of capillaries results in some of the histopathologic features characteristic of this disease: capillary necrosis and loss, perivascular inflammation and ischemia (rarely seen), and perifascicular atrophy (a late feature; see Fig. 78-1C and D). Although no direct comparison has been reported, the pathologic changes in juvenile and adult dermatomyositis appear to be similar, except that all the basic pathologic features are more prominent in the childhood form (see later). The factors that initiate complement activation in this disease are poorly understood; however, the consequences of complement-mediated damage are clearly visible in dermatomyositis.[83]

The endomysial inflammatory aggregates contain a high percentage of T cells, particularly activated CD8+ T cells, macrophages, and CD4+ T cells, and very few natural killer cells. Immunoelectron microscopic studies have provided evidence of the invasion, replacement, and probable destruction of non-necrotic muscle fibers by T cells and macrophages.[84] It is suggested that CD8 cytotoxic T lymphocytes (CTLs) recognize major histocompatibility complex (MHC) class I on muscle fibers and may mediate muscle fiber damage. Infiltrating CTLs express perforin-containing granules, which are characteristically oriented toward the target muscle fiber, indicating that muscle fiber injury may be partially mediated by perforin-dependent cytotoxic mechanisms

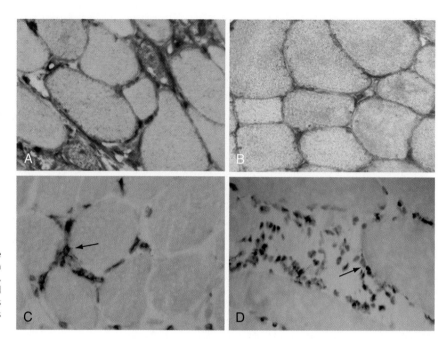

Figure 78-3 HLA-ABC, CD8 T cell, and granzyme B staining of polymyositis biopsy. HLA expression is evident on muscle fibers, infiltrating cells, and endothelial cells (**A**). HLA cell surface and sarcoplasmic staining is shown on muscle fibers (**B**), CD8 T cells (**C**), and granzyme B–positive cells (**D**) surrounding muscle fibers *(arrow)*.

(Fig. 78-3B and C).[85] In polymyositis and IBM, there is evidence of clonal proliferation of CD8 T cells, both within the muscle and in the peripheral circulation.[86,87] T cell lines from patients demonstrate cytotoxicity against autologous myotubes,[88] suggesting that the muscle fiber injury in polymyositis and IBM is mediated by CTLs. CTLs are known to mediate target cell damage by both perforin–granzyme B and Fas-FasL pathways. The overexpression of antiapoptotic molecules such as Bcl-2, FLIP (Fas-associated death domain–like IL-1 converting enzyme inhibitory protein), and human inhibitor of apoptosis protein–like protein in skeletal muscle of myositis patients suggests that perforin-granzyme B–mediated CTL damage may play a predominant role in muscle fiber injury and dysfunction in myositis.[89-91]

On the basis of the data just described, two different pathways have been proposed as major mediators of muscle damage and inflammation: one mediated through T lymphocytes (CTLs) directed against muscle fibers, predominating in polymyositis and IBM, and the other directed against vessels, predominating in dermatomyositis. However, several studies have shown that the degree of inflammation does not consistently correlate with the severity of the structural changes in the muscle fibers or with the severity of the clinical disease,[92] suggesting that nonimmune processes also play a role in disease pathogenesis. A role for nonimmune processes is supported by the following observations: First, marked structural changes in the muscle fibers occur in the absence of any inflammatory cells.[93,94] Second, there is a lack of correlation between the degree of inflammation and the degree of muscle weakness.[95] Third, some myositis patients do not respond, even to powerful anti-inflammatory therapy,[96,97] Fourth, steroid treatment may eliminate inflammatory cells in myositis muscle tissue, but this removal alone may not substantially improve the clinical disease, suggesting that immunosuppressive therapies modulate disease activity but do not change other mediators of the disease process.[98] Finally, the clinical disease may progress when identifiable inflammation has subsided,[99] suggesting

a role for nonimmune mechanisms in the pathogenesis of myositis. Thus, the exact contribution of immune-mediated pathways to muscle damage is currently unknown.

MHC CLASS I

Normal skeletal muscle cells do not constitutively express or display MHC class I molecules, although they can be induced to do so by proinflammatory cytokines such as interferon-γ or TNF-α.[93,100-102] In contrast, in human IIMs, the early and widespread appearance of MHC class I in nonnecrotic muscle cells is a striking feature, even in muscle cells distant from the lymphocytic infiltration.[93,94,103] MHC class I staining is usually observed on the sarcolemma of muscle fibers, but some fibers also show staining in both the sarcolemma and the sarcoplasm (see Fig. 78-3A and B). In some patients, the expression is restricted to a few clusters (often in early disease), whereas in others, almost every fiber is positively stained, particularly in late-phase and treatment-resistant cases. The biologic significance of these observations has been explored by generating a conditional transgenic mouse model overexpressing syngenic mouse MHC class I. The overexpression of MHC class I molecules in the skeletal muscle of mice results in the development of clinical, biochemical, histologic, and immunologic features that resemble human myositis and provide a close model of the human disease. The disease in these mice is inflammatory, limited to skeletal muscles, self-sustaining, more severe in females, and often accompanied by MSAs.[104]

A number of observations in human myositis patients and in the mouse model of myositis suggest that MHC class I molecules themselves may mediate muscle fiber damage and dysfunction in the absence of lymphocytes. For instance, in human myositis, the induction of MHC class I antigen in muscle fibers occurs early, preceding inflammatory cell infiltration.[105,106] MHC class I staining of human myositis biopsies shows both a cell surface and a sarcoplasmic reticulum pattern of internal reactivity, demonstrating that

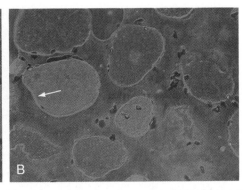

Figure 78-4 Nuclear factor κB(NFκB) expression in normal and myositis biopsy. Immunofluorescence staining with rabbit anti–NFκB and anti–rabbit Texas red and counterstaining with 4, 6-diamino-2-phenylindole (blue nuclei). Note the cytoplasmic expression of NFκB in normal muscle (**A**) and a subsarcolemmal pattern in the myositis biopsy (**B**; arrow). *(From Nagaraju K, Casciola-Rosen L, Lundberg I, et al: Activation of the endoplasmic reticulum stress response in autoimmune myositis: Potential role in muscle fiber damage and destruction. Arthritis Rheum 52:1824-1835, 2005.)*

some of the MHC class I molecules may be retained in the endoplasmic reticulum (ER) of these fibers.[69,94,107] Persistent MHC class I overexpression in muscle fibers may exist in the absence of an inflammatory infiltrate.[99] The controlled induction of MHC class I in the mouse model is followed by muscle weakness before mononuclear cell infiltration.[104] It has recently been shown that in vivo gene transfer of MHC class I plasmids attenuates muscle regeneration and differentiation.[108] Together, these observations, and particularly the obvious retention of MHC class I within the cell in both human and murine disease, indicate that the muscle fiber damage seen in myositis may not be solely mediated by immune attack (e.g., CTLs and autoantibodies); it may also be mediated through nonimmunologic mechanisms such as the ER stress response and hypoxia.

Because MHC class I assembly occurs in the ER, and because upregulation in myositis muscle fibers is widespread, even in the absence of visible inflammatory infiltrate, it is likely that ER stress plays a role in the muscle fiber damage and dysfunction associated with human myositis. The ER is intimately involved in the folding, exporting, and processing of newly synthesized proteins. When there is an imbalance between the protein load in the ER and the cell's ability to process that load, a series of signaling pathways that adapt cells to ER stress is activated. This ER stress response can be provoked by a variety of pathophysiologic conditions, including ischemia, hyperhomocysteinemia, viral infections, and mutations that impair protein folding, as well as by excess accumulation of protein in the ER.[109,110] Cells self-protect against ER stress by initiating at least four functionally distinct responses: (1) upregulation of the nuclear factor κB (NFκB) pathway (ER overload response); (2) upregulation of genes encoding ER chaperone proteins, such as Bip/GRP78 and GRP94, as a means of increasing protein folding activity and preventing protein aggregation; (3) translational attenuation to reduce the load of protein synthesis and to prevent the further accumulation of unfolded proteins (unfolded protein response); and (4) cell death, which occurs when the ER's functions are severely impaired. This cell death event is mediated by transcriptional activation of the gene for CHOP/GADD153, a member of the C/EBP family of transcription factors,[111] and by the activation of ER-associated caspase-12.[112]

In myositis, it appears that overexpression of MHC class I in myofibers initiates a series of cell autonomous changes that contribute to myofiber pathology. Recent investigations have indicated that overexpression of MHC class I on muscle fibers results in activation of the NFκB and ER stress response pathway in human inflammatory myopathies and in the mouse model of myositis.[69,113] NFκB can be activated within minutes by a variety of stimuli, including inflammatory cytokines such as TNF-α and IL-1, T cell activation signals, and stress inducers. It is likely that in human myositis, NFκB activates both classic (proinflammatory cytokines) and nonclassic (ER stress response) pathways.[69,113-116] Further, there is evidence that downstream target genes (e.g., MHC class I, intercellular adhesion molecule [ICAM], monocyte chemoattractant protein [MCP]-1) regulated by the NFκB pathway are very highly upregulated in myositis patients.[107,117,118] Recent studies have indicated that NFκB p65 is activated both in human myositis biopsies and in the mouse model,[69,113,119,120] suggesting that this pathway may be directly involved in muscle fiber damage (Fig.78-4). NFκB is a potential therapeutic target in myositis, and the use of NFκB pathway inhibitors significantly reduces the pathology associated with several autoimmune disease, including diabetes, multiple sclerosis, inflammatory bowel disease, and rheumatoid arthritis, suggesting that this pathway is a critical player in the effector phase of autoimmune pathology. Thus, it appears that MHC class I expression on muscle fibers links the immune and nonimmune mechanisms of muscle fiber damage.

CYTOKINES AND HYPOXIA

A number of other effector molecules produced in muscle tissue by inflammatory cells, endothelial cells, and muscle fibers are thought to play a role in the pathogenesis of myositis.[66] Most of the data assembled relate to cytokines, but some data related to chemokines are also available. The most consistently demonstrated cytokines in muscle tissue from patients with IIMs are cytokines with proinflammatory properties: IL-1α, IL-1β, TNF-α, and interferon-α. Recently, the DNA-binding high mobility group box 1 (HMGB1) was found to exhibit both an extranuclear and an extracellular pattern in the muscle tissue of patients with polymyositis and dermatomyositis. In addition to inducing the upregulation of MHC class I and II molecules on muscle fibers,

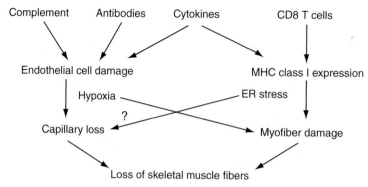

Figure 78-5 Mechanisms of muscle fiber damage in myositis. ER, endoplasmic reticulum; MHC, major histocompatibility complex.

cytokines may have a direct effect on muscle fiber function, as has been demonstrated for TNF-α.[121] The relative importance of the various cytokines and chemokines in patients with myositis is still uncertain, but these molecules offer possible targets for therapy in these conditions.

Microvessel involvement was first observed in dermatomyositis but has also become evident in polymyositis. The endothelial cells in both subsets show increased expression of adhesion molecules and proinflammatory cytokines such as IL-1α. This phenotype can be induced by tissue hypoxia, which may result from capillary loss and local tissue inflammation. Muscle tissue hypoxia can contribute to the clinical symptoms and muscle fatigue and might be associated with disease mechanisms in inflammatory myopathies.[66] The hypoxia hypothesis is supported by the clinical improvement observed after exercise, but a causal connection still needs to be established. Magnetic resonance spectroscopic analysis, before and after a work load, has demonstrated reduced levels of energy substrates that are important for muscle contraction, such as adenosine triphosphate and phosphocreatine, when compared with levels in healthy individuals. This finding supports the hypothesis that an acquired metabolic disturbance occurs in chronic inflammatory myopathies and that this disturbance can contribute to impaired muscle performance.

PROPOSED MECHANISMS OF MUSCLE DAMAGE

Currently available data suggest that both immune (cell-mediated and humoral) and nonimmune (ER stress, hypoxia) mechanisms play a role in muscle fiber damage and dysfunction in myositis. ER stress, hypoxia, and the NFκB pathway are highly active within the skeletal muscle of myositis patients, and the proinflammatory NFκB pathway connects the immune and nonimmune components contributing to muscle damage. The relative contribution of each of these pathways to muscle fiber damage is presently unclear (Fig. 78-5). Therefore, use of specific drugs to inhibit these pathways, either alone or in combination, would help define their roles in myositis and potentially serve as effective therapeutic agents.

CLINICAL FEATURES

The inflammatory myopathies may occur as distinct disease entities, or they may coexist with some other rheumatic disease. This observation is true for all three subsets of myositis,

but it is most often seen in polymyositis and dermatomyositis. The rheumatic diseases most often associated with inflammatory myopathies are systemic sclerosis, mixed connective tissue disease, Sjögren's syndrome, and SLE; however, rheumatoid arthritis may also be associated with inflammatory myopathies. IBM may be associated with Sjögren's syndrome, SLE, and others autoimmune diseases.[122,123] Because the clinical features of IBM differ somewhat from those of polymyositis and dermatomyositis, they are presented separately.

POLYMYOSITIS AND DERMATOMYOSITIS

The predominant symptoms in patients with polymyositis or dermatomyositis are muscle weakness and low muscle endurance. The weakness is most pronounced in proximal muscle groups—typically in the neck, pelvic, thigh, and shoulder muscles—with a symmetric distribution. Patients generally experience more problems performing repetitive movements than with single strength exercises, and they report difficulty walking uphill or upstairs, working with their arms above their shoulders, or rising from chairs. The onset is often subacute, occurring over a few weeks, or it may be insidious, developing over several months. If untreated, the muscle weakness progresses slowly, and in the most severe cases, patients may become wheelchair dependent. Problems with swallowing and nutrition may occur as a result of impaired contractility of the throat muscles, possibly leading to aspiration pneumonia. In rare cases, patients develop difficulty breathing because of weakness of the diaphragm or thoracic muscles, and they may require assisted ventilation. Other striated muscles may be involved, such as in the lower part of the esophagus (causing reflux problems) or the sphincter ani (causing incontinence).

Skin

Dermatomyositis is characterized by the presence of certain types of rashes[124]; the same types are often seen in both children and in adults. The most specific skin manifestations are Gottron's papules and the heliotrope rash (Fig. 78-6). Gottron's papules are slightly elevated violaceous, pink, or dusky red papules located over the dorsal side of the metacarpal or interphalangeal joints. These papules may also occur over the extensor side of the wrist, elbow, or knee joints. Gottron's papules are considered to be pathognomonic of dermatomyositis. A macular rash (without papules) with the same distribution as Gottron's papules is called Gottron's sign (see Fig. 78-6C and D). The heliotrope rash is

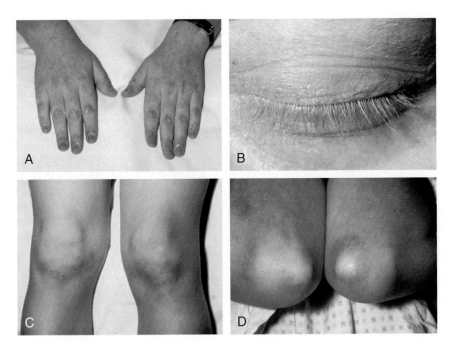

Figure 78-6 **Characteristic features of dermatomyositis skin changes. A,** Gottron's papules. **B,** Heliotrope rash. **C** and **D,** Gottron's sign on knee (**C**) and elbow (**D**). *(Courtesy of Dr. Paul Plotz.)*

a periorbital red or violaceous erythema of one or both eyelids, often with edema (see Fig. 78-6B). Linear erythema overlying the extensor surfaces of joints is also relatively specific to dermatomyositis (Fig. 78-7A). Many patients with dermatomyositis have photosensitive rashes, typically located on the face or scalp or over the neck (the so-called V sign), although this rash is not specific to dermatomyositis (Fig. 78-7B and C). Another common rash in dermatomyositis is located over the shoulders (shawl sign; Fig. 78-7D) or over the hips (holster sign). Pruritus is common. Patients with dermatomyositis often have skin lesions on their fingers, such as periungual erythema, nail-fold telangiectasias, and cuticular overgrowth (Fig. 78-8C). Other less common

skin manifestations are panniculitis, livedo reticularis, and nonscarring alopecia. Vasculitis may be seen in children with dermatomyositis but rarely in adults.

In general, the skin rash is moderate, with local erythema. In rare cases, a severe, diffuse erythema (erythroderma) may occur, occasionally with vesiculobullous lesions or ulcers. The skin rash may precede the muscle symptoms by months or even years, and in some patients, the skin manifestations may be the only clinical sign of dermatomyositis; this condition is often called amyopathic dermatomyositis or dermatomyositis sine myositis (see later). The pattern of the rash over the knuckles and dorsum of the hand is distinct, in that the rash generally affects the phalanges but

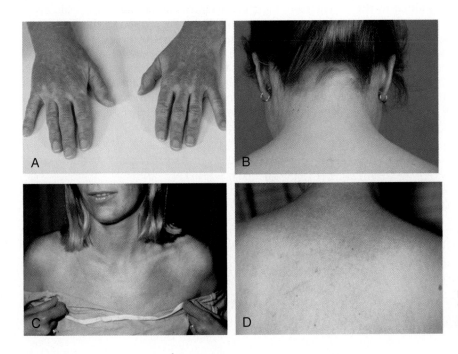

Figure 78-7 **Characteristic features of dermatomyositis skin changes. A,** Linear erythema. **B,** Scalp rash. **C,** V sign. **D,** Shawl sign. *(Courtesy of Dr. Paul Plotz.)*

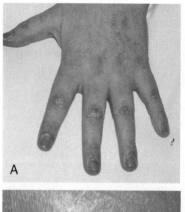

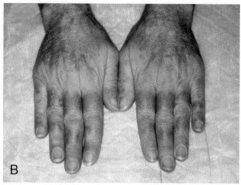

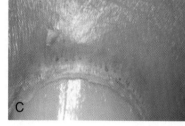

Figure 78-8 Erythematous rashes on the hand in dermatomyositis and systemic lupus erythematosus. A, Note the changes on the knuckles and dorsum of the hand in dermatomyositis (Gottron's sign). **B,** Rash is absent on the knuckles but present on the phalanges in lupus. **C,** Capillary nail-fold changes in dermatomyositis. *(Courtesy of Dr. Paul Plotz.)*

spares knuckles in SLE, and vice versa in dermatomyositis (Fig. 78-8A and B). However, no histopathologic skin features are specific for dermatomyositis; most of the features are also seen in patients with SLE. Thus, skin biopsy is rarely helpful in distinguishing between these two disorders. The cutaneous manifestations may fail to respond to immunosuppressive treatment, despite improvement in muscle symptoms. Thus, it is possible that different molecular pathways or disease mechanisms cause the skin rash and the muscle inflammation.

Calcinosis, which can be severe, is found mainly in juvenile dermatomyositis but is occasionally seen in adults. The calcinosis occurs predominantly in sites that have been subject to friction or trauma, such as the elbows or knees. Sometimes the calcinosis can be extensive and erupt, leading to ulcers. It is most often localized to the subcutaneous tissue but can also develop in the skin, fascia, or muscle and can be visualized by radiography, computed tomography (CT), or magnetic resonance imaging (MRI). The calcinosis seems to progress as long as there is active inflammatory disease. Also, once it has developed, it is often treatment resistant. There are data, however, suggesting that the progress of calcinosis can be inhibited by

effectively treating the inflammatory process in the skin and muscle.[125]

Another type of skin pathology seen in inflammatory myopathies is called mechanic's hands. This rash is often associated with the presence of antisynthetase autoantibodies and can be seen in both polymyositis and dermatomyositis. The rash is a hyperkeratotic, scaling, fissuring of the fingers, particularly on the radial side of the index fingers (Fig. 78-9).

Lungs

Lung involvement is frequent in polymyositis and dermatomyositis and is a major risk factor for morbidity and mortality. Clinical symptoms such as dyspnea and cough are common. Lung involvement can be caused by weakness of the respiratory muscles or inflammation of the lung tissue (interstitial lung disease). Weakness of the respiratory muscles may lead to restrictive lung disease, and involvement of the pharyngeal muscles is a risk factor for aspiration pneumonia. Interstitial lung disease, caused by inflammation in the small airways, is common in polymyositis and dermatomyositis and is often associated with antisynthetase autoantibodies;

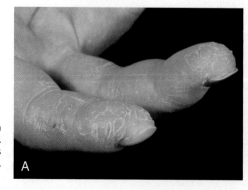

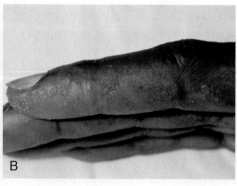

Figure 78-9 Mechanic's hands in a white **(A)** and a black **(B)** patient. Note the characteristic skin changes on the lateral side of the fingers. *(Courtesy of Dr. Paul Plotz.)*

it may be present in up to 70% of patients when investigated with sensitive techniques such as high-resolution CT and measurement of pulmonary function and diffusion capacity.[126] In most cases, the changes are present at the time of diagnosis of myositis; they rarely develop after immunosuppressive treatment has started. The severity of interstitial lung disease may vary from mild or even asymptomatic to rapidly progressive (Hamman-Rich like) with a fatal outcome. In most cases, the interstitial lung disease is mild and has a slowly progressive course. In some cases, improvement in lung function is seen with immunosuppressive treatment. The course and outcome vary, depending on the histopathology, suggesting that different disease mechanisms cause interstitial lung disease.

In general, the clinical course and histopathology of interstitial lung disease in myositis are no different from those in idiopathic interstitial lung disease. The most common histopathologic finding is nonspecific interstitial pneumonia, but other entities such as cryptogenic organizing pneumonia, bronchiolitis obliterans organizing pneumonia, diffuse alveolar damage, and usual interstitial pneumonia are also found. Some studies suggest that bronchiolitis obliterans organizing pneumonia responds favorably to corticosteroids, whereas histopathologic changes compatible with diffuse alveolar damage, usual interstitial pneumonia, or acute interstitial pneumonia respond poorly to corticosteroids or other immunosuppressive therapies and have a poor prognosis.

Arthritis

Joint pain and arthritis are common in patients with polymyositis or dermatomyositis. The most common form of arthritis is a symmetric arthritis of the small joints of the hands and feet. This arthritis is typically nonerosive but can sometimes be erosive and destructive. Most frequently, arthritis is seen in patients with anti–Jo-1 antibodies and other antisynthetase autoantibodies, but it is also seen in patients with overlapping syndromes of other rheumatic diseases.

Heart

Cardiovascular disease is a risk factor for death among patients with polymyositis and dermatomyositis. However, clinically evident heart involvement is rare, perhaps indicating that cardiac involvement may be overlooked in these conditions. Subclinical manifestations are frequently discovered when patients with polymyositis or dermatomyositis are evaluated. The most frequently reported subclinical manifestations are conduction abnormalities and arrhythmias detected by echocardiogram (ECG). The underlying pathophysiologic mechanisms that may lead to cardiac manifestations in patients with polymyositis or dermatomyositis are myocarditis and coronary artery disease, as well as involvement of the small vessels of the myocardium.

Examination with ECG is recommended in newly diagnosed patients with polymyositis or dermatomyositis. Serum tests such as CK-MB to detect cardiac involvement are unreliable in patients with inflammatory myopathies because CK-MB can be released from regenerating skeletal muscle fibers, a common feature in biopsies from patients with polymyositis or dermatomyositis. The CK-MB/total CK ratio may be greater than 3%, a threshold value that is used to define myocardial damage. A more specific marker for myocardial damage in myositis patients is increased serum levels of cardiac isoform troponin-I. The other cardiac troponin isoforms, troponin C and troponin T, are less specific and are also expressed in adult skeletal muscle; increased serum levels have been reported in various muscle disorders.

Gastrointestinal Tract

Difficulty swallowing is frequent in patients with inflammatory myopathies, particularly those with IBM. Muscle weakness occasionally becomes severe and causes problems with nutrition and aspiration pneumonia. The pathophysiology is related to weakness in the tongue, pharyngeal muscles, and sometimes the lower esophagus. Reflux that requires special care is common, occurring in 15% to 50% of patients. Constipation, diarrhea, and stomach pain are common symptoms and may result from disturbed motility of the gut or GI tract inflammation. Vasculitis in the blood vessels of the GI tract is rare but may be complicated by intestinal bleeding.

Antisynthetase Syndrome

A new classification system is based on the presence of MSAs, rather than clinical and histopathologic changes. The most common of these antibodies are the antisynthetase autoantibodies directed against aminoacyl-tRNA synthetases. A clinically distinct subset of myositis, often called antisynthetase syndrome, has been identified in patients with antisynthetase autoantibodies.[39,57] The most common of the antisynthetase autoantibodies is anti–Jo-1, which is directed against histidyl-tRNA synthetase. This autoantibody is present in approximately 20% of patients with polymyositis or dermatomyositis but is only rarely found in patients with IBM.[70] Antisynthetase syndrome is characterized by the presence of antisynthetase autoantibodies and a set of clinical features that includes myositis, interstitial lung disease, Raynaud's phenomenon, nonerosive symmetric polyarthritis of the small joints, and mechanic's hands (see Fig. 78-9). These patients often have fever at disease onset and during flares of disease. Antisynthetase syndrome can be seen in patients with polymyositis or dermatomyositis but is more often seen in patients without skin rashes other than mechanic's hands.

Amyopathic Dermatomyositis

A subset of dermatomyositis is called clinically amyopathic dermatomyositis. These patients have a skin rash, which is typical of dermatomyositis, but no clinical signs of muscle involvement.[127] The proposed definition is based on a skin biopsy consistent with dermatomyositis and a duration of 6 months or longer in the absence of clinical or laboratory evidence of myositis. Some of these patients do have subclinical myositis based on MRI or biopsy findings at presentation; others develop clinically overt myositis sometime later. Patients without clinically overt myositis, however, may develop extramuscular manifestations such as interstitial lung disease, which may be severe. Amyopathic dermatomyositis may be

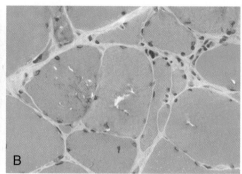

Figure 78-10 Trichrome and hematoxylin and eosin staining of inclusion body myositis biopsy. Note the red-rimmed inclusions (**A**) and marked variation in muscle fiber size (**A** and **B**). *(Courtesy of Dr. Paul Plotz.)*

associated with malignancies, as is the case for classic dermatomyositis. The frequency of this subset is uncertain, but some recent studies suggest that this form of dermatomyositis may be more common than previously thought.

Juvenile Dermatomyositis

The incidence of juvenile dermatomyositis (JDM) is between 1.7 and 3.0 per million children. The disease onset has two peaks—at age 6 and 11 years. JDM is more common in girls than in boys in Europe and North America; in Japan and Saudi Arabia, this difference is less prominent. The most common clinical manifestations at disease onset are muscle weakness, easy fatigability, skin rash, malaise, and in some cases fever.[125] The skin rash is often pathognomonic and similar to adult dermatomyositis, with the most typical skin manifestation being heliotrope discoloration of the upper eyelids, Gottron's papules, periungual erythema, and capillary loop abnormalities. Calcinosis, cutaneous ulceration, and lipodystrophy are more common in juvenile cases than in adults. Calcinosis is seen in 30% to 70% of children with JDM. The calcinosis is most often located at sites exposed to trauma and can be seen in the skin, fascia, or muscles. In some children, the calcinosis becomes prominent and causes contractures and ulcerations. Lipodystrophy occasionally develops, and other metabolic abnormalities, such as insulin resistance and hepatomegaly, are sometimes seen. Vasculopathy that affects the GI tract with ulceration, perforation, or hemorrhage is rare but seems to be more common in children than in adults with dermatomyositis. Because this can be a serious sign, screening for GI involvement should be included in the evaluation of patients with JDM. Interstitial lung disease is rarely seen in JDM cases.

The overall prognosis is variable, but some patients have a good prognosis. Patients with JDM may go into remission, allowing the discontinuation of immunosuppressive treatment. Side effects of immunosuppressive treatment, such as growth failure, are common. In many patients, however, the disease remains chronic, with persisting disease activity into adulthood.

INCLUSION BODY MYOSITIS

IBM is distinguished from polymyositis and dermatomyositis on the basis of both clinical and histopathologic features.[128,129] Sporadic IBM is a distinct entity from familial hereditary inclusion body myopathy, which shares some clinical and histopathologic features but lacks signs of inflammation in muscle tissue. IBM was identified in the 1960s as a subset of inflammatory myopathies, distinct from polymyositis, primarily on the basis of typical histopathologic features that include sarcoplasmic and nuclear inclusions and rimmed vacuoles.[16,17] A characteristic clinical phenotype was later identified, characterized by an insidious onset of muscle weakness over months to years, muscle weakness localized predominantly to the thigh muscles and finger flexors, and resistance to glucocorticoid treatment. IBM patients often have a history of frequent falling. Sporadic IBM cases are sometimes misdiagnosed as polymyositis, because the classic histopathologic changes (rimmed vacuoles and inclusions) may not be evident in early biopsies (Fig. 78-10). A slowly progressive clinical course, development of severe muscle atrophy in the thighs and forearms, and resistance to treatment with immunosuppressive drugs should raise the suspicion of IBM, and a second muscle biopsy should be considered.

In contrast to polymyositis and dermatomyositis, IBM is more frequent in men than in women, and it is seen mainly in individuals older than 50 years. The onset is more insidious than that of polymyositis or dermatomyositis. Patients with IBM rarely have pain. The most frequent initial symptoms are difficulty climbing stairs and walking uphill and frequent falls as a result of weakness in the knee extensor muscles. Muscle weakness may become prominent, and even walking across a threshold may become a problem. Difficulty swallowing may also be an early clinical feature, reflecting the involvement of the pharyngeal muscles. The course is slowly progressive, leading to muscle atrophy that can be striking, particularly in the thigh and forearm muscles. Severe weakness may develop, and many patients become wheelchair dependent. Extramuscular organ involvement is rare, although a subgroup of patients with IBM has sicca symptoms and may develop a secondary Sjögren's syndrome.[130] There are also occasional case reports of IBM in patients with other chronic inflammatory diseases, such as SLE, systemic sclerosis, and interstitial pneumonitis. Autoantibodies are rarely present in IBM patients.

IBM is usually resistant to treatment with glucocorticoids and other immunosuppressive agents. Because of this resistance to treatment, some have questioned whether IBM is an autoimmune disease or a degenerative muscle disease supported by the abnormal accumulation of proteins, such as amyloid-β, in muscle fibers. This issue is still under debate and subject to ongoing research in several institutions around the world.

MYOSITIS ASSOCIATED WITH MALIGNANCIES

An association between dermatomyositis and malignancies was observed in several early case reports. The clinical implications of this association, irrespective of the pathophysiologic mechanisms involved, are that it is imperative to screen for tumors in patients with dermatomyositis at the time of diagnosis and at relapse, particularly if the symptoms do not respond to conventional immunosuppressive treatment. The types of malignancies vary and include not only hematologic malignancies such as lymphoma but also solid tumors such as lung, ovarian, breast, and colon cancer. No specific form of cancer seems to be overrepresented in dermatomyositis. The screening for malignancies should include, at a minimum, a careful clinical examination, routine blood tests, chest radiograph, and mammography and a gynecologic examination for women. If any abnormalities are found, these should guide a more thorough investigation for malignancies.

CLASSIFICATION AND DIAGNOSTIC CRITERIA

At present, there are no prospectively validated diagnostic or classification criteria for myositis. Dividing diseases into homogeneous subsets serves several important functions, including allowing us to estimate disease incidence and prevalence, understand disease pathogenesis and natural history, and evaluate the patient's response to therapy and prognosis. More than 3 decades ago, Bohan and Peter proposed a set of five criteria to facilitate the diagnosis of IIM patients[14,15] (Table 78-4). They classified IIMs into five groups: primary idiopathic polymyositis, primary idiopathic dermatomyositis, IIMs associated with malignancy, childhood IIMs associated with vasculitis, and IIMs associated with collagen vascular diseases. Exclusion criteria include signs of central or peripheral neurologic disease; family history of muscle disease (although familial myositis has been reported in dozens of cases); and symptoms and signs suggestive of muscular dystrophy, granulomatous myositis, infections (including trichinosis, schistosomiasis, trypanosomiasis, staphylococcal infection, and toxoplasmosis), drug-induced myopathy, toxic myopathy, rhabdomyolysis, metabolic disorders, endocrinopathies, myasthenia gravis, or myositis after viral infection (influenza or rubella). A weakness of the Bohan and Peter classification is that it overdiagnoses polymyositis patients and loosely defines overlap syndromes.

Despite several drawbacks, these criteria have served well in diagnosing and defining patients for research purposes for the past 3 decades. IBM was later recognized as a separate disease entity characterized by a slow onset and progression and involving finger flexors or the quadriceps muscles.[128,129] It can occur as a stand-alone entity or with other connective tissue diseases, and patients are often resistant to steroid therapy. Other focal and diffuse forms of myositis, such as orbital myositis, focal nodular myositis, macrophagic myositis, and eosinophilic myositis, are relatively rare.

Since Bohan and Peter proposed their classification criteria, advances in clinical research have led to the identification of certain autoantibodies that are strikingly associated with some clinical phenotypes of myositis (see Table 78-3). The identification of clinical features associated with MSAs and MAAs has led to the proposal of a serologic approach

Table 78-4 Bohan and Peter Criteria for Polymyositis and Dermatomyositis

First exclude all other myopathies
Symmetric proximal muscle weakness
Increase in serum muscle enzymes, such as CK, AST, ALT, aldolase, and LDH
Abnormal electromyographic findings, such as short, small, polyphasic motor units; fibrillations; positive sharp waves; insertional irritability; and bizarre high-frequency repetitive discharges
Abnormal muscle biopsy findings, such as mononuclear infiltration, regeneration, degeneration, and necrosis
Skin rashes, such as the heliotrope rash, Gottron's sign, and Gottron's papules

ALT, alanine transaminase; AST, aspartate transaminase; CK, creatine kinase; LDH, lactate dehydrogenase.

to complement the Bohan and Peter classification system. Others have suggested that the Bohan and Peter criteria be modified to add MSA as a criterion.[131] However, the inclusion of MSA has some limitations: these antibodies are not present in all patients, the immunoprecipitation techniques that are the "gold standard" for identifying these antibodies are available in only a few commercial laboratories, and the enzyme-linked immunosorbent assays often used can give false-positive or false-negative results.

There is an extensive ongoing debate and dialogue within the scientific community about the nature of the diagnostic and classification criteria that could better define these disorders.[64,132,133] Some emphasize a focus on histopathologic features and others on autoantibody profiles. Certainly, the addition of autoantibody profiles, characteristic histopathologic and immunohistochemical features, and imaging techniques such MRI would significantly strengthen the current criteria and better define these disorders. The most frequently used subclassification is based on differences in clinical, immunologic, and histopathologic features and identifies three subtypes of inflammatory myopathies: polymyositis, dermatomyositis, and IBM[134] (Table 78-5).

PHYSICAL EXAMINATION

Although most patients present with muscle weakness or fatigue, the IIMs are systemic connective tissue diseases, and other organs are frequently involved; therefore, a full clinical examination should be conducted when patients present with muscle symptoms. This could also be helpful in distinguishing IIMs from noninflammatory myopathies.

The muscle problems reported by many patients consist not only of muscle weakness but also of muscle fatigue or reduced muscle function. Thus, the evaluation must differentiate between strength and fatigue by evaluating muscle strength and testing repetitive movements for muscle fatigue. In the early phases, atrophy is usually not a pronounced phenomenon in polymyositis or dermatomyositis. In later phases, a moderate symmetric atrophy of proximal muscles may be present. Asymmetric atrophies indicate conditions other than inflammatory myopathies. Patients with IBM often develop more severe atrophy of the quadriceps muscles and the flexor muscles of the forearms; they may also develop deformities in the finger joints and experience difficulty making fists.

Table 78-5 Clinical and Laboratory Features of Subgroups of Idiopathic Inflammatory Myopathies

Diagnostic Features	Dermatomyositis	Polymyositis	Inclusion Body Myositis
Clinical features			
Age	Children and adults	Adults*	Adults >50 yr
Disease onset	Subacute	Subacute	Chronic
Muscle weakness	Proximal	Proximal	Selective pattern†
Symmetry	Symmetric	Symmetric	Asymmetric
Systemic features	Yes‡	Yes‡	Yes§
Skin changes	Yes¶	No	No
Calcinosis	Yes¶	Rarely	No
Associated connective tissue disease	Yes**	Yes**	Yes††
Associated malignancy‡‡	Yes	Yes	Yes
Laboratory features			
Serum enzymes§§	Normal to high	Normal to high	Normal to high
Abnormal EMG¶¶	Yes	Yes	Yes
Abnormal muscle biopsy	Perifascicular atrophy, capillary depletion, patchy MHC class I expression and microinfarcts	CD8 T cell invasion of non-necrotic fibers and MHC class I expression on fibers	CD8 T cell invasion, MHC expression, vacuolated fibers, and tubulofilamentous inclusions in fibers

*Rarely in children.
†Early involvement of finger flexor, wrist flexor or wrist extensor weakness, and involvement of quadriceps femoris.
‡Some patients have dysphagia, synovitis, and interstitial lung disease.
§Some patients have dysphagia.
¶Gottron's sign and heliotrope rash.
¶Especially in children.
**Overlap with scleroderma, systemic lupus erythematosus, rheumatoid arthritis, Sjögren's syndrome, and mixed connective tissue disease (MCTD).
††Associated with Sjögren's syndrome but less frequently associated with other connective tissue diseases.
‡‡Dermatomyositis is more frequently associated with cancer than are polymyositis and inclusion body myositis and not overrepresented in PM or IBM.
§§Serum creatine kinase, aspartate transaminase, lactate dehydrogenase, and aldolase vary from normal to very high levels.
¶¶Myopathic motor unit potentials with spontaneous discharges in dermatomyositis, with and without spontaneous discharges in polymyositis, and mixed pattern of short- and long-duration motor unit potentials in inclusion body myositis.
EMG, electromyogram; MCH, major histocompatibility complex.

Muscle strength can be tested in various ways. A quick screening test for weakness in proximal lower leg muscles is to ask the patient to stand up from a sitting or squatting position without support. A more standardized test that is easy to perform in the clinic is the manual muscle test, with grading according to the Medical Research Council scale. There are many variants of this test, but a short form, addressing eight muscles on the dominant side, is recommended as part of the disease activity score by the International Myositis Assessment and Clinical Studies (IMACS).[135] In most patients with polymyositis or dermatomyositis, muscle strength as assessed by the manual muscle test is good in most of the tested muscle groups. Typically, moderate muscle weakness is seen in the neck flexors and hip girdle muscles. Testing that involves a number of repetitions is often a more sensitive method of detecting muscle impairment. The Functional Index in Myositis-2 is a myositis-specific outcome measure that assesses a number of repetitions. With this test, proximal muscle groups are more involved than are distal muscles. This index is often used by physical therapists.[136] In patients with IBM, knee extensors and finger flexors are often weak.

The skin should also be examined to detect changes, including nail-fold and scalp changes. Joints can be affected by arthritis, and heart and lung changes should be carefully looked for.

LABORATORY EVALUATIONS

Laboratory evaluations are critical components of both diagnosis and patient management. Combinations of laboratory tests are generally used during patient evaluations. Because

no laboratory test is highly specific for IIMs, the results of these tests are usually interpreted in the clinical context.

BIOCHEMICAL

Measuring serum levels of muscle enzymes is an important part of the evaluation of myositis patients. Increased levels of muscle-derived serum enzymes reflect ongoing damage to the muscle parenchyma. These measurements help differentiate IIMs from conditions such as steroid myopathy and denervation, in which atrophy is a prominent feature.[137] Measurement of the serum CK level is traditionally the first step in the assessment of patients with IIM. CK exists as MM (skeletal muscle), MB (cardiac muscle), and BB (brain) isoforms in serum. In comparison to other serum muscle enzymes, CK appears to be a relatively specific and sensitive indicator of the degree of muscle fiber injury. However, the range varies significantly among patients, with levels being near normal in some patients and elevated by several hundred-fold in others.

Generally, 80% to 90% of adult myositis patients show an increase in CK during the initial evaluation. However, a certain proportion of patients, especially those in advanced stages of the disease, show normal or relatively modest elevations in CK, in part because of a lack of muscle mass or the presence of inhibitors of CK activity.[138,139] Normal CK is relatively more common in dermatomyositis than in polymyositis. In the absence of CK elevation, it is usually easier to diagnose dermatomyositis than polymyositis because of the presence of skin rashes in the former. It is also known that CK levels are generally lower in IBM patients than in those with polymyositis or dermatomyositis. Therefore, a normal CK level does not exclude a diagnosis of IIM, particularly IBM or JDM.

Constantly elevated levels of CK are often a sign of inflammatory activity. A rise in CK level is generally correlated with overall disease activity over time, but not with strength or functional measures of disease activity.[140,141] CK measurements are usually not useful for monitoring disease exacerbations, and they should always be evaluated in the clinical context. CK levels may normalize without clinical improvement, or they may increase without clinical worsening; however, increasing levels point to a potential flare and warrant closer clinical evaluation. CK elevations are not specific for myositis, because this enzyme is also elevated in other muscle diseases, including muscular dystrophies, rhabdomyolysis, hypothyroidism, and many drug-induced myopathies. It is important to note that serum levels of CK-MB can be elevated in patients with myositis as a result of the regeneration of skeletal muscle fibers; they are not specific for heart involvement in these patients. The cardiac isoform troponin-I has the highest specificity as an indicator of myocardial involvement and is the most reliable serum marker for detecting myocardial damage in patients with inflammatory muscle disease.[142]

Measurement of other serum muscle enzymes, including aldolase, aspartate transaminase (AST), alanine transaminase (ALT), and lactate dehydrogenase (LDH), significantly improves the chance of diagnosing myositis, especially in patients with active disease and normal CK levels. Aldolase, LDH, and AST are better correlated with disease activity in JDM patients. The main disadvantage of these enzymes is that they are also elevated in liver diseases; therefore, the muscle source needs to be identified before interpreting the data.[143]

The serum myoglobin level is a sensitive index of muscle fiber membrane integrity and can therefore be used to assess the degree of disease activity. The advantage of the myoglobin assay is that it involves a nonenzymatic immunologic reaction; the disadvantages are that a significant range of serum myoglobin levels occurs in myositis patients because of circadian variation,[144] and the test is less readily available than CK for routine use. Elevation of other serum components such troponin, creatine, neopterin, manganese superoxide dismutase, hyaluronate, and soluble CD30 has been shown to correlate with disease activity, but assays of these components have not been validated for use in clinical practice, and they are not available for routine analyses.

IMMUNOLOGIC

The immune response to self-antigens is a common feature of several systemic autoimmune rheumatic diseases, including IIMs. ANAs are found in approximately 60% to 70% of myositis patients. The autoantibody response in IIMs is directed to ubiquitous nuclear and cytoplasmic antigens. The presence of these antibodies is usually assessed by an indirect immunofluorescence assay. ANAs are more frequently found in patients with polymyositis and dermatomyositis, especially those with overlap syndrome. These are less frequently seen in IBM patients or those with malignancy-associated myositis. High-titer ANA is a particularly valuable finding for differentiating IIMs from dystrophies. Many IIM patients show speckled nuclear ANA patterns, and about 10% of IIM patients also show exclusive cytoplasmic patterns in indirect immunofluorescence staining.[145] Many of the MSAs are associated with distinctive clinical features, such as skin rash or interstitial lung disease (Table 78-6). Certain MSAs, such as anti–Jo-1, are more frequently associated with polymyositis; others, such as Mi-2, are more frequent in dermatomyositis.

Table 78-6 Immunologic Features of Idiopathic Inflammatory Myopathies

Feature	Dermatomyositis	Polymyositis	Inclusion Body Myositis
B cell infiltration	+	–/+	–/+
T cell infiltration	+	+	+
CD8 T cell infiltration in non-necrotic fibers	–/+	+	+
Vascular membrane attack complex	+	–	–
Immunoglobulin deposition on blood vessels	+	–	–
MHC class I expression on muscle fibers	–/+*	+	+
Cytokines and chemokines	+	+	+
Cell adhesion molecules	+	+	+
Antinuclear antibodies	+	+	+†
Anti-Jo 1 antibodies‡,§	+	+	–/+
Anti–signal recognition particle antibodies§	–/+	+	–/+
Anti–Mi-2 antibodies¶	+	–/+	–/+
Anti–PM-Scl antibodies¶	+	+	–

*Mostly in perifascicular areas and necrotic fibers.
†Less frequently, but 20% higher than in normal population.
‡Frequency varies among ethnicities; more frequent in polymyositis (22%) than dermatomyositis (16%) or inclusion body myositis (5%).
§Present only in a proportion of polymyositis (14%), dermatomyositis (5%), and inclusion body myositis (3%) patients.
¶Present only in a proportion of polymyositis (9%), dermatomyositis (21%), and inclusion body myositis (8%) patients.
¶Present only in a proportion of polymyositis (7%) and dermatomyositis (6%) patients.

HISTOLOGIC

Muscle biopsy is the "gold standard" for the diagnosis of inflammatory myopathies and a critical component of the definitive diagnosis of IIMs.[146,147] For optimal biopsy results, it is important to select a muscle that is moderately weak. The histologic features can be grouped into general features that are common to all IIMs and specific features unique to a particular subgroup. The general features include necrosis, regeneration, degeneration, variation in fiber diameter, increase in connective tissue, and inflammation. The features specific to dermatomyositis include loss of capillaries, alterations in the morphology of capillaries, capillary necrosis with the deposition of complement products (e.g., membrane attack complex) on the vessel walls, and, rarely, muscle infarcts. Another specific histopathologic finding, albeit a late sign, is perifascicular atrophy. The infiltrates typically have a perivascular distribution. The inflammatory infiltrates are dominated by a high percentage of CD4 T cells and macrophages at the sites of inflammation, with B cells occasionally in evidence. Although perifascicular atrophy is the hallmark of the histologic changes seen in dermatomyositis, it may not be visible if a biopsy is acquired early in the course of the disease. In early dermatomyositis, the MHC class I expression is patchy, and the perifascicular areas are usually stained.

The features of polymyositis include the presence of macrophages and activated CD8 T cells in muscle fibers and the expression of MHC class I molecules on muscle fibers. Mononuclear cell invasion around non-necrotic muscle fibers in endomysial areas is a characteristic feature of IIMs. The histologic features of IBM resemble those of polymyositis but also include unique features, such as red-rimmed vacuoles and inclusions (cytoplasmic or nuclear) and amyloid deposits.[129] An increased number of cytochrome C oxidase–negative fibers can also be seen, but this change is not specific for IBM. In IBM, electron microscopy usually demonstrates 15- to 21-nm cytoplasmic and intranuclear tubulofilaments, which are not found in dermatomyositis or polymyositis. It is not uncommon to find biopsies that are negative for both rimmed vacuoles and tubulofilamentous inclusions. In this situation, if the suspicion for IBM is high, it is best to obtain another sample or to treat the patient with steroids. Nonresponsiveness to treatment further supports the diagnosis of IBM in an otherwise typical patient. Inflammation surrounding necrotic fibers is a feature of some muscular dystrophies (e.g., facioscapulohumeral muscular dystrophy, limb-girdle muscular dystrophy type 2B, and Duchenne's muscular dystrophy), where it is secondary to muscle cell degeneration. Thus, the presence of a mononuclear infiltration surrounding non-necrotic muscle fibers confirms the diagnosis of IBM or polymyositis. The common and unique immunologic and histologic features of the various subgroups are listed in Tables 78-6 and 78-7, respectively.

MOLECULAR

One of the more tangible deliverables of the human genome product has been the development and use of microarrays for messenger RNA (mRNA) profiling. In the commonly

Table 78-7 Histologic Features of Idiopathic Inflammatory Myopathies

Feature	Dermatomyositis	Polymyositis	Inclusion Body Myositis
Necrosis of muscle fibers	+	+	+
Variation in fiber diameter	+	+	+
Regeneration of muscle fibers	+	+	+
Proliferation of connective tissue	+	+	+
Infiltration of mononuclear cells*	+	+	+
Perivascular and perimysial inflammation	+	–/+	–/+
Endomysial inflammation	–/+	+	+
Perifascicular atrophy	+	–	–
Abnormally dilated capillaries	+	–/+	–
Reduced capillary density	+	–/+	–
Deposition of complement on vessel walls	+	–/+	–
Microinfarcts	+	–	–
Invasion of non-necrotic fibers by cytotoxic T lymphocytes and macrophages	–	+	+
Expression of MHC class I on muscle fibers	–/+	+	+
Rimmed vacuoles with amyloid deposits and tubulofilaments†	–	–	+
Angulated or atrophic and hypertrophic fibers	–	–	+
Ragged red or cytochrome oxidase–negative fibers	–	–	+

*Inflammation is absent in a small proportion of polymyositis and dermatomyositis biopsies.
†Also seen in chronic neurogenic conditions and distal myopathies.

used form of microarray, about 1 million DNA probes are placed on 1 cm^2 glass slides, allowing the query of each gene of the genome. Although all genes are shared among all cells, only certain genes are expressed (turned on) in any specific cell at any specific time. Messenger RNA expression profiling using microarrays allows genome-wide assessment of the response of each gene, with a comparison of normal and pathologic states.

Muscle is routinely biopsied as part of the clinical workup of muscle disease, and muscle histopathology is an important part of the diagnosis of inflammatory myopathies. Diagnostic muscle biopsies have been used for mRNA expression profiling in a series of studies, with comparisons between inflammatory myopathies (JDM, polymyositis, IBM) and dystrophic myopathies (Duchenne's muscular dystrophy).[148,149] These comparisons are important, because they differentiate between inflammation associated with downstream myofiber degeneration or regeneration (dystrophies) and inflammatory processes that may initiate the inflammatory myopathies.

Microarrays have provided considerable new insights into dermatomyositis. Early on, mRNA profiling in dermatomyositis showed a predominance of type 1 interferon-responsive pathways, suggesting the possible persistence of an antiviral response.[148] Particularly prevalent was the dramatic expression of the interferon-inducible MxA gene. This signature was confirmed and extended,[150] supporting an important role of the innate immune response, with prominent plasmacytoid dendritic cell infiltration in dermatomyositis compared with the other inflammatory myopathies. The beneficial effect of intravenous immunoglobulin (IVIG) in dermatomyositis has been queried by microarrays to define the drug-responsive genes, then compared to the lack of response in IBM.[151] This study suggested that IVIG suppressed a relatively small subset of inflammatory responses in dermatomyositis muscle, including complement (C1q) and inflammatory cell migration proteins (ICAM-1). Microarrays have helped elucidate an unexpectedly important role for innate immunity in dermatomyositis. They have also provided new insights into the humeral immunity in polymyositis and IBM. Specifically, mRNA expression profiling showed a high proportion of immunoglobulin transcripts as differentially expressed (59% of all detected genes in IBM, and 33% in polymyositis).[152] Plasma cells, defined as those terminally differentiated B cells expressing CD138 but not CD19 or CD20, were then shown to be a key differentiating cell type within IBM and polymyositis muscle.

IMAGING

MUSCLES

Ultrasonograophy, CT, and MRI are the three general imaging techniques used to evaluate skeletal muscle. MRI has emerged as the method of choice for the examination of soft tissue muscle abnormalities, because it efficiently visualizes and quantifies inflammation, fat infiltration, calcification, and alterations in muscle size and localizes pathologic changes in specific muscle groups (Fig. 78-11). MRI examinations can be done on large volumes and can be helpful guides for muscle biopsy sampling. MRI is a potential

outcome tool to be used in the longitudinal analysis of responses to therapy and in clinical trials, although its sensitivity to changes has not been validated.[153-156]

Ultrasonography is useful for detecting abnormal vascularization, and rates of blood flow can be monitored effectively with color Doppler imaging. The main disadvantage of ultrasonography is its inability to visualize deep-seated muscles in cross section. Moreover, image analyses are more subjective than with MRI and depend to a greater degree on the experience of the examiner.[157] Ultrasound muscle examinations are much more frequent in countries where physicians are responsible for performing such examinations and maintaining uniform standards for their evaluation. Ultrasonography provides a safe, noninvasive, easily portable, and relatively inexpensive approach to the evaluation of muscle abnormalities.[158]

CT is the modality of choice for identifying calcifications in soft tissues (e.g., JDM), but it is not useful for detecting inflammatory changes in muscle tissue. Cross-sectional CT images allow quantification of muscle atrophy and fat replacement in deep muscles that may not be generally accessible to ultrasonography.

A combination of MRI and P-31 magnetic resonance spectroscopy examinations produces the most comprehensive and accurate evaluation of patients.[153]

LUNGS

Radiography and high-resolution CT of the lungs are important for detecting lung involvement and should be considered at the time of myositis diagnosis, because the prevalence of interstitial lung disease is high. In contrast, conventional radiography may not always be sensitive enough to detect interstitial lung disease. These are also important tests for assessing the effects of immunosuppressive treatment.

ELECTROMYOGRAPHY

Electromyogram (EMG) changes are usually nonspecific but are a useful indicator of myopathic changes. The major abnormalities include abnormal electrical irritability, decrease in the mean duration of motor unit potentials or increase in the percentage of polyphasic motor unit potentials (short duration), and rapid firing of the motor unit potentials in relation to the level of activity. Later in the course of the disease, fibers are lost from some motor units, and recruitment is reduced. Abnormal electrical irritability in dermatomyositis and polymyositis involves increased insertional activity, trains of positive sharp waves, and fibrillation potentials. Spontaneous electrical activity is a reasonable measure of disease activity in dermatomyositis and polymyositis. EMG abnormalities correlate with alterations in muscle strength and serum muscle enzymes[159] and are a useful measure when serum levels and muscle strength are uninterpretable. The inflammation in IIMs is often patchy, and EMG is useful in determining which muscle should be sampled for biopsy. Because EMG can cause histopathologic changes that complicate the interpretation of the biopsy, it is best to perform EMG on one side and obtain the muscle biopsy from the same muscle on the contralateral side. Even for IBM, in which the disease is often asymmetric, this

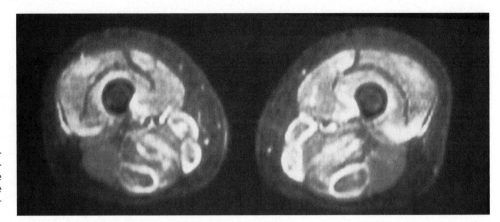

Figure 78-11 Magnetic resonance images (short tau inversion recovery) of the thigh. Note the symmetric inflammation in the affected muscle, seen as bright areas relative to unaffected muscle.

technique is useful as long as the contralateral muscle is also weak.

LUNG FUNCTION TESTS

Pulmonary function tests are an important means of obtaining an objective assessment of respiratory involvement. Typically, patients demonstrate a restrictive ventilatory impairment, with decreased total lung capacity, functional residual capacity, residual volume, forced expiratory volume in 1 second (FEV_1), and forced vital capacity (FVC), but with a normal or elevated FEV_1/FVC ratio and reduced diffusing capacity for carbon monoxide. Pulmonary function tests are also important in estimating disease severity and response to therapy, in concert with radiographic examination.

DIFFERENTIAL DIAGNOSIS

The differential diagnosis of IIMs and other myopathies is important because the clinical associations and response to therapeutic interventions differ significantly. There are a variety of myopathies that closely mimic IIMs (Table 78-8).

DYSTROPHIC MYOPATHIES

Dysferlinopathy

Genetic defects in the dysferlin gene result in limb-girdle muscular dystrophy type 2B and distal muscular dystrophy of the Miyoshi type. These diseases can appear in the late teens or early 20s, and the weakness in the limb-girdle type 2B phenotype first assumes a pelvifemoral distribution: the quadriceps muscle is affected first, followed by weakness in the arms in the later stages of the disease. A relatively acute onset with elevated levels of serum muscle enzymes points to polymyositis as a differential diagnosis. The weakness in the Miyoshi phenotype occurs predominantly in the gastrocnemius and soleus muscles, thereby affecting the ability to walk on the toes. The weakness is slowly progressive, with loss of ambulation generally occurring in the fourth decade, but earlier in some cases. Serum CK levels are very high during the active phase of the disease. In general, the muscle biopsy is dystrophic, with significant mononuclear cell infiltration and small sarcolemmal defects with thickened basal lamina structures over the defects.[160]

Facioscapulohumeral Muscular Dystrophy

A partial deletion of the D4Z4 repeats near the chromosome 4q telomere at 4q35 leads to the facioscapulohumeral phenotype. The initial weakness usually affects the facial muscles, and the onset is insidious. Shoulder weakness is commonly seen because of the weakness of the scapular fixator muscles. The weakness is generally slowly progressive, with typical myopathic changes on the EMG, such as brief, small-amplitude, polyphonic voluntary motor unit potentials. The presence of perivascular, endomysial, and perimysial inflammation is a common feature.[161] Serum CK levels are elevated and vary with age and sex.

Dystrophinopathies

These X-linked recessive disorders are caused by mutations in the dystrophin gene. Milder forms of Becker's muscular dystrophy manifest as myalgias, muscle cramps, exercise intolerance, mild limb-girdle weakness, and quadriceps myopathy. The severe Becker's phenotype that presents before age 8 years is indistinguishable from the Duchenne's phenotype. An elevation in serum CK levels is seen in asymptomatic patients. The mean age at loss of ambulation is usually in the fourth decade. Histologic features include variation in fiber size, central nuclei, regeneration, necrosis, hypercontracted fibers, and endomysial fibrosis. In Becker's dystrophy, the number of necrotic and regenerating fibers is decreased compared to the Duchenne phenotype, and the incidence of hypercontracted and central nuclei increases with age.[162] A plasma membrane defect in non-necrotic fibers and endomysial inflammation with macrophage, T cell, mast cell, and eosinophil infiltration are also characteristic features of this disease.

Proximal Myotonic Myopathy

CCTG expansion in intron 1 of the zinc finger transcription factor (ZNF9) gene results in type 2 myotonic dystrophy. The myotonia is usually absent or minimal but is detectable by EMG. The weakness is mainly proximal, with minimal or no facial involvement. Smooth muscle, cardiac, and diaphragmatic involvement is common in this disease. First-degree heart block is the most common abnormality, and sudden death is well documented.[163] Muscle biopsies show

Table 78-8 Differential Diagnosis of Inflammatory Myopathies

Disease	Key Diagnostic Features
Dystrophic Myopathies	
Dysferlinopathy (Miyoshi myopathy and LGMD2B)	Mutations in dysferlin gene Progressive proximal (LGMD2B) and distal (Miyoshi myopathy) muscle weakness Onset in late teens to early 20s Increased CK levels Inflammation in muscle biopsy Nonresponsiveness to steroids
Facioscapulohumeral muscular dystrophy	Partial deletion in D4Z4 repeats near chromosome 4q telomere at 4q35 Initial facial and shoulder girdle weakness progresses to pelvic girdle and extremities Normal serum CK levels or modest elevation
Becker's dystrophy	Mutations in dystrophin gene X-linked recessive disorders Limb-girdle weakness and cardiomyopathy High serum CK levels
Proximal myotonic myopathy	CCTG expansion in intron 1 of ZNF9 gene Autosomal dominant Proximal muscle weakness
Sarcoglycanopathy	Mutations in sarcoglycans (α, β, γ, and δ) Limb-girdle weakness and cardiomyopathy High serum CK levels
Metabolic Myopathies	
Acid maltase deficiency	Mutations in acid α-glucosidase Proximal muscle weakness Respiratory muscle involvement Abnormal irritability on EMG Increased serum CK levels
McArdle's disease	Mutations in myophosphorylase gene Exercise intolerance Fixed proximal muscle weakness Increased serum CK levels
Mitochondrial Myopathies	
	Mutations in complex I-IV, complex V, and coenzyme Q10 genes Myopathy with limb-girdle weakness Exercise intolerance and fatigue Increased serum CK levels
Endocrine Myopathies	
Cushing's syndrome	Insidious onset Proximal muscle weakness Normal serum CK, AST, and LDH levels
Thyrotoxic myopathy	Subacute onset of proximal muscle weakness Normal serum CK levels or modest elevation Respiratory muscle weakness
Infectious Myopathies	
HIV myopathy	Progressive myopathy Proximal symmetric muscle weakness Endomysial inflammation Increased serum CK levels
Parasitic Myopathies	
	Clinical features of idiopathic inflammatory myopthyies Focal or diffuse inflammation Myocarditis Increased serum CK levels
Drug-Induced Myopathies	
Zidovudine myopathy	Proximal muscle weakness Increased serum lactate levels Ragged red fibers and abnormal mitochondria in muscle Improves with drug discontinuation
Statin myopathy	Necrotizing myopathy Acute or subacute painful proximal myopathy Increased serum CK levels
Corticosteroid myopathy	Proximal and distal weakness Type 2 atrophy and vacuolar changes in muscle Increased serum CK levels
D-penicillamine, IFN-α, and procainamide-induced myopathy	Proximal muscle weakness and pain Inflammation and necrosis in muscle Skin changes Increased serum CK levels

AST, aspartate transaminase; CK, creatine kinase; EMG, electromyogram; IFN, interferon; LDH, lactate dehydrogenase; LGMD, limb-girdle muscular dystrophy.

Continued

Table 78-8 Differential Diagnosis of Inflammatory Myopathies—cont'd

Disease	Key Diagnostic Features
Neuromuscular Diseases	
Motoneuron disease	Upper and lower motoneuron signs
	Asymmetric weakness with denervation atrophy
	Fasciculations and fatigability
	Fibrillations and enlarged motor unit potentials on EMG
	Modest elevation in serum CK levels
Spinal muscular atrophy	Symmetric muscle weakness and atrophy
	Neurogenic changes on EMG and biopsy
	Normal serum CK levels
Myasthenia gravis	Abnormal weakness and fatigability
	Decremental EMG response
	Antiacetylcholine receptor antibodies
	Positive anticholinesterase drug test

nonspecific features, such as central nuclei, sarcoplasmic masses, and atrophy of type 1 fibers.

Sarcoglycanopathy

Mutations in sarcoglycans (α, β, γ, and δ) result in limb-girdle muscular dystrophy types 2C to 2F. Sarcoglycanopathies often start in childhood, with a median age of onset of 6 to 8 years. These diseases present initially as pelvic muscle weakness, including a waddling gait and difficulty performing common tasks, such as getting up from the floor, climbing the stairs, and running. The trunk muscles are prominently affected, and upper extremity involvement usually follows lower extremity involvement. Distal muscles are generally spared until later in the disease process.[164] These progressive disorders result in very high levels of serum CK early in the disease; the levels decrease when patients become wheelchair bound by 12 to 16 years of age. Dilated cardiomyopathy is often seen in these disorders, and muscle biopsies show marked regeneration and necrosis.

NEUROMUSCULAR DISORDERS

Motoneuron Diseases

These diseases, including amyotrophic lateral sclerosis (ALS), are progressive, degenerative disorders of motoneurons in the spinal cord, brainstem, and cerebral motor cortex that manifest clinically as amyotrophy and exaggerated reflexes. These diseases are characterized by a selective loss of function of upper or lower motoneurons, finally leading to a progressive loss of both types of motoneurons over time. EMG shows fibrillation and fasciculation potentials in the muscles of the lower and upper limbs or in the bulbar muscles. Muscle biopsies show the presence of denervation atrophy and secondary myopathic changes in chronically denervated muscles. IBM is the primary muscle disorder most likely to be confused with ALS, and muscle biopsy helps differentiate the two. Serum CK levels are slightly elevated, particularly in the early stages of the disease and in men who are physically active.

Spinal Muscular Atrophy

Late-onset forms of spinal muscular atrophy (SMA) are characterized by progressive muscle weakness and atrophy and reduced tendon reflexes. EMG and muscle testing reveal neurogenic changes in the muscle. Typical muscle biopsy findings include small and large groups of atrophic fibers in the chronic and severe forms of SMA, respectively. Histochemical changes show fiber type grouping, indicating reinnervation. Serum CK levels are slightly increased in juvenile-onset cases and normal in other forms of SMA. EMG shows abnormal spontaneous electrical activity (fibrillations, positive sharp waves, fasciculations), suggesting ongoing denervation.

Myasthenia Gravis

The clinical manifestations of myasthenia gravis include abnormal weakness that is worsened by repeated or sustained exertion and fatigability. Proximal muscles are usually more severely affected than distal muscles. This is a generalized disease that exhibits external ocular muscle involvement, positive anticholinesterase drug tests, and a decremental EMG response. Patients are often positive for antiacetylcholine receptor antibodies.

METABOLIC MYOPATHIES

Acid Maltase Deficiency

This autosomal recessive glycogen storage disease is caused by acid maltase gene mutations. The disease has infantile, childhood, and adult variants. The infantile form manifests in the first few months after birth as rapidly progressive weakness and hypotonia, with death occurring as a result of cardiorespiratory failure. The childhood form manifests as a myopathy in which the weakness is usually greater in the proximal than in the distal muscles; the disease progresses relatively slowly, and patients die of respiratory failure. The adult form presents in the 20s as a progressive myopathy that resembles polymyositis or limb-girdle muscular dystrophy, with additional respiratory symptoms. Serum muscle enzymes (CK, AST, and LDH) are increased in all three forms of the disease, and EMG indicates myopathy in all three cases. Histologic examination reveals a vacuolar myopathy, with the vacuoles displaying a high glycogen content and strongly positive staining for acid phosphatase; necrotic and regenerating fibers are uncommon.

McArdle's Disease

McArdle's disease is the most common of the nonlysosomal muscle glycogenoses. Exercise intolerance is the characteristic feature of this disease, and it often manifests as early fatigue, myalgia, and stiffness of exercising muscle that is relieved by resting. The EMG is normal in some patients; it shows nonspecific myopathic changes in others. Forearm ischemic exercise testing shows virtually no increase in venous lactate in most patients. Serum CK levels, however, are variably elevated in these patients. Muscle biopsies show subsarcolemmal deposits of glycogen at the periphery of the fibers.

MITOCHONDRIAL MYOPATHIES

Mitochondrial diseases are heterogeneous and often present a diagnostic challenge. It has been suggested that myopathy is due to mutations in mtDNA in the skeletal muscle.[165] The clinical course of the pure myopathy varies from rapidly progressive to almost reversible disease, with disease onset occurring from infancy through adulthood. The weakness is facioscapulohumeral and more proximal than distal, with involvement of the orbicularis and extraocular muscles. Patients often complain of exercise intolerance and fatigue and have recurrent episodes of myoglobinuria. Muscle biopsy plays a critical role in the diagnosis of these conditions, especially the use of special histochemical stains that detect succinate dehydrogenase, Cox staining, and Gomori trichrome staining.

ENDOCRINE MYOPATHIES

Cushing's Syndrome

Cushing's syndrome is an endogenous glucocorticoid excess disease that manifests as muscle weakness and wasting. Chronic corticosteroid treatment results in similar manifestations and significant loss of strength within a few weeks of treatment. Muscle biopsy shows increased vacuolations and glycogen accumulation in type 2 muscle. The onset of weakness is usually insidious. The weakness is primarily proximal, with more severe involvement in the legs than in the arms. These patients generally show normal serum muscle enzyme levels (CK, AST, and LDH). Muscle wasting can often be reversed if the glucocorticoid levels are returned to the normal range.

Hyper- and Hypothyroid Myopathy

Myopathic thyroid disease is characterized primarily by proximal muscle weakness and muscle wasting. When distal weakness occurs, it often follows proximal myopathy. Exercise intolerance, fatigue, and breathlessness are common complaints, and weakness of the respiratory muscles results in respiratory insufficiency and the need for ventilatory support. Patients often have difficulty rising from a sitting position or lifting their arms above their heads. Serum muscle enzymes (CK, AST, and ALT) are often normal or low in hyperthyroidism and elevated in hypothyroidism. EMG findings are variable, with short-duration motor unit potentials and increased polyphasic potentials in proximal muscles; fibrillations and fasciculations are uncommon. Muscle biopsy shows atrophy in fiber types, nerve terminal damage, fatty infiltration, and isolated fiber necrosis, with macrophage and lymphocyte infiltration.

INFECTIOUS MYOPATHIES

HIV Myopathy

Neuromuscular manifestations are common in human immunodeficiency virus (HIV)–induced myopathy. The clinical features typically include a myopathy of subacute onset that progresses slowly. The myopathy often starts as proximal symmetric muscle weakness with or without muscle wasting, similar to that in IIMs. Histologic features include muscle fiber necrosis, inflammation, and vacuolated muscle fibers, with a significant increase in serum CK levels. EMG shows spontaneous activity, with fibrillation potentials, positive sharp waves, and brief, low-amplitude polyphasic motor unit potentials.

HTLV-1 Myopathy

Myositis associated with human T-lymphotropic virus 1 (HTLV-1) has been noted in certain areas of the world (e.g., Japan, Jamaica). In these patients, symptoms of polymyositis and IBM occur either alone or in combination with tropical spastic paraparesis.[166] Typical features include weakness and increases in serum CK levels. Histologic findings include interstitial inflammation, muscle fiber necrosis in polymyositis, and endomysial inflammation, vacuoles, amyloid deposits, and tubulofilaments in IBM.

PARASITIC MYOPATHIES

Diseases caused by various parasites—protozoa (e.g., toxoplasmosis, trypanosomiasis, sarcocystosis, malaria), cestodes (e.g., cystocercosis, chinococcosis, coenurosis, sparganosis), and nematodes (trichinellosis, taxocariasis, racunculiasis)—can cause myositis. The clinical features include nonspecific complaints, such as myalgia and focal swelling, and typical features of polymyositis and dermatomyositis. Each parasitic infection shows typical changes on muscle biopsy (e.g., the presence of tachyzoites and toxoplasma cysts along with perimysial and endomysial inflammation). A combination of muscle biopsy and serologic findings is useful in making a diagnosis.

DRUG-INDUCED MYOPATHIES

Drugs can induce myopathic changes either by acting directly on the muscle or by indirectly influencing various factors required for muscle cell survival and growth.

Zidovudine Myopathy

Nucleoside analogues such as zidovudine are used to treat HIV because they act as false substrates for the viral reverse transcriptase. These drugs also cause myalgias, proximal muscle weakness, and fatigue and are sometimes associated with increased levels of serum CK. EMG shows typical myopathic changes. Histologically, muscle fibers show ragged red fibers; atrophic fibers show marked sarcoplasmic changes, with rod-body formation. Pronounced abnormalities in mitochondria, myofilaments, and tubules are also noted by electron microscopy. It has been suggested that these drugs also inhibit mitochondrial DNA polymerase, thus producing the mitochondrial abnormalities. Discontinuation of therapy improves muscle strength and function. In these patients, zidovudine-induced mitochondrial myopathy may coexist along with HIV-induced T cell–mediated inflammatory myopathy.[167]

Statin Myopathy

Statins are lipid-lowering drugs (e.g., lovastatin, simvastatin) that are known to cause necrotizing myopathy. These HMG-CoA reductase inhibitors generally suppress specific cholesterol synthesis and lower plasma concentrations of low-density lipoprotein. The clinical features of this condition include myalgia, cramps, and acute and subacute painful proximal myopathy, with histologic features varying from mild, discrete, and unspecific to muscle fiber necrosis, mononuclear cell infiltration, and myophagocytosis and regeneration. A mild increase in serum CK levels is also noted. Other agents that are known to cause necrotizing myopathy include fibric acid derivatives (clofibrate, gemfibrozil), nicotinic acid, organophosphate poisoning, and ε-aminocaproic acid.

Other Drugs

D-penicillamine is known to induce clinical features reminiscent of dermatomyositis; recovery usually occurs after withdrawal of the drug. Agents such as interferon-α that are used to treat viral hepatitis and certain malignant tumors are also known to induce clinical features that resemble polymyositis. Amphiphilic drugs such as chloroquine, hydroxyl chloroquine, and amiodarone are also known to induce cytoplasmic vacuoles, necrosis, and longitudinal branching of muscle fibers.[168] Drugs that affect microtubules, such as colchicines and vincristine, also induce myopathic changes, with the appearance of characteristic autophagic vacuoles in muscle fibers.

MANAGEMENT AND PROGNOSIS

The recommended treatment for patients with polymyositis or dermatomyositis is based on a combination of pharmacologic therapy and physical exercise. The optimal pharmacologic treatment in polymyositis and dermatomyositis is unclear. Very few controlled trials have been undertaken, so recommendations are based on clinical observations from case series. With these limitations in mind, a suggested outline of treatment for patients with polymyositis or dermatomyositis is depicted in Figure 78-12. In addition to providing treatment, it is important to give patients adequate information about their disease and its treatment. This educational component is best provided by a rheumatology team and patient support groups.

PHARMACOLOGIC TREATMENT

The initial pharmacologic treatment in polymyositis and dermatomyositis is high-dose glucocorticoids: 0.75 to 1 (up to 2) mg/kg body weight per day for 4 to 12 weeks. Most experts recommend that glucocorticoid treatment be combined with another immunosuppressive drug to reduce the side effects of the glucocorticoids and to boost the immunosuppressive effect. The most frequently used immunosuppressive agents are azathioprine and methotrexate. In the

extension phase of one of the few double-blind, placebo-controlled trials that have been reported, the combination of azathioprine and glucocorticoids, as compared with prednisone alone, was associated with better functional ability and a lower requirement for prednisone after 1 and 3 years.[169,170] The recommended azathioprine dosage is 2 mg/kg per day. The dosing regimen for methotrexate is similar to that for rheumatoid arthritis—up to 25 mg weekly, although there have been reports of higher doses. Pulmonary involvement related to myositis does not seem to be a contraindication for methotrexate.

The combination of methotrexate and azathioprine proved to be successful in a few patients with refractory myositis in a prospective, randomized, open-label crossover study comparing two aggressive approaches. There are also newer reports that mycophenolate mofetil might be effective. In patients with interstitial lung disease, cyclophosphamide could be of value. There are also a few reports that cyclosporine A or tacrolimus can be beneficial in these cases.[171,172] In treatment-resistant dermatomyositis, a high dose of IVIG was found to have a beneficial effect on muscle strength when compared with placebo; however, the therapeutic effect was temporary, and repeated infusions were required.[173] In patients with severe, rapidly progressive disease that might be life threatening, high-dose pulses of intravenous methylprednisolone have been reported to be beneficial.

Pharmacologic treatment, including tapering of the corticosteroid dose, should be guided by clinical outcome measures. As discussed earlier, the most appropriate outcome measures are muscle endurance and muscle strength. Side effects of glucocorticoids in these high doses are frequent. Prophylaxis against osteoporosis is recommended with vitamin D and calcium and, when clinically indicated, bisphosphonates. Steroid myopathy is another possible consequence of glucocorticoid treatment that is particularly problematic in patients with inflammatory myopathies. There is no specific test to verify steroid myopathy, but in the absence of active clinical disease, steroid myopathy could contribute to muscle weakness. If steroid myopathy is suspected, tapering of the glucocorticoid dose with careful evaluation of the clinical response is recommended. Glucocorticoids may also cause hypokalemia, and if this is not corrected, it may be associated with muscle weakness and incorrectly interpreted as myositis activity.

The depletion of B cells has recently emerged as a new strategy in autoimmune diseases. One approach is to use rituximab (monoclonal antibody against CD20). There are a few case series suggesting a beneficial effect of depleting B cells in patients with dermatomyositis or polymyositis.[174-176] A large international multicenter trial of B cell depletion is currently under way.

IBM is usually nonresponsive to glucocorticoids. There are occasional case reports of "stabilization" for a period of months, but this condition probably reflects the natural history of the disease. Prolonged administration of glucocorticoids to IBM patients may actually lead to worsening of clinical aspects of the disease, despite the improvement in CK levels and reduced T cell numbers in biopsies. Prednisone treatment also increases the number of amyloid-containing fibers.

A few small studies have shown some beneficial effect of methotrexate, anti–T lymphocyte globulin, or

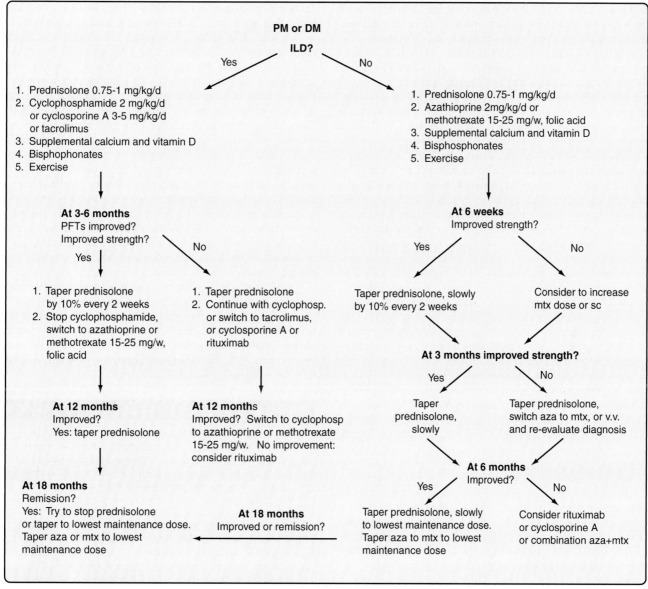

Figure 78-12 Treatment algorithm for adult patients with polymyositis (PM) or dermatomyositis (DM). ILD, interstitial lung disease; PFT, pulmonary function test.

mycophenolate. Anabolic steroids and oxandrolone may have some beneficial effects on muscle strength, although this benefit needs to be confirmed in larger studies. Most experts consider their use justified in combination with glucocorticoids for a limited period in patients who have inflammatory infiltrates on muscle biopsy, or in combination with a more aggressive immunosuppressive treatment (e.g., methotrexate, azathioprine) in patients with another connective tissue disease.

NONPHARMACOLOGIC TREATMENT

With immunosuppressive treatment, approximately 75% of patients improve, but very few recover normal muscle function, even in the absence of muscle inflammation. Combining exercise and immunosuppressive therapy is a safe approach and has clear beneficial effects on muscle function.[176a] The exercise regimen should be individualized and supervised by a physiotherapist to avoid the overuse of muscles. Physical exercise is now recommended as combination therapy with immunosuppressive treatment.

ASSESSING DISEASE ACTIVITY AND OUTCOME

The most important variable to measure in myositis patients is muscle performance or physical function. However, it is equally important to evaluate whether impaired muscle function reflects disease activity or irreversible muscle damage.

Muscle Examination

Manual Muscle Test. There are several tools to measure muscle performance, but the most often used method in clinical practice and clinical trials is the manual muscle test with the MRC scale (see earlier). The drawback is that these tools measure muscle strength but not muscle endurance, which is often a major problem in polymyositis or dermatomyositis. Further, they have not been validated in adults with inflammatory myopathies. Previously, the number of muscle groups tested using the manual muscle test varied, and different scales were used (5 or 10 grade). Recently, a consensus was reached to assess eight muscle groups on the dominant side using a 0- to 10-point scale, where 0 is no muscle contraction, 5 is ability to hold the test position without any added pressure, and 10 is ability to hold the test position against strong pressure. The points between these scores are based on gradual increased resistance against the examiner's pressure. The eight muscle groups tested are neck flexors, shoulder abduction (deltoid middle), biceps brachii, wrist extensors, knee extensors (quadriceps), dorsiflexion of ankle, gluteus maximus, and gluteus medius. The score achieved varies between 0 and 80.

Functional Index in Myositis. The Functional Index in Myositis and its revised form, the Functional Index in Myositis-2, were developed as outcome measures for patients with polymyositis or dermatomyositis. This test measures the number of repetitions that can be performed in defined muscle groups.[136,141] It is a more sensitive method of measuring impaired muscle function in patients with polymyositis or dermatomyositis.[136] The drawback is that it takes a longer time to perform than the manual muscle test, and it may be difficult to use in everyday clinical practice. Preferably, the Functional Index in Myositis-2 is administered by a physiotherapist and can be combined with the manual muscle test.

Extramuscular Involvement

In some patients, extramuscular symptoms predominate among the clinical features. These symptoms may require other assessment tools, such as those used to evaluate interstitial lung disease. For monitoring the effects of treatment of interstitial lung disease, high-resolution CT and pulmonary function tests are recommended.

Disease Activity and Damage

It is also important to distinguish whether symptoms are caused by active inflammatory disease or are a consequence of organ damage. IMACS, an international collaboration, made a consensus recommendation that

Table 78-9   Disease Activity Measure—Core Set

Physician's overall assessment of disease activity on a visual analog scale (VAS)
Patient's or parent's overall assessment of disease activity (VAS)
Functional assessment (health assessment questionnaire)
Muscle strength testing (manual muscle test)
Serum levels of at least two of four muscle enzymes (CK, LDH, AST, ALT)
Extramuscular score (myositis disease activity assessment VAS [MYOACT] or myositis intention to treat activity index [MITAX]), in which disease activity in seven organ systems (general symptoms, skin, joints, GI tract, pulmonary, heart, and muscles) is scored.

ALT, alanine transaminase; AST, aspartate transaminase; CK, creatine kinase; GI, gastrointestinal; LDH, lactate dehydrogenase.

outcome measures for patients with myositis include tools that measure disease activity, damage, and quality of life. The IMACS network developed one outcome measure to assess myositis disease activity and one to measure organ damage: the myositis disease activity assessment tool and the myositis damage index, respectively.[135] The disease activity outcome measure is a core set that consists of the six variables listed in Table 78-9. The damage index is recorded by the physician based on the patient's history and covers several organ systems that can be affected in patients with inflammatory myopathies. To assess the impact on general health, the generic short-form 36, a self-administered health-related quality of life questionnaire, is recommended. These outcome measures have been developed for clinical trials and research but can also be useful in clinical practice. More detailed information about these outcome measures can be found on the IMACS website: https://dir-apps.niehs.nih.gov/imacs.

IMACS has also reached a consensus on what constitutes improvement. Improvement is based on the disease activity core set and is defined as greater than 20% improvement in three of the six variables of the core set, with two or fewer of the variables (except the manual muscle test) worsening by less than 25%. However, this definition of improvement must be validated in longitudinal studies.

Future Directions

Application of new technologies, such as microarrays, to the inflammatory myopathies has provided new hypotheses regarding disease onset and progression and pointed to possible molecular pathways that can be targeted for therapeutic purposes. Particularly important are comparisons of specific subtypes of myositis both with one another and with other muscle diseases; this approach differentiates between downstream pathologic pathways that may be shared by all muscle diseases (myofiber necrosis, regeneration, fibrosis) and those that are farther upstream and more directly linked to disease cause. Importantly, large muscle biopsy microarray data sets inclusive of inflammatory myopathies are now in the public domain, permitting the analysis of this complex molecular data by researchers worldwide.[177] This should effectively parallelize research on the inflammatory myopathies and greatly speed our understanding of molecular pathogenesis and facilitate targeted therapeutics.

REFERENCES

1. Wagner E: Fall einer seltenen Muskelkrankheit. Arch Heilkd 4: 282, 1863.
2. Wagner E: Ein Fall von acuter polymyositis. Dtsch Arch Klin Med 40:241, 1887.
3. Jackson H: Myositis universalis acuta infectiosa with a case. Boston Med Surg J 116:498, 1887.
4. **Unverricht H: Polymyositis acuta progressiva. Z Klin Med 12: 533, 1887.**
5. Unverricht H: Dermatomyositis acuta. Dtsch Med Wochenschr 17:41, 1891.
6. Steiner WR: Dermatomyositis, with report of a case which presented a rare muscle anomaly but once described in man. J Exp Med 6:407, 1903.

7. Deleted in press.
8. Batten F: Case of dermatomyositis in a child, with pathological report. Br J Child Dis 9:247, 1912.
9. Pearson C: Polymyositis. Annu Rev Med 17:63, 1966.
10. Levison P: Polymyositis, acute and subchronic, with round-cell infiltration of muscles. Acta Psychiat Neurol 12:89, 1937.
11. Urechia CI, Dragomir L: Un cas de polymyosite. Monatsschr Psychiat Neurol 107:111, 1943.
12. Furtado D, Alvim F: Lisboa Med 22:259, 1945.
13. Banker BQ, Victor M: Dermatomyositis (systemic angiopathy) of childhood. Medicine (Baltimore) 45:261-289, 1966.
14. Bohan A, Peter JB: Polymyositis and dermatomyositis (first of two parts). N Engl J Med 292:344-347, 1975.
15. Bohan A, Peter JB: Polymyositis and dermatomyositis (second of two parts). N Engl J Med 292:403-407, 1975.
16. Yunis E, Samaha F: Inclusion body myositis. Lab Invest 25:240-248, 1971.
17. **Carpenter S, Karpati G, Heller I, Eisen A: Inclusion body myositis: A distinct variety of idiopathic inflammatory myopathy. Neurology 28:8-17, 1978.**
18. Oddis C, Conte C, Steen V: Incidence of polymyositis-dermatomyositis: A 20 year study of hospital diagnosed cases in Allegheny County, PA 1963-1982. J Rheumatol 17:1329-1334, 1990.
19. Mastaglia FL, Phillips BA: Idiopathic inflammatory myopathies: Epidemiology, classification, and diagnostic criteria. Rheum Dis Clin North Am 28:723-741, 2002.
20. Medsger TA Jr, Dawson WN Jr, Masi AT: The epidemiology of polymyositis. Am J Med 48:715-723, 1970.
21. Patrick M, Buchbinder R, Jolley D, et al: Incidence of inflammatory myopathies in Victoria, Australia, and evidence of spatial clustering. J Rheumatol 26:1094-1100, 1999.
22. Weitoft T: Occurrence of polymyositis in the county of Gavleborg, Sweden. Scand J Rheumatol 26:104-106, 1997.
23. Felice K, North W: Inclusion body myositis in Connecticut: Observations in 35 patients during an 8-year period. Medicine 80:320-327, 2001.
24. Phillips B: Prevalence of inclusion body myositis in western Australia. Muscle Nerve 23:970-972, 2000.
25. Badrising UA, Maat-Schieman M, van Duinen SG, et al: Epidemiology of inclusion body myositis in the Netherlands: A nationwide study. Neurology 55:1385-1387, 2000.
26. Amato A, Barohn R: Idiopathic inflammatory myopathies. Neurol Clin 15:615-648, 1997.
27. Foote R, Kimbrough S, Stevens J: Lupus myositis. Muscle Nerve 5:65-68, 1982.
28. Hill CL, Zhang Y, Sigurgeirsson B, et al: Frequency of specific cancer types in dermatomyositis and polymyositis: A population-based study. Lancet 357:96-100, 2001.
29. Buchbinder R, Forbes A, Hall S, et al: Incidence of malignant disease in biopsy-proven inflammatory myopathy: A population-based cohort study. Ann Intern Med 134:1087-1095, 2001.
30. Shamim EA, Miller FW: Familial autoimmunity and the idiopathic inflammatory myopathies. Curr Rheumatol Rep 2:201-211, 2000.
31. Shamim EA, Rider LG, Miller FW: Update on the genetics of the idiopathic inflammatory myopathies. Curr Opin Rheumatol 12:482-491, 2000.
32. Rider LG, Gurley RC, Pandey JP, et al: Clinical, serologic, and immunogenetic features of familial idiopathic inflammatory myopathy. Arthritis Rheum 41:710-719, 1998.
33. Rider LG, Shamim E, Okada S, et al: Genetic risk and protective factors for idiopathic inflammatory myopathy in Koreans and American whites: A tale of two loci. Arthritis Rheum 42:1285-1290, 1999.
34. O'Hanlon TP, Carrick DM, Arnett FC, et al: Immunogenetic risk and protective factors for the idiopathic inflammatory myopathies: Distinct HLA-A, -B, -Cw, -DRB1 and -DQA1 allelic profiles and motifs define clinicopathologic groups in caucasians. Medicine (Baltimore) 84:338-349, 2005.
35. O'Hanlon TP, Carrick DM, Targoff IN, et al: Immunogenetic risk and protective factors for the idiopathic inflammatory myopathies: Distinct HLA-A, -B, -Cw, -DRB1, and -DQA1 allelic profiles distinguish European American patients with different myositis autoantibodies. Medicine (Baltimore) 85:111-127, 2006.
36. O'Hanlon TP, Rider LG, Mamyrova G, et al: HLA polymorphisms in African Americans with idiopathic inflammatory myopathy: Allelic profiles distinguish patients with different clinical phenotypes and myositis autoantibodies. Arthritis Rheum 54:3670-3681, 2006.
37. Badrising UA, Schreuder GM, Giphart MJ, et al: Associations with autoimmune disorders and HLA class I and II antigens in inclusion body myositis. Neurology 63:2396-2398, 2004.
38. Furuya T: Association of HLA class 1 and class 2 alleles with myositis in Japanese patients. J Rheumatol 25:1109-1114, 1998.
39. **Love LA, Leff RL, Fraser DD, et al: A new approach to the classification of idiopathic inflammatory myopathy: Myositis-specific autoantibodies define useful homogeneous patient groups. Medicine (Baltimore) 70:360-374, 1991.**
40. Artlett CM, Cox LA, Jimenez SA: Detection of cellular microchimerism of male or female origin in systemic sclerosis patients by polymerase chain reaction analysis of HLA-Cw antigens. Arthritis Rheum 43:1062-1067, 2000.
41. Reed AM, Picornell YJ, Harwood A, Kredich DW: Chimerism in children with juvenile dermatomyositis. Lancet 356:2156-2157, 2000.
42. Reed AM, Ytterberg SR: Genetic and environmental risk factors for idiopathic inflammatory myopathies. Rheum Dis Clin North Am 28:891-916, 2002.
43. Travers RL, Hughes GR, Cambridge G, Sewell JR: Coxsackie B neutralisation titres in polymyositis/dermatomyositis. Lancet 1:1268, 1977.
44. Pearson CM: Editorial: Myopathy with viral-like structures. N Engl J Med 292:641, 1975.
45. Leff RL, Love LA, Miller FW, et al: Viruses in idiopathic inflammatory myopathies: Absence of candidate viral genomes in muscle. Lancet 339:1192-1195, 1992.
46. Behan WM, Behan PO, Draper IT, Williams H: Does *Toxoplasma* cause polymyositis? Report of a case of polymyositis associated with toxoplasmosis and a critical review of the literature. Acta Neuropathol (Berl) 61:246-252, 1983.
47. Calore EE, Minkovski R, Khoury Z, et al: Skeletal muscle pathology in 2 siblings infected with *Toxoplasma gondii*. J Rheumatol 27:1556-1559, 2000.
48. Bretagne S, Costa JM, Cosnes A, et al: Lack of *Toxoplasma gondii* DNA in muscles of patients with inflammatory myopathy and increased anti-*Toxoplasma* antibodies. Muscle Nerve 17:822-824, 1994.
49. Cossermelli W, Friedman H, Pastor EH, et al: Polymyositis in Chagas's disease. Ann Rheum Dis 37:277-280, 1978.
50. Buckner FS, Wilson AJ, Van Voorhis WC: Detection of live *Trypanosoma cruzi* in tissues of infected mice by using histochemical stain for beta-galactosidase. Infect Immun 67:403-409, 1999.
51. Atlas E, Novak SN, Duray PH, Steere AC: Lyme myositis: Muscle invasion by *Borrelia burgdorferi*. Ann Intern Med 109:245-246, 1988.
51a. Andersson J, Nyberg P, Dahlstedt A, et al: CBA/J mice infected with *Trypanosoma cruzi* as an experimental model for human polymyositis. Muscle Nerve 27:442-448, 2003.
52. Okada S: Global surface ultraviolet radiation intensity may modulate the clinical and immunologic expression of autoimmune muscle disease. Arthritis Rheum 48:2285-2293, 2003.
53. Sigurgeirsson B, Lindelof B, Edhag O, Allander E: Risk of cancer in patients with dermatomyositis or polymyositis: A population-based study. N Engl J Med 326:363-367, 1992.
54. Casciola-Rosen L: Autoimmune myositis: New concepts for disease initiation and propagation. Curr Opin Rheumatol 17:699-700, 2005.
55. Casciola-Rosen L, Nagaraju K, Plotz P, et al: Enhanced autoantigen expression in regenerating muscle cells in idiopathic inflammatory myopathy. J Exp Med 201:591-601, 2005.
56. Rosen A, Casciola-Rosen L: Stem cells in inflammatory disease. Curr Opin Rheumatol 18:618-619, 2006.
57. Love LA, Miller FW: Noninfectious environmental agents associated with myopathies. Curr Opin Rheumatol 5:712-718, 1993.
58. Sinzinger H, Rodrigues M: Atorvastatin and fibrinogen—a small subgroup shows extreme response. Atherosclerosis 145:415-417, 1999.
59. Sinzinger H, Schmid P, O'Grady J: Two different types of exercise-induced muscle pain without myopathy and CK-elevation during HMG-Co-enzyme-A-reductase inhibitor treatment. Atherosclerosis 143:459-460, 1999.
60. Argov Z: Drug-induced myopathies. Curr Opin Neurol 13:541-545, 2000.
61. Vassallo C, Passamonti F, Merante S, et al: Muco-cutaneous changes during long-term therapy with hydroxyurea in chronic myeloid leukaemia. Clin Exp Dermatol 26:141-148, 2001.
62. Gherardi RK, Coquet M, Cherin P, et al: Macrophagic myofasciitis lesions assess long-term persistence of vaccine-derived aluminium hydroxide in muscle. Brain 124:1821-1831, 2001.

63. Lyon MG, Bloch DA, Hollak B, Fries JF: Predisposing factors in polymyositis-dermatomyositis: Results of a nationwide survey. J Rheumatol 16:1218-1224, 1989.

64. Dalakas MC, Hohlfeld R: Polymyositis and dermatomyositis. Lancet 362:971-982, 2003.

65. Lundberg IE: The physiology of inflammatory myopathies: An overview. Acta Physiol Scand 171:207-213, 2001.

66. Lundberg IE: New possibilities to achieve increased understanding of disease mechanisms in idiopathic inflammatory myopathies. Curr Opin Rheumatol 14:639-642, 2002.

67. Nagaraju K: Immunological capabilities of skeletal muscle cells. Acta Physiol Scand 171:215-223, 2001.

68. Nagaraju K: Update on immunopathogenesis in inflammatory myopathies. Curr Opin Rheumatol 13:461-468, 2001.

69. Nagaraju K, Casciola-Rosen L, Lundberg I, et al: Activation of the endoplasmic reticulum stress response in autoimmune myositis: Potential role in muscle fiber damage and dysfunction. Arthritis Rheum 52:1824-1835, 2005.

70. Brouwer R, Hengstman GJ, Vree Egberts W, et al: Autoantibody profiles in the sera of European patients with myositis. Ann Rheum Dis 60:116-123, 2001.

71. Vazquez-Abad D, Rothfield NF: Sensitivity and specificity of anti-Jo-1 antibodies in autoimmune diseases with myositis. Arthritis Rheum 39:292-296, 1996.

72. Arnett FC, Targoff IN, Mimori T, et al: Interrelationship of major histocompatibility complex class II alleles and autoantibodies in four ethnic groups with various forms of myositis. Arthritis Rheum 39:1507-1518, 1996.

73. Mierau R, Dick T, Bartz-Bazzanella P, et al: Strong association of dermatomyositis-specific Mi-2 autoantibodies with a tryptophan at position 9 of the HLA-DR beta chain. Arthritis Rheum 39:868-876, 1996.

74. Targoff IN, Reichlin M: The association between Mi-2 antibodies and dermatomyositis. Arthritis Rheum 28:796-803, 1985.

75. Miller FW, Twitty SA, Biswas T, Plotz PH: Origin and regulation of a disease-specific autoantibody response: Antigenic epitopes, spectrotype stability, and isotype restriction of anti-Jo-1 autoantibodies. J Clin Invest 85:468-475, 1990.

76. Oddis CV, Okano Y, Rudert WA, et al: Serum autoantibody to the nucleolar antigen PM-Scl: Clinical and immunogenetic associations. Arthritis Rheum 35:1211-1217, 1992.

77. Blaszczyk M, Jablonska S, Szymanska-Jagiello W, et al: Childhood scleromyositis: An overlap syndrome associated with PM-Scl antibody. Pediatr Dermatol 8:1-8, 1991.

78. Hausmanowa-Petrusewicz I, Kowalska-Oledzka E, Miller FW, et al: Clinical, serologic, and immunogenetic features in Polish patients with idiopathic inflammatory myopathies. Arthritis Rheum 40:1257-1266, 1997.

79. Cambridge G, Ovadia E, Isenberg DA, et al: Juvenile dermatomyositis: Serial studies of circulating autoantibodies to a 56kD nuclear protein. Clin Exp Rheumatol 12:451-457, 1994.

80. Emslie-Smith AM, Engel AG: Microvascular changes in early and advanced dermatomyositis: A quantitative study. Ann Neurol 27:343-356, 1990.

81. Kissel JT, Mendell JR, Rammohan KW: Microvascular deposition of complement membrane attack complex in dermatomyositis. N Engl J Med 314:329-334, 1986.

82. Nagaraju K, Rider LG, Fan C, et al: Endothelial cell activation and neovascularization are prominent in dermatomyositis. J Autoimmune Dis 3:2, 2006.

83. Kissel JT, Halterman RK, Rammohan KW, Mendell JR: The relationship of complement-mediated microvasculopathy to the histologic features and clinical duration of disease in dermatomyositis. Arch Neurol 48:26-30, 1991.

84. Arahata K, Engel AG: Monoclonal antibody analysis of mononuclear cells in myopathies. III. Immunoelectron microscopy aspects of cell-mediated muscle fiber injury. Ann Neurol 19:112-125, 1986.

85. Goebels N, Michaelis D, Engelhardt M, et al: Differential expression of perforin in muscle-infiltrating T cells in polymyositis and dermatomyositis. J Clin Invest 97:2905-2910, 1996.

86. Mantegazza R, Andreetta F, Bernasconi P, et al: Analysis of T cell receptor repertoire of muscle-infiltrating T lymphocytes in polymyositis: Restricted V alpha/beta rearrangements may indicate antigen-driven selection. J Clin Invest 91:2880-2886, 1993.

87. Bender A, Ernst N, Iglesias A, et al: T cell receptor repertoire in polymyositis: Clonal expansion of autoaggressive CD8+ T cells. J Exp Med 181:1863-1868, 1995.

88. Hohlfeld R, Engel AG: Coculture with autologous myotubes of cytotoxic T cells isolated from muscle in inflammatory myopathies. Ann Neurol 29:498-507, 1991.

89. Behrens L, Bender A, Johnson MA, Hohlfeld R: Cytotoxic mechanisms in inflammatory myopathies: Co-expression of Fas and protective Bcl-2 in muscle fibres and inflammatory cells. Brain 120:929-938, 1997.

90. Nagaraju K, Casciola-Rosen L, Rosen A, et al: The inhibition of apoptosis in myositis and in normal muscle cells. J Immunol 164:5459-5465, 2000.

91. Li M, Dalakas MC: Expression of human IAP-like protein in skeletal muscle: A possible explanation for the rare incidence of muscle fiber apoptosis in T-cell mediated inflammatory myopathies. J Neuroimmunol 106:1-5, 2000.

92. DeVere R, Bradley WG: Polymyositis: Its presentation, morbidity and mortality. Brain 98:637-666, 1975.

93. Emslie-Smith AM, Arahata K, Engel AG: Major histocompatibility complex class I antigen expression, immunolocalization of interferon subtypes, and T cell-mediated cytotoxicity in myopathies. Hum Pathol 20:224-231, 1989.

94. Englund P, Nennesmo I, Klareskog L, Lundberg IE: Interleukin-1alpha expression in capillaries and major histocompatibility complex class I expression in type II muscle fibers from polymyositis and dermatomyositis patients: Important pathogenic features independent of inflammatory cell clusters in muscle tissue. Arthritis Rheum 46:1044-1055, 2002.

95. Plotz PH, Dalakas M, Leff RL, et al: Current concepts in the idiopathic inflammatory myopathies: Polymyositis, dermatomyositis, and related disorders. Ann Intern Med 111:143-157, 1989.

96. Adams E: A pilot study: Use of fludarabine for refractory dermatomyositis and polymyositis, and examination of endpoint measures. J Rheumatol 26:352-360, 1999.

97. Nawata Y, Kurasawa K, Takabayashi K, et al: Corticosteroid resistant interstitial pneumonitis in dermatomyositis/polymyositis: Prediction and treatment with cyclosporine. J Rheumatol 26:1527-1533, 1999.

98. Lundberg I, Kratz AK, Alexanderson H, Patarroyo M: Decreased expression of interleukin-1alpha, interleukin-1beta, and cell adhesion molecules in muscle tissue following corticosteroid treatment in patients with polymyositis and dermatomyositis. Arthritis Rheum 43:336-348, 2000.

99. Nyberg P, Wikman AL, Nennesmo I, Lundberg I: Increased expression of interleukin 1alpha and MHC class I in muscle tissue of patients with chronic, inactive polymyositis and dermatomyositis. J Rheumatol 27:940-948, 2000.

100. Engel AG, Arahata K, Emslie-Smith A: Immune effector mechanisms in inflammatory myopathies. Res Publ Assoc Res Nerv Ment Dis 68:141-157, 1990.

101. Nagaraju K, Raben N, Merritt G, et al: A variety of cytokines and immunologically relevant surface molecules are expressed by normal human skeletal muscle cells under proinflammatory stimuli. Clin Exp Immunol 113:407-414, 1998.

102. Hohlfeld R, Engel AG: HLA expression in myoblasts. Neurology 41:2015, 1991.

103. Karpati G, Pouliot Y, Carpenter S: Expression of immunoreactive major histocompatibility complex products in human skeletal muscles. Ann Neurol 23:64-72, 1988.

104. Nagaraju K, Raben N, Loeffler L, et al: Conditional up-regulation of MHC class I in skeletal muscle leads to self-sustaining autoimmune myositis and myositis-specific autoantibodies. Proc Natl Acad Sci U S A 97:9209-9214, 2000.

105. Tajima Y, Moriwaka F, Tashiro K: Temporal alterations of immunohistochemical findings in polymyositis. Intern Med 33:263-270, 1994.

106. Dalakas MC: Immunopathogenesis of inflammatory myopathies. Ann Neurol 37(Suppl 1):S74-S86, 1995.

107. Bartoccioni E, Gallucci S, Scuderi F, et al: MHC class I, MHC class II and intercellular adhesion molecule-1 (ICAM-1) expression in inflammatory myopathies. Clin Exp Immunol 95:166-172, 1994.

108. Pavlath GK: Regulation of class I MHC expression in skeletal muscle: Deleterious effect of aberrant expression on myogenesis. J Neuroimmunol 125:42-50, 2002.

109. Kaufman RJ: Stress signaling from the lumen of the endoplasmic reticulum: Coordination of gene transcriptional and translational controls. Genes Dev 13:1211-1233, 1999.

110. Mori K: Tripartite management of unfolded proteins in the endoplasmic reticulum. Cell 101:451-454, 2000.

111. Matsumoto M, Minami M, Takeda K, et al: Ectopic expression of CHOP (GADD153) induces apoptosis in M1 myeloblastic leukemia cells. FEBS Lett 395:143-147, 1996.

112. Nakagawa T, Zhu H, Morishima N, et al: Caspase-12 mediates endoplasmic-reticulum-specific apoptosis and cytotoxicity by amyloid-beta. Nature 403:98-103, 2000.

113. Vattemi G, Engel WK, McFerrin J, Askanas V: Endoplasmic reticulum stress and unfolded protein response in inclusion body myositis muscle. Am J Pathol 164:1-7, 2004.

114. **Lundberg I, Brengman JM, Engel AG: Analysis of cytokine expression in muscle in inflammatory myopathies, Duchenne dystrophy, and non-weak controls. J Neuroimmunol 63:9-16, 1995.**

115. Lundberg I, Ulfgren AK, Nyberg P, et al: Cytokine production in muscle tissue of patients with idiopathic inflammatory myopathies. Arthritis Rheum 40:865-874, 1997.

116. Kuru S, Inukai A, Liang Y, et al: Tumor necrosis factor-alpha expression in muscles of polymyositis and dermatomyositis. Acta Neuropathol (Berl) 99:585-588, 2000.

117. De Bleecker JL, Engel AG: Expression of cell adhesion molecules in inflammatory myopathies and Duchenne dystrophy. J Neuropathol Exp Neurol 53:369-376, 1994.

118. Nagaraju K, Raben N, Villalba ML, et al: Costimulatory markers in muscle of patients with idiopathic inflammatory myopathies and in cultured muscle cells. Clin Immunol 92:161-169, 1999.

119. Chevrel G, Granet C, Miossec P: Contribution of tumour necrosis factor alpha and interleukin (IL) 1beta to IL6 production, NF-kappaB nuclear translocation, and class I MHC expression in muscle cells: In vitro regulation with specific cytokine inhibitors. Ann Rheum Dis 64:1257-1262, 2005.

120. Monici MC, Aguennouz M, Mazzeo A, et al: Activation of nuclear factor-kappaB in inflammatory myopathies and Duchenne muscular dystrophy. Neurology 60:993-997, 2003.

121. Reid MB, Lannergren J, Westerblad H: Respiratory and limb muscle weakness induced by tumor necrosis factor-alpha: Involvement of muscle myofilaments. Am J Respir Crit Care Med 166:479-484, 2002.

122. Derk CT, Vivino FB, Kenyon L, et al: Inclusion body myositis in connective tissue disorders: Case report and review of the literature. Clin Rheumatol 22:324-328, 2003.

123. Yood RA, Smith TW: Inclusion body myositis and systemic lupus erythematosus. J Rheumatol 12:568-570, 1985.

124. Santmyire-Rosenberger B, Dugan EM: Skin involvement in dermatomyositis. Curr Opin Rheumatol 15:714-722, 2003.

125. Ramanan AV, Feldman BM: Clinical features and outcomes of juvenile dermatomyositis and other childhood onset myositis syndromes. Rheum Dis Clin North Am 28:833-857, 2002.

126. Fathi M, Dastmalchi M, Rasmussen E, et al: Interstitial lung disease, a common manifestation of newly diagnosed polymyositis and dermatomyositis. Ann Rheum Dis 63:297-301, 2004.

127. Gerami P, Schope JM, McDonald L, et al: A systematic review of adult-onset clinically amyopathic dermatomyositis (dermatomyositis sine myositis): A missing link within the spectrum of the idiopathic inflammatory myopathies. J Am Acad Dermatol 54:597-613, 2006.

128. Griggs RC: The current status of treatment for inclusion-body myositis. Neurology 66(2 Suppl 1):S30-S32, 2006.

129. Griggs RC, Askanas V, DiMauro S, et al: Inclusion body myositis and myopathies. Ann Neurol 38:705-713, 1995.

130. Lindvall B: Subclinical myositis is common in primary Sjogren's syndrome and is not related to muscle pain. J Rheumatol 29:717-725, 2002.

131. Bunn C, Mathews M: Two human tRNA(Ala) families are recognized by autoantibodies in polymyositis sera. Mol Biol Med 4:21-36, 1987.

132. Tanimoto K, Nakano K, Kano S, et al: Classification criteria for polymyositis and dermatomyositis. J Rheumatol 22:668-674, 1995.

133. Miller F, Rider L, Plotz P, et al: Diagnostic criteria for polymyositis and dermatomyositis. Lancet 362:1762-1763, 2003.

134. Dalakas M: Polymyositis, dermatomyositis and inclusion body myositis. N Engl J Med 325:1487-1498, 1991.

135. **Miller FW, Rider LG, Chung YL, et al: Proposed preliminary core set measures for disease outcome assessment in adult and juvenile idiopathic inflammatory myopathies. Rheumatology (Oxford) 40:1262-1273, 2001.**

136. Alexanderson H, Broman L, Tollback A, et al: Functional index-2: Validity and reliability of a disease-specific measure of impairment in patients with polymyositis and dermatomyositis. Arthritis Rheum 55:114-122, 2006.

137. Askari A, Vignos PJ Jr, Moskowitz RW: Steroid myopathy in connective tissue disease. Am J Med 61:485-492, 1976.

138. Kagen LJ, Aram S: Creatine kinase activity inhibitor in sera from patients with muscle disease. Arthritis Rheum 30:213-217, 1987.

139. Targoff IN: Laboratory testing in the diagnosis and management of idiopathic inflammatory myopathies. Rheum Dis Clin North Am 28:859-890, 2002.

140. Kroll M, Otis J, Kagen L: Serum enzyme, myoglobin and muscle strength relationships in polymyositis and dermatomyositis. J Rheumatol 13:349-355, 1986.

141. Josefson A, Romanus E, Carlsson J: A functional index in myositis. J Rheumatol 23:1380-1384, 1996.

142. Kiely P, Bruckner F, Nisbet J, Daghir A: Serum skeletal troponin 1 in inflammatory muscle disease: Relation to creatine kinase, CKMB and cardiac troponin 1. Ann Rheum Dis 59:750-751, 2000.

143. Helfgott SM, Karlson E, Beckman E: Misinterpretation of serum transaminase elevation in "occult" myositis. Am J Med 95:447-449, 1993.

144. Bombardieri S, Clerico A, Riente L, et al: Circadian variations of serum myoglobin levels in normal subjects and patients with polymyositis. Arthritis Rheum 25:1419-1424, 1982.

145. Targoff IN: Update on myositis-specific and myositis-associated autoantibodies. Curr Opin Rheumatol 12:475-481, 2000.

146. Dalakas MC: Muscle biopsy findings in inflammatory myopathies. Rheum Dis Clin North Am 28:779-798, 2002.

147. Hilton-Jones D: Inflammatory muscle diseases. Curr Opin Neurol 14:591-596, 2001.

148. Tezak Z, Hoffman EP, Lutz JL, et al: Gene expression profiling in DQA1*0501+ children with untreated dermatomyositis: A novel model of pathogenesis. J Immunol 168:4154-4163, 2002.

149. Greenberg SA, Sanoudou D, Haslett JN, et al: Molecular profiles of inflammatory myopathies. Neurology 59:1170-1182, 2002.

150. Greenberg SA, Pinkus JL, Pinkus GS, et al: Interferon-alpha/beta-mediated innate immune mechanisms in dermatomyositis. Ann Neurol 57:664-678, 2005.

151. Raju R, Dalakas MC: Gene expression profile in the muscles of patients with inflammatory myopathies: Effect of therapy with IVIG and biological validation of clinically relevant genes. Brain 128:1887-1896, 2005.

152. Greenberg SA, Bradshaw EM, Pinkus JL, et al: Plasma cells in muscle in inclusion body myositis and polymyositis. Neurology 65:1782-1787, 2005.

153. Park JH, Vital TL, Ryder NM, et al: Magnetic resonance imaging and P-31 magnetic resonance spectroscopy provide unique quantitative data useful in the longitudinal management of patients with dermatomyositis. Arthritis Rheum 37:736-746, 1994.

154. Fraser DD, Frank JA, Dalakas M, et al: Magnetic resonance imaging in the idiopathic inflammatory myopathies. J Rheumatol 18:1693-1700, 1991.

155. Fraser DD, Frank JA, Dalakas MC: Inflammatory myopathies: MR imaging and spectroscopy. Radiology 179:341-342, 1991.

156. Bartlett ML, Ginn L, Beitz L, et al: Quantitative assessment of muscles in thigh muscles using magnetic resonance imaging. Magn Reson Imaging 17:183-191, 1999.

157. Reimers CD, Finkenstaedt M: Muscle imaging in inflammatory myopathies. Curr Opin Rheumatol 9:475-485, 1997.

158. Olsen NJ, Qi J, Park JH: Imaging and skeletal muscle disease. Curr Rheumatol Rep 7:106-114, 2005.

159. Sandstedt PE, Henriksson KG, Larrsson LE: Quantitative electromyography in polymyositis and dermatomyositis. Acta Neurol Scand 65:110-121, 1982.

160. Selcen D, Stilling G, Engel AG: The earliest pathologic alterations in dysferlinopathy. Neurology 56:1472-1481, 2001.

161. Figarella-Branger D, Pellissier JF, Serratrice G, et al: [Immunocytochemical study of the inflammatory forms of facioscapulohumeral myopathies and correlation with other types of myositis]. Ann Pathol 9:100-108, 1989.

162. Kaido M, Arahata K, Hoffman EP, et al: Muscle histology in Becker muscular dystrophy. Muscle Nerve 14:1067-1073, 1991.

163. Holt JM, Lambert EH: Heart disease as the presenting feature in myotonia atrophica. Br Heart J 26:433-436, 1964.

164. Angelini C, Fanin M, Freda MP, et al: The clinical spectrum of sarcoglycanopathies. Neurology 52:176-179, 1999.

165. DiMauro S: Introduction: Mitochondrial encephalomyopathies. Brain Pathol 10:419-421, 2000.

166. Higuchi I, Hashimoto K, Matsuoka E, et al: The main HTLV-I-harboring cells in the muscles of viral carriers with polymyositis are not macrophages but CD4+ lymphocytes. Acta Neuropathol (Berl) 92:358-361, 1996.

167. Dalakas MC, Illa I, Pezeshkpour GH, et al: Mitochondrial myopathy caused by long-term zidovudine therapy. N Engl J Med 322:1098-1105, 1990.

168. Drenckhahn D, Lullmann-Rauch R: Experimental myopathy induced by amphiphilic cationic compounds including several psychotropic drugs. Neuroscience 4:549-562, 1979.

169. Bunch TW: Prednisone and azathioprine for polymyositis: Long-term followup. Arthritis Rheum 24:45-48, 1981.

170. Bunch TW, Worthington JW, Combs JJ, et al: Azathioprine with prednisone for polymyositis: A controlled, clinical trial. Ann Intern Med 92:365-369, 1980.

171. Vencovsky J: Cyclosporine A versus methotrexate in the treatment of polymyositis and dermatomyositis. Scand J Rheumatol 29:95-102, 2000.

172. Oddis CV, Sciurba FC, Elmagd KA, Starzl TE: Tacrolimus in refractory polymyositis with interstitial lung disease. Lancet 353:1762-1763, 1999.

173. Dalakas MC, Illa I, Dambrosia JM, et al: A controlled trial of high-dose intravenous immune globulin infusions as treatment for dermatomyositis. N Engl J Med 329:1993-2000, 1993.

174. Levine TD: Rituximab in the treatment of dermatomyositis: An open-label pilot study. Arthritis Rheum 52:601-607, 2005.

175. Lambotte O, Kotb R, Maigne G, et al: Efficacy of rituximab in refractory polymyositis. J Rheumatol 32:1369-1370, 2005.

176. Noss EH, Hausner-Sypek DL, Weinblatt ME: Rituximab as therapy for refractory polymyositis and dermatomyositis. J Rheumatol 33:1021-1026, 2006.

176a. Wiesinger GF, Quittan M, Aringer M, et al: Improvement of physical fitness and muscle strength in polymyositis/dermatomyositis patients by a training programme. Br J Rheumatol 37:196-200, 1998.

177. Bakay M, Wang Z, Melcon G, et al: Nuclear envelope dystrophies show a transcriptional fingerprint suggesting disruption of Rb-MyoD pathways in muscle regeneration. Brain 129:996-1013, 2006.

178. Benbassat J, Geffel D, Zlotnick A: Epidemiology of polymyositis-dermatomyositis in Israel, 1960-76. Isr J Med Sci 16:197-200, 1980.

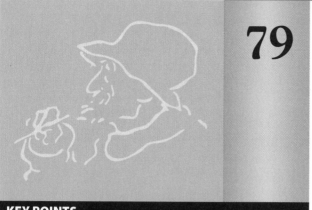

79 Overlap Syndromes

ROBERT M. BENNETT

KEY POINTS

Diffuse connective tissue diseases (DCTDs) are usually associated with autoimmunity to spliceosomal components (uridine ribonucleoprotein particles [U-RNPs], heterogeneous RNPs), nucleosomal components (nucleosomes, DNA, histones), or proteasomal components (HC9, LMP2).

Apoptotic modification of molecules often renders them more antigenic.

Epitope spreading often leads to a diversification of the antibody response in DCTDs.

The diagnosis of undifferentiated connective tissue disease (UCTD) is usually made in patients with Raynaud's phenomenon in combination with an unexplained synovitis or inflammatory myopathy.

About 55% of patients with UCTD fail to differentiate into a classic DCTD.

U1-RNP antibodies predict the differentiation into a mixed connective tissue disease (MCTD).

DNA antibodies predict the differentiation into systemic lupus erythematosus (SLE).

Nucleolar antibodies predict the differentiation into scleroderma.

Synthetase and PM-Scl antibodies predict the differentiation into a myositis overlap syndrome.

Myositis overlap syndromes are more common than the classic descriptions of polymyositis (PM) or dermatomyositis (DM).

In general, myositis overlap syndromes are more responsive to corticosteroids than the pure forms of PM and DM.

Arthritis and interstitial lung disease may antedate the appearance of myositis in patients with antisynthetase antibodies.

Patients with antibodies to synthetases, signal recognition particle, and nucleoporin are less responsive to corticosteroids.

Antibodies to U1-RNP, Pm-Scl, or Ku are associated with corticosteroid responsiveness.

The clinical overlap features of MCTD (i.e., scleroderma, SLE, idiopathic inflammatory myopathy) seldom occur concurrently; they develop sequentially over the course of months or years.

Raynaud's phenomenon is seen in nearly all patients with MCTD; if Raynaud's is absent, the diagnosis should be reconsidered.

About 25% of MCTD patients develop renal involvement—usually membranous glomerulonephritis; proliferative glomerulonephritis is uncommon in MCTD.

Serious central nervous system involvement is rare in MCTD; the most common finding is trigeminal neuropathy.

All patients with MCTD should be screened for pulmonary hypertension on an ongoing basis, because this is the most common cause of death in MCTD patients.

The management of overlap syndromes has not been the subject of controlled trials. Therefore, management is based on an analysis of clinical features and application of the usual management strategies for inflammatory arthritis, Raynaud's phenomenon, inflammatory muscle disease, serositis, interstitial lung disease, pulmonary hypertension, and the gastrointestinal features of scleroderma.

By definition, the clinical features of an overlap syndrome are quite diverse and often change over time. Thus, a reappraisal of management strategies is needed at each patient visit.

The clustering of symptoms and signs into readily recognizable groups has an important historic precedent in the classification of disease. With the progress of knowledge, such groups may become more precisely defined in terms of distinctive pathology or specific laboratory findings. According to current nosology, there are six diffuse connective tissue diseases (DCTDs):

1. Systemic lupus erythematosus (SLE)
2. Scleroderma
3. Polymyositis (PM)
4. Dermatomyositis (DM)
5. Rheumatoid arthritis (RA)
6. Sjögren's syndrome

All six classic DCTDs are descriptive syndromes without a "gold standard" for diagnosis. The diagnosis of a well-differentiated DCTD is usually readily apparent without recourse to extensive investigations. However, in the early stages, there are often common features such as Raynaud's phenomenon, arthralgias, myalgias, esophageal dysfunction, and positive tests for antinuclear antibodies (ANAs). When the diagnosis is not obvious, this is often referred to as an undifferentiated connective tissue disease (UCTD).[1] Only about 35% of such patients differentiate into a clinical picture consistent with the traditional description of a DCTD.[2] In some instances, one DCTD evolves into another DCTD over time.

The propensity for differentiation into a classic DCTD or the maintenance of an overlap state is often associated with distinctive serologic profiles and major histocompatibilty complex (MHC) linkages. Although most rheumatologists are more comfortable thinking in terms of the classic DCTD paradigms, a case can be made for using serologic profiles and human leukocyte antigen (HLA) typing to better understand the clinical features and prognoses. In this respect, a careful analysis of the overlap syndromes and

Table 79-1   Correlations between Autoantibodies and Clinical Features

Autoantigen	Clinical Associations
Rheumatoid factor	RA, erosive arthritis, cryoglobulinemia
Cyclic citrullinated peptide	RA
Nucleosome	SLE, scleroderma, MCTD
Proteasome	SLE, PM-DM, Sjögren's syndrome, multiple sclerosis
Smith snRNP	SLE
Histones H1, H2A, H2B, H3, H4	SLE, UCTD, RA, PBC, generalized morphea
Ribosomal P	SLE psychosis
Double-stranded DNA	SLE, glomerulonephritis, vasculitis
ACL/β_2-glycoprotein	SLE, thrombosis, thrombocytopenia, miscarriage
β_2-glycoprotein–independent ACL	MCTD (not associated with antiphospholipid syndrome)
68-kD peptide of U1-RNP	MCTD, Raynaud's phenomenon, pulmonary hypertension
U1-snRNP	MCTD, SLE, PM
hnRNP-A2 (also called RA-33)	MCTD, RA, erosive arthritis in SLE and scleroderma
Ro/La	Sjögren's syndrome, SLE, congenital heart block, photosensitivity, PBC
Fodrin	Sjögren's syndrome, glaucoma, moyamoya disease
Platelet-derived growth factor	Diffuse and limited scleroderma
Topoisomerase 1 (Scl-70)	Diffuse scleroderma with prominent organ involvement
Centromere	Limited scleroderma, CREST, Raynaud's phenomenon, pulmonary hypertension, PBC
Th/To	Limited scleroderma
U3-snRNP	Limited scleroderma
hnRNP-I	Scleroderma (early diffuse and limited)
RNA polymerases I and III	Scleroderma (diffuse with renovascular hypertension)
Fibrillarin	Severe generalized scleroderma
Ku	Myositis overlap, primary pulmonary hypertension, Graves' disease
U5-snRNP	Myositis overlap
PM-Scl	Myositis overlap with arthritis, skin lesions, mechanic's hands
Signal recognition particle	Myositis overlap (severe course with cardiac disease)
Antisynthetases (Jo-1, PL-7, PL-12)	Myositis overlap with arthritis and interstitial lung disease
Mi-2	DM
Proteinase-3	Wegener's granulomatosis, pulmonary capillaritis
Myeloperoxidase	Churg-Strauss syndrome, pauci-immune glomerulonephritis
Endothelial cell	Pulmonary hypertension, severe digital gangrene

ACL, anticardiolipin; CREST, syndrome of calcinosis, Raynaud's phenomenon, esophageal dysmotility, sclerodactyly, and telangiectasia; DM, dermatomyositis; hn, heterogeneous nuclear; MCTD, mixed connective tissue disease; PBC, primary biliary cirrhosis; PM, polymyositis; RA, rheumatoid arthritis; RNP, ribonucleoprotein particle; SLE, systemic lupus erythematosus; sn, small nuclear; UCTD, undifferentiated connective tissue disease.

their serologic associations has provided insights into the clinical heterogeneity of DCTDs and their management.[3] Numerous clinical correlations of autoantibodies have been reported and are summarized in Table 79-1.

EPIDEMIOLOGY

The reported prevalence of DCTDs is variable, depending on the study methodology, nature of referral bias, and patient ethnicity.[4] It is generally accepted that Sjögren's syndrome has the highest prevalence (500 to 3600 per 100,000) and that SLE is much less prevalent (about 15 to 50 per 100,000). Scleroderma, PM, and DM are relatively rare DCTDs, with prevalences less than 10 per 100,000. There is increasing realization that overlap syndromes of scleroderma and myositis are more common than the "pure" forms of the disease.[5,6] The only epidemiology studies of overlap syndromes are from Japan, where the reported prevalence of mixed connective tissue disease (MCTD) was 2.7 per 100,000.[7] The syndrome of MCTD usually occurs as an isolated finding, but there are reports of a familial occurrence.[8,9] Unlike SLE, precipitation by sun exposure has not been described in patients with MCTD. Likewise, drug exposure has not been related to the onset of MCTD, although the transient appearance of anti–ribonucleoprotein particle (RNP) antibodies has been seen at the initiation of procainamide therapy.[10] Vinyl chloride[11] and silica[12] are the only environmental agents that have been associated with MCTD.

AUTOIMMUNITY

There is compelling evidence that autoimmunity is often antigen driven by the components of subcellular particles—in particular, spliceosomes, nucleosomes, and proteasomes.[13]

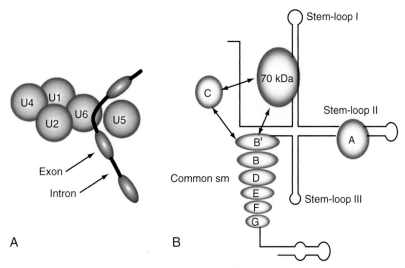

Figure 79-1   Spliceosome. A, The spliceosome is made up of five small nuclear RNAs (snRNAs) complexed with proteins to form a small nuclear ribonucleoprotein particle (snRNP). This subcellular structure is responsible for splicing introns from premessenger RNA to form messenger RNA. Antibodies to various spliceosomal constituents are a common feature of autoimmune rheumatic disorders, and they tend to be associated with different clinical profiles. **B,** The U1-snRNP particle of the spliceosome is composed of U1-RNA, RNP proteins (70-kD, A, and C), and common Smith (Sm) proteins (B'B, D, E, F, and G). The structure of U1-RNA consists of single-stranded RNA and double-stranded RNA called stem-loops I, II, III, and IV. The 70-kD protein can bind directly to stem-loop I of U1-RNA, and the A protein can bind directly to stem-loop II of U1-RNA through an RNA-binding domain known as the RNP-80 motif. The common Sm proteins bind as a complex to single-stranded RNA at the position shown. Because C protein does not have an RNA-binding domain, it cannot bind directly to U1-RNA. However, it does have a zinc-finger domain that facilitates its joining U1-snRNP through protein-protein interactions *(arrows)* of its zinc-finger domain with the 70-kD and common Sm proteins. **(B,** *From Hoffman RW, Greidinger EL: Mixed connective tissue disease. Curr Opin Rheumatol 12:386-390, 2000.)*

AUTOIMMUNITY TO SPLICEOSOMAL COMPONENTS

Certain components of the spliceosome are common targets of autoimmunity in the DCTDs.[14] Further, it appears that post-translational modifications of these molecules, as occur during apoptosis, are often associated with increased immunogenicity.[15] Spliceosomes are complex nuclear particles made up of some 300 distinct proteins and 5 RNAs, which are involved in the processing of premessenger RNA (pre-mRNA) into mature "spliced RNA"[16] (Fig. 79-1). There are two major spliceosomal subunits that are antigenic targets in autoimmunity: small nuclear RNPs and heterogeneous nuclear RNPs.[17]

The small nuclear RNPs contain small RNA species ranging in size from 80 to 350 nucleotides that are complexed with proteins. These RNAs contain a high content of uridine and are therefore called U-RNAs; five different U-RNAs were defined on the basis of immunoprecipitation (U1, U2, U4, U5, and U6).[18] Autoantibodies to these complexes are directed mainly to the protein components. Anti-Sm antibodies precipitate five proteins with molecular weights of 28,000 (B'B), 16,000 (D), 13,000 (E), 12,000 (F), and 11,000 (G); five of these polypeptides are common to the U1, U2, U4, U5, and U6 RNAs. Anti-RNP antibodies precipitate three proteins with molecular weights of 68,000 (70K), 33,000 (A'), and 22,000 (C); these polypeptides are uniquely associated with U1-RNA (see Fig. 79-1).[19] The clinical correlates considered to be distinctive of MCTD are associated with the 70-kD specificity, with an immunodominant epitope embracing amino acid residue 125 flanked by important conformational residues at positions 119 to 126. SLE is associated with anti-Sm antibodies.[20]

The heterogeneous nuclear RNPs are among the most abundant proteins in the eukaryotic cell nucleus.[17] They contain pre-mRNA associated with 30 small proteins that are all structurally related and have molecular weights of 33 to 43 kD. Nine heterogeneous nuclear RNP core proteins have been designated A1, A2, B1a, B1b, B1c, B2, C1, C2, and C3.[21] An antibody termed anti-RA33, which targets the 33-kD RNP-A2, is particularly interesting because it is found in the sera of about one third of patients with RA, SLE, and MCTD.[22] It also has associations with erosive arthritis in SLE, scleroderma, and MCTD[23] and predicts the eventual development of RA in patients with early polyarthritis.[24] Importantly, this association with anti-RA33 is not seen in scleroderma (sine erosions), PM, or overlaps of PM-scleroderma or PM-DM. The antigenic epitopes of heterogeneous nuclear RNP-A2 contain two RNA binding regions at the N-terminal end and a glycine-rich C-terminal region. Certain disease subsets target these two RNA binding regions differently. For instance, RA and SLE sera preferentially react with the second RNA binding domain, whereas MCTD sera target an epitope that spans both RNA binding domains.[25]

AUTOIMMUNITY TO NUCLEOSOMAL COMPONENTS

Nucleosomes are the compact building blocks of chromatin and consist of an octamer of two copies of histones H2A, H2B, H3, and H4, around wrapped approximately 146 base pairs of DNA (Fig. 79-2). During apoptosis, endonucleases cleave chromatin, with the liberation of nucleosomal particles. Following their release into the cytoplasm, nucleosomes migrate to the surface of the dying cell[26] and thus become accessible to B cell receptors. Apoptotic cells are normally inactivated by macrophages. The development of autoimmunity has been linked to defective phagocytosis

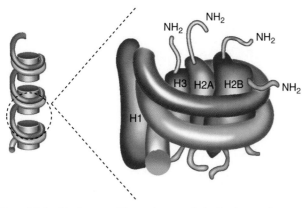

Figure 79-2 Nucleosome. The nucleosome is the fundamental repeating unit of chromatin. The central part of the nucleosome is composed of a tetramer made up of two molecules of histones H3 and H4, flanked by two dimers of histones H2A and H2B. This central core is surrounded by two superhelical turns consisting of 146 base pairs of histone-free DNA. Histone H1 is located at the point where DNA enters and exits the nucleosome. Antibodies to the nucleosome arise early in the evolution of systemic lupus erythematosus, before anti-DNA and antihistone antibodies. Thus, the nucleosome is thought to be an important early autoantigen in the development of epitope spreading. Nucleosome antibodies are also found in scleroderma and mixed connective tissue disease. *(From Amoura Z, Koutouzov S, Piette C, et al: The role of nucleosomes in lupus. Curr Opin Rheumatol 12:369-373, 2000.)*

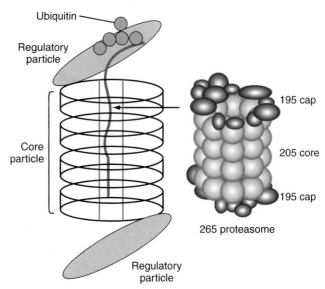

Figure 79-3 Proteasome. Most proteins in the cytosol and nucleus are degraded via the proteasome-ubiquitin pathway. The 26S proteasome is a huge complex of 2.5 mega-daltons (MD), made up of approximately 35 different subunits. It contains a proteolytic core complex, the 20S proteasome, and one or two 19S regulatory complexes that associate with the termini of the barrel-shaped 20S core. The function of proteasomes is twofold: (1) to degrade intracellular proteins that have been tagged with ubiquitin, and (2) to generate antigenic peptides for presentation by the MHC class I molecules. Antibodies to proteasomal subunits have been reported in several autoimmune diseases (especially systemic lupus erythematosus, polymyostis, and dermatomyositis), and elevated levels of proteasomes have been correlated with disease activity.

of apoptotically released constituents.[26] Nucleosomal antibodies are directed to antigenic determinants on the intact nucleosome rather than its individual components—DNA and histones.[27] In a study of 496 patients with 13 different DCTDs and 100 patients with hepatitis C, antinucleosome antibodies were found only in the sera of patients with SLE (71.7%), scleroderma (45.9%), and MCTD (45.0%).[28]

AUTOIMMUNITY TO PROTEASOMAL COMPONENTS

The 26S proteasome is a large subcellular particle involved in the degradation of proteins that have been tagged with ubiquitin, resulting in the generation of peptides for presentation by the MHC class I molecules[29] (Fig. 79-3). There is increasing evidence that it may be the target of an autoimmune response in DCTD.[30] Antibodies to proteasomal subunits have been reported in patients with autoimmune myosis, SLE, and primary Sjögren's syndrome. Iincreased levels of proteasome subunits have also been detected in the sera of patients with autoimmune myosis, SLE, primary Sjögren's syndrome, RA, and autoimmune hepatitis; they are correlated with disease activity.[31]

GENERATION OF AUTOIMMUNITY

The antibody response to just one component of an intracellular structure, such as a spliceosome, results in the uptake of the entire particle by antigen processing cells. Thus, all the proteins making up the particle are subject to antigen processing, with potential peptide presentation linked to their affinity for HLA class II antigens. Depending on the polymorphisms of the individual HLA molecules, there is a diversification of the antibody response to include some of these other antigens. This process is called *epitope spreading*, and it is considered pivotal in the development of the linked

antibody responses observed in different connective tissue diseases.[32] For instance, it has been shown that the induction of an immune response to one component of a U-RNP complex can induce a diversified autoantibody response to other components of the complex[33] (Fig. 79-4). In this way, an immune response becomes modified over time, and this change has been associated with changes in the clinical picture.[34]

The interaction between T cell receptors and peptides presented by HLA molecules is a critical event in the generation of autoimmunity. The 70-kD anti–U1-RNP antibody response is associated with the HLA-DR4 and DR2 phenotype.[35] DNA sequencing of HLA-DB genes has revealed that DR2- and DR4-positive patients share a common set of amino acids in the β chain at positions 26, 28, 30, 31, 32, 70, and 73.[36] Such amino acids form a pocket for antigen binding (Fig. 79-5). It is hypothesized that these two HLA subtypes represent a critical genetic specificity for the presentation of antigenic peptides to their cognate T cell receptors. The shared epitope on HLA-DR4/DR2 associated with an anti–U1-RNP response is different from the shared epitope associated with HLA-DR4/DR1 in RA patients.[37] The 68-kD polypeptide has several different epitopes, the most consistent sequence being KDK DRD RKR RSS RSR.[38] This region is preferentially targeted by MCTD serum but not by SLE serum.[39] The autoimmune response to the spliceosome in these three disorders is characterized by different degrees of epitope spreading. The widest range of antibodies, to both small nuclear RNPs and heterogeneous nuclear RNPs, is seen in SLE; a more restricted antispliceosomal antibody repertoire to both types of RNPs is seen in MCTD; and the antispliceosomal antibody repertoire is restricted to heterogeneous nuclear RNPs in RA.[40]

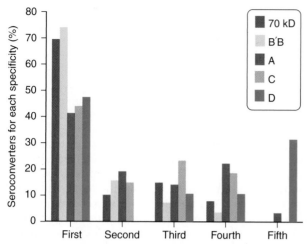

Figure 79-4 One hundred sixty-three patients with serial serum samples from 1989 to 1999 were identified from the University of Missouri Antibody Testing Laboratory. All sera tested were initially negative for U1-RNP peptide antibodies, but over the ensuing years, they developed antibodies to at least one U1-RNP peptide. The order in which seroconversion occurred was ranked from first through fifth for 70-kD, B'B, A, C, and D. For each individual peptide, the number of patients in each group divided by the total number of seroconverters for that peptide is shown. The first RNP antibodies to appear were most often directed against the 70-kD and B'B peptides. Antibodies to the A and C peptides usually developed after other RNP peptide antibodies, and antibodies to D often emerged only after immunity to multiple other U1-RNP proteins had appeared. Thus, there seems to be an orderly pattern of emergence of U1-RNP peptide antibodies, with the 70-kD and B'B molecules being important early immunogens in the development of human RNP immunity. *(From Hoffman RW, Greidinger EL: The appearance of U1 RNP antibody specificities in sequential autoimmune human antisera follows a characteristic order that implicates the U1-70 kD and B'B proteins as predominant U1 RNP immunogens. Arthritis Rheum 44:368-375, 2001.)*

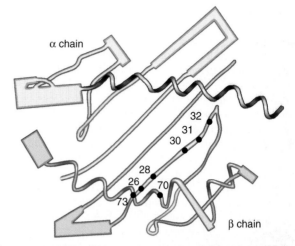

Figure 79-5 DR2- and DR4-positive patients with mixed connective tissue disease share a common set of amino acids in the β chain of both HLA class II molecules at positions 26, 28, 30, 31, 32, 70, and 73. These amino acids form a pocket for antigen binding and are thought to present a restricted set of processed peptides to cognate T cells. *(From Kallenberg CG: Overlapping syndromes, undifferentiated connective tissue disease, and other fibrosing conditions. Curr Opin Rheumatol 4:837-842, 1992.)*

In general, the autoimmune rheumatic diseases are characterized by the production of autoantibodies that recognize evolutionarily conserved molecules. The mechanisms whereby these "hidden" intracellular molecules become autoantigens is an area of ongoing research. The two main theories are apoptotic modification[41] and molecular mimicry.[42]

Apoptotic Modification

The biochemical hallmark of apoptosis is the cleavage of DNA into oligonucleotides that produce characteristic "DNA ladders" when separated on agarose gels. Interestingly, similar DNA ladders are found in the serum of lupus patients.[43] Although rheumatic disease autoantigens are not unified by a common structure or function, they have the common feature of becoming clustered and concentrated in the surface blebs of apoptotic cells. A population of smaller blebs contains fragmented endoplasmic reticulum and ribosomes, as well as the ribonucleoprotein Ro. Larger blebs (apoptotic bodies) contain nucleosomal DNA, Ro, La, and the small nuclear ribonucleoproteins.[44] Apoptosis also generates modified proteins, through cleavage with a class of enzymes called caspases.[45] During the process of apoptosis, several enzyme systems are upregulated, resulting in post-translational modifications of the cleaved proteins.[41] These modifications, which include citrullination, phosphorylation, dephosphorylation, transglutamination, and conjugation to ubiquitin, render the molecules more antigenic. For instance, the U1-70K protein is cleaved by the enzyme caspase-3, converting it into a C-terminally truncated fragment that contains a major B cell epitope that is preferentially recognized by autoimmune sera.[46] Over time, it is envisaged that this immune response is modified by epitope spreading, with the resulting generation of the distinctive clinical features of the classic DCTDs such as SLE and MCTD.[19,32]

Molecular Mimicry

The initial stimulus for a first antibody response may be a non-self-protein possessing a peptide region that mimics a self-epitope—so-called molecular mimicry.[47] Environmental stressors such as infections, toxins, drugs, and ultraviolet light may, under some circumstances, induce accelerated apoptosis.[41] A critical limitation to molecular mimicry is the necessity for the antigenic sequence to undergo T cell receptor recognition.[48] Helper T lymphocytes (CD4+) usually recognize peptides of 12 to 16 amino acids in the context of HLA class II molecules. However, in some instances, smaller peptides are recognized that may be *more* immunostimulatory than the parent ligand.[49] Such observations indicate that antigen recognition by T cells is highly degenerate and expands the potential for molecular mimicry because the universe of molecules containing a pentapeptide, for example, is manyfold greater than those containing a 12–amino acid residue peptide. Once an immune response to one component of an immunogenic molecular complex has been elicited, other proteins or epitopes of the complex may become antigenic by the process of epitope spreading.

UNDIFFERENTIATED CONNECTIVE TISSUE DISEASE

Rheumatologists frequently see patients who present with a weakly positive ANA test and nonspecific symptoms such as arthralgias, fatigue, and cold sensitivity. The critical question in such patients is whether they will develop a connective tissue disease or whether they have fibromyalgia.[50] The answer to this question is not always straightforward, because fibromyalgia is not a diagnosis of exclusion,[51] and it is a common comorbidity with well-defined connective tissue diseases.[52] In the early stages of a connective tissue disease, there may be only one or two suspicious clinical and laboratory features, and a definitive diagnosis cannot always be made. In such cases, a working diagnosis of UCTD may be appropriate.[1,53] Most patients with this diagnosis have Raynaud's phenomenon with or without an unexplained polyarthralgia and a positive ANA test.[54] A 5-year follow-up study of 665 patients with UCTD reported that only 34% developed a well-defined connective tissue disease: RA, 13.1%; Sjögren's, 6.8%; SLE, 4.2%; MCTD, 4.0%; scleroderma, 2.8%; systemic vasculitis, 3.3%; and PM-DM, 0.5%.[2] The highest probability of evolution into a well-defined connective tissue disease was within the first 2 years after onset of symptoms; a complete remission of symptoms occurred in 12.3%. Similar findings have been reported in other series.[55,56] An algorithm for evaluating patients with UCTD is given in Figure 79-6.

Certain combinations of features are predictive for the development of certain established connective tissue diseases[2]: polyarthritis plus U1-RNP antibodies predicts MCTD, sicca symptoms plus anti–SS-A/SS-B antibodies predicts Sjögren's syndrome, Raynaud's phenomenon plus a nucleolar ANA pattern predicts scleroderma, polyarthritis plus high levels of rheumatoid factor predicts RA, and fever or serositis plus a homogeneous ANA pattern or anti–double-stranded DNA antibodies predicts progression to SLE.

SCLERODERMA OVERLAPS

There is a wide variability in disease expression in scleroderma, ranging from diffuse cutaneous disease with a poor prognosis to limited cutaneous involvement with a generally good prognosis. Further, some patients with scleroderma have a prominent overlap with other connective tissue diseases.[57] In many cases, these overlaps occur in patients who do not have prominent skin involvement (sine scleroderma); many such patients have features of the CREST sydrome (calcinosis, Raynaud's phenomenon, esophageal dysmotility, sclerodactyly, and telangiectasia) or incomplete CREST. Approximately 90% of patients with scleroderma have a positive ANA test. Scleroderma-related antibodies include topoisomerase 1 (Scl-70), anticentromere (ACA), heterogeneous nuclear RNP-I, RA33, p23, p25, RNA polymerase I (RNAP-I), RNAP-III, U1-RNP, PM-Scl, fibrillarin, histone, Ku, endothelial cell, and Th/To[58] (see Table 79-1). Specific antibody profiles are associated with distinctive patterns of morbidity and mortality.[59] Patients with ACA, anti–U3 small nuclear RNP, and anti-Th/To antibodies tend to have the limited form of scleroderma, whereas anti–Scl-70, anti-ACA, and anti-RNAP are associated with diffuse skin involvement and systemic disease.[59-61] Patients with anti–PM-Scl antibodies may have a myositis-scleroderma overlap and a tendency to develop pulmonary interstitial disease.[62,63] Stimulatory antibodies for the platelet-derived growth factor receptor have recently been described as having a high specificity for scleroderma[64]; it will be interesting to see whether they are also present in scleroderma overlap

syndromes. About 60% of patients with scleroderma have obvious synovitis, and 35% are positive for rheumatoid factor.[65] Erosive arthritis in scleroderma has an association with anti-RA33; the scleroderma component in such overlap patients is often an incomplete form of CREST.[66] The characteristic vessel pathology in scleroderma is a bland intimal proliferation. Necrotizing vasculitis is rare but has been described in association with a CREST–Sjögren's syndrome overlap; such patients are often anti-Ro positive.[67]

The limited form of scleroderma has a well-documented overlap with primary biliary cirrhosis—often referred to as Reynold's syndrome.[68] The distinctive antibody association in this overlap syndrome is antimitochondrial antibodies.[69] Conversely, ACA antibodies have been found in 10% to 29% of patients with primary biliary cirrhosis; approximately half developed some features of the CREST syndrome.[70] Hence, a serologic overlap between the two syndromes is more prevalent than a clinical overlap.

Low-grade muscle involvement is not uncommon in scleroderma, being described in between 50% and 80% of patients.[71] A European review of 114 scleroderma overlap patients reported a 95% PM-Scl antibody positivity rate,[72] with 80% having inflammatory myositis. This "scleromyositis" differed from MCTD by the presence of coexistent features of DM (myalgia, myositis, Gottron's sign, heliotrope rash, calcinosis) but no features of SLE—as is characteristic of classic MCTD. Many of these patients had a deforming arthritis of the hands. In general, they had a chronic, benign course; most were steroid responsive. Scleroderma-lupus overlaps are less common. However, scleroderma patients often have ANAs other than ACA and Scl-70. In one report, anti–Scl-70 antibodies were found in 25% of SLE patients.[73]

MYOSITIS OVERLAPS

PM, DM, and inclusion body myositis (IBM) are the classic idiopathic inflammatory myopathies (IIMs), yet the same clinical picture and investigational findings may be found in patients with SLE, scleroderma, MCTD, and Sjögren's syndrome. Such overlaps, especially with scleroderma, are reportedly more common than classic PM.[5] When clinical overlaps emerge, they are most commonly associated with specific autoantibodies—namely, anti–PM-Scl, anti-Ku, U1-RNP, Jo-1, signal recognition particle (SRP), and aminoacyl–transfer RNA synthetase (ARS) antibodies.[74] The arthropathy associated with PM is characterized by deforming subluxations (particularly of the distal interphalangeal joints and thumbs), with only minor erosive changes.[75] Another myositis overlap syndrome is seen in patients with ARS antibodies.[76] This is a family of enzymes that catalyze the transfer of a specific amino acid to its cognate transfer RNA[77]; the most common association is with anti-Jo-1 (histidine–transfer RNA synthetase). The clinical syndromes associated with the various antisynthetase antibodies are similar, with remissions and exacerbations characterized by inflammatory myositis, fever (80%), Raynaud's phenomenon, and skin problems (mechanic's hands in 70%).[78] Arthropathy is seen in 50% to 90% of patients, and interstitial lung disease in 50% to 80%.[79] Interstitial lung disease may be a presenting clinical feature of patients with ARS antibodies, with myopathy occurring much later. The association of myositis in patients with anti–U1-RNP

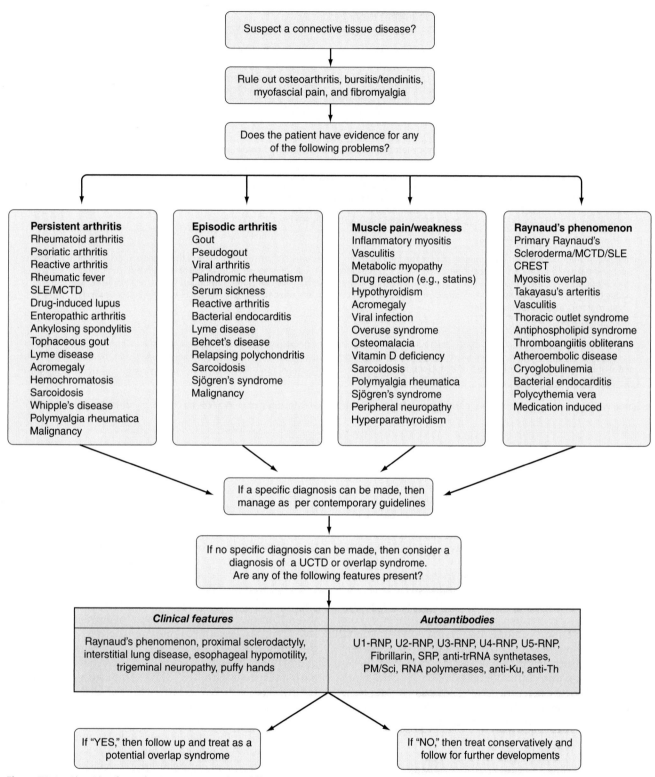

Figure 79-6 Algorithm for evaluating patients with undifferentiated connective tissue disease (UCTD). CREST, syndrome of calcinosis, Raynaud's phenomenon, esophageal dysmotility, sclerodactyly, and telangiectasia; MCTD, mixed connective tissue disease; SLE, systemic lupus erythematosus.

antibodies is usually seen in the context of MCTD. However, some patients with an inflammatory myositis, without Raynaud's phenomenon, have anti–U1-RNP antibodies in association with interstitial lung disease, arthritis, and neurologic symptoms.[80] Antibodies to SRP have been reported in 4% of 265 patients with scleroderma-PM overlap.[81]

Anti-SRP–positive patients usually have a severe, rapidly progressive myositis with prominent muscle fiber necrosis but not much inflammatory cell infiltration.[82]

A 2006 clinical and longitudinal study of 100 consecutive French Canadian patients with IIM concluded that the original Bohan and Peter classification of inflammatory

Table 79-2 Suggested Classification for Inflammatory Myopathies

Descriptions
Pure polymyositis (PM)
Pure dermatomyositis (DM)
Overlap myositis (OM): myositis with at least one clinical overlap feature or an overlap autoantibody
Cancer-associated myositis (CAM): clinical paraneoplastic features without an overlap autoantibody or anti–Mi-2

Bohan and Peter[83] Definition of Myositis
1. Symmetric proximal muscle weakness
2. Elevation of serum skeletal muscle enzymes
3. Electromyographic triad of short, small, polyphasic motor unit potentials; fibrillations, positive sharp waves, and insertional irritability; and bizarre, high-frequency repetitive discharges
4. Muscle biopsy abnormalities of degeneration, regeneration, necrosis, phagocytosis, and interstitial mononuclear infiltrate
5. Typical skin rash of DM, including heliotrope rash, Gottron's sign, and Gottron's papules
Definite myositis: 4 criteria (without the rash) for PM; 3 or 4 criteria (plus the rash) for DM
Probable myositis: 3 criteria (without the rash) for PM; 2 criteria (plus the rash) for DM
Possible myositis: 2 criteria (without the rash) for PM; 1 criterion (plus the rash) for DM

Definition of Clinical Overlap Features
Inflammatory myopathy plus at least one or more of the following clinical findings: polyarthritis, Raynaud's phenomenon, sclerodactyly, scleroderma proximal to metacarpophalangeal joints, typical SSc-type calcinosis in the fingers, lower esophageal or small-bowel hypomotility, D$_{LCO}$ lower than 70% of normal predicted value, interstitial lung disease on chest radiograph or computed tomography scan, discoid lupus, anti-native DNA antibodies plus hypocomplementemia, 4 or more of 11 American College of Rheumatology criteria for systemic lupus erythematosus, antiphospholipid syndrome

Definition of Overlap Autoantibodies
Antisynthetases (Jo-1, PL-7, PL-12, OJ, EJ, KS), scleroderma-associated autoantibodies (scleroderma-specific antibodies: centromeres, topoisomerase I, RNA polymerases I or III, Th; and antibodies associated with scleroderma overlap: U1-RNP, U2-RNP, U3-RNP, U5-RNP, Pm-Scl, Ku, and other autoantibodies (signal recognition particle, nucleoporins)

Definition of Clinical Paraneoplastic Features
Cancer within 3 yr of myositis diagnosis, plus absence of multiple clinical overlap features; plus, if cancer was cured, myositis was cured as well

Adapted from Troyanov Y, Targoff IN, Tremblay JL, et al: Novel classification of idiopathic inflammatory myopathies based on overlap syndrome features and autoantibodies: Analysis of 100 French Canadian patients. Medicine (Baltimore) 84:231-249, 2005.

myopathies should be abandoned, because 60% of patients with IIM were found to have an overlap syndrome.[5] In this study, the finding of an overlap syndrome was based on the presence of an inflammatory myopathy per the Bohan and Peter classification,[83] plus at least one clinical or autoantibody overlap feature (Table 79-2). The distinction between classic PM and DM and an overlap syndrome was reported to be of prognostic and therapeutic significance. Classic PM nearly always ran a chronic course, with 50% of patients being initially unresponsive to corticosteroid therapy. Pure DM was almost always chronic (92%), but 87% of patients had an initial response to corticosteroids. Myositis overlap syndromes (usually with scleroderma features) were almost always responsive to corticosteroids (~90% response rate). When overlap patients were divided according to antibody subsets, antisynthetase, SRP, and nucleoporin autoantibodies were markers for treatment-resistant myositis, whereas autoantibodies to U1-RNP, Pm-Scl, or Ku were markers for corticosteroid responsiveness.

MIXED CONNECTIVE TISSUE DISEASE

Mixed connective tissue disease was described by Sharp and his colleagues[84] in a 1971 paper reporting an overlap of SLE, scleroderma, and PM. This was the first overlap syndrome defined in terms of a specific antibody—namely, antibodies to a ribonuclease-sensitive extractable nuclear antigen. Over the last 30 years, many studies have explored the clinical correlates of this antibody system (now called U1-RNP).

SEROLOGIC FEATURES

The basic premise of the MCTD concept is that the presence of high-titer anti–U1-RNP antibodies modifies the expression of a DCTD in ways that are relevant to prognosis and treatment.[85] The first clue to diagnosing MCTD is usually a positive ANA test with a high-titer speckled pattern. The titer is often greater than 1:1000 and is sometimes greater than 1:10,000. This finding should prompt the measurement of antibodies to U1-RNP, Sm, Ro, and La. It is also pertinent to note whether the serum contains antibodies to double-stranded DNA and histones, because patients destined to follow a course most consistent with MCTD have sera with predominant U1-RNP reactivity. Antibodies to double-stranded DNA, Sm, and Ro are occasionally seen as a transient phenomenon in patients with MCTD. When they are found consistently, as the *predominant* antibody system, the clinical picture is usually more consistent with classic SLE. Antibodies to the 70-kD antigen are most closely associated with the clinical correlates of MCTD,[19] especially in its apoptotic form.[15]

CLINICAL FEATURES AND DIAGNOSIS

The central premise of the MCTD concept is that of an overlap syndrome that embraces features of SLE, scleroderma, and PM-DM.[86] These overlap features of MCTD seldom occur concurrently; it usually takes several years before enough overlapping features have appeared to

Table 79-3 Diagnostic Criteria for Mixed Connective Tissue Disease

	Alarcon-Segovia Criteria	Kahn Criteria
Serologic criteria	Anti-RNP at hemagglutination titer of ≥1:1600	High-titer anti-RNP corresponding to a speckled ANA of ≥1:1200 titer
Clinical criteria	1. Swollen hands 2. Synovitis 3. Myositis (biologically proven) 4. Raynaud's phenomenon 5. Acrosclerosis	1. Swollen fingers 2. Synovitis 3. Myositis 4. Raynaud's phenomenon
MCTD present if	Serologic criterion accompanied by 3 or more clinical criteria, one of which must be synovitis or myositis	Serologic criterion accompanied by Raynaud's phenomenon and at least 2 of the 3 remaining clinical criteria

ANA, antinuclear antibody; MCTD, mixed connective tissue disease; RNP, ribonucleoprotein particle.
From Alarcon-Segovia D, Cardiel MH: Comparison between 3 diagnostic criteria for mixed connective tissue disease: Study of 593 patients. J Rheumatol 16:328-334, 1989; Kahn MF, Appelboom T: Syndrom de Sharp. In Kahn MF, Peltier AP, Meyer O, Piette JC (eds): Les maladies systemiques, 3rd ed. Paris, Flammarion, 1991, pp 545-556.

Table 79-4 Differential Features of the Classic Diffuse Connective Tissue Diseases

Clinical Feature	SLE	RA	Scleroderma	PM	MCTD
Pleurisy, pericarditis	++++	+	+	−	+++
Erosive joint disease	±	++++	+	±	+
Raynaud's phenomenon	++	−	++++	+	++++
Inflammatory myositis	+	+	+	++++	+++
Sclerodactyly	±	−	++++	−	++
Nonacral skin thickening	−	−	+++	−	−
Interstitial pulmonary fibrosis	+	+	+++	++	+
Pulmonary hypertension	++	±	+	+	+++
Butterfly rash	++++	−	−	−	++
Oral ulcers	+++	−	−	−	++
Seizures, psychosis	+++	−	−	−	−
Trigeminal neuropathy	+	−	++	−	+++
Peripheral neuropathy	++	++	±	−	++
Transverse myelopathy	+++	+	−	−	++
Aseptic meningitis	+++	+	−	−	+++
Diffuse proliferative glomerulonephritis	++++	−	−	−	+
Membranous glomerulonephritis	+++	−	−	−	++
Renovascular hypertension	+	−	++++	−	+++
Inflammatory vasculitis	++	++	+	+	+
Noninflammatory vasculopathy	−	−	++++	−	+++
Esophageal dysmotility	+	±	++++	+	+++

MCTD, mixed connective tissue disease; PM, polymyositis; RA, rheumatoid arthritis; SLE, systemic lupus erythematosus.

be confident that MCTD is the most appropriate diagnosis.[87] The most common clinical associations with U1-RNP antibodies in the early phase of the disease are hand edema, arthritis, Raynaud's phenomenon, inflammatory muscle disease, and sclerodactyly.[88] There are no American College of Rheumatology (ACR) criteria for the diagnosis of MCTD, but a comparative study reported that two criteria sets, those of Alarcon-Segovia[89] and Kahn,[90] had the best sensitivity and specificity (62.5% and 86.2%, respectively) (Table 79-3). The sensitivity could be improved to 81.3% if the term *myalgia* was substituted for *myositis*.[90] In some patients initially diagnosed as having MCTD, the clinical picture evolves into one most consistent with SLE or RA; in one long-term follow-up, more than half the subjects continued to satisfy criteria for MCTD.[91] A comparison of the clinical and serologic features of MCTD, SLE, RA, scleroderma, and PM is given in Table 79-4.

Early Symptoms

In the early stages, most patients destined to develop MCTD cannot be differentiated from those with other classic DCTDs. The assumption that a diagnosis of MCTD implies the simultaneous presence of features usually seen in SLE, scleroderma, and PM is erroneous; it is unusual to see this overlap early in the course of MCTD, but with time, the overlapping features usually occur sequentially. Most patients complain of easy fatigability, poorly defined myalgias, arthralgias, and Raynaud's phenomenon; at this point, a diagnosis of RA, SLE, or UCTD seems most appropriate.[1] If such a patient is found to have swollen hands or puffy

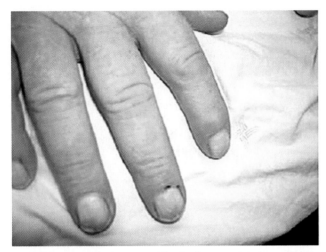

Figure 79-7 Hand of a man with mixed connective tissue disease. The fingers have a generally puffy appearance, with a fusiform proximal interphalangeal joint and swelling of the third finger from inflammatory arthritis. There is a periungual infarct at the nail fold of the third finger. *(Adapted from Pope JE: Other manifestations of mixed connective tissue disease. Rheum Dis Clin North Am 31:519-533, 2005.)*

fingers (Fig. 79-7) in association with a high-titer speckled ANA, he or she should be carefully followed for the evolution of overlap features. A high titer of anti-RNP antibodies in a patient with UCTD is a powerful predictor of eventual evolution into MCTD[19]; this highlights the importance of anti-RNP antibodies as a serologic marker for MCTD.[85] Less commonly, there is an acute onset of MCTD, providing few clues to the subsequent course; such presentations may include PM, acute arthritis, aseptic meningitis, digital gangrene, high fever, acute abdomen, and trigeminal neuropathy.

Fever

Fever may be a prominent feature of MCTD, with no obvious cause.[87] Fever of unknown origin may be the initial presentation of MCTD; however, after careful evaluation, the fever can usually be traced to a coexistent myositis, aseptic meningitis, serositis, lymphadenopathy, or intercurrent infection.

Joints

Joint pain and stiffness is an early symptom in nearly all patients who develop MCTD syndrome. It has become increasingly apparent that joint involvement in MCTD is more common and more severe than in classic SLE.[92] About 60% of patients eventually develop an obvious arthritis, often with deformities commonly seen in RA, such as ulnar deviation, swan neck, and boutonnière changes.[93] Radiographs usually show a characteristic absence of severe erosive changes; they often resemble Jaccoud's arthropathy. However, destructive arthritis, including arthritis mutilans, is a well-established association.[93] Small marginal erosions, often with a well-demarcated edge, are the most characteristic radiographic feature in patients with severe joint disease.[94] Some patients develop flexor tenosynovitis, bone edema, and pericapsular inflammation, reminiscent

of a seronegative spondyloarthropathy (Fig. 79-8). Positive rheumatoid factor is found in 50% to 70% of patients; indeed, patients may be diagnosed as having RA and fulfill the ACR criteria for that disease.[87] Joint histology in MCTD reveals a hyperplastic synovium with surface fibrinoid necrosis, increased vascularity, interstitial edema, and infiltration of macrophages, lymphocytes, neutrophils, and multinucleated giant cells.[95]

Skin and Mucous Membranes

Most patients with MCTD develop mucocutaneous changes sometime during the course of the syndrome. Raynaud's phenomenon is the most common problem and one of the earliest manifestations of MCTD.[96] It may be accompanied by puffy, swollen digits (see Fig. 79-7) and sometimes total hand edema.[92] In some patients, skin changes commonly associated with classic SLE are prominent findings, particularly malar rash and discoid plaques.[97] Other problems include buccal ulceration, sicca complex, orogenital ulceration, livedo vasculitis, subcutaneous nodules, and nasal septal perforation.

Muscle

Myalgia is a common symptom in patients with MCTD syndrome.[98] In most cases, there is no demonstrable weakness, electromyogram abnormalities, or muscle enzyme changes. It is often unclear whether the symptom represents a low-grade myositis, physical deconditioning, or an associated fibromyalgia syndrome. The inflammatory myopathy associated with MCTD is similar histologically to IIM,[99,100] with features of both the vascular involvement of DM and the cell-mediated changes of PM[101] (Fig. 79-9). In most patients, myositis occurs as an acute flare against a background of general disease activity. Such patients usually respond well to a short course of high-dose corticosteroid therapy. Another scenario is that of a low-grade inflammatory myopathy that is often insidious in onset; these patients often have a poor therapeutic response to corticosteroids. Some patients with PM associated with MCTD develop an impressive fever[87]; other patients may give a history of febrile myalgias that were diagnosed as "flu."

Heart

All three layers of the heart may be involved in MCTD.[102] An abnormal electrocardiogram (ECG) is noted in about 20% of patients. The most common ECG changes are right ventricular hypertrophy, right atrial enlargement, and interventricular conduction defects. Pericarditis is the most common clinical manifestation of cardiac involvement, being reported in 10% to 30% of patients; pericardial tamponade is rare. Involvement of the myocardium is increasingly recognized.[103,104] In some patients, myocardial involvement is secondary to pulmonary hypertension, which is often asymptomatic in its early stages and thus may be underdiagnosed.[105] The early detection of pulmonary hypertension is increasingly important because there are now more effective therapeutic options. In the setting of a community rheumatology practice, an elevation of the estimated right ventricular systolic pressure, consistent

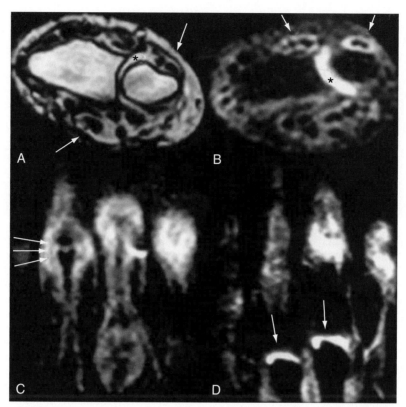

Figure 79-8 **Magnetic resonance images of the hands in two women aged 25 and 32 years with mixed connective tissue disease and hand arthritis. A,** Patient 1 has synovitis or effusion around the ulnar styloid *(asterisk)* and tenosynovitis of the flexor and extensor tendons *(arrows)* on a T1-weighted gadolinium-enhanced sequence in the axial plane. **B,** Patient 2 has intense synovitis of the radioulnar joint *(asterisk)* and extensor te-nosynovitis *(arrows)*, causing thickening of the dorsum of the hand on a T1-weighted short tau inversion recovery [STIR] sequence in the axial plane. **C,** In patient 1, synovitis or effusion and pericapsular edema are seen in the second proximal interphalangeal joint. The distended capsule is indicated by *arrows*. **D,** In patient 2, intracapsular synovial effusion or synovitis of the third and fourth metacarpophalangeal joints *(arrows)* are seen. (Both **C** and **D** are T1-weighted STIR sequences in the coronal plane.) *(From Cimmino MA, Iozzelli A, Garlaschi G, et al: Magnetic resonance imaging of the hand in mixed connective tissue disease. Ann Rheum Dis 62:380-381, 2003.)*

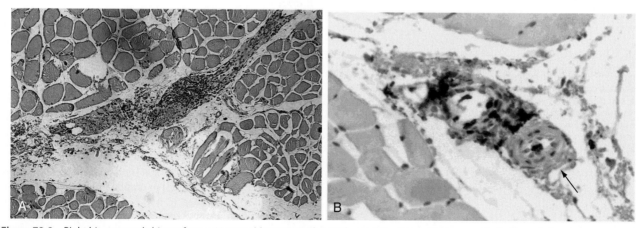

Figure 79-9 Right biceps muscle biopsy from a 64-year-old woman with mixed connective tissue disease complicated by an inflammatory myopathy and a "scleroderma" renal crisis. The biopsy shows a perivascular infiltrate consisting mainly of CD4[+] and CD8[+] lymphocytes **(A)**. There are scattered necrotic muscle fibers but no evidence of endomysial invasion by inflammation. The walls of many capillaries, arterioles, and venules had a thickened, pipe-stem appearance (see *arrow* in **B;** magnification ×230). *(From Greenberg SA, Amato AA: Inflammatory myopathy associated with mixed connective tissue disease and scleroderma renal crisis. Muscle Nerve 24:1562-1566, 2001.)*

with the diagnosis of pulmonary hypertension, was found in 13% of previously undiagnosed subjects.[106] This diagnosis should be suspected in patients with increasing exertional dyspnea. Two-dimensional echocardiography with Doppler flow studies is the most useful screening test.[107] A definitive diagnosis requires cardiac catheterization showing a mean resting pulmonary artery pressure greater than 25 mm Hg at rest.[108] The development of pulmonary hypertension has been correlated with a nail-fold capillary pattern similar to that seen in scleroderma, anti–endothelial cell antibodies, anticardiolipin antibodies, and anti–U1-RNP antibodies.[109,110]

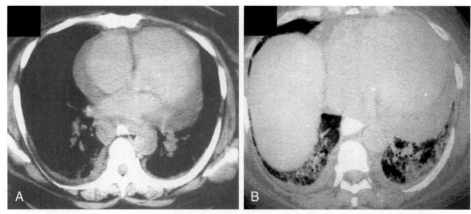

Figure 79-10 Computed tomography scans of a patient with mixed connective tissue disease and pulmonary hypertension (**A,** upper zones; **B,** lower zones). There are bilateral pleural effusions and enlarged bilateral mediastinal lymph nodes in the right paratracheal region and left prevascular areas. The pulmonary artery has a diameter greater than that of the ascending aorta, consistent with the diagnosis of pulmonary hypertension. Both hilar pulmonary arteries are also enlarged. A fairly large pericardial effusion is present. The lung windows show evidence of a diffuse abnormality, with linear opacities and some areas of ground-glass attenuation in the upper zones. At the lung bases, there are more confluent opacities, both reticular and ground glass, and some air-space consolidation. No honeycombing is identified, and there is no distortion of the lung architecture. *(From Saito Y, Terada M, Ishida T, et al: Pulmonary involvement in mixed connective tissue disease: Comparison with other collagen vascular diseases using high resolution CT. J Comput Assist Tomogr 26:349-357, 2002.)*

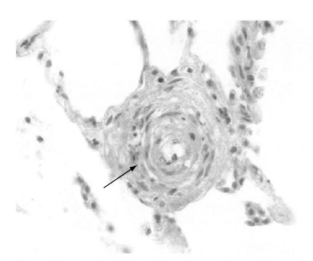

Figure 79-11 Intimal hyperplasia and smooth muscle hypertrophy without accompanying inflammation are the characteristic features of the vasculopathy of mixed connective tissue disease. When it occurs in the lung, as shown here, it may give rise to severe pulmonary hypertension. (Note the absence of pulmonary fibrosis.) The plexiform lesion *(arrow)* is a characteristic pathologic finding in this disease process. *(From Bull TM, Fagan KA, Badesch DB: Pulmonary vascular manifestations of mixed connective tissue disease. Rheum Dis Clin North Am 31:451-464, 2005.)*

Lung

Lung involvement occurs in up to 75% of patients and is usually asymptomatic in the early stages.[105] Early symptoms that should prompt a more thorough investigation are dry cough, dyspnea, and pleuritic chest pain.[111] Interstitial lung disease occurs in 30% to 50% of subjects.[112] High-resolution computed tomography is the most sensitive test to determine the presence of interstitial lung disease (Fig. 79-10), and lung scintigraphy with ^{99m}Tc-DTPA is proving to be a useful screening test that also shows sensitivity to improvement with immunosuppressive therapy.[105] The most common high-resolution computed tomography findings are septal thickening and ground-glass opacities with a peripheral or lower lobe predominance.[113] If untreated, interstitial lung disease is usually progressive, with the development of severe pulmonary fibrosis in 25% of subjects after 4 years of follow-up.[112] As noted earlier, pulmonary hypertension is the most severe form of pulmonary involvement in MCTD.[111] Unlike scleroderma, in which pulmonary hypertension is usually secondary to interstitial pulmonary fibrosis, pulmonary hypertension in MCTD is usually caused by a bland intimal proliferation and medial hypertrophy of pulmonary arterioles[111] (Fig. 79-11).

Kidney

In the initial description of MCTD, renal involvement was considered rare.[86] After some 3 decades of observation, it is now evident that renal involvement occurs in about 25% of patients.[92] However, high titers of anti–U1-RNP antibodies are relatively protective against the development of diffuse proliferative glomerulonephritis, irrespective of whether they occur in a setting of classic SLE or MCTD.[114] When patients with MCTD do develop renal changes, they usually take the form of a membranous glomerulonephritis.[115] This is often asymptomatic but may sometimes cause an overt nephrotic syndrome.[114] The development of diffuse proliferative glomerulonephritis or parenchymal interstitial disease has been rarely recorded in MCTD.[114] There is increasing recognition that MCTD patients are at risk of developing a renovascular hypertensive crisis similar to the scleroderma kidney.[92]

Gastrointestinal Tract

Gastrointestinal involvement is a major feature of the overlap with scleroderma, occurring in about 60% to 80% of patients.[92,116] The most common abdominal problem in MCTD is disordered motility in the upper gastrointestinal tract. There have been case reports of hemoperitoneum, hematobilia, duodenal bleeding, megacolon, pancreatitis, ascites, protein-losing enteropathy, primary biliary cirrhosis,

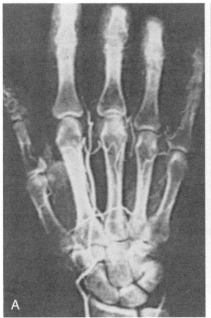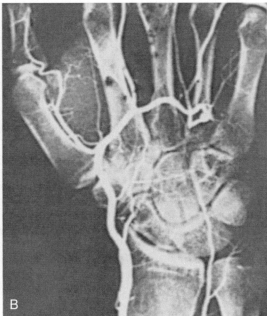

Figure 79-12 **A,** Digital angiogram showing multiple arterial occlusions with collateral formation. **B,** Digital angiogram showing ulnar artery occlusions. *(From Peller JS, Gabor GT, Porter JM, Bennett RM: Angiographic findings in mixed connective tissue disease: Correlation with fingernail capillary photomicroscopy and digital photoplethysmography findings. Arthritis Rheum 28:768, 1985.)*

portal hypertension, pneumatosis intestinalis, and autoimmune hepatitis.[92] Abdominal pain in MCTD may result from bowel hypomotility, serositis, mesenteric vasculitis, colonic perforation, and pancreatitis. Malabsorption syndrome can occur secondary to small bowel dilation with bacterial overgrowth. Liver involvement in the form of chronic active hepatitis and Budd-Chiari syndrome has been described. Pseudodiverticula, identical to those seen in SCC, may be seen along the antimesenteric border of the colon.

Nervous System

In keeping with Sharp's original description, central nervous system (CNS) involvement is not a conspicuous clinical feature of MCTD. There is general agreement that the most common problem is trigeminal neuropathy.[117] This is of some heuristic interest, because it is also the most frequent CNS manifestation of scleroderma. In a review of 81 cases of trigeminal neuropathy seen in a neurology clinic, the most frequently associated connective tissue diseases were UCTD (47%), MCTD (26%), and scleroderma (19%).[118] In a few instances, trigeminal neuropathy has been the presenting feature of MCTD. In contrast to CNS involvement in classic SLE, frank psychosis and convulsions have rarely been reported in MCTD.[119] Headaches are a relatively common symptom in MCTD; in the majority of patients, they are probably vascular in origin, with many of the components of classic migraine.[120] In a subset of these patients, signs of meningeal irritation develop, and examination of the cerebrospinal fluid reveals the changes of aseptic meningitis.[121] Aseptic meningitis in MCTD has also been described as a hypersensitivity reaction to nonsteroidal anti-inflammatory drugs, particularly sulindac and ibuprofen. There are isolated reports of transverse myelitis, cauda equina syndrome, cerebral hemorrhage, retinal vasculitis, optic neuropathy, progressive multifocal leukoencephalopathy, cold-induced brain ischemia, myasthenia gravis, polyradiculopathy, demyelinating disorder, and peripheral neuropathy.

Blood Vessels

Raynaud's phenomenon is an early feature in nearly all patients who are eventually diagnosed with MCTD.[96] A bland intimal proliferation and medial hypertrophy affecting medium and small vessels is the characteristic vascular lesion of MCTD[122] (see Fig. 79-11), and it is the characteristic pathology in pulmonary hypertension and renovascular crisis.[123] This vascular lesion differs from the usual changes encountered in SLE, in which a perivascular inflammatory infiltrate and fibrinoid necrosis are more characteristic. An angiographic study reported a high prevalence of medium-size vessel occlusion[124] (Fig. 79-12). Fingernail capillaroscopy is abnormal in most MCTD patients, with the same pattern of capillary dilation and dropout that has been reported in scleroderma.[124] In one study, all MCTD patients had a scleroderma-like capillaroscopy pattern; a "bushy organization" was noted in 73%—a finding reputed to have an 87% predictive value.[125] It appears that a scleroderma pattern on nail-fold capillaroscopy is a distinctive feature of MCTD that is not seen in classic SLE.[126] Anti–endothelial cell antibodies have been reported in 45% of patients with MCTD; the presence of these antibodies tends to correlate with pulmonary changes and spontaneous abortion.[127] Anti–U1-RNP antibodies may have a pathologic role in the small vessel pathology of MCTD because they induce the release of proinflammatory cytokines from cultured endothelial cells.[128]

Blood

Hematologic abnormalities are common in MCTD. Anemia is found in 75% of patients; the usual profile is most consistent with the anemia of chronic inflammation.[92] A positive Coombs test is seen in about 60% of patients, but an overt hemolytic anemia is uncommon.[129] As in SLE, a leukopenia affecting mainly the lymphocyte series is seen in about 75% of patients and tends to correlate with disease activity.[92] Less common associations are thrombocytopenia, thrombotic thrombocytopenic purpura, and red cell aplasia. Hypocomplementemia has been described in several studies,[92] but it is not as prevalent as in classic SLE and has not been correlated with any particular clinical situation. Positive tests for rheumatoid factor have been found in about 50% of patients.[130] The presence of rheumatoid factor is associated with more severe degrees of arthritis, especially if anti-A2/RA33 is also present.[40] Anticardiolipin antibodies or lupus anticoagulants have also been reported.[92] Unlike the anticardiolipin antibodies found in SLE, they are β_2-glycoprotein independent[131] and tend to be associated with thrombocytopenia rather than thrombotic events.[132]

PREGNANCY

Reports of maternal and fetal morbidity in MCTD are quite diverse.[133] In a comparison study of patients with MCTD and SLE, fertility rates were unaltered in both diseases, whereas parity and fetal wastage were increased in both.[134] Some studies have reported an exacerbation of MCTD during pregnancy and postpartum flares,[134] while others have not.[87,135] The mechanism for pregnancy complications is probably an autoimmune reaction against placental tissues, with immunostaining studies showing deposits of fibrinogen, immunoglobulin (Ig) G, IgM, IgA, and complement 3 (C3) localized to the trophoblast basement membrane.[136] Further, there is an association between anti–endothelial cell antibodies and spontaneous abortion in MCTD.[137] A single case of neonatal "lupus" has been reported, suggesting a pathogenic role for anti–U1-RNP antibodies.[138]

JUVENILE MIXED CONNECTIVE TISSUE DISEASE

MCTD may first become apparent in childhood. Some reports suggest that juvenile MCTD is relatively benign,[139-141] while others describe a mortality pattern similar to that of juvenile SLE, DM, and scleroderma.[142] Significant myocarditis, glomerulonephritis, thrombocytopenia, seizures, hemolytic uremic syndrome, acute coronary syndrome, and aseptic meningitis have been described.[143-145]

MANAGEMENT OF OVERLAP SYNDROMES

The rational management of overlap syndromes is confounded by the absence of controlled trials. Recommendations for management are based on conventional treatments for SLE, PM, DM, RA, and scleroderma.[146] General guidelines for treating specific features of the overlap syndromes are given in Table 79-5.

Pulmonary hypertension is the main cause of death in MCTD, and patients should be evaluated at regular intervals for its development, because early intervention is the key to effective management.[147] Recent advances in the treatment of pulmonary hypertension have led to reduced morbidity and mortality.[148] Effective management requires anticoagulation and vasodilator therapy, such as calcium channel blockers or prostacyclin analogues. Long-term treatment with intravenous epoprostenol or prostacyclin improves exercise capacity, hemodynamics, and survival in many patients,[149] as does therapy with inhaled iloprost.[150] There is evidence that some patients respond to a regimen of intravenous cyclophosphamide and corticosteroids.[151] Bosentan, an oral endothelin-1 antagonist, has been reported to improve dyspnea and slow disease progression.[152,153]

Many of the problems causing morbidity tend to be intermittent and responsive to corticosteroids, including aseptic meningitis, myositis, pleurisy, pericarditis, and myocarditis. Conversely, nephrotic syndrome, Raynaud's phenomenon, deforming arthropathy, acrosclerosis, and peripheral neuropathies are usually steroid resistant. Many scleroderma-like problems can be managed according to the usual practices in treating scleroderma, such as management of renal crisis with angiotensin-converting enzyme inhibitors, Raynaud's phenomenon with calcium channel blockers, and gastrointestinal reflux disease with proton pump inhibitors.[96]

As in SLE, it is worthwhile to consider the use of intravenous gammaglobulin[154,155] or danazol[156] in patients with steroid-resistant thrombocytopenia, refractory myositis, or hemolytic anemia.

Successful autologous peripheral blood stem cell transplantation has been reported in a patient with refractory mysositis and MCTD.[157] Over the long term, concern usually mounts over the total corticosteroid burden and the possibility of inducing an iatrogenic steroid myopathy, nosocomial infection, aseptic necrosis of bone, or accelerated osteoporosis. Routine evaluation of bone mineral density is warranted to detect early, presymptomatic osteoporosis and initiate therapy with antiresorptive agents. Unless contraindicated, all patients should take supplementary calcium and vitamin D. Postmenopausal patients should be offered estrogen-progesterone replacement therapy or raloxifene, unless there are specific contraindications; anecdotally, estrogen therapy has not been associated with flares of overlap connective tissue diseases. In patients requiring long-term corticosteroids, it is reasonable to use antimalarials[158,159] or methotrexate[160] in an attempt to minimize the cumulative steroid burden. As in SLE, the tumor necrosis factor inhibitor etanercept has been reported to exacerbate MCTD.[161] Digitalis is relatively contraindicated in patients with myocarditis, owing to the risk of inducing ventricular arrhythmias. Antimalarials should be used with caution in overlap patients with fascicular or bundle branch block, owing to the risk of causing complete heart block[162]; these drugs can also cause an idiosyncratic hepatitis.[163] Patients with severe hand deformities may be helped by soft tissue release operations and selected joint fusions.

The management of pregnancy presents several special problems. Doria and colleagues[164] have provided the following general advice: (1) patients should be correctly informed about the risk of becoming pregnant; (2) pregnancies should be planned when the disease is in remission, because doing so increases the probability of successful maternal and fetal outcome; (3) patients should be regularly monitored during gestation and post partum by a multidisciplinary team including a rheumatologist, obstetrician, and neonatologist; and (4) in the case of disease relapse, adequate treatment—even aggressive, if necessary—should be recommended, because active disease can be more detrimental to the fetus than drugs are.

Table 79-5 Guidelines for Managing Overlap Syndromes

Problem	Treatment
Fatigue, arthralgias, myalgias	NSAIDs, antimalarials, low-dose prednisone (<10 mg/day); trial use of modafinil
Arthritis	NSAIDs, antimalarials, methotrexate (?), TNF inhibition*
Raynaud's phenomenon	Keep warm, avoid finger trauma, avoid beta blockers, stop smoking; dihydropyridine calcium channel blocker (e.g., nifedipine), α-sympatholytic (e.g., prazosin); consider endothelin receptor antagonist (e.g., bosentan) in recalcitrant cases
Acute-onset digital gangrene	Local chemical sympathectomy (infiltration of lidocaine at base of involved digit), anticoagulation, topical nitrates; consider hospitalization for intra-arterial prostacyclin; start endothelin receptor antagonist therapy
Pleurisy	NSAID or short course of prednisone (≈20 mg/day)
Pericarditis	NSAID or short course of prednisone (≈20 mg/day); tamponade requires percutaneous or surgical drainage
Aseptic meningitis	Discontinue NSAIDs[†]; short course of high-dose prednisone (≈60 mg/day)
Myositis	Acute onset, severe: prednisone 60-100 mg/day Chronic, low grade: prednisone 10-30 mg/day[‡] Consider methotrexate or IVIG in recalcitrant cases
Membranous glomerulonephropathy	Mild: no treatment required Progressive proteinuria: trial of ACE inhibitor; trial of low-dose aspirin combined with dipyridamole Severe: trial of prednisone 15-60 mg/day plus monthly pulse cyclophosphamide or daily chlorambucil
Nephrotic syndrome	Steroids alone are seldom effective; low-dose aspirin combined with dipyridamole to prevent thrombotic complications; ACE inhibitor to reduce protein loss; trial of prednisone 15-60 mg/day plus monthly pulse cyclophosphamide or daily chlorambucil; dialysis or transplantation may be required
Scleroderma-like renal crisis	ACE inhibitor
Myocarditis	Trial of steroids and cyclophosphamide; avoid digoxin[§]
Incomplete heart block	Avoid chloroquine[¶]
Asymptomatic pulmonary hypertension	Trial of steroids and cyclophosphamide, low-dose aspirin and ACE inhibitors; consider endothelin receptor antagonist (oral bosentan)
Symptomatic pulmonary hypertension	Intravenous prostacyclin, ACE inhibitors, anticoagulation, endothelin receptor antagonist (oral bosentan); trial of sildenafil; heart-lung transplantation
Aseptic meningitis	Discontinue NSAIDs and give short course of high-dose prednisone (≈80 mg/day)
Vascular headache	Trial of propranolol, alternate-day aspirin 350 mg, or both; symptomatic use of a triptan (e.g., sumatriptan, eletriptan)
Autoimmune anemia, thrombocytopenia	High-dose steroids (e.g., prednisone 80 mg/day), with taper dependent on clinical course; consider danazol, IVIG, and immunosuppression in recalcitrant cases
Thrombotic thrombocytopenic purpura	Immediate infusion of fresh frozen plasma; may require plasma exchange and transfusion of platelet-depleted RBCs; consider splenectomy in recalcitrant cases
Dysphagia	Mild: no treatment With reflux: proton pump inhibitor; consider Nissen fundoplication Severe: calcium channel antagonist, alone or in combination with anticholinergic agent
Intestinal dysmotility	Prokinetic agents (e.g., metoclopramide) and erythromycin Small bowel bacterial overgrowth: tetracycline, erythromycin
Osteoporosis	Calcium, vitamin D supplements; estrogen replacement or raloxifene; biphosphonates; nasal calcitonin; carboxyl truncated PTH analogues such as hPTH-(1-34)
Heartburn, dyspepsia	Raise head of bed, discontinue smoking, lose weight, avoid caffeine; H_2 antagonists, H^+ proton pump blockers; trial of metoclopramide; consider *Helicobacter pylori* infection in recalcitrant cases
Trigeminal neuropathy	No effective therapy for numbness; trial of an antiepileptic (e.g., gabapentin) or tricyclic antidepressant (e.g., nortriptyline) for pain

*Has been associated with flares in MCTD and SLE.
[†]Sulindac and ibuprofen have been associated with a hypersensitivity aseptic meningitis.
[‡]Remain alert for steroid myopathy, aseptic necrosis of bone, and accelerated osteoporosis.
[§]Predisposes to ventricular arrhythmias.
[¶]Predisposes to complete heart block.
[¶]Cannot be used if esophagus is more than mildly involved.

ACE, angiotensin-converting enzyme; IVIG, intravenous immunoglobulin; NSAID, nonsteroidal anti-inflammatory drug; PTH, parathyroid hormone; RBC, red blood cell; TNF, tumor necrosis factor.

There is often a tendency to assume that all patients with overlap connective tissue diseases should be on long-term corticosteroids; this mistake is compounded by the assumption that all medical problems in these patients are related to their underlying disease. For instance, apparent flares of discomfort and pain in overlap syndromes may be due to myofascial pain syndrome or fibromyalgia and thus are unresponsive to corticosteroids.[165,166] Likewise, malaise and easy fatigability may be related to a reactive depression or the fact that the patient has become deconditioned. There is increasing recognition that a person's ability to deal effectively with a chronic rheumatic disease is a result of many variables, including level of education, level of aerobic fitness, associated depression, strong locus of internal control, and adequate social support framework. The management of patients with overlap syndromes requires a continual reassessment of an ever-changing pattern of clinical problems and a constant alertness to the development of iatrogenic disease. As with any disease of unknown cause, effective management of overlap syndromes presents a constant and evolving challenge.

PROGNOSIS

There is increasing evidence that the prognosis for overlap syndromes is often better than that for classic DCTDs.[5] For instance, Troyanov and coworkers[5] reported on the follow-up of 100 patients with IIM and found that the long-term course after treatment with prednisone (with a dose and duration that initially resulted in good symptomatic improvement) was very different. All PM patients (100%) and most DM patients (92%) progressed to chronic myositis, whereas only 58% of overlap patients developed persistent muscle disease. The tendency for overlap patients to develop chronic disease was more common in those with antisynthetase and nucleoporin antibodies (95%) and less common in those with antibodies to U1-RNP, Pm-Scl, or Ku (42%).

The original description of MCTD stressed two points: "a relatively good prognosis and an excellent response to corticosteroids."[86] With the benefit of more than 3 decades of experience, it is apparent that both these claims need to be qualified.[167] There is now unequivocal evidence that patients with high-titer U1-RNP antibodies have a low prevalence of serious renal disease and life-threatening neurologic problems; in this sense, MCTD compares favorably with classic SLE. However, not all patients with MCTD have a favorable prognosis, and death may occur from progressive pulmonary hypertension and its cardiac sequelae.[123] Rare causes of death are myocarditis,[103] renovascular hypertension, and cerebral hemorrhage.[168,169] A 29-year follow-up of 47 MCTD patients from Sharp's group at the University of Missouri reported a favorable course in 62% and continuing active disease in 38%. Eleven patients (23%) had a fatal outcome; death was related to pulmonary hypertension in 9 patients, and two deaths were unrelated to MCTD.[123] It is evident that the course of MCTD and other overlap syndromes is unpredictable; in many patients, the disease follows a relatively benign course, but major organ involvement ultimately dictates the morbidity and mortality of the disease.

REFERENCES

1. LeRoy EC, Maricq H, Kahaleh M: Undifferentiated connective tissue syndrome. Arthritis Rheum 23:341-343, 1980.
2. **Bodolay E, Csiki Z, Szekanecz Z, et al: Five-year follow-up of 665 Hungarian patients with undifferentiated connective tissue disease (UCTD). Clin Exp Rheumatol 21:313-320, 2003.**
3. Jury EC, D'Cruz D, Morrow WJ: Autoantibodies and overlap syndromes in autoimmune rheumatic disease. J Clin Pathol 54:340-347, 2001.
4. Gaubitz M: Epidemiology of connective tissue disorders. Rheumatology (Oxford) 45(Suppl 3):iii3-iii4, 2006.
5. **Troyanov Y, Targoff IN, Tremblay JL, et al: Novel classification of idiopathic inflammatory myopathies based on overlap syndrome features and autoantibodies: Analysis of 100 French Canadian patients. Medicine (Baltimore) 84:231-249, 2005.**
6. Maricq HR, Weinrich MC, Keil JE, et al: Prevalence of scleroderma spectrum disorders in the general population of South Carolina. Arthritis Rheum 32:998-1006, 1989.
7. Nakae K, Furusawa F, Kasukawa R, et al: A nationwide epidemiological survey on diffuse collagen diseases: Estimation of prevalence rate in Japan. In Kasukawa R, Sharp G (eds): Mixed Connective Tissue Disease and Anti-nuclear Antibodies. Amsterdam, Excerpta Medica, 1987, pp 9-13.
8. Ramos-Niembro F, Alarcon-Segovia D: Familial aspects of mixed connective tissue disease (MCTD). I. Occurrence of systemic lupus erythematosus in another member in two families and aggregation of MCTD in another family. J Rheumatol 5:433-440, 1978.
9. Horn JR, Kapur JJ, Walker SE: Mixed connective tissue disease in siblings. Arthritis Rheum 21:709-714, 1978.
10. Winfield JB, Koffler D, Kunkel HG: Development of antibodies to ribonucleoprotein following short term therapy with procainamide. Arthritis Rheum 18:531, 1975.
11. Kahn MF, Bourgeois P, Aeschlimann A, de Truchis P: Mixed connective tissue disease after exposure to polyvinyl chloride. J Rheumatol 16:533-535, 1989.
12. Sanchez-Roman J, Wichmann I, Salaberri J, et al: Multiple clinical and biological autoimmune manifestations in 50 workers after occupational exposure to silica. Ann Rheum Dis 52:534-538, 1993.
13. Fritzler MJ: Autoantibodies: Diagnostic fingerprints and etiologic perplexities. Clin Invest Med 20:50-66, 1997.
14. McClain MT, Ramsland PA, Kaufman KM, James JA: Anti-Sm autoantibodies in systemic lupus target highly basic surface structures of complexed spliceosomal autoantigens. J Immunol 168:2054-2062, 2002.
15. Hof D, Cheung K, de Rooij DJ, et al: Autoantibodies specific for apoptotic U1-70K are superior serological markers for mixed connective tissue disease. Arthritis Res Ther 7:R302-R309, 2005.
16. Nilsen TW: The spliceosome: The most complex macromolecular machine in the cell? Bioessays 25:1147-1149, 2003.
17. Caporali R, Bugatti S, Bruschi E, et al: Autoantibodies to heterogeneous nuclear ribonucleoproteins. Autoimmunity 38:25-32, 2005.
18. Lerner MR, Boyle JA, Hardin JA, Steitz JA: Two novel classes of small ribonucleoproteins detected by antibodies associated with lupus erythematosus. Science 211:400, 1981.
19. **Greidinger EL, Hoffman RW: Autoantibodies in the pathogenesis of mixed connective tissue disease. Rheum Dis Clin North Am 31:437-450, 2005.**
20. Mahler M, Stinton LM, Fritzler MJ: Improved serological differentiation between systemic lupus erythematosus and mixed connective tissue disease by use of an SmD3 peptide-based immunoassay. Clin Diagn Lab Immunol 12:107-113, 2005.
21. Wilk HE, Werr H, Friedrich D, et al: The core proteins of 35S hnRNP complexes: Characterization of nine different species. Eur J Biochem 146:71-81, 1985.
22. Steiner G, Skriner K, Hassfeld W, Smolen JS: Clinical and immunological aspects of autoantibodies to RA33/hnRNP-A/B proteins—a link between RA, SLE and MCTD. Mol Biol Rep 23:167-171, 1996.
23. Isenberg DA, Steiner G, Smolen JS: Clinical utility and serological connections of anti-RA33 antibodies in systemic lupus erythematosus. J Rheumatol 21:1260-1263, 1994.
24. Hassfeld W, Steiner G, Graninger W, et al: Autoantibody to the nuclear antigen RA33: A marker for early rheumatoid arthritis. Br J Rheumatol 32:199-203, 1993.

25. Skriner K, Sommergruber WH, Tremmel V, et al: Anti-A2/RA33 autoantibodies are directed to the RNA binding region of the A2 protein of the heterogeneous nuclear ribonucleoprotein complex: Differential epitope recognition in rheumatoid arthritis, systemic lupus erythematosus, and mixed connective tissue disease. J Clin Invest 100:127-135, 1997.

26. **Radic M, Marion T, Monestier M: Nucleosomes are exposed at the cell surface in apoptosis. J Immunol 172:6692-6700, 2004.**

27. Decker P: Nucleosome autoantibodies. Clin Chim Acta 366:48-60, 2006.

28. Amoura Z, Koutouzov S, Chabre H, et al: Presence of antinucleosome autoantibodies in a restricted set of connective tissue diseases: Antinucleosome antibodies of the IgG3 subclass are markers of renal pathogenicity in systemic lupus erythematosus. Arthritis Rheum 43:76-84, 2000.

29. Rivett AJ, Hearn AR: Proteasome function in antigen presentation: Immunoproteasome complexes, peptide production, and interactions with viral proteins. Curr Protein Pept Sci 5:153-161, 2004.

30. Chen M, von Mikecz A: Proteasomal processing of nuclear autoantigens in systemic autoimmunity. Autoimmun Rev 4:117-122, 2005.

31. Egerer K, Kuckelkorn U, Rudolph PE, et al: Circulating proteasomes are markers of cell damage and immunologic activity in autoimmune diseases. J Rheumatol 29:2045-2052, 2002.

32. **Deshmukh US, Bagavant H, Lewis J, et al: Epitope spreading within lupus-associated ribonucleoprotein antigens. Clin Immunol 117:112-120, 2005.**

33. Monneaux F, Muller S: Key sequences involved in the spreading of the systemic autoimmune response to spliceosomal proteins. Scand J Immunol 54:45-54, 2001.

34. Tuohy VK, Kinkel RP: Epitope spreading: A mechanism for progression of autoimmune disease. Arch Immunol Ther Exp (Warsz) 48:347-351, 2000.

35. Genth E, Zarnowski H, Mierau R, et al: HLA-DR4 and Gm(1,3;5,21) are associated with U1-nRNP antibody positive connective tissue disease. Ann Rheum Dis 46:189-196, 1987.

36. Kaneoka H, Hsu KC, Takeda Y, et al: Molecular genetic analysis of HLA-DR and HLA-DQ genes among anti-U1-70-kD autoantibody positive connective tissue disease patients. Arthritis Rheum 35:83-94, 1992.

37. Merryman PF, Crapper RM, Lee S, et al: Class II major histocompatibility complex gene sequences in rheumatoid arthritis: The third diversity region of both DR beta 1 and DR beta 2 genes in two DR1, DRw10-positive individuals specify the same inferred amino acid sequence as the DR beta 1 and DR beta 2 genes of a DR4(Dw14) haplotype. Arthritis Rheum 32:251-258, 1989.

38. James JA, Scofield RH, Harley JB: Basic amino acids predominate in the sequential autoantigenic determinants of the small nuclear 70K ribonucleoprotein. Scand J Immunol 39:557-566, 1994.

39. Barakat S, Briand JP, Abuaf N, et al: Mapping of epitopes on U1 snRNP polypeptide A with synthetic peptides and autoimmune sera. Clin Exp Immunol 86:71-78, 1991.

40. Hassfeld W, Steiner G, Studnicka-Benke A, et al: Autoimmune response to the spliceosome: An immunologic link between rheumatoid arthritis, mixed connective tissue disease, and systemic lupus erythematosus. Arthritis Rheum 38:777-785, 1995.

41. **Mahoney JA, Rosen A: Apoptosis and autoimmunity. Curr Opin Immunol 17:583-588, 2005.**

42. Mihara S, Suzuki N, Takeba Y, et al: Combination of molecular mimicry and aberrant autoantigen expression is important for development of anti-Fas ligand autoantibodies in patients with systemic lupus erythematosus. Clin Exp Immunol 129:359-369, 2002.

43. Rumore PM, Steinman CR: Endogenous circulating DNA in systemic lupus erythematosus: Occurrence as multimeric complexes bound to histone. J Clin Invest 86:69-74, 1990.

44. Casciola-Rosen LA, Anhalt G, Rosen A: Autoantigens targeted in systemic lupus erythematosus are clustered in two populations of surface structures on apoptotic keratinocytes. J Exp Med 179:1317-1330, 1994.

45. Casciola-Rosen L, Andrade F, Ulanet D, et al: Cleavage by granzyme B is strongly predictive of autoantigen status: Implications for initiation of autoimmunity. J Exp Med 190:815-826, 1999.

46. Greidinger EL, Foecking MF, Magee J, et al: A major B cell epitope present on the apoptotic but not the intact form of the U1-70-kDa ribonucleoprotein autoantigen. J Immunol 172:709-716, 2004.

47. Farris AD, Keech CL, Gordon TP, McCluskey J: Epitope mimics and determinant spreading: Pathways to autoimmunity. Cell Mol Life Sci 57:569-578, 2000.

48. Wucherpfennig KW: Structural basis of molecular mimicry. J Autoimmun 16:293-302, 2001.

49. Hemmer B, Kondo T, Gran B, et al: Minimal peptide length requirements for CD4+ T cell clones—implications for molecular mimicry and T cell survival. Int Immunol 12:375-383, 2000.

50. Daoud KF, Barkhuizen A: Rheumatic mimics and selected triggers of fibromyalgia. Curr Pain Headache Rep 6:284-288, 2002.

51. Wolfe F, Smythe HA, Yunus MB, et al: The American College of Rheumatology 1990 criteria for the classification of fibromyalgia: Report of the Multicenter Criteria Committee. Arthritis Rheum 33:160-172, 1990.

52. Fox RI: Sjogren's syndrome. Lancet 366:321-331, 2005.

53. Mosca M, Baldini C, Bombardieri S: Undifferentiated connective tissue diseases in 2004. Clin Exp Rheumatol 22(3 Suppl 33):S14-S18, 2004.

54. Williams HJ, Alarcon GS, Neuner R, et al: Early undifferentiated connective tissue disease. V. An inception cohort 5 years later: Disease remissions and changes in diagnoses in well established and undifferentiated connective tissue diseases. J Rheumatol 25:261-268, 1998.

55. Williams HJ, Alarcon GS, Joks R, et al: Early undifferentiated connective tissue disease (CTD). VI. An inception cohort after 10 years: Disease remissions and changes in diagnoses in well established and undifferentiated CTD. J Rheumatol 26:816-825, 1999.

56. Mosca M, Tavoni A, Neri R, et al: Undifferentiated connective tissue diseases: The clinical and serological profiles of 91 patients followed for at least 1 year. Lupus 7:95-100, 1998.

57. Pope JE: Scleroderma overlap syndromes. Curr Opin Rheumatol 14:704-710, 2002.

58. **Steen VD: Autoantibodies in systemic sclerosis. Semin Arthritis Rheum 35:35-42, 2005.**

59. Ho KT, Reveille JD: The clinical relevance of autoantibodies in scleroderma. Arthritis Res Ther 5:80-93, 2003.

60. Basu D, Reveille JD: Anti-Scl-70. Autoimmunity 38:65-72, 2005.

61. Miyawaki S, Asanuma H, Nishiyama S, Yoshinaga Y: Clinical and serological heterogeneity in patients with anticentromere antibodies. J Rheumatol 32:1488-1494, 2005.

62. Vandergheynst F, Ocmant A, Sordet C, et al: Anti-PM/Scl antibodies in connective tissue disease: Clinical and biological assessment of 14 patients. Clin Exp Rheumatol 24:129-133, 2006.

63. Mahler M, Raijmakers R, Dahnrich C, et al: Clinical evaluation of autoantibodies to a novel PM/Scl peptide antigen. Arthritis Res Ther 7:R704-R713, 2005.

64. Baroni SS, Santillo M, Bevilacqua F, et al: Stimulatory autoantibodies to the PDGF receptor in systemic sclerosis. N Engl J Med 354:2667-2676, 2006.

65. Misra R, Darton K, Jewkes RF, et al: Arthritis in scleroderma. Br J Rheumatol 34:831-837, 1995.

66. Zimmermann C, Steiner G, Skriner K, et al: The concurrence of rheumatoid arthritis and limited systemic sclerosis: Clinical and serologic characteristics of an overlap syndrome. Arthritis Rheum 41:1938-1945, 1998.

67. Oddis CV, Eisenbeis CH, Reidbord HE, et al: Vasculitis in systemic sclerosis: Association with Sjogren's syndrome and the CREST syndrome variant. J Rheumatol 14:942-948, 1987.

68. Leclech C, Friedel J, Jeandel C, et al: Reynolds' syndrome: The combination of scleroderma of CREST syndrome type and primary biliary cirrhosis. Ann Dermatol Venereol 114:857-859, 1987.

69. Akimoto S, Ishikawa O, Muro Y, et al: Clinical and immunological characterization of patients with systemic sclerosis overlapping primary biliary cirrhosis: A comparison with patients with systemic sclerosis alone. J Dermatol 26:18-22, 1999.

70. Makinen D, Fritzler M, Davis P, Sherlock S: Anticentromere antibodies in primary cirrhosis. Arthritis Rheum 26:914-917, 1984.

71. Ringel RA, Brick JE, Brick JF, et al: Muscle involvement in the scleroderma syndromes. Arch Intern Med 150:2550-2552, 1990.

72. Jablonska S, Blaszczyk M: Scleroderma overlap syndromes. Adv Exp Med Biol 455:85-92, 1999.

73. Gussin HA, Ignat GP, Varga J, Teodorescu M: Anti-topoisomerase I (anti-Scl-70) antibodies in patients with systemic lupus erythematosus. Arthritis Rheum 44:376-383, 2001.

74. Ghirardello A, Zampieri S, Tarricone E, et al: Clinical implications of autoantibody screening in patients with autoimmune myositis. Autoimmunity 39:217-221, 2006.

75. Oddis CV, Medsger TA, Cooperstein LA: A subluxing arthropathy associated with the anti-Jo-1 antibody in polymyositis/dermatomyositis. Arthritis Rheum 33:1640-1645, 1990.

76. Targoff IN: Idiopathic inflammatory myopathy: Autoantibody update. Curr Rheumatol Rep 4:434-441, 2002.

77. Mathews MB, Bernstein RM: Myositis autoantibody inhibits histidyl-tRNA synthetase: A model for autoimmunity. Nature 304:177-179, 1983.

78. Marguerie C, Bunn CC, Beynon HL, et al: Polymyositis, pulmonary fibrosis and autoantibodies to aminoacyl-tRNA synthetase enzymes. QJM 77:1019-1038, 1990.

79. Schmidt WA, Wetzel W, Friedlander R, et al: Clinical and serological aspects of patients with anti-Jo-1 antibodies—an evolving spectrum of disease manifestations. Clin Rheumatol 19:371-377, 2000.

80. Coppo P, Clauvel JP, Bengoufa D, et al: Inflammatory myositis associated with anti-U1-small nuclear ribonucleoprotein antibodies: A subset of myositis associated with a favourable outcome. Rheumatology (Oxford) 41:1040-1046, 2002.

81. Targoff IN, Johnson AE, Miller FW: Antibody to signal recognition particle in polymyositis. Arthritis Rheum 33:1361-1370, 1990.

82. Miller T, Al Lozi MT, Lopate G, Pestronk A: Myopathy with antibodies to the signal recognition particle: Clinical and pathological features. J Neurol Neurosurg Psychiatry 73:420-428, 2002.

83. Bohan A, Peter JB, Bowman RL, Pearson CM: Computer-assisted analysis of 153 patients with polymyositis and dermatomyositis. Medicine (Baltimore) 56:255-286, 1977.

84. Sharp GC, Irvin WS, LaRoque RL, et al: Association of autoantibodies to different nuclear antigens with clinical patterns of rheumatic disease and responsiveness to therapy. J Clin Invest 50:350-359, 1971.

85. Aringer M, Steiner G, Smolen JS: Does mixed connective tissue disease exist? Yes. Rheum Dis Clin North Am 31:411-420, 2005.

86. Sharp GC, Irvin WS, Tan EM, et al: Mixed connective tissue disease: An apparently distinct rheumatic disease syndrome associated with a specific antibody to an extractable nuclear antigen. Am J Med 52:148-159, 1972.

87. Bennett RM, O'Connell DJ: Mixed connective tisssue disease: A clinicopathologic study of 20 cases. Semin Arthritis Rheum 10: 25-51, 1980.

88. Venables PJ: Mixed connective tissue disease. Lupus 15:132-137, 2006.

89. Alarcon-Segovia D, Cardiel MH: Comparison between 3 diagnostic criteria for mixed connective tissue disease: Study of 593 patients. J Rheumatol 16:328-334, 1989.

90. Kahn MF, Appelboom T: Syndrom de Sharp. In Kahn MF, Peltier AP, Meyer O, Piette JC (eds): Les maladies systemiques, 3rd ed. Paris, Flammarion, 1991, pp 545-556.

91. van den Hoogen FH, Spronk PE, Boerbooms AM, et al: Long-term follow-up of 46 patients with anti-(U1)snRNP antibodies. Br J Rheumatol 33:1117-1120, 1994.

92. Pope JE: Other manifestations of mixed connective tissue disease. Rheum Dis Clin North Am 31:519-533, 2005.

93. Bennett RM: O'Connell DJ: The arthritis of mixed connective tissue disease. Ann Rheum Dis 37:397-403, 1978.

94. Udoff EJ, Genant HK, Kozin F, Ginsberg M: Mixed connective tissue disease: The spectrum of radiographic manifestations. Radiology 124:613-618, 1977.

95. Fujinami M, Saito K, Okawa-Takatsuji M, et al: Histological evaluation of destructive monoarthropathy in mixed connective tissue disease. Scand J Rheumatol 26:395-398, 1997.

96. Grader-Beck T, Wigley FM: Raynaud's phenomenon in mixed connective tissue disease. Rheum Dis Clin North Am 31:465-481, 2005.

97. Gilliam JN, Prystowsky SD: Conversion of discoid lupus erythematosus to mixed connective tissue disease. J Rheumatol 4:165-169, 1977.

98. Hall S, Hanrahan P: Muscle involvement in mixed connective tissue disease. Rheum Dis Clin North Am 31:509-517, 2005.

99. Oxenhandler R, Hart M, Corman L, et al: Pathology of skeletal muscle in mixed connective tissue disease. Arthritis Rheum 20:985-988, 1977.

100. Greenberg SA, Amato AA: Inflammatory myopathy associated with mixed connective tissue disease and scleroderma renal crisis. Muscle Nerve 24:1562-1566, 2001.

101. Vianna MA, Borges CT, Borba EF, et al: Myositis in mixed connective tissue disease: A unique syndrome characterized by immunohistopathologic elements of both polymyositis and dermatomyositis. Arq Neuropsiquiatr 62:923-934, 2004.

102. Lundberg IE: Cardiac involvement in autoimmune myositis and mixed connective tissue disease. Lupus 14:708-712, 2005.

103. Whitlow PL, Gilliam JN, Chubick A, Ziff M: Myocarditis in mixed connective tissue disease: Association of myocarditis with antibody to nuclear ribonucleoprotein. Arthritis Rheum 23:808-815, 1980.

104. Lash AD, Wittman AL, Quismorio FP Jr: Myocarditis in mixed connective tissue disease: Clinical and pathologic study of three cases and review of the literature. Semin Arthritis Rheum 15:288-296, 1986.

105. Sullivan WD, Hurst DJ, Harmon CE, et al: A prospective evaluation emphasizing pulmonary involvement in patients with mixed connective tissue disease. Medicine (Baltimore) 63:92-107, 1984.

106. Wigley FM, Lima JA, Mayes M, et al: The prevalence of undiagnosed pulmonary arterial hypertension in subjects with connective tissue disease at the secondary health care level of community-based rheumatologists (the UNCOVER study). Arthritis Rheum 52:2125-2132, 2005.

107. McGoon MD: The assessment of pulmonary hypertension. Clin Chest Med 22:493-508, 2001.

108. Chemla D, Castelain V, Herve P, et al: Haemodynamic evaluation of pulmonary hypertension. Eur Respir J 20:1314-1331, 2002.

109. Bodolay E, Csipo I, Gal I, et al: Anti-endothelial cell antibodies in mixed connective tissue disease: Frequency and association with clinical symptoms. Clin Exp Rheumatol 22:409-415, 2004.

110. Vegh J, Szodoray P, Kappelmayer J, et al: Clinical and immunoserological characteristics of mixed connective tissue disease associated with pulmonary arterial hypertension. Scand J Immunol 64:69-76, 2006.

111. Bull TM, Fagan KA, Badesch DB: Pulmonary vascular manifestations of mixed connective tissue disease. Rheum Dis Clin North Am 31:451-464, 2005.

112. Vegh J, Szilasi M, Soos G, et al: Interstitial lung disease in mixed connective tissue disease. Orv Hetil 146:2435-2443, 2005.

113. Kozuka T, Johkoh T, Honda O, et al: Pulmonary involvement in mixed connective tissue disease: High-resolution CT findings in 41 patients. J Thorac Imaging 2001; 16(2):94-98.

114. Kitridou RC, Akmal M, Turkel SB, Ehresmann GR, Quismorio FP, Jr, Massry SG: Renal involvement in mixed connective tissue disease: A longitudinal clinicopathologic study. Semin Arthritis Rheum 16:135-145, 1986.

115. Bennett RM, Spargo BH: Immune complex nephropathy in mixed connective tissue disease. Am J Med 63:534-541, 1977.

116. Marshall JB, Kretschmar JM, Gerhardt DC, et al: Gastrointestinal manifestations of mixed connective tissue disease. Gastroenterology 98:1232-1238, 1990.

117. Nitsche A, Leiguarda RC, Maldonado Cocco JA, et al: Neurological features in overlap syndrome. Clin Rheumatol 10:5-9, 1991.

118. Hagen NA, Stevens JC, Michet CJ Jr: Trigeminal sensory neuropathy associated with connective tissue diseases. Neurology 40:891-896, 1990.

119. Nadeau SE: Neurologic manifestations of connective tissue disease. Neurol Clin 20:151-178, 2002.

120. Bronshvas MM, Prystowsky SD, Traviesa DC: Vascular headaches in mixed connective tissue disease. Headache 18:154, 1978.

121. Okada J, Hamana T, Kondo H: Anti-U1RNP antibody and aseptic meningitis in connective tissue diseases. Scand J Rheumatol 32: 247-252, 2003.

122. Alpert MA, Goldberg SH, Singsen BH, et al: Cardiovascular manifestations of mixed connective tissue disease in adults. Circulation 68:1182-1193, 1983.

123. Burdt MA, Hoffman RW, Deutscher SL, et al: Long-term outcome in mixed connective tissue disease: Longitudinal clinical and serologic findings. Arthritis Rheum 42:899-909, 1999.

124. Peller JS, Gabor GT, Porter JM, Bennett RM: Angiographic findings in mixed connective tissue disease: Correlation with fingernail capillary photomicroscopy and digital photoplethysmography findings. Arthritis Rheum 28:768-774, 1985.

125. Granier F, Vayssairat M, Priollet P, Housset E: Nailfold capillary microscopy in mixed connective tissue disease: Comparison with systemic sclerosis and systemic lupus erythematosus. Arthritis Rheum 29:189-195, 1986.

126. Maricq HR, LeRoy EC, D'Angelo WA, et al: Diagnostic potential of in vivo capillary microscopy in scleroderma and related disorders. Arthritis Rheum 23:183, 1980.

127. Watanabe H, Kaise S, Takeda I, et al: Anti-endothelial cell antibodies in the sera of patients with mixed connective tissue disease—the clinical significance. Fukushima J Med Sci 43:13-28, 1997.

128. Okawa-Takatsuji M, Aotsuka S, Uwatoko S, et al: Increase of cytokine production by pulmonary artery endothelial cells induced by supernatants from monocytes stimulated with autoantibodies against U1-ribonucleoprotein. Clin Exp Rheumatol 17:705-712, 1999.
129. Segond P, Yeni P, Jacquot JM, Massias P: Severe autoimmune anemia and thrombopenia in mixed connective tissue disease. Arthritis Rheum 21:995, 1978.
130. Mimura Y, Ihn H, Jinnin M, et al: Rheumatoid factor isotypes in mixed connective tissue disease. Clin Rheumatol 4:572-574, 2006.
131. Mendonca LL, Amengual O, Atsumi T, et al: Most anticardiolipin antibodies in mixed connective tissue disease are beta2-glycoprotein independent. J Rheumatol 25:189-190, 1998.
132. Komatireddy GR, Wang GS, Sharp GC, Hoffman RW: Antiphospholipid antibodies among anti-U1-70 kDa autoantibody positive patients with mixed connective tissue disease. J Rheumatol 24:319-322, 1997.
133. Kitridou RC: Pregnancy in mixed connective tissue disease. Rheum Dis Clin North Am 31:497-508, 2005.
134. Kaufman RL, Kitridou RC: Pregnancy in mixed connective tissue disease: Comparison with systemic lupus erythematosus. J Rheumatol 9:549-555, 1982.
135. Kari JA: Pregnancy outcome in connective tissue diseases. Saudi Med J 22:590-594, 2001.
136. Ackerman J, Gonzalez EF, Gilbert-Barness E: Immunological studies of the placenta in maternal connective tissue disease. Pediatr Dev Pathol 2:19-24, 1999.
137. Bodolay E, Bojan F, Szegedi G, et al: Cytotoxic endothelial cell antibodies in mixed connective tissue disease. Immunol Lett 20:163-167, 1989.
138. Fujiwaki T, Urashima R, Urushidani Y, et al: Neonatal lupus erythematosus associated with maternal mixed connective tissue disease. Pediatr Int 45:210-213, 2003.
139. Tiddens HA, van der Net JJ, Graeff-Meeder ER, et al: Juvenile-onset mixed connective tissue disease: Longitudinal follow-up. J Pediatr 122:191-197, 1993.
140. van der Neti J, van der Hoeven H, Esseveld F, et al: Musculoskeletal disorders in juvenile onset mixed connective tissue disease. J Rheumatol 22:751-757, 1995.
141. Peskett SA, Ansell BM, Fizzman P, Howard A: Mixed connective tissue disease in children. Rheumatol Rehabil 17:245-248, 1978.
142. Michels H: Course of mixed connective tissue disease in children. Ann Med 29:359-364, 1997.
143. Yokota S, Imagawa T, Katakura S, et al: Mixed connective tissue disease in childhood: A nationwide retrospective study in Japan. Acta Paediatr Jpn 39:273-276, 1997.
144. Jang JJ, Olin JW, Fuster V: A teenager with mixed connective tissue disease presenting with an acute coronary syndrome. Vasc Med 9:31-34, 2004.
145. Braun J, Sieper J, Schwarz A, et al: Widespread vasculopathy with hemolytic uremic syndrome, perimyocarditis and cystic pancreatitis in a young woman with mixed connective tissue disease: Case report and review of the literature. Rheumatol Int 13:31-36, 1993.
146. Kim P, Grossman JM: Treatment of mixed connective tissue disease. Rheum Dis Clin North Am 31:549-565, 2005.
147. Bendayan D, Shitrit D, Kramer MR: Pulmonary arterial hypertension associated with autoimmune disease: A single medical center experience. Isr Med Assoc J 8:252-254, 2006.
148. McLaughlin VV: Medical management of primary pulmonary hypertension. Expert Opin Pharmacother 3:159-165, 2002.
149. Galie N, Manes A, Branzi A: Medical therapy of pulmonary hypertension: The prostacyclins. Clin Chest Med 22:529-537, 2001.
150. Vegh J, Soos G, Csipo I, et al: Pulmonary arterial hypertension in mixed connective tissue disease: Successful treatment with iloprost. Rheumatol Int 26:264-269, 2006.
151. Sanchez O, Sitbon O, Jais X, et al: Immunosuppressive therapy in connective tissue diseases-associated pulmonary arterial hypertension. Chest 130:182-189, 2006.
152. Cohen H, Chahine C, Hui A, Mukherji R: Bosentan therapy for pulmonary arterial hypertension. Am J Health Syst Pharm 61:1107-1119, 2005.
153. Rubin LJ, Badesch DB, Barst RJ, et al: Bosentan therapy for pulmonary arterial hypertension. N Engl J Med 346:896-903, 2002.
154. Godeau B, Chevret S, Varet B, et al: Intravenous immunoglobulin or high-dose methylprednisolone, with or without oral prednisone, for adults with untreated severe autoimmune thrombocytopenic purpura: A randomised, multicentre trial. Lancet 359:23-29, 2002.
155. Cherin P, Pelletier S, Teixeira A, et al: Results and long-term followup of intravenous immunoglobulin infusions in chronic, refractory polymyositis: An open study with thirty-five adult patients. Arthritis Rheum 46:467-474, 2002.
156. Blanco R, Martinez-Taboada VM, Rodriguez-Valverde V, et al: Successful therapy with danazol in refractory autoimmune thrombocytopenia associated with rheumatic diseases. Br J Rheumatol 36:1095-1099, 1997.
157. Myllykangas-Luosujarvi R, Jantunen E, Kaipiainen-Seppanen O, et al: Autologous peripheral blood stem cell transplantation in a patient with severe mixed connective tissue disease. Scand J Rheumatol 29:326-327, 2000.
158. Wallace DJ: Antimalarials—the "real" advance in lupus. Lupus 10:385-387, 2001.
159. D'Cruz D: Antimalarial therapy: A panacea for mild lupus? Lupus 10:148-151, 2001.
160. Sato EI: Methotrexate therapy in systemic lupus erythematosus. Lupus 10:162-164, 2001.
161. Richez C, Blanco P, Dumoulin C, Schaeverbeke T: Lupus erythematosus manifestations exacerbated by etanercept therapy in a patient with mixed connective tissue disease. Clin Exp Rheumatol 23:273, 2005.
162. Nolan RJ, Shulman ST, Victorica BE: Congenital complete heart block associated with maternal mixed connective tissue disease. J Pediatr 95:420-422, 1979.
163. Giner Galvan V, Oltra MR, Rueda D, et al: Severe acute hepatitis related to hydroxychloroquine in a woman with mixed connective tissue disease. Clin Rheumatol 9:971-972, 2006.
164. Doria A, Iaccarino L, Ghirardello A, et al: Pregnancy in rare autoimmune rheumatic diseases: UCTD, MCTD, myositis, systemic vasculitis and Behcet disease. Lupus 13:690-695, 2004.
165. Middleton GD, McFarlin JE, Lipsky PE: The prevalence and clinical impact of fibromyalgia in systemic lupus erythematosus. Arthritis Rheum 37:1181-1188, 1994.
166. Bennett R: The concurrence of lupus and fibromyalgia: Implications for diagnosis and management. Lupus 6:494-499, 1997.
167. Lundberg IE: The prognosis of mixed connective tissue disease. Rheum Dis Clin North Am 31:535, 2005.
168. Kuwana M, Kaburaki J, Okano Y, et al: Clinical and prognostic associations based on serum antinuclear antibodies in Japanese patients with systemic sclerosis. Arthritis Rheum 37:75-83, 1994.
169. Graf WD, Milstein JM, Sherry DD: Stroke and mixed connective tissue disease. J Child Neurol 8:256-259, 1993.

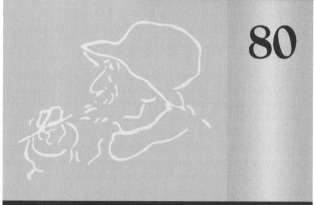

80

The Classification and Epidemiology of Systemic Vasculitis

JOHN H. STONE

KEY POINTS

Vasculitis is a heterogeneous group of disorders linked by the primary finding of inflammation within blood vessel walls. At least 20 forms of systemic vasculitis are recognized currently.

Vasculitides are classified first by the size of blood vessel involved—small (capillaries and postcapillary venules), medium (muscular arteries and arterioles), or large (the aorta and its major branches).

Additional considerations in classification include patient demographics, organ tropism, presence or absence of granulomatous inflammation, participation (or not) of immune complexes, finding of autoantibodies, and detection of infections associated with some vasculitides.

Different forms of vasculitis have widely divergent profiles with regard to age, gender, and ethnicity.

Associations between genes and vasculitis have been recognized increasingly in recent years. There also has been progress in the area of gene-environment interactions.

CLASSIFICATION

Few disorders in medicine are more challenging in diagnosis and treatment than the systemic vasculitides. These heterogeneous disorders are linked by the common finding of destructive inflammation within the walls of blood vessels. Current classification schemes recognize approximately 20 primary forms of vasculitis and several major categories of secondary vasculitis (e.g., other rheumatologic diseases, malignancy, and infection) (Table 80-1). Over the past half century, numerous comprehensive classification schemes have been attempted.[1] No attempt has been entirely satisfactory because understanding of these conditions continues to evolve. All vasculitis classification schemes are works in progress, susceptible to change as new information emerges.

Current classification schemes are understood best in light of their nosologic predecessors. The first "modern"

case of systemic vasculitis was recognized in the 1860s by Kussmaul and Maier.[2] That case, which involved medium-sized, muscular arteries, has served as the reference point for classifying many subsequently recognized forms of vasculitis. Because of the importance of that first report in the understanding and classification of vasculitis, the case is described in detail here.

FIRST MODERN CASE: "PERIARTERITIS NODOSA"

In 1866, Kussmaul and Maier reported the case of a 27-year-old tailor who died during a month-long hospital stay.[2,3] On presentation, the patient was strong enough to climb two flights of stairs to the clinic, but "afterward felt so weak that he immediately had to go to bed." He complained of numbness on the volar aspect of his thumb and the two neighboring fingers on the right hand. Over the ensuing days, "the general weakness increased so rapidly that he was unable to leave the bed, [and] the feeling of numbness also appeared in the left hand." Muscle paralysis progressed quickly: "Before our eyes, a young man developed a general paralysis of the voluntary muscles ... [He] had to be fed by attendants, and within a few weeks was robbed of the use of most of his muscles."[2,3]

The patient's weakness, caused by vasculitic neuropathy (mononeuritis multiplex), was accompanied by tachycardia, abdominal pains, and the appearance of cutaneous nodules over his trunk. His death was described as follows: "He was scarcely able to speak, lay with persistent severe abdominal and muscle pains, opisthotonically stretched, whimpering, and begged the doctors not to leave him ... Death occurred ... at 2 o'clock in the morning." At autopsy, grossly visible nodules were present along the patient's medium-sized arteries. Kussmaul and Maier suggested the name "periarteritis nodosa" for this disease because of the apparent localization of inflammation to the perivascular sheaths and outer layers of the arterial walls, leading to nodular thickening of the vessels. The name was later revised to polyarteritis nodosa (PAN), to reflect the widespread arterial involvement of this disease, and the fact that the inflammation in PAN extends through the entire thickness of the vessel wall.[4,5]

1401

Table 80-1 Classification Scheme of Vasculitides According to Size of Predominant Blood Vessels Involved

Primary Vasculitides
Predominantly Large Vessel Vasculitides
Takayasu's arteritis
Giant cell arteritis (temporal arteritis)
Cogan's syndrome
Behçet's disease*
Predominantly Medium Vessel Vasculitides
Polyarteritis nodosa
Cutaneous polyarteritis nodosa
Buerger's disease
Kawasaki disease
Primary angiitis of the central nervous system
Predominantly Small Vessel Vasculitides
Immune complex mediated
Goodpasture's disease (anti–glomerular basement membrane disease)†
Cutaneous leukocytoclastic angiitis ("hypersensitivity vasculitis")
Henoch-Schönlein purpura
Hypocomplementemic urticarial vasculitis
Essential cryoglobulinemia‡
Erythema elevatum diutinum
ANCA-associated disorders§
Wegener's granulomatosis‡
Microscopic polyangiitis‡
Churg-Strauss syndrome‡
Renal-limited vasculitis
Secondary Forms of Vasculitis
Miscellaneous Small Vessel Vasculitides
Connective tissue disorders‡ (rheumatoid vasculitis, lupus erythematosus, Sjögren's syndrome, inflammatory myopathies)
Inflammatory bowel disease
Paraneoplastic
Infection
Drug-induced vasculitis: ANCA-associated, other

*May involve small, medium, and large blood vessels.
†Immune complexes formed in situ, in contrast to other forms of immune complex–mediated vasculitis.
‡Frequent overlap of small and medium blood vessel involvement.
§Not all forms of these disorders are always associated with ANCA.
ANCA, antineutrophil cytoplasmic antibody.

POLYARTERITIS NODOSA AS A REFERENCE POINT

In addition to its status as the first form of vasculitis recognized, several features of PAN make it a logical reference point for the classification of inflammatory vascular disease. Other forms of vasculitis usually can be differentiated from PAN through their contrasts to one or more of the following PAN characteristics:

- The general confinement of the disease to medium-sized vessels*, as opposed to capillaries and postcapillary venules (small vessels) and the aorta and its major branches (large vessels)
- The exclusive involvement of arteries, with sparing of veins
- The tendency to form microaneurysms
- The absence of lung involvement

---

*The fact of vessel size overlap in vasculitis syndromes is acknowledged and discussed subsequently.

- The lack of granulomatous inflammation
- The absence of associated autoantibodies (e.g., antineutrophil cytoplasmic antibodies [ANCA], anti–glomerular basement membrane [anti-GBM] antibodies, or rheumatoid factor)
- The association of some cases with hepatitis B virus (HBV) infection

CLASSIFICATION BY VESSEL SIZE

Because the etiologies of most forms of vasculitis are unknown, the most valid basis for classifying the vasculitides is the size of the predominant blood vessels involved. Under such classification schemes, the vasculitides are categorized initially by whether the vessels affected are large, medium, or small (see Table 80-1). "Large" generally denotes the aorta and its major branches (and the corresponding vessels in the venous circulation in some forms of vasculitis, e.g., Behçet's disease). "Medium" refers to vessels that are smaller than the major aortic branches, yet still large enough to contain four elements: (1) an intima, (2) a continuous internal elastic lamina, (3) a muscular media, and (4) an adventitia. In clinical terms, medium vessel vasculitis (see Table 80-1) is generally macrovascular (i.e., involves vessels large enough to be observed in gross pathologic specimens or visualized by angiography). "Small vessel" vasculitis, which incorporates all vessels below macroscopic disease, includes capillaries, postcapillary venules, and arterioles. Such vessels all are typically less than 500 μ in outer diameter. Because glomeruli may be viewed simply as differentiated capillaries, forms of vasculitis that cause glomerulonephritis are considered to be small vessel vasculitides. Table 80-2 presents the typical clinical manifestations associated with small, medium, and large vessel vasculitides.

All discussions of vasculitis classification schemes involving vessel size must acknowledge the frequent occurrence of overlap. Although PAN primarily involves medium-sized arteries, palpable purpura—a manifestation of small vessel disease—can be observed in some cases. Despite the possibility of vessel size overlap within individual cases, the categorization of a patient's vasculitis as primarily large, medium, or small vessel in nature remains enormously useful in focusing the differential diagnosis and initiating plans for treatment.

ADDITIONAL CONSIDERATIONS IN CLASSIFICATION

Many other considerations are important in the classification of vasculitis (Table 80-3): (1) the patient's demographic profile (see Epidemiology section), (2) the disease's tropism for particular organs, (3) the presence or absence of granulomatous inflammation, (4) the participation of immune complexes in disease pathophysiology, (5) the finding of characteristic autoantibodies in the patients' serum (e.g., ANCA, anti-GBM antibodies, or rheumatoid factor), and (6) the detection of certain infections known to cause specific forms of vasculitis.

The organ tropisms of these disorders are illustrated by the following examples. Wegener's granulomatosis classically involves the kidneys, upper airways, and lungs. In contrast, Henoch-Schönlein purpura often affects the kidneys, but never the nose or sinuses and almost never the lungs.

Table 80-2 Typical Clinical Manifestations of Large, Medium, and Small Vessel Involvement by Vasculitis

Constitutional symptoms: fever, weight loss, malaise, arthralgias/arthritis (common to vasculitides of all vessel sizes)

Large	Medium	Small
Limb claudication	Cutaneous nodules	Purpura
Asymmetric blood pressures	Ulcers	Vesiculobullous lesions
Absence of pulses	Livedo reticularis	Urticaria
Bruits	Digital gangrene	Glomerulonephritis
Aortic dilation	Mononeuritis multiplex	Alveolar hemorrhage
Renovascular hypertension	Microaneurysms	Cutaneous extravascular necrotizing granulomas
	Renovascular hypertension	Splinter hemorrhages Uveitis/episcleritis/scleritis

Table 80-3 Considerations in the Classifications of Systemic Vasculitis

Size of predominant blood vessels affected

Epidemiologic features
    Age
    Gender
    Ethnic background

Pattern of organ involvement

Pathologic features
    Granulomatous inflammation
    Immune complex deposition versus pauci-immune
      histopathology
    Linear staining along glomerular basement membrane

Presence of ANCA, anti-GBM antibodies, or rheumatoid factor in serum

Demonstration of a specific associated infection (hepatitis B or hepatitis C)

ANCA, antineutrophil cytoplasmic antibody; GBM, glomerular basement membrane.

Table 80-4 Forms of Vasculitis Associated with Granulomatous Inflammation

Giant cell arteritis

Takayasu's arteritis

Cogan's syndrome

Wegener's granulomatosis

Churg-Strauss syndrome

Primary angiitis of the central nervous system*

Buerger's disease[†]

Rheumatoid vasculitis

*Sometimes granulomatous.
[†]Giant cells occur within inflammatory thrombi (and are diagnostic of Buerger's disease), but do not occur within the blood vessel wall.

angiitis or microscopic polyangiitis may be reclassified as having Wegener's granulomatosis if disease manifestations appear in new organs and granulomatous inflammation is found on biopsy specimens. Table 80-4 presents forms of vasculitis commonly associated with granulomatous inflammation.

Immune complexes are essential to the pathophysiology of some small and medium vessel vasculitides. Immune complex–mediated tissue injury does not produce a single clinical syndrome, but rather applies to many forms of vasculitis and overlaps with injuries caused by other immune mechanisms. Anti-GBM disease (Goodpasture's disease) is a unique form of immune complex disease in which the immune complexes form in situ rather than in the circulation.[6] Complexes of IgA1 are found in Henoch-Schönlein purpura. Immune complexes comprising IgG, IgM, complement components, and the hepatitis C virion characterize most cases of mixed cryoglobulinemia. HBV surface antigen/antibody complexes are present in the circulation and involved tissues of patients with HBV-associated PAN. Rheumatoid factor and complement proteins are found within organs involved by rheumatoid vasculitis.

In contrast, other small and medium vessel vasculitides, such as Wegener's granulomatosis, microscopic polyangiitis, and Churg-Strauss syndrome, are disorders associated with "pauci-immune" inflammation. "Pauci-immune" refers not to a lack of immunologic involvement in these disorders, but rather to the absence of significant immunoreactant deposition (immunoglobulin or complement) within diseased tissues. Many (but not all) patients with pauci-immune forms of vasculitis have ANCA in their serum. Three decades before the description of ANCA, Godman and Churg[7] observed pathologic links between these three entities, noting that the disorders "group themselves into a compass, [ranging from] necrotizing and granulomatous processes with angiitis, through mixed forms, to vasculitis without granulomata."

ANCA (see Chapter 82) are directed against antigens that reside within the primary granules of neutrophils and monocytes.[8] Two types of ANCA seem to be relevant to vasculitis: (1) ANCA directed against proteinase-3 (PR-3), a serine protease found within the primary granules of neutrophils and monocytes, and (2) ANCA directed against myeloperoxidase and another serine protease found within the same granules. Although rigorous serologic assays for these antibodies are helpful in diagnosis, evidence for a

In contrast to both of these forms of vasculitis, Cogan's syndrome is defined by the simultaneous occurrence of ocular inflammation (most often interstitial keratitis) and sensorineural hearing loss (and, in 10% of cases, a large vessel vasculitis). The histopathologic findings in these three disorders are equally distinctive, ranging from granulomatous inflammation of small to medium vessels (Wegener's granulomatosis), to IgA deposition in small vessels (Henoch-Schönlein purpura), to large vessel vasculitis centered on the adventitia (Cogan's syndrome).

The granulomatous features of some forms of vasculitis resemble chronic infections (e.g., infections caused by fungi or mycobacteria) or the inflammation induced by the presence of a foreign body. Granulomatous inflammation is more likely to be found in some organs (e.g., the lung) than in others (e.g., the kidney or skin). Some patients without evidence of granulomatous inflammation at early points in their courses later exhibit such features as their diseases unfold. Patients initially diagnosed with cutaneous leukocytoclastic primary etiologic role of these antibodies in human forms of pauci-immune vasculitis is still lacking. In contrast, anti-GBM antibodies have been proven to play a major role in the pathogenesis of Goodpastures's disease.[9] In RA, systemic rheumatoid vasculitis occurs only in patients who are rheumatoid factor positive. Rheumatoid factor is believed to play an essential role in the immune complex nature of that disease complication. Finally, although the causes of most forms of vasculitis are unknown, several infections have been linked definitively with specific forms of these diseases (e.g., HBV with some cases of PAN, and hepatitis C with type II mixed cryoglobulinemia).

HISTORICAL ATTEMPTS AT CLASSIFICATION AND NOMENCLATURE

For decades after this initial description of vasculitis, most forms of systemic inflammatory vascular disease were termed *periarteritis nodosa*. In the 1900s, two major factors led to the recognition of new forms of vasculitis: (1) The use of microscopy in the evaluation of pathologic specimens became routine, and (2) horse serum and sulfonamides came to be employed in the treatment of many medical conditions. These new therapies frequently induced small vessel vasculitides on the basis of serum sickness or "hypersensitivity" phenomena, which were observed readily through the microscope. In some cases, the histopathologicl findings of hypersensitivity reactions (e.g., serum sickness) were confused with periarteritis nodosa. The gradual recognition that these syndromes represented departures from PAN spurred interest in the first classification scheme for necrotizing angiitis.

In 1952, Zeek[10] identified five major categories of necrotizing angiitis. The Zeek Classification included (1) hypersensitivity angiitis, (2) allergic granulomatous angiitis (Churg-Strauss syndrome), (3) rheumatic arteritis (vasculitis associated with fulminant rheumatic fever), (4) periarteritis nodosa, and (5) temporal arteritis. This classification scheme omitted several forms of systemic vasculitis that were known but not yet described in the English medical literature (e.g., Wegener's granulomatosis and Takayasu's arteritis).

SOURCES OF CONFUSION IN CLASSIFICATION

Two forms of vasculitis, now termed *microscopic polyangiitis* and *cutaneous leukocytoclastic angiitis*, have been consistent sources of confusion in vasculitis nosology. In the current understanding of systemic vasculitides, these two conditions are separate entities. Microscopic polyangiitis affects capillaries, veins, and arteries (in contrast to PAN), and is recognized to be a disorder associated with ANCA in approximately 70% of cases.[11] In 1923, Wohlwill[12] observed unequivocal evidence of small vessel involvement in cases of vasculitis that he still considered part of the spectrum of "periarteritis nodosa." Davson and colleagues[13] remarked on two forms of "periarteritis nodosa" with differential effects on the kidney—one with a predilection for medium-sized, muscular arteries and the other with a predilection for small vessels, including glomerulonephritis. Davson and colleagues[13] termed this latter form *microscopic periarteritis nodosa*. Swayed by human and animal models of hypersensitivity that showed small vessel disease involving the

kidneys, lungs, and other organs,[14,15] Zeek chose to group microscopic periarteritis nodosa under the heading of *hypersensitivity vasculitis*.[10]

Over the next several decades, hypersensitivity vasculitis came to refer to an immune complex–mediated small vasculitis of the skin that spared internal organs and often followed drug exposures.[16] The Chapel Hill Consensus Conference (CHCC)[17] (see later) recommended eliminating the term *hypersensitivity* altogether because evidence for hypersensitivity is lacking in many cases. Participants in the CHCC preferred the term *cutaneous leukocytoclastic angiitis* because of the disorder's typical confinement to the skin and the usual predominant cell type—the neutrophil. Although cutaneous leukocytoclastic angiitis can mimic the skin features of microscopic polyangiitis, cutaneous leukocytoclastic angiitis does not involve the kidneys, lungs, peripheral nerves, and other internal organs, and is not associated with ANCA.

In 1990, the American College of Rheumatology (ACR) performed a study designed to establish criteria for the classification of vasculitis, through the identification of features that distinguished one form of vasculitis from others.[18,19] An important caveat: This study was *not* designed to establish criteria for diagnosis, but rather to facilitate research by permitting the inclusion of similar types of patients in studies. Patients with giant cell arteritis, Takayasu's arteritis, PAN, Wegener's granulomatosis, Churg-Strauss syndrome, Henoch-Schönlein purpura, and hypersensitivity vasculitis were included in this study.[16,20-25] The findings of the ACR study remain useful for the purposes of the study's original intention—the insurance of uniform inclusion criteria for patients in research studies. The passage of time and the development of new insights have shown the need for updates, however. First, because the study was performed before the days of reliable and widely available assays for ANCA, ANCA positivity was not considered as a possible classification criterion. Second, the ACR Classification Criteria study did not include microscopic polyangiitis as a separate disease, but rather lumped such patients under the heading of PAN.[22] Third, the study did not define classification criteria for such rarer forms of vasculitis as Cogan's syndrome and Behçet's disease. As noted subsequently, Behçet's disease is rare in North America, but not in countries bordering the Old Silk Route. Diagnostic criteria for this disease have been defined.[26]

In 1994, the CHCC reviewed the nomenclature of systemic vasculitides. Formal diagnostic criteria were not attempted, but definitions were created for 10 forms of vasculitis (in addition to the 7 forms of vasculitis included in the ACR study, microscopic polyangiitis, Kawasaki disease, and "essential" cryoglobulinemic vasculitis were defined). The CHCC emphasized the important role that ANCA play in the diagnosis of several forms of vasculitis and carefully distinguished microscopic polyangiitis from classic PAN. The conference defined classic PAN as necrotizing inflammation of medium-sized or small arteries without glomerulonephritis.[17] Microscopic polyangiitis was defined as a necrotizing vasculitis with few or no immune deposits that (1) affects small blood vessels (capillaries, venules, or arterioles), (2) often includes glomerulonephritis and pulmonary capillaritis, and (3) is often associated with either myeloperoxidase ANCA or proteinase 3 ANCA.

The classification of vasculitis continues to evolve. In the years since the CHCC, it has become clear that hepatitis C plays a major role in 90% of cases that formerly were termed *essential mixed cryoglobulinemia*. Some cases of this syndrome are not associated with hepatitis C infections, however, and probably have some other infectious etiology. Similarly, with the availability of the HBV vaccine, increasingly fewer cases of PAN are associated with this infection. Most PAN cases have no known cause. As emphasized by Churg,[27] cases of PAN currently termed *idiopathic* do not represent a single entity, but almost certainly include several different disorders. Some of these, as indicated by low serum complement levels and measurable immune complexes in the blood, are mediated by immune complex deposition. Others seem to be independent of this mechanism. Finally, although *cutaneous leukocytoclastic angiitis* may be preferable to *hypersensitivity vasculitis* in describing small vessel vasculitis confined to the skin, the term fails to acknowledge the few cases in which lymphocytic infiltrates predominate, even early in the inflammatory lesion.

EPIDEMIOLOGY

Accurate definition of the epidemiology of vasculitis confronts several challenges, as follows: (1) the uncommon nature of many forms of vasculitis, (2) the frequent difficulties in making the correct diagnosis of vasculitis (and in distinguishing one form of vasculitis from another), (3) the fact that the etiologies of most types of vasculitis remain unknown, and (4) historical uncertainty with regard to the classification of these conditions. Nevertheless, in recent years, the epidemiology of some forms of vasculitis has been defined with reasonable precision. Table 80-5 presents the major epidemiologic features of several forms of systemic vasculitis.

GEOGRAPHY

The epidemiologic features of systemic vasculitis vary tremendously by geography. This variation may reflect genetics, differences in environmental exposures dictated by continent and latitude, and the prevalence of other disease risk factors. Although Behçet's disease is rare in North Americans (affecting only approximately 1 in 300,000), the condition is perhaps several hundred times more common among inhabitants of countries that border the ancient Silk Route.[26,28] Similarly, although Takayasu's arteritis is rare in the United States—on the order of 3 new cases per 1 million people per year—the disease is reportedly the most common cause of renal artery stenosis in India, where the incidence may be 200 to 300/1 million/yr. Several studies indicate that the prevalence of giant cell arteritis in Olmsted County, Minnesota, is similar to that of Scandinavian countries, with an annual incidence rate of approximately 240 cases for every 1 million individuals older than age 50 years.[29] The similar prevalence calculations across these countries probably reflect shared genetic risk factors for this condition because many of the current inhabitants of Olmsted County are descended from Scandinavia and northern Europe. Based on 2000 U.S. Census data, the prevalence of giant cell arteritis in the United States is approximately 160,000 patients.

AGE, GENDER, AND ETHNICITY

Age is an important consideration in the epidemiology of vasculitis. Of patients with Kawasaki disease, 80% are younger than age 5 years.[30] In contrast, giant cell arteritis virtually never occurs in patients younger than age 50, and the mean age of patients with that disease is 72. Age also may affect disease severity and outcome. In Henoch-Schönlein purpura, most cases in children (who comprise 90% of all cases) have self-limited courses, resolving within several weeks. In adults, Henoch-Schönlein purpura may have a higher likelihood of chronicity and a greater likelihood of a poor renal outcome.[31]

The distribution of gender varies across many forms of vasculitis. Buerger's disease is the only form of vasculitis with a striking male predominance. The predilection of this disease for men may be explained by the greater prevalence of smoking among men in most societies. In contrast, Takayasu's arteritis has an overwhelming tendency to occur in women (a 9:1 female-to-male ratio), a fact that presently has no explanation. Pauci-immune forms of vasculitis, such as Wegener's granulomatosis, occur in men and women with approximately equal frequencies, but there is some evidence for a female predominance in patients with the limited form of the disease and a male predominance among patients with severe Wegener's granulomatosis.[32]

Table 80-5 Epidemiology of Selected Forms of Vasculitis

| Disease | Incidence | | Age/Gender/Ethnic Predispositions |
	United States	Elsewhere	
Giant cell arteritis	240/1 million (Olmsted County, MN)	220-270/1 million (Scandinavian countries)	Age >50, mean age 72/Females 3:1/Northern European ancestry
Takayasu's arteritis	3/1 million	200-300/1 million (India)	Age <40/Females 9:1/Asian
Behçet's disease	3/1 million	3000/1 million (Turkey)	Silk Route countries
Polyarteritis nodosa	7/1 million	7/1 million (Spain)	Slight male predominance
Kawasaki disease	100/1 million*	900/1 million (Japan)	Children of Asian ancestry
Wegener's granulomatosis	4/1 million	8.5/1 million (United Kingdom)	Whites >> Blacks
Henoch-Schönlein purpura	In children: 135-180/1 million; in adults: 13/1 million		Only 10% of cases occur in adults

*Among children younger than 5 years of age.
From Gonzalez-Gay MA, Garcia-Porrua: Epidemiology of the vasculitides. Rheum Dis Clin N Am 27:729-750, 2001.

For some forms of vasculitis, there are striking variations in tendencies to affect specific ethnic groups. Giant cell arteritis and Wegener's granulomatosis occur with an overwhelming predominance in whites.[33-35] Takayasu's arteritis and Kawasaki disease have higher incidences in patients of Asian ancestry.

GENES

Although genetic risk factors are undoubtedly important in the susceptibility to some forms of vasculitis, familial cases are rare (with the exception of giant cell arteritis; see later). The rarity of familial cases in vasculitis indicates that the genetics of these disorders are polygenic and complex. The strongest link between any single gene and vasculitis is the association of HLA-B51 with Behçet's disease. In Behçet's disease, 80% of Asian patients have the HLA-B51 gene.[28] The prevalence of HLA-B51 is significantly higher among patients with Behçet's disease in Japan than among nondisease controls (55% versus <15%). Among the sporadic cases of Behçet's disease involving white patients in the United States, however, HLA-B51 occurs in less than 15% of cases. In addition to increasing the risk of disease susceptibility in some patients, HLA-B51 increases disease severity. Patients with this gene are more likely to have posterior uveitis, central nervous system involvement, or other severe manifestations.

Reports of familial aggregation in giant cell arteritis are common. Genetic studies have indicated roles for HLA class II alleles such as HLA-DRB1*0401 and HLA-DRB1*0101, albeit the specific associations have varied from study to study.[36,37] Other work indicates that certain tumor necrosis factor microsatellite polymorphisms may contribute to disease susceptibility.[38]

The greatest progress in understanding the relationship of genetics to systemic vasculitis has come in the area of rheumatoid vasculitis. The contribution of the "shared epitope" found on class II HLA molecules (DR4) to the development of rheumatoid arthritis (RA) has been appreciated for 2 decades.[39] Possession of the shared epitope is now known to increase substantially the risk of extra-articular manifestations in RA, including vasculitis, at least in Northern European populations. A gene dosage effect for extra-articular RA with severe organ manifestations has been noted; patients with two copies of shared epitope alleles have a substantially higher risk of extra-articular disease manifestations, many of which are mediated by vasculitis.[40] One study reported an association between rheumatoid vasculitis and 0401/0404.[41]

In a case-control study of patients with severe extra-articular RA compared with RA patients without extra-articular disease manifestations, the presence of two HLA-DRB1*04 alleles encoding the shared epitope was associated with extra-articular RA (odds ratio 1.79; 95% confidence interval 1.04 to 3.08) and rheumatoid vasculitis (odds ratio 2.44; 95% confidence interval 1.22 to 4.89).[42] In a meta-analysis of HLA-DRB1 genotyping studies of patients with rheumatoid vasculitis,[43] rheumatoid vasculitis was found to be associated with the genotypes 0401/0401, 0401/0404, and 0401/0101.

An association between rheumatoid vasculitis and class I molecules also has been reported. An analysis of 159 patients with severe extra-articular RA (46 of whom had vasculitis) and 178 RA patients without extra-articular disease reported a strong association between the HLA-C3 allele and vasculitis.[44] Among vasculitis patients, the allele frequency of HLA-C3 was 0.411 compared with 0.199 in RA patients without extra-articular disease (P < .001). The odds ratio for vasculitis in patients with HLA-C3 was 4.15 (95% confidence interval 2.14 to 8.08).

The association between HLA-C3 and vasculitis was not due to linkage disequilibrium with HLA-DRB1, suggesting that these two genetic risk factors operate through different pathways. HLA-C3 was a strong predictor of vasculitis in patients lacking HLA-DRB1*04 shared epitope alleles, suggesting that HLA-C and HLA-DR genes influence the RA disease process through different pathways. Linkage disequilibrium with other genes in the MHC could not be excluded in this study, however.

In Wegener's granulomatosis, the allele frequency of a functional polymorphism, 620W, in the intracellular tyrosine phosphatase gene *PTPN22*, was found to be increased significantly among ANCA-positive patients compared with healthy controls.[45] Analyses of families with multiple autoimmune disorders have identified this allele as a risk factor for type 1 diabetes, seropositive RA, systemic lupus erythematosus, and autoimmune thyroid disease. In Wegener's granulomatosis, the allelic association was particularly strong among patients with generalized disease (i.e., vasculitis involving the kidney, lung, eye, and peripheral nervous system).

Study of the relationships between genes and systemic vasculitis is in its infancy. Substantial progress can be anticipated in this area in the future.

ENVIRONMENT

Several environmental and occupational exposures have been linked to the development of vasculitis. The strongest environmental exposure, now linked convincingly to Buerger's disease and to rheumatoid vasculitis, is cigarette smoking. Buerger's disease does not occur in the absence of cigarette smoking. The relationship between smoking and Buerger's disease is usually one of primary exposure (usually heavy), but cases related to second-hand smoke have been alleged.

In a case-control study of patients with recent-onset RA, the interactions between smoking, shared epitope genes, and antibodies to citrullinated proteins (i.e., anti–cyclic citrullinated peptide antibodies) were studied.[46] A dose-dependent relationship between smoking and the occurrence of anti–cyclic citrullinated peptide antibodies was found. The presence of shared epitope genes was a risk factor only for RA only among patients who were positive for anti–cyclic citrullinated peptide. A major gene-environment interaction between smoking and HLA-DR SE genes was evident in the large subgroup of patients who possessed anti–cyclic citrullinated peptide antibodies: The combination of smoking history and double copies of shared epitope alleles increased the risk of RA 21-fold. Smoking may trigger RA-specific immune reactions to citrullinated proteins in the context of shared epitope genes.

Associations have been reported, but not confirmed, between exposure to inhaled silica dust and some types of pauci-immune vasculitis.[47] Precise definitions of the relationships between exposures and vasculitis are complicated by difficulties in obtaining reliable measurements of the levels of such exposures, the likelihood of recall bias among patients who are diagnosed with vasculitis, and the choice of appropriate control groups.

Finally, estimates of disease prevalence in vasculitis may be subject to revision because of changing disease definitions. In the ACR Classification Criteria study, manifestations of small and medium vessel involvement were included in the criteria for PAN.[22] Four years later, the CHCC defined PAN as a form of arterial inflammation limited to medium-sized vessels, sparing capillaries, arterioles, and venules.[17] Under this definition, classic PAN is believed to be a rare condition. Applying the CHCC definition retrospectively, not a single case of classic PAN was reported over a 6-year period in the region of the Norwich Health Authority (United Kingdom), an area that included a population of more than 400,000.[48,49]

The epidemiologic differences among individual types of vasculitis raise compelling questions about the etiologies of these diseases. Ultimately, better insights into the pathogenesis of these conditions should explain these epidemiologic differences and facilitate the development of more refined classification schemes.

REFERENCES

1. Lie JT: Nomenclature and classification of vasculitis: Plus ça change, plus c'est la même chose. Arthritis Rheum 37:181-186, 1994.
2. **Kussmaul A, Maier R: Ueber eine bisher nicht beschriebene eigenthümliche Arterienerkrankung (Periarteritis nodosa), die mit Morbus Brightii und rapid fortschreitender allgemeiner Muskellähmung einhergeht. Dtsch Arch Klin Med 1:484-518, 1866.**
3. **Matteson E: Polyarteritis nodosa: Commemorative translation on the 130-year anniversary of the original article by Adolf Kussmaul and Rudolf Maier. Rochester, Minn, Mayo Foundation, 1996.**
4. Ferrari E: Ueber Polyarteritis acuta nodosa (sogenannte Periarteritis nodosa) und ihre Beziehungen zur Polymyositis und Polyneuritis acuta. Beitr Pathol Anat 34:350-386, 1903.
5. Dickson W: Polyarteritis acuta nodosa and periarteritis nodosa. J Pathol Bacterial 12:31-57, 1908.
6. Salama AD, Pusey CD: Immunology of anti-glomerular basement membrane disease. Curr Opin Nephrol Hypertension 11:279-286, 2002.
7. **Godman GC, Churg J: Wegener's granulomatosis: Pathology and review of the literature. Arch Pathol 58:533-553, 1954.**
8. **Hoffman GS, Specks U: Antineutrophil cytoplasmic antibodies. Arthritis Rheum 41:1521-1537, 1998.**
9. Salama AD, Levy JB, Lightstone L, et al: Goodpasture's disease. Lancet 358:917-920, 2001.
10. **Zeek PM: Periarteritis nodosa: A critical review. Am J Clin Pathol 22:777-790, 1952.**
11. Guillevin L, Durand-Gasselin B, Cevallos R, et al: Microscopic polyangiitis: Clinical and laboratory findings in 85 patients. Arthritis Rheum 42:421-430, 1999.
12. Wohlwill F: On the only microscopically recognizable form of periarteritis nodosa. Virchow's Archiv für pathologische Anatomie und Physiologie 246:377-411, 1923.
13. Davson J, Ball J, Platt R: The kidney in periarteritis nodosa. QJM 17:175-192, 1948.
14. Rich AR: The role of hypersensitivity in periarteritis nodosa. Bull Johns Hopkins Hosp 71:123-140, 1942.
15. Zeek P, Smith C, Weeter J: Studies on periarteritis nodosa, III: The differentiation between the vascular lesions of periarteritis nodosa and hypersensitivity. Am J Pathol 24:889-917, 1948.
16. Calabrese LH, Michel BA, Bloch DA, et al: The American College of Rheumatology 1990 criteria for the classification of hypersensitivity vasculitis. Arthritis Rheum 33:1094-1100, 1990.
17. **Jennette JC, Falk RJ, Andrassy K, et al: Nomenclature of systemic vasculitides: Proposal of an international consensus conference. Arthritis Rheum 37:187-192, 1994.**
18. Hunder GG, Arend WP, Bloch DA, et al: The American College of Rheumatology 1990 criteria for the classification of vasculitis: Introduction. Arthritis Rheum 33:1065-1067, 1990.
19. Bloch DA, Michel BA, Hunder GG, et al: The American College of Rheumatology 1990 criteria for the classification of vasculitis: Patients and methods. Arthritis Rheum 33:1068-1073, 1990.
20. Hunder GG, Bloch DA, Michel BA, et al: The American College of Rheumatology 1990 criteria for the classification of giant cell arteritis. Arthritis Rheum 33:1122-1128, 1990.
21. Arend WP, Michel BA, Bloch DA, et al: The American College of Rheumatology 1990 criteria for the classification of Takayasu's arteritis. Arthritis Rheum 33:1129-1134, 1990.
22. Lightfoot RW Jr, Michel BA, Bloch DA, et al: The American College of Rheumatology 1990 criteria for the classification of polyarteritis nodosa. Arthritis Rheum 33:1088-1093, 1990.
23. Leavitt RY, Fauci AS, Bloch DA, et al: The American College of Rheumatology 1990 criteria for the classification of Wegener's granulomatosis. Arthritis Rheum 33:1101-1107, 1990.
24. Masi AT, Hunder GG, Lie JT, et al: The American College of Rheumatology 1990 criteria for the classification of Churg-Strauss syndrome (allergic granulomatosis and angiitis). Arthritis Rheum 33:1094-1100, 1990.
25. Mills JA, Michel BA, Bloch DA, et al: The American College of Rheumatology 1990 criteria for the classification of Henoch-Schönlein purpura. Arthritis Rheum 33:1114-1121, 1990.
26. International Study Group for Behçet's disease: Criteria for diagnosis of Behçet's disease. Lancet 335:1078-1080, 1990.
27. Churg J: Nomenclature of vasculitic syndromes: A historical perspective. Am J Kidney Dis 18:148-153, 1991.
28. Sakane T, Tekeno M, Suzuki N, et al: Behçet's disease. N Engl J Med 341:1284-1291, 1999.
29. Salvarani C, Gabriel SE, O'Fallon WM, et al: The incidence of giant cell arteritis in Olmsted County, Minnesota: Apparent fluctuations in a cyclic pattern. Ann Intern Med 123:192-194, 1995.
30. Barron KS, Shulman ST, Rowley A, et al: Report of the National Institutes of Health Workshop on Kawasaki's Disease. J Rheumatol 26:170-190, 1999.
31. Blanco R, Martinez-Taboada VM, Rodriguez-Valverde V, et al: Henoch-Schönlein purpura in adulthood and childhood: Two different expressions of the same syndrome. Arthritis Rheum 40:859-864, 1997.
32. **The Wegener's Granulomatosis Etanercept Trial Research Group: Limited versus severe Wegener's granulomatosis: Baseline data on patients in the Wegener's Granulomatosis Etanercept Trial. Arthritis Rheum 48:2299-2309, 2003.**
33. Regan MJ, Green WR, Stone JH: Ethnic disparity in the incidence of temporal arteritis: A 32-year experience at an urban medical center. Arthritis Rheum 47:S108, 2002.
34. Falk RJ, Hogan S, Carey TS, et al: Clinical course of anti-neutrophil cytoplasmic autoantibody-associated glomerulonephritis and systemic vasculitis. The Glomerular Disease Collaborative Network. Ann Intern Med 113:656-663, 1990.
35. **Hoffman GS, Kerr GS, Leavitt RY, et al: Wegener's granulomatosis: An analysis of 158 patients. Ann Intern Med 116:488-498, 1992.**
36. Weyand CM, Hunder GG, Hickok KC, et al: HLA-DRB1 alleles in polymyalgia rheumatica, giant cell arteritis, and rheumatoid arthritis. Arthritis Rheum 37:514-520, 1994.
37. Rauzy O, Fort M, Nourhashemi F: Relation between HLA DRB1 alleles and corticosteroid resistance in giant cell arteritis. Ann Rheum Dis 57:380-382, 1998.
38. Mattey DL, Hajeer AH, Dababneh A, et al: Association of giant cell arteritis and polymyalgia rheumatica with different tumor necrosis factor microsatellite polymorphisms. Arthritis Rheum 43:1749-1755, 2000.
39. Gregersen PK, Silver J, Winchester RJ: The shared epitope hypothesis: An approach to understanding the molecular genetics of susceptibility to rheumatoid arthritis. Arthritis Rheum 30:1205-1213, 1987.
40. Weyand CM, Xie C, Goronzy JJ: Homozygosity for the HLA-DRB1 allele selects for extra-articular manifestations in rheumatoid arthritis. J Clin Invest 89:2033-2039, 1992.
41. Voskuhl AE, Hazes JMW, Schreuder GMT, et al: HLA-DRB!, DQA1, and DQB1 genotypes and risk of vasculitis in patients with rheumatoid arthritis. J Rheumatol 24:852-855, 1997.

42. Turesson C, Schaid DJ, Weyand CM, et al: The impact of HLA-DRB1 genes on extra-articular disease manifestations in rheumatoid arthritis. Arthritis Res Ther 7:R1386-R1393, 2005.

43. Gorman JD, David-Vaudey E, Pai M, et al: Particular HLA-DRB1 shared epitope genotypes are strongly associated with rheumatoid vasculitis. Arthritis Rheum 50:3476-3484, 2004.

44. Turesson C, Schaid DJ, Weyand CM, et al: Association of HLA-C3 and smoking with vasculitis in patients with rheumatoid arthritis. Arthritis Rheum 54:2776-2783, 2006.

45. Jagiello P, Aries P, Arning L, et al: The PTPN22 620W allele is a risk factor for Wegener's granulomatosis. Arthritis Rheum 52:4039-4043, 2005.

46. Klareskog L, Stolt P, Lundberg K, et al: A new model for an etiology of rheumatoid arthritis: Smoking may trigger HLA-DR (shared epitope)-restricted immune reactions to autoantigens modified by citrullination. Arthritis Rheum 54:38-46, 2006.

47. Hogan SL, Satterly KK, Dooley MA, et al: Silica exposure in anti-neutrophil cytoplasmic autoantibody-associated glomerulonephritis and lupus nephritis. J Am Soc Nephrol 12:134-142, 2001.

48. Watts R, Carruthers D, Scott D: Epidemiology of systemic vasculitis: Changing incidence or definition? Semin Arthritis Rheum 25:28-34, 1995.

49. Gonzalez-Gay MA: Garcia-Porrua J: Epidemiology of the vasculitides. Rheum Dis Clin N Am 27:729-750, 2001.

Relevant Websites

The Johns Hopkins Vasculitis Center: http://vasculitis.med.jhu.edu.

The Cleveland Clinic Foundation Center for Vasculitis: http://www.clevelandclinic.org/arthritis/vasculitis/default.htm.

The Vasculitis Foundation: http://www.vasculitisfoundation.org/.

The Vasculitis Clinical Research Consortium: http://rarediseasesnetwork.epi.usf.edu/vcrc/.

The National Institute of Allergy and Infectious Disease: http://niaid.nih.gov/dir/general.htm.

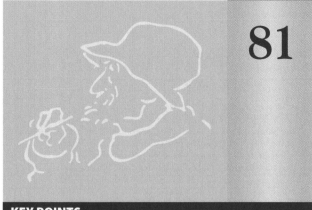

81

Giant Cell Arteritis, Polymyalgia Rheumatica, and Takayasu's Arteritis

DAVID B. HELLMANN

KEY POINTS

Giant cell arteritis affects adults older than 50 years.

The most common manifestations of giant cell arteritis are constitutional symptoms, headache, jaw claudication, and visual symptoms; almost all untreated patients have an elevated erythrocyte sedimentation rate.

The diagnosis of giant cell arteritis is usually confirmed by temporal artery biopsy.

Early treatment of giant cell arteritis can prevent blindness.

Polymyalgia rheumatica can occur by itself or with giant cell arteritis.

Polymyalgia rheumatica by itself responds to prednisone 10 to 20 mg/day, whereas giant cell arteritis requires an initial dose of prednisone of approximately 60 mg/day.

Takayasu's arteritis most frequently affects the aorta and its major branches in young women.

Giant cell arteritis (GCA) and polymyalgia rheumatica (PMR) are discussed together because they affect similar epidemiologic subsets of patients and often occur together in the same individual. Although GCA is a disease of older people and Takayasu's arteritis (TA) is a disease of younger people, their shared predilection for causing vasculitis of large arteries and their nearly identical histopathologic changes prompt their inclusion in the same chapter.

GIANT CELL ARTERITIS AND POLYMYALGIA RHEUMATICA

AMERICAN COLLEGE OF RHEUMATOLOGY CRITERIA

Classification criteria for the diagnosis of GCA have been proposed by the American College of Rheumatology (ACR) (Table 81-1).[1] Two classification schemes have been proposed for PMR (Table 81-2).[2,3]

DEFINITIONS

Giant Cell Arteritis

GCA is the most common form of systemic vasculitis in adults.[4] The disease affects primarily the extracranial branches of the carotid artery in patients older than 50 years. The most feared complication of GCA is irreversible loss of vision. Because the cause of GCA is unknown, various names—including temporal arteritis, cranial arteritis, and granulomatous arteritis—have been used to highlight different salient features.[5,6] All the names for this disease have both merits and shortcomings. The designation *temporal arteritis* or *cranial arteritis*, for example, conveys how frequently the temporal arteries or other cranial arteries are involved but fails to capture GCA's more widespread nature. Although *granulomatous arteritis* and GCA pay homage to an important pathologic finding, this focus is undeserved, because giant cells are absent in about half the cases and may be present in other forms of vasculitis. With no perfect name available, this chapter bows to convention and refers to this disease as GCA.

Polymyalgia Rheumatica

Polymyalgia rheumatica, a term suggested by Barber,[5] is a syndrome characterized by aching in the proximal portions of the extremities and torso. Because there are no specific diagnostic tests or pathologic findings, PMR is defined by its clinical features. The features included in most definitions of PMR are as follows: (1) aching and morning stiffness lasting half an hour or longer in the shoulder, hip girdle, neck, or some combination; (2) duration of these symptoms for 1 month or longer; (3) age older than 50 years; and (4) laboratory evidence of systemic inflammation, such as an elevated erythrocyte sedimentation rate (ESR).[2] Some definitions also include a rapid response to small doses of glucocorticoids, such as prednisone 10 mg/day.[7] The presence of another specific disease other than GCA, such as rheumatoid arthritis (RA), chronic infection, polymyositis, or malignancy, excludes the diagnosis of PMR.

EPIDEMIOLOGY

The incidence of GCA varies widely in different populations, from less than 0.1 per 100,000 to 33 per 100,000 persons aged 50 years and older.[8-19] The greatest risk factor for developing GCA is aging; the disease almost never occurs before age 50, and its incidence rises steadily thereafter. Nationality, geography, and race are also important, with the highest incidence figures found in Scandinavians and in Americans of Scandinavian descent. The lowest incidence of GCA is reported in Japanese, northern Indians, and African Americans. In western Europe, GCA is more common in the northern latitudes than the southern ones. The incidence of GCA has been increasing over the last 20 to 40 years, possibly because of greater physician awareness.[8] Some studies have reported seasonal variations and clustering of cases, with peaks about 7 years apart.[8,17,19] The prevalence of GCA in Olmsted County, Minnesota, home to many Scandinavian immigrants, is 200 per 100,000

Table 81-1 American College of Rheumatology Classification Criteria for Giant Cell Arteritis

Criterion*	Definition
Age at disease onset ≥50 yr	Development of symptoms or findings beginning at age 50 or older
New headache	New onset or new type of localized pain in the head
Temporal artery abnormality	Temporal artery tenderness to palpation or decreased pulsation, unrelated to arteriosclerosis of cervical arteries
Elevated erythrocyte sedimentation rate (ESR)	ESR ≥50 mm/hr by the Westergren method
Abnormal artery biopsy	Biopsy specimen with artery showing vasculitis characterized by a predominance of mononuclear cell infiltration or granulomatous inflammation, usually with multinucleated giant cells

*For purposes of classification, a patient with vasculitis is said to have giant cell (temporal) arteritis if at least three of these five criteria are present. The presence of any three or more criteria yields a sensitivity of 93.5% and a specificity of 91.2%.

From Hunder GG, Bloch DA, Michel BA, et al: The American College of Rheumatology 1990 criteria for the classification of giant cell arteritis. Arthritis Rheum 33:1125, 1990.

Table 81-2 Diagnostic Criteria* for Polymyalgia Rheumatica

Criteria of Chuang and Colleagues[2] (1982)
Age 50 yr or older
Bilateral aching and stiffness for 1 mo or more and involving two of the following areas: neck or torso, shoulders or proximal regions of the arms, and hips or proximal aspects of the thighs
Erythrocyte sedimentation rate (ESR) >40 mm/hr
Exclusion of all other diagnoses except giant cell arteritis

Criteria of Healey[3] (1984)
Pain persisting for at least 1 mo and involving two of the following areas: neck, shoulders, and pelvic girdle
Morning stiffness lasting >1 hr
Rapid response to prednisone (20 mg/day or less)
Absence of other diseases capable of causing the musculoskeletal symptoms
Age older than 50 yr
ESR >40 mm/hr

*For each set of criteria, all the findings must be present for polymyalgia rheumatica to be diagnosed.

From Salvarani C, Cantini F, Boiardi L, Hunder GG: Polymyalgia rheumatica and giant-cell arteritis. N Engl J Med 347:261, 2002.

population aged 50 years or older.[16] Autopsy studies suggest that GCA may be more common than is clinically apparent. Östberg[20] found arteritis in 1.6% of 889 postmortem cases in which sections of the temporal artery and two transverse sections of the aorta were examined.

Genetic susceptibility to the development of GCA was initially suggested by reports of GCA in families[21-23] and, more recently, by studies demonstrating an association with genes in the human leukocyte antigen (HLA) class II region.[24,25] Sixty percent of GCA patients have HLA-DRB1*04 haplotype variants, which have a common sequence motif in the second hypervariable region of the B1 molecule.[25] This motif differs from that found in patients with RA.[25] The low prevalence of these alleles in African Americans may explain why blacks develop GCA relatively infrequently. To date, GCA is the form of systemic vasculitis most closely associated with HLA class II genes.

The existence of environmental risk factors has been suggested by the geographic clustering of GCA cases. Smoking appears to increase the risk of developing GCA sixfold in women.[26] Circumstantial evidence links the development of GCA to a variety of infectious agents, including *Mycoplasma pneumoniae*, varicella-zoster virus, parvovirus B19, and parainfluenza virus type I.[17,18] The results of examining temporal artery biopsy specimens with polymerase chain reaction methods to detect parvovirus B19 or herpesvirus DNA have been negative or inconsistent.[27,28] The reported association between GCA and *Chlamydia pneumoniae* infection has not withstood close scrutiny.[29]

Gender and health status also influence the development of GCA. Women are affected about twice as often as men.[17] Having diabetes reduces the risk of developing GCA by 50% in women.[2] Although patients with GCA have an increased risk of developing thoracic aortic aneurysms, they do not have overall higher mortality rates.[17]

PMR is two to three times more common than GCA.[17,18,30,31] In Olmsted County, Minnesota, 245 cases of PMR were diagnosed during the 22-year period from 1970 through 1991, providing an average annual incidence rate of 52.5 cases per 100,000 persons aged 50 years or older.[31] The prevalence of PMR (active plus remitted cases) was approximately 600 per 100,000 persons aged 50 years and older.[31] PMR is associated with the same HLA-DR4 genes as GCA.[24,25,32]

CAUSE, PATHOLOGY, AND PATHOGENESIS

The causes of GCA and PMR are unknown. Because pathologic studies have provided important clues to the pathogenesis, they are discussed first.

In GCA, inflammation is found most often in medium-size muscular arteries that originate from the arch of the aorta.[17,20,33-36] The inflammation tends to affect the arteries in a segmental fashion (possibly leading to "skip lesions" within arteries), but long portions of arteries may be involved.[37] In patients who died during the active phase of GCA, the greatest frequency of severe involvement was noted in the superficial temporal arteries, vertebral arteries, and ophthalmic and posterior ciliary arteries.[38] The internal carotid, external carotid, and central retinal arteries were affected somewhat less frequently.[38] In other postmortem studies, lesions were commonly found in the proximal and distal aorta and internal and external carotid, subclavian, brachial, and abdominal arteries.[20] Because GCA affects vessels with an internal elastic lamina and vasa vasorum, and because intracranial arteries lose these structures after penetrating the dura, it is not surprising that GCA rarely involves intracranial arteries.[38-41] In some patients with GCA, follow-up biopsy or autopsy surveys showed the persistence of mild chronic inflammation, even though symptoms had resolved.[42]

Early in the disease, collections of lymphocytes are confined to the region of the internal or external elastic lamina or adventitia. The inflammation may be limited to the vasa vasorum in some cases.[43] Intimal thickening with prominent cellular infiltration is a hallmark of more advanced cases.

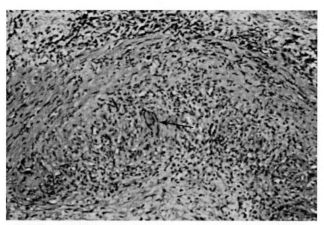

Figure 81-1 **Giant cell arteritis.** In this transverse section of the temporal artery, the adventitia is at the top and the intima is at the bottom center. A multinucleated giant cell *(arrow)* is present at the junction of the media and intima. There is extensive disruption of all layers of the vessel wall (hematoxylin and eosin, ×100). *(Courtesy of Dr. J. T. Lie.)*

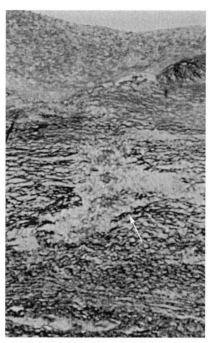

Figure 81-2 **Giant cell arteritis involving the proximal aorta in a patient who died of a ruptured ascending aorta.** This section of the ascending aorta is distal to the ruptured portion and shows destruction of elastic fibers *(arrow)* (elastic van Gieson stain, ×64). Neighboring sections stained with hematoxylin and eosin showed infiltrations of mononuclear leukocytes in the areas of disrupted fibers.

In heavily involved areas, all layers are affected (Fig. 81-1). Transmural inflammation of portions of the arterial wall (including the elastic laminae) and granulomas containing multinucleated histiocytic and foreign body giant cells, histiocytes, lymphocytes (which are predominantly CD4+ T cells), and some plasma cells and fibroblasts are found.[35,44-47] Eosinophils may be seen, but polymorphonuclear leukocytes are rare. Thrombosis may develop at sites of active inflammation; later, these areas may recanalize. The inflammatory process is usually most marked in the inner portion of the media adjacent to the internal elastic lamina. Fragmentation and disintegration of elastic fibers occur, closely associated with an accumulation of giant cells (Fig. 81-2). However, giant cells are seen in only about half of routinely examined specimens; therefore, they are not required to make the diagnosis if other features are compatible. In contrast to some other forms of systemic vasculitis (e.g., polyarteritis nodosa, microscopic polyangiitis, Wegener's granulomatosis), fibrinoid necrosis is rarely if ever observed in GCA.[43]

Immunohistochemical studies demonstrate inflammatory changes that are specific for each layer of the affected artery.[18,45-52] Dendritic cells, which can present antigen and activate T cells, are found in the adventitia.[53-55] The adventitia is also infiltrated by CD4+ T cells that secrete interferon-γ (IFN-γ) and interleukin-2 (IL-2), and macrophages that secrete IL-1, IL-6, and transforming growth factor-β (TGF-β). This cytokine pattern is characteristic of a T helper type 1 (Th1)–mediated reaction.[35,49] The adventitial T cells show evidence of clonal expansion. The media is populated mostly by macrophages that, in contrast to those in other layers, produce matrix metalloproteinases and oxygen free radicals. Closer to the intima, the macrophages secrete nitric oxide and unite to form syncytia—the giant cells—which produce platelet-derived growth factor (PDGF) and substances that stimulate intimal proliferation.[35,56]

Although microscopic examination of arteries in PMR are usually normal, immunohistochemical studies of apparently uninvolved temporal arteries reveal upregulation of the same macrophage-related inflammatory cytokines found in GCA.[35,49] The T cell cytokine IFN-γ is abundantly expressed in GCA and is absent in arteries from patients having only PMR.[49] Pathologically, relatively little else has been found in PMR. Granulomatous myocarditis and hepatitis have been noted.[57] Muscle biopsy specimens may be normal or show nonspecific type II muscle atrophy.[58] However, a number of reports have shown the presence of lymphocytic synovitis in the knees, sternoclavicular joints, and shoulders and evidence of a similar reaction in sacroiliac joints.[59-63] Synovitis (mostly subclinical) was shown in bone scans demonstrating an increased uptake of technetium pertechnetate in the joints of 24 of 25 patients with PMR.[60] More sensitive studies using magnetic resonance imaging (MRI) and ultrasonography have convincingly demonstrated that in PMR, the principal foci of inflammation are the bursae surrounding the shoulder more than the glenohumeral joint itself.[64] Sera from patients with GCA, PMR, or both demonstrate evidence of systemic inflammation, with increased levels of circulating immune complexes during active disease[65,66] and elevated levels of IL-6 and IL-1.[48]

These observations, together with the results from experiments in which temporal arteries from patients with GCA have been implanted into mice with severe combined immunodeficiency (SCID), have been used to propose a model of the immunopathogenesis of GCA[35,45,55] (Fig. 81-3). The key initiating event might be the activation of dendritic cells located in the adventitia, the only arterial layer normally penetrated by the vasa vasorum. In large and medium-size arteries, immunohistochemical studies reveal that the dendritic cells in temporal arteries have a specific phenotype and express fascin and CD11c.[35,53,54,66] In GCA, activation of Toll-like receptors (TLRs) on dendritic cells appears to be the initial triggering event.[53,54,67] Of the many different types of TLRs, TRL-2 and TLR-4 might be the most important in GCA. Experiments in the GCA-SCID mouse model have shown that blood-borne

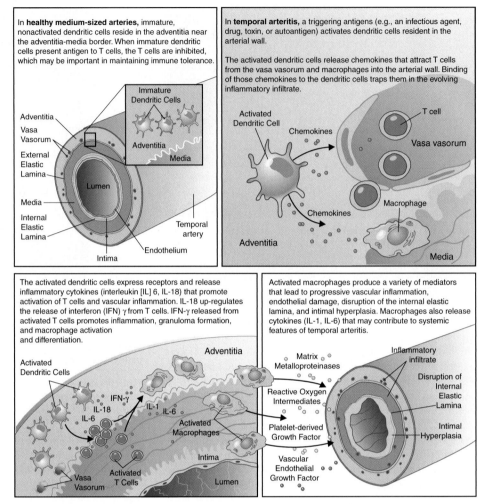

In **healthy medium-sized arteries,** immature, nonactivated dendritic cells reside in the adventitia near the adventitia-media border. When immature dendritic cells present antigen to T cells, the T cells are inhibited, which may be important in maintaining immune tolerance.

In **temporal arteritis,** a triggering antigens (e.g., an infectious agent, drug, toxin, or autoantigen) activates dendritic cells resident in the arterial wall.

The activated dendritic cells release chemokines that attract T cells from the vasa vasorum and macrophages into the arterial wall. Binding of those chemokines to the dendritic cells traps them in the evolving inflammatory infiltrate.

The activated dendritic cells express receptors and release inflammatory cytokines (interleukin [IL] 6, IL-18) that promote activation of T cells and vascular inflammation. IL-18 up-regulates the release of interferon (IFN) γ from T cells. IFN-γ released from activated T cells promotes inflammation, granuloma formation, and macrophage activation and differentiation.

Activated macrophages produce a variety of mediators that lead to progressive vascular inflammation, endothelial damage, disruption of the internal elastic lamina, and intimal hyperplasia. Macrophages also release cytokines (IL-1, IL-6) that may contribute to systemic features of temporal arteritis.

Figure 81-3 **Model for the pathogenesis of giant cell arteritis.** *(From Shermling RH: An 81-year-old women with temporal arteritis. JAMA 295:2525-2534, 2006.)*

lipopolysaccharide serves as an effective TLR ligand in temporal arteries.[54] Other constituents of microorganisms or some self-antigens (e.g., oxidized lipids) may also be TLR ligands that activate the arterial dendritic cells.

Once its TLRs have been engaged, dendritic cells differentiate from the resting to the active state and release cytokines such as IL-6 and IL-18, which recruit, activate, and retain CD4+ T cells in the blood vessel. The crucial role of dendritic cells in activating T cells and maintaining vasculitis has been demonstrated in the GCA-SCID mouse model: depleting the dendritc cells markedly reduces the T cell infiltrate and suppresses the vasculitis.[54] In turn, these activated CD4+ T cells clonally expand and secrete IFN-γ, which causes macrophages to migrate, differentiate, and form granulomas. Production of matrix metalloproteinases and lipid peroxidation agents by macrophages in the media results in the destruction of elastic laminae. The vessel attempts to counter the tissue destruction by elaborating a variety of growth factors, including PDGF, vascular endothelial growth factor (VEGF), and TGF-β, which prompt smooth muscle cells in the media to revert from a contractile phenotype to a secretory one and migrate to the intima. Proliferation of the intimal smooth muscle cells results in occlusion of the lumen.[35,45,53]

PMR appears to result from a similar but less intense adaptive immune response in blood vessels (as evidenced by the in situ production of many inflammatory cytokines).[49] According to this model, both PMR and GCA begin with the activation of dendritic cells at the adventitia-media border.[53,67] However, the distinguishing feature of PMR is the absence of T cells producing IFN-γ. Without IFN-γ to stimulate the recruitment and differentiation of macrophages, the level of arterial inflammation in PMR remains subclinical. Thus, the development of GCA appears to require both vascular dendritic cell activation and a disease-inducing repertoire of T cells.[35,53,67] The constitutional symptoms of PMR and GCA are attributed to the high levels of inflammatory cytokines (e.g., IL-1, IL-6) found in the sera. Whether these serum cytokine elevations result from blood vessel inflammation alone or from some other source of inflammation is not yet clear. The attractiveness of this model is increased by its ability to explain why subsets of clinical features occur together.

CLINICAL FEATURES

The mean age at onset of GCA and PMR is approximately 70 years, with a range of about 50 to 90 years of age.[17] Younger patients with PMR have been described occasionally. Women are affected about twice as often as men.[4,31] Although the onset of the disease is usually insidious, typically evolving over weeks or months, in one third of cases, the disease begins so abruptly that some patients recall the very day they became ill.[17,57]

Table 81-3 Symptoms of Giant Cell Arteritis

Symptom	Frequency (%)
Headache	76
Weight loss	43
Fever	42
Fatigue	39
Any visual symptom	37
Anorexia	35
Jaw claudication	34
Polymyalgia rheumatica	34
Arthralgia	30
Unilateral visual loss	24
Bilateral visual loss	15
Vertigo	11
Diplopia	9

Modified from Smetana GW, Shmerling RH: Does this patient have temporal arteritis? JAMA 287:92, 2002. Data from a review of 2475 patients reported in the literature.

Giant Cell Arteritis

Classic Manifestations. The most common manifestations of GCA are constitutional symptoms, headache, visual symptoms, jaw claudication, and PMR[17] (Table 81-3). Almost all patients experience one or more constitutional symptoms, including fatigue, weight loss, malaise, and fever.

Besides constitutional symptoms, headache is the most common symptom in GCA, being present in nearly three quarters of patients.[68] The pain is typically described as boring in quality, of moderate severity, and most commonly appreciated in the temporal area. However, the description of the headache varies enormously. It can be mild to so severe that the patient seeks immediate relief by presenting to the emergency department. The pain may localize to any part of the skull, including the occiput (owing to involvement of the occipital artery).[17,20] The most consistent characteristic is that the patient experiences the headache as something new and unusual. In untreated patients, the headache may subside over weeks, even though the disease activity continues. Often, the headache of GCA is not associated with any particular findings on physical examination. Abnormalities of the temporal artery—including enlargement, nodular swelling, tenderness, or loss of pulse—develop in only about half of patients (Fig. 81-4). Some patients note tenderness of the scalp, which can be aggravated by brushing or combing the hair.

Visual symptoms are common in GCA, especially loss of vision and diplopia. Vision loss can be unilateral or (less commonly) bilateral, transient or permanent, and partial or complete.[69,70] Vision loss lasting more than a few hours usually does not reverse. Loss of vision often reflects an anterior ischemic optic neuropathy caused by occlusive arteritis of the posterior ciliary artery, the chief blood supply to the head of the optic nerve. The posterior ciliary artery is a branch of the ophthalmic artery (which derives, in turn, from the internal carotid artery). Less frequently, vision loss in GCA stems from a retinal artery occlusion. Regardless of the site of the culprit lesion, vision loss in GCA is usually profound, with more than 80% of patients unable to see hand waving.[69] GCA patients who

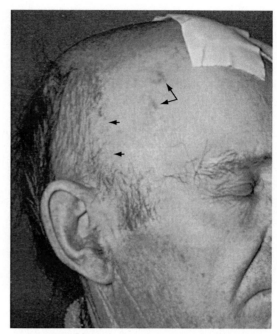

Figure 81-4 Giant cell arteritis (GCA) involving the temporal artery. Short segments of curved artery were erythematous and tender *(long arrows)*. The bandage on the scalp covers a similar artery that was biopsied and showed GCA. A previous biopsy specimen of a proximal segment of the right temporal artery, which was normal on physical examination, was normal histologically. The faint scar from that biopsy can be seen above and anterior to the right ear *(short arrows)*.

present with fever or other systemic symptoms are less likely to develop vision loss.[71-73] One possible explanation of this protective effect of fever and other systemic manifestations is that patients with prominent systemic inflammation demonstrate more extensive angiogenesis in temporal artery biopsies.[74] The angiogenesis associated with increased inflammation may result in the development of collateral circulation that reduces the chance of ischemic events.[36,74]

The early funduscopic appearance in the setting of blindness caused by anterior ischemic optic neuropathy is that of ischemic optic neuritis: slight pallor and edema of the optic disk, with scattered cotton-wool patches and small hemorrhages[69] (Fig. 81-5). Later, optic atrophy occurs. Rarely, blindness may be the initial symptom; however, it tends to follow other symptoms by several weeks or even months. Ophthalmoscopic examination in patients without eye involvement is generally normal. In most reports, the incidence of blindness is 20% or less.[7,30,39,66,69,75] In a series of 245 patients from the modern era, 34 (14%) had some permanent loss of vision.[75] In 32 of these patients, the deficit developed before glucocorticoid therapy was begun; in the other 2, vision loss occurred after therapy was started. Vision loss progressed in 3 of the 32 after therapy was initiated, and it improved in 5. At 5 years' follow-up, among the patients who had visual deficits caused by GCA at the time glucocorticoids were started, the risk of additional loss of vision was 13% over the follow-up period. If no loss had occurred at the beginning of glucocorticoid therapy, there was only a 1% risk of new loss of vision over the subsequent 5 years.

Another potential ocular complication of GCA is ophthalmoplegia. Diplopia usually results from ocular motor

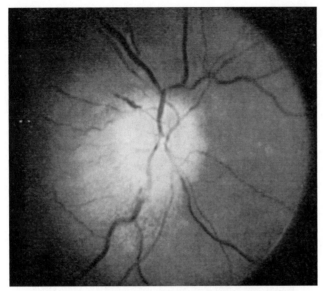

Figure 81-5 Ophthalmoscopic view of the acute phase of ischemic optic neuropathy seen in patients with giant cell arteritis and loss of vision. The optic disk is pale and swollen, the retinal veins are dilated, and a flame-shaped hemorrhage is visible. *(Courtesy of Dr. J. Trautmann.)*

Table 81-4 Atypical Manifestations of Giant Cell Arteritis

Fever of unknown origin
Respiratory symptoms (especially cough)

Otolaryngeal manifestations
    Glossitis
    Lingual infarction
    Throat pain
    Hearing loss

Large artery disease
    Aortic aneurysm
    Aortic dissection
    Limb claudication
    Raynaud's phenomenon

Neurologic manifestations
    Peripheral neuropathy
    Transient ischemic attack, stroke
    Dementia
    Delirium

Myocardial infarction

Tumor-like lesions
    Breast mass
    Ovarian and uterine mass

Syndrome of inappropriate antidiuretic hormone secretion
Microangiopathic hemolytic anemia

nerve palsies caused by ischemia and usually resolves after therapy is started. Oculomotor nerve involvement in GCA usually spares the pupil.[69] Rarely, arterial lesions cause infarction of the occipital cortex and vision loss.

Intermittent claudication may occur in the muscles of mastication (jaw claudication), the extremities, and occasionally the muscles of the tongue or those involved in swallowing.[17] In the jaw muscles, the discomfort is noted especially when chewing meat and may involve the muscles on one side of the mandible more than those on the other. In some instances, facial artery involvement results in spasm of the jaw muscles. More marked vascular narrowing may lead to gangrene of the scalp or tongue.

Atypical Manifestations. Approximately 40% of patients present with disease manifestations that are considered atypical[55,76-78] (Table 81-4). In these patients, headache, jaw claudication, visual symptoms, and PMR do not occur or are less prominent.

Fever occurs in up to 40% of patients with GCA, but it is usually low grade and overshadowed by other classic symptoms. However, 15% of GCA patients may present with fever of unknown origin (FUO) in which the temperature spikes are high, dominating the clinical picture.[7,57] Although GCA causes only 2% of all cases of FUO, it is responsible for 16% of all such fevers in individuals older than 65 years.[57] Approximately two thirds of patients experience shaking chills and drenching sweats, features often attributed to infection or malignancy. The median temperature is 39.1°C, and the maximum 39.8°C. The white blood cell count in GCA-induced FUO is usually normal or nearly so (at least before the initiation of prednisone).

Neurologic problems occur in approximately 30% of patients.[40,41,79] These are diverse, but most common are neuropathies and transient ischemic attacks or strokes. Hemiparesis or brainstem events are due to narrowing or occlusion of the carotid or vertebrobasilar artery. GCA preferentially involves the posterior circulation; the 3:2 ratio of anterior to posterior strokes and transient ischemic attacks seen in the normal population reaches nearly 1:1 in patients with GCA.[40] Delirium, reversible dementia, and myelopathy have also been reported.[40] However, the assignment of an exact cause to ischemic central nervous system events is often challenging, given the older population in which GCA occurs. The neuropathies of GCA include mononeuropathies and peripheral polyneuropathies and may affect the upper or lower extremities. Presumably, they are secondary to the involvement of nutrient arteries, but little pathologic documentation is available. Among the vasculitides, GCA has a nearly unique propensity for involving the C5 nerve root, resulting in loss of shoulder abduction.[40] Mononeuropathies affecting the hands and feet, so typical of polyarteritis and other forms of vasculitis, develop less often in GCA.

Prominent respiratory tract symptoms occur in about 10% of patients.[80] These include cough with or without sputum, sore throat, and hoarseness. When these symptoms are severe or an initial manifestation of GCA, they may direct the attention of the examining physician away from the underlying arteritis. Vasculitis may induce these symptoms by causing ischemia or hyperirritability of the affected tissues. Otolaryngeal manifestations of GCA include throat pain, dental pain, tongue pain, glossitis, and ulceration or infarction of the tongue.[80,81]

Clinical evidence of large artery involvement occurs in 10% to 15% of cases at presentation and in up to 27% eventually.[34,36,62,63,82-85] Positron emission tomography (PET) studies using fluorodeoxyglucose (FDG) revealed that subclinical involvement of large arteries occurs in the vast majority of GCA patients. One PET study, for example, showed that 88% of 35 patients had increased FDG uptake in large arteries, with subclavian involvement in 74% and aortic involvement in 54%.[86]

Generally, clinically evident disease can be divided into early (within a year of diagnosis) and late (years after diagnosis) stages. Usually, early disease consists chiefly of large artery stenosis resulting in upper extremity claudication; bruits over the carotid, subclavian, axillary, and brachial arteries; absent or decreased pulses in the neck or arms; and Raynaud's phenomenon (Fig. 81-6).[85] Angiographic features that suggest GCA are smooth-walled arterial stenoses or occlusions alternating with areas of normal or increased caliber in the absence of irregular plaques and ulcerations, located especially in the carotid, subclavian, axillary, and brachial arteries. Late disease most frequently involves thoracic aortic aneurysm.[85] The tendency for aneurysm to develop late was confirmed in one series of 41 patients in which the average time between diagnosis of GCA and recognition of this complication was 7 years.[65] Thoracic aortic aneurysm is 17 times more likely to develop in patients with GCA than in persons without this disease. To place this risk in context, thoracic aortic aneurysms are twice as likely to complicate GCA as lung cancer is to result from smoking.[83] Abdominal aortica aneurysm is also 2.4 times more common in patients with GCA.[34,65] In aggregate, nearly one out of five patients (18%) with GCA develops an aortic aneurysm or dissection.[85] Patients with large artery disease often do not have headache or other classic manifestation of GCA, and less than 50% have an abnormal temporal artery biopsy. Computed tomography (CT) angiography and magnetic resonance angiography (MRA) are the imaging modalities most commonly used to detect large artery disease in GCA.

In women, GCA may present as a breast or ovarian mass. The mass lesions in these tissues result from granulomatous inflammation in and around the arteries.[84] Angina pectoris, congestive heart failure, and myocardial infarction secondary to coronary arteritis occur rarely.

Clinical Subsets. Studies suggest that GCA is not just one disease but rather a number of clinical subsets that are explained by the differential expression of inflammatory cytokines.[87,88] Ischemic events, including blindness, stroke, and large artery disease, occur more commonly in patients who express high levels of IFN-γ and low levels of IL-6.[88] In contrast, patients who produce high levels of IL-6 are more likely to have strong inflammatory features (such as fever and constitutional symptoms) and are less likely to develop vision loss or other ischemic events.[88-91]

Polymyalgia Rheumatica

As in GCA, PMR patients are characteristically in good health before their disease begins.[17] Systemic manifestations, such as malaise, low-grade fever, and weight loss, are present in more than half the patients and may be the initial symptoms. High, spiking fevers are uncommon in PMR in the absence of GCA.[57] Arthralgias and myalgias may develop abruptly or evolve insidiously over weeks or months.[2] Malaise, fatigue, and depression, along with aching and stiffness, may be present for months before the diagnosis is made. In most patients, the shoulder girdle is the first to become symptomatic; in the remainder, the hip or neck is involved at the onset. The discomfort may begin in one shoulder or hip but usually becomes bilateral within weeks. Symptoms center on the proximal limb, axial musculature, and

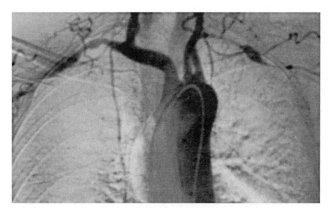

Figure 81-6 **Giant cell arteritis of large arteries.** Arch aortogram. Both subclavian and axillary arteries are affected. Smooth-walled segmental constrictions alternate with areas of normal caliber or aneurysmal dilation. *(From Klein RG, Hunder GG, Stanson AW, Sheps SG: Large artery involvement in giant cell [temporal] arteritis. Ann Intern Med 83:806, 1975.)*

tendinous attachments. Morning stiffness resembling that of RA and "gelling" after inactivity are usually prominent. If the symptoms are severe, aching is more persistent. Although movement of the joints accentuates the pain, it is often felt in the proximal extremities rather than in the joints.[2] Distal joint pain and swelling occur in some cases, including diffuse distal extremity swelling with pitting edema.[92] Pain at night is common, and movement during sleep may awaken the patient. Muscle strength is generally unimpaired, although pain with movement makes the interpretation of strength-testing maneuvers difficult. Pain with movement also makes it difficult for patients to get out of bed or the bathtub. In the later stages of the syndrome, muscle atrophy may develop, and contracture of the shoulder capsule may result in limitation of passive as well as active motion.

As noted, the presence of bursal inflammation and synovitis in PMR has been described by many authors and is undoubtedly the cause of many of the findings in this condition.[64] A careful examination may reveal transient synovitis of the knees, wrists, and sternoclavicular joints. The shoulders and hips are covered by heavy muscles, and minimal effusions of slight synovitis are not palpable on physical examination. Synovitis has been documented by biopsies, synovial analysis, joint scintiscans, ultrasonography, and MRI.[57-63,93]

Relationship between Polymyalgia Rheumatica and Giant Cell Arteritis

There is abundant evidence that PMR and GCA are related and should be considered different manifestations of a common disease process.[17,35] The associations with age, ethnicity, geographic region, and HLA class II alleles are the same in both disorders. Moreover, both disorders involve overproduction of many of the same inflammatory cytokines. Between 30% and 50% of patients with GCA develop PMR. Approximately 10% to 15% of patients who appear to have only PMR have positive temporal artery biopsies. In the absence of symptoms of GCA (e.g., headache, jaw claudication, visual symptoms, high fever), PMR by itself does not appear to cause vision loss and responds to low doses of glucocorticoids (see later).[17]

LABORATORY STUDIES

Except for the findings on arterial biopsy, laboratory results in PMR and GCA are similar[30] (Table 81-5). A mild to moderate normochromic anemia is usually present in both diseases during their active phases. Leukocyte and differential counts are generally normal. A markedly elevated ESR and C-reactive protein (CRP) level are characteristic of both. An ESR higher than 100 mm/hr (Westergren method) is common, but untreated biopsy-proven cases of GCA may be associated with normal or nearly normal levels. In a study of 167 GCA patients, 10.8% presented with an ESR of less than 50 mm/hr, and 3.6% had a rate of less than 30 mm/hr.[94] Rare individuals appear to be unable to develop an elevated ESR during any inflammatory process, including active GCA.[94] The ESR is also liable to be relatively low or normal in patients who have been receiving corticosteroids for another condition.[95] Thus, a normal ESR does not exclude GCA, especially in a patient with otherwise classic symptoms and findings. Platelet counts are often increased.

Nonspecific changes in plasma proteins are often present and include a decrease in the concentration of albumin and an increase in α_2-globulins, fibrinogen, and other acute-phase reactant proteins. Slight increases in gammaglobulins and complement may be present. Results of tests for antinuclear antibodies and rheumatoid factor are generally negative.

Liver function test results are mildly abnormal in approximately one third of patients with GCA and in a slightly smaller fraction of those with PMR.[30,66] An increased alkaline phosphatase level is the most common abnormality, but increases in aspartate transaminase and prolonged prothrombin time may also be found.[96] Liver biopsy specimens are generally normal; granulomatous hepatitis has been observed.[57] Renal function and urinalysis are usually normal. Red blood cell casts are found in some instances, but their presence does not correlate with clinical large artery involvement.[37]

Levels of serum creatine kinase and other enzymes reflecting muscle damage are normal. Electromyograms are usually normal, and muscle biopsy shows normal histologic features or only the mild atrophy characteristic of disuse.[58]

Synovial fluid analyses reported in GCA or PMR showed evidence of mild inflammation, including increased synovial fluid leukocyte counts, with a mean of 2900 cells/mm³ but a range from 300 to 20,000 cells/mm³, with 40% to 50%

Table 81-5 Physical Findings and Laboratory Abnormalities in Giant Cell Arteritis

Feature	Frequency (%)
Any temporal artery abnormality	65
Prominent or enlarged temporal artery	47
Absent temporal artery pulse	45
Scalp tenderness	31
Any funduscopic abnormality	31
Abnormal erythrocyte sedimentation rate (ESR)	96
ESR >50 mm/hr	83
ESR >100 mm/hr	39
Anemia	44

Modified from Smetana GW, Shmerling RH: Does this patient have temporal arteritis? JAMA 287:92, 2002.

being polymorphonuclear leukocytes.[61,93] Synovial fluid complement levels are usually normal.[97] In some instances, synovial biopsy has shown lymphocytic synovitis.[59-63]

Serum IL-6 levels are elevated in patients with PMR and GCA and appear to closely parallel the inflammatory activity.[98] Levels of factor VIII or von Willebrand's factor are elevated in patients with GCA and PMR.[99,100]

DIFFERENTIAL DIAGNOSIS

The diagnosis of GCA should be considered in any patient older than 50 years who experiences loss of vision, diplopia, new form of headache, jaw claudication, PMR, FUO, unexplained constitutional symptoms, anemia, and a high ESR. GCA can cause so many forms of cranial discomfort (e.g., headache, scalp tenderness, jaw claudication, pain of the throat, gums, and tongue) that the disease should also be considered in any patient older than 50 who develops new, unexplained "above-the-neck" pain. The protean manifestations of GCA means that it should also be considered in the differential diagnosis of an older patient presenting with dry cough, stroke, arm claudication, or acute C5 radiculopathy accompanied by other classic symptoms or findings of GCA.

Only a few individual symptoms or findings substantially increase or decrease the likelihood of a patient having this disease[68] (Table 81-6). For example, jaw claudication, diplopia, abnormal temporal artery signs, scalp tenderness, and ESR greater than 50 mm/hr increase the likelihood that a patient has GCA.[68] In one series of 373 patients, the presence of either jaw claudication or diplopia increased the likelihood of a positive biopsy by more than threefold; the presence of both jaw claudication and double vision had a 100% positive predictive value for a diagnostic temporal artery biopsy.[101] Conversely, the absence of headache or temporal artery abnormalities on physical examination, the presence of synovitis, and a normal ESR reduce the likelihood of GCA.

A large number of disorders can mimic GCA. There are many causes of monocular vision loss besides vasculitis, including arteriosclerosis-induced thromboembolic disease.[69] Patients with nonarteritic vision loss do not have other GCA-related symptoms, signs, or findings. The funduscopic examination may help by revealing Hollenhorst plaques in cases caused by cholesterol emboli. Anterior ischemic optic neuropathy, the most common cause of vision loss in GCA, can also be caused by arteriosclerosis. Nonarteritic optic neuropathy invariably produces a small optic disk and cup-to-disk ratio, whereas GCA-related optic neuropathy results in an optic disk of variable size.[69] Thus, a normal size or large cup in a patient with anterior ischemic optic neuropathy suggests GCA until proved otherwise.[69]

Constitutional symptoms with anemia and an elevated ESR in an older person may also be produced by occult infections (e.g., tuberculosis, bacterial endocarditis, human immunodeficiency virus [HIV]) or malignancy (especially lymphoma and multiple myeloma). These diagnoses highlight the value of selective serologic tests, imaging studies, and immunoelectrophoresis in appropriate patients. Systemic amyloidosis can closely mimic GCA, being one of the few disorders other than GCA that causes jaw claudication.[102] The amyloid deposits in the temporal artery may not be detected

Table 81-6 Likelihood Ratios* for Symptoms, Signs, and Laboratory Findings in Giant Cell Arteritis

Finding	Positive Likelihood Ratio (95% CI)	Negative Likelihood Ratio (95% CI)
Symptoms		
Jaw claudication	4.2 (2.8-6.2)	0.72 (0.65-0.81)
Diplopia	3.4 (1.3-8.6)	0.95 (0.91-0.99)
Weight loss	1.3 (1.1-1.5)	0.89 (0.79-1.0)
Any headache	1.2 (1.1-1.4)	0.7 (0.57-0.85)
Fatigue	NS	NS
Anorexia	NS	NS
Arthralgia	NS	NS
Polymyalgia rheumatica	NS	NS
Fever	NS	NS
Visual loss	NS	NS
Signs		
Beaded temporal artery	4.6 (1.1-18.4)	0.93 (0.88-0.99)
Tender temporal artery	2.6 (1.9-3.7)	0.82 (0.74-0.92)
Any temporal artery abnormality	2.0 (1.4-3.0)	0.53 (0.38-0.75)
Scalp tenderness	1.6 (1.2-2.1)	0.93 (0.86-1.0)
Synovitis	0.41 (0.23-0.72)	1.1 (1.0-1.2)
Optic atrophy	NS	NS
Laboratory Results		
ESR abnormal	1.1 (1.0-1.2)	0.2 (0.08-0.51)
ESR >50 mm/hr	1.2 (1.0-1.4)	0.35 (0.18-0.67)
ESR >100 mm/hr	1.9 (1.1-3.3)	0.8 (0.68-0.95)
Anemia	NS	NS

*Based on literature review, with the number of patients for each variable ranging from 68 to 2475.

CI, confidence interval; ESR, erythrocyte sedimentation rate; NS, not significant.

Modified from Smetana GW, Shmerling RH: Does this patient have temporal arteritis? JAMA 287:92, 2002.

unless the specimen is stained with Congo red. Polyarthritis in an older patient is much more likely caused by RA than by GCA. In one study of 520 GCA patients, less than 2% developed polyarthritis before GCA was diagnosed.[102,103]

Criteria for the classification of GCA have been formulated and can help differentiate this arteritis from other forms of vasculitis[1] (see Table 81-1). Takayasu's arteritis, like GCA, can affect the aorta and the major arterial branches to the head and arms. Takayasu's arteritis, however, is a disease of young women. Wegener's granulomatosis can affect the temporal artery and, along with systemic amyloidosis, is an exception to the rule that jaw claudication is pathognomonic for GCA. Wegener's granulomatosis, however, almost always produces telltale involvement of the respiratory tract or kidneys and is associated with antineutrophil cytoplasmic antibodies. Polyarteritis nodosa can also affect the temporal artery and should be considered if the biopsy does not contain giant cells and the patient has other features atypical for GCA, such as mesenteric arteritis. Fibrinoid necrosis of the vasa vasorum occurs in polyarteritis but rarely, if ever, in GCA. Primary angiitis of the central nervous system differs from GCA in that it affects the intracranial arteries.

The diagnosis of PMR is clinical and depends on eliciting the symptoms and findings noted earlier. Two sets of criteria for the diagnosis have been proposed[2,3] (see Table 81-2). Several disorders can mimic PMR. Distinguishing early RA from PMR can be difficult, especially in the 15%

of patients who are rheumatoid factor negative and in those few RA patients who have not yet developed prominent synovitis of the small joints of the hands and feet. Patients with polymyositis complain much more of weakness than of pain—the opposite symptom pattern reported by patients with PMR. In addition, in polymyositis, levels of muscle enzymes are elevated, and electromyograms are abnormal. Although patients with neoplasms may have generalized musculoskeletal aching, there is no association between PMR and malignant neoplasia. Therefore, a search for an underlying tumor is not necessary unless some clinical evidence for a tumor is present or the patient has an atypically poor response to low-dose prednisone.

Some patients with chronic infections, such as bacterial endocarditis, may have findings simulating PMR, and blood cultures should be obtained in patients with fever.[104] Patients with fibromyalgia usually do not have typical morning stiffness and have laboratory test results that are normal or nearly so. Rarely, the stiffness of early Parkinson's disease can be confused with PMR if the bradykinesia and tremor of Parkinson's disease are subtle or absent. Lumbar spinal stenosis sometimes causes patients to complain of pain and stiffness in the hip girdle area. The absence of symptoms above the waist helps differentiate it from PMR. Cholesterol-lowering statin drugs can produce myalgia with or without muscle enzyme elevations but rarely mimic PMR. Hypothyroidism in the elderly can mimic many conditions, including PMR.[104] A peculiar syndrome of remitting, seronegative synovitis with pitting edema (designated RS$_3$PE syndrome) may be difficult to differentiate from PMR,[104] and they may be related disorders. Patients with the RS$_3$PE syndrome develop acute symmetric polysynovitis of distal joints with pitting edema of the hands and feet. The RS$_3$PE syndrome and PMR both respond to nonsteroidal anti-inflammatory drugs (NSAIDs) and low-dose prednisone.[17,105]

DIAGNOSTIC EVALUATION IN GIANT CELL ARTERITIS

Temporal artery biopsy is the "gold standard" for diagnosing GCA.[17,106] Because GCA does not involve the artery in a continuous fashion, temporal artery biopsy should be directed to the symptomatic side, if evident. Removing a small (1- to 2-cm) section of temporal artery is usually adequate in patients who have palpable abnormalities of the vessel.[107] Otherwise, the surgeon should try to excise a 4- to 6-cm sample, and the pathologist should examine multiple sections.[17] In skilled hands, temporal artery biopsy is virtually free of morbidity or mortality. Scalp necrosis can rarely complicate active GCA but has not developed as a consequence of temporal artery biopsy.[106]

Temporal artery biopsies performed at institutions experienced in treating GCA are sensitive and have a high negative predictive value. At the Mayo Clinic, the sensitivity of temporal artery biopsy is approximately 90% to 95%, meaning that only 5% to 10% of patients with negative biopsies will subsequently be proved (by additional biopsy, angiography, or autopsy) to have GCA and require corticosteroid therapy.[106,108] The sensitivity figures noted previously include some patients who underwent bilateral temporal artery biopsy. Estimates of the value of bilateral biopsies vary. Of 234 cases of biopsy-proven GCA, unilateral biopsy was

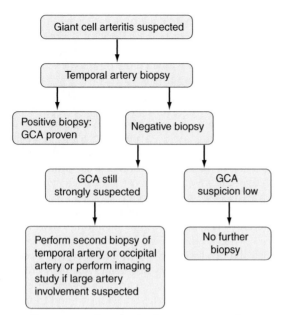

Figure 81-7 Algorithm for diagnosing giant cell arteritis (GCA).

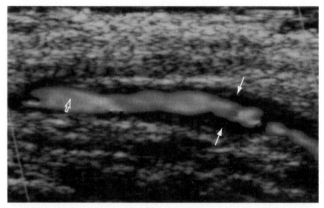

Figure 81-8 Color duplex ultrasound examination of a swollen, tender temporal artery in a patient with giant cell arteritis. The variably thickened artery wall is visible as a clear "halo" *(solid arrows)* around the lumen in the center *(open arrow)*.

positive in 86%, and the second biopsy was positive in 14%.[105] Other studies indicate that a second temporal artery biopsy improves the diagnostic yield by only 3% to 5%.[109,110]

Management of a patient with a negative unilateral biopsy depends on how strongly the patient's clinical picture suggests GCA (Fig. 81-7). When GCA is still strongly suspected, a second biopsy should be considered. Patients with chiefly occipital headache may be best diagnosed by biopsy of the occipital artery.[111] Patients who have signs of subclavian and axillary disease manifested by arm claudication, unequal arm blood pressures, and supraclavicular or axillary bruits may be diagnosed by angiogram, MRA, or CT scan.[88] Typically, patients with extracranial GCA have smooth, tapered stenosis or occlusion of the subclavian, axillary, and proximal brachial arteries. In one series, temporal artery biopsy was positive in only 58% of patients with larger artery involvement.[88] MRI and CT are the best-established methods for detecting aortic involvement by GCA.[17]

Other imaging techniques have been proposed to assist in the diagnosis of GCA. Color duplex ultrasonography showed abnormalities of the temporal artery in 28 of 30 patients with GCA (sensitivity of 93%).[112] The most characteristic finding was a dark halo around the lumen of the temporal artery (Fig. 81-8). However, the diagnostic value of ultrasonography remains controversial.[113] One study found that ultrasonography did not improve the diagnostic accuracy of a carefully performed physical examination.[114] High-resolution MRI of the superficial temporal artery has shown promise in small series bur remains experimental.[115] PET has shown promise in detecting occult involvement of the aorta and great vessels by GCA, but its specifity has not been established.[86,116,117]

TREATMENT AND COURSE

Most authorities recommend starting glucocorticoid therapy as soon as the diagnosis of GCA is strongly suspected. The main goal of treatment is to prevent loss of vision. Because

vision loss is almost always permanent, it seems prudent to initiate corticosteroid therapy as early as possible, even before the biopsy is performed. Fortunately, the diagnostic yield of temporal artery biopsy is not altered by corticosteroid therapy for at least 2 weeks and perhaps longer.[118,119]

Initial Treatment for Giant Cell Arteritis

An initial dose of prednisone 40 to 60 mg/day or equivalent is adequate in nearly all cases.[17] Dividing the dose for the first 1 to 2 weeks may accelerate the rate of improvement. If the patient does not respond promptly, the dose should be increased. One double-blind, placebo-controlled, randomized trial involving 27 GCA patients suggested that initiating treatment with intravenous methylprednisolone (15 mg/kg of ideal weight per day) for 3 days allowed more rapid tapering of oral corticosteroids and increased the likelihood of achieving a sustained remission.[120] The small size of that study and the possible overreliance on laboratory tests to define relapse raise questions about the generalizability of these results. High-dose, intravenous-pulse methylprednisolone (1000 mg/day) for 3 days has also been tried in patients with recent loss of vision. Unfortunately, the loss remains permanent in the vast majority of patients.[121] The occlusive nature of the vasculitis argues against any role of acute thrombolytic therapy in the treatment of blindness.[47]

Because all patients with GCA require months of glucocorticoid therapy, measures to prevent osteoporosis should be started early, as outlined in Table 81-7. In addition, because traditional risk factors for atherosclerosis (e.g., smoking, hypertension, diabetes, hypercholesterolemia) might increase the risk of vision loss or stroke in GCA,[72] reducing or eliminating these risk factors is an important part of overall management.

Subsequent Treatment for Giant Cell Arteritis

The initial effective dose of prednisone should be continued until all reversible symptoms, signs, and laboratory abnormalities have reverted to normal.[17] This usually takes 2 to 4 weeks. After that, the dose can be gradually reduced by a maximum of 10% of the total dose each week or every 2 weeks.[17] The decision to reduce prednisone should be based on a composite assessment of the patient's symptoms, signs,

Table 81-7 Measures to Prevent Corticosteroid-Induced Osteoporosis in Giant Cell Arteritis or Polymyalgia Rheumatica

Avoid or stop smoking
Reduce alcohol consumption if excessive
Participate in weight-bearing exercise
Supplement diet with calcium (1000 to 1500 mg/day)
Supplement diet with vitamin D (800 IU/day)

Measure bone mineral density (BMD) at lumbar spine and hip
   If BMD is normal, repeat BMD annually
   If BMD is not normal (i.e., T score below −1), prescribe
     bisphosphonate

Modified from American College of Rheumatology Ad Hoc Committee on Glucocorticoid-Induced Osteoporosis: Recommendations for the prevention and treatment of glucocorticoid-induced osteoporosis. Arthritis Rheum 44:1496, 2001.

and laboratory markers of inflammation. The ESR and serum concentration of CRP are generally the most convenient and helpful laboratory markers of inflammation. The ESR is reliable only if performed promptly after the blood sample is obtained. Serum levels of IL-6 appear to be the most sensitive marker of activity of GCA, but this test is not widely available.[122] CRP may be slightly more sensitive than ESR in detecting flares.[122] At some point during drug tapering, the ESR or CRP may rise above normal again, and further reductions of prednisone should be temporarily interrupted. If, over the next week or so, the patient does not develop signs or symptoms of active GCA, reductions in prednisone (at smaller decrements and at longer intervals) can usually be resumed. Doses of 10 to 20 mg/day or more are often required for several months before further reductions are possible However, making the prednisone dose a slave to the levels of inflammatory markers without regard to the patient's overall clinical context risks corticosteroid-related side effects. Gradual reductions allow the identification of the minimal suppressive dose and help avoid exacerbations resulting from too-rapid tapering. Even with a gradual reduction of prednisone, more than 50% of patients experience flares of disease activity during the first year.[123,124] These exacerbations can usually be handled by increasing the prednisone 10 mg above the last dose at which the disease was controlled.

GCA tends to run a self-limited course for several months to several years, commonly 1 or 2 years.[17] Glucocorticoids can eventually be reduced and discontinued in some patients. Many patients require low doses of prednisone for several years or more to control musculoskeletal symptoms.

The nearly universal experience of serious side effects associated with daily corticosteroids has prompted the search for alternative steroid-sparing treatments. Unfortunately, to date, none has been convincingly effective. Alternate-day prednisone, for example, is not effective initial therapy for GCA.[125] The combination of weekly low-dose oral methotrexate and prednisone was steroid sparing in one placebo-controlled, double-blind treatment trial[124] but not in another.[123] These conflicting results argue against using methotrexate in combination with prednisone as initial therapy for GCA. Methotrexate may be worth adding to the treatment regimen of a patient who has experienced several exacerbations despite slow tapering of prednisone. Although it was appealing to think that anti–tumor necrosis factor

(TNF) agents might be effective in a granulomatous vasculitic process, a recent trial demonstrated that infliximab is not effective in GCA.[126] Similarly, cytotoxic drugs, dapsone, antimalarials, and cyclosporine have not been clearly shown to be effective, but they may be considered in patients who cannot achieve an acceptably low dose of prednisone.[17]

No prospective, double-blind trials have tested the potential adjuncitve role of aspirin or anticoagulants in the treatment of GCA. However, aspirin is theoretically appealing because, in experimental models of GCA, it inhibits IFN-γ production more effectively than prednisone.[127] In addition, two retrospective studies found that GCA patients taking low-dose aspirin or anticoagulant therapy had a three- to fivefold lower risk of developing an ischemic event such as vision loss.[128,129] Together, these studies suggest that it is reasonable to add low-dose aspirin in GCA patients who do not have an excessive risk of gastrointestinal bleeding.

Arm claudication from GCA affecting the subclavian and axillary arteries usually improves or resolves with corticosteroid therapy. Rare GCA patients with severe upper extremity claudication unresponsive to corticosteroid therapy may benefit from balloon angioplasty. In one series of 10 patients, all improved initially after angioplasty; but 50% developd symptomatic restenosis over 24 months.[130] In all cases, recurrent stenosis developed in vascular lesions that were greater than 3 cm long.[130]

Thoracic aortic aneurysm is greatly increased in patients with GCA.[83] Although it can be present at the outset, aneurysms are usually noted late in the disease course, an average of 7 years after onset. Some authorities have recommended annual chest radiographs to detect thoracic aortic aneurysms.[83]

Treatment for Polymyalgia Rheumatica

Patients with PMR without symptoms or signs or biopsy evidence of GCA are usually treated initially with prednisone 10 to 20 mg/day or equivalent.[131] Salicylates and NSAIDs have been used but are less appealing; salicylates and NSAIDs adequately control symptoms in only a minority of patients with milder symptoms and add to overall adverse drug reactions when they are used with glucocorticoids.[2,10,132] Prednisone therapy usually results in rapid (often overnight) and dramatic improvement of the musculoskeletal aching and stiffness and a more gradual return of the ESR and CRP level to normal.[133] A minority of patients with isolated PMR fail to respond to prednisone 20 mg/day after 1 week and may require up to 30 mg/day as initial treatment.[134] Studies suggest that these resistant cases are more likely to have ESRs greater than 50 mm/hr and very high levels of IL-6.[134] Failure to respond to prednisone 30 mg/day for 1 week should prompt a search for an alternative diagnosis (Fig. 81-9). Lower doses of prednisone may not suppress an underlying arteritis if it is present. Thus, the patient must be observed carefully even though the aching improves. In patients with PMR, the dose should be reduced gradually as soon as symptoms permit. Pretreatment ESR, CRP, and IL-6 concentrations and initial responses to therapy appear to be helpful in dividing patients into subsets with different treatment requirements.[131,133] If the laboratory test results become normal while the patient is receiving a smaller dose, the likelihood of an underlying active vasculitis seems

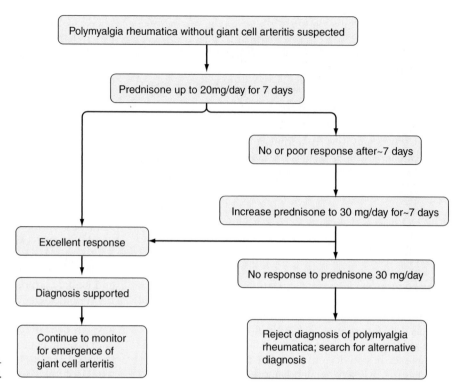

Figure 81-9   Algorithm for diagnosing poly-myalgia rheumatica without giant cell arteritis.

to be much less, and the risk of vascular complications is smaller. However, this is not true in all instances, because active arteritis has been observed even though the ESR improved.[135]

Once the symptoms, signs, and laboratory abnormalities of PMR have resolved (usually after 2 to 3 weeks of therapy), the daily dose of prednisone can be slowly tapered. Some experts recommend tapering prednisone by 2.5 mg every week until 10 mg/day is reached, at which point the decrements should be reduced by 1 mg each month.[133] Flares are common, necessitating a dose increase to achieve remission before attempting a slower taper. The minority of patients with PMR succeed in tapering off prednisone in less than 1 year.[132] Many require at least 2 years of low-dose prednisone.[136]

Some, but not all, studies suggest that oral methotrexate (10 mg once a week for 48 weeks) can reduce the long-term

Table 81-8   American College of Rheumatology Classification Criteria for Takayasu's Arteritis*

Onset before age 40 yr
Limb claudication
Decreased brachial artery pulse
Unequal arm blood pressure (>10 mm Hg)
Subclavian or aortic bruit
Angiographic evidence of narrowing or occlusion of aorta or its primary branches, or large limb arteritis

*The presence of three or more of the six criteria is sensitive (91%) and specific (98%) for the diagnosis of Takayasu's arteritis.

American College of Rheumatology 1990 criteria for the classification of Takayasu arteritis. Arthritis Rheum 33:1129, 1990. From Hellmann DB: Takayasu arteritis. In Imboden JB, Hellmann DB, Stone JH (eds): Current Rheumatology Diagnosis and Treatment. New York, Lange Medical Books/McGraw-Hill, 2004, p 245.

need for corticosteroids in patients with PMR.[137] It is not yet known whether the small but statistically significant reduction in prednisone use achieved with methotrexate results in a clinically important reduction in prednisone-related side effects.

TAKAYASU'S ARTERITIS

Takayasu's arteritis (TA), also known as pulseless disease or occlusive thromboaortopathy, is a form of vasculitis of unknown cause that chiefly affects the aorta and its major branches, most frequently in young women.[138-143] The disease is named for the Japanese ophthalmologist who in 1908 described a young woman with peculiar retinal arteriovenous anastomoses caused by retinal ischemia from large vessel vasculitis.[144]

AMERICAN COLLEGE OF RHEUMATOLOGY CRITERIA

The ACR classification criteria for the diagnosis of TA are listed in Table 81-8.[145]

EPIDEMIOLOGY

Although TA has been described worldwide, it occurs most commonly in Japan, China, India, and Southeast Asia; the disease is also prevalent in Mexico.[146] Whereas the incidence of TA in Japan is nearly 150 per million per year, it is only 0.2 to 2.6 per million in western Europe and North America.[146] TA affects women eight times more frequently than men. The median age of onset is 25 years; however, approximately 25% of cases begin before age 20, and 10% to 20% present after age 40.[138,146,147] Immunogenetic studies in Japanese patients suggest an association with several HLAs, especially HLA-Bw52, Dw12, DR2, and DQw1.[146] Different

HLA associations have been found in Koreans and Indians. No HLA association has been found in North American patients. In Mexican patients, TA has been associated with previous exposure to *Mycobacterium tuberculosis*.[146]

CAUSE AND PATHOGENESIS

The cause of TA is unknown. The nearly identical pathology in TA and GCA has invited speculation that the model of immunopathogenesis of GCA described earlier (see Fig. 81-3) applies to TA as well.[35,34,148] Like GCA, TA is thought to result from an autoimmune process that targets large elastic-containing arteries. Both feature panarteritis involving infiltration of dendritic cells, T cells (including αß, γδ, and cytotoxic), natural killer cells, and macrophages. In TA, the majority of lymphocytes are perforin-secreting killer lymphocytes, such as T cells and natural killer cells.[149-153] The T cell receptors in TA, as in GCA, are oligoclonal, suggesting that the vasculitis is driven in both diseases by a T cell response to a specific but unknown antigen.[149,150] Chronic inflammation of the vessel wall leads to aneurysm formation, stenosis, or thrombosis more frequently in TA than in GCA. Dissection occurs in TA but is rare and less frequent than in syphilitic aortitis.[152,153] The late phase of TA, like that of GCA, is characterized by intima proliferation with superimposed atherosclerosis, medial necrosis with scarring, and adventitial fibrosis. As in GCA, the inflammatory involvement in TA can be continuous or segmental, with skip areas of normal vessel interposed between involved areas.[152] It is possible that the humoral immune system may play some role in the pathogenesis of TA; most TA patients possess anti–endothelial cell antibodies that can damage vessels by inducing endothelial inflammatory cytokine production, adhesion molecules, and apoptosis.[154,155]

The geographic clustering of cases has suggested that genetics and environmental factors participate in the pathogenesis of TA.[146] However, immunogenetic studies (detailed earlier) have not identified any other universally shared genetic risk factors. The young age of onset and the female predominance in TA and in systemic lupus erythematosus have invited speculation about the influence of female hormones in promoting an autoimmune disease process. In some countries, the apparent association of TA with high rates of exposure to tuberculosis has suggested an infectious cause. An animal model of TA has been produced in mice using a herpesvirus that infects the smooth muscle cells of the media. In that model, the media of large elastic arteries serves as an immunoprivileged site that allows the herpesvirus to propagate a chronic inflammatory response in the aorta and its major branches.[156]

CLINICAL FEATURES

Symptoms and Signs

Although the presenting manifestations of TA are protean, the vast majority of patients present with symptoms and signs of vascular insufficiency (from stenosis, occlusion, or aneurysm), systemic inflammation, or both[138,141] (Table 81-9). In a North American series of 60 patients followed at the National Institutes of Health, the most common presenting vascular symptoms were claudication (35%), reduced or absent pulse (25%), carotid bruit (20%), hypertension (20%), carotidynia (20%) lightheadedness (20%), and asymmetrical arm blood pressures (15%).[138] Stroke, aortic regurgitation, and visual abnormalities were present at onset in less than 10% of patients. The extreme manifestations of retinal ischemia noted in Takayasu's original patient are rarely seen now.[138] Permanent loss of vision, the major concern in GCA, rarely develops in TA.

Claudication affects the arms at least twice as frequently as the legs. For many young women, arm claudication first reveals itself as arm pain or fatigue experienced while trying to hold a hair dryer. Overall, bruit is the most common sign, eventually found in 80% of patients. Although bruit over the carotid artery is most frequent, it can also be found in the supraclavicular, infraclavicular, axillary, flank, chest, abdominal, and femoral areas. One third of patients have multiple bruits.[138] Unequal arm blood pressures eventually develop in half of all patients. Headache, which is common in TA, does not correlate with carotid or vertebral disease, which develops in nearly 40% of patients.[138]

Constitutional, musculoskeletal, and other symptoms of systemic inflammation are also common presenting complaints.[138,141-143,157,158] About one in five TA patients presents with fever and malaise, which can be accompanied by night sweats and weight loss. A few patients who have minimal or no signs of vascular insufficiency may appear to have FUO for weeks or months before the diagnosis of TA becomes evident. A minority of patients present with myalgia or arthralgia (see Table 81-9). Some patients have striking

Table 81-9 Clinical Features of Takayasu's Arteritis

Feature	At Presentation (%)	Ever Present (%)
Vascular	50	100
Bruit		80
Claudication (upper extremity)	30	62
Claudication (lower extremity)	15	32
Hypertension	20	33
Unequal arm blood pressures	15	50
Carotidynia	15	32
Aortic regurgitation		20
Central nervous system	30	57
Lightheadedness	20	35
Visual abnormality	10	30
Stroke	5	10
Musculoskeletal	20	53
Chest wall pain	10	30
Joint pain	10	30
Myalgia	5	15
Constitutional	33	43
Malaise	20	30
Fever	20	25
Weight loss	15	20
Cardiac	15	38
Aortic regurgitation	8	20
Angina	2	12
Congestive heart failure	2	10

Data based on a study of 60 North American patients reported by Kerr GS, et al: Takayasu arteritis. Ann Intern Med 120:919, 1994. From Hellmann DB: Takayasu arteritis. In Imboden JB, Hellmann DB, Stone JH (eds): Current Rheumatology Diagnosis and Treatment. New York, Lange Medical Books/McGraw-Hill, 2004, p 243.

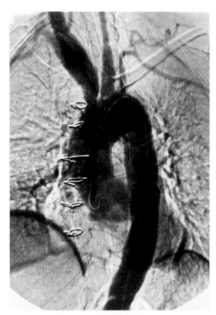

Figure 81-10 Angiogram showing multiple changes of Takayasu's arteritis, including dilation of the aortic root (with surgical wires from previous aortic valve replacement), aneurysmal dilation of the innominate and right carotid arteries, and occlusion of the distal left common carotid artery. *(From Hellmann DB, Flynn JA. Clinical presentation and natural history of Takayasu's arteritis and other inflammatory anrteritides. In Perler BA, Becker GJ [eds]: Vascular Intervention: A Clinical Approach. New York, Thieme Medical and Scientific Publisher, 1998, pp 249-256.)*

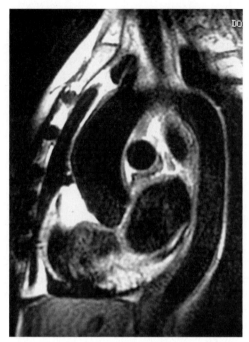

Figure 81-11 Magnetic resonance image (sagittal section) through the chest showing thickening of the ascending and descending thoracic aorta in a 26-year-old woman with Takayasu's arteritis. *(From Hellmann DB: Takayasu arteritis. In Imboden J, Hellmann DB, Stone JH [eds]: Current Rheumatology: Diagnosis & Treatment. New York, McGraw-Hill, 2004, p 244.)*

midthoracic back pain, perhaps as a result of aortic inflammation irritating nociceptive nerve fibers.

Cardiac involvement occurs eventually in nearly one third of patients (see Table 81-9).[138] Aortic regurgitation develops in 20% of patients as a result of aortic root dilation. Aortic regurgitation is important because it frequently progresses and may lead to left ventricular dilation with secondary mitral regurgitation and congestive heart failure. Aortic valve replacement is often required eventually. Angina can develop as a result of coronary artery disease. TA of the coronary arteries most often produces ostial lesions but can also produce either diffuse vasculitis of the coronary arteries or aneurysms.[159-164] Myocarditis also occurs in TA and causes potentially reversible congestive heart failure. Pericarditis is very rare. TA is, along with Behçet's disease, one of the few forms of vasculitis that can affect the large pulmonary arteries. Although TA of the pulmonary arteries is rare (<3%), affected patients can present with cough, chest wall pain, dyspnea, or hemoptysis.

Unlike polyarteritis or Wegener's granulomatosis, TA rarely causes peripheral neuropathies. Cutaneous manifestations develop in less than 10% of patients with TA.[138] Erythema nodosum is most common, but purpura, livedo reticularis, and ulceration may rarely occur. As in GCA, a minority of TA patients with active disease have a persistent, dry cough.

Laboratory Findings

At presentation, the ESR is more frequently elevated (80%) than the CRP (≈50%).[141] Mild anemia and hypergammaglobulinemia are common. The white blood cell count is usually normal or slightly elevated. The platelet count is elevated in one third of patients and may exceed 500,000/μL in those with active disease. The serum creatinine and urinalysis are

usually normal. Any renal abnormalities are usually secondary to hypertension; unlike antineutrophil cytoplasmic antibody–associated vasculitis, TA rarely causes glomerulonephritis.

Imaging Studies

Vascular abnormalities in TA can be imaged by conventional angiography, MRI, MRA, CT angiography, or ultrasonography[38,138,165] (Figs. 81-10 to 81-12). Each imaging technique has advantages and disadvantages (Table 81-10).

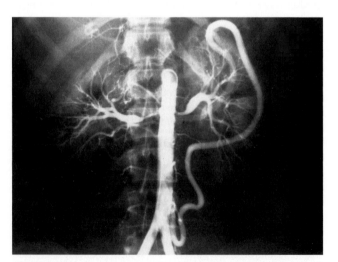

Figure 81-12 Angiogram showing bilateral renal artery stenosis. A large left colic branch of the inferior mesenteric artery provides collateral circulation to the gut. *(From Hellmann DB, Flynn JA: Clinical presentation and natural history of Takayasu's arteritis and other inflammatory anrteritides. In Perler BA, Becker GJ [eds]: Vascular Intervention: A Clinical Aprroach. New York, Thieme Medical and Scientific Publisher, 1998, pp 249-256.)*

Table 81-10 Comparison of Imaging Techniques in Takayasu's Arteritis

Technique	Advantages	Disadvantages
Conventional angiography	"Gold standard" image quality Allows CAP measurement Allows angioplasty at same time	Invasive Radiation exposure Does not visualize vessel wall thickness
Magnetic resonance angiography	Excellent image quality Noninvasive No ionizing radiation exposure Visualizes vascular wall thickness	Image quality not "gold standard" Cannot use in patients with pacemaker CAP measurement not possible
Ultrasonography	Noninvasive No ionizing radiation exposure Can visualize vessel wall edema	Image quality not "gold standard" Image quality affected by obesity Operator dependent CAP measurement not possible
Computed tomography angiography	Excellent image quality	Ionizing radiation exposure CAP measurement not possible Intravenous contrast agent required
Positron emission tomography	Can measure intensity of vascular inflammation	Ionizing radiation exposure Vascular anatomy not well seen CAP measurement not possible Intravenous contrast agent required

CAP, central arterial blood pressure.

Table 81-11 Frequency of Blood Vessel Involvement in Takayasu's Arteritis

Blood Vessel	% Abnormal
Aorta	65
Aortic arch or root	35
Abdominal aorta	47
Thoracic aorta	17
Subclavian artery	93
Common carotid artery	58
Renal artery	38
Vertebral artery	35
Celiac axes	18
Common iliac artery	17
Pulmonary artery	5

Data based on a study of 60 North America patients reported by Kerr GS, et al: Takayasu arteritis. Ann Intern Med 120:919, 1994. From Hellmann DB: Takayasu arteritis. In Imboden JB, Hellmann DB, Stone JH (eds): Current Rheumatology Diagnosis and Treatment. New York, Lange Medical Books/McGraw-Hill, 2004, p 245.

The earliest detectable abnormality in TA is thickening of the vessel wall from inflammation. MRI, ultrasonography, and, to a lesser degree, CT can detect this early vessel wall thickening.[36] Conventional angiography is invasive and provides the least sensitive method for visualizing wall thickness; however, conventional angiography is the "gold standard" for precisely delineating the stenoses, occlusions, and aneurysms that characterize the latter stages of TA.[36] Also, only conventional angiography allows the direct measurement of central arterial blood pressure, which may be otherwise unobtainable in patients with stenotic lesions affecting all four extremities. PET scanning is showing promise in TA as in GCA in detecting the extent and intensity of vascular inflammation,[36,166] but the value of PET scanning is not firmly established. Although MRA does not provide the same level of detail as conventional angiography, it comes close. Because MRA is not invasive and does not involve ionizing radiation, it has become the preferred imaging method for following patients with TA.

The most common sites of lesions in TA are the aorta (65%) and the left subclavian arteries (93%)[138] (Table 81-11). The left subclavian artery is affected slightly more frequently than the right. Carotid, renal, and vertebral arteries are also commonly affected.[138] Lesions may be stenotic (93%), occluded (57%), dilated (16%), or aneurysmal (7%).[139] Stenotic lesions are about four times more common

than aneurysmal lesions.[138] Stenotic segments often extend a few centimeters and may be followed by areas of dilation (see Fig. 81-10). The majority of patients (53%) have vascular lesions above and below the diaphragm.[139] However, the frequency distribution of aortic lesions varies considerably from country to country.[138]

DIAGNOSIS AND DIAGNOSTIC TESTS

As previously noted, the ACR has established classification criteria for the diagnosis of TA (see Table 81-8). In clinical practice, the diagnosis of TA is almost always secured by an imaging procedure (see Table 81-10) that demonstrates the characteristic abnormalities of the aorta and its major branches (Fig. 81-13). Rarely, the diagnosis is first suggested when a pathologist finds granulomatous inflammation in a section of aorta or other larger artery that was removed or biopsied during a vascular surgery procedure. Unfortunately,

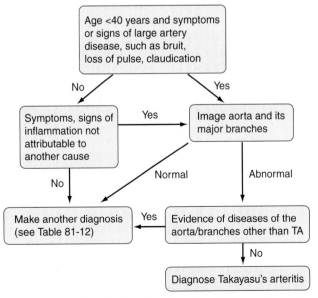

Figure 81-13 Algorithm for the diagnosis of Takayasu's arteritis. TA, Takayasu's arteritis.

Table 81-12 Differential Diagnosis of Takayasu's Arteritis: Other Diseases that Can Affect the Aorta

Disease Type	Specific Entities
Rheumatic	Giant cell arteritis, Cogan's syndrome, relapsing polychrondritis, ankylosing spondylitis, rheumatoid arthritis, systemic lupus erythematosus, Buerger's disease, Behçet's disease
Infectious	Syphilis, tuberculosis
Other	Atherosclerosis, ergotism, radiation-induced damage, retroperitoneal fibrosis, inflammatory bowel disease, sarcoidosis, neurofibromatosis, congenital coarctation, Marfan's syndrome, Ehlers-Danlos syndrome

From Hellmann DB: Takayasu arteritis. In Imboden JB, Hellmann DB, Stone JH (eds): Current Rheumatology Diagnosis and Treatment. New York, Lange Medical Books/McGraw-Hill, 2004, p 243.

Table 81-13 Comparison of Giant Cell Arteritis and Takayasu's Arteritis

Feature	Giant Cell	Takayasu's
Female-male ratio	2:1	8:1
Age range (yr)	≥50	<40
Average age of onset (yr)	72	25
Visual loss	10%-30%	Rare
Involvement of aorta or its major branches	25%	100%
Pathology	Granulomatous arteritis	Granulomatous arteritis
Pulmonary artery involvement	No	Possible
Renal hypertension	Rare	Common
Claudication	Uncommon	Common
Ethnic groups with highest incidence	Scandinavians	Asians
Corticosteroid responsive	Yes	Yes
Bruits present	Minority	Majority
Surgical intervention needed	Rarely	Commonly

the diagnosis of TA is often delayed; the delay averaged 44 months in one large series.[139] The most frequent impediment to a speedy diagnosis is a physician's failure to consider TA in the differential diagnosis. Although the rarity of TA helps explain its omission from diagnostic consideration, another reason is that some patients have striking features of inflammation that camouflage or overshadow the somewhat more familiar vascular abnormalities. Indeed, a few patients with TA present chiefly with FUO. Most of these patients have other, albeit subtle, manifestations of TA such as bruits, diminished pulses, unequal arm blood pressures, or aortic regurgitation. In other patients with more striking vascular abnormalities, the physician may be lured into focusing on familiar and dramatic abnormalities such as anemia or thrombocytopenia. Thus, instead of ordering an imaging test that would explain the patient's unequal and low blood pressure in her left arm, the physician mistakenly diverts the patient to a hematologist, gastroenterologist, or oncologist for additional blood tests and procedures that further delay the diagnosis.

Many of these delays can be prevented by remembering that TA should be included in the differential diagnosis of any person younger than 40 years who presents with FUO, aortic regurgitation, hypertension, or absent pulse. Delays in diagnosis can also be reduced by carefully searching for unequal or absent upper extremity pulses and by listening for bruits not only over the carotid arteries but also above and below the clavicle (for subclavian artery bruits) and over the abdomen and flanks (for renal and other mesenteric artery bruits). Recognizing that anemia and thrombocytosis can be manifestations of active inflammatory disorders, such as vasculitis, can also help speed the diagnosis of TA.

Once an imaging test demonstrates disease of the aorta or its major branches, the differential diagnosis narrows to a set of disorders that are usually easily differentiated (Table 81-12). Most rheumatic diseases that can affect the aorta are distinguished by their associated features. For example, Cogan's syndrome typically produces ocular inflammation (especially keratitis) and vestibuloauditory dysfunction. The one rheumatic disease that can, on rare occasions, be difficult to distinguish from TA is GCA (Table 81-13). Usually, the patient's age and the distribution of lesions allow their rapid differentiation, but distinguishing TA beginning after age 40 from GCA affecting chiefly the major branches of

the aorta can be difficult or even impossible. The similarity of treatment (see later) diminishes the practical importance of solving this diagnostic dilemma.

Infections of the aorta are rare in most countries. Tertiary syphilis can be excluded by a negative fluorescent treponemal antibody test (the rapid plasma reagin test is falsely negative in about one quarter of patients with late syphilis). Other diseases of the aorta (see Table 81-13) are readily separated from TA by the history and physical examination.

TREATMENT

Medical Therapy

Corticosteroids are the cornerstone of treatment of active TA.[138,139,148,167] Prednisone, at a dose of 0.5 to 1 mg/kg per day, is indicated for the treatment of active disease. Criteria for active disease include new onset or worsening of two or more of the following: (1) fever or other systemic features (in the absence of other cause), (2) elevated ESR, (3) symptoms or signs of vascular ischemia or inflammation (e.g., claudication, absent pulse, carotidynia), and (4) typical angiographic lesions.[138] Although about 85% of TA patients present with active disease, about 15% do not.[141] The initial dose of prednisone is continued for 4 to 12 weeks before commencing a gradual taper, as is done when treating GCA (see earlier). Although nearly two thirds of patients achieve remission, more than half later relapse. Relapses are especially common as the prednisone dose falls below 20 mg per day.

Relapses can be treated by increasing the prednisone dose or adding an immunosuppressive agent. No agent used for TA has been evaluated in a double-blind, placebo-controlled trial. However, open trials have suggested that weekly oral methotrexate (started at 0.3 mg/kg per week, with the initial dose not to exceed 15 mg/wk) is a moderately effective corticosteroid-sparing drug.[168] Methotrexate can be gradually increased to 25 mg/wk. The emphasis is on lowering the corticosteroid dose, because methotrexate seldom allows the elimination of prednisone completely; most patients continue to require at least 5 to 10 mg/day of prednisone.

Small studies and series suggest that other corticosteroid-sparing drugs include azathioprine (2 mg/kg per day), mycophenolate mofetil (2000 mg/day), and cyclophosphamide (2 mg/kg per day).[138,148,169,170] The toxicity of cyclophosphamide in young women is so high that it is rarely used in TA.[138,148]

The experience using TNF inhibitors for TA has been encouraging but limited.[170] In one series, anti-TNF therapy achieved improvement in 14 of 15 patients who had failed other therapies; 10 of 15 patients were able to discontinue corticosteroids.[170]

To prevent osteoporosis, patients on chronic corticosteroids should take calcium, vitamin D, and a bisphosphonate and perform weight-bearing exercises. Modifiable risk factors for atherosclerosis—especially hypertension, smoking, inactivity, diabetes, and hyperlipidemia—should be treated maximally.

Surgical Therapy

TA is the form of vasculitis most frequently requiring revascularization procedures.[138,148,171-173] Unfortunately, medical therapy rarely reduces or reverses stenotic lesions. Treating stenotic or aneurysmal lesions may require bypass surgery (especially of stenotic cervicobrachial arteries, coronary arteries, or renal arteries), aortic valve replacement (for aortic regurgitation), or percutaneous transluminal angioplasty (especially for stenotic renal arteries causing hypertension).

A review of the experience with vascular interventions in TA allows several general recommendations.[148] First, the mere presence of stenosis does not necessitate intervention. The gut, for example, has such rich collaterals that even critical stenoses of the celiac, superior, or inferior mesenteric arteries usually produce no symptoms and require no surgical intervention. Moreover, many patients with arm claudication will develop collateral circulation and improve substantially over time with medical therapy alone. For upper extremity vascular insufficiency, patiently waiting for a response to medical therapy usually pays higher dividends than undertaking rapid surgical intervention. Second, whenever possible, surgical intervention should be deferred until TA is in remission; procedures done during active disease often produce disappointing results. Third, bypass surgery yields better results than angioplasty. With bypass graft procedures, autologous vessels give better results than synthetic grafts (restenosis rates of 9% versus 36%)[148] Patients who undergo aortic surgery are liable to develop anastomotic aneurysms; such aneurysms developed in nearly 14% of patients followed for 20 years.[148,171] Although angioplasty gives good short-term results, long-term results are often disappointing except for very short stenotic segments. The experience with conventional stents has been mostly disappointing.[148]

OUTCOME AND PROGNOSIS

Twenty percent of TA patient have a self-limited disease. The rest have a relapsing-remitting or progressive course requiring chronic corticosteroid therapy. Nearly two thirds of patients experience new angiographic lesions.[148] In one study from the National Institutes of Health, 74% of patients experienced some form of morbidity, and 47% were permanently disabled.[138] No parameters at disease onset have been shown to predict mortality.[148] The survival is 92.9% at 5 years, 87.2% at 10 years,[141] and 73.5% at 20 years.[148,171] Congestive heart failure and renal failure are the most common causes of death.[171] Pregnancy appears to be relatively well tolerated in the presence of good medical care and in the absence of abdominal aortic involvement.[138,174,175]

Future Directions

Two of the most pressing issues in TA are how to measure active disease and how to safely minimize the use and toxicity of corticosteroids. Serologic tests such as the ESR are helpful but lack sensitivity and specificity; active disease as reflected in inflammatory pathology has been found in patients with normal ESRs.[148] Efforts are under way to determine whether imaging techniques can help assess disease activity. Unfortunately, although "edema-weighted" MRI and MRA appear to have high specificity, the positive predictive value for active disease is poor.[36,176] Studies are under way to assess the ability of PET scanning, serum proteomic markers, and serum levels of inflammatory cytokines to detect active disease. The success of using biologic agents to treat RA and the good preliminary experience using infliximab for TA offer hope that new therapies will be more effective and less toxic than corticosteroids.

REFERENCES

1. Hunder GG, Bloch DA, Michel BA, et al: The American College of Rheumatology 1990 criteria for the classification of giant cell arteritis. Arthritis Rheum 33:1122, 1990.
2. Chuang T-Y, Hunder GG, Ilstrup DM, Kurland LT: Polymyalgia rheumatica: A 10-year epidemiologic and clinical study. Ann Intern Med 97:672, 1982.
3. **Healey LA: Long-term follow-up of polymyalgia rheumatica: Evidence for synovitis. Semin Arthritis Rheum 13:322, 1984.**
4. **Hunder GG, Allen GL: Giant cell arteritis: A review. Bull Rheum 29:980, 1978-1979.**
5. Barber HS: Myalgic syndrome with constitutional effects: Polymyalgia rheumatica. Ann Rheum Dis 16:230, 1957.
6. Hunder GG: The early history of giant cell arteritis and polymalgia rheumatica. Mayo Clin Proc 81:1071, 2006.
7. Healey LA, Wilske KR: The Systemic Manifestations of Temporal Arteritis. New York, Grune & Stratton, 1978.
8. Salvarani C, Gabriel SE, O'Fallon WM, Hunder GG: The incidence of giant cell arteritis in Olmsted County, Minnesota: Apparent fluctuations in cyclic pattern. Ann Intern Med 123:192, 1995.
9. Baldursson O, Steinsson K, Bjornsson J, Lie JT: Giant cell arteritis in Iceland: An epidemiologic and histologic analysis. Arthritis Rheum 37:1007, 1994.
10. Nordborg E, Bengtsson B-A: Epidemiology of biopsy-proven giant cell arteritis (GCA). J Intern Med 227:233, 1990.
11. Jonasson F, Cullen JF, Elton RA: Temporal arteritis: A 14-year epidemiologic, clinical and prognostic study. Scot Med J 24:111, 1979.
12. Boesen P, Sorensen SF: Giant cell arteritis, temporal arteritis and polymyalgia rheumatica in a Danish county: A prospective investigation, 1982-1985. Arthritis Rheum 30:294, 1987.
13. Barrier J, Pion P, Massari R, et al: Epidemiologic approach to Horton's disease in Department of Loire-Atlantique: 110 cases in 10 years (1970-1979). Rev Med Interne 3:13, 1983.
14. Smith CA, Fidler WJ, Pinals RS: The epidemiology of giant cell arteritis: Report of a ten-year study in Shelby County, Tennessee. Arthritis Rheum 26:1214, 1983.
15. Friedman G, Friedman B, Benbassat J: Epidemiology of temporal arteritis in Israel. Isr J Med Sci 18:241, 1986.

16. Machado EBV, Michet CJ, Ballard DJ, et al: Trends in incidence and clinical presentation of temporal arteritis in Olmsted County, Minnesota, 1950-1985. Arthritis Rheum 31:745, 1988.
17. **Salvarani C, Cantini F, Boiardi L, Hunder GG: Polymyalgia rheumatica and giant cell arteritis. N Engl J Med 347:261, 2002.**
18. Levine SM, Hellmann DB: Giant cell arteritis. Curr Opin Rheumatol 14:3, 2002.
19. Smeeth L, Cook C, Hall AJ: Incidence of diagnosed polymyalgia rheumatica and temporal arteritis in the United Kingdom, 1990-2001. Ann Rheum Dis 65:1093, 2006.
20. Östberg G: On arteritis with special reference to polymyalgia arteritica. Acta Pathol Microbiol Scand (A) Suppl 237:1, 1973.
21. Hunder GG, Lie JT, Goronzy JJ, Weyand CM: Pathogenesis of giant cell arteritis. Arthritis Rheum 36:757, 1993.
22. Liang GC, Simkin PA, Hunder GG, et al: Familial aggregation of polymyalgia rheumatica and giant cell arteritis. Arthritis Rheum 17:19, 1974.
23. Mathewson JA, Hunder GG: Giant cell arteritis in two brothers. J Rheumatol 13:190, 1986.
24. Weyand CM, Hunder NN, Hicok KC, et al: The HLA-DRB1 locus as a genetic component in giant cell arteritis: Mapping of a disease-linked sequence motif to the antigen binding site of the HLA-DR molecule. J Clin Invest 90:2355, 1992.
25. Weyand CM, Hunder NN, Hicok KC, et al: HLA-DRB1 alleles in polymyalgia rheumatica, giant cell arteritis, and rheumatoid arthritis. Arthritis Rheum 37:514, 1994.
26. Duhaut P, Pinede L, Demolombe-Rague S, et al: Giant cell arteritis and cardiovascular risk factors. Arthritis Rheum 41:1960, 1998.
27. Rodriguez-Pla A, Bosch-Gil JA, Echevarria-Mayo JE, et al: No detection of parvovirus B19 or herpesvirus DNA in giant cell arteritis. J Clin Virol 31:11, 2004.
28. Álvarez-Lafuente R, Fernández-Gutiérrez B, Jover JA, et al: Human parvovirus B19, varicella zoster virus, and human herpes virus 6 in temporal artery biopsy specimens of patients with giant cell arteritis: Analysis with quantitative real time polymerase chain reaction. Ann Rheum Dis 64:780, 2005.
29. Regan MJ, Wood BJ, Hsieh YH, et al: *Chlamydia pneumoniae* and temporal arteritis: Failure to detect the organism by PCR in 180 cases and controls. Arthritis Rheum 46:1056, 2002.
30. Calamia KT, Hunder GG: Clinical manifestations of giant cell arteritis. Clin Rheum Dis 6:389, 1980.
31. Salvarani C, Gabriel SE, O'Fallon WM, Hunder GG: Epidemiology of polymyalgia rheumatica in Olmsted County, Minnesota, 1970-1991. Arthritis Rheum 38:369, 1995.
32. Sakkas LI, Loqueman N, Panayi GS, et al: Immunogenetics of polymyalgia rheumatica. Br J Rheumatol 29:331, 1990.
33. Klein RG, Hunder GG, Stanson AW, Sheps SG: Large artery involvement in giant cell (temporal) arteritis. Ann Intern Med 83:806, 1975.
34. Bongartz T, Matteson EL: Large-vessel involvement in giant cell arteritis. Curr Opin Rheumatol 18:10, 2006.
35. Weyand CM, Goronzy JJ: Medium- and large-vessel vasculitis. N Engl J Med 349:160, 2003.
36. Seo P, Stone JH: Large-vessel vasculitis. Arthritis Rheum (Arthritis Care Res) 51:128, 2004.
37. Klein RG, Campbell RJ, Hunder GG, Carney JA: Skip lesions in temporal arteritis. Mayo Clin Proc 51:504, 1976.
38. Wilkinson IMS, Russell RWR: Arteries of the head and neck in giant cell arteritis: A pathological study to show the pattern of arterial involvement. Arch Neurol 27:378, 1972.
39. Casselli RJ, Hunder GG, Whisnant JP: Neurologic disease in biopsy-proven giant cell (temporal) arteritis. Neurology 38:352, 1988.
40. Caselli RJ, Hunder GG: Neurologic aspects of giant cell (temporal) arteritis. Rheum Dis Clin North Am 19:941, 1993.
41. Reich KA, Giansiracusa DF, Strongwater SL: Neurologic manifestations of giant cell arteritis. Am J Med 89:67, 1990.
42. Evans JM, Batts KP, Hunder GG: Persistent giant cell arteritis despite corticosteroid treatment. Mayo Clin Proc 69:1060, 1994.
43. Esteban M-J, Front C, Hernández-Rodríguez J, et al: Small-vessel vasculitis surrounding a spared temporal artery. Arthritis Rheum 44:1387, 2001.
44. Cid MC, Campo E, Ercilla G, et al: Immunohistochemical analysis of lymphoid and macrophage cell subsets and the immunological activation markers in temporal arteritis. Arthritis Rheum 32:884, 1989.
45. Weyand CM, Goronzy JJ: Arterial wall injury in giant cell arteritis. Arthritis Rheum 42:844, 1999.
46. Brach A, Gusler A, Martinez-Taboada, et al: Giant cell vasculitis is a T cell-dependent disease. Mol Med 3:530, 1997.
47. Weyand CM, Wagner, AD, Bjornsson J, et al: Correlation of the topographical arrangement and the functional pattern of tissue-infiltrating macrophages in giant cell arteritis. J Clin Invest 98:1642, 1996.
48. Wagner AD, Garonzy JJ, Weyand CM: Functional profile of tissue-infiltrating and circulating CD68+ cells in giant cell arteritis: Evidence for two components of the disease. J Clin Invest 4:1134, 1994.
49. Weyand CM, Hicok KC, Hunder GG, et al: Tissue cytokine patterns in patients with polymyalgia rheumatica and giant cell arteritis. Ann Intern Med 121:484, 1994.
50. Weyand CM, Tetzlaff N, Bjornsson J, et al: Disease patterns and tissue cytokine profiles in giant cell arteritis. Arthritis Rheum 40:19, 1997.
51. Grunewald J, Andersson R, Rydberg L, et al: CD4+ and CD8+ T cell expansions using selected TCR V and J gene segments at the onset of giant cell arteritis. Arthritis Rheum 37:1221, 1994.
52. Shiiki H, Shimokama T, Watanabe T: Temporal arteritis: Cell composition and the possible pathogenetic role of cell-mediated immunity. Hum Pathol 20:1057, 1989.
53. Weyand CM, Ma-Krupa W, Pryshchep O, et al: Vascular dendritic cells in giant cell arteritis. Ann N Y Acad Sci 1062:195, 2005.
54. Ma-Krupa W, Jeon MS, Spoerl S, et al: Activation of arterial wall dendritic cells and breakdown of self-tolerance in giant cell arteritis. J Exp Med 199:173, 2004.
55. Shmerling RH: An 81-year-old woman with temporal arteritis. JAMA 295:2525, 2006.
56. Kaiser M, Weyand CM, Bjornsson J, et al: Platelet-derived growth factor, intimal hyperplasia, and ischemic complications in giant cell arteritis. Arthritis Rheum 41:623, 1998.
57. **Calamia KT, Hunder GG: Giant cell arteritis (temporal arteritis) presenting as fever of undetermined origin. Arthritis Rheum 24:1414, 1981.**
58. Brooke MH, Kaplan H: Muscle pathology in rheumatoid arthritis, polymyalgia rheumatica, and polymyositis: A histochemical study: Arch Pathol 94:101, 1972.
59. Salvarani C, Canlini F, Oliveri I, et al: Proximal bursitis in active polymyalgia rheumatica. Ann Intern Med 127:27, 1997.
60. O'Duffy JD, Hunder GG, Wahner HW: A follow-up study of polymyalgia rheumatica: Evidence of chronic axial synovitis. J Rheumatol 7:685, 1980.
61. Healey LA: Long-term follow-up of polymyalgia rheumatica: Evidence for synovitis. Semin Arthritis Rheum 13:322, 1984.
62. Douglas WA, Martin BA, Morris JH: Polymyalgia rheumatica: An arthroscopic study of the shoulder joint. Ann Rheum Dis 42:311, 1983.
63. Chow CT, Schumacher HR Jr: Clinical and pathologic studies of synovitis in polymyalgia rheumatica. Arthritis Rheum 27:1107, 1984.
64. Cantini F, Salvarani C, Olivieri I, et al: Inflamed shoulder structures in polymyalgia rheumatica with normal erythrocyte sedimentation rate. Arthritis Rheum 44:1155, 2001.
65. Papaioannou CC, Gupta RC, Hunder GG, McDuffie FC: Circulating immune complexes in giant cell arteritis polymyalgia rheumatica. Arthritis Rheum 23:1021, 1980.
66. Smith AJ, Kyle V, Cawston TE, Hazleman BL: Isolation and analysis of immune complexes from sera of patients with polymalgia rheumatica and giant cell arteritis. Ann Rheum Dis 46:468, 1987.
67. Ma-Krupa W, Kwan M, Goronzy JJ, Weyand CM: Toll-like receptors in giant cell arteritis. Clin Immunol 115:38, 2005.
68. Smetana GW, Shmerling RH: Does this patient have temporal arteritis? JAMA 287:92, 2002.
69. Miller NR: Visual manifestations of temporal arteritis. In Stone JH, Hellmann DB (eds): Rheumatic Disease Clinics of North America. Philadelphia, WB Saunders, 2001, p 781.
70. Mehler MF, Rabinowich L: The clinical neuro-ophthalmologic spectrum of temporal arteritis. Am J Med 85:839, 1988.
71. Nesher G, Berkun Y, Mates M, et al: Risk factors for cranial ischemic complications in giant cell arteritis. Medicine 83:114, 2004.
72. Gonzalez-Gay MA, Piñeiro A, Gomez-Gigirey A, et al: Influence of traditional risk factors of atherosclerosis in the development of severe ischemic complications in giant cell arteritis. Medicine 83:342, 2004.
73. Salvarani C, Cimino L, Macchioni P, et al: Risk factors for visual loss in an Italian population-based cohort of patients with giant cell arteritis. Arthritis Rheum 53:293, 2005.

74. Cid MC, Hernandez-Rodriguez J, Esteban MJ, et al: Tissue and serum angiogenic activity is associated with low prevalence of ischemic complications in patients with giant-cell arteritis. Circulation 106:1664, 2002.

75. Aiello PD, Trautmann JC, McPhee TJ, et al: Visual prognosis in giant cell arteritis. Ophthalmology 100:550, 1993.

76. Healy LA, Wilske KR: Presentation of occult giant cell arteritis. Arthritis Rheum 23:641, 1980.

77. Hellmann DB: Occult manifestations of giant cell arteritis. Med Rounds 2:296, 1989.

78. Sonnenblick M, Nesher G, Rosin A: Nonclassical organ involvement in temporal arteritis. Semin Arthritis Rheum 19:183, 1989.

79. Hollenhorst RW, Brown JR, Wagener HP, Shick RM: Neurologic aspects of temporal arteritis. Neurology 10:490, 1960.

80. Larson TS, Hall S, Hepper NGG, Hunder GG: Respiratory tract symptoms as a clue to giant cell arteritis. Ann Intern Med 101:594, 1984.

81. **Hamilton CR, Shelley WM, Tumulty PA: Giant cell arteritis: Including temporal arteritis and polymyalgia rheumatica. Medicine 50:1, 1971.**

82. Evans JM, Bowles CA, Bjornsson J, et al: Thoracic aortic aneurysm and rupture in giant cell arteritis. Arthritis Rheum 37:1539, 1994.

83. Evans JM, O'Fallon WM, Hunder GG: Increased incidence of aortic aneurysm and dissection in giant cell (temporal) arteritis: A population based study. Ann Intern Med 122:502, 1995.

84. Gonzalez-Gay MA, Garcia-Porrua C, Piñeiro A, et al: Aortic aneurysm and dissection in patients with biopsy-proven giant cell arteritis from northwestern Spain: A population-based study. Medicine 83:335, 2004.

85. Nuenninghoff DM, Hunder GG, Christianson TJ, et al: Incidence and predictors of large-vessel complication (aortic aneurysm, aortic dissection, and/or large-artery stenosis) in patients with giant cell arteritis: A population-based study over 50 years. Arthritis Rheum 48:3522, 2003.

86. Blockmans D, de Ceuninck L, Vanderschueren S, et al: Repetitive 18F-fluorodeoxyglucose positron emission tomography in giant cell arteritis: A prospective study of 35 patients. Arthritis Rheum 55:131, 2006.

87. Kariv R, Sidi Y, Gur H: Systemic vasculitis presenting as a tumorlike lesion: Four case reports and an analysis of 79 reported cases. Medicine 79:349, 2000.

88. Brack A, Martinez-Taboada V, Stanson A, et al: Disease pattern in cranial and large-vessel giant cell arteritis. Arthritis Rheum 42:311, 1999.

89. Liozon E, Herrmann F, Ly K, et al: Risk factors for visual loss in giant cell (temporal) arteritis: A prospective study of 174 patients. Am J Med 111:211, 2001.

90. González-Gay MA, Blanco R, Rodríguez-Valverde V, et al: Permanent visual loss and cerebrovascular accidents in giant cell arteritis: Predictors and response to treatment. Arthritis Rheum 41:1497, 1998.

91. Cid MC, Font C, Oristrell J, et al: Association between strong inflammatory response and low risk of developing visual loss and other cranial ischemic complications in giant cell (temporal) arteritis. Arthritis Rheum 41:26, 1998.

92. Salvarani C, Gabriel S, Hunder GG: Distal extremity swelling with pitting edema in polymyalgia rheumatica: Report of nineteen cases. Arthritis Rheum 39:73, 1996.

93. Chou C-T, Schumacher HR Jr: Clinical and pathologic studies of synovitis in polymyalgia rheumatica. Arthritis Rheum 27:1107, 1984.

94. Salvarani C, Hunder GG: Giant cell arteritis with low erythrocyte sedimentation rate: Frequency of occurrence in a population-based study. Arthritis Care Res 45:140, 2001.

95. Wise CM, Agudelo CA, Chmelewski WL, et al: Temporal arteritis with low erythrocyte sedimentation rate: A review of five cases. Arthritis Rheum 34:1571, 1991.

96. Dickson ER, Maldonado JE, Sheps SG, Cain JA Jr: Systemic giant-cell arteritis with polymyalgia rheumatica: Reversible abnormalities of liver function. JAMA 224:1496, 1973.

97. Bunch TW, Hunder GG, McDuffie FC, et al: Synovial fluid complement determination as a diagnostic aid in inflammatory joint disease. Mayo Clin Proc 49:715, 1974.

98. Roche NE, Fulbright JW, Wagner AD, et al: Correlation of interleukin-6 production and disease activity in polymyalgia rheumatica and giant cell arteritis. Arthritis Rheum 36:1286, 1993.

99. Persellin ST, Daniels TM, Rings LJ, et al: Factor VIII-von Willebrand factor in giant cell arteritis and polymyalgia rheumatica. Mayo Clin Proc 60:457, 1985.

100. Olsson A, Elling P, Elling H: Serologic and immunohistochemical determination of von Willebrand factor antigen in serum and biopsy specimens from patients with arteritis temporalis and polymyalgia rheumatica. Clin Exp Rheumatol 8:55, 1990.

101. Younge BR, Cook BE Jr, Bartley GB, et al: Initiation of glucocorticoid therapy: Before or after temporal artery biopsy? Mayo Clin Proc 79:483, 2004.

102. Gertz MA, Kyle RA, Griffing WL, Hunder GG: Jaw claudication in primary systemic amyloidosis. Medicine (Baltimore) 65:173, 1986.

103. Ginsburg WW, Cohen MD, Hall SB, et al: Seronegative polyarthritis in giant cell arteritis. Arthritis Rheum 28:1362, 1985.

104. Gonzalez-Gay MA, Garcia-Porrua C, Salvarani C, et al: The spectrum of conditions mimicking polymyalgia rheumatica in northwestern Spain. J Rheumatol 27:2179, 2000.

105. McCarty DJ, O'Duffy D, Pearson L, Hunter JB: Remitting seronegative symmetrical synovitis with pitting edema: RS3PE syndrome. JAMA 254:2763, 1985.

106. Hall S, Hunder GG: Is temporal artery biopsy prudent? Mayo Clin Proc 59:793, 1984.

107. Gonzalez-Gay MA: The diagnosis and management of patients with giant cell arteritis. J Rheumatol 32:1186, 2005.

108. Hall S, Lie JT, Kurland LT, et al: The therapeutic impact of temporal artery biopsy. Lancet 2:1217, 1983.

109. Boyev LR, Miller NR, Green WR: Efficacy of unilateral versus bilateral temporal artery biopsies for the diagnosis of giant cell arteritis. Am J Ophthalmol 128:211, 1999.

110. Pless M, Rizzo JF III, Lamkin JC, Lessell S: Concordance of bilateral temporal artery biopsy in giant cell arteritis. J Neuroophthalmol 20:216, 2000.

111. Jundt JW, Mock D: Temporal arteritis with normal erythrocyte sedimentation rates presenting as occipital neuralgia. Arthritis Rheum 34:217, 1991.

112. Schmidt WA, Kraft HE, Vorpahl L, et al: Color duplex ultrasonography in the diagnosis of temporal arteritis. N Engl J Med 337:1336, 1997.

113. Hunder GG, Weyand CM: Sonography in giant cell arteritis. N Engl J Med 337:1385, 1997.

114. Salvarani C, Silingardi M, Ghirarduzzi A, et al: Is duplex ultrasonography useful for the diagnosis of giant-cell arteritis? Ann Intern Med 137:232, 2002.

115. Bley T, Wieben O, Uhl M, et al: High-resolution MRI in giant cell arteritis: Imaging of the wall of the superficial temporal artery. AJR Am J Roentgenol 184:283, 2005.

116. Blockmans D, Stroobants S, Maes A, Mortelmans L: Positron emission tomography in giant cell arteritis and polymyalgia rheumatica: Evidence for inflammation of the aortic arch. Am J Med 108:246, 2000.

117. Turlakow A, Yeung HWD, Pui J, et al: Fludeoxyglucose positron emission tomography in the diagnosis of giant cell arteritis. Arch Intern Med 161:1003, 2001.

118. Ray-Chaudhuri N, Kiné DA, Tijani SO, et al: Effect of prior steroid treatment on temporal artery biopsy findings in giant cell arteritis. Br J Ophthalmol 86:530, 2002.

119. Achkar AA, Lie JT, Hunder GG, et al: How does previous corticosteroid treatment affect the biopsy findings in giant cell (temporal) arteritis? Ann Intern Med 120:987, 1994.

120. **Mazlumzadeh M, Hunder GG, Easley KA, et al: Treatment of giant cell arteritis using induction therapy with high-dose glucocorticoids: A double-blind, placebo-controlled, randomized prospective clinical trial. Arthritis Rheum 54:3310-3318, 2006.**

121. Hayreh SS: Steroid therapy for visual loss in patients with giant-cell arteritis: Lancet 355:1572, 2000.

122. Weyand CM, Fulbright JW, Hunder GG, et al: Treatment of giant cell arteritis: Interleukin-6 as a biologic marker of disease activity. Arthritis Rheum 43:1041, 2000.

123. **Hoffman GS, Cid MC, Hellmann DB, et al: A multicenter, randomized, double-blind, placebo-controlled trial of adjuvant methotrexate treatment for giant cell arteritis. Arthritis Rheum 46:1309, 2002.**

124. Jover JA, Hernández-Garcia C, Morado IC, et al: Combined treatment of giant-cell arteritis with methotrexate and prednisone: A randomized, double-blind, placebo-controlled trial. Ann Intern Med 134:106, 2001.

125. Hunder GG, Sheps SG, Allen GL, Joyce JW: Daily and alternate-day corticosteroid regimens in treatment of giant cell arteritis: Comparison in a prospective study. Ann Intern Med 82:613, 1975.

126. Hoffman GS, Cid MC, Rendt-Zagar KE, et al: Infliximab for maintenance of glucocorticosteroid-induced remission of giant cell arteritis: A randomized trial. Ann Intern Med 146:621, 2007.

127. Weyand CM, Kaiser M, Yang H, et al: Therapeutic effects of acetylsalicylic acid in giant cell arteritis. Arthritis Rheum 46:457, 2002.

128. Nesher G: Low-dose aspirin and prevention of cranial ischemic complications in giant cell arteritis. Arthritis Rheum, 50:1332, 2004.

129. Lee MS, Smith SD, Galor A, Hoffman GS: Antiplatelet and anticoagulant therapy in patients with giant cell arteritis. Arthritis Rheum 54:3306, 2006.

130. Both M, Aries PM, Müller-Hülsbeck S, et al: Balloon angioplasty of arteries of the upper extremities in patients with extracranial giant-cell arteritis. Ann Rheum Dis 65:1124, 2006.

131. Weyand CM, Fulbright JW, Evans JM, et al: Corticosteroid requirements in polymyalgia rheumatica. Arch Intern Med 159:577, 1999.

132. Gabriel SE, Sunku J, Salvarani C, et al: Adverse outcomes of antiinflammatory therapy among patients with polymyalgia rheumatica. Arthritis Rheum 40:1873, 1997.

133. Schreiber S, Buyse M: The CRP initial response to treatment as prognostic factor in patients with polymyalgia rheumatica. Clin Rheumatol 14:315, 1995.

134. Weyand CM, Fulbright JW, Evans JM, et al: Corticosteroid requirements in polymyalgia rheumatica. Arch Intern Med 159:577, 1999.

135. Rynes RI, Mika P, Bartholomew LE: Development of giant cell (temporal) arteritis in a patient "adequately" treated for polymyalgia rheumatica. Ann Rheum Dis 36:88, 1977.

136. Narvaez J, Nolla-Sole JM, Clavaguera MT, et al: Longterm therapy in polymyalgia rheumatica: Effect of coexistent temporal arteritis. J Rheumatol 26:1945, 1999.

137. Caporali R, Cimmino MA, Ferraccioli G, et al: Prednisone plus methotrexate for polymyalgia rheumatica: A randomized, double-blind, placebo-controlled trial. Ann Intern Med 141:493, 2004.

138. Kerr GS, Hallahan CW, Giordano J, et al: Takyasu arteritis. Ann Intern Med 120:919, 1994.

139. Vanoli M, Daina E, Salvarani C, et al: Takayasu's arteritis: A study of 104 Italian patients. Arthritis Rheum 53:100, 2005.

140. Nakao K, Ikeda M, Kimata S-C, et al: Takayasu's arteritis: Clinical report of eighty-four cases and immunological studies of seven cases. Circulation 35:1141, 1967.

141. Park M-C, Lee S-W, Park Y-B, et al: Clinical characteristics and outcomes of Takayasu's arteritis: Analysis of 108 patients using standardized criteria for diagnosis activity assessment, and angiographic classification. Scand J Rheumatol 34:284, 2005.

142. Shelhamer JH, Volkman DJ, Parrillo JE, et al: Takayasu's arteritis and its therapy. Ann Intern Med 103:121, 1985.

143. Lupi-Herrera E, Sanchez-Torres G, Marcushamer J, et al: Takayasu's arteritis: Clinical study of 107 cases. Am Heart J 93:94, 1977.

144. Takayasu M: A case of a peculiar change in the central retinal vessels. Acta Soc Ophthalmol Jpn 12:554, 1908.

145. Arend WP, Michel BA, Bloch DA, et al: The American College of Rheumatology 1990 criteria for the classification of Takayasu arteritis. Arthritis Rheum 33:1129, 1990.

146. González-Gay MA: García-Porrúa: Epidemiology of the vasculitides. Rheum Dis Clin North Am 27:729, 2001.

147. Hellmann DB: Takayasu's arteritis. In Imboden J, Hellmann D, Stone J (eds): Current Rheumatology Diagnosis & Treatment, 1st ed. New York, Lange Medical Books/McGraw-Hill, 2004, pp 242-247.

148. Liang P, Hoffman GS: Advances in the medical and surgical treatment of Takayasu arteritis. Curr Opin Rheumatol 17:16, 2005.

149. Seko Y, Sato O, Takagi A, et al: Restricted usage of T-cell receptor Vα-Vβ genes in infiltrating cells in aortic tissue of patients with Takayasu's arteritis. Circulation 93:1788, 1996.

150. Seko Y, Minota S, Kawasaki A, et al: Perforin-secreting killer cell infiltration and expression of a 65-kD heat-shock protein in aortic tissue of patients with Takayasu's arteritis. J Clin Invest 93:750, 1994.

151. Seko Y, Sugishita K, Sata O, et al: Expression of costimulatory molecules (4-1BBL and Fas) and major histocompatibility class I chain-related A (MICA) in aortic tissue with Takayasu's arteritis. Vasc Res 41:84, 2004.

152. Tavora F, Burke A: Review of isolated ascending aortitis: Differential diagnosis, including syphilitic, Takayasu's and giant cell aortitis. Pathology 38:302, 2006.

153. Tavora F, Jeudy J, Gocke C, Burke A: Takayasu aortitis with acute dissection and hemopericardium. Cardiovasc Pathol 14:320, 2005.

154. Park MC, Park YB, Jung SY, et al: Anti-endothelial cell antibodies and antiphospholipid antibodies in Takayasu's arteritis: Correlations of their titers and isotype distributions with disease activity. Clin Exp Rheumatol 24:S10, 2006.

155. Chauhan SK, Tripathy NK, Nityanand S: Antigenic targets and pathogenicity of anti-aortic endothelial cell antibodies in Takayasu arteritis. Arthritis Rheum 54:2326, 2006.

156. Dal Canto AJ, Swanson PE, O'Guin AK, et al: IFN-gamma action in the media of the great elastic arteries, a novel immunoprivileged site. J Clin Invest 107:R15, 2001.

157. Ueda H, Morooka S, Oto I, et al: Clinical observation of 52 cases of aortitis syndrome. Jpn Heart J 10:277, 1969.

158. Ishikawa K: Natural history and classification of occlusive thromboaortopathy (Takayasu's disease). Circulation 57:27, 1978.

159. Talwar KK, Kuman K, Chopra P, et al: Cardiac involvement in nonspecific aortoarteritis (Takayasu's arteritis). Am Heart J 122:1666, 1991.

160. Matsubara O, Kuwata T, Nemoto T, et al: Coronary artery lesions in Takayasu arteritis: Pathological considerations. Heart Vessels Suppl 7:26, 1992.

161. Malik IS, Harare O, Al-Nahhas A, et al: Takayasu's arteritis: Management of left main stem stenosis. Heart 89:e9, 2003.

162. Byrne JA, Cotton JM, Thomas M: Bilateral ostial coronary artery stenoses: An important presentation of Takayasu's arteritis. Heart 85:555, 2001.

163. Amano J, Suzuki A: Coronary artery involvement in Takayasu's arteritis: Collective review and guideline for surgical treatment. J Thorac Cardiovasc Surg 102:554, 1991.

164. Endo M, Tomizawa Y, Nishida H, et al: Angiographic findings and surgical treatment of coronary artery involvement in Takayasu arteritis. J Thorac Cardiovasc Surg 125:570, 2003.

165. Andrews J, Al-Nahhas A, Pennell DJ, et al: Non-invasive imaging in the diagnosis and management of Takayasu's arteritis. Ann Rheum Dis 63:995, 2004.

166. Walter MA, Melzer RA, Schindler C, et al: The value of [¹⁸F]FDG-PET in the diagnosis of large-vessel vasculitis and the assessment of activity and extent of disease. Eur J Nucl Med Mol Imaging 32:674, 2005.

167. Ishikawa K: Effects of prednisone therapy on arterial angiopgrahic features in Takayasu's disease. Am J Cardiol 68:410, 1991.

168. Hoffman GS, Leavitt RY, Kerr GS, et al: Treatment of glucocorticoid-resistant or relapsing Takayasu arteritis with methotrexate. Arthritis Rheum 37:578, 1994.

169. Koening CL, Langford CA: Novel therapeutic strategies for large vessel vasculitis. Rheum Dis Clin North Am 32:173, 2006.

170. Hoffman GS, Merkel PA, Brasington RD, et al: Anti-tumor necrosis factor therapy in patients with difficult to treat Takayasu arteritis. Arthritis Rheum 50:2296, 2004.

171. Miyata T, Sato O, Koyama H, et al: Long-term survival after surgical treatment of patients with Takayasu's arteritis. Circulation 108:1474, 2003.

172. Bloss RS, Duncan JM, Cooley DA, et al: Takayasu's arteritis: Surgical consideration. Ann Thorac Surg 27:574, 1979.

173. Matsuura K, Ogino H, Kobayashi J, et al: Surgical treatment of aortic regurgitation due to Takayasu arteritis: Long-term morbidity and mortality. Circulation 112:3707, 2005.

174. Sharma BK, Jain S, Visishta K: Outcome of pregnancy in Takayasu arteritis. Int J Cardiol 75(Suppl):S159, 2000.

175. Ishikawa K, Matsuura S: Occlusive thromboaortopathy (Takayasu's disease) and pregnancy: Clinical course and management of 33 pregnancies and deliveries. Am J Cardiol 50:1293, 1982.

176. Tso E, Flamm SD, White RD, et al: Takayasu arteritis: Utility and limitations of magnetic resonance imaging in diagnosis and treatment. Arthritis Rheum 46:1634, 2002.

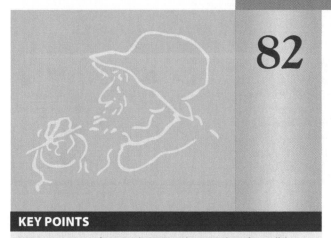

82

Antineutrophil Cytoplasmic Antibody–Associated Vasculitis

LEONARD H. CALABRESE •
EAMONN S. MOLLOY • GEORGE F. DUNA

KEY POINTS

Wegener's granulomatosis (WG), microscopic polyangiitis (MPA), and Churg-Strauss syndrome (CSS) are forms of vasculitis that affect small to medium vessels and share a number of clinical, pathologic, and laboratory features.

Antineutrophil cytoplasmic antibodies (ANCAs) may be involved in the pathogenesis of these vasculitides in at least some patients.

Testing for ANCAs is a useful tool in the diagnosis of small vessel vasculitis, but its role in disease monitoring is more controversial.

WG can affect any organ or tissue but has a predilection for the upper and lower respiratory tracts and the kidneys. WG is most commonly associated with ANCA positivity by immunofluorescence and positive testing for the proteinase 3 antigen.

MPA can be distinguished from other forms of small vessel vasculitis by the absence of granuloma formation, the relative lack of upper airway involvement, and the predominance of perinuclear ANCA staining by immunofluorescence and positive testing for the myeloperoxidase antigen.

CSS can be distinguished from other forms of small vessel vasculitis on the basis of a prior history of adult-onset asthma or allergic rhinitis and tissue eosinophilia with necrotizing vasculitis and extravascular granuloma formation.

Combination therapy with glucocorticoids and oral cyclophosphamide is required for the treatment of severe systemic small vessel vasculitis; methotrexate may be substituted for cyclophosphamide in non-organ- or non-life-threatening disease.

Upon induction of disease remission, cyclophosphamide should be switched to less toxic immunosuppressive agents for the maintenance of remission.

In recent years, considerable progress has been made in understanding the nature of and relationships among the major classes of primary vasculitic syndromes. The discovery of antineutrophil cytoplasmic antibody (ANCA), its development as a diagnostic tool, and the identification of its role in the nosology of the vasculitides are of major clinical and theoretical importance. Three diseases—Wegener's granulomatosis (WG), microscopic polyangiitis (MPA), and Churg-Strauss syndrome (CSS)—are now considered together owing to their shared pathologic, clinical, and laboratory features.[1] These diseases also share histologic features, preferentially involving small vessels (venules, capillaries, arterioles), and have a similar glomerular lesion (focal necrosis, crescents, absence or paucity of immunoglobulin [Ig] deposition). All three diseases also share clinical features, including a propensity to present as pulmonary

or renal syndromes. Finally, all share a varying prevalence of ANCA positivity. The epidemiology of these disorders reveals a collective incidence approaching 2 per 100,000 people in the United States and approximately 1 in 10,000 in Sweden.[1] Although each disease, in its characteristic form, can be distinguished from the others on clinical and histologic grounds, the distinctions are often blurred. Thus, their consideration as a group is reasonable from a pathologic as well as a clinical perspective.

ANTINEUTROPHIL CYTOPLASMIC ANTIBODY

BACKGROUND

ANCAs were first described in 1982 by Davies and colleagues[2] in eight patients with necrotizing pauci-immune glomerulonephritis who were suspected of having viral infections. A few years later, Hall and colleagues[3] identified ANCA in four patients with systemic vasculitis. In 1985, van der Woude and colleagues[4] were the first to suggest an association between ANCA and WG. Since that time, subsequent studies have established a close association between ANCA and three major vasculitis syndromes: WG, MPA, and CSS.[1] ANCAs were originally described based on their immunofluorescence patterns and were divided into cytoplasmic (c-ANCA) and perinuclear (p-ANCA) categories. The antigens responsible for these patterns and closely allied with the vasculitic syndromes have also been identified: proteinase 3 (PR3) for c-ANCA, and myeloperoxidase (MPO) for p-ANCA. ANCA testing is now an established diagnostic tool for systemic vasculitis, and its potential role in the pathogenesis of disease and as a target for therapy is still evolving. These issues have recently been comprehensively reviewed.[5]

METHODOLOGY

As noted previously, ANCAs were originally defined by indirect immunofluorescence assay (IFA) performed on ethanol-fixed neutrophils as substrate and broadly categorized as c-ANCA or p-ANCA (Fig. 82-1). In patients with vasculitis (WG, MPA, or CSS), specific immunochemical assays have demonstrated two major antigenic specificities responsible for these immunofluorescent patterns. In the case of c-ANCA reactivity, PR3 is responsible for more than 90% of such reactions, although other antigens may occasionally contribute, including bactericidal permeability-inducing protein (BPI) and, rarely, MPO.[1,5] The p-ANCA pattern is much less closely correlated with MPO, which was found in less than 10% of 620 consecutive p-ANCA–positive sera

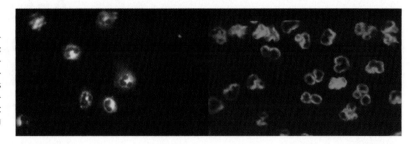

Figure 82-1 Immunofluorescence of diffuse or cytoplasmic antineutrophil cytoplasmic antibody (c-ANCA; *left*), which is highly correlated with antibodies to proteinase 3 (PR3), and the less-specific perinuclear pattern (p-ANCA, *right*), which is indicative of antibodies to myeloperoxidase (MPO). Although immunofluorescence was once the standard for ANCA testing, current standards require confirmatory antigen-specific testing for PR3 and MPO. *(Courtesy of Dr. C. G. M. Kallenberg.)*

samples by IFA in one laboratory.[6] Other antigens capable of producing p-ANCA reactivity include elastase, azurocidin, cathepsin G lysozyme, and lactoferrin.[7] Antinuclear antibodies (ANAs) may also yield a p-ANCA pattern, further compromising IFA as a diagnostic technique.

To circumvent the lack of correlation between immunofluorescent patterns and the antigens of interest (PR3 and MPO), as well as the inherent interobserver variability of IFA, antigen-specific assays have been developed and are readily available. Clinicians ordering ANCA assays need to ensure that ANCA positivity by IFA testing is confirmed by antigen-specific testing for both PR3 and MPO. With these criteria (PR3-ANCA indicating c-ANCA, with confirmatory antigenic testing for PR3; and MPO-ANCA indicating p-ANCA, with confirmatory antigenic testing for MPO), the test is highly specific for the vasculitic syndromes under discussion, even when tested in patients with connective tissue disease.[8] Guidelines for testing and reporting of ANCA have been published.[9]

DISEASE ASSOCIATIONS

Vasculitis

A large number of investigations have attempted to establish the sensitivity of PR3-ANCA and MPO-ANCA in systemic vasculitis, and these have been extensively reviewed.[7] In general, PR3-ANCA and MPO-ANCA are detected in a limited number of disorders, including the three small vessel vasculitic syndromes as well as the renal-limited form of vasculitis called idiopathic necrotizing crescentic glomerulonephritis. The sensitivity of ANCA varies in these disorders from 50% to more than 90%. A large, multicenter cooperative European trial attempting to standardize ANCA testing has been reported and is summarized in Figure 82-2.[10] The results of this trial emphasize that a significant number of patients with idiopathic small vessel vasculitis are ANCA negative; therefore, a negative test does not rule out the diagnosis in patients with a high pretest probability of disease. In WG, the disorder most highly associated with PR3-ANCA, the test is most likely to be positive in patients with triad (upper respiratory, lung, kidney) disease that is active and untreated.[7] Similar correlations of end-organ damage and disease activity with ANCA positivity are less clear in the other vasculitic syndromes.

The specificity of ANCA testing appears to depend on both technical factors and the nature of the control populations tested. If IFA results are combined with antigen-specific assays, the specificity of both PR3-ANCA and MPO-ANCA is exceedingly high (see Fig. 82-1). In the European cooperative study of Hagen and colleagues,[10] 184 disease controls were studied, including various forms of glomerulonephritis

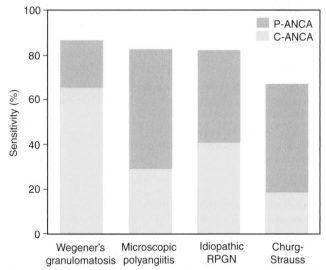

Figure 82-2 Frequency of antineutrophil cytoplasmic antibody (ANCA) reactivity in associated vasculitic conditions, divided on the basis of proteinase 3 (PR3) ANCA and myeloperoxidase (MPO) ANCA. c-ANCA, cytoplasmic ANCA; p-ANCA, perinuclear ANCA ; RPGN, rapidly progressive glomerulonephritis.

and granulomatous disease, and specificity for the ANCA-associated small vessel vasculitides exceeded 99%. A study by Merkel and colleagues,[8] using IFA confirmed by antigen-specific assay, examined a large cohort of well-characterized connective tissue disease patients and also reported specificity in excess of 99%. An earlier study of ANCA, which also included a large number of disease controls, demonstrated high specificity as well.[11] Salient points from these large, controlled studies include the unreliability of IFA testing, even when performed by highly trained and experienced personnel, and that IFA alone is less specific than IFA combined with antigen-specific testing for PR3 and MPO. Collectively, clinicians using ANCA to diagnose vasculitis must demand substantial experience from their laboratories and require IFA testing be supplemented by antigen-specific determinations. Even when these technical criteria are met, it must still be appreciated that ANCA, like any laboratory test, provides optimal diagnostic value only when applied in a clinical context.

In general, the specificity of ANCA influences disease phenotype, at least by association. In addition to the predilection of PR3 patients to develop WG and those with MPO to develop MPA, a direct comparison of patient populations reveals that PR3-positive patients have more extrarenal manifestations, granuloma formation, and relapses. Even among patients with MPA, those with PR3 specificity are more likely to have severe disease or to die. Despite substantial overlap, there appear to be distinct clinical and pathologic differences among patients with PR3-ANCA and those with MPO-ANCA, suggesting possible differences in pathogenic mechanisms.[12]

Other Diseases

ANCAs have been reported in a wide variety of other conditions.[7] Although ANCA positivity can occur in a number of conditions that mimic systemic vasculitis, the vast majority of such cases are negative for PR3 and MPO.[13] Patients with connective tissue diseases, including rheumatoid arthritis (RA),[8,14,15] systemic lupus erythematosus (SLE),[8] and myositis,[8] occasionally display ANCA positivity, but these are largely non-MPO and non-PR3 types. Patients with infections such as those seen in cystic fibrosis,[16] endocarditis,[17] and human immunodeficiency virus (HIV), among others,[7] are occasionally ANCA positive. This may be of particular clinical importance, because infections can mimic systemic vasculitis. As with connective tissue diseases reported to be ANCA positive, most reports of ANCA in infectious diseases are largely non-PR3 and non-MPO, underscoring the importance of confirming IFA by antigen-specific testing.

ANCAs are often encountered in inflammatory bowel disease and are more frequent in ulcerative colitis than in Crohn's disease.[18,19] The antigenic target is non-PR3 or non-MPO and is largely unknown, although a multitude of targets have been reported, including cathepsin G, lactoferrin, elastase lysozyme, and BPI.[18-20] Other forms of gastrointestinal (GI) disease reported to be ANCA positive (of the non-PR3, non-MPO variety) include sclerosing cholangitis and autoimmune hepatitis.[21,22]

Drugs may be a particularly important cause of false-positive ANCA reactions, especially because hydralazine, propylthiouracil, D-penicillamine, and minocycline may be associated with high-titer MPO-ANCA reactivity, with or without an associated vasculitic syndrome. Minocycline has also been associated with a reversible autoimmune syndrome and MPO-ANCA.[23]

PATHOPHYSIOLOGY

Although ANCAs are firmly entrenched in the diagnostic process for vasculitis, their role in the pathophysiology of these conditions is less so. Teleologic objections to a central role include the observation that ANCAs are not detected in a sizable portion of patients with well-documented small vessel vasculitis.[24] Despite such considerable limitations, mounting evidence suggests that ANCA may either induce or augment vascular inflammation. These data have been critically reviewed by several groups.[5,25,26]

A variety of in vitro observations favor a pathogenic role for ANCA in some forms of vasculitis. For instance, in neutrophils, both MPO and PR3 are transported from primary granules to the cell membrane during activation and are part of the physiologic response to inflammatory mediators (e.g., tumor necrosis factor-α [TNF-α] and interleukin [IL]-8).[27-29] Evidence of surface expression of PR3 on circulating neutrophils and MPO release within renal lesions has been reported in WG.[27,28] The binding of PR3-ANCA, MPO-ANCA, and other ANCAs to their cognate targets on

neutrophils augments a variety of activation-related neutrophilic functions, including degranulation, respiratory burst, nitric oxide production, chemotaxis, adhesion molecule expression, and binding to cultured endothelial cells.[27,29-31] Such binding appears to be dependent not only on binding of ANCA via the antigen-binding site but also on engagement of the Fcγ receptor.[32] Collectively, these events may contribute to vascular damage. ANCAs also stabilize cell adhesion and promote migration and flow of neutrophils through endothelium.[33]

Whether PR3 is synthesized and expressed on endothelial cells is controversial, but PR3 does appear to be capable of passive binding to the cell surface and thus serves as a target for PR3-ANCA. Binding of PR3-ANCA to endothelial cells has been demonstrated to lead to upregulation of adhesion molecule expression and production of IL-8, both of which might contribute to vessel inflammation and injury.[27,32] ANCAs are able to positively or negatively affect the proteolytic activity of PR3 or MPO, depending on epitope restriction.[7,34] Thus, if these enzymes play a homeostatic role in the inflammatory response, ANCAs might have a modulatory effect.

The activity of ANCAs in vivo has been demonstrated in animal models of vascular inflammation,[35,36] but these have been criticized on methodologic grounds and for the lack of similarity to human disease. More recently, a murine model has strengthened the argument that ANCAs actually cause vasculitis.[37] Anti-MPO antibodies alone have induced glomerulonephritis with crescent formation and systemic vasculitis in mice lacking functional T or B cells, as well as in an immunocompetent wild-type strain C57BL/6J, thus offering strong support for a direct pathogenic role. Further work with this model has demonstrated the central role of neutrophils in these glomerular lesions.[38]

Despite the observation that ANCAs are not present in all patients with systemic small vessel vasculitic syndromes, a number of studies have reported correlations between the presence and magnitude of ANCA and a variety of disease manifestations. Among these clinical correlates supported by many (but not all) investigations are disease activity and severity,[39,40] risk of relapse,[41,42] target organ distribution, and response to therapy.[40]

Most of these data stem from studies of PR3-ANCA in patients with WG; supporting data from other diseases such as MPA and CSS are much more limited. Despite such limitations, there is evidence that MPO-ANCA may play a similar role, including the display of MPO on the neutrophil cell membrane and its subsequent engagement, leading to degranulation, endothelial cell adhesion, and injury.[43,44] The pathophysiologic significance of non-PR3- and non-MPO-ANCA is much less clear, but other antigen autoantibody systems, such as lactoferrin, may also lead to inflammatory damage at the neurophil-endothelial interface.[45,46] Collectively, these studies indirectly support ANCA's direct role in the pathogenesis of small vessel vasculitis. Figure 82-3 is a schematic representation of the pathogenic role of ANCA in vascular inflammation.

DISEASE ACTIVITY

Although the specificity and diagnostic value of ANCA testing are well established, there is still considerable controversy about the relative worth of such serology in monitoring

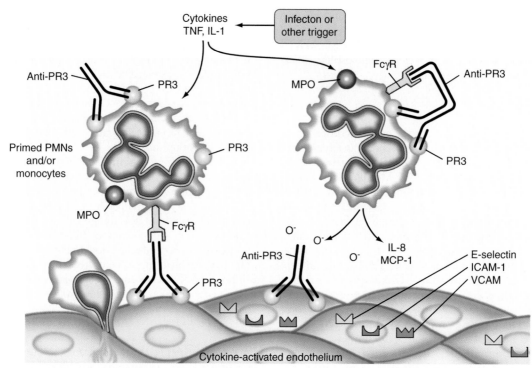

Figure 82-3 Schematic representation of the immune mechanisms hypothetically involved with antineutrophil cytoplasmic antibody (ANCA) enhancement of vascular injury. An infectious trigger or other environmental stimulus leads to a burst of cytokines, which primes the neutrophils or monocytes and may lead to the local upregulation of adhesion molecules on endothelium. The priming process within the inflammatory cells leads to enhanced expression of ANCA antigens on the cell surface. Activated neutrophils or monocytes may degranulate and release reactive oxygen species and lysosomal enzymes, leading to endothelial injury and further activation of the endothelial cell surface. The magnitude of this effect is influenced by the specificity of ANCA for proteinase 3 (PR3) or myeloperoxidase (MPO), as well as different epitopes of these respective antigens. The reaction may be further influenced by the immunoglobulin G (IgG) and Fcγ receptor phenotype engaged. Products released from degranulated inflammatory cells become bound to endothelial cells and further serve as targets of ANCA. Release of chemotactic chemokines such as interleukin-8 (IL-8) and macrophage chemoattractant protein-1 (MCP-1) serve to augment chemotaxis and inflammatory cell transmigration, in conjunction with other adhesion molecules. Thus, the scheme provides the prerequisites for endothelial and vascular injury induced by ANCA: the presence of ANCA, the expression of target antigens for ANCA on primed neutrophils and monocytes, the interaction between primed neutrophils and endothelium via adhesion molecules, and, finally, the activation of endothelial cells and ultimate efflux of inflammatory cells to the extravascular and perivascular tissues. FcγR, Fcγ receptor; ICAM-1, intercellular adhesion molecule-1; PMN, polymorphonuclear leukocyte; TNF, tumor necrosis factor.

disease activity.[7] In a pooled analysis of published data, only 48% of the rises in ANCA titers as measured by IFA were followed by relapse, and only 51% of all relapses were preceded by a rise in ANCA.[47] Therefore, a rise in the ANCA titer should not be the sole basis for therapeutic decision making.

A study of 100 ANCA-positive patients with vasculitis followed serially over a 2-year period found that 92% of flares were associated with rises in ANCA. The predictive values were higher for enzyme-linked immunosorbent assay (ELISA) than for IFA with regard to both PR3 and MPO. Although a substantial number of patients with rising ANCA levels did not flare, it was rare to see a flare in the absence of increased ANCA, which affirms this test's strong negative predictive value in this setting. For all tests with high sensitivity, their greatest clinical utility is when they are negative.[48]

WEGENER'S GRANULOMATOSIS

WG is a granulomatous necrotizing vasculitis characterized by a predilection to affect the upper and lower respiratory tracts and, in most cases, the kidneys. The disease was first described in 1931 by Heinz Klinger,[49] a German medical student. In 1936 and 1939, Friedrich Wegener,[50,51] a young pathologist, provided detailed information about three patients with a similar illness. Both Klinger and Wegener were struck by the

unusual distribution of disease in their patients. Involvement of the upper and lower airways was quite unlike the pattern seen in periarteritis nodosa. What later came to be known as WG remained relatively absent from the American literature until the 1950s, when Godman and Churg[52] published a detailed clinicopathologic description of the disorder. In 1973, Fauci and Wolff,[53] at the National Institutes of Health (NIH), recorded their observations of 18 patients with WG treated with a combination of steroids and cyclophosphamide. Sustained remissions and prolonged survival resulted, marking the beginning of a new era in the treatment of WG.

EPIDEMIOLOGY

No rigorous epidemiologic studies of WG have been published. The NIH experience suggests that WG affects both sexes equally, occurs in patients of all ages (mean age, 41 years; range, 9 to 78 years), and is more common in Caucasian patients (97%).[54] Based on the National Hospital Discharge Survey, the estimated prevalence of WG in the 1986–1990 period was approximately 3 per 100,000 persons.[55] Both sexes were equally represented. Only 0.1% of patients were younger than 19 years (versus 15% in the NIH series). Most patients were Caucasian (80.9%). Seasonal differences in dates of hospitalization were not readily apparent.

It is likely that the prevalence of WG has been underestimated. Only since the early 1990s have we recognized the existence of mild and more indolent forms of the disease and the variability in its clinical presentation and course of illness. Future epidemiologic studies should take such factors into consideration and extend beyond the hospital setting.

PATHOGENESIS

The cause of WG is unknown. Sporadic efforts have been made to identify a genetic predisposition to WG, and a higher prevalence of human leukocyte antigen (HLA)-DR1[56] and HLA-DQw7[57] has been reported among a small number of patients with WG. However, larger studies failed to identify any unique genetic markers.[58]

Several attempts to link infectious diseases to the development of WG have been unconvincing. Reports that the onset of disease occurs mostly in winter (a period of presumed increased respiratory illness)[59] have not been confirmed in larger series.[54,55] Analysis of bronchoalveolar lavage fluid and open lung biopsy specimens in patients with recent-onset disease did not reveal bacteria, fungi, mycoplasma, respiratory viruses, or virus-like inclusions.[60]

Although the association of PR3-ANCA antibodies and WG is now well established, the pathogenic role of these antibodies remains unclear. Many of the arguments supporting a pathogenic role were described previously. In addition, several clinical, in vitro, and ex vivo studies provide indirect evidence that these autoantibodies are more than an epiphenomenon. Clinical studies have documented that PR3-ANCA antibodies are highly specific for WG (90% to 97%).[4,10] They are almost always present in active, generalized WG[54,61] and may be produced by pulmonary lymphoid tissue in patients with active disease but not in those in remission.[62] In vitro and ex vivo studies have shown that activation of polymorphonuclear cells and monocytes leads to the translocation of PR3 from the intracellular compartment to the cell surface, where it becomes accessible to circulating antibodies.[63] ANCAs enhance neutrophil activation, degranulation, and respiratory burst, as well as adherence and damage to endothelial cells.[29,31,43] Endothelial cells might also be a direct target for ANCA: PR3 is present in the cytoplasm of untreated human cultured endothelial cells, and stimulation with TNF leads to a time-dependent translocation of PR3 to the cell surface.[64] These observations suggest, but do not prove, that ANCAs are directly involved in the pathogenesis of WG.

Evidence of T cell involvement in WG is less direct than that supporting the pathogenic effect of ANCA. Biopsies of various tissues reveal the presence of polymorphonuclear and mononuclear infiltrates, the latter consisting of plasma cells, monocytes, and T cells, with a predominance of CD4+ cells.[65,66] Increasing levels of soluble IL-2 receptors, sometimes preceding disease relapse, indicate the presence of activated T cells.[67,68] In addition, autoreactive PR3-specific T cells are present in higher percentages in patients with WG compared with controls.[69] The role of PR3-autoreactive T cells in ANCA production, disease activity, and pathogenesis of the granulomatous lesions remains to be established.

Also, as previously mentioned, a recently described animal model of vasculitis has provided substantial support for a direct pathogenic role of ANCA by producing lesions in the kidney and lung highly reminiscent of WG and MPA through

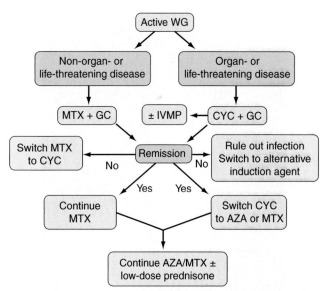

Figure 82-4 Wegener's granulomatosis (WG) treatment algorithm. AZA, azathioprine; CYC, cyclophosphamide (oral); GC, glucocorticoids; IVMP, intravenous methylprednisolone; MTX, methotrexate.

the action of anti-MPO antibodies alone.[37] In this important model, the production of lesions similar to human disease in the absence of other confounding immunologic variables adds an important argument for causation by ANCA.

CLINICAL FEATURES

As stated earlier, WG is characterized by a predilection for the upper and lower respiratory tracts and the kidneys. Relatively mild forms of WG without renal involvement have been described. The course of illness may be indolent or rapidly progressive. Mild and indolent disease may go unrecognized for months to years, leading to delays in diagnosis and the institution of appropriate therapy. Neither clinical nor laboratory markers are able to distinguish which patients will continue to have limited, nonrenal forms of disease and which patients will experience progression in the future. A general approach to the diagnosis of WG is shown in Figure 82-4.

Unexplained constitutional symptoms are often part of the initial presentation. Fever is present in about one fourth of patients at disease onset and occurs in up to half of cases during the course of illness.[54] Weight loss exceeding 10% of usual body weight has been reported in 15% of patients at onset and 35% of patients overall.[54]

The clinical features of WG are presented in the following sections using an organ-oriented approach. For each organ system, we discuss the signs and symptoms of disease, differential diagnoses (when appropriate), clinical and laboratory methods to diagnose and assess disease activity, and aspects of disease-related morbidity.

Upper Airway Manifestations

Upper airway disease is the most common presenting feature of WG, occurring in more than 70% of patients at onset and ultimately developing in more than 90%.[54,70,71]

Otologic manifestations may be part of the initial presentation in about 25% of patients with WG and may occur in up to 60% during the course of disease.[54,70-72] Serous otitis

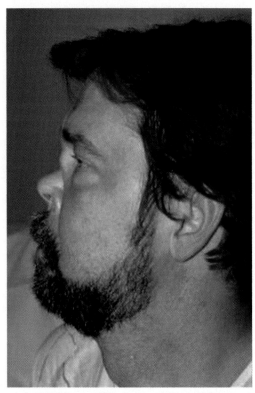

Figure 82-5 Saddle-nose deformity in a patient with Wegener's granulomatosis. *(Courtesy of Dr. G. Hoffman.)*

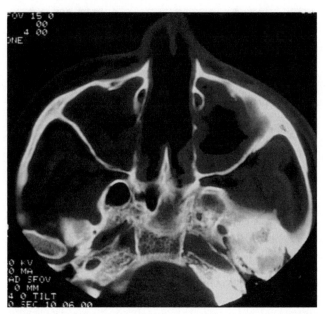

Figure 82-6 Computed tomography scan of the sinuses, revealing the presence of chronic sinusitis.

media is the most common ear problem encountered (25% to 44%). It may be complicated by the presence of a suppurative infection in up to 25% of cases. Significant degrees of hearing loss (mostly conductive) may result in 14% to 42% of patients.[54,70-72] Inner ear manifestations include sensorineural hearing loss and, rarely, vertigo.[71,72]

Nasal disease is a prominent presenting feature in about 33% of cases, but it eventually develops in 64% to 80% of patients.[54,70,71] Symptoms and signs of nasal involvement in WG include mucosal swelling with nasal obstruction, crusted nasal ulcers and septal perforations, serosanguineous discharge, epistaxis (11% to 32%), and external saddle-nose deformity (9% to 29%) (Fig. 82-5).[54,70,71]

Sinusitis is present at initial presentation in about 50% to 67% of patients with WG and is seen in 85% during the course of disease.[54,70] A simple computed tomography (CT) scan of the sinuses (Fig. 82-6) is often anatomically more informative than plain radiographs, especially in the setting of destructive or erosive bony changes. Most patients with sinus or nasal disease eventually develop a secondary infection of these tissues; *Staphylococcus aureus* is the predominant organism identified from cultures.[70]

Although laryngotracheal disease in WG may be asymptomatic, the clinical presentation can range from subtle hoarseness to stridor and life-threatening upper airway obstruction.[54,71,73] The most characteristic lesion is subglottic stenosis (Fig. 82-7), which occurs in up to 16% of patients.[54,73] It is important to note that in pediatric and adolescent patients with WG, the frequency of subglottic stenosis is dramatically increased, reaching an alarming prevalence of 48%.[73,74] Direct laryngoscopy may reveal either active erythematous, friable mucosa or bland scar.[71] Tracheal tomograms, CT, and

magnetic resonance imaging (MRI) may be useful adjuncts in the diagnosis of subglottic stenosis. Langford and coworkers[75] reported that in 49% of patients, subglottic stenosis occurred in the absence of other features of active disease; in 49%, it developed during treatment with systemic immunosuppressive therapy for other disease features.

Pulmonary Manifestations

Pulmonary involvement is one of the cardinal features of WG. Pulmonary manifestations occur in 45% of cases at presentation and in 87% during the course of disease.[54] Cough, hemoptysis, and pleuritis are the most common pulmonary symptoms. However, it is important to realize that up to one third of patients with radiographically demonstrable pulmonary lesions may not have lower airway symptoms. The most common radiographic findings include pulmonary infiltrates (67%) and nodules (58%).[54] The pulmonary infiltrates in WG may be quite fleeting, appearing and resolving in some cases before the institution of therapy.[53] Persistent, diffuse

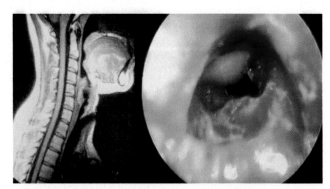

Figure 82-7 Subglottic stenosis in a patient with Wegener's granulomatosis. Magnetic resonance imaging *(left)* and endoscopic view *(right)*. *(Right, courtesy of Dr. G. S. Hoffman; from Hoffman GS, Kerr GS, Leavitt RY, et al: Wegener granulomatosis: An analysis of 158 patients. Ann Intern Med 116:488-498, 1992.)*

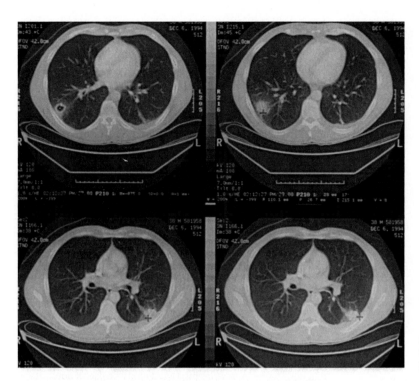

Figure 82-8 Computed tomography scan of the lungs, revealing the presence of nodules. The right-sided pulmonary nodule is cavitary.

interstitial infiltrates are rare (<1%) and should suggest other diagnoses. Pulmonary nodules in WG are usually multiple and bilateral and often cavitate (50%).[76-78] CT of the chest may reveal infiltrates and nodules (Fig. 82-8) that were undetected by conventional radiographs in 43% to 63% of cases.[77-79] Less common pulmonary manifestations of WG include pleural effusions, diffuse pulmonary hemorrhage, and mediastinal or hilar lymph node enlargement or mass.[80,81] Diffuse pulmonary hemorrhage has been reported in up to 8% of cases and carries a high fatality rate (50%).[53,77,82]

In patients presenting with pulmonary symptoms, it is imperative to make every effort to exclude the presence of infection in a timely fashion, because pneumonia in an immunocompromised host can result in up to 50% mortality. Bronchoscopy is often needed to satisfactorily exclude infection or establish a microbiologic diagnosis by performing the appropriate stains and cultures. Pneumonia may account for up to 40% of serious infections in patients with WG and may be the cause of death in a significant proportion of cases (16%).[54,76]

Pulmonary morbidity in WG is significant. Pulmonary function tests may reveal obstructive defects in up to 55% of patients, generally caused by endobronchial lesions and scarring.[83] Restrictive defects with reduced lung volumes and carbon monoxide diffusion capacity are observed in 30% to 40% of patients.[83] In more than 17% of patients, serial pulmonary function tests document moderate to severe degrees of progressive pulmonary insufficiency, perhaps as a result of fibrosis following active disease, pneumonia, cyclophosphamide-induced pneumonitis, or some combination of these.[54]

Renal Manifestations

The presence or absence of renal disease defines the subsets of generalized and limited WG, respectively.[84,85] The exact frequency of renal involvement in WG is difficult to ascertain. Limited WG may go undiagnosed in patients with mild disease. By excluding such patients, published series may overestimate the frequency of renal disease in WG. Early renal disease may be clinically silent; that is, kidney biopsies may, on rare occasions, reveal focal inflammatory changes in patients with normal urinary sediment and renal function.[53,84,86] In addition, patients who appear to have limited WG at one time may later develop glomerulonephritis. This observation mandates caution in patients thought to have limited WG and dictates the need for careful and close monitoring of renal status in all patients.

When renal disease is defined by pathologic findings on kidney biopsy or the presence of an active urinary sediment and functional abnormalities, it is estimated to occur in 11% to 18% of patients at presentation and in 77% to 85% during the course of disease.[54,70] Extrarenal manifestations often precede renal disease. Once present, renal disease may progress from asymptomatic and mild to fulminant glomerulonephritis within days or weeks, resulting in end-stage renal failure.[70] If untreated, mean survival time for this subset of patients is about 5 months.[87] Even when appropriate therapy is instituted, initial and recurrent renal damage may lead to chronic renal insufficiency in up to 42% of patients, often requiring dialysis (11%) and renal transplantation (5%).[54]

The role of microscopic urinalysis in the evaluation of patients with suspected or proven WG cannot be overemphasized. It remains the most useful tool to assess for the presence of active glomerulonephritis. The freshly collected urinary sediment should be carefully examined. The presence of red blood cell casts approaches a 100% positive predictive value for glomerulonephritis. In the absence of red blood cell casts, the presence of hematuria should lead to consideration of lower urinary tract involvement by the vasculitic process, which is uncommon, or the presence of cyclophosphamide-induced cystitis.

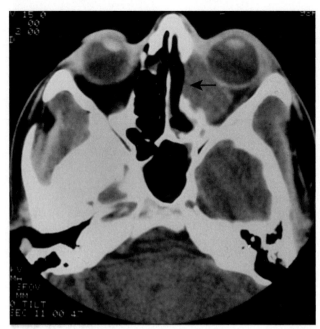

Figure 82-9 Computed tomography scan of the orbits, revealing the presence of a retro-orbital mass (orbital pseudotumor).

Ocular Manifestations

Ocular manifestations reportedly occur in 28% to 58% of patients with WG and may be part of the initial presentation in 8% to 16% of cases.[88,89] Any compartment of the eye can be affected. Keratitis, conjunctivitis, scleritis, episcleritis, nasolacrimal duct obstruction, uveitis, retro-orbital pseudotumor with proptosis (Fig. 82-9), retinal vessel occlusion, and optic neuritis have all been described.[88,89] Vision loss may occur in as many as 8% of patients.[54,90] Although most ocular findings are nonspecific, proptosis is a diagnostically helpful finding,[54,70] but it is a poor prognostic sign; about half of patients with proptosis in one series lost vision due to optic nerve ischemia.[54] A complete ophthalmologic examination is an important part of the diagnostic evaluation. In patients with proptosis, CT or MRI of the orbits and sinuses may provide useful anatomic information.[89,91]

Ocular disease may also occur as a complication of therapy. Glucocorticoid-related cataracts occurred in 21% of patients in one series.[54] Glucocorticoid and cyclophosphamide therapy has been associated with opportunistic ocular infections including cytomegalovirus retinitis and herpes zoster ophthalmicus.[92]

Cutaneous Manifestations

Cutaneous manifestations have been reported in 40% to 50% of patients with WG and may be part of the initial presentation in 13% to 25% of cases.[93] The cutaneous manifestations of WG include ulcers, palpable purpura, subcutaneous nodules, papules, and vesicles. Although cutaneous lesions rarely dominate the clinical picture, they do tend to parallel disease activity in other organs. The presence of active skin lesions is thus a reliable clinical marker for active systemic disease and should prompt the clinician to evaluate other organ systems thoroughly.

Musculoskeletal Manifestations

Musculoskeletal symptoms are common in patients with WG, occurring in 32% to 53% of patients at presentation and in 67% to 76% during the course of disease.[54,70,94] Although most patients experience only arthralgias and myalgias, arthritis is observed in up to 28% of patients.[70,94] When synovitis is present, several patterns can be observed, including monarticular disease, migratory oligoarthritis, and symmetric or asymmetric polyarthritis of small and large joints.[54,94] Symmetric polyarthritis of small and large joints may be mistaken for RA.[54,94] A positive test for rheumatoid factor may be observed in as many as 50% to 60% of patients, often contributing to an incorrect diagnosis.[54,94] In contrast to RA, the symmetric polyarthritis of WG is generally nonerosive and nondeforming.[54,70,94]

Neurologic Manifestations

Neurologic involvement is rarely a presenting feature of WG, but it may develop during the course of disease in 22% to 50% of cases.[54,70,76,95] Multiple neurologic complications may occur in up to 11% of patients. Peripheral neuropathy is the most common single neurologic manifestation of WG (10% to 16%).[54,70,76,95] Mononeuritis multiplex is the most frequent clinical pattern (12% to 15%), followed by a distal and symmetric polyneuropathy (2%).[54,95] Electromyography and nerve conduction studies may be useful in demonstrating the extent and distribution of involvement and can often identify an overlapping mononeuropathy multiplex that is not apparent on clinical examination. Biopsy of the involved nerve or nerves reveals the presence of vasculitis, but biopsy is rarely necessary to establish the diagnosis or make therapeutic decisions.

The overall frequency of central nervous system (CNS) involvement is difficult to estimate because the symptoms, signs, and clinical presentations of CNS disease have been variably defined and accrued in different series. In addition, significant classification overlap exists among the symptoms and signs of CNS, ocular, and sinus disease and treatment complications. Chronic pachymeningitis (Fig. 82-10), cerebral vasculitis, pituitary involvement, cerebral hemorrhage or thrombosis, and cranial neuropathies can all occur.[96] Cranial neuropathy occurs in 6% to 9% of patients.[54,95] Cerebrovascular events, occurring in up to 4% of cases, may include cerebral or brainstem infarction, subdural hematoma, and subarachnoid hemorrhage.[54,76,95] Diffuse meningeal and periventricular white matter disease, presumably reflecting CNS vasculitis, has been reported in patients presenting with diffuse and focal CNS symptoms.[96-98]

In patients presenting with symptoms and signs of CNS disease, several diagnostic tests may be considered. CT or MRI of the brain may document the presence of infarcts, hemorrhage, mass lesions, diffuse meningeal enhancement, or periventricular white matter lesions. In some cases, lumbar puncture is necessary to exclude CNS infections and subarachnoid hemorrhage. Cerebral angiography is a test of low diagnostic yield in WG because, in most instances, relatively small vessels are involved.[95,97,98]

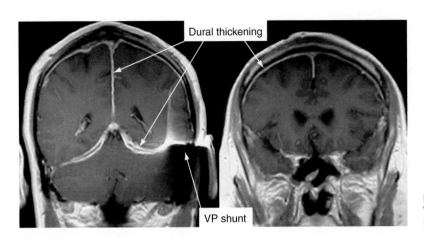

Figure 82-10 Pachymeningitis in a patient with Wegener's granulomatosis. Magnetic resonance imaging findings.

Gastrointestinal Manifestations

The frequency of GI involvement in WG is difficult to estimate, perhaps because it is frequently asymptomatic and may be unrecognized. The literature consists mainly of individual case reports of patients with dramatic or unusual GI presentations. Abdominal pain, diarrhea, and bleeding are the most frequently reported symptoms, and they relate to the presence of ulcerations in the small intestines, large intestines, or both (enterocolitis).[99] Small and large bowel perforations have been described, with dramatic and often fatal presentations.[99] Other unusual presentations include cholecystitis, unexplained ascites, nonhealing perianal ulcers, recurrent acute pancreatitis, and pancreatic mass with extrahepatic obstruction.[99] Steroid-induced peptic ulcers may occur, but a biopsy is required to distinguish such lesions from those due to vasculitis. Unexplained elevations of liver enzymes have also been described and may resolve with therapy.[70] In autopsy series of patients with WG, the spleen was commonly involved; the majority of cases demonstrated splenic lesions with a combination of necrosis, vasculitis, and granuloma formation.[87] However, clinically apparent splenic disease is rare.

The occurrence of GI complaints in a patient with a known or suspected diagnosis of WG (or other systemic vasculitides) represents a medical emergency.[100] In patients with abdominal pain and systemic vasculitis, especially those receiving glucocorticoids, the lack of physical signs on abdominal examination should not lead to a false sense of security. Plain abdominal radiographs may detect the presence of free air, indicative of perforation. Arteriography may not be helpful because WG most often affects small vessels, which are beyond the resolution of this technique.[100] Endoscopic studies (colonoscopy, gastroscopy) may document the presence of ulcerations. Endoscopic biopsies usually demonstrate nonspecific inflammatory changes and may, on rare occasions, reveal granulomatous necrotizing vasculitis, thus establishing a histopathologic diagnosis. Histologic diagnosis is more commonly made on examination of surgical specimens because of the greater amount of tissue available.[101]

Genitourinary Manifestations

Virtually every segment of the genitourinary tract distal to the kidneys may be involved in WG. The literature consists mostly of individual case reports, suggesting that such manifestations are uncommon. Ureteral obstruction by an extrinsic inflammatory mass has been reported.[102] Hemorrhagic cystitis is more commonly seen in relation to cyclophosphamide therapy, but it may be due to involvement of the bladder wall by necrotizing vasculitis.[103] In an autopsy series, granulomatous or necrotizing prostatitis was found in 7.4% of patients with WG.[87] Other genitourinary manifestations include necrotizing urethritis, orchitis, epididymitis, and penile necrosis.[99]

Microscopic examination of freshly voided urine is the most important diagnostic test. The presence of hematuria in the absence of red blood cell casts (after adequate review by the clinician) should prompt an evaluation of the lower genitourinary tract. Cystoscopy is preferred because it allows direct visualization of abnormal structures and the performance of diagnostic biopsies. This is also important in patients receiving long-term cyclophosphamide therapy. Urinary tract infections should always be considered and the appropriate cultures obtained.

Cardiac Manifestations

The frequency of cardiac involvement in WG ranges from 6% to 12% in clinical series[54,70] and may reach 30% in autopsy series.[87] Pericarditis is the most frequently reported cardiac manifestation in WG.[104] Patients may present with asymptomatic pericardial effusions or complain of chest pain associated with a pericardial friction rub on physical examination. In the setting of advanced renal disease, the differential diagnosis includes uremic and infectious causes of pericarditis. Pericardial tamponade has rarely been reported and may require pericardiocentesis, pericardiectomy, or both.[54,105,106] Pericarditis is also the most common pathologic finding in the heart, accounting for about 50% of histologically documented cardiac disease in WG.[107] Necrotizing vasculitis and granuloma formation may involve the pericardium in a focal or diffuse pattern.[107] Other cardiac manifestations of WG include myocardial ischemia due to coronary vasculitis, myocarditis, endocarditis, and valvulitis; arrhythmias; and conduction defects.[104]

ASSOCIATED CONDITIONS

Recent evidence suggests that there is an increased rate of venous thromboembolic events in patients with WG.[108] A rate of 7 symptomatic events (mainly deep vein thrombosis and pulmonary embolus) per 100 patient-years of observation was recorded. This may be an underestimate, because ultrasonography to detect asymptomatic thromboses was not performed. Nevertheless, it is significantly greater than the rates seen in patients with SLE, RA, or the general population.[108] These results were corroborated by another recent report that showed an increased rate of venous thromboembolic events in patients with WG, MPA, and renal-limited vasculitis.[109] No evidence of an underlying thrombophilic disorder was found in patients tested. This has implications for the differential diagnosis of pulmonary symptoms in WG patients and complicates the approach to treatment, particularly in the setting of pulmonary hemorrhage.

It has also been postulated that, similar to other rheumatic disorders such as RA and SLE, WG is associated with accelerated atherosclerosis.[110] WG has been associated with biomarkers of coronary artery disease such as endothelial dysfunction, arterial stiffness, and carotid intimal-medial thickness.[110,111] Additional data are necessary to clearly delineate the risk of atherosclerotic disease in WG, but it is prudent to address traditional cardiac risk factors in WG patients.

LABORATORY DIAGNOSIS

General laboratory abnormalities in untreated patients may include leukocytosis, normocytic normochromic anemia, thrombocytosis, and elevated erythrocyte sedimentation rate. These are imperfect markers of disease activity and should always be interpreted in relation to organ-specific clinical and laboratory evidence of active disease. The role of ANCA testing in the evaluation of WG and other systemic vasculitides has already been discussed. The sensitivity of PR3-ANCA is about 90% in active WG and 40% when the disease is in remission.[4,61,112] The specificity of PR3-ANCA in the diagnosis of WG exceeds 95%.[4,61,112] In general, the presence of high-titer ANCA by IFA combined with confirmatory antigen-specific assay for either PR3 or MPO in the setting of a high index of suspicion for vasculitis (i.e., high pretest probability) is sufficient for diagnosis, even in the absence of tissue confirmation.

PATHOLOGY

Inflammatory lesions in WG typically include necrosis, granulomatous changes, and vasculitis.[49-51,53,54,70,87] The diagnostic yield of a biopsy varies with the size of the pathologic specimen and how completely it is sectioned and studied.

The small amount of tissue available in head and neck biopsies (mostly from nasal and paranasal sinuses) may make it difficult to identify all the pathologic features of WG.[113-115] Vasculitis, necrosis, and granulomatous inflammation are each encountered in roughly one third to one half of pathologic specimens.[113-115] Vasculitis and necrosis are seen together in only one fifth of biopsies.[114,115] The frequency of combined vasculitis and granulomatous inflammation is also about one fifth.[114,115] Most important, the complete diagnostic triad is seen in only 3% to 16% of biopsies.[114,115] Thus, head and neck biopsies most often reveal findings compatible with, but rarely characteristic of, WG. Awareness of these limitations is required for the correct interpretation of head and neck biopsy results in patients suspected of having WG.

The diagnostic yield of lung biopsies similarly reflects the sample size of pulmonary tissue obtained.[54,66] Transbronchial biopsies are rarely diagnostic (<7%), whereas open lung biopsies reveal various combinations of vasculitis, granulomas, and necrosis in about 90% of cases (Fig. 82-11).[54,66] Nonetheless, bronchoscopy and transbronchial biopsy remain valuable in the diagnosis or exclusion of bacterial, mycobacterial, or fungal infections that can mimic or complicate WG. Capillaritis (Fig. 82-12), a pathologic finding, has been described in 35% to 45% of WG cases in surgical biopsy and autopsy series.[116,117] In one study, capillaritis was found in all 11 patients with WG presenting with diffuse pulmonary hemorrhage.[118] However, the finding of capillaritis is not diagnostically specific. Capillaritis has been described in SLE, immune complex–associated vasculitides, dermatomyositis, RA, Henoch-Schönlein purpura, and even bronchopneumonias.[82]

Pathologically, renal disease in WG is characterized by the presence of focal and segmental glomerulonephritis (Fig. 82-13).[53,54,70,76,86,87] Fibrinoid necrosis and proliferative changes are seen in varying degrees. In patients with

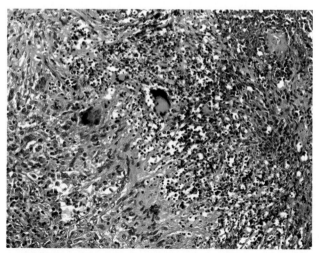

Figure 82-11 Giant cells within areas of collagenous necrosis *(right)* and histiocytic infiltrate *(middle and left)* in a lung nodule in a patient with Wegener's granulomatosis (hematoxylin and eosin, ×20). *(Courtesy of Dr. C. Farver.)*

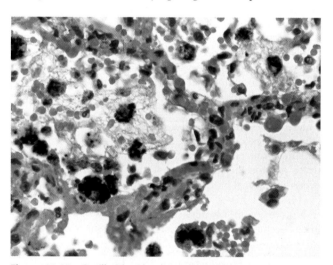

Figure 82-12 **Capillaritis.** Alveolar septae with congestion, neutrophilic infiltrate, and fibrinoid necrosis of capillary walls. Adjacent alveolar spaces contain hemosiderin-laden macrophages, consistent with a history of pulmonary hemorrhage (hematoxylin and eosin, ×40). *(Courtesy of Dr. C. Farver.)*

irreversible renal impairment, epithelial crescents and sclerotic lesions are commonly encountered.[54,70,87] True vasculitis of medium-sized renal arteries is only occasionally noted (3% to 15%), and granulomatous changes are equally rare (3%).[52-54,70,76] Immune complex deposition, as demonstrated by immunofluorescence or electron microscopy, is distinctly unusual.[54,86,119] The results of kidney biopsies are thus more often compatible with, rather than diagnostic of, WG.

TREATMENT

To manage WG effectively, the clinician must establish the diagnosis without delay, recognize the variability in clinical course and severity, critically monitor disease activity, and anticipate disease- and treatment-related morbidity. Therapeutic decision making should be based on a critical assessment of disease activity. Meticulous attention should be paid to complications of therapy, which often lead to permanent morbidity and, sometimes, mortality. In addition, certain complications (infections, drug reactions or toxicity, drug-induced pneumonitis, renal impairment) may be confused with active disease. The significant toxicity of currently available therapeutic agents has been the main driving force for the development of new drugs and innovative approaches to the treatment of WG and other systemic vasculitides. An overview of the approach to treatment of WG is shown in Figure 82-4.

Glucocorticoids

In WG, glucocorticoids are most commonly used in combination with cytotoxic agents. Although palliation of limited, indolent disease may be achieved with glucocorticoids alone, disease progression and relapses usually occur. Patients with generalized WG uniformly fail to achieve remission with glucocorticoid therapy alone. Treatment is generally initiated at a high dose, such as prednisone 1 mg/kg per day or more. High doses are maintained until all manifestations

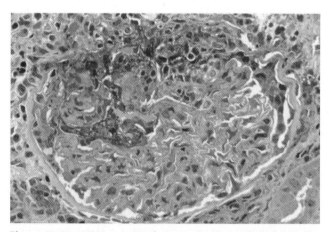

Figure 82-13 ANCA-associated crescentic glomerulonephritis. This toluidine blue–stained plastic section demonstrates a glomerulus with a cellular crescent. There is partial obliteration of Bowman's space by a proliferation of epithelial cells and macrophages. All types of crescentic glomerulonephritis appear similar by light microscopy, and immunofluorescence is needed to distinguish among pauci-immune, immune complex, and anti–glomerular basement membrane subtypes. *(Courtesy of Dr. J. Myles.)*

of active disease have abated (e.g., stabilization of renal function, resolution of pulmonary infiltrates). Drug tapering should begin after WG is well under control, usually about 1 month after the initiation of treatment. The literature does not provide a consensus opinion about the strategy for tapering glucocorticoids. In the initial seminal studies of WG, prednisone was reduced on an alternate-day basis.[54,70,120] Currently, however, the favored approach is to taper prednisone on a daily basis, with varying regimens reported.[121-123] Another approach during the initiation of therapy is to use intravenous "pulse" or "bolus" methylprednisolone (e.g., 1 g daily for 3 days) for immediately life-threatening disease (e.g., diffuse pulmonary hemorrhage, rapidly progressive glomerulonephritis). However, the optimal dose and frequency of intravenous glucocorticoids have not been studied in a controlled fashion for systemic vasculitis. In addition, the short-lasting effects of pulse glucocorticoids do not obviate the need for maintenance therapy.

Before the advent of glucocorticoids, the mean survival time of patients with WG was 5 months. Glucocorticoids alone modestly increased the mean survival time to 12 months.[124] Five-year survival rates greater than 80% were not seen until the introduction of aggressive combination therapy with glucocorticoids and daily cyclophosphamide.

Cyclophosphamide

Combination therapy with daily oral cyclophosphamide and glucocorticoid has been considered the standard therapy for WG.[53,54,70] Oral cyclophosphamide is generally initiated at doses of 2 mg/kg per day. In life-threatening situations (pulmonary hemorrhage or rapidly progressive glomerulonephritis), doses of 3 to 5 mg/kg per day can be used for 3 to 4 days, then reduced to the more conventional range. The leukocyte count is used to guide subsequent dosage adjustments (discussed later). Tapering and discontinuation of the glucocorticoid generally precede attempts to taper cyclophosphamide. The traditional approach to the treatment of systemic WG is to continue cyclophosphamide for at least 1 year after the patient has achieved complete remission.

Orally administered cyclophosphamide is well absorbed and completely metabolized within 24 hours by the liver; the multiple active and inactive metabolites are excreted mostly in the urine. One of these metabolites, acrolein, is known to be responsible for hemorrhagic cystitis, bladder fibrosis, and bladder cancer. High oral fluid intake should be encouraged to dilute this bladder irritant and reduce the incidence of such complications. The time from initial use of cyclophosphamide to detection of bladder cancer may be as short as 7 months or as long as 10 to 15 years, even after the drug has been discontinued.[54,125] Urine cytology is an insensitive diagnostic tool to detect bladder cancer. Cystoscopy is therefore necessary in any cyclophosphamide-treated patient with nonglomerular hematuria. Lifelong surveillance for bladder cancer, as well as hematologic malignancies, is indicated in all patients who have been treated with chronic daily cyclophosphamide therapy.[54,125] Dose-related bone marrow suppression is a common drug-related toxicity, and blood counts should be closely observed during the course of treatment. Leukopenia is the most frequent sign of marrow suppression and should guide dosage adjustments in these patients. The risk of infection is increased even in the absence of leukopenia. Total leukocyte counts of less than 3500/mm³ or absolute neutrophil counts of 1500/mm³ or less should be avoided. Based on data from recent pharmacokinetic investigations, the dose of cyclophosphamide should be adjusted downward by 25% to 30% in the presence of significant renal impairment.[126] Cyclophosphamide is formally contraindicated during pregnancy, and birth control should be strongly advised in women of childbearing age. When the drug is used in men considering fatherhood, they should be counseled regarding sperm banking.

In a large series of 158 patients with WG followed at the NIH for up to 24 years (mean follow-up, 8 years), 84% of patients received standard therapy with daily cyclophosphamide and glucocorticoid.[54] This regimen produced marked improvement in 91% of patients and complete remission in 75%. Disease relapse was seen in 50% of patients in this study, with permanent morbidity from disease occurring in 86% of that group. This included chronic renal insufficiency (42%), hearing loss (35%), cosmetic and functional nasal deformities (28%), tracheal stenosis (13%), and vision loss (8%), with many patients experiencing more than one type of morbidity. Permanent morbidity as a result of treatment with cyclophosphamide and glucocorticoid occurred in 42% of patients and included cystitis (43%), bladder cancer (2.8%—33 times the expected rate), lymphoma (1.5%—11 times the expected rate), myelodysplasia (2%), infertility (>57% of women), cataracts (21%), fractures (11%), and aseptic necrosis (3%). Moreover, 46% of patients experienced serious infectious episodes that required hospitalization and intravenous antibiotics.[54]

The awareness of this significant disease- and treatment-related morbidity in WG patients, and the recognition of more indolent forms of disease without any significant pulmonary or renal abnormalities, led to efforts to identify effective and less toxic therapeutic interventions. Approaches have focused largely on minimizing cumulative cyclophosphamide exposure, including the use of intermittent high-dose intravenous cyclophosphamide, alternative induction agents for less severe disease (e.g., methotrexate), and a staged therapeutic approach. The last of these considers the treatment of WG in two parts: remission induction and remission maintenance. The aim is to treat active disease aggressively to induce remission, typically with cyclophosphamide and glucocorticoid, as outlined earlier, and then switch from cyclophosphamide to a less toxic agent for remission maintenance. This takes advantage of the potency of cyclophosphamide as a remission-inducing agent and the lower toxicity of antimetabolites.

Studies of intermittent high-dose intravenous (pulse) cyclophosphamide were motivated by its demonstrated efficacy in the treatment of lupus nephritis and the anticipation of reduced toxicity. Pulse cyclophosphamide is only rarely associated with hemorrhagic cystitis and has not been associated with bladder cancer. Several small randomized trials of 0.7 g/m² every 3 weeks have suggested an efficacy comparable to daily oral cyclophosphamide in achieving initial remission in WG, with fewer associated infections, especially *Pneumocystis carinii* pneumonia, and lower mortality than oral therapy, albeit with a trend toward a greater risk of disease relapse.[127,128] Several criticisms of these investigations have been voiced, including an unacceptable overall mortality rate in one trial[127] and a lack of statistical power in the

other.[128] To minimize bladder toxicity, some investigators recommend the use of mesna (sodium 2-mercaptoethane sulfate).[129] This can be given intravenously at the time of cyclophosphamide infusion, but owing to a short half-life, it must be administered orally 2 and 4 hours after the infusion to be effective. In addition to having its own toxicities, the technique is cumbersome; thus, many favor a high oral intake of fluids as an alternative. A multicenter randomized, controlled trial has been performed comparing oral and pulse cyclophosphamide for the treatment of WG. Until the results of this study are available, the pulse method cannot be recommended as standard treatment for WG.

Azathioprine

Azathioprine is a derivative of thioguanine, a purine antimetabolite. It has long been used for the prevention of transplant rejection and the treatment of many rheumatic diseases (e.g., RA, SLE) and other inflammatory conditions (e.g., inflammatory bowel disease). Azathioprine is a prodrug and is metabolized to 6-mercaptopurine. 6-Mercaptopurine is further metabolized by thiopurine methyltransferase (TPMT) and hypoxanthine phosphoribosyl transferase. Deficiency of TPMT leads to preferential formation of toxic metabolites and lower drug tolerance. Low levels of TPMT activity occur in 11% of the population, with very low levels occurring in 0.3%. Therefore, in an effort to reduce the incidence of azathioprine toxicity, some recommend TPMT screening before the initiation of azathioprine therapy, particularly at higher doses.[130]

The mechanism of action of azathioprine is related to the reduction of intracellular purine synthesis, thereby inhibiting DNA replication. This leads to a decrease in circulating B and T lymphocytes and a reduction in immunoglobulin synthesis. Recent evidence also points to the ability of azathioprine metabolites to disrupt T cell activation pathways. The most common side effects at the doses used to treat rheumatic diseases are GI intolerance, bone marrow suppression, and infection, with a potential risk for malignancy in the long term. A hypersensitivity syndrome may occur in up to 5% of patients, typically manifested by rash, fever, myalgias, malaise, and GI symptoms. Mild elevation of liver enzymes can occur, but cirrhosis has not been reported.

Azathioprine has been evaluated in a multicenter randomized, controlled trial for the maintenance of remission in patients with WG and MPA.[122] Remission was induced with standard therapy (oral cyclophosphamide and glucocorticoid) in 144 of 155 patients enrolled. Upon remission, patients were randomized to receive either azathioprine 2 mg/kg per day or oral cyclophosphamide 1.5 mg/kg per day in conjunction with prednisolone 10 mg/day. At 12 months, both groups were treated with azathioprine 1.5 mg/kg per day in combination with prednisolone 7.5 mg/day. At 18 months, relapse rates were similar in both groups (azathioprine, 15.5%; cyclophosphamide, 13.7%) suggesting that the two drugs are equally efficacious for remission maintenance in WG and MPA. The adverse event rates did not differ between treatment groups, perhaps reflecting the late onset of many of the toxicities associated with cyclophosphamide. This study demonstrated that cyclophosphamide can safely be switched to azathioprine upon the induction of remission in WG.

Methotrexate

Low-dose methotrexate (MTX), such as 0.05 to 0.3 mg/kg per week, has been used to treat a variety of autoimmune diseases. MTX-related toxicity is most often mild and can be diminished by either dose reduction or temporary discontinuation of the drug. Folic or folinic acid supplementation may also reduce the incidence of certain MTX side effects, although it is unclear whether this compromises its therapeutic efficacy in RA.[131,132] Mild elevations of liver enzymes are common during MTX therapy, but cirrhosis rarely occurs with careful monitoring and in the absence of risk factors. MTX appears to be less oncogenic than cyclophosphamide. Nonetheless, reversible lymphoproliferative disorders have occurred during MTX therapy for other rheumatic diseases.[133,134] MTX is teratogenic and causes a high rate of malformation and abortion. Therefore, birth control is mandatory in females and is advised in males who are taking the drug.

MTX has been evaluated for both remission induction and remission maintenance in WG. In a prospective open-label study of 42 patients at the NIH, the sequential use of cyclophosphamide followed by MTX was effective at maintaining remission. Although 52% of patients suffered relapses at a median interval of 15 months, some while still on therapy, none of the relapses met prespecified criteria for severe disease.[135,136] Another prospective open-label study reported a relapse rate of 36.6% among 71 patients at a mean interval of 19.4 months, at which time the mean MTX dose was 18 mg/wk.[137] A limitation of this strategy is the danger of using MTX in settings of changing renal function or when the baseline value is greater than 2 mg/dL. In these situations, azathioprine is a safer option.

In an effort to find an effective and safe alternative to cyclophosphamide for the induction of remission in WG, the NIH initiated an open-label study of weekly low-dose MTX plus glucocorticoid in 42 patients with biopsy-proven WG.[138,139] Although none of the patients included in this study had immediately life-threatening disease (serum creatinine >2.5 mg/dL or acute pulmonary hemorrhage), 50% had active glomerulonephritis. Twenty-six patients (62%) had previously received treatment with a glucocorticoid, a cytotoxic agent, or both. These patients were enrolled because of either persistent or relapsing disease, serious toxicity from prior use of cytotoxic drugs, or both. Weekly administration of MTX (0.15 to 0.30 mg/kg per week) and glucocorticoid produced remission in 71% of patients after a median of 4.2 months. Nonetheless, relapses occurred in 36% after a median of 29 months. Treatment was not free of serious side effects: four patients developed *Pneumocystis carinii* pneumonia, and two of them died. This stresses the need for vigilance in monitoring for opportunistic infections, particularly in patients receiving daily steroids and a cytotoxic agent. Pneumonia prophylaxis should be standard in such patients.

A recently completed unblinded, multicenter, randomized, controlled trial compared the efficacy and safety of MTX and oral cyclophosphamide for remission induction in nonsevere WG and MPA.[140] Patients were newly diagnosed, without severe organ- or life-threatening manifestations. MTX and cyclophosphamide treatment led to similar remission rates within 6 months (89.8% and 93.5%, respectively), despite a slow escalation of the MTX dose from 15 mg/wk to 20 to 25 mg/wk over a 12-week period. However, time to remission was longer in the MTX group, particularly in those patients with more extensive disease or pulmonary involvement at baseline. Relapse occurred in 69.5% of MTX-treated patients and 46.5% of cyclophosphamide-treated patients, with a median interval from remission to relapse of 13 and 15 months, respectively. These higher than expected relapse rates may reflect the fact that treatment was discontinued in both groups at 12 months. Contrasting these results with the low relapse rates observed in the previously cited study[122] (in which immunosuppressive therapy was continued for 18 months) supports the practice of long-term continuation of maintenance therapy in WG. However, the optimal duration has yet to be determined.

Other Maintenance Therapies

Other agents that have been proposed for the maintenance of remission in WG include mycophenolate mofetil and leflunomide. Open-label studies with small numbers of patients suggest that these agents may be efficacious in preventing relapse in WG[141-143]; however, their use should be considered only if patients are either intolerant of or refractory to azathioprine and MTX.

Antimicrobial Agents

Since the original report by Wegener,[51] it has been postulated that airway stimulation is necessary for disease expression. Upper or lower airway symptoms are present at disease onset in 90% of patients.[54] Neutrophilic alveolitis and increased concentration of IgG c-ANCA in bronchoalveolar lavage fluid are seen in patients with active WG, but not in those in remission.[60,62] Most patients with WG develop respiratory tract infections at some point during the course of their disease. Secondary infection of the paranasal sinuses occurs most frequently with *S. aureus*.[70] An observational cohort study of 57 patients with biopsy-proven WG suggested that chronic nasal carriage of *S. aureus* identifies a subgroup of patients who are more prone to relapse.[144] Whether infectious organisms can induce a relapse of disease activity and whether relapses can be prevented by antibiotic prophylaxis remain the subject of speculation. A reduced rate of relapse was found in a placebo-controlled trial of trimethoprim-sulfamethoxazole (TMP-SMX) for the prevention of relapse in WG; however, this reduction was accounted for by upper airway disease alone.[145] In another prospective study in which infection was carefully ruled out and concomitant immunosuppressive therapy was unchanged for the previous 3 months, no patient had sustained improvement.[54] In a controlled trial, TMP-SMX was clearly inferior to MTX for the maintenance of remission in patients with generalized WG.[146] Because TMP-SMX seemed to increase the chance of relapse, the authors recommended against using TMP-SMX alone or TMP-SMX plus prednisone for the maintenance of remission in generalized WG.

Intravenous Immunoglobulin

Treatment with intravenous immunoglobulin (IVIG) has been used in a wide variety of autoimmune disorders, with variable results. In systemic inflammatory diseases, several mechanisms of action have been postulated and reviewed.[147] Of relevance to WG, anti-idiotypic antibodies present in IVIG preparations may bind to idiotypic determinants on pathogenic autoantibodies, downregulate B cell receptors for antigen, or bind to T cell receptors and influence their activation and regulatory properties.[147,148]

The investigational use of IVIG in the treatment of WG was prompted by the detection of anti-idiotype antibody reactivity with ANCA in IVIG preparations.[148] Several small, open trials and numerous anecdotes have been published on the use of IVIG, but Jayne and colleagues[149] recently published a small controlled trial. In this study, 17 patients were randomized to receive IVIG and 17 to receive placebo. Treatment responses were observed in 14 of 17 in the IVIG group and 6 of 17 in the placebo group, as measured by a vasculitis activity scale. This modest treatment effect was observed for only 3 months following a single infusion. Significant decreases in C-reactive protein were seen for up to 1 month in the IVIG group but then returned to pretreatment levels. No differences were observed in ANCA levels or cumulative exposure to immunosuppressive drugs. Reversible increases in serum creatinine occurred in four patients from the IVIG group. Thus, IVIG might be an alternative treatment for some forms of systemic vasculitis with persistent disease activity after standard therapy.

Tumor Necrosis Factor Inhibitors

Evidence from animal models and in vitro studies in humans suggest that TNF-α plays a prominent role in the pathogenesis of ANCA-associated vasculitis. These data, combined with encouraging results from uncontrolled studies,[150-153] provided reason for optimism that anti-TNF therapy might be a safe and effective therapy in WG. However, 180 patients with WG were enrolled in a multicenter randomized, controlled trial of etanercept versus placebo in addition to standard therapy. That study found that etanercept did not add to the efficacy of standard therapy in terms of either remission induction or remission maintenance.[121] Further, an increased rate of solid malignancy was observed in the etanercept (and cyclophosphamide) group. Although there is some reason to believe that infliximab might have greater efficacy than etanercept in the treatment of WG, the design of any future trial evaluating infliximab in this setting would require careful consideration of safety issues, including infection and malignancy. At present, anti-TNF therapy cannot be recommended for use in WG.

Rituximab

Rituximab is a chimeric mouse-human monoclonal anti-CD20 antibody that selectively depletes B cells. It has demonstrated efficacy in the treatment of RA, SLE, and other autoimmune conditions, as well as B cell non-Hodgkin's lymphoma. Rituximab has been proposed for the treatment of WG based on the role of B cells in ANCA production, antigen presentation, T cell costimulation, and proinflammatory cytokine production. A number of uncontrolled studies have suggested that rituximab may be efficacious in refractory ANCA-associated vasculitis.[154-156] However, in two of these studies, contemporaneous changes in other immunosuppressive therapies made it difficult to delineate the degree of efficacy attributable to rituximab.[154,155] Further, little benefit was achieved in another series of refractory patients with predominantly granulomatous disease manifestations.[157] A randomized, controlled trial comparing rituximab and oral cyclophosphamide for remission induction in WG is currently in progress.

Apheresis

Several small controlled trials suggest that apheresis might be of therapeutic efficacy in a subset of patients with advancing oliguric renal failure.[158] These studies are methodologically diverse, and no definitive conclusions can be drawn. A recently completed multicenter randomized, controlled study compared apheresis with intravenous methylprednisolone as add-on therapy to standard treatment with oral cyclophosphamide and glucocorticoids in patients with severe renal disease,[159] and final results are awaited. At present, apheresis in addition to standard therapy is reasonable in patients presenting with severe renal involvement with initial creatinine levels greater than 6 mg/dL who fail to respond to standard therapy.

Other Immunosuppressive Therapies

Other immunosuppressive therapies, including 15-deoxyspergualin,[160,161] antithymocyte globulin,[162] and cyclosporine[163,164] have been examined in uncontrolled studies in WG, with variable degrees of efficacy reported. Many of these agents have significant toxicities and should be considered only for cases refractory to the established treatments already discussed.

Surgical Intervention

WG is an illness that requires a multidisciplinary approach. For instance, the management of subglottic stenosis in WG is complex and often requires individualized multimodality interventions to achieve satisfactory results. To plan strategies for treatment, it is extremely important to assess whether stenosis is due to active inflammation, noninflammatory scar tissue, or both. However, systemic immunosuppressive therapy is typically ineffective for subglottic stenosis and is best avoided if there is no evidence of active disease affecting other organ systems. Patients with severe subglottic stenosis may need temporary, and sometimes permanent, tracheostomy. Laryngotracheoplasty and microvascular laryngotracheal reconstruction have been used with success in WG patients with subglottic stenosis.[73] However, it can be treated effectively by a combination of mechanical dilation and intralesional glucocorticoid injection, although the procedure may need to be repeated.[73,75] In a study of 20 patients with subglottic stenosis, this strategy led to tracheostomy reversal in 6 patients and avoidance of tracheostomy in the remainder.[75] Other reports demonstrate the sustained efficacy of this approach, with better outcomes seen in patients who had not undergone previous surgery.[165]

Patients with WG might also need tympanostomies and drainage tubes for chronic otitis media, irrigation and drainage procedures (maxillary windows, Caldwell-Luc procedure) for impacted sinuses with persistent or recurrent infections, and ocular surgery for orbital pseudotumors or nasolacrimal duct obstruction. Urgent surgical intervention may be needed in patients with severe pulmonary hemorrhage or GI vasculitis. Regardless of whether surgery is indicated, aggressive medical therapy is required to suppress active inflammatory processes and prevent further damage.

In patients with end-stage renal failure, kidney transplantation is generally successful when recipients have been in sustained remission at the time of surgical engraftment. Although disease can recur in the transplanted kidney, renal survival is comparable to that associated with other conditions leading to renal failure.[166-171]

PROGNOSIS

As discussed earlier, untreated systemic WG had a dismal prognosis, with a mean survival of approximately 5 months.[87] Monotherapy with glucocorticoids prolonged mean survival time to just over 12 months.[124] Combination therapy with oral cyclophosphamide and glucocorticoid dramatically changed the prognosis of WG, with remission anticipated in most patients and an 80% survival rate at 8 years; however, rates of adverse events and disease relapse were significant.[53,54,70] A number of strategies have been implemented to address these issues, which may explain, in part, the recent data suggesting that greater than 95% survival among 82 WG patients with a median follow-up of 4.5 years is achievable.[172] However, recent data from cohorts of patients followed in a controlled setting underline the fact that WG patients still experience significant disease- and treatment-related morbidity.[90] This provides added impetus for continued collaborative efforts to identify safer and more effective treatments for patients with WG.

MICROSCOPIC POLYANGIITIS

MPA was first recognized as a distinct entity by Davson and colleagues[173] in 1948. They described it as a subgroup of polyarteritis nodosa, distinguished by the presence of segmental necrotizing glomerulonephritis.

MPA was not included in the American College of Rheumatology classification scheme, and it is assumed that most of these patients were labeled as having polyarteritis or, less frequently, WG. The Chapel Hill international consensus criteria defined MPA as a necrotizing vasculitis with few or no deposits affecting small vessels (i.e., capillaries, venules, or arterioles)[174]; it is often associated with necrotizing glomerulonephritis and pulmonary capillaritis. MPA is occasionally referred to as *microscopic polyarteritis*, but MPA is preferred because it distinguishes the syndrome more clearly.

CLINICAL FEATURES

The general clinical features of MPA, collected from four large clinical series,[175-178] are summarized in Table 82-1 and reflect the propensity for widespread target-organ involvement. The disease tends to affect males more frequently than females, with male-to-female ratios ranging from 1.0[176] to 1.8.[177] The age of onset is generally in the fourth or fifth decade but can range from early childhood to old age.[179] The onset may be hyperacute, with rapidly progressive glomerulonephritis and pulmonary hemorrhage, presenting

as the pulmonary renal syndrome; alternatively, it can be insidious, with several years of intermittent constitutional symptoms, purpura, mild renal disease, and even periodic bouts of hemoptysis.

Renal Manifestations

The universal presence of renal disease in most large series[175-178] reflects both the common involvement of the kidney and the ascertainment bias of reporting by nephrology groups. Clearly, MPA can be seen in the absence of renal disease, although it is less common. The course of the renal disease is also variable, but a rapidly progressive course has been reported in series by nephrology groups. Dialysis has been required in 25% to 45% of patients in several large series.[175,177] The renal lesion of MPA is that of necrotizing glomerulonephritis. The characteristic features of this lesion are segmental necrosis, crescent formation (extracapillary proliferation), slight or no endocapillary proliferation, slight or no immune deposits by immunohistology, and slight or no electron-dense deposits by electron microscopy.[180] This lesion is clearly distinct from immune complex–mediated glomerulonephritis and anti–glomerular basement membrane antibody–mediated disease, but it is not distinguishable from the glomerular lesion of WG or idiopathic rapidly progressive crescentic glomerulonephritis (see Fig. 82-13).

Pulmonary Manifestations

Lung involvement is common in MPA and is present in more than half of reported cases in most series. Diffuse alveolar hemorrhage (DAH) is the most serious form of lung involvement and has been reported in 12% to 29% of patients in several series.[175-178] The clinical manifestations may range from mild dyspnea and anemia without any hemoptysis to massive hemorrhage and bleeding with profound hypoxia, but the onset is acute in most patients. The radiographic features of DAH are nonspecific, demonstrating alveolar infiltration ranging from patchy to diffuse. The characteristic finding of alveolar infiltrates in the absence of congestive heart failure or infection is helpful, but the clinical differentiation of these disorders in an acutely ill patient may be difficult. The absence of frank hemoptysis should never dissuade serious consideration of possible, even massive, DAH, because it may be absent in up to one third of patients.[181] An alternative presentation of lung involvement in MPA is that of interstitial fibrosis based on recurrent episodes of DAH. This generally occurs after a prolonged (i.e., many years) history of such events.[181]

The characteristic histopathology of MPA is pulmonary capillaritis (see Fig. 82-12). In this lesion, there is disruption of the alveolar interstitium, leading to loss of integrity of the constituent capillary network and resulting in red blood cell leakage into the alveolar spaces. The alveolar wall expands and becomes edematous and ultimately undergoes fibrinoid necrosis. Characteristically, there is prominent neutrophilic leukocytosis of the alveolar septum, often accompanied by leukocytoclasia. Immunohistology, similar to in the kidney, rarely demonstrates immune deposits. Other findings include capillary thrombosis, type II epithelial cell hyperplasia, and lymphoplasmacytic infiltration.[181] This clinical and histologic picture can be seen in a variety of conditions

Table 82-1 Clinical Features of Microscopic Polyangiitis

Clinical Feature	Percentage*
Constitutional symptoms	76-79
Fever	50-72
Renal disease	100
Arthralgias	28-65
Purpura	40-44
Pulmonary disease (hemorrhage, infiltrates, effusion)	50
Neurologic disease (central, peripheral)	28
Ear, nose, throat involvement	30

*Percentage of a population totaling 150 patients from four studies.[175-178]

and is commonly observed in WG, SLE, and in an isolated form.[181,182] When DAH occurs in an isolated form, it may be in the presence or absence of MPO-ANCA.[181]

Other Manifestations

Other clinical features of MPA are similar to the other major forms of ANCA-associated small vessel vasculitis, as well as classic polyarteritis nodosa. Arthralgia, myalgia, and fever are common (see Table 82-1). Skin involvement is common and most frequently manifests as palpable purpura. Peripheral neuropathy is observed in a minority of patients and appears to be less common than in the other ANCA-associated syndromes. Involvement of the ears, nose, and throat is infrequent and, when present, should raise the suspicion of WG, with granulomas either overlooked or missed by sampling error on biopsy.

DIAGNOSIS

The diagnosis of MPA can be problematic. There is great variability in the presenting manifestations as well as the intensity of the illness. Clearly, MPA should be considered in any patient with the general features of a systemic vasculitis, such as prolonged unexplained fever, unexplained multisystem organ involvement (especially renal and pulmonary), and palpable purpura. MPA is prominent in the differential diagnosis of pulmonary renal syndromes, along with WG, SLE, and anti–glomerular basement membrane disease.

Although the diagnosis of MPA can sometimes be based on clinical and laboratory findings, it is preferable to secure the diagnosis with histology. The most accessible and rewarding tissues are skin, kidney, and lung. It must be emphasized that in none of these organs is there a specific histopathologic picture of MPA. However, the presence of pulmonary capillaritis, necrotizing pauci-immune glomerulonephritis, or leukocytoclastic vasculitis in skin can secure the diagnosis in a patient with the appropriate degree of pretest probability and the necessary exclusions. As noted, MPO-ANCA is present in 60% to 85% of patients, but occasionally, patients may be PR3-ANCA positive. Diagnosis of MPA based solely on a positive MPO-ANCA test in a patient with low probability is fraught with risk, considering the gravity of the therapy.

DIFFERENTIAL DIAGNOSIS

Differentiating MPA from classic polyarteritis is often based on the pattern of renal disease, which differs dramatically between the two. In classic polyarteritis, the glomerulus is largely spared, and extraglomerular vascular disease (i.e., vascular nephropathy) is common. Pulmonary involvement is uncommon in classic disease, and hemorrhage is virtually never encountered. Hypertension and peripheral neuropathy are much more common in classic polyarteritis as well. From the laboratory perspective, classic polyarteritis is rarely PR3- or MPO-ANCA positive, and MPA is rarely associated with hepatitis B. Angiographically, classic polyarteritis nodosa is far more frequently associated with microaneurysms, which are rare in MPA.[183]

Differentiation from WG may be difficult because of the random nature of the granulomas in this condition. Prominent involvement of the upper respiratory tract or the presence of PR3-ANCA should raise the possibility of WG, because the occurrence of these findings are unusual, though not unheard of, in MPA.

TREATMENT AND PROGNOSIS

The treatment of MPA is based on the same therapeutic principles as those outlined for WG (see Fig. 82-4). The majority of information on the therapy and prognosis of this disorder is based on retrospective analyses of case series.[175,177,184] Most investigators agree that in the presence of serious renal or pulmonary disease, combined therapy with high-dose glucocorticoid and cyclophosphamide is indicated. A recent study by the French Vasculitis Study Group,[185] representing the longest follow-up of a cohort including MPA (88.3 months), reaffirmed that combined glucocorticoid and cyclophosphamide is beneficial, especially in severe disease. In this complex study representing a pooled analysis of four prospective trials of different therapeutic agents, there was an overall mortality of 30% throughout approximately 7 years of follow-up. Mortality, not surprisingly, was seen in those with a high incidence of renal, GI, cardiovascular, or CNS involvement. Survival rates were superior among the most severely ill patients treated with combination of glucocorticoid and cyclophosphamide versus those treated with glucocorticoid alone. There are limited data supporting a role of apheresis in those with advanced renal disease, including those who are dialysis dependent.[186,187] There are also reports of successful therapy with IVIG.[149,188] Although the rate of relapse appears to be lower in MPA than in WG,[122] careful follow-up is required, including monitoring of clinical symptoms and renal function with serial examination of the urinary sediment.

CHURG-STRAUSS SYNDROME

The syndrome defined by Churg and Strauss in 1951 has undergone several redefinitions but is still characterized by three histopathologic features: necrotizing vasculitis, infiltration by eosinophils, and extravascular granulomas.[189] Using only pathologic features to define the disease made it a diagnostic rarity. Thus, in 1984, Lanham and colleagues[190] suggested that the diagnosis be based on clinical and pathologic grounds requiring three criteria: asthma, peak eosinophil count greater than 1500 cells/mL, and systemic vasculitis involving two or more organs. In 1994, the international consensus conference held in Chapel Hill, North Carolina,[174] defined the disease as an eosinophil-rich and granulomatous inflammation involving the respiratory tract and necrotizing vasculitis involving the medium-sized vessels associated with asthma and eosinophilia. Each component of these definitions (histopathology, eosinophilia in blood and tissues, asthma) helps define the disease, but none of these features individually is specific for CSS, and not every patient has all the features. Although most cases can be clearly defined, the concept of partial or incomplete CSS remains necessary.[191]

PATHOGENESIS

The cause of CSS is unknown, but its association with allergy and atopic disorders is a dominant factor. Nearly 70% of patients have a history of allergic rhinitis, often associated with nasal polyposis; the association with asthma, usually adult onset, is part of most case definitions. Both peripheral blood and tissue eosinophilia is a major constituent of the syndrome, and the majority of patients tested have elevated IgE levels.[190] A link between the use of leukotriene receptor antagonists and CSS has been suggested,[192] but the epidemiologic link between this class of drugs and vasculitis is not proved.[193]

Some clinical and pathologic features of CSS are shared with the other ANCA-associated syndromes, suggesting a possible pathogenic role for ANCA in CSS. Arguing against such a role is the fact that up to 60% of patients with CSS in some series may be ANCA negative.[194,195] At this point, it is best to define CSS by its unique clinical and pathologic features, regardless of ANCA status.[196]

CSS has been reported to occur in asthmatics following the use of either lipoxygenase inhibitors or cysteinyl leukotriene receptor type 1 antagonists, thereby raising the concern that leukotriene inhibition might function as a causative factor.[197,198] Alternative explanations include an unmasking effect when these drugs are provided to a population with severe airway disease, followed by steroid tapering.[199] A simple unmasking effect is unlikely, however, in patients who were not on steroids or did not taper the dose of steroids before the onset of CSS. To date, there are few data to suggest causality, but it is probably prudent to avoid these agents in patients with CSS until more definitive studies become available.

CLINICAL FEATURES

CSS is thought by some observers to be characterized by three distinct phases. A prodrome, dominated by allergic features, is common in patients ultimately diagnosed with CSS. Allergic rhinitis and asthma often precede the diagnosis of vasculitis by 3 to 7 years.[190,200] It is interesting and important to note that asthma can abruptly abate as the patient moves into the vasculitic phase of the illness. Tissue infiltration by eosinophils, in the form of eosinophilic pneumonia (Löffler's syndrome) and eosinophilic gastroenteritis, may also occur in the prodrome. Because these patients may have marked constitutional symptoms and high blood eosinophilia, this stage may be difficult to distinguish from the onset of frank vasculitis on other than histologic grounds. The vasculitic

stage comes next, and the clinical picture is dependent on the distribution of target organs. Finally, the vasculitic stage abates, and allergic disease dominates the clinical picture. Clearly, not all patients exhibit a sequential staging of the illness and may present with only one or two manifestations.

The literature suggests that ANCA may influence the expression of the disease in certain organs. ANCA positivity, for example, is associated with a higher incidence of renal disease (particularly rapidly progressive glomerulonephritis), alveolar hemorrhage, mononeuritis multiplex, and purpura. In contrast, ANCA-negative patients were more likely to suffer from cardiomyopathy, nonhemorrhagic pulmonary infiltrates, nasal polyposis, and eosinophilic gastritis or enteritis.[194,195,201]

Pulmonary Manifestations

Pulmonary infiltrates may occur in the prodromal phase, vasculitic phase, or both, and their appearance is generally nonspecific. Their radiographic appearance is variable, but lobar, interstitial, and nodular patterns have all been described, with most abnormalities being fleeting in nature. Pleural effusions were reported in 27% of patients in one series[190] and are typically rich in eosinophils. Pulmonary hemorrhage is a grave complication and may occur with or without renal involvement.

Neurologic Manifestations

Peripheral neurologic involvement often dominates the clinical picture and has been reported in the majority of patients.[183,190,200] It was found in 62% of patients in one series.[190] The pattern of involvement may be that of mononeuritis multiplex or symmetric or asymmetric polyneuropathy. Less commonly, cranial neuropathy is observed.[200] CNS involvement is uncommon and tends to dominate in the latter stages of the illness.[191] Collectively, involvement of the peripheral nervous system is so common that in any patient with asthma who develops neurologic symptoms, CSS should be considered.

Renal Manifestations

Kidney involvement is less common in CSS than in MPA or WG and, when present, is rarely the cause of death. CSS shares the same renal lesion (necrotizing crescentic pauci-immune glomerulonephritis) with the other ANCA-associated diseases. A noteworthy feature of CSS is its propensity to involve the lower urinary tract, including the prostate gland.[202] We have seen extremely high levels of prostate-specific antigen in the setting of active CSS normalize during successful treatment. Such lower urinary tract involvement may lead to obstruction.

Other Manifestations

CSS may involve a wide variety of other target organs, including the skin, heart, skeletal muscle, joints, eye, and GI tract.[190] Skin involvement often leads to confusion, because Churg-Strauss granuloma may be seen in other disorders. Palpable purpura has been observed in nearly 50% of CSS patients, and the histopathology may be quite nonspecific. Alternatively, inflammatory nodules with characteristic histopathology (necrotizing vasculitis, eosinophilic infiltration, and extravascular granulomas) are less commonly encountered.[203]

GI involvement may precede the vasculitic phase or coincide with it. Diarrhea, pain, and bleeding are not uncommon. Similar to classic polyarteritis, abdominal complications may dominate.[204,205] Cardiac disease is common in postmortem series[189] and may contribute heavily to morbidity and mortality.[190] The cardiac pathology most frequently demonstrates granulomatous nodules in the epicardium, which may lead to ventricular dysfunction and congestive heart failure.[189] Coronary arteritis may also occur. Last, a variety of ocular complications have been described, including conjunctivitis, episcleritis, panuveitis, and marginal corneal ulcerations.[202]

PATHOLOGY

As noted previously, the pathologic features of CSS are necrotizing vasculitis, eosinophilic tissue infiltration, and extravascular granulomas (Fig. 82-14). Unfortunately, depending on the timing and tissue sampling, not all these features may be present.[191] Necrotizing vasculitis of small

vessels accompanied by tissue infiltration with eosinophils is not specific for CSS and may also be seen in WG and polyarteritis nodosa.[191] The extravascular Churg-Strauss granuloma, in its fully developed form, is highly specific for the condition. Its distinctive features include an eosinophilic core, which differentiates it from the basophilic granuloma (unfortunately, also referred to as Churg-Strauss granuloma), but it is frequently seen in numerous other disorders.[191]

It has also been suggested that ANCA status may influence the pathologic expression of disease. ANCA positivity is associated with necrotizing vasculitis; eosinophilic infiltrates, granulomas, and fibrosis are associated with the absence of ANCA.[194,195,201]

LABORATORY TESTS

Peripheral eosinophilia at levels in excess of 1500 cells/mm^3 often occurs in the prodromal stages of CSS, associated with rhinitis and asthma. Occasionally, patients have been described without significant blood eosinophilia but with prominent tissue eosinophilia.[206] There is no definite correlation between eosinophilia and disease activity, for eosinophils often rapidly decrease on initiation of glucocorticoid therapy.

ANCAs have been reported in about 40% of patients,[194,195] the majority of which are MPO-ANCA. A negative ANCA test should not dissuade the clinician from the diagnosis of CSS if there is a high probability.

DIAGNOSIS AND DIFFERENTIAL DIAGNOSIS

The diagnosis of CSS should be based on the documentation of necrotizing vasculitis with eosinophils occurring in a patient with adult-onset asthma or allergic rhinitis. The presence of extravascular granulomas adds to the specificity but is not essential. High-yield sites for biopsy include nerve and muscle in patients with clinical evidence of involvement at those sites.

Differentiation of CSS from WG, MPA, and classic polyarteritis nodosa is generally straightforward (Table 82-2). Significant peripheral eosinophilia is uncommon in the other conditions, although this point is often poorly appreciated; the misconception stems from early reports describing WG

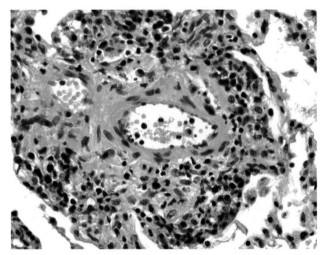

Figure 82-14 Churg-Strauss syndrome. Transmural eosinophilic infiltrate with scattered plasma cells and lymphocytes involving a small artery in the lung of a patient with Churg-Strauss syndrome (hematoxylin and eosin, ×40). *(Courtesy of Dr. C. Farver.)*

Table 82-2 Differential Diagnostic Features of the Antineutrophil Cytoplasmic Antibody–Associated Vasculitides

Feature	Wegener's Granulomatosis	Microscopic Polyangiitis	Polyarteritis Nodosa	Churg-Strauss Syndrome	Comments
Pulmonary infiltrates or nodules	+++	++	−	+++	Asthma and eosinophilia in CSS
Alveolar hemorrhage	++	++	−	+	
Glomerulonephritis	+++	+++	−	++	Progressive renal failure uncommon in CSS
Upper airway disease	+++	+	+	++	ENT disease usually favors WG
Skin, purpura	+	+++	−	++	
Peripheral nervous system involvement	++	+	++	+++	Often a prominent feature of CSS
Central nervous system involvement	+	+	+	++	

CSS, Churg-Strauss syndrome; ENT, ear, nose, and throat; WG, Wegener's granulomatosis.

that were contaminated with unrecognized CSS patients. Microaneurysms can be seen in both classic polyarteritis and CSS and thus do little to differentiate the conditions. Asthma is uncommon in polyarteritis, as is glomerulonephritis.

CSS may be difficult to differentiate from eosinophilic infiltrative diseases. Acute (Löffler's syndrome) and chronic eosinophilic pneumonia are not associated with extrapulmonary disease. Hypereosinophilic syndrome may, however, be associated with eosinophilic infiltration of numerous target organs and may be difficult to differentiate from CSS. In this disorder, there is no true vasculitis, and eosinophil counts are often much higher, possibly in excess of 100,000 cells/mm^3.

PROGNOSIS AND TREATMENT

Some investigators consider the outcome of patients with CSS to be similar to that of patients with polyarteritis nodosa, but several factors limit these observations. The largest series comparing such patient populations is, by its own admission, contaminated by patients with both the microscopic and the classic forms of polyarteritis, owing to the more recent recognition of the former.[207] Other investigators have asserted that CSS is a more benign disease.[202,208,209] The work of Guillevin and colleagues[210] has helped clarify this debate and has demonstrated that, as with polyarteritis, the outcome of patients with CSS is dependent on disease severity, which can be assessed clinically. Overall, the 5-year survival rate for patients with CSS was 78.9%, but five factors were associated with poor outcome: azotemia (creatinine level >1.58 mg/dL), proteinuria (>1 g/day), GI tract involvement, cardiomyopathy, and CNS involvement. Relative risk of death increased in the presence of these risk factors. Absence of these complications, such as disease limited to muscle and nerve, carried the best prognosis.

Therapeutic trials are limited, but they have demonstrated that both glucocorticoid alone and glucocorticoid combined with cyclophosphamide are efficacious.[211,212] Based on these data and the prognostic studies of Guillevin and colleagues, it appears reasonable to treat patients with limited disease with glucocorticoid alone and reserve combined therapy for those with immediately life-threatening or major organ–threatening disease. Patients who should be considered for combined therapy include, but are not limited to, those with any of the five prognostic factors listed earlier. The principles of such therapy are similar to those outlined for the treatment of WG.

REFERENCES

1. Jennette JC, Falk RJ: Small-vessel vasculitis. N Engl J Med 337:1512-1523, 1997.
2. Davies DJ, Moran JE, Niall JF, et al: Segmental necrotizing glomerulonephritis with antineutrophil antibody: Possible arbovirus aetiology. BMJ 285:606, 1982.
3. Hall JB, Wadham BM, Wood CJ, et al: Vasculitis and glomerulonephritis: A subgroup with an antineutrophil cytoplasmic antibody. Aust N Z J Med 14:277, 1984.
4. van der Woude FJ, Rasmussen N, Lobatto S, et al: Autoantibodies against neutrophils and monocytes: Tool for diagnosis and marker of disease activity in Wegener's granulomatosis. Lancet 1:425, 1985.
5. Bosch X, Guilabert A, Font J: Antineutrophil cytoplasmic antibodies. Lancet 368:404-418, 2006.
6. Ulmer M, Rautmann A, Gross WL: Immunodiagnostic aspects of autoantibodies against myeloperoxidase. Clin Nephrol 37:161, 1992.
7. Hoffman GS, Specks U: Antineutrophil cytoplasmic antibodies [see comment]. Arthritis Rheum 41:1521-1537, 1998.
8. Merkel PA, Polisson RP, Chang Y, et al: Prevalence of antineutrophil cytoplasmic antibodies in a large inception cohort of patients with connective tissue disease. Ann Intern Med 126:866-873, 1997.
9. Savige J, Gillis D, Benson E, et al: International consensus statement on testing and reporting of antineutrophil cytoplasmic antibodies (ANCA). Am J Clin Pathol 111:507-513, 1999.
10. Hagen EC, Daha MR, Hermans J, et al: Diagnostic value of standardized assays for anti-neutrophil cytoplasmic antibodies in idiopathic systemic vasculitis. EC/BCR Project for ANCA Assay Standardization [see comments]. Kidney Int 53:743-753, 1998.
11. Niles JL, Pan GL, Collins AB, et al: Antigen-specific radioimmunoassays for anti-neutrophil cytoplasmic antibodies in the diagnosis of rapidly progressive glomerulonephritis. J Am Soc Nephrol 2:27-36, 1991.
12. Specks U: ANCA subsets: Influence on disease phenotype. Cleve Clin J Med 69(Suppl 2):SII56-SII59, 2002.
13. Vassilopoulos D, Niles JL, Villa-Forte A, et al: Prevalence of antineutrophil cytoplasmic antibodies in patients with various pulmonary diseases or multiorgan dysfunction. Arthritis Rheum 49:151-155, 2003.
14. de Bandt M, Meyer O, Haim T, Kahn MF: Antineutrophil cytoplasmic antibodies in rheumatoid arthritis patients. Br J Rheumatol 35:38-43, 1996.
15. Rother E, Schochat T, Peter HH: Antineutrophil cytoplasmic antibodies (ANCA) in rheumatoid arthritis: A prospective study. Rheumatol Int 15:231-237, 1996.
16. Efthimiou J, Spickett G, Lane D: Antineutrophil cytoplasmic antibodies, cystic fibrosis, and infection. Lancet 337:1037, 1991.
17. Soto A, Jorgensen C, Oksman F, et al: Endocarditis associated with ANCA [see comments]. Clin Exp Rheumatol 12:203-204, 1994.
18. Abad E, Tural C, Mirapeix E, Cuxart A: Relationship between ANCA and clinical activity in inflammatory bowel disease: Variation in prevalence of ANCA and evidence of heterogeneity. J Autoimmun 10:175-180, 1997.
19. Freeman H, Roeck B, Devine D, Carter C: Prospective evaluation of neutrophil autoantibodies in 500 consecutive patients with inflammatory bowel disease. Can J Gastroenterol 11:203-207, 1997.
20. Mulder AH, Broekroelofs J, Horst G, et al: Anti-neutrophil cytoplasmic antibodies (ANCA) in inflammatory bowel disease: Characterization and clinical correlates. Clin Exp Immunol 95:490-497, 1994.
21. Gur H, Shen G, Sutjita M, et al: Autoantibody profile of primary sclerosing cholangitis. Pathobiology 63:76-82, 1995.
22. Targan SR, Landers C, Vidrich A, Czaja AJ: High-titer antineutrophil cytoplasmic antibodies in type-1 autoimmune hepatitis [see comments]. Gastroenterology 108:1159-1166, 1995.
23. Elkayam O, Yaron M, Caspi D: Minocycline induced arthritis associated with fever, livedo reticularis, and pANCA. Ann Rheum Dis 55:769-771, 1996.
24. Hoffman GS: Classification of the systemic vasculitides: Antineutrophil cytoplasmic antibodies, consensus and controversy. Clin Exp Rheumatol 16:111-115, 1998.
25. Csernok E: Anti-neutrophil cytoplasmic antibodies and pathogenesis of small vessel vasculitides. Autoimmun Rev 2:158-164, 2003.
26. Reumaux D, Duthilleul P, Roos D: Pathogenesis of diseases associated with antineutrophil cytoplasm autoantibodies. Hum Immunol 65:1-12, 2004.
27. Cid MC: New developments in the pathogenesis of systemic vasculitis. Curr Opin Rheumatol 8:1-11, 1996.
28. Csernok E, Ernst M, Schmitt W, et al: Activated neutrophils express proteinase 3 on their plasma membrane in vitro and in vivo. Clin Exp Immunol 95:244-250, 1994.
29. Falk RJ, Terrell RS, Charles LA, Jennette JC: Anti-neutrophil cytoplasmic autoantibodies induce neutrophils to degranulate and produce oxygen radicals in vitro. Proc Natl Acad Sci U S A 87:4115-4119, 1990.
30. De Bandt M, Meyer O, Hakim J, Pasquier C: Antibodies to proteinase-3 mediate expression of intercellular adhesion molecule-1 (ICAM-1, CD 54). Br J Rheumatol 36:839-846, 1997.
31. Keogan MT, Rifkin I, Ronda N, et al: Anti-neutrophil cytoplasm antibodies (ANCA) increase neutrophil adhesion to cultured human endothelium. Adv Exp Med Biol 336:115-119, 1993.

32. Ralston DR, Marsh CB, Lowe MP, et al: Antineutrophil cytoplasmic antibodies induce monocyte IL-8 release: Role of surface proteinase-3, α1-antitrypsin, and Fcγ receptors. J Clin Invest 100:1416, 1997.

33. Radford DJ, Luu NT, Hewins P, et al: Antineutrophil cytoplasmic antibodies stabilize adhesion and promote migration of flowing neutrophils on endothelial cells. Arthritis Rheum 44:2851-2861, 2001.

34. Griffin SV, Chapman PT, Lianos EA, Lockwood CM: The inhibition of myeloperoxidase by ceruloplasmin can be reversed by anti-myeloperoxidase antibodies. Kidney Int 55:917-925, 1999.

35. Brouwer E, Huitema MG, Klok PA, et al: Antimyeloperoxidase-associated proliferative glomerulonephritis: An animal model. J Exp Med 177:905, 1993.

36. Kobayashi K, Shibata T, Sugisaki T: Aggravation of rat nephrotoxic serum nephritis by anti-myeloperoxidase antibodies. Kidney Int 47:454-463, 1995.

37. Xiao H., Heeringa P., Hu P., et al: Antineutrophil cytoplasmic autoantibodies specific for myeloperoxidase cause glomerulonephritis and vasculitis in mice. J Clin Invest 110:955-963, 2002.

38. Xiao H, Heeringa P, Liu Z, et al: The role of neutrophils in the induction of glomerulonephritis by anti-myeloperoxidase antibodies. Am J Pathol 167:39-45, 2005.

39. Cohen Tervaert JW, van der Woude FJ, Fauci AS, et al: Association between active Wegener's granulomatosis and anticytoplasmic antibodies. Arch Intern Med 149:2461, 1989.

40. Jayne DR, Gaskin G, Pusey CD, Lockwood CM: ANCA and predicting relapse in systemic vasculitis. QJM 88:127-133, 1995.

41. Slot MC, Tervaert JW, Boomsma MM, Stegeman CA: Positive classic antineutrophil cytoplasmic antibody (C-ANCA) titer at switch to azathioprine therapy associated with relapse in proteinase 3-related vasculitis. Arthritis Rheum 51:269-273, 2004.

42. Tervaert JW, Stegeman CA, Kallenberg CG: Serial ANCA testing is useful in monitoring disease activity of patients with ANCA-associated vasculitides. Sarcoidosis Vasc Diffuse Lung Dis 13:241-245, 1996.

43. Charles LA, Caldas ML, Falk RJ, et al: Antibodies against granule proteins activate neutrophils in vitro. J Leukoc Biol 50:539-546, 1991.

44. Ewert BH, Becker ME, Jennette JC, et al: Antimyeloperoxidase antibodies induce neutrophil adherence to cultured human endothelial cells. Ren Fail 17:125, 1995.

45. Oseas R, Yang HH, Baehner RL, et al: Lactoferrin: A promoter of polymorphonuclear leukocyte adhesiveness. Blood 57:939, 1981.

46. Peen E, Sundqvist T, Skogh T: Leucocyte activation by anti-lactoferrin antibodies bound to vascular endothelium. Clin Exp Immunol 103:403-407, 1996.

47. Davenport A, Lock RJ, Wallington T: Clinical significance of the serial measurement of autoantibodies to neutrophil cytoplasm using a standard indirect immunofluorescence test. Am J Nephrol 15:201-207, 1995.

48. Boomsma MM, Stegeman CA, van der Leij MJ, et al: Prediction of relapses in Wegener's granulomatosis by measurement of antineutrophil cytoplasmic antibody levels: A prospective study. Arthritis Rheum 43:2025-2033, 2000.

49. Klinger H: Grenzformen der periarteritis nodosa. Frankfurt Z Pathol 42:455, 1931.

50. Wegener F: Über eine eigenartige rhinogene granulomatose mit besonderer beteiligung des arterien systems und der nieren. Beitr Pathol Anat Allg Pathol 36: 1939.

51. Wegener F: Über eine generalisierte, septische gefäberkrankungen. Verh Dtsch Pathol Ges 29:202, 1936.

52. Godman GC, Churg J: Wegener's granulomatosis: Pathology and review of the literature. Arch Pathol Lab Med 6:533, 1954.

53. Fauci AS, Wolff SM: Wegener's granulomatosis: Studies in eighteen patients and a review of the literature. Medicine 52:535, 1973.

54. Hoffman GS, Kerr GS, Leavitt RY, et al: Wegener granulomatosis: An analysis of 158 patients [see comments]. Ann Intern Med 116:488-498, 1992.

55. Cotch MF, Hoffman GS, Yerg DE, et al: The epidemiology of Wegener's granulomatosis: Estimates of the five-year period prevalence, annual mortality, and geographic disease distribution from population-based data sources. Arthritis Rheum 39:87-92, 1996.

56. Papiha SS, Murty GE, Ad'Hia A, et al: Association of Wegener's granulomatosis with HLA antigens and other genetic markers. Ann Rheum Dis 51:246, 1992.

57. Spencer SJ, Burns A, Gaskin G, et al: HLA class II specificities in vasculitis with antibodies to neutrophil cytoplasmic antigens. Kidney Int 41:1059-1063, 1992.

58. Murty GE, Mains BT, Middleton D, et al: HLA antigen frequencies and Wegener's granulomatosis. Clin Otolaryngol 16:448, 1991.

59. Falk RJ, Hogan S, Carey TS, Jennette JC: Clinical course of antineutrophil cytoplasmic autoantibody-associated glomerulonephritis and systemic vasculitis. The Glomerular Disease Collaborative Network [see comments]. Ann Intern Med 113:656-663, 1990.

60. Hoffman GS, Sechler JM, Gallin JI, et al: Bronchoalveolar lavage analysis in Wegener's granulomatosis: A method to study disease pathogenesis. Am Rev Respir Dis 143:401-407, 1991.

61. Specks U, Wheatley CL, McDonald TJ, et al: Anticytoplasmic autoantibodies in the diagnosis and follow-up of Wegener granulomatosis. Mayo Clin Proc 64:28, 1989.

62. Baltaro RJ, Hoffman GS, Sechler JM, et al: Immunoglobulin G antineutrophil cytoplasmic antibodies are produced in the respiratory tract of patients with Wegener's granulomatosis. Am Rev Respir Dis 143:275-278, 1991.

63. Csernok E, Schmitt WH, Ernst M, et al: Membrane surface proteinase 3 expression and intracytoplasmic immunoglobulin on neutrophils from patients with ANCA-associated vasculitides. Adv Exp Med Biol 336:45-50, 1993.

64. Mayet WJ, Csernok E, Szymkowiak C, et al: Human endothelial cells express proteinase 3, the target antigen of anticytoplasmic antibodies in Wegener's granulomatosis. Blood 82:1221-1229, 1993.

65. Gephardt GN, Ahmad M, Tubbs RR: Pulmonary vasculitis (Wegener's granulomatosis): Immunohistochemical study of T and B cell markers. Am J Med 74:700, 1985.

66. Travis WD, Hoffman GS, Leavitt RY, et al: Surgical pathology of the lung in Wegener's granulomatosis: Review of 87 open lung biopsies from 67 patients. Am J Surg Pathol 15:315-333, 1991.

67. Schmitt WH, Heesen C, Csernok E, et al: Elevated serum levels of soluble interleukin-2 receptor in patients with Wegener's granulomatosis: Association with disease activity. Arthritis Rheum 35:1088-1096, 1992.

68. Stegeman CA, Cohen Tervaert JW, Huitema MG, Kallenberg CG: Serum markers of T cell activation in relapses of Wegener's granulomatosis. Clin Exp Immunol 91:415-420, 1993.

69. Brouwer E, Stegeman CA, Huitema MG, et al: T cell reactivity to proteinase 3 and myeloperoxidase in patients with Wegener's granulomatosis (WG). Clin Exp Immunol 98:448-453, 1994.

70. Fauci AS, Haynes BF, Katz P, et al: Wegener's granulomatosis: Prospective clinical and therapeutic experience with 85 patients for 21 years. Ann Intern Med 98:76, 1983.

71. Murty GE: Wegener's granulomatosis: Otorhinolaryngological manifestations. Clin Otolaryngol 15:385, 1990.

72. McCaffrey TV, McDonald TJ, Facer GW, et al: Otologic manifestations of Wegener's granulomatosis. Otolaryngol Head Neck Surg 88:586, 1980.

73. Lebovics RS, Hoffman GS, Leavitt RY, et al: The management of subglottic stenosis in patients with Wegener's granulomatosis. Laryngoscope 102:1341-1345, 1992.

74. Rottem M, Fauci AS, Hallahan CW, et al: Wegener granulomatosis in children and adolescents: Clinical presentation and outcome. J Pediatr 122:26-31, 1993.

75. Langford CA, Sneller MC, Hallahan CW, et al: Clinical features and therapeutic management of subglottic stenosis in patients with Wegener's granulomatosis. Arthritis Rheum 39:1754-1760, 1996.

76. Anderson G, Coles ET, Crane M, et al: Wegener's granuloma: A series of 265 British cases seen between 1975 and 1985. A report by a sub-committee of the British Thoracic Society Research Committee. QJM 83:427, 1992.

77. Cordier JF, Valeyre D, Guillevin L, et al: Pulmonary Wegener's granulomatosis: A clinical and imaging study of 77 cases. Chest 97:906, 1990.

78. Kuhlman JE, Hruban RH, Fishman EK: Wegener granulomatosis: CT features of parenchymal lung disease. J Comput Assist Tomogr 15:948, 1991.

79. Papiris SA, Manoussakis MN, Drosos AA, et al: Imaging of thoracic Wegener's granulomatosis: The computed tomographic appearance. Am J Med 93:529, 1992.

80. George TM, Cash JM, Farver C, et al: Mediastinal mass and hilar adenopathy: Rare thoracic manifestations of Wegener's granulomatosis. Arthritis Rheum 40:1992-1997, 1997.

81. Lohrmann C, Uhl M, Kotter E, et al: Pulmonary manifestations of Wegener granulomatosis: CT findings in 57 patients and a review of the literature. Eur J Radiol 53:471-477, 2005.
82. Travis WD, Carpenter HA, Lie JT: Diffuse pulmonary hemorrhage: An uncommon manifestation of Wegener's granulomatosis. Am J Surg Pathol 11:702, 1987.
83. Rosenberg DM, Weinberger SE, Fulmer JD, et al: Functional correlates of lung involvement in Wegener's granulomatosis: Use of pulmonary function tests in staging and follow-up. Am J Med 69:387, 1980.
84. Carrington CB, Liebow AA: Limited forms of angiitis and granulomatosis of Wegener's type. Am J Med 41:497, 1966.
85. Cassan SM, Coles DT, Harrison EG: The concept of limited forms of Wegener's granulomatosis. Am J Med 49:366, 1970.
86. Horn RG, Fauci AS, Rosenthal AS, et al: Renal biopsy pathology in Wegener's granulomatosis. Am J Pathol 74:423, 1974.
87. Walton EW: Giant-cell granuloma of the respiratory tract (Wegener's granulomatosis). BMJ 2:265, 1958.
88. Harper SL, Letko E, Samson CM, et al: Wegener's granulomatosis: The relationship between ocular and systemic disease. J Rheumatol 28:1025-1032, 2001.
89. Pakrou N, Selva D, Leibovitch I: Wegener's granulomatosis: Ophthalmic manifestations and management. Semin Arthritis Rheum 35:284-292, 2006.
90. **Seo P, Min YI, Holbrook JT, et al: Damage caused by Wegener's granulomatosis and its treatment: Prospective data from the Wegener's Granulomatosis Etanercept Trial (WGET). Arthritis Rheum 52:2168-2178, 2005.**
91. **Courcoutsakis NA, Langford CA, Sneller MC, et al: Orbital involvement in Wegener granulomatosis: MR findings in 12 patients. J Comput Assist Tomogr 21:452-458, 1997.**
92. Bullen CL, Liesegang TJ, McDonald TJ, et al: Ocular complications of Wegener's granulomatosis. Ophthalmology 90:279, 1983.
93. Carlson JA, Cavaliere LF, Grant-Kels JM: Cutaneous vasculitis: Diagnosis and management. Clin Dermatol 24:414-429, 2006.
94. Noritake DT, Weiner SR, Bassett LW, et al: Rheumatic manifestations of Wegener's granulomatosis. J Rheumatol 14:949, 1987.
95. Nishino H, Rubino FA, DeRemee RA, et al: Neurological involvement in Wegener's granulomatosis: An analysis of 324 consecutive patients at the Mayo Clinic. Ann Neurol 33:4, 1993.
96. **Seror R, Mahr A, Ramanoelina J, et al: Central nervous system involvement in Wegener granulomatosis. Medicine (Baltimore) 85:54-65, 2006.**
97. Stumvoll M, Schnauder G, Overkamp D, et al: Systemic vasculitis positive for circulating anti-neutrophil cytoplasmic antibodies and with predominantly neurological presentation. Clin Invest 71:613-615, 1993.
98. Weinberger LM, Cohen ML, Remler BF, et al: Intracranial Wegener's granulomatosis. Neurology 43:1831, 1993.
99. Duna GF, Galperin C, Hoffman GS: Wegener's granulomatosis. Rheum Dis Clin North Am 21:949-986, 1995.
100. Hoffman GS, Kerr GS: Gastrointestinal Emergencies: Vasculitis and the Gut. Georg Thieme Verlag, 1990.
101. Lie JT: Vasculitis and the gut: Unwitting partners or strange bedfellows. J Rheumatol 18:647-648, 1991.
102. Hensle TW, Mitchell ME, Crooks KK, et al: Urologic manifestations of Wegener granulomatosis. Urology 12:553, 1978.
103. Hansen BJ, Hørby J, Hansen HJ: Wegener's granulomatosis in the bladder. Br J Urol 65:108, 1990.
104. Korantzopoulos P, Papaioannides D, Siogas K: The heart in Wegener's granulomatosis. Cardiology 102:7-10, 2004.
105. Grant SCD, Levy RD, Venning MC, et al: Wegener's granulomatosis and the heart. Br Heart J 71:82, 1994.
106. Meryhew NL, Bache RJ, Messner RP: Wegener's granulomatosis with acute pericardial tamponade. Arthritis Rheum 31:300, 1988.
107. Forstot JZ, Overlie PA, Neufeld GK, et al: Cardiac complications of Wegener granulomatosis: A case report of complete heart block and review of the literature. Semin Arthritis Rheum 10:148, 1980.
108. Merkel PA, Lo GH, Holbrook JT, et al: Brief communication: High incidence of venous thrombotic events among patients with Wegener granulomatosis: The Wegener's Clinical Occurrence of Thrombosis (WeCLOT) Study. Ann Intern Med 142:620-626, 2005.
109. Weidner S, Hafezi-Rachti S, Rupprecht HD: Thromboembolic events as a complication of antineutrophil cytoplasmic antibody-associated vasculitis. Arthritis Rheum 55:146-149, 2006.
110. **Bacon P.A.: Endothelial cell dysfunction in systemic vasculitis: New developments and therapeutic prospects. Curr Opin Rheumatol 17:49-55, 2005.**
111. de Leeuw K, Sanders JS, Stegeman C, et al: Accelerated atherosclerosis in patients with Wegener's granulomatosis. Ann Rheum Dis 64:753-759, 2005.
112. Kerr GS, Fleisher TA, Hallahan CW, et al: Limited prognostic value of changes in antineutrophil cytoplasmic antibody titer in patients with Wegener's granulomatosis [see comments]. Arthritis Rheum 36:365-371, 1993.
113. Colby TV, Tazelaar HD, Specks U, et al: Nasal biopsy in Wegener's granulomatosis. Hum Pathol 22:101, 1991.
114. Delbuono EA, Flint A: Diagnostic usefulness of nasal biopsy in Wegener's granulomatosis. Hum Pathol 22:107, 1991.
115. Devaney KO, Travis WD, Hoffman G, et al: Interpretation of head and neck biopsies in Wegener's granulomatosis: A pathologic study of 126 biopsies in 70 patients. Am J Surg Pathol 14:555, 1990.
116. Myers JL, Katzenstein ALA: Wegener's granulomatosis presenting with massive pulmonary hemorrhage and capillaritis. Am J Surg Pathol 11:895, 1987.
117. Yoshikawa Y, Watanabe T: Pulmonary lesions in Wegener's granulomatosis: A clinicopathologic study of 22 autopsy cases. Hum Pathol 17:401, 1986.
118. Travis WD, Colby TV, Lombard C, Carpenter HA: A clinicopathologic study of 34 cases of diffuse pulmonary hemorrhage with lung biopsy confirmation. Am J Surg Pathol 14:1112, 1990.
119. Andrassy K, Erb A, Koderisch J, et al: Wegener's granulomatosis with renal involvement: Patient survival and correlations between initial renal function, renal histology, therapy and renal outcome. Clin Nephrol 35:139, 1991.
120. Fauci AS: Alternate-day corticosteroid therapy. Am J Med 64:729, 1978.
121. **Etanercept plus standard therapy for Wegener's granulomatosis. N Engl J Med 352:351-361, 2005.**
122. **Jayne D, Rasmussen N, Andrassy K, et al: A randomized trial of maintenance therapy for vasculitis associated with antineutrophil cytoplasmic autoantibodies. N Engl J Med 349:36-44, 2003.**
123. Regan MJ, Hellmann DB, Stone JH: Treatment of Wegener's granulomatosis. Rheum Dis Clin North Am 27:863-886, 2001.
124. Hollander D, Manning RT: The use of alkylating agents in the treatment of Wegener's granulomatosis. Ann Intern Med 67:393, 1967.
125. Talar-Williams C, Hijazi YM, Walther MM, et al: Cyclophosphamide-induced cystitis and bladder cancer in patients with Wegener granulomatosis. Ann Intern Med 124:477-484, 1996.
126. Haubitz M, Bohnenstengel F, Brunkhorst R, et al: Cyclophosphamide pharmacokinetics and dose requirements in patients with renal insufficiency. Kidney Int 61:1495-1501, 2002.
127. Guillevin L, Cordier J, Lhote F, et al: A prospective, multicenter, randomized trial comparing steroids and pulse cyclophosphamide versus steroids and oral cyclophosphamide in the treatment of generalized Wegener's granulomatosis. Arthritis Rheum 40:2187, 1997.
128. Haubitz M, Schellong S, Gobel U, et al: Intravenous pulse administration of cyclophosphamide versus daily oral treatment in patients with antineutrophil cytoplasmic antibody-associated vasculitis and renal involvement: A prospective, randomized study. Arthritis Rheum 41:1835-1844, 1998.
129. Richmond R, McMillan TW, Luqmani RA: Optimisation of cyclophosphamide therapy in systemic vasculitis. Clin Pharmacokinet 34:79-90, 1998.
130. Clunie GP, Lennard L: Relevance of thiopurine methyltransferase status in rheumatology patients receiving azathioprine. Rheumatology (Oxford) 43:13-18, 2004.
131. Whittle SL, Hughes RA: Folate supplementation and methotrexate treatment in rheumatoid arthritis: A review. Rheumatology (Oxford) 43:267-271, 2004.
132. Khanna D, Park GS, Paulus HE, et al: Reduction of the efficacy of methotrexate by the use of folic acid: Post hoc analysis from two randomized controlled studies. Arthritis Rheum 52:3030-3038, 2005.
133. Georgescu L, Quinn GC, Schwartzman S, Paget SA: Lymphoma in patients with rheumatoid arthritis: Association with the disease state or methotrexate treatment. Semin Arthritis Rheum 26:794-804, 1997.
134. Mariette X, Cazals-Hatem D, Warszawki J, et al: Lymphomas in rheumatoid arthritis patients treated with methotrexate: A 3-year prospective study in France. Blood 99:3909-3915, 2002.

135. Langford CA, Talar-Williams C, Barron KS, Sneller MC: Use of a cyclophosphamide-induction methotrexate-maintenance regimen for the treatment of Wegener's granulomatosis: Extended follow-up and rate of relapse. Am J Med 114:463-469, 2003.

136. Langford CA, Talar-Williams C, Barron KS, Sneller MC: A staged approach to the treatment of Wegener's granulomatosis: Induction of remission with glucocorticoids and daily cyclophosphamide switching to methotrexate for remission maintenance. Arthritis Rheum 42:2666-2673, 1999.

137. Reinhold-Keller E, Fink CO, Herlyn K, et al: High rate of renal relapse in 71 patients with Wegener's granulomatosis under maintenance of remission with low-dose methotrexate. Arthritis Rheum 47:326-332, 2002.

138. Langford CA, Talar-Williams C, Sneller MC: Use of methotrexate and glucocorticoids in the treatment of Wegener's granulomatosis: Long-term renal outcome in patients with glomerulonephritis. Arthritis Rheum 43:1836-1840, 2000.

139. Sneller MC, Hoffman GS, Talar-Williams C, et al: An analysis of forty-two Wegener's granulomatosis patients treated with methotrexate and prednisone. Arthritis Rheum 38:608-613, 1995.

140. De Groot K, Rasmussen N, Bacon PA, et al: Randomized trial of cyclophosphamide versus methotrexate for induction of remission in early systemic antineutrophil cytoplasmic antibody-associated vasculitis. Arthritis Rheum 52:2461-2469, 2005.

141. Langford CA, Talar-Williams C, Sneller MC: Mycophenolate mofetil for remission maintenance in the treatment of Wegener's granulomatosis. Arthritis Rheum 51:278-283, 2004.

142. Metzler C, Fink C, Lamprecht P, et al: Maintenance of remission with leflunomide in Wegener's granulomatosis. Rheumatology (Oxford) 43:315-320, 2004.

143. Nowack R, Gobel U, Klooker P, et al: Mycophenolate mofetil for maintenance therapy of Wegener's granulomatosis and microscopic polyangiitis: A pilot study in 11 patients with renal involvement. J Am Soc Nephrol 10:1965-1971, 1999.

144. Stegeman CA, Tervaert JW, Sluiter WJ, et al: Association of chronic nasal carriage of Staphylococcus aureus and higher relapse rates in Wegener granulomatosis [see comments]. Ann Intern Med 120:12-17, 1994.

145. Stegeman CA, Tervaert JW, de Jong PE, Kallenberg CG: Trimethoprim-sulfamethoxazole (co-trimoxazole) for the prevention of relapses of Wegener's granulomatosis. Dutch Co-Trimoxazole Wegener Study Group [see comments]. N Engl J Med 335:16-20, 1996.

146. de Groot K, Reinhold-Keller E, Tatsis E, et al: Therapy for the maintenance of remission in sixty-five patients with generalized Wegener's granulomatosis: Methotrexate versus trimethoprim/sulfamethoxazole. Arthritis Rheum 39:2052, 1996.

147. Ronda N, Hurez V, Kazatchkine MD: Intravenous immunoglobulin therapy of autoimmune and systemic inflammatory diseases. Vox Sang 64:65, 1993.

148. Rossi F, Jayne DR, Lockwood CM, Kazatchkine MD: Anti-idiotypes against anti-neutrophil cytoplasmic antigen autoantibodies in normal human polyspecific IgG for therapeutic use and in the remission sera of patients with systemic vasculitis. Clin Exp Immunol 83:298-303, 1991.

149. Jayne DR, Chapel H, Adu D, et al: Intravenous immunoglobulin for ANCA-associated systemic vasculitis with persistent disease activity. QJM 93:433-439, 2000.

150. Bartolucci P, Ramanoelina J, Cohen P, et al: Efficacy of the anti-TNF-alpha antibody infliximab against refractory systemic vasculitides: An open pilot study on 10 patients. Rheumatology (Oxford) 41:1126-1132, 2002.

151. Booth A, Harper L, Hammad T, et al: Prospective study of TNF-alpha blockade with infliximab in anti-neutrophil cytoplasmic antibody-associated systemic vasculitis. J Am Soc Nephrol 15:717-721, 2004.

152. Booth AD, Jefferson HJ, Ayliffe W, et al: Safety and efficacy of TNF-alpha blockade in relapsing vasculitis. Ann Rheum Dis 61:559, 2002.

153. Lamprecht P, Voswinkel J, Lilienthal T, et al: Effectiveness of TNF-alpha blockade with infliximab in refractory Wegener's granulomatosis. Rheumatology (Oxford) 41:1303-1307, 2002.

154. Eriksson P: Nine patients with anti-neutrophil cytoplasmic antibody-positive vasculitis successfully treated with rituximab. J Intern Med 257:540-548, 2005.

155. Keogh KA, Wylam ME, Stone JH, Specks U: Induction of remission by B lymphocyte depletion in eleven patients with refractory antineutrophil cytoplasmic antibody-associated vasculitis [see comments]. Arthritis Rheum 52:262-268, 2005.

156. Keogh KA, Ytterberg SR, Fervenza FC, et al: Rituximab for refractory Wegener's granulomatosis: Report of a prospective, open-label pilot trial. Am J Respir Crit Care Med 173:180-187, 2006.

157. Aries PM, Hellmich B, Voswinkel J, et al: Lack of efficacy of rituximab in Wegener's granulomatosis with refractory granulomatous manifestations. Ann Rheum Dis 65:853-858, 2006.

158. Klemmer PJ, Chalermskulrat W, Reif MS, et al: Plasmapheresis therapy for diffuse alveolar hemorrhage in patients with small-vessel vasculitis. Am J Kidney Dis 42:1149-1153, 2003.

159. Watts R, Harper L, Jayne D, et al: Translational research in autoimmunity: Aims of therapy in vasculitis. Rheumatology (Oxford) 44:573-576, 2005.

160. Birck R, Warnatz K, Lorenz HM, et al: 15-Deoxyspergualin in patients with refractory ANCA-associated systemic vasculitis: A six-month open-label trial to evaluate safety and efficacy. J Am Soc Nephrol 14:440-447, 2003.

161. Schmitt WH, Birck R, Heinzel PA, et al: Prolonged treatment of refractory Wegener's granulomatosis with 15-deoxyspergualin: An open study in seven patients. Nephrol Dial Transplant 20:1083-1092, 2005.

162. Schmitt WH, Hagen EC, Neumann I, et al: Treatment of refractory Wegener's granulomatosis with antithymocyte globulin (ATG): An open study in 15 patients. Kidney Int 65:1440-1448, 2004.

163. Allen NB, Caldwell DS, Rice JR, McCallum RM: Cyclosporin A therapy for Wegener's granulomatosis. Adv Exp Med Biol 336:473-476, 1993.

164. Haubitz M, Koch KM, Brunkhorst R: Cyclosporin for the prevention of disease reactivation in relapsing ANCA-associated vasculitis. Nephrol Dial Transplant 13:2074-2076, 1998.

165. Hoffman GS, Thomas-Golbanov CK, Chan J, et al: Treatment of subglottic stenosis, due to Wegener's granulomatosis, with intralesional corticosteroids and dilation. J Rheumatol 30:1017-1021, 2003.

166. Briggs JD, Jones E: Renal transplantation for uncommon diseases. Scientific Advisory Board of the ERA-EDTA Registry. European Renal Association-European Dialysis and Transplant Association. Nephrol Dial Transplant 14:570-575, 1999.

167. Deegens JK, Artz MA, Hoitsma AJ, Wetzels JF: Outcome of renal transplantation in patients with pauci-immune small vessel vasculitis or anti-GBM disease. Clin Nephrol 59:1-9, 2003.

168. Elmedhem A, Adu D, Savage CO: Relapse rate and outcome of ANCA-associated small vessel vasculitis after transplantation. Nephrol Dial Transplant 18:1001-1004, 2003.

169. Haubitz M, Kliem V, Koch KM, et al: Renal transplantation for patients with autoimmune diseases: Single-center experience with 42 patients. Transplantation 63:1251-1257, 1997.

170. Nachman PH, Segelmark M, Westman K, et al: Recurrent ANCA-associated small vessel vasculitis after transplantation: A pooled analysis. Kidney Int 56:1544-1550, 1999.

171. Wrenger E, Pirsch JD, Cangro CB, et al: Single-center experience with renal transplantation in patients with Wegener's granulomatosis. Transpl Int 10:152-156, 1997.

172. Villa-Forte A, Clark TM, Mascha E, et al: Wegener's granulomatosis: Customized treatment using cyclophosphamide and methotrexate. A 12 year single-practice experience. Arthritis Rheum 54:S495, 2006.

173. Davson J, Ball J, Platt R: The kidney in periarteritis nodosa. QJM 17:175, 1948.

174. Jennette JC, Falk RJ, Andrassy K, et al: Nomenclature of systemic vasculitides: Proposal of an international consensus conference. Arthritis Rheum 37:187-192, 1994.

175. Adu D, Howie AJ, Scott DGI, et al: Polyarteritis and the kidney. QJM 62:221, 1987.

176. D'Agati V, Chander P, Nash M, et al: Idiopathic microscopic polyarteritis nodosa: Ultrastructural observations on the renal vascular and glomerular lesions. Am J Kidney Dis 7:95, 1986.

177. Savage COS, Winearls CG, Evans DJ, et al: Microscopic polyarteritis: Presentation, pathology and prognosis. QJM 56:467, 1985.

178. Serra A, Cameron JS, Turner M, et al: Vasculitis affecting the kidney: Presentation, histopathology and long-term outcome. QJM 53:181, 1984.

179. Lhote F, Cohen P, Guillevin L: Polyarteritis nodosa, microscopic polyangiitis and Churg-Strauss syndrome. Lupus 7:238-258, 1998.

180. Rosen S, Falk RJ, Jennette JC: Polyarteritis Nodosa Including Microscopic Form and Renal Vasculitis. New York, Igaku-Shoin, 1991.
181. Schwarz MI: The nongranulomatous vasculitides of the lung. Semin Respir Crit Care Med 19:47, 1998.
182. Jennings CA, King TE Jr: Diffuse alveolar hemorrhage with underlying isolated pauci-immune pulmonary capillaritis. Am J Respir Crit Care Med 155:1101, 1997.
183. Guillevin L, Lhote F, Amouroux J, et al: Antineutrophil cytoplasmic antibodies, abnormal angiograms and pathological findings in polyarteritis nodosa and Churg-Strauss syndrome: Indications for the classification of vasculitides of the polyarteritis nodosa group. Br J Rheumatol 35:958-964, 1996.
184. Rodgers H, Gutherie JA, Brownjohn AM, et al: Microscopic polyarteritis: Clinical features and treatment. Postgrad Med J 65:515, 1989.
185. **Gayraud M, Guillevin L, le Toumelin P, et al: Long-term followup of polyarteritis nodosa, microscopic polyangiitis, and Churg-Strauss syndrome: Analysis of four prospective trials including 278 patients. Arthritis Rheum 44:666-675, 2001.**
186. Hasegawa M, Kawamura N, Murase M, et al: Efficacy of granulocytapheresis and leukocytapheresis for the treatment of microscopic polyangiitis. Ther Apher Dial 8:212-216, 2004.
187. Pusey CD, Rees AJ, Evans DJ, et al: Plasma exchange in focal necrotizing glomerulonephritis without anti-GBM antibodies. Kidney Int 40:757, 1991.
188. Jayne DRW: Intravenous immunoglobulins in the therapy of systemic vasculitis. Transfus Sci 13:317, 1992.
189. Churg J, Strauss L: Allergic granulomatosis, allergic angiitis and periarteritis nodosa. Am J Pathol 27:277, 1951.
190. Lanham JG, Elkon KB, Pusey CD, et al: Systemic vasculitis with asthma and eosinophilia: A clinical approach to the Churg-Strauss syndrome. Medicine 63:65, 1984.
191. Lanham JG, Churg J: Churg-Strauss Syndrome. New York, Igaku Shoin, 1991.
192. Wechsler ME, Garpestad E, Flier SR, et al: Pulmonary infiltrates, eosinophilia and cardiomyopathy following corticosteroid withdrawal in patient with asthma receiving zafirlukast. JAMA 279:455, 1998.
193. Keogh KA, Specks U: Churg-Strauss syndrome. Semin Respir Crit Care Med 27:148-157, 2006.
194. **Sable-Fourtassou R, Cohen P, Mahr A, et al: Antineutrophil cytoplasmic antibodies and the Churg-Strauss syndrome. Ann Intern Med 143:632-638, 2005.**
195. Sinico RA, Di Toma L, Maggiore U, et al: Prevalence and clinical significance of antineutrophil cytoplasmic antibodies in Churg-Strauss syndrome. Arthritis Rheum 52:2926-2935, 2005.
196. Hoffman GS, Langford CA: Are there different forms of life in the antineutrophil cytoplasmic antibody universe? Ann Intern Med 143:683-685, 2005.
197. Bielory L, Gewirtz M, Hinrichs C, Lal P: Asthma and vasculitis: Controversial association with leukotriene antagonists. Ann Allergy Asthma Immunol 87:274-282, 2001.
198. Jamaleddine G, Diab K, Tabbarah Z, et al: Leukotriene antagonists and the Churg-Strauss syndrome. Semin Arthritis Rheum 31:218-227, 2002.
199. Weller PF, Plaut M, Taggart V, Trontell A: The relationship of asthma therapy and Churg-Strauss syndrome: NIH workshop summary report. J Allergy Clin Immunol 108:175-183, 2001.
200. Sehgal M, Swanson JW, DeRemee RA, et al: Neurologic manifestations of Churg-Strauss syndrome. Mayo Clin Proc 70:337, 1995.
201. Kallenberg CG: Churg-Strauss syndrome: Just one disease entity? Arthritis Rheum 52:2589-2593, 2005.
202. Chumbley LC, Harrison EG, DeRemee RA: Allergic granulomatosis and angiitis (Churg-Strauss syndrome). Mayo Clin Proc 52:477, 1977.
203. Crotty CP, DeRemee RA, Winkelmann RK: Cutaneous clinicopathologic correlation of allergic granulomatosis. J Am Acad Dermatol 5:571, 1981.
204. Guillevin L, Cohen P, Gayraud M, et al: Churg-Strauss syndrome: Clinical study and long-term follow-up of 96 patients. Medicine (Baltimore) 78:26-37, 1999.
205. Pagnoux C, Mahr A, Cohen P, Guillevin L: Presentation and outcome of gastrointestinal involvement in systemic necrotizing vasculitides: Analysis of 62 patients with polyarteritis nodosa, microscopic polyangiitis, Wegener granulomatosis, Churg-Strauss syndrome, or rheumatoid arthritis-associated vasculitis. Medicine (Baltimore) 84:115-128, 2005.
206. Shields CL, Shields JA, Rozanski TI: Conjunctival involvement in Churg-Strauss syndrome. Am J Ophthalmol 102:601, 1986.
207. Guillevin L, Le THD, Godeau P, et al: Clinical findings and prognosis of polyarteritis nodosa and Churg-Strauss angiitis: A study in 165 patients. Br J Rheumatol 27:258, 1988.
208. Cohen R, Conn D, Ilstrup D: Clinical features, prognosis and response to treatment in polyarteritis. Mayo Clin Proc 55:146, 1980.
209. Finan MC, Winkelmann RK: The cutaneous extravascular necrotizing granuloma (Churg-Strauss granuloma) and systemic disease: A review of 27 cases. Medicine 62:142, 1983.
210. Guillevin L, Lhote F, Gayraud M, et al: Prognostic factors in polyarteritis nodosa and Churg-Strauss syndrome: A prospective study in 342 patients. Medicine (Baltimore) 75:17-28, 1996.
211. Guillevin L, Gain O, Lhote F, et al: Lack of superiority of steroids plus plasma exchange to steroids alone in the treatment of polyarteritis nodosa and Churg-Strauss syndrome: A prospective, randomized trial in 78 patients. Arthritis Rheum 35:208, 1992.
212. Guillevin L, Jarrousse B, Lok C, et al: Longterm followup after treatment of polyarteritis nodosa and Churg-Strauss angiitis with comparison of steroids, plasma exchange and cytophosphamide to steroids and plasma exchange: A prospective randomized trial of 71 patients. J Rheumatol 18:567, 1991.

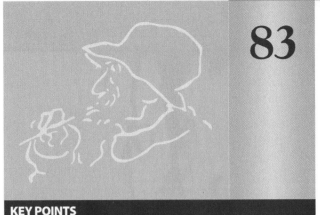

83

Polyarteritis and Related Disorders

JOHN S. SERGENT

KEY POINTS

Although in the past the term *polyarteritis* often was used in a generic sense to cover many types of vasculitis, today the term is used to describe an illness characterized by vasculitis of medium-sized arteries with few or no immune deposits. By that definition, polyarteritis nodosa (PAN) is a rare disease, although its actual incidence and prevalence are uncertain.

The typical patient is a man (male-to-female ratio approximately 2:1) in the fifth or sixth decade who presents with an insidious illness over several weeks or months.

The most common and characteristic features of PAN include purpuric skin lesions, mononeuritis multiplex, symptoms of mesenteric ischemia, and renal involvement.

Renal disease in PAN usually is manifested by hypertension and mild proteinuria with or without azotemia.

Occasional patients may have PAN limited entirely to the skin, known as cutaneous PAN. Most of these patients do not develop systemic disease.

Buerger's disease, also known as thromboangiitis obliterans, was previously thought of as a disease of men that began in the lower extremities, but today is increasingly recognized as a disease of both sexes and of the upper and lower extremities.

In addition to digital ischemia, superficial phlebitis, often migratory, may be a presenting manifestation.

The role of tobacco use in Buerger's disease is not understood, but the only effective treatment of the disease is total abstention from all tobacco exposure. Even so, many patients still require multiple amputations over time.

POLYARTERITIS NODOSA

Polyarteritis nodosa (PAN) is a necrotizing vasculitis of medium-sized arteries. Immune deposits are minimal or absent. Test results for antineutrophil cytoplasmic antibodies (ANCAs) are typically negative.

PAN has undergone an impressive change in its definition. For many years, the term was used in a generic sense to include most cases of generalized vasculitis, but as understanding improved, the definitions became more specific. What was formerly "PAN complicating rheumatoid arthritis" is now termed *rheumatoid vasculitis*, and most cases of "polyarteritis nodosa with lung involvement" are now termed *Churg-Strauss vasculitis*.

The most important shift in thinking about PAN came about with the finding that patients with microscopic PAN have ANCAs directed against myeloperoxidase (MPO). This disease is much more common than classic PAN of medium-sized arteries (see Chapter 82), and as a result of the separation of the two, PAN, as currently defined, is a rare disease. In my experience, it accounts for less than 5% of all cases of systemic vasculitis and is severalfold less common than Wegener's granulomatosis, although the actual incidence is unknown.

Patients with classic PAN can be any age, including children, but the peak onset is in the fifth or sixth decade. There is approximately a 2:1 male-to-female preponderance in most studies.[1] There are reports of polyarteritis that follow infections[2-7]; vaccination[8,9]; serous otitis media[10]; and the use of various drugs, especially amphetamines,[11] minocycline,[12,13] and interferon.[14] No etiology is apparent in most cases. It is possible that some of the associations mentioned could be random events, or that PAN already was present before the exposure. Hepatitis B has been strongly linked to polyarteritis and is discussed separately later.

Onset may be abrupt and catastrophic, but the typical patient has a period of weeks or months of systemic symptoms, including fever, abdominal pain, weight loss, and arthralgias. During this period the diagnosis is usually not apparent, and individuals are often treated for presumed diagnoses ranging from infections to systemic juvenile rheumatoid arthritis. In this setting, sudden events may occur, such as intestinal ischemia, digital gangrene, ischemic skin ulcers, infarction of a kidney or other major organ, or sudden loss of multiple nerves (mononeuritis multiplex). Table 83-1 shows the estimated frequency of various findings in PAN; virtually all are due to ischemia of the area involved.

PATHOLOGY

PAN is a patchy disease, with areas of impressive necrosis and inflammation interspersed with unaffected vessels (Fig. 83-1).[14-16] There is a propensity for aneurysm formation, especially in the mesenteric circulation. Other target organs include the kidney, the peripheral nerves, and the heart. There is strong correlation between the amount of fibrinoid necrosis and the number of neutrophils in the vessel wall and surrounding tissues.[16,17]

Because of this irregular distribution, obtaining a diagnostic biopsy specimen can be difficult. If purpura is present, a skin biopsy may be diagnostic, although a generous sample may be required. Punch biopsy may show only hemorrhage and nonspecific inflammation. In individuals with few or no localizing findings but in whom PAN is highly suspected, "blind" muscle biopsy is often performed, although about half the patients later shown to have PAN have a negative biopsy finding.

Table 83-1 Selected Clinical Manifestations of Polyarteritis Nodosa

Clinical Feature	Frequency (%)
Muscle pain or weakness	69
Weight loss	67
Mononeuritis multiplex	42
Polyneuropathy	36
Azotemia	40
Hypertension	37
Testicular pain	29
Skin ulcers or infarcts	27
Livedo reticularis	25

From Lightfoot RW, Michel BA, Bloch DA, et al: The American College of Rheumatology 1990 criteria for the classification of polyarteritis nodosa. Arthritis Rheum 33:1088, 1990.

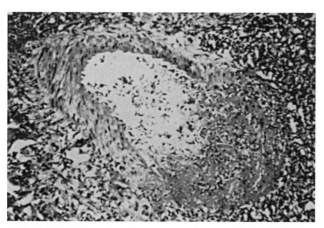

Figure 83-1 Polyarteritis. Right lower portion of arterial wall shows fibrinoid necrosis and formation of a "microaneurysm." Intense infiltration of leukocytes is present in and around the artery wall. (Hematoxylin and eosin, ×40.) *(Courtesy of Dr. J. T. Lie.)*

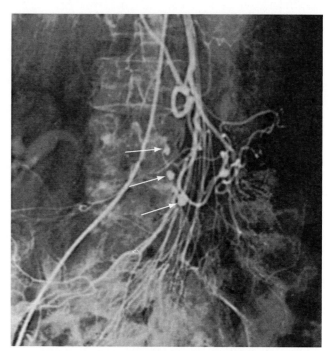

Figure 83-2 Superior mesenteric arteriogram in a patient with polyarteritis. Several small aneurysms *(arrows)* are present in branches of the superior mesenteric artery. *(Courtesy of Dr. A. W. Stanson.)*

Mesenteric arteriography showing widespread aneurysms[18] is an impressive diagnostic finding (Fig. 83-2). Mesenteric arteriography is probably the procedure of choice in patients with significant abdominal pain.

Probably the most popular biopsy site today is the sural nerve.[19] In patients with neuropathy, especially if sural nerve conduction is abnormal, the biopsy finding is positive more than 80% of the time. Other areas in which biopsy is occasionally performed include the testicle, especially if it is painful or if a mass is palpable, and the kidney.

Laboratory findings in PAN are nonspecific. Anemia and leukocytosis are typical, and almost all patients have an elevated erythrocyte sedimentation rate (ESR). Evidence of mild liver dysfunction, such as an elevated alkaline phosphatase, may be seen. There are no specific serologic findings, and ANCAs are absent, almost by definition (see Chapter 82).

SYSTEMS INVOLVED IN POLYARTERITIS NODOSA

Cutaneous manifestations occur in one third of patients, usually seen as areas of palpable purpura, sometimes with ulceration (Fig. 83-3). Frequent sites include the fingers, the ankles around the malleoli, and the pretibial areas. In severe

cases, there may be widespread digital cyanosis secondary to ischemia. Splinter hemorrhages and livedo reticularis (Fig. 83-4) also are commonly observed.[20]

Hypertension, owing to arteritis in the renal circulation, is present in approximately one third of cases and is occasionally severe. New-onset hypertension in a patient with systemic symptoms, such as fever, weight loss, and joint pain, should be a clue that vasculitis, specifically PAN, may be present.

The term *mononeuritis multiplex* is applied to the widespread development of neuropathy involving large, mixed motor and sensory nerves. The loss of each involved nerve may be sudden, although many patients describe paresthesias or weakness of the involved area before the total loss of nerve function. Frequently affected nerves include the peroneal, median, ulnar, and sural nerves.[21] The nerve injury is

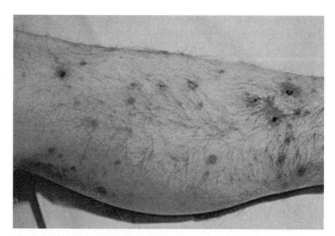

Figure 83-3 Polyarteritis involving the skin. Sharply circumscribed skin infarcts are 1 to 1.5 cm in diameter and are in various stages of healing.

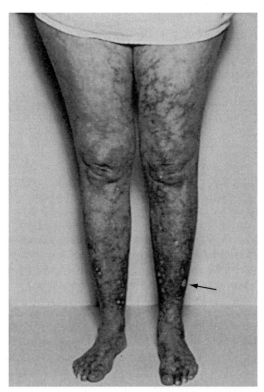

Figure 83-4 Polyarteritis involving the skin of the legs. Livedo reticularis is most prominent over the left anterior region of the thigh, but also is visible over the right thigh, legs below knees, and dorsa of feet. Petechiae and ulcers (arrow) are present on anterior and medial portions of the lower legs.

Table 83-2 Prednisone Therapy in Polyarteritis Nodosa

Disease control (4-8 wk)	Administer prednisone, 1 mg/kg/day in divided doses
Consolidation (1 mo)	Gradually change to a single daily dose, 1 mg/kg/day
Rapid tapering (1-2 mo)	Decrease by 5-10 mg every 2-4 wk, observing closely, until dose is 15-20 mg/day
Slow tapering (1-2 mo)	Decrease dose in increments of 1-2 mg/day at intervals of 1-2 wk, continuing close observation

due to ischemia and eventual infarction. The nerve injuries may progress in an asymmetric manner over days to weeks and are a major cause of long-term morbidity. Less often, a slowly progressive sensory neuropathy in a stocking-glove distribution develops.

Abdominal pain, owing to mesenteric vasculitis, is usually dull and constant, but it is often worsened by eating. Some patients exhibit classic findings of mesenteric ischemia, including food avoidance and rapid weight loss. Mesenteric infarction and bowel perforation are infrequent but catastrophic manifestations.

The liver is frequently involved at autopsy, but clinical involvement is uncommon. Occasional patients present with appendiceal or biliary tract involvement, usually cholecystitis, and there are reports of spontaneous splenic rupture as a complication of rupture of vasculitic aneurysms.

The testicle also is a frequent site of involvement in autopsy series, and testicular pain is occasionally seen. In addition, in a few patients, the diagnosis was made from prostatic tissue after presentation with symptoms of prostatic hypertrophy or prostatitis.

Kidney involvement usually manifests only as hypertension, often with mild-to-moderate azotemia. There is no glomerulitis, and the urinalysis usually shows only moderate proteinuria with modest hematuria, or the sediment may be entirely normal. Occasional patients have sudden severe flank pain, however, as a result of renal infarction or spontaneous rupture of intrarenal aneurysms, a life-threatening event.[22]

The musculoskeletal symptoms of PAN are typically nonspecific, with widespread arthralgias and myalgias. Joint pain is occasionally severe and debilitating, although signs of frank arthritis are uncommon.

COURSE

Without treatment, PAN is probably nearly universally fatal, although because of changing definitions, new serologic tests, and the universal treatment of patients in this era, the true natural history is unknown. It is highly probable, however, that most patients would die within 1 to 2 years if left untreated.

THERAPY

Although occasional patients seem to have limited disease that remains stable with minimal therapy, the risk of major organ involvement necessitates aggressive therapy in nearly all patients after the diagnosis is made. Treatment consists of prednisone, 1 mg/kg/day in divided doses, and, in most cases, an additional agent, usually a cytotoxic drug.

The prednisone dose should be maintained until the patient is clinically stable with no evidence of ongoing active disease. The precise method of steroid reduction is a matter open to individual variation and interpretation; a typical regimen is outlined in Table 83-2.

Although there are no studies comparing corticosteroids alone with corticosteroids with a second drug, virtually all rheumatologists would add a second drug to corticosteroids if major organs are threatened, or if the prednisone dose required to suppress disease activity is regarded as unacceptably high. Guillevin and coworkers[23] have described five prognostic factors that predict a high probability of mortality and are considered indications for another immunosuppressive drug in addition to prednisone: (1) proteinuria greater than 1 g/day, (2) azotemia, (3) cardiomyopathy, (4) gastrointestinal involvement, and (5) central nervous system disease. With none of these factors, 5-year mortality is 12%. With two or more, 5-year mortality is 46%.

Cyclophosphamide has been the drug of choice of Fauci and coworkers[24] at the National Institutes of Health. Many physicians regard the diagnosis of PAN as an indication for cyclophosphamide therapy. Alternatives to cyclophosphamide are chlorambucil, azathioprine, methotrexate, dapsone, cyclosporine, plasma exchange, and others.[25-28]

Table 83-3 Treatment of Polyarteritis Nodosa

Drug	Dose	Comment
Oral prednisone	1 mg/kg/day	Mainstay of therapy
Methylprednisolone	1 g/day for 3-5 days	Used in fulminant disease
Cyclophosphamide	2-4 mg/kg/day orally	Used with major organ involvement or inability to withdraw steroids
Cyclophosphamide	10-15 mg/kg/mo intravenously	Alternative to oral therapy, less toxic
Chlorambucil	0.1 mg/kg/day	Alternative to cyclophosphamide
Azathioprine	2-4 mg/kg/day	Less toxic and possibly less effective than cyclophosphamide
Methotrexate	15-25 mg orally weekly	Less effective, but often used after 1-2 yr of therapy with more potent agents
Plasmapheresis		No proven benefit
Intravenous immunoglobulin		Proven benefit in vasculitis caused by parvovirus B19; may benefit others
Monoclonal antibody		Limited experience
Interferon alfa		Used in vasculitis secondary to hepatitis B
Immunoadsorption[27]		Investigational

Alkylating agents work quickly and are regarded as the agent of choice for seriously ill patients. Cyclophosphamide is used most commonly, although chlorambucil may be equally effective. Both agents have oncogenic potential. Cyclophosphamide has a disproportionate increase in bladder cancer, whereas chlorambucil has a higher incidence of secondary leukemia (see Chapter 57).

If cyclophosphamide is chosen, the usual dose is 2 mg/kg, although doses of 4 mg/kg are sometimes used for short periods. When such an agent is instituted, most rheumatologists maintain patients with the alkylating agent for 1 to 2 years. An alternative is intermittent intravenous cyclophosphamide, usually given in doses of 10 to 15 mg/kg monthly, which is less toxic and may be equally effective.[27]

The use of high-dose intravenous methylprednisolone (≤1 g/day) is recommended occasionally in cases of fulminant vasculitis.[28] Table 83-3 compares some agents that have been used in PAN.

There are case reports of polyarteritis associated with familial Mediterranean fever that have been treated successfully with colchicine, with or without corticosteroids.[29] More recently, case reports have shown apparently favorable responses to anti–tumor necrosis factor therapy.[30]

PROGNOSIS

In a rare disease whose definition has undergone considerable changes and whose treatment is not standard, it is difficult to be confident about the prognosis. With a combination of prednisone and an alkylating agent, however, it seems that approximately 80% of PAN patients survive, with most entering a long-term remission.[31] In classic PAN, the usual approach is to maintain prednisone at 1 mg/kg for 1 to 2 months, then slowly taper over 4 to 6 months. Some physicians favor converting patients to an alternate-day steroid regimen; others maintain daily steroids during the period of dose reduction.

These crucial first 6 months of therapy require careful monitoring for toxicity of the drugs and for evidence of disease relapse. Most rheumatologists follow blood counts, urinalyses, serum chemistries, and the ESR on at least monthly intervals. At the end of 6 months or so, the goal is to have the patient in remission (no active disease) and taking little or no steroids. Patients generally are maintained with cyclophosphamide for a full year, and then it is tapered and withdrawn over 3 to 6 months.

CUTANEOUS POLYARTERITIS NODOSA

Cutaneous (or limited) PAN refers to a small group of patients who have cutaneous manifestations of the disease, with characteristic histopathologic features, but no systemic features.[31] By definition, the patients have no fever, weight loss, or evidence of disease in any internal organs. Cases have been associated with streptococcal infection,[32] minocycline,[33] and hepatitis C,[34] but the etiology is unknown in most. The disease affects individuals of all ages, including children, but the peak age at onset seems to be in the 30s.

PATHOLOGY

Biopsy specimens of lesions show necrotizing vasculitis with transmural inflammation of small and medium-sized arteries.[35] As is true of systemic PAN, the definition of cutaneous PAN has changed over the years, so that many examples in the literature would be classified today as hypersensitivity angiitis, microscopic PAN, or other entities.

CLINICAL FEATURES

The typical patient develops crops of tender subcutaneous nodules over the lower legs, often with scattered lesions elsewhere. Larger nodules may become necrotic, and painful ulcers develop about 50% of the time.[36] In addition to the lower legs, lesions occur on the arms, the buttocks, the trunk, and occasionally the head and neck. The lesions usually occur in crops, appearing within a few days of each other. Untreated, they persist 1 to 6 months; occasional lesions persist for years. Livedo reticularis is common, and most patients complain of some joint pain, especially in joints adjacent to the lesions. No synovitis is present, however, and there are no other associated physical findings.

DIAGNOSIS

The results of laboratory studies are typically normal, other than mild elevation of the ESR and occasionally mild leukocytosis. There are a few reports of positive test results for ANCAs, although there are no studies to date to determine whether the presence of these antibodies describes a different set of patients who may evolve in time into microscopic PAN.

TREATMENT AND COURSE

Acute lesions usually respond to corticosteroids, although moderate-to-high doses may be required. For that reason, combined with the tendency of the disease to relapse and remit for many years, a variety of other agents have been used, with variable success, including anti-inflammatory drugs, sulfapyridine, methotrexate,[37] dapsone,[38] intravenous immune globulin,[39] tamoxifen,[40] and thalidomide.[41]

The prognosis is generally good, although the painful cutaneous ulcers can be disabling. Most patients have recurrent disease for many years,[42] however, and frustration with the disease and with the treatment regimen is high. Rarely, patients with cutaneous PAN develop features of systemic PAN, even after many years.[43]

COGAN'S SYNDROME

Cogan's syndrome is a rare disease, consisting of interstitial keratitis, audiovestibular symptoms, and, in most cases, systemic manifestations. It has been reported in several hundred patients since Cogan's description of four cases in 1945.[44] Cogan's syndrome is a disease of young people, for the most part, with a median age at onset of 25 years in one large study.[45,46]

CLINICAL FEATURES

The initial manifestations are usually ocular or audiovestibular, with more than 75% of patients developing eye and ear complications within 4 months of each other. In classic Cogan's syndrome, with interstitial keratitis as the ocular manifestation, systemic vasculitis occurs rarely; other systemic manifestations, especially aortitis with aneurysm formation or aortic insufficiency, occur in about 10% of patients.

Atypical Cogan's syndrome, in which the ocular manifestation is something other than interstitial keratitis, has a higher frequency of aortic and other systemic manifestations and a correspondingly worse prognosis.[47] Atypical manifestations of eye disease in Cogan's syndrome include episcleritis, scleritis, iritis, uveitis, and chorioretinitis. Rare cases of optic neuritis also are reported.

The eye symptoms usually begin with photophobia, redness, and local irritation. The audiovestibular symptoms are abrupt in onset with partial or total hearing loss, vertigo, and ataxia. The vestibular symptoms usually improve with time, but the hearing loss rarely returns to normal.

About half of patients have constitutional features, including weight loss, fever, lymphadenopathy, hepatosplenomegaly, and rash. Aortitis, causing aneurysms and aortic insufficiency, is the most serious manifestation of Cogan's syndrome and accounts for most deaths. The aortic manifestations may follow the ophthalmic and audiovestibular features by months to several years. Rarely, patients develop widespread vasculitis, including purpura and skin necrosis.[48]

PATHOLOGY

The aortic and other vascular lesions are characterized by a mixture of acute and chronic inflammation, often most prominent in the region of the internal elastic lamina. Granulomas containing giant cells have been reported, but many lesions contain a mixture of neutrophils, eosinophils, mononuclear cells, and fibrosis.

DIAGNOSIS

The diagnosis of Cogan's syndrome is entirely clinical because there are no definitive serologic or histologic markers. As would be expected, most patients have leukocytosis, anemia, thrombocytosis, and an elevated ESR during active phases of their disease. Patients with aortitis show aortic root dilation and aortic insufficiency on echocardiography or aortography. Cases have been reported with anti–endothelial cell antibodies[49] and anti-MPO antibodies.[50] The significance of these antibodies, if any, is unknown.

TREATMENT AND COURSE

No prospective studies of treatment regimens have been done in this rare disease. The interstitial keratitis usually responds to topical corticosteroids. It is common practice to treat acute audiovestibular symptoms with high doses of corticosteroids. Generally, patients respond quickly or not at all so that after 2 to 4 weeks, the clinician can determine whether long-term therapy is indicated. High-dose corticosteroids, cytotoxic drugs,[47] methotrexate,[51] and cyclosporine[52] have been used to treat the vasculitis.

The course varies. Some patients have a single episode and are free of active disease thereafter. The more typical course is one of waxing and waning symptoms for months to years. Virtually all patients sustain some permanent hearing loss, and nearly half are left totally deaf. Aortic valve replacement and surgical repair of aortic aneurysms may be required.

BUERGER'S DISEASE

Buerger's disease, also known as thromboangiitis obliterans, is an inflammatory vaso-occlusive disease that primarily affects the lower extremities in young adult male cigarette smokers, although women and older adults also are affected. The average age at onset is 35 years. More recent reports have emphasized a higher percentage of female patients, older age at onset, and perhaps a declining overall incidence.[53]

The role of tobacco, especially cigarette smoking, is clear, but the pathogenesis remains unknown. No consistent HLA association has been shown.[54] Antibodies against collagen, elastin, and laminin have been reported in some patients.[55,56] One study showed high levels of anti–endothelial cell antibodies in patients with active disease, but not in patients in remission.[57] ANCAs directed against MPO, lactoferrin, and elastase also have been associated with severe disease.[58]

PATHOLOGY

In most cases, Buerger's disease is limited to small arteries and veins in the distal extremities. There are numerous reports of visceral involvement, however, including mesenteric, coronary, and pulmonary arteries. Active lesions show a segmental inflammatory response with transmural infiltration of polymorphonuclear leukocytes and lymphocytes and preservation of the internal elastic membrane.[59] Thrombosis is prominent, and microabscesses are seen in the vessel wall and surrounding tissue. The infiltrating cells are enriched in CD3 T cells, and CD68 macrophages and S-100 dendritic cells have been reported to be increased during disease activity.[60]

CLINICAL FEATURES

Buerger's disease typically begins with bilateral pain and ischemia in both lower extremities, although the upper extremities may be the site of initial symptoms. At onset, the symptoms may be mild, such as paresthesias or pain only with exposure to cold. Most cases rapidly evolve, however, into a painful condition with digital cyanosis, splinter hemorrhages, vesicles, and severe claudication. Digital ulcers often occur, especially after minor trauma.[61] The disease typically begins distally, with symptoms worse in the tips of the fingers and toes, but it tends to progress to larger, more proximal vessels over several years. Proximal leg claudication is uncommon, however. Superficial phlebitis occurs in about one third of patients and may be the first symptom. Elevated plasma homocysteine levels have been associated with poor prognosis.[62]

DIAGNOSIS

Characteristic angiographic changes include multiple bilateral areas of narrowing or occlusion in the digital, palmar, plantar, ulnar, radial, tibial, and peroneal arteries. Small collateral vessels around the occlusion often take on a corkscrew appearance. More proximal lesions resemble atherosclerotic occlusion. Although these findings are typical, they are not pathognomonic; in the absence of pathologic confirmation, the disease must be differentiated from premature atherosclerosis; hyperviscosity syndrome; scleroderma and other rheumatic diseases; Takayasu's arteritis; embolic disease including cholesterol emboli and atrial myxomas; ergot toxicity; and thoracic outlet syndrome.

TREATMENT AND COURSE

Treatment consists of abstinence from all forms of tobacco. In severely addicted individuals unable to stop smoking, nicotine substitutes may be employed[63]—it is hoped for only a brief period.

Affected limbs must be protected from trauma and cold. Ulcers and cellulitis often require antibiotics and careful débridement. Calcium channel blockers and pentoxifylline reportedly have been beneficial in some patients, as has intra-arterial streptokinase.[64] Most patients show little or no response to any of these measures, however. Sympathectomy likewise seems to provide little or no long-term benefit and is not usually recommended. Therapy using the transfer of the gene for vascular endothelial growth factor is under investigation.[65]

In individuals with Buerger's disease who continue to smoke, about half require amputation, often multiple times as more proximal vessels are involved. If smoking is stopped, most patients stabilize, with amputation required in a few. The ischemic limb may be a source of pain and ulceration

for many years, however. Although most patients are men, the course in affected women is no different from that in men.[66,67]

VASCULITIS CAUSED BY VIRAL INFECTIONS

The vasculitis resulting from human immunodeficiency virus infection is discussed in Chapter 103. Many other viruses have been reported to be associated with vasculitis, but the cases are so infrequent as to render the diagnosis in doubt. Two viruses, hepatitis B and parvovirus B19, clearly have an association with vasculitis, however.

HEPATITIS B VASCULITIS

Hepatitis B vasculitis, described simultaneously in 1970 by investigators in the United States and in France,[2,3] is seen in individuals with chronic hepatitis B antigenemia, most of whom have active liver disease. The manifestations vary considerably, from diffuse small vessel vasculitis predominantly in the skin to larger vessel lesions typical of PAN.[64] Clinical symptoms may include the entire spectrum of vasculitic manifestations, from purpura and other rashes to abdominal pain, hypertension, renal disease, and stroke. Patients with cryoglobulinemia almost always have concomitant hepatitis C infection (see Chapter 85).

Treatment of these patients with immunosuppressive drugs has been only moderately successful; many patients die as a result of vasculitis or liver disease. Trepo and colleagues[68] and more recently Guillevin and coworkers[69] have reported good results using a combination of plasmapheresis, corticosteroid therapy, and antiviral therapy. Successful treatment with interferon-alfa also has been reported.

PARVOVIRUS B19 VASCULITIS

Although the most common rheumatic manifestation of parvovirus B19 infection is arthritis (see Chapter 104), occasional patients, usually children, have been reported to develop an impressive vasculitis, usually resembling PAN, in the setting of chronic parvovirus B19 infection.[70,71] These children have responded well to intravenous immune globulin therapy, suggesting that they may have a specific immune deficit regarding an inability to mount a normal immune response to parvovirus B19, although there was no other evidence suggesting generalized immunodeficiency.

REFERENCES

1. Cohen RD, Conn DL, Ilstrup DM: Clinical features, prognosis, and response to treatment in polyarteritis. Mayo Clin Proc 55:146, 1980.
2. **Gocke DJ, Morgan C, Lockshin M, et al: Association between polyarteritis nodosa and Australia antigen. Lancet 2:1149, 1970.**
3. Trepo C, Thivolet J: Hepatitis associated antigens and periarteritis nodosa (PAN). Vox Sang 19:410, 1970.
4. Goodman MD, Porter DD: Cytomegalovirus vasculitis with fatal colonic hemorrhage. Arch Pathol 96:281, 1973.
5. Massari M, Salvarani C, Portioli I, et al: Polyarteritis nodosa and HIV infection: No evidence of a direct pathogenic role of HIV. Infection 24:159, 1996.
6. **Calabrese LH: Vasculitis and infection with the human immunodeficiency virus. Rheum Dis Clin N Am 17:131, 1991.**

7. Caldeira T, Meireles C, Cunha F, et al: Systemic polyarteritis nodosa associated with acute Epstein-Barr virus infection. Clin Rheumatol 26:1733-1735, 2007.

8. Wharton CF, Pieroni R: Polyarteritis after influenza vaccination. BMJ 2:331, 1974.

9. Bani-Sadr F, Gueit I, Humbert G: Vasculitis related to hepatitis A vaccination. Clin Infect Dis 22:596, 1996.

10. Sergent JS, Christian CL: Necrotizing vasculitis after acute serous otitis media. Ann Intern Med 81:195, 1974.

11. Bingham C, Beaman M, Nicholls AJ, et al: Necrotizing renal vasculopathy resulting in chronic renal failure after ingestion of methamphetamine and 3,4-methylenedioxymethamphetamine ("ecstasy"). Nephrol Dial Transplant 13:2654, 1998.

12. Culver B, Itkin A, Pischel K: Case report and review of minocycline-induced cutaneous polyarteritis nodosa. Arthritis Care Res 53:468, 2005.

13. Katada Y, Harada Y, Azuma N, et al: Minocycline-induced vasculitis fulfilling the criteria of polyarteritis nodosa. Mod Rheumatol 16: 256-259, 2006.

14. Garcia-Diaz J, Garcia-Sanchez M, Busteros J, et al: Polyarteritis nodosa after interferon treatment for chronic hepatitis C. J Clin Virol 32:181, 2005.

15. Moskowitz RW, Baggenstoss AH, Slocumb CH: Histopathologic classification of periarteritis nodosa: A study of 56 cases confirmed at necropsy. Mayo Clin Proc 38:345, 1963.

16. Antonovych TT, Sabnis GG, Tuur SM, et al: Morphologic differences between polyarteritis and Wegener's granulomatosis using light, electron and immunohistochemical techniques. Mod Pathol 24:349, 1989.

17. Cid MC, Grau JM, Casademont J, et al: Immunohistochemical characterization of inflammatory cells and immunologic activation markers in muscle and nerve biopsy specimens from patients with polyarteritis nodosa. Arthritis Rheum 37:1055, 1994.

18. Ewald EA, Griffin D, McCune WJ: Correlation of angiographic abnormalities with disease manifestations and disease severity in polyarteritis nodosa. J Rheumatol 14:952, 1987.

19. Wees SJ, Sunivoo IN, Oh SJ: Sural nerve biopsy in systemic necrotizing vasculitis. Am J Med 71:525, 1981.

20. Lightfoot RW, Michel BA, Bloch DA, et al: The American College of Rheumatology 1990 criteria for the classification of polyarteritis nodosa. Arthritis Rheum 33:1088, 1990.

21. Chang RW, Bell CL, Hallet M: Clinical characteristics and prognosis of vasculitic mononeuropathy multiplex. Arch Neurol 41:618, 1984.

22. Smith DL, Wernick R: Spontaneous rupture of a renal artery aneurysm in polyarteritis nodosa: Critical review of the literature and report of a case. Am J Med 87:464, 1989.

23. Guillevin L, Lhote F, Gayraud M, et al: Prognostic factors in polyarteritis nodosa and Churg-Strauss syndrome: A prospective study in 342 patients. Medicine (Balt) 75:17, 1996.

24. Fauci AS, Katz P, Haynes BF, et al: Cyclophosphamide therapy of severe systemic necrotizing vasculitis. N Engl J Med 301:235, 1979.

25. Clements PJ, Davis J: Cytotoxic drugs and their clinical application to rheumatic diseases. Semin Arthritis Rheum 15:231, 1986.

26. Guillevin L, Lhote F: Treatment of polyarteritis nodosa and microscopic polyangiitis. Arthritis Rheum 41:2100, 1998.

27. Gayraud M, Guillevin L, Cohen P, et al: Treatment of good-prognosis polyarteritis nodosa and Churg-Strauss syndrome: Comparison of steroids and oral or pulse cyclophosphamide in 25 patients. Br J Rheumatol 36:1290, 1997.

28. Fort JG, Abruzzo JL: Reversal of progressive necrotizing vasculitis with intravenous pulse cyclophosphamide and methylprednisolone. Arthritis Rheum 31:1194, 1998.

29. Balbir-Gurman A, Nahir A, Braun-Moscovici Y: Vasculitis in siblings with familial Mediterranean fever: A report of three cases and review of the literature. Clin Rheumatol 26:1183, 2007.

30. Wu K, Throssell D: A new treatment for polyarteritis nodosa. Nephrol Dial Transplant 21:1710, 2006.

31. Moreland LW, Ball GV: Cutaneous polyarteritis nodosa. Am J Med 88:426, 1990.

32. Albornoz MA, Benedetto AV, Korman M, et al: Relapsing cutaneous polyarteritis nodosa associated with streptococcal infections. Int J Dermatol 37:664, 1998.

33. Schaffer JV, Davidson DM, McNiff JM, et al: Perineuclear antineutrophil cytoplasmic antibody-positive cutaneous polyarteritis nodosa associated with minocycline therapy for acne vulgaris. J Am Acad Dermatol 44:1908, 2001.

34. Soufir N, Descamps V, Crickx B, et al: Hepatitis C virus infection in cutaneous polyarteritis nodosa: A retrospective study of 16 cases. Arch Dermatol 135:1001, 1999.

35. Chen KR: Cutaneous polyarteritis nodosa. Am J Med 88:426, 1990.

36. Diaz-Perez JL, Winkelmann RK: Cutaneous polyarteritis nodosa. Arch Dermatol 110:407, 1974.

37. Jorrizzo JL, White WL, Wise CM, et al: Low-dose weekly methotrexate for unusual neutrophilic vascular reactions: Cutaneous polyarteritis nodosa and Behçet's disease. J Am Acad Dermatol 24:973, 1991.

38. Gibson LE, Su WP: Cutaneous vasculitis. Rheum Dis Clin N Am 16:309, 1990.

39. Uziel Y, Silverman ED: Intravenous immunoglobulin therapy in a child with cutaneous polyarteritis nodosa. Clin Exp Rheumatol 16:187, 1998.

40. Cvancara JL, Meffert JJ, Elston DN: Estrogen-sensitive cutaneous polyarteritis nodosa: Response to tamoxifen. J Am Acad Dermatol 39:643, 1998.

41. Cejudo-Rodriguez C, Hernandez V, Rodriguez R, et al: Thalidomide in mild and severe recurrent cutaneous polyarteritis nodosa. Ann Allergy Asthma Immunol 82:128, 1999.

42. Kelleman D, Kempf W, Burg G, et al: Cutaneous polyarteritis nodosa. Vasa 27:54, 1998.

43. Dervar CL, Bellamy N: Necrotizing mesenteric vasculitis after long-standing cutaneous polyarteritis nodosa. J Rheumatol 19:1308, 1992.

44. Cogan DG: Syndrome of nonsyphilitic interstitial keratitis and vestibuloauditory symptoms. Arch Ophthalmol 33:144, 1945.

45. Vollertsen RS, McDonald TJ, Younge BR, et al: Cogan's syndrome: 18 cases and a review of the literature. Mayo Clin Proc 61:344, 1986.

46. Haynes BF, Kaiser-Kupfer MI, Mason P, et al: Cogan syndrome: Studies in thirteen patients, long-term follow-up, and a review of the literature. Medicine (Balt) 59:426, 1980.

47. VanDoornum S, McColl G, Walter M, et al: Prolonged prodrome, systemic vasculitis, and deafness in Cogan's syndrome. Ann Rheum Dis 60:69, 2001.

48. Vollertsen RS: Vasculitis and Cogan's syndrome. Rheum Dis Clin N Am 16:433, 1990.

49. Ottaviani F, Cadoni G, Marinelli L, et al: Anti-endothelial cell autoantibodies in patients with sudden hearing loss. Laryngoscope 109:1084, 1999.

50. Yamanishi Y, Ishioka S, Takeda M, et al: Atypical Cogan's syndrome associated with antineutrophil cytoplasmic antibodies. Br J Rheumatol 35:601, 1996.

51. Richardson B: Methotrexate therapy for hearing loss in Cogan's syndrome. Arthritis Rheum 37:1559, 1994.

52. Hammer M, Witte T, Mugge A, et al: Complicated Cogan's syndrome with aortic insufficiency and coronary stenosis. J Rheumatol 21:552, 1994.

53. Olin JW, Young JR, Graor RA, et al: The changing clinical spectrum of thromboangiitis obliterans (Buerger's disease). Circulation 82(Suppl IV):3, 1990.

54. Olin JW: Thromboangiitis obliterans. Curr Opin Rheumatol 6:44, 1994.

55. Aclar R, Papa MZ, Halpern Z, et al: Cellular sensitivity to collagen in thromboangiitis obliterans. N Engl J Med 308:1113, 1983.

56. Hada M, Sakihama T, Kamiya K, et al: Cellular and humoral immune responses to vascular components in thromboangiitis obliterans. Angiology 44:533, 1993.

57. Eichhorn J, Sima D, Lindschau C, et al: Antiendothelial cell antibodies in thromboangiitis obliterans. Am J Med Sci 315:17, 1998.

58. Halacheva KS, Manolova IM, Petkov DP, et al: Study of antineutrophil cytoplasmic antibodies in patients with thromboangiitis obliterans (Buerger's disease). Scand J Immunol 48:544, 1998.

59. Lie JT: Diagnostic histopathology of major systemic and pulmonary vasculitic syndromes. Rheum Dis Clin N Am 16:269, 1990.

60. Kobayashi M, Ito M, Nakagawa A, et al: Immunohistochemical analysis of arterial cell wall infiltration in Buerger's disease (endartheritis obliterans). J Vasc Surg 29:451, 1999.

61. Joyce JW: Buerger's disease (thromboangiitis obliterans). Rheum Dis Clin N Am 16:463, 1990.

62. Olin JW, Childs MB, Bathrolomex JR, et al: Anticardiolipin antibodies and homcysteine levels in patients with thromboangiitis obliterans. Arthritis Rheum 39:547, 1996.

63. Kawallata H, Kanekura T, Gushi A, et al: Successful treatment of digital ulceration in Buerger's disease with nicotine chewing gum. Br J Dermatol 140:187, 1999 (letter).

64. Hussein EA, el Douri A: Intra-arterial streptokinase as adjuvant therapy for complicated Buerger's disease: Early trials. Int Surg 78:54, 1993.

65. Isner JM, Baumgartner I, Rauch G, et al: Treatment of thromboangiitis obliterans (Buerger's disease) by intramuscular gene transfer of vascular endothelial growth factor: Preliminary clinical results. J Vasc Surg 28:964, 1998.

66. Sasaki S, Sakuma M, Kunihara T, et al: Current trends in thromboangiitis obliterans (Buerger's disease) in women. Am J Surg 177:316, 1999.

67. **Sergent JS, Lockshin MD, Christian CL, et al: Vasculitis with hepatitis B antigenemia. Medicine (Balt) 55:1, 1976.**

68. Trepo C, Ouzan D, Delmont J, et al: Superiorite d'un nouveau traitement etiopathogenique curateur des periarteritis noueuses induites par le virus de l'hepatite B grace a l'association corticotherapie breve, vidarabine, echanges plasmatiques. Presse Med 17:1527, 1988.

69. Guillevin L, Mahr A, Cohen P, et al: Short-term corticosteroids then lamivudine and plasma exchanges to treat hepatitis B virus-related polyarteritis nodosa. Arthritis Rheum 51:482, 2004.

70. Gattorno M, Picco P, Vignola S, et al: Brother and sister with different vasculitides. Lancet 353:728, 1999.

71. Finkel TH, Torok TJ, Ferguson PJ, et al: Chronic parvovirus B19 infection and systemic necrotizing vasculitis: Opportunistic infection or aetiological agent? Lancet 343:1255, 1994.

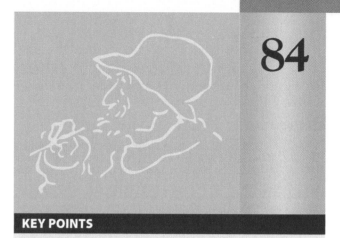

84

Isolated Angiitis of the Central Nervous System

JOHN S. SERGENT

KEY POINTS

Isolated angiitis of the central nervous system (CNS) may manifest with myriad symptoms, but headache, waxing and waning altered mental status, and transient ischemic attack–like events are most common.

Patients with CNS angiitis typically have no evidence of vasculitis elsewhere.

No laboratory markers (e.g., C-reactive protein, erythrocyte sedimentation rate) are useful in making the diagnosis.

Diagnosis is often based on angiography in the appropriate clinical setting, although brain biopsy is the only definitive diagnostic test.

CNS angiitis is a very rare disease, and its manifestations can be mimicked by many other diseases.

When CNS angiitis is confirmed, the preferred treatment is cyclophosphamide and prednisone, although residual morbidity is high.

Isolated angiitis of the central nervous system (CNS) is a rare disorder with a large differential diagnosis, making it a particularly difficult clinical challenge. Involvement of the CNS by other forms of vasculitis, especially common in disorders such as giant cell arteritis, Takayasu's arteritis, and Wegener's granulomatosis, is considered to be secondary CNS angiitis. By definition, in primary CNS angiitis, the vasculitis is limited to the central nervous system.

EPIDEMIOLOGY

Most reported series of CNS angiitis are small, and single case reports describe unusual features or associations; the disease seems to be most frequent in the fourth and fifth decades, with case reports describing individuals of all ages, ranging from children to the elderly. Vasculitis resembling isolated CNS angiitis has been described in association with human immunodeficiency virus (HIV) infection,[1-3] varicella zoster,[4] amyloid angiopathy,[5,6] sarcoidosis,[7] parvovirus B19 infection,[8] ulcerative colitis,[9] drugs,[10] and lymphomas.[11] In children, there are numerous reports of familial hemophagocytic lymphohistiocytosis mimicking vasculitis.[12] Moshous and associates[13] reported a 4-year-old girl with perforin deficiency who had CNS vasculitis with no evidence of hemophagocytosis, and who was cured with a stem cell transplant from an HLA-identical brother.[13] Other considerations in the differential diagnosis include granulomatous infections, such as tuberculosis[14] and brucellosis.[15]

PATHOLOGY

CNS angiitis was first described in 1959 by Cravioto and Fegin[16] as a granulomatous vasculitis. For many years, the term *granulomatous angiitis of the central nervous system* was used. Pathologic studies have shown, however, that granulomas are not always present, with some cases showing only vascular necrosis or a lymphocytic or mixed cellular infiltrate.[17] The site of involvement in the CNS also varies, ranging from small leptomeningeal vessels to large arteries and veins.

CLINICAL FEATURES

A typical patient presents with a 1- to 3-month history of headache and various other symptoms such as intermittent confusion and focal neurologic symptoms, including transient ischemic attacks and strokes. Seizures occur in a few patients, and some patients progress rapidly to dementia.[18] Paraplegia and other spinal cord syndromes are rare manifestations. Table 84-1 shows the author's estimate of the approximate frequency of the various presenting features of the disease.

LABORATORY FINDINGS

The "gold standard" for the diagnosis of primary CNS angiitis is a brain and leptomeningeal biopsy. Inflammatory indices, including the erythrocyte sedimentation rate and C-reactive protein, are typically normal or only mildly elevated. Patients may be mildly anemic, but other tests, including antineutrophil cytoplasmic antibodies, antinuclear antibodies, rheumatoid factor, and complement levels, are almost always normal.

RADIOGRAPHIC FEATURES

Although angiographic features may be characteristic of the disease, they are not specific, and many entities can cause angiographic changes identical to those seen in primary CNS angiitis. Because of this fact, and because of the rarity of the disease, the clinician is urged to be wary of relying on radiography to make the diagnosis. In the author's experience, only a few patients considered by the radiologist to have primary CNS angiitis have turned out to have the disease on further examination. With that caveat, the typical angiographic findings include stenosis or occlusion of multiple arteries, with occasional series reporting aneurysmal dilation as well (Fig. 84-1). Beading, usually in association with areas of stenosis, occasionally is found.[19]

Table 84-1 Estimated Presenting Symptoms
of Central Nervous System Angiitis

Symptom	Frequency (%)
Headache	70
Episodic confusion	50
Focal signs	50
Seizures	30
Dementia	Rare*

*Many patients become demented late in the course.

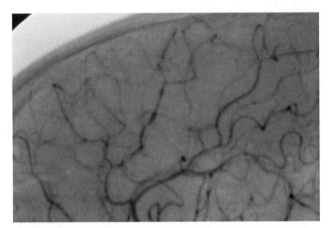

Figure 84-1 Angiogram of a patient with primary CNS angiitis showing multiple small aneurysms.

DIFFERENTIAL DIAGNOSIS

The differential diagnosis of CNS angiitis is large, and clinicians should be especially wary of the diagnosis in the setting of migraine,[20] severe hypertension,[21] various vasoactive drugs,[22,23] lymphoma,[24] and coagulopathies, especially if antiphospholipid antibodies are present.[25] Infections known to have CNS manifestations mimicking vasculitis include syphilis,[26] brucellosis,[27] varicella zoster,[28] and HIV.[29] Vasculitis in the setting of these conditions should always be considered secondary.

CLINICAL COURSE

Although apparently benign forms of CNS angiitis are reported,[30] most untreated cases and many that are treated have a devastating outcome, including dementia, severe paralysis, and death.

TREATMENT

Treatment is empiric, and in severe cases the largest experience would suggest an approach similar to treatment of polyarteritis nodosa or Wegener's granulomatosis using cyclophosphamide and corticosteroids. That regimen is followed by remission in more than half of cases, but significant morbidity is common.[31]

A particularly challenging problem is a patient with angiographic findings of CNS angiitis who presents with acute focal disease. Calabrese and colleagues[32] termed this condition the *reversible cerebral vasoconstriction syndrome* and suggested a conservative approach using corticosteroids and calcium channel blockers. The author's experience would definitely support this approach, especially in the setting of any other potentially precipitating conditions, such as migraine, the postpartum period, or various drugs.

REFERENCES

1. Nogueras C, Sala M, Sasal M, et al: Recurrent stroke as a manifestation of primary angiitis of the central nervous system in a patient infected with human immunodeficiency virus. Arch Neurol 59:468, 2002.
2. Ake JA, Erickson JC, Lowry KJ: Cerebral aneurysmal arteriopathy associated with HIV infection in an adult. Clin Infect Dis 43:e46-e50, 2006.
3. Nieuwhof CMG, Damoiseaux J, Tervaert JW, et al: Successful treatment of cerebral vasculitis in an HIV-positive patient with anti-CD25 treatment. Ann Rheum Dis 65:1677-1678, 2006.
4. Al-Abdulla NA, Kelley JS, Green WR, et al: Herpes zoster vasculitis presenting as giant cell arteritis with choroidal infarction. Retina 23:567-569, 2003.
5. Scolding NJ, Fady J, Kirby PA, et al: AB-related angiitis: Primary angiitis of the central nervous system associated with cerebral amyloid angiopathy. Brain 128:500-515, 2005.
6. Wong SH, Robbins PD, Knuckey NW, et al: Cerebral amyloid angiopathy presenting with vasculitic pathology. J Clin Neurosci 13:291-294, 2006.
7. Brisman JL, Hinduja A, McKinney JS, et al: Successful emergent angioplasty of neurosarcoid vasculitis presenting with strokes. Surg Neurol 66:402-404, 2006.
8. Bilge I, Sadikoglu B, Emre S, et al: Central nervous system vasculitis secondary to parvovirus B19 infection in a pediatric renal transplant patient. Pediatr Nephrol 20:529-533, 2005.
9. Pandian JD, Henderson RD, O'Sullivan JD, et al: Cerebral vasculitis in ulcerative colitis. Arch Neurol 63:780, 2006.
10. Vanek C, Samuels MH: Central nervous system vasculitis caused by propylthiouracil therapy: A case report and literature review. Thyroid 15:80-84, 2005.
11. Albrecht R, Krebs B, Reusche E, et al: Signs of rapidly progressive dementia in a case of intravascular lymphomatosis. Eur Arch Psychiatry Clin Neurosci 255:232-235, 2005.
12. Turtzo LC, Lin DD, Hartung H, et al: A neurologic presentation of familial hemophagocytic lymphohistiocytosis which mimicked septic emboli to the brain. J Child Neurol 22:863-868, 2007.
13. Moshous D, Feyen O, Lankisch P, et al: Primary necrotizing lymphocytic central nervous system vasculitis due to perforin deficiency in a four-year-old girl. Arthritis Rheum 56:995-999, 2007.
14. Poltera AA: Thrombogenic intracranial vasculitis in tuberculous meningitis: A 20 year "post mortem" survey. Acta Neurol Belg 77:12-24, 1977.
15. Adaletli I, Albayram S, Gurses B, et al: Vasculopathic changes in the cerebral arterial system with neurobrucellosis. AJNR Am J Neuroradiol 27:384-386, 2006.
16. Cravioto ID, Fegin I: Non-infectious granulomatous angiitis with a predilection for the nervous system. Neurology 9:599-609, 1959.
17. MacLaren K, Gillespie J, Shrestha S, et al: Primary angiitis of the central nervous system: Emerging variants. QJM 98:643-654, 2005.
18. Lie JT: Primary (granulomatous) angiitis of the central nervous system: A clinicopathologic analysis of 15 new cases and a review of the literature. Hum Pathol 23:164-171, 1992.
19. Kadkhodayan Y, Alreshaid A, Moran CJ, et al: Primary angiitis of the central nervous system at conventional angiography. Radiology 233:878-882, 2004.
20. Kurth T: Migraine and ischaemic vascular events. Cephalalgia 27:965-975, 2007.
21. Garner BF, Burns P, Bunning BD, et al: Acute blood pressure elevation can mimic arteriographic appearance of cerebral vasculitis—a postpartum case with relative hypertension. J Rheumatol 17:93, 1990.
22. Lake CR, Gallant S, Mason E, et al: Adverse drug effects attributed to phenylpropanolamine: A review of 142 case reports. Am J Med 89:195, 1990.
23. De Silva DA, Wong MC, Lee MP, et al: Amphetamine-associated ischemic stroke: Clinical presentation and proposed pathogenesis. J Stroke Cerebrovasc Dis 16:185-186, 2007.
24. Holmoy T, Nakstad PH, Fredo HL, et al: Intravascular large B-cell lymphoma presenting as cerebellar and cerebral infarction. Arch Neurol 64:754-755, 2007.

25. Rahemtullah A, Van Cott EM: Hypercoagulation testing in ischemic stroke. Arch Pathol Lab Med 131:890-901, 2007.

26. Asdaghi N, Muayqil T, Scozzafava J, et al: Teaching case report: The re-emergence in Canada of meningovascular syphilis: 2 patients with headache and stroke. Can Med Assoc J 176:1699-1700, 2007.

27. Karsen H, Akdeniz H, Karahocagil MK, et al: Toxic-febrile neurobrucellosis, clinical findings and outcome of treatment of four cases based on our experience. Scand J Infect Dis 6:1-6, 2007.

28. **Gilden D: Varicella zoster virus and central nervous system syndromes. Herpes 11(Suppl 2):89A-94A, 2004.**

29. **Tipping B, deVilliers L, Wainwright H, et al: Stroke in patients with human immunodeficiency virus infection. J Neurol Neurosurg Psychiatry 78:1320-1324, 2007.**

30. Jolly M, Curran JJ, Ellman M: Benign angiopathy of the central nervous system. J Clin Rheumatol 10:80-82, 2004.

31. Calabrese LH: Vasculitis of the central nervous system. Rheum Dis Clin N Am 21:1059-1076, 1995.

32. **Calabrese LH, Dodick DW, Schwedt TJ, et al: Narrative review: Reversible cerebral vasoconstriction syndromes. Ann Intern Med 146:34-44, 2007.**

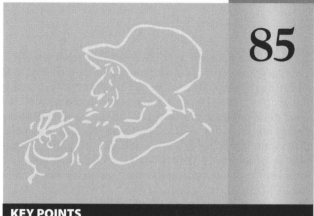

85

Immune Complex–Mediated Small Vessel Vasculitis

JOHN H. STONE

KEY POINTS

Vasculitides mediated by immune complexes (ICs) are a clinically heterogeneous group of disorders linked by inefficient or dysregulated clearance of ICs.

The most common types of IC-mediated vasculitis are hypersensitivity vasculitis, Henoch-Schönlein purpura (HSP), and mixed cryoglobulinemia. Rarer forms of this condition include hypocomplementemic urticarial vasculitis and erythema elevatum diutinum.

Connective tissue disorders such as systemic lupus erythematosus and rheumatoid arthritis can also be associated with IC-mediated vasculitis.

Cutaneous involvement of small blood vessels is the most prominent feature in the majority of cases, but extracutaneous involvement occurs in some forms.

The classic cutaneous finding in small vessel vasculitis is palpable purpura, but a variety of other skin lesions may be found: pustules, vesicles, urticaria, and small ulcerations.

The terms *vasculitis* and *angiitis* are used interchangeably when referring to inflammation involving small blood vessels (capillaries, venules, arterioles).

Direct immunofluorescence studies of involved blood vessels demonstrate characteristic types and patterns of immunoglobulin (Ig) and complement deposition.

Hypersensitivity vasculitis usually results from a reaction to a medication or an infection.

HSP is associated with purpura, arthritis, glomerulonephritis, and colicky abdominal pain. IgA deposition is found within blood vessel walls.

Cryoglobulinemic vasculitis is associated with long-standing hepatitis C virus infection in 90% of cases. The term *mixed cryoglobulinemia* is sometimes used for this disorder because the immunoreactants involved in the disease include both IgG and IgM.

The inflammation within blood vessel walls that characterizes vasculitis frequently leads to cellular destruction, damage to the vascular structures, compromise of blood flow to organs, and organ dysfunction. It has been known for decades that immune complex (IC)–mediated mechanisms play critical roles in many forms of systemic vasculitis, particularly those that involve primarily small blood vessels. As described in Chapter 80, the use of horse serum and sulfonamides as therapeutic agents for infectious diseases in the early 1900s frequently led to small vessel vasculitis on the basis of serum sickness or hypersensitivity phenomena. *Hypersensitivity*

angiitis, often confused with the pauci-immune form of vasculitis now termed *microscopic polyangiitis* (see Chapter 82),[1] was one of five disorders included in the original classification of the vasculitides in 1952.[2]

This chapter focuses on forms of small vessel vasculitis that are mediated by IC deposition. These disorders include hypersensitivity vasculitis, Henoch-Schönlein purpura (HSP), mixed cryoglobulinemia, urticarial vasculitis, and erythema elevatum diutinum. In addition, forms of vasculitis associated with connective tissue diseases, particularly systemic lupus erythematosus (SLE) and rheumatoid vasculitis, are discussed briefly. Anti–glomerular basement membrane disease and the pauci-immune forms of vasculitis, such as those associated with antineutrophil cytoplasmic antibodies, are discussed elsewhere (see Chapter 82). Throughout this chapter, the terms *vasculitis* and *angiitis* are used interchangeably when referring to inflammation involving small blood vessels (capillaries, venules, arterioles).

Because all forms of IC-mediated vasculitis share certain elements of pathogenesis, have many cutaneous findings in common, and have overlapping differential diagnoses, these aspects of the disorders are considered together. The epidemiology, cause, distinctive pathophysiologic mechanisms, unique clinical features, and approaches to treatment are discussed separately for each condition.

PATHOGENESIS

ARTHUS REACTION

The Arthus reaction, described after the injection of horse serum into rabbits, forms the basis of our understanding of IC-mediated diseases.[3] The formation of ICs in the Arthus reaction initiates complement activation and an influx of inflammatory cells, followed by thrombus formation and hemorrhagic infarction in the areas of most intense inflammation. ICs, formed by the combination of antibody and antigen, are continuously created (and usually cleared swiftly and efficiently) by the reticuloendothelial system as a means of neutralizing foreign antigens. Under some circumstances, however, ICs escape clearance and become deposited within joints, blood vessels, and other tissues, inciting inflammation and causing disease. ICs deposited in the blood vessel walls lead to vasculitis. Similarly, those deposited within small blood vessels of the kidney—the glomeruli—cause glomerulonephritis.[4]

IMMUNOGENICITY

The fate of formed ICs is governed by several major factors, including antigen load, antibody response, efficiency of the reticuloendothelial system, physical properties of the blood vessels (including flow dynamics and previous endothelial damage), and solubility of the ICs themselves. The ratio of antibody to antigen determines the solubility of ICs. Large ICs, formed when antibody and antigen are present in approximately equal proportions, are identified and removed easily by the reticuloendothelial system. In contrast, small ICs are formed in conditions of antibody excess. Small ICs remain in the serum and do not elicit an immune response within tissues. However, when there is a slight antigen excess, ICs precipitate from the serum and become trapped within certain vascular beds. Following the deposition of ICs in tissue, a cascade of pathologic events ensues: complement fixation, neutrophil recruitment, local inflammation, lysosomal release, oxygen free radical generation, and tissue injury.

CUTANEOUS MANIFESTATIONS

Small blood vessels generally include capillaries, postcapillary venules, and nonmuscular arterioles—vessels that are typically less than 50 µm in diameter. These are found principally within the superficial papillary dermis (Fig. 85-1). Medium-sized blood vessels, those between 50 and 150 µm in diameter, contain muscular walls and are located principally in the deep reticular dermis, near the junction of the dermis and subcutaneous tissues. Vessels larger than 150 µm in diameter are not commonly found in the skin.

Figure 85-1, which demonstrates the location and size of blood vessels involved in various types of cutaneous vasculitis, illustrates the types of blood vessels affected by several forms of IC-mediated disease. A blood vessel's size correlates closely with its depth in the skin layers: the larger the vessel, the deeper its location. Although telltale signs of vasculitis may be evident on inspection of the skin's surface, the epidermis is avascular. Therefore, the pathologic findings in cutaneous vasculitides lie within the dermis and subcutaneous tissues.

Palpable purpura, synonymous with small vessel vasculitis, is the most common cutaneous finding in IC-mediated vasculitis (Fig. 85-2). Purpuric lesions result from the extravasation of erythrocytes through damaged blood vessel walls into tissue. Many other skin manifestations are possible in these conditions, including vesicles, pustules, urticaria, superficial ulcerations, nonpalpable lesions (macules and patches), and splinter hemorrhages (Fig. 85-3). These lesions frequently occur in combination, and careful examination usually reveals a purpuric component. Purpuric lesions *do not blanch* when pressure is applied to the skin. Following resolution, purpuric lesions may leave postinflammatory hyperpigmentation, particularly if repeated bouts occur (see Fig. 85-3F).

In IC-mediated vasculitis, purpuric lesions are usually distributed in a symmetric fashion over dependent regions of the body, particularly the lower legs, because of the increased hydrostatic pressure in these areas. Purpuric lesions are not always palpable to the touch, and the existence of palpable purpura does not necessarily imply an IC-mediated pathophysiology; pauci-immune forms of vasculitis, such as Wegener's granulomatosis, microscopic polyangiitis, and Churg-Strauss syndrome, for example, may present with identical skin findings (albeit distinctive histopathology; see Chapter 82).

PATHOLOGIC FEATURES

Full pathologic assessment of cutaneous vasculitis involves examination of a skin biopsy specimen by both light microscopy and direct immunofluorescence (DIF). DIF is a particularly critical procedure in the evaluation of small vessel vasculitides. DIF studies must be planned at the time the biopsy is performed, because they require a fresh skin biopsy sample.

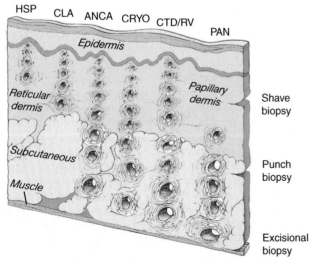

Figure 85-1 Size of the blood vessels involved in forms of cutaneous vasculitis. The types of vasculitis with an immune complex–mediated pathogenesis include Henoch-Schönlein purpura (HSP), cutaneous leukocytoclastic angiitis (CLA), mixed cryoglobulinemia (CRYO), and connective tissue disease/rheumatoid vasculitis (CTD/RV). ANCA, antineutrophil cytoplasmic antibody; PAN, polyarteritis nodosa.

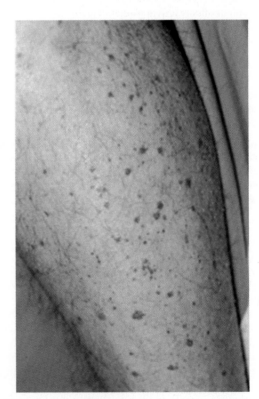

Figure 85-2 Hypersensitivity vasculitis. Palpable purpura in a patient with hypersensitivity vasculitis.

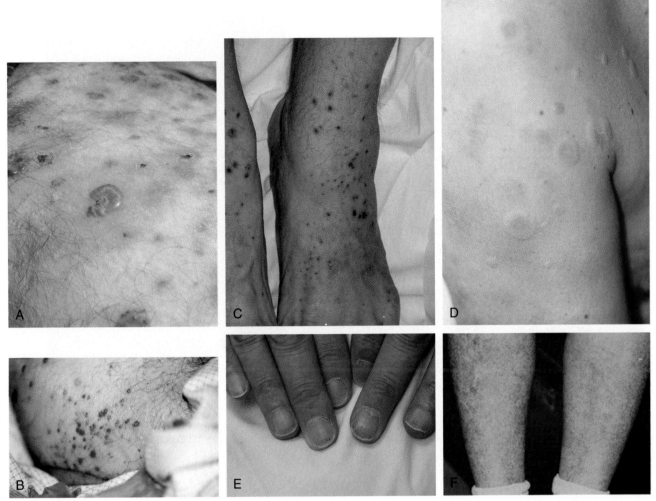

Figure 85-3   Other cutaneous findings of immune complex–mediated small vessel vasculitis. **A**, Vesicles. **B**, Pustules. **C**, Superficial ulcerations. **D**, Urticaria. **E**, Splinter hemorrhages. **F**, Hyperpigmentation.

LIGHT MICROSCOPY

Figure 85-4A displays the light microscopy findings of cutaneous vasculitis. The optimal time for skin biopsy is 24 to 48 hours after the appearance of a lesion. Biopsies should be obtained from a nonulcerated site. For ulcerated lesions—usually more of an issue with medium vessel vasculitides—biopsies should be taken from the ulcer's edge. The cellular infiltrates in cutaneous vasculitis are usually made up of a combination of neutrophils and lymphocytes, but most cases demonstrate a predominance of one cell type or the other. Lymphocyte-rich infiltrates may be seen in specimens taken from either new (<12 hours) or old (>48 hours) lesions, regardless of the underlying type of vasculitis. Even in connective tissue disorders such as Sjögren's syndrome, the typical finding is a leukocytoclastic vasculitis rather than a lymphocytic vasculitis.[5]

The essential histologic feature in any form of cutaneous vasculitis is the disruption of blood vessel architecture by an inflammatory infiltrate within and around the vessel walls. Endothelial swelling and proliferation, leukocytoclasis (degranulation of neutrophils, leading to the production of nuclear "dust"; see Fig. 85-4), and extravasation of erythrocytes may be evident in the biopsy but are not essential to the diagnosis.

DIRECT IMMUNOFLUORESCENCE

Although the diagnosis of cutaneous vasculitis rests on routine histology, the features revealed by hematoxylin and eosin stains do not distinguish between pauci-immune and IC-mediated disorders. DIF studies complement the histologic information, provide the only way of diagnosing HSP with certainty, and yield important clues regarding the nature of the underlying disease. The performance of *separate* biopsies for histologic and DIF analyses is recommended if sufficient lesions exist. With DIF studies, frozen sections are incubated with fluorescein-labeled anti–human immunoglobulin (Ig) G, IgM, IgA, and C3. The staining patterns of these immunoreactants may provide insight not only into the diagnosis but also into the pathophysiology of certain conditions. Figure 85-4B displays the typical DIF findings in a skin lesion from a patient with IC-mediated vasculitis.

DIFFERENTIAL DIAGNOSIS

The differential diagnosis of IC-mediated small vessel vasculitis is shown in Table 85-1. There are three main groups of disorders in the differential diagnosis of IC-mediated small vessel vasculitis: other forms of IC-mediated disorders, forms

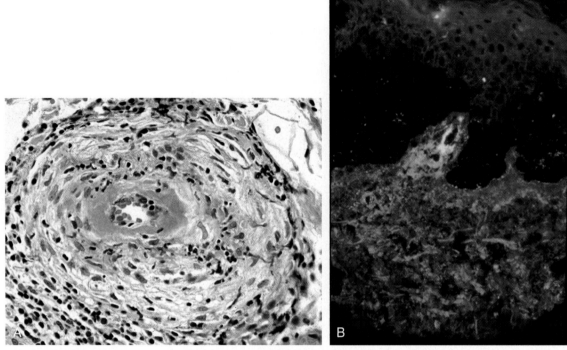

Figure 85-4 Skin biopsy findings in immune complex–mediated small vessel vasculitis. **A,** Light microscopy findings. **B,** Direct immunofluorescence findings.

of small vessel vasculitis that are not mediated through ICs, and vasculitis mimickers that involve small blood vessels. A diagnostic algorithm that includes the critical laboratory and radiographic tests is shown in Figure 85-5.

CLINICAL SYNDROMES

HYPERSENSITIVITY VASCULITIS (CUTANEOUS LEUKOCYTOCLASTIC ANGIITIS)

The term *hypersensitivity vasculitis* (see Chapter 80) refers generally to an IC-mediated small vessel vasculitis of the skin that spares internal organs and usually follows drug exposures or infections. The Chapel Hill Consensus Conference recommended eliminating the term *hypersensitivity vasculitis* in favor of *cutaneous leukocytoclastic angiitis*, because of the disorder's usual confinement to the skin and its predominant cell type, the neutrophil.[1] However, *hypersensitivity vasculitis* remains firmly embedded in the medical literature. The disease is characterized pathologically by IC deposition in capillaries, postcapillary venules, and arterioles. A similar illness—serum sickness—is a systemic illness that includes rash and prominent arthralgias or arthritis; it occurs 1 to 2 weeks after exposure to a drug or foreign antigen.

In 1990, the American College of Rheumatology (ACR) performed a study designed to identify features that distinguished one form of vasculitis from others.[6] The resulting ACR classification criteria for hypersensitivity vasculitis are shown in Table 85-2.[7] A long list of medications, infections, and other exposures may lead to the syndrome of hypersensitivity vasculitis. The key historical element in evaluating a patient with possible hypersensitivity vasculitis is identifying exposures that may have triggered the reaction.

However, in approximately half of all patients with this disorder, no inciting agent can be identified. Thorough efforts are also required to exclude disease in organs other than the skin, the finding of which would implicate another form of vasculitis (see Fig. 85-5). For example, although hypersensitivity vasculitis can mimic the skin features of microscopic polyangiitis, it does not involve the kidneys, lungs, peripheral nerves, or other internal organs and is not associated with antineutrophil cytoplasmic antibodies.

Removal of the inciting agent is the most critical therapy for hypersensitivity vasculitis when the likely agent can be identified. In patients who have been exposed to multiple medications, determining the inciting agent may be difficult and may require the withdrawal of multiple agents simultaneously until the syndrome clears, typically in 1 to 2 weeks.

The prognosis for patients with hypersensitivity vasculitis depends on the inciting cause. Treatment with glucocorticoids is reserved for patients with extensive disease and can usually be discontinued within several weeks. Patients who experience repeated disease flares may need low-dose glucocorticoids to prevent recurrences. Colchicine (0.6 mg twice daily) and dapsone (100 mg/day) have also been used successfully in some patients.

HENOCH-SCHÖNLEIN PURPURA

HSP is an IC-mediated form of small vessel vasculitis that is strongly associated with IgA deposition within blood vessel walls. Many cases of HSP are reported to occur after upper respiratory tract infections. Multiple bacterial, viral, and other infectious agents have been suggested as the cause of HSP, but the true cause remains unknown. The 1990 ACR criteria for the classification of HSP are shown in Table 85-3.[8]

Table 85-1 Differential Diagnosis of Immune Complex–Mediated Vasculitis

Other Immune Complex–Mediated Vasculitides
Hypersensitivity vasculitis
Henoch-Schönlein purpura
Mixed cryoglubilinemia
Urticarial vasculitis
Erythema elevatum diutinum
Connective tissue disease, rheumatoid vasculitis
Pauci-Immune Vasculitides
Wegener's granulomatosis
Churg-Strauss syndrome
Microscopic polyangiitis
Miscellaneous Small Vessel Vasculitides
Behçet's disease
Malignancy associated
Infection
Inflammatory bowel disease
Vasculitis Mimickers
Hemorrhage
Pigmented purpuric dermatoses
Scurvy
Immune thrombocytopenic purpura
Thrombosis
Antiphospholipid syndrome
Thrombotic thrombocytopenic purpura
Livedoid vasculopathy (atrophie blanche)
Warfarin-induced skin necrosis
Purpura fulminans
Disseminated intravascular coagulation
Embolism
Cholesterol emboli
Atrial myxoma
Vascular wall pathology
Calciphylaxis
Amyloidosis
Infection
Infective endocarditis
Leprosy (Lucio's phenomenon)

The hallmarks of HSP include an upper respiratory tract infection followed by a syndrome characterized by a purpuric rash, arthralgias, abdominal pain, and renal disease. HSP is usually viewed as a disease of childhood, and the majority of cases affect children younger than 5 years. However, adults can also be affected by HSP and have a greater tendency toward a prolonged disease course (with recurrent bouts of purpura) than do children.[9] Colicky abdominal pain, presumably secondary to gastrointestinal vasculitis, is a common characteristic of HSP and frequently occurs within a week after the onset of rash. Sometimes the gastrointestinal symptoms of HSP precede the onset of purpura, leading to a diagnostic quandary and occasionally to exploratory surgery. Endoscopy may demonstrate purpura in the upper or lower intestinal tract. Mild glomerulonephritis is common and generally self-limited, although some patients develop end-stage renal disease.

In children with mild manifestations, the clinical history alone may be sufficient to confirm the diagnosis. In more serious cases (e.g., in the presence of renal involvement) or when there is sufficient doubt about the diagnosis, biopsy of an involved organ is essential. Unlike in other forms of IC-mediated disease, however, DIF reveals florid IgA deposition. In the proper clinical setting, this finding is

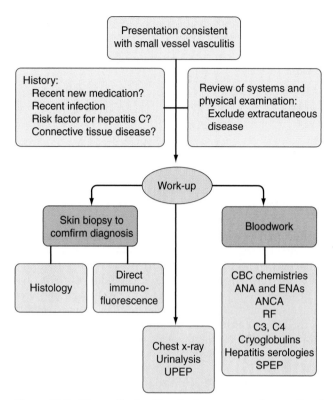

Figure 85-5 Diagnostic algorithm for immune complex–mediated small vessel vasculitis. The critical diagnostic test is usually a skin biopsy with hematoxylin and eosin (H&E) staining and direct immunofluorescence. ANA, antinuclear antibody; ANCA, antineutrophil cytoplasmic antibody; CBC, complete blood count; ENA, extractable nuclear antigen; RF, rheumatoid factor; SPEP, serum protein electrophoresis; UPEP, urine protein electrophoresis.

diagnostic of HSP. Other forms of small vessel vasculitis may have small quantities of IgA within blood vessels, but IgA is not the predominant immunoreactant in such cases.

In mild cases of HSP, no specific therapy is necessary. Even for patients with glomerulonephritis, it has been difficult to demonstrate that treatment with glucocorticoids or immunosuppressive agents significantly alters the outcome. Despite this, it is prudent to treat aggressive renal involvement with an immunosuppressive regimen, including high-dose glucocorticoids and another immunosuppressive agent such as cyclophosphamide, azathioprine, or mycophenolate mofetil, depending on disease severity.

Table 85-2 American College of Rheumatology 1990 Criteria* for the Classification of Hypersensitivity Vasculitis

Age >16 yr
Use of a possible offending medication in temporal relation to symptoms
Palpable purpura
Maculopapular rash
Biopsy of a skin lesion showing neutrophils around an arteriole or venule

*The presence of three or more criteria has a sensitivity of 71% and specificity of 84% for the diagnosis of hypersensitivity vasculitis.

From Calabrese LH, Michel BA, Bloch DA, et al: American College of Rheumatology 1990 criteria for the classification of hypersensitivity vasculitis. Arthritis Rheum 33:1108-1113, 1990.

Table 85-3 American College of Rheumatology 1990 Criteria* for the Classification of Henoch-Schönlein Purpura

Palpable purpura
Age at onset <20 yr
Bowel angina
Vessel wall granulocytes on biopsy

*The presence of two criteria identified Henoch-Schönlein purpura with a sensitivity of 87% and a specificity of 88% in a group of individuals with forms of systemic vasculitis.

From Mills JA, Michel BA, Bloch DA, et al: The American College of Rheumatology 1990 criteria for the classification of Henoch-Schönlein purpura. Arthritis Rheum 33:1114-1121, 1990.

Recurrences of skin disease, often consisting of multiple episodes occurring over many months, are not unusual. Generally, however, even in patients with recurrent disease, the rule is for the disorder to subside and to resolve completely over a few months to a year. In a minority of patients, some evidence of permanent renal damage persists in the form of proteinuria and hematuria. Less than 5% of patients develop renal failure as a result of HSP.

CRYOGLOBULINEMIC VASCULITIS

Cryoglobulins are immunoglobulins characterized by a tendency to precipitate from serum under conditions of cold.[10] Such proteins, detectable to a varying degree in a wide array of inflammatory conditions, do not always cause disease. In some patients, however, cryoglobulins bind to circulating antigen (e.g., portions of the hepatitis C virion), deposit in the walls of small and medium-sized blood vessels, and activate complement, leading to cryoglobulinemic vasculitis.

In contrast to most other forms of IC-mediated vasculitis, cryoglobulinemia has a tendency to involve medium-sized blood vessels as well as small ones. Thus, the syndrome of cryoglobulinemic vasculitis can be associated with the development of large cutaneous ulcers, digital ischemia, and livedo racemosa—findings characteristic of disturbances in medium-sized vessels. The Chapel Hill Consensus Conference provided a consensus definition for mixed cryoglobulinemia (Table 85-4).[1]

Three major types of cryoglobulinemia are recognized, defined by the specific kinds of immunoglobulins with which they are associated (Table 85-5). Type I, characterized by a monoclonal gammopathy (generally IgG or IgM),

Table 85-4 Chapel Hill Consensus Conference Definitions of Immune Complex–Mediated Forms of Vasculitis

Disease	Definition
Cutaneous leukocytoclastic angiitis	Isolated cutaneous leukocytoclastic angiitis without systemic vasculitis or glomerulonephritis
Henoch-Schönlein purpura	Vasculitis with immunoglobulin A–dominant immune deposits, affecting small blood vessels (capillaries, venules, arterioles); typically involves skin, gut, and glomeruli and is associated with arthralgias or arthritis
Essential cryoglobulinemia	Vasculitis with cryoglobulin immune deposits, affecting small blood vessels (capillaries, venules, arterioles) and associated with cryoglobulins in serum; skin and glomeruli often involved

From Jennette JC, Falk RJ, Andrassy K, et al: Nomenclature of systemic vasculitides: Proposal of an international consensus conference. Arthritis Rheum 37:187-192, 1994.

differs substantially from types II and III in its clinical presentation and disease associations. Type I cryoglobulinemia, associated with Waldenström's macroglobulinemia or, less frequently, multiple myeloma, is more likely to cause syndromes related to hyperviscosity (dizziness, confusion, headache, and stroke) than necrotizing vasculitis. In contrast to the monoclonal nature of type I cryoglobulinemia, types II and III are known as *mixed cryoglobulinemias* because they are composed of both IgG and IgM. In type II cryoglobulinemia, more than 90% of cases are caused by hepatitis C infection, and the cryoproteins consist of monoclonal IgM and polyclonal IgG. Cases of type II cryoglobulinemia not associated with hepatitis C are sometimes termed *mixed essential cryoglobulinemia*, because their cause is not known. Type III cryoglobulinemia, typically associated with polyclonal IgG and polyclonal IgM, is associated with many forms of chronic inflammation, including infection and autoimmune disease.

Type II and III cryoglobulinemias often present with a triad of signs and symptoms: purpura, arthralgias, and myalgias. The purpura may be extensive and confluent (Fig. 85-6), sometimes involving the trunk, upper extremities, and even the face; in most cases, however, the rash is confined to the lower extremities. Other organ systems commonly involved

Table 85-5 Types of Cryoglobulins

Cryoglobulin	RF Positivity	Monoclonality	Associated Diseases
Type I	No	Yes (IgG or IgM)	Hematopoietic malignancy (multiple myeloma, Waldenström's macroglobulinemia)
Type II	Yes	Yes (polyclonal IgG, monoclonal IgM)	Hepatitis C Other infection Sjögren's syndrome SLE
Type III	Yes	No (polyclonal IgG and IgM)	Hepatitis C Other infection Sjögren's syndrome SLE

Ig, immunoglobulin; RF, rheumatoid factor.

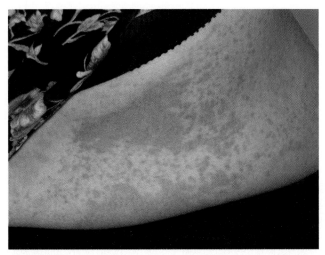

Figure 85-6 **Confluent purpura in mixed cryoglobulinemia.** Extensive purpuric lesions are often so numerous that they form confluent areas of cutaneous involvement.

in mixed cryoglobulinemia are the kidneys and peripheral nerves. Mixed cryoglobulinemia may cause a membranoproliferative glomerulonephritis that resembles lupus nephritis histopathologically. It may also cause a vasculitic neuropathy, usually with sensory symptoms predominating over motor symptoms.

Skin biopsy is the most straightforward method of confirming the diagnosis. Light microscopy of purpuric lesions demonstrates leukocytoclastic vasculitis. In addition, DIF studies reveal various types of immunoglobulin and complement deposition, depending on the type. In type II cryoglobulinemia, for example, DIF reveals IgG and IgM deposition, as well as complement components. Serologic testing may also yield clues to the presence of mixed cryoglobulinemia. To assay for serum cryoglobulins, the blood is collected in a prewarmed apparatus, allowed to clot at 37°C before processing, and then refrigerated at 4°C for several days. The percentage of the serum occupied by the cryoprecipitate is referred to as the "cryocrit." The difficulties involved in performing cryoglobulin assays often lead to false-negative results. Nonspecific serologic testing may also implicate mixed cryoglobulinemia. As noted, cryoglobulins detected are not always associated with disease.

A strong clue is the presence of an extremely low level of C4, reduced out of proportion to C3. In addition, the monoclonal component of type II cryoglobulins almost invariably has rheumatoid factor activity (i.e., binds to the Fc portion of IgG). Thus, essentially all patients with type II cryoglobulinemia have high titers of rheumatoid factor. As markers of clinical disease activity, C4 levels, rheumatoid factor titers, and cryocrits all fare poorly, often remaining abnormal in the face of clinically improved disease.

Treatment of the underlying cause of the cryoglobulins is the only approach that leads to a long-term response. Immunosuppression alone is insufficient to treat cryoglobulinemic vasculitis that is driven by malignancy or chronic infection. In the case of hepatitis C–associated cryoglobulinemic vasculitis, for example, the optimal therapy consists of effective control of the underlying viral infection (typically with interferon-α and ribavirin).[11] In patients who experience severe consequences of cryoglobulinemia such

as mononeuritis multiplex, glomerulonephritis, or extensive cutaneous ulceration, immunosuppression with high-dose glucocorticoids and cyclophosphamide may be necessary to prevent further damage. In some cases of active vasculitis, the introduction of antiviral therapy before controlling the inflammation with immunosuppression is believed to trigger disease exacerbation by altering the antigen-antibody ratio unfavorably.

The prognosis of patients with cryoglobulinemia generally depends on the underlying cause. The outcome of type I cryoglobulinemia relates closely to the success in treating the cause. Type II or III cryoglobulinemia secondary to hepatitis C can be treated effectively if the viral infection is responsive to therapy. If patients do not tolerate antiviral therapy well or if the treatment is ineffective, they may require low to moderate doses of prednisone to control the disease.

URTICARIAL VASCULITIS

In contrast to common urticaria, the lesions of urticarial vasculitis (UV) last more than 48 hours, do not blanch when pressure is applied to the skin, and may leave postinflammatory hyperpigmentation. Unlike common urticaria, the lesions of UV are frequently associated with moderate pain, burning, and tenderness in addition to pruritus. Whereas common urticaria typically resolves completely within 24 to 48 hours, the lesions of UV may take days to resolve completely, often leaving residual hyperpigmentation; they may worsen without therapy.

Three different syndromes of UV are recognized: normocomplementemic UV, hypocomplementemic UV, and the hypocomplementemic urticarial vasculitis syndrome (HUVS). Normocomplementemic UV is typically a self-limited subset of hypersensitivity vasculitis. In chronic cases, normocomplementemic UV must be distinguished carefully from neutrophilic urticaria, a persistent form of urticaria not associated with vasculitis. In contrast, hypocomplementemic UV is more likely to be a chronic disorder that has certain overlapping features with SLE: low serum complements, autoantibodies, and an interface dermatitis characterized by immunoreactant deposition (complement and immunoglobulins) at the dermal-epidermal junction in a pattern essentially identical to the lupus band test. Finally, HUVS is a severe form of the disease associated with extracutaneous disease and an array of organ system findings atypical of SLE.[12] For example, HUVS may be associated with uveitis, chronic obstructive pulmonary disease (COPD), and angioedema.

The skin lesions in UV tend to be centripetal, favoring the trunk and proximal extremities more than dependent regions. The lesions are painful and associated with a burning sensation rather than the pruritus of common urticaria. Biopsy of an urticarial wheal in UV demonstrates evidence of leukocytoclastic vasculitis, including injury to the endothelial cells of the postcapillary venules, erythrocyte extravasation, leukocytoclasis, fibrin deposition, and a perivascular neutrophilic (or, less commonly, lymphocytic) infiltrate. DIF demonstrates IC deposition around blood vessels in the superficial dermis and a striking deposition of immunoglobulins and complement along the dermal-epidermal junction. In the proper setting, these findings (interface dermatitis as well as immunoreactant deposition within blood vessels) are diagnostic of hypocomplementemic UV. HUVS, in contrast, is a clinical diagnosis based on the presence of UV and the occurrence of typical features in extracutaneous organ systems.

Some cases of hypocomplementemic UV respond to therapies commonly used for the treatment of SLE, including low-dose prednisone, hydroxychloroquine, dapsone, or other immunomodulatory agents. Serious cases of HUVS, particularly those presenting with glomerulonephritis or other forms of serious organ involvement, may require high doses of glucocorticoids and cytotoxic agents. Both COPD and cardiac valve abnormalities are associated with HUVS and may require specific treatment as well.

The prognosis of UV is linked to the disorder with which it is associated. SLE, COPD, angioedema, and valvular abnormalities are all known to occur in association with this disorder and may strongly influence both quality and quantity of life.

ERYTHEMA ELEVATUM DIUTINUM

Erythema elevatum diutinum (EED) is a rare, distinctive form of leukocytoclastic vasculitis limited to the skin. The disorder is distinctive because of the unusual distribution of skin lesions (found symmetrically over the extensor surfaces of joints) and the prompt response to sulfone medications. The cutaneous findings are typical of any small vessel vasculitis, with a predominance of papules, plaques, and nodules. Early lesions are often pink or yellowish and then become red or purple (Fig. 85-7). The natural history of untreated lesions is to persist for years, becoming doughy or hard with time. The lesions have a predilection for the skin overlying the small joints of the hands and the knees; they can also affect the buttocks. The trunk is generally spared.

The principal histopathologic findings of EED are leukocytoclastic vasculitis with fibrinoid necrosis. Although an IC basis is suspected in this disorder, DIF studies are not distinctive. EED has been associated with various connective tissue diseases (CTDs), rheumatoid arthritis, other forms of vasculitis such as Wegener's granulomatosis, human immunodeficiency virus infections, and paraproteinemias (particularly IgA). EED typically responds promptly to dapsone or sulfapyridine, but chronic therapy may be required because skin lesions recur after cessation of treatment.

CONNECTIVE TISSUE DISEASE–ASSOCIATED VASCULITIS

Vasculitis rarely occurs in CTDs without overt manifestations of the underlying disorder. The forms of CTD typically complicated by vasculitis include those related to SLE: lupus itself, mixed CTD, Sjögren's syndrome, and overlap CTD. Although vasculitis clearly occurs in some CTD settings, it is commonly overdiagnosed to explain perplexing disease features in patients with known rheumatic illnesses. For example, neuropsychiatric SLE is generally not caused by a true vasculitis but rather by other mechanisms that remain poorly defined. Whenever possible, the clinical hypothesis of vasculitis should be confirmed by biopsy.

Cutaneous vasculitis in CTDs is associated almost invariably with hypocomplementemia and high titers of antinuclear antibodies (ANAs). DIF examination of skin lesions shows granular IgG and C3 deposition in and around dermal vessels, with or without IgM, reflecting the contribution of ICs to disease pathogenesis. The phenomenon of the "in vivo ANA" is also observed in keratinocytes and dermal cells in DIF studies (Fig. 85-8).[13]

Vasculitis in patients with SLE-related disorders is more likely than other forms of vasculitis to be associated with a lymphocytic predominance. One variant of CTD-associated cutaneous vasculitis, the so-called benign hypergammaglobulinemia of Waldenström, is usually a true lymphocytic

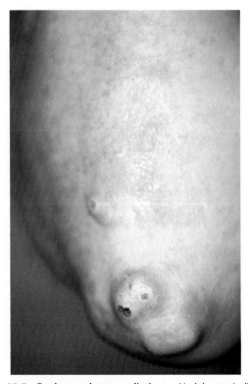

Figure 85-7 Erythema elevatum diutinum. Nodules typically form over the extensor surfaces of the knuckles and other joints.

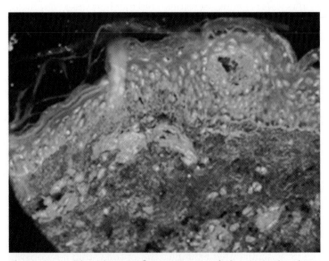

Figure 85-8 Direct immunofluorescence study in connective tissue disease–associated vasculitis, revealing an "in vivo antinuclear antibody" phenomenon. This phenomenon is caused by the binding of immunoreactants to targets within the nuclei of epidermal cells.

vasculitis. Patients with this disorder invariably have anti-Ro antibodies, and many have subclinical Sjögren's syndrome.

Lymphocytic vasculitis typically demonstrates less disruption of blood vessel architecture than does leukocytoclastic vasculitis, perhaps because lymphocytes contain fewer of the destructive enzymes found within neutrophil granules. Fibrinoid necrosis, for example, is very rare in lymphocytic vasculitis. True lymphocytic vasculitis is nearly always confined to the small blood vessels of the superficial papillary dermis.

RHEUMATOID VASCULITIS

Rheumatoid vasculitis (RV) must be distinguished from the isolated digital (periungual) vasculitis that, in the absence of severe involvement, does not require intensive, vasculitis-specific therapy. Isolated digital vasculitis in patients with rheumatoid arthritis, characterized by splinter-like lesions in the periungual region (Bywaters' lesions), is not necessarily associated with a poorer prognosis than rheumatoid arthritis without digital vasculitic lesions and does not require specific therapy for vasculitis. In contrast, RV is a potentially devastating complication that may involve both medium and small blood vessels and requires the most aggressive therapeutic interventions. Many clinical manifestations of RV are indistinguishable from polyarteritis nodosa, although microaneurysms are less common in RV. RV classically occurs in patients with nodular, rheumatoid factor–positive, joint-destructive disease who have few clinical indications of active synovitis at the time vasculitis begins. However, RV occasionally complicates early disease.

The most common presentation of RV includes purpuric lesions with or without evidence of concomitant medium vessel vasculitis. DIF examination of the skin lesions shows granular IgM and C3 deposition in vessels, consistent with an IC-mediated pathophysiology in which rheumatoid factor, complement, and cryoglobulins may all participate. Deep cutaneous ulcers near the malleoli are a hallmark of RV and require scrupulous local care as well as judicious immunosuppression. Mononeuritis multiplex often complicates RV.

REFERENCES

1. **Jennette JC, Falk RJ, Andrassy K, et al: Nomenclature of systemic vasculitides. Proposal of an international consensus conference. Arthritis Rheum 37:187-192, 1994.**
2. Zeek PM: Periarteritis nodosa: A critical review. Am J Clin Pathol 22:777-790, 1952.
3. Arthus M: Injections repetees de serum de cheval cuez le lapin. Seances et Memoire de la Societe de Biologie 55:817-825, 1903.
4. Nangaku M, Couser WG: Mechanisms of immune-deposit formation and the mediation of immune renal injury. Clin Exp Nephrol 9:183-191, 2005.
5. Ramos-Casals M, Anaya JM, Garcia-Carrasco M, et al: Cutaneous vasculitis in primary Sjogren syndrome: Classification and clinical significance of 52 patients. Medicine (Baltimore) 83:96, 2004.
6. **Hunder GG, Arend WP, Bloch DA, et al: The American College of Rheumatology 1990 criteria for the classification of vasculitis: Introduction. Arthritis Rheum 33:1065-1067, 1990.**
7. Calabrese LH, Michel BA, Bloch DA, et al: American College of Rheumatology 1990 criteria for the classification of hypersensitivity vasculitis. Arthritis Rheum 33:1108-1113, 1990.
8. Mills JA, Michel BA, Bloch DA, et al: The American College of Rheumatology 1990 criteria for the classification of Henoch-Schönlein purpura. Arthritis Rheum 33:1114-1121, 1990.
9. Blanco R, Martinez-Taboada VM, Rodriguez-Valverde V, et al: Henoch-Schonlein purpura in adulthood and childhood: Two different expressions of the same syndrome. Arthritis Rheum 40:859-864, 1997.
10. Wintrobe MM, Buell MV: Hyperproteinemia associated with multiple myeloma: With report of a case in which an extraordinary hyperproteinemia was associated with thrombosis of the retinal veins and symptoms suggesting Raynaud's disease. Bull Johns Hopkins Hosp 52:156, 1933.
11. Ferri C, Mascia MT: Cryoglobulinemic vasculitis. Curr Opin Rheumatol 18:54-63, 2006.
12. Davis MD, Brewer JD: Urticarial vasculitis and hypocomplementemic urticarial vasculitis syndrome. Immunol Allergy Clin North Am 24:183-213, 2004.
13. Wahl CE, Bouldin MB, Gibson LE: Erythema elevatum diutinum: Clinical, histopathologic, and immunohistochemical characteristics of six patients. Am J Dermatopathol 27:397-400, 2005.

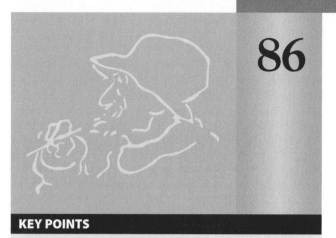

86 Behçet's Disease

B. ASHER LOUDEN • JOSEPH L. JORIZZO

KEY POINTS

Behçet's disease is a complex multisystem disease characterized by oral aphthae and other features.

Diagnosis is based on the criteria set forth by the International Study Group, including oral aphthae, genital aphthae, ocular lesions, cutaneous lesions, and a positive pathergy test.

Cutaneous lesions should display a neutrophilic vascular reaction on histopathologic examination.

Treatment is based on the degree of systemic involvement and ranges from topical corticosteroids to thalidomide to systemic immunosuppressive agents and tumor necrosis factor-α inhibitors.

Prognosis is variable, and patients typically have periods of exacerbations and remissions.

Behçet's disease is a chronic, complex multisystem disease characterized clinically by oral aphthae and at least two of the following: genital aphthae, cutaneous lesions, and ophthalmic, neurologic, or rheumatologic manifestations. The first description of Behçet's disease was probably by Hippocrates in the fifth century BC,[1] and the first modern account was presented in 1937 by the Turkish dermatologist Hulusi Behçet, who reported on a patient with recurrent oral and genital aphthae and uveitis.[2]

EPIDEMIOLOGY

Behçet's disease is seen worldwide, with the highest prevalence reported in Turkey (80 to 370 patients per 100,000 inhabitants)[3] and Japan (13.6 per 100,000).[4] Other regions with high prevalence include the Middle East and the Mediterranean (i.e., the "Silk Route").[5] It is relatively uncommon in northern Europe and the United States (0.1 to 7.5 patients per 100,000 inhabitants).[3,5] Patients commonly fulfill the diagnostic criteria in their mid-20s to 30s.[6] In the past, Behçet's disease was thought to predominantly affect males, but current epidemiologic data show a more equal male-to-female ratio.[7] Overall, males are more affected in the Middle East, whereas females predominate in northern Europe and the United States.[7]

CAUSE AND PATHOGENESIS

Although the pathogenesis of Behçet's disease remains unclear, many factors have been implicated. Heredity, immunologic factors, infectious agents, and inflammatory mediators likely contribute.

GENETICS

A familial pattern of Behçet's disease has been reported, but there are regional differences throughout the world. Familial occurrence is more common in Korea, Israel, Turkey, and Arab countries, compared with Japan, China, and Europe.[7] Studies have shown a significant association between the human leukocyte antigen (HLA)-B51 and Behçet's disease.[8,9] The relative risk of HLA-B51–positive individuals' developing Behçet's disease varies, depending on geographic region.[7] The causative role of HLA-B51 in Behçet's remains unclear. It may be that HLA-B51 is not directly involved in causing the disease but is closely linked to disease-related genes.[10] Candidate genes have been localized to chromosome 6 and include the major histocompatibility complex class I chain-related gene A (MICA) and, more specifically, the MICA6 allele; perth block (PERB); new organization associated with HLA-B (NOB); and transporter associated with antigen processing genes (TAP).[10,11]

Although Behçet's disease has many features in common with the spondyloarthropathies, especially those associated with inflammatory bowel disease (IBD), the disorder in IBD patients generally evolves in a pattern resembling reactive arthritis, with an erosive axial arthritis; erosive arthritis and HLA-B27 are not associated with Behçet's disease.[12] Patients who are HLA-DR1 and HLA-DQw1 positive may have an innate resistance to the development of Behçet's disease.[13]

IMMUNE MECHANISMS

Immune mechanisms play a major role in Behçet's disease. Heat shock proteins, cytokines, alterations in neutrophil and macrophage activity, and autoimmune mechanisms have all been implicated.[10] Heat shock proteins are released in response to stress and may be involved in stimulating a T helper type 1 immune response through interaction with Toll-like receptors.[14] Most of the T lymphocytes thought to be involved in this reaction are of the γδ type.[15] Cytokines such as interleukin (IL)-1, IL-8, and tumor necrosis factor-α (TNF-α) seem to be involved in the pathogenesis, and elevated levels may be a marker of disease activity.[10] It should be appreciated, however, that plasma TNF-α levels may rise and fall as an acute-phase reactant along with C-reactive protein and the erythrocyte sedimentation rate. The production of these proinflammatory cytokines, which are responsible for the chronic inflammation observed, may be the result of activated macrophages.[10,16] In addition to macrophage activation, neutrophil chemotaxis and phagocytosis are increased in the lesions of Behçet's disease.[10,17] This increased activity of neutrophils leads to tissue injury in the form of the neutrophilic vascular reaction seen in lesions, such as aphthae, pustular cutaneous lesions, and erythema nodosum–like lesions. Circulating immune complexes also play a role in precipitating the characteristic neutrophilic vascular reaction.[18] Finally, the role of endothelial cell dysfunction in the pathogenesis of Behçet's disease has been suggested by decreased levels of prostacyclin in the serum of Behçet's disease patients. Other abnormalities in the endothelium and in clotting factors have also been found.[19]

INFECTIOUS AGENTS

Several studies have suggested a role for various infectious agents in the pathogenesis of Behçet's disease; however, no organisms have been consistently isolated. Antistreptococcal antibodies have been isolated in the serum of patients with Behçet's disease.[20] Higher concentrations of *Streptococcus sanguis* have also been found in the oral flora of patients with Behçet's disease and may play a role in the development of aphthae, which is often the initial manifestation.[21] In addition to streptococcal antigens, other bacteria such as *Escherichia coli* and *Staphylococcus aureus* may have a role in Behçet's disease through the activation of lymphocytes.[22]

Herpes simplex virus (HSV) DNA has been isolated from the nuclei of peripheral blood lymphocytes by polymerase chain reaction (PCR) assay in patients with Behçet's disease.[13] HSV has also been detected by PCR in biopsy samples of genital and intestinal ulcers of Behçet's patients.[22] Other studies, however, have shown no difference in the detection of HSV in Behçet's patients with and without oral aphthae.[23]

In summary, although the cause and pathogenesis of Behçet's disease are not completely understood, they likely involve an infectious or environmental trigger and subsequent inflammatory response in a genetically predisposed individual. The recent article by Zouboulis and May[10] provides an excellent overview of the pathogenesis of Behçet's disease.

CLINICAL FEATURES

APHTHAE

Oral aphthae, or canker sores (Fig. 86-1), are often the initial feature of Behçet's disease and constitute a requisite diagnostic feature (although it should be pointed out that a number of investigators believe that this disease can occur in the absence of oral aphthae). Oral ulcerations usually occur in crops of more than 3 to 10s of lesions, but individual lesions may occur on the buccal mucosa, gingiva, lips, and tongue. Aphthae tend to be painful and shallow, and they heal without scarring over 1 to 3 weeks.[24] Genital ulcers typically occur on the scrotum and penis in males and on the vulva or vaginal mucosa in females. These aphthae are similar in appearance to oral lesions, but they have a greater tendency to scar and may recur less frequently.[24] Lesions in the oral mucosa are generally easy to distinguish from oral HSV, but with genital lesions, HSV should be excluded by viral culture or PCR before they are accepted as a diagnostic criterion.

CUTANEOUS LESIONS

Several cutaneous manifestations of Behçet's disease have been described: erythema nodosum–like lesions, pyoderma gangrenosum–like lesions, Sweet's syndrome–like lesions, cutaneous small vessel vasculitis, and pustular vasculitic lesions (Fig. 86-2), including lesions induced by trauma—the so-called pathergy lesion.[24] Specimens from all these lesions demonstrate a neutrophilic vascular reaction on histopathologic analysis.[25] Acneiform or pseudofolliculitis lesions should be considered nonspecific, nondiagnostic findings because of their common occurrence in acne vulgaris and folliculitis.

OPHTHALMIC FEATURES

A variety of ocular manifestations have been reported in Behçet's patients, including anterior and posterior uveitis, retinal vasculitis, and hypopyon, with secondary glaucoma, cataract formation, decreased visual acuity, and synechiae formation.[26] Ocular involvement occurs in 83% to 95% of men and 67% to 73% of women with Behçet's disease.[26] Although ocular involvement is not commonly the presenting feature of Behçet's disease, it is a major source of serious morbidity, and close ophthalmologic evaluation and follow-up are critical to prevent blindness in these patients.[27] BenEzra and Cohen[28] suggested that if ocular disease does not present within a few years of diagnosis, it is unlikely to be a major problem.

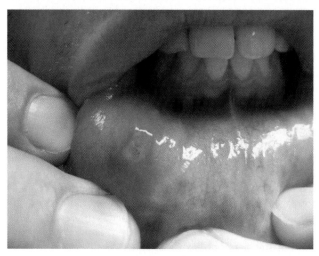

Figure 86-1 Oral aphtha.

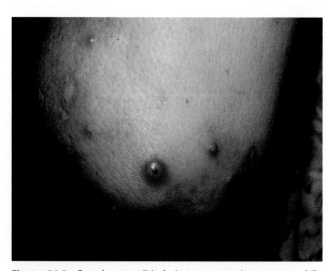

Figure 86-2 Pustular vasculitis lesions representing a neutrophilic vascular reaction.

ARTHRITIS

The arthritis of Behçet's disease is typically a nonerosive, inflammatory, symmetric or asymmetric oligoarthritis, although polyarticular and monarticular forms are also seen. The most commonly involved joints are the knees, wrists, ankles, and elbows.[29] The prevalence of arthritis among different populations ranges from 40% to 60%, and joint erosions are not observed.[27] Dilsen and colleagues[30] reported that 10% of patients with Behçet's disease had a sacroiliitis. However, HLA-B27–positive patients were not excluded from their series, and occult IBD was not excluded, as required by O'Duffy.[40] Other studies have shown no significant difference in the occurrence of sacroiliitis between patients with Behçet's disease and the normal population. HLA-B27–positive patients with erosive sacroiliitis should be included in the Reiter's syndrome or enteropathic arthritis disease spectrum, given the erosive, axial nature of the arthritis in the HLA-B27 pattern. This contrasts with the classically nonerosive, nonaxial nature of the arthritis in Behçet's disease. Oral aphthae, ocular lesions, erythema nodosum–like lesions, pustular vasculitis, and pyoderma gangrenosum all occur in patients with IBD.

OTHER SYSTEMIC MANIFESTATIONS

Central nervous system involvement is most commonly characterized by brainstem or corticospinal tract syndromes (neuro-Behçet's syndrome), venous sinus thrombosis, increased intracranial pressure secondary to venous sinus thrombosis or aseptic meningitis, isolated behavioral symptoms, or isolated headache.[31] Rarely, ruptured aneurysms, peripheral neuropathy, optic neuritis, and vestibular involvement can occur.[31] Poor prognosis is associated with a progressive course, parenchymal or brainstem involvement, and cerebrospinal fluid abnormalities.[32] Cranial and peripheral nerve involvement may also occur.

Patients with Behçet's disease may have gastrointestinal lesions resembling orogenital aphthae. These occur most commonly in the ileocecal region and in the ascending colon, transverse colon, or esophagus.[33] Large aphthae may lead to perforation. Presenting symptoms include abdominal pain, diarrhea, and melena. It is important to distinguish IBD from Behçet's disease (discussed later).[33] Aphthae may also affect the bladder.

Pulmonary abnormalities are uncommon in Behçet's disease. Pulmonary artery aneurysms occur most frequently, followed by other complications secondary to vasculitis affecting the small pulmonary vessels. Aneurysm, thrombosis, hemorrhage, and infarction can result[34] and can cause death in patients with Behçet's disease.

Renal manifestations vary from minimal changes to proliferative glomerulonephritis and rapidly progressive crescentic glomerulonephritis. The pathogenesis likely involves immune complex deposition.[35]

Cardiac complications include myocardial infarction, pericarditis, arterial and venous thromboses, and aneurysm formation. Thromboses more commonly involve the venous system, sometimes leading to superior and inferior vena cava obstruction.[25] Cardiac manifestations, either occlusive or aneurysmal, are postulated to occur due to a vasculitis of the vasa vasorum, which induces a thickening of the media and splitting of elastic fibers.[36]

HISTOPATHOLOGY

Histopathologic analysis of specimens from the cutaneous lesions seen in Behçet's disease reveals a neutrophilic vascular reaction or even fully developed leukocytoclastic vasculitis. Microscopic examination of dermal capillary or venule walls shows neutrophilic infiltrates, nuclear dust, and extravasation of erythrocytes, with or without fibrinoid necrosis.[37] Immune complex–mediated vasculitis is the likely mechanism in the development of Behçet's disease.[38] A previously reported finding of lymphocytic vasculitis in patients with Behçet's disease is thought to represent an older lesion.[25]

Biopsy specimens of synovial membranes reveal a neutrophilic reaction, with occasional plasma cells and lymphocytes. Immunofluorescence microscopy may show immunoglobulin G (IgG) deposition along the synovial membrane.[27] Reports of synovial fluid analysis in patients with Behçet's disease show leukocyte counts ranging from 300 to 36,200 cells/mm^3, with a predominance of neutrophils and normal glucose levels.[39] Synovitis is included as one of the O'Duffy-Goldstein criteria for the diagnosis of Behçet's disease.[40]

DIAGNOSIS

The diagnosis of Behçet's disease can be difficult to confirm, particularly in patients with only a limited number of common features of the disease. Clinicians and investigators must rely on clinical criteria, because there are no pathognomonic laboratory findings. Several sets of diagnostic criteria have been proposed, including those by O'Duffy and Goldstein,[40] Mason and Barnes,[41] and a Japanese study group.[42] In 1990, the International Study Group established a set of criteria based on the presence of recurrent oral aphthae and two additional findings from the following list: recurrent genital aphthae, cutaneous lesions, ocular involvement, and a positive pathergy test result (Table 86-1).[43] These criteria were found to have a sensitivity of 91% and a specificity of 96%.[43]

Although not required by the International Study Group criteria, IBD, systemic lupus erythematosus, Reiter's syndrome, and herpetic infections should first be excluded, because the presenting manifestations of these conditions are often similar to those of Behçet's disease. Recurrent aphthous stomatitis and complex aphthosis, defined as recurrent oral and genital aphthae or almost constant, multiple (three or more) oral aphthae, should also be considered in the differential diagnosis of patients presenting with oral or genital aphthae.[44]

The O'Duffy-Goldstein criteria mandate the presence of recurrent oral aphthae plus at least two of the following: genital aphthae, synovitis, posterior uveitis, cutaneous pustular vasculitis, and meningoencephalitis. Patients who have only two of these findings, one being recurrent oral aphthae, are considered to have an incomplete form of Behçet's disease. Another concern with regard to the International Study Group criteria is the inclusion of acneiform lesions, which are a common nonspecific finding in both adolescents and adults. Therefore, our group advocates histologic confirmation of vessel-based histology to exclude acne lesions and the use of both the O'Duffy and the International Study Group criteria to exclude patients with IBD and enteropathic arthritis.[45]

Table 86-1 International Study Group Criteria for the Diagnosis of Behçet's Disease*

Recurrent Oral Ulceration

Minor aphthous, major aphthous, or herpetiform ulceration observed by physician or patient that recurred at least three times in one 12-month period
Plus two of the following criteria:

Recurrent Genital Ulceration

Aphthous ulceration or scarring observed by physician or patient

Eye Lesions

Anterior uveitis, posterior uveitis, or cells in vitreous on slit-lamp examination
or
Retinal vasculitis observed by ophthalmologist

Skin Lesions

Erythema nodosum observed by physician or patient, pseudofolliculitis, or papulopustular lesions
or
Acneiform nodules observed by physician in postadolescent patients not on corticosteroid treatment

Positive Result on Pathergy Testing

Read by physician at 24 to 48 hr

*Findings applicable only in the absence of other clinical explanations.
Data from International Study Group for Behçet's Disease: Criteria for the diagnosis of Behçet's disease. Lancet 335:1078-1080, 1990.

The initial evaluation should include referral for ophthalmologic consultation to identify insidious ocular involvement. Patients who have arthralgias, gastrointestinal symptoms, or neurologic abnormalities may require radiographic studies and evaluation by appropriate subspecialists. Cutaneous pustular lesions, erythema nodosum–like lesions, and pyoderma gangrenosum–like lesions should be biopsied (for both histologic evaluation and culture) to confirm the clinical diagnosis.

A diagnostic algorithm for patients presenting with characteristic oral aphthae is presented in Figure 86-3.

TREATMENT

Therapeutic options should be based on the degree of systemic involvement (Table 86-2).[24]

MUCOCUTANEOUS DISEASE

Patients with oral and genital aphthae can be treated with intralesional, superpotent topical or aerosolized (not inhaled) corticosteroids. Topical tacrolimus can also be used, often in combination with superpotent topical corticosteroids. Other palliative therapies include oral tetracycline solutions, topical anesthetics, and rinses containing chlorhexidine gluconate. Oral colchicine, 0.6 mg two to three times daily, can decrease the size and frequency of mucocutaneous lesions.[46,47] Doses can be adjusted according to the degree of gastrointestinal upset experienced by the patient. Dapsone in a dose of 50 to 150 mg/day is often helpful alone[48] or in combination with colchicine.[44] Patients must be monitored for the development of hemolytic anemia and methemoglobinemia; the glucose-6-phosphate dehydrogenase level should be checked in all patients before beginning therapy with dapsone.

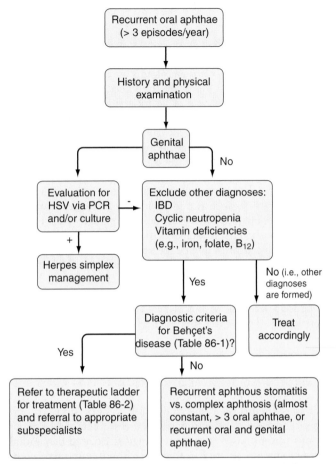

Figure 86-3 Diagnostic algorithm for patients presenting with characteristic oral aphthae. HSV, herpes simplex virus; IBD, inflammatory bowel disease; PCR, polymerase chain reaction.

SEVERE MUCOCUTANEOUS DISEASE

Patients who fail to respond to conservative therapy as outlined for mucocutaneous disease may require thalidomide. Its mechanism of action is thought to be mediated by modulation of TNF-α and other cytokines. Previous studies have shown that thalidomide is a relatively safe and effective agent for the treatment of Behçet's disease.[49,50] Thalidomide is known to cause severe birth defects, and all patients and prescribing physicians must adhere to the System for Thalidomide Education and Prescribing Safety (STEPS) protocol, including monthly follow-up visits.[51] Patients receiving thalidomide can be monitored with nerve conduction studies for the development of peripheral neuropathy, if doing so is warranted based on the clinical neurologic evaluation.

Low-dose oral methotrexate (2.5 to 25 mg/wk) and low-dose prednisone are alternatives for patients with severe mucocutaneous involvement.[47,52] Patients receiving methotrexate should be monitored for the development of hepatotoxicity and leukopenia. The risk of rebound upon the tapering or discontinuation of systemic prednisone greatly limits its use for mucocutaneous disease alone. In addition, interferon-α is effective for severe mucocutaneous lesions and some systemic manifestations.[53,54] A review of the safety and efficacy of interferon-α by Zouboulis and Orfanos[53] recommended a 3-month high-dose regimen of 9 million units three times per week, followed by a low, maintenance dose of 3 million units three times per week.

Table 86-2 Treatment of Behçet's Disease

Mucocutaneous Disease Only
Topical, intralesional, or aerosolized corticosteroids
Topical sucralfate
Local anesthetics
Topical tacrolimus
Colchicine (0.6-1.8 mg/day)
Dapsone (50-150 mg/day)
Combinations of these agents

Severe Mucocutaneous Disease
Thalidomide (50-150 mg/day)
Methotrexate (2.5-25 mg/wk)
Prednisone
Interferon-α (3 million-9 million U/wk)

Systemic Disease
Prednisone
Azathioprine (50-200 mg bid)
Chlorambucil (4-6 mg/day)
Cyclophosphamide
Cyclosporine
Mycophenolate mofetil (1-1.5 g bid)
Intravenous immunoglobulin
Anti–TNF-α agents (adalimumab, etanercept, infliximab)

SYSTEMIC DISEASE

Patients with systemic disease, such as ocular and cardiovascular abnormalities, require immunosuppressive therapy, particularly in view of the risk of morbidity and mortality resulting from untreated disease. Systemic corticosteroids may be used alone or in combination with other immunosuppressive agents such as azathioprine, interferon-α, cyclosporine, cyclophosphamide, and chlorambucil.[47,55] The standard of care for eye disease is prednisone plus azathioprine.[56] If this combination is not successful, one of the aforementioned immunosuppressive agents can be substituted for azathioprine.[55] Several of these immunosuppressive agents have associated hematologic toxicity, as well as the potential for the development of associated malignancies; therefore, close monitoring is essential. There have also been reports of Behçet's disease treated with anti–TNF-α agents. A double-blind, placebo-controlled trial showed that etanercept was successful in suppressing most of the mucocutaneous manifestations of Behçet's disease.[57] Other reports support the efficacy of adalimumab and infliximab.[58,59] Larger studies looking at the long-term efficacy and safety of these agents are in progress.

PROGNOSIS

Behçet's disease has a variable clinical course in most patients, with a pattern of exacerbations and remissions. A delay in diagnosis after the initial manifestation of Behçet's disease is not uncommon. Most patients present initially with mucocutaneous manifestations, and evidence of ocular and neurologic involvement may appear several years after diagnosis. Patients with the finding of complex aphthosis may represent a forme fruste of Behçet's disease, and they should be monitored for the development of additional abnormalities fulfilling the diagnostic criteria through regular follow-up and referral to appropriate specialists.[44] Mortality in Behçet's disease is low and is usually related to pulmonary or central nervous system involvement or to

bowel perforation.[7] The most common cause of morbidity is ocular involvement; manifestations such as posterior uveitis and retinal vasculitis can cause blindness.

REFERENCES

1. Feigenbaum A: Description of Behçet's syndrome in the Hippocratic third book of endemic diseases. Br J Ophthalmol 40:355, 1956.
2. Behçet H: Uber rezidivierende Aphthose durch ein Virus verursachte Geschwure am Mund, am Auge, und an den Genitalien. Dermatol Wochenschr 105:1152-1157, 1937.
3. Zoubloulis CC: Epidemiology of Adamantiades-Behçet's disease [abstract]. Ann Med Interne (Paris) 150:488-498, 1999.
4. Kontogiannis V, Powell RJ: Behçet's disease. Postgrad Med J 76: 629-637, 2000.
5. Dilsen N: History and development of Behçet's disease [abstract]. Rev Rhum Engl Ed 63:512-519, 1996.
6. Hegab S, Al-Mutawa S: Immunopathogenesis of Behçet's disease. Clin Immunol 96:174-186, 2000.
7. Zouboulis CC: Epidemiology of Adamantiades-Behçet's disease. In Bang D, Lang E-S, Lee S (eds): Behçet's Disease: Proceedings of the 8th and 9th International Conference on Behçet's Disease. Seoul, Design Mecca, 2000, pp 43-47.
8. Yazici H, Chamberlain MA, Schreuder I, et al: HLA antigens in Behçet's disease: A reappraisal by a comparative study of Turkish and British patients. Ann Rheum Dis 39:344-348, 1980.
9. Ohno S, Ohguchi M, Hirose S, et al: Close association of HLA-BW51 with Behçet's disease. Arch Ophthalmol 100:1455-1458, 1982.
10. Zouboulis CC, May T: Pathogenesis of Adamantiades-Behçet's disease. Adv Exp Med Biol 528:161-171, 2003.
11. Zierhut M, Mizuki N, Ohno S, et al: Immunology and functional genomics of Behçet's disease. Cell Mol Life Sci 60:1903-1922, 2003.
12. O'Duffy JD, Taswell HF, Elveback LR: HLA antigens in Behçet's disease. J Rheumatol 3:1-3, 1976.
13. Jorizzo JL: Behçet's disease: An update based on the 1985 International Conference in London. Arch Dermatol 122:556-558, 1986.
14. Direskeneli H, Saruhan-Direskeneli G: The role of heat shock proteins in Behçet's disease. Clin Exp Rheumatol 21(4 Suppl 30):S44-S48, 2003.
15. Hasan A, Fortune F, Wilson A, et al: Role of gamma delta T cells in the pathogenesis and diagnosis of Behçet's disease. Lancet 347: 789-794, 1996.
16. Sahin S, Lawrence R, Direskeneli H, et al: Monocyte activity in Behçet's disease. Br J Rheumatol 35:424-429, 1996.
17. Takeno M, Kariyone A, Yamashita N, et al: Excessive function of peripheral blood neutrophils from patients with Behçet's disease and from HLA-B51 transgenic mice. Arthritis Rheum 38:426-433, 1955.
18. Gupta RC, O'Duffy JD, McDuffie FC, et al: Circulating immune complexes in active Behçet's disease. Clin Exp Immunol 34:213-218, 1978.
19. Saylan T, Mat C, Fresko I, et al: Behçet's disease in the Middle East. Clin Dermatol 17:209-223, 1999.
20. Mizushima Y: Behçet's disease. Curr Opin Rheumatol 3:32-35, 1991.
21. Isogai E, Ohno S, Kotake S, et al: Chemiluminescence of neutrophils from patients with Behçet's disease and its correlation with an increased proportion of uncommon serotypes of Streptococcus sanguis in the oral flora. Arch Oral Biol 35:43-48, 1990.
22. Direskeneli H: Behçet's disease: Infectious aetiology, new autoantigens, and HLA-B51. Ann Rheum Dis 60:996-1002, 2001.
23. Lee S, Bang D, Cho YH: Polymerase chain reaction reveals herpes simplex virus DNA in saliva of patients with Behçet's disease. Arch Dermatol Res 288:179-183, 1996.
24. Ghate JV, Jorizzo JL: Behçet's disease and complex aphthosis. J Am Acad Dermatol 40:1-8, 1999.
25. Jorizzo JL, Abernethy JL, White WL, et al: Mucocutaneous criteria for the diagnosis of Behçet's disease: An analysis of clinicopathologic data from multiple international centers. J Am Acad Dermatol 32:968-976, 1995.
26. Bhisitkul RB, Foster CS: Diagnosis and ophthalmological features of Behçet's disease. Int Ophthalmol Clin 36:127-134, 1996.
27. Kaklamani VG, Vaiopoulos G, Kaklamanis PG: Behçet's disease. Semin Arthritis Rheum 27:197-215, 1998.
28. BenEzra D, Cohen E: Treatment and visual prognosis in Behçet's disease. Br J Ophthalmol 70:589-592, 1986.

29. Moral F, Hamuryudan V, Yurdakul S, et al: Inefficacy of azapropazone in the acute arthritis of Behçet's syndrome: A randomized, double blind, placebo controlled study. Clin Exp Rheumatol 13:493-495, 1995.

30. Dilsen N, Konice M, Aral O: Why Behçet's disease should be accepted as a seronegative arthritis. In Lehner T, Barnes CG (eds): Recent Advances in Behçet's Disease. International Congress and Symposium Series no. 103. London, Royal Society of Medicine Services, 1986, pp 281-284.

31. Siva A, Kantarci OH, Saip S, et al: Behçet's disease: Diagnostic and prognostic aspects of neurological involvement. J Neurol 248:95-103, 2001.

32. Akman-Demir G, Serdaroglu P, Tasçi B (Neuro-Behçet Study Group): Clinical patterns of neurological involvement in Behçet's disease: Evaluation of 200 patients. Brain 122:2171-2181, 1999.

33. Sakane T, Takeno M, Suzuki N, et al: Behçet's disease. N Engl J Med 341:1284-1291, 1999.

34. Uzun O, Akpolat T, Erkan L: Pulmonary vasculitis in Behçet's disease. Chest 127:2243-2253, 2005.

35. El Ramahi KM, Al Dalaan A, Al Shaikh A, et al: Renal involvement in Behçet's disease: Review of 9 cases. J Rheumatol 25:2254-2260, 1998.

36. Du LTH, Wechsler B, Piette J, et al: Long-term prognosis of arterial lesions in Behçet's disease. In Wechsler B, Godeau P (eds): Behçet's Disease: Proceedings of the 6th International Conference on Behçet's Disease. Paris, France, 30 June-1 July, 1993. Amsterdam, Elsevier Science, 1993, pp 557-562.

37. Ackerman AB: Behçet's disease. In Ackerman AB, Chongchitnant N, Sanchez J, et al (eds): Histologic Diagnosis of Inflammatory Skin Diseases: An Algorithmic Method Based on Pattern Analysis, 2nd ed. Baltimore, Williams & Wilkins, 1997, pp 229-232.

38. Lakhanpal S, Tani K, Lie JT, et al: Pathologic features of Behçet's syndrome: A review of Japanese autopsy registry data. Hum Pathol 16:790, 1985.

39. Yurdakul S, Yazici H, Tuzun Y, et al: The arthritis of Behçet's disease: A prospective study. Ann Rheum Dis 42:505-515, 1983.

40. **O'Duffy JD, Goldstein NP: Neurologic involvement in seven patients with Behçet's disease. Am J Med 61:17-18, 1976.**

41. Mason RM, Barnes CG: Behçet's syndrome with arthritis. Ann Rheum Dis 28:95-103, 1969.

42. Behçet's Disease Research Committee of Japan: Behçet's disease: A guide to diagnosis of Behçet's disease. Jpn J Ophthalmol 18:291-294, 1974.

43. **International Study Group for Behçet's Disease: Criteria for the diagnosis of Behçet's disease. Lancet 335:1078-1080, 1990.**

44. Letsinger JA, McCarty MA, Jorizzo JL: Complex aphthosis: A large case series with evaluation algorithm and therapeutic ladder from topicals to thalidomide. J Am Acad Dermatol 52:500-508, 2005.

45. Jorizzo JL: Behçet's disease. In Fitzpatrick TB, Eisen AZ, Wolff K, et al (eds): Dermatology in General Medicine, 5th ed. New York, McGraw-Hill, 1999, pp 2161-2165.

46. **Yurdakul S, Mat C, Tuzun Y, et al: A double-blind trial of colchicine in Behçet's syndrome. Arthritis Rheum 44:2686-2692, 2001.**

47. Kaklamani VG, Kaklamanis PG: Treatment of Behçet's disease: An update. Semin Arthritis Rheum 30:299-312, 2001.

48. Sharquie KE, Najim RA, Abu-Raghif AR: Dapsone in Behçet's disease: A double-blind, placebo-controlled, cross-over study. J Dermatol 29:267-279, 2002.

49. **Hamuryudan V, Mat C, Saip S, et al: Thalidomide in the treatment of the mucocutaneous lesions of Behçet's syndrome: A randomized double-blinded, placebo controlled trial. Ann Intern Med 128: 443-450, 1998.**

50. De Wazieres B, Gil H, Vuitton DA, et al: Treatment of recurrent orogenital ulceration with low doses of thalidomide. Clin Exp Rheumatol 17:393, 1999.

51. Housman TS, Jorizzo JL, McCarty AM, et al: Low-dose thalidomide therapy for refractory cutaneous lesions of lupus erythematosus. Arch Dermatol 139:50-54, 2003.

52. Jorizzo JL, White WL, Wise CM, et al: Low-dose weekly methotrexate for unusual neutrophilic vascular reactions: Cutaneous polyarteritis nodosa and Behçet's disease. J Am Acad Dermatol 24:973-978, 1991.

53. Zouboulis CC, Orfanos CE: Treatment of Adamantiades-Behçet disease with systemic interferon alpha. Arch Dermatol 134:1010-1016, 1998.

54. O'Duffy JD, Calamia K, Cohen S, et al: Alpha interferon treatment of Behçet's disease. J Rheumatol 25:1938-1944, 1998.

55. Green JJ, Jorizzo JL: Behçet disease. In Lebwohl M, Heymann WR, Berth-Jones J, Coulson I (eds): Treatment of Skin Disease: Comprehensive Therapeutic Strategies, 1st ed. London, Harcourt, 2002, pp 86-89.

56. **Yazici H, Pazarli H, Barnes CG, et al: A controlled trial of azathioprine in Behçet syndrome. N Engl J Med 322:281-285, 1990.**

57. **Melikoglu M, Fresko I, Mat C, et al: Short-term trial of etanercept in Behçet's disease: A double blind, placebo controlled study. J Rheumatol 32:98-105, 2005.**

58. Alexis AF, Strober BE: Off-label dermatologic uses of anti-TNF-α therapies. J Cutan Med Surg 9:296-302, 2005.

59. Van Laar JA, Missotten T, van Daele PL, et al: Adalimumab; a new modality for Behçet's disease? ARD Online First 1-8, 2006. Available at http://ard.bmj.com.

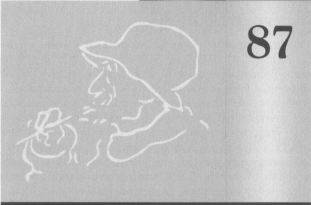

87

Gout and Hyperuricemia ▶

ROBERT L. WORTMANN

KEY POINTS

Hyperuricemia is defined as a serum urate level greater than 6.8 mg/dL.

Acute gouty arthritis can be treated with nonsteroidal anti-inflammatory drugs (NSAIDs), colchicine, corticosteroids, or adrenocorticotropic hormone. The effectiveness of treatment depends more on how quickly the therapy is initiated than which agent is used.

Before starting a specific urate-lowering agent, the patient should be treated with low-dose colchicine or NSAID in an attempt to prevent further attacks.

Regardless of whether a xanthine oxidase inhibitor or uricosuric agent is used to treat hyperuricemia, the patient should receive the lowest dose that maintains the serum urate level below 6.8 mg/dL—preferably between 5 and 6 mg/dL.

Individuals who are hyperuricemic should be screened for hypertension, coronary artery disease, diabetes, obesity, and alcoholism.

Using a specific urate-lowering agent to manage asymptomatic hyperuricemia is not recommended. However, associated conditions such as hypertension, coronary artery disease, diabetes, obesity, and alcoholism should be managed in these patients as well as in those with symptomatic gout.

Gout has been called the "king of diseases" and the "disease of kings." Today, the term *gout* is used to represent a heterogeneous group of diseases found exclusively in humans that include the following characteristics:

- Elevated serum urate concentration (hyperuricemia)
- Recurrent attacks of acute arthritis in which monosodium urate monohydrate crystals are demonstrable in synovial fluid leukocytes
- Aggregates of sodium urate monohydrate crystals (tophi) deposited chiefly in and around joints, which sometimes lead to deformity and crippling
- Renal disease involving glomerular, tubular, and interstitial tissues and blood vessels
- Uric acid nephrolithiasis

These manifestations can occur in various combinations.[1,2]

Hyperuricemia denotes an elevated level of urate in the blood. This occurs in an absolute (or physiochemical) sense when the serum urate concentration exceeds the limit of solubility of monosodium urate in the serum, which is 6.8 mg/dL at 37°C. Thus, a value greater than 6.8 mg/dL indicates supersaturation of body fluids. The serum urate concentration is elevated in a relative sense when it exceeds the upper limit of an arbitrary normal range, which is usually defined as the mean serum urate value plus two standard deviations in a sex- and age-matched healthy population. In most epidemiologic studies, the upper limit has been rounded off at 7 mg/dL in men and 6 mg/dL in women. A serum urate value in excess of 7 mg/dL begins to carry an increased risk of gouty arthritis or renal stones.

EPIDEMIOLOGY

Hyperuricemia is fairly common, with prevalence ranging between 2.6% and 47.2% in various populations.[3,4] A variety of factors appears to be associated with high serum urate concentrations. In adults, serum urate levels correlate strongly with the serum creatinine and urea nitrogen levels, body weight, height, age, blood pressure, and alcohol intake.[5] In epidemiologic studies, body bulk (as estimated by body weight, surface area, or body mass index) has proved to be one of the most important predictors of hyperuricemia in people of many different races and cultures, with rare exceptions.[6-8]

Serum urate concentrations vary with age and sex. Children normally have a concentration in the range of 3 to 4 mg/dL because of high renal uric acid clearance.[9] At puberty, serum urate concentrations increase by 1 to 2 mg/dL in males, and this higher level is generally sustained throughout life. In contrast, females exhibit little change in the serum urate concentration until menopause, when concentrations increase and approach those seen in adult men. The mechanism of lower serum urate levels in women is a consequence of sex hormones and is related to a higher fractional excretion of urate secondary to lower tubular urate postsecretory reabsorption.[10]

The incidence of gout varies among populations, with an overall prevalence ranging from less than 1% to 15.3%.[5]

This upper limit appears to be increasing.[11,12] The prevalence increases substantially with age and with increasing serum urate concentration. The annual incidence rate of gout is 4.9% for urate levels greater than 9 mg/dL, 0.5% for values between 7 and 8.9 mg/dL, and 0.1% for values less than 7 mg/dL.[13] For serum urate values greater than 9 mg/dL, the cumulative incidence of gout reaches 22% after 5 years.

ENVIRONMENTAL FACTORS

An association between alcohol consumption and gout has been recognized for centuries. The risk of developing gout varies by the type of alcohol ingested.[14] Beer, which is purine rich, carries the highest risk; this risk is substantially greater than that for liquor. Moderate wine drinking does not increase the risk of gout. The quantity of alcohol also strongly correlates with gout. Compared with men who did not consume alcohol, the relative risk of gout was 1.32 for an alcohol intake of 10.0 to 14.9 g/day, 1.49 for 15.0 to 29.9 g/day, 1.96 for 30.0 to 49.9 g/day, and 2.53 for 50 g/day and higher.

Diet also influences hyperuricemia and gout. Serum urate levels increase with meat or seafood intake and decrease with dairy intake.[15] Men in the highest quintile of seafood consumption have a 51% higher risk of developing gout, and those in the highest quintile of meat intake have a 41% higher risk. However, consumption of oatmeal and purine-rich vegetables (e.g., peas, mushrooms, lentils, spinach, and cauliflower) is not associated with an increased risk for gout. The consumption of milk one or more times a day or yogurt consumption at least once every other day is associated with lower serum urate levels.

CLINICAL FEATURES

Throughout its natural history, gout passes through three stages: (1) asymptomatic hyperuricemia, (2) episodes of acute gouty arthritis separated by asymptomatic intervals (termed intercritical or interval gout), and (3) chronic gouty arthritis, the period when tophi often become apparent.

The basic pattern of clinical gout begins with acute attacks of intensely painful arthritis. The first attack is usually monarticular and associated with few constitutional symptoms. Later, attacks may become polyarticular and are associated with fever. Attacks vary in duration but are time limited. Over time, attacks recur at shorter intervals, last longer, and eventually resolve incompletely. This leads to the development of chronic arthritis that slowly progresses to a crippling disease on which acute exacerbations are superimposed.

ASYMPTOMATIC HYPERURICEMIA

Asymptomatic hyperuricemia is a condition in which the serum urate level is high, but gout—manifested by arthritis or uric acid nephrolithiasis—has not yet occurred. Most people with hyperuricemia remain asymptomatic throughout their lifetimes. The tendency toward acute gout increases with the serum urate concentration. The risk of nephrolithiasis increases with the serum urate level and with the magnitude of urinary uric acid excretion. The phase of asymptomatic hyperuricemia ends with the first attack of gouty arthritis or urolithiasis. In most instances, this occurs after at least 20 years of sustained hyperuricemia. Between 10% and 40% of gouty subjects have one or more attacks of renal colic before the first articular event.

ACUTE GOUTY ARTHRITIS

The first attack of acute gouty arthritis usually occurs between age 40 and 60 years in men and after age 60 in women. Onset before age 25 should raise the possibility of an unusual form of gout, perhaps one related to a specific enzymatic defect that causes marked purine overproduction, an inherited renal disorder, or the use of cyclosporine.

A single joint is involved in about 85% to 90% of first attacks, with the first metatarsophalangeal joint being the most commonly affected site. The initial attack is polyarticular in 3% to 14%. Acute gout is predominantly a disease of the lower extremities, but eventually, any joint of any extremity may be involved. Ninety percent of patients experience acute attacks in the great toe at some time during the course of their disease. Next in order of frequency are the insteps, ankles, heels, knees, wrists, fingers, and elbows. Acute attacks rarely affect the shoulders, hips, spine, sacroiliac joints, sternoclavicular joints, acromioclavicular joints, or temporomandibular joints.[16,17] Acute gouty bursitis, tendinitis, or tenosynovitis can also occur.[18,19] Urate deposition and subsequent gout appear to have a predilection for previously damaged joints, such as in Heberden's nodes of older women.[20]

Some patients report a history of short, trivial episodes of "ankle sprains," sore heels, or twinges of pain in the great toe before the first dramatic gouty attack. In most patients, however, the initial attack occurs with explosive suddenness and commonly begins at night after the individual has gone to sleep feeling well. Within a few hours of onset, the affected part becomes hot, dusky red, swollen, and extremely tender. Occasionally, lymphangitis may develop. Systemic signs of inflammation may include leukocytosis, fever, and elevation of the erythrocyte sedimentation rate. Radiographs usually show only soft tissue swelling during early episodes.

The course of untreated acute gout is highly variable. Mild attacks may subside in several hours or persist for only a day or two and never reach the intensity described for the classic attack. Severe attacks may last days to weeks. The skin over the joint often desquamates as the erythema subsides. With resolution, the patient becomes asymptomatic and enters the intercritical period.

Drugs may precipitate acute gout by either increasing or decreasing serum urate levels acutely. The occurrence of gout after the initiation of antihyperuricemic therapy is well established. In fact, the more potent the urate-lowering effect, the more likely there is to be an acute attack.[21] Drug-induced gout secondary to increased serum urate levels occurs on occasion with diuretic therapy, intravenous heparin, and cyclosporine.[22-24] Diuretic therapy in the elderly appears to be a particularly important precipitating factor for gouty arthritis. Other provocative factors include trauma, alcohol ingestion, surgery, dietary excess, hemorrhage, foreign protein therapy, infections, and radiographic contrast exposure.[25,26] The risk of a patient with gout developing an attack during hospitalization is 20%.[27]

Table 87-1 Criteria for the Classification of Acute Gouty Arthritis

The presence of characteristic urate crystals in the joint fluid, or a tophus proved to contain urate crystals by chemical means or polarized light microscopy, or the presence of 6 of the following 12 clinical, laboratory, and radiographic phenomena:

More than one attack of acute arthritis

Maximal inflammation developed within 1 day

Attack of monarticular arthritis

Joint redness observed

First metatarsophalangeal joint painful or swollen

Unilateral attack involving first metatarsophalangeal joint

Unilateral attack involving tarsal joint

Suspected tophus

Hyperuricemia

Asymmetric swelling within a joint (radiograph)

Subcortical cysts without erosions (radiograph)

Negative culture of joint fluid for microorganisms during attack of joint inflammation

Adapted from Wallace SL, Robinson H, Masi AT, et al: Preliminary criteria for the classification of acute arthritis of primary gout. Arthritis Rheum 20: 895-900, 1977.

The definitive diagnosis of gout is best established by aspiration of the joint and identification of intracellular needle-shaped crystals that have negative birefringence with compensated polarized light microscopy. However, criteria have been proposed for a presumptive diagnosis.[28] These include the triad of acute monarticular arthritis, hyperuricemia, and a dramatic response to colchicine therapy, and a set of criteria proposed by the American College of Rheumatology (Table 87-1).[29] There are limitations to using either of these schemes. First, although the diagnosis of acute gouty arthritis can be strongly suggested by the typical presentation, not all inflammation of the great toe (podagra) in hyperuricemic patients is caused by gout.[30] Second, some patients with gout are normouricemic at the time of an acute attack, a phenomenon related to alcohol use or a consequence of interleukin (IL)-6 generation by the acute inflammatory process.[31-33] Third, diseases other than gout can occasionally improve with colchicine therapy; these include pseudogout, hydroxyapatite calcific tendinitis, sarcoid arthritis, erythema nodosum, serum sickness, rheumatoid arthritis, and familial Mediterranean fever.[34] Finally, the simultaneous presence of both gout and septic arthritis can be confusing clinically, with the former masking the latter.[35]

INTERCRITICAL GOUT

The terms *intercritical gout* and *interval gout* have been applied to the periods between gouty attacks. Some patients never have a second attack. However, most patients suffer a second attack within 6 months to 2 years. In Gutman's series,[36] 62% had recurrences within the first year, 16% in 1 to 2 years, 11% in 2 to 5 years, and 4% in 5 to 10 years; 7% had experienced no recurrence in 10 or more years. The frequency of gout attacks usually increases over time in untreated patients. Later attacks have a less

explosive onset, are polyarticular, become more severe, last longer, and abate more slowly. Nevertheless, recovery is complete. Radiographic changes may develop during the intercritical period despite no sign of tophi on physical examination. These changes are more likely in patients with more severe hyperuricemia and more frequent acute attacks.[27,37]

The diagnosis of gout in a hyperuricemic patient with a history of acute attacks of monarthritis may be difficult or inconclusive during the intercritical phase. Aspiration of an asymptomatic joint, however, can be a useful adjunct in the diagnosis of gout if urate crystals are demonstrated. Joint fluids obtained from gouty patients during the intercritical phase revealed monosodium urate crystals in 12.5% to 90% of joints.[38] Such crystals in asymptomatic joints are often associated with mild synovial fluid leukocytosis, which suggests the potential to contribute to joint damage even in the intervals between attacks.

CHRONIC GOUTY ARTHRITIS

Eventually, the patient may enter a phase of chronic polyarticular gout with no pain-free intercritical periods. At this stage, gout may be easily confused with other types of arthritis or other conditions.[39-41] The time from the initial attack to the beginning of chronic symptoms or visible tophaceous involvement is highly variable in studies of untreated patients. Hensch[42] reported intervals ranging from 3 to 42 years, with an average of 11.6 years between the first attack and the development of chronic arthritis.[42] Ten years after the first attack, about half the individuals were still free of obvious tophi, and most of the remainder had only minimal deposits. Thereafter, the proportion of those with nontophaceous involvement slowly declined, to 28% after 20 years. Two percent of the patients had severe crippling disease some 20 years after the initial attack.

The rate of formation of tophaceous deposits correlates with both the degree and the duration of hyperuricemia. The principal determinant is the serum urate level.[27] Gutman[43] found the mean serum urate concentration to be 9.1 mg/dL in 722 patients without tophi, 10 to 12 mg/dL in 456 patients with minimal to moderate tophi, and greater than 11 mg/dL in 11 patients with extensive tophaceous involvement. The rate of tophus formation also increases with the severity of renal disease and the use of diuretics.[22]

Tophaceous gout is the consequence of the chronic inability to eliminate urate as rapidly as it is produced. As the urate pool expands, deposits of urate crystals appear in cartilage, synovial membranes, tendons, soft tissues, and elsewhere. Tophi are rarely present at the time of an initial attack of primary gout[44,45]; they are more likely to be present in gout secondary to myeloproliferative diseases, in juvenile gout-complicating glycogen storage diseases (GSDs), in Lesch-Nyhan syndrome, or after allograft transplantation in patients treated with cyclosporine.[34,46]

Tophi can occur in a variety of locations. Tophaceous deposits may produce irregular, asymmetric, moderately discrete tumescence of the fingers (Fig. 87-1), hands, knees, or feet. Tophi also form along the ulnar surfaces of the forearm, as saccular distentions of the olecranon bursa (Fig. 87-2), in the antihelix of the ear (Fig. 87-3), or as fusiform enlargements of the Achilles tendon (Fig. 87-4). The process of tophaceous deposition advances insidiously. Although the tophi themselves are relatively painless, acute inflammation can occur around them. Eventually, extensive destruction of the joints and large subcutaneous tophi may lead to grotesque deformities, particularly of the hands and feet, and to progressive crippling (Fig. 87-5). The tense, shiny, thin

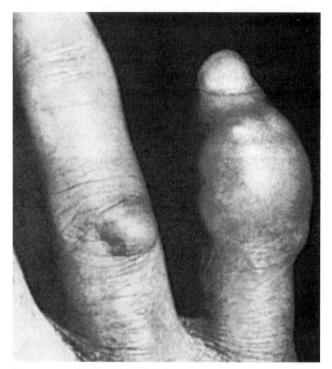

Figure 87-1   Tophus of the fifth digit, with a smaller tophus over the fourth proximal interphalangeal joint.

skin overlying the tophus may ulcerate and extrude white, chalky, or pasty material composed of urate crystals. Secondary infection of tophi is rare.

Typical radiographic changes, particularly erosions with sclerotic margins and overhanging edges of bone, occur with the development of tophi (Fig. 87-6).[47] These may be difficult to distinguish from erosions of other causes, but the presence of a thin, overhanging calcified edge is strong evidence of gout. Calcifications can be seen in some tophi, and bony ankylosis may rarely occur. Ultrasonography, magnetic resonance imaging, and computed tomography can demonstrate tophi, with the last providing the most specific images.[48]

Tophi can produce a marked limitation of joint movement by involvement of the joint structure directly or of a tendon serving the joint. Any joint can be involved, although those of the lower extremity are affected primarily. Spinal joints do not escape urate deposition,[41,49] but acute gouty spondylitis is unusual. Symptoms related to nerve or spinal cord compression by tophi have rarely been observed. Tophi rarely occur in myocardium, valves, cardiac conduction system, various parts of the eye, and larynx.[50,51]

GENETICS OF GOUT

Since antiquity, gout has been recognized as a familial disorder. The familial incidences reported range from 11% to 80%.[34] In two large series, one English and one American, about 40% of gouty subjects gave a positive family history of gout. These wide discrepancies may be attributed in part to variations in diligence and pursuit of genealogic data. When all available data are considered, they suggest that serum urate concentrations are controlled by polygenic traits. Several rare forms of hyperuricemia and gout, such as hypoxanthine phosphoribosyltransferase deficiency,

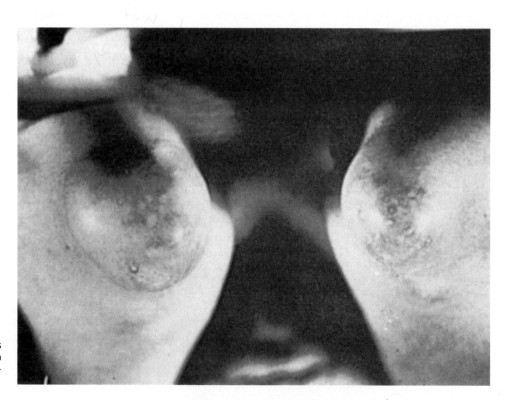

Figure 87-2   Saccular tophaceous enlargements of the oclecranon bursae, with small cutaneous deposits of urate.

phosphoribosyl-1-pyrophosphate synthetase overactivity, and familial hyperuricemia nephropathy, have a genetic basis and are discussed later.

ASSOCIATED CONDITIONS

The association of gout with obesity and overeating is well recognized.[52] In 6000 subjects, hyperuricemia was found in only 3.4% of those with a relative weight at or below the 20th percentile, in 5.7% of those between the 21st and 79th percentiles, and in 11.4% of those at or above the 80th percentile.[53]

Hypertriglyceridemia has been reported in 75% to 80% of patients with gout,[54] and hyperuricemia is found in more than 80% of patients with hypertriglyceridemia.[34] However, studies have been unable to show a correlation between serum urate and cholesterol values or a unique lipid

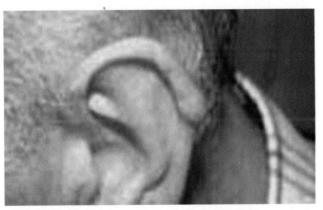

Figure 87-3 Tophus of the helix of the ear adjacent to the auricular tubercle. (From Swash M: Hutchinson's Clinical Methods, 21st ed. Philadelphia, WB Saunders, 2001.)

phenotype.[55] Gouty patients who drink alcohol excessively have mean serum triglyceride levels that are higher than those of their obesity-matched controls and of non–alcohol drinking gouty patients.[56]

Hyperuricemia has been reported in 2% to 50% of patients with diabetes mellitus, and gouty arthritis has been reported in less than 0.1% to 9%.[57] Abnormal glucose tolerance tests have been noted in 7% to 74% of patients with gout, depending, in part, on the criteria used.[58]

Hyperuricemia has been reported in 22% to 38% of patients with untreated hypertension. This figure increases to 67% when diuretic therapy and renal disease are present.[34] Hyperuricemia may be an indication of a potential risk for hypertension in adolescent males.[59] Hypertension is present in one fourth to one half of patients with classic gout, but the presence of hypertension is unrelated to the duration of gout.[52,53] Elevated serum urate concentrations are associated with increased tubular reabsorption of sodium.[58] The serum urate concentration also correlates inversely with renal blood flow and urate clearance and correlates directly with both renovascular and total resistance. Therefore, the association between hypertension and hyperuricemia may be related to the reduction of renal blood flow in hypertension. In addition, uric acid causes smooth muscle proliferation in vitro and vascular disease in animal models through a mechanism that involves complex intracellular signaling, mitogen-activated protein kinase activation, and platelet-derived growth factor expression.[60,61]

The association between hyperuricemia and the manifestations of atherosclerosis has led to speculation that hyperuricemia is a risk factor for coronary artery disease. Some studies show no clear associations between blood pressure, blood glucose, or serum cholesterol and serum urate concentration when adjustments are made for the effects of age,

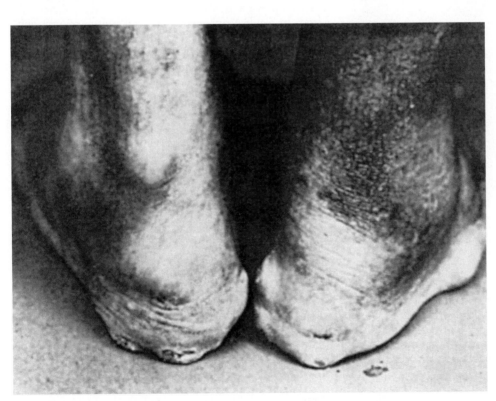

Figure 87-4 Tophi of Achilles tendons and their insertions in a patient with gout.

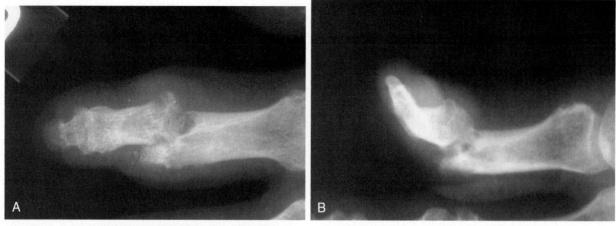

Figure 87-5 Radiographs (**A** and **B**) demonstrating severe destructive changes in tophaceous gout.

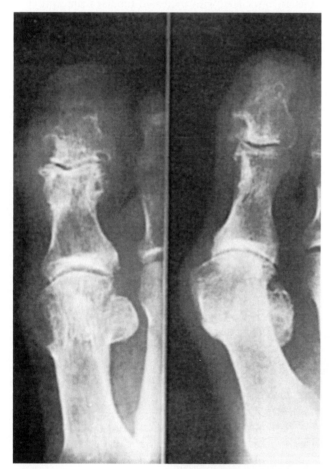

Figure 87-6 Radiographs show changes typical of bony tophi, including soft tissue distortion, erosions with sclerotic margins, and overwhelming edges. Joint space narrowing is minimal, despite the large erosions. *(From Nakayama DA, Barthelemy C, Carrera G, et al: Tophaceous gout: A clinical and radiographic assessment. Arthritis Rheum 27:468, 1984.)*

sex, and relative weight[53,62-65]; the serum urate concentrations of persons with coronary heart disease are not significantly different from the mean levels of the population.[65,66] Other studies, however, maintain that hyperuricemia is an independent risk factor for coronary artery disease.[67,68]

The term *metabolic syndrome* has been applied to a cluster of abnormalities, including resistance to insulin-stimulated glucose uptake, hyperinsulinemia, hypertension, and dyslipoproteinemia, that are characterized by high levels of plasma triglycerides and high-density lipoprotein cholesterol. Hyperuricemia closely correlates with the degree of insulin resistance[65-71] and, therefore, is a likely feature of metabolic syndrome. Metabolic syndrome has been associated with coronary artery disease, and hyperuricemia as a component of metabolic syndrome may explain the previously recognized association between coronary artery disease and hyperuricemia. A recent study concluded that the relationship between hyperuricemia and acute myocardial infarction is independent, but that patients who experience gouty arthritis are at an increased risk for myocardial infarction. This association could not be explained by renal function, metabolic syndrome, diuretic use, or traditional cardiovascular risk factors.[72]

Alcohol consumption has long been associated with hyperuricemia and gout. In susceptible persons, alcohol use can precipitate acute gouty arthritis. An epidemiologic study in Saudi Arabia, where alcohol consumption is quite rare, revealed an 8.42% prevalence of hyperuricemia but no cases of gout among the study group.[73] Both a decrease in the renal excretion of uric acid and an increase in uric acid production seem to be important factors in this association.[74] Ethanol increases uric acid production by accelerating the turnover of adenosine triphosphate (ATP). Among alcoholic beverages, beer may have more potent effects on uric acid production because of its high guanosine content.[14]

There appears to be a significant increased prevalence of hypothyroidism among both female and male patients with gouty arthritis.[75] Hyperuricemia may also be more prevalent in patients with hypothyroidism. Thyroid replacement therapy is associated with a decrease in serum urate concentration caused by an increased uric acid diuresis—a change not explained solely by a change in creatinine clearance.[76] Although the cause of hyperuricemia and gout in patients with hypothyroidism is unknown, it is speculated that urate metabolism is mediated by thyroid-stimulating hormone receptors in extrathyroidal tissues, including the kidney, and that these modulate urate homeostasis.

Studies of acutely ill patients in intensive care units indicate that markedly increased serum urate concentrations, in the vicinity of 20 mg/dL, are associated with hypotensive events and a poor prognosis.[77] This finding may be related to two factors. First, ischemic tissue may foster the degradation

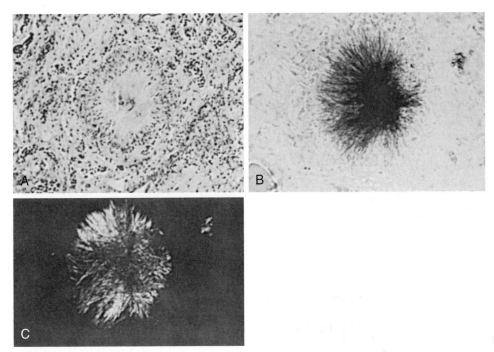

Figure 87-7 **A,** Urate deposit in the medulla of the kidneys as seen in an alcohol-fixed section stained with hematoxylin and eosin (×250). **B,** Adjacent section of the deposit shown in **A,** stained with methenamine silver (×250). **C,** Adjacent section of the deposit shown in **A** seen with polarized light (×250).

of ATP to purine end products, thereby enhancing the production of urate. The finding of increased plasma ATP degradation products associated with hyperuricemia and adult respiratory distress syndrome supports this possibility.[78] Second, the conversion of hypoxanthine to uric acid by xanthine oxidase during ischemia produces oxidant radicals, which are themselves associated with tissue injury.[79] It is possible that inhibition of xanthine oxidase with allopurinol may be a useful therapy in this setting.

Maternal serum urate concentrations normally decrease during pregnancy until the 24th week and then increase until 12 weeks after delivery.[80] An increase in the serum urate level occurs in preeclampsia and toxemia of pregnancy, owing to a decrease in the renal clearance of urate.[81] Perinatal mortality is markedly increased when maternal plasma urate levels are raised, usually in association with early-onset preeclampsia. The highest mortality rate is seen with serum urate concentrations higher than 6 mg/dL and diastolic blood pressures greater than 110 mm Hg. Labor itself is associated with an increased serum urate level, and it remains elevated for 1 to 2 days after delivery.

Gout is rarely seen in patients with rheumatoid arthritis, systemic lupus erythematosus, or ankylosing spondylitis.[18,82-84] The basis for the decreased concurrence of these disorders is unclear, although the long-term use of nonsteroidal anti-inflammatory drugs (NSAIDs) or corticosteroids may mask the clinical features of gout in some of these patients.

RENAL DISEASE

After gouty arthritis, renal problems appear to be the most frequent complication of hyperuricemia. Twenty percent to 40% of patients with gout have albuminuria, which is usually mild and often intermittent. Hyperuricemia alone may be implicated as the cause of chronic kidney disease only when the concentration of urate chronically exceeds 13 mg/dL in men or 10 mg/dL in women.[85] Before the routine treatment of asymptomatic hypertension, renal failure accounted for 10% of the deaths in patients with gout. Whether moderate hyperuricemia has a direct harmful effect on renal function is unclear. Some evidence suggests that urate damages the kidneys and leads to hypertension.[60,61]

The term *urate nephropathy* is used to describe the deposition of urate crystals in the interstitium of the medulla and pyramids, with a surrounding giant cell reaction—a distinctive histologic finding characteristic of the gouty kidney (Fig. 87-7). Factors such as coexistent hypertension, chronic lead exposure, ischemic heart disease, and primary preexisting renal insufficiency probably play important roles in the pathogenesis of this pathology. Although urate nephropathy appears to exist as a distinct entity, it is not believed to be an important contributor to renal function in most gouty patients.[34,86]

In contrast, *uric acid nephropathy* is the term used to describe acute renal failure resulting from the precipitation of large quantities of uric acid crystals in the collecting ducts and ureters. This complication most commonly occurs in patients with leukemia and lymphoma as a result of rapid malignant cell turnover, often during chemotherapy.[87,88] This syndrome (also termed *acute tumor lysis syndrome*) has been more clearly defined as hyperuricemia, lactic acidosis, hyperkalemia, hyperphosphatemia, and hypocalcemia and is most commonly observed in patients with aggressive, rapidly proliferating tumors, including lymphoproliferative disorders and metastatic medulloblastoma. Uric acid nephropathy is less commonly found with other neoplasms, after epileptic seizures, after vigorous exercise with heat stress, and after angiography and coronary artery bypass surgery.[34]

In the tumor lysis syndrome, the large amount of nucleic acid in nucleotides liberated with massive cytolysis is converted rapidly to uric acid. Typically, there is marked hyperuricemia, with a mean serum urate level of 20 mg/dL (range, 12 to 80 mg/dL). The pathogenesis of acute renal failure in uric acid nephropathy is related to the precipitation of uric acid in the distal tubules and collecting ducts, the sites of maximal acidification and concentration of urine. Oliguria, or even anuria, as well as azotemia may occur. There may be "gravel" or "sand" noted in the urine. The ratio of urinary uric acid to creatinine in these patients typically exceeds 1; in patients with most other causes of acute renal failure, the ratio is 0.4 ± 0.3.[88]

Nephrolithiasis occurs in 10% to 25% of patients with primary gout, a prevalence greater than that in the general population. The likelihood of stones in a given patient with gout increases with the serum urate concentration and with amounts of urinary uric acid excretion.[89,90] It exceeds 50% with a serum urate value above 13 mg/dL or with urinary uric acid excretion rates in excess of 1100 mg every 24 hours.

Uric acid calculi account for approximately 10% of all stones in patients in the United States; elsewhere, rates range from as low as 5% up to 40% in Israel and Australia.[34] Uric acid stones can occur in patients with no history of gouty arthritis, and only 20% in this group are hyperuricemic. Other renal stone disease is associated with hyperuricemia and gout. Gouty subjects also have an increased incidence of stones that contain calcium. In addition, about 30% of patients with recurrent calcium stone disease have either an increased urinary uric acid excretion rate or hyperuricemia. A causative link between uric acid and recurrent calcium oxalate stones is provided by reports of reduced stone frequency in patients treated with allopurinol.

Finally, the report of uric acid as the major constituent of a stone obtained from a patient with no apparent abnormalities of uric acid metabolism should suggest the possibility that the constituent is actually 2,8-dihydroxyadenine and that the patient has adenine phosphoribosyltransferase deficiency.[91] This is because x-ray diffraction is required to distinguish uric acid from 2,8-dihydroxyadenine.

Familial juvenile hyperuricemic nephropathy (FJHN), sometimes called familial juvenile gouty nephropathy, was first described in 1960.[92] This disorder is inherited as an autosomal dominant trait with a high degree of penetrance and is usually associated with gout. Renal disease typically develops in the second decade of life and progresses to end-stage renal failure by midlife.[93-95] Histologic examination of kidney tissue reveals tubulointerstitial inflammation and splitting of thickened tubular basement membranes. The primary diagnostic criterion is a reduced fractional excretion of urate (defined as uric acid clearance factored by creatinine clearance × 100 equal to 5% or less; normal is 8% to 18%).[96] The dramatically low fractional excretion of urate and the early onset of disease are conspicuous characteristics of FJHN and distinguish it from other autosomal dominant hyperuricemic disorders that usually appear later in life (Table 87-2). Genotype mapping has linked the gene for FJHN to chromosome 16p12-p11.[94]

Autosomal dominant medullary cystic kidney disease (ADMCKD) is another hereditary nephropathy that usually includes gout among its constellation of symptoms. The onset of renal dysfunction occurs later than in those with

Table 87-2 Genetics of Renal Diseases Associated with Gout

Condition	Inheritance	Chromosomal Location	Gene
FJHN	AD	16p12.3	Uromodulin
		17cenq21.3	Hepatic nuclear factor 1β
MCKD type 1	AD	1q21	?
MCKD type 2	AD, AR	16p12.3	Uromodulin

AD, autosomal dominant; AR, autosomal recessive; FJHN, familial juvenile hyperuricemic nephropathy; MCKD, medullary cystic kidney disease.

FJHN. Renal histology reveals numerous corticomedullary and intramedullary cysts in the kidneys and increased medullary connective tissue. At least two loci appear to be responsible for ADMCKD. One, termed ADMCKD1, is located on chromosome 1; the other, ADMCKD2, is a 16p locus. ADMCKD2 and FJHN loci map to approximately the same region of chromosome 16p.[97]

The chromosome 16p12 locus that harbors the candidate interval for FJHN and ADMCKD2 contains six candidate genes, including the uromodulin gene (*UMOD*).[98-100] *UMOD* encodes the Tamm-Horsfall protein, a glycosylphosphatidylinositol-anchored glycoprotein localized to the thick ascending limb of the loop of Henle. Amorphous deposits of uromodulin are present in the renal interstitium of patients with medullary cystic kidney disease.[101] Four different mutations in exon 4 have been identified in the *UMOD* gene. Because mutations in the same gene are responsible for both FJHN and ADMCKD, the two entities appear to be allelic variants in *UMOD* that cause decreased urinary concentrations of Tamm-Horsfall protein, with resulting hyperuricemia and progressive renal failure.[102]

LEAD INTOXICATION

Hyperuricemia and gout are well-recognized complications of chronic lead intoxication, with the prevalence of gout in patients with plumbism ranging between 6% and 50%.[103] Although a renal defect is recognized, it has not been well defined.[104,105] Some patients with primary gout have increased blood lead levels compared with age- and sex-matched controls, despite the absence of a history of overt lead exposure.[106] This suggests that occult chronic lead intoxication may play a causative role in some cases of primary gout (up to 36% of some gout populations).[103] In addition, patients with gout who have renal impairment seem to have an increased quantity of mobilized lead compared with gouty patients with normal renal function.[107] These observations suggest an important role for lead in the pathogenesis of gouty nephropathy.

CYCLOSPORINE-INDUCED HYPERURICEMIA AND GOUT

Cyclosporine interferes with the renal excretion of uric acid. Hyperuricemia and gout occur with increased frequency among transplant recipients treated with cyclosporine and are even more common when diuretics are used concomitantly.[46,108] However, serum urate levels do not correlate directly with cyclosporine levels or with the degree of hypertension or renal insufficiency. The onset of gout may occur soon after transplantation, with a mean of about 17 months. Gouty attacks may be typical and monarticular, or they may affect unusual sites such as the shoulder, hip, or sacroiliac joints. Polyarticular attacks and an accelerated course, with early development of tophi, may also be observed. Nephrolithiasis develops in about 3% of renal transplant patients. All calculi from azathioprine-treated patients are composed of calcium compounds, whereas 60% of the calculi from those treated with cyclosporine contain uric acid.[109]

PURINE METABOLISM

Uric acid is a purine base composed of a six-membered pyrimidine ring fused to a five-membered imidazole ring (Fig. 87-8). Purine nucleosides are composed of a purine base plus a pentose joined to the base by an N-glycosyl bond between carbon atom 1 of the pentose and nitrogen atom 9 of the purine base. There are two series of nucleosides: the ribonucleosides, which contain D-ribose as the sugar component, and the deoxyribonucleosides, which contain 2′-deoxy-D-ribose (Fig. 87-9). Purine nucleotides and deoxynucleotides consist of a nucleoside of deoxynucleoside with a phosphate group and ester linkage with carbon 5 of the pentose (Fig. 87-10). The nucleosides and deoxynucleosides exist as 5′-monophosphates, 5′-diphosphates, and 5′-triphosphates (Fig. 87-11). These compounds serve as building blocks for RNA and DNA; as precursors of the cyclic nucleotides adenosine-3′,5′-cyclic-phosphate and

guanosine-3′,5′-cyclic-phosphate; as a source of chemical energy; and as precursors of various purine cofactors and coenzymes, such as nicotinamide adenine dinucleotide.

Xanthine oxidase is a flavoprotein containing both iron and molybdenum that oxidizes a wide variety of purines and pteridines. A soluble form of the enzyme that has dehydrogenase activity (xanthine dehydrogenase, or D-form) is highly active in the liver and small intestine and is responsible for the formation of uric acid as the final metabolic product in human purine metabolism. This enzyme converts hypoxanthine to xanthine and xanthine to uric acid (Fig. 87-12).

Purines can be synthesized de novo in cells. The initial and rate-limiting step of this biosynthetic process is the conversion of phosphoribosylpyrophosphate (PRPP) to 5′-phosphoribosylamine. This step is catalyzed by the enzyme amidophosphoribosyltransferase, and it is regulated by the concentrations of nucleoside monophosphates and PRPP. Adenylic acid (AMP) and guanylic acid (GMP) are feedback inhibitors of the enzyme. Under normal conditions,

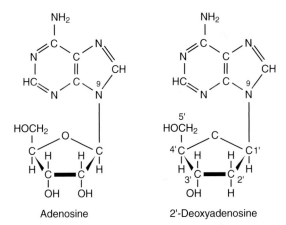

Figure 87-9 Structures of adenosine and 2′-deoxyadenosine as examples of nucleosides and 2′-deoxynucleosides, respectively.

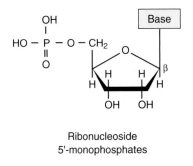

Ribonucleoside
5′-monophosphates

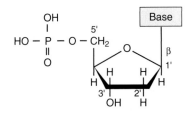

2′-Deoxyribonucleoside
5′-monophosphates

Figure 87-10 General structures of nucleosides and deoxynucleoside 5′-monophosphates.

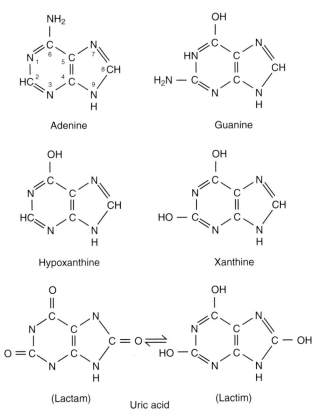

Figure 87-8 **Structure of uric acid.** All purine bases may exist in the lactam form in a reversible manner, as shown for uric acid.

depletion of PRPP decreases the rate of purine biosynthesis de novo, and elevation of PRPP is associated with an increased rate of purine biosynthesis.

The first branch point in the pathway leading to the de novo synthesis of AMP and GMP (see Fig. 87-12) occurs

$$\text{Hypoxanthine} + H_2O + 2O_2 \longrightarrow$$
$$\text{Xanthine} + 2O^{2-} + 2H^+$$

$$\text{Hypoxanthine} + H_2O + O_2 \longrightarrow \text{Xanthine} + H_2O_2$$

$$\text{Xanthine} + H_2O + 2O_2 \longrightarrow \text{Uric Acid} +$$
$$2O^{2-} + 2H^+$$

or

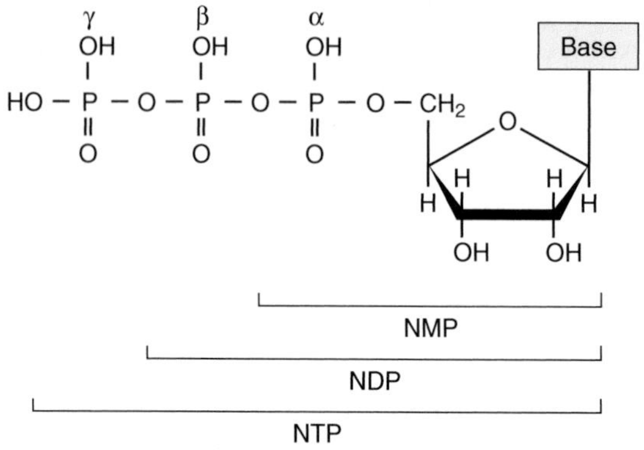

Figure 87-11 Comparison of the structures of nucleosides, monophosphates, diphosphates, and triphosphates.

with the synthesis of inosinic acid (IMP). IMP is used to form AMP and GMP, and these steps may be governed by the intracellular concentration of guanylic acid triphosphate (GTP). GTP is a substrate of adenylosuccinate synthetase and an inhibitor of IMP dehydrogenase. As IMP is formed, it is used for the synthesis of xanthylic acid, GMP, guanylic acid diphosphate, and GTP. As GTP reaches a critical concentration in the cell, it may increase the activity of adenylosuccinate synthetase, allowing IMP to be effectively used in the synthesis of AMP. When accelerated purine biosynthesis results in the production of surplus IMP, there is a rapid conversion of the excess ribonucleotide to uric acid rather than a continued expansion of the pools of adenyl and guanyl nucleotides.

Nucleotide breakdown is regulated in a complex manner. Regulation of nucleotide degradation is critically controlled by AMP deaminase and 5'-nucleotidase activities. Release of inhibition of AMP deaminase results in accelerated production of uric acid. Regulation of dephosphorylation is complex, involving three soluble 5'-nucleotidase activities. The nucleosides formed by nucleotidase reactions are converted to the bases adenine, guanine, or hypoxanthine. These bases can be "salvaged" by reconversion to nucleosides catalyzed by purine nucleoside phosphorylase activity (hypoxanthine and guanine) or conjugated with PRPP to form ribonucleotides by phosphoribosyltransferase activities. If not salvaged, they are degraded to uric acid.

Exogenous purines also significantly contribute to the total body urate pool. The magnitude of this contribution

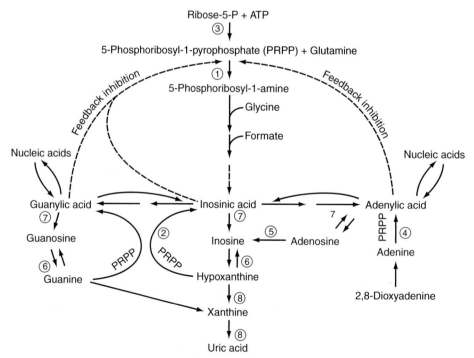

Figure 87-12 Outline of purine metabolism: (1) amidophosphoribosyltransferase, (2) hypoxanthine-guanine phosphoribosyltransferase, (3) phosphoribosylpyrophosphate (PRPP) synthetase, (4) adenine phosphoribosyltransferase, (5) adenosine deaminase, (6) purine nucleoside phosphorylase, (7) 5'-nucleotidase, (8) xanthine oxidase. *(From Seegmiller JE, Rosenbloom RM, Kelley WN: Enzyme defect associated with sex-linked human neurological disorder and excessive purine synthesis. Science 155:1682, 1967.)*

depends on the amount and type of purine in the diet, but it is often considerable. When healthy young men were given an isocaloric, purine-free formula diet, serum urate values declined in 10 days from about 4.9 to 3.1 ± 0.4 mg/dL, and urinary excretion of uric acid declined from between 500 and 600 to 336 ± 39 mg/day.[110] Urinary uric acid excretion declines to constant low values after 5 to 7 days of dietary purine elimination or severe restriction. Mean values then range from 336 ± 39 to 426 ± 81 mg every 24 hours. These values reflect the continued synthesis and turnover of endogenous purines. Urinary uric acid excretion accounts for only part of the daily disposition of uric acid, however. The true rate of endogenous purine turnover cannot accurately be determined by the measurement of urinary uric acid excretion; it requires the use of isotope-dilution techniques in subjects in whom the exogenous contribution has been reduced to a minimum by severe dietary purine restriction.

URIC ACID ELIMINATION AND EXCRETION

Most uric acid is eliminated from the body by renal and extrarenal routes. Less than 2% of the turnover of the total body urate pool can be attributed to tissue uricolysis. Extrarenal routes include saliva, gastric juice, pancreatic secretions, and bowel. These routes account for about one third of the uric acid normally turned over each day. The percentage of extrarenal excretion increases, however, when serum urate concentrations rise above 12 to 14 mg/dL.

Until recently, a four-component model has been used to describe the renal handling of urate and uric acid: glomerular filtration, tubular reabsorption, secretion, and postsecretory reabsorption. Although these processes were once considered sequential, it is now apparent that they are coexistent and carried out via transporters. The renal clearance of urate uses specific organic anion transporters (OATs), including URAT 1 (Fig. 87-13). URAT 1 and

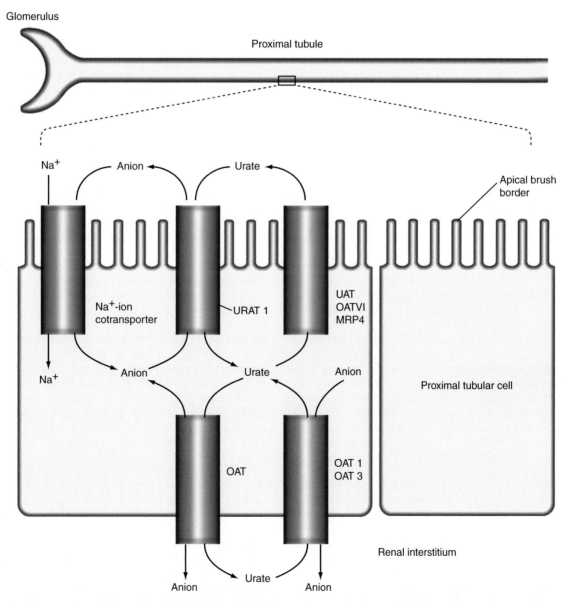

Figure 87-13 Urate transport in the proximal tubule. MRP4, multiple drug resistance protein 4, an ATP-driven efflux pathway; OAT, organic anion transporter; OATV, voltage-driven organic anion transporter; URAT, urate transporter.

Table 87-3 Drugs that Are Uricosuric in Humans

Acetohexamide	Glycerol guaiacolate
Amflutizole	Glycine
Ascorbic acid	Glycopyrrolate
Azapropazone	Iodopyracet
Azauridine	Iopanoic acid
Benzbromarone	Losartan
Calcitonin	Meclofenamic acid
Calcium ipodate	Orotic acid
Citrate	Outdated tetracyclines
Dicumarol	Phenolsulfonphthalein
Diflunisal	Probenecid
Estrogens	Salicylates
Fenofibrate	Sulfinpyrazone

other OATs carry urate into the proximal tubular cells from the luminal (apical) side. Once inside the cell, urate must pass to the other side, a process controlled by the voltage-dependent carrier hUAT. As a result of the activities of URAT 1 and other transporters, 8% to 12% of the urate filtered by the glomerulus is excreted as uric acid.

URAT 1 is a novel transporter expressed at the apical brush border of the proximal nephron.[105] Uricosuric compounds (Table 87-3) directly inhibit URAT 1 from the apical side of the tubular cell (so-called cis-inhibition).[67,91] In contrast, antiuricosuric compounds (those that promote hyperuricemia) serve as the exchange anions from inside the cell, thereby stimulating anion exchange and urate reabsorption (trans-stimulation).[111] There appears to be a transporter on the proximal tubule brush borders that mediates the absorption of pyrozinoate, pyruvate, lactate, nicotinate, β-hydroxybutyrate, and acetoacetate by a sodium-dependent process.[106,107,112] However, these anions are also substrates for URAT 1.[67] Consequently, when levels of these anions increase in plasma, their glomerular filtration and reabsorption into proximal tubular cells are increased. The resulting intraepithelial concentrations, in turn, induce increased urate reabsorption via URAT 1–dependent anion exchange.

Sodium-dependent loading of proximal tubular cells also results in increased urate reabsorption. However, the identity of the relevant sodium-dependent anion cotransporters remains speculative.[108] This mechanism probably accounts for the hyperuricemia that accompanies reduced extracellular fluid volume[113] or states accompanied by elevated levels of parathyroid hormone,[114] angiotensin II,[114] or insulin.[65]

Recognition of the role of URAT 1 in urate reabsorption and anion exchange helps explain why monovalent ions such as salicylates and probenecid can induce hyperuricemia at low doses and are uricosuric at high doses.[115,116] This occurs by the trans-inhibition of URAT 1 at low doses, causing antiuricosuric effects,[107] and cis-inhibition at higher doses, resulting in increased uricosuria.[67,117]

Urate gains access to the proximal tubular cells from the renal interstitium through OAT 1 and OAT 3 transporters.[118,119] This process is driven by the sodium-dependent

uptake of divalent anions, such as α-ketoglutarate.[120] Each appears to play a part in the efflux and influx of urate.[119,121,122] Additional proteins believed to be involved in the renal handling of urate include the urate transporter channel (UAT, also called galectin-9), the voltage-driven organic anion transporter-1 (OATV-1), and the apical ATP-driven anion transporter multiple drug resistance protein 4 (MRP4).[123-125]

A variety of additional factors influence the renal clearance of urate, including urine flow, estrogens, surgery, and the autonomic nervous system. Uric acid excretion increases by more than 25% as urine flow doubles in response to oral and intravenous fluid loading in humans. Changes in clearance are at least partially responsible for lower concentrations of serum urate in children and in women before menopause.[7,9] An increase in the excretion of uric acid in urine occurs in patients undergoing abdominal surgery, with little or no change taking place in the serum urate concentration. Factors such as anesthesia, increased endogenous steroids, intravenous fluids, intestinal manipulation, and vagotomy have been suggested as possibly affecting urate clearance. Several anticholinergic agents increase the renal clearance of urate, indicating that the parasympathetic nervous system plays a role in controlling the renal excretion of uric acid.

PHYSICAL PROPERTIES OF URIC ACID

The weakly acidic nature of uric acid results from ionization of hydrogen ions at position 9 (pKa1 = 5.75) and position 3 (pKa2 = 10.3). The ionized forms of uric acid readily form salts, which are monosodium and disodium or potassium urates. In extracellular fluids, in which sodium is the principal cation, approximately 98% of uric acid is in the form of monosodium salt at a pH of 7.4. When the solubility limits of body fluids are exceeded, the crystals that occur in the synovial fluid or the tophi of gouty patients are composed of monosodium urate monohydrate. As mentioned earlier, actual determinations of solubility of monosodium urate in human plasma (or serum) indicate that saturation occurs at concentrations of about 7 mg/dL. Considerably higher concentrations of monosodium urate in plasma can be achieved in supersaturated solutions. Stable supersaturated solutions of monosodium urate up to 40 to 90 mg/dL have been observed in patients with leukemia or lymphoma after aggressive therapy with cytotoxic drugs in the absence of allopurinol therapy.[88] The factors responsible for enhanced urate solubility in such patients are not clear and may include both the natural tendency for urate to form stable supersaturated solutions and an increase in plasma of substances capable of solubilizing urate. Studies of urate binding disclose that no more than 4% to 5% of urate is bound to plasma protein, indicating that the binding of uric acid to plasma proteins at 37°C is probably of little physiologic significance.

As the urine is acidified along the renal tubule, a portion of urinary urate is converted to uric acid. The solubility of uric acid in aqueous solutions is substantially less than that of urate. At pH 5, urine is saturated with uric acid at 15 mg/dL; at pH 7, urine accommodates 158 to 200 mg/dL in solution. The limited solubility of uric acid in urine of pH 5 is of particular significance in patients with gout, many of whom display a tendency toward the excretion of unusually acidic urine.

Monosodium urate occurs as a monohydrate and forms needle- or rod-shaped crystals in tissue and joint fluids. Urate crystals are insoluble in ethanol, sparingly soluble in water, and markedly soluble in formalin. Free uric acid crystallizes from pure solutions in an orthorhombic system, forming rhombic plates. Crystals formed in urine incorporate pigments and exist in a variety of crystalline forms. Tissue deposits are composed of monosodium urate monohydrate, whereas urinary stones are largely composed of uric acid. Both urate and uric acid crystals are birefringent, with strong negative elongation when viewed under compensated polarized light. These features should permit ready identification of urate crystals in synovial fluid, leukocytes, or tissue deposits and, therefore, constitute an important diagnostic aid.[114]

CLASSIFICATION AND PATHOGENESIS OF HYPERURICEMIA AND GOUT

The concentration of urate in body fluids is determined by the balance between production and elimination. Accordingly, hyperuricemia may be caused by an excessive rate of urate production, a decrease in the renal excretion of uric acid, or a combination of both events.

Hyperuricemia and gout may be classified as follows (Table 87-4):

Primary: These cases appear to be innate, neither secondary to an acquired disorder nor the result of a subordinate manifestation of an inborn error that leads initially to a major disease unlike gout. Some cases of primary gout have a genetic basis; others do not.

Secondary: These cases develop in the course of another disease or as a consequence of drug use.

Idiopathic: In these cases, a more precise classification cannot be assigned.

Further subdivisions within each major category are based on the identification of overproduction, underexcretion, or both, as responsible for the hyperuricemia. Evidence of overproduction of urate is provided by determination of the 24-hour urinary uric acid excretion. For adults ingesting a purine-free diet, a total excretion of up to 600 mg/day is considered within the normal range.[113] For patients on regular diets, a value in excess of 1000 mg/day is clearly abnormal and an indication of overproduction, and values between 800 and 1000 mg/day are considered borderline. It has been suggested that overproduction of uric acid can be assessed simply by determining the ratio of uric acid to creatinine in the urine or the $C_{urate}/C_{creatinine}$ ratio. However, comparison of these two ratios with the 24-hour urinary uric acid excretion reveals a poor correlation in most patients.[126,127] Exceptions include patients with specific enzymatic deficiencies or with rapid cell lysis during chemotherapy for leukemia or lymphoma.

PRIMARY GOUT

Renal mechanisms are responsible for the hyperuricemia in most cases of gout. Genetic factors exert an important control in the renal clearance of urate.[115] A careful comparison of uric acid clearances and excretion rates over

Table 87-4 Classification of Hyperuricemia and Gout

Type	Metabolic Disturbance	Inheritance
Primary		
Molecular defects undefined		
Underexcretion (90% of primary gout)	Not established	Polygenic
Overproduction (10% of primary gout)	Not established	Polygenic
Associated with specific enzyme defects		
PRPP synthetase variants; increased activity	Overproduction of PRPP and uric acid	X-linked
HPRT deficiency, partial	Overproduction of uric acid; increased purine biosynthesis de novo driven by surplus PRPP; Kelley-Seegmiller syndrome	X-linked
Secondary		
Associated with increased purine biosynthesis de novo		
HPRT deficiency, "virtually complete"	Overproduction of uric acid; increased purine biosynthesis de novo driven by surplus PRPP; Lesch-Nyhan syndrome	X-linked
Glucose-6-phosphatase deficiency or absence	Overproduction plus underexcretion of uric acid; glycogen storage disease type I (von Gierke's disease)	Autosomal recessive
Fructose-1-phosphate aldolase deficiency	Overproduction plus underexcretion of uric acid	Autosomal recessive
Associated with increased ATP degradation		
Associated with increased nucleic acid turnover	Overproduction of uric acid	Most not familial
Associated with decreased renal excretion of uric acid	Decreased filtration of uric acid, inhibited tubular secretion of uric acid, or enhanced tubular reabsorption of uric acid	Some autosomal dominant; some not familial; most unknown
Idiopathic		Unknown

ATP, adenosine triphosphate; HPRT, hypoxanthine phosphoribosyltransferase; PRPP, phosphoribosylpyrophosphate.

a wide but comparable range of filtered loads of urate indicates that most gouty subjects have a lower ratio of urate to inulin clearance (C_{urate}/C_{inulin} ratio) than do nongouty subjects.[113,115,128] The excretion rates and the capacity of the excretory mechanism for uric acid are the same for gouty subjects and nongouty individuals (Fig. 87-14). The excretion curve, however, is shifted. Gouty subjects require serum urate values 2 or 3 mg/dL higher than those of controls to achieve equivalent uric acid excretion rates. Theoretically, the shift in the excretion curve in gouty subjects may result from reduced filtration of urate, enhanced reabsorption, or decreased secretion. Patients classified as exhibiting an overproduction of uric acid represent less than 10% of the gouty population.

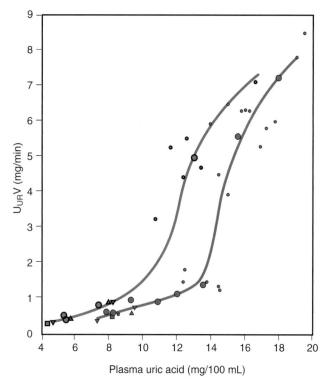

Figure 87-14   Rate of uric acid excretion at various plasma urate levels in nongouty *(blue symbols)* and gouty *(red symbols)* subjects. Large symbols represent mean values; small symbols represent individual data of a few mean values selected to illustrate the degree of scatter within groups. Studies were conducted under basal conditions, after RNA feeding, and after infusions of lithium urate. *(From Wyngaarden JB: Gout. Adv Metabol Dis 2:2, 1965. Data from references 90, 113, 116, and 117.)*

SECONDARY GOUT

Numerous secondary causes of hyperuricemia and gout can be attributed to a decrease in the renal excretion of uric acid. A reduction in the glomerular filtration rate leads to a decrease in the filtered load of urate and, consequently, to hyperuricemia. Patients with renal disease are hyperuricemic on this basis. Other factors, such as decreased secretion of urate, have been postulated in patients with some types of renal disease (e.g., polycystic kidney disease, lead nephropathy). Gout is a rare complication of the secondary hyperuricemia that results from renal insufficiency. When it occurs in this setting, there is likely to be a positive family history.

Diuretic therapy currently represents one of the most important causes of secondary hyperuricemia in humans. Diuretic-induced volume depletion leads to a decreased filtered load and enhanced tubular reabsorption of urate. A number of other drugs lead to hyperuricemia by a renal mechanism. These agents include low-dose aspirin, pyrazinamide, nicotinic acid, ethambutol, ethanol, and cyclosporine.

Decreased renal excretion of uric acid is thought to be an important mechanism for the hyperuricemia associated with several disease states. Volume depletion may be an important factor in patients with hyperuricemia associated with adrenal insufficiency or nephrogenic diabetes insipidus. An accumulation of organic acids leads to hyperuricemia. This is the case in starvation, alcoholic ketosis, diabetic ketoacidosis, maple syrup urine disease, and lactic acidosis of any cause (e.g., hypoxemia, respiratory insufficiency,

chronic beryllium disease, acute alcohol intoxication). The renal basis of the hyperuricemia in conditions such as chronic lead intoxication, hypoparathyroidism, pseudohypoparathyroidism, and hypothyroidism remains unclear.

Secondary gout can also result from urate overproduction. Four specific defects cause urate overproduction as a consequence of accelerated de novo purine biosynthesis: hypoxanthine phosphoribosyltransferase (HPRT) deficiency, PRPP synthetase overactivity, glucose-6-phosphatase deficiency, and fructose-1-phosphate aldolase deficiency.

A complete deficiency of the enzyme HPRT, known as Lesch-Nyhan syndrome, is characterized by choreoathetosis, striking growth, mental retardation, spasticity, self-mutilation, and marked hyperuricemia with excessive uric acid production and uric acid crystalluria (Figs. 87-15 and 87-16).[118,119,129] Adolescent and adult patients with a "partial" rather than a "complete" deficiency of HPRT—called Kelley-Seegmiller syndrome—present with uric acid calculi or gouty arthritis but do not have the devastating neurologic and behavioral features characteristic of children with a complete enzyme deficiency.[121] Both the complete and partial deficiencies are inherited in an X chromosome–linked manner.

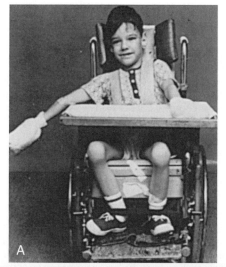

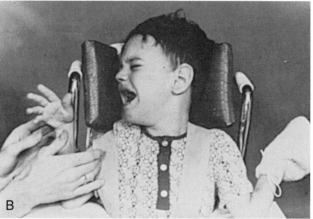

Figure 87-15   A, Patient with hypoxanthine phosphoribosyltransferase deficiency. **B,** Example of self-multilating behavior. Note the patient's agitated appearance and the attempt to bite his fingers after the wrapping is removed from his hands.

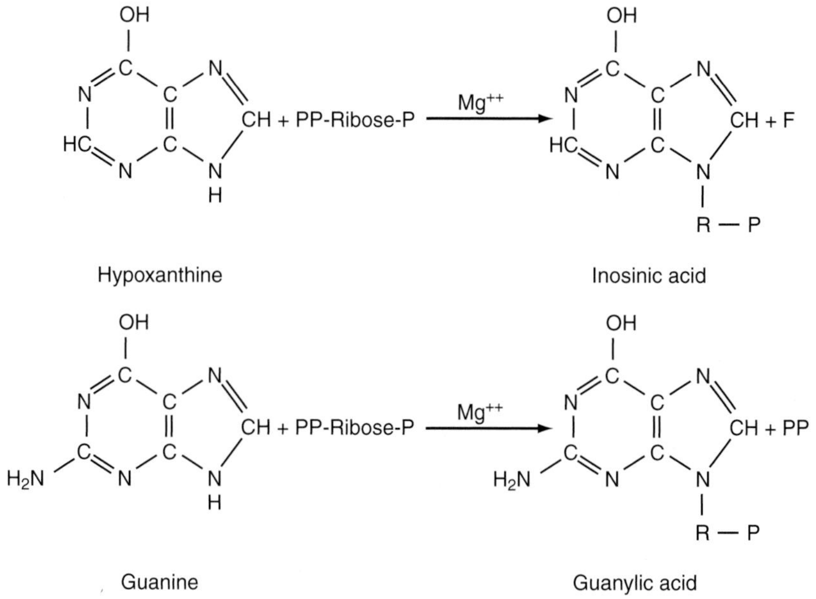

Figure 87-16 Reactions catalyzed by hypoxanthine-guanine phosphoribosyltransferase.

The level of HPRT activity in patients with each syndrome is the same within a family, but it often differs among families, with values ranging from 0.01% to almost 70% of normal. More than 50 different mutations have been defined.[34,122] Among these, major and minor deletions and rearrangements, as well as base substitutions, are represented. The excessive production of urate that characterizes partial HPRT deficiency results from accelerated de novo purine biosynthesis. This is caused by decreased consumption of PRPP and decreased reuse of hypoxanthine through at least three mechanisms. First, the deficiency leads to enhanced purine synthesis by virtue of decreased concentrations of either IMP or GMP, because these nucleotides are normally important inhibitors of de novo purine synthesis. Second, the loss of hypoxanthine reuse leads to decreased consumption of PRPP and increased intracellular concentrations of this compound. These increased concentrations of PRPP increase de novo purine biosynthesis by providing more substrate for amidophosphoribosyltransferase, the enzyme that catalyzes the presumed limiting step of this pathway. Third, in the absence of HPRT activity, hypoxanthine cannot be salvaged and is therefore oxidized to urate.

Increased PRPP synthetase activity causes accelerated PRPP formation (Fig. 87-17). This, in turn, results in increased de novo purine biosynthesis and excessive overproduction of urate.[123,124] Transmitted by X-linked inheritance, this disorder causes male subjects to exhibit clinical gout typically between 21 and 39 years of age; they can have renal calculi with an onset as early as 18 years of age.[125]

Patients with glucose-6-phosphatase deficiency (von Gierke's disease, or GSD type I) uniformly exhibit an increased production of uric acid as well as an accelerated rate of de novo purine biosynthesis. A major cause of increased uric acid synthesis is accelerated breakdown of ATP.[130]

In patients with hereditary fructose intolerance caused by fructose-1-phosphate aldolase deficiency, hyperuricemia develops in part because of accelerated purine nucleotide catabolism. In homozygotes, vomiting and hypoglycemia after fructose ingestion can proceed to hepatic failure and proximal tubular dysfunction. Ingestion of fructose causes an accumulation of fructose-1-phosphate, the substrate for the enzyme, which in turn results in ATP depletion. Both lactic acidosis and renal tubular acidosis also contribute to urate retention. Heterozygous carriers develop hyperuricemia, and perhaps one third develop gout.[131]

In most patients with secondary hyperuricemia caused by an overproduction of uric acid, the predominant abnormality appears to be an increased turnover of nucleic acids. A number of diseases, including the myeloproliferative and lymphoproliferative disorders, multiple myeloma, secondary polycythemia, pernicious anemia, certain hemoglobinopathies, thalassemia, other hemolytic anemias, infectious mononucleosis, and some carcinomas, may be associated with increased marrow activity or increased turnover and an associated increased turnover of nucleic acids. The increased turnover of nucleic acid, in turn, leads to hyperuricemia, hyperuricaciduria, and a compensatory increase in the rate of de novo purine biosynthesis.

D-Ribose 5'-phosphate

α 5-Phospho-D-ribosyl-1-pyrophosphate (PP-ribose-P)

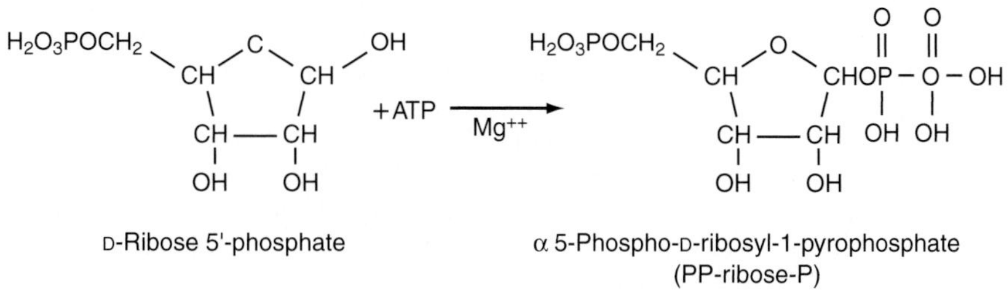

Figure 87-17 Reaction catalyzed by phosphoribosylpyrophosphate synthetase.

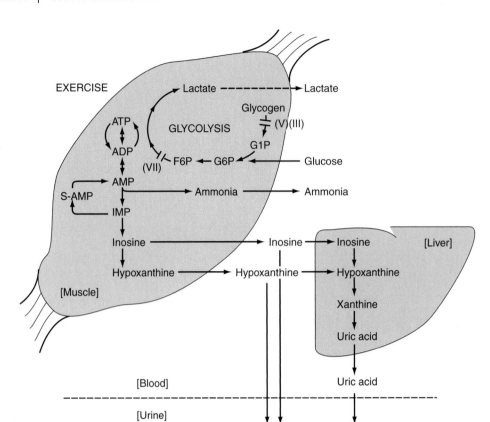

Figure 87-18 Mechanism of myogenic hyperuricemia in glycogen storage diseases (GSDs). In the three GSDs associated with metabolic myopathy, there is impairment of the metabolic pathways, providing the substrate necessary for adenosine triphosphate (ATP) synthesis. Thus, when ATP is consumed by muscle contraction, accelerated degradation of ATP may occur. *(Adapted from Mineo I, Kono N, Hara N, et al: Myogenic hyperuricemia: A common pathophysiologic feature of glycogenosis types III, V, and VII. N Engl J Med 317:75, 1987.)*

An important cause of overproduction of uric acid in secondary hyperuricemia appears to be related to the acceleration of ATP degradation to uric acid. This can occur with excessive alcohol consumption, myocardial infarction, acute smoke inhalation, respiratory failure, status epilepticus, and strenuous exercise.[34] The resulting increase in serum urate levels can be substantial with extreme exercise, as occurs in status epilepticus. Myogenic hyperuricemia has been reported in patients with muscle involvement either in the basal state or after exercise in three GSDs[121]: debranching enzyme deficiency (GSD type III), myophosphorylase deficiency (GSD type V), and muscle phosphofructokinase deficiency (GSD type VII) (Fig. 87-18).[132] Excessive formation of ATP degradation products can also occur in carnitine palmitoyltransferase deficiency, myoadenylate deaminase deficiency, and medium-chain acyl-coenzyme A dehydrogenase deficiency.[133-135]

ACUTE GOUT ATTACKS

During the initial phase of an acute gout attack, there is an influx of polymorphonuclear leukocytes into the synovial fluid. Inflammatory cytokines stimulate the synovial lining layer to become hyperplastic and infiltrated with neutrophils, monocyte-macrophages, and lymphocytes. These inflammatory responses are triggered by monosodium urate crystals that are either formed de novo or released from preformed deposits in or around the joint. Debris or other factors within the synovial cavity may also provide an initial nucleus for early crystal development.[136] Mast cells

may play a critical role in the initial event. They contain preformed proinflammatory substances, including histamine, cytokines, and enzymes, all of which may contribute to the promotion of downstream inflammatory cascades. Depletion of endogenous mast cells has been found to significantly inhibit neutrophil influx in a murine monosodium urate crystal–induced peritonitis model.[137]

It appears, however, that innate immunity—the system that provides the first line of defense against infectious agents—plays a critical role in the initial inflammatory response in acute gout.[138] Monosodium urate crystals activate both the classic and the alternative complement pathways, leading to the production of C5a, which is chemotactic for leukocytes, and the formation of C5b-C9, the membrane attack complex.[139] In addition, uncoated monosodium urate crystals can activate macrophages, synovial lining cells, and neutrophils through Toll-like receptor (TLR) 2 and TLR4 signal transduction.[140-142] TLRs are found in the cell membrane and survey the extracellular environment for pathogens. Activation of TLR2 and TLR4 not only induces crystal phagocytosis but also is critical for the expression of proinflammatory cytokines, including nuclear factor κB. An intracellular adapter protein, myeloid differentiation factor 88 (MyD88) and another pattern recognition protein, CD14, functionally interact with TLR2 and TLR4 and mediate these inflammatory responses.[143-145] Thus, monosodium urate crystals serve as a "warning signal," just like the pathogen-associated molecular pattern does in activating innate immune responses.

The intracellular NALP3 (or calopyrin) inflammasome also appears to play a major role in the acute inflammatory response to monosodium urate crystals.[146] NALP3 is expressed primarily in leukocytes.[147] When NALP3 is activated, the adapter protein ASC (apoptosis-associated speck-like protein containing a CARD) connects it with caspase-1, resulting in the production of interleukin (IL)-1β and IL-18.

A significant component of the early inflammatory response involves vasodilation, with increased blood flow, increased permeability to plasma proteins, and recruitment of leukocytes into the tissues. Initial endothelial activation, with expression of adhesion molecules such as E-selectin, intercellular adhesion molecule (ICAM)-1, and vascular cell adhesion molecule (VCAM)-1, is caused by factors such as IL-1 and tumor necrosis factor-α (TNF-α) released by mast cells.[137] Endothelial activation is then amplified by substances released by leukocytes upon entering the tissues and encountering crystals. Leukocyte recruitment is also enhanced by local generation of chemotactic factors, such as C5a, and chemokines, such as S100A8, S100A9, CXCL8, CXCL2, and IL-8.[148,149]

Uncoated crystals can activate neutrophils but may also cause membranolysis. A number of interstitial fluid proteins bind monosodium urate crystals. These include immunoglobulins (IgG and IgM), adhesion proteins (fibronectin), and complement components. The coating of crystals may protect against cell lysis[150] but may activate inflammatory cascades, such as complement and kininogen, and promote direct interactions with specific cell surface receptors, such as leukocyte integrin CD11b/CD18 (CR3) and the FC receptor CD16.[139,150,151] These, in turn, cause the release of soluble cellular products, which further amplify the inflammatory response, leading to both local arthritis and a systemic acute-phase response.

A number of neutrophil surface receptors are believed to be involved in mediating responses to monosodium urate crystals, including CR3 (CD11b/CD18) and FcγRIII (CD16), which bind crystal-bound iC3b and IgG, respectively.[151,152] As a consequence of neutrophil interaction with monosodium urate crystals, a large variety of mediators that promote vasodilation, erythema, and pain associated with the acute gout attack are synthesized and released. These include reactive oxygen species such as superoxide, hydrogen peroxide, and singlet oxygen; nitric oxide; leukotriene B_4; prostaglandin E_2; antimicrobial peptides; enzymes; IL-1; and the chemokines S100A8, S100A9, and IL-8.[153-156]

Monocytes also amplify the inflammatory response in acute gout. Following exposure to monosodium urate crystals, monocytes become activated and produce a number of proinflammatory substances, including IL-1, TNF-α, IL-6, IL-8, and prostaglandin E_2.[157-159]

The acute gout attack is usually self-limited, resolving in 7 to 10 days even in the absence of anti-inflammatory therapy. This can be explained by several factors. Proteins coating monosodium urate crystals may significantly modify leukocyte responses during the course of the inflammatory reaction. Coating with either apolipoprotein-B-100 or apolipoprotein-E can reduce the responsiveness of neutrophils to monosodium urate crystals.[160] Apolipoprotein-E has been detected on the surface of monosodium urate

crystals recovered from patients with gout and is probably synthesized locally in synovium. Melanocortins, such as adrenocorticotropic hormone (ACTH) and melanocyte-stimulating hormone, may contribute to the resolution of an acute attack.[161] Further, spontaneous resolution of the acute attack may involve the induction of transcription factor peroxisome proliferator-activated receptor-γ (PPAR-γ), which functions as an important negative regulator of the inflammatory response.[162] PPAR-γ expression can be detected in monocytes after exposure to monosodium urate crystals and is capable of inhibiting the production of IL-1ß and TNF-α and cellular infiltration.

Differentiated macrophages also play an important role in the resolution of an acute gout attack. Monosodium urate crystals can be found in asymptomatic joints of patients in the intercritical phase of gout.[38] The crystals are typically found within macrophages and almost never within neutrophils. Thus, macrophage–monosodium urate crystal interaction can occur without triggering an inflammatory response and appears to reflect a differential response of monocytes and macrophages to the crystals.[163,164]

Following exposure to monosodium urate crystals, undifferentiated peripheral blood monocytes secrete proinflammatory cytokines (IL-1ß, TNF-α, and IL-6), induce endothelial activation, and promote neutrophil adhesion to endothelial cells. However, differentiation of monocytes into mature macrophages leads to loss of the capacity to release proinflammatory cytokines capable of activating endothelial cell adhesion molecule expression. This loss of the ability to secrete proinflammatory cytokines such as TNF-α is accompanied by an increased capacity to release transforming growth factor-β1 (TGF-ß1). High levels of TGF-ß1 are present in the synovial fluid of patients with acute gout, and TGF-ß1 is a key soluble factor in the suppression of monosodium urate–induced inflammation by differentiated macrophages.[165,166]

TOPHACEOUS GOUT

Histologically, tophi are granulomas of mono- and multinucleated macrophages surrounding a core of debris and monosodium urate crystals, encased by dense connective tissue. Within the tophus, macrophages express late or mature differentiation markers and show high levels of apoptosis. However, in perivascular regions, most of the mononucleated monocyte-macrophages express surface markers of recent migration.[167] Therefore, development of gouty tophi is a dynamic process consisting of low-level continuous recruitment, proinflammatory activation, maturation, and turnover of monocyte-macrophages.[157,167]

Tophi are frequently associated with erosion of cartilage and bone (see Fig. 87-5). Monocyte-macrophages within the gouty tophus produce matrix metalloproteinase (MMP)-2 (gelatinase-A) and MMP-9 (gelatinase-B), enzymes that are capable of degrading type IV and type V collagen, elastin, and gelatine.[167] Resident stromal cells also produce MMPs on exposure to monosodium urate crystals, with chondrocytes producing MMP-3 (stromelysin 1) and synovial fibroblasts producing MMP-1 (collagenase).[168,169] These enzymes likely play a role in the degradation of tissues adjacent to the tophus.

TREATMENT OF GOUT

The therapeutic aims in gout are as follows:

1. To terminate the acute attack as promptly and gently as possible
2. To prevent recurrences of acute gouty arthritis
3. To prevent or reverse complications of the disease resulting from the deposition of sodium urate or uric acid crystals in joints, kidneys, or other sites
4. To prevent or reverse associated features of the illness that are deleterious, such as obesity, hypertriglyceridemia, and hypertension

ASYMPTOMATIC HYPERURICEMIA

The presence of hyperuricemia is rarely an indication for specific antihyperuricemic drug therapy. Rather, the finding of hyperuricemia should cause the following questions to be addressed:

1. What is the cause of the hyperuricemia?
2. Are associated findings present?
3. Has damage to tissues or organs occurred as a result?
4. What, if anything, should be done?

Hyperuricemia may be the initial clue to the presence of a previously unsuspected disorder. In 70% of hyperuricemic patients, an underlying cause can be readily defined by history and physical examination. The nature of the underlying cause may be useful in predicting the potential consequences, if any, of the elevated serum urate concentration. Therefore, an underlying cause should be sought in every patient with hyperuricemia.

Whether to treat hyperuricemia uncomplicated by articular gout, urolithiasis, or nephropathy is an exercise in clinical judgment, and universal agreement is lacking. When considering whether to treat asymptomatic hyperuricemia with urate-lowering agents, the following data are pertinent:

- Although there is intriguing data from animal models to the contrary,[170] there is no good evidence that renal function is adversely affected by elevated serum urate concentrations.
- The renal disease that accompanies hyperuricemia is most often related to inadequately controlled hypertension.
- Although debate exists regarding whether hyperuricemia is an independent risk factor for coronary artery disease,[65-68] there is no evidence that correction of hyperuricemia has an effect on the development of heart disease.

Thus, it seems prudent not to treat hyperuricemia with specific antihyperuricemic agents until symptoms develop. Rare exceptions include individuals with a known hereditary cause of uric acid overproduction or patients at risk for acute uric acid nephropathy.

It is, however, strongly recommended that the cause of hyperuricemia be determined and any associated factors related to the process, such as obesity, hyperlipidemia, alcoholism, and, especially, hypertension, be addressed. Fenofibrate and losartan might be appropriate agents for the treatment of hypertriglyceridemia and hypertension, respectively, in hyperuricemic individuals, because each has modest uricosuric effects.[171,172]

ACUTE GOUTY ARTHRITIS

The acute gouty attack may be successfully terminated by any of several drugs. For practical purposes, the choice in most situations is among colchicine, an NSAID, a corticosteroid preparation, or ACTH. The timing of therapy initiation is more important than the choice of drug.[173] With any of these agents, the sooner the drug is started, the more rapidly a complete response will be attained. Generally, colchicine is preferred for patients in whom the diagnosis of gout is not confirmed, whereas NSAIDs are preferred when the diagnosis is secure. If a patient cannot take medications by mouth or has active peptic ulcer disease, the choice is among intravenous colchicine, intra-articular glucocorticoid, or parenteral glucocorticoid. Local application of ice packs may help control the pain of an acute attack.[174] In some cases, analgesics, including narcotics, may be added as well. Drugs that affect serum urate concentrations, including antihyperuricemic agents, should not be changed (either started or stopped) during an acute attack. Just as sudden fluctuations in serum urate levels tend to precipitate an acute attack, an inflammatory reaction that is already in progress may be substantially worsened by a major change in the serum urate concentration.

Colchicine

Colchicine can be administered orally or intravenously.[175] In the past, the traditional oral dosing schedule was 0.5 or 0.6 mg taken hourly until one of three things occurred: joint symptoms eased; nausea, vomiting, or diarrhea developed; or the patient had taken a maximum of 10 doses. If 10 doses were taken without benefit, the clinician questioned the accuracy of the diagnosis. Today, many clinicians recommend that doses be taken every 2 to 6 hours to reduce side effects.[176]

Peak plasma concentrations occur within 2 hours of oral administration. Although its plasma half-life is 4 hours, levels can be detected in neutrophils 10 days after ingestion. Colchicine has a low therapeutic index, with steady-state plasma concentrations after acute treatment ranging from 0.5 to 3.0 ng/mL and with toxic effects occurring at approximately 3 ng/mL.[177] Therefore, in most patients, the side effects precede or coincide with the improvement in joint symptoms. These side effects develop in 50% to 80% of patients and include increased peristalsis, cramping abdominal pain, diarrhea, nausea, and vomiting. The drug must be stopped promptly at the first sign of gastrointestinal side effects.[178]

Colchicine derives its effectiveness from its ability to interfere with acute inflammatory reactions in a variety of ways. Colchicine blocks the processing of IL-1β[146] and inhibits E-selectin–mediated adhesiveness to neutrophils.[155] Its action diminishes neutrophil L-selectin expression, random motility, chemotaxis, phospholipase A_2 activation, and IL-1 expression, as well as the stimulated elaboration of platelet-activating factor, crystal-induced chemotactic factor, and leukotriene B_4. Colchicine also inhibits endothelial cell ICAM-1 expression and mast cell histamine release and downregulates TNF-α receptors on macrophages and endothelial cells.

Colchicine can also be given intravenously, but this route is often discouraged because adverse outcomes, including death, can occur with inappropriate dosing.[179,180] When used properly, the drug abolishes the acute attack with a low incidence of gastrointestinal side effects (provided the patient is not also taking oral colchicine). An initial dose of 1 or 2 mg can be followed by one or two additional 1-mg doses administered at 6-hour intervals, if needed. The total dose of intravenous colchicine should not exceed 4 mg. Colchicine should be diluted with 20 mL of normal saline before administration and given slowly into a secure venous access to minimize sclerosis of the vein. Extravasation can lead to severe local necrosis. In addition, oral colchicine should be discontinued, and no additional colchicine should be given for at least 7 days because of the slow excretion of this drug.

Nonsteroidal Anti-inflammatory Drugs

In a patient with an established diagnosis of uncomplicated gout, the preferred agent is an NSAID, and indomethacin has been the traditional choice. Although this drug may be effective in doses as low as 25 mg four times a day, an initial dose of 50 to 75 mg, followed by 50 mg every 6 to 8 hours, with a maximum dose of 200 mg in the first 24 hours, has generally been recommended. To prevent relapse, it is reasonable to continue this dose for an additional 24 hours, then to taper to 50 mg every 6 to 8 hours for the next 2 days. Clinical trials have shown that oral naproxen, fenoprofen, ibuprofen, sulindac, piroxicam, and ketoprofen, as well as intramuscular ketorolac, are also effective. In fact, all members of this family of drugs can be highly effective in the treatment of acute gouty arthritis, including the cyclooxygenase-2 (COX-2) selective agents.[181]

Corticosteroids

Intra-articular glucocorticoids are useful in the treatment of acute gout limited to a single joint or bursa.[173,182] Oral, intramuscular, or intravenous glucocorticoids can also provide relief, but these agents are usually reserved for patients who are intolerant of colchicine or NSAIDs or who have medical conditions such as peptic ulcer disease or renal disease that contraindicate their use. Doses of glucocorticoids have been systematically studied, and generally, high doses (prednisone 20 to 60 mg/day) are needed. Lower doses may not be effective, as evidenced by gout flares occurring in organ transplant patients who are taking maintenance prednisone at doses of 7.5 to 15 mg a day.[183] Anecdotally, rebound attacks have been reported as steroids were withdrawn.

Adrenocorticotropic Hormone

Single injections of intramuscular ACTH gel (25 to 80 IU) can terminate an acute gout attack.[184] More often, however, repeated administration is required every 24 to 72 hours. This treatment is effective postoperatively and may be more effective than glucocorticoids, possibly related to the mechanism of action. In addition to stimulating the adrenal cortex to produce corticosteroids, ACTH interferes with the acute inflammatory response through activation of melanocortin receptor-3.[161]

Prophylaxis

The practice of giving small daily doses of colchicine as prophylaxis to prevent acute attacks is up to 85% effective.[185] Colchicine 0.6 mg one to three times a day is generally well tolerated, although the drug may produce a reversible axonal neuromyopathy.[186] This complication causes proximal muscle weakness with or without painful paresthesia and elevated serum levels of creatine phosphokinase. This is most often seen in patients with hypertension, renal dysfunction, or liver disease who are also using diuretics. Rhabdomyolysis may also occur in these settings and is more common in individuals who are also taking a statin (HMG-CoA reductase inhibitor) or cyclosporine.[187]

In patients who are unable to tolerate even one colchicine tablet per day, indomethacin or another NSAID has been used prophylactically at low doses (e.g., 25 mg indomethacin twice a day or naproxen 250 mg/day), with some success.[188] Maintenance doses of colchicine or an NSAID may make the difference between frequent incapacitation and uninterrupted daily activities. Prophylaxis is usually continued until the serum urate value has been maintained well within the normal range and there have been no acute attacks for 3 to 6 months. It is important to warn patients that colchicine discontinuation may be followed by an exacerbation of acute gouty arthritis and advise them what to do should an attack occur. Finally, prophylactic treatment is not recommended unless the clinician also uses urate-lowering agents. Prophylactic colchicine may block the acute inflammatory response but does not alter the deposition of crystals in tissues. When deposition continues without the warning signs of recurrent bouts of acute arthritis, tophi and destruction to cartilage and bone can occur without notice.

CONTROL OF HYPERURICEMIA

Elimination of hyperuricemia with antihyperuricemic agents can prevent as well as reverse urate deposition. Today, opinion differs as to when in the course of gout the clinician should start antihyperuricemic therapy. Some physicians regard the first gouty attack as a late event in a disorder marked by years of antecedent silent deposition of urate crystals in cartilage and other connective tissue. Others believe that because tophi and symptomatic chronic gouty arthritis develop in only a minority of cases and ordinarily develop very slowly after many years of recurrent acute attacks, unnecessary or premature medication can be avoided without demonstrable penalty. In practice, it is the rare patient who never experiences a second attack.[36] The probability of such a benign course is greatest in patients who have only minimally elevated serum urate concentrations and normal 24-hour urinary uric acid values. Arguably, a case can be made for initiating antihyperuricemia therapy after the second attack in most patients.[189]

Antihyperuricemic drugs provide a definitive method for controlling hyperuricemia. Although it is important to treat and prevent acute attacks of gouty arthritis with anti-inflammatory agents, it is the long-term control of hyperuricemia that ultimately modifies the manifestations of the gouty diathesis. Once started, treatment with specific urate-lowering agents is lifelong, and the dose must be sufficient to maintain the serum urate level below 6.8 mg/dL, and preferably between 5 and 6 mg/dL. Lowering the serum urate level from 11 mg/dL to 7.5 mg/dL may seem encouraging, but this change does not reverse the process. It merely slows the rate at which crystals continue to deposit. Generally, the lower the serum urate level achieved during antihyperuricemic therapy, the faster the reduction in tophaceous deposits.[190] The 5 to 6 mg/dL target is recommended because it is far enough below the saturation level of 6.8 mg/dL that it provides some margin for fluctuations in serum levels and avoids excessive exposure to the medication, which might increase the chance of toxicity.

Reduction to target levels may be achieved pharmacologically by the use of xanthine oxidase inhibitors or uricosuric agents. Xanthine oxidase, the enzyme that catalyzes the oxidation of hypoxanthine to xanthine and xanthine to uric acid, is inhibited by allopurinol and oxypurinol. Probenecid, sulfinpyrazone, and benzbromarone are uricosuric agents that reduce serum urate concentrations by enhancing the renal excretion of uric acid. These antihyperuricemic drugs do not have anti-inflammatory properties.

For those patients with gout who excrete less than 800 mg of uric acid per day and have normal renal function, reduction of the serum urate concentration can be achieved equally well with a xanthine oxidase inhibitor or a uricosuric drug. These agents are equally effective in preventing the deterioration of renal function in patients with primary gout.[191] In most cases, allopurinol is the drug of choice because it can be used with fewer restrictions compared with uricosuric agents.

In general, the ideal candidate for uricosuric agents is a gouty patient who is younger than 60 years and has normal renal function (creatinine clearance >80 mL/min), uric acid excretion of less than 800 mg per 24 hours on a general diet, and no history of renal calculi. Patients prescribed uricosuric agents should be counseled to avoid salicylate use at doses greater than 81 mg/day.[192]

In certain situations, an inhibitor of xanthine oxidase is clearly the drug of choice in a gouty patient. Gouty individuals who excrete larger quantities of uric acid in their urine or who have a history of renal calculi of any type should be treated with allopurinol (Table 87-5). The incidence of renal calculi is about 35% in patients with primary gout who excrete more than 700 mg/day of uric acid.[90] There is also a greater risk for uric acid stones on initiation of uricosuric therapy. In addition, patients with tophi generally should receive allopurinol to decrease the load of urate that must be handled by the kidney. Patients with gout and mild renal insufficiency can be given either type of agent,

but probenecid and sulfinpyrazone would not be expected to work when the glomerular filtration rate is less than 50 mL/min. Allopurinol is effective in the presence of renal insufficiency, but doses may have to be decreased in that situation. A final indication for a xanthine oxidase inhibitor is the failure of uricosuric agents to produce a serum urate concentration lower than 6 mg/dL or patient intolerance of the uricosuric agent. Allopurinol and a uricosuric drug may be used in combination for a patient with tophaceous gout in whom it is not possible to reduce the serum urate below 6 mg/dL with a single agent. In most settings, if allopurinol does not cause the serum urate to drop below 6 mg/dL, it is the result of insufficient dosing or poor patient compliance.

Xanthine Oxidase Inhibitors

Allopurinol is presently the only xanthine oxidase inhibitor approved for use, but others are under development. Allopurinol is a substrate for xanthine oxidase and is converted to oxypurinol by that enzyme activity. Oxypurinol is also an inhibitor of xanthine oxidase. Allopurinol is metabolized in the liver and has a half-life of 1 to 3 hours, but oxypurinol, which is excreted in the urine, has a half-life of 12 to 17 hours. Because of these pharmacokinetic properties, allopurinol is dosed on a daily basis, and the dosage required to reduce serum urate levels is lower in patients with decreased glomerular filtration rates.

In 1984, guidelines for allopurinol dosing based on creatinine clearance were published (Table 87-6).[193] It is now apparent that these guidelines are useful for selecting the initial dosage of allopurinol, but they do not provide the effective maintenance dose for many individuals, and following them does not protect against cutaneous hypersensitivity reactions.[194-196]

Allopurinol should be used at the lowest dose that lowers the serum urate level below 5 to 6 mg/dL. The most commonly prescribed dose is 300 mg/day, but this is insufficient to adequately reduce serum urate to the target level in 21% to 55% of individuals.[21,197,198] Thus, higher doses, with a maximum of 800 mg/day, may be required. The sudden

Table 87-5 Indications for Allopurinol

Hyperuricemia associated with increased uric acid production
Urinary uric acid excretion of 1000 mg or more in 24 hr
Hyperuricemia associated with HPRT deficiency or PRPP synthetase overactivity
Uric acid nephropathy
Nephrolithiasis
Prophylaxis before cytolytic therapy
Intolerance or reduced efficacy of uricosuric agents
Gout with renal insufficiency (GFR <60 mL/min)
Allergy to uricosurics

GFR, glomerular filtration rate; HPRT, hypoxanthine phosphoribosyltransferase; PRPP, phosphoribosylpyrophosphate.

Table 87-6 Maintenance Doses of Allopurinol Based on Creatinine Clearance Measurement*

Creatinine Clearance (mL/min)	Allopurinol Dose (mg)
0	100 every 3 days
10	100 every 2 days
20	100 daily
40	150 daily
60	200 daily
80	250 daily
100	300 daily
120	350 daily
140	400 daily

*These doses represent those that might be selected when initiating therapy with allopurinol. However, urate levels should be checked and the dosage adjusted so that the patient is taking the lowest dose that maintains the serum urate level below 5 to 6 mg/dL.

From Hande KR, Noone RM, Stone WJ: Severe allopurinol toxicity: Description and guidelines for presentation in patients with renal insufficiency. Am J Med 76:47, 1984.

lowering of serum urate concentrations that accompanies the initiation of allopurinol therapy may trigger acute gout attacks. This risk can be minimized by beginning prophylactic colchicine or NSAID (see the previous discussion) 2 weeks before the first dose of allopurinol. Alternatively, the clinician can start allopurinol at a dose of 50 to 100 mg/day and increase it by similar increments weekly until the desired target is reached.

About 20% of patients who take allopurinol report side effects, with 5% discontinuing the medication. Common side effects include gastrointestinal intolerance and skin rashes. The occurrence of a rash does not necessarily mean the drug should be discontinued. If the rash is not severe, the allopurinol can be withheld temporarily and resumed after the rash has cleared. Oxypurinol has been tried in patients who are sensitive to allopurinol, but its use is limited by poor gastrointestinal absorption and a high prevalence of cross-reactivity with allopurinol. Oral and intravenous protocols for desensitization to allopurinol have been successful in some patients following cutaneous reactions.[188,199]

Other adverse reactions include fever, toxic epidermal necrolysis, alopecia, bone marrow suppression with leukopenia or thrombocytopenia, agranulocytosis, aplastic anemia, granulomatous hepatitis, jaundice, sarcoid-like reaction, and vasculitis. The most severe reaction is the allopurinol hypersensitivity syndrome, which may include fever, skin rash, eosinophilia, hepatitis, progressive renal insufficiency, and death.[193,200] Autopsies reveal diffuse vasculitis involving multiple organs. This is most likely to develop in individuals with preexisting renal dysfunction and those taking diuretics.

Allopurinol is involved in relatively few drug-drug interactions. Its use potentiates the actions of other agents that are inactivated by xanthine oxidase. The most important of these are azathioprine and 6-mercaptopurine. In addition, allopurinol can reduce the activity of hepatic microsomal drug-metabolizing enzymes and prolong the half-lives of warfarin and theophylline. Rash may be more common in patients using allopurinol and ampicillin, and bone marrow suppression may be increased in those also taking cyclophosphamide.

Phase III studies with febuxostat have been completed.[21] Febuxostat is a potent xanthine oxidase inhibitor that differs from allopurinol in that it is of another chemical class and is a selective inhibitor of enzyme activity. These properties indicate that it would be an excellent alternative for individuals who are intolerant of or hypersensitive to allopurinol. In addition, the dosage of febuxostat does not need to be adjusted in individuals with mild to moderate renal insufficiency.

Uricosuric Agents

Administration of a uricosuric agent increases the rate of renal uric acid excretion.[201] In the kidney, there are separate transport systems for the secretion and reabsorption of organic ions, including uric acid. Because urate is reabsorbed by a renal tubular brush border anion transporter, the reabsorption of urate can be inhibited when uricosuric agents are present in the lumen and compete with urate for the transporter. This inhibition of reabsorptive anion transporter requires high doses of uricosuric agents. Because the

secretory transport system is quantitatively much smaller than that for reabsorption and is located in the basolateral membrane of the tubule, when uricosuric agents are taken in very low doses, they actually decrease the renal excretion of uric acid and raise serum urate levels by inhibiting the secretory transport system.

Probenecid and sulfinpyrazone are the most widely used uricosuric agents available in the United States; benzbromarone is used for this purpose in other countries as well. However, many other agents can reduce serum urate levels by enhancing the renal excretion of uric acid (see Table 87-3).

Probenecid is readily absorbed from the gastrointestinal tract. Its half-life in plasma is dose dependent, varying from 6 to 12 hours. This can be prolonged by the concomitant use of allopurinol. Probenecid is metabolized in vivo, with less than 5% of the administered dose recovered in the urine. The maintenance dosage of probenecid ranges from 500 mg to 3 g per day and is administered two or three times a day. Acute gouty attacks may accompany the initiation of this medication, and, as with all uricosuric agents, patients using probenecid are at increased risk for developing renal calculi. With long-term use, up to 18% of individuals develop gastrointestinal complaints, and 5% develop hypersensitivity and rash. Although serious toxicity is rare, approximately one third of individuals eventually become intolerant of probenecid and discontinue its use. Probenecid alters the metabolism of several other agents by several mechanisms (Table 87-7). Concomitant use of probenecid can increase the potency of some agents by decreasing their renal excretion, delaying their metabolism, or impairing their hepatic uptake. It may decrease the effectiveness of other medications by reducing their volume of distribution.

Sulfinpyrazone is completely absorbed from the gastrointestinal tract and has a half-life of 1 to 3 hours. Most of the drug is excreted in the urine as the parahydroxyl metabolite,

Table 87-7 Effects of Probenecid on Metabolism of Other Drugs

Decreased Renal Excretion
p-Aminohippuric acid
Phenolsulfonphthalein
Salicylic acid and its acyl and phenolic glucuronides
Phlorizin and its glucuronide
Acetazolamide
Dapsone and its metabolites
Sulfinpyrazone and its parahydroxyl metabolite
Indomethacin
Ampicillin
Penicillin
Cephradine
Reduced Volume of Distribution
Ampicillin
Ancillin
Nafcillin
Cephaloridine
Impairment of Hepatic Uptake
Bromsulfophthalein
Indocyanine green
Rifampicin
Delayed Metabolism
Heparin

which is also uricosuric. Sulfinpyrazone is usually given at a dosage of 300 to 400 mg/day divided into three or four doses. The rates of tolerability and types of adverse reactions are similar to those with probenecid.

Benzbromarone is more potent than probenecid and sulfinpyrazone.[191] It is well tolerated and effective in cyclosporine-treated renal transplant patients. It can be used in those with moderate renal dysfunction (creatinine clearance approximately 25 mL/min).

COMPLIANCE WITH TREATMENT

Because the disease processes involved in gout are so well understood, the diagnosis can be definitively established. Once gout is diagnosed, the available therapies are so effective that it should be a readily treated and easily managed disease. However, too many patients, including those who are accurately diagnosed, do not do well. Failure of antihyperuricemic therapy to attain the target urate level is usually due to improper prescribing or poor compliance.[194] Compliance is often a problem when treating chronic asymptomatic conditions, and associated alcoholism can be a factor. Perhaps more important is the fact that patients may need to take up to three different medications on three different schedules to control their symptoms and treat the disease.

It is believed that if patients understand why they are taking medications, they are more likely to be compliant. Toward this end, an analogy has been developed that helps some patients become more compliant.[202] In this analogy, urate crystals are compared to matches. The patient is told that "when the match strikes," it causes a gout attack. To "put out the fire," the patient takes an NSAID or colchicine. Although this resolves the attack, "the matches are still there." To eliminate future attacks, the patient is given prophylactic colchicine, "which makes the matches damp and harder to strike," and allopurinol (or a uricosuric agent), "which actually removes the matches from the body."

MANAGEMENT OF GOUT AFTER ORGAN TRANSPLANTATION

The management of patients with gout after organ transplantation requires careful consideration. The use of glucocorticoids, azathioprine, or cyclosporine and the precarious status of renal function in many patients pose complex problems. Colchicine and NSAIDs may be inappropriate for the management of acute gouty arthritis in this setting because of their potential toxicities. Intra-articular glucocorticoid injections may be most helpful, and one may be forced to rely more heavily on pain medications in this setting. Prophylactic colchicine can be used in patients with normal renal function, but treatment must be monitored closely. The combination of colchicine and cyclosporine has induced rhabdomyolysis.[187]

When considering chronic therapy, it is helpful to lower the doses of cyclosporine and eliminate the use of diuretics, if possible. Uricosuric agents can be used safely, but their usefulness declines if renal function is poor. Allopurinol can be used in patients with abnormal renal function, but the dose may need to be reduced. Allopurinol, however, may have a severe interaction with azathioprine. Azathioprine is metabolized by xanthine oxidase, and because allopurinol inhibits that enzyme, the breakdown of azathioprine is slowed, increasing the effective dose. If care is not taken, significant bone marrow toxicity can result. If azathioprine and allopurinol are used together, they can be started at 25 and 50 mg/day, respectively.[203] Complete blood counts and serum urate level concentrations are then monitored weekly, and the allopurinol dose is adjusted to bring the serum urate concentration to less than 6 mg/dL. As an alternative to azathioprine, mycophenolate mofetil has been used effectively with allopurinol in some transplant patients.[204]

Urate oxidase has been used to drastically lower serum urate levels and shrink tophi in a small number of patients with gout after cardiac transplantation.[205] This treatment has been associated with significant allergic reactions, including anaphylaxis, bronchospasm, and hemolytic anemia, but newer preparations of uricase formulated with polyethylene glycol may avoid those complications and prove more effective.[206]

ANCILLARY FACTORS

In addition to anti-inflammatory agents, colchicine prophylaxis, and antihyperuricemic therapy, other factors may be decisive in determining whether recurrent attacks, chronic gouty arthritis, kidney stones, or nephropathy develops. Today, dietary purine restriction solely to control serum urate levels is rarely advised. A totally purine-free diet reduces the urinary excretion of uric acid by only 200 to 400 mg/day and lowers the mean serum urate value by about 1 mg/dL. In addition, the antihyperuricemic agents available today are so effective that this type of dietary manipulation is rarely needed. Nevertheless, beneficial results have been reported with a diet of moderate calorie and carbohydrate restriction and a proportionally increased intake of protein and unsaturated fat.[207] Some subjects with gout are susceptible to acute attacks after the consumption of alcoholic beverages or rich foods. Others describe idiosyncratic responses, such as acute gout after eating a particular food, but such relationships are rare and questionable. A diet designed to avoid indiscretions known to precipitate acute gouty attacks in a particular individual is recommended.

In addition, diet is very important with regard to other medical problems.[208] Many gouty patients are overweight, and restoration of ideal body weight through regulated calorie restriction is recommended. In addition, at least 75% of patients with primary gout have hypertriglyceridemia. The initial step in managing hypertriglyceridemia is reduction to ideal body weight and elimination of alcohol ingestion.

Many patients with gout consume liberal amounts of alcohol. Acute excesses may lead to exacerbations of hyperuricemia secondary to temporary hyperlactacidemia, and chronic ingestion of alcohol may stimulate increased purine production.[74] The added purine load resulting from regular ingestion of beer may also be a contributing factor. Patients should be warned about the deleterious effects of excessive alcohol intake. Compliance with medication is also much worse among patients who consume alcohol.

About one third of gouty subjects are hypertensive. The complications of hypertension are potentially more serious than those of hyperuricemia, and the clinician should not hesitate to use whatever drugs are necessary to control the hypertension. Many hypertensive gouty patients require a thiazide diuretic. If this medication is needed to control hypertension, it should be used, with the recognition that the dosage of concomitant antihyperuricemic therapy may need to be adjusted to maintain appropriate control of serum urate levels.

REFERENCES

1. Wyngaarden JD, Kelley WN: Gout and Hyperuricemia. New York, Grune & Stratton, 1976.
2. Wortmann RL, Schumacher HR Jr, Becker MA, Ryan LM: Crystal-Induced Arthropathies: Gout, Pseudogout, and Apatite-Associated Syndromes. New York, Informa Healthcare, 2006.
3. Currie W: Prevalence and incidence of the diagnosis of gout in Great Britain. Ann Rheum Dis 38:101, 1979.
4. Klemp P, Stansfield S, Castle B, Robertson M: Gout is on the increase in New Zealand. Ann Rheum Dis 56:22, 1997.
5. **Mikuls TR, Saag KG: New insights into gout epidemiology. Curr Opin Rheumatol 18:199, 2006.**
6. Darmawan J, Valkenburg HA, Muirden KD, Wigley RD: The epidemiology of gout and hyperuricemia in a rural population in Java. J Rheumatol 19:1595, 1992.
7. Park YB, Park YS, Lee WK, et al: Clinical manifestations of Korean female gouty patients. Clin Rheumatol 19:142, 2000.
8. Chang H-Y, Pan W-H, Yeh W-T, et al: Hyperuricemia and gout in Taiwan: Results of the nutritional and health survey in Taiwan. J Rheumatol 28:1640, 2001.
9. Cameron JS, Moro F, Simmonds HA: Gout, uric acid, and purine metabolism in pediatric nephrology. Pediatr Nephrol 17:105, 1993.
10. Marinello E, Giuseppe RS, Marcolongo R: Plasma follicle-stimulating hormone, luteinizing hormone, and sex hormones in patients with gout. Arthritis Rheum 28:127, 1985.
11. Arromlee E, Michet CJ, Crowson CS, et al: Epidemiology of gout: Is the incidence rising? J Rheumatol 29:2403, 2002.
12. Wallace KL, Riedel AA, Joseph-Ridge N, Wortmann RL: Increased prevalence of gout and hyperuricemia over 10 years among older adults in a managed care population. J Rheumatol 31:1582, 2004.
13. Campion EW, Glynn RJ, deLabry LO: Asymptomatic hyperuricemia: The risks and consequences. Am J Med 82:421, 1987.
14. Choi H, Atkinson KK, Karlson E, et al: Alcohol intake and risk incidence of gout in men: A prospective study. Lancet 363:1277, 2004.
15. Choi HK, Liu S: Intake of purine-rich foods, protein, and dairy products and relationship to serum levels of uric acid: The Third National Health and Nutrition Examination Survey. Arthritis Rheum 52:283, 2005.
16. Parhami N, Feng H: Gout in the hip joint. Arthritis Rheum 36:1026, 1993.
17. Musgrave DS, Ziran BH: Monoarticular acromioclavicular joint gout. Am J Orthop 29:544, 2000.
18. Weinzweig J, Gletcher JW, Lindburg RM: Flexor tendonitis and median nerve compression caused by gout in a patient with rheumatoid arthritis. Plast Reconstr Surg 106:1570, 2000.
19. Townsend D, Vasu P: Gouty tenosynovitis—more common than we think? N Z Med J 117:1188, 2004.
20. Lally EV, Zimmerman B, Ho G, Kaplan SR: Urate-mediated inflammation in nodal osteoarthritis: Clinical and roentgenographic correlations. Arthritis Rheum 32:86, 1989.
21. Becker MA, Schumacher HR, Wortmann RL, et al: A study comparing safety and efficiency of oral febuxostat and allopurinol in subjects with hyperuricemia and gout. N Engl J Med 353:2450, 2005.
22. Hunter DJ, York M, Chaisson CE, et al: Recent diuretic use and the risk of recurrent gout attacks: The online case-crossover gout study. J Rheumatol 33:1341, 2006.
23. Khalifa P, Sereni D, Boissonnas A, et al: Attacks of gout and thromboembolic disease: Role of heparin therapy. Ann Intern Med 136:582, 1985.
24. Howe S, Edwards NL: Controlling hyperuricemia and gout in cardiac transplant recipients. J Musculoskel Med 12:15, 1995.
25. Kalia KK, Moossy JJ: Carpal tunnel release complicated by acute gout. Neurosurgery 33:1102, 1993.
26. Williamson SC, Roger DJ, Petrera P, Glockner F: Acute gouty arthropathy after total knee arthroplasty: A case report. J Bone Joint Surg Am 76:126, 1994.
27. **Nakayama DA, Barthelemy C, Carrera G, et al: Tophaceous gout: A clinical and radiographic assessment. Arthritis Rheum 27:468, 1984.**
28. Wallace SL, Bernstein D, Diamond H: Diagnostic value of the colchicine therapeutic trial. JAMA 1999:525, 1967.
29. Wallace SL, Robinson H, Masi AT, et al: Preliminary criteria for the classification of acute arthritis of primary gout. Arthritis Rheum 20:897, 1977.
30. Bonal J, Schumacher HR: Podagra is more than gout. Bull Rheum Dis 34:1, 1984.
31. Vandenberg MK, Moxley G, Breitbach SA, et al: Gout attacks in chronic alcoholics occur at lower serum urate levels than in nonalcoholics. Rheumatology 21:700, 1994.
32. Tsutani H, Yoshio N, Takanori U: Interleukin 6 reduces serum urate concentrations. J Rheumatol 27:554, 2000.
33. Urano W, Yamanaka H, Tsutani H, et al: The inflammatory process in the mechanism of decreased serum uric acid concentration during acute gouty arthritis. J Rheumatol 29:1950, 2002.
34. Wortmann RL, Kelley WN: Gout and hyperuricemia. In Ruddy S, Harris ED Jr, Sledge CB (eds): Kelley's Textbook of Rheumatology, 6th ed. Philadelphia, WB Saunders, 2001.
35. Rogachefsky RA, Carneiro R, Altman RD, et al: Gout presenting as infectious arthritis. J Bone Joint Surg Am 76:269, 1994.
36. Gutman AB: Gout. In Beeson PB, McDermott W (eds): Textbook of Medicine, 12th ed. Philadelphia, WB Saunders, 1958, p 595.
37. **McCarthy GM, Barthelemy CR, Verum JA, et al: Influence of antihyperuricemia therapy and radiographic progression of gout. Arthritis Rheum 34:1489, 1991.**
38. Pascual E, Battle-Gualda E, Martinez A, et al: Synovial fluid analysis for diagnosis of intercritical gout. Ann Intern Med 131:756, 1999.
39. Schapira D, Stahl S, Izhak OB, et al: Chronic tophaceous gouty arthritis mimicking rheumatoid arthritis. Semin Arthritis Rheum 29:56, 1999.
40. Kini S, Mittal G, Balakrishna C, et al: An unusual systemic presentation of gout. JAPI 48:354, 2000.
41. Barrett K, Miller M, Wilson JT: Tophaceous gout of the spine mimicking epidural infection: Case report and review of the literature. Neurosurgery 48:1170, 2001.
42. Hensch PS: The diagnosis of gout and gouty arthritis. J Lab Clin Med 220:48, 1936.
43. Gutman AB: The past four decades of progress in the knowledge of gout, with an assessment of the present status. Arthritis Rheum 16:431, 1973.
44. Wernick R, Winkler C, Campbell S: Tophi as the initial manifestation of gout: Report of six cases and review of the literature. Arch Intern Med 152:873, 1992.
45. King CW, Helm TN, Narins RB: Intradermal tophaceous gout. Cutis 67:205, 2001.
46. Beathge BA, Work J, Landreneau MD, et al: Tophaceous gout in patients with renal transplants treated with cyclosporine A. J Rheumatol 20:718, 1993.
47. Barthelemy CR, Nakayama DA, Carrera GF, et al: Gouty arthritis: A prospective radiographic evaluation of sixty patients. Skeletal Radiol 11:1, 1984.
48. Gentili A: The advanced imaging of gouty tophi. Curr Rheum Rep 8:231, 2006.
49. St George E, Liller CEM, Hutfield R: Spinal cord compression: An unusual neurologic complication of gout. Rheumatology 40:711, 2001.
50. Gawoski JM, Balogh K, Landis WJ: Aortic valvular tophus: Identification by x-ray diffraction of urate and calcium phosphates. J Clin Pathol 38:873, 1985.
51. Habermann W, Kiesler K, Eherer A, et al: Laryngeal manifestations of gout: A case of a subglottic tophus. Auris Nasus Larynx 28:265, 2001.
52. Choi HK, Atkinson K, Karlson EW, et al: Obesity weight change, hypertension, diuretic use, and risk of gout in white men: The Health Professionals Follow-up Study. Arch Intern Med 165:742, 2005.
53. Myers A, Epstein FH, Dodge HJ, et al: The relationship of serum uric acid to risk factors in coronary heart disease. Am J Med 45:520, 1968.
54. Takahashi S, Yamamoto T, Moriwaki Y, et al: Impaired lipoprotein metabolism in patients with primary gout: Influence of alcohol intake and body weight. Br J Rheumatol 33:731, 1994.
55. Collantes E, Tinahones FJ, Cisnal A, et al: Variability of lipid phenotypes in hyperuricemic hyperlipidemic patients. Clin Rheumatol 13:244, 1994.

56. Tsutsumi S, Yamamoto T, Moriwaki Y, et al: Decreased activities of lipoprotein lipase and hepatic triglyceride lipase in patients with gout. Metabolism 50:952, 2001.
57. Mikkelsen WM: The possible association of hyperuricemia and/or gout with diabetes mellitus. Arthritis Rheum 8:853, 1965.
58. Denis G, Launay MP: Carbohydrate intolerance in gout. Metabolism 18:770, 1969.
59. Feig DI, Johnson RJ: Hyperuricemia in childhood primary hypertension. Hypertension 42:247, 2003.
60. Cappuccio FP, Stazzullo P, Farinaro E, Trevisan M: Uric acid metabolism and tubular sodium handling: Results from a population based study. JAMA 270:354, 1993.
61. Kang DH, Nakagawa T, Feng L, et al: A role for uric acid in the progression of renal disease. J Am Soc Nephrol 13:1288, 2002.
62. Mazzali M, Kanellis J, Han L, et al: Hyperuricemia induces primary renal arteriolopathy in rats by a blood pressure-independent mechanism. Am J Physiol Renal Physiol 282:F991, 2002.
63. Brand FN, McGee DL, Kannel WB, et al: Hyperuricemia as a risk factor for coronary heart disease: The Framingham Heart Study. Am J Epidemiol 121:11, 1985.
64. Gelber AC, Klag MJ, Mead LA, et al: Gout and risk for subsequent coronary heart disease: The Meharry-Hopkins Study. Arch Intern Med 157:1436, 1997.
65. Culleton BF, Larson MG, Kannel WB, Levy D: Serum uric acid and the risk for cardiovascular disease and death: The Framingham Heart Study. Ann Intern Med 131:7, 1999.
66. Grundy SM, Balady GJ, Criqui MH, et al: Primary prevention of coronary heart disease: Guidance from Framingham. A statement of health care professionals from the AHA task force on risk reduction. Circulation 97:1876, 1998.
67. Fang J, Alderman MH: Serum uric acid and cardiovascular mortality: The NHANES I Epidemiologic Follow-up Study, 1971-1992. JAMA 283:2404, 2000.
68. Verdecchia P, Schillaci G, Reboldi GP, et al: Relation between serum uric acid and risk of cardiovascular disease in hypertension: The PIUMA Study. Hypertension 36:1072, 2000.
69. Chou P, Lin K-C, Lin Y-H, et al: Gender differences in the relationship of serum uric acid with fasting serum insulin and plasma glucose in patients without diabetes. J Rheumatol 28:571, 2001.
70. Takahashi S, Moriwaki Y, Tsutsuni Z, et al: Increased visceral fat accumulation further aggravates the risks of insulin resistance in gout. Metabolism 50:393, 2001.
71. Ford ES, Giles WH, Dietz WH: Prevalence of metabolic syndrome among US adults: Findings of the Third National Health and Nutrition Examination Survey. JAMA 287:356, 2002.
72. Krishnan E, Baker JF, Furst DE, Schumacher HR: Gout and the risk of acute myocardial infarction. Arthritis Rheum 54:2688, 2006.
73. Al-Arfaj AS: Hyperuricemia in Saudi Arabia. Rheumatol Int 20:61, 2001.
74. Puig JG, Fox IH: Ethanol-induced activation of adenine nucleotide turnover: Evidence for a role of acetate. J Clin Invest 74:936, 1984.
75. Giordano N, Santacroce C, Mattii G, et al: Hyperuricemia and gout in thyroid endocrine disorders. Clin Exp Rheumatol 19:661, 2001.
76. Nordstrom DM, Merenich JA: The relationship of gout to hyperthyroidism [abstract]. Arthritis Rheum 32:S68, 1989.
77. Woolliscroft JO, Fox IH: Increased body fluids purines during hypotensive events: Evidence for ATP degradation. Am J Med 81:472, 1986.
78. Grum CM, Simon RH, Dantzker DR, Fox IH: Biochemical indicators of cellular hypoxia in critically ill patients: Evidence for ATP degradation. Chest 88:763, 1985.
79. McCord J: Oxygen-derived free radicals in postischemic tissue injury. N Engl J Med 312:159, 1985.
80. Lind T, Godfrey KA, Otun H: Changes in serum uric acid concentrations during normal pregnancy. Br J Obstet Gynaecol 91:128, 1984.
81. Liedholm H, Montan S, Aberg A: Risk grouping of 113 patients with hypertensive disorders during pregnancy, with respect to serum urate, proteinuria and time of onset of hypertension. Acta Obstet Gynecol Scand 118(Suppl):43, 1984.
82. Wooten MD, Lipsmeyer E: Gout accompanying rheumatoid arthritis: A comparison of affected women and men. J Clin Rheumatol 4:220, 1998.
83. Wall BA, Agudelo CA, Weinblatt ME, et al: Acute gout and systemic lupus erythematosus: Report of 2 cases and literature review. J Rheumatol 9:305, 1982.
84. Wong DMT, Chambers LM: Coexistent acute gouty arthritis and ankylosing spondylitis: A rare occurrence. J Rheumatol 21:773, 1994.
85. **Fessel WJ: Renal outcomes of gout and hyperuricemia. Am J Med 67:74, 1979.**
86. Yu TF, Berger L: Renal function in gout: Its association with hypertensive vascular disease and intrinsic renal disease. Am J Med 72:95, 1982.
87. Cohen LF, Balow JE, Poplack DG, et al: Acute tumor lysis syndrome: A review of 37 patients with Burkitt's lymphoma. Am J Med 68:486, 1980.
88. Kelton J, Kelley WN, Holmes EW: A rapid method for the diagnosis of acute uric acid nephropathy. Arch Intern Med 138:612, 1978.
89. Gutman AB, Fu TF: Uric acid nephrolithiasis. Am J Med 45:756, 1968.
90. Yu TF, Gutman AB: Uric acid nephrolithiasis in gout: Predisposing factors. Ann Intern Med 67:1133, 1967.
91. Simmonds HA, Sahota AS, Van Acker KJ: Adenine phosphoribosyltransferase deficiency and 2, 8-dihydroxyadenine lithiasis. In Scriver CR, Beaudet AC, Sly WS, Valle D (eds): The Metabolic and Molecular Bases of Inherited Disease, 7th ed. New York, McGraw-Hill, 1995, pp 1655-1670.
92. Rosenbloom FM, Kelley WN, Carr AA, Seegmiller JE: Familial nephropathy and gout in a kindred. Clin Res 15:270, 1967.
93. McBride MB, Simmonds HA, Moro F: Genetic gout in childhood: Familial juvenile hyperuricemic nephropathy or "familial renal disease". J Inherit Metab Dis 20:351, 1997.
94. Kamatani N, Moritani M, Yamanaka H, et al: Localization of a gene for familial juvenile hyperuricemic nephropathy causing under-excretion type gout to 16p12 by genome-wide linkage analysis of a large family. Arthritis Rheum 43:925, 2000.
95. Stacey JM, Turner JJO, Harding B, et al: Genetic mapping studies of familial juvenile hyperuricemic nephropathy on chromosome 16p13-p11. J Clin Endocrinol Metab 88:464, 2003.
96. Van Goor W, Kooiker CJ, Mees FJD: An unusual form of renal disease associated with gout and hypertension. J Clin Pathol 24:354, 1971.
97. Hart TC, Gorry MC, Hart PS, et al: Mutations of the UMOD gene are responsible for medullary cystic kidney disease 2 and familial juvenile hyperuricemic nephropathy. J Med Genet 39:882, 2002.
98. Wolf MTF, Mucha BE, Attanasio M, et al: Mutations in the uromodulin gene in MCKD type 2 patients cluster in exon 4 which codes three EGF-like domains. Kidney Int 64:1580, 2003.
99. Bleyer AJ, Trachtman H, Sandhu J, et al: Renal manifestations of a mutation in the uromodulin (Tamm- Horsfall protein) gene. Am J Kidney Dis 42:E20, 2003.
100. Kudo E, Kamatani N, Tezuka O, et al: Familial juvenile hyperuricemic nephropathy: Detection of mutations in the uromodulin gene in five Japanese families. Kidney Int 65:1589, 2004.
101. **Turner JJ, Stacey JM, Harding B, et al: Uromodulin mutations cause familial juvenile hyperuricemic nephropathy. J Clin Endocrinol Metab 88:1398, 2003.**
102. Rezende-Lima W, Parreira KS, Garcia-Gonzalez M, et al: Homozygosity for uromodulin disorders: FJHN and MCKD-type 2. Kidney Int 66:558, 2004.
103. Halla JT, Ball GV: Saturnine gout: A review of 42 patients. Semin Arthritis Rheum 11:307, 1982.
104. Lin J-L, Tan D-T, Ho H-H, et al: Environmental lead exposure and urate excretion in the general population. Am J Med 113:563, 2002.
105. Marsden PA: Increased body lead burden—cause or consequence of chronic renal insufficiency? N Engl J Med 348:345, 2002.
106. Batuman V: Lead nephropathy, lead, and hypertension. Am J Med Sci 305:241, 1993.
107. Lin JL, Huang PT: Body lead stores and urate excretion in men with chronic renal disease. J Rheumatol 21:705, 1994.
108. Burack DA, Griffith BP, Thompson ME, Kahl LE: Hyperuricemia and gout among heart transplant recipients receiving cyclosporine. Am J Med 92:141, 1992.
109. Cantarell MC, Capdevila L, Morlans M, Piera L: Uric acid calculus in renal transplant patients treated with cyclosporine. Clin Nephrol 35:288, 1992.
110. Griebsch A, Zollner N: Effects of ribonucleotides given orally on uric acid production in man. In Sperling O, de Vries A, Wyngaarden JD (eds): Purine Metabolism in Man, Vol 41B. New York, Plenum Press, 1974, p 443.

111. Calabrese G, Simmonds HA, Cameron JS, Davies PM: Precocious familial gout with reduced fractional urate clearance and normal purine enzymes. QJM 75:441, 1990.

112. Reynolds PP, Knapp MJ, Baraf HSB, Holmes EW: Moonshine and lead: Relationship to the pathogenesis of hyperuricemia in gout. Arthritis Rheum 26:1057, 1983.

113. Seegmiller JE, Grauze AO, Howell RR, et al: The renal excretion of uric acid in gout. J Clin Invest 41:1094, 1962.

114. Segal JB, Albert D: Diagnosis of crystal-induced arthritis by synovial fluid examination: Lessons from an imperfect test. Arthritis Care Res 12:376, 1999.

115. Emmerson BT, Nagel SL, Duffy DL, Martin NG: Genetic control of the renal clearance of urate: A study of twins. Ann Rheum Dis 51:375, 1992.

116. Nugent CA, Tyler FH: The renal excretion of uric acid in patients with gout and in nongouty subjects. J Clin Invest 38:1890, 1959.

117. Latham W, Rodnan GP: Impairment of uric acid excretion in gout. J Clin Invest 41:1955, 1962.

118. Lesch M, Nyhan WL: A familial disorder of uric acid metabolism and central nervous system function. Am J Med 36:561, 1964.

119. Kelley WN: Hypoxanthine guanine phosphoribosyltransferase deficiency in the Lesch-Nyhan syndrome and gout. Fed Proc 27:1060, 1968.

120. Caspi D, Lubert E, Graff E, et al: The effect of mini-dose aspirin on renal function and uric acid handling in elderly patients. Arthritis Rheum 43:103, 2000.

121. Kelley WN, Rosenbloom EM, Henderson JF, et al: A specific enzyme defect in gout associated with overproduction of uric acid. Proc Natl Acad Sci U S A 57:1735, 1967.

122. Chang SJ, Chang JG, Chen CJ, et al: Identification of a new single nucleotide substitution on the hypoxanthine-guanine phosphoribosyltransferase gene (HPRT[Tsou]) from a Taiwanese aboriginal family with severe gout. J Rheumatol 26:1802, 1999.

123. Sperling O, Eilam G, Persky-Brosh S, et al: Accelerated erythrocyte 5′-phosphoribosylpyrophosphate synthesis: A familial abnormality associated with excessive uric acid production and gout. Biochem Med 6:310, 1972.

124. Becker MA, Losman JM, Itkin P, et al: Gout with superactive phosphoribosylpyrophosphate synthetase due to increased enzyme catalytic rate. J Lab Clin Med 99:495, 1982.

125. Takeuchi F, Hanaoka F, Yano E, et al: The mode of genetic transmission of a gouty family with increased phosphoribosylpyrophosphate synthetase activity. Hum Genet 58:322, 1981.

126. Wortmann RL, Fox IH: Limited value of uric acid to creatinine ratios in estimating uric acid excretion. Ann Intern Med 93:822, 1980.

127. Moriwaki Y, Yamamoto T, Takahashi S, et al: Spot urine uric acid to creatinine ratio used in the estimation of uric acid excretion in primary gout. J Rheumatol 28:1306, 2001.

128. Vecchio PC, Emmerson BT: Gout due to renal disease. Br J Rheumatol 31:63, 1992.

129. Seegmiller JE, Rosenbloom RM, Kelley WN: An enzyme defect associated with a sex-linked human neurological disorder and excessive purine synthesis. Science 155:1682, 1967.

130. Cohen JL, Vinik A, Faller J, Fox IH: Hyperuricemia in glycogen storage disease type I: Contributions by hypoglycemia and hyperglucagonemia to increased urate production. J Clin Invest 75:251, 1985.

131. Seegmiller JE, Dixon RM, Kemp GJ, et al: Fructose-induced aberration of metabolism in familial gout identified by 31p magnetic resonance spectroscopy. Proc Natl Acad Sci USA 87:8326, 1990.

132. Mineo I, Kono N, Hara N, et al: Myogenic hyperuricemia: A common pathophysiologic feature of glycogenosis types III, V, and VII. N Engl J Med 317:75, 1987.

133. Bertorini TE, Shively V, Taylor B, et al: ATP degradation products after ischemic exercise: Hereditary lack of phosphorylase or carnitine palmitoyltransferase. Neurology 35:1355, 1985.

134. Sabina RL, Swain JL, Olanow CW, et al: Myoadenylate deaminase deficiency: Functional and metabolic abnormalities associated with disruption of the purine nucleotide cycle. J Clin Invest 73:720, 1984.

135. Davidson-Mundt A, Luder AS, Greene CL: Hyperuricemia in medium-chain acyl coenzyme A dehydrogenase deficiency. J Pediatr 120:444, 1992.

136. McGill NW, Dieppe PA: Evidence for a promoter of urate crystal formation in gouty synovial fluid. Ann Rheum Dis 50:558, 1991.

137. Getting SJ, Flower RJ, Parente L, et al: Molecular determinants of monosodium urate crystal-induced murine peritonitis: A role for endogenous mast cells and a distinct requirement for endothelial-derived selectins. J Pharmacol Exp Ther 283:123, 1997.

138. Takeda K, Akira S: Toll-like receptors in innate immunity. Int Immunol 17:1, 2005.

139. Tramontini N, Huber C, Liu-Bryan R, et al: Central role of complement membrane attack complex in monosodium urate crystal-induced neutrophilic rabbit knee synovitis. Arthritis Rheum 50:2633, 2004.

140. Liu-Bryan R, Pritzker K, Firestein GS, et al: TLR2 signaling in chondrocytes drives calcium pyrophosphate dihydrate and monosodium urate crystal-induced nitric oxide generation. J Immunol 174:5016, 2005.

141. Liu-Bryan R, Scott P, Sydlaske A, et al: Innate immunity conferred by TLR2, TLR4 and MyD88 expression is pivotal for monosodium urate crystal-induced inflammation. Arthritis Rheum 52:2936, 2005.

142. Parker LC, Whyte MK, Dower SK, Sabroe I: The expression and roles of Toll-like receptors in the biology of the human neutrophil. J Leukoc Biol 77:886, 2005.

143. Iwaki D, Mitsuzawa H, Murakami S, et al: The extra-cellular toll-like receptor 2 domain directly binds peptidoglycan derived from *Staphylococcus aureus*. J Biol Chem 277:24315, 2002.

144. Fujihara M, Muroi M, Tanamoto K, et al: Molecular mechanisms of macrophage activation and deactivation by lipopolysaccharide: Roles of the receptor complex. Pharmacol Ther 100:171, 2003.

145. Chen C-J, Shi Y, Hearn A, et al: MyD88-dependent IL-1 receptor signaling is essential for gouty inflammation stimulated by monosodium urate crystals. J Clin Invest 116:2262, 2006.

146. Martinon F, Petrilli V, Mayor A, et al: Gout-associated uric acid crystals activate the NALP3 inflammasome. Nature 440:237, 2006.

147. Martinon F, Tschopp J: NLRs join TLRs as innate sensors of pathogens. Trends Immunol 26:447, 2005.

148. Nishimura A, Akahoshi T, Takahashi M, et al: Attenuation of monosodium urate crystal-induced arthritis in rabbits by a neutralizing antibody against interleukin-8. J Leukoc Biol 62:444, 1997.

149. Terkeltaub R, Baird S, Sears P, et al: The murine homolog of the interleukin-8 receptor CXCR-2 is essential for the occurrence of neutrophilic inflammation in the air pouch model of acute urate crystal-induced gouty synovitis. Arthritis Rheum 41:900, 1998.

150. Kam M, Perl-Treves D, Caspi D, Addadi L: Antibodies against crystals. FASEB J 6:2608, 1992.

151. Barabe F, Gillvert C, Liao N, et al: Crystal-induced neutrophil activation. VI. Involvement of Fc gamma RIIIB (CD16) and CD11b in response to inflammatory microcrystals. FASEB J 12:209, 1998.

152. Onello E, Traynor-Kaplan A, Sklar L, Terkeltaub R: Mechanism of neutrophil activation by an unopsonized inflammatory particulate: Monosodium urate crystals induce pertussis toxin-insensitive hydrolysis of phosphatidylinositol 4,5-bisphosphate. J Immunol 146:4289, 1991.

153. Hachicha M, Naccache PH, McColl SR: Inflammatory microcrystals differentially regulate the secretion of macrophage inflammatory protein 1 and interleukin 8 by human neutrophils: A possible mechanism of neutrophil recruitment to sites of inflammation in synovitis. J Exp Med 182:2019, 1995.

154. Gilbert C, Poubelle PE, Borgeat P, et al: Crystal-induced neutrophil activation. VIII. Immediate production of prostaglandin E2 mediated by constitutive cyclooxygenase 2 in human neutrophils stimulated by urate crystals. Arthritis Rheum 48:1137, 2003.

155. Ryckman C, Gilbert C, De Medicis R, et al: Monosodium urate monohydrate crystals induce the release of the proinflammatory protein S100A8/A9 from neutrophils. J Leukoc Biol 76:433, 2004.

156. Desaulniers P, Marois S, Pare G, et al: Characterization of an activation factor released from human neutrophils after stimulation by tricyclic monosodium urate crystals. J Rheumatol 33:928, 2006.

157. di Giovine FS, Malawista SE, Thornton E, Duff GW: Urate crystals stimulate production of tumor necrosis factor alpha from human blood monocytes and synovial cells: Cytokine mRNA and protein kinetics, and cellular distribution. J Clin Invest 87:1375, 1991.

158. Terkeltaub R, Zachariae C, Santoro D, et al: Monocyte-derived neutrophil chemotactic factor/interleukin-8 is a potential mediator of crystal-induced inflammation. Arthritis Rheum 34:894, 1991.

159. Pouliot M, James MJ, McColl SR, et al: Monosodium urate microcrystals induce cyclooxygenase-2 in human monocytes. Blood 91:1769, 1998.

160. Terkeltaub RA, Dyer CA, Martin J, Curtiss LK: Apolipoprotein (apo) E inhibits the capacity of monosodium urate crystals to stimulate neutrophils: Characterization of intraarticular apo E and demonstration of apo E binding to urate crystals in vivo. J Clin Invest 87:20, 1991.

161. Getting SJ, Christian HC, Flower RJ, Perritti M: Activation of melanocortin type 3 receptor as a molecular mechanism for adrenocorticotropic hormone efficacy in gouty arthritis. Arthritis Rheum 46:2765, 2002.

162. Akahoshi T, Namai R, Murakami Y, et al: Rapid induction of peroxisome proliferator-activated receptor gamma expression in human monocytes by monosodium urate monohydrate crystals. Arthritis Rheum 48:231, 2003.

163. Yagnik DR, Hillyer P, Marshall D, et al: Noninflammatory phagocytosis of monosodium urate monohydrate crystals by mouse macrophages: Implications for the control of joint inflammation in gout. Arthritis Rheum 43:1779, 2000.

164. Landis RC, Yagnik DR, Florey O, et al: Safe disposal of inflammatory monosodium urate monohydrate crystals by differentiated macrophages. Arthritis Rheum 46:3026, 2002.

165. Liote F, Prudhommeaux F, Schiltz C, et al: Inhibition and prevention of monosodium urate monohydrate crystal-induced acute inflammation in vivo by transforming growth factor beta 1. Arthritis Rheum 39:1192, 1996.

166. Yagnik DR, Evans BJ, Florey O, et al: Macrophage release of transforming growth factor beta 1 during resolution of monosodium urate monohydrate crystal-induced inflammation. Arthritis Rheum 50:2273, 2004.

167. Schweyer S, Hennerlein B, Radzun HJ, Fayyazi A: Continuouis recruitment, co-expression of tumour necrosis factor-alpha and matrix metalloproteinases, and apoptosis of macrophages in gout tophi. Virchows Arch 437:534, 2000.

168. Hseich MS, Ho HC, Chou DT, et al: Expression of matrix metalloproteinase-9 (gelatinase B) in gouty arthritis and stimulation of MMP-9 by urate crystals in macrophages. J Cell Biochem 89:791, 2003.

169. Liu R, Liote F, Rose DM, et al: Proline-rich tyrosine kinase 2 and Src kinase signaling transduce monosodium urate crystal-induced nitric oxide production and matrix metalloproteinase 3 expression in chondrocytes. Arthritis Rheum 50:247, 2004.

170. Nakagawa T, Mazzali M, Kang DH, et al: Hyperuricemia causes glomerular hypertrophy in the rat. Am J Nephrol 23:2, 2002.

171. Yamamoto T, Moriwaki Y, Tukahashi S, et al: Effect of finafibrate on plasma concentration and urinary excretion of purine bases and oxypurinal. J Rheumatol 28:2294, 2001.

172. Wurzner G, Gester JC, Chiolero A, et al: Comparative effects of losartan and irbesartan on serum uric acid in hypertensive patients with hyperuricemia and gout. J Hypertens 19:1855, 2001.

173. Schlesinger N, Baker DG, Schumacher HR Jr: How well have diagnostic tests and therapies for gout been evaluated? Curr Opin Rheumatol 11:441, 1999.

174. Schlesinger N, Detry MA, Holland BK, et al: Local ice therapy during bouts of acute gouty arthritis. J Rheumatol 29:331, 2002.

175. Lange U, Schumann C, Schmidt KL: Current aspects of colchicine therapy: Classical indications and new therapeutic uses. Eur J Med Res 6:150, 2001.

176. Kim KY, Schumacher H, Hunsche E, et al: A literature review of the epidemiology and treatment of acute gout. Clin Ther 25:1593, 2003.

177. Molad Y: Update on colchicine and its mechanism of action. Curr Rheum Rep 4:252, 2002.

178. Iacobuzio-Donahue CA, Lee EL, Abraham SC, et al: Colchicine toxicity: Distinct morphologic findings in gastrointestinal biopsies. Am J Surg Pathol 25:1067, 2001.

179. Wallace SL, Singer JZ: Review: Systemic toxicity associated with the intravenous administration of colchicine: Guidelines for use. J Rheumatol 15:495, 1988.

180. Evans TI, Wheeler MT, Small RE, et al: A comprehensive investigation of inpatient colchicine use shows more education is needed. J Rheumatol 23:143, 1996.

181. Schumacher HR, Boice HA, Daikh J, et al: Randomized double blind trial of etoricoxib and indomethacin in treatment of acute gouty arthritis. BMJ 324:1488, 2002.

182. Fernandez C, Moguera R, Gonzalez JA, et al: Treatment of acute attacks of gout with a small dose of intraarticular triamcinolone acetonide. J Rheumatol 26:2285, 1999.

183. Clive DM: Renal transplant-associated hyperuricemia and gout. J Am Soc Nephrol 11:974, 2000.

184. Ritter L, Kerr LD, Valeriano-Marcet J, Spirea H: ACTH revisted: Effective treatment for acute crystal induced synovitis in patients with multiple medical problems. J Rheumatol 21:696, 1994.

185. Yu TF, Gutman AB: Efficacy of colchicine prophylaxis: Prevention of recurrent gouty arthritis over a mean period of five years in 208 gouty subjects. Ann Intern Med 55:179, 1961.

186. Kunck RW, Duncan G, Watson D, et al: Colchicine myopathy and neuropathy. N Engl J Med 316:1562, 1987.

187. Chattopadhyay I, Shetty HMG, Routledge PA, et al: Colchicine induced rhabdomyolysis. Postgrad Med J 77:191, 2001.

188. Fam AG: Difficult gout and new approaches for control of hyperuricemia in the allopurinol-allergic patient. Curr Rheum Rep 3:29, 2001.

189. Ferraz MB, O'Brien B: A cost effectiveness analysis of urate lowering drugs in nontophaceous recurrent gouty arthritis. J Rheumatol 22:908, 1995.

190. Perez-Ruiz F, Calabozo M, Pijoan JI, et al: Effect of urate-lowering therapy on the velocity of size reduction of tophi in chronic gout. Arthritis Care Res 47:356, 2002.

191. Perez-Ruiz F, Calabozo C, Herrero-Betes A, et al: Improvement in renal function in patients with chronic gout after proper control of hyperuricemia and gouty bouts. Nephron 86:287, 2000.

192. Harris M, Bryant LR, Danaher P, Alloway J: Effect of low dose daily aspirin on serum urate levels and urinary excretion in patients receiving probenecid for gouty arthritis. J Rheumatol 27:2873, 2000.

193. Hande KR, Noone RM, Stone WJ: Severe allopurinol toxicity: Description and guidelines for presentation in patients with renal insufficiency. Am J Med 76:47, 1984.

194. Stamp L, Sharples K, Gow P, et al: The optional use of allopurinol: An audit of allopurinol use in South Auckland. Aust N Z J Med 30:567, 2000.

195. Perez-Ruiz F, Hernando I, et al: Correction of allopurinol dosing should be based on clearance of creatinine, but not plasma creatinine levels: Another insight to allopurinol-related toxicity. J Clin Rheumatol 11:129, 2005.

196. Dalbeth N, Kumar S, Stamp L, Gow P: Dose adjustment of allopurinol according to creatinine clearance does not provide adequate control of hyperuricemia in patients with gout. J Rheumatol 33:1646, 2006.

197. Perez-Ruiz F, Alonso-Ruiz A, et al: Efficacy of allopurinol and benzbromarone for the control of hyperuricemia: A pathogenic approach to the treatment of primary chronic gout. Ann Rheum Dis 57:545, 1998.

198. Li-Yu J, Clayburne G, et al: Treatment of chronic gout: Can we determine when urate stores are depleted enough to prevent attacks of gout? J Rheumatol 28:577, 2001.

199. Fam AG, Dunne SM, Lazzetta J, et al: Efficacy and safety of desensitization to allopurinol following cutaneous reactions. Arthritis Rheum 44:231, 2001.

200. Singer JZ, Wallace SL: The allopurinol hypersensitivity syndrome: Unnecessary morbidity and mortality. Arthritis Rheum 29:82, 1986.

201. Weiner IM, Mudge GH: Inhibitors of tubular transport of organic compounds. In Gillman AG, Rail TW, Niew AW, Taylor P (eds): The Pharmacologic Basis of Therapeutics, 8th ed. New York, Pergamon Press, 1990, p 920.

202. Wortmann RL: The treatment of gout: The use of an analogy. Am J Med 105:513, 1998.

203. Perez-Ruiz F, Alonso-Ruiz A, Calabozo M, Duruelo J: Treatment of gout after transplantation. Br J Rheumatol 37:580, 1998.

204. Jacobs F, Mamzer-Bruneel MF, Skhir H, et al: Safety of the mycophenolate mofetil-allopurinol combination in kidney transplant recipients with gout. Transplantation 64:1087, 1997.

205. Rozenberg S, Koeger AC, Bourgeois P: Urate-oxidase for gouty arthritis in cardiac transplant recipients. J Rheumatol 20:2171, 1993.

206. Bomalaski JS, Holtsberg FW, Ensor CM, et al: Uricase formulated with polyethyleneglycol (uricase-PEG 20): Biochemical rationale and preclinical studies. J Rheumatol 29:1942, 2002.

207. Dessein PH, Shipton EA, Stanwix AE, et al: Beneficial effects of weight loss associated with moderate calorie/carbohydrate restriction, and increased proportional intake of protein and unsaturated fat on serum urate and lipoprotein levels in gout: A pilot study. Ann Rheum Dis 59:539, 2000.

208. Fam AG: Gout, diet and the insulin resistance syndrome. J Rheumatol 29:1350, 2002.

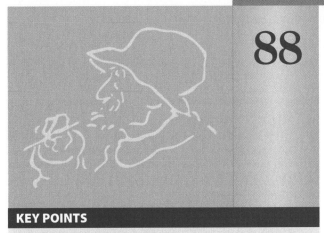

88

Diseases Associated with Articular Deposition of Calcium Pyrophosphate Dihydrate and Basic Calcium Phosphate Crystals ▪◀

ROBERT TERKELTAUB

KEY POINTS

Autosomal dominant familial chondrocalcinosis in several kindreds has been linked to certain mutations in *ANKH*, a gene encoding an inorganic pyrophosphate (PP_i) transporter.

Both dysregulated chondrocyte differentiation and PP_i metabolism are central to the pathogenesis of chondrocalcinosis.

NALP3 (cryopyrin) inflammasome activation and consequent caspase-1 activation and interleukin-1β processing and secretion drive cell responses to calcium pyrophosphate dihydrate (CPPD) crystals and CPPD crystal-induced inflammation.

Degenerative arthropathy due to CPPD crystal deposition disease often involves joints uncommonly affected by primary osteoarthritis, such as the metacarpophalangeal, wrist, and elbow joints.

Diagnosis of CPPD deposition disease before age 50, particularly if CPPD deposition is widespread, should prompt consideration of a primary metabolic or familial disorder.

In the elderly, CPPD deposition may present as diffuse pain, sometimes with fever of unknown origin, mimicking infection, polymyalgia rheumatica, and rheumatoid arthritis.

Radiographic chondrocalcinosis is not detectable in all joints affected by CPPD crystal deposition disease.

Joint cartilage and synovial fluid CPPD and basic calcium phosphate (BCP) crystals commonly coexist in affected joints.

BCP crystals are not birefringent, although the aggregated particles of BCP crystals demonstrate edge birefringence.

PROPOSED CRITERIA FOR DISEASE

The proposed diagnostic criteria for calcium pyrophosphate dihydrate (CPPD) deposition disease are summarized in Table 88-1. The diagnosis is based on detection of CPPD crystals by one or more methods. These methods include standard radiography, which detects calcifications characteristic of CPPD, as well as compensated polarized light microscopic analysis of synovial fluids or tissue sections for the detection of typical CPPD crystals. On occasion, specialized approaches to crystal analysis, including x-ray energy spectroscopy and powder diffraction analysis[1,2] or atomic force

microscopy,[3] may be helpful in establishing or confirming CPPD crystal deposition. When assessing deposited crystals in calcifications, determination of the calcium-to-phosphate ratio, as well as the spacing of x-ray powder diffraction lines, provides the most specific information.

Consensus clinical diagnostic criteria for articular basic calcium phosphate (BCP) crystal deposition disorders do not exist. Importantly, BCP crystals (unlike urate and CPPD) do not demonstrate intrusive birefringence, although the aggregated particles of BCP crystals demonstrate edge birefringence. Hence, diagnosis is predicated on (1) radiographic detection of calcifications characteristic of BCP crystals, (2) synovial fluid crystals that stain strongly for the calcium-binding dye alizarin red S (which only weakly stains CPPD crystals), and (3) BCP crystals confirmed by transmission electron microscopy or specialized crystal analytic approaches (including those mentioned earlier for CPPD and discussed later).

EPIDEMIOLOGY

Studies of the prevalence of both CPPD crystal deposition disease and various forms of articular BCP crystal deposition disease have been based predominantly on characteristic plain radiographic features in limited numbers of joints. This is an incompletely sensitive and specific approach. Other studies have been based on results of synovial fluid analyses and pathologic findings on examination of articular cartilages. As such, the true prevalence of both CPPD crystal deposition disease and pathologic articular BCP crystal deposition is not known.

Women may be more commonly affected by CPPD crystal deposition disease than are men.[4] Chondrocalcinosis, including asymptomatic disease, increases in prevalence with age.[5,6] Idiopathic or sporadic chondrocalcinosis is rare before age 50, particularly in the absence of a history of joint trauma or knee meniscectomy.

In a classic study, knee meniscal calcification was detected in 16% of women aged 80 to 89 and in 30% of women older than 89,[7] figures comparable to those obtained in other studies.[8,9] For example, in a radiographic survey study of hands, wrists, pelvis, and knees of patients admitted to a geriatrics ward, there was a 44% prevalence of chondrocalcinosis

Table 88-1   Proposed Diagnostic Criteria for Calcium Pyrophosphate Dihydrate (CPPD) Crystal Deposition Disease

Criteria
I. Demonstration of CPPD crystals, obtained by biopsy or aspirated synovial fluid, by definitive means (e.g., characteristic x-ray diffraction powder pattern)
II. A. Identification of monoclinic or triclinic crystals showing a weak positive birefringence (or no birefringence) by compensated polarized light microscopy
B. Presence of typical calcifications on radiographs (as discussed in text): heavy punctate and linear calcifications in fibrocartilage, articular (hyaline) cartilage, and joint capsules, especially if bilaterally symmetric
III. A. Acute arthritis, especially of knees or other large joints
B. Chronic arthritis, especially of knee, hip, wrist, carpus, elbow, shoulder, and metacarpophalangeal joints, particularly if accompanied by acute exacerbations

Diagnostic Categories
A. Definite: criterion I or IIA must be fulfilled
B. Probable: criterion IIA or IIB must be fulfilled
C. Possible: criterion IIIA or IIIB suggests possible underlying CPPD deposition disease

Adapted from McCarty DJ: Crystals and arthritis. Dis Month 6:255, 1994.

in patients older than 84, a 36% prevalence in 75- to 84-year-olds, and a prevalence of 15% in 65- to 74-year-olds.[10] Most elderly patients with chondrocalcinosis of the knee also have detectable chondrocalcinosis in other joints.[7]

In a random sample of Beijing residents older than 60 years, radiographic chondrocalcinosis was compared with the findings among whites in the American Framingham Osteoarthritis Study.[11] The Chinese had a much lower prevalence of knee chondrocalcinosis, and wrist chondrocalcinosis was particularly rare in elderly Chinese.[11] These findings were unexpected, because there is an excess of knee osteoarthritis (OA) in Beijing,[12] and chondrocalcinosis and OA are commonly associated in the knee joint.

CAUSE

The loose avascular connective tissue matrices of articular hyaline cartilage, fibrocartilaginous menisci, and certain ligaments and tendons are particularly susceptible to calcification. Calcium-containing crystals deposited in the pericellular matrix of cartilage are often in the form of CPPD (chemical formula $Ca_2P_2O_7\cdot H_2O$; calcium-phosphate ratio, 1.0). This disorder is commonly termed *chondrocalcinosis* or *pyrophosphate arthropathy*; when associated with acute arthritis, it is called *pseudogout*. Crystals of BCP, including partially carbonate-substituted hydroxyapatite ($Ca_5[PO_4]_3OH\cdot 2H_2O$; calcium-phosphate ratio, 1.67), also may be deposited pathologically in articular cartilage, particularly in OA. Importantly, physiologic (and noninflammatory) deposition of hydroxyapatite (HA) is essential, because HA is the principal mineral phase laid down in growth cartilage and in bone.

Inflammatory conditions also may result from deposition of HA and the closely related BCP crystals octacalcium phosphate ($Ca_8H_2[PO_4]_6\cdot 5H_2O$; calcium-phosphate ratio, 1.33) and tricalcium phosphate or whitlockite ($Ca_3[PO_4]_2$; calcium-phosphate ratio, 1.5) in periarticular structures, such as the rotator cuff (calcific tendinitis) and subacromial

bursa of the shoulder. CPPD and BCP crystal deposition disease are by far the most prevalent arthropathies associated with calcium-containing crystals. Articular calcium oxalate crystal deposition, which is less common, is reviewed in Chapter 112. Supersaturation of certain solutes in body fluids may culminate in the deposition of distinct crystals and calculi, exemplified by pathologic crystallization within extracellular fluids, such as the biliary and urinary tracts. In addition, pathologic calcification can occur in the extracellular matrix of certain connective tissues, such as the artery wall in subjects with atherosclerosis or chronic renal failure and in the synovium and articular cartilage in gout. Articular cartilage, unlike growth plate cartilage, is specialized to avoid the process of matrix calcification. However, the matrix of articular hyaline cartilage, like that of fibrocartilaginous menisci, is prone to pathologic calcification,[13] particularly in association with certain changes in extracellular matrix composition caused by aging and OA.[14]

PATHOGENESIS

Joint cartilage calcification reflects a complex interplay between organic and inorganic biochemistry, aging, molecular genetics, inflammation, oxidative stress, and dysregulated chondrocyte growth factor responsiveness and differentiation. Pathologic cartilage calcification can reflect deficiencies of certain physiologic calcification inhibitors or upregulation of mediators that actively drive stereotypical patterns of tissue injury, culminating in calcification within degenerating cartilage.[15,16]

Alterations in the concentrations of calcium, inorganic phosphate (P_i), inorganic pyrophosphate (PP_i), and the solubility products of these ions are clearly at work in promoting CPPD and BCP crystal formation.[13-16] The levels of ambient magnesium and the composition of the chondrocyte extracellular matrix influence the dynamics of CPPD crystal formation and help determine whether predominantly monoclinic or triclinic CPPD crystals are formed.[14,15] Significantly, monoclinic CPPD crystals are more inflammatory than triclinic CPPD crystals.[17]

Besides the physical effects of calcium, P_i, and PP_i on crystal nucleation and propagation, these solutes exert a variety of mineralization-regulating effects on gene expression, differentiation, and viability in chondrocytes, mediated partly by calcium-sensing receptors and sodium-dependent phosphate cotransport in chondrocytes.[18-23] Noxious effects of excess PP_i on chondrocytes, including induction of matrix metalloproteinase-13 (MMP-13) expression[24] and the promotion of apoptosis,[25] support the terminology *pyrophosphate arthropathy* to describe the chronic cartilage degenerative manifestations of CPPD crystal deposition disease.

DYSREGULATED INORGANIC PYROPHOSPHATE METABOLISM AND THE ROLE OF NUCLEOTIDE PYROPHOSPHATASE PHOSPHODIESTERASE 1

PP_i is a potent inhibitor of the nucleation and propagation of BCP crystals.[15,16] Concordantly, maintenance of physiologic extracellular PP_i levels by chondrocytes and certain other cells suppresses calcification with HA, as illustrated in mouse models of deficient PP_i generation and transport[19,26,27] and a variant of human infantile arterial calcification associated with periarticular calcification.[28] The relatively distinctive capacity of chondrocytes to produce copious amounts of extracellular PP_i is double edged, because supersaturation of cartilage extracellular matrix with PP_i is a major factor in promoting CPPD crystal deposition.[16,29,30] Further, excess PP_i generation can promote BCP crystal deposition by providing a source for increased extracellular P_i generation via PP_i hydrolysis by tissue-nonspecific alkaline phosphatase (TNAP).[16,29] Depending on cartilage adenosine triphosphate (ATP) and PP_i concentrations and the level of activity of P_i-generating ATPases and TNAP, CPPD and HA crystal formation may be jointly promoted in cartilage, an event that commonly occurs clinically in OA (discussed later). In addition, alterations in PP_i transport by the multiple-pass plasma membrane protein ANKH[16,24,26] are implicated in the pathogenesis of chondrocalcinosis (discussed later with regard to familial chondrocalcinosis). Increased ANKH expression in OA cartilage is a factor in secondary chondrocalcinosis (Fig. 88-1).[24]

Sporadic aging-associated CPPD crystal deposition disease is consistently linked with excess chondrocyte PP_i-generating nucleotide pyrophosphatase phosphodiesterase (NPP) activity and augmented PP_i generation by chondrocytes.[16,29-32] In this context, the NPP family isoenzymes NPP1 and NPP3 actively generate PP_i by hydrolysis of nucleoside triphosphates, including ATP.[16,29,30] A substantial portion of ATP used by chondrocytes to generate extracellular PP_i is provided by the mitochondria.[16] In idiopathic chondrocalcinosis, cartilage NPP activity and PP_i levels may average approximately double those of normal subjects.[33]

NPP1 (formerly known as plasma cell membrane glycoprotein-1, or PC-1) plays a central role in sustaining and augmenting extracellular PP_i in chondrocytes and certain other cells.[16,29,30] NPP1 is one of three highly homologous NPP family isoenzymes (NPP1 to NPP3) that share NPP catalytic activity and modular type II transmembrane ectoenzyme structures.[16,34] NPP1 plays the greatest role by far in augmenting extracellular PP_i in chondrocytes.[29,30] Significantly, marked and total NPP1 deficiency states in vivo and in vitro are associated with up to 50% less plasma and extracellular PP_i.[18,28]

Increased NPP1 expression is associated with both calcification and apoptosis in degenerative human cartilages.[29] Direct upregulation of NPP1 in chondrocytic cells stimulates calcification as well as apoptosis.[25] These effects are not shared by NPP3, which likely has other intracellular "housekeeping" functions in chondrocytes.[25,29] NPP2, which is also expressed in normal cartilage, functions more actively in physiology as lysophospholipase D,[35] and NPP2 only modestly stimulates chondrocytes to calcify in vitro.[29]

The chondrocyte growth factor transforming growth factor-β (TGF-β) stimulates NPP1 expression and NPP1 subcellular movement to the plasma membrane, which drives the elevation of extracellular PP_i.[30,36] Interleukin (IL)-1β suppresses both NPP1 expression and extracellular PP_i in chondrocytes and blocks the effects of TGF-β on PP_i.[30,36] The capacity of TGF-β to raise chondrocyte PP_i increases with aging, as does TGF-β–stimulated NPP activity,[37] whereas growth-promoting effects of TGF-β decrease with aging in articular chondrocytes.[32] The anabolic chondrocyte growth factor insulin-like growth factor-1 (IGF-1) normally suppresses extracellular PP_i in chondrocytes.[38] Moreover, chondrocyte IGF-1 resistance is characteristic

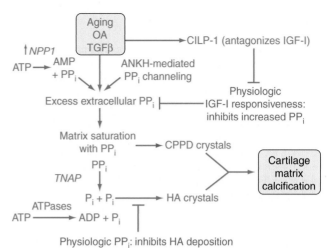

Figure 88-1 Proposed inorganic pyrophosphate (PPi)–dependent mechanisms stimulating calcium pyrophosphate dihydrate (CPPD) and hydroxyapatite (HA) crystal deposition in aging and osteoarthritis (OA). Roles of adenosine triphosphate (ATP) and PP_i metabolism and inorganic phosphate (P_i) generation in pathologic cartilage calcification. This model accounts for the association of extracellular PP_i excess with both CPPD and basic calcium phosphate (BCP) crystal deposition in OA and chondrocalcinosis, as well as the paradoxical association of extracellular PP_i deficiency (from defective ANKH or nucleotide pyrophosphatase phosphodiesterase 1 [NPP1] expression) with pathologic calcification of articular cartilage with HA crystals in vivo. Factors driving pathologic calcification are indicated in *green*, and physiologic factors suppressing calcification in *red*. Excess PP_i generation in cartilage in idiopathic CPPD deposition disease of aging and in OA is mediated in part by increased NPP1. In idiopathic chondrocalcinosis of aging, mean cartilage PP_i and NPP catalytic activity levels are double normal. NPP1 is markedly increased at sites of meniscal cartilage calcification in vivo, and NPP1 directly induces PP_i elevation and matrix calcification by chondrocytes in vitro. Depending on the extracellular availability of substrate PP_i, the activity of the pyrophosphatase tissue-nonspecific alkaline phosphatase (TNAP), the availability of substrate ATP, the activity of ATPases, and other factors, such as substantial local Mg^{2+} concentrations, HA crystal deposition (as opposed to CPPD deposition) may be stimulated. In this model, excess extracellular PP_i also may result from heightened "leakiness" of intracellular PP_i via increased ANKH expression in OA and abnormal ANKH function in familial chondrocalcinosis. Also illustrated is the role of increased expression of cartilage intermediate layer protein-1 (CILP-1) in cartilage calcification in OA and aging, which inhibits the capacity of insulin-like growth factor-1 (IGF-1) to suppress the elevation of extracellular PP_i. ADP, adenosine diphosphate; AMP, adenosine monophosphate; TGF, transforming growth factor.

of OA and aging cartilage.[39] IGF-1 induces the expression of cartilage intermediate layer protein (CILP; see Fig. 88-1), a secreted cartilage matrix molecule whose expression increases with aging and in OA and is most abundant in the middle zone of articular cartilage, where CPPD crystal deposition is most prevalent.[40] Significantly, the CILP-1 but not the CILP-2 isoform promotes increased extracellular PP_i in chondrocytes indirectly by antagonizing IGF-1 at the receptor level.[39]

CALCIUM PYROPHOSPHATE DIHYDRATE DEPOSITION DISEASE SECONDARY TO PRIMARY METABOLIC DISORDERS

Hypophosphatasia, hypomagnesemic conditions (including the Gitelman's variant of Bartter's syndrome), hemochromatosis, and hyperparathyroidism are the best-characterized primary metabolic disorders linked to secondary CPPD crystal deposition disease.[41] Increased joint fluid PP_i levels in each of these condition suggests at least one common thread in the pathogenesis of chondrocalcinosis via cartilage PP_i excess.[42] Magnesium is a cofactor for pyrophosphatase activity, and iron excess can suppress pyrophosphatase activity. Hypercalcemia may promote CPPD crystal deposition in hyperparathyroidism by effects beyond cartilage matrix supersaturation with ionized calcium, such as calcium functioning as a cofactor in NPP1 catalytic activity, as well as chondrocyte-activating effects mediated by the calcium-sensing receptor.[20,21,23,43] In addition, normal articular chondrocytes express parathyroid hormone (PTH) and PTH-related protein receptors, and functional responses of chondrocytes to PTH can promote proliferation, altered matrix synthesis, and mineralization.[44,45]

Hypophosphatasia is due to deficient activity of the ecto-enzyme TNAP, whose activities include hydrolysis of PP_i to generate P_i.[19] TNAP is a major physiologic antagonist of the NPP1-mediated elevation of extracellular PP_i.[19] Conversely, physiologic NPP1-induced PP_i generation antagonizes the essential prominineralizing effects of TNAP mediated by P_i generation,[19] and cartilage PP_i excess presumably drives chondrocalcinosis in hypophosphatasia. NPP1 knockout mice and mice homozygous for the NPP1 truncation mutant *ttw* demonstrate marked articular cartilage calcification with HA and OA, as well as ankylosing spinal ligament hyperostosis and synovial joint ossific fusion.[19,27] Extracellular PP_i levels and mineralization disturbances in soft tissues (but not long bones) of NPP1 knockout and TNAP knockout mice are mutually corrected by crossbreeding to double knockout mice.[19]

FAMILIAL CALCIUM PYROPHOSPHATE DIHYDRATE CRYSTAL DEPOSITION DISEASE AND THE ROLE OF ANKH

Familial chondrocalcinosis is clinically heterogeneous. For example, prominent CPPD and HA crystal deposits and cartilage and periarticular calcifications in association with OA were described in a kindred not yet linked to a specific chromosomal locus.[46] A syndrome of spondyloepiphyseal dysplasia tarda, brachydactyly, precocious OA, and intra-articular calcifications with CPPD or HA crystals (or both), as well as periarticular calcifications, was linked to mutation of the procollagen type II gene in natives of the Chiloé Island region of Chile, a population with a high prevalence of familial CPPD deposition disease.[47] Families multiply affected with diffuse idiopathic skeletal hyperostosis (DISH) or chondrocalcinosis have been identified in the Azores Islands, suggesting that the concurrence of DISH and chondrocalcinosis reflects an unknown, shared pathogenic mechanism.[48]

Two major chromosomal linkages, 8q and 5p, have been identified in studies of familial CPPD deposition disease. Linkage of chromosome 8q with both early-onset OA and chondrocalcinosis in a New England family was given the designation CCAL1.[49] Chromosome 5p–linked chondrocalcinosis (CCAL2) is broadly distributed and has been studied in greater detail than 8q chondrocalcinosis.[50-53] Linkage of familial CPPD crystal deposition disease to the gene *ANKH* on chromosome 5p has been established in these studies.[50-53] A search for ANKH mutations in 95 subjects with sporadic chondrocalcinosis uncovered a unique mutation in only one subject.[52]

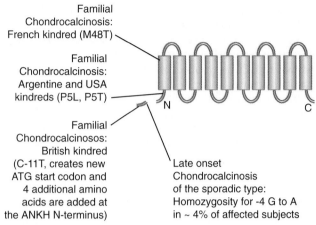

Figure 88-2 **Model for multiple-pass membrane protein structure of ANKH and for *ANKH* mutations associated with chromosome 5p–linked autosomal dominant familial chondrocalcinosis and heritable late-onset chondrocalcinosis.** The figure schematizes the putative multiple-pass transmembrane protein structure of ANKH, which appears to promote bidirectional inorganic pyrophosphate (PP_i) movement between the cytosol and the extracellular space. The gradient for ANKH-stimulated PP_i movement in chondrocytes (which generate abundant PP_i by both high specific activity of nucleotide pyrophosphatase phosphodiesterase 1 [NPP1] and robust matrix biosynthesis) is from the intracellular to the extracellular space. Distinct mutations in *ANKH* promote differences in age of onset and phenotypes in familial chondrocalcinosis. The figure summarizes sites of known *ANKH* mutations clustered near the N-terminus that are associated with chromosome 5p–linked autosomal dominant familial chondrocalcinosis (calcium pyrophosphate dihydrate [CPPD] crystal deposition disease). The figure also depicts the –4 G to A transition in the 5'-untranslated region of *ANKH*, for which homozygosity is seen in about 4% of late-onset chondrocalcinosis of the sporadic type, suggesting a heritable subset of otherwise typical late-onset chondrocalcinosis. As a group, these N-terminally clustered *ANKH* mutations linked to human chondrocalcinosis promote chronic low-grade extracellular PP_i excess, resulting in CPPD crystal formation. However, some of the *ANKH* mutations are distinct in their effects on chondrocyte differentiation, and the M48T *ANKH* mutant in a French kindred appears to be functionally unique because it is associated with increased intracellular PP_i.

ANKH encodes a multiple-pass transmembrane protein that functions in PP_i channeling (Fig. 88- 2).[26,31,54,55] ANKH promotes bidirectional movement of PP_i at the plasma membrane in vitro,[54] but the gradient for ANKH-stimulated PP_i movement in chondrocytes (which generate abundant PP_i by both robust NPP1 expression and intense matrix biosynthetic activity) is from the intracellular to the extracellular space.[16] Indeed, transport of PP_i generated intracellularly by NPP1[24] is a primary means of regulating extracellular PP_i levels.[16] Modeling of the PP_i channeling function of ANKH has proposed 10 or 12 membrane-spanning domains in ANKH with an alternating inside-out orientation and with a central channel to accommodate the passage of PP_i (see Fig. 88-2).[26,55] Mutations at different locations in ANKH can affect function and the skeleton, including autosomal dominant chondrocalcinosis[51-54] and certain other phenotypes, such as murine progressive ankylosis in the *ank/ank* mouse and human craniometaphyseal dysplasia associated with apparent decreased capacity to transport PP_i within bone.[26,54,55] Clinical heterogeneity even for chondrocalcinosis associated with ANKH mutations[51-54] suggests that different functional effects of ANKH are mediated by specific regions of the molecule. All the N-terminally clustered ANKH mutations identified to cause familial chondrocalcinosis appear to increase PP$_i$ transport.[54] However, some of the ANKH mutations have distinct effects on chondrocyte differentiation,[56] and the M48T ANKH mutant in a French kindred appears to be functionally unique by association with increased intracellular PP$_i$.[57]

In 5p familial chondrocalcinosis, a subtle "gain of function" of intrinsic ANKH PP$_i$ channeling activity may lead to chronic, low-grade chondrocyte PP$_i$ "leakiness," thereby causing matrix supersaturation with PP$_i$, CPPD crystal deposition, and cartilage degeneration.[31,51] Expression of wild-type ANKH is highly regulated, and ANKH is increased in OA and chondrocalcinotic cartilage.[24] Thus, secondary alterations in chondrocyte expression of both wild-type ANKH and NPP1 likely drive PP$_i$ supersaturation in cartilage in idiopathic or sporadic and OA-associated CPPD crystal deposition disease (see Fig. 88-1). Moreover, homozygosity for a single nucleotide substitution (–4 G to A) in the ANKH 5'-untranslated region that promotes increased ANKH messenger RNA expression was present in about 4% of British subjects previously thought to have idiopathic or sporadic chondrocalcinosis of aging.[56]

INFLAMMATION, ALTERED CHONDROCYTE DIFFERENTIATION, AND TRANSGLUTAMINASE 2 IN JOINT CARTILAGE CALCIFICATION

Regulated changes in chondrocyte differentiation and viability appear to be part of a mechanistically unified process that promotes joint cartilage CPPD and HA crystal deposition as well as OA. Such changes include the development of foci of chondrocyte maturation, with the presence of hypertrophy, as seen in histopathology of the knee cartilage in Figure 88-3; apoptosis of chondrocytes also is typically found adjacent to cartilage calcifications.[58,59] Articular chondrocyte hypertrophy, promoted synergistically by mediators (including those depicted in Fig. 88-4), is associated with heightened PP$_i$ generation, increased production of calcifying cell fragments known as matrix vesicles, and certain other calcification-promoting changes in differentiation, including alteration of extracellular matrix composition.[60,61] For example, hypertrophic chondrocytes express less type II collagen and aggrecan and further modify their extracellular matrix via increased aggrecanase and MMP activities, as well as expression of type X collagen, osteopontin, and several other stereotypical bone and growth plate proteins that regulate calcification (see Chapter 3). Altered TGF-β signal transduction in aging[32] and OA may be involved in promoting chondrocyte hypertrophy, because expression of a truncated, kinase-defective TGF-β receptor type II promotes hypertrophy and terminal chondrocyte differentiation, along with cartilage degeneration in vivo.[62]

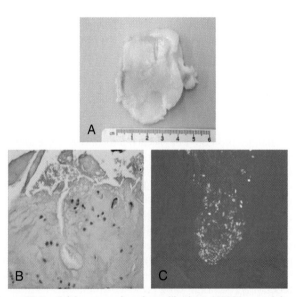

Figure 88-3 Calcium pyrophosphate dihydrate (CPPD) crystal deposition arthropathy of the knee joint. **A,** Femoral condyle. There are extensive foci of chalky white particulate deposits within the articular cartilage. This is characteristic of CPPD crystal deposition. **B,** Histology of CPPD crystal deposition within the hyaline articular cartilage. The hypertrophic chondrocytes adjacent to the crystal aggregates are within enlarged chondrons (hematoxylin and eosin, ×250). **C,** Polarized light microscopy of CPPD crystal aggregates within the hyaline articular cartilage. The individual crystals have rod and rhomboid shapes and are positively birefringent (×250). *(Courtesy of Dr. Ken Pritzker, Mount Sinai Hospital Pathology Department, University of Toronto, Ontario, Canada.)*

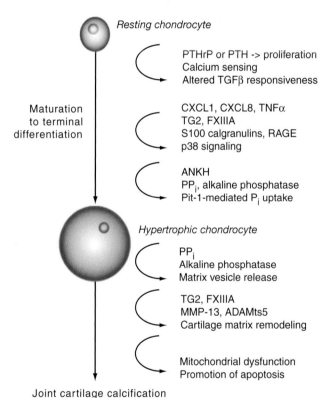

Figure 88-4 **Coordinated forces promoting chondrocyte maturation to hypertrophy in joint cartilage calcification.** The top portion of the figure depicts some of the major synergistic forces promoting chondrocyte maturation to hypertrophy that are likely to be operative in osteoarthritis and aging. Hypertrophic and apoptotic chondrocytes are observed adjacent to calcific crystal deposits in joint cartilages. The lower portion of the figure shows that chondrocyte hypertrophy is a differentiation state specialized for calcification, based in part on alteration of the extracellular matrix composition (with attendant dysregulation of matrix repair), enhanced release of matrix vesicles to promote mineral seeding, increased generation of inorganic pyrophosphate (PP$_i$) and inorganic phosphate (P$_i$), and increased transglutaminase 2 (TG2) and factor XIIIA expression. The increased susceptibility of hypertrophic chondrocytes to apoptotic death is also significant because of the prominineralizing effects of chondrocyte apoptosis.

Local upregulation of PTH-related protein expression may be one of the shared features driving sequential chondrocyte proliferation and altered differentiation in growth plate chondrocytes and articular chondrocytes.[44,45] In addition, P_i taken up by Pit-1 sodium-dependent cotransport and calcium sensing can modulate chondrocyte hypertrophic differentiation and apoptosis.[16,22,63-65] Chondrocyte apoptosis also promotes calcification, partly through the calcifying potential of apoptotic bodies functioning as "inside-out" matrix vesicles on release from dying chondrocytes.[25,66-68] Mitochondrial dysfunction, a central factor in tissue aging and an apparent mediator of OA progression in aging,[69,70] can also stimulate cartilage matrix degeneration and calcification. Mitochondria are remarkably specialized to regulate calcification, and apoptosis is critically regulated by mitochondrial function.[69] Moreover, chondrocyte ATP depletion is driven by the suppression of mitochondrial oxidative phosphorylation by nitric oxide (NO) as OA evolves in aging (see Chapter 89), thereby promoting increased ATP scavenging by NPP activity and consequent augmentation of extracellular PP_i.[70]

Inflammation-associated chondrocyte hypertrophy is driven by multiple cytokines and calgranulins, oxidative stress, P_i transport, and receptor for advanced glycation end products (RAGE) signaling, and it is modulated by transglutaminase 2 (TG2) release. This process appears to drive chondrocalcinosis and the progression of OA. For example, IL-1β, which is increased in OA cartilage, stimulates articular chondrocytes to calcify the matrix.[37,60] NO stimulates both apoptosis and calcification in chondrocytes.[66,67,69] IL-1β stimulates inducible NO synthase expression and increased NO generation, as well as expression of other cytokines and MMPs, which can alter extracellular matrix collagen and proteoglycan composition to potentially favor calcification (see Chapters 3 and 89). IL-1 also induces TG family enzymes factor XIIIA and TG2, which cross-link numerous extracellular proteins by transamidation.[37,60] IL-1β (as well as tumor necrosis factor[TNF]-α, donors of NO, and the potent oxidant peroxynitrite) also induces increased chondrocyte TG activity.[37]

TG2 and factor XIIIA are markers of growth plate chondrocyte hypertrophy.[37,60] Significantly, there is marked upregulation of TG2 and factor XIIIA expression in hypertrophic cells in the superficial and deep zones of knee OA articular cartilage and the central (chondrocytic) zone of OA menisci.[37] Moreover, increased factor XIIIA and TG2 activity directly stimulates calcification by chondrocytes.[37] IL-1–induced increases in TG activity, related to OA severity and age, occur in chondrocytes from human knee menisci.[37] TG2 is essential for IL-1β to stimulate articular chondrocytes to calcify their matrix in vitro.[60] In addition, the closely related inflammatory chemokines CXCL1 and CXCL8, which are both increased in OA cartilage, stimulate increased TG activity attributed specifically to TG2.[71] CXCL1 and CXCL8 stimulate chondrocyte hypertrophic differentiation and calcification in a manner that requires TG2.[71]

Distinct TG2-independent and TG2-dependent mechanisms promote articular chondrocyte hypertrophy and calcification in vitro, and increased TG2 release is sufficient to promote chondrocyte hypertrophy.[60] TG2 acts as a molecular switch to induce chondrocyte hypertrophy in a β1 integrin–mediated manner, associated with rapid phosphorylation of p38 kinase and dependent on TG2 being in the guanosine triphosphate–bound conformational state.[72] TG2 transamidation activity is not required for TG2 to induce chondrocyte hypertrophy, but TG2 transamidation activity does modulate chondrocyte differentiation and function. For example, TG2 promotes the activation of TGF-β.[73]

The multiligand RAGE mediates several chronic vascular and neurologic degenerative diseases accompanied by low-grade inflammation.[74] RAGE ligands include S100/calgranulins, a class of small, calcium-binding polypeptides, several of which are expressed by chondrocytes. Normal human knee cartilage demonstrates constitutive RAGE and S100A11 expression, and both RAGE and S100A11 expression are increased in OA cartilage.[74,75] CXCL8 and TNF-α induce S100A11 release in cultured chondrocytes.[74] Further, S100A11 induces chondrocyte hypertrophy in vitro.[74] CXCL1-induced and TNF-α–induced chondrocyte hypertrophy require RAGE, mitogen-activated protein kinase (MAPK)-3, and p38 MAPK signaling.[74]

ARTICULAR AND PERIARTICULAR BASIC CALCIUM PHOSPHATE CRYSTAL DEPOSITION

CPPD and BCP crystal deposition can develop in different zones of articular cartilage and probably in distinct phases of cartilage degenerative disease, such as ongoing loss of viability in hypertrophic chondrocytes. In addition, abundant cartilage NO production may promote mitochondrial dysfunction, chondrocyte extracellular ATP depletion,[70] and lowering of extracellular PP_i, favoring HA over CPPD crystal deposition.[76] The observation that OA and HA crystal deposition in articular cartilage (and arteries)[26,28] are both promoted by extracellular PP_i deficiency strikingly illustrates the deleterious effects of deprivation of physiologic extracellular PP_i levels.[16] Yet it is noted that joint fluid PP_i and NPP levels are elevated in HA-associated shoulder arthropathy (Milwaukee shoulder syndrome),[77] consistent with the model in Figure 88-1.

Pathologic BCP crystal deposition may occur in periarticular sites as well as numerous organs and soft tissues.[11] Significantly, the shoulder is the most common articular region affected by symptomatic BCP crystal deposition, in part reflecting unique shoulder structure and function. Degenerative changes promoted by biomechanical stress promote calcific tendinitis in the body of the rotator cuff.[78] Such tendon calcifications can remain asymptomatic and may eventually resorb, but the degenerative changes can predispose to tendon rupture. Osteopontin, a factor that normally restrains BCP crystal deposition (and is regulated by PP_i and P_i),[18] can be detected in fibroblast-like cells and multinucleated macrophages surrounding areas of calcification in calcific tendinitis.[79] In this regard, osteopontin promotes oxidative stress, MMP activation, macrophage recruitment, and osteoclast activation.[18] The presence of multinucleated cells with cathepsin K expression and osteoclast-like functions at sites of tendon calcification[80] suggests a mechanism for both resorption of BCP crystal deposits and tendon degeneration.

CRYSTAL-INDUCED INFLAMMATION

Some of the crystals deposited in cartilage can subclinically travel to joint fluid and synovium, and the crystals can directly stimulate chondrocytes, synovial lining cells, and intra-articular leukocytes.[81-83] Inflammation triggered by CPPD and HA crystals thereby contributes to cartilage degradation and can cause worsening of OA.[81-83] Many proinflammatory mechanisms active in gout (see Chapter 87) likely mediate the synovitis and cartilage degeneration associated with CPPD and HA crystal deposition.[81-83] In this regard, CPPD and HA crystals activate cells partly via nonspecific activation of signal transduction pathways (e.g., MAPK activation) and induce cellular release of cyclooxygenase- and lipoxygenase-derived metabolites of arachidonic acid and cytokines, including TNF-α, IL-1, and CXCL8.[81-83] Innate immune recognition of extracellular CPPD crystals by Toll-like receptor 2 (TLR2)[84] and CPPD crystal-induced activation of the intracellular NALP3 (cryopyrin) inflammasome, resulting in caspase-1 activation and IL-1β processing and release, drive cell responses to CPPD crystals in vitro and CPPD crystal-induced inflammation in vivo.[85] The ingress of neutrophils into the joint is central in triggering acute crystal-induced synovitis, and effects on neutrophil-endothelial interaction likely represent a major locus for both the prophylactic effects of nanomolar concentrations of colchicine and the therapeutic effects of higher concentrations of colchicine in acute disease.[86] At relatively high (micromolar) concentrations, colchicine selectively suppresses crystal-induced NALP3 inflammasome activation.[85] CXCL8 and related chemokines that bind the CXCL8 receptor CXCR2 (including CXCL1) appear to be critical in initiating and perpetuating neutrophil ingress in acute crystal-induced inflammation.[87] Despite the fact that BCP and CPPD crystals share the capacity to activate certain cell signaling pathways and to induce several MMPs,[88] BCP crystals generally trigger much less neutrophil influx into the joint than do CPPD crystals. Concordantly, free intra-articular BCP crystals likely induce less proinflammatory cytokine expression than do CPPD and monosodium urate crystals.[89-91]

CLINICAL FEATURES

CALCIUM PYROPHOSPHATE DIHYDRATE DEPOSITION DISEASE

Most elderly individuals with CPPD deposition disease in the United States have a primary (idiopathic or sporadic) disorder (Table 88-2). Idiopathic chondrocalcinosis generally appears only after the fifth decade of life, but patients with a history of repetitive joint trauma or knee meniscectomy may present with nonsystemic (monarticular) chondrocalcinosis before age 50. Familial forms of CPPD crystal deposition disease have been widely documented, as discussed later. Familial chondrocalcinosis often manifests in the third or fourth decade of life, but in some cases, familial disease is detected before age 20 or first presents clinically at an advanced age. CPPD crystal deposition disease is a common manifestation of a variety of hereditary and metabolic conditions (including hyperparathyroidism, dialysis-dependent renal failure, and hemochromatosis)[41] in which CPPD-related arthropathy can present earlier than age 50. For unclear reasons, hemochromatosis can present predominantly as CPPD crystal deposition disease or as OA (see Chapter 111). The weight of evidence from controlled studies suggests that hypothyroidism (with the probable

Table 88-2 Causes of Calcium Pyrophosphate Dihydrate Crystal Deposition Disease

High Prevalence
Idiopathic in association with aging (most frequent)
Complication of primary osteoarthritis
Long-term consequence of mechanical joint trauma or knee meniscectomy
Moderate Prevalence
Familial
Associated with systemic metabolic disease (hyperparathyroidism, dialysis-dependent renal failure, hemochromatosis, hypomagnesemia)
Low Prevalence (Largely Based on Case Reports)
X-linked hypophosphatemic rickets
Familial hypocalciuric hypercalcemia
Ochronosis
Gout
Articular amyloidosis
Myxedematous hypothyroidism
Osteochondrodysplasias and spondyloepiphyseal dysplasias
Neuropathic joints
Wilson's disease

exception of myxedematous hypothyroidism) is not associated with a significantly increased prevalence of CPPD crystal deposition disease, although both disorders are clearly more prevalent with aging.[41,92,93] It has been suggested that initiation of thyroxine supplementation therapy may trigger pseudogout.[94]

The clinical manifestations of CPPD deposition disease vary widely (Table 88-3).[95] Quite commonly, the disease is asymptomatic. Alternatively, it can mimic OA (pseudo-osteoarthritis), gout (pseudogout), or acute-onset or insidious rheumatoid arthritis (pseudo–rheumatoid arthritis; Fig. 88-5), or it may present as pseudoneuropathic arthropathy. Patients with CPPD crystal deposition disease also commonly present with episodes of hemarthrosis, often

Table 88-3 Common Clinical Presentations of Calcium Pyrophosphate Dihydrate (CPPD) Crystal Deposition Disease

Asymptomatic or incidental finding (e.g., asymptomatic knee fibro-cartilage chondrocalcinosis in the elderly)
Recurrent acute inflammatory monarticular arthritis or pseudogout (e.g., wrist or knee, including provocation by trauma, concurrent medical or surgical illness, or intra-articular hyaluronan)
Pseudoseptic arthritis
Recurrent acute hemarthrosis
Chronic degenerative arthritis (pseudo-osteoarthritis or pseudoneuropathic arthritis)
Chronic symmetric inflammatory polyarthritis (pseudo–rheumatoid arthritis)
Systemic illness (pseudo–polymyalgia rheumatica, fever of unknown origin)
Destructive arthritis in dialysis-dependent renal failure
Carpal tunnel syndrome
Tumoral and pseudotophaceous CPPD crystal deposits
Central nervous system disease complicating ligamentum flavum or transverse ligament of atlas involvement (cervical canal stenosis, cervical myelopathy, meningismus, foramen magnum syndrome, odontoid fracture)

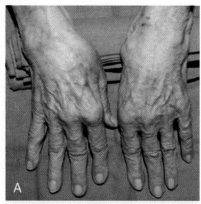

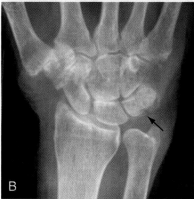

Figure 88-5 Idiopathic, symmetric pseudorheumatoid calcium pyrophosphate dihydrate (CPPD) deposition arthropathy in an elderly woman. This 84-year-old woman presented with a history of past right carpal tunnel syndrome and chronic symmetric proliferative synovitis of both wrists and second and third metacarpophalangeal (MCP) joints. Physical findings included synovial and dorsal extensor tenosynovial swelling of the wrists and synovial swelling at the second to third MCP joints **(A)**. Changes on hand and wrist plain radiographs were consistent with the diagnosis of CPPD deposition disease. Those in the right wrist **(B)** included cystic changes in multiple carpal bones, including the scaphoid and lunate; linear calcification on the ulnar side of the carpus *(arrow)*, typical for the chondrocalcinosis of CPPD deposition; and mild narrowing of the radiocarpal joint, indicative of cartilage loss.

post-traumatic and in the knee.[96] It is not clear how the form of CPPD deposited (i.e., monoclinic versus triclinic crystals) and host factors contribute to these wide differences in clinical manifestation. Overall, only a small fraction of patients with CPPD deposition disease have prolonged, recurring polyarticular inflammation. Progressive degenerative arthropathy is more common. Although CPPD deposition disease appears to be a common and significant public health problem in the elderly, the disease impact and the long-term course of CPPD-associated degenerative arthropathy in an unselected population have not been adequately evaluated.

ACUTE SYNOVITIS

Pseudogout is a major cause of acute monarticular or oligoarticular arthritis in the elderly. The attacks typically involve a large joint—most often the knee, less often the wrist or ankle, and, unlike gout, rarely the first metatarsophalangeal joint. Acute attacks of inflammatory pseudogout in patients with CPPD deposition disease typically have a sudden onset and can be excruciatingly painful, with pronounced periarticular erythema, warmth, and swelling,

comparable to gout. In addition, in some attacks of pseudogout, arthritis can be migratory or additive, polyarticular, and bilateral. Polyarticular pseudogout is particularly common in association with familial chondrocalcinosis and hyperparathyroidism.

Pseudogout can be provoked by minor trauma or intercurrent medical or surgical conditions, including pneumonia, myocardial infarction, cerebrovascular accident, and pregnancy. Parathyroid surgery for hyperparathyroidism frequently triggers pseudogout attacks. In addition, pseudogout of the knee can be precipitated by arthroscopy or by intraarticular administration of hyaluronan,[97-99] which could reflect proinflammatory mechanisms triggered through the hyaluronan receptor CD44.[100,101] Parenteral administration of granulocyte colony-stimulating factor[102] and bisphosphonates[103,104] also can trigger pseudogout, the former likely by ignition of smoldering subclinical intra-articular inflammation and the latter (theoretically) via pyrophosphatase inhibition, because bisphosphonates are nonhydrolyzable analogues of PP_i.

Acute and subacute pseudogout can be associated with fever, chills, elevated erythrocyte sedimentation rate, and systemic leukocytosis, particularly with polyarticular involvement and in the elderly.[105] Leukocyte counts in the synovial fluid are substantially elevated, and intraleukocytic CPPD crystals are most often (but not universally) detectable by compensated polarized light microscopy in pseudogout. The attacks typically last for 7 to 10 days, but they can also be clustered and last for weeks to months. Occasionally, the leukocyte count in pseudogout can exceed $50,000/mm^3$ (pseudoseptic arthritis).

CHRONIC DEGENERATIVE AND INFLAMMATORY ARTHROPATHIES

Acute pseudogout attacks may be interspersed with chronic arthropathy in CPPD crystal deposition disease. Chronic degenerative arthropathy in CPPD deposition disease commonly affects certain joints that are typically spared in primary OA (e.g., metacarpophalangeal joints, wrists, elbows, glenohumeral joints). The development of cartilage degenerative changes in joints both typical and atypical for primary OA suggests one or more systemic abnormalities.

Degenerative cartilage disease associated with sporadic CPPD crystal deposition disease may present as destructive arthropathy of the knees, hips, or shoulders, particularly in elderly women (Figs. 88-6 and 88-7). CPPD crystal arthropathy–associated degenerative disease can be less or more destructive than that observed in primary OA. For example, patients with primary OA and CPPD crystals have been reported to require knee replacement surgery more often than those with primary OA without crystals.[106] In another study, 60% of patients undergoing joint replacement had CPPD or BCP crystals (commonly both types) in their knee synovial fluid and higher mean radiographic scores correlated with the presence of calcium-containing crystals.[107] However, prospective analysis of CPPD deposition disease that involved primarily the knee suggested that radiographic worsening of degenerative changes may be slow.[108] Also, the disease may not appear to progress clinically in the involved knee after substantial periods of follow-up in a subset of patients, although clinical involvement may spread to other

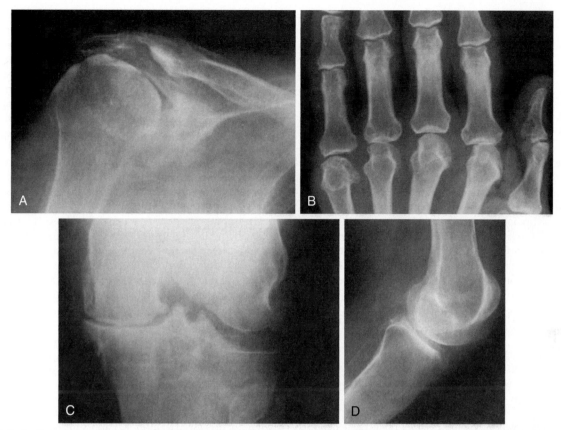

Figure 88-6 Radiographic features of calcium pyrophosphate dihydrate arthropathy. **A,** Destructive shoulder arthropathy. **B,** Metacarpophalangeal joint arthropathy. **C,** Knee degenerative joint disease with large subchondral bone cyst. **D,** Wraparound patella (same patient shown in **A**).

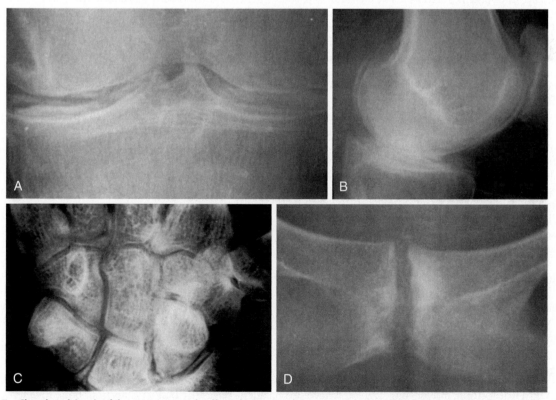

Figure 88-7 Chondrocalcinosis of the most commonly affected joints in calcium pyrophosphate dihydrate deposition disease. **A,** Lineal calcifications observed in knee menisci and fibrocartilage. **B,** Lateral view showing calcification of the articular cartilage as a line parallel to the femoral condyles. **C,** Calcification of intercarpal joints and triangular ligament. **D,** Calcification of the symphysis pubis fibrocartilage associated with subchondral bone erosions and subchondral increased bone density.

joints in the same time frame.[108] Most patients develop changes in the radiographic extent of chondrocalcinosis over time,[108] but there is no clear correlation between the extent of calcification and the progression of CPPD deposition arthropathy. There may be a relatively good prognosis for those with CPPD deposition disease in the knee presenting as acute pseudogout attacks alone.[108]

Pseudorheumatoid involvement in a small subset of patients with CPPD deposition disease presents as a chronic, bilateral, symmetric, deforming inflammatory polyarthropathy (see Fig. 88-5). Many of these patients have bilateral wrist and metacarpophalangeal joint involvement. Wrist tenosynovitis, carpal tunnel syndrome, cubital tunnel syndrome, and tendon rupture may develop. Ingestion of CPPD crystals by synovial lining cells, and lysosomal catabolism of such ingested crystals, stimulates synovial proliferation, in part via solubilization of the crystalline calcium. Such effects may contribute to regional synovial and periarticular tenosynovial proliferation promoted by CPPD crystal deposition.[82]

OTHER FORMS OF CALCIUM PYROPHOSPHATE DIHYDRATE CRYSTAL DEPOSITION

Concentrated (tumoral or pseudotophaceous) CPPD crystal deposition can occur in periarticular structures, including tendons, ligaments, bursae, and occasionally bone.[95,109] CPPD deposits in tendons (e.g., Achilles, triceps, obturator tendons) are usually fine and linear on radiographs. Pseudotophaceous deposits of CPPD crystals have been detected in the temporal bone, around the knee and hip, and in the acromioclavicular, temporomandibular, elbow, and small hand joints.[109] Peripheral tumoral CPPD crystal deposits sometimes present with acute arthritic attacks. Rarely, tumoral CPPD deposits around the knee can mimic osteonecrosis.[110] Tumoral CPPD crystal deposition typically is associated with tissue chondroid metaplasia and behaves like a benign but locally aggressive chondroid tumor, with some of the connective tissue invasion and destruction likely mediated by CPPD crystal-induced cell activation.

Axial skeletal CPPD crystal deposition occasionally involves the intervertebral disks, sacroiliac joints, and lumbar facet joints, and radiographic findings such as linear calcification and spinal ankylosis may appear.[111] Meningismus and clinical manifestations resembling herniated intervertebral disk, ankylosing spondylitis, and acute pseudogout of the lumbar facet joints have been observed.[111,112] In addition, CPPD deposits within the ligamentum flavum or the transverse ligament of the atlas can be sizable and can progress, causing cervical canal stenosis, cervical myelopathy, and foramen magnum syndrome.[113-115] Odontoid fracture due to the calcification of the atlantoaxial joint may occur in CPPD deposition disease.[113-116] Thus, CPPD deposition disease can be a factor in the differential diagnosis of patients with neurologic disturbances and painful cervical masses, especially in the elderly.

FAMILIAL CHONDROCALCINOSIS

Familial CPPD deposition disease has been described in numerous countries and ethnic groups, including kindreds from Czechoslovakia, Holland, France, England, Germany, Sweden, Israel, the United States, Canada, and Japan; it

may be most prevalent in Chile and Spain.[117] In one English kindred with CPPD disease linked to *ANKH* mutation on chromosome 5p, recurrent childhood seizures were strongly associated with the later development of CPPD deposition disease.[118] With linkages to chromosome 5p,[54,55] some families manifest early-onset polyarthritis, which can include ankylosing intervertebral and sacroiliac joint disease. In others, a late-onset chondrocalcinosis occurs, and the disease can be oligoarticular, mild in intensity and destructiveness, and nearly indistinguishable from idiopathic CPPD deposition disease.[118] Kindreds from Argentina and the Alsace region of France with linkages to chromosome 5p shared similar phenotypic features of chondrocalcinosis, including early age at onset (third decade of life), common but not universal premature OA, some cases of pseudo–rheumatoid arthritic peripheral joint disease, and radiographic evidence of fibrocartilage and hyaline cartilage calcifications typical of CPPD deposition.[50] The most commonly affected joints in these kindreds were the knees and wrists, with involvement of the pubic symphysis and intervertebral disks also described.[50]

BASIC CALCIUM PHOSPHATE CRYSTAL DEPOSITION AT THE JOINT

Unlike the case for urate and CPPD crystal deposition, acute synovitis due to HA crystal deposition is unusual.[119] However, acute inflammatory syndromes, including subacromial bursitis (see Chapter 40) and a form of pseudopodagra described in young women,[120] may occur in association with periarticular HA crystal deposition in bursae, tendons, ligaments, and soft tissues. Patients with advanced chronic renal failure, particularly those on dialysis, may develop symptomatic articular and periarticular BCP crystal deposition (Fig. 88-8), which may be destructive and involve the axial skeleton.[121-123] In some cases of dialysis-dependent renal failure, destructive arthropathy associated with BCP crystal deposition may resemble or be associated with CPPD deposition disease,[123] and monosodium urate crystal deposits in the joint may also occur in this setting. Hyperparathyroidism can promote BCP-associated arthropathy[124] and periarticular disease, including calcific bursitis. Clinically significant periarticular HA crystal deposition also may occur in certain post-traumatic conditions and in the systemic autoimmune diseases scleroderma and dermatomyositis.[125]

BCP crystal deposition has a predilection for the shoulder, where it may manifest as calcific tendinitis of the rotator cuff (see Chapter 40) or as a destructive process associated with rotator cuff tear, which is most prevalent in the elderly and more common in females.[126] Abundant intra-articular BCP crystalline material is typically present in the distinctive noninflammatory syndrome of rotator cuff tear and marked cartilage degeneration—an entity termed Milwaukee shoulder syndrome, cuff tear arthropathy, or apatite-associated destructive arthritis.[46,77,127-129] Mechanical instability of the shoulder due to rotator cuff tear may be the driving force in many of these patients, with consequent release of BCP crystals from bone fragments into the joint space, promoting secondary synovitis and connective tissue destruction. The process may be bilateral but is generally worse on the side of the dominant hand. Substantial

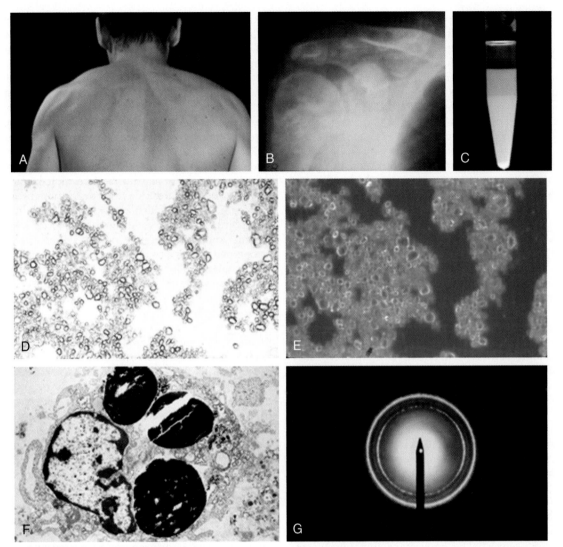

Figure 88-8 Hydroxyapatite crystal-associated calcific bursitis of the shoulder in a patient with chronic renal failure and secondary hyperparathyroidism. **A,** Chronic soft tissue swelling involving the right shoulder due to calcific right shoulder subacromial bursitis in a middle-aged man with a history of chronic renal failure on hemodialysis. Note the convex contour of the right shoulder compared with the left. **B,** Radiograph showing extensive calcification within both the rotator cuff and the expanded subacromial bursa surrounding the right shoulder joint. An incidental finding is resorption of the distal end of the clavicle, consistent with secondary hyperparathyroidism in this patient. **C,** Subacromial bursa fluid from the right shoulder. Note the milk-white appearance, with a chalky sediment of particulate material in the fluid after centrifugation, consistent with crystal deposition disease. **D,** Microscopic appearance of bursa fluid aggregates of basic calcium phosphate crystals in the absence of special stains. The particles are irregular but have approximately spherical profiles (unstained, ×250). **E,** Appearance of the bursa fluid under polarized light microscopy. Importantly, the aggregated particles of basic calcium phosphate crystals demonstrate edge birefringence but do not display intrusive birefringence (unstained, ×250). **F,** Electron photomicrograph of a mononuclear phagocyte from this bursa fluid that contained phagocytosed electron-dense (dark black) spherical aggregates of crystals of basic calcium phosphate hydroxyapatite in three phagolysosomes oriented vertically to the right of the nucleus. Hundreds of tiny needle-shaped hydroxyapatite crystals are clumped in each of these dense aggregates. For perspective, the size of the mononuclear phagocyte is about 20 μm, and an individual (nonaggregated) hydroxyapatite crystal is about 0.04 × 0.01 × 0.01 μm in size (transmission electron microscopy, ×1000). **G,** Electron diffraction pattern of hydroxyapatite crystal aggregates. The diffraction rings are indicative of a powder pattern (i.e., small crystals). The position of the bright rings with d-spacings = 3.44 and 2.81 Å are characteristic of hydroxyapatite (calcium apatite). *(Courtesy of Dr. Ken Pritzker, Mount Sinai Hospital Pathology Department, University of Toronto, Ontario, Canada.)*

glenohumeral joint effusions are typically seen, and synovial fluid is often blood stained but contains, at most, relatively low numbers of mononuclear leukocytes. Joints other than the shoulder, such as the knee and hip, can be affected by a condition similar to Milwaukee shoulder syndrome, sometimes in an individual with shoulder involvement.[46,126,127] In contrast to primary OA, lateral tibiofemoral compartment involvement is common in BCP-associated destructive knee arthropathy. Concurrent CPPD deposition, biomechanical abnormalities, chronic renal failure, and neuropathic factors

appear to be predisposing factors. A kindred with familial OA and apparent Milwaukee shoulder-knee syndrome had an unusual type of degenerative joint disease with both intra-articular and periarticular calcifications.[46]

Studies of synovial fluids and cartilage specimens from OA indicated that intra-articular BCP crystalline material, including HA in the pericellular matrix of chondrocytes, is frequently detectable in the disease.[58,107] Synovial fluid HA crystals are frequently present in conjunction with CPPD crystals in OA, particularly in advanced disease of the knee at the time of total joint replacement.[107,128] Subchondral bone shards in OA cartilage that are composed of BCP crystalline material may contribute to a fraction of such crystal-positive specimens. In addition, the movement of crystals from articular cartilage to synovium[82,83] can promote calcific synovial crystal deposits at or just beneath the synovial surface, and synovium-derived rice bodies can give rise to BCP crystal deposits released into the joint space.[129,130] Therefore, it is difficult to quantify the precise prevalence of HA crystal deposits in articular cartilage in OA. Both HA and CPPD crystal-induced synovial proliferation, cytotoxic effects on chondrocytes, and synovial and chondrocyte MMP expression can promote OA progression.[82,83]

DIAGNOSIS AND DIAGNOSTIC TESTS

DIFFERENTIAL DIAGNOSIS

CPPD deposition disease can imitate a number of other conditions, and vice versa (see Table 88-3); therefore, attention to the diagnostic criteria for CPPD deposition disease is mandatory (see Table 88-1). Conversely, it is important to note that radiographic evidence of chondrocalcinosis is a common finding in the aged and does not necessarily indicate that the patient's symptomatic articular problem is due to CPPD deposition disease, which is often asymptomatic. The demonstrable presence of CPPD crystals in synovial fluid or in tissues using compensated polarized light microscopy (as discussed earlier for distinguishing gout from pseudogout) is definite evidence of CPPD deposition disease. Although weakly birefringent relative to urate crystals, and often rhomboid in shape, CPPD crystals can be rod-shaped and intracellular, resembling urate crystals. Thus, the use of compensated polarized light microscopy is essential to confirm the presence of positively birefringent CPPD crystals, although it should be noted that some CPPD crystals are nonbirefringent.[131] The appearance and number of CPPD crystals can change with storage. Therefore, clinicians should examine relatively fresh specimens collected in vials free of calcium-chelating anticoagulants such as EDTA.

The ability of pseudogout to mimic septic arthritis (pseudo–septic arthritis), and vice versa, underscores the diagnostic importance of arthrocentesis with appropriate synovial fluid crystal analysis and, in many instances, concomitant exclusion of joint infection. Significantly, crystal deposits can be "enzymatically strip-mined" by inflammation associated with joint sepsis. Hence, CPPD crystals (as well as other crystals) may be observed in the joint fluid and within synovial fluid leukocytes in an infected joint.

Chronic arthritis in CPPD deposition disease has several clinical and plain radiographic features that help differentiate it from OA. These include involvement at sites uncommon for primary OA, such as the wrist, metacarpophalangeal joints, elbow, or shoulder, as well as heavy punctate and linear calcifications in fibrocartilage, articular (hyaline) cartilage, and joint capsules on radiographs, especially if they are bilateral and symmetric (see Figs. 88-6 and 88-7). It should be noted that faint or atypical calcifications may be due to BCP-related vascular calcifications. It was thought that deposition of nonpathologic dicalcium

phosphate dihydrate ($CaHPO_4 \cdot 2H_2O$; calcium-phosphate ratio, 1.0), or brushite, crystals could cause some atypical calcifications, but brushite crystals can arise as an artifact of preparation of calcified tissue for pathologic analysis.[132]

Patients with arthritis in whom CPPD deposition disease is part of the differential diagnosis can be adequately screened radiographically by obtaining an anteroposterior view of each knee, an anteroposterior view of the pelvis (to detect symphysis pubis involvement, which is quite common), and posteroanterior views of both hands that include visualization of both wrists (see Figs. 88-6 and 88-7). Calcific deposits may or may not be detectable by radiographic screening of these areas in CPPD deposition disease. In this case, radiographic evidence other than chondrocalcinosis may point to the correct diagnosis.[133] For example, radiographic findings suggestive of CPPD deposition disease, as opposed to primary OA, include radiocarpal or marked patellofemoral joint space narrowing, especially if isolated (such as the patella "wrapped around" the femur), as well as scaphoid-lunate widening and femoral cortical erosion superior to the patella. Severe progressive degeneration in the knee, with subchondral bony collapse (microfractures), fragmentation, and formation of intra-articular radiodense bodies, is a feature of CPPD presenting as a pseudoneuropathic joint. CPPD deposition disease involving the metacarpophalangeal joints can be distinguished radiographically from rheumatoid arthritis by metacarpal squaring associated with "beaklike" osteophytes and subchondral cyst formation. Tendon calcifications (e.g., Achilles, triceps, obturator tendons) are a valuable differential diagnostic feature of CPPD deposition. Osteophyte formation is more variable with CPPD deposition disease than with OA.

Diagnosis of CPPD deposition disease in a patient younger than 50 years, particularly if CPPD deposition is widespread, should prompt consideration of a primary metabolic or familial disorder (see Table 88-2). In the elderly, presentation of CPPD deposition as diffuse pain and fever of unknown origin[105] can mimic infection, polymyalgia rheumatica, and rheumatoid arthritis. A false-positive rheumatoid factor test is common in the elderly (>30% positivity). Thus, patients with pseudorheumatoid CPPD deposition disease are often seropositive for rheumatoid factor.

BCP crystals may be detected as nonbirefringent globular clumps within leukocytes in some synovial and bursal fluids (see Fig. 88-8), and BCP crystal clumps stain with the calcium-binding dye alizarin red S under light microscopy.[119,128] CPPD crystals can also be detected using alizarin red S, but they stain more weakly than BCP crystals. The relative paucity of osteophytes (so-called atrophic degenerative arthritis) and the sizable glenohumeral joint effusions with abundant synovial fluid BCP crystalline material associated with Milwaukee shoulder syndrome help distinguish it from primary OA of the glenohumeral joint. However, destructive, neuropathic shoulder arthropathy due to syringomyelia or alcoholism sometimes merits consideration in the differential diagnosis of Milwaukee shoulder syndrome.[134] Oxalate crystal deposition arthropathy can be a major differential diagnostic consideration with BCP-associated arthritis and periarticular calcifications in dialysis-dependent renal failure.[135] The differential diagnosis of calcific tendinitis of the shoulder is discussed in Chapter 40.

DIAGNOSTIC TESTS

A thorough laboratory evaluation of a newly diagnosed CPPD disease patient routinely includes serum levels of calcium, phosphorus, magnesium, alkaline phosphatase, ferritin, iron and total iron binding capacity, and thyroid-stimulating hormone (Fig. 88-9). Conventional radiography is usually the first method to evaluate patients with suspected chondrocalcinosis, but the findings may not correlate with pathologic and clinical manifestations. For example, the correlation between radiographic and pathologic findings was only 39.2% in a study of patients via knee arthroscopy.[136] Other imaging approaches to the diagnosis of CPPD deposition disease with the potential to improve sensitivity include computed tomography, magnetic resonance imaging (MRI), and ultrasonography, which can detect CPPD (as well as BCP) crystals, particularly in the knee.[133,137,138] However, standard, nonenhanced MRI is less sensitive in detecting knee meniscal fibrocartilage calcification than hyaline cartilage calcification.[139] Specialized techniques beyond alizarin red S staining, such as x-ray diffraction, Raman spectroscopy, Fourier transform intrared spectroscopy, atomic force microscopy, or transmission electron microscopy showing electron-dense clumps of needle-like crystals, may be needed to confirm BCP crystal deposition (see Fig. 88-8).[2,3]

If synovial fluid specimens are not fresh (or have not been stored at 4°C),[140] Gram stain and Diff Quick staining methods for crystal analysis have been suggested as a means of obtaining information beyond that available from compensated polarized light microscopy.[141,142] Demonstration of CPPD crystals in articular tissues (see Fig. 88-3) can be difficult in specimens stained with hematoxylin and eosin, because the acidity of hematoxylin solutions promotes decalcification. However, the decalcifying effect of hematoxylin can be diminished by limiting the staining period with Mayer's hematoxylin to 3 minutes.[143]

TREATMENT

CALCIUM PYROPHOSPHATE DIHYDRATE DEPOSITION DISEASE

As in gout (see Chapter 87), therapeutic approaches to patients with CPPD deposition disease involve treatment and prophylaxis of acute arthritic attacks, as well as therapy to lessen chronic and anatomically progressive sequelae of crystal deposition (Table 88-4). Although reduced meniscal calcification was reported over a 10-year period in association with the administration of oral magnesium to a patient with secondary CPPD deposition disease due to hypomagnesemia,[144] there is no specific treatment for idiopathic CPPD deposition disease. Metabolic disorders that secondarily cause CPPD crystal deposition obviously require treatment. However, the potential benefits of preventing chondrocalcinotic cartilage degeneration with the appropriate treatment of hemochromatosis and hyperparathyroidism are unclear, because the ability to detect chondrocalcinosis radiographically is usually indicative of advanced crystal deposition disease.

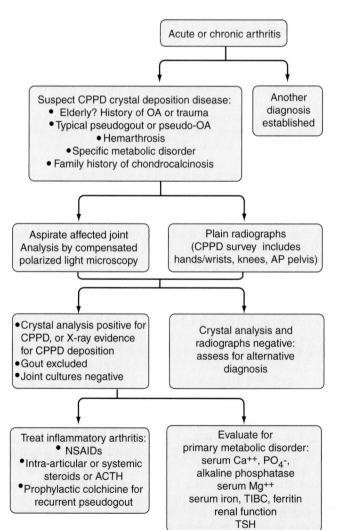

Figure 88-9 Algorithm for the evaluation and treatment of calcium pyrophosphate dihydrate (CPPD) deposition disease.

Table 88-4 Therapeutics for Calcium Pyrophosphate Dihydrate (CPPD) Crystal Deposition Disease

Proven Benefits
NSAIDs or COX-2 inhibitors
Intra-articular corticosteroids
Systemic corticosteroids
ACTH
Prophylactic low-dose colchicine

Possible Benefits Already Observed Clinically
Methotrexate for refractory chronic inflammation and recurrent pseudogout
Oral magnesium (for patients with hypomagnesemia)

Theoretical Benefits
Phosphocitrate
Caspase-1 or IL-1 antagonism for CPPD crystal-induced inflammation
Hydroxychloroquine for refractory chronic inflammation
TLR2 antagonism for CPPD-associated degenerative arthropathy
Oral calcium supplementation to suppress PTH levels
ANKH anion channel blockade (probenecid)
NPP1 inhibition
TG2 inhibition
Polyphosphates
Promotion of crystal dissolution by alkaline phosphatase or polyamines

ACTH, adrenocorticotropic hormone; COX-2, cyclooxygenase-2; IL-1, interleukin-1; NPP1, nucleotide pyrophosphatase phosphodiesterase 1; NSAID, nonsteroidal anti-inflammatory drug; PTH, parathyroid hormone; TG2, transglutaminase 2; TLR2, Toll-like receptor 2.

Episodes of pseudogout generally respond to nonsteroidal anti-inflammatory drugs (NSAIDs), including cyclooxygenase-2 inhibitors, or intra-articular steroids, although the response is sometimes slower than in gout. Adrenocorticotropic hormone[145] and systemic glucocorticoids,[146] generally given as described for acute gout (see Chapter 87), are effective in most cases of acute pseudogout. The response to colchicine bolus is less consistent than that usually seen in acute gout. Intravenous colchicine is not recommended for pseudogout and can be quite dangerous in elderly patients; however, pseudogout episodes can be diminished in frequency by low-dose daily colchicine prophylaxis, as for gouty arthritis. Although most acute pseudogout attacks in the knee are self-limited, resolution can sometimes be enhanced by simple arthrocentesis and thorough drainage of the joint effusion; there are currently no data on measures such as tidal irrigation.

Hydroxychloroquine may be of some benefit in patients with refractory, chronic polyarticular CPPD deposition disease and may reduce the flares of pseudogout.[147] Methotrexate was particularly promising in this setting in an exploratory study limited to five consecutive patients who were used as their own controls (before methotrexate treatment).[148] However, at this time, there is insufficient evidence to recommend hydroxychloroquine and methotrexate as standard therapies for refractory inflammation in CPPD crystal deposition disease.

Effective cartilage-preserving therapy is still lacking in idiopathic, chronic, progressive CPPD deposition disease. Some reports have suggested that OA patients with cartilage calcification respond to arthroscopic irrigation and daily low-dose colchicine,[149-151] but further substantiation is needed. There is currently no evidence to support arthroscopic débridement as a treatment modality for CPPD deposition disease. There is insufficient evidence of beneficial effects of intra-articular hyaluronan therapy in CPPD deposition disease of the knee, and the risks of precipitating pseudogout appear to be significant with this treatment modality, as noted earlier.

BASIC CALCIUM PHOSPHATE CRYSTAL ARTHROPATHIES

NSAIDs and local glucocorticoid injection are effective treatment options for BCP crystal-associated calcific tendinitis and subacromial bursitis (see Chapter 40) (Table 88-5). BCP crystal-associated inflammation of the rotator cuff and subacromial bursa of the shoulder can be successfully treated using needle aspiration, irrigation, and steroid injections. Ultrasound-guided techniques, which promote resorption of rotator cuff and bursal calcifications, can enhance the success of such approaches.[152,153]

FUTURE THERAPEUTIC APPROACHES

One factor that may account for the low prevalence of chondrocalcinosis in China is high oral calcium intake, which suppresses PTH production by the parathyroid. Specifically, calcium levels in tap water in Beijing were 12- to 20-fold higher than in Framingham, whereas no difference was found in magnesium levels in the aforementioned study of Chinese versus U.S. chondrocalcinosis

Table 88-5 Therapeutics for Articular and Periarticular Basic Calcium Phosphate Crystal Deposition

Proven Benefits
NSAIDs or selective COX-2 inhibitors
Local corticosteroid injection
Local irrigation
Ultrasonography
Theoretical Benefits
Phosphocitrate
Modulators of ANKH (e.g., probenecid), NPP1, or TG2

COX-2, cyclooxygenase-2; NPP1, nucleotide pyrophosphatase phosphodiesterase 1; NSAID, nonsteroidal anti-inflammatory drug; TG2, transglutaminase 2.

prevalence by Zhang and coworkers.[11] Oral calcium intake suppresses PTH production, and deficient calcium intake in aging is a major public health problem in Western countries. Primary hyperparathyroidism as well as chondrocalcinosis are rare in mainland China.[154] It is possible that chondrocalcinosis is more of an environmentally mediated finding than previously recognized, influenced by subclinical variability in calcium intake and parathyroid function. Given the current lack of effective, rational therapies to prevent or lessen idiopathic CPPD crystal deposition, further study of the potential prophylactic and therapeutic benefits of dietary calcium supplementation is warranted.

The potential to develop therapies for both CPPD and BCP crystal-associated arthropathies based on new molecular targets has been advanced by the identification of ANKH, NPP1, and TG2 as specific molecular mediators of cartilage calcification. Intriguingly, the anion transport inhibitor probenecid suppresses ANKH-induced and TGF-β–induced increases in extracellular PP_i in vitro.[26,54,155] Prevention of CPPD deposition by polyphosphates or promotion of CPPD dissolution by depot alkaline phosphatase and by pyrophosphatase activation-promoting polyamines could provide alternative therapeutic approaches.[156,157] However, in the past, incomplete CPPD crystal dissolution by intra-articular lavage in patients with chondrocalcinosis of the knees with disodium EDTA and magnesium ions was a therapeutic failure, in that insignificant amounts of CPPD were removed and all subjects developed postlavage attacks of pseudogout mediated by crystal shedding.[158]

The PP_i analogue phosphocitrate, a natural compound in mammalian mitochondria and in the urinary tract, is a potent inhibitor of HA crystal formation.[159] Phosphocitrate inhibits NO-induced calcification of cartilage[67] and also inhibits both HA and CPPD crystal-associated cell stimulation, including induction of MMP-3 in fibroblasts.[160] Systemic phosphocitrate treatment suppresses ankylosing ossification in murine progressive ankylosis of ank/ank mice.[161] Moreover, an analogue of phosphocitrate (CaNaPC) decreased both the abundant meniscal cartilage HA deposition and the continual progression of OA in the Hartley guinea pig model of spontaneous knee OA.[162] The CaNaPC treatment did not exert therapeutic effects in a rabbit knee hemimeniscectomy model of OA in which there was an absence of intra-articular calcification.[162] Such results suggest that phosphocitrate acts on calcification-mediated mechanisms of dysregulation of joint biomechanics and cartilage degeneration without exerting nonspecific chondroprotective effects.

Further clinical development of phosphocitrate would be of interest, but it has been slowed in part by its low bioavailability unless given parenterally.[159]

The use of bisphosphonates as PP_i analogues can be beneficial in some cases of soft tissue calcification with HA, as illustrated in disease associated with NPP1 deficiency.[16,163] Last, the identified roles of TLR2 in chondrocyte responsiveness to CPDD crystals,[84] of TLR4 in HA crystal-induced inflammatory responses,[164] and of NALP3 inflammasome-mediated caspase-1 activation and IL-1β processing in CPPD crystal-induced inflammation[85] suggest that certain mediators of innate immunity, including TLR2, TLR4, caspase-1, and IL-1β, may be therapeutic targets for human forms of CPPD and HA crystal-driven inflammation and connective tissue destruction.

OUTCOME AND PROGNOSIS

The presence of CPPD crystals in primary knee OA had been proposed as a predictive factor for more frequent knee replacement surgery.[106] Moreover, mean radiographic scores directly correlate with the presence of calcium-containing crystals in OA patients at the time of total joint arthroplasty.[107] However, degenerative cartilage disease associated with sporadic CPPD crystal deposition disease may be less destructive than that observed in primary OA. For example, a prospective analysis of CPPD deposition disease of the knee suggested that radiographic worsening of degenerative arthritis was slow to occur.[108] Typically, changes in the radiographic extent of chondrocalcinosis are observed over time,[108] but there is no clear correlation between the extent of calcification and progression of CPPD deposition arthropathy.

In the Boston OA Knee Study (BOKS) and in the Health, Aging, and Body Composition (Health ABC) Study,[165] the relationship between chondrocalcinosis and the progression of knee OA was prospectively evaluated longitudinally using MRI. In BOKS, knees with chondrocalcinosis had a decreased risk of cartilage loss compared with knees without chondrocalcinosis; there was no difference in risk in the Health ABC Study. Stratification by the presence of intact or damaged knee menisci produced comparable results within each cohort.[165] In a Thai study, CPPD crystal deposition disease was identified radiographically or by synovial fluid analysis in 52.9% of 102 patients undergoing total knee arthroplasty.[166] Patients with and without chondrocalcinosis did not differ in the ability to perform daily activities or treatment, and those with chondrocalcinosis did not undergo knee arthroplasty at an earlier age than those without chondrocalcinosis.[166]

In the setting of OA, the processes leading to matrix calcification were once thought to reflect passive secondary consequences of advanced cartilage pathology. Moreover, joint inflammation induced by deposited crystals was thought to be the primary determinant of the clinical impact of chondrocalcinosis on the progression of OA. The aforementioned studies[165,166] and advances in our understanding of the pathogeneses of OA and chondrocalcinosis paint a different picture. In essence, the dysregulated cartilage matrix repair that generates cartilage calcification may be as effective (or in some cases more effective) at slowing cartilage tissue failure than other phenotypes of cartilage repair in OA.

REFERENCES

1. Pritzker KP, Cheng PT, Grynpas MD, et al: Crystal associated diseases: Role of scanning electron microscopy in diagnosis. Scanning Microsc 2:1471-1478, 1988.
2. Pritzker KP, Cheng PT, Renlund RC: Calcium pyrophosphate crystal deposition in hyaline cartilage: Ultrastructural analysis and implications for pathogenesis. J Rheumatol 15:828-835, 1988.
3. Luisiri P, Blair J, Ellman MH: Calcium pyrophosphate dihydrate deposition disease presenting as tumoral calcinosis (periarticular pseudogout). J Rheumatol 23:1647-1650, 1996.
4. Felson DT, Anderson JJ, Naimark A, et al: The prevalence of chondrocalcinosis in the elderly and its association with knee osteoarthritis: The Framingham Study. J Rheumatol 16:1241-1245, 1989.
5. Zitnan D, Sitaj S: Chondrocalcinosis articularis. Section I. Clinical and radiological study. Ann Rheum Dis 22:142-169, 1963.
6. Ellman MH, Brown NL, Levin B: Prevalence of knee chondrocalcinosis in hospital and clinic patients aged 50 or older. J Am Geriatr Soc 29:189-192, 1981.
7. Ellman MH, Levin B: Chondrocalcinosis in elderly persons. Arthritis Rheum 18:43-47, 1975.
8. Mitrovic DR, Stankovic A, Iriarte-Borda O, et al: The prevalence of chondrocalcinosis in the human knee joint: An autopsy survey. J Rheumatol 15:633-641, 1988.
9. McCarty DJ Jr, Hogan JM, Gatter RA, et al: Studies on pathological calcifications in human cartilage. I. Prevalence and types of crystal deposits in the menisci of two hundred fifteen cadavera. J Bone Joint Surg Am 48:309-325, 1966.
10. Wilkins E, Dieppe P, Maddison P, et al: Osteoarthritis and articular chondrocalcinosis in the elderly. Ann Rheum Dis 42:280-284, 1983.
11. Zhang Y, Terkeltaub R, Nevitt M, et al: Lower prevalence of chondrocalcinosis in Chinese subjects in Beijing than in white subjects in the United States: The Beijing Osteoarthritis Study. Arthritis Rheum 54:3508-3512, 2006.
12. Zhang Y, Xu L, Nevitt MC, et al: Comparison of the prevalence of knee osteoarthritis between the elderly Chinese population in Beijing and whites in the United States: The Beijing Osteoarthritis Study. Arthritis Rheum 44:2065-2071, 2001.
13. Mandel N, Mandel G: Calcium pyrophosphate crystal deposition in model systems. Rheum Dis Clin North Am 14:321-340, 1988.
14. Hunter GK, Grynpas MD, Cheng PT, et al: Effect of glycosaminoglycans on calcium pyrophosphate crystal formation in collagen gels. Calcif Tissue Int 41:164-170, 1987.
15. Cheng PT, Pritzker KP: Pyrophosphate, phosphate ion interaction: Effects on calcium pyrophosphate and calcium hydroxyapatite crystal formation in aqueous solutions. J Rheumatol 10:769-777, 1983.
16. Terkeltaub R: Inorganic pyrophosphate (PP_i) generation and disposition in pathophysiology. Am J Physiol Cell Physiol 281:C1-C11, 2001.
17. Swan A, Heywood B, Chapman B, et al: Evidence for a causal relationship between the structure, size, and load of calcium pyrophosphate dihydrate crystals, and attacks of pseudogout. Ann Rheum Dis 54:825-830, 1995.
18. Johnson K, Goding J, van Etten D, et al: Linked deficiencies in extracellular inorganic pyrophosphate and osteopontin expression mediate pathologic calcification in PC-1 null mice. Am J Bone Miner Res 18:994-1004, 2003.
19. Hessle L, Johnson KA, Anderson HC, et al: Tissue-nonspecific alkaline phosphatase and plasma cell membrane glycoprotein-1 are central antagonistic regulators of bone mineralization. Proc Natl Acad Sci U S A 99:9445-9449, 2002.
20. Chang W, Tu C, Chen TH, et al: Expression and signal transduction of calcium-sensing receptors in cartilage and bone. Endocrinology 140:5883-5893, 1999.
21. Chang W, Tu C, Pratt S, et al: Extracellular Ca^{2+} sensing receptors modulate matrix production and mineralization in chondrogenic RCJ3.1C5.18 cells. Endocrinology 143:1467-1474, 2002.
22. Adams CS, Mansfield K, Perlot RL, et al: Matrix regulation of skeletal cell apoptosis: Role of calcium and phosphate ions. J Biol Chem 276:20316-20322, 2001.
23. Wang D, Canaff L, Davidson D, et al: Alterations in the sensing and transport of phosphate and calcium by differentiating chondrocytes. J Biol Chem 276:33995-34005, 2001.
24. Johnson K, Terkeltaub R: Upregulated ANK expression in osteoarthritis can promote both chondrocyte MMP-13 expression and calcification via chondrocyte extracellular PP_i excess. Osteoarthritis Cartilage 12:321-335, 2004.

25. Johnson K, Pritzker K, Goding J, et al: The nucleoside triphosphate pyrophosphohydrolase (NTPPPH) isozyme PC-1 directly promotes cartilage calcification through chondrocyte apoptosis and increased calcium precipitation by mineralizing vesicles. J Rheumatol 28: 2681-2691, 2001.

26. Ho A, Johnson M, Kingsley DM: Role of the mouse ANK gene in tissue calcification and arthritis. Science 289:265-270, 2000.

27. Okawa A, Nakamura I, Goto S, et al: Mutation in NPPS in a mouse model of ossification of the posterior longitudinal ligament of the spine. Nat Genet 19:271-273, 1998.

28. Rutsch F, Ruf N, Vaingankar S, et al: Mutations in ENPP1 are associated with "idiopathic" infantile arterial calcification. Nat Genet 34:379-381, 2003.

29. Johnson K, Hashimoto S, Lotz M, et al: Up-regulated expression of the phosphodiesterase nucleotide pyrophosphatase family member PC-1 is a marker and pathogenic factor for knee meniscal cartilage matrix calcification. Arthritis Rheum 44:1071-1081, 2001.

30. Johnson K, Vaingankar S, Chen Y, et al: Differential mechanisms of inorganic pyrophosphate production by plasma cell membrane glycoprotein-1 and B10 in chondrocytes. Arthritis Rheum 42:1986-1997, 1999.

31. Zaka R, Stokes D, Dion AS, et al: P5L mutation in ANK results in an increase in extracellular PP_i during proliferation and non-mineralizing hypertrophy in stably transduced ATDC5 cells. Arthritis Res Ther 8:R164, 2006.

32. Rosen F, McCabe G, Quach J, et al: Differential effects of aging on human chondrocyte responses to transforming growth factor beta: Increased pyrophosphate production and decreased cell proliferation. Arthritis Rheum 40:1275-1281, 1997.

33. Pattrick M, Hamilton E, Hornby J, et al: Synovial fluid pyrophosphate and nucleoside triphosphate pyrophosphatase: Comparison between normal and diseased and between inflamed and non-inflamed joints. Ann Rheum Dis 50:214-218, 1991.

34. Terkeltaub R: Physiologic and pathologic functions of the NPP nucleotide pyrophosphatase/phosphodiesterase family focusing on NPP1 in calcification. Purinergic Signaling 2:371-377, 2006.

35. Tokumura A, Majima E, Kariya Y, et al: Identification of human plasma lysophospholipase D, a lysophosphatidic acid-producing enzyme, as autotaxin, a multifunctional phosphodiesterase. J Biol Chem 277: 39436-39442, 2002.

36. Lotz M, Rosen F, McCabe G, et al: Interleukin 1 beta suppresses transforming growth factor-induced inorganic pyrophosphate [PP_i] production and expression of the PP_i-generating enzyme PC-1 in human chondrocytes. Proc Natl Acad Sci U S A 92:10364-10368, 1995.

37. Johnson K, Hashimoto S, Lotz M, et al: IL-1 induces pro-mineralizing activity of cartilage tissue transglutaminase and factor XIIIa. Am J Pathol 159:149-163, 2001.

38. Olmez U, Ryan LM, Kurup IV, et al: Insulin-like growth factor-1 suppresses pyrophosphate elaboration by transforming growth factor beta1-stimulated chondrocytes and cartilage. Osteoarthritis Cartilage 2:149-154, 1994.

39. Johnson K, Farley D, Hu S-I, et al: One of two chondrocyte-expressed isoforms of cartilage intermediate layer protein functions as an IGF-I antagonist. Arthritis Rheum 48:1302-1314, 2003.

40. Lorenzo P, Bayliss MT, Heinegard D: A novel cartilage protein (CILP) present in the mid-zone of human articular cartilage increases with age. J Biol Chem 273:23463-23468, 1998.

41. Jones AC, Chuck AJ, Arie EA, et al: Diseases associated with calcium pyrophosphate deposition disease. Semin Arthritis Rheum 22: 188-202, 1992.

42. Doherty M, Belcher C, Regan M, et al: Association between synovial fluid levels of inorganic pyrophosphate and short term radiographic outcome of knee osteoarthritis. Ann Rheum Dis 55:432-436, 1996.

43. Burton DW, Foster M, Johnson KA, et al: Chondrocyte calcium-sensing receptor expression is up-regulated in early guinea pig knee osteoarthritis and modulates PTHrP, MMP-13, and TIMP-3 expression. Osteoarthritis Cartilage 13:5395-5404, 2005.

44. Terkeltaub R, Lotz M, Johnson K, et al: Parathyroid hormone related protein (PTHrP) expression is abundant in osteoarthritic cartilage, and the PTHrP 1-173 isoform is selectively induced by TGFβ in articular chondrocytes, and suppresses extracellular inorganic pyrophosphate generation. Arthritis Rheum 41:2152-2164, 1998.

45. Goomer R, Johnson K, Burton D, et al: A tetrabasic C-terminal motif determines intracrine regulatory effects of PTHrP 1-173 on PP_i metabolism and collagen synthesis in chondrocytes. Endocrinology 141:4613-4622, 2000.

46. Pons-Estel BA, Gimenez C, Sacnun M, et al: Familial osteoarthritis and Milwaukee shoulder associated with calcium pyrophosphate and apatite crystal deposition. J Rheumatol 27:471-480, 2000.

47. Reginato AJ, Passano GM, Neumann G, et al: Familial spondyloepiphyseal dysplasia tarda, brachydactyly, and precocious osteoarthritis associated with an arginine 75→cysteine mutation in the procollagen type II gene in a kindred of Chiloe Islanders. I. Clinical, radiographic, and pathologic findings. Arthritis Rheum 37:1078-1086, 1994.

48. Bruges-Armas J, Couto AR, et al: Ectopic calcification among families in the Azores: Clinical and radiologic manifestations in families with diffuse idiopathic skeletal hyperostosis and chondrocalcinosis. Arthritis Rheum 54:1340-1349, 2006.

49. Baldwin CT, Farrer LA, Adair R, et al: Linkage of early-onset osteoarthritis and chondrocalcinosis to human chromosome 8q. Am J Hum Genet 56:692-697, 1995.

50. Andrew LJ, Brancolini V, Serrano de la Pena L, et al: Refinement of the chromosome 5p locus for familial calcium pyrophosphate dihydrate deposition disease. Am J Hum Genet 64:136-145, 1999.

51. Williams CJ, Pendleton A, Bonavita G, et al: Mutations in the amino terminus of ANKH in two US families with calcium pyrophosphate dihydrate crystal deposition disease. Arthritis Rheum 48:2627-2631, 2003.

52. Pendleton A, Johnson MD, Hughes A, et al: Mutations in ANKH cause chondrocalcinosis. Am J Hum Genet 71:933-940, 2002.

53. Williams JC, Zhang Y, Timms A, et al: Autosomal dominant familial calcium pyrophosphate dihydrate deposition disease is caused by mutation in the transmembrane protein ANKH. Am J Hum Genet 71:985-991, 2002.

54. Gurley KA, Reimer RJ, Kingsley DM: Biochemical and genetic analysis of ANK in arthritis and bone disease. Am J Hum Genet 79: 1017-1029, 2006.

55. Nurnberg P, Thiele H, Chandler D, et al: Heterozygous mutations in ANKH, the human ortholog of the mouse progressive ankylosis gene, result in craniometaphyseal dysplasia. Nat Genet 28:37-41, 2001.

56. Zhang Y, Johnson K, Russell RG, et al: Association of sporadic chondrocalcinosis with a 4-basepair G-to-A transition in the 5'-untranslated region of ANKH that promotes enhanced expression of ANKH protein and excess generation of extracellular inorganic pyrophosphate. Arthritis Rheum 52:1110-1117, 2005.

57. Lust G, Faure G, Netter P, et al: Increased pyrophosphate in fibroblasts and lymphoblasts from patients with hereditary diffuse articular chondrocalcinosis. Science 214:809-810, 1981.

58. Kirsch T, Swoboda B, Nah H: Activation of annexin II and V expression, terminal differentiation, mineralization and apoptosis in human osteoarthritic cartilage. Osteoarthritis Cartilage 8:294-302, 2000.

59. Masuda I., Ishikawa K., Usuku G.: A histologic and immunohistochemical study of calcium pyrophosphate dihydrate crystal deposition disease. Clin Orthop 263:272-287, 1991.

60. Johnson K, Van Etten D, Nanda N, et al: Distinct transglutaminase II/TG2-independent and TG2-dependent pathways mediate articular chondrocyte hypertrophy. J Biol Chem 278:18824-18832, 2003.

61. Kirsch T, Nah HD, Shapiro IM, et al: Regulated production of mineralization competent matrix vesicles in hypertrophic chondrocytes. J Cell Biol 137:1149-1160, 1997.

62. Serra R, Johnson M, Filvaroff EH, et al: Expression of a truncated, kinase-defective TGF-beta type II receptor in mouse skeletal tissue promotes terminal chondrocyte differentiation and osteoarthritis. J Cell Biol 139:541-552, 1997.

63. Cecil DL, Rose DM, Terkeltaub R, et al: Role of interleukin-8 in PiT-1 expression and CXCR1-mediated inorganic phosphate uptake in chondrocytes. Arthritis Rheum 52:144-154, 2005; erratum in Arthritis Rheum 54:2320, 2006.

64. Wang W, Xu J, Du B, et al: Role of the progressive ankylosis gene (ANK) in cartilage mineralization. Mol Cell Biol 25:312-323, 2005.

65. Adams CS, Shapiro IM: The fate of the terminally differentiated chondrocyte: Evidence for microenvironmental regulation of chondrocyte apoptosis. Crit Rev Oral Biol Med 13:465-473, 2002.

66. Hashimoto S, Ochs RL, Rosen F, et al: Chondrocyte-derived apoptotic bodies and calcification of articular cartilage. Proc Natl Acad Sci U S A 95:3094-3099, 1998.

67. Cheung HS, Ryan LM: Phosphocitrate blocks nitric oxide-induced calcification of cartilage and chondrocyte-derived apoptotic bodies. Osteoarthritis Cartilage 7:409-412, 1999.

68. Kirsch T, Wang W, Pfander D: Functional differences between growth plate apoptotic bodies and matrix vesicles. J Bone Miner Res 18:1872-1881, 2003.

69. Terkeltaub R, Johnson K, Murphy A, et al: The mitochondrion in osteoarthritis. Mitochondrion 1:301-319, 2002.

70. Johnson K, Svensson CI, Etten DV, et al: Mediation of spontaneous knee osteoarthritis by progressive chondrocyte ATP depletion in Hartley guinea pigs. Arthritis Rheum 50:1216-1225, 2004.

71. Merz D, Liu R, Johnson K, et al: IL-8/CXCL8 and growth-related oncogene alpha/CXCL1 induce chondrocyte hypertrophic differentiation. J Immunol 171:4406-4415, 2003.

72. Johnson KA, Terkeltaub RA: External GTP-bound transglutaminase 2 is a molecular switch for chondrocyte hypertrophic differentiation and calcification. J Biol Chem 280:15004-15012, 2005.

73. Rosenthal AK, Gohr CM, Henry LA, et al: Participation of transglutaminase in the activation of latent transforming growth factor beta1 in aging articular cartilage. Arthritis Rheum 43:1729-1733, 2000.

74. Cecil DL, Johnson K, Rediske J, et al: Inflammation-induced chondrocyte hypertrophy is driven by receptor for advanced glycation end products. J Immunol 175:8296-8302, 2005.

75. Loeser RF, Yammani RR, Carlson CS, et al: Articular chondrocytes express the receptor for advanced glycation end products: Potential role in osteoarthritis. Arthritis Rheum 52:2376-2385, 2005.

76. Johnson K, Jung AS, Andreyev A, et al: Mitochondrial oxidative phosphorylation is a downstream regulator of nitric oxide effects on chondrocyte matrix synthesis and mineralization. Arthritis Rheum 43:1560-1570, 2000.

77. Rachow JW, Ryan LM, McCarty DJ, et al: Synovial fluid inorganic pyrophosphate concentration and nucleotide pyrophosphohydrolase activity in basic calcium phosphate deposition arthropathy and Milwaukee shoulder syndrome. Arthritis Rheum 31:408-413, 1988.

78. Sano H, Ishii H, Trudel G, et al: Histologic evidence of degeneration at the insertion of 3 rotator cuff tendons: A comparative study with human cadaveric shoulders. J Shoulder Elbow Surg 8:574-579, 1999.

79. Takeuchi E, Sugamoto K, Nakase T, et al: Localization and expression of osteopontin in the rotator cuff tendons in patients with calcifying tendinitis. Virchows Arch 438:612-617, 2001.

80. Nakase T, Takeuchi E, Sugamoto K, et al: Involvement of multinucleated giant cells synthesizing cathepsin K in calcified tendinitis of the rotator cuff tendons. Rheumatology (Oxford) 39:1074-1077, 2000.

81. Liu R, O'Connell M, Johnson K, et al: Extracellular signal-regulated kinase 1/extracellular signal-regulated kinase 2 mitogen-activated protein kinase signaling and activation of activator protein 1 and nuclear factor kappaB transcription factors play central roles in interleukin-8 expression stimulated by monosodium urate monohydrate and calcium pyrophosphate crystals in monocytic cells. Arthritis Rheum 43:1145-1155, 2000.

82. Morgan MP, McCarthy GM: Signaling mechanisms involved in crystal-induced tissue damage. Curr Opin Rheumatol 14:292-297, 2002.

83. Sun Y, Wenger L, Brinckerhoff CE, et al: Basic calcium phosphate crystals induce matrix metalloproteinase-1 through the Ras/mitogen-activated protein kinase/c-Fos/AP-1/metalloproteinase 1 pathway: Involvement of transcription factor binding sites AP-1 and PEA-3. J Biol Chem 277:1544-1552, 2002.

84. Liu-Bryan R, Pritzker K, Firestein GS, et al: TLR2 signaling in chondrocytes drives calcium pyrophosphate dihydrate and monosodium urate crystal-induced nitric oxide generation. J Immunol 174:5016-5023, 2005.

85. Martinon F, Petrilli V, Mayor A, et al: Gout-associated uric acid crystals activate the NALP3 inflammasome. Nature 440:237-241, 2006.

86. Cronstein BN, Molad Y, Reibman J, et al: Colchicine alters the quantitative and qualitative display of selectins on endothelial cells and neutrophils. J Clin Invest 96:994-1002, 1995.

87. Terkeltaub R, Baird S, Sears P, et al: The murine homolog of the interleukin-8 receptor CXCR-2 is essential for the occurrence of neutrophilic inflammation in the air pouch model of acute urate crystal-induced gouty synovitis. Arthritis Rheum 41:900-909, 1998.

88. Halverson PB, Carrera GF, McCarty DJ: Milwaukee shoulder syndrome: Fifteen additional cases and a description of contributing factors. Arch Intern Med 150:677-682, 1990.

89. Carroll GJ, Stuart RA, Armstrong JA, et al: Hydroxyapatite crystals are a frequent finding in osteoarthritic synovial fluid, but are not related to increased concentrations of keratan sulfate or interleukin 1 beta. J Rheumatol 18:861-866, 1991.

90. Alwan WH, Dieppe PA, Elson CJ, et al: Hydroxyapatite and urate crystal induced cytokine release by macrophages. Ann Rheum Dis 48:476-482, 1989.

91. Di Giovine FS, Malawista SE, Nuki G, et al: Interleukin 1 (IL 1) as a mediator of crystal arthritis: Stimulation of T cell and synovial fibroblast mitogenesis by urate crystal-induced IL 1. J Immunol 138:3213-3218, 1987.

92. Chaisson CE, McAlindon TE, Felson DT, et al: Lack of association between thyroid status and chondrocalcinosis or osteoarthritis: The Framingham Osteoarthritis Study. J Rheumatol 23:711-715, 1996.

93. Job-Deslandre C, Menkes CJ, Guinot M, et al: Does hypothyroidism increase the prevalence of chondrocalcinosis? Br J Rheumatol 32:197-198, 1993.

94. Benito-Lopez P, Ramos-Rolon G, Ysamat-Marfa R, et al: Pseudogout caused by thyroid hormone replacement therapy. Rev Clin Esp 163:349-350, 1981.

95. Canhao H, Fonseca JE, Leandro MJ, et al: Cross-sectional study of 50 patients with calcium pyrophosphate dihydrate crystal arthropathy. Clin Rheumatol 20:119-122, 2001.

96. Stevens LW, Spiera H: Hemarthrosis in chondrocalcinosis (pseudogout). Arthritis Rheum 15:651-653, 1972.

97. Disla E, Infante R, Fahmy A, et al: Recurrent acute calcium pyrophosphate dihydrate arthritis following intraarticular hyaluronate injection. Arthritis Rheum 42:1302-1303, 1999.

98. Bernardeau C, Bucki B, Liote F: Acute arthritis after intra-articular hyaluronate injection: Onset of effusions without crystals. Ann Rheum Dis 60:518-520, 2000.

99. Kroesen S, Schmid W, Theiler R: Induction of an acute attack of calcium pyrophosphate dihydrate arthritis by intra-articular injection of hylan G-F 20. Clin Rheumatol 19:147-149, 2000.

100. Fujii K, Tanaka Y, Hubscher S, et al: Crosslinking of CD44 on rheumatoid synovial cells augment interleukin 6 production. Lab Invest 79:1439-1446, 1999.

101. Mikecz K, Dennis K, Shi M, et al: Modulation of hyaluronan receptor (CD44) function in vivo in a murine model of rheumatoid arthritis. Arthritis Rheum 42:659-668, 1999.

102. Sandor V, Hassan R, Kohn E: Exacerbation of pseudogout by granulocyte colony-stimulating factor. Ann Intern Med 125:781, 1996.

103. Malnick SD, Ariel-Ronen S, Evron E, et al: Acute pseudogout as a complication of pamidronate. Ann Pharmacother 31:499-500, 1997.

104. Gallacher SJ, Boyle IT, Capell HA: Pseudogout associated with the use of cyclical etidronate therapy. Scott Med J 36:49, 1991.

105. Mavrikakis ME, Antoniades LG, Kontoyannis SA, et al: CPPD crystal deposition disease as a cause of unrecognised pyrexia. Clin Exp Rheumatol 12:419-421, 1994.

106. Reuge L, Lindhoudt DV, Geerster J: Local deposition of calcium pyrophosphate crystals in evolution of knee osteoarthritis. Clin Rheumatol 20:428-431, 2001.

107. Derfus BA, Kurian JB, Butler JJ, et al: The high prevalence of pathologic calcium crystals in pre-operative knees. J Rheumatol 29:570-574, 2002.

108. Doherty M, Dieppe P, Watt I: Pyrophosphate arthropathy: A prospective study. Br J Rheumatol 32:189-196, 1993.

109. Yamakawa K, Iwasaki H, Ohjimi Y, et al: Tumoral calcium pyrophosphate dihydrate crystal deposition disease. Pathology 197:499-506, 2001.

110. Kwak SM, Resnick D, Haghighi P: Calcium pyrophosphate dihydrate crystal deposition disease of the knee simulating spontaneous osteonecrosis. Clin Rheumatol 18:390-393, 1999.

111. el Maghraoui A, Lecoules S, Lechavalier D, et al: Acute sacroiliitis as a manifestation of calcium pyrophosphate dihydrate crystal deposition disease. Clin Exp Rheumatol 17:477-478, 1999.

112. Fujishiro T, Nabeshima Y, Yasui S, et al: Pseudogout attack of the lumbar facet joint: A case report. Spine 27:396-398, 2002.

113. Pascal-Moussellard H, Cabre P, Smadja D, et al: Myelopathy due to calcification of the cervical ligamenta flava: A report of two cases in French West Indian patients. Euro Spine J 8:238-240, 1999.

114. Cabre P, Pascal-Moussellard H, Kaidomar S, et al: Six cases of ligamentum cervical flavum calcification in blacks in the French West Indies. Joint Bone Spine 68:158-165, 2001.

115. Assaker R, Louis E, Boutry N, et al: Foramen magnum syndrome secondary to calcium pyrophosphate crystal deposition in the transverse ligament of atlas. Spine 26:1396-1400, 2001.

116. Kakitsubata Y, Boutin RD, Theodorou DJ, et al: Calcium pyrophosphate dihydrate crystal deposition in and around the atlantoaxial joints: Association with type 2 odontoid fractures in nine patients. Radiology 216:213-219, 2000.

117. Balsa A, Martin-Mola E, Gonzalez T, et al: Familial articular chondrocalcinosis in Spain. Ann Rheum Dis 49:531-535, 1990.

118. Doherty M, Hamilton E, Henderson J, et al: Familial chondrocalcinosis due to calcium pyrophosphate dihydrate crystal deposition in English families. Br J Rheumatol 30:10-15, 1991.

119. Schumacher HR, Smolyo AP, Tse RL, et al: Arthritis associated with apatite crystals. Ann Intern Med 87:411-416, 1977.

120. Fam AG, Rubenstein J: Hydroxyapatite pseudopodagra: A syndrome of young women. Arthritis Rheum 32:741-747, 1989.

121. Grinlinton FM, Vuletic JC, Gow PJ: Rapidly progressive calcific periarthritis occurring in a patient with lupus nephritis receiving chronic ambulatory peritoneal dialysis. J Rheumatol 17:1100-1103, 1990.

122. Ferrari AJ, Rothfuss S, Schumacher HR Jr: Dialysis arthropathy: Identification and evaluation of a subset of patients with unexplained inflammatory effusions. J Rheumatol 24:1780-1786, 1997.

123. Braunstein EM, Menerey K, Martel W, et al: Radiologic features of a pyrophosphate-like arthropathy associated with long-term dialysis. Skeletal Radiol 16:437-441, 1987.

124. ter Borg EJ, Eggelmijer F, Jaspers PJ, et al: Milwaukee shoulder associated with primary hyperparathyroidism. J Rheumatol 22:561-562, 1995.

125. Fam AG, Pritzker KP: Acute calcific periarthritis in scleroderma. J Rheumatol 19:1580-1585, 1992.

126. Halverson PB, Carrera GF, McCarty DJ: Milwaukee shoulder syndrome: Fifteen additional cases and a description of contributing factors. Arch Intern Med 150:677-682, 1990.

127. Doherty M, Holt M, MacMillan P: A reappraisal of "analgesic hip." Ann Rheum Dis 45:272-276, 1986.

128. Paul H, Reginato AJ, Schumacher HR: Alizarin red S staining as a screening test to detect calcium compounds in synovial fluid. Arthritis Rheum 26:191-200, 1983.

129. van Linthoudt D, Beutler A, Clayburne G, et al: Morphometric studies on synovium in advanced osteoarthritis: Is there an association between apatite-like material and collagen deposits? Clin Exp Rheumatol 15:493-497, 1997.

130. Li-Yu J, Clayburne GM, Sieck MS, et al: Calcium apatite crystals in synovial fluid rice bodies. Ann Rheum Dis 61:387-390, 2002.

131. Ivorra J, Rosas J, Pascual E: Most calcium pyrophosphate crystals appear as non-birefringent. Ann Rheum Dis 58:582-584, 1999.

132. Keen CE, Crocker PR, Brady K, et al: Intraosseous secondary calcium salt crystal deposition: An artefact of acid decalcification. Histopathology 27:181-185, 1995.

133. Steinbach LS, Resnick D: Calcium pyrophosphate dihydrate crystal deposition disease: Imaging perspective. Curr Probl Diagn Radiol 29:209-229, 2000.

134. Hatzis N, Kaar TK, Wirth MA, et al: Neuropathic arthropathy of the shoulder. J Bone Joint Surg Am 80:1314-1319, 1998.

135. Maldonado I, Prasad V, Reginato AJ: Oxalate crystal deposition disease. Curr Rheumatol Rep 4:257-264, 2002.

136. Fisseler-Eckhoff A, Muller KM: Arthroscopy and chondrocalcinosis. Arthroscopy 8:98-104, 1992.

137. Sofka CM, Adler RS, Cordasko FA: Ultrasound diagnosis of chondrocalcinosis in the knee. Skeletal Radiol 31:43-45, 2002.

138. Foldes K: Knee chondrocalcinosis: An ultrasonographic study of the hyaline cartilage. J Clin Imaging 26:194-196, 2002.

139. Abreu M, Johnson K, Chung CB, et al: Calcification in calcium pyrophosphate dihydrate (CPPD) crystalline deposits in the knee: Anatomic, radiographic, MR imaging, and histologic study in cadavers. Skeletal Radiol 33:392-398, 2004.

140. Galvez J, Saiz E, Linares LF, et al: Delayed examination of synovial fluid by ordinary and polarized light microscopy to detect and identify crystals. Ann Rheum Dis 61:444-447, 2002.

141. Petrocelli A, Wong AL, Sweezy RL: Identification of pathologic synovial fluid crystals on Gram stains. J Clin Rheumatol 4:103-105, 1998.

142. Selvi E, Manganelli S, Catenaccio M, et al: Diff Quik staining method for detection and identification of monosodium urate and calcium pyrophosphate crystals in synovial fluids. Ann Rheum Dis 60:194-198, 2001.

143. Ohira T, Ishikawa K: Preservation of calcium pyrophosphate dihydrate crystals: Effect of Mayer's haematoxylin staining period. Ann Rheum Dis 60:80-82, 2001.

144. Smilde TJ, Haverman JF, Schipper P, et al: Familial hypokalemia/hypomagnesemia and chondrocalcinosis. J Rheumatol 21:1515-1519, 1994.

145. Ritter J, Kerr LD, Valeriano-Marcet J, et al: ACTH revisited: Effective treatment for acute crystal induced synovitis in patients with multiple medical problems. J Rheumatol 21:696-699, 1994.

146. Roane DW, Harris MD, Carpenter MT, et al: Prospective use of intramuscular triamcinolone acetonide in pseudogout. J Rheumatol 24:1168-1170, 1997.

147. Rothschild B, Yakubov LE: Prospective 6-month, double-blind trial of hydroxychloroquine treatment of CPPD. Compr Ther 23:327-331, 1997.

148. Chollet-Janin A, Finckh A, Dudler J, et al: Methotrexate as an alternative therapy for chronic calcium pyrophosphate deposition disease: An exploratory analysis. Arthritis Rheum 56:688-692, 2007.

149. Kalunian KC, Ike RW, Seeger LL, et al: Visually-guided irrigation in patients with early knee osteoarthritis: A multicenter randomized, controlled trial. Osteoarthritis Cartilage 8:412-418, 2000.

150. Das SK, Mishra K, Ramakrishnan S, et al: A randomized controlled trial to evaluate the slow-acting symptom modifying effects of a regimen containing colchicine in a subset of patients with osteoarthritis of the knee. Osteoarthritis Cartilage 10:247-252, 2002.

151. Das SK, Ramakrishnan S, Mishra K, et al: A randomized controlled trial to evaluate the slow-acting symptom modifying effects of colchicine in osteoarthritis of the knee: A preliminary report. Arthritis Care Res 47:280-284, 2002.

152. Farin PU, Rasenen H, Jaroma H, et al: Rotator cuff calcifications: Treatment with ultrasound-guided percutaneous needle aspiration and lavage. Skeletal Radiol 25:551-554, 1996.

153. Ebenbicher G, Erdogmus C, Resch K, et al: Ultrasound therapy for calcific tendonitis of the shoulder. N Engl J Med 340:1533-1538, 1999.

154. Bilezikian P, Meng X, Shi Y, et al: Primary hyperparathyroidism in women: A tale of two cities—New York and Beijing. Int J Fertil Womens Med 45:158-165, 2000.

155. Rosenthal AK, Ryan LM: Probenecid inhibits transforming growth factor-beta 1 induced pyrophosphate elaboration by chondrocytes. J Rheumatol 21:896-900, 1994.

156. Cini R, Chindamo D, Catenaccio M, et al: Dissolution of calcium pyrophosphate crystals by polyphosphates: An in vitro and ex vivo study. Ann Rheum Dis 60:962-967, 2001.

157. Shinozaki T, Pritzker KP: Polyamines enhance calcium pyrophosphate dihydrate crystal dissolution. J Rheumatol 22:1907-1912, 1995.

158. Bennett RM, Lehr JR, McCarty DJ: Crystal shedding and acute pseudogout: An hypothesis based on a therapeutic failure. Arthritis Rheum 19:93-97, 1976.

159. Cheung HS: Phosphocitrate as a potential therapeutic strategy for crystal deposition disease. Curr Rheumatol Rep 3:24-28, 2001.

160. Nair D, Misra RP, Sallis JD, et al: Phosphocitrate inhibits a basic calcium phosphate and calcium pyrophosphate dihydrate crystal-induced mitogen-activated protein kinase cascade signal transduction pathway. J Biol Chem 272:18920-18925, 1997.

161. Krug HE, Mahowald ML, Halverson PB, et al: Phosphocitrate prevents disease progression in murine progressive ankylosis. Arthritis Rheum 36:1603-1611, 1993.

162. Cheung HS, Sallis JD, Demadis KD, et al: Phosphocitrate blocks calcification-induced articular joint degeneration in a guinea pig model. Arthritis Rheum 54:2452-2461, 2006.

163. Hashiba H, Aizawa S, Tamura K, et al: Inhibitory effects of etidronate on the progression of vascular calcification in hemodialysis patients. Ther Apher Dial 8:241-247, 2004.

164. Grandjean-Laquerriere A, Tabary O, Jacquot J, et al: Involvement of Toll-like receptor 4 in the inflammatory reaction induced by hydroxyapatite particles. Biomaterials 28:400-404, 2007.

165. Neogi T, Nevitt M, Niu J, et al: Lack of association between chondrocalcinosis and increased risk of cartilage loss in knees with osteoarthritis: Results of two prospective longitudinal magnetic resonance imaging studies. Arthritis Rheum 54:1822-1828, 2006.

166. Viriyavejkul P, Wilairatana V, Tanavalee A, et al: Comparison of characteristics of patients with and without calcium pyrophosphate dihydrate crystal deposition disease who underwent total knee replacement surgery for osteoarthritis. Osteoarthritis Cartilage 13:232-235, 2006.

Web Sites

Familial Chondrocalcinosis Recruitment Page for Wellcome Trust Centre for Human Genetics: http://www.well.ox.ac.uk/brown/chondro.shtml.

Teaching resource page for radiographic images of BCP and CPPD arthropathies: http://www.orthopaedicweblinks.com/Teaching_Resources/Radiology/more3.html.

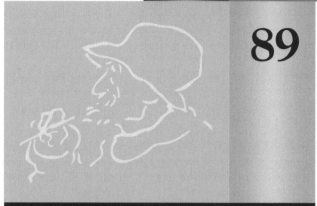

89

Pathogenesis of Osteoarthritis

PAUL E. DI CESARE •
STEVEN B. ABRAMSON •
JONATHAN SAMUELS

KEY POINTS

Osteoarthritis is a degenerative joint disease, occurring primarily in older individuals, characterized by erosion of the articular cartilage, hypertrophy of bone at the margins (i.e., osteophytes), subchondral sclerosis, and a range of biochemical and morphologic alterations of the synovial membrane and joint capsule.

Risk factors for developing osteoarthritis include age, joint location, obesity, genetic predisposition, joint malalignment, trauma, and gender.

Morphologic changes in early osteoarthritis include articular cartilage surface irregularity, superficial clefts within the tissue, and altered proteoglycan distribution.

Morphologic changes in late osteoarthritis include deepened clefts, increase in surface irregularities, and eventual articular cartilage ulceration, exposing the underlying bone. Chondrocytes form clusters or clones in an attempt at self-repair. Marginal osteophytes form.

The matrix metalloproteinase family of proteinases degrade proteoglycans (aggrecanases) and collagen (collagenases).

A suboptimal repair response of normal articular cartilage to injury typically results in secondary osteoarthritis.

Chondrocytes can sense and respond to mechanical and physicochemical stimuli via several regulatory pathways.

Mediators classically associated with inflammation during the course of osteoarthritis include interleukin-1β and tumor necrosis factor-α.

Nitric oxide, produced by the inducible isoform of nitric oxide synthase, is a major catabolic factor produced by chondrocytes in response to proinflammatory cytokines.

The expression of inducible cyclooxygenase-2 is increased in osteoarthritis chondrocytes.

Low-grade inflammatory processes occur in osteoarthritic synovial tissues and contribute to disease pathogenesis.

Several biomarkers have been correlated with osteoarthritis.

Most current treatments aim to improve the signs and symptoms of osteoarthritis.

Osteoarthritis is a degenerative joint disease that occurs primarily in older individuals and is characterized by erosion of the articular cartilage, hypertrophy of bone at the margins (i.e., osteophytes), subchondral sclerosis, and a range of biochemical and morphologic alterations of the synovial membrane and joint capsule. Pathologic changes in the late stages of osteoarthritis include softening, ulceration, and focal disintegration of the articular cartilage. Secondary synovial inflammation also may occur. Typical clinical symptoms are pain and stiffness, particularly after prolonged activity.

In industrialized societies, osteoarthritis is the leading cause of physical disability, increases in health care usage, and impaired quality of life. The impact of arthritic conditions is expected to grow as the population increases and ages in the coming decades.[1] Despite its prevalence, the precise etiology, pathogenesis, and reasons for progression of osteoarthritis are not understood, primarily owing to confounding factors in human epidemiologic studies, which include individual variations in physical activity, diet, and medical history; the poor correlation between symptoms of osteoarthritis and radiographic lesions; and the inability to detect early disease. The arthritic human tissue that is subjected to study typically is obtained at surgery from patients with severe osteoarthritis and does not exhibit the features that occur early in the disease process. Many studies focus on a single tissue type from affected or at-risk joints and lack general relevance. Without a clear-cut picture of how osteoarthritis arises at the cellular or molecular level, many clinicians still consider it a result of "wear and tear"—an inevitable consequence of aging.

Although the etiology of osteoarthritis is incompletely understood, the accompanying biochemical, structural, and metabolic changes in joint cartilage have been well documented. It is now known that cytokines, mechanical trauma, and altered genetics are involved in its pathogenesis, and that these factors can initiate a degradative cascade that results in many of the characteristic alterations of articular cartilage in osteoarthritis. More recently, it has become apparent that osteoarthritis is a disease process that affects the entire joint structure, including cartilage, synovial membrane, subchondral bone, ligaments, and periarticular muscles. Osteoarthritis is better thought of as a group of overlapping disorders, of various etiologies and arising from a combination of systemic factors (e.g., genetics) and local factors (e.g., biomechanically or biochemically mediated events), which gradually converge to produce a condition with definable morphologic and clinical outcomes.[2]

Osteoarthritis may be classified as primary or secondary according to its cause or major predisposing factor; both types have in common altered cartilage physiology. Primary osteoarthritis is the most common type and has no identifiable etiology or predisposing cause. Secondary osteoarthritis, although it has an identifiable underlying cause, is pathologically indistinguishable from primary osteoarthritis. The most common causes of secondary osteoarthritis are metabolic conditions (e.g., calcium crystal deposition, hemochromatosis, acromegaly), anatomic factors (e.g., leg-length inequality, developmental hip dislocation), traumatic events (e.g., major joint trauma, chronic joint injury, joint surgery), or the sequelae of inflammatory disorders (e.g., ankylosing spondylitis, septic arthritis). In cases of secondary osteoarthritis arising from inflammatory joint disease, cartilage degeneration most likely results initially from degradative enzymes released from the synovium or leukocytes within the joint space, and later from the mechanical attrition of a biomechanically altered extracellular matrix. Distinguishing between primary and secondary osteoarthritis may be difficult because the clinical presentation and symptoms are often similar.

ETIOLOGIC FACTORS IN OSTEOARTHRITIS

Major factors that affect the degree of risk for developing osteoarthritis include age, joint location, obesity, genetic predisposition, joint malalignment, trauma, and gender.

AGE

Age is the risk factor most strongly correlated with osteoarthritis.[3,4] Osteoarthritis is the most common chronic disease that develops in later life. More than 80% of individuals older than 75 years are affected, and osteoarthritis increases progressively with age at all joint sites. Radiologic changes of osteoarthritis increase as individuals age,[5] although these changes do not always correlate with clinical symptoms or disability.[6,7] Although an age-related disease, osteoarthritis is not an inevitable consequence of aging.

Age-related morphologic and structural changes in articular cartilage include fraying, softening, and thinning of the articular surface; decreased size and aggregation of matrix proteoglycans; and loss of matrix tensile strength and stiffness. These age-related tissue changes are most often caused by a decrease in chondrocytes' ability to maintain and repair the tissue, as chondrocytes themselves undergo age-related decreases in mitotic and synthetic activity, exhibit decreased responsiveness to anabolic growth factors, and synthesize smaller and less uniform large aggregating proteoglycans and fewer functional link proteins. Cultured chondrocytes have been shown to exhibit an age-related decline in response to insulin-like growth factor (IGF)-I, a growth factor that stimulates the production of proteoglycans, collagen, and integrin cell receptors. Progressive chondrocyte senescence (as reflected in expression of the senescence-associated enzyme β-galactosidase), erosion of chondrocyte telomere length, and mitochondrial degeneration secondary to oxidative damage also contribute to the age-related reduction in chondrocyte function.[3]

There also seems to be a direct correlation between chondrocyte apoptosis and cartilage degradation leading to osteoarthritis. Age seems to be an independent factor that predisposes articular chondrocytes to apoptosis because the expression levels of specific proapoptotic genes (Fas, Fas ligand, caspase-8, and p53) is higher in aged cartilage.[8,9]

JOINT LOCATION

Although osteoarthritis occurs most commonly in weight-bearing joints,[10] age affects joints differentially.[11] A study comparing tensile fracture stress of cartilage in the femoral head and in the talus showed that it decreased progressively with age in the former, but not in the latter.[12] Joint-specific, age-related viability in articular cartilage may explain why osteoarthritis is more common in hip and knee joints with increasing age, but occurs rarely in the ankle. Alterations in chondrocyte responsiveness to cytokines also seem to vary depending on the joint. Studies show that knee joint chondrocytes exhibit more interleukin (IL)-1 receptors than ankle joint chondrocytes, and that knee chondrocytes express mRNA for matrix metalloproteinase (MMP)-8, whereas ankle chondrocytes do not.[13-15]

OBESITY

Obesity is another important risk factor for osteoarthritis.[16-18] Greater body mass index in women and men has been shown to be associated with an increased risk of knee, but not hip, osteoarthritis.[6,19,20] In a study that examined 715 paired radiographs (index and 4-year follow-up), Hart and colleagues[21] reported that obesity significantly increased the risk of knee symptoms and radiographic osteophytes.

An increase in mechanical forces across weight-bearing joints is probably the primary factor leading to joint degeneration. Obesity not only increases the forces at weight-bearing joints, but also may change posture, gait, and physical activity level, any or all of which may contribute further to altered joint biomechanics.[22] Most obese patients, particularly women, exhibit varus knee deformities that result in increased joint reactive forces in the medial compartment of the knee, accelerating the degenerative process.[23]

Particularly in elderly obese individuals, heavy physical activity is an additional risk factor for the development of knee osteoarthritis, whereas light-to-moderate activity does not seem to increase risk for knee osteoarthritis and may alleviate symptomatic knee osteoarthritis by reducing body mass index.[6,19,20] Similarly, weight loss can reduce radiographic knee osteoarthritis progression and clinical symptoms. More recent evidence indicates that in obese patients with osteoarthritis, significant weight loss dramatically improves functional status, with short-term results equivalent to the results of patients who have undergone joint replacement.[24]

The discovery of the "obesity gene" and its product leptin may have important implications for the onset and progression of osteoarthritis and increase understanding of the link between obesity and osteoarthritis. The fact that women have a greater proportion of total body fat and higher levels of adipose-derived systemic leptin concentrations than men may partially account for the gender disparity in osteoarthritis patients. Leptin is produced not only by adipose cells, but also by osteoblasts and chondrocytes, however, suggesting that local leptin production may play a role in osteoarthritis. Significant levels of leptin were observed in the cartilage and osteophytes of subjects with osteoarthritis, but in the cartilage of healthy subjects, few chondrocytes produced leptin. Leptin also has been shown to induce anabolic activity in the chondrocytes of rats and ultimately may confer structural joint changes.[25,26] Further work is required to determine whether leptin is an important systemic or local factor in the link between obesity and osteoarthritis.

GENETIC PREDISPOSITION

Because of the prevalence of osteoarthritis in the general population and its extensive clinical heterogeneity, the genetic contribution to its pathogenesis has been difficult to analyze.[27,28] In the 1960s, Kellgren and associates[29] reported that generalized nodal osteoarthritis, characterized by multiple joint involvement, including the presence of Heberden's nodes and knee osteoarthritis, was twice as likely to occur in first-degree relatives as in controls. Population studies of patients with radiographic evidence of osteoarthritis followed in two major cohorts (the Framingham Study and the Baltimore Longitudinal Study on Aging) clearly support a significant genetic contribution to osteoarthritis, with evidence for a major recessive gene and a multifactorial component, representing either polygenic or environmental factors.[30,31]

Twin pair and family risk studies have indicated that the heritable component of osteoarthritis may be 50% to 65%.[28,32,33] Family, twin, and population studies have indicated differences among genetic influences that determine the site of osteoarthritis (hip, spinal, knee, hand).[31,34,35] Further evidence supporting a genetic predisposition to osteoarthritis is the demonstration of a significantly higher concordance for osteoarthritis between monozygotic twins than between dizygotic twins. Genetic studies have identified multiple gene variations associated with an increased risk of osteoarthritis.[36]

Structural genes are important for the maintenance and repair of articular cartilage and for the regulation of chondrocyte proliferation and gene expression. In some cases (e.g., chondrodysplasias), structural genes are the identifiable causes of osteoarthritis. Several candidate genes encoding for structural proteins of the extracellular matrix of the articular cartilage have been associated with early-onset osteoarthritis.[37,38] Although likely of limited importance in most cases of osteoarthritis, the discovery of a point mutation (Arg519Cys in exon 31) in the cDNA coding for type II collagen in several generations of a family with spondyloepiphyseal dysplasia and polyarticular osteoarthritis[37,38] has focused attention on this area.

In addition to the point mutation in type II collagen, which was identified in the family mentioned in the previous paragraph,[38] inherited forms of osteoarthritis may be caused by mutations in several other genes that are expressed in cartilage, including genes encoding types IV, V, and VI collagens and cartilage oligomeric matrix protein (COMP).[39] It was reported more recently that mice deficient in the type IX collagen gene and the matrilin 3 gene (equivalent condition in humans not yet reported) developed age-dependent, osteoarthritis-like changes in the knee and temporal mandibular joints.[40,41] Candidate genes in osteoarthritis have been identified that are not structural proteins. The haplotype of a vitamin D receptor that plays a vital role in controlling bone mineral density seems to be associated with a twofold risk of knee osteoarthritis,[42-44] although the vitamin D receptor locus is very close to the COL2A1 locus on chromosome 12q, and so the association may be due to linkage disequilibrium with the latter.[27]

The locus of the IGF-I gene has been associated with radiographic osteoarthritis, as has an aggrecan polymorphic allele with hand osteoarthritis.[27] Evidence from animal models indicates that disorders characterized by calcium crystal deposition may predispose to osteoarthritis. The defect in the progressive ankylosis (ank) mouse is in a gene that encodes a transmembrane protein that controls levels of inorganic phosphate, an inhibitor of matrix calcification.[45] Analysis of the joints in the ank mouse reveals hydroxyapatite crystals in articular cartilage, with accompanying joint space narrowing, cartilage erosion, and osteophyte formation—all hallmarks of osteoarthritis.

In more recent population studies, genome-wide linkage scans have highlighted seven chromosomal regions that may harbor osteoarthritis susceptibility genes.[46] Chromosome 2q was positive in several scans, suggesting that this chromosome is likely to harbor one or more susceptibility genes. In a study of affected sibling pairs, a region of linkage stretching from 2q12 to 2q21 was reported for osteoarthritis of the distal interphalangeal joint, and a previous study of affected sibling pairs in the United Kingdom showed a broader region of linkage, stretching from 2q12 to 2q31.[46,47] Two IL-1 genes (IL1α and IL1β) and the gene encoding IL-1Ra (IL1RN) are located on chromosome 2q13 within a 430-kb genomic fragment.

Given the importance of IL-1 in the perpetuation of cartilage damage in osteoarthritis, it is possible that a proportion of the genetic susceptibility to osteoarthritis may be encoded for by variation in the activity of ILs, and that for chromosome 2q this susceptibility could reside within the IL-1 gene clusters. Loughlin and colleagues[46] have provided evidence, however, that the IL-1 gene cluster harbors susceptibility for knee osteoarthritis, but not for hip osteoarthritis. These and other epidemiologic studies have highlighted potential differences in the degree of osteoarthritis heritability among different joint groups and between the two sexes.[48]

Genomic and postgenomic technology, in addition to defining susceptibility genotypes, is expected to lead to the discovery of genes and gene products that are overexpressed in osteoarthritis tissues and that contribute to disease pathogenesis and progression.[49-51] Studies of differential gene expression in diseased tissue, in addition to elucidating pathogenic processes that lead to novel therapies, could have two other benefits: (1) identification of unique biomarkers that can be used for osteoarthritis diagnosis or management and (2) identification of candidate susceptibility genotypes, such as polymorphic variations of cytokines or growth factors, which may predispose to disease progression.[52]

JOINT MALALIGNMENT AND TRAUMA

Joint malalignment or trauma may lead to rapid development of osteoarthritis, or it may initiate a slow process that results in symptomatic osteoarthritis years later. Probably as a result of progressive reduction in periarticular blood flow and the resultant decrease in rate of remodeling at the osteochondral junction, joints become increasingly congruent with age.[53,54] Altered joint geometry may interfere with nutrition of the cartilage, or it may alter load distribution, either of which may result in altered biochemical composition of the cartilage, regardless of age.[55,56] Local factors, such as stresses related to joint use and joint deformity, also influence the development of osteoarthritis.

Joint incongruence (e.g., poorly reduced intra-articular fractures, developmental dysplasia of the hip, recurrent dislocation of the patella) can lead to early-onset osteoarthritis.[57] Repetitive, high-impact sports are strongly associated with joint injury and increase the risk for lower limb osteoarthritis.[58,59] Repetitive trauma at a subfracture level has been shown to accelerate remodeling in the zone of calcified cartilage, with reduplication of the tidemark and thinning of the noncalcified zone, resulting in stiffening of the subchondral bone, increased wear of the overlying cartilage, and ultimately development of osteoarthritis.[60] Regular exercise is important in maintaining articular cartilage structure and metabolic function. Recreational running and low-impact activities have not been shown to increase the risk of osteoarthritis in previously normal joints.

Articular cartilage is remarkably resistant to damage by shear forces; it is, however, highly vulnerable to repetitive impact loading.[61] When joints are subjected to in vitro cyclic loads that are easily borne by subchondral bone, cartilage degeneration still results.[62] This vulnerability accounts for the high frequency of osteoarthritis in shoulders and elbows of pneumatic drill operators and baseball pitchers, ankles of ballet dancers, metacarpophalangeal joints of boxers, and knees of basketball players. The risk for knee osteoarthritis among participants in sports may be more closely related to previous knee injury, however, than to participation in sports alone.[63]

The major forces on articular cartilage, in addition to weight bearing, are due to the contraction of the muscles that stabilize or move the joint.[64] In normal walking, 4 to 5 times the body weight may be transmitted through the knee, and in squatting 10 times the body weight may be transmitted.[43] Articular cartilage is believed to be too thin to be an effective shock absorber under these high loads. What protects the joint under physiologic conditions of impact loading is joint motion, with the associated lengthening of muscles under tension and deformation of the subchondral bone.[44,65]

Cancellous subchondral bone functions as a major shock absorber owing to its material properties.[60] Two thirds of subchondral bone stiffness derives from bony trabeculae, and about one third derives from intraosseous fluid.[66] In the normal unloaded joint, the opposing surfaces are not congruous, but under loading, the cartilage and the bone deform so that a larger proportion of the opposing surfaces comes into contact, which increases joint congruity and results in a force distribution over the largest possible area.[67] Excessive loads may cause microfractures of subchondral trabeculae that heal via callus formation and remodeling, resulting in stiffer than normal bone that is less effective as a shock absorber, and predisposing articular cartilage to degeneration.

Whether subchondral sclerosis precedes the onset of osteoarthritis or is a change secondary to cartilage degeneration is unknown. Indirect evidence supports the theory that biomechanical changes in subchondral bone may be important in osteoarthritis.[66,68,69] Foss and Byers[70] reported cases of femoral osteoporosis (which is associated with softening and greater compliance of the subchondral bone) that may have protected the hip from osteoarthritis. Conversely, in vitro studies have shown that stiffening of the cancellous bone with methacrylate, reducing its deformability, leads to cartilage degeneration with repetitive impact loading.[71]

GENDER

Women are about twice as likely as men to develop osteoarthritis. Although women have a lower prevalence of osteoarthritis than men before age 50 years, there is a marked increase in prevalence among women after age 50, particularly in the knee.[72] Radiographic and interview data from the National Health and Nutrition Examination Survey (NHANES III), a representative cross-sectional health examination survey of the U.S. population, reported that the lifetime prevalence of radiographic knee osteoarthritis was 37.4%, and that the prevalence of symptomatic knee osteoarthritis was 12.1% in adults 60 years old and older; prevalence was greater among women than men (42.1% versus 31.2%), and women had significantly more Kellgren-Lawrence grade 3-4 changes (12.9% versus 6.5% in men).[73] Women have a greater number of joints involved and are more likely to exhibit clinical symptoms of morning stiffness, joint swelling, and nocturnal pain.

The gender differences in osteoarthritis incidence after age 50 may be the result of postmenopausal estrogen deficiency. Articular chondrocytes possess functional estrogen receptors (ERs), suggesting that these cells can be regulated by estrogen. Nuclear ERs have been detected in articular chondrocytes of humans,[74,75] rats,[75,76] monkeys,[75,77] and pigs,[78] and in human growth plate chondrocytes.[79] Chondrocytes express two isoforms of ER—ER-α and ER-β—that may have different organ-specific roles; ER-α is expressed more predominantly in cortical bone, and ER-β is expressed more predominantly in cartilage[75] and cancellous bone.[80] One direct effect of estrogen on cultured chondrocytes is upregulation of ER,[77] and an increase in ER has been associated with increased proteoglycan synthesis in rats.[76]

More recent epidemiologic studies have linked estrogen replacement therapy (ERT) with a lower than expected risk of knee and hip osteoarthritis in postmenopausal women. Clinical investigations of the association between osteoarthritis and hormonal level in women have involved measurement of circulating estrogen levels in postmenopausal women, general radiographic evaluation of postmenopausal women, and examination of the effect of ERT on such variables as knee osteoarthritis and cartilage volume.[81-84]

In a study of more than 4000 women 65 years old or older that assessed pelvis radiographs for hip osteoarthritis, Nevitt and colleagues[81] showed that women using oral estrogen were at a significantly reduced risk of hip osteoarthritis. Estrogen users for 10 years or longer had a greater reduction in risk of developing hip osteoarthritis than users for less than 10 years. Zhang and coworkers,[83] using weight-bearing radiographs in female participants in the Framingham Osteoarthritis Study ($N = 831$, mean age 73 years, age range 63 to 93 years) to study the rate of knee osteoarthritis, reported a modest but nonsignificant greater protective effect for radiographically detected osteoarthritis in women who were on ERT. They categorized their sample into three groups according to estrogen use at biennial examination: never-users ($n = 349$), past users ($n = 162$), and current users ($n = 40$). When incident and progressive radiographic knee osteoarthritis cases were combined, current ERT users were found to have 60% less risk for knee osteoarthritis than never-users.

In a cross-sectional study of postmenopausal women from the Chingford Study ($N = 606$) using standard anteroposterior radiographs of hands and knees, ERT was shown to have a significant protective effect against knee osteoarthritis and a similar but not significant effect for hand osteoarthritis.[85] Women who had discontinued ERT for more than 1 year had no overall protective effect of the ERT for osteoarthritis. Wluka and colleagues[84] reported on the longer term use of ERT and its association with knee cartilage volume (measured by magnetic resonance imaging) in postmenopausal women; results showed that after adjusting for confounders, women using long-term ERT had more knee cartilage than controls. Beneficial effects of ERT on the severity of knee osteoarthritis in ovariectomized monkeys also have been shown.[86]

Further clinical evidence of the role of estrogen in osteoarthritis came from a case-control study to determine whether an association exists between ER gene polymorphisms and generalized osteoarthritis.[87] The investigators analyzed 65 women with generalized osteoarthritis and compared them with 318 healthy female controls for the Pvu II and Xba I restriction fragment length polymorphisms of ER gene. The result showed that the ER genotype PpXx, with the combination of the Pvu II and Xba I restriction fragment length polymorphisms, was a significant risk factor for generalized osteoarthritis and was most prevalent in younger patients with severe radiographic changes. Overall, these human and animal studies show that women taking ERT may have a lower incidence of osteoarthritis, although prospective randomized trials to confirm these observations have not been done.

CHANGES IN OSTEOARTHRITIS

MORPHOLOGIC CHANGES

In early osteoarthritis, the articular cartilage surface becomes irregular, and superficial clefts within the tissue become apparent. Proteoglycan distribution is altered, as revealed by histochemical staining. As the condition worsens, the clefts deepen, surface irregularities increase, and the articular cartilage eventually ulcerates, exposing the underlying bone. Attempts at local self-repair can be seen as an initial increase in the number of chondrocytes in the form of clusters or clones, with 50 or more cells in a cluster (Fig. 89-1).[43] Marginal osteophytes form, representing production of new bone capped by newly formed, irregularly shaped hyaline and fibrocartilage.

BIOCHEMICAL CHANGES

The biochemical changes that occur in the articular cartilage vary from early to later stages in the disease process. In early osteoarthritis, the water content of the articular cartilage significantly increases, causing the tissue to swell and altering its biomechanical properties. This phenomenon suggests that there has been weakening of the collagen network; the type II collagen fibers have a smaller diameter than the fibers in normal cartilage, and the normally tight weave in the midzone is relaxed and distorted.[88-93]

In later stages of osteoarthritis, type I collagen concentration within the extracellular matrix increases, and the proteoglycan concentration decreases to 50% or less than normal, with less aggregation and shorter glycosaminoglycan side chains.[93,94] Keratan sulfate concentration decreases, and the ratio of chondroitin-4-sulfate to chondroitin-6-sulfate increases, reflecting synthesis by chondrocytes of a proteoglycan profile more typical of immature cartilage.[95] Proteoglycan concentration in the cartilage diminishes progressively until the end stages, when histologic staining detects little or no proteoglycan.[96]

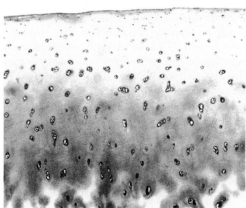

Normal

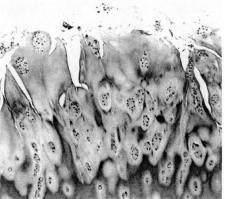

Osteoarthritis

Figure 89-1 Histologic sections of normal *(left)* and osteoarthritic *(right)* articular cartilage obtained from the femoral head. The osteoarthritic cartilage has surface irregularities, with clefts to the radial zone and cloning of chondrocytes.

Calcium crystals (e.g., calcium pyrophosphate dihydrate [CPPD], basic calcium phosphate crystals) are commonly found in the cartilage of the elderly, and often crystal arthropathy coexists with osteoarthritis.[97] It is unclear, however, whether these crystals are directly involved in the pathogenesis of osteoarthritis or are merely a by-product or marker of the disease.[98,99] That calcium crystals play a role in causing or worsening osteoarthritis is supported by clinical and laboratory studies, but the relationship is complex.[100]

Pyrophosphate is produced from adenosine triphosphate by the exoenzyme nucleoside pyrophosphohydrolase.[101] In normal cartilage basal zones, there is strong staining for alkaline phosphatase and matrix vesicles indicative of cartilage calcification.[102] Human osteoarthritic cartilage cultured in vitro also produces large quantities of alkaline phosphatase and pyrophosphate.[102] Synovial fluid from osteoarthritis patients shows high levels of pyrophosphate, similar to those in CPPD crystal deposition disease, levels that correlate directly with severity of joint damage.[103,104] Young or proliferating chondrocytes are a major source of pyrophosphate, whereas resting chondrocytes from normal adult cartilage secrete little pyrophosphate.[101] It has been theorized that the increased pyrophosphate secretion in osteoarthritis cartilage may be an indication of increased chondrocyte metabolic activity toward matrix repair.[105] The presence of CPPD may alter the biomechanical properties of the cartilage extracellular matrix and lead to cartilage breakdown. Hemochromatosis (hemosiderin), Wilson's disease (copper), ochronotic arthropathy (homogentisic acid polymers), gouty arthritis (crystals of monosodium urate), and CPPD crystal deposition disease are further examples of conditions in which the abnormal entity may alter the cartilage extracellular matrix, leading to either direct or indirect chondrocyte injury by increasing the stiffness of the tissue and precipitating the development of osteoarthritis.

METABOLIC CHANGES

As the severity of osteoarthritis progresses, the synthesis and secretion of matrix-degrading enzymes by chondrocytes markedly increase.[96,106] Early cartilage degeneration in osteoarthritis is most likely the result of the action of enzymes from the matrix metalloproteinase (MMP) family of proteinases that degrade proteoglycans (aggrecanases) and collagen (collagenases).[107-109] Collagenases typically make the first cleavage in triple-helical collagen, allowing its further degradation by other proteases. Aggrecanases in conjunction with other MMPs degrade aggrecan. Serine-dependent and cysteine-dependent proteases (e.g., plasminogen activator/plasmin system and cathepsin B) and membrane-type MMPs act primarily as MMP activators.[110-112] The control of these enzymes is complex, with regulation occurring at three different levels: synthesis and secretion, activation of latent enzyme, and inactivation by proteinase inhibitors.[113]

In osteoarthritis, the expression and production of proteinases is increased. Native collagen has been shown to be cleaved by MMP-1, MMP-8, and MMP-13; the resultant fragments may be susceptible to cleavage by other enzymes such as MMP-2 (gelatinase A), MMP-9 (gelatinase B), MMP-3 (stromelysin 1), and cathepsin B. Of the three major MMPs that degrade native collagen, MMP-13 may be the most important in osteoarthritis because it preferentially degrades type II collagen.[114] It also has been shown that expression of MMP-13 greatly increases in osteoarthritis.[115] Overall, collagenase activity also markedly increases in human osteoarthritic cartilage cultures, suggesting that it is a major factor in osteoarthritis progression and cartilage matrix degradation.[116,117]

MMPs can degrade other cartilage extracellular matrix molecules in addition to collagen. If combined with plasmin (which has the capability of activating many MMPs), MMPs can rapidly destroy cartilage altogether. In osteoarthritis, collagenase, stromelysin, and gelatinase are secreted as proenzymes by the chondrocyte, upregulated by IL-1 or tumor necrosis factor (TNF).[118,119] These proenzymes, each exhibiting a zinc-binding catalytic sequence, contain three histidine residues and a glutamine residue, all of which must be activated by proteolytic cleavage of their amino terminal sequence.

The aggrecanases belong to a family of extracellular proteases known as the ADAMTS (a disintegrin and metalloproteinase with thrombospondin motifs).[120] Two aggrecanases, ADAMTS-4 and ADAMTS-5, seem to be major enzymes in cartilage degradation in arthritis.[121] Recombinant ADAMTS-4 and ADAMTS-5 cleave aggrecan at five distinct sites along the core protein, and all resultant fragments have been identified in cartilage explants undergoing matrix degradation. Aggrecanase proteolytic activity can be modulated by altered expression, by activation via proteolytic cleavage at a furin-sensitive site, by binding to the aggrecan substrate through the C-terminal thrombospondin motif, by activation through post-translational processing of a portion of the C-terminus, and by inhibition of activity by the endogenous inhibitor tissue inhibitor of metalloproteinases (TIMP)-3.

ADAMTS-4 and ADAMTS-5 activity also has been detected in joint capsule and synovium and may be upregulated in arthritic synovium either at the message level or through post-translational processing. In addition to aggrecan, aggrecanases have been shown to degrade the nonaggregated chondroitin-sulfate proteoglycans brevican and versican. Most recently, it has been shown that ADAMTS-7 and ADAMTS-12 bind to and degrade COMP (a prominent noncollagenous protein in cartilage), and that the latter is highly upregulated in osteoarthritic cartilage.[122,123] ADAMTS-4, ADAMTS-19, and ADAMTS-20 also have been shown to degrade COMP in vitro; however, their in vivo activity in osteoarthritis has yet to be determined.[124,125]

The G_1 region of aggrecan is highly resistant to proteases; however, a glutamate-alanine bond within the extended region between G_1 and G_2 is remarkably susceptible to proteolytic degradation.[126] Low concentrations of stromelysin readily cleave the region between G_1 and G_2 domains, resulting in disruption of the proteoglycan aggregate structure and increased loss of proteoglycans from the extracellular matrix. A specific hyaluronidase has not been found in articular cartilage, but one or several lysosomal enzymes that can cleave hyaluronic acid and chondroitin-6-sulfate have been implicated.[110]

The decrease in chondroitin sulfate chain length in osteoarthritic cartilage may be due to digestion by synovial fluid hyaluronidase, which may diffuse into the matrix as its permeability increases.[95] Evidence to support this theory is the finding that the hyaluronic acid concentration in osteoarthritis cartilage is low, even though its rate of synthesis is considerably greater than normal.[96,106] These degradative enzymes serve to disrupt the proteoglycan aggregate. The early result of the MMP-induced tissue degradation is thinning of the collagen fibers, loosening of the tight collagen network, and the consequent cartilage matrix swelling seen in osteoarthritis.

Many investigators consider IL-1 a prime mediator in cartilage matrix degradation (Fig. 89-2). IL-1 is synthesized by mononuclear cells (including synovial lining cells) in the inflamed joint and by chondrocytes as an autocrine activity.[127-129] IL-1 stimulates the synthesis and secretion of many degradative enzymes in cartilage, including latent collagenase, latent stromelysin, latent gelatinase, and tissue plasminogen activator.[130-132] With regard to aggrecanases, it seems that ADAMTS-5 is constitutively expressed, whereas IL-1 and TNF can induce ADAMTS-4.[133] Plasminogen, synthesized by the chondrocyte or entering the matrix by diffusion from the synovial fluid, is the substrate for tissue plasminogen activator.

The balance of active and latent enzymes is controlled to some extent by at least two enzyme inhibitors: TIMP and plasminogen activator inhibitor-1.[108,134,135] TIMP and plasminogen activator inhibitor-1 are synthesized in increased amounts under the regulation of transforming growth factor (TGF)-β.[136,137] If insufficient concentrations of or degraded TIMP or plasminogen activator inhibitor-1 are present in the matrix along with active enzymes, increased matrix degradation occurs. Expression profiling of all known members of the MMP, ADAMTS, and TIMP gene families in normal cartilage and cartilage from patients with osteoarthritis has revealed that several members are regulated in osteoarthritis. Genes that showed increased expression in osteoarthritis were MMP-13, MMP-28, and ADAMTS-16 (all at $P < .001$); MMP-9, MMP-16, ADAMTS-2, and ADAMTS-14 (all at $P < .01$); and MMP-2, TIMP-3, and ADAMTS-12 (all at $P < .05$). Genes with decreased expression in osteoarthritis were MMP-1, MMP-3, and ADAMTS-1 (all at $P < .001$); MMP-10, TIMP-1, and ADAMTS-9 (all at $P < .01$); and TIMP-4, ADAMTS-5, and ADAMTS-15 (all at $P < .05$).[138] These results illustrate the complexity of the events that occur within the extracellular matrix regarding regulation of tissue-degrading enzymes.

Early osteoarthritis is characterized by increases in the synthesis of proteoglycans, collagen, noncollagenous proteins, hyaluronate, and DNA (indicating cell replication and accounting for the observed chondrocyte clones or clusters).[96,106] Anabolic and catabolic processes increase as cells attempt to repair or maintain tissue integrity[90]; this

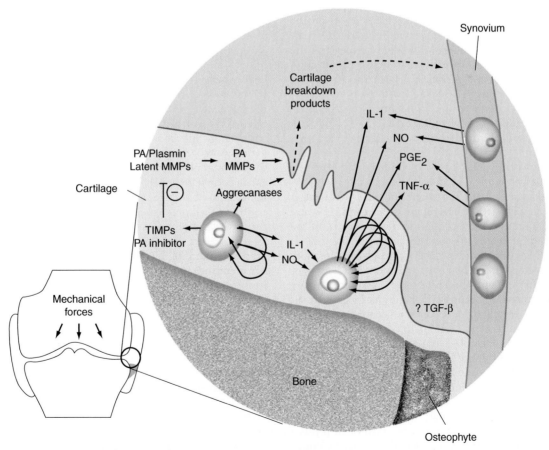

Figure 89-2 Schematic of pathogenic mechanisms of osteoarthritis. Mechanical stress initiates altered metabolism characterized by the release of matrix metalloproteinases (MMPs), proinflammatory cytokines, and mediators such as nitric oxide (NO) and prostaglandin E_2 (PGE$_2$). Cartilage breakdown products play a role by stimulating the release of cytokines from synovial lining cells, and by inducing MMP production by chondrocytes. Perpetuation of cartilage damage is amplified by the autocrine and paracrine actions of interleukin (IL)-1β and tumor necrosis factor (TNF)-α produced by chondrocytes. PA, plasminogen activator; TGF-β, transforming growth factor-β.

explains why osteoarthritis typically is slowly progressive and sometimes remains static by morphologic criteria. Eventually, osteoarthritis progresses when the cell number declines, proteoglycan synthesis declines sharply, and the chondrocytic anabolic repair processes cannot keep pace with catabolic processes, resulting in the further degeneration of cartilage extracellular matrix.[90,96]

The imbalance between proteoglycan synthesis and degradation is important in the pathogenesis of cartilage breakdown.[139] Osteoarthritis cartilage is deficient in TIMP content. Increased proteoglycan synthesis in early osteoarthritis is compromised further by the fact that osteoarthritic chondrocytes synthesize proteoglycans in a manner different from that of normal chondrocytes with respect to the composition and distribution of their glycosaminoglycans, the size of the proteoglycan subunit, and their ability to aggregate with hyaluronic acid.[90,92,95,111,140]

MATRIX CHANGES

Much of what is known about changes in the extracellular matrix in early osteoarthritis comes from animal models (e.g., rabbit partial meniscectomy model, canine anterior cruciate ligament–deficient model).[141,142] These animal models represent secondary osteoarthritis, produced by internal derangement of the joint, and may not precisely simulate the state of affairs in primary osteoarthritis. New models for spontaneous osteoarthritis include a postmenopausal rat model, the groove model, and a joint-specific bone morphogenetic receptor–deficient mouse. Of particular interest is an iodoacetate model, validated as the first pain model of osteoarthritis, in which intra-articular injection of iodoacetate in rats has been shown to lead to cartilage degeneration associated with pain and manifesting as time-dependent and concentration-dependent alterations in hind limb weight bearing.[143,144] That not all animal models of osteoarthritis are equivalent becomes clear when one considers the differences in therapeutic response between young and old animals and between spontaneous and surgical models.[145]

In the dog model, the first alteration seen within days after joint destabilization is an increase in cartilage water content.[146] Initially, water content increases locally, in the tibial plateau and femoral condyle cartilage, but it soon spreads to the entire joint cartilage. Proteoglycans are more readily extractable from the matrix of experimental animals than from that of controls. These matrix changes also are seen in spontaneously occurring dog and steer osteoarthritis and in experimentally induced rabbit osteoarthritis.[146-148]

The increase in water content in osteoarthritic cartilage is due to loss of the collagen network's elastic restraint, enabling the hydrophilic proteoglycans to swell more than normally.[149] In early-stage osteoarthritis, proteoglycan concentration may increase, and the cartilage consequently may become thicker than normal and exhibit increased staining for proteoglycans.[150-152] Shortly after the increase in cartilage water, newly synthesized proteoglycans are characterized by a higher proportion of chondroitin sulfate and a lower proportion of keratan sulfate, and proteoglycan aggregation is impaired.[142,146] These abnormal changes in extracellular matrix occur before fibrillation or any other gross morphologic changes are evident and result in a generalized decrease in stiffness that occurs in grossly normal cartilage adjacent to fibrillated areas.[153] As osteoarthritis progresses, focal cartilage ulcerations develop. Proteoglycan loss is accompanied by a decrease in its ability to aggregate, persistence in abnormal glycosaminoglycan composition, and a decrease in chondroitin sulfate chain length. When proteoglycan loss reaches a critical threshold, water content, which initially increased, decreases to less than normal.[154]

BIOMECHANICAL CHANGES

Two long-standing biomechanical theories of the pathogenesis of osteoarthritis hold that mechanical stresses injure chondrocytes, causing them to release degradative enzymes, and that mechanical stresses initially damage the collagen network (as opposed to the cells per se),[155,156] leading to a breakdown of the matrix. Extracellular matrix breakdown in osteoarthritic cartilage leads to (1) loss of compressive stiffness and elasticity, resulting in greater mechanical stress on chondrocytes, and (2) an increase in hydraulic permeability, resulting in loss of interstitial fluid during compression and increased diffusion of solutes through the matrix (including the movement of degradative enzymes and their inhibitors). One important consequence is disruption of normal fluid film joint lubrication and loading dynamics owing to alterations in inflammatory synovial fluid.[157-159] Joint friction, wear, lubrication, and contact mechanics are further negatively affected by the loss of cartilage proteoglycans.[160-163]

OSTEOPHYTE FORMATION

Osteophytes—bony proliferations at the joint margins and in the floor of cartilage lesions—are partly responsible for the pain and restriction of joint movement in osteoarthritis. Human osteoarthritic joint osteophytes synthesize cartilage with significant amounts of type I collagen and nonaggregating proteoglycans.[164] In experimentally induced osteoarthritis, osteophytes may develop even though the articular cartilage appears grossly normal.[165] Because osteophytes may increase joint surface available for load bearing, they may contribute to some cases of regression of the early osteoarthritis cartilage changes.[166]

It has been theorized that osteophytes occur as a result of penetration of blood vessels into the basal layers of degenerating cartilage, or as a result of abnormal healing of stress fractures in the subchondral trabeculae near the joint margins.[167,168] In the osteoarthritis dog model, periarticular osteophyte formation begins in the marginal zone, where synovium merges with periosteum and articular cartilage, 3 days after induction of knee instability.[169] TGF-β is a known anabolic growth factor that increases the expression of several types of collagen and proteoglycans.[170] When introduced into the joint in experimental animals, however, TGF-β induces osteophyte formation,[171] and TGF-β expression is observed in osteophytes in patients with osteoarthritis.[172]

Bony proliferation may result from venous congestion. In human hip osteoarthritis, phlebography has shown the formation of medullary varices, presumably resulting from changes in the medullary sinusoids, which may be compressed by subchondral cysts and thickened subchondral trabeculae.[173,174] Subchondral cysts in osteoarthritis may be created by entry of synovial fluid under pressure through defects in the cartilage or may develop in necrotic areas of subchondral bone.[175,176] The increased venous pressure caused by the cysts and remodeled trabeculae may account for some of the pain in osteoarthritis. Immobilization and glucocorticoids (but not bisphosphonates) have been shown to decrease the size and prevalence of osteophytes in experimental models of osteoarthritis.[177]

BIOMECHANICS AND DISEASE MECHANISMS OF OSTEOARTHRITIS

RESPONSE OF CARTILAGE TO MECHANICAL INJURY

The response of normal articular cartilage to injury typically results in suboptimal repair; these injuries often can result in secondary osteoarthritis.[178,179] In contrast to tissues that have the ability to regenerate injured regions with new cells and extracellular matrices that closely resemble the original tissue, articular cartilage produces a repair tissue with neither the original structure nor properties of normal cartilage.[180-183] Chondrocytes in areas surrounding an injured zone are unable to migrate, proliferate, repopulate, or regenerate repair tissue with similar structure, function, and biomechanical properties of normal hyaline cartilage.[154,180,184]

That articular cartilage lacks regenerative power has a long history of documentation.[185] Redfern[186] reported that articular cartilage wounds healed with fibrous tissue, which he believed arose from chondrocyte intercellular substance. Fisher[187] and Ito[188] in the 1920s proposed that cartilage repair is effected by fibrous tissue resulting from proliferation of cells from bone marrow, synovial membrane, and occasionally surrounding articular cartilage. It was later observed that the fibrous tissue subsequently transforms into fibrocartilage, with occasional foci of imperfect hyaline cartilage.[189-192] The common findings of these investigators was that articular cartilage lacks regenerative potential, and that the regenerative fibrous tissue and fibrocartilage tissue must have originated from undifferentiated mesenchymal tissue arising from bone marrow, synovium, or the superficial layer of articular cartilage.[185]

One reason the reparative process of cartilage significantly differs from the reparative processes of other tissues is that it is avascular. The healing response in vascularized tissues consists of three main phases: necrosis, inflammation, and repair.[178,183] Cartilage undergoes the initial phase of necrosis in response to injury, although typically less cell death occurs than in vascularized tissues because of chondrocytes' relative insensitivity to hypoxia.[178,183] The inflammatory phase, primarily mediated (in other tissues) by the vascular system, is largely absent in partial-thickness injuries (i.e., lesions that do not cross the tidemark), and the repair phase is severely limited given the lack of vascularity and a preceding inflammatory response. No local hyperemia results, no fibrin network is produced, no subsequent clot develops to act as a scaffold for the ingrowth of repair tissue, no mediators or cytokines are released that can stimulate cellular migration and proliferation, and no inflammatory cells that have mitotic and

reparative potential are recruited.[154,183] In lesions that do not cross the tidemark, the burden of repair falls on the chondrocytes[183] in a process that has been termed *intrinsic repair*.[193] Although fetal cartilage is capable of mitotic activity and replication, adult chondrocytes have little potential for replication and intrinsic repair.[191,192] Articular cartilage lesions that cross the tidemark may undergo extrinsic repair via differentiation and proliferation of mesenchymal stem cells from para-articular connective tissues, although most often a fibrocartilaginous tissue results.[193]

There are three categories of articular cartilage injury: (1) microdamage or repetitive trauma to the matrix and cells; (2) partial-thickness or superficial injuries or chondral fractures, articular surface injuries that do not penetrate the subchondral plate; and (3) osteochondral (full-thickness or deep penetrating) injuries, which extend through the tidemark and into the underlying subchondral bone.[178,180,183] The host response to each type of injury differs in timing and quality of repair.

Microdamage to the chondrocytes or extracellular matrix or both without gross disruption of the articular surface can be caused by a single severe impact or repetitive blunt trauma.[178,180,183] Repetitive loading of rabbit cartilage produces a surface loss of proteoglycans and an increase in chondrocyte metabolic activity.[194] Proteoglycans become more easily extractable from the articular cartilage, with a greater percentage of nonaggregated forms.[154] Several investigators have observed that cellular, metabolic, and biochemical changes after repetitive blunt trauma resemble the changes in the early stages of osteoarthritis—increased hydration, cellular degeneration or death, disruption of the collagen ultrastructure resulting in marked variation in the size and arrangements of fibers, fissuring and ulceration of the articular surface, thickening of the subchondral bone, and softening of the cartilage with loss of its compressive and tensile stiffness.[154,180,195-197] Trauma induces the release of degradative enzymes and proinflammatory factors (e.g., nitric oxide, TNF, IL-1) that frequently cause degradation of the surrounding matrix.[194,198,199] Eventually, the material properties of the cartilage are altered—cartilage matrix thins and subchondral bone stiffens—which often accelerate the degenerative process.[154] The point at which accumulated microdamage becomes irreversible is unknown, although it has been shown that lost proteoglycans and matrix components may be restored if damage to chondrocytes and the collagen network is limited, and the repetitive trauma is halted.[180]

Necrosis of neighboring chondrocytes follows chondral fractures and superficial lacerations, injuries that do not cross the tidemark.[178,183,200] Within 48 to 72 hours, surviving chondrocytes bordering the defect exhibit increased synthesis rates of extracellular matrix molecules and type II collagen, sometimes accompanied by cell proliferation and formation of clusters or clones in the periphery of the injured zone.[154,183,200,201] The increased metabolism and mitotic activity is transient, however, and is followed by a decrease in metabolic rate back to normal levels, typically resulting in a suboptimal repair.[154,183] Chondrocytes proliferating on the border of the injured zone do not migrate into the defect, which remains unfilled by the newly synthesized matrix.[154,180,184] In some cases, superficial lacerations in otherwise normal joints may not progress to full-thickness loss of cartilage or osteoarthritis.[154]

Lesions that cross the articular cartilage tidemark and disrupt the underlying subchondral plate elicit the three-phase repair response normally encountered in vascularized tissues. A hematoma forms in the defect that becomes organized into a fibrin clot, activating an inflammatory response. Transformation of the fibrin clot into vascular fibroblastic repair tissue[183,201] is accompanied by release of cytokines important in stimulating a repair response (e.g., TGF-β, platelet-derived growth factor, IGF, bone morphogenetic proteins).[181] These cytokines help set in motion the recruitment, proliferation, and differentiation of undifferentiated cells into a fibrin network that serves as a scaffold for fibrocartilaginous repair tissue.[181,202,203] The origin of these mesenchymal stem cells has been determined to be the underlying bone marrow, rather than the adjacent residual articular surface.[201,203,204] These cells progressively differentiate into chondroblasts, chondrocytes, and osteoblasts and synthesize cartilage and bone matrices. At 6 to 8 weeks postinjury, the repair tissue contains a high proportion of chondrocyte-like cells surrounded by a matrix consisting of proteoglycans and type II collagen, with a lesser amount of type I collagen.[204-206] Cells in the deeper layers of the defect differentiate into osteoblasts and subsequently undergo endochondral ossification to heal the subchondral bone defect.[154]

This regenerative tissue eventually undergoes a transformation to a more fibrocartilaginous repair accompanied by a shift in the synthesis of collagen from type II to type I.[184,200,202,203,206] Typically, within 1 year from injury, the repair tissue resembles a mixture of fibrocartilage and hyaline cartilage, with a substantial component (20% to 40%) of type I collagen.[205] The size of the osteochondral defect is an important factor in the quality of repair; as a general rule, the smaller the defect, the better the repair.[207] Depending on the joint, there exists a critical size defect that does not repair. Fibrocartilaginous repair is susceptible to early degenerative changes because it lacks the biomechanical properties to withstand normal physiologic joint loads.[203,205]

MECHANOTRANSDUCTION AND GENE EXPRESSION

Chondrocytes can sense and respond to mechanical and physicochemical stimuli via several regulatory pathways (e.g., upstream signaling, transcription, translation, posttranslational modification, vesicular transport).[208] Physical forces also may influence the synthesis, assembly, and degradation of the extracellular cartilage matrix. Normal stimuli help chondrocytes maintain the extracelluar matrix; abnormal stimuli can disrupt this balance.

Mechanotransduction influences the cell-mediated feedback between physical stimuli, the molecular structure of newly synthesized matrix molecules, and the resulting biomechanical tissue properties.[209] Cell-matrix interactions are believed to be an important mediator in mechanotransduction in chondrocytes. In a study on the expression of COMP to long-term cyclic compression, it was found that with uniaxial unconfined dynamic compression, COMP expression was significantly upregulated; incubation with

anti–α$_1$ integrin blocking antibodies abolished the mechanosensitivity of COMP expression.[210] Studies of cyclic and static unconfined compression of bovine articular cartilage explants showed that cyclic loading increased protein synthesis by 50% above free-swelling controls, but had an inhibitory influence on proteoglycan synthesis. Static compression was associated with a dose-dependent decrease in biosynthetic activity.[211] Fibronectin and COMP were the most affected noncollagenous extracellular proteins; static compression caused a significant increase in fibronectin synthesis versus free-swelling control levels, and cyclic compression caused a significant increase in synthesis of COMP and fibronectin. These results support the theory that chondrocytes can remodel extracellular matrix in response to alterations in functional demand.

Human articular chondrocytes use the α5β1 integrin as a mechanoreceptor. Mechanical stimulation initiates a signal cascade involving stretch-activated ion channels, the actin cytoskeleton, and tyrosine phosphorylation of the focal adhesion complex molecules pp125 focal adhesion kinase and paxillin, and β-catenin.[212] Autocrine secretion of IL-4 ensues. After binding to its type II receptors, IL-4 induces membrane hyperpolarization of chondrocytes from normal human knee joint articular cartilage. The result is an anabolic response, manifested by increased levels of aggrecan mRNA after mechanical stimulation and decreased levels of MMP-3. Mechanically induced release of the chondroprotective cytokine IL-4 from chondrocytes acts in an autocrine and a paracrine manner and represents an important regulator of articular cartilage structure and function; dysfunction of this pathway may be implicated in osteoarthritis.

Although the mechanoreceptor in osteoarthritis chondrocytes also is the α5β1 integrin, downstream signaling pathways in osteoarthritic chondrocytes differ and may contribute to changes in chondrocyte behavior, leading to increased cartilage breakdown.[213] Integrins and integrin-associated signaling pathways are at least partly regulated by mechanical stimulation by activation of plasma membrane apamin-sensitive, Ca^{2+}-activated K$^+$ channels; the result is membrane hyperpolarization after cyclical mechanical stimulation.[214] Chondrocytes from normal articular cartilage exhibit membrane hyperpolarization response to cyclic pressure-induced strain, whereas chondrocytes from osteoarthritic cartilage respond by membrane depolarization and exhibit no changes in aggrecan or MMP-3 mRNA after mechanical stimulation.[215,216] These findings suggest that chondrocytes derived from osteoarthritic cartilage have a different signaling pathway via the α5β1 integrin in response to mechanical stimulation; these may play a role in the phenotypic changes seen in diseased cartilage.

Another study used cDNA array analysis to compare the expression profiles of mRNA from hydrostatic pressurized and nonpressurized human chondrosarcoma cells.[217] Several immediate-early and regulating cell cycle and growth genes were upregulated in response to high pressure, whereas a decrease was observed in osteonectin, fibronectin, and collagen types VI and XVI mRNA.

Fluid flow during dynamic compression of cartilage explants can stimulate proteoglycan and protein synthesis independent of changes in cell shape. A study using a tissue shear-loading model to uncouple fluid flow from cell and matrix deformation showed that deformation of cells and pericellular matrix alone stimulated protein synthesis by approximately 50% and proteoglycan synthesis by approximately 25%; even in the absence of macroscopic tissue-level fluid flow, chondrocytes can respond to a change in shape.[218] The magnitude and duration of specific loads also can cause chondrocyte death and collagen damage; chondrocytes in the superficial zone seem to be more vulnerable to load-induced injury than chondrocytes in the middle and deep zones.[219,220]

Indian hedgehog (Ihh) protein is a key signaling molecule that controls chondrocyte proliferation and differentiation. Ihh also may be an essential mediator of mechanotransduction in cartilage. Cyclic mechanical stress was shown to induce Ihh expression by chondrocytes.[221]

ROLE OF INFLAMMATORY MEDIATORS IN DISEASE PROGRESSION

Among the many biochemical pathways that are activated within joint tissues during the course of osteoarthritis are mediators classically associated with inflammation, notably IL-1β and TNF-α. These cytokines autocatalytically stimulate their own production and induce chondrocytes to produce proteases, chemokines, nitric oxide, and eicosanoids such as prostaglandins and leukotrienes. The action of these inflammatory mediators within cartilage is predominantly to drive catabolic pathways, inhibit matrix synthesis, and promote cellular apoptosis. Although osteoarthritis is not conventionally considered an inflammatory disease, "inflammatory" mediators perpetuate disease progression and represent potential targets for disease modification.

INFLAMMATORY MOLECULES PRODUCED BY ARTICULAR CARTILAGE

Cytokines and Chemokines

A characteristic feature of established osteoarthritis is the increased production of proinflammatory cytokines, such as IL-1β and TNF-α, by articular chondrocytes. IL-1β and TNF-α exert comparable catabolic effects on chondrocyte metabolism, decreasing proteoglycan collagen synthesis and increasing aggrecan release via the induction of degradative proteases.[109,222-227] IL-1β and TNF-α also induce chondrocytes and synovial cells to produce other inflammatory mediators, such as IL-8, IL-6, nitric oxide, and prostaglandin E_2. The actions of both cytokines are mediated partly by the activation of the transcription factor nuclear factor κB, which increases further their own expression and that of other catabolic proteins, such as inducible nitric oxide synthase (iNOS) and cyclooxygenase-2 (COX-2), creating an autocatalytic cascade that promotes self-destruction of articular cartilage (see Fig. 89-2).[228,229]

IL-1β and TNF-α are synthesized intracellularly as precursors, converted through proteolytic cleavage to their mature forms by caspases—membrane-bound IL-1β-converting enzyme (ICE) and TNF-α-converting enzyme (TACE)—and released extracellularly in their active forms.[230] The expression of ICE and TACE has been shown to be upregulated in osteoarthritis cartilage.[260-262] Inhibitors of ICE and TACE are of interest as future therapeutic small-molecule antagonists of downstream IL-1β and TNF-α expression; studies with an ICE inhibitor are now under way in two murine models.

The actions of IL-1 depend on the engagement of two specific cell surface receptors (IL-1R), designated type I and type II. The type I receptor, which spans the plasma membrane, is responsible for signal transduction, whereas the type II receptor is a "decoy" receptor, expressed at the cell membrane, but unable to signal. A deficit of the ratio of IL-1Ra (the competitive inhibitor to the IL-1/IL-1R complex) to IL-1 has been described in osteoarthritis synovial tissue, which may permit increased IL-1 activity.[231,232] Addition of IL-1Ra, or soluble types I and II IL-1 receptors, to osteoarthritis explant cultures blocks prostaglandin E_2 synthesis, collagenase production, and nitric oxide production[227,233]; addition of these antagonists in culture also results in an increase in aggrecan content, likely by inhibiting degradation of newly synthesized molecules.[234] Encouraging results with IL-1Ra also have been reported in vivo, where gene therapy or the intra-articular administration of IL-1Ra has been shown to retard the progression of osteoarthritis in experimental animal models.[235,236]

Other lines of evidence also point to IL-1β as an essential link in the pathogenesis of cartilage damage, including proteoglycan loss produced by intra-articular injection of IL-1.[235] Clinical trials using IL-1β antagonists are few and have been inconclusive. One multicenter trial with double-blinded doses of intra-articular IL-1Ra to 14 osteoarthritis patients resulted in decreased pain without significant adverse events or acute injection reactions.[237] No long-term studies of structure-modifying effects of such therapies have been reported, however. Osteoarthritic cartilage also is the site of increased production of CXC and CC chemokines. These include IL-8, monocyte chemoattractant protein-1, and RANTES (regulated on activation, normally T cell expressed and secreted), also known as CCL5, chemokine and the receptors CCR-2 and CCR-5.[238-240]

The expression of chemokines is low or undetectable in normal chondrocytes unless stimulated with cytokines such as IL-1 or IL-17.[241] Chemokines are detected by immunohistochemistry in the superficial and mid zones of the tissue, as has been shown for other inflammatory mediators, such as iNOS, IL-1β, and TNF-α.[239] RANTES induces expression of its own receptor, CCR-5, suggesting an autocrine/paracrine pathway of the chemokine within the cartilage. Monocyte chemoattractant protein-1 and RANTES promote chondrocyte catabolic activities, including induction of nitric oxide synthase, increased MMP-3 expression, inhibition of proteoglycan synthesis, and enhancement of proteoglycan release.[239,242] Consistent with these effects, treatment of normal articular cartilage with RANTES increases the release of glycosaminoglycans and profoundly reduces the intensity of safranin O staining.[239]

Proteinases

A presumed key action of cytokines and chemokines produced in osteoarthritis is to promote cartilage proteolysis via the induction of a wide array of proteases, in particular MMPs. The two main families of MMPs are (1) the collagenases that break down type II collagen (especially MMP-1, MMP-8, MMP-13, and MMP-28) and proteoglycans

(MMP-3, which also cleaves pro-MMPs into their active forms) and (2) the aggrecanases, also known as ADAMTS family, which mediate aggregan degradation in cartilage.[138,149] Both families of MMPs are expressed in osteoarthritis cartilage at lesional sites, and it is presumed that they play a major role in degradation of the extracellular matrix.

A comprehensive analysis of specific metalloproteinases that are overexpressed by osteoarthritis cartilage and synovium has revealed several MMPs and ADAMTSs that may be candidates as targets for disease modification.[243] Among the most interesting is MMP-13, which is overexpressed in murine and human osteoarthritis cartilage and is the most efficient protease capable of cleaving type II collagen.[202,244] Similarly, the aggrecanase ADAMTS-5 has surfaced as the aggrecanase required for aggrecan loss in experimental osteoarthritis[245] and inflammatory joint disease.[246] It has been shown that mice lacking ADAMTS-5 are protected from developing osteoarthritis.[245]

The expression and degradation of noncollagenous proteins and nonaggregating proteoglycans also are altered in osteoarthritis cartilage and may have a direct or indirect effect on modulating the catabolic state of the chondrocyte.[247] These groups of molecules are likely to have important structural and biologic functions.[248,249] From their interactions with other extracellular matrix constituents, they can influence the supramolecular assembly of the cartilage matrix and as a result affect the physical properties of the tissue; by interacting directly with chondrocytes or neighboring cells or both, they can provide biologic signals on matrix properties and influence cellular function.[250]

There is increased expression of fibronectin, osteonectin, and osteopontin in osteoarthritis cartilage compared with normal cartilage.[251] In addition, proteolytic processes generate fragments of extracellular matrix proteins, including fibronectin and type II collagen, which seem to exert catabolic and proteolytic activities. Homandberg and others[252-254] have shown that fragments of fibronectin (but not the intact fibronectin molecule) induce the production of metalloproteinases and other catabolic factors in cartilage, in a process that partly depends on IL-1 induction. More recent studies indicate that fibronectin fragments stimulate type II collagen cleavage via enhanced MMP-13 and MMP-3 production.[255] The chondrolytic effects of the fragments were blocked by the addition of either a preferential MMP-13 inhibitor or IL1-Ra. Type II collagen fragments also can induce matrix resorption when abundant enough.[255,256]

Nitric Oxide

Nitric oxide, produced by the inducible isoform of nitric oxide synthase (iNOS), is a major catabolic factor produced by chondrocytes in response to proinflammatory cytokines such as IL-1β and TNF-α.[238] Considerable evidence indicates that the overproduction of nitric oxide by chondrocytes plays a role in the perpetuation of cartilage destruction in osteoarthritis (Fig. 89-3).[257-259] Increased concentrations of nitrites have been shown in the synovial fluid of patients with osteoarthritis, and iNOS has been shown in osteoarthritis synoviocytes and chondrocytes by in situ hybridization and immunohistochemistry.[85,260,261] Although normal cartilage does not express iNOS or produce nitric oxide without stimulation by cytokines such as IL-1, osteoarthritis cartilage explants spontaneously produce large amounts of nitric oxide.[257] iNOS also is upregulated from chondrocytes by cartilage compression.[262,263]

Nitric oxide exerts multiple effects on chondrocytes that promote articular cartilage degradation,[264] including (1) inhibition of collagen and proteoglycan synthesis,[264] (2) activation of metalloproteinases,[265] (3) increased susceptibility to injury by other oxidants (e.g., hydrogen peroxide),[266] and (4) apoptosis.[233] Several studies have implicated nitric oxide as an important mediator in chondrocyte apoptosis, a feature common in progressive osteoarthritis.[266,267] Immunohistochemistry of joint tissue obtained from patients with osteoarthritis reveals colocalization of iNOS protein and apoptosis in articular cartilage cells.[268] There is evidence that apoptosis results from the formation of peroxynitrite, a toxic free radical produced by the reaction of nitric oxide and superoxide anion. Peroxynitrite reacts with tyrosine residues on proteins, which can be detected by antibodies to nitrotyrosine. Immunostaining of osteoarthritis cartilage reveals

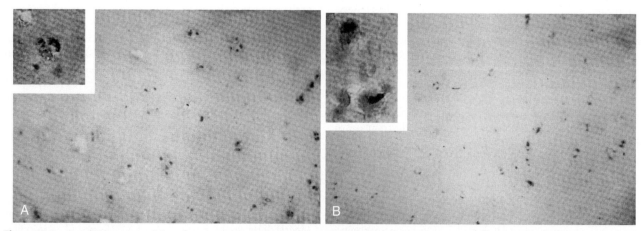

Figure 89-3   A and B, Immunostaining of osteoarthritic cartilage specimen for inducible nitric oxide synthase **(A)** and interleukin-1β **(B).** Note intense staining of chondrocytes in the superficial zones for both inflammatory proteins. *(From Melchiorri C, et al: Enhanced and coordinated in vivo expression of inflammatory cytokines and nitric oxide synthase by chondrocytes from patients with osteoarthritis. Arthritis Rheum 41:2165-2174, 1998.)*

that chondrocytes that are highly positive for IL-1β also stain for nitrotyrosine, consistent with overproduction of peroxynitrate and oxidative damage.[261]

The importance of nitric oxide has been corroborated in animal models of osteoarthritis. In the Pond-Nuki canine model, the inhibition of nitric oxide reduced the progression of cartilage lesions.[269] The protective effect of nitric oxide inhibition also was reflected in decreased levels in articular cartilage of metalloproteinases, caspase-2, and IL-1β, and in decreased chondrocyte apoptosis.[270] Osteoarthritis pathology, including cartilage lesions and osteophyte formation, was reduced in the mutant mice.

Nitric oxide also may play protective roles, however, as protease activity and proteoglycan degradation are enhanced when nitric oxide production is blocked.[271] In murine models, the development of surgically induced osteoarthritis can be accelerated in mice that are knocked out for ICE or iNOS—suggesting that a certain level of these molecules may be necessary to maintain a healthy joint, and that complete pharmacologic suppression may be detrimental.[272]

Transforming Growth Factor-β₁

In most respects, TGF-α acts as a counterregulatory molecule that opposes the effects of inflammatory mediators in cartilage. TGF-β$_1$ has been shown to downregulate proteolytic MMP-1, MMP-13, IL-1, and TNF receptors on osteoarthritis chondrocytes.[273] TGF-β$_2$ selectively suppresses the cleavage of type II collagen by collagenases in osteoarthritis cartilage in culture and limits MMP and proinflammatory cytokine expression.[222] Studies using the murine knee osteoarthritis model indicate that TGF-β$_3$ protects articular cartilage; histologic staining for this molecule revealed a lack of TGF-β$_3$ in damaged cartilage compared with normals. Although premature osteophyte chondrocyte clusters express high levels of TGF-β$_3$, other data suggest that bone morphogenetic protein-2 is more responsible for late osteophyte development.[274] TGF-β$_1$ also may exert selected catabolic effects via the stimulation of ADAMTS-4 expression.[273]

Hyaluronic Acid

Hyaluronic acid has been investigated as a marker of cartilage degradation that can be detected in synovial fluid and serum,[275] but it also seems to play a role in limiting the progression of arthritis. A study by Karna and colleagues[276] found that hyaluronic acid in vitro counteracts the ability of IL-1β to inhibit collagen biosynthesis. At the transcriptional and post-transcriptional levels, chondrocyte cultures with IL-1β upregulated collagen synthesis markers, whereas hyaluronic acid negated this effect. The same group found that hyaluronic acid similarly protects against IL-1-induced inhibition of collagen synthesis in human skin fibroblasts at the level of the IGF-I receptor.[277]

Prostaglandins

The expression of inducible COX-2 is increased in osteoarthritis chondrocytes, which spontaneously produce prostaglandin E$_2$ ex vivo.[240] The effects of prostaglandins on chondrocyte metabolism are complex and include enhanced type II collagen synthesis, activation of metalloproteinases,

and promotion of apoptosis.[278] In cartilage explants, IL-1β induces COX-2 expression, and prostaglandin E$_2$ production coordinates with proteoglycan degradation. COX-2 inhibition prevents IL-1β-induced proteoglycan degradation, which can be reversed by the addition of prostaglandin E$_2$ to cultures.[279] In contrast, in vitro evidence has accumulated that selected nonsteroidal anti-inflammatory drugs may interfere with proteoglycan synthesis.[280] Another study concluded that 30% of prostaglandin E$_2$ expression in osteoarthritis synovial tissue stems from the COX-1 pathway.[4] Whether any differences exist between the effects of COX-1-derived and COX-2-derived prostaglandins on cartilage metabolism is unknown.

ALTERATIONS IN BONE

The inflammatory mediators produced by bone in osteoarthritis are less well understood than those produced by cartilage and synovium. Biomechanical and biochemical factors seem to influence the remodeling, but the underlying pathogenesis has yet to be identified. Nitric oxide plays a role in bone cell function, which could have implications for osteoarthritis insofar as it contributes to alterations in subchondral bone. The endothelial isoform endothelial cell nitric oxide synthase is constitutively expressed in bone, where it seems to play a key role in regulating osteoblast activity and bone formation. Endothelial cell nitric oxide synthase also mediates the effects of mechanical loading on the skeleton, where it acts along with prostaglandins to promote bone formation and suppress bone resorption.[281]

In contrast, such proinflammatory cytokines as IL-1 and TNF induce iNOS in bone cells, and nitric oxide derived from this pathway potentiates bone loss.[238] Osteophyte formation and subchondral bone remodeling likely result from local production of anabolic growth factors such as IGF-I and mostly TGF-β, which is highly expressed in osteophytes of the femoral head in osteoarthritis patients.[282,283] Areas of increased radionuclide uptake ("hot spots") on bone scintigraphy also have been reported to identify osteoarthritis joints more likely to progress by radiographic criteria or to require surgical intervention or both over a 5-year period.[216]

ALTERATIONS IN SYNOVIAL TISSUE

One reason that osteoarthritis is classified as a noninflammatory arthritis is that the synovial fluid leukocyte count in osteoarthritis is typically less than 2000 cells/mm.[3] Although such parameters can be misleading, low-grade inflammatory processes nevertheless occur in osteoarthritic synovial tissues and contribute to disease pathogenesis, and some degree of synovitis has been observed even in early osteoarthritis (Fig. 89-4).[284] This localized synovitis may be subclinical because arthroscopic studies suggest that localized proliferative and inflammatory changes of the synovium occur in 50% of osteoarthritis patients, and the activated synovium may produce proteases and cytokines that accelerate damage to the adjacent cartilage.[285]

Many of the clinical symptoms and signs seen in osteoarthritis joints (e.g., joint swelling and effusion, stiffness, occasionally redness) reflect synovial inflammation. Synovial histologic changes include synovial hypertrophy and

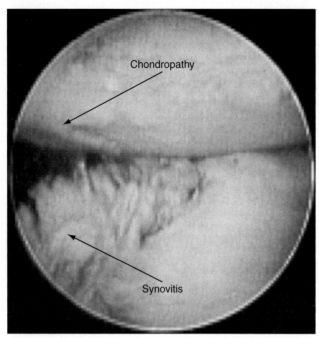

Figure 89-4 Arthroscopic view of osteoarthritic lesion of the femoral condyle (designated chondropathy). Note that proliferative synovitis is localized to the area of the osteoarthritic lesion. *(Courtesy of Maxime Dougados.)*

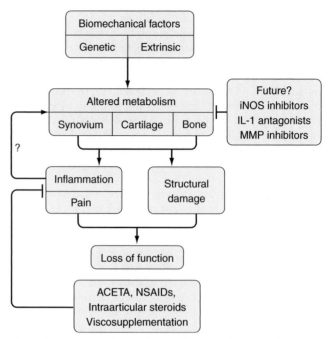

Figure 89-5 Multiple factors that predispose to, initiate, and perpetuate osteoarthritis. In the future, structure-modifying treatments will be targeted to the biochemical processes that promote disease progression. ACETA, acetaminophen; IL-1, interleukin-1; iNOS, inducible nitric oxide synthase; MMP, matrix metalloproteinase; NSAIDs, nonsteroidal anti-inflammatory drugs.

hyperplasia with an increased number of lining cells, often accompanied by infiltration of the sublining tissue with scattered foci of lymphocytes. In contrast to rheumatoid arthritis, synovial inflammation in osteoarthritis is mostly confined to areas adjacent to pathologically damaged cartilage and bone. This activated synovium can release proteinases and cytokines that may accelerate destruction of nearby cartilage.[283]

As described earlier, the metalloproteinases that degrade cartilage are produced not only by the cartilage itself, but also by the synovium. Although cartilage destruction might be directed by the chondrocytes, some degree of synovitis exists in patients even with mild osteoarthritis. A comprehensive analysis by Davidson and coworkers[243] reported several proinflammatory genes significantly elevated in the synovium that had not previously been reported. Cartilage breakdown products, derived from the articular surface as a result of mechanical or enzymatic destruction of the cartilage, can provoke the release of collagenase and other hydrolytic enzymes from synovial cells and macrophages (Fig. 89-5).[286,287] Cartilage breakdown products also are believed to result in mononuclear cell infiltration and vascular hyperplasia in the synovial membrane in osteoarthritis.[288-290]

A consequence of these low-grade inflammatory processes is the induction of synovial IL-1β and TNF-α, which are likely contributors to the degradative cascade.[238] There also are reports of increased numbers of immune cells in synovial tissue, including activated B cells and T lymphocytes, and evidence that osteoarthritis patients express cellular immunity to the cartilage proteoglycan link protein and C1 domain.[291,292] A more recent study of 10 patients with early osteoarthritis (arthroscopic specimens) and 15 patients undergoing total knee arthroplasty revealed that

synovial tissues from early osteoarthritis had higher levels of IL-1β and TNF-α and increased mononuclear cell infiltration compared with late osteoarthritis.[293] In addition, although less prominent than in rheumatoid arthritis, deposits of immunoglobulin and complement can be found in the collagenous network of the superficial zone of articular cartilage in osteoarthritis, suggesting that deposition of immune complexes, perhaps containing breakdown products of the cartilage as antigens, may play a role in the chronicity of the inflammatory reaction in the joint.[294] It is probable that any acquired immune-driven component of osteoarthritis is secondary, and not likely to be of major importance in future treatment strategies.

Patients with distal or proximal interphalangeal osteoarthritis are generally asymptomatic when the disease is nonerosive and become symptomatic during inflammatory episodes (associated with erosive osteoarthritis changes).[295] Other evidence that erosive osteoarthritis is more inflammatory comes from a study of rapidly destructive hip osteoarthritis, in which levels of MMP-3 and MMP-9 were especially elevated, not only in patients' synovial cells, but also in their synovial fluid, plasma, and sera.[296,297] In addition, in vitro studies have implicated MMP-10 expression in synovial fibroblasts from diseased osteoarthritis human tissue and in osteoarthritis synovial fluid and chondrocytes stimulated with catabolic IL-1 and oncostatin M.[298]

Osteoarthritis patients have been shown to express cellular immunity to the cartilage proteoglycan link protein, and C1 domain and immune complexes containing antibodies to type II collagen have been detected in the superficial layer of osteoarthritis cartilage.[299] Histologic changes in osteoarthritis synovium usually show mild or moderate synovitis characterized by an increase in the number of inflammatory mononuclear cells in the sublining tissue, including activated B cells and T lymphocytes.[302-307] Along the lines of acute episodes of osteoarthritis, the inflammation may result from crystal-induced synovitis (either calcium apatite or CPPD).

"Milwaukee shoulder syndrome" is a rapidly destructive form of osteoarthritis with evidence of inflammation in the synovial membrane, but minimal synovial fluid leukocytosis. It is typically associated with rotator cuff degeneration, severe shoulder osteoarthritis, and hydroxyapatite crystal deposition in the synovial membrane.[306] The synovial fluid typically contains few cells and high levels of active collagenase. It is theorized that crystals released from the degenerating tendons trigger the release of collagenase from synovial mononuclear cells, which leads to cartilage breakdown; cartilage breakdown products further activate release of enzymes from the synovium. This inflammation typically is associated with increases in synovial IL-1 and TNF that further potentiate the degradative cascade.[307]

BIOMARKERS OF OSTEOARTHRITIS

Several biomarkers have been correlated with osteoarthritis, but they often lack any known pathophysiologic or biochemical function that would classify them as inflammatory mediators.[308] Such markers, including C-reactive protein (CRP) and COMP, have been used to assess the diagnosis, severity, and prognosis of osteoarthritis. The formation of the National Institutes of Health (NIH)–funded osteoarthritis Biomarkers Network, a consortium of five NIH-designated sites, has proposed the "BIPED" biomarker classification with five separate categories of surrogate markers: burden of disease, investigative, prognostic, efficacy of intervention, and diagnostic.[283] Some established markers for burden of disease and for prognosis for hip and knee osteoarthritis include serum COMP, serum hyaluronic acid, and urinary CTX-II.[309]

One study of 62 patients with knee osteoarthritis compared magnetic resonance imaging findings at baseline and 1 year and levels of serum hyaluronic acid, osteocalcin, cartilage glycoprotein 39, COMP, and urine C-telopeptide of type II collagen. This study suggested that a single measurement of serum hyaluronic acid or short-term increases in urine CTX-II would identify patients at greatest risk for progression of osteoarthritis.[310]

Elevated levels of the inflammatory marker CRP seem to be predictive of radiographic progression of long-term knee osteoarthritis.[238] In a study of 1025 women, higher levels of serum CRP were associated with a statistically significant increase in prevalent and incident knee osteoarthritis and greater knee osteoarthritis severity. Women with bilateral knee osteoarthritis had higher CRP levels than women with unilateral knee osteoarthritis. Compared with women who did not develop knee osteoarthritis, the women who did had a higher baseline CRP than at their index test 2.5 years earlier.[311] In another study comprising women (44 to 67 years old), CRP levels were statistically greater in 105 women with knee osteoarthritis than in 740 women without osteoarthritis. These and other studies report that CRP levels are modestly but significantly increased in women with early knee osteoarthritis, and that higher levels are predictive of osteoarthritis that will progress over time.[85]

Several studies have identified COMP levels as helpful assessors of the potential for, presence of, and progression of osteoarthritis.[312] This noncollagenous extracellular matrix protein, synthesized by cartilage and synovium with TGF-β_1 stimulation,[313] is abundant in articular cartilage.[314-317] The degradation and the tissue distribution of COMP exhibit marked differences in normal and osteoarthritic human knee articular cartilage. COMP in normal cartilage is predominantly localized to the interterritorial matrix throughout all zones of the matrix, with increased staining in the deeper cartilaginous zones. COMP in osteoarthritic cartilage is predominantly localized to the superficial zones of fibrillated cartilage, with little to no immunostaining in the midzones and poor staining in the deeper cartilaginous zones. In areas of fibrocartilaginous repair in osteoarthritis, the repair matrix stained poorly for proteoglycans, but strongly for COMP; some fibrocartilaginous cells stained positively for COMP, suggesting that these cells were actively synthesizing COMP.[318] Synovial fluid COMP levels were found to be higher in individuals with knee pain or injury,[319] anterior cruciate ligament or meniscal injury,[319,320] and osteoarthritis[319,321] than in demographically matched healthy individuals. Similarly, serum levels of COMP are often higher in patients with more rapidly progressive joint damage[240,242,322] with some studies showing this specifically in hip osteoarthritis[247,295] and knee osteoarthritis.[241]

Hyaluronic acid has been investigated as a marker of cartilage degradation that can be detected in synovial fluid and serum.[275] The level of hyaluronic acid in synovial fluid and serum may be reflective of cartilage metabolism, even though most circulating hyaluronic acid originates from extracartilaginous sources. It has become clear that hyaluronic acid levels reflect synovial activity, whereas proteoglycan levels reflect cartilage turnover.[275,323] In addition, higher serum hyaluronic acid levels have been correlated with the number of joints involved and degree of clinical disability. These findings support the theory that serum hyaluronic acid levels reflect synovial hyperactivity. An animal model in which the anterior cruciate ligament was transected to induce osteoarthritis also showed an increase in serum hyaluronic acid level within 7 days after joint injury, an increase sustained at 13 weeks; the increase in synovial fluid hyaluronic acid levels correlated with serum levels.[324] Serum hyaluronic acid levels, which also may serve as a predictor of osteoarthritis disease progression,[247,325] correlated with radiographic evidence of disease progression over a 5-year period, as patients whose disease progressed had higher levels than at the outset.[309]

SUMMARY

Osteoarthritis, although classically conceived of as a degenerative consequence of aging, is a disease with an increasingly well-characterized molecular pathophysiology. Biomechanical factors, particularly in the context of genetic predisposition, obesity, and malalignment, result in chemical alterations within the joint that promote cartilage degradation. Early, anabolic changes, characterized by proliferation of chondrocytes and increased matrix production, are followed by a predominantly catabolic state, characterized by decreased matrix synthesis, increased proteolytic degradation of matrix, and chondrocyte apoptosis.

Many of the features of the chondrocyte in the catabolic state are related to the production of inflammatory mediators by synovium and chondrocytes that act locally to perpetuate cartilage degradation. Although current treatments improve the signs and symptoms of disease, further characterization of the altered metabolism in synovium, cartilage, and bone that promote disease progression should lead to future treatments that prevent structural damage in osteoarthritis (see Fig. 89-5).

REFERENCES

1. Herndon JH, Davidson SM, Apazidis A: Recent socioeconomic trends in orthopaedic practice. J Bone Joint Surg Am 83A: 1097-1105, 2001.
2. Sarzi-Puttini P, Cimmino MA, Scarpa R, et al: Osteoarthritis: An overview of the disease and its treatment strategies. Semin Arthritis Rheum 35(1 Suppl 1):1-10, 2005.
3. Peyron JG: The epidemiology of osteoarthritis. In Moskowitz RW, Howell DS, Goldberg YM, et al (eds): Osteoarthritis: Diagnosis and Management. Philadelphia, WB Saunders, 1984, pp 9-27.
4. Martin JA, Buckwalter JA: Aging, articular cartilage chondrocyte senescence and osteoarthritis. Biogerontology 3:257-264, 2002.
5. Lawrence JS: Rheumatism in Populations. London, Heinemann Medical, 1977.
6. Forman MD, Kaplan DA, Muller GF, et al: The epidemiology of osteoarthritis of the knee. In Peyron JG (ed): Epidemiology of Osteoarthritis. Paris, Ciba-Geigy, 1980, p 243.
7. Brandt KD, Flusser D: Osteoarthritis. In Bellamy N (ed): Prognosis in the Rheumatic Diseases. Lancaster, UK, Kluwer Academic Publishers, 1991, p 11.
8. Todd Allen R, Robertson CM, Harwood FL, et al: Characterization of mature vs aged rabbit articular cartilage: Analysis of cell density, apoptosis-related gene expression and mechanisms controlling chondrocyte apoptosis. Osteoarthritis Cartilage 12:917-923, 2004.
9. Robertson CM, Pennock AT, Harwood FL, et al: Characterization of pro-apoptotic and matrix-degradative gene expression following induction of osteoarthritis in mature and aged rabbits. Osteoarthritis Cartilage 14:471-476, 2006.
10. Cole AA, Kuettner KE: Molecular basis for differences between human joints. Cell Mol Life Sci 59:19-26, 2002.
11. Kerin A, Patwari P, Kuettner K, et al: Molecular basis of osteoarthritis: Biomechanical aspects. Cell Mol Life Sci 59:27-35, 2002.
12. Kempson GE: Age-related changes in the tensile properties of human articular cartilage: A comparative study between the femoral head of the hip joint and the talus of the ankle joint. Biochim Biophys Acta 1075:223-230, 1991.
13. Huch K, Kuettner KE, Dieppe P: Osteoarthritis in ankle and knee joints. Semin Arthritis Rheum 26:667-674, 1997.
14. Hauselmann HJ, Mok SS, Fleechtenmacher J, et al: Chondrocytes from human knee and ankle joints show differences in response to IL-1 and IL-1 receptor inhibitor. Orthop Trans 17:710, 1993.
15. Chubinskaya S, Huch K, Mikecz K, et al: Chondrocyte matrix metalloproteinase-8: Up-regulation of neutrophil collagenase by interleukin-1 beta in human cartilage from knee and ankle joints. Lab Invest 74:232-240, 1996.
16. Anderson JJ, Felson DT: Factors associated with osteoarthritis of the knee in the first national Health and Nutrition Examination Survey (HANES I): Evidence for an association with overweight, race, and physical demands of work. Am J Epidemiol 128:179-189, 1988.
17. **Felson DT, Zhang Y, Hannan MT, et al: The incidence and natural history of knee osteoarthritis in the elderly. The Framingham Osteoarthritis Study. Arthritis Rheum 38:1500-1505, 1995.**
18. Hunter DJ, March L, Sambrook PN: Knee osteoarthritis: The influence of environmental factors. Clin Exp Rheumatol 20:93-100, 2002.
19. **Kellgren JH, Lawrence JS, Bier F: Genetic factors in generalized osteoarthritis. Ann Rheum Dis 22:237-255, 1963.**
20. Saville PD, Dickson J: Age and weight in osteoarthritis of the hip. Arthritis Rheum 11:635-644, 1968.
21. Hart DJ, Doyle DV, Spector TD: Incidence and risk factors for radiographic knee osteoarthritis in middle-aged women: The Chingford Study. Arthritis Rheum 42:17-24, 1999.
22. Jadelis K, Miller ME, Ettinger WH Jr, et al: Strength, balance, and the modifying effects of obesity and knee pain: Results from the Observational Arthritis Study in Seniors (OASIS). J Am Geriatr Soc 49:884-891, 2001.
23. Leach RE, Baumgard S, Broom J: Obesity: Its relationship to osteoarthritis of the knee. Clin Orthop 93:271-273, 1973.
24. Bliddal H, Christensen R: The management of osteoarthritis in the obese patient: Practical considerations and guidelines for therapy. Obes Rev 7:323-331, 2006.
25. Teichtahl AJ, Wluka AE, Proietto J, et al: Obesity and the female sex, risk factors for knee osteoarthritis that may be attributable to systemic or local leptin biosynthesis and its cellular effects. Med Hypotheses 65:312-315, 2005.
26. Dumond H, Presle N, Terlain B, et al: Evidence for a key role of leptin in osteoarthritis. Arthritis Rheum 48:3118-3129, 2003.
27. Newman B, Wallis GA: Is osteoarthritis a genetic disease? Clin Invest Med 25:139-149, 2002.
28. Loughlin J: Genetic epidemiology of primary osteoarthritis. Curr Opin Rheumatol 13:111-116, 2001.
29. Kellgren J, Lawrence J, Bier F: Genetic factors in generalized osteoarthrosis. Ann Rheum Dis 22:237-255, 1963.
30. Felson DT, Couropmitree NN, Chaisson CE, et al: Evidence for a Mendelian gene in a segregation analysis of generalized radiographic osteoarthritis: The Framingham Study. Arthritis Rheum 41:1064-1071, 1998.
31. Hirsch R, Lethbridge-Cejku M, Hanson R, et al: Familial aggregation of osteoarthritis: Data from the Baltimore Longitudinal Study on Aging. Arthritis Rheum 41:1227-1232, 1998.
32. MacGregor AJ, Antoniades L, Matson M, et al: The genetic contribution to radiographic hip osteoarthritis in women: Results of a classic twin study. Arthritis Rheum 43:2410-2416, 2000.
33. Cicuttini FM, Spector TD: What is the evidence that osteoarthritis is genetically determined? Baillieres Clin Rheumatol 11:657-669, 1997.
34. Spector TD, Cicuttini F, Baker J, et al: Genetic influences on osteoarthritis in women: A twin study. BMJ 312:940-943, 1996.
35. Bijkerk C, Houwing-Duistermaat JJ, Valkenburg HA, et al: Heritabilities of radiologic osteoarthritis in peripheral joints and of disc degeneration of the spine. Arthritis Rheum 42:1729-1735, 1999.
36. Reginato AM, Olsen BR: The role of structural genes in the pathogenesis of osteoarthritic disorders. Arthritis Res 4:337-345, 2002.
37. Knowlton RG, Katzenstein PL, Moskowitz RW, et al: Genetic linkage of a polymorphism in the type II procollagen gene (COL2A1) to primary osteoarthritis associated with mild chondrodysplasia. N Engl J Med 322:526-530, 1990.
38. Ala-Kokko L, Baldwin CT, Moskowitz RW, et al: Single base mutation in the type II procollagen gene (COL2A1) as a cause of primary osteoarthritis associated with a mild chondrodysplasia. Proc Natl Acad Sci U S A 87:6565-6568, 1990.
39. Jimenez SA, Williams CJ, Karasick D: Hereditary osteoarthritis. In Brandt KD, Doherty M, Lohmander LS (eds): Osteoarthritis. Oxford, Oxford University Press, 1998, pp 31-49.
40. Hu K, Xu L, Cao L, et al: Pathogenesis of osteoarthritis-like changes in the joints of mice deficient in type IX collagen. Arthritis Rheum 54:2891-2900, 2006.
41. van der Weyden L, Wei L, Luo J, et al: Functional knockout of the matrilin-3 gene causes premature chondrocyte maturation to hypertrophy and increases bone mineral density and osteoarthritis. Am J Pathol 169:515-527, 2006.
42. Glowacki J, Hurwitz S, Thornhill TS, et al: Osteoporosis and vitamin-D deficiency among postmenopausal women with osteoarthritis undergoing total hip arthroplasty. J Bone Joint Surg Am 85A: 2371-2377, 2003.
43. Sokoloff L: The Biology of Degenerative Joint Disease. Chicago, University of Chicago Press, 1969.
44. **Radin EL, Paul IL: Does cartilage compliance reduce skeletal impact loads? The relative force-attenuating properties of articular cartilage, synovial fluid, periarticular soft tissues and bone. Arthritis Rheum 13:139-144, 1970.**
45. Ho AM, Johnson MD, Kingsley DM: Role of the mouse ank gene in control of tissue calcification and arthritis. Science 289:265-270, 2000.

46. Loughlin J, Dowling B, Mustafa Z, et al: Association of the interleukin-1 gene cluster on chromosome 2q13 with knee osteoarthritis. Arthritis Rheum 46:1519-1527, 2002.
47. Leppavuori J, Kujala U, Kinnunen J, et al: Genome scan for predisposing loci for distal interphalangeal joint osteoarthritis: Evidence for a locus on 2q. Am J Hum Genet 65:1060-1067, 1999.
48. Loughlin J: Genome studies and linkage in primary osteoarthritis. Rheum Dis Clin N Am 28:95-109, 2002.
49. Attur MG, Patel IR, Patel RN, et al: Autocrine production of IL-1 beta by human osteoarthritis-affected cartilage and differential regulation of endogenous nitric oxide, IL-6, prostaglandin E2, and IL-8. Proc Assoc Am Physicians 110:65-72, 1998.
50. Attur MG, Dave MN, Clancy RM, et al: Functional genomic analysis in arthritis-affected cartilage: Yin-yang regulation of inflammatory mediators by alpha 5 beta 1 and alpha V beta 3 integrins. J Immunol 164:2684-2691, 2000.
51. Meng J, Ma X, Ma D, et al: Microarray analysis of differential gene expression in temporomandibular joint condylar cartilage after experimentally induced osteoarthritis. Osteoarthritis Cartilage 13:1115-1125, 2005.
52. Moos V, Rudwaleit M, Herzog V, et al: Association of genotypes affecting the expression of interleukin-1beta or interleukin-1 receptor antagonist with osteoarthritis. Arthritis Rheum 43:2417-2422, 2000.
53. Bullough PG: The geometry of diarthrodial joints, its physiologic maintenance, and the possible significance of age-related changes in geometry-to-load distribution and the development of osteoarthritis. Clin Orthop 156:61-66, 1981.
54. Lane LB, Villacin A, Bullough PG: The vascularity and remodelling of subchondral bone and calcified cartilage in adult human femoral and humeral heads: An age- and stress-related phenomenon. J Bone Joint Surg Br 59B:272-278, 1977.
55. Day WH, Swanson SA, Freeman MA: Contact pressures in the loaded human cadaver hip. J Bone Joint Surg Br 57B:302-313, 1975.
56. Slowman SD, Brandt KD: Composition and glycosaminoglycan metabolism of articular cartilage from habitually loaded and habitually unloaded sites. Arthritis Rheum 29:88-94, 1986.
57. Schumacher HR: Secondary osteoarthritis. In Moskowitz RW, Howell DS, Goldberg VM, et al (eds): Osteoarthritis: Diagnosis and Management. Philadelphia, WB Saunders, 1984, p 235.
58. Conaghan PG: Update on osteoarthritis, Part 1: Current concepts and the relation to exercise. Br J Sports Med 36:330-333, 2002.
59. Donahue JM, Oegema TR Jr, Thompson RG Jr: The zone of calcified cartilage: The focal point of changes following blunt trauma to articular cartilage. Trans Orthop Res Soc 11:233, 1986.
60. Radin EL: Mechanical factors in the etiology of osteoarthrosis. In Peyron JG (ed): Epidemiology of Osteoarthrosis. Paris, Ciba-Geigy, 1981, p 136.
61. Linn FC, Radin EL: Lubrication of animal joints, 3: The effect of certain chemical alterations of the cartilage and lubricant. Arthritis Rheum 11:674-682, 1968.
62. Radin EL, Paul IL: Response of joints to impact loading, I: In vitro wear. Arthritis Rheum 14:356-362, 1971.
63. Thelin N, Holmberg S, Thelin A: Knee injuries account for the sports-related increased risk of knee osteoarthritis. Scand J Med Sci Sports 16:329-333, 2006.
64. Reilly DT, Martens M: Experimental analysis of the quadriceps muscle force and patellofemoral joint reaction force for various activities. Acta Orthop Scand 43:126-137, 1972.
65. Hill AV: Production and absorption of work by muscle. Science 131:897-903, 1960.
66. Ochoa JA, Heck DA, Brandt KD, et al: The effect of intertrabecular fluid on femoral head mechanics. J Rheumatol 18:580-584, 1991.
67. Bullough P, Goodfellow J, O'Conner J: The relationship between degenerative changes and load-bearing in the human hip. J Bone Joint Surg Br 55B:746-758, 1973.
68. Todd RC, Freeman MA, Pirie CJ: Isolated trabecular fatigue fractures in the femoral head. J Bone Joint Surg Br 54:723-728, 1972.
69. Fazzalari NL, Vernon-Roberts B, Darracott J: Osteoarthritis of the hip: Possible protective and causative roles of trabecular microfractures in the head of the femur. Clin Orthop 216:224-233, 1987.
70. Foss MV, Byers PD: Bone density, osteoarthrosis of the hip, and fracture of the upper end of the femur. Ann Rheum Dis 31:259-264, 1972.
71. Radin EL: Mechanical aspects of osteoarthrosis. Bull Rheum Dis 26:862-865, 1976.
72. Wluka AE, Cicuttini FM, Spector TD: Menopause, oestrogens and arthritis. Maturitas 35:183-199, 2000.
73. Dillon CF, Rasch EK, Gu Q, et al: Prevalence of knee osteoarthritis in the United States: Arthritis data from the Third National Health and Nutrition Examination Survey 1991-94. J Rheumatol 33:2271-2279, 2006.
74. Ushiyama T, Ueyama H, Inoue K, et al: Expression of genes for estrogen receptors alpha and beta in human articular chondrocytes. Osteoarthritis Cartilage 7:560-566, 1999.
75. Pelletier G, El-Alfy M: Immunocytochemical localization of estrogen receptors alpha and beta in the human reproductive organs. J Clin Endocrinol Metab 85:4835-4840, 2000.
76. Ng MC, Harper RP, Le CT, et al: Effects of estrogen on the condylar cartilage of the rat mandible in organ culture. J Oral Maxillofac Surg 57:818-823, 1999.
77. Richmond RS, Carlson CS, Register TC, et al: Functional estrogen receptors in adult articular cartilage: Estrogen replacement therapy increases chondrocyte synthesis of proteoglycans and insulin-like growth factor binding protein 2. Arthritis Rheum 43:2081-2090, 2000.
78. Claassen H, Hassenpflug J, Schunke M, et al: Immunohistochemical detection of estrogen receptor alpha in articular chondrocytes from cows, pigs and humans: In situ and in vitro results. Ann Anat 183:223-227, 2001.
79. Nilsson LO, Boman A, Savendahl L, et al: Demonstration of estrogen receptor-beta immunoreactivity in human growth plate cartilage. J Clin Endocrinol Metab 84:370-373, 1999.
80. Bord S, Vedi S, Beavan SR, et al: Megakaryocyte population in human bone marrow increases with estrogen treatment: A role in bone remodeling? Bone 27:397-401, 2000.
81. Nevitt MC, Cummings SR, Lane NE, et al: Association of estrogen replacement therapy with the risk of osteoarthritis of the hip in elderly white women. Study of Osteoporotic Fractures Research Group. Arch Intern Med 156:2073-2080, 1996.
82. Sowers MF, Hochberg M, Crabbe JP, et al: Association of bone mineral density and sex hormone levels with osteoarthritis of the hand and knee in premenopausal women. Am J Epidemiol 143:38-47, 1996.
83. Zhang Y, McAlindon TE, Hannan MT, et al: Estrogen replacement therapy and worsening of radiographic knee osteoarthritis: The Framingham Study. Arthritis Rheum 41:1867-1873, 1998.
84. Wluka AE, Davis SR, Bailey M, et al: Users of oestrogen replacement therapy have more knee cartilage than non-users. Ann Rheum Dis 60:332-336, 2001.
85. Spector TD, Hart DJ, Nandra D, et al: Low-level increases in serum C-reactive protein are present in early osteoarthritis of the knee and predict progressive disease. Arthritis Rheum 40:723-727, 1997.
86. Ham KD, Loeser RF, Lindgren BR, et al: Effects of long-term estrogen replacement therapy on osteoarthritis severity in cynomolgus monkeys. Arthritis Rheum 46:1956-1964, 2002.
87. Ushiyama T, Ueyama H, Inoue K, et al: Estrogen receptor gene polymorphism and generalized osteoarthritis. J Rheumatol 25:134-137, 1998.
88. **Maroudas AI: Balance between swelling pressure and collagen tension in normal and degenerate cartilage. Nature 260:808-809, 1976.**
89. Maroudas A: Transport through articular cartilage and some physiological implications. In Ali SY, Elves MW, Leaback DH (eds): Normal and Osteoarthrotic Articular Cartilage. London, Institute of Orthopaedics, 1974, p 33.
90. Mankin HJ, Brandt KD: Biochemistry and metabolism of articular cartilage in osteoarthritis. In Moskowitz RW, Howell DS, Goldberg VM, et al (eds): Osteoarthritis: Diagnosis and Medical/Surgical Management, 2nd ed. Philadelphia, WB Saunders, 1992, pp 109-154.
91. Herbage D, Huc A, Chabrand D, et al: Physicochemical study of articular cartilage from healthy and osteoarthritic human hips: Orientation and thermal stability of collagen fibres. Biochim Biophys Acta 271:339-346, 1972.
92. Muir H: Current and future trends in articular cartilage research and osteoarthritis. In Kuettner KE, Schleyerbach R, Hascall VC (eds): Articular Cartilage and Biochemistry. New York, Raven Press, 1986, pp 423-440.

93. **Mankin HJ, Lippiello L: Biochemical and metabolic abnormalities in articular cartilage from osteo-arthritic human hips. J Bone Joint Surg Am 52:424-434, 1970.**
94. Inerot S, Heinegard D, Audell L, et al: Articular-cartilage proteoglycans in aging and osteoarthritis. Biochem J 169:143-156, 1978.
95. Bollet AJ, Nance JL: Biochemical findings in normal and osteoarthritic articular cartilage, II: Chondroitin sulfate concentration and chain length, water, and ash contents. J Clin Invest 44:1170-1177, 1966.
96. Mankin HJ, Dorfman H, Lippiello L, et al: Biochemical and metabolic abnormalities in articular cartilage from osteo-arthritic human hips, II: Correlation of morphology with biochemical and metabolic data. J Bone Joint Surg Am 53A:523-537, 1971.
97. Jaovisidha K, Rosenthal AK: Calcium crystals in osteoarthritis. Curr Opin Rheumatol 14:298-302, 2002.
98. Rosenthal AK: Calcium crystal deposition and osteoarthritis. Rheum Dis Clin N Am 32:401-412, vii, 2006.
99. Wu CW, Terkeltaub R, Kalunian KC: Calcium-containing crystals and osteoarthritis: Implications for the clinician. Curr Rheumatol Rep 7:213-219, 2005.
100. Ryan LM, Cheung HS: The role of crystals in osteoarthritis. Rheum Dis Clin N Am 25:257-267, 1999.
101. Howell DS, Muniz OE, Morales S: 5′ Nucleotidase and pyrophosphate (Ppi)-generating activities in articular cartilage extracts in calcium pyrophosphate deposition disease (CPPD) and in primary osteoarthritis (OA). In Peyron JG (ed): Epidemiology of Osteoarthritis. Paris, Ciba-Geigy, 1980, p 99.
102. Howell DS, Muniz O, Pita JC, et al: Extrusion of pyrophosphate into extracellular media by osteoarthritic cartilage incubates. J Clin Invest 56:1473-1478, 1975.
103. Altman RD, Muniz OE, Pita JC, et al: Articular chondrocalcinosis: Microanalysis of pyrophosphate (PPi) in synovial fluid and plasma. Arthritis Rheum 16:171-178, 1973.
104. Silcox DC, McCarty DJ Jr: Elevated inorganic pyrophosphate concentrations in synovial fluids in osteoarthritis and pseudogout. J Lab Clin Med 83:518-531, 1974.
105. Tenenbaum J, Muniz O, Schumacher HR, et al: Comparison of phosphohydrolase activities from articular cartilage in calcium pyrophosphate deposition disease and primary osteoarthritis. Arthritis Rheum 24:492-500, 1981.
106. **Ryu J, Treadwell BV, Mankin HJ: Biochemical and metabolic abnormalities in normal and osteoarthritic human articular cartilage. Arthritis Rheum 27:49-57, 1984.**
107. Mort JS, Billington CJ: Articular cartilage and changes in arthritis: Matrix degradation. Arthritis Res 3:337-341, 2001.
108. Murphy G, Docherty AJP: Molecular studies on the connective tissue metalloproteinases and their inhibitor TIMP. In Galuert AM (ed): The Control of Tissue Damage. Oxford, Elsevier, 1988, p 223.
109. Mankin HJ, Thrasher AZ: Water content and binding in normal and osteoarthritic human cartilage. J Bone Joint Surg Am 57:76-80, 1975.
110. Sandy JD, Lark MW: Proteolytic degradation of normal and osteoarthritic cartilage matrix. In Brandt KD, Doherty M, Lohmander LS (eds): Osteoarthritis. Oxford, Oxford University Press, 1998, p 84.
111. Morales TI, Kuettner KE: The properties of the neutral proteinase released by primary chondrocyte cultures and its action on proteoglycan aggregate. Biochim Biophys Acta 705:92-101, 1982.
112. Sapolsky AI, Howell DS: Further characterization of a neutral metalloprotease isolated from human articular cartilage. Arthritis Rheum 25:981-988, 1982.
113. Hedbom E, Hauselmann HJ: Molecular aspects of pathogenesis in osteoarthritis: The role of inflammation. Cell Mol Life Sci 59:45-53, 2002.
114. Knauper V, Lopez-Otin C, Smith B, et al: Biochemical characterization of human collagenase-3. J Biol Chem 271:1544-1550, 1996.
115. Tetlow LC, Adlam DJ, Woolley DE: Matrix metalloproteinase and proinflammatory cytokine production by chondrocytes of human osteoarthritic cartilage: Associations with degenerative changes. Arthritis Rheum 44:585-594, 2001.
116. Ehrlich MG, Mankin HJ, Jones H, et al: Collagenase and collagenase inhibitors in osteoarthritic and normal cartilage. J Clin Invest 59:226-233, 1977.
117. Ehrlich MG, Houle PA, Vigliani G, et al: Correlation between articular cartilage collagenase activity and osteoarthritis. Arthritis Rheum 21:761-766, 1978.
118. Xie DL, Hui F, Meyers R, et al: Cartilage chondrolysis by fibronectin fragments is associated with release of several proteinases: Stromelysin plays a major role in chondrolysis. Arch Biochem Biophys 311:205-212, 1994.
119. Campbell IK, Piccoli DS, Butler DM, et al: Recombinant human interleukin-1 stimulates human articular cartilage to undergo resorption and human chondrocytes to produce both tissue- and urokinase-type plasminogen activator. Biochim Biophys Acta 967:183-194, 1988.
120. **Tang BL: ADAMTS: A novel family of extracellular matrix proteases. Int J Biochem Cell Biol 33:33-44, 2001.**
121. Arner EC: Aggrecanase-mediated cartilage degradation. Curr Opin Pharmacol 2:322-329, 2002.
122. Liu CJ, Kong W, Ilalov K, et al: ADAMTS-7: A metalloproteinase that directly binds to and degrades cartilage oligomeric matrix protein. FASEB J 20:988-990, 2006.
123. Liu CJ, Kong W, Xu K, et al: ADAMTS-12 associates with and degrades cartilage oligomeric matrix protein. J Biol Chem 281:15800-15808, 2006.
124. Dickinson SC, Vankemmelbeke MN, Buttle DJ, et al: Cleavage of cartilage oligomeric matrix protein (thrombospondin-5) by matrix metalloproteinases and a disintegrin and metalloproteinase with thrombospondin motifs. Matrix Biol 22:267-278, 2003.
125. Stracke JO, Fosang AJ, Last K, et al: Matrix metalloproteinases 19 and 20 cleave aggrecan and cartilage oligomeric matrix protein (COMP). FEBS Lett 478(1-2):52-56, 2000.
126. Hardingham T, Bayliss M: Proteoglycans of articular cartilage: Changes in aging and in joint disease. Semin Arthritis Rheum 20(3 Suppl 1):12-33, 1990.
127. Campbell IK, Wojta J, Novak U, et al: Cytokine modulation of plasminogen activator inhibitor-1 (PAI-1) production by human articular cartilage and chondrocytes: Down-regulation by tumor necrosis factor alpha and up-regulation by transforming growth factor-β basic fibroblast growth factor. Biochim Biophys Acta 1226:277-285, 1994.
128. Ollivierre F, Gubler U, Towle CA, et al: Expression of IL-1 genes in human and bovine chondrocytes: A mechanism for autocrine control of cartilage matrix degradation. Biochem Biophys Res Commun 141:904-911, 1986.
129. Rath NC, Oronsky AL, Kerwar SS: Synthesis of interleukin-1-like activity by normal rat chondrocytes in culture. Clin Immunol Immunopathol 47:39-46, 1988.
130. Kandel RA, Dinarello CA, Biswas C: The stimulation of collagenase production in rabbit articular chondrocytes by interleukin-1 is increased by collagens. Biochem Int 15:1021-1031, 1987.
131. Dodge GR, Poole AR: Immunohistochemical detection and immunochemical analysis of type II collagen degradation in human normal, rheumatoid, and osteoarthritic articular cartilages and in explants of bovine articular cartilage cultured with interleukin 1. J Clin Invest 83:647-661, 1989.
132. Ratcliffe A, Tyler JA, Hardingham TE: Articular cartilage cultured with interleukin 1: Increased release of link protein, hyaluronate-binding region and other proteoglycan fragments. Biochem J 238:571-580, 1986.
133. **Tortorella MD, Malfait AM, Deccico C, et al: The role of ADAM-TS4 (aggrecanase-1) and ADAM-TS5 (aggrecanase-2) in a model of cartilage degradation. Osteoarthritis Cartilage 9:539-552, 2001.**
134. Dean DD, Woessner JF Jr: Extracts of human articular cartilage contain an inhibitor of tissue metalloproteinases. Biochem J 218:277-280, 1984.
135. Yamada H, Stephens RW, Nakagawa T, et al: Human articular cartilage contains an inhibitor of plasminogen activator. J Rheumatol 15:1138-1143, 1988.
136. Malemud CJ: The role of growth factors in cartilage metabolism. Rheum Dis Clin N Am 19:569-580, 1993.
137. Morales TI: Transforming growth factor-beta and insulin-like growth factor-1 restore proteoglycan metabolism of bovine articular cartilage after depletion by retinoic acid. Arch Biochem Biophys 315:190-198, 1994.
138. Kevorkian L, Young DA, Darrah C, et al: Expression profiling of metalloproteinases and their inhibitors in cartilage. Arthritis Rheum 50:131-141, 2004.
139. Dean DD, Azzo W, Martel-Pelletier J, et al: Levels of metalloproteases and tissue inhibitor of metalloproteases in human osteoarthritic cartilage. J Rheumatol 14(Spec No):43-44, 1987.

140. Teshima R, Treadwell BV, Trahan CA, et al: Comparative rates of proteoglycan synthesis and size of proteoglycans in normal and osteoarthritic chondrocytes. Arthritis Rheum 26:1225-1230, 1983.
141. Moskowitz RW, Davis W, Sammarco J, et al: Experimentally induced degenerative joint lesions following partial meniscectomy in the rabbit. Arthritis Rheum 16:397-405, 1973.
142. Muir H: Heberden Oration, 1976. Molecular approach to the understanding of osteoarthrosis. Ann Rheum Dis 36:199-208, 1977.
143. Bove SE, Calcaterra SL, Brooker RM, et al: Weight bearing as a measure of disease progression and efficacy of anti-inflammatory compounds in a model of monosodium iodoacetate-induced osteoarthritis. Osteoarthritis Cartilage 11:821-830, 2003.
144. Pomonis JD, Boulet JM, Gottshall SL, et al: Development and pharmacological characterization of a rat model of osteoarthritis pain. Pain 114:339-346, 2005.
145. Ameye LG, Young MF: Animal models of osteoarthritis: Lessons learned while seeking the "Holy Grail." Curr Opin Rheumatol 18:537-547, 2006.
146. McDevitt CA, Muir H: Biochemical changes in the cartilage of the knee in experimental and natural osteoarthritis in the dog. J Bone Joint Surg Br 58:94-101, 1976.
147. Brandt KD: Enhanced extractability of articular cartilage proteoglycans in osteoarthrosis. Biochem J 143:475-478, 1974.
148. Moskowitz RW, Howell DS, Goldberg VM, et al: Cartilage proteoglycan alterations in an experimentally induced model of rabbit osteoarthritis. Arthritis Rheum 22:155-163, 1979.
149. Maroudas A, Katz EP, Wachtel EJ, et al: Physiochemical properties and functional behavior of normal and osteoarthritic human cartilage. In Schleyerbach R, Kuettner KE, Hascall VC (eds): Articular Cartilage Biochemistry. New York, Raven Press, 1986, pp 311-330.
150. Adams ME, Brandt KD: Hypertrophic repair of canine articular cartilage in osteoarthritis after anterior cruciate ligament transection. J Rheumatol 18:428-435, 1991.
151. Bywaters EGL: Metabolism of joint tissue. J Pathol Bacteriol 44:247, 1937.
152. Johnson LD: Kinetics of osteoarthritis. Lab Invest 8:1223, 1959.
153. Kempson GE, Spivey CJ, Swanson SA, et al: Patterns of cartilage stiffness on normal and degenerate human femoral heads. J Biomech 4:597-609, 1971.
154. Mankin HJ, Mow VC, Buckwalter JA, et al: Form and function of articular cartilage. In Simon S (ed): Orthopaedic Basic Science. Chicago, American Academy of Orthopaedic Surgeons, 1994, pp 1-44.
155. Bollet AJ: Connective tissue polysaccharide metabolism and the pathogenesis of osteoarthritis. Adv Intern Med 13:33-60, 1967.
156. Freeman MAR: Discussion on pathogenesis of osteoarthrosis. In Ali SY, Elves MW, Leaback DH (eds): Normal and Osteoarthrotic Articular Cartilage. London, Institute of Orthopaedics, 1974, p 301.
157. Hlavacek M: The role of synovial fluid filtration by cartilage in lubrication of synovial joints, I: Mixture model of synovial fluid. J Biomech 26:1145-1150, 1993.
158. **Mow VC, Ateshian GA, Spilker RL: Biomechanics of diarthrodial joints: A review of twenty years of progress. J Biomech Eng 115(4B):460-467, 1993.**
159. Unsworth A: Tribology of human and artificial joints. Proc Inst Mech Eng [H] 205:163-172, 1991.
160. Hlavacek M: The role of synovial fluid filtration by cartilage in lubrication of synovial joints, IV: Squeeze-film lubrication: The central film thickness for normal and inflammatory synovial fluids for axial symmetry under high loading conditions. J Biomech 28:1199-1205, 1995.
161. Hlavacek M, Novak J: The role of synovial fluid filtration by cartilage in lubrication of synovial joints, III: Squeeze-film lubrication: Axial symmetry under low loading conditions. J Biomech 28:1193-1198, 1995.
162. Hlavacek M: Squeeze-film lubrication of the human ankle joint with synovial fluid filtrated by articular cartilage with the superficial zone worn out. J Biomech 33:1415-1422, 2000.
163. Hlavacek M: The influence of the acetabular labrum seal, intact articular superficial zone and synovial fluid thixotropy on squeeze-film lubrication of a spherical synovial joint. J Biomech 35:1325-1335, 2002.
164. Malemud CJ, Goldberg VM, Moskowitz RW, et al: Biosynthesis of proteoglycan in vitro by cartilage from human osteochondrophytic spurs. Biochem J 206:329-341, 1982.

165. Marshall JL, Olsson SE: Instability of the knee: A long-term experimental study in dogs. J Bone Joint Surg Am 53:1561-1570, 1971.
166. Danielsson LG: Incidence and prognosis of coxarthrosis. 1964. Clin Orthop 287:13-18, 1993.
167. Trueta J: Studies of the Development and Decay of the Human Frame. Philadelphia, WB Saunders, 1968.
168. Swanson SAV, Freeman MAR: The mechanics of synovial joints. In Simpson DC (ed): Modern Trends in Biomechanics, Vol 1. London, Butterworths, 1970, p 239.
169. Gilbertson EM: Development of periarticular osteophytes in experimentally induced osteoarthritis in the dog: A study using microradiographic, microangiographic, and fluorescent bone-labelling techniques. Ann Rheum Dis 34:12-25, 1975.
170. Shuler FD, Georgescu HI, Niyibizi C, et al: Increased matrix synthesis following adenoviral transfer of a transforming growth factor beta1 gene into articular chondrocytes. J Orthop Res 18:585-592, 2000.
171. Bakker AC, van de Loo FA, van Beuningen HM, et al: Overexpression of active TGF-beta-1 in the murine knee joint: Evidence for synovial-layer-dependent chondro-osteophyte formation. Osteoarthritis Cartilage 9:128-136, 2001.
172. Uchino M, Izumi T, Tominaga T, et al: Growth factor expression in the osteophytes of the human femoral head in osteoarthritis. Clin Orthop 377:119-125, 2000.
173. Bernstein MA: Experimental production of arthritis by artificially produced passive congestion. J Bone Joint Surg 15:661, 1933.
174. Phillips RS: Phlebography in osteoarthritis of the hip. J Bone Joint Surg Br 48:280-288, 1966.
175. Landells JW: The bone cysts of osteoarthritis. J Bone Joint Surg 35:643, 1953.
176. Palmoski MJ, Brandt KD: Immobilization of the knee prevents osteoarthritis after anterior cruciate ligament transection. Arthritis Rheum 25:1201-1208, 1982.
177. Myers SL, Brandt KD, Burr DB, et al: Effects of a bisphosphonate on bone histomorphometry and dynamics in the canine cruciate deficiency model of osteoarthritis. J Rheumatol 26:2645-2653, 1999.
178. Chen FS, Frenkel SR, Di Cesare PE: Repair of articular cartilage defects, Part I: basic science of cartilage healing. Am J Orthop 28:31-33, 1999.
179. Frenkel SR, Di Cesare PE: Degradation and repair of articular cartilage. Front Biosci 4:D671-D685, 1999.
180. Buckwalter JA, Mow VC, Ratcliffe A: Restoration of injured or degenerated articular cartilage. J Am Acad Orthop Surg 2:192-201, 1994.
181. Buckwalter JA, Lohmander S: Operative treatment of osteoarthrosis: Current practice and future development. J Bone Joint Surg Am 76:1405-1418, 1994.
182. Coletti JM Jr, Akeson WH, Woo SL: A comparison of the physical behavior of normal articular cartilage and the arthroplasty surface. J Bone Joint Surg Am 54:147-160, 1972.
183. **Mankin HJ: The response of articular cartilage to mechanical injury. J Bone Joint Surg Am 64:460-466, 1982.**
184. Hamerman D: Prospects for medical intervention in cartilage repair. In Woessner JF, Howell D (eds): Joint Cartilage Degradation: Basic and Clinical Aspects. New York, Marcel Dekker, 1993, pp 529-546.
185. Campbell CJ: The healing of cartilage defects. Clin Orthop 64:45-63, 1969.
186. Redfern P: On the healing of wounds in articular cartilage. Clin Orthop 64:4-6, 1969.
187. Fisher T: Some researches into the physiological principles underlying the treatment of injuries and diseases of the articulations. Lancet 2:541-548, 1923.
188. Ito LK: The nutrition of articular cartilage and its method of repair. Br J Surg 12:31-42, 1924.
189. Carlson H: Reactions of rabbit patellary cartilage following operative defects. Acta Orthop Scand Suppl 28:1-118, 1957.
190. Gilmer WS Jr, Calandruccio R: Proliferation, regeneration, and repair of articular cartilage of immature animals. J Bone Joint Surg Am 44A:431-455, 1962.
191. Mankin HJ: Localization of tritiated thymidine in articular cartilage of rabbits, II: Repair in immature cartilage. J Bone Joint Surg Am 44A:688-698, 1962.
192. Mankin HJ: Localization of tritiated thymidine in articular cartilage of rabbits, III: Mature articular cartilage. J Bone Joint Surg Am 45A:529-540, 1963.

193. Grande DA, Singh IJ, Pugh J: Healing of experimentally produced lesions in articular cartilage following chondrocyte transplantation. Anat Rec 218:142-148, 1987.

194. Radin EL, Ehrlich MG, Chernack R, et al: Effect of repetitive impulsive loading on the knee joints of rabbits. Clin Orthop 131:288-293, 1978.

195. Beim GM, Fu FH: Classification and treatment of DJD of the knee. Orthop Spec Ed 2:31-35, 1996.

196. Dekel S, Weissman SL: Joint changes after overuse and peak overloading of rabbit knees in vivo. Acta Orthop Scand 49:519-528, 1978.

197. Lee SH, Abramson SA: Stepped-care guide to osteoarthritis therapy. Orthop Spec Ed 2:7-10, 1996.

198. Farrell AJ, Blake DR, Palmer RM, et al: Increased concentrations of nitrite in synovial fluid and serum samples suggest increased nitric oxide synthesis in rheumatic diseases. Ann Rheum Dis 51:1219-1222, 1992.

199. Yoshimi T, Kikuchi T, Obara T, et al: Effects of high-molecular-weight sodium hyaluronate on experimental osteoarthrosis induced by the resection of rabbit anterior cruciate ligament. Clin Orthop 298:296-304, 1994.

200. Cheung HS, Cottrell WH, Stephenson K, et al: In vitro collagen biosynthesis in healing and normal rabbit articular cartilage. J Bone Joint Surg Am 60:1076-1081, 1978.

201. DePalma AF, McKeever CD, Subin DK: Process of repair of articular cartilage demonstrated by histology and autoradiography with tritiated thymidine. Clin Orthop 48:229-242, 1966.

202. Mitchell N, Shepard N: The resurfacing of adult rabbit articular cartilage by multiple perforations through the subchondral bone. J Bone Joint Surg Am 58:230-233, 1976.

203. Shapiro F, Koide S, Glimcher MJ: Cell origin and differentiation in the repair of full-thickness defects of articular cartilage. J Bone Joint Surg Am 75:532-553, 1993.

204. Cheung HS, Lynch KL, Johnson RP, et al: In vitro synthesis of tissue-specific type II collagen by healing cartilage, I: Short-term repair of cartilage by mature rabbits. Arthritis Rheum 23:211-219, 1980.

205. Furukawa T, Eyre DR, Koide S, et al: Biochemical studies on repair cartilage resurfacing experimental defects in the rabbit knee. J Bone Joint Surg Am 62:79-89, 1980.

206. Hjertquist SO, Lemperg R: Histological, autoradiographic and microchemical studies of spontaneously healing osteochondral articular defects in adult rabbits. Calcif Tissue Res 8:54-72, 1971.

207. Convery FR, Akeson WH, Keown GH: The repair of large osteochondral defects: An experimental study in horses. Clin Orthop 82:253-262, 1972.

208. Mobasheri A, Carter SD, Martin-Vasallo P, et al: Integrins and stretch activated ion channels: Putative components of functional cell surface mechanoreceptors in articular chondrocytes. Cell Biol Int 26:1-18, 2002.

209. Grodzinsky AJ, Levenston ME, Jin M, et al: Cartilage tissue remodeling in response to mechanical forces. Annu Rev Biomed Eng 2:691-713, 2000.

210. Giannoni P, Siegrist M, Hunziker EB, et al: The mechanosensitivity of cartilage oligomeric matrix protein (COMP). Biorheology 40:101-109, 2003.

211. Wong M, Siegrist M, Cao X: Cyclic compression of articular cartilage explants is associated with progressive consolidation and altered expression pattern of extracellular matrix proteins. Matrix Biol 18:391-399, 1999.

212. Lee HS, Millward-Sadler SJ, Wright MO, et al: Integrin and mechanosensitive ion channel-dependent tyrosine phosphorylation of focal adhesion proteins and beta-catenin in human articular chondrocytes after mechanical stimulation. J Bone Miner Res 15:1501-1509, 2000.

213. Salter DM, Millward-Sadler SJ, Nuki G, et al: Differential responses of chondrocytes from normal and osteoarthritic human articular cartilage to mechanical stimulation. Biorheology 39(1-2):97-108, 2002.

214. Millward-Sadler SJ, Wright MO, Lee H, et al: Integrin-regulated secretion of interleukin 4: A novel pathway of mechanotransduction in human articular chondrocytes. J Cell Biol 145:183-189, 1999.

215. Millward-Sadler SJ, Wright MO, Davies LW, et al: Mechanotransduction via integrins and interleukin-4 results in altered aggrecan and matrix metalloproteinase 3 gene expression in normal, but not osteoarthritic, human articular chondrocytes. Arthritis Rheum 43:2091-2099, 2000.

216. Millward-Sadler SJ, Wright MO, Lee H, et al: Altered electrophysiological responses to mechanical stimulation and abnormal signalling through alpha5beta1 integrin in chondrocytes from osteoarthritic cartilage. Osteoarthritis Cartilage 8:272-278, 2000.

217. Sironen RK, Karjalainen HM, Torronen K, et al: High pressure effects on cellular expression profile and mRNA stability: A cDNA array analysis. Biorheology 39(1-2):111-117, 2002.

218. Jin M, Frank EH, Quinn TM, et al: Tissue shear deformation stimulates proteoglycan and protein biosynthesis in bovine cartilage explants. Arch Biochem Biophys 395:41-48, 2001.

219. Chen CT, Bhargava M, Lin PM, et al: Time, stress, and location dependent chondrocyte death and collagen damage in cyclically loaded articular cartilage. J Orthop Res 21:888-898, 2003.

220. Lin PM, Chen CT, Torzilli PA: Increased stromelysin-1 (MMP-3), proteoglycan degradation (3B3- and 7D4) and collagen damage in cyclically load-injured articular cartilage. Osteoarthritis Cartilage 12:485-496, 2004.

221. Wu Q, Zhang Y, Chen Q: Indian hedgehog is an essential component of mechanotransduction complex to stimulate chondrocyte proliferation. J Biol Chem 276:35290-35296, 2001.

222. Tchetina EV, Kobayashi M, Yasuda T, et al: Chondrocyte hypertrophy can be induced by a cryptic sequence of type II collagen and is accompanied by the induction of MMP-13 and collagenase activity: Implications for development and arthritis. Matrix Biol 26:247-258, 2007.

223. Pelletier JP, Martel-Pelletier J, Abramson SB: Osteoarthritis, an inflammatory disease: Potential implication for the selection of new therapeutic targets. Arthritis Rheum 44:1237-1247, 2001.

224. Martel-Pelletier J, di Battista JA, Lajeunesse D: Biochemical factors in joint articular tissue degradation in osteoarthritis. In Reginster JY, Pelletier JP, Martel-Pelletier J, et al (eds): Osteoarthritis: Clinical and Experimental Aspects. Berlin, Springer-Verlag, 1999, pp 156-187.

225. Caron JP, Fernandes JC, Martel-Pelletier J, et al: Chondroprotective effect of intraarticular injections of interleukin-1 receptor antagonist in experimental osteoarthritis: Suppression of collagenase-1 expression. Arthritis Rheum 39:1535-1544, 1996.

226. van de Loo FA, Joosten LA, van Lent PL, et al: Role of interleukin-1, tumor necrosis factor alpha, and interleukin-6 in cartilage proteoglycan metabolism and destruction: Effect of in situ blocking in murine antigen- and zymosan-induced arthritis. Arthritis Rheum 38:164-172, 1995.

227. Attur MG, Dave M, Cipolletta C, et al: Reversal of autocrine and paracrine effects of interleukin 1 (IL-1) in human arthritis by type II IL-1 decoy receptor: Potential for pharmacological intervention. J Biol Chem 275:40307-40315, 2000.

228. Vaillancourt F, Morquette B, Shi Q, et al: Differential regulation of cyclooxygenase-2 and inducible nitric oxide synthase by 4-hydroxynonenal in human osteoarthritic chondrocytes through ATF-2/CREB-1 transactivation and concomitant inhibition of NF-kappaB signaling cascade. J Cell Biochem 100:1217-1231, 2007.

229. Lianxu C, Hongti J, Changlong Y: NF-kappaBp65-specific siRNA inhibits expression of genes of COX-2, NOS-2 and MMP-9 in rat IL-1beta-induced and TNF-alpha-induced chondrocytes. Osteoarthritis Cartilage 14:367-376, 2006.

230. Kronheim SR, Mumma A, Greenstreet T, et al: Purification of interleukin-1 beta converting enzyme, the protease that cleaves the interleukin-1 beta precursor. Arch Biochem Biophys 296:698-703, 1992.

231. Slack J, McMahan CJ, Waugh S, et al: Independent binding of interleukin-1 alpha and interleukin-1 beta to type I and type II interleukin-1 receptors. J Biol Chem 268:2513-2524, 1993.

232. Martel-Pelletier J, Alaaeddine N, Pelletier JP: Cytokines and their role in the pathophysiology of osteoarthritis. Front Biosci 4:D694-D703, 1999.

233. Alaaeddine N, DiBattista JA, Pelletier JP, et al: Osteoarthritic synovial fibroblasts possess an increased level of tumor necrosis factor-receptor 55 (TNF-R55) that mediates biological activation by TNF-alpha. J Rheumatol 24:1985-1994, 1997.

234. Kobayashi H, Saito T, Koshino T: Immunolocalization of carboxy-terminal type II procollagen peptide in regenerated articular cartilage of osteoarthritic knees after reduction of mechanical stress. Osteoarthritis Cartilage 10:870-878, 2002.

235. Fernandes JC, Martel-Pelletier J, Pelletier JP: The role of cytokines in osteoarthritis pathophysiology. Biorheology 39(1-2):237-246, 2002.

236. Pelletier JP, Caron JP, Evans C, et al: In vivo suppression of early experimental osteoarthritis by interleukin-1 receptor antagonist using gene therapy. Arthritis Rheum 40:1012-1019, 1997.

237. Chevalier X, Giraudeau B, Conrozier T, et al: Safety study of intraarticular injection of interleukin 1 receptor antagonist in patients with painful knee osteoarthritis: A multicenter study. J Rheumatol 32:1317-1323, 2005.

238. Pelletier JP, Martel-Pelletier J, Abramson SB: Osteoarthritis, an inflammatory disease: Potential implication for the selection of new therapeutic targets. Arthritis Rheum 44:1237-1247, 2001.

239. Alaaeddine N, Olee T, Hashimoto S, et al: Production of the chemokine RANTES by articular chondrocytes and role in cartilage degradation. Arthritis Rheum 44:1633-1643, 2001.

240. Amin AR, Attur M, Patel RN, et al: Superinduction of cyclooxygenase-2 activity in human osteoarthritis-affected cartilage: Influence of nitric oxide. J Clin Invest 99:1231-1237, 1997.

241. Honorati MC, Bovara M, Cattini L, et al: Contribution of interleukin 17 to human cartilage degradation and synovial inflammation in osteoarthritis. Osteoarthritis Cartilage 10:799-807, 2002.

242. Yuan GH, Masuko-Hongo K, Sakata M, et al: The role of C-C chemokines and their receptors in osteoarthritis. Arthritis Rheum 44:1056-1070, 2001.

243. Davidson RK, Waters JG, Kevorkian L, et al: Expression profiling of metalloproteinases and their inhibitors in synovium and cartilage. Arthritis Res Ther 8:R124, 2006.

244. Neuhold LA, Killar L, Zhao W, et al: Postnatal expression in hyaline cartilage of constitutively active human collagenase-3 (MMP-13) induces osteoarthritis in mice. J Clin Invest 107:35-44, 2001.

245. Glasson SS, Askew R, Sheppard B, et al: Deletion of active ADAMTS5 prevents cartilage degradation in a murine model of osteoarthritis. Nature 434:644-648, 2005.

246. East CJ, Stanton H, Golub SB, et al: ADAMTS-5 deficiency does not block aggrecanolysis at preferred cleavage sites in the chondroitin sulfate-rich region of aggrecan. J Biol Chem 282:8632-8640, 2007.

247. Aigner T, McKenna L: Molecular pathology and pathobiology of osteoarthritic cartilage. Cell Mol Life Sci 59:5-18, 2002.

248. Scher DM, Stolerman ES, Di Cesare PE: Biologic markers of arthritis. Am J Orthop 25:263-272, 1996.

249. Heinegard D, Oldberg A: Structure and biology of cartilage and bone matrix noncollagenous macromolecules. FASEB J 3:2042-2051, 1989.

250. Roughley PJ: Articular cartilage and changes in arthritis: Noncollagenous proteins and proteoglycans in the extracellular matrix of cartilage. Arthritis Res 3:342-347, 2001.

251. Attur MG, Dave MN, Stuchin S, et al: Osteopontin: An intrinsic inhibitor of inflammation in cartilage. Arthritis Rheum 44:578-584, 2001.

252. Arner EC, Tortorella MD: Signal transduction through chondrocyte integrin receptors induces matrix metalloproteinase synthesis and synergizes with interleukin-1. Arthritis Rheum 38:1304-1314, 1995.

253. Homandberg GA, Hui F, Wen C, et al: Fibronectin-fragment-induced cartilage chondrolysis is associated with release of catabolic cytokines. Biochem J 321(Pt 3):751-757, 1997.

254. Homandberg GA, Meyers R, Williams JM: Intraarticular injection of fibronectin fragments causes severe depletion of cartilage proteoglycans in vivo. J Rheumatol 20:1378-1382, 1993.

255. Yasuda T, Poole AR: A fibronectin fragment induces type II collagen degradation by collagenase through an interleukin-1-mediated pathway. Arthritis Rheum 46:138-148, 2002.

256. Fichter M, Korner U, Schomburg J, et al: Collagen degradation products modulate matrix metalloproteinase expression in cultured articular chondrocytes. J Orthop Res 24:63-70, 2006.

257. Amin AR, Di Cesare PE, Vyas P, et al: The expression and regulation of nitric oxide synthase in human osteoarthritis-affected chondrocytes: Evidence for up-regulated neuronal nitric oxide synthase. J Exp Med 182:2097-2102, 1995.

258. Pelletier JP, Mineau F, Ranger P, et al: The increased synthesis of inducible nitric oxide inhibits IL-1ra synthesis by human articular chondrocytes: Possible role in osteoarthritic cartilage degradation. Osteoarthritis Cartilage 4:77-84, 1996.

259. McInnes IB, Leung BP, Field M, et al: Production of nitric oxide in the synovial membrane of rheumatoid and osteoarthritis patients. J Exp Med 184:1519-1524, 1996.

260. Hayashi T, Abe E, Yamate T, et al: Nitric oxide production by superficial and deep articular chondrocytes. Arthritis Rheum 40:261-269, 1997.

261. Loeser RF, Carlson CS, Del Carlo M, et al: Detection of nitrotyrosine in aging and osteoarthritic cartilage: Correlation of oxidative damage with the presence of interleukin-1beta and with chondrocyte resistance to insulin-like growth factor 1. Arthritis Rheum 46:2349-2357, 2002.

262. Fermor B, Weinberg JB, Pisetsky DS, et al: The influence of oxygen tension on the induction of nitric oxide and prostaglandin E2 by mechanical stress in articular cartilage. Osteoarthritis Cartilage 13:935-941, 2005.

263. Piscoya JL, Fermor B, Kraus VB, et al: The influence of mechanical compression on the induction of osteoarthritis-related biomarkers in articular cartilage explants. Osteoarthritis Cartilage 13:1092-1099, 2005.

264. Abramson SB, Attur M, Amin AR, et al: Nitric oxide and inflammatory mediators in the perpetuation of osteoarthritis. Curr Rheumatol Rep 3:535-541, 2001.

265. Hirai Y, Migita K, Honda S, et al: Effects of nitric oxide on matrix metalloproteinase-2 production by rheumatoid synovial cells. Life Sci 68:913-920, 2001.

266. Clancy RM, Abramson SB, Kohne C, et al: Nitric oxide attenuates cellular hexose monophosphate shunt response to oxidants in articular chondrocytes and acts to promote oxidant injury. J Cell Physiol 172:183-191, 1997.

267. Lotz M: The role of nitric oxide in articular cartilage damage. Rheum Dis Clin N Am 25:269-282, 1999.

268. van't Hof RJ, Hocking L, Wright PK, et al: Nitric oxide is a mediator of apoptosis in the rheumatoid joint. Rheumatology (Oxf) 39:1004-1008, 2000.

269. Pelletier JP, Jovanovic D, Fernandes JC, et al: Reduced progression of experimental osteoarthritis in vivo by selective inhibition of inducible nitric oxide synthase. Arthritis Rheum 41:1275-1286, 1998.

270. van den Berg WB, van de Loo F, Joosten LA, et al: Animal models of arthritis in NOS2-deficient mice. Osteoarthritis Cartilage 7:413-415, 1999.

271. Clements KM, Burton-Wurster N, Lust G: The spread of cell death from impact damaged cartilage: Lack of evidence for the role of nitric oxide and caspases. Osteoarthritis Cartilage 12:577-585, 2004.

272. Clements KM, Price JS, Chambers MG, et al: Gene deletion of either interleukin-1beta, interleukin-1beta-converting enzyme, inducible nitric oxide synthase, or stromelysin 1 accelerates the development of knee osteoarthritis in mice after surgical transection of the medial collateral ligament and partial medial meniscectomy. Arthritis Rheum 48:3452-3463, 2003.

273. Moulharat N, Lesur C, Thomas M, et al: Effects of transforming growth factor-beta on aggrecanase production and proteoglycan degradation by human chondrocytes in vitro. Osteoarthritis Cartilage 12:296-305, 2004.

274. Blaney Davidson EN, Vitters EL, van der Kraan PM, et al: Expression of transforming growth factor-beta (TGFbeta) and the TGFbeta signalling molecule SMAD-2P in spontaneous and instability-induced osteoarthritis: Role in cartilage degradation, chondrogenesis and osteophyte formation. Ann Rheum Dis 65:1414-1421, 2006.

275. Hedin PJ, Weitoft T, Hedin H, et al: Serum concentrations of hyaluronan and proteoglycan in joint disease: Lack of association. J Rheumatol 18:1601-1605, 1991.

276. Karna E, Miltyk W, Palka JA, et al: Hyaluronic acid counteracts interleukin-1-induced inhibition of collagen biosynthesis in cultured human chondrocytes. Pharmacol Res 54:275-281, 2006.

277. Nawrat P, Surazynski A, Karna E, et al: The effect of hyaluronic acid on interleukin-1-induced deregulation of collagen metabolism in cultured human skin fibroblasts. Pharmacol Res 51:473-477, 2005.

278. Amin AR, Abramson SB: The role of nitric oxide in articular cartilage breakdown in osteoarthritis. Curr Opin Rheumatol 10:263-268, 1998.

279. Hardy MM, Seibert K, Manning PT, et al: Cyclooxygenase 2-dependent prostaglandin E2 modulates cartilage proteoglycan degradation in human osteoarthritis explants. Arthritis Rheum 46:1789-1803, 2002.

280. Dingle JT: The effect of nonsteroidal antiinflammatory drugs on human articular cartilage glycosaminoglycan synthesis. Osteoarthritis Cartilage 7:313-314, 1999.

281. van't Hof RJ, Ralston SH: Nitric oxide and bone. Immunology 103:255-261, 2001.

282. Bettica P, Cline G, Hart DJ, et al: Evidence for increased bone resorption in patients with progressive knee osteoarthritis: Longitudinal results from the Chingford study. Arthritis Rheum 46:3178-3184, 2002.

283. Abramson S, Krasnokutsky S: Biomarkers in osteoarthritis. Bull Hosp Jt Dis 64(1-2):77-81, 2006.

284. Rizkalla G, Reiner A, Bogoch E, et al: Studies of the articular cartilage proteoglycan aggrecan in health and osteoarthritis: Evidence for molecular heterogeneity and extensive molecular changes in disease. J Clin Invest 90:2268-2277, 1992.

285. Ayral X, Pickering EH, Woodworth TJ, et al: Synovitis predicts the arthroscopic progression of medial tibiofemoral knee osteoarthritis (OA). Ann Rheum Dis 60:57, 2001.

286. Evans CH: Cellular mechanisms of hydrolytic enzyme release in proteoglycan. Semin Arthritis Rheum 11:93, 1981.

287. Evans CH, Mears DC, McKnight JL: A preliminary ferrographic survey of the wear particles in human synovial fluid. Arthritis Rheum 24:912-918, 1981.

288. Haraoui B, Pelletier JP, Cloutier JM, et al: Synovial membrane histology and immunopathology in rheumatoid arthritis and osteoarthritis: In vivo effects of antirheumatic drugs. Arthritis Rheum 34:153-163, 1991.

289. Farahat MN, Yanni G, Poston R, et al: Cytokine expression in synovial membranes of patients with rheumatoid arthritis and osteoarthritis. Ann Rheum Dis 52:870-875, 1993.

290. Smith MD, Triantafillou S, Parker A, et al: Synovial membrane inflammation and cytokine production in patients with early osteoarthritis. J Rheumatol 24:365-371, 1997.

291. Krenn V, Hensel F, Kim HJ, et al: Molecular IgV(H) analysis demonstrates highly somatic mutated B cells in synovialitis of osteoarthritis: A degenerative disease is associated with a specific, not locally generated immune response. Lab Invest 79:1377-1384, 1999.

292. Nakamura H, Yoshino S, Kato T, et al: T-cell mediated inflammatory pathway in osteoarthritis. Osteoarthritis Cartilage 7:401-402, 1999.

293. Benito MJ, Veale DJ, FitzGerald O, et al: Synovial tissue inflammation in early and late osteoarthritis. Ann Rheum Dis 64:1263-1267, 2005.

294. Cooke TD: Significance of immune complex deposits in osteoarthritic cartilage. J Rheumatol 14(Spec No):77-79, 1987.

295. Verbruggen G, Veys EM: Numerical scoring systems for the anatomic evolution of osteoarthritis of the finger joints. Arthritis Rheum 39:308-320, 1996.

296. Masuhara K, Nakai T, Yamaguchi K, et al: Significant increases in serum and plasma concentrations of matrix metalloproteinases 3 and 9 in patients with rapidly destructive osteoarthritis of the hip. Arthritis Rheum 46:2625-2631, 2002.

297. Tchetverikov I, Lohmander LS, Verzijl N, et al: MMP protein and activity levels in synovial fluid from patients with joint injury, inflammatory arthritis, and osteoarthritis. Ann Rheum Dis 64:694-698, 2005.

298. Barksby HE, Milner JM, Patterson AM, et al: Matrix metalloproteinase 10 promotion of collagenolysis via procollagenase activation: Implications for cartilage degradation in arthritis. Arthritis Rheum 54:3244-3253, 2006.

299. Mort JS, Caterson B, Poole AR, et al: The origin of human cartilage proteoglycan link-protein heterogeneity and fragmentation during aging. Biochem J 232:805-812, 1985.

300. Roughley PJ, Lee ER: Cartilage proteoglycans: Structure and potential functions. Microsc Res Tech 28:385-397, 1994.

301. Neame PJ, Sandy JD: Cartilage aggrecan: Biosynthesis, degradation and osteoarthritis. J Fla Med Assoc 81:191-193, 1994.

302. Perkins SJ, Nealis AS, Dudhia J, et al: Immunoglobulin fold and tandem repeat structures in proteoglycan N-terminal domains and link protein. J Mol Biol 206:737-753, 1989.

303. Williams AF, Barclay AN: The immunoglobulin superfamily—domains for cell surface recognition. Annu Rev Immunol 6:381-405, 1988.

304. Rosenberg LC: Structure and function of dermatan sulfate proteoglycans in articular cartilage. In Kuettner KE, Schleyerbach R, Peyron JG, et al (eds): Articular Cartilage and Osteoarthritis. New York, Raven Press, 1992, pp 45-62.

305. Noyori K, Jasin HE: Inhibition of human fibroblast adhesion by cartilage surface proteoglycans. Arthritis Rheum 37:1656-1663, 1994.

306. McCarty DJ, Halverson PB, Carrera GF, et al: "Milwaukee shoulder"—association of microspheroids containing hydroxyapatite crystals, active collagenase, and neutral protease with rotator cuff defects, I: Clinical aspects. Arthritis Rheum 24:464-473, 1981.

307. Shlopov BV, Smith GN Jr, Cole AA, et al: Differential patterns of response to doxycycline and transforming growth factor beta1 in the down-regulation of collagenases in osteoarthritic and normal human chondrocytes. Arthritis Rheum 42:719-727, 1999.

308. Lohmander LS, Felson D: Can we identify a 'high risk' patient profile to determine who will experience rapid progression of osteoarthritis? Osteoarthritis Cartilage 12(Suppl A):S49-S52, 2004.

309. Sharif M, George E, Dieppe PA: Correlation between synovial fluid markers of cartilage and bone turnover and scintigraphic scan abnormalities in osteoarthritis of the knee. Arthritis Rheum 38:78-81, 1995.

310. Bruyere O, Genant H, Kothari M, et al: Longitudinal study of magnetic resonance imaging and standard x-rays to assess disease progression in osteoarthritis. Osteoarthritis Cartilage 15:98-103, 2007.

311. Sowers M, Jannausch M, Stein E, et al: C-reactive protein as a biomarker of emergent osteoarthritis. Osteoarthritis Cartilage 10:595-601, 2002.

312. Jordan JM: Update on cartilage oligomeric matrix protein as a marker of osteoarthritis. J Rheumatol 32:1145-1147, 2005.

313. Black RA, Rauch CT, Kozlosky CJ, et al: A metalloproteinase disintegrin that releases tumor-necrosis factor-alpha from cells. Nature 385:729-733, 1997.

314. Oldberg A, Antonsson P, Lindblom K, et al: COMP (cartilage oligomeric matrix protein) is structurally related to the thrombospondins. J Biol Chem 267:22346-22350, 1992.

315. DiCesare PE, Morgelin M, Mann K, et al: Cartilage oligomeric matrix protein and thrombospondin 1: Purification from articular cartilage, electron microscopic structure, and chondrocyte binding. Eur J Biochem 223:927-937, 1994.

316. Hedbom E, Antonsson P, Hjerpe A, et al: Cartilage matrix proteins: An acidic oligomeric protein (COMP) detected only in cartilage. J Biol Chem 267:6132-6136, 1992.

317. Morgelin M, Heinegard D, Engel J, et al: Electron microscopy of native cartilage oligomeric matrix protein purified from the Swarm rat chondrosarcoma reveals a five-armed structure. J Biol Chem 267:6137-6141, 1992.

318. DiCesare P, Hauser N, Lehman D, et al: Cartilage oligomeric matrix protein (COMP) is an abundant component of tendon. FEBS Lett 354:237-240, 1994.

319. Lohmander LS, Saxne T, Heinegard DK: Release of cartilage oligomeric matrix protein (COMP) into joint fluid after knee injury and in osteoarthritis. Ann Rheum Dis 53:8-13, 1994.

320. Lohmander LS, Ionescu M, Jugessur H, et al: Changes in joint cartilage aggrecan after knee injury and in osteoarthritis. Arthritis Rheum 42:534-544, 1999.

321. Neidhart M, Hauser N, Paulsson M, et al: Small fragments of cartilage oligomeric matrix protein in synovial fluid and serum as markers for cartilage degradation. Br J Rheumatol 36:1151-1160, 1997.

322. Amin AR: Regulation of tumor necrosis factor-alpha and tumor necrosis factor converting enzyme in human osteoarthritis. Osteoarthritis Cartilage 7:392-394, 1999.

323. Goldberg RL, Huff JP, Lenz ME, et al: Elevated plasma levels of hyaluronate in patients with osteoarthritis and rheumatoid arthritis. Arthritis Rheum 34:799-807, 1991.

324. Manicourt DH, Cornu O, Lenz ME, et al: Rapid and sustained rise in the serum level of hyaluronan after anterior cruciate ligament transection in the dog knee joint. J Rheumatol 22:262-269, 1995.

325. Sinigaglia L, Varenna M, Binelli L, et al: Urinary and synovial pyridinium crosslink concentrations in patients with rheumatoid arthritis and osteoarthritis. Ann Rheum Dis 54:144-147, 1995.

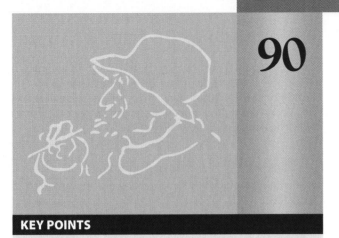

90

Clinical Features of Osteoarthritis 📹

JÉRÉMIE SELLAM •
FRANCIS BERENBAUM

KEY POINTS

Osteoarthritis is a common and disabling musculoskeletal disorder with increasing prevalence and socioeconomic impact.

Classically, clinical symptoms and signs constitute the primary diagnostic aid.

The natural history of osteoarthritis varies widely—the diagnosis encompasses subgroups in which rapid, progressive destructive disease can occur.

Imaging modalities useful in diagnosis include plain radiographs, although increasingly musculoskeletal ultrasound and particularly magnetic resonance imaging are being evaluated for clinical trial outcome and ultimately routine clinical use.

The etiology of osteoarthritis is unclear, but comprises a multigene, environmental disorder.

Treatment should be with a team approach and should include management of physical function, pain, and inflammation, and may require integration with orthopaedic surgical teams.

There are few reliable clinical prognostic features as yet available; there is an urgent need for appropriate widely applicable biomarkers to identify patients with poor prognosis and patients with subtypes of disease that may require closer observation and earlier intervention.

Osteoarthritis is the most common chronic joint disorder. It usually results in pain and deformity, ultimately leading to chronic disability. It is rapidly becoming a significant medical and financial burden in a world whose population is aging.[1,2] Osteoarthritis affects retired and working individuals and has a broad health economic impact.[3] The disease is classically defined as a focal lesion of the articular cartilage, combined with a hypertrophic reaction (sclerosis) in the subchondral bone and new bone formation (osteophytes) at the joint margins. Muscle weakness, lax ligaments, misalignment, low-grade synovitis, and meniscal degeneration often occur, however, so that all three major tissues of a diarthrodal joint are usually implicated. Optimal management requires early diagnosis and awareness of the risk factors that can affect the prognosis.

PREVALENCE

The prevalence of osteoarthritis depends on the precise definition used and the region of interest. Forty-eight percent of knees at autopsy have histologic evidence of osteoarthritis, whereas only 10% of these patients previously reported any clinical manifestations of knee osteoarthritis.[4] In general and consistent with this observation, radiologic osteoarthritis

is more prevalent than symptomatic osteoarthritis. The Rotterdam study on a population-based cohort 55 years old and younger found that 67% of women and 55% of men had radiographic hand osteoarthritis.[5,6] Radiographic osteophytes are seen in only 50% of the distal interphalangeal joints of individuals with hand osteoarthritis in which Heberden's nodes are detected on clinical examination, however, suggesting that clinical and radiographic measures may not be synchronous.[7] The knee is the most clinically significant site affected—the prevalence increases with age so that 53% of women older than 80 years and 33% of men older than 80 years have radiographic knee osteoarthritis.[8] Clinically symptomatic knee osteoarthritis is less frequent (16% of 80-year-old women and 5.4% of 80-year-old men). About 11% of individuals older than 64 years have symptomatic knee osteoarthritis.[9]

More recent data are compatible with the aforementioned studies. The age-standardized and sex-standardized incidence of hand osteoarthritis is 100/100,000 person-years, the age-standardized and sex-standardized incidence of hip osteoarthritis is 88/100,000 person-years, and the age-standardized and sex-standardized incidence of knee osteoarthritis is 240/100,000 person-years.[10] Hand, hip, and knee osteoarthritis become more frequent with age, and more women are affected than men after age 50. The incidence of knee osteoarthritis is 1% per year in women 70 to 89 years old.[10]

NATURAL HISTORY OF OSTEOARTHRITIS

The natural history of osteoarthritis varies greatly. Osteoarthritis generally develops progressively over several years, although symptoms may remain stable for prolonged periods within that time frame. Previous trauma, causing articular, meniscal, or ligamental damage or joint incongruity, can reveal or accelerate the disorder, especially in knee osteoarthritis. The correlation between clinical outcome and radiographic course is poor at the individual level. Although symptoms can improve, the radiographic picture rarely does—radiographic deterioration is observed in 30% to 60% of patients.[11]

Symptoms and structural progression are significantly correlated when groups of patients are compared. Although osteoarthritis is considered to be a degenerative chronic process, inflammatory flares can occur during the course of the disease. Inflammatory arthritis, infection, and crystal arthropathies should be excluded in such cases. Flares are not clearly defined, but are characterized by episodes of increased pain (possibly nocturnal), sudden increases in pain with increased morning stiffness, and the development of synovial effusions. Inflammatory flares should be detected and properly defined clinically because they seem to be associated with altered rates of joint space narrowing.[11] Joints occasionally may be destroyed rapidly, and such destruction is associated with a poor prognosis. Regional localization of such events has attracted discrete clinical syndromes including those affecting hips ("rapid destructive hip arthropathy"), shoulders ("Milwaukee shoulder"), the spine ("pseudotuberculosis spondylodiscitis"), and knees.

CLINICAL MANIFESTATIONS

The general symptoms and signs of osteoarthritis are considered first. A detailed description of characteristic features of regional osteoarthritis syndromes is given later.

SYMPTOMS OF OSTEOARTHRITIS

Symptoms are often initially insidious and can be highly variable, depending on the joint affected, the severity of joint involvement, and the number of joints affected.[12]

Pain

Pain is the first and predominant symptom of osteoarthritis that sends a patient to the general practitioner. Pain typically is worsened by activities such as long distance walking for weight-bearing joints and is alleviated by rest, in contrast to inflammatory disorders.

Pain begins within a few minutes of starting an activity and may persist for hours after the activity has ceased. The pain sometimes can have an onset several hours after physical activities, especially in young patients. Although osteoarthritis pain is unusual during the night or at rest, there are exceptions, including in patients with mild osteoarthritis using joints for several hours especially during sport, in advanced osteoarthritis with destructive arthropathy, and in an acute inflammatory flare of osteoarthritis mimicking inflammatory arthropathy. Associated bursitis also can be a source of pain. Pain intensity and joint damage on radiographs are poorly correlated. Finally, there is no agreement as to whether a decrease in atmospheric pressure or a change in the weather increases osteoarthritis pain.[13,14]

Stiffness and Loss of Movement and Function

Stiffness also may occur in the morning, after a period of inactivity, or particularly in the evening. Morning stiffness generally resolves after less than 10 minutes, in contrast to the prolonged (usually >30 minutes) stiffness seen in inflammatory disorders.

Loss of movement and function reflected in limited range of motion observed at physical examination is sometimes the main reason for a visit to the practitioner. Patients report limitations in their ability to perform day-to-day activities, such as kneeling for knee osteoarthritis, or cutting one's toenails for hip osteoarthritis.[15] Osteoarthritis also can hamper stair climbing, walking, and performing household chores. Limited joint function is caused by several mechanisms, including pain, decreased motion related to reduced joint space, diminished muscle strength, and instability. Joint proprioceptor sensitivity may be altered; its relationship to disability is less clear as yet, but is probably not caused by pain alone.[16]

Lastly, symptomatic osteoarthritis may be associated with depression and disturbed sleep, which are additional contributors to disability. Osteoarthritis, wherever it occurs, typically causes pain, alters function, and leads to a significant deterioration in the quality of life.[17]

PHYSICAL EXAMINATION

A physical examination should be done to confirm and characterize joint involvement and to exclude pain and functional syndromes arising from other causes, especially periarticluar structures and inflammatory arthritis. A normal examination does not rule out the diagnosis of osteoarthritis, however, especially disease of early nature or of modest severity.

Joint enlargement results from joint effusion or bony swelling or both, which are mainly observed in advanced disease. Bony swelling is easily recognized in superficial joints, such as the finger joints or knees. A synovial effusion may be seen during osteoarthritis flares, but also can occur during chronic phases as a persistent feature. It is most easily detected in knees by the evidence of patellar shock (tap) or by the elicitation of a fluid thrill (wave test).

Joints are usually tender during active motion testing and under pressure. Limited passive movement can be the first and only physical sign of symptomatic osteoarthritis. Bursitis, tendinitis, muscle spasm, and, especially for the knee, a torn meniscus, can cause the same pain syndrome and must be sought carefully during examination.[18] Crepitus, an audible or palpable sensation of crunching or crackling, is commonly felt on passive or active mobilization of an osteoarthritis joint. This sensation is due to the irregularity of the opposing cartilage surfaces or intra-articular debris.

Joint deformities reflect advanced disease with joint destruction involving the cartilage and surrounding bone and soft tissue, the articular capsule, and the ligaments. This destruction contributes to misalignment, joint instability, and limb (usually manifest as leg) shortening. Misalignment also is a cause of compartmental knee osteoarthritis (e.g., varus angulation of the knee responsible for medial tibiofemoral damage and valgus angulation for lateral tibiofemoral damage). Fingers also can be misaligned in the presence of Heberden's or Bouchard's nodes.

The physical examination should include examination of the legs with the patient standing (i.e., to facilitate detection of varus or valgus malalignment). The knees are farther apart than the feet in the frontal plane in cases of varus alignment, whereas the knees are closer together than the feet in cases of valgus alignment. Varus and valgus alignments are responsible for medial and lateral tibiofemoral osteoarthritis. Both can affect the range of motion and accelerate joint space narrowing; they may enhance the development of osteoarthritis.[19-22] The presence of anterior laxity also should be evaluated because a decrease in anteroposterior laxity is associated with decreased joint space.[23]

A joint can lock if loose bodies or fragments of cartilage get into the joint space. This occurrence is rare, but care should be taken to distinguish between the stiffness experienced after prolonged immobilization of a limb and true mechanical locking, which suggests a meniscus lesion. Musculature and joint laxity should be evaluated because periarticular muscle spasms may occur. The circumference of the quadriceps should be measured and compared with that of the opposite side—this may be particularly informative in asymmetric disease. A weak quadriceps femoris is a known disability factor in knee osteoarthritis. This weakness can more convincingly explain the knee "giving way" than the often suggested ligament instability. A lax joint is defined by the excess displacement or rotation of the tibia with respect to the femur in the varus-valgus direction. Joint laxity increases functional disability owing to weak muscles.[24]

Soft tissues and bursa areas should be examined in parallel because they can be amenable to local treatment, such as corticosteroid injections. Gait also must be assessed because hip or knee osteoarthritis results in a characteristic gait. It also is useful for examining the consequence of the pain. The appropriate use of a cane may be assessed during examination.

Caution should be exercised in attributing pain to the correct region (e.g., patients with hip osteoarthritis may report pain in the knee region because of referred pain or biomechanical dysfunction). In these cases, moving the knee causes no pain, whereas hip movement is painful, and the range of hip motion is limited. Patients with hip osteoarthritis also have symptoms mimicking a cruralgia. Careful neurologic and spine examination usually rules out this diagnosis.

IMAGING

The diagnosis of osteoarthritis in patients presenting with knee, hip, or hand pain is based on a comprehensive assessment of the joint, including evaluation of symptoms and signs that favor this diagnosis and exclude other diagnoses. The diagnosis of osteoarthritis is often obvious after an interview and physical examination. In straightforward presentations, radiologic investigation often is unnecessary to confirm the diagnosis of hand or forefoot osteoarthritis. Some regions and clinical scenarios require a radiologic examination, however, to exclude other diseases, including avascular osteonecrosis, Paget's disease, algoneurodystrophy, inflammatory arthropathies, and stress fractures. Less commonly involved locations, such as the ankle, shoulder, or elbow, also require radiologic examination. Radiographic assessment not only is helpful to diagnose osteoarthritis, but also is useful to establish the severity of joint damage; to monitor disease activity, progression, and response to therapy; and to look for complications of the disorder or the treatment.[25]

Standard radiographs are the most common investigations, depending on the region involved. Weight-bearing radiographs are mandatory for knee and hip osteoarthritis. A standard radiograph cannot diagnose early osteoarthritis, however. The radiologic features of osteoarthritis at various sites are shown in Figure 90-1. Osteophytes at the joint margin,

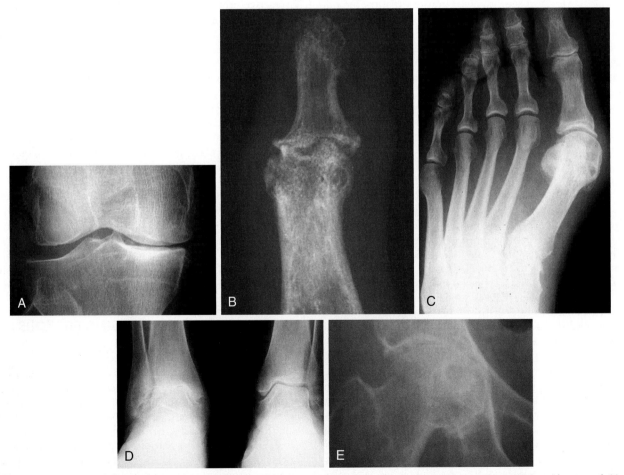

Figure 90-1 **A-E,** Radiologic features of osteoarthritis. **A,** Medial femoro-tibial knee osteoarthritis. **B,** Distal interphalangeal joint with osteoarthritis. **C,** Osteoarthritis of the first metatarsophalangeal joint. **D,** Right ankle osteoarthritis. **E,** Hip osteoarthritis. *(Figures provided by www.lecofer.org.)*

indicating new bone formation, are the most characteristic feature of osteoarthritis and usually precede joint space narrowing.[25,26] Subchondral bone sclerosis and joint space narrowing are classically seen in more advanced osteoarthritis. Clinical symptoms and radiographic findings are poorly correlated, however; many joints with radiographic evidence of osteoarthritis remain asymptomatic, and the joints of many patients with severe symptoms can appear only marginally affected on x-ray.[25] Demineralization is not a classic feature of osteoarthritis, and its presence strongly suggests an inflammatory arthropathy. Joint space narrowing not only is related to a decreased volume of articular cartilage, but also to meniscal cartilage lesions and cartilage extrusion.[27]

Although standard x-rays are useful for monitoring the evolution of osteoarthritis, there are no clear guidelines about the optimal frequency of radiographs that can best inform practice. Classically, evolving radiographic features include progressive joint space narrowing, subchondral sclerosis, and joint line osteophytosis. These are the radiologic features of the most common form of osteoarthritis—"hypertrophic" osteoarthritis with bone construction. The other form, "atrophic" osteoarthritis, is rare, characterized by an absence of osteophytes and sclerosis; it usually involves the hip.

Other investigations are rarely performed to confirm the diagnosis of osteoarthritis, but they are sometimes useful to exclude alternative possibilities in a difficult differential diagnosis. All the tissues involved in osteoarthritis, including cartilage lesions, fluid effusion, subchondral bone marrow edema, low-grade synovitis, and meniscus or ligament lesions, can be seen by magnetic resonance imaging (MRI).[28] MRI is useful for excluding tumor, algoneurodystrophy, or avascular osteonecrosis. The pain and progression of knee osteoarthritis seem to be associated with the bone marrow edema seen on MRI, but this is controversial.[29-35] Although the usual term used is *bone marrow edema*, autopsy examinations have revealed that necrosis, fibrosis, and abnormal remodeled trabeculae are the most common features.[30]

The presence of bone resorption also is clearly recognized as part of osteoarthritis progression.[29,36-38] The meniscus tears seen by MRI are common in middle-aged and older adults, with or without knee pain. Although MRI accurately detects meniscus damage or injury of the anterior cruciate ligament, which are known to be associated with increased osteoarthritis progression, this finding does not influence therapeutic management and should not lead to aggressive procedures.[37,39] MRI is now being used to assess the quantity and function of cartilage, synovium, and bone. The routine use of MRI in osteoarthritis clinical practice is not yet recommended, however; it should be used only for clinical research purposes at this time.

Ultrasound is presently useful only for detecting joint effusions, including a minimal effusion that is below the limit of detection on clinical examination, and changes in cartilage, such as fibrillation of cartilage or cleft formation and the proliferation of synovium and osteophytes.[40-43] Popliteal cysts also can be visualized by ultrasound, and potential complications, including compression of adjacent vascular structures, can be detected. Many studies are presently evaluating the advantages of this procedure in terms of early diagnosis and evaluation of pain symptoms, severity, and prognosis.[44-46] Ultrasonography has been studied extensively in knee osteoarthritis; it may be useful for detecting inflammatory flares of osteoarthritis in individual cases.[45,47]

Ultrasonography also may be useful in hand osteoarthritis, to differentiate between erosive and nonerosive osteoarthritis.[48] Ultrasonography can be used to perform aspirations and injections within the joint and periarticular tissue.[49] Ultrasound imaging is limited, however, by its inability to visualize the whole cartilage surface. Artifacts caused by the position of the probe can lead to misinterpretation. Ultrasonography is presently used in clinical trials, but it is likely to have a place in clinical practice for diagnosing the early phase of osteoarthritis. The examination and the interobserver and intraobserver variations must be standardized before it can be used widely in daily practice.

Arthroscopy visualizes cartilage, synovial membranes, osteophytes, and meniscal lesions. This approach, similar to MRI, may detect findings of dubious significance (e.g., meniscal lesions are frequent in patients >60 years old, but rarely the cause of pain). Dissection of the meniscus could be highly deleterious by accelerating the progression of osteoarthritis.[50]

LABORATORY TESTS

Blood tests are not routinely indicated in cases of uncomplicated chronic pain arising from clearly defined osteoarthritis. The erythrocyte sedimentation rate and concentration of the C-reactive protein are usually within the normal range for age. Low titers of rheumatoid factors can be found, reflecting the median age of patients with osteoarthritis and not differing in that respect from control populations. Some laboratory tests may be done to rule out a metabolic arthropathy (e.g., gout) or inflammatory arthritis, or to investigate the adverse effects of drugs pending the characteristics of the presentation. Synovial fluid should be examined if another arthropathy or septic arthritis is suspected. Crystal analysis by polarized light microscopy is an important part of this assessment. Analysis of synovial fluid reveals a white blood cell count of less than 2000/mm^3, sterile, without any crystals.[51]

Biochemical markers of cartilage or bone turnover or remodeling are not currently assayed in the day-to-day management of osteoarthritis because no single marker is yet adequate for predicting or monitoring osteoarthritis in an individual patient. In the future, biomarkers probably will be used in daily clinical practice, in combination with other risk factors such as clinical or imaging findings, to predict the clinical course of osteoarthritis.[52]

ETIOLOGY AND PREDISPOSING FACTORS
SECONDARY OSTEOARTHRITIS

Because osteoarthritis may follow almost any established joint disorder, osteoarthritis is considered to be primary if it is idiopathic and secondary in cases of previous injury or disease of the target joint. Table 90-1 lists disorders responsible for secondary osteoarthritis. It is not always easy to distinguish between primary and secondary osteoarthritis, however, because a significant proportion of subjects who develop secondary osteoarthritis have some predisposition to osteoarthritis that may operate independent of the prior condition. An interview and a physical examination may help the physician to identify an etiology. Along with these clinical features, radiographs can help diagnose some secondary osteoarthritis conditions, such as chondrocalcinosis and Paget's disease.

PREDISPOSING FACTORS

A risk factor must fulfill several criteria, including a time relationship, a strong statistical association after exclusion of confounding factors, consistent published findings, and biologic plausibility. The predisposing risk factors to idiopathic osteoarthritis act by increasing the susceptibility of

Table 90-1 Etiologies of Secondary Osteoarthritis

Metabolic
Crystal-associated arthritis (gout, calcium pyrophosphate dihydrate arthropathy, pseudogout)
Acromegaly
Ochronosis
Hemachromatosis
Wilson's disease
Anatomic
Slipped femoral epiphysis
Epiphyseal dysplasias
Blount's disease
Legg-Calvé-Perthes disease
Congenital dislocation of the hip
Unequal leg lengths
Hypermobility syndromes
Traumatic
Major joint trauma
Fracture through a joint or osteonecrosis
Joint surgery (e.g., meniscectomy)
Chronic injury (occupational arthropathy)
Inflammatory
Any inflammatory arthropathy
Septic arthritis

joints to injury, by directly damaging joints, or by impairing the process of repair of damaged joint tissue. Table 90-2 shows the main risk factors identified to date. Clinicians must differentiate between factors of occurrence and factors of progression. Clinicians also should distinguish "not modifiable" risk factors, which are valuable from a pathophysiologic point of view and in groups, and "modifiable" risk factors, which are potentially more valuable for individuals in routine practice.

Obesity

Obesity seems to be independently implicated in the pathogenesis of osteoarthritis and is one of the strongest risk factors for knee osteoarthritis because it precedes knee osteoarthritis by many years. Obesity is less strongly associated with hip osteoarthritis. Obesity not only is associated with weight-bearing activities that cause cartilage breakdown, but also with non–weight-bearing joints secondary to different systemic factors (Fig. 90-2).[53] Elevated blood glucose and C-reactive protein (high-sensitivity assays) are associated with the risk of knee osteoarthritis and its progression in women. The link between obesity and osteoarthritis seems stronger in women than in men.

Systemic Risk Factors

Patient age is the best recognized risk factor because the incidence of radiographic and symptomatic osteoarthritis increases sharply with age; this is probably mediated by increases in systemic and local factors, including obesity, ligament laxity, and impaired neuromuscular joint protective mechanisms.[54-56] Women are at greater risk than men of developing hand, knee, and generalized osteoarthritis.[10,57-59] In contrast, the frequency of hip osteoarthritis increases at about the same rate in women and men, but the disease seems to progress more rapidly in women.[11] This difference

Table 90-2 Risk Factors for the Occurrence or Progression of Osteoarthritis in Knees, Hips, and Hands

Disease Progression	Location		
	Knee	**Hip**	**Hand**
Occurrence of osteoarthritis	Age[151] Female[151] Physical activity[84,154,155] BMI[84,156] Bone density[157] Previous injury[62,84,155,156,158-160] Hormone replacement therapy[156,161,162] Vitamin D[163] Smoking (protective)[164] Alignment[82] Quadriceps strength[99] Intense sport activities[98,165]	Age[149] Physical activity[166,167] BMI[166,168] Previous injury[169] Intense sport activities[99]	Age[149] Grip strength[170] BMI[171] Occupation[172] Intense sport activities[172]
Progression of osteoarthritis	Age[173] Vitamin D[163] Hormone replacement therapy[174] Alignment[83] Hydrarthrodial osteoarthritis[171] Synovitis[175] Intense sport activities[98] Subchondral bone edema on MRI[29]	Age Symptomatic activity[58] Gender[58] Intense sport activities[98]	Unknown

BMI, body mass index; MRI, magnetic resonance imaging.

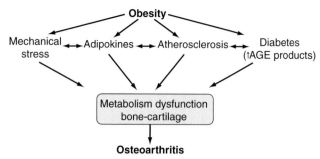

Figure 90-2 Hypothesis concerning the relationship between obesity and osteoarthritis. AGE, advanced glycation end-products.

between men and women suggests that sex hormones are involved. Involvement of sex hormones also is suggested by the fact that the occurrence of hip and knee radiographic osteoarthritis is associated with a lack of postmenopausal estrogen replacement. This link seems less clear for osteoarthritis symptoms.[60]

A link between bone mineral density and the occurrence of osteoarthritis has been reported, but it remains to be elucidated further. Although individuals with a high bone density are more likely to develop osteoarthritis, disease progression may be associated with local and general bone loss.[61-63] The prevalence of osteoarthritis in different ethnic groups and races has been extensively studied. There is some bias—differences in weight and daily and occupational activities could explain the variability between African-American, white, and Chinese subjects.[11]

Some specific genetic factors have been identified in a few families with osteoarthritis.[64-73] The phenotype of these patients is not similar to that of idiopathic osteoarthritis, however, having features of chondrodysplasia rather than osteoarthritis.[67,74] Gene association still poses difficult interpretation because idiopathic osteoarthritis is a polygenic disease with various phenotypes. Future studies on the genetic factors of osteoarthritis are likely to lead to new insights into the pathogenesis of osteoarthritis.[73,75,76]

Local Mechanical Risk Factors

Joint Deformity. Joint deformity is associated with the development of osteoarthritis. Congenital abnormalities, such as acetabular dysplasia and slipped capital femoral epiphysis of the hip, can be considered as etiologies of secondary osteoarthritis. They act by causing the load distribution within the joint to be abnormal.[77-81] Angular misalignment is the most potent risk factor for deterioration of the joint structure because it increases the degree of focal loading, creating a vicious cycle of joint damage, contributing to the development and progression of single compartment osteoarthritis of the knee.[36] About 65% of the weight-bearing load is transmitted through the medial compartment in a normally aligned knee, which explains the greater frequency of tibiofemoral medial knee osteoarthritis.[81] Varus misalignment increases the risk of joint space narrowing threefold to fourfold.[82] Long-standing obesity seems to increase the risk of structural radiographic progression in cases of moderate misalignment, presumably owing to the combined effect of the focus of load from misalignment and the excess load from increased weight.[83]

Acute Injury and Repetitive Joint Loading. Acute joint injuries, especially anterior cruciate ligament damage or tears of the knee meniscus, are associated with knee osteoarthritis and its progression.[84-88] There is a combined effect of the injury itself and its biomechanical consequences, which alter load distribution on the joint.[88] An acute knee injury is more likely to lead to osteoarthritis if there is an associated systemic risk factor of osteoarthritis. The development and progression of osteoarthritis may not be prevented, however, even if the damaged anterior cruciate ligament is surgically repaired, and the risk of developing osteoarthritis is 10-fold greater.[89,90] Osteoarthritis often manifests as a slight reduction of joint space about 10 to 20 years after anterior cruciate ligament injury, but usually without any major clinical symptoms.

Meniscus damage may play an important role in osteoarthritis pathophysiology. Whether meniscus damage or cartilage degradation occurs first is unknown, however. A torn meniscus and extrusion seem to be strong risk factors for the development and progression of knee osteoarthritis. Meniscectomy increases the risk of knee osteoarthritis twofold, and more if it is combined with anterior cruciate ligament damage or other ligament injury. There is a significant risk of radiographic tibiofemoral osteoarthritis 21 years after the surgical removal of a meniscus following knee injury, with the relative risk estimated to be 14-fold.[87] Mixed patellofemoral and tibiofemoral osteoarthritis is common in individuals who have undergone a meniscectomy.[91] Obesity dramatically increases the risk of developing osteoarthritis after medial or lateral meniscectomy.[92] Partial meniscus resection is associated with less radiographic osteoarthritis over time than is total meniscectomy.[92] Radiographic changes can be observed after 15 to 20 years.

Repetitive activities with joint overuse increase the risk of developing osteoarthritis, particularly in the knee, hip, and distal interphalangeal joints. Obesity amplifies this effect on the knee.[93,94] Professional and elite sporting activities also are associated with the development of osteoarthritis, even without major injury.[95,96] Reasonable recreational sports activities leading to low-grade repetitive impact, such as recreational running, are not likely to be harmful for most individuals, in terms of the occurrence or progression of hip and knee osteoarthritis in the absence of sudden impacts.[97,98]

Muscle Strength and Weakness. Quadriceps weakness is a primary risk factor for knee pain, disability, and the progression of knee osteoarthritis.[99] Data are conflicting, however, as to whether quadriceps strength has a preventive or aggravating effect on osteoarthritis progression. Although quadriceps weakness has been associated with the development of radiographic knee osteoarthritis, quadriceps muscle strength also is associated with faster progression in deformed knees, suggesting that local biomechanical factors influence the load distribution.[11]

Consequence of Identification of a Risk Factor. Some of the most important risk factors of osteoarthritis identified to date are "nonmodifiable"; these include female gender, joint malformation, and previous trauma. These nonmodifiable risk factors may help, however, to target measures designed to prevent osteoarthritis in clearly defined sub-populations at high risk of developing osteoarthritis. The finding of a modifiable risk factor of osteoarthritis does not mean that prevention or treatment of it can influence the ultimate osteoarthritis profile. Physical exercise and weight reduction have been shown to affect pain and function in knee osteoarthritis, but it is unclear that modifying footwear is effective, or that muscle strengthening leads to structural progression in patients with misaligned or lax knees.[100]

OSTEOARTHRITIS ASSESSMENT, CATEGORIZATION, AND OUTCOMES

Most available diagnostic or prognostic criteria are much more useful in clinical trials than in routine clinical practice. Assessment in clinical trials must be separated from assessment in routine practice. There are a variety of clinical and radiologic diagnostic criteria, different scoring systems according to the target joint for a clinical or a radiologic definition of osteoarthritis, and more recently emerging guidelines for conducting clinical trials.[101,102]

CRITERIA FOR DEFINING OSTEOARTHRITIS

The groups of patients with osteoarthritis who participate in clinical trials testing new therapies should be as homogeneous as possible, and need to fulfill a set of criteria that includes the clinical and radiologic items proposed by the American College of Rheumatology (ACR) (Table 90-3).[103-105] Osteoarthritis also should be classified as primary or secondary, specifying the cause of the secondary osteoarthritis. International guidelines proposed by the Osteoarthritis Research Society International suggest that secondary osteoarthritis should be excluded.[101]

The sensitivity and specificity of the ACR hip criteria are estimated to be 91% and 89%, whereas the sensitivity and specificity of ACR knee criteria are estimated to be 91% and 86%. The osteoarthritic changes seen on x-ray have not been found to add to the ACR diagnostic criteria for hand osteoarthritis; the sensitivity is 92%, and the specificity is 98%. The ACR criteria are very specific. These criteria are useful for differentiating patients with osteoarthritis from patients with inflammatory disorders because the sensitivity is less impressive, but not for differentiating patients with early osteoarthritis from healthy controls. Their use in population-based research is less clearly defined, and the prevalence of osteoarthritis is underestimated compared with a definition based on radiographic criteria.[106-109]

The radiologic definition of osteoarthritis is used in epidemiologic studies and in many clinical studies. The most commonly used grading system is that of Kellgren and Lawrence, based on the presence of osteophytes, joint space narrowing, subchondral sclerosis, and bony cysts.[110] This system divides osteoarthritis into five grades (0 to 4), giving a global score at various joint sites compared with a radiographic atlas. A score of 2 or more traditionally has been considered to be a definitive radiographic diagnosis of osteoarthritis and has been widely used in research. The Kellgren and Lawrence grade 1 (doubtful) is more likely to evolve to a patent osteoarthritis than is grade 0, suggesting that it corresponds to an early disease

Table 90-3 American College of Rheumatology Radiologic and Clinical Criteria for Knee and Hip Osteoarthritis

		Osteoarthritis if the Items Are Present
Hand	**Clinical** 1. Hand pain, aching, or stiffness for most days or prior months 2. Hard tissue enlargement of ≥2 of 10 selected joints* 3. Metacarpophalangeal joint swelling in ≥2 joints 4. Hard tissue enlargement of ≥2 distal interphalangeal joints 5. Deformity of ≥2 of 10 selected hand joints*	1, 2, 3, 4 or 1, 2, 3, 5
Hip	**Clinical and Radiographic** 1. Hip pain for most days or prior months 2. ESR of <20 mm at the first hour 3. Femoral or acetabular osteophytes on radiographs 4. Hip joint space narrowing on radiographs	1, 2, 3 or 1, 2, 4 or 1, 3, 4
Knee	**Clinical** 1. Knee pain for most days or prior months 2. Crepitus on active joint motion 3. Morning stiffness lasting ≤30 min 4. Age ≥38 yr 5. Bony enlargement of knee on examination	1, 2, 3, 4 or 1, 2, 5 or 1, 4, 5
	Clinical and Radiographic 1. Knee pain for most days or prior months 2. Osteophytes at joint margins on radiographs 3. Synovial fluid typical of osteoarthritis (laboratory) 4. Age ≥40 years 5. Crepitus on active joint motion 6. Morning stiffness lasting ≤30 min	1, 2 or 1, 3, 5, 6 or 1, 4, 5, 6

*Ten selected joints include bilateral second and third interphalangeal proximal joints, second and third prximal interphalangeal joints, and first carpometacarpal joint.
ESR, erythrocyte sedimentation rate.

subgroup.[111] Because the Kellgren and Lawrence grading system relies predominantly on osteophyte size to determine osteoarthritis severity, the atrophic form of osteoarthritis, which consists mainly of joint space narrowing, is underestimated. Many studies have shown a lack of agreement between knee pain and radiographic osteoarthritis produced by the Kellgren and Lawrence grading, with radiographic osteoarthritis detected in 15% to 53% of subjects with knee pain.[25] Similar results have been obtained for hip osteoarthritis.[112]

MRI and biochemical markers should be included in such criteria in the future.[52,75,113] Many questions remain, such as the type of target joint to be studied in clinical trials on hand osteoarthritis. The definition of the trapeziometacarpal joint as a separate entity in hand osteoarthritis is controversial. It is often associated with interphalangeal osteoarthritis, but may be involved alone in cases of constitutional hypermobility.[114-118]

OSTEOARTHRITIS CLINICAL ASSESSMENT

The assessment of a patient with osteoarthritis should include discrete evaluations of pain and function. A patient's overall, global pain, or disability assessment can be evaluated using a visual analog scale such as a 5-point Likert scale (none, mild, moderate, severe, very severe) or a 100-mm visual analog scale. Pain also can be assessed indirectly by estimating the symptomatic treatment required, such as the number of days per week that drugs are required or their consistent dose usage.[119] Single questions about pain can be used, but the activity causing pain should be specified (e.g., resting, nocturnal, stair climbing, weight bearing). One of the instruments widely used to assess pain and disability is the Western Ontario and McMaster Universities (WOMAC) composite index.[120] It is used mainly for the knee. In addition to the WOMAC questionnaire pain subscale (Table 90-4), a 0-to-100 mm visual analog scale is sometimes used to answer the question: "What pain do you have after activities in your daily life?"

Functional disability resulting from knee or hip osteoarthritis usually is evaluated using the WOMAC function subscale, which is a questionnaire of 17 items related to daily activities, and the Lequesne's algofunctional index (Table 90-5), which is an index including questions related to pain, performance, and function impairment.[121] The Health Assessment Questionnaire also can be used.[122]

The Knee Osteoarthritis Outcome Score (KOOS) has been validated more recently (http://www.koos.nu).[123,124] It is a 42-item, self-administered, knee-specific questionnaire covering several types of knee injury and osteoarthritis. It consists of five subscales (pain, other symptoms, function in daily living, function in sport and recreation, and knee-related quality of life). Standardized answer options are given (five Likert boxes), and the response to each question is scored from 0 to 4. A score of 0 to 100 is calculated for each subscale; 100 is the best result.[125] A difference of 10 points is considered to be clinically significant. The Foot and Ankle Outcome Score (FAOS) and Hip disability and Osteoarthritis Outcome Score (HOOS) also are available.[126,127] The FAOS has been used mainly in patients with lateral ankle instability, Achilles tendinosis, and plantar fasciitis.

Impaired function in hand osteoarthritis can be assessed in clinical trials using the Functional Index for Hand Osteoarthritis (FIHOA), and the Australian/Canadian Osteoarthritis Hand Index (AUSCAN) has been validated more recently (Table 90-6).[128-131] The FIHOA is a 10-item, investigator-administered questionnaire that is relevant and reliable and has been well validated externally and

Table 90-4   WOMAC Questionnaire

Pain Subscale (5 Questions)

How much pain do you have…
- Walking on a flat surface?
- Going up or down stairs?
- At night while in bed?
- Sitting or lying?
- Standing upright?

Stiffness Subscale (2 Questions)

How severe is your stiffness after first waking in the morning?
How severe is your stiffness after sitting, lying down, or resting later in the day?

Function Subscale (17 Questions)

What degree of difficulty do you have with…
- Descending stairs?
- Ascending stairs?
- Rising from sitting?
- Standing?
- Bending to floor?
- Walking on a flat surface?
- Getting in or out of a car?
- Going shopping?
- Putting on socks or stockings?
- Rising from bed?
- Taking off socks or stockings?
- Lying in bed?
- Getting in and out of the bath?
- Sitting?
- Getting on or off the toilet?
- Heavy domestic duties?
- Light domestic duties?

WOMAC, Western Ontario and McMaster Universities.

Table 90-5   Lequesne's Algofunctional Index

Pain or Discomfort	Points*
During nocturnal bed rest	
None or insignificant	0
Only on movement or in certain positions	1
With no movement	2
Morning stiffness or regressive pain after rising	
≤1 min	0
>1 min, but <15 min	1
After standing for 30 min	0 or 1
While walking	
None	0
Only after walking some distance	1
After initial walking and increasingly with continued walking	2
With prolonged sitting (2 hr)	0 or 1
Maximum distance walked (even with pain)	
Unlimited	0
>1 km (>0.6 mile) but limited	1
About 1 km (0.6 mile) in about 15 min	2
500-600 m (1640-2952 ft or 0.31-0.56 mile) in about 8-15 min	3
300-500 m (987-1640 ft)	4
100-300 m (328-985 ft)	5
<100 m (<328 ft)	6
With one walking stick or crutch	1
With two walking sticks or crutches	2
Day-to-day activities	
Put on socks by bending forward	0 or 2
Pick up an object from the floor	0 or 2
Climb up and down a standard flight of stairs	0 or 2
Get into and out of a car	0 or 2

*0, without difficulty; 1 (or 0.5 or 1.5), with difficulty; 2, unable.

Table 90-6 Functional Index for Hand Osteoarthritis

Are you able to turn a key in a lock?
Are you able to cut meat with a knife?
Are you able to cut cloth paper with a pair of scissors?
Are you able to fit a full bottle with the hand?
Are you able to clench your fist?
Are you able to tie a knot?
For women: are you able to sew?
For men: are you able to use a screwdriver?
Are you able to fasten buttons?
Are you able to write for a long period of time?
Would you accept a handshake without reluctance?

Developed by Dreiser RL, Maheu E, Guillou GB: Sensitivity to change of the functional index for hand osteoarthritis. Osteoarthritis Cartilage 8(Suppl A): S25-S28, 2000.

internally.[132] The AUSCAN is a self-administered questionnaire investigating pain, stiffness, and function. This index has been designed specifically for use with hand osteoarthritis patients with acceptable reliability, construct validity, and responsiveness.[130]

EVALUATING STRUCTURAL SEVERITY

Imaging

Structural severity is still difficult to evaluate. Standard plain radiographs have been extensively evaluated and remain the "gold standard" in clinical trials, even though this method has many weaknesses.[35,133] Structural progression has not yet been accurately defined, despite the fact that it is crucial for evaluating an osteoarthritic drug that has the potential to modify structure. MRI and ultrasonography should be useful tools for investigating alterations of joint structure in the future. MRI also can be used to study cartilage, subchondral bone, and synovial tissue simultaneously.

Biologic Markers

Many laboratories are working to find surrogate biomarkers that can reveal a correlation between joint space narrowing and the concentration of specific biologic parameters in the blood or urine.[113] These biologic markers include components of matrix proteins, including several collagens and cross-linked derivative peptides and matrix metalloproteinases. There is no consensus yet as to the optimal biomarker.

Time to Total Joint Replacement

Total joint replacement can be considered as the best end point for clinical trials evaluating disease-modifying osteoarthritis drugs. Great efforts are being made to validate a composite index, which could define states of severity and "need for total joint replacement."[134] Many parameters other than the severity of the disease itself influence the decision for surgery, however, including socioeconomic factors and access to health services.[135-138]

CLINICAL SUBSETS OF OSTEOARTHRITIS

DISTRIBUTION

General Considerations

Osteoarthritis tends to affect the distal interphalangeal joints, thumb base, knee, hip, and intervertebral facet joints. More than one joint is commonly involved, and there is a significant association between contralateral joints that is stronger than the association between different joint groups. Knee and hip osteoarthritis are each associated with hand osteoarthritis; the association between knee and hand osteoarthritis is stronger.[139-143] Wrists, elbows, metacarpophalangeal joints, and shoulders are usually less likely to be affected by osteoarthritis.

Knee

Osteoarthritis can involve the medial tibiofemoral, the lateral tibiofemoral, and the femoropatellar compartments. The lateral tibiofemoral compartment is involved mainly in women who have a genu valgum deformity. The precise location of pain can indicate which compartment of the joint is involved. Patients also sometimes report knee instability—the knee "gives way." This instability is likely linked to decreased muscle strength rather than true meniscus damage. Posterior pain can be due to an abundant effusion. Physical examination for knee osteoarthritis should begin by investigating the gait, using a slow walk to check for an extension defect. Thereafter, any misalignment (genu valgus or genu varus) should be sought, and the presence of bone swelling should be noted (Fig. 90-3A).

A popliteal (Baker's) cyst communicating with the joint space is common and may be complicated less often by distal vascular thrombosis. Acute cyst rupture may mimic venous thrombus and should be considered in "Doppler negative" leg swelling in the acute setting. Local tenderness along the joint line is characteristic of femorotibial osteoarthritis. Crepitus is detected on passive motion of the patella or knee flexion-extension testing. The range of motion may be normal or limited by structural alterations or abundant effusion. Periarticular structure examination may reveal anserine bursitis or infrapatellar or prepatellar bursitis. Trochanteric bursitis also can cause pain radiating through the tensor fascia lata and iliotibial band to the lateral part of the knee. An acute tear of the anterior cruciate ligament may cause pain, but is unusual in middle-aged subjects. A positive Lachman's test may be elicited. The circumference of the quadriceps muscle should be noted to detect any atrophy. Finally, the hip should be examined routinely because it may refer pain to the knee.

The syndrome of femoropatellar osteoarthritis is very specific: Pain occurs mainly during climbing or descending stairs; pain during walking on level ground is usually a symptom originating in the femorotibial compartment. Involvement of the femoropatellar compartment can cause anterior or posterior pain or both. Femoropatellar pain is produced by the patella pressing on the femoral condyles, or after patella subluxation or blocking elevation of patella during quadriceps contraction when the knee is extended. Femoropatellar osteoarthritis is usually better tolerated than femorotibial osteoarthritis, but severe disability is possible. The

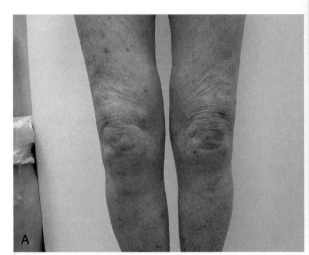
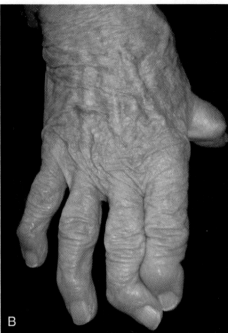

Figure 90-3 **A,** Bone swelling in knee osteoarthritis: Right knee effusion with flexion deformity. **B,** Heberden's nodes in hand osteoarthritis responsible for misalignment and disfigurement of fingers. *(Figures provided by www.lecofer.org.)*

femoropatellar compartment is investigated using a specific x-ray axial incidence with variable degrees of knee flexion.

Radiographs should include bilateral, comparative images of both knees. The femorotibial compartment is evaluated by a standard standing anteroposterior radiograph of the extended knee to take into account any weight-bearing effect. The "schuss" view is useful for assessing the posterior part of the femorotibial compartment, where early decrease in joint space may be evident.[144] Squaring of the femoral condyle, intercondylar spurring, and varus or valgus misalignment of the affected limb can occur. Radiographs of the hip, knee, and ankle made on one long film with the patient standing may identify angular deformity. The patient must be able to place his or her full weight on the affected limb for a true measurement of limb deformity. A mechanical axis of 0 to 3 degrees of varus is considered to be within normal limits.[145]

Hand Osteoarthritis

Hand osteoarthritis results in pain and reduced hand mobility and grip force, limiting activity and restricting participation in personal, occupational, and group functions. Women are more likely to have hand osteoarthritis than men, and genetic factors explain familial aggregation.[146] It can affect the distal interphalangeal, proximal interphalangeal, and first carpometacarpal joints of the hand. The metacarpophalangeal joints are less commonly involved, but if implicated, consideration should be given to complicating factors, such as a coincident or causal metabolic arthropathy.

Patients with hand osteoarthritis express three primary complaints: pain, disfigurement, and disability, with impaired manual dexterity a significant consequence, especially with involvement of the first metacarpophalangeal joint. Bony enlargements of the proximal interphalangeal joints are called Bouchard's nodes, whereas enlargements of the distal interphalangeal joints are called Heberden's nodes (Fig. 90-3B). They can be associated with mucinous cysts.

As the disease progresses there is characteristic loss of mobility. In contrast, hypermobility may protect joints from radiographic osteoarthritis of the proximal interphalangeal joints.[147] The disease course is usually insidious, sometimes with acute inflammatory phases mimicking inflammatory arthropathies. Sagittal deviation of the distal phalanges is frequent. Osteoarthritis frequently involves the first carpometacarpal joints, causing intense pain, tenderness, squared deformation of the radial base of the thumb, and fixed adduction that leads to severe disability. de Quervain's tenosynovitis can be associated throughout the disease process and exacerbate this functional limitation.

Posteroanterior radiographs of both hands, including the wrists, should reveal characteristic features of osteoarthritis. Erosions of the interphalangeal distal joints on radiographs (seagull erosions) are prominent features in a subset of osteoarthritis patients.[148] This disorder is more frequent in middle-aged women and has an acute, inflammatory clinical presentation, leading to joint deformity and occasional ankylosis. The fingers are often significantly completely deformed within a few years, with firm bony swelling and consequent reduced joint motion—at advanced stages, flares and pain tend to subside. Patients with erosive osteoarthritis may have signs of inflammation in the interphalangeal joints. Synovitis can occur; in such cases, the differential diagnosis should consider psoriatic or less likely rheumatoid arthritis. Very rarely, multicentric reticular histiocytosis can manifest with similar features.

Hip Osteoarthritis

In hip osteoarthritis, hip pain is classically present during weight bearing; it is located in the buttocks and the groin region, and may radiate down to the anterior thigh. Less commonly, the sole presenting feature may be knee pain.

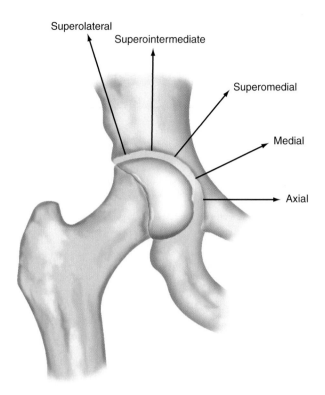

Superolateral
Superointermediate
Superomedial
Medial
Axial

Figure 90-4 Patterns of osteoarthritis of the hip. *(From Harris E, Budd R, Firestein G, et al [eds]: Kelley's Textbook of Rheumatology, 7th ed. Philadelphia, WB Saunders, 2005.)*

Patients often report significant disability during activities of daily living (e.g., finding it difficult to reach their feet to cut their toenails or to tie their shoelaces) (see Table 90-5). Flares are frequent, with pain at night and morning stiffness, sometimes associated with the presence of an effusion. Advanced osteoarthritis is often preceded by a progressive phase with increasing aggravation of symptoms (between 3 months and 3 years). The symptoms seldom improve except in concentric hip osteoarthritis with marked osteophytosis.

Limited range of movement is the main physical sign of hip osteoarthritis, although it is not always present. Limited movement may be seen in early disease only when extension is tested. Groin pain can be reproduced by palpation during physical examination. This pain also can be reproduced by passive movement of the hip, especially on internal rotation and flexion. Quadriceps muscle weakness is a further common finding. The main differential diagnoses are cruralgia (in which neurologic signs are usually present), psoas and iliopsoas lesions, and trochanteric bursitis (characterized by pain at the external surface of the hip and thigh). Consideration also should be given to intrapelvic lesions if clinical examination is entirely normal in the face of a convincing history.

Radiologic examination should be bilateral and comparative, including a false profile view.[149] Osteoarthritis can involve several compartments of the hip (Fig. 90-4; see Fig. 90-1). The superior-external pole is most often involved (superior-lateral, superior-intermediate and superior-medial). Medial osteoarthritis is much rarer, occurs mainly in women, and progresses slowly. Hip osteoarthritis may be rapidly destructive, defined by Lequesne and Ray[150] as joint space narrowing at greater than 2 mm/yr (i.e., a loss of >50% of the joint space within 1 year). Bone sclerosis and osteophytes are rare in such patients. A hip joint replacement usually is considered within a few

months of the first symptoms being recognized. The common etiologies of secondary hip osteoarthritis include congenital dysplasia, avascular osteonecrosis, and previous trauma.

Spinal Osteoarthritis

Spine and peripheral osteoarthritis share anatomic similarities and common pathophysiologic processes. The posterior facet articulations are true diarthrodial joints and as such are susceptible to osteoarthritis. Common regions of involvement include the cervical and lumbar spine, but the dorsal spine only exceptionally because of the stability provided by the thoracic cage. Osteophytes of the vertebrae can narrow the foramina and compress nerve roots. Patients also report, in addition to pain, radicular symptoms with pain, weakness, and numbness of the arms or legs.

Foot and Ankle Osteoarthritis

Osteoarthritis commonly attacks the first metatarsophalangeal joint. Patients have difficulty walking, and the overlying skin can appear inflamed. Deformation in valgus is frequent (hallux valgus), and there may be ankylosis of the joint (hallux rigidus). There are usually radiologic features of foot and ankle osteoarthritis, even in subjects younger than 40 years old.[151] The tarsal joints may be involved in cases of pes planus. Tibiotalar and subtalar osteoarthritis are generally due to trauma, misalignment, or neuropathic arthropathy.

Shoulder Osteoarthritis

Osteoarthritis is less common in the shoulder than in weight-bearing joints. Pain occurs at movement, but pain at night also is common. Examination reveals limitation of passive movement, with rotation particularly being reduced. Shoulder osteoarthritis sometimes follows lesions of the rotator cuff, which promote ascension of the humeral head. Radiographs can show a distinction between eccentric osteoarthritis and noneccentric osteoarthritis, which is useful for therapeutic decision making. The long-term outcome of a shoulder prosthesis is better in cases of eccentric osteoarthritis. Milwaukee shoulder is a particular form of shoulder osteoarthritis characterized by hydroxyapatite deposits and severe destruction of the joint.[152] The differential diagnosis includes acromioclavicular disease, in which pain is elicited on direct palpation of this particular joint. The acromioclavicular joints are often affected in individuals such as construction workers subject to direct weight bearing to the shoulder area. Shoulder osteoarthritis also can develop after vascular osteonecrosis, causing the humeral head to become aspheric.

Elbow Osteoarthritis

Elbow osteoarthritis is rare and generally considered to be the result of repeated vibration exposure, trauma, or metabolic arthropathy, such as pseudogout.

Temporomandibular Joint Osteoarthritis

Radiologic signs of osteoarthritis are common, but orofacial pain and radiographic signs of osteoarthritis are poorly correlated.[153]

REFERENCES

1. Badley EM, Wang PP: Arthritis and the aging population: Projections of arthritis prevalence in Canada 1991 to 2031. J Rheumatol 25:138-144, 1998.
2. March LM, Bachmeier CJ: Economics of osteoarthritis: A global perspective. Baillieres Clin Rheumatol 11:817-834, 1997.
3. Fautrel B, Clarke AE, Guillemin F, et al: Valuing a hypothetical cure for rheumatoid arthritis using the contingent valuation methodology: The patient perspective. J Rheumatol 32:443-453, 2005.
4. Gordon GV, Villanueva T, Schumacher HR, et al: Autopsy study correlating degree of osteoarthritis, synovitis and evidence of articular calcification. J Rheumatol 11:681-686, 1984.
5. Dahaghin S, Bierma-Zeinstra SM, Ginai AZ, et al: Prevalence and pattern of radiographic hand osteoarthritis and association with pain and disability (the Rotterdam study). Ann Rheum Dis 64:682-687, 2005.
6. Dahaghin S, Bierma-Zeinstra SM, Reijman M, et al: Prevalence and determinants of one month hand pain and hand related disability in the elderly (Rotterdam study). Ann Rheum Dis 64:99-104, 2005.
7. Cicuttini FM, Baker J, Hart DJ, et al: Relation between Heberden's nodes and distal interphalangeal joint osteophytes and their role as markers of generalised disease. Ann Rheum Dis 57:246-248, 1998.
8. Felson DT, Naimark A, Anderson J, et al: The prevalence of knee osteoarthritis in the elderly. The Framingham Osteoarthritis Study. Arthritis Rheum 30:914-918, 1987.
9. Felson DT, Zhang Y: An update on the epidemiology of knee and hip osteoarthritis with a view to prevention. Arthritis Rheum 41:1343-1355, 1998.
10. Oliveria SA, Felson DT, Reed JI, et al: Incidence of symptomatic hand, hip, and knee osteoarthritis among patients in a health maintenance organization. Arthritis Rheum 38:1134-1141, 1995.
11. Arden N, Nevitt MC: Osteoarthritis: Epidemiology. Best Pract Res Clin Rheumatol 20:3-25, 2006.
12. Peat G, Croft P, Hay E: Clinical assessment of the osteoarthritis patient. Best Pract Res Clin Rheumatol 15:527-544, 2001.
13. Wilder FV, Hall BJ, Barrett JP: Osteoarthritis pain and weather. Rheumatology (Oxf) 42:955-958, 2003.
14. Verges J, Montell E, Tomas E, et al: Weather conditions can influence rheumatic diseases. Proc West Pharmacol Soc 47:134-136, 2004.
15. McAlindon TE, Cooper C, Kirwan JR, et al: Determinants of disability in osteoarthritis of the knee. Ann Rheum Dis 52:258-262, 1993.
16. Bennell KL, Hinman RS, Metcalf BR, et al: Relationship of knee joint proprioception to pain and disability in individuals with knee osteoarthritis. J Orthop Res 21:792-797, 2003.
17. CDC: Prevalence of disabilities and associated health conditions among adults: United States, 1999. MMWR Morb Mortal Wkly Rep 50:120-125, 2001.
18. Cibere J, Bellamy N, Thorne A, et al: Reliability of the knee examination in osteoarthritis: Effect of standardization. Arthritis Rheum 50:458-468, 2004.
19. Sharma L: The role of proprioceptive deficits, ligamentous laxity, and malalignment in development and progression of knee osteoarthritis. J Rheumatol Suppl 70:87-92, 2004.
20. Brouwer GM, van Tol AW, Bergink AP, et al: Association between valgus and varus alignment and the development and progression of radiographic osteoarthritis of the knee. Arthritis Rheum 56:1204-1211, 2007.
21. Sharma L: The role of varus and valgus alignment in knee osteoarthritis. Arthritis Rheum 56:1044-1047, 2007.
22. Cahue S, Dunlop D, Hayes K, et al: Varus-valgus alignment in the progression of patellofemoral osteoarthritis. Arthritis Rheum 50:2184-2190, 2004.
23. Dayal N, Chang A, Dunlop D, et al: The natural history of anteroposterior laxity and its role in knee osteoarthritis progression. Arthritis Rheum 52:2343-2349, 2005.
24. van der Esch M, Steultjens M, Knol DL, et al: Joint laxity and the relationship between muscle strength and functional ability in patients with osteoarthritis of the knee. Arthritis Rheum 55:953-959, 2006.
25. Cibere J: Do we need radiographs to diagnose osteoarthritis? Best Pract Res Clin Rheumatol 20:27-38, 2006.
26. Spector TD, Cooper C: Radiographic assessment of osteoarthritis in population studies: Whither Kellgren and Lawrence? Osteoarthritis Cartilage 1:203-206, 1993.
27. Raynauld JP, Martel-Pelletier J, Berthiaume MJ, et al: Quantitative magnetic resonance imaging evaluation of knee osteoarthritis progression over two years and correlation with clinical symptoms and radiologic changes. Arthritis Rheum 50:476-487, 2004.
28. Peterfy CG: Scratching the surface: Articular cartilage disorders in the knee. Magn Reson Imaging Clin N Am 8:409-430, 2000.
29. **Felson DT, Chaisson CE, Hill CL, et al: The association of bone marrow lesions with pain in knee osteoarthritis. Ann Intern Med 134:541-549, 2001.**
30. Conaghan PG, Felson D, Gold G, et al: MRI and non-cartilaginous structures in knee osteoarthritis. Osteoarthritis Cartilage 14(Suppl A):A87-A94, 2006.
31. Sowers MF, Hayes C, Jamadar D, et al: Magnetic resonance-detected subchondral bone marrow and cartilage defect characteristics associated with pain and x-ray-defined knee osteoarthritis. Osteoarthritis Cartilage 11:387-393, 2003.
32. Garnero P, Peterfy C, Zaim S, et al: Bone marrow abnormalities on magnetic resonance imaging are associated with type II collagen degradation in knee osteoarthritis: A three-month longitudinal study. Arthritis Rheum 52:2822-2829, 2005.
33. Link TM, Steinbach LS, Ghosh S, et al: Osteoarthritis: MR imaging findings in different stages of disease and correlation with clinical findings. Radiology 226:373-381, 2003.
34. Torres L, Dunlop DD, Peterfy C, et al: The relationship between specific tissue lesions and pain severity in persons with knee osteoarthritis. Osteoarthritis Cartilage 14:1033-1040, 2006.
35. Raynauld JP, Martel-Pelletier J, Berthiaume MJ, et al: Long term evaluation of disease progression through the quantitative magnetic resonance imaging of symptomatic knee osteoarthritis patients: Correlation with clinical symptoms and radiographic changes. Arthritis Res Ther 8:R21, 2006.
36. **Felson DT, McLaughlin S, Goggins J, et al: Bone marrow edema and its relation to progression of knee osteoarthritis. Ann Intern Med 139(5 Pt 1):330-336, 2003.**
37. Conaghan P: Is MRI useful in osteoarthritis? Best Pract Res Clin Rheumatol 20:57-68, 2006.
38. Pessis E, Drape JL, Ravaud P, et al: Assessment of progression in knee osteoarthritis: Results of a 1 year study comparing arthroscopy and MRI. Osteoarthritis Cartilage 11:361-369, 2003.
39. Bhattacharyya T, Gale D, Dewire P, et al: The clinical importance of meniscal tears demonstrated by magnetic resonance imaging in osteoarthritis of the knee. J Bone Joint Surg Am 85:4-9, 2003.
40. Grassi W, Filippucci E, Farina A: Ultrasonography in osteoarthritis. Semin Arthritis Rheum 34(6 Suppl 2):19-23, 2005.
41. Grassi W, Lamanna G, Farina A, et al: Sonographic imaging of normal and osteoarthritic cartilage. Semin Arthritis Rheum 28:398-403, 1999.
42. Aisen AM, McCune WJ, MacGuire A, et al: Sonographic evaluation of the cartilage of the knee. Radiology 153:781-784, 1984.
43. Adler RS: Future and new developments in musculoskeletal ultrasound. Radiol Clin North Am 37:623-631, 1999.
44. Jung YO, Do JH, Kang HJ, et al: Correlation of sonographic severity with biochemical markers of synovium and cartilage in knee osteoarthritis patients. Clin Exp Rheumatol 24:253-259, 2006.
45. D'Agostino MA, Conaghan P, Le Bars M, et al: EULAR report on the use of ultrasonography in painful knee osteoarthritis, Part 1: Prevalence of inflammation in osteoarthritis. Ann Rheum Dis 64:1703-1709, 2005.
46. Naredo E, Cabero F, Palop MJ, et al: Ultrasonographic findings in knee osteoarthritis: A comparative study with clinical and radiographic assessment. Osteoarthritis Cartilage 13:568-574, 2005.
47. Conaghan P, D'Agostino MA, Ravaud P, et al: EULAR report on the use of ultrasonography in painful knee osteoarthritis, Part 2: Exploring decision rules for clinical utility. Ann Rheum Dis 64:1710-1714, 2005.
48. Iagnocco A, Filippucci E, Ossandon A, et al: High resolution ultrasonography in detection of bone erosions in patients with hand osteoarthritis. J Rheumatol 32:2381-2383, 2005.
49. Iagnocco A, Filippucci E, Meenagh G, et al: Ultrasound imaging for the rheumatologist, III: Ultrasonography of the hip. Clin Exp Rheumatol 24:229-232, 2006.
50. Ike RW: Diagnostic arthroscopy. Baillieres Clin Rheumatol 10:495-517, 1996.
51. Dougados M: Synovial fluid cell analysis. Baillieres Clin Rheumatol 10:519-534, 1996.

52. Kraus VB: Do biochemical markers have a role in osteoarthritis diagnosis and treatment? Best Pract Res Clin Rheumatol 20:69-80, 2006.

53. Pottie P, Presle N, Terlain B, et al: Obesity and osteoarthritis: More complex than predicted! Ann Rheum Dis 65:1403-1405, 2006.

54. Newman AB, Haggerty CL, Goodpaster B, et al: Strength and muscle quality in a well-functioning cohort of older adults: The Health, Aging and Body Composition Study. J Am Geriatr Soc 51:323-330, 2003.

55. Hurley MV: The role of muscle weakness in the pathogenesis of osteoarthritis. Rheum Dis Clin N Am 25:283-298, vi, 1999.

56. Sharma L, Lou C, Felson DT, et al: Laxity in healthy and osteoarthritic knees. Arthritis Rheum 42:861-870, 1999.

57. Kellgren JH, Moore R: Generalized osteoarthritis and Heberden's nodes. BMJ 1:181-187, 1952.

58. **Dougados M, Gueguen A, Nguyen M, et al: Radiological progression of hip osteoarthritis: Definition, risk factors and correlations with clinical status. Ann Rheum Dis 55:356-362, 1996.**

59. Ledingham J, Dawson S, Preston B, et al: Radiographic progression of hospital referred osteoarthritis of the hip. Ann Rheum Dis 52:263-267, 1993.

60. **Nevitt MC, Felson DT, Williams EN, et al: The effect of estrogen plus progestin on knee symptoms and related disability in postmenopausal women: The Heart and Estrogen/Progestin Replacement Study, a randomized, double-blind, placebo-controlled trial. Arthritis Rheum 44:811-818, 2001.**

61. Hart DJ, Cronin C, Daniels M, et al: The relationship of bone density and fracture to incident and progressive radiographic osteoarthritis of the knee: The Chingford Study. Arthritis Rheum 46:92-99, 2002.

62. Zhang Y, Hannan MT, Chaisson CE, et al: Bone mineral density and risk of incident and progressive radiographic knee osteoarthritis in women: The Framingham Study. J Rheumatol 27:1032-1037, 2000.

63. Sowers M, Zobel D, Weissfeld L, et al: Progression of osteoarthritis of the hand and metacarpal bone loss: A twenty-year followup of incident cases. Arthritis Rheum 34:36-42, 1991.

64. Riyazi N, Kurreeman FA, Huizinga TW, et al: The role of interleukin 10 promoter polymorphisms in the susceptibility of distal interphalangeal osteoarthritis. J Rheumatol 32:1571-1575, 2005.

65. Mier RJ, Holderbaum D, Ferguson R, et al: Osteoarthritis in children associated with a mutation in the type II procollagen gene (COL2A1). Mol Genet Metab 74:338-341, 2001.

66. Pun YL, Moskowitz RW, Lie S, et al: Clinical correlations of osteoarthritis associated with a single-base mutation (arginine519 to cysteine) in type II procollagen gene: A newly defined pathogenesis. Arthritis Rheum 37:264-269, 1994.

67. Ritvaniemi P, Korkko J, Bonaventure J, et al: Identification of COL2A1 gene mutations in patients with chondrodysplasias and familial osteoarthritis. Arthritis Rheum 38:999-1004, 1995.

68. Min JL, Meulenbelt I, Riyazi N, et al: Association of the Frizzled-related protein gene with symptomatic osteoarthritis at multiple sites. Arthritis Rheum 52:1077-1080, 2005.

69. Ingvarsson T, Stefansson SE, Gulcher JR, et al: A large Icelandic family with early osteoarthritis of the hip associated with a susceptibility locus on chromosome 16p. Arthritis Rheum 44:2548-2555, 2001.

70. Riyazi N, Meulenbelt I, Kroon HM, et al: Evidence for familial aggregation of hand, hip, and spine but not knee osteoarthritis in siblings with multiple joint involvement: The GARP study. Ann Rheum Dis 64:438-443, 2005.

71. Kalichman L, Kobyliansky E, Malkin I, et al: Search for linkage between hand osteoarthritis and 11q12-13 chromosomal segment. Osteoarthritis Cartilage 11:561-568, 2003.

72. Hoaglund FT, Steinbach LS: Primary osteoarthritis of the hip: Etiology and epidemiology. J Am Acad Orthop Surg 9:320-327, 2001.

73. Li Y, Xu L, Olsen BR: Lessons from genetic forms of osteoarthritis for the pathogenesis of the disease. Osteoarthritis Cartilage 15:1101-1105, 2007.

74. Mundlos S, Spranger J: Genetic disorders of connective tissues. Curr Opin Rheumatol 3:832-837, 1991.

75. Petersson IF, Jacobsson LT: Osteoarthritis of the peripheral joints. Best Pract Res Clin Rheumatol 16:741-760, 2002.

76. Bukulmez H, Matthews AL, Sullivan CM, et al: Hip joint replacement surgery for idiopathic osteoarthritis aggregates in families. Arthritis Res Ther 8:R25, 2006.

77. Harris WH: Etiology of osteoarthritis of the hip. Clin Orthop 213:20-33, 1986.

78. Lane NE, Lin P, Christiansen L, et al: Association of mild acetabular dysplasia with an increased risk of incident hip osteoarthritis in elderly white women: The study of osteoporotic fractures. Arthritis Rheum 43:400-404, 2000.

79. Lane NE, Nevitt MC, Cooper C, et al: Acetabular dysplasia and osteoarthritis of the hip in elderly white women. Ann Rheum Dis 56:627-630, 1997.

80. Smith RW, Egger P, Coggon D, et al: Osteoarthritis of the hip joint and acetabular dysplasia in women. Ann Rheum Dis 54:179-181, 1995.

81. Andriacchi TP: Dynamics of knee malalignment. Orthop Clin North Am 25:395-403, 1994.

82. Sharma L, Song J, Felson DT, et al: The role of knee alignment in disease progression and functional decline in knee osteoarthritis. JAMA 286:188-195, 2001.

83. Felson DT, Goggins J, Niu J, et al: The effect of body weight on progression of knee osteoarthritis is dependent on alignment. Arthritis Rheum 50:3904-3909, 2004.

84. Cooper C, Snow S, McAlindon TE, et al: Risk factors for the incidence and progression of radiographic knee osteoarthritis. Arthritis Rheum 43:995-1000, 2000.

85. Sowers M, Lachance L, Jamadar D, et al: The associations of bone mineral density and bone turnover markers with osteoarthritis of the hand and knee in pre- and perimenopausal women. Arthritis Rheum 42:483-489, 1999.

86. Gelber AC, Hochberg MC, Mead LA, et al: Joint injury in young adults and risk for subsequent knee and hip osteoarthritis. Ann Intern Med 133:321-328, 2000.

87. Roos H, Lauren M, Adalberth T, et al: Knee osteoarthritis after meniscectomy: Prevalence of radiographic changes after twenty-one years, compared with matched controls. Arthritis Rheum 41:687-693, 1998.

88. Englund M, Paradowski PT, Lohmander LS: Association of radiographic hand osteoarthritis with radiographic knee osteoarthritis after meniscectomy. Arthritis Rheum 50:469-475, 2004.

89. Wilder FV, Hall BJ, Barrett JP Jr, et al: History of acute knee injury and osteoarthritis of the knee: A prospective epidemiological assessment. The Clearwater Osteoarthritis Study. Osteoarthritis Cartilage 10:611-616, 2002.

90. Pelletier JP, Martel-Pelletier J, Raynauld JP: Most recent developments in strategies to reduce the progression of structural changes in osteoarthritis: Today and tomorrow. Arthritis Res Ther 8:206, 2006.

91. Englund M, Lohmander LS: Patellofemoral osteoarthritis coexistent with tibiofemoral osteoarthritis in a meniscectomy population. Ann Rheum Dis 64:1721-1726, 2005.

92. **Englund M, Lohmander LS: Risk factors for symptomatic knee osteoarthritis fifteen to twenty-two years after meniscectomy. Arthritis Rheum 50:2811-2819, 2004.**

93. Coggon D, Croft P, Kellingray S, et al: Occupational physical activities and osteoarthritis of the knee. Arthritis Rheum 43:1443-1449, 2000.

94. Felson DT, Hannan MT, Naimark A, et al: Occupational physical demands, knee bending, and knee osteoarthritis: Results from the Framingham Study. J Rheumatol 18:1587-1592, 1991.

95. Spector TD, Harris PA, Hart DJ, et al: Risk of osteoarthritis associated with long-term weight-bearing sports: A radiologic survey of the hips and knees in female ex-athletes and population controls. Arthritis Rheum 39:988-995, 1996.

96. Buckwalter JA, Lane NE: Athletics and osteoarthritis. Am J Sports Med 25:873-881, 1997.

97. Lane NE, Oehlert JW, Bloch DA, et al: The relationship of running to osteoarthritis of the knee and hip and bone mineral density of the lumbar spine: A 9 year longitudinal study. J Rheumatol 25:334-341, 1998.

98. Lequesne MG, Dang N, Lane NE: Sport practice and osteoarthritis of the limbs. Osteoarthritis Cartilage 5:75-86, 1997.

99. Slemenda C, Brandt KD, Heilman DK, et al: Quadriceps weakness and osteoarthritis of the knee. Ann Intern Med 127:97-104, 1997.

100. Roddy E, Doherty M: Changing life-styles and osteoarthritis: What is the evidence? Best Pract Res Clin Rheumatol 20:81-97, 2006.

101. **Maheu E, Altman RD, Bloch DA, et al: Design and conduct of clinical trials in patients with osteoarthritis of the hand: Recommendations from a task force of the Osteoarthritis Research Society International. Osteoarthritis Cartilage 14:303-322, 2006.**

102. Altman R, Brandt K, Hochberg M, et al: Design and conduct of clinical trials in patients with osteoarthritis: Recommendations from a task force of the Osteoarthritis Research Society: Results from a workshop. Osteoarthritis Cartilage 4:217-243, 1996.

103. **Altman R, Alarcon G, Appelrouth D, et al: The American College of Rheumatology criteria for the classification and reporting of osteoarthritis of the hip. Arthritis Rheum 34:505-514, 1991.**

104. **Altman R, Asch E, Bloch D, et al: Development of criteria for the classification and reporting of osteoarthritis: Classification of osteoarthritis of the knee. Diagnostic and Therapeutic Criteria Committee of the American Rheumatism Association. Arthritis Rheum 29:1039-1049, 1986.**

105. **Altman R, Alarcon G, Appelrouth D, et al: The American College of Rheumatology criteria for the classification and reporting of osteoarthritis of the hand. Arthritis Rheum 33:1601-1610, 1990.**

106. McAlindon T, Dieppe P: Osteoarthritis: Definitions and criteria. Ann Rheum Dis 48:531-532, 1989.

107. Schouten JS, Valkenburg HA: Classification criteria: Methodological considerations and results from a 12 year following study in the general population. J Rheumatol Suppl 43:44-45, 1995.

108. Croft P, Cooper C, Coggon D: Case definition of hip osteoarthritis in epidemiologic studies. J Rheumatol 21:591-592, 1994.

109. Bierma-Zeinstra S, Bohnen A, Ginai A, et al: Validity of American College of Rheumatology criteria for diagnosing hip osteoarthritis in primary care research. J Rheumatol 26:1129-1133, 1999.

110. Kellgren JH, Jeffrey M, Ball J: Atlas of Standard Radiographs. Oxford, Blackwell Scientific, 1963.

111. Lachance L, Sowers MF, Jamadar D, et al: The natural history of emergent osteoarthritis of the knee in women. Osteoarthritis Cartilage 10:849-854, 2002.

112. Birrell F, Lunt M, Macfarlane G, et al: Association between pain in the hip region and radiographic changes of osteoarthritis: Results from a population-based study. Rheumatology (Oxf) 44:337-341, 2005.

113. Garnero P: Osteoarthritis: Biological markers for the future? Joint Bone Spine 69:525-530, 2002.

114. Armstrong AL, Hunter JB, Davis TR: The prevalence of degenerative arthritis of the base of the thumb in post-menopausal women. J Hand Surg Br 19:340-341, 1994.

115. Acheson RM, Chan YK, Clemett AR: New Haven survey of joint diseases, XII: Distribution and symptoms of osteoarthrosis in the hands with reference to handedness. Ann Rheum Dis 29:275-286, 1970.

116. Jonsson H, Valtysdottir ST, Kjartansson O, et al: Hypermobility associated with osteoarthritis of the thumb base: A clinical and radiological subset of hand osteoarthritis. Ann Rheum Dis 55:540-543, 1996.

117. Spacek E, Poiraudeau S, Fayad F, et al: Disability induced by hand osteoarthritis: Are patients with more symptoms at digits 2-5 interphalangeal joints different from those with more symptoms at the base of the thumb? Osteoarthritis Cartilage 12:366-373, 2004.

118. Egger P, Cooper C, Hart DJ, et al: Patterns of joint involvement in osteoarthritis of the hand: The Chingford Study. J Rheumatol 22:1509-1513, 1995.

119. Constant F, Guillemin F, Herbeth B, et al: Measurement methods of drug consumption as a secondary judgment criterion for clinical trials in chronic rheumatic diseases. Am J Epidemiol 145:826-833, 1997.

120. **Bellamy N, Buchanan WW, Goldsmith CH, et al: Validation study of WOMAC: A health status instrument for measuring clinically important patient relevant outcomes to antirheumatic drug therapy in patients with osteoarthritis of the hip or knee. J Rheumatol 15:1833-1840, 1988.**

121. **Lequesne MG, Mery C, Samson M, et al: Indexes of severity for osteoarthritis of the hip and knee: Validation—value in comparison with other assessment tests. Scand J Rheumatol Suppl 65: 85-89, 1987.**

122. Fries JF, Spitz P, Kraines RG, et al: Measurement of patient outcome in arthritis. Arthritis Rheum 23:137-145, 1980.

123. **Roos EM, Roos HP, Ekdahl C, et al: Knee injury and Osteoarthritis Outcome Score (KOOS)—validation of a Swedish version. Scand J Med Sci Sports 8:439-448, 1998.**

124. Roos EM, Roos HP, Lohmander LS, et al: Knee Injury and Osteoarthritis Outcome Score (KOOS)—development of a self-administered outcome measure. J Orthop Sports Phys Ther 28:88-96, 1998.

125. Roos EM, Lohmander LS: The Knee Injury and Osteoarthritis Outcome Score (KOOS): From joint injury to osteoarthritis. Health Qual Life Outcomes 1:64, 2003.

126. Roos EM, Brandsson S, Karlsson J: Validation of the foot and ankle outcome score for ankle ligament reconstruction. Foot Ankle Int 22:788-794, 2001.

127. Nilsdotter AK, Lohmander LS, Klassbo M, et al: Hip disability and Osteoarthritis Outcome Score (HOOS)—validity and responsiveness in total hip replacement. BMC Musculoskelet Disord 4:10, 2003.

128. Bellamy N, Campbell J, Haraoui B, et al: Clinimetric properties of the AUSCAN Osteoarthritis Hand Index: An evaluation of reliability, validity and responsiveness. Osteoarthritis Cartilage 10:863-869, 2002.

129. Bellamy N, Campbell J, Haraoui B, et al: Dimensionality and clinical importance of pain and disability in hand osteoarthritis: Development of the Australian/Canadian (AUSCAN) Osteoarthritis Hand Index. Osteoarthritis Cartilage 10:855-862, 2002.

130. Allen KD, Jordan JM, Renner JB, et al: Validity, factor structure, and clinical relevance of the AUSCAN Osteoarthritis Hand Index. Arthritis Rheum 54:551-556, 2006.

131. Dreiser RL, Maheu E, Guillou GB: Sensitivity to change of the functional index for hand osteoarthritis. Osteoarthritis Cartilage 8(Suppl A):S25-S28, 2000.

132. Dreiser RL, Maheu E, Guillou GB, et al: Validation of an algofunctional index for osteoarthritis of the hand. Rev Rhum Engl 62(Suppl 1):43S-53S, 1995.

133. Ravaud P, Dougados M: Radiographic assessment in osteoarthritis. J Rheumatol 24:786-791, 1997.

134. Gossec L, Hawker G, Davis AM, et al: OMERACT/OARSI initiative to define states of severity and indication for joint replacement in hip and knee osteoarthritis. J Rheumatol 34:1432-1435, 2007.

135. Steel N, Melzer D, Gardener E, et al: Need for and receipt of hip and knee replacement—a national population survey. Rheumatology (Oxf) 45:1437-1441, 2006.

136. March L, Cross M, Tribe K, et al: Cost of joint replacement surgery for osteoarthritis: The patients' perspective. J Rheumatol 29:1006-1014, 2002.

137. Escalante A, Espinosa-Morales R, del Rincon I, et al: Recipients of hip replacement for arthritis are less likely to be Hispanic, independent of access to health care and socioeconomic status. Arthritis Rheum 43:390-399, 2000.

138. Fielden JM, Cumming JM, Horne JG, et al: Waiting for hip arthroplasty: Economic costs and health outcomes. J Arthroplasty 20: 990-997, 2005.

139. Hirsch R, Lethbridge-Cejku M, Scott WW Jr, et al: Association of hand and knee osteoarthritis: Evidence for a polyarticular disease subset. Ann Rheum Dis 55:25-29, 1996.

140. Hochberg MC, Lane NE, Pressman AR, et al: The association of radiographic changes of osteoarthritis of the hand and hip in elderly women. J Rheumatol 22:2291-2294, 1995.

141. Croft P, Cooper C, Wickham C, et al: Is the hip involved in generalized osteoarthritis? Br J Rheumatol 31:325-328, 1992.

142. Cushnaghan J, Dieppe P: Study of 500 patients with limb joint osteoarthritis, I: Analysis by age, sex, and distribution of symptomatic joint sites. Ann Rheum Dis 50:8-13, 1991.

143. Cooper C, Egger P, Coggon D, et al: Generalized osteoarthritis in women: Pattern of joint involvement and approaches to definition for epidemiological studies. J Rheumatol 23:1938-1942, 1996.

144. Vignon E, Piperno M, Le Graverand MP, et al: Measurement of radiographic joint space width in the tibiofemoral compartment of the osteoarthritic knee: Comparison of standing anteroposterior and Lyon schuss views. Arthritis Rheum 48:378-384, 2003.

145. Iorio R, Healy WL: Unicompartmental arthritis of the knee. J Bone Joint Surg Am 85A:1351-1364, 2003.

146. **Spector TD, Cicuttini F, Baker J, et al: Genetic influences on osteoarthritis in women: A twin study. BMJ 312:940-943, 1996.**

147. Kraus VB, Li YJ, Martin ER, et al: Articular hypermobility is a protective factor for hand osteoarthritis. Arthritis Rheum 50:2178-2183, 2004.

148. Utsinger PD, Resnick D, Shapiro RF, et al: Roentgenologic, immunologic, and therapeutic study of erosive (inflammatory) osteoarthritis. Arch Intern Med 138:693-697, 1978.

149. Lequesne M: The false profile view of the hip: Role, interest, economic considerations. Joint Bone Spine 69:109-113, 2002.

150. Lequesne M, Ray G: [Rapid idiopathic destructive coxarthrosis: Prospective etiologic study of 27 cases]. Rev Rhum Mal Osteoartic 56:115-119, 1989.

151. van Saase JL, van Romunde LK, Cats A, et al: Epidemiology of osteo-arthritis: Zoetermeer survey: Comparison of radiological osteoarthritis in a Dutch population with that in 10 other populations. Ann Rheum Dis 48:271-280, 1989.

152. Halverson PB, McCarty DJ, Cheung HS, et al: Milwaukee Shoulder syndrome: Eleven additional cases with involvement of the knee in seven (basic calcium phosphate crystal deposition disease). Semin Arthritis Rheum 14:36-44, 1984.

153. Engel E, Lachmann S, Axmann-Krcmar D: The prevalence of radiologic TMJ findings and self-reported orofacial pain in a patient group wearing implant dentures. Int J Prosthodont 14:120-126, 2001.

154. McAlindon TE, Wilson PW, Aliabadi P, et al: Level of physical activity and the risk of radiographic and symptomatic knee osteoarthritis in the elderly: The Framingham study. Am J Med 106:151-157, 1999.

155. Felson DT, McAlindon T, Anderson JJ: Defining radiographical osteoarthritis for the whole knee. Osteoarthritis Cartilage 5:220-241, 1997.

156. Hart D, Doyle DV, Spector T: Incidence and risk factors for radiographic knee osteoarthritis in middle-aged women: The Chingford study. Arthritis Rheum 42:17-24, 1999.

157. Felson DT, Lawrence RC, Hochberg MC, et al: Osteoarthritis: New insights, Part 2: Treatment approaches. Ann Intern Med 133:726-737, 2000.

158. Felson DT, Lawrence RC, Dieppe P: Level of physical activity and the risk of radiographic and symptomatic knee osteoarthritis in the elderly: The Framingham Study. Am J Med 106:151-157, 1999.

159. McAlindon T, Wilson PG, Aliabadi P: Level of physical activity and the risk of radiographic and symptomatic knee osteoarthritis in th ederly: The Framingham Study. Am J Med 106:151-157, 1999.

160. Rohrbough JT, Mudge MK, Schilling RC, et al: Radiographic osteoarthritis in the hands of rock climbers. Am J Orthop 27:734-738, 1998.

161. Nevitt M, Cummings SR, Lane NE: Association of estrogen replacement therapy with the risk of osteoarthritis of the hip in elderly white women: Study of Osteoporotic Fractures Research Group. Arch Intern Med 156:2056-2080, 1996.

162. Zhang Y, McAlindon TE, Hannan MT, et al: Estrogen replacement therapy and worsening of radiographic knee osteoarthritis: The Framingham Study. Arthritis Rheum 41:1867-1873, 1998.

163. McAlindon TE, Felson DT, Zhang Y, et al: Relation of dietary intake and serum levels of vitamin D to progression of osteoarthritis of the knee among participants in the Framingham Study. Ann Intern Med 125:353-359, 1996.

164. Felson DT, Zhang Y, Hannan MT, et al: Risk factors for incident radiographic knee osteoarthritis in the elderly: The Framingham Study. Arthritis Rheum 40:728-733, 1997.

165. Lane NE: Physical activity at leisure and risk of osteoarthritis. Ann Rheum Dis 55:682-684, 1996.

166. Flugsrud GB, Nordsletten L, Espehaug B, et al: Risk factors for total hip replacement due to primary osteoarthritis: A cohort study in 50,034 persons. Arthritis Rheum 46:675-682, 2002.

167. Coggon D, Kellingray S, Inskip H, et al: Osteoarthritis of the hip and occupational lifting. Am J Epidemiol 147:523-528, 1998.

168. Croft P: The occurrence of osteoarthritis outside Europe. Ann Rheum Dis 55:661-664, 1996.

169. Cooper C, Inskip H, Croft P, et al: Individual risk factors for hip osteoarthritis: Obesity, hip injury, and physical activity. Am J Epidemiol 147:516-522, 1998.

170. Chaisson CE, Zhang Y, Sharma L, et al: Grip strength and the risk of developing radiographic hand osteoarthritis: Results from the Framingham Study. Arthritis Rheum 42:33-38, 1999.

171. Carman WJ, Sowers M, Hawthorne VM, et al: Obesity as a risk factor for osteoarthritis of the hand and wrist: A prospective study. Am J Epidemiol 139:119-129, 1994.

172. Lawrence J: Rheumatism in Populations. London, Heineman, 1977.

173. Dougados M, Gueguen A, Nguyen M, et al: Longitudinal radiologic evaluation of osteoarthritis of the knee. J Rheumatol 19:378-384, 1992.

174. Nevitt MC, Felson DT: Sex hormones and the risk of osteoarthritis in women: Epidemiological evidence. Ann Rheum Dis 55:673-676, 1996.

175. Ayral X, Dougados M, Listrat V, et al: Arthroscopic evaluation of chondropathy in osteoarthritis of the knee. J Rheumatol 23:698-706, 1996.

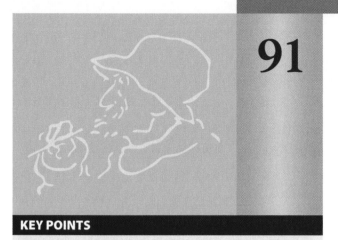

91

Management of Osteoarthritis

CARLOS J. LOZADA

KEY POINTS

Osteoarthritis (OA) is the most common form of arthritis.

Pain is the most common symptom in patients with OA.

The management plan should be individualized, accounting for factors such as sources of pain and extent of accompanying inflammatory features.

Nonpharmacologic interventions such as weight loss and exercise should be an integral part of the management plan for OA.

Currently available pharmacologic interventions are directed at symptomatic relief

Investigation continues into potential disease-modifying interventions in OA.

Osteoarthritis (OA) is the most common form of arthritis. It is often referred to by other names such as *arthrosis, osteoarthrosis*, or simply *arthritis*. Because its incidence increases with age, OA is becoming a more important health issue with the "graying" of the world's population.

OA can be defined radiographically or clinically. The most useful definition, however, includes symptoms as well as radiographic changes. If a purely radiographic definition is used, it can be demonstrated that almost all individuals older than 75 years have OA.[1] Although the epidemiology of OA is well covered in Chapter 90, it has been estimated that between 10% and 30% of those affected with OA are significantly disabled, making OA the leading cause of chronic disability in the United States.[2] This leads to heavy direct and indirect costs.

Traditional treatment paradigms for OA have conceded the inexorable progression of the disease and concentrated on pain management.[3] The importance of training physicians in the management of OA has been underscored by the development of treatment guidelines, but with the relatively rapid evolution in the field of rheumatology, some of these guidelines have required revision. A simplistic but potentially useful algorithm is provided in Figure 91-1. As the population ages, there will be increasing societal pressure on physicians, particularly rheumatologists, to improve the available treatments for OA.[4-6] Researchers have now turned to the investigation of agents that might delay the progression of OA. Potential future interventions include the use of collagenase inhibitors, polysaccharides, and growth factor and cytokine manipulation.[7]

PATIENT ASSESSMENT

Appropriate management of OA begins with an accurate diagnosis. As with most rheumatic illnesses, obtaining a good history is of paramount importance. Symptoms should

be carefully described, particularly pain. Duration, location, and any alleviating or exacerbating factors should be ascertained. Distinct features such as stiffness or gelling and the description of events such as "locking" or "giving way" of a joint can help direct the physical examination.

The physical examination seeks to confirm the diagnostic suspicion and establish the causes of symptoms. Laboratory evaluations are not helpful in establishing the diagnosis of OA but can help in excluding alternative diagnoses. They are also useful in determining which therapeutic approaches are appropriate for a particular patient, because conditions such as renal insufficiency or anemia can be identified.

Radiographs are not necessary for diagnosis in the majority of patients but can identify coexistent conditions such as chondrocalcinosis that may require further workup or modification of the therapeutic plan.

SOURCE OF PAIN

The main symptom in OA is pain. It has many potential sources in and around the joint. These include focal synovitis, synovial effusions, subchondral bone pain receptors, and periarticular tendons and bursae. Factors complicating the determination of the source of pain may include varus or valgus deformity, weight issues, and the emotional impact of chronic pain. Once the source or sources of pain are accurately identified, a treatment plan can be formulated.

MANAGEMENT

The management of OA can be divided into nonpharmacologic interventions (Table 91-1), pharmacologic interventions, and surgical options. Pharmacologic interventions can be further subdivided into symptomatic therapy and potential structure- or disease-modifying therapy.

NONPHARMACOLOGIC INTERVENTIONS

Psychosocial Interventions

As in other types of arthritis, patient education is an important first step in OA therapy. The patient should be an integral part of the decision-making team. To do this effectively, the patient should understand the nature of OA, including its natural history and treatment options. It is often reassuring for the patient to realize that OA is a very common, slowly progressive ailment and is not typically as disabling or deforming as the inflammatory arthritides. A significant number of patients have already tried nonprescription medications or nutriceutical remedies before seeing a physician and will want to discuss these options. Physicians should emphasize

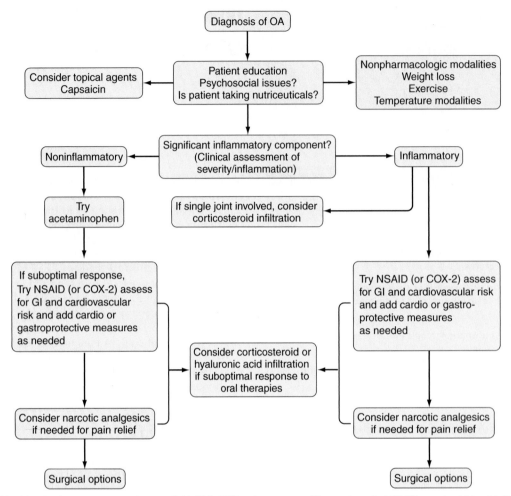

Figure 91-1 Algorithm for the management of osteoarthritis (OA). COX, cyclooxygenase; GI, gastrointestinal; NSAID, nonsteroidal anti-inflammatory drug.

Table 91-1 Nonpharmacolgic Management of Osteoarthritis

Conventional Options
Patient education
Arthritis self-help courses
Weight loss
Temperature modalities
Exercise
Orthotics
Modified activities of daily living

Unconventional Options
Transcutaneous electrical nerve stimulation
Pulsed electromagnetic fields
Static magnets
Acupuncture
Spa therapy
Yoga

that treatment includes nonpharmacologic as well as pharmacologic interventions. Organizations such as the Arthritis Foundation can be valuable sources of information geared toward patients and can provide helpful reading materials.

Some patients may develop significant emotional disturbances related to the pain and changes in normal daily activities that can stem from OA. These may include mood disorders, such as depression, or sleep disorders. A suspicion of either condition should lead to an evaluation by a psychiatrist or a primary physician who regularly manages these types of disorders.

Weight Loss

Obesity is an important risk factor in the development of OA of the knee.[8,9] Further, higher body mass index (BMI) has been associated with an increased risk of progression of OA of the knee.[10] This can be compounded by malalignment—namely, varus and valgus deformities that modulate the effect of weight on knee OA.[11] In one study, BMI was associated with OA severity in those with varus deformity but not in those with valgus.

Regimens of weight loss and exercise have been associated with improvement in pain and disability in OA of the knee.[12] Weight loss alone has been associated with a decrease in the odds of developing symptomatic knee OA.[13] One study suggested that a reduction in the percentage body fat, rather than weight, may be significant in reducing pain from OA of the knee.[14] The symptom-relieving effects of weight loss have been shown to last as long as 1 year.[15] The combination of weight loss and exercise can be superior to either intervention alone.[16]

Temperature Modalities

Topical applications of heat or cold can be a helpful adjunct to the therapeutic plan. These are more effectively used in superficial joints, such as the knees, than in deep ones, such as the hip. An acute injury, such as a sprained ankle, calls for cold applications for the first 2 to 3 days.[17] In a setting of chronic pain, most patients prefer warm applications, although if superior pain relief is obtained from cold applications, these can be continued.

Warm applications can be in the form of warm soaks or heating pads. Individual sessions should not exceed a temperature of 45°C or last more than approximately 30 minutes.[18] The application of warmth should be avoided over certain areas, such as close to the testicles, and in patients with poor vascular supply, neuropathy, or cancer. Benefits of warm applications include decreased pain and stiffness, along with relief of muscle spasm and prevention of contractures.

Exercise

Periarticular structures, particularly muscles, influence the expression of OA. This is likely due to their role in providing stability to the joints and in dampening some of the forces acting across joints. Quadriceps muscle weakness has been postulated as a risk factor for OA of the knee.[19] Quadriceps strengthening exercises have been advanced as fundamental to the management of conditions such as chondromalacia patellae.[20]

Both the dynamic and isometric exercise arms of a 16-week study of patients with knee OA showed equivalent improvement in symptoms and physical functioning.[21] Walking can be beneficial, and supervised fitness-walking regimens can improve function in those with OA of the knee.[20] Home-based exercise interventions also significantly improve symptoms in those with knee OA.[22,23] Finally, community-based aquatic exercise programs, such as aquatic aerobics, have merit.[24]

Orthotics and Bracing

Orthotics—ranging from insoles to braces—can be effective in providing symptomatic relief and are probably underused by most physicians. Studies have demonstrated that lateral wedged insoles provide substantial relief to those with medial compartment knee OA, particularly those with varus deformity.[25] In some studies, those with milder symptoms obtained greater benefit.[26] Knee braces have been evaluated as well. Valgus bracing of patients with medial compartment OA can reduce pain and increase levels of activity.[27] In one study, medial taping of the patella reduced the pain of those with patellofemoral compartment OA by 25%.[28]

Heel lifts have been tried in those with hip OA. In one uncontrolled study, most patients reported diminished symptoms. Time to improvement lengthened with the radiographic stage of OA.[29] For those with calcaneal spurs or foot joint OA in general, appropriate athletic-type footwear is recommended. A good athletic shoe should provide medial arch support and calcaneal cushioning, as well as good mediolateral stability.

Those with carpometacarpal joint arthritis should initially be offered conservative management, including the use of splints. In one trial, 70% of patients treated with a 7-month intervention that included the use of splints were able to improve their symptoms considerably and avoid surgical intervention.[30]

Cane

The appropriate use of a cane can be an important adjunct, particularly in OA of the hip. It has been estimated that a cane can provide up to a 40% reduction in hip contact forces during ambulation.[31] The cane should be used in the hand contralateral to the affected hip or knee[32] and should be advanced with the affected limb while walking. The appropriate cane size is that which results in about a 20-degree flexion of the elbow during use.[33] A useful approximation is a cane that is equal to the distance from the floor to the patient's greater trochanter.

Modification in Activities of Daily Living

Physician advice and occupational therapy can provide useful insights into modifications of daily activities to reduce OA symptoms. These interventions can range from using an elevated toilet seat or shower bench in someone with lower extremity OA to using appliances designed to open jars in patients with hand OA. Assistance from occupational therapists can be valuable.

Other Interventions

Other modalities have been tried in OA. These are unconventional and include magnetic field application, acupuncture, and yoga-based regimens. These are not accepted as standard therapy for OA, but some deserve further study. A significant number of these interventions are being used by patients on their own and should be formally studied not only for evidence of any benefit but also to ensure that there are no harmful effects.

Studies of transcutaneous electrical nerve stimulation (TENS) have generally been small. A recent review of TENS studies in OA of the knee concluded that a trend toward symptom improvement existed, warranting larger, well-controlled studies.[34] In one randomized, controlled study, patients had initial symptom reduction, but at 1 year follow-up, only two patients continued to use the device.[35] TENS use for 3 weeks was compared with 3 weekly hyaluronic acid injections in 60 patients with OA of the knee. Pain relief was observed in both groups through the 6 months of follow-up. There was superior improvement in the Western Ontario McMaster Osteoarthritis Index (WOMAC) physical function subscale score for the hyaluronic acid group.[36]

Pulsed electromagnetic fields have been tested in double-blind, placebo-controlled trials. These fields are applied through the daily use of a brace-type device. In one study, a primary end point of pain reduction was not achieved.[37] Another study did not meet its primary end point but reported an improvement in knee stiffness in subjects younger than 65 years, without an accompanying reduction in pain.[38]

The use of static magnets in chronic knee pain has become quite popular with some patients. In one double-blind, randomized, placebo-controlled trial of 43 patients, the WOMAC pain and physical function subscales, along with a 50-foot walk, demonstrated a statistically significant benefit of static magnets at 2 weeks.[39] Another 29-patient double-blind, placebo-controlled trial in knee OA reported a benefit over placebo after 4 hours of use, but there were no significant differences between groups at 6 weeks of continued treatment.[40] The potential mechanism for any effect remains unclear, and larger, longer-term studies are needed before any clinical benefit can be postulated.

Acupuncture is being formally tested in a National Institutes of Health (NIH)–sponsored multicenter clinical trial. It has been difficult to develop appropriate controls to test acupuncture's clinical efficacy. Most recent studies have tried to employ "sham" methods in the control arm, such as the use of blunted, telescopic needles.[41] Early clinical trials[42,43] and one literature review[44] concluded that acupuncture shows promise in the treatment of knee pain from OA. A double-blind, randomized, placebo-controlled trial of acupuncture as adjunctive therapy in OA of the knee enrolled 570 patients in two outpatient clinics. Reduction in knee pain in the true acupuncture group was superior to that in the sham acupuncture group at 26 weeks by WOMAC function score, WOMAC pain score, and patient global assessment. Twenty-five percent of the patients in each of the acupuncture groups were unavailable for analysis at 26 weeks, however.[45]

The most recent and largest randomized, double-blind, placebo-controlled trial of acupuncture in knee OA showed a benefit of both sham and "traditional" methods of acupuncture over physiotherapy and as-needed nonsteroidal anti-inflammatory drugs (NSAIDs); however, there were no significant differences between the sham and "traditional" arms of the studies in terms of OA symptom relief. The beneficial pain-relieving effect seen in slightly more than half the patients in each of these arms appeared to be secondary to the use of the needles themselves rather than the specific locations where they were placed.

Spa therapy also has advocates. It has been touted for low back pain and for lower extremity OA.[46] However, randomized, controlled studies are lacking.[47] Yoga has also shown some symptomatic benefit in OA of the hands, based on limited testing.[48]

PHARMACOLOGIC INTERVENTIONS

Topical Agents

Topical agents for the management of OA are available without a prescription in the United States (Table 91-2). The two most widely used types are preparations containing capsaicin and those containing topical NSAIDs.

Capsaicin is a pungent ingredient found in red peppers (such as hot chili peppers). The mechanism of action is thought to be through selective stimulation of unmyelinated type C afferent neurons, causing the release of substance P. This release reversibly depletes the stores of substance P, a neurotransmitter of peripheral pain sensations.[49] Capsaicin preparations are available in concentrations of 0.025% or 0.075% in either ointment or, more recently, "roll-on" form, and they can be applied up to four times daily. They have been tested in controlled, double-blind studies in OA of the hands and knees.[50,51] Patient response is quite variable, with

Table 91-2 Symptom-Relieving Pharmacologic Therapies for Osteoarthritis

Topical
Capsaicin
Topical nonsteroidal anti-inflammatory drug (NSAID) preparations

Systemic
Acetaminophen
Nonselective NSAIDs
Cyclooxygenase-2 (COX-2)–specific inhibitors
Tramadol
Narcotic analgesics

Intra-articular
Corticosteroids
Hyaluronic acid derivatives

some obtaining significant pain relief and others not being able to tolerate the burning or stinging sensation produced by its application. Usually, the counterirritant sensation decreases gradually with repeated use, but pain relief remains. Although very safe overall, capsaicin products can be quite irritating if they come in contact with mucosal surfaces, particularly the eyes. Patients should wear disposable gloves, if possible, when applying the agents. There may be some reddening of the skin where the compound is applied.

Topical NSAID preparations are popular worldwide for the treatments of OA.[52,53] Safety concerns about traditional oral NSAIDs were the driving force in the use of these topical agents,[54] although questions remain as to their absorption and the degree of relief obtained. Results of placebo-controlled trials in OA of the knee have been conflicting. Some demonstrated symptomatic relief with topical application of gels containing NSAIDs, such as diclofenac,[55,56] whereas others showed only trends favoring the NSAID or no difference at all. In one recent trial, diclofenac gel was compared with placebo in 238 patients with OA of the knee over 3 weeks. The primary outcome was average pain with movement on days 1 to 14. The group on diclofenac gel had statistically superior improvement in this variable compared with those on placebo. WOMAC scores for function, pain, and disability were also significantly superior to placebo at weeks 2 and 3.[57] Patients were also randomized to receive eltenac or placebo gel over 4 weeks. Eltenac is a nonselective NSAID that is structurally similar to diclofenac. The primary end point was global pain on a visual analog scale (VAS). At 4 weeks, there was a trend, but no statistical difference, favoring the eltenac gel. Two patients in the active treatment group and two in the placebo group had local itching, reddening, or both in the application area.

There are also menthol- and salicylate-based over-the-counter topical preparations, but there are no published trials supporting their use in OA.

Systemic Agents

Non-narcotic Analgesics. Acetaminophen (paracetamol) has often been touted as the initial systemic intervention for the management of OA. This is mainly due to its favorable side effect profile but also to a perception of its equivalent efficacy to NSAIDs. This perception derives from studies of OA in which patients were not stratified in terms of degree of symptoms. In one study, acetaminophen 4 g/day was equivalent to ibuprofen 1200 or 2400 mg/day, with the notable exception of pain at rest.[58] A meta-analysis of 10 randomized, controlled trials concluded that acetaminophen is effective in the relief of pain associated with OA. However, the effect was small, and there was no improvement in overall WOMAC score. This suggests that acetaminophen may be effective for the relief of pain and should not be expected to have a strong effect on stiffness or function.[59] More recently, it has been noted that NSAIDs may have superior efficacy in patients with more symptomatic or inflammatory presentations, because acetaminophen has no anti-inflammatory effects at approved doses.[60] A recent database review concluded that the available evidence suggests that NSAIDs have superior efficacy in symptomatic relief in those with hip or knee OA and also in those with moderate to severe levels of pain from OA.[61] Particular concerns in patients taking acetaminophen include the concomitant use of alcohol or over-the-counter products containing acetaminophen. Either of these situations can lead to the possibility of hepatic toxicity through toxic metabolites.

Nonsteroidal Anti-inflammatory Drugs. NSAIDs are the most commonly prescribed medications for the treatment of OA. Nonselective NSAIDs work through nonspecific inhibition of cyclooxygenase isoforms 1 and 2 (COX-1 and COX-2). COX-1 is constitutively expressed in renal and gastrointestinal (GI) tissues, among others. COX-2 is inducible in inflammatory responses. The major side effects of NSAIDs are GI toxicities (gastritis, peptic ulcer disease) and renal toxicities (interstitial nephritis, prostaglandin inhibition-related renal insufficiency). Because GI tissues have a higher expression of COX-1, a selective COX-2 inhibitor might spare patients the GI side effects. Unfortunately, COX-2 is expressed in renal tissue, and COX-2–specific drugs, such as traditional NSAIDs, have potential adverse renal effects. This is especially true in those with baseline renal insufficiency. Concerns about cardiovascular risks led to the voluntary withdrawal of rofecoxib from the market in the United States. There have also been concerns about celecoxib at a dose of 200 mg twice daily, owing to an increased relative risk for myocardial infarction in an adenomatous polyp trial[62]; this, however, has not been confirmed in six observational studies.[63] All NSAIDs and COX-2–specific agents have received "black box" warnings in their package inserts addressing cardiovascular risk. Alternative mechanisms of action of NSAIDs, such as interference with receptors in the cell membrane phospholipid bilayers, have been proposed.[64] Further discussion of NSAIDs can be found in Chapter 56.

Nonselective NSAIDs are widely used for the management of OA. They include ibuprofen, naproxen, diclofenac, and others. NSAIDs are usually analgesic at lower doses but have both analgesic and anti-inflammatory effects at their higher recommended doses. They are prescribed either in fixed doses or "as needed" and are quite effective as symptom modifiers; however, they have no structure- or disease-modifying effects. NSAIDs should be used in the smallest dose that provides satisfactory symptom relief, because GI toxicity has been linked to dosage. Adverse GI events have also been linked to patient age, previous history of peptic ulcers or bleeding, and the presence of comorbid conditions such as heart disease.

To reduce the potential for adverse GI events, misoprostol can be added to the therapeutic regimen. It is a prostaglandin E_2 analogue that has been shown to reduce the GI side effects of NSAIDs when used at 200 μg three times a day.[65] Diarrhea is a potential side effect. The use of a concomitant proton pump inhibitor may reduce upper GI endoscopic ulceration rates from NSAIDs, although no study has attempted to show a decrease in events such as symptomatic ulcers or bleeds.[66] Over-the-counter doses of H_2 blockers and antacids have not been shown to reduce either endoscopic or serious clinical GI events. COX-2–specific inhibitors are the latest drugs used in an attempt to reduce the GI adverse event profile of OA therapy.

COX-2–specific inhibitors are highly selective for COX-2 in vitro. Currently, only three such agents are available: celecoxib, rofecoxib, and valdecoxib. Others are in various stages of investigation. All the available agents can reportedly reduce the rate of endoscopic ulceration by more than 50% when compared with nonselective NSAIDs. Rofecoxib and celecoxib also significantly reduce the rates of symptomatic ulcers, bleeds, perforations, and obstructions in patients not concurrently on aspirin.[67,68] It remains unclear how substantial the benefits of these compounds are to patients taking aspirin. Because COX-2–specific agents can inhibit endothelial prostacyclin but do not affect platelet thromboxane, cardiovascular safety remains an area of investigation.[69,70]

Combination COX-lipoxygenase inhibitors are in development. It remains to be seen how these will compare with traditional NSAIDs and with COX-2 inhibitors in terms of both safety and efficacy.[71] Animal studies have hinted at the possibility of a structure- and disease-modifying effect.[72]

Narcotic Analgesics. Although several options exist for the management of pain in OA, some patients obtain suboptimal pain relief. If a patient has failed to respond to other nonpharmacologic and pharmacologic modalities and has no additional identifiable causes of pain (such as fibromyalgia), a narcotic analgesic should be considered.

The pain of OA is generally responsive to narcotic analgesics. Because of concerns about potential addiction, appropriate patient selection is important. Narcotic analgesics such as codeine and propoxyphene have been used effectively in patients with OA, especially in combination with non-narcotic analgesics (e.g., acetaminophen). Potential side effects include nausea, constipation, and somnolence.

Tramadol is an oral medication with mild suppressive effects on the μ opioid receptor. It also inhibits the uptake of norepinephrine and serotonin[73] and is not thought to have significant addictive tendencies.[74] It is available alone or in combination with acetaminophen and is not a controlled-schedule medication in the United States.[75] Tramadol has been used for the symptomatic relief of OA.[76] Seizures and allergic reactions are potential side effects.[77] The incidence of nausea can be reduced by slowly escalating the dose until the desired pain relief is achieved.

One study compared tramadol and acetaminophen to the combination of codeine and acetaminophen.[78] Patients with OA or chronic low back pain were randomized to receive tramadol and acetaminophen (37.5 mg and 325 mg, respectively) or codeine and acetaminophen (30 mg and 300 mg, respectively) for 4 weeks. Pain relief and changes in pain intensity were equivalent in both groups. Those on codeine and acetaminophen had a significantly higher incidence of somnolence (24% versus 17%) and constipation (21% versus 11%). The tramadol-acetaminophen combination also provides symptomatic relief as add-on therapy in OA patients receiving NSAIDs or COX-2 agents as baseline therapy.[79]

Extended-release narcotic analgesics have been tested in clinical trials in OA. This approach is intended to achieve a lower level of peak to trough variability in the plasma concentration of the narcotic. An extended-release, once-a-day preparation of tramadol relieves pain in OA of the knee and hip.[80] Extended-release oxymorphone dosed twice a day also provides relief in those with moderate to severe pain from OA of the hip or knee, as demonstrated by a VAS and the WOMAC composite index, as well as the subscales for pain, stiffness, and physical function.[81]

Transdermal fentanyl, a narcotic analgesic, has been used in the treatment of moderately to severely symptomatic knee and hip OA. It relieved pain and improved function in clinical trials as judged by a VAS and the WOMAC physical function subscale.[82]

Intra-articular Agents

Corticosteroids. Although there is no role for systemic corticosteroids in OA, local intra-articular corticoid preparations have a long history in the management of OA. Corticosteroids have been shown to downregulate the expression of adhesion molecules. This, in turn, can reduce cellular infiltration into the joint and subsequent inflammation. Corticosteroid injections slow macrophage-like cell infiltration of the synovium in OA.[83] The dose of steroid injected is determined by the volume of the joint being injected, with larger joints such as the knee receiving higher doses. The risk of joint infection is very low if proper technique is employed. Postinjection flares due to corticosteroid crystal synovitis can occur.

There is a relative dearth of information from clinical trials of intra-articular corticosteroid injections. However, in one trial, symptomatic benefit from corticosteroid injection for OA of the knee was demonstrated in a double-blind trial at 1 and 4 weeks post injection.[84] Another trial attempted to assess the possible disease-modifying effects of corticosteroids by randomizing 68 patients to corticosteroid or saline injections of the knee every 3 months for 2 years. At the study's end, there was no significant difference in rate of joint space narrowing; thus, no case could be made for a disease-modifying effect of corticosteroid injections. There was a trend favoring pain relief in the corticosteroid group as measured by the pain subscale of the WOMAC.[85] A review of published studies of intra-articular corticosteroid injections in OA concluded that the short-term symptomatic benefits have been well established, with few adverse events, but long-term benefits have not been confirmed.[86]

The specific corticosteroid compound used, the frequency of injections, and other factors related to the use of corticosteroid injections in OA vary widely and are heavily influenced by the training program the rheumatologist attended and where he or she practices.[87] In general, corticosteroid injections are believed to be most effective in patients with evidence of inflammation, effusions, or both. Because of concerns over possible deleterious effects, usually no more than four corticosteroid injections per year are given in a particular joint. Further discussion of arthrocentesis can be found in Chapter 47.

Hyaluronic Acid Derivatives. Synthetic and naturally occurring hyaluronic acid derivatives are administered intra-articularly. Two of these agents—Hyalgan and Synvisc—are approved for use in the United States for OA of the knee. Multiple injections are required, with the injections spaced 1 week apart. One medication (Synvisc) requires three injections per course of treatment; the other (Hyalgan) five injections. Although often mentioned as potential structure-modifying agents, these products are presently considered symptom-modifying drugs. Their molecular weights vary (from <100,000 to >1 million Svedberg units), depending on the preparation. They reportedly reduce pain for prolonged periods and may improve mobility.[88] Improvement in overall physical functioning has also been reported.[89] The mechanisms of action are not known. However, there is evidence of an anti-inflammatory effect (particularly at high molecular weight), a short-term lubricant effect, an analgesic effect by direct buffering of synovial nerve endings, and a stimulating effect on synovial lining cells, leading to the production of normal hyaluronic acid.[90]

In one study, three weekly hyaluronic acid intra-articular injections provided comparable pain relief to a single corticosteroid intra-articular injection at 1-week follow-up; at 45 days' follow-up, hyaluronic acid was superior to the corticosteroid.[91] In a Canadian study, 102 patients with OA of the knee were randomized to three weekly intra-articular injections of hylan G-F (Synvisc), hylan G-F plus an NSAID, or NSAID alone. At 26 weeks, both groups receiving hylan G-F were significantly better than the group receiving NSAIDs alone.[92]

Substantial clinical responses to the saline injections used as placebo in hyaluronic acid trials have sometimes made data interpretation challenging. In a double-blind, placebo-controlled trial, 495 patients with knee OA were randomized to receive five intra-articular injections of hyaluronic acid (Hyalgan) given 1 week apart, placebo, or naproxen (500 mg orally twice a day) and followed for 26 weeks.[93] Patients in the group receiving hyaluronic acid had significantly greater improvement in pain on the 50-foot walk compared with placebo, and more of them had a 20-mm or greater reduction in pain as judged by a VAS. At the conclusion of the trial, more hyaluronic acid–treated patients (47.6%) had slight pain or were pain free compared with placebo-treated (33.1%) or naproxen-treated (36.9%) patients. As expected, GI adverse events were significantly more common in the naproxen group than the hyaluronic acid and placebo groups.

Hyaluronic acid preparations have been tested in other randomized trials, with symptomatic relief of OA of the ankles, shoulders, and hips being reported.[94-96] One multicenter, randomized, double-blind study, reported as an abstract, revisited the issue of disease modification with hyaluronic acid. Patients received three courses of three intra-articular knee injections of either hyaluronan or saline over the course of 1 year. Joint space width was assessed using standing, weight-bearing radiographs; 273 patients completed the trial and had complete data collection. This study failed to demonstrate a disease-modifying effect for hyaluronan therapy, because the primary end point was not met. Both the active treatment group and the placebo group had similar joint space narrowing during the study period. In those with a joint space width of 4.6 mm or greater at entry, hyaluronan use led to slightly less joint space narrowing than saline (placebo 0.55 mm ± 1.04, hyaluronan 0.13 mm ± 1.05; $P = .02$).[97] These results have not been confirmed in other trials. Hyaluronic acid products continue to be actively investigated in shoulder joint OA, periarthritis,[98] and adhesive capsulitis.[99]

NUTRICEUTICALS

Two nutritional supplements—glucosamine and chondroitin sulfate—have received significant attention (Table 91-3). Health food stores and the lay press have been touting them as "cures for arthritis." The mechanism of action of glucosamine sulfate is uncertain. Some in vitro experiments have shown stimulation of the synthesis of cartilage glycosaminoglycans and proteoglycans.[100,101] Others have shown that glucosamine and N-acetylglucosamine inhibit interleukin (IL)-1β– and tumor necrosis factor-α (TNF-α)–induced nitric oxide production in normal human articular chondrocytes.[102] N-acetylglucosamine also suppresses the production of IL-1β and stimulates IL-6 and COX-2.

Glucosamine

Urinary excretion of glucosamine (and other glycosaminoglycans) has been investigated and found to be elevated in both OA and rheumatoid arthritis.[103] Supplementation with glucosamine sulfate, an intermediate in mucopolysaccharide synthesis, has been tried both orally and intramuscularly as therapy for OA. Glucosamine sulfate (400 mg injected intramuscularly twice weekly for 6 weeks) reduced the severity of disease as judged by the Lequesne index when compared with placebo.[104] A randomized, double-blind, parallel-group study in knee OA compared 500 mg oral glucosamine sulfate three times a day to 400 mg ibuprofen three times a day for 4 weeks. The response to ibuprofen was more rapid, but at 4 weeks, there was no statistically significant difference in the response rate (reduction of at least 2 points in the Lequesne index).[105] No group in the study received higher, anti-inflammatory doses of ibuprofen. An NIH-sponsored trial is currently under way in the United States to more thoroughly study the symptom-relieving and possible structure-modifying properties of glucosamine. Meanwhile, some already advocate the use of glucosamine as part of the first line of therapy for symptomatic OA.[106]

Glucosamine has also been compared with acetaminophen in an industry-sponsored trial. In the GUIDE trial, 318 patients with knee OA were randomized to glucosamine sulfate soluble powder 1500 mg once a day, acetaminophen 1000 mg three times a day, or placebo for 6 months. The main efficacy parameter was the 6-month change in the Lequesne index. At 6 months, the glucosamine group achieved significantly greater efficacy versus placebo. Those on acetaminophen failed to achieve a statistically significant benefit versus placebo by either the Lequesne index or WOMAC. There was no statistically significant difference between those on glucosamine and those on placebo based on WOMAC outcomes.[107] Another clinical trial

Table 91-3 Nutriceuticals for Osteoarthritis

Glucosamine
Chondroitin sulfate
Ginger extracts
Avocado and soy unsaponifiables
Cat's claw
Shark cartilage
S-adenosyl methionine

randomized 80 patients with knee OA to either glucosamine sulfate 1500 mg/day or placebo for 6 months. There was no difference between glucosamine and placebo in the primary variable of patients' global assessment of pain in the affected knee.[108] Another trial used a unique Internet-based recruiting system and followed 205 patients with knee OA randomized to glucosamine sulfate 1500 mg/day or placebo for 12 weeks.[109] The primary end point was the pain subscale of the WOMAC. At study conclusion, there was no difference in the groups with regard to pain, physical function, or overall WOMAC scores. Stratification by severity of OA, glucosamine product used, or use of NSAIDs did not alter the results. The Cochrane review of glucosamine therapy in OA analyzed a pool of 20 studies and 2570 patients. Pain and function improved by 28% and 21%, respectively, by the Lequesne index, compared with placebo. There was no improvement in the overall WOMAC pain and function scales. There has been speculation that these inconsistencies in study results may be due to a lack of standardization in glucosamine preparations.[110]

A recent discontinuation trial has added to the uncertainty about glucosamine's efficacy. It found that 137 patients who had been clinically classified as moderate responders to glucosamine sulfate were equally likely to experience an OA flare whether they continued or discontinued the glucosamine. No statistically significant differences between the groups were noted in pain and WOMAC function scores after 6 months.[111]

Combination products containing both glucosamine and chondroitin have become quite popular in the United States, despite a dearth of clinical trial data. One small, placebo-controlled trial randomized patients with knee OA to receive a regimen of glucosamine hydrochloride (1000 mg), chondroitin sulfate (800 mg), and manganese ascorbate (152 mg) twice a day or placebo.[112] Patients were evaluated at baseline and then every 2 months for 6 months using the Lequesne index of OA severity. At 4 and 6 months, those with mild to moderate radiographic OA of the knee showed significant improvement by the Lequesne index compared with those on placebo. In those with severe radiographic OA of the knee, no significant symptomatic benefit could be demonstrated. The study did not evaluate patients for structure or disease modification.

Results of the NIH-sponsored Glucosamine/Chondroitin Arthritis Intervention Trial (GAIT) were recently published.[113] In that study, 1583 patients with OA of the knee were randomized to placebo, glucosamine hydrochloride 1500 mg/day, chondroitin sulfate 1200 mg/day, celecoxib 200 mg/day, or glucosamine hydrochloride and chondroitin sulfate. The primary end point was the percentage of patients achieving at least 20% improvement on the

WOMAC pain subscale at 6 months. The only statistically significant response was seen in those on celecoxib versus placebo (70.1% versus 60.1%; $P = .008$). Patients were then stratified for baseline severity by WOMAC pain scores, most of them falling into the mild OA pain category. In a subgroup analysis, in those with moderate to severe OA pain (WOMAC pain 301 to 400 mm), the combination of glucosamine hydrochloride and chondroitin sulfate was more efficacious than placebo as measured by a dichotomous response rate (positive = 50% improvement in pain): 79.2% versus 54.3% ($P = .002$).

From these results, it appears that patient selection may be important in maximizing any potential benefit from glucosamine or chondroitin therapy. The NIH study also had a particularly high placebo response rate, which may reflect the enrollment of patients with less symptomatic OA, and that may have affected the results. The GAIT study also used a glucosamine hydrochloride preparation instead of the glucosamine sulfate used in most other studies, particularly those that have demonstrated efficacy. This raises the question of whether the choice of glucosamine hydrochloride negatively affected efficacy in the trial. However, one small (142 patients) Chinese trial randomized patients with OA of the knee to glucosamine sulfate 1500 mg/day or glucosamine hydrochloride 1440 mg/day for 1 month.[114] No efficacy differences were noted, with a clear majority of patients in each treatment arm achieving symptomatic improvement by Lequesne scores. The study had no placebo arm. Safety assessments continued for 2 additional weeks, with no significant adverse events reported. At present, it is still unclear whether glucosamine hydrochloride preparations have the same potential clinical benefits as glucosamine sulfate preparations. Additional investigations are needed.

Two European trials tried to address the subject of disease modification with glucosamine. In one study, 212 patients with OA of the knee were randomized to receive placebo or glucosamine sulfate (1500 mg/day) and were followed prospectively for 3 years.[115] Fluoroscopically positioned, standing anteroposterior radiographs of the knees were taken at enrollment, 1 year, and 3 years. At 3 years, the treatment group had a joint space reduction of 0.06 mm, whereas the placebo group had a reduction of 0.31 mm. Whether this is a clinically meaningful difference in joint space is unclear. Those taking glucosamine also showed symptomatic benefit on the order of 20% to 25%, whereas those taking placebo had a slight worsening of symptoms, as judged by the WOMAC. There were no significant adverse events attributed to the use of the glucosamine sulfate. A second group of researchers randomized 202 patients to receive placebo or glucosamine sulfate (1500 mg/day) for 3 years.[116] The width of the narrowest medial joint space of the tibiofemoral joint was measured serially, using visual assessments with a 0.1-mm graduated magnifying glass on standardized full-extension, weight-bearing anteroposterior radiographs of each knee. At 3 years, there was a significant difference in joint space width, with a decrease of 0.19 mm in the placebo group and an increase of 0.04 mm in the glucosamine sulfate group. Also, significantly greater improvements in the WOMAC score and the Lequesne index were seen in the glucosamine group. The favorable results of these studies have been questioned because of the radiographic technique used to assess joint space. At issue is whether the joint space seen on standing films of the knee might be significantly affected by the symptoms of OA (i.e., pain) and whether a semiflexed film would be preferable. In one study, investigators obtained baseline radiographs (after analgesic or NSAID washout) using both standing-extended and semiflexed, fluoroscopically positioned techniques in 19 patients with knee OA.[117] Radiographs were then repeated 2 to 8 weeks later after reinstitution of analgesic or NSAID therapy. Joint space width increased with effective pain relief in highly symptomatic patients if measured by standing-extended radiographs. Using the semiflexed technique, there were no significant changes in joint space width related to severity of pain or responsiveness to pain therapy. This suggests that data obtained using the standing-extended radiographic technique may need to be revisited, because the results may represent a therapeutic intervention's effect on symptoms (pain) rather than a disease-modifying effect. More recent, ongoing trials have changed to the semiflexed, fluoroscopically positioned knee radiograph to assess potential disease modification.[118]

Chondroitin Sulfate

Oral chondroitin sulfate, a glycosaminoglycan composed of units of glucosamine with attached sugar molecules (molecular mass of around 14,000), has also been used as therapy for hip and knee OA. Its mechanism of action is unknown. A double-blind, placebo-controlled study included a 3-month treatment phase followed by a 2-month treatment-free phase. The major outcome parameter was NSAID consumption. Those receiving chondroitin sulfate used fewer NSAIDs than the controls both at the completion of treatment and in the treatment-free phase.[119] Another study compared chondroitin sulfate to diclofenac sodium. One group received chondroitin sulfate (400 mg three times a day) and the other diclofenac sodium (50 mg three times a day). Each group was also changed over to placebo at some point. The chondroitin group received the active drug for 3 months, whereas the diclofenac group received it only for 1 month before being switched to placebo. For months 4 through 6, both groups took only placebo. The diclofenac group had a quicker response to therapy, whereas the chondroitin group had a more prolonged improvement as measured by the Lequesne index, VAS for pain, four-point scale for pain, and paracetamol use (rescue medication).[112,120] This study raises questions because of the different lengths of treatment with active drug in each group. Further studies are needed.

One study evaluated chondroitin sulfate as a disease-modifying intervention. Three hundred patients were enrolled and randomized to chondroitin sulfate 800 mg daily or placebo for 2 years.[121] Joint space width was assessed using anteroposterior semiflexed radiographs. Pain and function were assessed as secondary end points. In the placebo group, the mean change in joint space width was 0.07 mm/year, while in the treatment group, the mean change was 0.00. A similar difference was noted when the minimum joint space width was evaluated. The differences were statistically significant (mean joint space width, $P = .04$; minimum joint space width, $P = .05$), but the clinical relevance remains unclear. The changes in radiographic progression were not matched by similar differences when pain and function were analyzed. The treatment group achieved improvement in all

WOMAC subscales of pain, function, and stiffness, but a statistically significant difference could not be shown. It has been suggested that the overall low baseline WOMAC scores created difficulties in assessing for clinical improvement.

Ginger extracts have been popular "natural" remedies for OA for some time.[122] Most of the world's ginger comes from China, and its "medicinal" use dates back more than 2000 years. Ginger actually contains very small amounts of salicylate.[123] In some animal models, ginger has been shown to have inhibitory effects on COX and lipoxygenase.[124] One study with 247 evaluable patients revealed a small but statistically significant reduction in knee pain on standing (63% versus 50%; $P = .048$) after taking ginger.[125] Reduction in knee pain after a 50-foot walk was also significant. Use of acetaminophen was reduced in the ginger-extract group, but the difference was not statistically significant. The extract was well tolerated, except for GI events such as dyspepsia, nausea, and eructation, which were increased over placebo. The question remains whether benefits observed represent a clinically relevant effect.

Some of the more unusual agents proposed as structure or disease modifiers in OA are oral preparations of avocado and soy unsaponifiables (ASUs). These compounds are derived from unsaponifiable residues of avocado and soya oils mixed in a 1:2 ratio. In vitro studies on cultured chondrocytes showed partial reversal of IL-1β effects. The roles of IL-1β in OA are thought to include inhibition of prostaglandin synthesis by chondrocytes and stimulation of matrix metalloproteinases (MMPs) and nitric oxide production. MMPs and nitric oxide can degrade cartilage matrix and cause chondrocyte apoptosis. Use of ASUs also reportedly results in inhibited production of IL-6, IL-8, and MMPs and stimulation of collagen synthesis. Increased aggrecan synthesis has been reported as well.[126] The mechanism of action is unknown, as is the active ingredient in ASUs.[127] Symptomatic benefit in double-blind human trials in OA of the hip and knee has been reported.[128] However, a double-blind, placebo-controlled trial in OA of the hip failed to show disease modification in the overall population, although a post hoc analysis reported benefit in those with more advanced OA at baseline. Some abstract presentations have suggested structure or disease modification in human hip OA.[129]

Other Supplements

Other nutritional supplements, such as cat's claw and shark cartilage, have become entrenched in regional and international popular cultures. Many people take them, despite limited or no data to support their use. A small, placebo-controlled trial showed improvement of OA pain with activity in those taking cat's claw extracts.[130] Shark cartilage contains a small amount of chondroitin sulfate.[131] S-adenosyl methionine (SAMe), a methyl group donor and oxygen radical scavenger, is often touted as a remedy for OA, although little evidence of its effectiveness has been published.[132,133] In one double-blind, placebo-controlled study, two centers reported differing results. One center reported reductions in overall pain and rest pain, whereas the other showed no significant difference between the test group and placebo group.[134] Another small, double-blind, placebo-controlled crossover study of 61 patients compared oral SAMe 1200 mg/day to oral celecoxib 200 mg/day for 16 weeks. After the first month of phase I, celecoxib provided superior pain relief that was statistically significantly. By the end of the second month, however, there was no statistically significant difference between the groups.[135] There is insufficient evidence to recommend the use of these products in the treatment of OA.

OTHER POTENTIAL STRUCTURE- OR DISEASE-MODIFYING THERAPIES

The term *chondroprotective* has been used to describe structure- or disease-modifying agents. This is a misnomer, however, because the goal is to protect the entire joint (not only the cartilage) from the arthritic process. A workshop of the Osteoarthritis Research Society recommended that the term *structure-modifying drugs* be used for medications that previously would have been classified as chondroprotective.[136] These drugs are intended to prevent, retard, stabilize, or even reverse the development of OA. Recently, the term *disease-modifying osteoarthritis drug* has been used for any such agent (Table 91-4). Such a disease-modifying effect in OA would require prolonged observation, given the typically slow progression of OA. Therefore, clinical trials in this area have been challenging, with most being designed for at least 2½ to 3 years of follow-up. Progress in the methodology used to assess structure and disease modification may shorten the length of these trials. Radiographic assessments of joint space, such as fluoroscopically positioned anteroposterior radiographs of the knee or magnetic resonance imaging, may be useful in this regard.[137]

Unfortunately, to date, no drug has been conclusively proved to be structure or disease modifying. Although this chapter focuses on medication-based therapies, other approaches, such as osteochondral grafts of chondrocytes, donation of stem cells, or both, with eventual differentiation into bone and cartilage, are in various stages of development.[138] Potential structure- or disease-modifying interventions under investigation include collagenase inhibitors, polysaccharides, and growth factor and cytokine manipulation.

Tetracyclines, apart from any antimicrobial effect, are inhibitors of tissue metalloproteinases, perhaps owing to their ability to chelate calcium and zinc ions. There has also been research into the potential role of nitric oxide in the mechanism of action of the tetracyclines.[139] Minocycline, a tetracycline-family antibiotic, has been used in the management of rheumatoid arthritis.[140] Doxycycline, another tetracycline derivative, has been shown to inhibit articular cartilage

Table 91-4 Potential Structure- and Disease-Modifying Drugs in Osteoarthritis

Tetracyclines
Metalloproteinase or collagenase inhibitors
Glucosamine
Diacerein
Growth factor and cytokine manipulation (interleukin-1 receptor antagonist [IL-1Ra], transforming growth factor-β)
Gene therapy (IL-1Ra, IL-1RII)
Chondrocyte and stem cell transplantation

collagenase activity.[141,142] Doxycycline has also reduced the severity of OA in canine models. In one study, there was preservation of medial femoral condyle cartilage in treated dogs compared with the untreated group. Other lesions, such as medial trochlear ridge cartilage damage, superficial fibrillation of the medial tibial plateau, and osteophytosis, were unaffected by treatment. Collagenolytic activity and gelatinolytic activity, however, were reduced to 20% and 25% of their previous levels, respectively, compared with untreated dogs. In an in vitro model, doxycycline not only reduced collagenase and gelatinase activity in cartilage but also prevented proteoglycan loss, cell death, and deposition of type X collagen matrix.[143]

A multicenter, double-blind, placebo-controlled trial using doxycycline for structure or disease modification in obese female subjects with OA of the knee has been completed. In this study, 431 obese women with unilateral OA of the knee were treated with doxycycline 100 mg twice daily or placebo. The primary end point was radiographic progression. The minimum joint space width was assessed by fluoroscopically positioned anteroposterior, semiflexed, standing radiographs. Pain and function were evaluated as secondary end points. Progression of minimum joint space width at 30 months was 0.3 ± 0.60 mm in the treatment group and 0.45 ± 0.70 mm in the placebo group ($P = .017$). Imaging of the contralateral knee was also performed at baseline and at 30 months. Progression in the contralateral knees was no different between the groups.[144] Secondary outcomes of pain and function were also recorded by WOMAC, VAS, 50-foot walk pain, and global assessment. Mean overall scores for pain were not significantly different between the groups. However, the frequency with which patients reported 20% or greater increase in knee pain was less in the treatment group ($P < .05$). Although a small disease-modifying effect was demonstrated in the target knee, no such effect could be demonstrated in the contralateral knee. Thus, the implications of these findings for clinical practice are uncertain. Other compounds with collagenase-inhibiting properties are being developed and investigated as structure- or disease-modifying agents not only in OA but also in rheumatoid arthritis.[145]

Glycosaminoglycan polysulfuric acid (GAGPS; Arteparon or Adequan) has been purported to work by reducing the activity of collagenase. It is a highly sulfated glycosaminoglycan, with a molecular weight ranging from 2000 to 16,000,[146] derived from bovine tracheal cartilage. In a canine model of OA, GAGPS was administered intra-articularly twice weekly for 4 weeks.[147] Four weeks after completion of the GAGPS treatment, medial femoral condylar lesions had developed to a lesser degree in the treated group than in saline-treated dogs. Swelling, an indicator of collagen network integrity, remained near control levels in the treatment group. In humans, OA of the knee was studied in a 5-year trial. There was improvement in multiple measured parameters, including less time lost from work.[148] Another double-blind, placebo-controlled trial evaluated GAGPS in 80 patients with OA of the knee; patients received two series of five intra-articular injections of 25 mg (0.5 mL) GAGPS at 1-week intervals. At 14 weeks, 31% of the GAGPS group had improvement as judged by the Lequesne index, compared with 15% in the placebo group.[149] Potential allergy and heparin-like effects

were observed. GAGPS is available in the United States for equine, but not human, use.

Another extract, a glycosaminoglycan-peptide complex (GP-C) known as Rumalon, has been investigated. It is a highly sulfated polysaccharide derived from bovine tracheal cartilage and bone marrow and is administered intramuscularly.[150] It has been shown to increase the levels of tissue inhibitor of metalloproteinases (TIMP).[151] A randomized, placebo-controlled trial selected patients with hip or knee OA to receive 10 courses of injections of placebo or GP-C (2 mL) over 5 years (two courses per year). Each course consisted of 15 injections given twice weekly. GP-C failed to demonstrate a structure- or disease-modifying effect.[152] In addition, there were no statistical differences favoring the active treatment group when measured by the Lequesne index, pain on passive motion, or consumption of NSAIDs. GP-C is available in parts of Europe and South America.

Pentosan polysulfate (Cartrofen) is a purified extract of beech hemicellulose administered intramuscularly or orally as a calcium salt. It can inhibit granulocyte elastase and has inhibited the catabolism of aggrecan in cartilage explants.[153] Experimental studies in animal models suggest that it helps preserve cartilage proteoglycan content and retards cartilage degradation.[154,155] However, a recent blinded, placebo-controlled study using an oral preparation in a dog model failed to demonstrate either a symptomatic benefit or a structure- or disease-modifying effect.[156]

Diacerein and its active metabolite rhein are anthraquinones related to senna compounds.[157] They inhibit the synthesis of IL-1β in human OA synovium in vitro, as well as the expression of IL-1 receptors on chondrocytes.[158] No effects have been reported on TNF or its receptors. Collagenase production and articular damage have been reduced in animal models.[159-161] Early human clinical trials have shown improved pain scores compared with placebo and comparable efficacy to NSAIDs but a slower onset of action. Diarrhea is the main potential side effect. On the strength of these prior trials, diacerein has been proposed as a slow-acting symptom-modifying and perhaps structure- or disease-modifying drug for OA.

A double-blind, randomized, placebo-controlled trial looking at the efficacy and safety of diacerein enrolled 484 patients with symptomatic knee OA.[162] They were randomized to receive placebo, diacerein 25 mg twice a day, diacerein 50 mg twice a day, or diacerein 75 mg twice a day. Using intent-to-treat analysis, diacerein 100 mg/day was significantly superior to placebo ($P < .05$) by the primary end point—patients' assessment of pain on movement at week 24 (-18.3 ± 19.3 mm versus -10.9 ± 19.3 mm). It was also superior based on WOMAC and disability scores. However, no statistical difference was detected in the primary end point between placebo and 50 mg/day diacerein (-15 ± 21.0 mm) or 150 mg/day diacerein (-14.3 ± 23.7 mm).

There have also been investigations into the potential structure- or disease-modifying attributes of diacerein in OA.[163] In one study, 507 patients with OA of the hip (according to American College of Rheumatology criteria) were randomized to receive either diacerein (50 mg orally twice a day) or placebo for 3 years. Patients were followed with yearly pelvic radiographs to assess hip joint space. Using completer analysis, the diacerein patients showed a significantly lower rate of radiographic progression (0.18 versus 0.23 mm/yr). Using intent-to-treat analysis, a smaller proportion of those taking diacerein had significant joint space loss (defined as loss of ≥0.5 mm) during the study (50.7% versus 60.4%). Unfortunately, almost 50% of the patients failed to complete the 3-year study. In the placebo group, the principal reason for discontinuation was lack of efficacy, whereas in the diacerein group, it was adverse effects such as diarrhea. Curiously, the symptom-relieving effect of diacerein observed in prior studies could not be confirmed in this one. A recent meta-analysis of clinical trials of diacerein in OA concluded that available clinical evidence supports pain relief in hip and knee OA. There was no analysis of a disease-modifying effect.[164]

Potential methods of intervention in OA include growth factor and cytokine manipulation.[165] Cytokines, such as IL-1 and TNF-α, are produced by the synovium and contribute to inflammation within osteoarthritic joints.[166] Moreover, there may be deficient expression of naturally occurring anti-inflammatory compounds such as IL-1 receptor antagonist (IL-1Ra) by the chondrocytes of patients with OA.[167] In some cases, increased nitric oxide production by OA articular chondrocytes may inhibit IL-1Ra synthesis.[168] In a dog model of OA, IL-1Ra therapy reduced the expression of collagenase-1 in cartilage.[169] The severity of cartilage lesions is also diminished.[170] In a rabbit model of OA, transfer of the IL-1Ra gene to joints prevented OA progression.[171] The effect of IL-1 blockade in humans with OA through the use of IL-1Ra is currently being investigated. Induction of repair in partial-thickness articular cartilage lesions by the timed release of transforming growth factor-β using liposomes has been attempted in an animal model. There was an increase in the cellularity of the defects, which were populated by cells of mesenchymal origin from the synovial membrane. The repaired cartilage resembled hyaline cartilage, and its integrity persisted up to 1 year after surgery.[172] Combination therapy is another alternative. In a study of canine induced OA, sodium pentosan polysulfate, when combined with insulin-like growth factor 1, reduced stromelysin activity and increased TIMP.[173]

Gene therapy has been attempted as well. The control of genes such as TIMP and MMPs would, in theory, provide the opportunity to modulate the patient's disease. As previously noted, gene expression of IL-1Ra has already been tried in rabbits and dogs, as well as in an equine model of OA using an adenovirus vector.[174] Use of gene transfer–mediated overexpression of IL-1β decoy receptor has also been contemplated.[175] Chondrocyte and stem cell transplants into articular cartilage defects have been tried as well. Chondrocytes transplanted (expressing a previously transfected β-galactosidase gene) into human cartilage explants survived up to 45 days in vitro in one trial.[176,177] Transfection of chondrocytes with the galactosidase gene has been successful both before and after transplantation.

SURGICAL INTERVENTION

Surgical interventions in OA usually consist of osteotomies or joint replacements. Osteotomies can be effective pain-relieving interventions and can delay the need for joint replacement surgery in selected patients. These tend to be younger subjects with OA.

Joint replacement surgery (joint arthroplasty) is effective in providing pain relief and restoring function in many patients with OA. Hip and knee joint replacements are most common. Indications for surgery include pain that is refractory to the previously discussed interventions and significant impairment of the patient's daily life. Therefore, patients should be the key decision makers, because they are the ones who must weigh the severity of symptoms and impairment. Patients undergoing replacement surgery should be deemed able to undertake the rehabilitation necessary to regain reasonable use of the joint involved. Infections are rare but do occur. Joint replacements have a typical life span of between 10 and 15 years. Revision surgery may be necessary, particularly in a relatively young patient who outlives the useful life of the prosthesis.

Other potential rationales for surgical intervention in OA include removal of loose bodies, stabilization of joints, redistribution of joint forces (e.g., osteotomy), and relief of neural impingement (e.g., spinal stenosis, herniated disk). The value of arthroscopic debridement or lavage in OA has been questioned. A recent randomized, blinded trial failed to demonstrate significant symptomatic benefit in OA of the knee.

SUMMARY

The treatment of OA includes a variety of possible non-pharmacologic and pharmacologic interventions. Treatment should be tailored to the individual and consists of a combination of modalities. These provide symptom relief but have no proven effect on the progression of disease. Structure and disease modification has yet to be achieved in OA. Trials that are under way could determine whether this is a realistic goal. Claims of structure or disease modification in OA should not be made for any drugs until well-designed, double-blind, placebo-controlled trials demonstrate that this is so. Some of the drugs being tested for structure and disease modification can provide symptom relief and can be added to our armamentarium in that capacity, even if it turns out they are not successful as structure- or disease-modifying agents. It is hoped that with the advent of disease-modifying OA drugs, treatment will eventually consist of a combination of symptom-relieving and disease-modifying interventions.

REFERENCES

1. Lawrence JS, Bremmer JM, Bier F: Osteo-arthrosis: Prevalence in the population and relationship between symptoms and x-ray changes. Ann Rheum Dis 25:1-24, 1966.
2. Peyron JG, Altman RD: The epidemiology of osteoarthritis. In Moskowitz RW, Howell DS, Goldberg M, Mankin HI (eds): Osteoarthritis: Diagnosis and Medical/Surgical Management, 2nd ed. Philadelphia, WB Saunders, 1992, pp 15-37.
3. Lozada CJ, Altman RD: Osteoarthritis: A comprehensive approach to management. J Musculoskeletal Med 14:26-38, 1997.
4. Hochberg MC, Altman RD, Brandt RD, et al: Guidelines for the medical management of osteoarthritis. I. Osteoarthritis of the hip. Arthritis Rheum 38:1535-1540, 1995.
5. Hochberg MC, Altman RD, Brandt KD, et al: Guidelines for the medical management of osteoarthritis. II. Osteoarthritis of the knee. Arthritis Rheum 38:1541-1546, 1995.
6. **American College of Rheumatology Subcommittee on Osteoarthritis Guidelines: Recommendations for the medical management of osteoarthritis of the hip and knee: 2000 update. Arthritis Rheum 43:1905-1915, 2000.**

7. Lozada CJ, Altman RD: Management of osteoarthritis. In Koopman WJ (ed): Arthritis and Allied Conditions, 13th ed. Baltimore, Williams & Wilkins, 1997, pp 2013-2025.

8. Coggon D, Reading I, Croft P, et al: Knee osteoarthritis and obesity. Int J Obes Relat Metab Disord 25:622-627, 2001.

9. Sturmer T, Gunther KP, Brenner H: Obesity, overweight and patterns of osteoarthritis: The Ulm Osteoarthritis Study. J Clin Epidemiol 53:307-313, 2000.

10. **Cooper C, Snow S, McAlindon TE, et al: Risk factors for the incidence and progression of radiographic knee osteoarthritis. Arthritis Rheum 43:995-1000, 2000.**

11. Sharma L, Lou C, Cahue S, Dunlop DD: The mechanism of the effect of obesity in knee osteoarthritis: The mediating role of malalignment. Arthritis Rheum 43:568-575, 2000.

12. Messier SP, Loeser RF, Mitchell MN, et al: Exercise and weight loss in obese older adults with knee osteoarthritis: A preliminary study. J Am Geriatr Soc 48:1062-1072, 2000.

13. **Felson DT, Zhang Y, Anthony JM, et al: Weight loss reduces the risk for symptomatic knee osteoarthritis in women. Ann Intern Med 116:535-539, 1992.**

14. Toda Y, Toda T, Takemura S, et al: Change in body fat, but not body weight or metabolic correlates of obesity, is related to symptomatic relief of obese patients with knee osteoarthritis after a weight control program. J Rheumatol 25:2181-2186, 1998.

15. Christensen R, Astrup A, Bliddal H, et al: Sustained weight loss as a treatment of osteoarthritis in obese patients: Long-term results from a randomized trial. Ann Rheum Dis 64(Suppl III):66, 2005.

16. Messier SP, Loeser RF, Miller GD, et al: Exercise and dietary weight loss in overweight and obese older adults with knee osteoarthritis: The arthritis, diet and activity promotion trial. Arthritis Rheum 50:1501-1510, 2005.

17. Swezey RL: Essentials of physical management and rehabilitation in arthritis. Semin Arthritis Rheum 3:349-368, 1974.

18. Lehman JF, DeLateur BJ: Diathermy and superficial heat, laser, and cold therapy. In Kottke FJ, Lehman JF (eds): Krusen's Handbook of Physical Medicine and Rehabilitation, 4th ed. Philadelphia, WB Saunders, 1990, pp 283-367.

19. Slemenda C, Heilman DK, Brandt KD, et al: Reduced quadriceps strength relative to body weight: A risk factor for knee osteoarthritis in women? Arthritis Rheum 41:1951-1959, 1998.

20. Bentley G, Dowd G: Current concepts of etiology and treatment of chondromalacia patellae. Clin Orthop 189:209-228, 1984.

21. Topp R, Woolley S, Hornyak J III, et al: The effect of dynamic versus isometric resistance training on pain and functioning among adults with osteoarthritis of the knee. Arch Phys Med Rehabil 83:1187-1195, 2002.

22. Kovar PA, Allegrante JP, MacKenzie R, et al: Supervised fitness walking in patients with osteoarthritis of the knee. Ann Intern Med 116:529-534, 1992.

23. Thomas KS, Muir KR, Doherty M, et al: Home based exercise programme for knee pain and knee osteoarthritis: Randomised controlled trial. BMJ 325:752, 2002.

24. Belza B, Topolski T, Kinne S, et al: Does adherence make a difference? Results from a community-based aquatic exercise program. Nurs Res 51:285-291, 2002.

25. Kerrigan DC, Lelas JL, Goggins J, et al: Effectiveness of a lateral-wedge insole on knee varus torque in patients with knee osteoarthritis. Arch Phys Med Rehabil 83:889-893, 2002.

26. Keating EM, Faris PM, Ritter MA, Kane J: Use of lateral heel and sole wedges in the treatment of medial osteoarthritis of the knee. Orthop Rev 22:921-924, 1993.

27. Pollo FE, Otis JC, Backus SI, et al: Reduction of medial compartment loads with valgus bracing of the osteoarthritic knee. Am J Sports Med 30:414-421, 2002.

28. Cushnaghan J, McCarthy C, Dieppe P: Taping the patella medially: A new treatment for osteoarthritis of the knee joint? BMJ 308:753-755, 1994.

29. Ohsawa S, Ueno R: Heel lifting as a conservative therapy for osteoarthritis of the hip: Based on the rationale of Pauwels' intertrochanteric osteotomy. Prosthet Orthot Int 21:153-158, 1997.

30. Berggren M, Joost-Davidsson A, Lindstrand J, et al: Reduction in the need for operation after conservative treatment of osteoarthritis of the first carpometacarpal joint: A seven year prospective study. Scand J Plast Reconstr Surg Hand Surg 35:415-417, 2001.

31. Brand RA, Crowninshield RD: The effect of cane use on hip contact force. Clin Orthop 147:181-184, 1980.

32. Chan GN, Smith AW, Kirtley C, Tsang WW: Changes in knee moments with contrateral versus ipsilateral cane usage in females with knee osteoarthritis. Clin Biomech 20:396-404, 2005.

33. **Blount WP: Don't throw away the cane. J Bone Joint Surg Am 38:695-708, 1956.**

34. Osiri M, Welch V, Brosseau L, et al: Transcutaneous electrical nerve stimulation for knee osteoarthritis. Cochrane Database Syst Rev 4: CD002823, 2000.

35. Taylor P, Hallett M, Flaherty L: Treatment of osteoarthritis of the knee with transcutaneous electrical nerve stimulation. Pain 11:233-240, 1981.

36. Paker N, Tekdos D, Kesiktas N, Soy D: Comparison of the therapeutic efficacy of TENS versus intra-articular hyaluronic acid injection in patients with knee osteoarthritis: A prospective, randomized study. Adv Ther 23:342-353, 2006.

37. Pipitone N, Scott DL: Magnetic pulse treatment for knee osteoarthritis: A randomised, double-blind, placebo-controlled study. Curr Med Res Opin 17:190-196, 2001.

38. Thamsborg G, Florescu A, Oturai P, et al: Treatment of knee osteoarthritis with pulsed electromagnetic fields: A randomized, double-blind, placebo-controlled study. Osteoarthritis Cartilage 13: 575-581, 2005.

39. Hinman MR, Ford J, Heyl H: Effects of static magnets on chronic knee pain and physical function: A double-blind study. Altern Ther Health Med 8:50-55, 2002.

40. Wolsko PM, Eisenberg DM, Simon LS, et al: Double-blind, placebo-controlled trial of static magnets for the treatment of osteoarthritis of the knee: Results of a pilot study. Altern Ther Health Med 10:36-43, 2004.

41. White AR, Filshie J, Cummings TM: International Acupuncture Research Forum: Clinical trials of acupuncture: Consensus recommendations for optimal treatment, sham controls and blinding. Complement Ther Med 9:237-245, 2001.

42. Tillu A, Tillu S, Vowler S: Effect of acupuncture on knee function in advanced osteoarthritis of the knee: A prospective, non-randomised controlled study. Acupunct Med 20:19-21, 2002.

43. Berman BM, Singh BB, Lao L, et al: A randomized trial of acupuncture as an adjunctive therapy in osteoarthritis of the knee. Rheumatology (Oxford) 38:346-354, 1999.

44. Ezzo J, Hadhazy V, Birch S, et al: Acupuncture for osteoarthritis of the knee: A systematic review. Arthritis Rheum 44:819-825, 2001.

45. Berman BM, Lao L, Langenberg P, et al: Effectiveness of acupuncture as adjunctive therapy in osteoarthritis of the knee: A randomized, controlled trial. Ann Intern Med 141:901-910, 2004.

46. Guillemin F, Virion JM, Escudier P, et al: Effect on osteoarthritis of spa therapy at Bourbonne-les-Bains. Joint Bone Spine 68:499-503, 2001.

47. Ernst E, Pittler MH: [How effective is spa treatment? A systematic review of randomized studies]. Dtsch Med Wochenschr 123:273-277, 1998.

48. Garfinkel M, Schumacher HR Jr: Yoga. Rheum Dis Clin North Am 26:125-132, 2000.

49. Rains C, Bryson HM: Topical capsaicin: A review of its pharmacological properties and therapeutic potential in post-herpetic neuralgia, diabetic neuropathy and osteoarthritis. Drugs Aging 7:317-328, 1995.

50. McCarthy GM, McCarty DJ: Effect of topical capsaicin in the therapy of painful osteoarthritis of the hands. J Rheumatol 19: 604-607, 1992.

51. Deal CL, Schnitzer TJ, Lipstein E, et al: Treatment of arthritis with topical capsaicin: A double-blind trial. Clin Ther 13:383-395, 1991.

52. Dreiser RL, Tisne-Camus M: DHEP plasters as a topical treatment of knee osteoarthritis: A double-blind placebo-controlled study. Drugs Exp Clin Res 19:117-123, 1993.

53. Rolf C, Engstrom B, Beauchard C, et al: Intra-articular absorption and distribution of ketoprofen after topical plaster application and oral intake in 100 patients undergoing knee arthroscopy. Rheumatology 38:564-567, 1999.

54. Goodman LS, Gilman A: The Pharmacological Basis of Therapeutics. New York, Pergamon Press, 1990.

55. Grace D, Rogers J, Skeith K, Anderson K: Topical diclofenac versus placebo: A double blind, randomized clinical trial in patients with osteoarthritis of the knee. J Rheumatol 26:2659-2663, 1999.

56. Niethard FU, Gold MS, Solomon GS, et al: Efficacy of topical diclofenac diethylamine gel in osteoarthritis of the knee. J Rheumatol 32:2384-2392, 2005.

57. Sandelin J, Harilainen A, Crone H, et al: Local NSAID gel (eltenac) in the treatment of osteoarthritis of the knee: A double blind study comparing eltenac with oral diclofenac and placebo gel. Scand J Rheumatol 26:287-292, 1997.
58. **Bradley JD, Brandt KD, Katz BP, et al: Comparison of an antiinflammatory dose of ibuprofen, an analgesic dose of ibuprofen, and acetaminophen in the treatment of patients with osteoarthritis of the knee. N Engl J Med 325:87-91, 1991.**
59. Zhang W, Jones A, Doherty M: Does paracetamol (acetaminophen) reduce the pain of osteoarthritis? A meta-analysis of randomized controlled trials. Ann Rheum Dis 63:901-907, 2005.
60. Pincus T, Koch GG, Sokka T, et al: A randomized, double-blind crossover clinical trial of diclofenac plus misoprostol versus acetaminophen in patients with osteoarthritis of the hip or knee. Arthritis Rheum 44:1587-1598, 2001.
61. Towheed TE, Maxwell L, Judd MG, et al: Acetaminophen for osteoarthritis. Cochrane Database Syst Rev CD004257, 2006.
62. Solomon SD, McMurrray JV, Pfeffer MA, et al: Cardiovascular risk associated with celecoxib in a clinical trial for colorectal adenoma prevention. N Engl J Med 352:1071-1080, 2005.
63. Solomon DH: Selective cyclooxygenase 2 inhibitors and cardiovascular events. Arthritis Rheum 52:1968-1978, 2005.
64. Abramson SB, Weissmann G: The mechanism of action of nonsteroidal antiinflammatory drugs. Arthritis Rheum 32:1, 1989.
65. Graham DY, Agrawal NM, Roth SH: Prevention of NSAID-induced gastric ulcer with misoprostol: Multicenter, double-blind, placebo-controlled trial. Lancet 2:1277-1280, 1988.
66. **Hawkey CJ, Karrasch JA, Szczepanski L, et al: Omeprazole compared with misoprostol for ulcers associated with nonsteroidal antiinflammatory drugs: Omeprazole versus Misoprostol for NSAID-Induced Ulcer Management (OMINUM) Study Group. N Engl J Med 338:727-734, 1998.**
67. Bombardier C, Laine L, Reicin A, et al: Comparison of upper gastrointestinal toxicity of rofecoxib and naproxen in patients with rheumatoid arthritis: VIGOR Study Group. N Engl J Med 343:1520-1528, 2000.
68. Silverstein FE, Faich G, Goldstein JL, et al: Gastrointestinal toxicity with celecoxib vs nonsteroidal anti-inflammatory drugs for osteoarthritis and rheumatoid arthritis: The CLASS study-randomized controlled trial: Celecoxib Long-term Arthritis Safety Study. JAMA 284:1247-1255, 2000.
69. Cheng Y, Austin SC, Rocca B, et al: Role of prostacyclin in the cardiovascular response to thromboxane A2. Science 296:539-541, 2002.
70. Mukherjee D, Nissen SE, Topol EJ: Risk of cardiovascular events associated with selective COX-2 inhibitors. JAMA 286:954-959, 2001.
71. Jovanovic DV, Fernandes JC, Martel-Pelletier J, et al: In vivo dual inhibition of cyclooxygenase and lipoxygenase by ML-3000 reduces the progression of experimental osteoarthritis: Suppression of collagenase 1 and interleukin-1beta synthesis. Arthritis Rheum 44:2320-2330, 2001.
72. Boileau C, Martel-Pelletier J, Jouzeau JY, et al: Licofelone (ML-3000), a dual inhibitor of 5-lipoxygenase and cyclooxygenase, reduces the level of cartilage chondrocyte death in vivo in experimental dog osteoarthritis: Inhibition of pro-apoptotic factors. J Rheumatol 29:1446-1453, 2002.
73. Raffa RB, Friederichs E, Reimann W, et al: Opioid and non-opioid components independently contribute to the mechanism of action of tramadol, an "atypical" opioid analgesic. J Pharmacol Exp Ther 260:275-285, 1992.
74. Katz WA: Pharmacology and clinical experience with tramadol in osteoarthritis. Drugs 52(Suppl 3):39-47, 1996.
75. Silverfield JC, Kamin M, Wu SC, et al: Tramadol/acetaminophen combination tablets for the treatment of osteoarthritis flare pain: A multicenter, outpatient, randomized, double-blind, placebo-controlled, parallel-group, add-on study. Clin Ther 24:282-297, 2002.
76. Roth SH: Efficacy and safety of tramadol HCl in breakthrough musculoskeletal pain attributed to osteoarthritis. J Rheumatol 25:1358-1363, 1998.
77. Goeringer KE, Logan BK, Christian GD: Identification of tramadol and its metabolites in blood from drug-related deaths and drug-impaired drivers. J Anal Toxicol 21:529-537, 1997.
78. Mullican WS, Lacy JR: TRAMAP-ANAG-006 Study Group: Tramadol/acetaminophen combination tablets and codeine/acetaminophen combination capsules for the management of chronic pain: A comparative trial. Clin Ther 23:1429-1445, 2001.
79. **Emkey R, Rosenthal N, Wu SC, et al: Efficacy and safety of tramadol/acetaminophen tablets (Ultracet) as add-on therapy for osteoarthritis pain in subjects receiving a COX-2 nonsteroidal antiinflammatory drug: A multicenter, randomized, double-blind, placebo-controlled trial. J Rheumatol 31:150-156, 2004.**
80. Gana TJ, Pascual ML, Fleming RR, et al: Extended release tramadol in the treatment of osteoarthritis: A multicenter, randomized, double-blind, placebo-controlled clinical trial. Curr Med Res Opin 22:1391-13401, 2006.
81. Kivitz A, Ma C, Ahdieh H, Galer BS: A 2-week, multicenter, randomized, double-blind, placebo-controlled, dose-ranging, phase III trial comparing the efficacy of oxymorphone extended release and placebo in adults with pain associated with osteoarthritis of the hip or knee. Clin Ther 28:352-364, 2006.
82. Langford R, McKenna F, Ratcliffe S, et al: Transdermal fentanyl for improvement of pain and functioning in osteoarthritis: A randomized, placebo-controlled trial. Arthritis Rheum 54:1829-1837, 2006.
83. Young L, Katrib A, Cuello C, et al: Effects of intraarticular glucocorticoids on macrophage infiltration and mediators of joint damage in osteoarthritis synovial membranes: Findings in a double-blind, placebo-controlled study. Arthritis Rheum 44:343-350, 2001.
84. Ravaud P, Moulinier L, Giraudeau B, et al: Effects of joint lavage and steroid injection in patients with osteoarthritis of the knee: Results of a multicenter, randomized, controlled trial: Arthritis Rheum 42:475-482, 1999.
85. **Raynauld JP, Buckland-Wright C, Ward R, et al: Safety and efficacy of long term intraarticular steroid injections in osteoarthritis of the knee: A randomized, double-blind, placebo-controlled trial. Arthritis Rheum 48:370-377, 2003.**
86. Bellamy N, Campbell J, Robinson V, et al: Intraarticular corticosteroid for treatment of osteoarthritis of the knee. Cochrane Database Syst Rev CD005328, 2006.
87. Centeno LM, Moore ME: Preferred intraarticular corticosteroids and associated practice: A survey of members of the American College of Rheumatology. Arthritis Care Res 7:151-155, 1994.
88. Peyron JG: Intraarticular hyaluronan injections in the treatment of osteoarthritis: State-of-the art review. J Rheumatol 20(Suppl 39):10-15, 1993.
89. Petrella RJ, DiSilvestro MD, Hildebrand C: Effects of hyaluronate sodium on pain and physical functioning in osteoarthritis of the knee: A randomized, double-blind, placebo-controlled clinical trial: Arch Intern Med 162:292-298, 2002.
90. Kuiper-Geertsma DG, Bijlsma JW: Intra-articular injection of hyaluronic acid as an alternative option to corticosteroid injections for arthrosis. Ned Tijdschr Geneeskd 144:2188-2192, 2000.
91. Leardini G, Mattara L, Franceschini M, Perbellini A: Intra-articular treatment of knee osteoarthritis: A comparative study between hyaluronic acid and 6-methyl prednisolone acetate. Clin Exp Rheumatol 9:375-381, 1991.
92. Adams ME, Atkinson MH, Lussier AJ, et al: The role of viscosupplementation with hylan G-F 20 (Synvisc) in the treatment of osteoarthritis of the knee: A Canadian multicenter trial comparing hylan G-F 20 alone, hylan G-F 20 with non-steroidal anti-inflammatory drugs (NSAIDs) and NSAIDs alone. Osteoarthritis Cartilage 3:213-225, 1995.
93. **Altman RD, Moskowitz R: Intraarticular sodium hyaluronate (Hyalgan) in the treatment of patients with osteoarthritis of the knee: A randomized clinical trial. Hyalgan Study Group. J Rheumatol 25:2203-2212, 1998.**
94. Salk RS, Chang TJ, D'Costa WF, et al: Sodium hyaluronate in the treatment of osteoarthritis of the ankle: A controlled, randomized, double-blind pilot study. J Bone Joint Surg Am 88:295-302, 2006.
95. Altman RD, Moskowitz R, Joacobs S, et al: A double-blind randomized trial of intra-articular injection of sodium hyaluronate for the treatment of chronic shoulder pain [abstract 1206]. Arthritis Rheum 52(Suppl), 2005.
96. Qvistgaard E, Christensen R, Torp-Pedersen S, Bliddal H: Intra-articular treatment of hip osteoarthritis: A randomized trial of hyaluronic acid, corticosteroid, and isotonic saline. Osteoarthritis Cartilage 14:163-170, 2006.

97. Jubb RW, Beinat L, Dacre J, et al: A one-year randomized, placebo (saline) controlled clinical trial of 500-730 kDa sodium hyaluronate (Hyalgan) on the radiological change in osteoarthritis of the knee. Int J Clin Pract 57:467-474, 2003.

98. Itokazu M, Matsunaga T: Clinical evaluation of high-molecular-weight sodium hyaluronate for the treatment of patients with periarthritis of the shoulder. Clin Ther 17:946-955, 1995.

99. Rovetta G, Monteforte P: Intraarticular injection of sodium hyaluronate plus steroid versus steroid in adhesive capsulitis of the shoulder. Int J Tissue React 20:125-130, 1998.

100. Karzel K, Domenjoz R: Effects of hexosamine derivatives and uronic acid derivatives on glycosaminoglycan metabolism of fibroblast cultures. Pharmacology 5:337-345, 1971.

101. Bassleer C, Reginster JY, Franchimont P: Effects of glucosamine on differentiated human chondrocytes cultivated in clusters [abstract]. Rev Esp Reumatol 20(Suppl 1):96, 1993.

102. Shikhman AR, Kuhn K, Alaaeddine N, Lotz M: N-acetylglucosamine prevents IL-1 beta-mediated activation of human chondrocytes. J Immunol 166:5155-5160, 2001.

103. Krajickova J, Macek J: Urinary proteoglycan degradation product excretion in patients with rheumatoid arthritis and osteoarthritis. Ann Rheum Dis 47:468-471, 1988.

104. Reichelt A, Forster KK, Fischer M, et al: Efficacy and safety of intramuscular glucosamine sulfate in osteoarthritis of the knee: A randomised, placebo-controlled, double-blind study. Arzneimittelforschung Drug Res 44:75-80, 1994.

105. Muller-Fabender H, Bach GL, Haase W, et al: Glucosamine sulfate compared to ibuprofen in osteoarthritis of the knee. Osteoarthritis Cartilage 2:61-69, 1994.

106. Hochberg MC: What a difference a year makes: Reflections on the ACR recommendations for the medical management of osteoarthritis. Curr Rheumatol Rep 3:473-478, 2001.

107. Herrero-Beaumont G, Roman JA, Trabado MC, et al: Effects of glucosamine sulfate on 6-month control of knee osteoarthritis symptoms vs. placebo and acetaminophen: Results from the Glucosamine Unum in Die Efficacy (GUIDE) trial [abstract 1203]. Arthritis Rheum 52(Suppl):S460, 2005.

108. Hughes R, Carr A: A randomized, double-blind, placebo-controlled trial of glucosamine sulphate as an analgesic in osteoarthritis of the knee. Rheumatology 41:279-284, 2002.

109. McAlindon T, Formica M, LaValley M, et al: Effectiveness of glucosamine for symptoms of knee osteoarthritis: Results from an Internet-based randomized, double-blind, controlled trial. Am J Med 117:643-649, 2004.

110. Towheed T, Maxwell L, Anastassiades T, et al: Glucosamine therapy for treating osteoarthritis. Cochrane Database Syst Rev CD002946, 2005.

111. Cibere J, Kopec JA, Thorne A, et al: Randomized double-blind, placebo-controlled glucosamine discontinuation trial in knee osteoarthritis. Arthritis Care Res 51:738-745, 2004.

112. Das A Jr, Hammad TA: Efficacy of a combination of FCHG49 glucosamine hydrochloride, TRH122 low molecular weight sodium chondroitin sulfate and manganese ascorbate in the management of knee osteoarthritis. Osteoarthritis Cartilage 8:343-350, 2000.

113. **Clegg DO, Reda DJ, Harris CL, et al: Glucosamine, chondroitin sulfate, and the two in combination for painful knee osteoarthritis. N Engl J Med 354:795-808, 2006.**

114. Qiu GX, Weng XS, Zhang K, et al: A multi-center, randomized, controlled clinical trial of glucosamine hydrochloride/sulfate in the treatment of knee osteoarthritis. Zhonghua Yi Xue Za Zhi 85: 3067-3070, 2005.

115. Reginster JY, Deroisy R, Rovati LC, et al: Long-term effects of glucosamine sulphate on osteoarthritis progression: A randomised, placebo-controlled clinical trial. Lancet 357:251-256, 2001.

116. Pavelka K, Gatterova J, Olejarova M, et al: Glucosamine sulfate use and delay of progression of knee osteoarthritis: A 3-year, randomized, placebo-controlled, double-blind study. Arch Intern Med 162: 2113-2123, 2002.

117. Mazzuca SA, Brandt KD, Lane KA, et al: Knee pain reduces joint space width in conventional standing anteroposterior radiographs of osteoarthritic knees. Arthritis Rheum 46:1223-1227, 2002.

118. Le Graverand MP, Mazzuca S, Lassere M, et al: Assessment of the radiographic positioning of the osteoarthritic knee in serial radiographs: Comparison of three acquisition techniques. Osteoarthritis Cartilage 14(Suppl A):A37-A43, 2006.

119. Mazieres B, Loyau G, Menkes CJ, et al: Chondroitin sulfate in the treatment of gonarthrosis and coxarthrosis: 5-month results of a multicenter double-blind controlled prospective study using placebo. Rev Rhum 59:466-472, 1992.

120. Morreale P, Manopulo R, Galati M, et al: Comparison of the anti-inflammatory efficacy of chondroitin sulfate and diclofenac sodium in patients with knee osteoarthritis. J Rheumatol 23:1385-1391, 1996.

121. Michel BA, Stucki G, Frey D, et al: Chondroitins 4 and 6 sulfate in osteoarthritis of the knee: A randomized, controlled trial. Arthritis Rheum 52:779-786, 2005.

122. Srivasta KC, Mustafa T: Ginger (Zingiber officinale) in rheumatism and musculoskeletal disorders. Med Hypotheses 39:342-348, 1992.

123. Swain AR, Duton SP, Truswell AS: Salicylates in foods. J Am Diet Assoc 85:950-960, 1985.

124. Mustafa T, Srivastava KC, Jensen KB: Drug development. Report 9. Pharmacology of ginger, Zingiber officinale. J Drug Dev 6:25-89, 1993.

125. Altman RD, Marcussen KC: Effects of a ginger extract on knee pain in patients with osteoarthritis. Arthritis Rheum 44:2531-2538, 2001.

126. Henrotin YE, Sanchez C, Deberg MA, et al: Avocado/soybean unsaponifiables increase aggrecan synthesis and reduce catabolic and proinflammatory mediator production by human osteoarthritic chondrocytes. J Rheumatol 30:1825-1834, 2003.

127. Henroitin YE, Labasse AH, Jaspar JM, et al: Effects of three avocado/soybean unsaponifiable mixtures on metalloproteinases, cytokines and prostaglandin E2 production by human articular chondrocytes. Clin Rheumatol 17:31-39, 1998.

128. Maheu E, Mazieres B, Valat JP, et al: Symptomatic efficacy of avocado/soybean unsaponifiables in the treatment of osteoarthritis of the knee and hip: A prospective, randomized, double-blind, placebo-controlled, multicenter clinical trial with six-month treatment period and two-month follow-up demonstrating a persistent effect. Arthritis Rheum 41:81-91, 1998.

129. Lequesne M, Maheu E, Cadet C, et al: Structural effect of avocado/soybean unsaponifiables (ASU) on joint space loss in hip osteoarthritis (HOA) over 2 years: A placebo controlled trial. Arthritis Rheum 47:50-58, 2002.

130. Piscoya J, Rodriguez Z, Bustamante SA, et al: Efficacy and safety of freeze-dried cat's claw in osteoarthritis of the knee: Mechanisms of action of the species Uncaria guianensis. Inflamm Res 50:442-448, 2001.

131. Nadanaka S, Clement A, Masayama K, et al: Characteristic hexasaccharide sequences in octasaccharides derived from shark cartilage chondroitin sulfate D with a neurite outgrowth promoting activity. J Biol Chem 273:3296-3307, 1998.

132. Barcelo HA, Wiemeyer JC, Sagasta CL, et al: Experimental osteoarthritis and its course when treated with S-adenosyl-L-methionine. Rev Clin Esp 187:74-78, 1990.

133. Montrone F, Fumagalli M, Sarzi Puttini P, et al: Double-blind study of S-adenosyl-methionine versus placebo in hip and knee arthrosis. Clin Rheumatol 4:484-485, 1985.

134. Bradley JD, Flusser D, Katz BP, et al: A randomized, double blind, placebo controlled trial of intravenous loading with S-adenosylmethionine (SAM) followed by oral SAM therapy in patients with knee osteoarthritis. J Rheumatol 21:905-911, 1994.

135. Najm WI, Reinsch S, Hoehler F, et al: S-adenosyl methionine (SAMe) versus celecoxib for the treatment of osteoarthritis symptoms: A double-blind, cross-over trial. BMC Musculoskeletal Disord 5:6, 2004.

136. Altman R, Brandt K, Hochberg M, et al: Design and conduct of clinical trials in patients with osteoarthritis: Recommendations from a task force of the Osteoarthritis Research Society. Osteoarthritis Cartilage 4:217-243, 1996.

137. Lozada CJ, Altman RD: Chondroprotection in osteoarthritis. Bull Rheum Dis 46:5-7, 1997.

138. Brittberg M, Lindahl A, Nilsson A, et al: Treatment of deep cartilage defect in the knee with autologous chondrocyte transplantation. N Engl J Med 331:889-895, 1994.

139. Amin AR, Attur MG, Thakker GD, et al: A novel mechanism of action of tetracyclines: Effects on nitric oxide synthases. Proc Natl Acad Sci U S A 93:14014-14019, 1996.

140. Tilley BC, Alarcon GS, Heyse SP, et al: Minocycline in rheumatoid arthritis: A 48-week, double-blind, placebo-controlled trial. Ann Intern Med 122:81-89, 1995.

141. Cole AD, Chubinskaya S, Luchene LJ, et al: Doxycycline disrupts chondrocyte differentiation and inhibits cartilage matrix degradation. Arthritis Rheum 32:1727-1734, 1994.

142. Yu LP Jr, Smith GN Jr, Hasty KA, Brandt KD: Doxycycline inhibits type XI collagenolytic activity of extracts from human osteoarthritic cartilage and of gelatinase. J Rheumatol 18:1450-1452, 1991.

143. Brandt KD, Yu LP, Amith G, et al: Therapeutic effect of doxycycline (doxy) in canine osteoarthritis (OA). Osteoarthritis Cartilage 1:14, 1993.

144. Brandt KD, Mazzuca SA, Katz BP, et al: Effects of doxycycline on progression of osteoarthritis: Results of a randomized, placebo-controlled, double-blind trial. Arthritis Rheum 52:2105-2025, 2005.

145. Lewis EJ, Bishop J, Bottomley D, et al: Ro32-3555, an orally active collagenase inhibitor, prevents cartilage breakdown in vitro and in vivo. Br J Pharmacol 121:540-546, 1997.

146. Burkhardt D, Ghosh P: Laboratory evaluation of antiarthritic drugs as potential chondroprotective agents. Semin Arthritis Rheum 17 (Suppl 1):3-34, 1987.

147. Altman RD, Dean DD, Muniz OE, Howell DS: Prophylactic treatment of canine osteoarthritis with glycosaminoglycan polysulfuric acid ester. Arthritis Rheum 32:759-766, 1989.

148. Rejholec V: Long-term studies of antiosteoarthritic drugs: An assessment. Semin Arthritis Rheum 17(Suppl 1):35-53, 1987.

149. Pavelka K Jr, Sedlackova M, Gatterova J, et al: Glycosaminoglycan polysulfuric acid (GAGPS) in osteoarthritis of the knee. Osteoarthritis Cartilage 3:15-23, 1995.

150. Moskowitz RW, Reese JH, Young RG, et al: The effects of Rumalon, a glycosaminoglycan peptide complex, in a partial meniscectomy model of osteoarthritis in rabbits. J Rheumatol 18:205-209, 1991.

151. Howell DS, Altman RD: Cartilage repair and conservation in osteoarthritis. Rheum Dis Clin North Am 19:713-724, 1993.

152. Pavelka K, Gatterova J, Gollerova V, et al: A 5-year randomized controlled, double-blind study of glycosaminoglycan polysulphuric acid complex (Rumalon) as a structure modifying therapy in osteoarthritis of the hip and knee. Osteoarthritis Cartilage 8:335-342, 2000.

153. Munteanu SE, Ilic MZ, Handley CJ: Calcium pentosan polysulfate inhibits the catabolism of aggrecan in articular cartilage explant cultures. Arthritis Rheum 43:2211-2218, 2000.

154. Golding JC, Ghosh P: Drugs for osteoarthrosis. I. The effects of pentosan polysulphate (SP54) on the degradation and loss of proteoglycans from articular cartilage in a model of osteoarthrosis induced in the rabbit knee joint by immobilization. Curr Ther Res 32:173-184, 1983.

155. Smith MM, Ghosh P, Numata Y, et al: The effects of orally administered calcium pentosan polysulfide on inflammation and cartilage degradation produced in rabbit joints by intra-articular injection of a hyaluronate-polylysine complex. Arthritis Rheum 37:125-136, 1994.

156. Innes JF, Barr AR, Sharif M: Efficacy of oral calcium pentosan polysulphate for the treatment of osteoarthritis of the canine stifle joint secondary to cranial cruciate ligament deficiency. Vet Rec 146:433-437, 2000.

157. Spencer CM, Wilde MI: Diacerein. Drugs 53:98-108, 1997.

158. Martel-Pelletier J, Mineau F, Jolicoeur FC, et al: In vitro effects of diacerhein and rhein on interleukin 1 and tumor necrosis factor-alpha systems in human osteoarthritic synovium and chondrocytes. J Rheumatol 25:753-762, 1998.

159. Carney SL, Hicks CA, Tree B, Broadmore RJ: An in vivo investigation of the effect of anthraquinones on the turnover of aggrecans in spontaneous osteoarthritis in the guinea pig. Inflamm Res 44:182-186, 1995.

160. Brun PH: Effect of diacetylrhein on the development of experimental osteoarthritis: A biochemical investigation [letter]. Osteoarthritis Cartilage 5:289-291, 1997.

161. Brandt K, Smith G, Kang SY, et al: Effects of diacerein in an accelerated canine model of osteoarthritis. Osteoarthritis Cartilage 5:438-449, 1997.

162. Pelletier JP, Yaron M, Haraoui B, et al: Efficacy and safety of diacerein in osteoarthritis of the knee. Arthritis Rheum 43:2339-2348, 2000.

163. Dougados M, Nguyen M, Berdah L, et al: Evaluation of the structure-modifying effects of diacerein in hip osteoarthritis: ECHODIAH, a three-year, placebo-controlled trial: Evaluation of the Chondro-modulating Effect of Diacerein in OA of the Hip. Arthritis Rheum 44:2539-2547, 2001.

164. Rintelen B, Neumann K, Leeb BF: A meta-analysis of controlled clinical studies with diacerein in the treatment of osteoarthritis. Arch Intern Med 166:1899-1906, 2006.

165. Pelletier JP, Roughley PJ, DiBattista JA, et al: Are cytokines involved in osteoarthritic pathophysiology? Semin Arthritis Rheum 20(Suppl 2):12-25, 1991.

166. Smith MD, Triantafillou S, Parker A, et al: Synovial membrane inflammation and cytokine production in patients with early osteoarthritis. J Rheumatol 24:365-371, 1997.

167. Attur MG, Dave M, Cipolletta C, et al: Reversal of autocrine and paracrine effects of interleukin 1 (IL-1) in human arthritis by type II IL-1 decoy receptor: Potential for pharmacological intervention. J Biol Chem 275:40307-40315, 2000.

168. Pelletier JP, Mineau F, Ranger P, et al: The increased synthesis of inducible nitric oxide inhibits IL-1ra synthesis by human articular chondrocytes: Possible role in osteoarthritic cartilage degradation. Osteoarthritis Cartilage 4:77-84, 1996.

169. Caron JP, Fernandes JC, Martel-Pelletier J, et al: Chondroprotective effect of intraarticular injections of interleukin-1 receptor antagonist in experimental osteoarthritis: Suppression of collagenase-1 expression. Arthritis Rheum 39:1535-1544, 1996.

170. Pelletier JP, Caron JP, Evans C, et al: In vivo suppression of early experimental osteoarthritis by interleukin-1 receptor antagonist using gene therapy. Arthritis Rheum 40:1012-1019, 1997.

171. Fernandes J, Tardif G, Martel-Pelletier J, et al: In vivo transfer of interleukin-1 receptor antagonist gene in osteoarthritic rabbit knee joints: Prevention of osteoarthritis progression. Am J Pathol 154:1159-1169, 1999.

172. Hunziker EB, Rosenberg L: Induction of repair in partial thickness articular cartilage lesions by timed release of TGF-beta. Transactions of the 40th Annual Meeting of the Orthopaedic Research Society, 1994, Vol 19, Sec 1, p 236.

173. Rogachefsky RA, Dean DD, Howell DS, Altman RD: Treatment of canine osteoarthritis with insulin-like growth factor-1 (IGF-1) and sodium pentosan polysulfate. Osteoarthritis Cartilage 1:105-114, 1993.

174. Frisbie DD, Ghivizzani SC, Robbins PD, et al: Treatment of experimental equine osteoarthritis by in vivo delivery of the equine interleukin-1 receptor antagonist gene. Gene Ther 9:12-20, 2002.

175. Attur MG, Dave MN, Leung MY, et al: Functional genomic analysis of type II IL-1beta decoy receptor: Potential for gene therapy in human arthritis and inflammation. J Immunol 168:2001-2010, 2002.

176. Doherty PJ, Zhang H, Tremblay L, et al: Resurfacing of articular cartilage explants with genetically-modified human chondrocytes in vitro. Osteoarthritis Cartilage 6:153-159, 1998.

177. Moseley JB, O'Malley K, Petersen NJ, et al: A controlled trial of arthroscopic surgery for osteoarthritis of the knee. N Engl J Med 347:81-88, 2002.

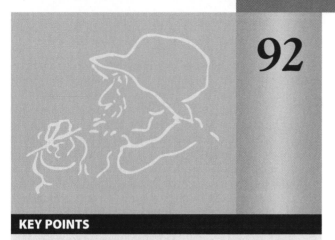

92 Metabolic Bone Disease

NANCY E. LANE

KEY POINTS

Osteoporosis is a disease defined by low bone density and deterioration of microarchitecture, which reduces bone strength and increases fracture risk.

Nearly half of all white women and about one quarter of men will suffer an osteoporotic fracture in their lifetimes.

Major clinical risk factors for osteoporotic fractures include older age, low weight, family history of hip fracture, fracture occurring after age 50, glucocorticoid use, and inability to rise from a chair without assistance.

Postmenopausal and age-related bone loss results from an uncoupling of bone remodeling such that bone resorption is greater than bone formation, resulting in a net loss of bone.

Receptor activator of nuclear factor κB ligand (RANKL), produced mainly by osteoblasts in estrogen-deficiency bone loss, is a major stimulator of osteoclast maturation and activity.

Polymorphisms in antagonists of the wnt/B catenin signaling pathway that result in a gain of function (e.g., LRP5) are associated with a reduced risk of osteoporosis.

Nearly 50% of osteoporosis in men results from secondary causes.

Vitamin D deficiency can result in osteoporosis and fractures.

Biochemical markers measured in the serum, including C and N telopeptide cross-links of type I collagen, correlate with osteoclast activity on the bone surface.

Treatment of high-turnover osteoporosis from estrogen deficiency with antiresorptive agents (estrogen, raloxifene, and bisphosphonates—alendronate, risedronate, zoledronic acid, ibandronate) and an anabolic agent (recombinant human parathyroid hormone 1-34) can reduce incident vertebral fractures.

Bisphosphonates and estrogen can reduce new-incident hip fractures.

C and N telopeptide cross-links of type I collagen serum levels are lowered with treatment with antiresorptive agents (estrogen, raloxifene, bisphosphonates).

The workup for osteoporosis is directed toward excluding secondary causes of bone loss and includes a determination of serum calcium, phosphorus, supersensitive thyroid-stimulating hormone, 25-hydroxyvitamin D (25-OHD), and intact parathyroid hormone (PTH) levels; urine calcium and creatinine levels; complete blood count; and alkaline phosphatase and liver function tests.

PTH increases osteoblast maturation and life span, increases trabecular bone mass and cortical thickness, and improves bone strength.

PTH treatment (Fortéo 20 μg/day) for 18 to 20 months reduced vertebral fractures by nearly 70% and nonvertebral fractures by nearly 50%.

Antiresorptive therapy is needed after a full course of PTH to maintain the newly formed bone mass.

Glucocorticoid-induced bone loss results from increased osteoclast activity and reduced osteoblast activity.

Glucocorticoid bone loss is most severe in the first 6 months of the therapy, but bone loss continues slowly thereafter.

Prevention of glucocorticoid bone loss with bisphosphonates is effective and prevents fractures.

Aromatase inhibitors reduce serum estrogen and result in rapid bone loss in postmenopausal women on adjuvant breast cancer therapy.

Gonadotropin-releasing hormone agonists decrease testosterone and estrogen levels and cause bone loss in men being treated for prostate cancer.

Osteoporosis is characterized by low bone density and a deterioration of bone microarchitecture that reduces bone strength and increases the risk of fracture. The hallmark of osteoporosis is the loss of bone mineral and bone matrix that results in maintenance of a normal mineral-to-matrix ratio. Bone consists of an organic matrix (collagen and noncollagenous proteins) and an inorganic mineral component (calcium and phosphate in hydroxyapatite crystals; see Chapter 4). Normally, bone turnover is tightly coupled with osteoclast-mediated bone resorption followed by osteoblast-stimulated bone formation. This delicate balance in bone remodeling results in no net change in skeletal mass. Osteoblasts synthesize osteoid—bone matrix that subsequently undergoes mineralization and becomes mature bone matrix. The skeleton contains approximately 80% cortical bone, which is concentrated in the appendicular skeleton and femoral neck, and 20% more metabolically active trabecular bone, which is located in the spine, epiphyses, and pelvis. Osteoporosis is characterized by reduced bone mass. Osteomalacia encompasses disorders in which there is decreased mineralization of bone matrix. Paget's disease is a skeletal disorder characterized by increased rates of bone turnover with the development of disorganized woven bone.

OSTEOPOROSIS

EPIDEMIOLOGY AND CLINICAL SIGNS

Osteoporosis, the most common metabolic bone disease, affects 200 million individuals worldwide. Approximately 28 million Americans have osteoporosis or are at risk for it.

Osteoporosis, or "porous bone," is a "disease characterized by low bone mass and structural deterioration of bone tissue, leading to bone fragility and an increased susceptibility to fractures, especially of the hip, spine and wrist."[1] Although usually asymptomatic, osteoporosis can produce loss of height, pain, dowager's hump, and increased risk of fracture. After 50 years of age, there is an exponential rise in fractures, such that 40% of women and 13% of men develop one or more osteoporotic fractures in their lifetimes. In the United States alone, there are more than 1.5 million osteoporotic fractures annually, including 250,000 hip, 250,000 wrist, and 500,000 vertebral fractures. Hip fractures are associated with a 12% to 24% mortality rate in women and a 30% mortality rate in men within the first year of fracture, and 50% of patients are unable to ambulate independently and require long-term nursing home care.[2] These numbers will continue to grow exponentially as the elderly population of industrialized nations increases.

Bone accretion occurs during adolescence, when there is a large increment in bone mass. Peak bone density is normally achieved after puberty and into the third decade of life. However, by age 22, most individuals have achieved their peak bone mass. At menopause, an acceleration of bone loss usually occurs over approximately 5 to 8 years, with an annual 2% to 3% loss of trabecular bone and a 1% to 2% loss of cortical bone. Both men and women lose bone with age. Over a lifetime, women lose approximately 50% of trabecular and 30% of cortical bone; men generally lose two thirds of these amounts.[3] Osteoporosis was previously thought to be a silent disease that was part of the normal aging process. However, the advent of bone densitometry has made it possible to accurately and reproducibly identify patients at risk for osteoporosis so that prevention and treatment strategies can be instituted to reduce fractures. With a health care expenditure of $13.8 billion annually for osteoporosis-related fractures and a projected threefold rise in these costs over the next 40 years in the United States, the institution of effective prevention and treatment strategies to reduce fractures is of great importance.[1,4]

PATHOPHYSIOLOGY OF MENOPAUSAL AND AGE-RELATED BONE LOSS

Bone is constantly undergoing remodeling, whereby areas of bone resorption produced by osteoclastic action are replaced by bone laid down by osteoblasts. Osteoporosis results from an imbalance between bone resorption and formation. The initiation of bone remodeling is still being debated; however, the osteocytes, or terminally differentiated osteoblasts, located within the bone matrix and connected to one another and the bone surface may release chemical mediators that attract osteoclasts to the bone surface (Fig. 92-1). Osteoclasts originate from the colony-forming unit granulocyte-monocytes, are attracted to the bone surface, attach to bone matrix, and resorb bone tissue. Generally, bone resorption is rapid, and a resorption pit is formed within 10 to 14 days. After resorption is complete, osteoblasts, derived from the bone marrow stromal cells, attach to the resorbed bone surface and produce osteoid, which is then mineralized. Bone formation can take up to 3 or 4 months. Therefore, a normal bone remodeling cycle in adults can last 4 to 6 months (see Fig. 92-1A). A number of metabolic changes

such as estrogen deficiency, immobilization, metabolic acidosis, hyperparathyroidism, and systemic and local inflammatory diseases can increase osteoclast number and activity, uncoupling bone turnover. This results in greater bone resorption than bone formation and a net loss of bone tissue. New data show that a number of local factors in bone affect the regulation of bone formation and resorption and the coupling of these processes. These include prostaglandins, insulin-like growth factors (IGFs), interleukins (IL-1, IL-6, and IL-11), tumor necrosis factor (TNF), receptor activator of nuclear factor κB ligand (RANKL), and transforming growth factor (TGF).[5] Animal studies have shown that IL-1, IL-6, and TNF knockout mice do not lose bone with estrogen deficiency.[6] In addition, inflammatory arthritis animal models find that TNF, IL-1, and IL-6 are all strong stimulators of osteoclastic bone resorption. This link between the immune system and the maintenance of bone mass is intriguing, but additional work is required before we can understand its significance.

A number of mechanisms underlie primary osteoporosis, including a low peak bone mass as a young adult and rapid bone loss during menopause. Factors contributing to age-related bone loss include impaired calcium absorption with age, a compensatory rise in parathyroid hormone (PTH) levels, and greater resorption than formation of bone. Estrogen deficiency is associated with the release of cytokines IL-1, IL-6, TNF, and RANKL, which leads to the recruitment and stimulation of osteoclasts in the marrow and increased production of bone-resorptive cytokines, which may contribute to menopause-related bone loss.[5] Estrogen therapy, however, inhibits IL-1 release, and in oophorectomized rats, an inhibitor of IL-1 (the IL-1 receptor antagonist) suppresses bone loss.[6] IL-6 levels also increase with age in human marrow cultures[7] and in peripheral monocytes. IL-1 and TNF induce the production of IL-6 from osteoblasts and stromal cells. Further evidence supporting a role of IL-6 in bone turnover includes data showing that oophorectomized IL-6 knockout transgenic mice do not lose bone. Two other proteins have been identified that influence osteoclast activity: osteoprotegerin (OPG) and RANKL, which are produced by osteoblasts.[8] Estrogen deficiency increases osteoblast production of RANKL, which stimulates maturation and activity of osteoclasts by attaching to RANKL on the surface of immature and mature osteoclasts. Simultaneously, estrogen deficiency decreases osteoblast production of OPG, the decoy receptor that reduces RANKL production and activity. Adenoviral delivery of OPG ameliorates bone resorption in a mouse ovariectomy model of osteoporosis.[8] Both preclinical animal models and clinical trials of women with low bone mass have been completed and demonstrate that inhibition of RANKL with a monoclonal antibody (RANKL inhibitor) prevents estrogen-deficiency bone loss.[9]

In addition, a number of genetic, nutritional, and lifestyle risk factors predispose to the development of osteoporosis. Caucasians and Asians are at risk for low bone mass and osteoporosis, whereas African Americans have a higher bone density and one third to one half the number of fractures.[1,8,9] Some studies show that African Americans have lower vitamin D and urinary calcium levels, higher PTH levels, and skeletal resistance to the effects of PTH on bone.[10-12] Studies in twins and families show that up to 80% of the variance in bone mass is accounted for by genetic

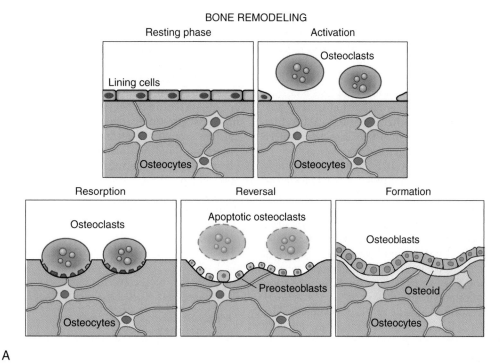

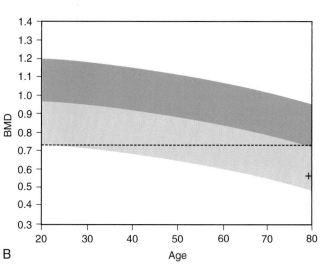

BMD (Total [L]) = 0.596 g/cm^2

Region	BMD	T		Z	
Neck	0.444	3.65 52% (25.0)		1.42	74%
Troch	0.491	2.10 70% 25.0		0.41	92%
Inter	0.720	2.45 65% (35.0)		0.72	87%
TOTAL	0.596	2.83 63% (25.0)		0.87	85%
Ward's	0.263	4.03 36% (25.0)		1.08	67%

T = peak BMD matched
Z = age matched   NHA   02/01/97

Figure 92-1 **A,** Bone remodeling cycle. Osteocytes most likely release chemicals to the bone surface that attract osteoclasts. Osteoclasts attach to the bone matrix, create a tight ring, and release acid that lowers the pH and dissolves the mineral from the bone matrix. After the mineral is released, the demineralized matrix is broken down. The osteoclast leaves the bone surface, and an osteoblast is attracted to the area of the bone that was resorbed. The resorption phase is about 10 to 14 days. Osteoblasts produce new bone, or osteoid, that fills in the resorption pit. Also, some of the osteoblasts are left within the bone matrix as osteocytes. The osteoid mineralizes over about 3 months, and the bone remodeling cycle is complete. **B** and **C,** The bone density of a postmenopausal woman is compared with that of both young, normal controls and age- and gender-matched controls. The T-score and Z-score represent the number of standard deviations below young, normal controls and age-matched controls, respectively. Because the bone density provides a gradient of fracture risk, therapies can be instituted to prevent the development of osteoporosis or to treat patients at increased risk for fracture.

factors.[13] A maternal history of hip fracture, for example, is associated with a twofold increased risk of a hip fracture.[14] Data from Uitterlinden and colleagues[15] show that the gene encoding collagen type IA1 is associated with low bone density with increasing age and an increased risk of fracture. In the *ss* allele group, bone density was 12% lower at the femoral neck and 20% lower at the lumbar spine than that in the *SS* group, indicating an increased gene-dose effect with increasing age. However, COLIA1 is associated with a lower baseline bone density and not an increased rate of

bone loss. Further, genetically determined architectural features of bone, such as a long hip axis length, may contribute to increased fracture risk; conversely, a short hip axis length confers some protective effect.[16] Recently, a family has been described whose members have very high bone mass but are otherwise phenotypically normal. This family has a mutation (an amino acid change) in the low-density lipoprotein receptor-related protein 5 (LRP5). Using in situ hybridization to a rat tibia, expression of LRP5 was detected in areas of bone involved in remodeling. Additional studies have reported that this LRP5 mutation increases wnt signaling, which may alter bone mass through a primary defect of bone formation. Individuals with this mutation demonstrate normal levels of bone resorption, but specific markers of bone formation are strikingly elevated. The observation that LRP5 is expressed at high levels in osteoblasts is consistent with its having a role in this area. Further work is now required to determine whether other mutations in the chromosome containing the LRP5 segment are associated with a variation in bone density in the general population.[17,18]

Other risk factors for osteoporosis, as enumerated in Table 92-1, include low body weight and reduced gonadal steroid levels.[13] Lifestyle factors that may contribute to the development of osteoporosis include cigarette smoking, excessive alcohol intake, reduced physical activity, and inadequate calcium intake, according to some reports. Cigarette smokers have poorer health than nonsmokers, impaired calcium absorption, lower estrogen levels, earlier menopause, and more fractures, and they exercise less; smoking cessation reverses this risk of osteoporosis.

In a large, prospective study of 9516 women older than 65 years, the following lifestyle factors significantly increased the risk of hip fracture: no walking for exercise, intake of more than two cups of coffee daily, current use of long-acting benzodiazepines and anticonvulsant drugs, current weight less than weight at age 25 years, height greater than 5 feet 7 inches, age older than 80 years, fracture since age 50 years, inability to stand from a chair without using arms, poor depth perception, and self-evaluation of health as fair to poor.[14] Low bone density in conjunction with a fall or trauma predisposes an individual to a fracture. Poor health and compromise of neuromuscular function increase the risk of osteoporosis and falls, which in turn increase the risk of hip fracture.[14] Importantly, elderly Caucasian women with both a low bone mass and more than two risk factors have a nearly 20-fold increased risk for fracture.

Secondary causes of bone loss that can affect women and men of all ages and races are listed in Table 92-2. Glucocorticoid therapy is the most common secondary cause of bone loss. Osteoporotic fractures develop in an estimated 30% to 50% of glucocorticoid-treated patients.[19] Glucocorticoid therapy causes bone loss through a number of different mechanisms, such as producing a negative calcium balance through impaired intestinal calcium absorption, increasing urinary calcium excretion, decreasing bone formation, increasing bone resorption by stimulating osteoclast activity by macrophage colony-stimulating factor, and suppressing endogenous gonadal steroid production.[19] Therapy with glucocorticoids leads to an early and, in some instances, dramatic loss of trabecular bone, with less effect on cortical bone.

Table 92-1 Risk Factors for Osteoporosis

Primary
Previous fracture after age 30
Family history of hip fracture
Cigarette smoking
Weight <127 lb
Low bone mineral density
Secondary
Nonmodifiable
White race
Advanced age
Frailty or poor health
Dementia
Modifiable
Low calcium intake
Eating disorder
Low testosterone levels (men)
Premenopausal estrogen deficiency (amenorrhea >1 yr or menopause at age <45 yr)
Excessive alcohol intake
Physical inactivity
Impaired vision
Neurologic disorder
Lack of sunlight exposure

Table 92-2 Medical Disorders and Medications Associated with Bone Loss and Osteoporosis

Primary osteoporosis
Juvenile osteoporosis
Postmenopausal osteoporosis
Involutional osteoporosis
Endocrine abnormalities
Glucocorticoid excess
Thyroid hormone excess (supraphysiologic)
Hypogonadism (including from prolactinoma or anorexia nervosa)
Hyperparathyroidism
Hypercalciuria
Processes affecting bone marrow
Multiple myeloma
Leukemia
Gaucher's disease
Systemic mastocytosis
Immobilization
Space flight
Gastrointestinal diseases
Gastrectomy
Primary biliary cirrhosis
Celiac disease
Renal insufficiency
Chronic respiratory diseases
Connective tissue disorders
Osteogenesis imperfecta
Homocysteinuria
Ehlers-Danlos syndrome
Rheumatologic disorders
Ankylosing spondylitis
Rheumatoid arthritis
Systemic lupus erythematosus
Medications
Anticonvulsants
Heparin
Methotrexate
Cyclophosphamide (Cytoxan) and GnRH agonists (hypogonadism)
Lithium
Cyclosporine
Aluminum
Excessive alcohol
Premenopausal tamoxifen
Aromatase inhibitors

Modified from LeBoff MS: Calcium and metabolic bone disease. In Medical Knowledge Self Assessment Program. Philadelphia, American College of Physicians, 1995.

GnRH, gonadotropin-releasing hormone.

In hyperthyroidism (Graves' disease or toxic nodule) or supraphysiologic therapy with thyroid hormone, the ensuing accelerated bone turnover may produce a reduction in bone mass when the thyroid-stimulating hormone level is suppressed, even when thyroid hormone levels are within the normal range.[20] Athletic amenorrhea, anorexia nervosa, and other hypogonadal states, including the use of gonadotropin-releasing hormone agonists,[21,22] may result in bone loss. In addition to estrogen deficiency, women with anorexia nervosa have low levels of IGF-1 and reduced levels of adrenal androgen dehydroepiandrostenedione, which may contribute to the development of osteoporosis.[23]

Osteoporosis in Men

Osteoporosis in men was not recognized 20 years ago but is now a major public health problem owing to men's longer life spans. The epidemiology of osteoporosis in men is just now being evaluated. Fracture risk occurs in adolescence and young adulthood and then increases after the age of 70. Long bone fractures occur more commonly in young men, while hip and spine fractures are more prevalent in men older than 70 years. The increase in fractures in older men is just as significant as it is in women, but it occurs about 10 years later in life, with an age-adjusted incidence of hip fractures in men of about one third to one half that of women.[24] Elderly men who sustain hip fractures have a greater risk of dying or being permanently disabled compared with women.[24] Risk factors for osteoporosis in men include older age, low bone mineral density (BMD), history of a low-trauma fracture as an adult, and a family history of osteoporotic fractures.

There are a number of secondary causes of osteoporosis in men; for instance, hypogonadism causes an increase in bone turnover and rapid bone loss as gonadal function declines with age. At this time, severe hypogonadism from androgen deprivation therapy for prostate cancer is common in elderly men. The exact role of estrogen and androgens in male skeletal health is not yet known. Although estrogen is needed for the young male skeleton, serum estrogen levels are highly correlated with bone remodeling, BMD, and rate of BMD loss in older men; the associations are stronger than with testosterone. However, serum testosterone levels are also highly correlated with indices of bone resorption and formation. The roles of estrogen and testosterone in the male skeleton need additional investigation.[25] Some of the other common causes of osteoporosis in men that are not as frequent in women are alcoholism, gastrointestinal disorders, including hepatic disorders, and malabsorption.[24]

Osteoporosis in Rheumatic Diseases and Other Conditions

Recently, studies have reported significant bone loss in patients with systemic inflammatory diseases such as rheumatoid arthritis, systemic lupus erythematosus (SLE), and ankylosing spondylitis. Patients with rheumatoid arthritis experience periarticular and generalized bone loss, with an increased incidence of fractures compared with the general population.[26] T lymphocytes, tissue macrophages, and synovial-like fibroblasts release inflammatory cytokines (IL-1, TNF, IL-6) and inhibitory wnt signaling proteins such as dkk-1 and RANKL, which stimulate preosteoclasts in the bone marrow and synovium to actively resorb bone; in addition, osteoblast maturation is altered.[27,28] In an animal model of inflammatory arthritis induced with collagen, animals pretreated with OPG did not have bone loss within the periarticular bone or the presence of erosions.[29] Additional factors that may contribute to osteoporosis in patients with rheumatic diseases include decreased mobility, glucocorticoid therapy, and systemic inflammation.[30] Some data, however, show that low-dose glucocorticoid therapy in women with rheumatoid arthritis does not have adverse skeletal effects, possibly because of a decrease in disease activity in association with the suppression of inflammatory cytokines and improved physical activity and function.[31,32] Ankylosing spondylitis is also associated with fractures and reduced bone density in the spine and proximal femur, even early in the disease.[33] Patients with SLE have a high rate of osteoporotic fractures in the presence of low to normal bone mass, suggesting that systemic inflammation alters bone turnover. Increased serum levels of TNF can reduce osteoblast maturation and increase osteoclast maturation and activity; in addition, other inflammatory factors such as oxidized low-density lipoproteins and inflammatory high-density lipoproteins can direct mesenchymal stem cells to differentiate into adipocytes instead of osteoblasts and impair bone mass.[34] Infiltrative processes in the marrow, such as multiple myeloma, mastocytosis, and Gaucher's disease, may produce osteoporosis. Patients with Gaucher's disease show an accumulation of glucocerebrosides in macrophages in the spleen, liver, and bone marrow, which causes hepatosplenomegaly, anemia, thrombocytopenia, bone infarcts and infections, fractures, and aseptic necrosis.[35]

The immunosuppressant drug cyclophosphamide (Cytoxan) induces amenorrhea and hypogonadism, which may increase the risk of bone loss. Women who undergo premature menopause from cyclophosphamide therapy can have estrogen-deficiency bone loss in their 30s. Young women with SLE who try to preserve ovarian function while undergoing cyclophosphamide therapy by taking gonadotropin-releasing hormone agonists may also experience estrogen-deficiency bone loss. In rodent models, the immunosuppressive drug cyclosporine produces a time- and dose-dependent bone loss[36]; in contrast, azathioprine (Imuran) and rapamycin (sirolimus) do not appear to adversely affect skeletal homeostasis.[37] Therapy with both cyclosporine and prednisone in transplant recipients is associated with early accelerated bone loss after the initiation of treatment and the development of osteoporosis and fractures with continued exposure.[38]

Vitamin D deficiency may also manifest as osteopenia and fractures, but this condition is both preventable and treatable.[39] Vitamin D insufficiency is common in older patients and in those with SLE who do not get an adequate amount of sunlight or use very potent sunscreens. Also, patients with malabsorption syndromes and liver disease can be vitamin D deficient. Unlike the situation in osteoporosis, very low vitamin D levels are often characterized by a mineralization defect and osteomalacia. Vitamin D deficiency is reported to be present in up to 50% of women with hip fractures.[39]

ASSESSMENT OF BONE DENSITY AND OSTEOPOROTIC RISK

Osteoporosis may first be diagnosed when a radiograph shows signs of demineralization or a spinal film shows evidence of compression fractures of vertebral bodies. Because an estimated 25% to 50% of bone mass must be lost to show osteopenia on radiographs, conventional radiography is an insensitive technique for diagnosing bone loss. Radiographs may demonstrate signs of secondary causes of osteoporosis, such as the presence of subperiosteal resorption in hyperparathyroidism, characteristic lytic changes or bone infarcts in Gaucher's disease, local sites of lytic destruction in malignancy, and pseudofractures in osteomalacia. Bone densitometry makes it possible to measure the amount of bone in the relevant fracture sites of the spine, forearm, and proximal femur, as well as the total body.

Techniques for evaluating bone mass include dual-energy x-ray absorptiometry (DEXA) and quantitative computed tomography (CT) scanning of the spine.[1,2] Bone density evaluations using DEXA incorporate the attenuation of soft tissue and bone by x-rays to calculate the BMD. DEXA is both precise and safe, with a very low radiation exposure. With reproducibility errors of approximately 0.6% to 1.5%, this technique is able to detect small changes over time.[2,40,41] Further, newer DEXA techniques measure bone density rapidly, in 0.5 to 2.5 minutes. It is possible to determine the BMD of the central trabecular portion of the spine using DEXA, excluding osteophytes or extraskeletal calcifications that may falsely raise the bone density in the standard anteroposterior projection. With quantitative CT scanning, it is possible to directly measure the loss of trabecular bone in the central region of the spine, but the procedure entails a comparatively high radiation exposure and time, and precision errors are usually higher than those associated with DEXA.

Figure 92-1B and C show the BMD in a postmenopausal patient compared with that of young, healthy controls to determine whether there is reduction in BMD compared with peak bone mass (percentage of young healthy controls expressed as a T-score) and with age-matched controls to assess whether BMD is diminished relative to an age-matched cohort (percentage of age-matched controls expressed as a Z-score). There is an inverse relationship between bone density and the gradient of risk for fracture.[42] Prospective studies show that bone densitometry identifies patients with an increased gradient of risk for fracture. In 8134 women, a 1–standard deviation (SD) decrement in the bone density of the spine and the femoral neck compared with age-adjusted controls was associated with a 1.6- and 2.6-fold increased risk of hip fracture, respectively.[43] Measurement of bone density in the hip is more predictive of hip fracture than is measurement at another site. Studies show that in women older than 65 years, hip bone density is predictive of spine and hip fracture and that conventional spine density does not add to the diagnostic utility of a single hip bone density test in assessing the risk of fracture.

Although bone densitometry provides a quantitative measure of bone mass, in vitro studies using ultrasonography indicate that this technique also provides information about the mechanical properties of bone, including both density and elasticity. These qualities are strong predictors of bone strength. Ultrasound techniques include speed-of-sound and broadband ultrasound attenuation methods; the speed-of-sound technique reflects bone density and elasticity, and broadband ultrasound attenuation is an indicator of bone density, bone structure, and composition. Approved for clinical use by the U.S. Food and Drug Administration (FDA), both ultrasound techniques have been shown to discriminate between normal and osteoporotic patients at increased fracture risk.[44] The T-score parameters used by some ultrasound machines do not correspond to T-score levels as measured by DEXA. Although ultrasonography is a radiation-free technique that may provide information about the risk of fracture and bone quality, the reproducibility of this technique and the measurement sites of mainly cortical bone or low-weight-bearing locations may make it unsuitable for monitoring small changes in bone over time. Therefore, ultrasound measurements cannot reliably be used to monitor response to osteoporosis therapies. Further data are necessary to validate the clinical utility of ultrasonography.

On the basis of the guidelines of the Scientific Advisory Board of the National Osteoporosis Foundation, bone densitometry is useful in determining which patients might benefit from therapy to protect the skeleton, including patients who have a deficiency of gonadal hormones (postmenopausal women younger than 65 years with one or more risk factors or older than 65 years regardless of risk factors), postmenopausal fracture, evidence of osteopenia or a vertebral abnormality on radiographs, hyperparathyroidism, or exposure to supraphysiologic doses of glucocorticoids (Table 92-3). Bone densitometry is also used to decide when to commence therapy for osteoporosis and to assess the clinical response to therapeutic interventions.[40] Screening normal premenopausal women is not cost-effective.

The World Health Organization (WHO)[1,45] has published criteria for osteoporosis based on bone density:

1. Osteopenia (low bone mass) is defined as a bone density measurement between 1 and 2.5 SD below the young-adult mean (T-score between −1 and −2.5).
2. Osteoporosis is defined as a bone density measurement less than 2.5 SD below that of young, healthy controls (T-score <2.5).
3. Established osteoporosis is defined as a T-score of less than 2.5 and the presence of a fracture.

Therapy to prevent bone loss is recommended if the T-score is −1.5 or less in a patient with risk factors or previous fracture, or if the T-score is −2 or less with no risk factors.

Table 92-3 Indications for Bone Densitometry

All postmenopausal women <65 yr who have one or more additional risk factors for osteoporosis (besides menopause)
All women >65 yr regardless of additional risk factors
To document reduced bone density in patients with vertebral abnormalities or osteopenia on radiographs
Estrogen-deficient women at risk for low bone density who are considering use of estrogen or an alternative therapy, if bone density would influence the decision
Women who have been on estrogen replacement therapy for prolonged periods or to monitor the efficacy of a therapeutic intervention or interventions for osteoporosis
To diagnose low bone mass in glucocorticoid-treated individuals
To document low bone density in patients with asymptomatic primary or secondary hyperparathyroidism

Treatment of osteoporosis is recommended for those in groups 2 and 3 as defined by the preceding list. T-score cutoffs for diagnosis and treatment do not apply to secondary osteoporosis.[45]

The current WHO guidelines require a BMD measurement before a patient can be treated for osteoporosis. Recently, WHO developed new guidelines for osteoporosis treatment that can be applied without a BMD measurement. Other guidelines still in development will provide patients and their health care providers with a 5- and 10-year osteoporotic fracture risk determination based on clinical risk factors and BMD (if obtained). These new WHO guidelines should be available soon, and they are intended to increase the number of individuals treated for this disabling disease.[46]

Markers of Bone Turnover

The development of sensitive biochemical markers of bone turnover makes it possible to analyze changes in bone formation and resorption at a given point in time and obtain additional information about a patient's risk of bone loss and fracture. Only three bone formation markers are currently available. Osteocalcin, a noncollagenous matrix protein in bone, is produced exclusively by osteoblasts; it correlates with histomorphometric bone measurements. In most conditions, bone resorption and formation are tightly coupled, and osteocalcin levels reflect bone turnover. The other markers of bone formation are bone-specific alkaline phosphatase (BSAP), an enzyme that is activated as osteoblasts mature, and amino-terminal propeptide of type I procollagen, a protein whose synthesis is very high in maturing osteoblasts.[47]

Sensitive indicators of bone resorption derived from the degradation of mature collagen include the urine and serum markers of type I collagen cross-links, including amino-terminal telopeptide of type I collagen (N telopeptides, or NTX) or carboxy-terminal telopeptide of type I collagen (C telopeptides, or CTX). Urinary pyridinoline cross-link, NTX, and CTX levels correlate with histomorphometric determinations of bone resorption; these biomarkers increase with menopause and are high in patients with a variety of disorders characterized by accelerated bone turnover, including Paget's disease, osteoporosis, and rheumatoid arthritis.[48,49] Urinary excretion of N telopeptides is inversely related to total hip and spinal bone density and, according to some studies, may be a more specific index of bone resorption than urinary pyridinoline levels.[50] The Epidimiologie de l'Ostioporose Study (EPIDOS) in elderly women showed that elevated C telopeptide and deoxypyridinoline levels are associated with an increased risk of hip fracture independent of BMD (odds ratio of 2). When it is coupled with a T-score less than −2.5, there is an increased risk of fracture, with an odds ratio of 4.8 over a 2.5-year follow-up period.[51] Also, Seibel and colleagues[52] reported that baseline urine resorption markers, urinary pyridinoline cross-links, were predictive of a new vertebral fracture in women over 1 year of follow-up. In clinical studies, antiresorptive agents such as estrogen and bisphosphonates induce a significant decrease (30% to 70%) first in markers of resorption and then in bone formation markers, often within 3 to 6 months. Resorption markers decrease before

formation markers and correlate with either maintenance of or increase in BMD. A significant change in bone markers can be observed within months of antiresorptive therapy, before there are changes in BMD.[52] Both bone formation and resorption marker changes over 6 to 12 months have been found to predict future fracture risk. In a study of alendronate to reduce osteoporotic fractures, patients who had more than a 30% reduction in bone alkaline phosphatase had the greatest reduction in risk for new vertebral and nonvertebral fractures. Interestingly, studies have found that reductions in markers of bone turnover, either resorption or formation markers, are associated with a reduction in fracture risk. However, long-term, prospective studies of large numbers of women are necessary to determine whether selective biochemical markers of bone turnover can predict changes in BMD or fracture risk and whether these tests should be used in standard clinical practice.

Most bone turnover marker data are derived from large studies of antiresorptive agents. However, a bone-building anabolic agent, PTH, has been approved for the treatment of osteoporosis. PTH's action is to stimulate osteoblast activity; therefore, osteocalcin and other markers of bone formation increase rapidly, within a few weeks of the initiation of treatment. However, activation of the osteoblast over time results in RANKL production, which stimulates osteoclast activity. With continued PTH treatment, markers of osteoclast activity also increase, reaching levels equal to those of formation markers. Because the overall result is an increase in bone mass, the bone turnover markers during PTH therapy reflect significant bone remodeling on both trabecular and cortical bone surfaces. A few small studies have found that increases in both bone formation and resorption markers predict an increase in bone mass with PTH treatment.[53-55]

Evaluation for Secondary Bone Loss

The workup for osteoporosis is directed toward excluding secondary causes of bone loss and includes a determination of serum calcium, phosphorus, supersensitive thyroid-stimulating hormone, 25-hydroxyvitamin D (25-OHD), and intact PTH, as well as urine calcium and creatinine levels. Also, a complete blood cell count, alkaline phosphatase and liver function tests, erythrocyte sedimentation rate (in some cases), and serum and urine protein electrophoresis for patients older than 50 years may be necessary (Table 92-4). In men, additional testing for secondary causes of osteoporosis includes serum testosterone and luteinizing hormone.

Further tests to rule out neoplastic or endocrinologic disorders and a bone biopsy (a decalcified bone specimen is obtained after a double tetracycline label with two different fluorescent labels) should be considered in certain patients with progressive bone loss and in those in whom osteoporosis is unlikely. Identification and appropriate therapy for underlying secondary causes of osteoporosis are important. For example, treatment of vitamin D deficiency is best accomplished with vitamin D supplements. Parathyroidectomy in patients with hyperparathyroidism characterized by hypercalcemia, hypercalciuria, nephrolithiasis, age younger than 50 years, or low cortical BMD (Z-score ≤ 2) was associated with a large (4% to 12.8%) increase in bone density over 4 years.[56] Bone density was, however, stable for up to

Table 92-4 Workup for Osteoporosis

For All Patients
Laboratory tests, including SMA, CBC, supersensitive TSH; ± PTH, alkaline phosphatase, 25-hydroxyvitamin D levels, and either measurement or estimate of 24-hr urinary calcium; ± serum and urine protein electrophoresis and ESR
For Selected Patients*
Definitive tests for endocrine, neoplastic, and gastrointestinal disorders Bone biopsy under calcified sections with double tetracycline label In some patients, markers of bone turnover to identify those at risk for increased bone loss

*Children, premenopausal women, men younger than 60 yr, African Americans, patients with rapidly progressive disease.

CBC, complete blood cell count; ESR, erythrocyte sedimentation rate; PTH, parathyroid hormone; SMA, sequential multiple analysis; TSH, thyroid-stimulating hormone.

Adapted from Primer on the Metabolic Bone Diseases and Disorders of Mineral Metabolism, 6th ed. Published by the American Society of Bone and Mineral Research, 2006.

Table 92-5 Calcium Requirements Recommended by the National Academy of Sciences (1997)

Age Group	Optimal Daily Calcium Intake (mg)
Infants	
Birth-6 mo	400
6 mo-1 yr	600
Children 1-8 yr	500-800
Adolescents 9-18 yr	
9-10 yr	800-1200
11-18 yr	1200-1500
Pregnant and nursing females	1300
Men and women	
19-50 yr	1000
>50 yr (± hormone replacement therapy)	1200-1500

Modified from Atkinson SA, Abrams SA, Dawson-Hughes B, et al: Calcium. In Young V (ed): Dietary Reference Intake for Calcium, Phosphorus, Magnesium, Vitamin D and Fluoride. Washington, DC, National Academy Press, 1997, pp 91-143.

6 years in patients with mild hyperparathyroidism.[57] In addition, treatment of hyperthyroidism, hypercortisolism, and a variety of other disorders that may cause osteoporosis can produce increments in bone mass. Reduction in the systemic inflammation associated with rheumatic diseases, such as TNF blocking agents for rheumatoid arthritis or ankylosing spondylitis or glucocorticoid-sparing agents for SLE (e.g., azathioprine [Imuran], mycophenolate mofetil [CellCept]), can also produce increments in bone mass.

TREATMENT

Calcium

The goals of therapy for osteoporosis are to reduce bone resorption and enhance bone formation, if possible. Bone loss occurs when the calcium intake and absorption are insufficient to balance the daily calcium losses. Prospective data show that calcium stabilizes bone.[58]

Table 92-5 shows the current recommendations for optimal calcium intake for women and men from the 1997 report of the Institute of Medicine to the National Academy of Sciences.[59] In the absence of kidney stones or an underlying disorder of calcium metabolism, these calcium intakes are safe. To prevent negative calcium balance, premenopausal women require 1000 mg and postmenopausal women 1200 mg of total elemental calcium daily.[60] Children have increasing calcium requirements during adolescence, and data show increased bone accretion with increased calcium intake in prepubescent and pubertal children. Calcium carbonate contains 40% elemental calcium and should be taken with meals because of poor absorption in achlorhydric patients in the absence of food. Calcium citrate, which contains 24% elemental calcium, has better bioavailability and is more readily absorbed.[61] It is also absorbed well on an empty stomach in patients with achlorhydria.

Estrogen

Hormone replacement therapy (HRT) was once the mainstay of treatment in osteoporosis because estrogen inhibits bone resorption, produces a small rise in bone density, and reduces the risk of fracture by approximately 50% in

retrospective observational studies. Cardiovascular disease is the leading cause of death in postmenopausal women. Previous data from longitudinal observational studies suggested that estrogen replacement had a beneficial effect on reducing primary and secondary cardiac events in postmenopausal women. However, in 1998, data from the 4-year Heart and Estrogen/Progestin Replacement Study were published.[62] In this study, 2763 postmenopausal women with a previous history of heart disease were randomized to receive estrogen (0.625 mg) plus progestin (2.5 mg) or placebo alone. Results showed no reduction in the overall rate of coronary heart disease or cardiac events in the treatment group; in fact, an early increase in risk for cardiac events was noted, possibly related to increased coagulability.[63]

In addition, a large, multicenter, longitudinal study by the Women's Health Initiative (WHI)—in which 162,000 women aged 50 to 79 years were randomized into a placebo group, an HRT group (if the uterus was intact), or an estrogen-only group (if the uterus was absent)—was terminated early due to an increased risk of breast and cardiovascular events. The research goals for the WHI study were to determine the effects of HRT, diet modification, and calcium and vitamin D supplements on heart disease, osteoporosis, and colorectal cancer risk. After a mean follow-up of 5.3 years in an 8.5-year study, the HRT group had an increased risk of seven more cardiac events per 10,000 women taking the drug for a year, eight more invasive breast cancers, eight more strokes, and eight more pulmonary emboli, but six fewer colorectal cancers and five fewer hip fractures.[64]

At this time, the general recommendation is that HRT should be used only for vasomotor symptoms that occur at the time of menopause. When these symptoms abate, it is recommended that estrogen replacement (combined estrogen and progestin for women with an intact uterus) be stopped, because the perceived cardiovascular benefits have not been substantiated, and the cardiovascular disease and breast cancer risk make the benefit-to-risk ratio unacceptable for most women. It is important to acknowledge that the estrogen-only arm of the WHI study in women without a uterus did not show an increased risk of heart disease or breast cancer.

If a woman and her physician decide that she is going to take HRT or estrogen alone for vasomotor symptoms, in those with an increased risk of coagulability, transdermal estrogen replacement should be used.

Selective Estrogen Receptor Modulators

The ideal estrogen replacement therapy would confer the beneficial effects of estrogen on bone and cardiovascular disease without increasing the risk of breast or uterine cancer. Selective estrogen receptor modulators (SERMs) are a nonsteroidal class of drugs that bind to the estrogen receptor and differ from one another in their actions on estrogen-responsive tissues, acting selectively as agonists or antagonists. Tamoxifen, the first available SERM, is an estrogen antagonist that binds to the estrogen receptor and also has estrogen-agonist effects on bone, lipids, clotting factors, and endometrium. Tamoxifen therapy in women with breast cancer produced a small increase in bone density of the spine over 2 years, with no effect on radial bone density, in association with reductions in both low-density lipoprotein and total cholesterol.[65] The Breast Cancer Prevention Trial studied 13,388 women at increased risk for breast cancer, comparing treatment with tamoxifen (20 mg daily) to placebo for 5 years.[66] Tamoxifen reduced the risk of invasive and noninvasive breast cancer by 50%, and a decreased risk of fracture was observed as well: 45% reduction at the hip and 29% at the spine. An increased incidence of low-grade endometrial cancer was noted, but there was no change in the risk of ischemic heart disease.[66]

Raloxifene,[67] now FDA-approved for the prevention and treatment of osteoporosis, is a SERM that acts as an estrogen agonist on bone, with antagonist effects on the breast and uterus.[68] Raloxifene (60 mg/day over a 2-year study period) increased BMD in the lumbar spine by 2.4%, in the total hip by 2.4%, and in the total body by 2%, with a reduction in fracture risk at 2 years similar to that seen with estrogen or alendronate (5 mg) treatment. Over the 2-year study period, raloxifene produced a significant reduction in vertebral fractures: fractures were present in 1.6% of raloxifene-treated women, compared with 2.9% of those in the placebo group; fractures recurred in 7.6% of treated women with a previous fracture, compared with 14.3% of those in the placebo group.[69] Endometrial thickness is not increased by raloxifene, but menopausal symptoms may be made worse. Raloxifene has been shown to decrease low-density lipoprotein cholesterol by 12%, with a nonsignificant increase in high-density lipoprotein cholesterol; cardiovascular protection has not yet been determined.[70] However, raloxifene, unlike estrogen, does not affect C-reactive protein, which is associated with a risk of cardiovascular disease.[71,72] Raloxifene also decreased the incidence of breast cancer by 76% in patients enrolled in a clinical study of osteoporosis, with breast cancer incidence studied as a secondary end point.[67] A study that evaluated the effects of raloxifene on cardiovascular disease found no effect.[73] One study compared tamoxifen and raloxifene, and another study evaluated raloxifene versus placebo, in the prevention of breast cancer. The first study reported that both tamoxifen and raloxifene reduced the risk of developing breast cancer, and the second found that raloxifene reduced the risk of estrogen receptor–positive breast cancer compared with placebo in postmenopausal women.[74,75] At this time, there is very little information on the use of raloxifene in men, so it is not recommend for male patients.

Testosterone

Men with osteoporosis, hypogonadism, and symptoms of low libido may benefit from testosterone replacement therapy. This can be administered as testosterone cypionate or enanthate (50 to 400 mg intramuscularly every 2 to 4 weeks) or as a transdermal testosterone replacement patch that is applied to the scrotal area (Testoderm, 4 to 6 mg/day) or elsewhere (Androderm, 2.5 or 5 mg/day).[76] Most studies find that bone mass increases with testosterone replacement when levels of testosterone were very low at the initiation of therapy.

Calcitonin

Calcitonin, a 32–amino acid peptide synthesized by the C cells of the thyroid gland, is a potent inhibitor of osteoclast-mediated bone resorption. Although human and salmon calcitonin are commercially available, salmon calcitonin is most commonly used because of its greater potency. Based on data showing an increase in total body calcium, parenteral calcitonin was approved by the FDA for the treatment of osteoporosis in 1984, and calcitonin in a nasal spray was approved for the treatment of postmenopausal osteoporosis in 1995. Parenteral calcitonin (100 IU subcutaneously or intramuscularly three times a week or daily) can maintain bone density or produce a small increase in bone mass in the spine and, in some instances, the forearm, particularly in patients with a high bone turnover.[77] Nasal spray calcitonin is absorbed through the nasal mucosa and is approximately 40% as potent as the parenterally administered drug (e.g., 50 to 100 IU of injectable calcitonin is comparable to 200 IU of nasal spray calcitonin).[78] In osteoporotic women more than 5 years past menopause, nasal calcitonin (200 IU/day) increases spinal bone density 2% to 3% compared with placebo, with no effect on proximal femur bone mass; higher doses are necessary in the early menopausal period.[78,79] Nasal spray calcitonin therapy in patients with osteoporosis is associated with a 36% reduction in vertebral fractures over 5 years.[79]

The adverse effects of parenteral calcitonin include nausea, flushing, and local irritation at the injection site. Calcitonin given intranasally is well tolerated, with rhinitis and nasal symptoms such as dryness and crusting being potential side effects. Patients treated with parenteral or intranasal calcitonin may also obtain a beneficial analgesic response in the presence of osteoporotic fractures.

Bisphosphonates

Bisphosphonates are analogues of pyrophosphate, with a P-C-P rather than a P-O-P core; they are absorbed by the hydroxyapatite of bone and suppress bone resorption. Modification of the side chains can result in the development of a variety of compounds with differing abilities to inhibit bone resorption (Table 92-6). Some bisphosphonates are administered intermittently because of a long skeletal half-life and prolonged retention in bone. These compounds must be taken on an empty stomach because gastrointestinal absorption is less than 10%.

Table 92-6 Ability of Bisphosphonates to Inhibit Metaphyseal Bone Resorption in Vivo

Chemical Modification	Examples	Antiresorptive Potency
First generation: short alkyl or halide side chain	Etidronate Clodronate	1 10
Second generation: NH₂-terminal group	Tiludronate* Pamidronate Alendronate	10 100 100-1000
Third generation: cyclic side chain	Risedronate Ibandronate Zoledronate	1000-10,000 1000-10,000 10,0000

*Tiludronate has a cyclic side chain, not an NH₂-terminal group, but it is generally classified as a second-generation compound based on its time of development and potency.

Adapted from Watts NB: Treatment of osteoporosis with bisphosphonates [review]. Endocrinol Metab Clin North Am 27:419-439, 1998.

Bisphosphonates have been used for the treatment of patients with Paget's disease of bone, hypercalcemia of malignancy, and osteoporosis and for the prevention and treatment of glucocorticoid-induced osteoporosis. Etidronate (Didronel) administered intermittently (400 mg/day for 2 weeks in 3-month cycles) produced an approximately 5% increase in bone density of the spine and a 50% reduction in vertebral fractures at 2 years. Longer follow-up did not reveal a significant reduction in vertebral fractures compared with baseline, except in a post hoc analysis of patients with three or more fractures and low bone density.[80] Etidronate is not approved by the FDA for the treatment of osteoporosis.

Alendronate (Fosamax) is FDA-approved for the prevention and treatment of osteoporosis. Data in postmenopausal women with bone density at least 2.5 SD below peak bone mass show that alendronate (10 mg/day) compared with placebo produces an 8.8% and 7.8% increase in bone density in the spine and femoral trochanter, respectively, and a 5.9% increase in the femoral neck after 3 years of therapy[81]; there are smaller rises (2.3% to 4.4%) in bone density in the spine and proximal femur in women within 0.5 to 3 years of menopause. Fosamax treatment in women with osteoporosis (T-score <2.5) yields a significant reduction in spine and hip fractures compared with the placebo-treated patients.[82] Treatment with alendronate (5 mg/day over 2 years) increased BMD in the lumbar spine by 2.9% and in the hip by 1.3%; in contrast, estrogen-progestin therapy increased BMD in these locations by 4% and 1.8%, respectively.[83] Alendronate did not reduce the incidence of clinical fractures in women who had low bone mass but not osteoporosis, although longer studies may be necessary.[84] Alendronate treatment is also effective in increasing bone mass in the spine, hip, and total body and helps prevent vertebral fractures and height loss in men with osteoporosis.[85] Adverse effects of bisphosphonates include gastrointestinal symptoms, such as stomach pain and esophagitis (caution is advised in patients with active symptoms or a history of ulcer disease), myalgias and arthralgias, and, rarely, osteonecrosis of the jaw. A once-a-week preparation of alendronate (70 mg) is the most commonly used dose for the treatment of osteoporosis.[86] This preparation increased spinal and hip bone mass similarly to alendronate 10 mg/day over a 2-year study period.

Risedronate, another oral bisphosphonate, administered at a dose of 5 mg/day increased bone mass and reduced the risk of new vertebral fractures 50% better than placebo.[87-89] Another study performed to assess the effect of risedronate on hip fractures found that women with osteoporosis (defined by a femoral neck T-score of ≤ −4.0) had a significant reduction in the risk of hip fracture.[90] Risedronate has been approved for the prevention and treatment of osteoporosis (35 mg once a week)[91] and for the treatment of Paget's disease (30 mg/day for 2 months, with retreatment if relapse occurs after 2 months).[92] Studies show that risedronate may be well tolerated even in patients with mild gastrointestinal symptoms. Bisphosphonates may also reduce bone pain.

Ibandronate (Boniva), another aminobisphosphonate, is approved for the treatment and prevention of postmenopausal osteoporosis. In phase III studies of ibandronate (2.5 mg/day) versus placebo in postmenopausal women with osteoporosis, incident vertebral fractures were reduced about 50%. Another study compared ibandronate 150 mg once a month to the daily 2.5-mg dose and found similar gains in lumbar spine and hip BMD. The FDA approved ibandronate 150 mg/month for the treatment of osteoporosis based on this bridging study.[93] Recently, intravenous ibandronate in a dose of 3 mg every 3 months was found to be similar to ibandronate 2.5 mg/day in terms of increasing lumbar spine and hip BMD, and the FDA has approved intravenous ibandronate for this indication. There are no data on hip fractures for this compound.[94]

Studies of other new bisphosphonates in the prevention and treatment of osteoporosis are under way. Zoledronic acid (Zometa), a potent bisphosphonate, is approved for the treatment of hypercalcemia of malignancy. A phase II, dose-ranging study of zoledronic acid for the treatment of postmenopausal osteoporosis has been completed. A dose of 4 mg given at the beginning of the study increased lumbar spine bone mass by nearly 5%, and biochemical markers of bone resorption remained suppressed nearly 70% below baseline levels at the 12-month point.[94a] In a recently reported phase III study of intravenous zoledronic acid at a dose of 5 mg/year for 3 years, the absolute risk of new vertebral fractures was reduced by 70%, and the risk of incident hip fracture was reduced by 40% compared with placebo-treated women.[95] It is expected that intravenous zoledronic acid will be approved for the treatment of postmenopausal osteoporosis in the near future. Zoledronic acid at a dose of 4 mg intravenously every 4 weeks is currently approved for the prevention and treatment of bone metastases in patients with breast cancer and multiple myeloma.

Parathyroid Hormone

Small randomized studies have determined that the 1-34 fragment of the PTH protein can significantly increase bone mass in the spine, with small losses or no gain at the skeletal sites rich in cortical bone. Small randomized studies have also been performed to assess the anabolic effects of PTH on changes in bone mass. PTH 1-34 (400 to 500 IU/day subcutaneously) with 1,25-dihydroxyvitamin D (0.25 mg/day) produced large increases in spinal bone density, although there was a small loss of cortical bone. The use of parenteral PTH (40 μg/day) alone in women who had endometriosis treated with gonadotropin-releasing hormone agonists for

12 months produced a 7.5% rise in lateral spinal bone density and prevented bone loss from the femoral neck, trochanter, and total body, despite severe estrogen deficiency over this time interval.[96] Lindsay and coworkers[97] showed that PTH 1-34 (25 μg/day) increases bone density and decreases vertebral fractures in postmenopausal women taking estrogen replacement therapy. Over a 3-year period, bone density increased 13% in the vertebrae, 2.7% in the hip, and 8% in the total body. Markers of bone formation increased by 55%, and markers of bone resorption increased 20%, demonstrating the uncoupling of bone turnover with an overall increase in formation.

In 2001, a recombinant human PTH (rhPTH) composed of the 34 amino acids from the amino-terminal end of the hormone, known as Forteo, was approved for the treatment of postmenopausal osteoporosis. In a large international, multicenter study, osteoporotic women with fracture were randomized to receive rhPTH 20 μg/day, 40 μg/day, or placebo for an average of 21 months. Lumbar spine bone mass increased between 9% and 13% in the rhPTH-treated subjects compared with the placebo-treated ones; hip bone mass also increased slightly. Most important, the risk of new vertebral fractures was reduced nearly 70% in both sets of rhPTH-treated subjects, and nonvertebral low-trauma fractures were reduced nearly 50% compared with placebo-treated patients.[98] This study was initially supposed to continue for 3 years; however, it was stopped at approximately 21 months because of preclinical evidence of malignant bone tumors in animal models. Additional studies of osteoporosis in men treated with rhPTH 1-34 have reported significant gains in bone mass.[99] Forteo is given as a daily injection. Individuals using this medication may experience headache, nausea, and flushing with initiation of treatment, but these side effects generally become less severe after a few weeks.

A number of recent studies have evaluated whether rhPTH 1-34 or rhPTH 1-84 is more effective in combination with an antiresorptive agent (either bisphosphonates or raloxifene) than rhPTH alone in increasing BMD and reducing fractures.[100-103] Interestingly, two studies found that the combination of PTH and alendronate was less effective in stimulating bone gain at the lumbar spine in both osteopenic women and men over 1 to 1.5 years.[100,101] Another interesting study found that if PTH was cycled with alendronate for 3 months, followed by alendronate only for 3 months, the gain in lumbar spine BMD was similar to that in patients given the two medications continuously for 15 months.[102]

PTH stimulates new bone formation, increases bone mass, and reduces new vertebral and nonvertebral fractures, but when the medication is discontinued, the bone gained is rapidly lost. Black and coworkers[103] performed a study in which patients were given PTH for 1 year, followed by 1 year of alendronate treatment. Interestingly, the BMD gain after 1 year of PTH was about 6%; when followed by alendronate, nearly 6% BMD was gained at the spine. These data suggest that although PTH is an effective monotherapy for increasing bone mass, especially in the spine, the gain in BMD should be maintained with a potent antiresorptive agent for a number of years. Recent data from Deal and colleagues[104] indicate that lumbar spine BMD gained after PTH therapy is maintained with raloxifene treatment.

PTH is the first bone anabolic agent approved for the treatment of osteoporosis. Patients give themselves a subcutaneous injection daily for 18 to 24 months. Other routes of administration are now being studied, including an intranasal route and a skin patch.

Vitamin D

Physiologic doses of vitamin D are important to ensure normal bone mineralization. Individuals 50 years of age and older should take at least 600 IU of vitamin D daily as a multivitamin or combined with a calcium supplement. Hypovitaminosis D is common in the elderly population, with one study demonstrating that 57% of patients in a general medical ward were vitamin D deficient.[105] Low vitamin D levels increase the risk of bone loss and fracture. LeBoff and associates[39] found that 50% of patients admitted with acute femur fractures had vitamin D deficiency (25-OHD level <12 ng/mL), and 36.7% had secondary hyperparathyroidism. Data show seasonal variations in vitamin D levels; low 25-OHD levels during the winter and spring are associated with decreases in bone density. The importance of vitamin D to skeletal health was shown when elderly women in a nursing home treated with only 800 IU/day of vitamin D had a 40% reduction in incident hip fractures over 18 months, compared with placebo-controlled subjects.[105a] Although this dramatic effect on fractures in an elderly population may represent a correction of vitamin D insufficiency, this study underscores that adequate vitamin D replacement can effectively diminish fractures in older individuals. Insufficient calcium and low 25-OHD levels are common in ambulatory patients and should be identified and treated before antiresorptive or other therapies for osteoporosis are initiated.

Although 200 IU of vitamin D prevents bone loss in the spine, data show that a higher daily intake (800 IU) is necessary to diminish bone loss in the hip during the winter and spring. Daily treatment with 700 IU of cholecalciferol and 500 mg of calcium carbonate reduced the rate of bone loss significantly in the femoral neck, spine, and total body and decreased the incidence of nonvertebral fractures by 50%.[106] Therefore, to maintain skeletal health, patients require a vitamin D intake that results in a serum 25-OHD level of at least 30 ng/mL. To achieve this level in patients who do not receive regular sunlight, the daily intake of vitamin D needs to be higher. Replacement with 1,25-dihydroxyvitamin D $(1,25[OH]_2D)$ is not recommended, because hypercalcemia and hypercalciuria are common and require regular and costly monitoring.

PREVENTIVE MEASURES

Because bone loss is not completely reversible with existing therapies, prevention is essential for optimizing skeletal health. Strategies directed at increasing peak bone mass, reducing risk factors for bone loss (e.g., hypogonadism, decreased body fat, cigarette smoking, inactivity, excessive alcohol intake), and reversing the secondary causes of osteoporosis may prevent bone loss. Patients should be advised to consume adequate vitamin D and calcium and participate in a regular weight-bearing exercise program. Weight-bearing exercise increases muscle strength and may stabilize or modestly increase bone density. Emerging data show that increased calcium intake and exercise can add to bone accretion during adolescence and that interventions such as vitamin D and calcium supplementation can reduce fractures in older patients. Thus, it is highly recommended that preventive strategies or therapies be instituted at any age to diminish the risk of fractures, which rises exponentially with age.

GLUCOCORTICOID-INDUCED OSTEOPOROSIS

Bone loss is a common sequela of therapy with glucocorticoids,[107] and glucocorticoid use increases the risk of fractures in patients with rheumatic diseases.[19] The severity of the bone loss in glucocorticoid-treated patients varies, with an approximately 3% to 20% decrease in bone density over 1 to 2 years. Glucocorticoid therapy is associated with increased fractures of the ribs and vertebrae, sites that contain predominantly trabecular bone, and it triples the risk of hip fracture in one third of patients after 5 to 10 years of treatment.[108,109] In adults, alternate-day glucocorticoid therapy does not prevent bone loss. In patients with rheumatic diseases, concerns over the development of glucocorticoid-induced osteoporosis often limit the dose and duration of glucocorticoid therapy.

The lowest possible glucocorticoid dose should be used, along with general preventive strategies such as a regular weight-bearing exercise program, adequate calcium and vitamin D intake, and reduction of other risk factors that might contribute to the development of osteoporosis. However, data show that even patients on prednisone 5 mg/day have accelerated bone loss compared with controls. General prophylactic measures to prevent glucocorticoid-induced osteoporosis are shown in Table 92-7. Intestinal calcium absorption is impaired in glucocorticoid-treated patients, and early studies showed that this could be offset with vitamin D (40 to 100 μg/day two to three times a week) or 25-OHD, which produced an increase in bone density of the forearm. However, the administration of supraphysiologic doses of vitamin D requires careful monitoring of the serum and urinary calcium concentrations in patients at high risk for bone loss (with a normal urinary calcium level and no history of nephrolithiasis). An alternative approach in patients at risk for osteoporosis and receiving long-term glucocorticoid therapy is to raise the 25-OHD level into the upper-normal range (>30 ng/mL) to ensure adequate intestinal calcium absorption. This can usually be accomplished by administering vitamin D at 800 IU/day.

Because of the enhanced bone resorption in patients treated with glucocorticoids, investigators have examined the effects of inhibitors of bone resorption. The use of bisphosphonates in patients receiving chronic glucocorticoid therapy is quite beneficial for both the prevention and treatment of osteoporosis. The use of alendronate 5 or 10 mg/day for 1 year in patients receiving glucocorticoid therapy increased lumbar spine BMD by 2.1% and 2.9%, respectively, and increased femoral neck BMD by 1.2% and 1%, respectively ($P < .001$).[109] After 1 year of treatment, there was an insignificant reduction in new vertebral fractures, but after 2 years of treatment, there was a nearly 40% reduction in new vertebral fracture risk. Risedronate 5 mg/day was also effective in the prevention and treatment of

Table 92-7 Recommendations for the Prevention and Treatment of Glucocorticoid-Induced Osteoporosis

Prevention
Patients starting GC therapy at a dose equivalent to prednisone ≥5 mg/day for 3 mo or longer should:
Modify risk factors for osteoporosis (stop smoking, decrease excessive alcohol consumption)
Start regular weight-bearing physical exercise
Initiate intake of calcium (total 1500 mg/day) and vitamin D (400-800 IU/day)
Consider BMD testing to predict risk of fracture and bone loss
Initiate bisphosphonate therapy (alendronate 5 mg/day or 35 mg/wk, or risedronate 5 mg/day or 35 mg/wk)

Treatment
Patients on long-term GC therapy should be tested for osteoporosis using BMD measurement. If the T-score is < −1, consider:
Risk factor modification, including reducing risk of falls
Regular weight-bearing physical exercises
Calcium and vitamin D supplementation
Replacement of gonadal steroids, if deficient
Bisphosphonate therapy (alendronate 10 mg/day or 70 mg/wk, or risedronate 5 mg/day or 35 mg/wk); if bisphosphonates are contraindicated or not tolerated, consider calcitonin as second-line agent, intravenous bisphosphonate (pamidronate or zolendronate), or PTH 1-34
Repeat BMD measurement annually or biannually

BMD, bone mineral density; GC, glucocorticoid; PTH, parathyroid hormone.
Adapted from Recommendations for the prevention and treatment of glucocorticoid-induced osteoporosis: 2001 update. Arthritis Rheum 44: 1496-1503, 2001.

glucocorticoid-induced bone loss.[110,111] Both alendronate and risedronate are approved by the FDA to reduce bone loss in glucocorticoid-treated patients.

In a prospective pilot study in glucocorticoid-treated patients, intravenous infusions of pamidronate (30 mg every 3 months) increased spinal bone density 3.4% in 1 year.[112] Studies of new, more potent bisphosphonates for the prevention and treatment of glucocorticoid-induced bone loss are in progress.

Traditionally, postmenopausal women on glucocorticoids have been treated with HRT, and there are some data that this prevents bone loss in these women.[113] However, because the earlier cited WHI results showed unacceptable cardiovascular and cancer risks associated with HRT therapy, it is no longer the standard of care. Studies of SLE subjects treated with dehydroepiandrosterone (DHEA) found an increase in lumbar spine and hip bone mass compared with placebo-treated patients.[114,115] The mechanism of DHEA's effect on bone mass is not yet known. Investigators have suggested the bone mass preservation results from DHEA metabolism to estrogen or by direct effects on IGF-1 bone-promoting factors. Additional studies are now in progress to determine whether this agent is effective for the prevention of bone loss in glucocorticoid-treated SLE patients.

In addition, men on glucocorticoids can have a lowering of testosterone levels.[116] They are generally asymptomatic, but if men on glucocorticoids have evidence of low serum testosterone levels and symptoms of low libido, they can be safely treated with testosterone. Bone mass increases have been observed in men with low testosterone levels on glucocorticoids who were treated with testosterone.[117] However, because of the risks associated with testosterone treatment, it is more prudent to treat these patients with a bisphosphonate medication.

Although glucocorticoids alter bone metabolism via a number of different mechanisms, inhibition of osteoblast life span and activity is the most significant. Whereas calcium and vitamin D supplementation and antiresorptive therapies can prevent bone loss as well as reduce fracture risk, they do not significantly alter osteoblast activity in the presence of glucocorticoids. Because a bone anabolic agent, rhPTH 1-34, can increase osteoblast activity and increase bone mass in postmenopausal osteoporosis, Lane and colleagues[118] tested the hypothesis that rhPTH 1-34 could override the suppressive effects of glucocorticoids on osteoblast activity and reverse the bone loss. Data from a 12-month randomized trial of rhPTH 1-34 in postmenopausal women with osteoporosis currently taking glucocorticoids and estrogen replacement therapy showed an 11% increase in lumbar BMD, compared with no change in the estrogen-only group. After 1 year of treatment and 1 year of follow-up, total and femoral neck BMD increased nearly 5%, with little change in the estrogen-only group. In this study, quantitative CT of the lumbar spine, a measure of only trabecular bone, found a nearly 35% increase in PTH-treated patients compared with the estrogen-only group after 12 months of therapy.[119] This information demonstrates that the major effect of PTH is to increase bone mass by thickening the existing trabeculae. In addition, 1 year of rhPTH 1-34 treatment increased the vertebral cross-sectional area, most likely by thickening of the periosteal envelope.[120] Studies are now under way comparing rhPTH 1-34 to alendronate for the treatment of osteoporosis. Currently, there is no fracture information for PTH and glucocorticoid-induced bone loss.

To prevent bone loss in patients with pulmonary diseases requiring glucocorticoid therapy, treatment with inhaled glucocorticoids has been studied.[121,122] Inhaled glucocorticoids appear to uncouple bone turnover and increase bone loss; however, this is dose dependent. Less than 800 μg/day of inhaled budesonide dipropionate does not increase the risk of osteoporosis, but more than 800 μg/day does. New inhaled steroids are more potent than older ones; for instance, Advair 200 μg/day is equivalent to nearly 5 mg/day of prednisone.[122] Therefore, patients on chronic steroid inhalers should be screened for bone loss.

Because patients receiving glucocorticoids may lose a dramatic amount of bone, it is important to monitor the efficacy of a treatment intervention, assess the need for further diagnostic evaluation for other causes of bone loss, and consider alternative treatment strategies if a given therapy is ineffective in preventing bone loss or fractures. In patients at increased risk of fracture, therapy with a potent bisphosphonate is highly recommended to slow bone loss and the rate of new fractures. Alendronate and risedronate are available for use, and future studies of more potent bisphosphonates and PTH are expected.

OSTEOMALACIA

Osteomalacia is characterized by impaired mineralization of bone matrix. Calcium, phosphate, and vitamin D are necessary for the mineralization of bone. Normally, there is a steep inverse relationship between the serum calcium and PTH concentrations. A small decrease in the serum calcium concentration leads to a rise in PTH release, which promotes distal renal calcium reabsorption, proximal tubulorenal phosphorus excretion, and resorption of calcium from bone. Vitamin D is produced in the skin in the presence of ultraviolet light or absorbed in the intestine from dietary or supplemental sources. Activation of vitamin D to 25-OHD occurs in the liver and to $1,25(OH)_2D$ in the proximal tubules of the kidney. PTH, hypocalcemia, and hypophosphatemia stimulate the renal 1-hydroxylase enzyme that converts 25-OHD to $1,25(OH)_2D$, which in turn indirectly enhances intestinal calcium absorption.

Osteomalacia results from reduced availability of calcium or phosphate for incorporation into the hydroxyapatite of bone or from deficient absorption or activation of vitamin D.[123,124] The term *rickets* applies to the defective mineralization of bone and the cartilaginous growth plate in growing children. As shown in Table 92-8, osteomalacia or rickets may result from decreased availability of vitamin D as a consequence of insufficient ultraviolet light exposure, insufficient vitamin intake, or malabsorption in patients with gastrointestinal or biliary disorders. Reduced levels of 25-OHD are caused by severe liver disease, increased renal excretion of vitamin D metabolites due to nephrotic syndrome, or accelerated metabolism of 25-OHD caused by anticonvulsant drugs. Decreased activation of $1,25(OH)_2D$

Table 92-8 Causes of Osteomalacia and Rickets

Vitamin D Deficiency or Dysfunction
Reduced Availability
Nutritional deficit
Reduced exposure to ultraviolet light
Malabsorption (gastrointestinal or biliary disease, surgical resection)
Alteration in Metabolism
Reduced 25-hydroxyvitamin D from liver or gastrointestinal disease, nephrotic syndrome, anticonvulsant drugs
Reduced 1,25-dihydroxyvitamin D from renal disease, vitamin D–dependent rickets type I
Alteration in Action on Target Tissues
Vitamin D–dependent rickets type II
Phosphate Deficiency
Decreased availability—dietary deficiency, phosphate-binding antacids
Decreased renotubular phosphate reabsorption
Familial—X-linked hypophosphatemic rickets, adult-onset vitamin D–resistant osteomalacia
Acquired—hypophosphatemic osteomalacia (phosphate diabetes), oncogenic osteomalacia
Generalized renotubular disorders
Acidosis
Renotubular acidosis
Ureterosigmoidostomy
Carbonic anhydrase inhibitors (acetazolamide)
Miscellaneous Mineralization Defects
Inhibitors of mineralization—fluoride, bisphosphonates (e.g., etidronate), chronic renal failure (aluminum)
Hypophosphatasia

Modified from LeBoff MS, Brown EM: Metabolic bone disease. In Hare JW (ed): Signs and Symptoms in Endocrine and Metabolic Disorders. Philadelphia, JB Lippincott, 1986, pp 239-260.

is seen in patients with renal insufficiency due to increased phosphate levels; the resultant lower ionized calcium levels lead to secondary or tertiary hyperparathyroidism.

A careful history is important in the diagnosis of osteomalacia or vitamin D insufficiency. For example, a history of a malabsorptive process such as gastrectomy, intestinal resection, sprue, primary biliary cirrhosis, or pancreatic deficiency may lead to the identification of vitamin D deficiency and osteomalacia.[124] Patients with osteomalacia may present with generalized pain involving the pelvis, spine, ribs, or lower extremities or with skeletal deformities such as bowing of the long bones, kyphoscoliosis, or pelvic abnormalities. Another clinical sign of osteomalacia in adults is proximal muscle weakness, which may result in an antalgic or waddling gait and difficulty ambulating.

Pain may be elicited by deep palpation of the tibia, ribs, or pubic ramus.[124] One of the radiographic signs of osteomalacia is the presence of pseudofractures, or Looser's zones, which are transverse lines of rarefaction through the cortices, with incomplete healing in the ribs, scapulae, long bones (Fig. 92-2), or pubic rami. Pseudofractures, however, may be indistinguishable from those associated with osteogenesis imperfecta or Paget's disease. Other radiographic findings in osteomalacia are vertebral fractures or protrusio acetabuli. Vitamin D deficiency may result in irreversible cortical bone loss.[124] In subtle cases of osteomalacia, a bone biopsy with a double tetracycline label may be necessary; characteristic histomorphometric findings in this disorder include increased osteoid and delayed mineralization of bone.

Rickets causes abnormalities of the epiphyseal growth plate, and the clinical signs include an inability to ambulate, growth disturbances, bowing of the long bones, and short stature. Bony deformities of the skull and ribs may develop, with widened cranial sutures (craniotabes), thickened costochondral junctions (rachitic rosary), or indentation of the margins of the ribs (Harrison's grooves).

The biochemical parameters in patients with osteomalacia reflect the underlying pathophysiologic process and the compensatory biologic responses. In vitamin D deficiency states, the serum calcium levels are usually normal or slightly decreased, because PTH levels rise rapidly as a compensatory response to impaired calcium absorption.[125]

In renal insufficiency phosphate retention, impaired renal production of $1,25(OH)_2D$, hypocalcemia, and skeletal resistance to PTH are thought to lead to the development of hyperparathyroidism and resultant renal osteodystrophy, mixed osteomalacia, and osteitis fibrosa cystica.[126] Also, aluminum intoxication may present with pure osteomalacia or adynamic bone disease.[125,127] Chronic vitamin D deficiency may increase the secretory demands of the parathyroid glands, thereby producing secondary or, in some instances, tertiary hyperparathyroidism. In patients with osteomalacia without hepatobiliary disease, alkaline phosphatase levels are often elevated.[124]

Osteomalacia may be associated with a deficiency of phosphate, principally in patients with decreased renotubular reabsorption of phosphate. Familial hypophosphatemic vitamin D–resistant rickets in children or osteomalacia in adults usually presents with renal phosphate leak, hypophosphatemia, rachitic or osteomalacial changes, and inappropriately normal or low-normal $1,25(OH)_2D$ level for the degree of hypophosphatemia. This X-linked dominant disorder may present in young children with the inability to walk, followed by progressive bowing and skeletal deformities, without signs of proximal myopathy. The genetic locus for X-linked hypophosphatemic rickets has been mapped to Xp22.1, and the gene is named *PHEX* (phosphate-regulating gene with homology to endopeptidases on the X chromosome).[128]

Oncogenic osteomalacia or rickets is a vitamin D–resistant process associated with certain neoplasias, principally small, benign mesenchymal or endodermal tumors and, infrequently, certain malignant tumors (e.g., multiple myeloma; prostatic, oat cell, breast carcinomas).[129,130] Such patients typically present with decreased renotubular phosphate reabsorption, hypophosphatemia, muscle weakness, diminished $1,25(OH)_2D$ levels, and normocalcemia. The benign tumors tend to be small and difficult to identify on physical examination or radiographs. Surgical removal of these tumors results in a rise in the phosphate and $1,25(OH)_2D$ levels and resolution of the skeletal process. Osteomalacia may also be associated with generalized renotubular disorders and the use of certain drugs that contain inhibitors of mineralization (e.g., fluoride, etidronate, aluminum). The evaluation of a patient suspected of having osteomalacia is outlined in Table 92-9.

Osteomalacia is often a treatable disease, but the diagnosis may be overlooked. Vitamin D deficiency can be treated with physiologic doses of vitamin D, but higher doses (1000 to 2000 IU/day) may hasten the healing of bone. In the presence of intestinal malabsorption, and until the underlying malabsorptive process is corrected, very large doses of

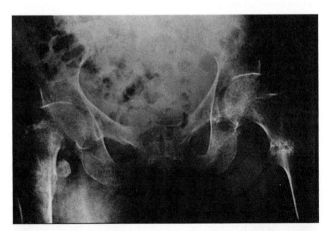

Figure 92-2 **Osteomalacia and fractures in a 65-year-old woman with malabsorption.** Shown are a pseudofracture of the left lesser trochanter and an avulsion of the right lesser trochanter. This patient also had previous bilateral pubic rami fractures.

Table 92-9 Workup for Osteomalacia

Calcium, phosphorus, alkaline phosphatase, urinary calcium levels; 25-hydroxyvitamin D and intact parathyroid hormone levels

In selected patients:
   1,25-Dihydroxyvitamin D levels (e.g., renal insufficiency, vitamin D–resistant osteomalacia or rickets)
   Vitamin D absorption test: obtain 25-hydroxyvitamin D levels at 0, 4, and 8 hr (e.g., some cases of malabsorption)
   Tubular reabsorption of phosphate (e.g., vitamin D–resistant osteomalacia or rickets)
   Bone biopsy with double tetracycline labels

vitamin D (50,000 IU once a week to three or more times a week) are often required. Careful monitoring of the serum and urinary calcium levels and 25-OHD concentrations is necessary to prevent vitamin D intoxication. Use of the active metabolite of 25-OHD (Calderol) may occasionally be necessary in resistant patients or in those with severe liver disease who cannot achieve activation of this metabolite. The potential advantages of using 25-OHD are more stable bioavailability, shorter half-life, and greater potency than the parent compound,[124] although the cost is greater.

In patients with hypophosphatemia and disorders of renotubular phosphate reabsorption, mineralization of bone occurs with phosphate therapy and moderately high doses of $1,25(OH)_2D$, the latter being necessary to prevent the secondary hyperparathyroidism associated with phosphate therapy. In patients with renal insufficiency or failure, a phosphate binder (calcium acetate or calcium carbonate) should be used after meals to decrease intestinal phosphate absorption. Calcium citrate therapy should not be used because it augments aluminum absorption. In those with renal failure, $1,25(OH)_2D$ therapy administered orally[125,131] (or intravenously in some dialysis patients) suppresses parathyroid cell secretion and proliferation; a threefold elevation of the PTH level is advocated by some investigators to prevent adynamic bone disease.[126] Analogues of $1,25(OH)_2D$ that do not produce hypercalcemia but decrease levels of PTH are now available and may be useful in patients with renal insufficiency.

PAGET'S DISEASE OF BONE

Paget's disease affects approximately 2% to 3% of the population older than 50 years and is uncommon in individuals younger than 40 years.[132] Paget's disease of bone is characterized by enhanced resorption of bone by giant, multinucleated osteoclasts, followed by the formation of disorganized woven bone by osteoblasts. The resultant bone is expanded, weak, and vascular, so that affected bones may become enlarged and deformed, and the overlying skin may feel warm to the touch.[133]

CAUSE

The cause of Paget's disease is uncertain, although data showing the presence of viral inclusion particles in giant pagetic osteoclasts support a viral cause, possibly associated with measles, respiratory syncytial, or canine distemper virus. Paget's disease tends to aggregate in families in an autosomal dominant pattern, and 40% of patients have at least one other family member affected.[106] Recently, in a family with juvenile Paget's disease, the disease was found to be associated with a polymorphism in the OPG allele.[134] Studies of additional families with this mutation may lead to the discovery of the cause of Paget's disease.

CLINICAL FEATURES

Many patients with Paget's disease are asymptomatic, and the disease is detected by the incidental finding of an elevated alkaline phosphatase level or characteristic radiographic abnormality. Other patients present with a range of symptoms that include bone pain, skeletal deformities (bowing

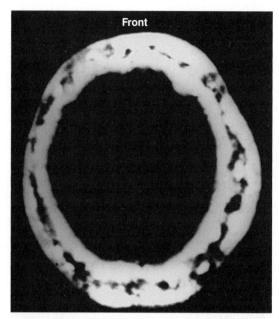

Figure 92-3 **Paget's disease of the skull in a woman with signs of increasing head size and progressive hearing loss.** The alkaline phosphatase level was 2100 U/L. This computerized axial tomogram shows marked thickening of the inner and outer skull tables, with osteoblastic pagetoid changes. Audiologic evaluation revealed bilateral hearing loss.

of long bones, enlarged skull, pelvic alterations), pathologic fractures, increased cardiac output (with extensive disease), and nerve compression. Paget's disease typically includes a lytic phase, a combined lytic and blastic phase, and a sclerotic or "burned out" phase occurring late in the disease process.

Radiographic signs of the three stages of Paget's disease may be present at different sites in the same patient.[132] The skeletal sites commonly involved with Paget's disease include the skull (Fig. 92-3), vertebrae, pelvis, sacrum, and lower extremities. Degenerative joint disease may develop adjacent to the bones and cause pain that may obscure the symptoms associated with Paget's disease.[132] Ten percent to 30% of patients with Paget's disease may experience fractures that present initially as asymptomatic or painful short fissure fractures traversing the bony cortex (Fig. 92-4). Complete fractures of the bones, such as the "chalk stick" fracture, also occur; fractures of the long bones may be a serious complication because the increased vascularity of pagetic bone may lead to excessive blood loss. Healing of fractures in pagetic bone usually occurs normally, although there have been reports of nonunion. A rare complication of Paget's disease of bone is sarcomatous degeneration in less than 1% of patients (with osteogenic sarcomas or, less commonly, fibrosarcomas or chondrosarcomas); these patients generally have a poor prognosis. The development of a sarcoma may be heralded by the presence of a soft tissue mass, localized pain, and rise in the alkaline phosphatase level.

Neurologic symptoms generally result from compression of the nerves by pagetic bone. Hearing loss is common and is caused by sensory loss and conduction abnormalities due to pagetic involvement of the bones of the inner ear. Paget's disease of the skull may also produce ocular and other cranial nerve palsies. Compression of the base of the skull may lead to basilar invagination, cerebellar dysfunction, or obstructive hydrocephalus, with symptoms of nausea, ataxia,

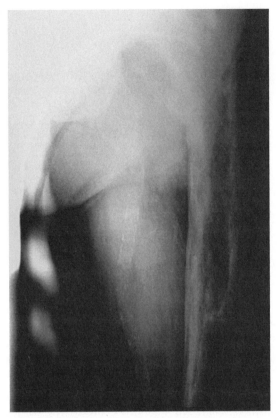

Figure 92-4 Paget's disease of the proximal femur. Note the coarse trabeculae, thickened cortices, lateral fissure fracture, and expanding lytic region characteristic of the "blade-of-grass" lesion.

incontinence, gait disturbances, and dementia. Neurologic compromise of the thoracic or lumbar spine may lead to spinal cord compression or, in the latter instance, cauda equina syndrome.

LABORATORY FINDINGS

Biochemical indices in patients with Paget's disease usually show normal serum calcium and phosphate levels, although hypercalcemia may develop with immobilization when there is an uncoupling of bone resorption and formation. Patients with Paget's disease may also be hypercalcemic if they coincidentally acquire primary hyperparathyroidism, which can further increase bone remodeling and worsen the disease process. Secondary hyperparathyroidism may develop in approximately 10% to 15% of patients with Paget's disease, presumably because of inadequate calcium intake to meet the skeletal demands of the heightened bone remodeling.[132]

Alkaline phosphatase levels of bone origin (BSAP) are commonly elevated in patients with significant Paget's disease because of the increased osteoblastic activity combined with bone breakdown. In the absence of liver disease, the alkaline phosphatase level typically correlates with the extent of the pagetic involvement of bone, although it may be more elevated in Paget's disease of the skull (see Fig. 92-3).

Unexpectedly, circulating osteocalcin levels do not reflect disease activity in patients with Paget's disease as well as bone specific alkaline phosphatase levels reflect disease activity. Markers of bone resorption, such as urinary collagen cross-links like N telopeptides and C telopeptides are also

Table 92-10	Indications for Treatment of Paget's Disease of Bone
Pain
Hypercalcemia
Fractures
High-output cardiac failure (rare)
Skull involvement
Neurologic compromise
Periarticular disease
Prevention of progression of Paget's disease

elevated in active Paget's disease. Other laboratory abnormalities in patients with Paget's disease include hypercalciuria, hyperuricuria, and hyperuricemia, possibly related to the increased turnover of osteoclasts. Serum uric acid levels should be measured periodically because of the association of Paget's disease with gouty arthritis.

DIAGNOSIS

Bone scans are valuable tools for assessing the extent of Paget's disease and are, therefore, useful as part of the initial evaluation.[133] As diagnostic tests, however, bone scans in general are sensitive but not specific for a number of skeletal processes. Radiographs show characteristic radiologic findings such as transverse lucent areas, osteoporosis circumscripta, enlargement of the bones, expanding lytic changes, the "blade-of-grass" lesion shown in Figure 92-4, thickened cortices, a coarse trabecular pattern, or sclerotic changes.

In patients with involvement of the skull and changes in mental status, a skull radiograph, magnetic resonance imaging (MRI), or QCT may be useful to diagnose platybasia and flattening of the base of the skull, basilar invagination, or the infrequent complication of hydrocephalus. Audiologic evaluation may reveal hearing loss in patients with pagetic involvement of the skull.

TREATMENT

The indications for treatment of Paget's disease (Table 92-10) include pain, hypercalcemia, fractures, high-output cardiac failure (rare), and neurologic compromise. Therapy can also be used to prevent the progression of deformity or risk of nerve compression when there is pagetic involvement of the skull, a vertebral body, or a weight-bearing bone (femur) or when disease is present adjacent to a major articular joint.

Treatment of symptomatic Paget's disease is usually directed at suppression of the enhanced bone resorption and skeletal turnover with calcitonin or bisphosphonates.[132,135] Response to therapy is monitored by the reduction of symptoms and maintenance of the alkaline phosphatase level in a mid-normal range, with retreatment once values rise 25% above normal.

Calcitonin

Salmon calcitonin and human calcitonin inhibit the function of osteoclasts, which are active in the pagetic process; both types of calcitonin preparations come in an injectable form and are FDA-approved for patients with Paget's disease.[136] Salmon calcitonin therapy is usually initiated at a low dose to ensure patient tolerance and then increased to a daily dose of 100 Medical Research Council units (intramuscularly or subcutaneously). After 6 months of therapy, the patient may be maintained on 50 to 100 Medical Research Council units daily.[132] Approximately two thirds of patients show a decrease in alkaline phosphatase levels of 50% or more in 2 to 6 months. Some patients experience resistance to the effects of calcitonin, which can be reversed in some instances by switching from salmon calcitonin to human calcitonin. Calcitonin is a safe drug.

Calcitonin is useful in patients with expanding lytic lesions, particularly of a weight-bearing bone, or for preoperative therapy before elective orthopedic procedures. The use of calcitonin nasal spray has few systemic side effects but is not FDA-approved for the treatment of Paget's disease.

Bisphosphonates

Several bisphosphonates are currently approved by the FDA for the treatment of Paget's disease; they include etidronate (Didronel), pamidronate (Aredia), alendronate (Fosamax), tiludronate, risedronate (Actonel), and zoledronic acid (Zometa).

Etidronate is an orally administered drug that produces a clinical and biochemical response similar to that of calcitonin.[136] The therapeutic dose for Paget's disease is 5 mg/kg per day (400 mg/day, or a minimum of 200 mg/day for smaller patients) for 6 months; the drug is then stopped for 6 months before being reinstituted in 6-month cycles of therapy.[137] As mentioned previously, higher doses of etidronate are associated with defective mineralization of bone and osteomalacia, with symptoms of pain and fractures. Measurements of alkaline phosphatase levels at 3- to 6-month intervals are useful to ensure the suppression of bone turnover; an estimated 25% of patients may become resistant to etidronate.[132] However, newer, more potent bisphosphonates are very effective for the treatment of Paget's disease.

Parenteral pamidronate is also approved for the treatment of symptomatic Paget's disease of bone in patients with a threefold or greater elevation of alkaline phosphatase concentrations. This more potent bisphosphonate is useful in patients who become resistant to etidronate and in those with more severe disease. An advantage of this therapy is that alkaline phosphatase levels may be reduced to the normal range, with a sustained response for a prolonged period (up to a year or more).[132,138]

The FDA-recommended dose of pamidronate for patients with Paget's disease is 30 mg/day as a 4-hour infusion on 3 sequential days (total dose 90 mg), with retreatment possible if necessary. Other regimens for the treatment of Paget's disease include 60 mg of pamidronate daily (infused over 3 hours) once a week for 1 or 2 weeks in patients with alkaline phosphatase levels between 300 and 400 U/L. For more extensive disease, three or four infusions of pamidronate every 1 to 2 weeks may be necessary. To assess the efficacy of these regimens for Paget's disease, clinical symptoms should be reviewed and alkaline phosphatase levels measured 2 to 3 months later.[138]

Some patients treated with pamidronate may experience a transient fever, musculoskeletal and flulike symptoms, and hypocalcemia; calcium supplementation (500 mg twice daily in vitamin D–replete patients) can offset the hypocalcemia that results from the suppression of bone resorption. Pamidronate is available only as a parenteral drug, which restricts its use.[138]

Oral alendronate has been approved for the treatment of Paget's disease at a dose of 40 mg/day for 6 months. Therapy with alendronate is recommended for patients with at least a twofold elevation in alkaline phosphatase levels or for those with specific indications for therapy (see Table 92-10). The use of alendronate produces a normalization of, or a 60% or greater reduction in, the alkaline phosphatase level in approximately 85% of patients. Studies indicate that this therapy is more effective than etidronate. (All bisphosphonates must be taken correctly to minimize gastrointestinal side effects.)[139]

Risedronate is another potent bisphosphonate (see Table 92-6) that is FDA-approved for the treatment of Paget's disease. Siris and colleagues[139] treated 162 patients with moderate to severe Paget's disease with oral risedronate (30 mg/day for 84 days, followed by 112 days without treatment). This cycle was repeated if the serum alkaline phosphatase level did not normalize or increased more than 25% from its nadir value. After the first and second cycles, the serum alkaline phosphatase level decreased 65% and 69%, respectively, and urine markers decreased 50% and 66.9%, respectively. The serum alkaline phosphatase level normalized in 53.8% of patients, and a significant decrease in bone pain was noted. Risedronate is well tolerated and has few adverse effects, including a flulike syndrome, gastrointestinal symptoms, and, rarely, iritis. Other groups have shown a decrease in serum alkaline phosphatase levels of 79% and 86%, with an 85% and 100% decrease in urine markers.[140] There is no evidence of osteomalacia in bone biopsies from patients treated with 30 mg of risedronate. Patients who have become resistant to etidronate appear to respond to risedronate. Patients must be instructed to have an adequate intake of calcium and vitamin D while taking risedronate. Recently, zoledronic acid was also found to be effective in the treatment of Paget's disease, and approval is pending from the FDA.[141]

In addition to antiresorptive therapies, nonsteroidal anti-inflammatory drugs (NSAIDs) and aspirin are useful modalities to alleviate the joint pain and other symptoms that result from degenerative joint disease. Finally, surgical intervention is sometimes warranted in patients with Paget's disease and bony deformities, pathologic fractures, nerve compression, or degenerative arthritis. Orthopedic procedures, such as total joint replacement and osteotomies, are associated with a reduced risk of intraoperative bleeding or other complications if patients are treated medically (e.g., with calcitonin or other bisphosphonates) to reduce the disease activity and vascularity for at least 6 weeks before the procedure.

OTHER MEDICATION-INDUCED OSTEOPOROSIS

Aromatase inhibitors in women undergoing breast cancer treatment are associated with bone loss. Postmenopausal women maintain a low level of circulating estrogen because of aromatization of androgens to estrogen in tissues such as fat and muscle by cytochrome P-450 enzyme. Inhibition of this enzyme is now used in postmenopausal women with breast cancer. There are two classes of aromatase inhibitors: nonsteroidal reversible inhibitors (anastrozole and letrozole) and steroidal reversible inhibitors (exemestane). Because these agents prevent the conversion of androgen to estrogen, this results in very low serum estrogen levels and increased bone remodeling. Fracture rates in clinical trials of aromatase inhibitors compared with either tamoxifen or placebo ranged from 3% to 7%.[142] In a 2-year study, significantly higher markers of bone turnover and nearly twice the lumbar spine bone loss and fracture rates were observed with anastrazole compared with tamoxifen.[142] Although the data are just beginning to be collected regarding skeletal health in women treated for breast cancer with aromatase inhibitors, it is important to obtain a history of clinical risk factors for osteoporosis and a BMD measurement of the hip and spine. Preventive treatment should be initiated in women with normal or low bone mass and no history of fractures. Treatment of women with low bone mass (T score ≤−2) should be initiated with potent antiresorptive agents, and BMD should be monitored at least every 2 years. If a woman continues to lose bone mass on aromatase inhibitors despite compliance with potent antiresorptive agents, and if the patient has not had radiation to the skeleton as part of the breast cancer protocol, rhPTH 1-34 treatment can be used to build up bone mass. At this time, studies are ongoing to evaluate the efficacy of zoledronic acid and an inhibitor of RANKL for the prevention of bone loss in women treated for breast cancer with aromatase inhibitors.[143]

Gonadotropin-releasing hormone antagonists are used to treat women with endometriosis and men with prostate cancer. These compounds induce bone loss by lowering estrogen levels, resulting in accelerated bone turnover. A study of more than 50,000 men with prostate cancer treated with androgen-deprivation therapy consisting of either gonadotropin-releasing hormone agonists or orchiectomy found an increased risk of fracture or hospitalization due to fracture. Although the overall risk of fracture associated with androgen-deprivation therapy was only modestly increased overall, the risk of fracture was significantly associated with the number of doses of gonadotropin-releasing hormone agonists. Other studies have reported that androgen-deprivation therapy increases bone loss at all sites, with a 2% to 8% annual loss in the lumbar spine and a 2% to 6% loss in the hip after 1 year.[143a] Given the high incidence of prostate cancer and the increasing use of this treatment, assessment of bone mass and the prevention of additional bone mass loss are probably appropriate. Oncologists currently recommend that BMD be measured at the time of initiation of androgen-deprivation therapy and that clinical risk factors for osteoporosis be reviewed, including history of fracture after age 30, family history of hip fracture, smoking history, use of glucocorticoids, low testosterone level, and rheumatoid arthritis. If the patient has a low BMD (T-score <−2.5) or a T-score between −1 and −2.5 and other risk factors, treatment with calcium and vitamin D supplementation and a bisphosphonate (zoledronic acid, alendronate, risedronate, pamidronate) should be initiated. BMD of the lumbar spine and hip should be measured at least once a year while patients are maintained on androgen-deprivation therapy.[144,145]

REFERENCES

1. National Osteoporosis Foundation: Osteoporos Int 4(Suppl):S7-S80, 1998.
2. Riggs BL, Melton LJI: The prevention and treatment of osteoporosis. N Engl J Med 327:620-627, 1992.
3. Riggs BL, Wahner HW, Dunn WL, et al: Differential changes in bone mineral density of the appendicular and axial skeleton with aging: Relationship to spinal osteoporosis. J Clin Invest 67:328, 1981.
4. National Osteoporosis Foundation: Physician's Guide to Prevention and Treatment of Osteoporosis. Belle Mead, NJ, Excerpta Medica, 1998.
5. Manolagas SC, Jilka RL: Bone marrow, cytokines, and bone remodeling. N Engl J Med 332:305-311, 1995.
6. Kimble RB, Kitazawa R, Vannice JL, et al: Persistent bone-sparing effect of interleukin-1 receptor antagonist: A hypothesis on the role of IL-1 in ovariectomy-induced bone loss. Calcif Tissue Int 55:260-265, 1996.
7. Cheleuitte D, Mizuno S, Glowacki J: In vitro secretion of cytokines by human bone marrow: Effects of age and estrogen status. J Clin Endocrinol Metab 83:2043-2051, 1998.
8. Boyce BF, Hughes RD, Wright KR: Recent advances in bone biology provide insights in the pathogenesis of bone disease. Lab Invest 79:83-94, 1999.
9. McClung MR, Lewiecki EM, Cohen SB, et al: Denosumab in postmenopausal women with low bone mineral density. N Engl J Med 354:821-831, 2006.
10. Nevitt MC: Epidemiology of osteoporosis. Osteoporosis 20:535-554, 1994.
11. El-Hajj Fuleihan G, Gundberg CM, Gleason R, et al: Racial differences in parathyroid hormone dynamics. J Clin Endocrinol Metab 79:1642-1647, 1994.
12. Bell NH, Shary J, Stevens J: Demonstration that bone mass is greater in black than in white children. J Bone Miner Res 6:719-723, 1991.
13. Sambrook PN, Kelly PJ, Morrison NA, et al: Scientific review: Genetics of osteoporosis. Br J Rheumatol 33:1007-1011, 1994.
14. **Cummings SR, Nevitt MC, Browner WS, et al: Risk factors for hip fracture in white women. N Engl J Med 332:767-773, 1995.**
15. Uitterlinden AG, Burger H, Huang Q, et al: Relation of alleles of the collagen type 1α1 gene to bone density and the risk of osteoporotic fractures in postmenopausal women. N Engl J Med 338:1016-1021, 1998.
16. Faulkner KG, Cummings SR, Black D, et al: Simple measurement of femoral geometry predicts hip fracture: The study of osteoporotic fractures. J Bone Miner Res 8:1211-1217, 1993.
17. Little RD, Carulli JP, Del Mastro RG, et al: A mutation in the LDL receptor-related protein 5 gene results in the autosomal dominant high-bone mass trait. Am J Hum Genet 70:11-19, 2002.
18. Boyden LM, Mao J, Belsky J, et al: High bone density due to a mutation in LDL-receptor protein 5. N Engl J Med 346:1513-1521, 2002.
19. Lane NE, Lukert BP: The science and therapy of glucocorticoid-induced osteoporosis. Endocrinol Metab Clin North Am 27:465-483, 1998.
20. Ross DS, Neer RM, Ridgway EC: Subclinical hyperthyroidism and reduced bone density as a possible result of prolonged suppression of the pituitary-thyroid axis with L-thyroxine. Am J Med 82:1167-1170, 1987.
21. Biller BMK, Saxe V, Herzog DB, et al: Mechanisms of osteoporosis in adult and adolescent women with anorexia nervosa. J Clin Endocrinol Metab 68:548-551, 1989.
22. Friedman AJ, Daly M, Juneau-Norcross M, et al: A prospective, randomized trial of gonadotropin-releasing hormone agonist plus estrogen-progestin add-back regimens for women with leiomyomata uteri. J Clin Endocrinol Metab 76:1439-1445, 1993.
23. Gordon CM, Grace E, Emans SJ, et al: Changes in bone turnover markers and menstrual function after short-term oral DHEA in young women with anorexia nervosa. J Bone Miner Res 14:136-145, 1999.
24. Orwoll ES: Osteoporosis in men: Primer on the Metabolic Bone Diseases and Disorders of Mineral Metabolism, 6th ed. American Society of Bone and Mineral Research, 2006, pp 290-292.
25. Leder BZ, leBlanc A, Schoenfeld DA, et al: Differential effects of androgens and estrogens on bone turnover in normal men. J Clin Endocrinol Metab 88:204-210, 2003.
26. Sambrook PN, Ansell BM, Foster S, et al: Bone turnover in early rheumatoid arthritis. II. Longitudinal bone density studies. Ann Rheum Dis 44:580-584, 1985.

27. Rehman Q, Lane NE: Therapeutic approaches for preventing bone loss in inflammatory arthritis. Arthritis Res 3:221-227, 2001.

28. Gravallese EM, Goldring SR: Cellular mechanisms and the role of cytokines in bone erosions in rheumatoid arthritis. Arthritis Rheum 43:2143-2151, 2000.

29. Kong YY, Yoshida H, Sarosi I, et al: OPGL is a key regulator of osteoclastogenesis, lymphocyte development and lymph-node organogenesis. Nature 397:316-323, 1999.

30. **American College of Rheumatologists Task Force on Osteoporosis Guidelines: Recommendations for the prevention and treatment of glucocorticoid-induced osteoporosis: 2001 update. Arthritis Rheum 44:1496-1503, 2001.**

31. Hansen M, Florescu A, Stoltenberg M, et al: Bone loss in rheumatoid arthritis: Influence of disease activity, duration of the disease, functional capacity, and corticosteroid treatment. Scand J Rheumatol 25:367-376, 1996.

32. LeBoff MS, Wade JP, Mackowiak S, et al: Low dose prednisone does not affect calcium homeostasis or bone density in postmenopausal women with rheumatoid arthritis. J Rheumatol 18:339-344, 1991.

33. Hunter T, Dubo HI: Spinal fractures complicating ankylosing spondylitis: A longterm follow-up study. Arthritis Rheum 26:751-759, 1983.

34. Lane NE. Osteoporosis and osteonecrosis in systemic lupus erythematous. Nat Clin Pract Rheumatol 2:562-569, 2006.

35. Stowens DW, Teitelbaum SL, Kahn AJ, et al: Skeletal complications of Gaucher disease. Medicine 64:310-322, 1985.

36. Movsowitz C, Epstein S, Fallon M, et al: Cyclosporin-A in vivo produces severe osteopenia in the rat: Effect of dose and duration of administration. Endocrinology 123:2571-2577, 1988.

37. Bryer HP, Isserow JA, Armstrong EC, et al: Azathioprine alone is bone sparing and does not alter cyclosporin A-induced osteopenia in the rat. J Bone Miner Res 10:132-138, 1995.

38. Rich GM, Mudge GH, Laffel GL, et al: Cyclosporine A and prednisone-associated osteoporosis in heart transplant recipients. J Heart Lung Transplant 11:950-958, 1992.

39. LeBoff MS, Kohlmeier L, Hurwitz S, et al: Occult vitamin D deficiency in postmenopausal US women with acute hip fracture. JAMA 281:1505-1511, 1999.

40. Johnston CC Jr, Slemenda CW, Melton LJ III: Clinical use of bone densitometry. N Engl J Med 324:1105-1109, 1991.

41. El-Hajj Fuleihan G, Testa MA, Angell JE, et al: Reproducibility of DXA absorptiometry: A model for bone loss estimates. J Bone Miner Res 10:1004-1014, 1995.

42. Melton LJ, Atkinson EJ, O'Fallon WM, et al: Long-term fracture prediction by bone mineral assessed at different skeletal sites. J Bone Miner Res 8:1227-1233, 1993.

43. Cummings SR, Black DM, Nevitt MC, et al: Bone density at various sites for prediction of hip fractures: The Study of Osteoporotic Fractures Research Group. Lancet 341:72-75, 1993.

44. Stewart A, Reid DM, Porter RW: Broadband ultrasound attenuation and dual energy x-ray absorptiometry in patients with hip fractures: Which technique discriminates fracture risk? Calcif Tissue Int 54:466, 1994.

45. Kanis JA, Melton LJ III, Christiansen C, et al: Perspective: The diagnosis of osteoporosis. J Bone Miner Res 9:1137-1141, 1994.

46. Kanis JA, Borgstrom F, De Laet C, et al: Assessment of fracture risk. Osteoporos Int 16:581-589, 2005.

47. Hannon RA, Eastell R: Bone markers and current laboratory assays. Cancer Treat Rev 32(Suppl 1):7, 2004.

48. Uebelhart D, Schlemmer A, Johansen JS, et al: Effect of menopause and hormone replacement therapy on the urinary excretion of pyridinium cross-links. J Clin Endocrinol Metab 72:367-373, 1991.

49. Delmas PD, Schlemmer A, Gineyts E, et al: Rapid publication: Urinary excretion of pyridinoline crosslinks correlates with bone turnover measured on iliac crest biopsy in patients with vertebral osteoporosis. J Bone Miner Res 6:639-644, 1991.

50. Rosen HN, Dresner-Pollak R, Moses AC, et al: Specificity of urinary excretion of cross-linked N-telopeptides of type I collagen as a marker of bone turnover. Calcif Tissue Int 54:26-29, 1994.

51. Garnero P, Hausherr E, Chapuy MC, et al: Markers of bone resorption predict hip fracture risk in elderly women: The EPIDOS Prospective Study. J Bone Miner Res 11:1531-1538, 1996.

52. Seibel MJ, Naganathan V, Barton I, Grauer A: Relationship between pretreatment bone resorption and vertebral fracture incidence in postmenopausal osteoporotic women treated with risedronate. J Bone Miner Res 19:323-329, 2004.

53. Lane NE, Sanchez S, Genant HK, et al: Short-term increases in bone turnover markers predict parathyroid hormone-induced spinal bone mineral density gains in postmenopausal women with glucocorticoid-induced osteoporosis. Osteoporos Int 11:434-442, 2000.

54. Buxton EC, Yao W, Lane N: Changes in serum receptor activator of nuclear factor-kappaB ligand, osteoprotegerin, and interleukin-6 levels in patients with glucocorticoid-induced osteoporosis treated with human parathyroid hormone (1-34). J Clin Endocrinol Metab 89:3332-3336, 2004.

55. Cosman F, Nieves J, Woeflert I: Alendronate does not block the anabolic effect of PTH in postmenopausal osteoporotic women. J Bone Miner Res 13:1051-1055, 1998.

56. Silverberg SJ, Gartenberg F, Jacobs TP, et al: Increased bone mineral density after parathyroidectomy in primary hyperparathyroidism. J Clin Endocrinol Metab 80:729-734, 1995.

57. Silverberg SJ, Gartenberg F, Jacobs TP, et al: Longitudinal measurements of bone density and biochemical indices in untreated primary hyperparathyroidism. J Clin Endocrinol Metab 80:723-728, 1995.

58. Dawson-Hughes B, Dallal GE, Krall EA, et al: A controlled trial of the effect of calcium supplementation on bone density in postmenopausal women. N Engl J Med 323:878-883, 1990.

59. Atkinson SA, Abrams SA, Dawson-Hughes B, et al: Calcium. In Young V (ed): Dietary Reference Intake for Calcium, Phosphorus, Magnesium, Vitamin D and Fluoride. Washington, DC, National Academy Press, 1997, pp 91-143.

60. Optimal calcium intake: NIH Consensus Conference. JAMA 272:1942-1947, 1994.

61. Nicar MJ, Pak CYC: Calcium bioavailability from calcium carbonate and calcium citrate. J Clin Endocrinol Metab 61:391-393, 1985.

62. **Hulley S, Grady D, Bush T, et al: Randomized trial of estrogen plus progestin for secondary prevention of coronary heart disease in postmenopausal women. JAMA 280:605-613, 1998.**

63. Grady D, Herrington D, Bittner V, et al: Cardiovascular disease outcomes during 6.8 years of hormone therapy: Heart and Estrogen/Progestin Replacement Study follow-up (HERS II). JAMA 288:58-66, 2002.

64. Writing Group for the Women's Health Initiative Investigators: Risk and benefits of estrogen plus progestin in healthy postmenopausal women: Principal results from the Women's Health Initiative randomized controlled trial. JAMA 288:321-333, 2002.

65. Love RR, Mazess RB, Barden HS, et al: Effects of tamoxifen on bone mineral density in postmenopausal women with breast cancer. N Engl J Med 326:852-856, 1992.

66. Fisher B, Costantino JP, Wicherham DL, et al: Tamoxifen for prevention of breast cancer: Report of the National Surgical Adjuvant Breast and Bowel Project P-1 Study. J Natl Cancer Inst 90:1371-1388, 1998.

67. Cummings SR, Eckert S, Krueger KA, et al: The effect of raloxifene on risk of breast cancer in postmenopausal women: Results from the MORE randomized trial. Multiple Outcomes of Raloxifene Evaluation. JAMA 281:2189-2197, 1999.

68. Delmas P, Bjarnason NH, Mitlak B, et al: Effects of raloxifene on bone mineral density, serum cholesterol concentrations, and uterine endometrium in postmenopausal women. N Engl J Med 337:1641-1647, 1997.

69. **Ettinger B, Black D, Mitlak B, et al: Reduction of vertebral fracture risk in postmenopausal women with osteoporosis treated with raloxifene: Results from 3 year randomized clinical trial (MORE). JAMA 282:637-645, 1999.**

70. Walsh BW, Kuller LH, Wild RA, et al: Effects of raloxifene on serum lipids and coagulation factors in healthy postmenopausal women. JAMA 279:1445-1451, 1998.

71. Walsh BW, Paul S, Wild RA, et al: The effects of hormone replacement therapy and raloxifene on C-reactive protein and homocystein in healthy postmenopausal women: A randomized controlled trial. J Clin Endocrinol Metab 85:214-218, 2000.

72. Ridker PM, Buring JE, Shin J, et al: Prospective study of C-reactive protein and the risk of future cardiovascular events among apparently healthy women. Circulation 98:731-733, 1998.

73. Barrett-Connor E, Mosca L, Collins P, et al: Raloxifene Use for the Heart (RUTH) Trial Investigators. Effects of raloxifene on cardiovascular events and breast cancer in postmenopausal women. N Engl J Med 355:125-137, 2006.

74. Vogel VG, Costantino JP, Wickerham DL, et al: National Surgical Adjuvant Breast and Bowel Project (NSABP). Effects of tamoxifen vs raloxifene on the risk of developing invasive breast cancer and other disease outcomes: The NSABP Study of Tamoxifen and Raloxifene (STAR) P-2 trial. JAMA 295:2727-2741, 2006.

75. Bradbury J: CORE breast-cancer prevention trial. Lancet Oncol 6:8, 2005.

76. Tenover JL: Male hormone replacement therapy including "Andropause." Endocrinol Metab Clin North Am 27:969-988, 1998.

77. Gennari C, Chierichetti SM, Bigazzi S, et al: Comparative effects on bone mineral content of calcium and calcium plus salmon calcitonin given in two different regimens in postmenopausal osteoporosis. Curr Ther Res 38:455-464, 1985.

78. Overgaard K, Riis BJ, Christiansen C, et al: Nasal calcitonin for treatment of established osteoporosis. Clin Endocrinol 30:435-442, 1989.

79. Chesnut C, Silverman S, Andriono K, et al: A randomized trial of nasal spray salmon calcitonin in postmenopausal women with established osteoporosis: The Prevent Recurrence of Osteoporotic Fractures Study. PROOF Study Group. Am J Med 109:267-276, 2000.

80. Harris ST, Watts NB, Jackson RD, et al: Four-year study of intermittent cyclic etidronate treatment of postmenopausal osteoporosis: Three years of blinded therapy followed by one year of open therapy. Am J Med 95:557-567, 1993.

81. Liberman UA, Weiss SR, Broll J, et al: Effect of oral alendronate on bone mineral density and the incidence of fractures in postmenopausal osteoporosis. N Engl J Med 333:1437-1443, 1995.

82. **Black DM, Cummings SR, Karpt DB, et al: Randomized trial of effect of alendronate on risk of fracture in women with existing vertebral fractures. Lancet 348:1535-1541, 1996.**

83. Hosking D, Chilvers CE, Christiansen C, et al: Prevention of bone loss with alendronate in postmenopausal women under 60 years of age. N Engl J Med 338:485-492, 1998.

84. Cummings SR, Black DM, Thompson DE, et al: Effect of alendronate on risk of fracture in women with low bone density but without vertebral fractures. JAMA 280:2077-2082, 1998.

85. Orwoll E, Ettinger M, Weiss S, et al: Alendronate for the treatment of osteoporosis in men. N Engl J Med 343:604-610, 2000.

86. Schnitzer T, Bone HG, Crepaldi G, et al: Therapeutic equivalence of alendronate 70 mg once-weekly and alendronate 10 mg daily in the treatment of osteoporosis. Aging 12:1-12, 2000.

87. Harris ST, Watts NB, Genant HK, et al: Effects of risedronate treatment on vertebral and nonvertebral fractures in women with postmenopausal osteoporosis: A randomized controlled trial. Vertebral Efficacy with Risedronate Therapy (VERT) Study Group. JAMA 282:1344, 1999.

88. Heaney RP, Zizic TM, Fogelman I, et al: Risedronate reduces the risk of first vertebral fracture in osteoporotic women. Osteoporos Int 13:501-505, 2002.

89. Reginster J-Y, Minne HW, Sorensen O, et al: Randomized trial of the effects of risedronate on vertebral fractures in women with postmenopausal osteoporosis. Osteoporos Int 11:83-91, 2000.

90. McClung MR, Geusens P, Miller PD, et al: Effect of risedronate on the risk of hip fracture in elderly women. N Engl J Med 344:333-340, 2001.

91. Delaney M, Harwitz S, Shaw J, LeBoff MS: Bone density changes with once weekly risedronate in postmenopausal women. J Clin Densitom 6:45-50, 2003.

92. Miller PD, Brown JP, Siris ES: A randomized double-blind trial of risedronate and etidronate in the treatment of Paget's disease of bone. Am J Med 106:513-520, 1999.

93. Reginster JY, Adami S, Lakatos P, et al: Efficacy and tolerability of once-monthly oral ibandronate in postmenopausal osteoporosis: 2 year results from the MOBILE study. Ann Rheum Dis 65:654-661, 2006.

94. Delmas PD, Adami S, Strugala C, et al: Intravenous ibandronate injections in postmenopausal women with osteoporosis: One-year results from the dosing intravenous administration study. Arthritis Rheum 54:1838-1846, 2006.

94a. Reid IR, Brown JP, Burckhardt P, et al: Intravenous zoledronic acid in postmenopausal women with low bone density. N Engl J Med 36:653-661, 2002.

95. **Black DM, Delmas PD, Eastell R, et al: Once-yearly zoledronic acid for treatment of postmenopausal osteoporosis. N Engl J Med 356:1809-1822, 2007.**

96. Finkelstein JS, Klibanski A, Arnold A, et al: Prevention of estrogen deficiency-related bone loss with human parathyroid hormone (1-34). JAMA 280:1067-1073, 1998.

97. Lindsay R, Nieves J, Formica C, et al: Randomized controlled study of effect of parathyroid hormone on vertebral-bone mass and fracture incidence among postmenopausal women on oestrogen with osteoporosis. Lancet 350:550-555, 1997.

98. **Neer RM, Arnaud CD, Zanchetta JR, et al: Effect of parathyroid hormone (1-34) on fractures and bone mineral density in postmenopausal women with osteoporosis. N Engl J Med 344:1434-1441, 2001.**

99. Kurland ES, Cosman F, McMahon DJ, et al: Parathyroid hormone as a therapy for idiopathic osteoporosis in men: Effects on bone mineral density and bone markers. J Clin Endocrinol Metab 85:2129-2134, 2000.

100. Black DM, Greenspan SL, Ensrud KE, et al: The effects of parathyroid hormone and alendronate alone or in combination in postmenopausal osteoporosis. N Engl J Med 349:1207-1215, 2003.

101. Finkelstein JS, Hayes A, Hunzelman JL, et al: The effects of parathyroid hormone, alendronate, or both in men with osteoporosis. N Engl J Med 349:1216-1226, 2003.

102. Cosman F, Nieves J, Zion M, et al: Daily and cyclic parathyroid hormone in women receiving alendronate. N Engl J Med 353:566-575, 2005.

103. Black DM, Bilezikian JP, Ensrud KE, et al: One year of alendronate after one year of parathyroid hormone (1-84) for osteoporosis. N Engl J Med 353:555-565, 2005.

104. Deal C, Omizo M, Schwartz EN, et al: Combination teriparatide and raloxifene therapy for postmenopausal osteoporosis: Results from a 6-month double-blind placebo-controlled trial. J Bone Miner Res 20:1905-1911, 2005.

105. Thomas MK, Lloyd-Jones DM, Thadhani RI, et al: Hypovitaminosis D in medical inpatients. N Engl J Med 338:777-783, 1998.

105a. Chapay MC, Arlot ME, Duboeuf F, et al: Vitamin D and calcium to prevent hip fractures in elderly women. N Engl J Med 327:1637-1642, 1992.

106. Dawson-Hughes B, Harris SS, Krall EA, et al: Effect of calcium and vitamin D supplementation on bone density in men and women 65 years of age or older. N Engl J Med 337:670-676, 1997.

107. van Staa TP: The pathogenesis, epidemiology and management of glucocorticoid-induced osteoporosis. Calcif Tissue Int 79:129-137, 2006.

108. Adinoff AD, Hollister JR: Steroid-induced fractures and bone loss in patients with asthma. N Engl J Med 309:265-268, 1983.

109. **Saag HG, Emkey R, Schnitzer TJ, et al: Aledronate for the prevention and treatment of glucocorticoid-induced osteoporosis. N Engl J Med 339:292-299, 1998.**

110. Cohen S, Levy RM, Keller M, et al: Risedronate therapy prevents corticosteroid-induced bone loss. Arthritis Rheum 42:2309-2318, 1999.

111. Reid DM, Hughes RA, Laan R, et al: Efficacy and safety of daily risedronate in the treatment of corticosteroid-induced osteoporosis in men and women: A randomized trial. J Bone Miner Res 15:1006-1013, 2000.

112. Boutsen Y, Jamart J, Esselinckx W, Devogelaer JP: Primary prevention of glucocorticoid-induced osteoporosis with intravenous pamidronate and calcium: A prospective controlled 1-year study comparing a single infusion, an infusion given once every 3 months, and calcium alone. J Bone Miner Res 16:104-112, 2001.

113. Lukert BP, Johnson BE, Robinson RG: Estrogen and progesterone replacement therapy reduces glucocorticoid-induced bone loss. J Bone Miner Res 7:1063-1069, 1992.

114. Petri MA, Lahita RG, Van Vollenhoven RF, et al: Effects of prasterone on corticosteroid requirements of women with systemic lupus erythmatosus: A double blind, randomized, placebo-controlled trial. Arthritis Rheum 46:1820-1829, 2002.

115. Meese PJ, Ginzler EM, Gluck OS, et al: Improvement in bone mineral density in steroid-treated SLE patients during treatment with prasterone (DHEA). Arthritis Rheum 43(Suppl I):S206, 2000.

116. Reid IR, Ibbertson HK, France JT, et al: Plasma testosterone concentrations in asthmatic men treated with glucocorticoids. BMJ 291:574, 1985.

117. Reid IR, Wattie DJ, Evans MC, et al: Testosterone therapy in gluco-corticoid-treated men. Arch Intern Med 156:1173-1178, 1996.

118. **Lane NE, Sanchez S, Modin GW, et al: Parathyroid hormone treatment can reverse corticosteroid-induced osteoporosis. J Clin Invest 102:1627-1633, 1998.**

119. Lane NE, Sanchez S, Genant HK, et al: Bone mass continues to increase at the hip after parathyroid hormone treatment is discontinued in postmenopausal women with glucocorticoid-induced osteoporosis. J Bone Miner Res 15: 994, 2001.

120. Rehman Q, Lang T, Lane NE: Daily treatment with parathyroid hormone is associated with an increase in vertebral cross-sectional area in postmenopausal women with glucocorticoid-induced osteoporosis. Osteoporos Int 41:374-382, 2003.

121. Wang WQ, Ip MS, Tsang KW, Lam KS: Antiresorptive therapy in asthmatic patients receiving high-dose inhaled steroids: A prospective study for 18 months. J Allergy Clin Immunol 101:445-450, 1998.

122. Sosa M, Saavedra P, Valero C, et al: Inhaled steroids do not decrease bone mineral density but increase risk of fractures: Data from the GIUMO Study Group. J Clin Densitom 9:154-158, 2006.

123. Frame B, Parfitt AM: Osteomalacia: Current concepts. Ann Intern Med 89:966-982, 1978.

124. Holick MF, Garabedian M: Vitamin D: Photobiology, metabolism, mechanism of action, and clinical applications. In Primer on the Metabolic Bone Diseases and Disorders of Mineral Metabolism, 2006, pp 106-114.

125. Streeten EA, Levine MA: Hyperparathyroidism and hypoparathyroidism. In Rakel RE (ed): Conn's Current Therapy. Philadelphia, WB Saunders, 2000, pp 627-634.

126. Hruska KA, Teitelbaum SL: Renal osteodystrophy. N Engl J Med 333:166-174, 1995.

127. Felsenfeld AJ, Llach F: Parathyroid gland function in chronic renal failure. Kidney Int 43:771-789, 1993.

128. Econs MJ, Rowe PS, Francis F, et al: Fine structure mapping of the human X-linked hypophosphatemic rickets gene locus. J Clin Endocrinol Metab 79:1351-1354, 1994.

129. Ryan EA, Reiss E: Oncogenous osteomalacia: Review of the world literature of 42 cases and report of two new cases. Am J Med 77: 501-512, 1984.

130. Drezner MK, Lyles KW, Haussler MR, et al: Evaluation of a role for 1,25-dihydroxyvitamin D_3 in the pathogenesis and treatment of X-linked hypophosphatemic rickets and osteomalacia. J Clin Invest 66:1020-1032, 1980.

131. Quarles LD, Davidai GA, Schwab SJ, et al: Oral calcitriol and calcium: Efficient therapy for uremic hyperparathyroidism. Kidney Int 34:840-844, 1988.

132. Siris ES: Extensive personal experience: Paget's disease of bone. J Clin Endocrinol Metab 80:335-338, 1995.

133. Siris ES, Chines AA, Altman RD, et al: Risedronate in the treatment of Paget's disease of bone: An open label, multicenter study. J Bone Miner Res 13:1032-1038, 1998.

134. Whyte MP, Obrecht SE, Finnegan PM, et al: Osteoprotegrin deficiency and juvenile Paget's disease. N Engl J Med 347:175-184, 2002.

135. LeBoff MS, El-Hajj Fuleihan G, Brown EM: Osteoporosis and Paget's disease of bone. In Branch WT (ed): Office Practice of Medicine, 3rd ed. Philadelphia, WB Saunders, 1994, pp 700-714.

136. DeRose J, Singer FR, Avramides A, et al: Response of Paget's disease to porcine and salmon calcitonins: Effects of long-term treatment. Am J Med 56:858-866, 1974.

137. Krane SM: Etidronate disodium in the treatment of Paget's disease of bone. Ann Intern Med 96:619-625, 1982.

138. Gallacher SJ, Boyce BF, Patel U, et al: Clinical experience with pamidronate in the treatment of Paget's disease of bone. Ann Rheum Dis 50:930-933, 1991.

139. Siris E, Weinstein RS, Altman R, et al: Comparative study of alendronate versus etidronate for the treatment of Paget's disease of bone. J Clin Endocrinol Metab 81:961-967, 1996.

140. Hosking DJ, Eusabio RA, Chines AA: Paget's disease of bone: Reduction of disease activity with oral risedronate. Bone 22:51-55, 1998.

141. **Reid IR, Miller P, Lyles K, et al: Comparison of a single infusion of zoledronic acid with risedronate for Paget's disease. N Engl J Med 353:898-908, 2005.**

142. Eastell R, Hannon RA, Cuzick J, et al: Effect of an aromatase inhibitor on BMD and bone turnover markers: 2-year results of the Anastrozole, Tamoxifen, Alone or in Combination (ATAC) trial (18233230). J Bone Miner Res 21:1215-1223, 2006.

143. Eastell R, Hannon R: Long-term effects of aromatase inhibitors on bone. J Steroid Biochem Mol Biol 95:151-154, 2005.

143a. Smith MR, Boyce SP, Moyneur E, et al: Risk of clinical fractures after GNRH agonist therapy for prostate cancer. J Urol 175:136-139, 2006.

144. Diamond TH, Higano CS, Smith MR, et al: Osteoporosis in men with prostate carcinoma receiving androgen-deprivation therapy: Recommendations for diagnosis and therapies. Cancer 100:892, 2004.

145. Shahinian VB, Kuo YF, Freeman JL, Goodwin JS: Risk of fracture after androgen deprivation for prostate cancer. N Engl J Med 352:154-164, 2005.

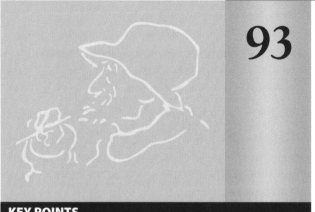

93

Proliferative Bone Diseases

REUVEN MADER

KEY POINTS

Although diffuse idiopathic skeletal hyperostosis (DISH) usually is defined by the presence of large flowing osteophytes connecting at least four vertebrae, typically in the thoracic spine, the disease often involves the cervical and lumbar spine and peripheral joints, especially entheses.

The etiology of DISH is unclear, but it is associated with a variety of metabolic abnormalities, many of which are also seen in type 2 diabetes.

Treatment of spinal DISH is mostly symptomatic, but patients and physicians need to be aware of the increased fracture risk of these patients.

Patients with DISH are at increased risk for heterotopic bone formation after joint surgery, and appropriate prophylactic measures should be carried out.

Because of the metabolic abnormalities associated with DISH, many of which also are cardiac risk factors, the discovery of the disease, such as an incidental finding on chest x-ray, should prompt careful evaluation of known cardiovascular risk factors.

Hypertrophic osteoarthropathy can be seen in many conditions, but growth factors such as platelet-derived growth factor and vascular endothelial growth factor are implicated as the common etiology of most, if not all, cases.

Hypertrophic osteoarthropathy usually responds dramatically to effective treatment of the primary disease, such as surgical resection of a lung carcinoma.

Proliferative bone diseases encompass a variety of conditions characterized by exuberant bone and entheseal ossifications and calcifications. New bone formation is the main feature in diffuse idiopathic skeletal hyperostosis (DISH) and hypertrophic osteoarthropathy (HOA) and is a common finding in osteoarthritis. New bone formation also may accompany some seronegative spondyloarthropathies, such as ankylosing spondylitis, psoriatic arthritis, and sternoclavicular syndrome, also known as SAPHO (synovitis, acne, pustulosis, hyperostosis, and osteomyelitis). New bone formation also has been described in endocrine diseases, however, such as thyroid disorders, acromegaly, and hypoparathyroidism (Table 93-1).[1-3] Osteoarthritis, seronegative spondyloarthropathies, and endocrine disorders are discussed elsewhere in this book.

DIFFUSE IDIOPATHIC SKELETAL HYPEROSTOSIS

DISH is a condition characterized by calcification and ossification of soft tissues, mainly ligaments and entheses. This condition was described by Forestier and Rotes-Querol

in 1950,[4] and was termed *senile ankylosing hyperostosis*. There is a marked predilection to the axial skeleton, particularly the thoracic spine. Recognition that the condition is not limited to the spine and may involve peripheral joints led researchers to coin the name DISH, a term now widely used.[5]

DISH is characterized by the production of coarse, flowing osteophytes involving, in particular, the right side of the thoracic spine with preservation of the intervertebral disk space, and by ossification of the anterior longitudinal ligament. Calcification and ossification of the posterior longitudinal ligament seem to be additional skeletal manifestations of DISH. Other entheseal regions might be affected, such as the peripatellar ligaments, Achilles tendon insertion, plantar fascia, olecranon, and others.[6-8]

The diagnosis usually is based on the definition suggested by Resnick and Niwayama.[5] This radiographic approach requires the presence of flowing, coarse osteophytes on the right side of the thoracic spine, connecting at least four contiguous vertebrae, or ossification of the anterior longitudinal ligament, preserved intervertebral disk height in the involved segment, and the absence of apophyseal joint ankylosis and sacroiliac joint involvement (Table 93-2).[8] Another set of criteria, for epidemiologic purposes, was suggested by Utsinger.[7] These criteria consider also peripheral enthesopathies. A definite diagnosis of DISH is established by criteria similar to those suggested by Resnick and Niwayama. A probable diagnosis of DISH is possible, however, with continuous ossification or calcification, or both, of the anterolateral aspect of at least two contiguous vertebral bodies and bilateral well-corticated enthesopathies in the heel, olecranon, and patella.

EPIDEMIOLOGY

DISH is more common in men than women. An autopsy study reported that in a series of 75 spines studied at autopsy, 28% had DISH.[9] The reported prevalence of DISH varies according to age, ethnic origin, geographic location, and clinical setting (i.e., hospital-based versus population-based). In a study of a North American metropolitan hospital population, the prevalence in men and women older than 50 years of age was reported to be 25% and 15%, respectively, and the prevalence in men and women older than 70 years was 35% and 26%, respectively.[10] Similar figures were reported for patients from Budapest.[11] Higher figures were reported for Jews older than 40 years living in Jerusalem, reaching a prevalence of 46% for men older than 80.[12] A much smaller prevalence was reported from Korea, barely reaching 9% in the older age group.[13] Native Africans had a prevalence of 13.6% in patients older than 70 years of age with no difference

Table 93-1 Proliferative Bone Diseases

Diffuse idiopathic skeletal hyperostosis
Hypertrophic osteoarthropathy
Thyroid disorders
Acromegaly
Hypoparathyroidism
Seronegative spondyloarthropathies (i.e., psoriatic arthritis, ankylosing spondylitis, SAPHO)
Osteoarthritis

SAPHO, synovitis, acne, pustulosis, hyperostosis, and osteomyelitis.

Table 93-2 Suggested Diagnostic Criteria for Diffuse Idiopathic Skeletal Hyperostosis

Flowing calcification and ossification along the anterolateral aspect of at least four contiguous vertebral bodies
Preservation of intervertebral disk height in the involved vertebral segment and absence of extensive radiographic changes of degenerative disk disease
Absence of apophyseal joint bony ankylosis and sacroiliac joint erosion, sclerosis, or intra-articular osseous fusion

Table 93-3 Conditions Associated with Diffuse Idiopathic Skeletal Hyperostosis

Non–insulin-dependent diabetes mellitus
Obesity
High waist circumference ratio
Dyslipidemia
Hypertension
Hyperuricemia
Hyperinsulinemia
Elevated insulin-like growth factor-1
Elevated growth hormone
Use of retinoids
Genetic predisposition

between men and women.[14] In population-based, as opposed to hospital-based, studies, the reported prevalence was slightly greater than 10% in patients older than 70 years of age.[15] Mild DISH was found in human remains dating back 4000 years. In human remains from the 6th to 8th century, the prevalence of DISH was higher in men than in women, reaching 3.7%. Although these studies were performed on different and relatively young populations, it seems that the prevalence of DISH is increasing.[16,17]

ETIOLOGY AND PATHOGENESIS

The etiology of DISH is unknown. Several metabolic, genetic, and constitutional factors were reported to be associated with this condition, however, including obesity, a high waist circumference ratio, hypertension, diabetes mellitus, hyperinsulinemia, dyslipidemia, elevated growth hormone levels, elevated insulin-like growth factor (IGF)-I, hyperuricemia, use of retinoids, and genetic factors (Table 93-3).[18-28]

The association of DISH with excess body weight is well known since the early descriptions by Forestier and others.[9,29] This association was reiterated in a study in which patients with DISH were compared with healthy individuals and patients with spondylosis.[30] The association of DISH with diabetes mellitus was reported in several studies.[23,26] It was reported more recently that the prevalence of DISH is no higher in diabetic patients than in nondiabetic subjects suggesting re-evaluation of diabetes as a risk factor for the development of DISH.[31] More often, DISH was reported to be associated with more complex metabolic and endocrine derangements, with or without overt type 2 diabetes mellitus, comprising glucose intolerance, hyperinsulinemia, dyslipidemia, hyperuricemia, and elevated levels of growth hormone and IGF-I.[18-20,23]

Hyperinsulinemia has a profound effect on ligaments and entheses, which is independent of age and obesity. The differentiation of mesenchymal cells in ligaments into chondrocytes and the subsequent enchondral ossification is promoted by insulin.[24] The enthesis provides the growth plate for tendons and ligaments in children and persists into adulthood. This particular structure is composed of collagen fibers, fibroblasts, chondrocytes, and calcified matrix, which is probably a target for the ossification process promoted by insulin.[19] Bone morphogenetic protein-2 is a potent osteogenic factor that promotes differentiation of mesenchymal stem cells into osteoblasts and chondroblasts. It stimulates cell proliferation, alkaline phosphatase (ALP) activity, and collagen synthesis.[32,33] Its ability to promote mineralization is inhibited by matrix Gla protein, which is highly expressed in bone and cartilage. Matrix Gla protein deficiency or its altered carboxylation may cause a high level of bone morphogenetic protein-2 activity that leads to hyperostosis.[27]

The enthesis also may be under the influence of other growth-promoting peptides. Elevated growth hormone levels were reported in DISH. Growth hormone is capable of inducing osteoblast cell proliferation and may promote local production of IGF-I, which mediates the action of growth hormone and can stimulate ALP activity in osteoblasts.[20,27,34,35] ALP promotes the calcification process during bone formation and is considered a good indicator for the maturation stages of osteoblasts.[36] There is no explanation yet as to why the new bone formation is localized mainly at the ligamentous and entheseal sites. In male DISH patients, growth hormone serum levels were not elevated in the serum, but were much higher in the synovial fluid.[37] In the spine, vertebral blood supply could be a factor in the onset or progression of DISH.[38] Intraerythrocyte growth hormone levels may exceed serum growth hormone levels and could be transported to the vertebral site by the mechanism described by Denko and colleagues.[39]

The expression of various genes involved in cell division and growth is regulated by nuclear factor κB (NFκB), which is capable of regulating the differentiation of multipotential cells. It was shown that activation of environmental factors such as platelet-derived growth factor (PDGF)-BB and transforming growth factor (TGF)-β1 in ligament cells stimulates the activation of NFκB, which influences the osteoblastic differentiation of mesenchymal cells. This event is accompanied by elevation of ALP activity in cells of patients with DISH and serves as an indicator of maturation stages of the osteoblast.[36] Inflammatory cytokines such as PDGF-BB, TGF-β1, and others may be related to the onset of non–insulin-dependent diabetes mellitus and may be the link between this condition and the occurrence of DISH.[40,41]

Vitamin A and its derivatives have been implicated in the pathogenesis of DISH owing to their ability to promote new bone formation. Levels of vitamin A were reported to be higher in patients with DISH compared with controls, and some reports showed DISH-like manifestations in young patients treated with vitamin A or its derivatives.[42,43] The role of vitamin A is unclear, however, because more recent studies did not show an increased prevalence of DISH among patients treated with vitamin A in various dosages and for various lengths of time.[22,25,28] Larger prospective studies are needed to elucidate the role played by this vitamin in the etiology of DISH.

Familial clustering of DISH or families with very early presentation of DISH suggest a genetic background for this disorder.[44,45] Ossification of the posterior longitudinal ligament is closely related to DISH, and the two conditions can coexist. *COL6A1*, which is the candidate gene for ossification of the posterior longitudinal ligament, was reported to be significantly associated with DISH in Japanese, but not in Czech, patients.[46,47] This finding would suggest that other factors might play an important role in the genetic predisposition for the development of DISH.

There are no convincing explanations for the predilection of the hyperostotic process to affect the anterolateral aspect of the thoracic spine. The limited range of motion of the thoracic spine has been cited as a possible cause for the predilection to this site. This assumption cannot explain the involvement of the extremely mobile cervical spine or the lumbar spine, however. The less frequent involvement of the left side of the thoracic spine was ascribed to the pulsation of the aorta. This assumption was based on a few reports that described left-sided bridging osteophytes in cases with a right-sided aorta, suggesting that the aortic pulsations interfere with the production of the osteophytes.[48,49] Calcifications, ossification, and subsequent stiffening of ligaments and joint capsules have important pathogenetic implications.

Osteoarthritis may have pathogenetic features in common with the peripheral joint manifestions of DISH. It was suggested that in the small non–weight-bearing joints in osteoarthritis, the process is caused by an increased intra-articular pressure and subsequent development of "crash" forces.[50] This development was attributed to thickening of the collateral ligaments of these joints that enforce a constraint movement, and not to primary damage to the cartilage. It seems reasonable that the joints affected by DISH may develop the same "crash" forces operating in small osteoarthritis joints, as a result of this mechanism. This mechanism might explain the involvement of "atypical" joints, not commonly affected by osteoarthritis, and the hypertrophic osteoarthritic changes in the commonly affected joints.

CLINICAL MANIFESTATIONS

The lack of specific symptoms and signs of DISH, and the radiographic diagnostic criteria have raised doubts about DISH as a separate entity.[51] Although the disease may be asymptomatic, it was reported to be associated with morning stiffness, dorsolumbar pain, and reduced range of motion in most patients.[7,8] Patients with DISH may have extremity pain involving peripheral large and small joints and

peripheral entheses, such as the heel, Achilles tendon, shoulder, patella, and olecranon. Pain in the axial skeleton may involve all three segments of the spine and the costosternal and sternoclavicular joints. The level of pain and disability is significantly higher compared with healthy subjects, but is not different from patients with ankylosing spondylitis.[30] Complaints of pain referable to the thoracic spine are common and are accompanied by a reduced chest expansion.

Although similar in some aspects to osteoarthritis of the spine, DISH is a distinct clinical entity with different characteristics.[52] Classically, the portions of the spine that are involved in osteoarthritis are the lower portions of the cervical spine and the lumbar spine. Thoracic spine involvement is uncommon in osteoarthritis or occurs in late stages of the disease, as opposed to the common involvement of the thoracic spine in DISH. Thoracic spine involvement in DISH is characterized by preserved intervertebral height, whereas in spinal osteoarthritis, reduced intervertebral disk height is common. These differences in the radiologic appearance and anatomic spinal distribution probably have to do with the different pathogenetic mechanisms described earlier. It is presumed that the primary target for the osteoarthritic process is the cartilage represented in the spine by the intervertebral disks and the cartilage of the facet joints.

The wear-and-tear forces operating in the extremely mobile lower cervical and lumbar portions of the spine might explain the frequent involvement of these segments in osteoarthritis, whereas the thoracic spine is the least mobile of the spinal segments. The main targets of the disease in DISH are the spinal ligaments and entheses (Fig. 93-1).[5,53] These abnormalities are not limited to the thoracic spine and may involve the lumbar spine and the cervical spine (Fig. 93-2).

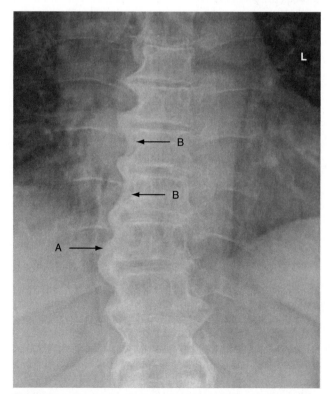

Figure 93-1 Large, flowing, right-sided osteophytes of the thoracic spine (A). Note the translucent area between the vertebral body and the ossified ligamentous tissue (B).

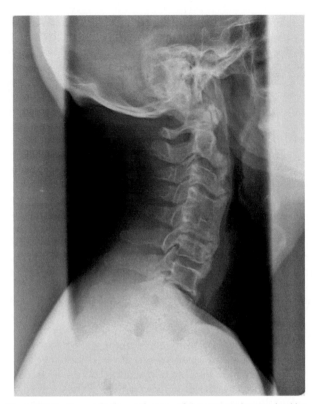

Figure 93-2 Severe bulky ossification of the anterior longitudinal ligament of the cervical spine.

Table 93-4 Clinical Manifestations of Diffuse Idiopathic Skeletal Hyperostosis in the Cervical Spine

Spontaneous
Dysphagia
Hoarseness
Stridor
Ossification of posterior longitudinal ligament
Myelopathy
Aspiration pneumonia
Sleep apnea
Atlantoaxial complications (pseudarthrosis, subluxation)
Thoracic outlet syndrome

Induced
Endoscopic problems
Intubation difficulties
Fractures

From Mader R: Clinical manifestations of diffuse idiopathic skeletal hyperostosis of the cervical spine. Semin Arthritis Rheum 32:130-135, 2002.

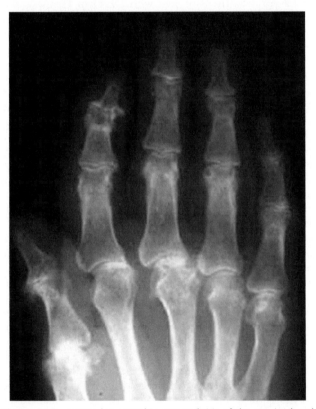

Figure 93-3 Severe hypertrophic osteoarthritis of the proximal and distal interphalangeal joints. Of particular interest is the involvement of the metacarpophalangeal joints with enlarged metacarpal heads, osteophytes, joint space narrowing, and subchondral sclerosis.

In the lumbar spine, the large bridging osteophytes are not uniformly one-sided.[54] These sites of ossification, and the subsequent production of large osteophytes, may result in spinal stenosis[55] and spinal stiffening, which increases the risk of fractures.[56,57] These fractures may be unrecognized, unstable, and associated with treatment delays and permanent neurologic deficits. Severe complications may develop, especially when the cervical spine is affected, including dysphagia, hoarseness, stridor, ossification of the posterior longitudinal ligament, myelopathy, aspiration pneumonia, sleep apnea, atlantoaxial complications, thoracic outlet syndrome, esophageal obstruction, endoscopic and intubation difficulties, and fractures (Table 93-4).[58] The high prevalence of coexisting intervertebral disk damage in young patients with DISH suggests an important role for DISH in the pathogenesis of spondylosis in this group of patients.[59]

Clinical manifestations similar or identical to those of osteoarthritis are prominent features of DISH in the peripheral joints. The peripheral joints affected by DISH have features that distinguish them from primary osteoarthritis, however. One is the more frequent involvement of joints that are not usually affected in osteoarthritis, such as the metacarpophalangeal joints, elbows, and shoulders (Fig. 93-3).[60-63] Another feature is a more severe hypertrophic disease that may result in a reduced range of motion in the affected joints.[64]

As described previously, the primary event in DISH is thickening, calcification, or ossification of ligaments and entheses. In particular, enthesopathy affecting the peripheral joints has been described.[65] The radiographic appearance of peripatellar, cruciate ligament insertion, and pericapsular osseous enthesopathies are some examples of the contribution of DISH to stiffening of the soft tissues surrounding a joint (Fig. 93-4).[66] Entheseal ossification at various sites other than joints, such as the heel, ribs, and pelvis, is a common finding in DISH. These enthesopathies may become symptomatic exhibiting pain and swelling in the affected region. A high probability for the presence of spinal DISH was noted for ossification of the iliolumbar and sacrotuberous ligaments, and with bony overgrowth of the inferior acetabular rim.[65-67] The tendency for new bone formation puts the patient at risk for the development of heterotopic ossification after joint surgery.

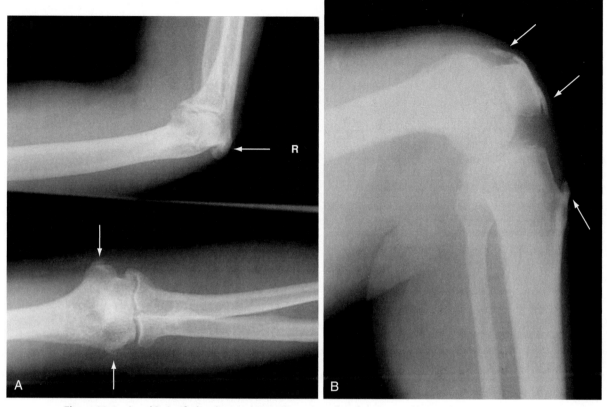

Figure 93-4 **A** and **B,** Ossified enthesopathies in the peripatellar, olecranon, and humeral epicondyles *(arrows).*

Patients with DISH often have higher body weight and body mass index, waist circumference, and systolic blood pressure.[30] These factors, and the metabolic abnormalities described earlier, put patients at an increased risk for cardiovascular diseases.[68,69] The diagnosis of DISH should be suspected in patients with osteoarthritis in atypical locations (e.g., elbow), in patients with hypertrophic osteoarthritis, and in patients with large enthesopathies and entrapment neuropathies of uncertain origin. This is particularly true for patients with the associated diseases and metabolic abnormalities discussed before. It was shown that chest radiographs might serve as a screening tool for the diagnosis of DISH with a sensitivity of 77% and specificity of 97%.[70]

TREATMENT CONSIDERATIONS

Treatment of DISH should address several issues. Treatment is expected to alleviate pain and stiffness; prevent, retard, or arrest progression; correct the associated metabolic disorders; and prevent spontaneous or induced complications (Table 93-5).

Specific therapeutic interventions in DISH have not been systematically explored; this is probably related to the inclusion of DISH in the spectrum of osteoarthritis, and the assumption that the same therapeutic interventions for osteoarthritis are suitable for DISH. It was suggested more recently that serum levels of growth hormone and IGF-I might be a useful surrogate marker for assessing DISH progression and remission.[34] It was estimated that a period of at least 10 years is needed for the pathologic process to evolve completely.[71] This notion implies that a long observation

Table 93-5 Therapeutic Targets in Diffuse Idiopathic Skeletal Hyperostosis

Symptomatic relief of pain and stiffness
Prevent, retard, or arrest progression
Treatment of associated metabolic disorder
Prevent spontaneous complications
Prevent traumatic complications
Prevent complications that might emerge during diagnostic or therapeutic procedures

From Mader R: Current therapeutic options in the management of diffuse idiopathic skeletal hyperostosis. Exp Opin Pharmacother 6:1313-1316, 2005.

period is needed to show that a therapeutic intervention might prevent the development of the disease, arrest its progression, or, it is hoped, reverse the pathologic changes.

There are few reports about remedies to alleviate the symptoms of the disease, but some investigators have reported on the beneficial effects of light exercise, heat, analgesics, and nonsteroidal anti-inflammatory drugs (NSAIDs).[31,72] More recently, the use of locally acting NSAIDs for the treatment of osteoarthritis was shown to be as effective as the same product by oral route, suggesting that locally acting NSAIDs also might be successfully employed for the symptomatic relief of pain and stiffness in the peripheral joints of patients with DISH.[73,74] Treatment of symptomatic enthesopathies might be necessary to alleviate local pain and swelling; this can be achieved by local soft applications such as insoles for plantar spurs or protective bandages at other sites. Infiltration of local anesthetic with long-acting corticosteroids might offer at least temporary relief in severely symptomatic

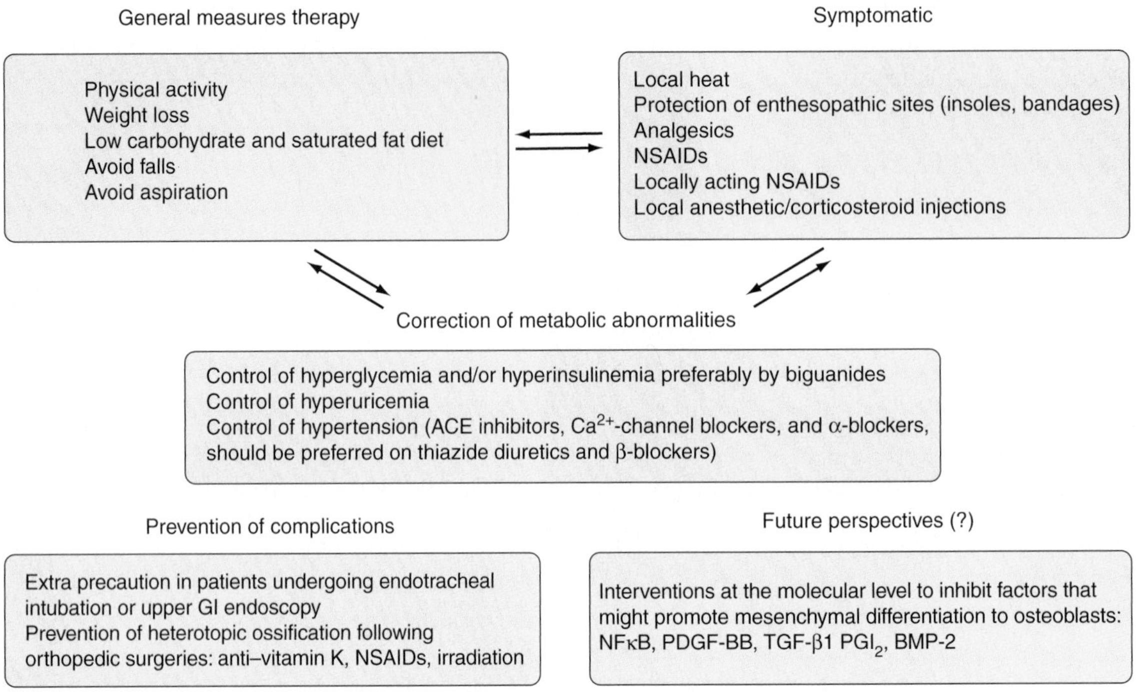

General measures therapy

Symptomatic

Physical activity
Weight loss
Low carbohydrate and saturated fat diet
Avoid falls
Avoid aspiration

Local heat
Protection of enthesopathic sites (insoles, bandages)
Analgesics
NSAIDs
Locally acting NSAIDs
Local anesthetic/corticosteroid injections

Correction of metabolic abnormalities

Control of hyperglycemia and/or hyperinsulinemia preferably by biguanides
Control of hyperuricemia
Control of hypertension (ACE inhibitors, Ca^{2+}-channel blockers, and α-blockers, should be preferred on thiazide diuretics and β-blockers)

Prevention of complications

Future perspectives (?)

Extra precaution in patients undergoing endotracheal intubation or upper GI endoscopy
Prevention of heterotopic ossification following orthopedic surgeries: anti–vitamin K, NSAIDs, irradiation

Interventions at the molecular level to inhibit factors that might promote mesenchymal differentiation to osteoblasts: $NF\kappa B$, PDGF-BB, TGF-β1 PGI_2, BMP-2

Figure 93-5 Therapeutic options in diffuse idiopathic skeletal hyperostosis. ACE, angiotensin-converting enzyme; BMP-2, bone morphogenetic protein-2; $NF\kappa B$, nuclear factor κB; NSAIDs, nonsteroidal anti-inflammatory drugs; PDGF-BB, platelet-derived growth factor-BB; PGI_2, prostaglandin I_2; TGF-β1, transforming growth factor-β1. *(From Mader R: Current therapeutic options in the management of diffuse idiopathic skeletal hyperostosis. Expert Opin Pharmacother 6:1313-1316, 2005.)*

cases. When multiple sites are involved, the same therapeutic modalities mentioned for osteoarthritis may be used.

The coexistence of many cardiovascular risk factors places patients with DISH at a higher risk for cardiovascular complications. It seems appropriate to screen these patients for known cardiovascular risk factors and to treat when appropriate. General measures such as weight reduction, adequate physical activity, and a diet low in saturated fat and carbohydrates all might be important in preventing or arresting the progression of DISH. Some of these factors may have pathogenetic implications and may become therapeutic targets. Based on present understanding, therapeutic interventions should aim at a reduction of insulin secretion and insulin resistance. In patients with non–insulin-dependent diabetes mellitus, the use of biguanides, which decrease insulin resistance, may offer an advantage over the use of sulfonylureas, which increase insulin secretion. When coexisting hypertension should be treated, medications that might improve insulin resistance, such as angiotensin-converting enzyme inhibitors, calcium channel blockers, and α-blockers, should be preferred to medications that might worsen insulin resistance, such as thiazide diuretics and β-blockers.[75] Some growth factors that might have a role in the development of DISH, such as $NF\kappa B$, PDGF-BB, TGF-β1, growth hormone, and IGF-I, may become targets someday for specific therapeutic interventions.

Some complications can be avoided if taken into consideration. Aspiration pneumonia can be partially avoided if instructions in proper deglutition and preservation of an upright position after meals are carefully explained to the patient. Physicians familiar with DISH can avoid or minimize damage to the cervical spine or to soft tissues in patients who might need certain diagnostic or therapeutic interventions, such as upper gastrointestinal endoscopy or endotracheal

Table 93-6 Future Considerations in Diffuse Idiopathic Skeletal Hyperostosis

Establish and validate diagnostic criteria that consider also the peripheral manifestations of the disease
Clarify the natural course and prognosis
Study the systemic nature and the impact on quality of life and life expectancy
Seek a better understanding of the pathogenetic basis for the disease
Offer a disease-modifying therapeutic approach

intubation. It is reasonable to adopt the common measures to prevent falls and trauma, especially in elderly patients. Heterotopic ossification after orthopaedic surgeries, in particular hip arthroplasty, is common in patients with DISH.[54] Several therapeutic interventions aimed at abolishing heterotopic ossification, such as administration of NSAIDs, anti–vitamin K, and irradiation, have been reported with variable success.[76-78] Patients in the high-risk group to develop this complication, such as patients with DISH, should be considered candidates for one of these regimens. The therapeutic options are summarized in Figure 93-5.[79] Many tasks lay ahead to define better, understand the pathogenesis, and delineate future effective interventions for this disorder (Table 93-6).

HYPERTROPHIC OSTEOARTHROPATHY

HOA is a well-known entity characterized by skin and bone proliferation. The hallmark and main visual manifestation is a bulbous deformity of the distal end of the digits, also known as clubbing or drumsticks. Periostosis is a progressive process with predilection for the tubular bones, principally the tibia and fibula. Periostosis is bilateral; is symmetric; and spares the medullary cavity, the axial skeleton, and the skull. The prevalence of the condition is unknown, but it was found in skeletal human remains dating thousands of years ago.[80] It may be primary or secondary to many other diseases.

ETIOLOGY

Primary HOA is an autosomal dominant disorder characterized by periostosis, clubbing, thickening of the skin of the face and scalp, seborrhea, and hyperhidrosis. It is also termed *pachydermoperiostosis*. There is a male predominance with a male-to-female ratio of 9:1 with one peak of presentation in the first year of life and the other in adolescence.[81]

Secondary forms of HOA may manifest as isolated clubbing or with the full spectrum of the disease. Clubbing may be unilateral or bilateral and has been reported to occur in a variety of diseases, including pulmonary, cardiac, gastrointestinal, neurologic, infectious, vascular, and other diseases (Table 93-7).[82-86]

PATHOGENESIS

HOA is characterized by excessive collagen deposition, endothelial hyperplasia, edema, and new bone formation involving mainly the distal extremity and eventually progressing proximally. Various hypotheses have been generated in an attempt to explain the development of HOA. Most cases with secondary HOA have severe lung or cyanotic heart diseases. It was suggested that megakaryocytes are fragmented into platelets during their passage in the lung capillaries. In severe lung diseases or right-to-left shunts, megakaryocytes or platelet aggregates bypass the pulmonary capillary bed, however, and lodge in the peripheral vasculature of the digits.

It was shown that locally released growth factors, such as vascular endothelial growth factor (VEGF) and PDGF, were remarkably increased in tissue samples obtained from digits of patients with HOA.[87] It is feasible that these substances might be responsible for the distal overgrowth of collagen and bone. VEGF was found to be produced by a lung tumor in a patient with HOA. In this case, serum levels of VEGF were very high, and resection of the tumor reversed the digital clubbing and reduced the serum VEGF levels.[88] Activation of platelets and endothelial cells was supported by an increase in circulating von Willebrand factor antigen.[89] Other growth factors have been associated with digital clubbing, including hepatocyte growth factor, which was found to be increased in the serum of patients with lung cancer and HOA compared with patients with lung cancer without HOA.[90]

CLINICAL MANIFESTATIONS

Often HOA is asymptomatic, and sometimes it is the patient who notes the changes in the shape of the fingers. Symptomatic patients complain about a deep-seated pain in the lower extremity and over the long tubular bones, which is exacerbated by palpation. Large joint effusions are common, and the synovial fluid is thick with few white blood cells.[91,92] Skin hypertrophy may be confined to the nail beds or involve the face or larger areas overlying the tubular bones or joints.

The most common and apparent clinical manifestation is digital clubbing. The bulbous deformity of the fingertips

Table 93-7 Etiologies of Hypertrophic Osteoarthropathy

Unilateral
Hemiplegia
Patent ductus arteriosus
Aneurysms
Bilateral
Pulmonary Diseases
Cystic fibrosis
Pulmonary fibrosis
Primary or secondary lung tumors
Lung and pleural infections
Pleural tumors
Heart Diseases
Cyanotic diseases
Infective endocarditis
Gastrointestinal Diseases
Cirrhosis
Hepatic carcinoma
Intestinal and esophageal malignant tumors
Inflammatory bowel diseases
Intestinal polyposis
Other Diseases
Various malignancies
POEMS syndrome
Rheumatic diseases
Thymoma
AIDS
Thalassemia

AIDS, acquired immunodeficiency syndrome; POEMS, polyneuropathy, organomegaly, endocrinopathy, M component, and skin changes.

is accompanied by a convex nail (watch-crystal nail). The skin around the nail bed becomes shiny and thin with disappearance of the creases (Fig. 93-6). Palpation of the base of the nail bed yields the sensation of a "floating" nail within the soft tissue. Cases of advanced clubbing can be identified easily. Several methods were developed, however, to diagnose early phases of the condition. Among those techniques, the digital index and the phalangeal depth ratio have been most widely used.[93,94] The digital index measures the ratio between the perimeter of the nail bed and the perimeter at the distal interphalangeal joint of the 10 fingers. A ratio greater than 10 suggests clubbing. The phalangeal depth ratio measures the ratio between the depth of the distal phalanx and the depth of the distal interphalangeal joint of the index finger. A ratio greater than 1 is considered abnormal.

There are no specific laboratory tests to diagnose HOA. Radiographs of the fingers and toes may show acro-osteolysis, and periostitis manifest by cortical thickening of long bones is often observed. The process may involve few or multiple sites and can be regular or irregular in appearance. Characteristically, there is no reduction in joint space or erosions. Radioisotope bone scanning can be useful for diagnosis and for evaluating the extent of the process. Increased uptake can be seen in the cortex of long bones sometimes in the form of splints (Fig. 93-7).

TREATMENT CONSIDERATIONS

Asymptomatic cases need no treatment. NSAIDs are sometimes useful in symptomatic patients. Case reports have suggested that significant pain relief was observed after treatment

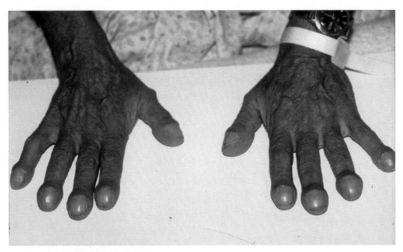

Figure 93-6   Severe clubbing in a patient with advanced lung cancer.

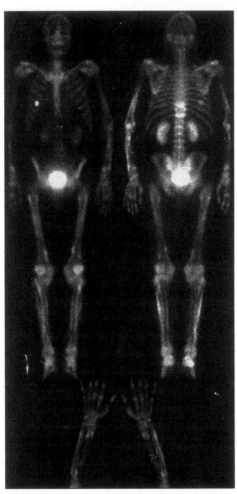

Figure 93-7   Increased non-nodular cortical bone uptake in a patient with bronchogenic carcinoma. *(From Vandemergel X, Blocket D, Decaux G: Periostitis and hypertrophic osteoarthropathy: Etiologies and bone scan patterns in 115 cases. Eur J Intern Med 15:375-380, 2004; with permission from the European Federation of Internal Medicine.)*

with octreotide or pamidronate.[95-97] In secondary cases of HOA, all features and symptoms promptly regress with successful treatment of the primary disease, such as correction of a heart malformation, removal of tumors, and therapy of infective endocarditis or inflammatory bowel disease.

REFERENCES

1. Lambert RG, Becker EJ: Diffuse skeletal hyperostosis in idiopathic hypoparathyroidism. Clin Radiol 40:212-215, 1989.
2. Fatourechi V, Ahmed DDF, Schwartz KM: Thyroid acropachy: Report of 40 patients treated at a single institution in a 26 years period. J Clin Endocrinol Metab 87:5435-5441, 2002.
3. Scarpan R, De Brasi D, Pivonello R, et al: Acromegalic axial arthropathy: A clinical case control study. J Clin Endocrinol Metab 89:598-603, 2004.
4. **Forestier J, Rotes-Querol J: Senile ankylosing hyperostosis of the spine. Ann Rheum Dis 9:321-330, 1950.**
5. **Resnick D, Niwayama G: Radiographic and pathologic features of spinal involvement in diffuse idiopathic skeletal hyperostosis (DISH). Radiology 119:559-568, 1976.**
6. Resnick D, Guerra J Jr, Robinson CA, et al: Association of diffuse idiopathic skeletal hyperostosis (DISH) and calcification and ossification of the posterior longitudinal ligament. AJR Am J Roentgenol 131:1049-1053, 1978.
7. Utsinger PD: Diffuse idiopathic skeletal hyperostosis. Clin Rheum Dis 11:325-351, 1985.
8. Resnick D, Niwayama G: Diagnosis of Bone and Joint Disorders, 2nd ed. Philadelphia, WB Saunders, 1988, pp 1563-1615.
9. Boachie-Adjei O, Bullough PG: Incidence of ankylosing hyperostosis of the spine (Forestier's disease) at autopsy. Spine 12:739-743, 1987.
10. Weinfeld RM, Olson PN, Maki DD, et al: The prevalence of diffuse idiopathic skeletal hyperostosis (DISH) in two large American Midwest metropolitan hospital populations. Skeletal Radiol 26:222-225, 1997.
11. Kiss C, O'Neill TW, Mituszova M, et al: Prevalence of diffuse idiopathic skeletal hyperostosis in Budapest, Hungary. Rheumatology 41:1335-1336, 2002.
12. Bloom RA: The prevalence of ankylosing hyperostosis in a Jerusalem population—with description of a method of grading the extent of the disease. Scand J Rheumatol 13:181-189, 1984.
13. Kim SK, Choi BR, Kim CG, et al: The prevalence of diffuse idiopathic skeletal hyperostosis in Korea. J Rheumatol 31:2032-2035, 2004.
14. Cassim B, Mody GM, Rubin DL: The prevalence of diffuse idiopathic skeletal hyperostosis in African Blacks. Br J Rheumatol 29:131-132, 1990.
15. Julkunen H, Heinonen OP, Knekt P, et al: The epidemiology of hyperostosis of the spine together with its symptoms and related mortality in a general population. Scand J Rheumatol 4:23-27, 1975.
16. Arriaza BT: Seronegative spondyloarthropathies and diffuse idiopathic skeletal hyperostosis in ancient northern Chile. Am J Phys Anthropol 91:263-278, 1993.
17. Vidal P: A paleoepidemiologic study of diffuse idiopathic skeletal hyperostosis. Joint Bone Spine 67:210-214, 2000.
18. Littlejohn GO, Smythe HA: Marked hyperinsulinemia after glucose challenge in patients with diffuse idiopathic skeletal hyperostosis. J Rheumatol 8:965-968, 1981.
19. Littlejohn GO: Insulin and new bone formation in diffuse idiopathic skeletal hyperostosis. Clin Rheumatol 4:294-300, 1985.

20. **Denko CW, Boja B, Moskowitz RW: Growth promoting peptides in osteoarthritis and diffuse idiopathic skeletal hyperostosis—insulin, insulin-like growth factor-I, growth hormone. J Rheumatol 21: 1725-1730, 1994.**
21. Nesher G, Zuckner J: Rheumatologic complications of vitamin A and retinoids. Semin Arthritis Rheum 24:291-296, 1995.
22. Van Dooren-Greebe RJ, Lemmens JAM, De Boo T, et al: Prolonged treatment of oral retinoids in adults: No influence on the frequency and severity of spinal abnormalities. Br J Dermatol 134:71-76, 1996.
23. Vezyroglou G, Mitropoulos A, Kyriazis N, et al: A metabolic syndrome in diffuse idiopathic skeletal hyperostosis: A controlled study. J Rheumatol 23:672-676, 1996.
24. Akune T, Ogata N, Seichi A, et al: Insulin secretory response is positively associated with the extent of ossification of the posterior longitudinal ligament of the spine. J Bone Joint Surg Am 83:1537-1544, 2001.
25. Ling TC, Parkin G, Islam J, et al: What is the cumulative effect of long term, low dose isotretinoin on the development of DISH? Br J Dermatol 144:628-650, 2001.
26. Kiss C, Szilagyi M, Paksy A, et al: Risk factors for diffuse idiopathic skeletal hyperostosis: A case control study. Rheumatology (Oxf) 41:27-30, 2002.
27. **Sarzi-Puttini P, Atzeni F: New developments in our understanding of DISH (diffuse idiopathic skeletal hyperostosis). Curr Opin Rheumatol 16:287-292, 2004.**
28. Katugampola RP, Finlay AY: Oral retinoid therapy for disorders of keratinization: Single-centre retrospective 25 years' experience on 23 patients. Br J Dermatol 154:267-276, 2006.
29. Forestier J, Lagier R: Ankylosing hyperostosis of the spine. Clin Orthop 74:65-83, 1971.
30. **Mata S, Fortin PR, Fitzcharles MA, et al: A controlled study of diffuse idiopathic skeletal hyperostosis: Clinical features and functional status. Medicine 76:104-117, 1997.**
31. Sencan D, Elden H, Nacitarhan V, et al: The prevalence of diffuse idiopathic skeletal hyperostosis in patients with diabetes mellitus. Rheumatol Int 25:518-521, 2005.
32. Tanaka H, Nagai E, Murata H, et al: Involvement of bone morphogenic protein-2 (BMP-2) in the pathological ossification process of the spinal ligament. Rheumatology 40:1163-1168, 2001.
33. Kobacz K, Ullrich R, Amoyo L, et al: Stimulatory effects of distinct members of the bone morphogenetic protein family on ligament fibroblasts. Ann Rheum Dis 65:169-177, 2006.
34. Denko CW, Malemud CJ: Role of growth hormone/insulin-like growth factor-1 paracrine axis in rheumatic diseases. Semin Arthritis Rheum 35:24-34, 2005.
35. **Denko CW, Malemud CJ: Body mass index and blood glucose: Correlations with serum insulin, growth hormone, and insulin-like growth factor-1 levels in patients with diffuse idiopathic skeletal hyperostosis (DISH). Rheumatol Int 26:292-297, 2006.**
36. Kosaka T, Imakiire A, Mizuno F, et al: Activation of nuclear factor κB at the onset of ossification of the spinal ligaments. J Orthop Sci 5:572-578, 2000.
37. Denko CW, Boja B, Moskowitz RW: Growth factors, insulin-like growth factor-1 and growth hormone, in synovial fluid and serum of patients with rheumatic disorders. Osteoarthritis Cartilage 4:245-249, 1996.
38. el Miedany YM, Wassif G, el Baddini M: Diffuse idiopathic skeletal hyperostosis (DISH): Is it of vascular etiology? Clin Exp Rheumatol 18:193-200, 2000.
39. Denko CW, Boja B, Malemud CJ: Intra-erythrocyte deposition of growth hormone in rheumatic diseases. Rheumatol Int 23:11-14, 2003.
40. Inaba T, Ishibashi S, Gotoda T, et al: Enhanced expression of platelet-derived growth factor-beta receptor by high glucose: Involvement of platelet-derived growth factor in diabetic angiopathy. Diabetes 45:507-512, 1996.
41. Pfeiffer A, Middelberg-Bisping K, Drewes C, et al: Elevated plasma levels of transforming growth factor-beta 1 in NIDDM. Diabetes Care 19:1113-1117, 1996.
42. Abiteboul M, Arlet J, Sarrabay MA, et al: Etude du metabolisme de la vitamine A au cours de la maladie hyperostosique de Forestier et Rote's-Querol. Rev Rhum Ed Fr 53:143-145, 1986.
43. Nesher G, Zuckner J: Rheumatologic complications of vitamin A and retinoids. Semin Arthritis Rheum 24:291-296, 1995.
44. Gorman C, Jawad ASM, Chikanza I: A family with diffuse idiopathic hyperostosis. Ann Rheum Dis 64:1794-1795, 2005.
45. Bruges-Armas J, Couto AM, Timms A, et al: Ectopic calcification among families in the Azores: Clinical and radiologic manifestations in families with diffuse idiopathic skeletal hyperostosis and chondrocalcinosis. Arthritis Rheum 54:1340-1349, 2006.
46. Havelka S, Vesela M, Pavelkova A, et al: Are DISH and OPLL genetically related? Ann Rheum Dis 60:902-903, 2001.
47. Tsukahara S, Miyazawa N, Akagawa H, et al: COL6A1, the candidate gene for ossification of the posterior longitudinal ligament, is associated with diffuse idiopathic skeletal hyperostosis in Japanese. Spine 30:2321-2324, 2005.
48. Ciocci A: Diffuse idiopathic skeletal hyperostosis (DISH) and situs viscerum inversus: Report of a single case. Clin Exp Rheumatol 5:159-160, 1987.
49. Carile L, Verdone F, Aiello A, et al: Diffuse idiopathic skeletal hyperostosis and situs viscerum inversus. J Rheumatol 16:1120-1122, 1989.
50. Smythe HA: The mechanical pathogenesis of generalized osteoarthritis. J Rheumatol 10(Suppl 9):11-12, 1983.
51. Hutton C: DISH…a state not a disease? Br J Rheumatol 28:277-280, 1989.
52. Mader R: Diffuse idiopathic skeletal hyperostosis: A distinct clinical entity. Isr Med Assoc J 5:506-508, 2003.
53. Fornasier VL, Littlejohn GO, Urowitz MB, et al: Spinal entheseal new bone formation: The early changes of spinal diffuse idiopathic skeletal hyperostosis. J Rheumatol 10:934-947, 1983.
54. **Belanger TA, Rowe DE: Diffuse idiopathic skeletal hyperostosis: Musculoskeletal manifestations. J Am Acad Orthop Surg 9:258-267, 2001.**
55. Laroche M, Moulinier L, Arlet J, et al: Lumbar and cervical stenosis: Frequency of the association, role of the ankylosing hyperostosis. Clin Rheumatol 11:533-535, 1992.
56. Paley D, Schwartz M, Cooper P, et al: Fracture of the spine in diffuse idiopathic skeletal hyperostosis. Clin Orthop 267:22-23, 1991.
57. Le Hir PX, Sautet A, Le Gars L, et al: Hyperextension vertebral body fractures in diffuse idiopathic skeletal hyperostosis: A cause of intra-vertebral fluid-like collections on MR imaging. AJR Am J Roentgenol 173:1679-1683, 1999.
58. **Mader R: Clinical manifestations of diffuse idiopathic skeletal hyperostosis of the cervical spine. Semin Arthritis Rheum 32:130-135, 2002.**
59. Di Girolamo C, Pappone N, Rengo C, et al: Intervertebral disc lesions in diffuse idiopathic skeletal hyperostosis (DISH). Clin Exp Rheumatol 19:310-312, 2001.
60. Littlejohn JO, Urowitz MB, Smythe HA, et al: Radiographic features of the hand in diffuse idiopathic skeletal hyperostosis (DISH). Diagn Radiol 140:623-629, 1981.
61. Beyeler C, Schlapbach P, Gerber NJ, et al: Diffuse idiopathic skeletal hyperostosis (DISH) of the shoulder: A cause of shoulder pain? Br J Rheumatol 29:349-353, 1990.
62. Utsinger PD, Resnick D, Shapiro R: Diffuse skeletal abnormalities in Forestier's disease. Arch Intern Med 136:763-768, 1976.
63. Resnick D, Shapiro RF, Weisner KB, et al: Diffuse idiopathic skeletal hyperostosis (DISH): Ankylosing hyperostosis of Forestier and Rote's-Querol. Semin Arthritis Rheum 7:153-187, 1978.
64. Schlapbach P, Beyeler C, Gerber NJ, et al: The prevalence of palpable finger joints nodules in diffuse idiopathic skeletal hyperostosis (DISH): A controlled study. Br J Rheumatol 31:531-534, 1992.
65. Littlejohn JO, Urowitz MB: Peripheral enthesopathy in diffuse idiopathic skeletal hyperostosis (DISH): A radiologic study. J Rheumatol 9:568-572, 1982.
66. **Resnick D, Shaul SR, Robins JM: Diffuse idiopathic skeletal hyperostosis (DISH): Forestier's disease with extraspinal manifestations. Radiology 115:513-524, 1975.**
67. Haller J, Resnick D, Miller GW, et al: Diffuse idiopathic skeletal hyperostosis: Diagnostic significance of radiographic abnormalities of the pelvis. Radiology 172:835-839, 1989.
68. Mader R, Dubenski N, Lavi I: Morbidity and mortality of hospitalized patients with diffuse idiopathic skeletal hyperostosis. Rheumatol Int 26:132-136, 2005.
69. Miyazawa N, Akiyama I: Diffuse idiopathic skeletal hyperostosis associated with risk factors for stroke. Spine 31:E225-E229, 2006.
70. Mata S, Hill RO, Joseph L, et al: Chest radiographs as a screening tool for diffuse idiopathic skeletal hyperostosis. J Rheumatol 20:1905-1910, 1993.

71. Mader R: Diffuse idiopathic skeletal hyperostosis: Isolated involvement of cervical spine in a young patient. J Rheumatol 31:620-621, 2004.
72. El Garf A, Khater R: Diffuse idiopathic skeletal hyperostosis (DISH): A clinicopathological study of the disease pattern in Middle Eastern populations. J Rheumatol 11:804-807, 1984.
73. Tugwell PS, Wells, Shainhouse JZ: Equivalence study of a topical diclofenac solution (pennsaid) compared with oral diclofenac in symptomatic treatment of osteoarthritis of the knee: A randomized controlled trial. J Rheumatol 31:2002-2012, 2004.
74. Roth SH, Shainhouse JZ: Efficacy and safety of a topical diclofenac solution (pennsaid) in the treatment of primary osteoarthritis of the knee: A randomized, double-blind, vehicle-controlled clinical trial. Arch Intern Med 164:2017-2023, 2004.
75. Lithell HOL: Effect of antihypertensive drugs on insulin, glucose, and lipid metabolism. Diabetes Care 14:203-209, 1991.
76. Cella JP, Salvati EA, Sculco TP: Indomethacin for the prevention of heterotopic ossification following total hip arthroplasty: Effectiveness, contraindications, and adverse effects. J Arthroplasty 3:229-234, 1988.
77. Guillemin F, Mainard D, Rolland H, et al: Antivitamin K prevents heterotopic ossification after hip arthroplasty in diffuse idiopathic skeletal hyperostosis: A retrospective study in 67 patients. Acta Orthop Scand 66:123-126, 1995.
78. Knelles D, Barthel T, Karrer A, et al: Prevention of heterotopic ossification after total hip replacement: A prospective, randomized study using acetylsalicylic acid, indomethacin and fractional or single-dose irradiation. J Bone Joint Surg Br 79:596-602, 1997.
79. Mader R: Current therapeutic options in the management of diffuse idiopathic skeletal hyperostosis. Exp Opin Pharmacother 6:1313-1316, 2005.
80. Martinez-Lavin M, Mansilla J, Pineda C, et al: Evidence of hypertrophic osteoarthropathy in human skeletal remains from PreHispanic era in Mesoamerica. Ann Intern Med 12:238-241, 1994.
81. Martinez-Lavin M, Pineda C, Valdez T, et al: Primary hypertrophic osteoarthropathy. Semin Arthritis Rheum 17:156-162, 1988.
82. Spicknall KE, Zirwas MJ, English JC: Clubbing: An update on diagnosis, differential diagnosis, pathophysiology, and clinical relevance. J Am Acad Dermatol 52:1020-1028, 2005.
83. **Martinez-Lavin M: Hypertrophic osteoarthropathy. Curr Opin Rheumatol 9:83-86, 1997.**
84. Stridhar KS, Lobo CF, Altman RD: Digital clubbing and lung cancer. Chest 114:1535-1537, 1998.
85. Vongpatanasin W, Brickner ME, Hillis LD, et al: The Eisenmenger syndrome in adults. Ann Intern Med 128:745-755, 1998.
86. Botton E, Saraux A, Laselve H, et al: Musculoskeletal manifestations in cystic fibrosis. Joint Bone Spine 70:327-335, 2003.
87. **Atkinson S, Fox SB: Vascular endothelial growth factor (VEGF)—A platelet-derived growth factor (PDGF) plays a central role in the pathogenesis of digital clubbing. J Pathol 203:721-728, 2004.**
88. Olan F, Portela M, Navarro C, et al: Circulating vascular endothelial growth factor concentrations in a case of pulmonary hypertrophic osteoarthropathy: Correlation with disease activity. J Rheumatol 31:614-616, 2004.
89. Matucci-Cerinic M, Martinez-Lavin M, Rojo F, et al: Von Willebrand factor antigen in hypertrophic osteoarthropathy. J Rheumatol 19:765-767, 1992.
90. Hojo S, Fujita J, Yamadori I, et al: Hepatocyte growth factor and digital clubbing. Intern Med 36:44-46, 1997.
91. Schumacher HR Jr: Articular manifestations of hypertrophic pulmonary osteoarthropathy in bronchogenic carcinoma. Arthritis Rheum 19:629-636, 1976.
92. Schumacher HR Jr: Hypertrophic osteoarthropathy: Rheumatologic manifestations. Clin Exp Rheumatol 10(Suppl 7):35-40, 1992.
93. Vazquez-Abad D, Pineda C, Martinez-Lavin M: Digital clubbing: A numerical assessment of the deformity. J Rheumatol 16:518-520, 1989.
94. Myers KA, Farquhar DRE: Does this patient have clubbing? JAMA 286:341-347, 2001.
95. Garske LA, Bell SC: Pamidronate results in symptom control of hypertrophic pulmonary osteoarthropathy in cystic fibrosis. Chest 121:1363-1364, 2002.
96. Amital H, Applbaum YH, Vasiliev L, et al: Hypertrophic pulmonary osteoarthropathy: Control of pain and symptoms with pamidronate. Clin Rheumatol 23:330-332, 2004.
97. Angel-Moreno Maroto A, Martinez-Quintana E, Suarez-Castellano L, et al: Painful hypertrophic osteoarthropathy successfully treated with ocreotide: The pathogenetic role of vascular endothelial growth factor (VEGF). Rheumatology 44:1326-1327, 2005.

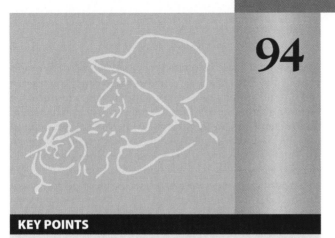

94

Osteonecrosis

CHRISTOPHER CHANG •
ADAM GREENSPAN •
M. ERIC GERSHWIN

KEY POINTS

Knowledge of risk factors and early detection is crucial to the successful management of osteonecrosis.

Abnormalities in lipid metabolism might play a role in the pathogenesis of osteonecrosis.

The most common causes of nontraumatic osteonecrosis are corticosteroid use and alcohol consumption.

The final common pathway in the pathogenesis of osteonecrosis is the disruption of blood supply to a segment of bone.

The femoral head is the most common site of osteonecrosis.

Osteonecrosis affects younger patients than osteoarthritis and has significantly greater long-term morbidity.

Nonsurgical treatment of osteonecrosis does not change the natural history of the disease.

Magnetic resonance imaging is currently the optimal study for early diagnosis and identification of the extent of osteonecrosis.

Although there are many variations on surgical treatment of femoral head osteonecrosis, most hips eventually require total hip arthroplasty.

Osteonecrosis literally means "bone death" (*ossis* [Latin] = bone; *necrosis* = killing or causing to die). Other synonyms include avascular necrosis, ischemic necrosis of bone, aseptic necrosis, osteochrondritis dissecans, and subchondral avascular necrosis. Hippocrates first described the concept of bone death,[1] and the first description of osteonecrosis appeared in a case of sepsis-induced bone death in 1794 by Russell.[2] Approximately a century later, in 1888, it was recognized that bone necrosis could occur in the absence of infection.[3] The first report of osteonecrosis occurring in a deep-sea diver appeared in 1936.[4] Osteonecrosis occurs as a result of partial or complete reduction in blood flow, although multiple mechanisms might be responsible for this disruption.[5,6]

EPIDEMIOLOGY

The prevalence of osteonecrosis is unknown, but it is estimated that there are 10,000 to 20,000 new patients with osteonecrosis diagnosed per year in the United States. It occurs in 15% to 80% of patients with femoral neck fractures.[7] Of the 500,000 hip replacements done in the United States every year, about 10% are thought to be the result of osteonecrosis.[8] The disease primarily affects men, with a notable exception of cases related to systemic lupus erythematosus, which has a female predominance. Osteonecrosis predominantly occurs in the third to fifth decades of life.[9] As a result of this age distribution, long-term morbidity can be significant.

ETIOLOGY

Osteonecrosis has been linked to numerous conditions (Table 94-1). In many of these conditions, a causal relationship has yet to be determined. In others, the association is tenuous and may consist only of anecdotal or case reports. One accepted risk factor is corticosteroid use, first described in 1957.[10] Corticosteroids also are associated with significant side effects when used for prolonged periods, and a high index of suspicion should be maintained for osteonecrosis.

In one study, 2500 to 3300 cases of nontraumatic osteonecrosis were reported in 1988, with 34.7% related to corticosteroid use, 21.7% associated with alcohol consumption, and the rest idiopathic. Although the risk of osteonecrosis with steroid use is low, the morbidity associated with the resulting hip deformity is significant. The time interval between steroid use and the development of osteonecrosis varies among individuals. In one study of 22 patients diagnosed with stage I osteonecrosis by magnetic resonance imaging (MRI), the interval between the use of steroids and diagnosis ranged from 1 to 16 months.[11] The cumulative dose of steroids in this study ranged from 1800 to 15,505 mg (mean 5928 mg) of prednisolone or the equivalent. In other studies, cumulative doses of steroids associated with osteonecrosis ranged from 480[12] to 4320 mg[13] of dexamethasone dose equivalence.

Although corticosteroid-related osteonecrosis is dose related, additional host-inherent risk factors play a role. The incidence of osteonecrosis in a group of patients receiving glucocorticoid replacement therapy for primary or secondary adrenal insufficiency was 2.4%. In a study of renal transplantation, 26 patients who developed osteonecrosis had a higher cumulative oral dose of prednisone after 1 month and 3 months compared with 28 control transplant patients who did not develop osteonecrosis.[14] A separate study estimated the incidence of osteonecrosis in renal transplant patients on steroids to be 5%.[15] It is unknown why certain patients on steroids develop osteonecrosis and others do not. The minimum dosage or duration of use that can lead to osteonecrosis also is unknown. Patients with systemic lupus erythematosus and organ transplantation who are receiving corticosteroids are particularly prone to developing osteonecrosis. There is no evidence that topical, inhaled, or intranasal route of administration can lead to osteonecrosis. Although data are limited to case reports, a link between intra-articular administration of corticosteroids

Table 94-1 Conditions Associated with Osteonecrosis

Dietary, Drugs, and Environmental Factors
Corticosteroids[145,146]
Cigarette smoking[22]
Dysbaric osteonecrosis[4,147]
Alcohol consumption[22,148]
Lead poisoning[149,150]
Bisphosphonates[98,151]

Musculoskeletal Conditions—Compromise in Structural Integrity
Trauma[152]
Legg-Calvé-Perthes disease[29,153]
Congenital hip dislocation[154,155]
Hereditary dysostosis
Slipped capital femoral epiphysis[156,157]

Metabolic Diseases—Abnormality in Fat or Other Metabolic Component
Gaucher's disease[158]
Fat embolism[159,160]
Pancreatitis[62,64,161,162]
Chronic liver disease[163]
Pregnancy[37,164]
Fabry's disease[165,166]
Gout[167]
Hyperparathyroidism[168]
Hyperlipidemia[159,160]
Hypercholesterolemia[167]
Diabetes[169]

Hematologic Conditions—Abnormalities in Components of Blood
Hemoglobinopathies
Sickle cell anemia[38,170,171]
Thalassemia[172]
Disseminated intravascular coagulation[85,173-176]
Hemophilia[41-43]
Thrombophilia[177]
Marrow infiltrative disorders
Hypofibrinolysis[178]
Thrombophlebitis/venous thrombosis[179]

Rheumatologic Conditions
Antiphospholipid antibody syndrome[180]
Rheumatoid arthritis[181]
Systemic lupus erythematosus[61,97,182-184]
Inflammatory bowel disease[185,186]
Necrotizing arteritis[187]
Mucocutaneous lymph node syndrome[188]
Polymyositis[189]
Sarcoidosis[63]
Mixed connective tissue disease
Infectious diseases
HIV infection[190]
Osteomyelitis[191]
Meningococcemia[173,176,192]

Oncologic Disorders and Their Treatment
Organ transplantation[193-198]
Radiation exposure[199-204]
Regional deep hyperthermia[205]
Acute lymphoblastic leukemia[206,207]

HIV, human immunodeficiency virus.

has been reported.[16] Parenteral steroids pose a higher risk because of lipid absorption and a longer half-life.

Other therapeutic interventions associated with osteonecrosis include dialysis, bisphosphonate usage, and radiation therapy. A retrospective chart review of patients with osteonecrosis in bone specimens of the maxilla and mandible identified 23 cases associated with use of the newer generation bisphosphonates zoledronate, pamidronate, or alendronate, after exclusion of patients who did not have metastatic bone cancer in the same site and who also were treated with radiation therapy.[17] Of the 23 patients, 18 were treated with the intravenous form, and the other 5, who had osteoporosis or Paget's disease, were treated with the oral form.

The association between alcohol consumption and osteonecrosis was first described in 1922.[18] A study of patients with idiopathic osteonecrosis revealed that the risk of osteonecrosis increased with increasing daily consumption of alcohol. None of these patients were on corticosteroids, and the data were compared with hospital controls. The relative risk of developing osteonecrosis for three broad categories of alcohol consumption (<400 mL/wk, 400 to 1000 mL/wk, and >1000 mL/wk) was 3-fold, 10-fold, and 18-fold respectively. The data were adjusted for confounding variables such as cigarette smoking.[19] Another study showed that liver damage was unnecessary for the development of osteonecrosis in alcohol-consuming patients, although abnormal liver enzymes, such as elevated serum γ-glutamyl transferase activity, have been noted.[20] In another study of nearly 1200 patients who were treated medically for alcoholism, the incidence of osteonecrosis was 5.3%. Most of the cases involved the femoral head (82 of 92 lesions), and the other 10 sites involved the humeral head.[21] It is generally accepted that the use of steroids and chronic alcohol usage would lead to an additive risk.

Cigarette smoking is associated with osteonecrosis,[19,22,23] although there is no clear cause-and-effect relationship. A significant relative risk of 3.0 was observed for current smokers, but a dose-dependent relationship was not seen, and the risk is much less than steroids.

Musculoskeletal conditions in which osteonecrosis has been observed include slipped capital femoral epiphysis, Ehlers-Danlos syndrome, Legg-Calvé-Perthes disease, hereditary dysostosis, and congenital hip dislocation. Legg-Calvé-Perthes disease is a disorder first described in 1910[24-26] affecting children 3 to 12 years old. Femoral head osteonecrosis is a feature of the disease and has been linked to trauma,[27,28] congenital hip dislocation,[29] and transient synovitis.[30] Bilateral involvement commonly occurs, and associated clinical manifestations include abnormal growth and stature,[31,32] delayed skeletal maturation,[33] disproportionate skeletal growth,[32] congenital anomalies,[34] and abnormal hormone levels.[35,36]

Metabolic disorders, such as Cushing's syndrome, Gaucher's disease, disorders of lipid and glucose metabolism, pancreatitis, and pregnancy, also are associated with osteonecrosis. Although the association with pregnancy is rare, most cases occur in primigravid patients, with onset of pain in the late second to third trimesters. Diagnosis can be delayed until months after delivery. Women who developed osteonecrosis tended to have a small body frame and a large weight gain during pregnancy.[37]

Hematologic conditions, such as sickle cell anemia, hemophilia, and intravascular coagulation, have been associated with osteonecrosis. The long-term morbidity of osteonecrosis in patients with sickle cell anemia is dismal.[38] Deformities occur in 80% of these patients and persist into adulthood. Common deformities include decreased mobility, abnormal gait, and leg-length discrepancy.[39] Osteonecrosis in hemophilia patients has been described,[40-45] but the numbers are small, and no statistically reliable causal link can be established.

Finally, a type of osteonecrosis known as dysbaric osteonecrosis has been described in construction workers in the Elhe tunnel exposed to high-pressure environments.[46] The prevalence of dysbaric osteonecrosis is 4.2% in divers and 17% in compressed air workers.[47] Patients with dysbaric osteonecrosis may have more than one lesion, and common sites besides the femoral head include the tibia and the humeral head and shaft. The condition is not related to decompression sickness, and although proper decompression procedures can reduce "the bends," they do not have any effect on development of osteonecrosis. Osteonecrosis can occur months or years after the last exposure to high pressures.

CLINICAL FEATURES

The primary presenting symptom in osteonecrosis is pain. In osteonecrosis of the femoral head, the pain is located in the hip joint and may radiate to the groin, anterior thigh, or knee. The severity of the pain can vary, depending on the size of the infarct and whether the onset of the disease is insidious or sudden. In trauma, where there is sudden and severe disruption of blood flow, and in Gaucher's disease, dysbarism, or hemoglobinopathy, where the infarcts are large, pain can be intense and occur suddenly. In other conditions, pain can occur insidiously. The pain of osteonecrosis usually is increased with use of the joint, but in advanced disease, the pain is persistent even at rest. Limitation of range of motion except that associated with accompanying pain is usually a progressive and late symptom. The risk of developing osteonecrosis in the contralateral hip when one side is affected ranges from 31% to 55%.

In addition to the femoral head, osteonecrosis can affect other sites, including the humeral head,[48-51] femoral condyles[52-54] and proximal tibiae,[53,55-59] wrists and ankles,[60] bones of the hands and feet,[61] vertebrae,[62-64] jaw,[65,66] and bony structures of the face.[67] Osteonecrosis of the humeral head is the second most commonly seen location, and pain is usually in the shoulder with limited range of motion and weakness. Pain in the ankle is the main presenting symptom in atraumatic osteonecrosis of the talus, and in some cases, disease had already progressed to Ficat and Arlet stage III by the time of presentation.[60] Kienböck's disease involves osteonecrosis of the lunate, and patients present with pain in the radiolunate joint, along with weakness and limitation of motion. Kienböck's disease seems to be related to manual labor.

The Ficat and Arlet method of staging osteonecrosis consists of four stages. Stages I and II are reversible, whereas stage III, which involves subchondral collapse, and stage IV, which involves joint space narrowing and destruction of cartilage, are irreversible. The Marcus staging system consists of six stages; the first two are reversible, and the subsequent four are irreversible. The modified Steinberg staging system is based on the Marcus system and also consists of six stages. Within each stage, the extent of head involvement is subdivided into three subclasses—A involves less than 25%; B, 26% to 50%; and C, greater than 50% of the head.

Table 94-2 presents similarities and differences between the staging systems. The Association of Research Circulation Osseous (ARCO) has proposed a modification to the Ficat and Arlet system, adding a stage 0 for patients with negative imaging studies but who are at high risk for developing osteonecrosis. In addition, stages I to III are stratified further to take into account lesion size, location, and extent of collapse.[68] In 2001, the Japanese Ministry of Health, Labor, and Welfare proposed revised criteria for the diagnosis and staging of osteonecrosis of the femoral head. Diagnostic criteria included the following: (1) collapse of the femoral head without joint space narrowing or acetabular abnormality on plain radiography, (2) demarcating sclerosis in the femoral head without joint space narrowing or acetabular abnormality, (3) "cold in hot" on bone scans, (4) low-intensity band on T1-weighted MRI, and (5) trabecular and marrow necrosis on histology. If a patient fulfills two of the five criteria, the diagnosis is established. The working group also proposed four types of lesions based on extensiveness, and defined stages of disease based on diagnostic imaging.

PATHOGENESIS

To understand why the femoral head is preferentially affected in osteonecrosis, it is important to understand the anatomy of the femoral head and its blood supply. Three arterial networks supply the femoral head and neck. The extracapsular arterial ring consists of the lateral femoral circumflex artery and the medial femoral circumflex artery, which arise from the profunda femoris. The medial femoral circumflex artery and its branches supply most of the blood to the head and neck of the femur. The lateral circumflex artery gives rise to transverse branches, which supply the femoral head. The medial and lateral circumflex arteries anastomose with the superior and inferior gluteal branches of the internal iliac artery, providing collateral circulation between the femoral artery and the internal iliac artery. Retinacular arteries are ascending cervical branches of the extracapsular ring and form an intra-articular ring at the level of the cartilage. Epiphyseal arterial branches arise from this ring and penetrate the head and neck of the femur, including the epiphyses. The artery of the ligament of the head of the femur is a branch of the obturator artery and may be the sole supplier of blood to the proximal fragment of the head.

These anatomic features render the femoral head particularly prone to ischemia. Numerous theories abound concerning the pathogenesis of the various risk factors associated with osteonecrosis of the femoral head. Table 94-3 presents a potential pathway for some of the disease entities associated with osteonecrosis. The common end result is the disruption of the blood supply, which can result from vascular, intravascular, or extravascular factors.

Histologically, after an infarct, a rim of bony thickening or sclerosis begins to form at the margins of the infarcted area. If the necrotic lesion is within the weight-bearing region of the femoral head, subchondral fractures follow. The repair process is inadequate and itself compromises the structural integrity of the bone. With repeated microfractures and continued weight bearing, the original fracture cannot heal completely, and new fractures appear. The secondary fracture propagates along the junction between subchondral bone and the necrotic segment. As time goes

Table 94-2 Various Staging Systems for Osteonecrosis

Ficat and Arlet		
Stage	**Radiographic Appearance**	**Reversible**
I	Normal	Yes
II	Cystic or osteosclerotic lesions; normal contour of bone; no subchondral fracture	Yes
III	Crescent sign or subchondral collapse	No
IV	Joint space narrowing; secondary distal tibial, femoral, humeral changes (cysts, marginal osteophytes, and cartilage destruction)	No
Marcus		
Stage	**Radiographic Appearance**	**Reversible**
I	Subtle, mottled densities in weight-bearing segments of femoral head	Yes
II	Well-demarcated area of infarction	Yes
III	Crescent sign, signifying collapse or separation of the subchondral trabeculae from the articular cartilage	No
IV	Collapse of the avascular segment; fractures may be seen on articular surfaces	No
V	Osteoarthritis of the hip; joint space narrowing; presence of cystic areas and small osteophytes in subchondral bone	No
VI	Marked degenerative changes; joint space narrowing; collapse of the femoral head	No
Modified Steinberg		
Stage	**Radiographic Appearance**	**Reversible**
I	Normal radiograph, but abnormal bone scan or MRI	Yes
II	Lucent and sclerotic changes	Yes
III	Subchondral fracture without flattening	No
IV	Subchondral fracture with flattening or segmental depression of femoral head	No
V	Joint space narrowing or acetabular changes	No
VI	Advanced degenerative changes	No
Specific Disease Investigation Committee of the Japanese Ministry of Health, Labor, and Welfare		
Stage	**Radiographic Appearance**	**Reversible**
1	Normal radiographs, but positive findings on MRI, bone scintigraphy, or histology	Yes
2	Demarcating sclerosis without collapse	Yes
3A	Collapse of the femoral head, <3 mm (crescent sign) without joint space narrowing; mild osteophyte formation	No
3B	Same as 3A except that femoral head collapse is >3 mm	No
4	Osteoarthritic changes	No

MRI, magnetic resonance imaging.

on, the femoral head becomes flattened and eventually collapses. A nonspherical head articulating with the acetabulum produces friction and erosion and loss of cartilage. The cycle repeats itself, and the structure of the joint deteriorates, with the appearance of degenerative changes and eventually total joint destruction.[69]

The association between alcohol and osteonecrosis has led investigators to study the effects of alcohol on rabbit bone marrow.[73] Alcohol consumption was associated with reduced superoxide dismutase activity. Histologically, the rabbit bone marrow showed adipogenesis, and fatty infiltration of the liver was found; this led to increases in fat cell hypertrophy and proliferation and a decrease in hematopoiesis in the subchondral femoral head. Osteocytes contained triglyceride deposits, and there was an increase in empty osteocyte lacunae. Alcohol also primarily affected differentiation of bone marrow stromal cells into adipocytes, and this was a dose-dependent response. Intracellular lipid deposits led to death of osteocytes.

In rats fed a diet of alcohol and glucose, lower bone mineral content and density were detected compared with controls. In hamsters, alcohol led to thinning of the trabeculae of the distal part of the femur. Cytologic effects included mitochondrial swelling in osteoblasts and osteocytes. Partial osteonecrosis of the femoral head was detected in Merino sheep that were injected with ethanol. In humans, alcohol causes increased plasma calcium levels, decreased osteocalcin and circulating parathyroid hormone levels, reduced serum calcitriol, reduced bone volume, and increased osteoclast number. Alcohol also has deleterious effects on muscle, including increased oxygen free radical–related damage to muscle, reduced myocardial contractility, defective mitochondrial function, and increased tissue enzymes.[75]

A study investigated the effects of alcohol on the ability of mesenchymal stem cells to differentiate into osteogenic lineages. The bone marrow in the proximal head of femurs was isolated during hip replacement surgery from 33 patients with either femoral neck fractures or alcohol-induced osteonecrosis. The cells from femurs of patients with alcohol-induced osteonecrosis showed a reduced ability to differentiate into osteoblasts.[76] A subsequent study compared the mesenchymal stem cells from patients with hip osteoarthritis and nontraumatic osteonecrosis associated with steroid use or alcohol use and idiopathic osteonecrosis. In alcohol-induced osteonecrosis and idiopathic osteonecrosis, the ability of mesenchymal stem cells to differentiate into osteoblasts was decreased, but in steroid-induced osteonecrosis, it was elevated, although not to a statistically significant level. The adipogenic differentiation ability was similar in all four groups.[77]

In corticosteroid-induced osteonecrosis, the pathogenic mechanism parallels that of alcohol-induced osteonecrosis. In both cases, fatty infiltration of osteocytes has been postulated to occur.[70,72,74] Table 94-4 lists lipid-altering effects of corticosteroids and alcohol. In addition, interosseous venous stasis affects the interosseous microcirculation, which can lead to hemodynamic and structural changes in the femoral head. The resulting decrease in blood flow leads to osteonecrosis. In chickens treated with steroids, fatty infiltration of the liver and fat cell hypertrophy and proliferation in the femoral head occurred concurrently 1 week after the initiation of steroids. As in the case of alcohol-induced

Table 94-3 Proposed Mechanism of Disease of Common Conditions Associated with Osteonecrosis

Condition	Mechanism of Action			
	1—Secondary to	2—Secondary to	3—Secondary to	4—Secondary to
Trauma	Direct vascular injury			
Sickle cell anemia	Vascular occlusion	Abnormal shape of erythrocytes		
Legg-Calvé-Perthes disease	Mechanical instability of femoral epiphyseal plate	Delayed expression of type X collagen during epiphyseal ossification	Alteration in expression of insulin-like growth factor	
Corticosteroids	Sinusoidal collapse	Increase in intracortical pressure	Increase in femoral head fat content	Hyperlipidemia
Pregnancy	Fat embolism	Acute fatty liver in third trimester of pregnancy	Increased plasma lipid levels in second trimester of pregnancy	
Diabetes	Fat embolism			
Pancreatitis	Fat embolism			
Hereditary dysostosis	Collapse of femoral head	Femoral head subchondral cyst formation	Abnormal endochondral ossification of epiphyseal plate	
Dysbaric osteonecrosis	Occlusion of end arterioles	Formation of intravascular gas bubbles or accumulation of nitrogen gas in the bone marrow		
Intravascular coagulation	Arteriolar thrombosis	Increase in plasma fibrinopeptide A		
Legg-Calvé-Perthes disease	Collapse of subchondral bone	Widening of joint space	Loss of endochondral ossification in the periosseous epiphyseal cartilage and physeal plate	Ischemia
Dialysis	Decreased bone strength	Increased subchondral bone resorption and formation of disorganized bone matrix	Increased bone turnover	Hyperparathyroidism
Ehlers-Danlos syndrome	Hip dislocation			
Gaucher's disease	Vascular compromise	Mass compression	Lipid-laden Gaucher cell infiltration of bone marrow	
Alcohol	Increased concentration of fat emboli in metaphyses of femur	Venous stasis	Absence of vascular sinusoids in bone marrow	Increased blood cortisol levels

Table 94-4 Lipid-Altering Effects of Steroids and Alcohol

Fatty liver
Swelling and necrosis of fat cells
Lipid-filled osteocytes
Hyperlipidemia
Adipogenesis of marrow stromal cells
Fatty infiltration of bone marrow
Fat emboli

osteonecrosis, adipocytes contained triglyceride vesicles. In rabbits treated with steroids, it was found that intraosseous pressure was increased, and the size of bone marrow fat cells was larger than in control rabbits.[78] A histologic study of acetabular and proximal femoral bone in osteonecrosis of the femoral head revealed that osteonecrosis is more extensive in corticosteroid-induced compared with alcohol-induced or idiopathic osteonecrosis. The reason for this is unknown.[79]

In sickle cell anemia, the sickle cells lead to a hyperviscosity syndrome, which blocks vessels and decreases blood delivery to the femoral head.[80] Hyperviscosity also can be seen in hyperlipoproteinemia and Legg-Calvé-Perthes disease.[81] The mechanism for bisphosphonate-induced osteonecrosis might be related to the ability of bisphosphonates to inhibit bone remodeling and decrease interosseous blood flow.[82]

GENETICS OF OSTEONECROSIS

The role of host factors or genetics in the pathogenesis of osteonecrosis is unknown. Studies to identify gene polymorphisms stemmed from the realization that endothelial nitric oxide synthase has beneficial effects on three systems that have been implicated in the development of osteonecrosis—skeletal, vascular, and thrombotic. Comparative analysis of the 26-base pair repeat polymorphism in intron 4 and the Glu298Asp polymorphism in exon 7 was performed between patients with idiopathic, steroid-induced, or alcohol-related osteonecrosis and matched control subjects. The frequency of the 4a allele was higher in patients with idiopathic osteonecrosis compared with control subjects. In addition, the frequency of the 4a/b genotype was higher in all patients with osteonecrosis compared with control subjects.

The 4a allele is known to be associated with reduced synthesis of endothelial nitric oxide synthase, suggesting that nitric oxide may provide a protective effect against the development of osteonecrosis.[83] Forty one percent of patients with osteonecrosis compared with only 20% of controls were homozygous for the 4G/4G mutation in the plasminogen activator inhibitor-1 gene.[84] The mutation causes increased hypofibrolytic plasminogen activator inhibitor activity, resulting in decreased stimulated plasminogen activator activity. This observation gives support to the role that procoagulants might play in the pathogenesis of osteonecrosis.

Alcohol-induced or steroid-induced hyperlipemia, which results in increased serum free fatty acids and prostaglandins, can potentially trigger vascular inflammation and coagulation. Other triggers for intravascular coagulation include atherosclerosis and arteriolar fibroid degeneration. Jones[85] proposed these changes as a possible pathologic mechanism for the development or progression of osteonecrosis from stage 1A to 1B, arguing that an inability to clear procoagulants from the blood or tissue leads to persistent levels of tissue thromboplastin, leading to arteriolar thrombosis, vascular stasis, free fatty acid–induced endothelial damage, and hypercoagulability. Studies of the levels of procoagulants in patients with osteonecrosis showed that 82% of patients with osteonecrosis had at least one abnormal procoagulant level and 47% had at least two abnormal procoagulant levels compared with 30% and 2.5% in normal controls. The procoagulants measured included free protein S, protein C, lipoprotein A, homocysteine, plasminogen activator inhibitor, stimulated tissue plasminogen activator, anticardiolipin antibodies (IgG and IgM), and resistance to activated protein C.[86]

Changes in the vasculature itself may lead to a compromise in blood flow. Examples include structural damage to arteriolar walls, degeneration of the tunica media, smooth muscle cell necrosis, and disruption of the internal elastic lamina. These changes can lead to eventual hemorrhagic infarction[87] and were shown in a series of 24 core biopsy specimens from osteonecrotic femoral heads; the changes did not occur in 11 femoral heads with osteoarthrosis.[88]

In Legg-Calvé-Perthes disease, obstruction to venous drainage elevates intraosseous pressure and consequently elevates intra-articular pressures. In a study of patients with Legg-Calvé-Perthes disease, bone scintigraphy using Tc 99m methylene diphosphonate (Tc 99m MDP) was employed to measure arterial and venous flow in the diseased hip. Although arterial flow was normal, there was a significant disturbance in venous drainage.[89] This disturbance was reproduced in a dog model in which injection of silicone was used to obstruct venous flow distal to the hip.[90] Ischemia as a result of venous drainage obstruction can cause a cessation of endochondral ossification in the preosseous epiphyseal cartilage and the physeal plate. Widening of the joint space ensues followed by revascularization of the epiphysis and deposition of new immature bone. A weakened or unstable femoral epiphyseal plate results, and the subchondral bone becomes prone to segmental collapse and fracture.[91]

The pathologic mechanism in dysbaric osteonecrosis is unclear. The most intuitive explanation is that formation of gas bubbles in the vessels causes occlusion and ischemia. Multiple other factors might contribute to the disease,

however, including thromboembolic events such as platelet aggregation, erythrocyte clumping, lipid coalescence, intraosseous vessel compression as a result of extravascular gas bubbles, formation of fibrin thrombi, and narrowing of arterial lumens owing to myointimal thickening caused by gas bubbles. The interaction between gas and blood can lead to the formation of vessel-occluding substances. All these events may lead to redistribution of blood flow.

The increased vulnerability of bone to compression disorders has been explained by several factors, including the relative rigidity of bone and inability to absorb increased gas pressure, inherent poor vascularization, and gas supersaturation of fatty marrow.[92] A sheep model for dysbaric osteonecrosis has been developed. Exposure to compressed air at pressures of 2.6 to 2.9 atm for 24 hours results in extensive bone and marrow necrosis. The authors proposed that the initial event involving elevated intramedullary pressures leads to formation of nitrogen bubbles in the fatty marrow of the long bones. Radiography shows medullary opacities and endosteal thickening. Later neovascularization of previously ischemic fatty marrow occurs, followed by new bone formation. Osteonecrosis occurs in subchondral cortical bone with marrow fibrosis and osteocyte loss.[93]

Alteration in osteoblast function could contribute to the pathogenesis of osteonecrosis. Osteoblastic cells were obtained from bone biopsy specimens from the intertrochanteric region of the femur and of the iliac crest of 13 patients with osteonecrosis and 8 patients with hip osteoarthritis. Cell replication was measured based on proliferation rate in secondary culture. Levels of alkaline phosphatase activity, collagen synthesis, and the sensitivity to 1,25-dihydroxyvitamin D_3 were measured. The results indicated that although differentiation was not affected, the proliferation rate of osteoblastic cells was reduced in samples obtained from patients with osteonecrosis compared with patients with osteoarthritic hips.[94] Osteocyte death or apoptosis also is a feature of osteonecrosis. In a rat model, ischemia caused an induction in the expression of stress proteins oxygen-regulated protein (ORP150) and hemoxygenase 1 (HO1). Induction of ischemia in these rats caused DNA fragmentation and the presence of apoptotic bodies in chondrocytes, bone marrow cells, and osteocytes.[95]

Osteonecrosis occurs not as a result of a single factor, but as a result of an interrelated combination of factors. This is the basis for the accumulated cell stress hypothesis, first proposed by Kenzora and Glimcher in 1983.[96] The contributing factors can vary for different etiologies of osteonecrosis. Although lipid anomalies might be the primary pathologic event in steroid-induced osteonecrosis, other factors, such as the production of inflammatory mediators, can play a role, explaining why the incidence varies depending on the underlying disorder for which steroids are being used. The prevalence of osteonecrosis in healthy patients being treated with steroids for head trauma was 0% compared with a rate of 52% in patients with systemic lupus erythematosus treated with steroids.[97] In dysbaric osteonecrosis, the primary factor may be gas bubbles and increased interosseous pressures, but lipid abnormalities may play a lesser role. The hypothesis suggests that when the damaging effects of multiple events are added together, cells are unable to recover from the chronic stress, and osteonecrosis ensues.

DIAGNOSIS AND DIAGNOSTIC TESTS

A high index of suspicion is crucial to the diagnosis of osteonecrosis. Pain is usually the presenting symptom, but the disease may be quite advanced by the time patients present with pain, especially when the progression is insidious. In addition to obtaining a complete history, including identification of potential risk factors such as trauma, a complete examination of the affected joint must be performed. The examination should include direct observation for any obvious abnormalities, such as leg-length discrepancies, masses, and abnormal orientation. Additionally, the hip should be palpated for tenderness and to identify any masses not detected on direct visualization. The hip should be examined for range of motion, muscle strength, and gait. The Harris hip score is frequently used for evaluating hip function and is useful in monitoring effectiveness of treatment. The Harris hip score is a multidimensional observational assessment based on eight items, which address pain, walking function, daily activity, and range of motion. Scores range from 0 (maximum disability) to 100 (no disability). Figure 94-1 is an algorithm for the diagnosis of osteonecrosis.

When the diagnosis is suspected, it can be confirmed either by imaging studies or by arthroscopy. Earlier employed imaging techniques, such as radiography, were inadequate in establishing the diagnosis because in very early stages of osteonecrosis radiographs are often completely normal. The earliest radiographic sign of osteonecrosis is the presence of a radiolucent crescent (so-called crescent sign) (Fig. 94-2),

which is the result of structural collapse of a necrotic segment of subchondral trabecular bone. At this stage, the disease already would have progressed to an irreversible stage, however. Subsequently, the radiographs show sclerotic changes (Fig. 94-3). The appearance of radiographic "density" is secondary to compression of bone trabeculae after microfracture of the nonviable bone, calcification of detritic marrow, and repair of the necrotic area by deposition of new bone, the so-called creeping substitution. Flattening of the articular surface of bone is the sign of further bone collapse (Fig. 94-4). To show best the radiographic appearance of osteonecrosis in the hips, and for better visualization of the extent of the necrotic lesion, anteroposterior and frog-leg lateral films should be obtained.

Skeletal scintigraphy (radionuclide bone scan) using technetium-labeled diphosphonates also has been used to diagnose osteonecrosis. The use of this technique in the early diagnosis of this condition depends on the fact that osteoblastic activity and blood flow are increased in the early stages of osteonecrosis. In an advanced stage of disease, the appearance may be one of increased activity in a subchondral distribution owing to osteoblastic activity at the reactive interface around the necrotic segment; however, the center of the osteonecrotic lesion may show much less radionuclide activity (Fig. 94-5), or even complete lack of activity, reflecting decreased metabolism in the necrotic focus as a result of interruption of blood supply.[6]

In addition to bone scintigraphy, single-photon emission computed tomography (SPECT) maximizes sensitivity.

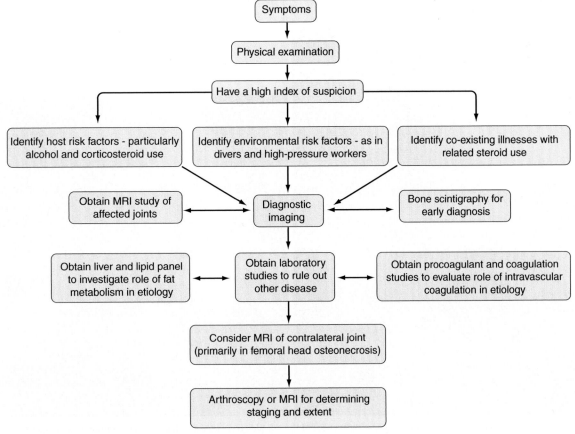

Figure 94-1 Algorithm for the diagnosis of osteonecrosis. MRI, magnetic resonance imaging.

A study comparing conventional radiography, MRI, computed tomography (CT), and Tc 99m MDP three-phase bone scan in diagnosing bisphosphonate-associated osteonecrosis of the jaw showed that CT and MRI were the best at defining the extent of the disease, but that bone scan was the best at identifying disease at an early stage. Bone scan could be an excellent screening tool for the diagnosis of osteonecrosis before further characterization of the lesions using CT or MRI.[98]

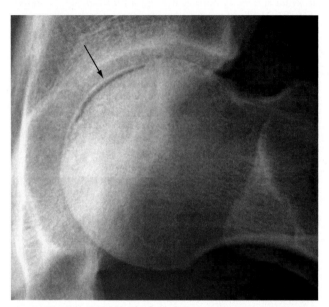

Figure 94-2 A radiolucent crescent in the subchondral region of the left femoral head *(arrow)* is an early radiographic sign of osteonecrosis.

CT allows more detailed examination of the femoral head. A star-shaped structure, formed by weight-bearing bone trabeculae, gave the appearance of an asterisk on CT scan (the asterisk sign).[99-101] This asterisk undergoes a characteristic change in ischemic bone necrosis of the femoral head, and this change was considered important for early detection of osteonecrosis. At a later stage, the collapse of necrotic bone can be well shown (Fig. 94-6).

More recently, MRI has become the "gold standard" for imaging of osteonecrosis, and the staging systems for osteonecrosis are based on changes seen on MRI appearance (Table 94-5). MRI of osteonecrosis can show changes earlier than radiography or CT. It is able to detect bone marrow edema, an early feature of osteonecrosis that is invisible on radiography or CT in early stages.

The typical MRI findings are intermediate or low signal intensity on T1-weighted images and high signal on T2-weighted images (Fig. 94-7). As the disease progresses, the subchondral necrotic lesion is surrounded by a low signal line on T1-weighted images, and a high signal line is seen in T2-weighted images that is central to the low signal line. This produces the "double-line" sign (Fig. 94-8).[102] In advanced osteonecrosis, the necrotic segment exhibits low signal intensity on T1-weighted and T2-weighted images (Fig. 94-9). MRI is done in the sagittal, coronal, and axial planes, and includes T1-weighted and T2-weighted sequences. There is excellent correlation between histologic findings and MRI appearance (see Table 94-5).

MRI is an important tool in determining the extent of femoral head involvement in osteonecrosis. Three techniques are used to determine this. The first is estimating head involvement. This method was first proposed by Steinberg

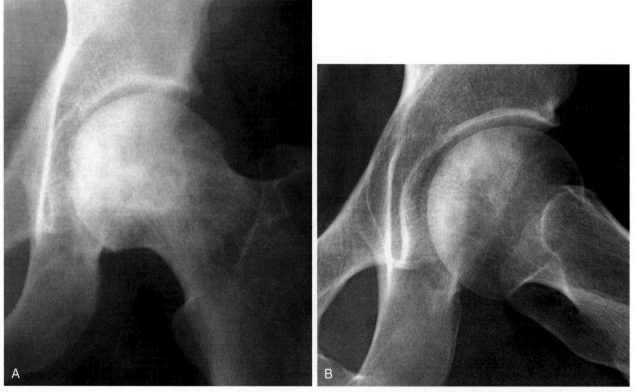

Figure 94-3 **A** and **B,** Anteroposterior **(A)** and frog-lateral **(B)** views of the left hip show sclerotic changes of the femoral head typical of advanced osteonecrosis.

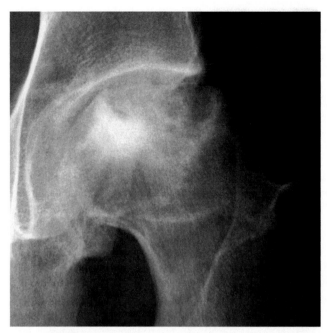

Figure 94-4 Increased density of the femoral head, loss of the normal spherical shape, and flattening of the superior aspect are characteristic radiographic features of osteonecrosis.

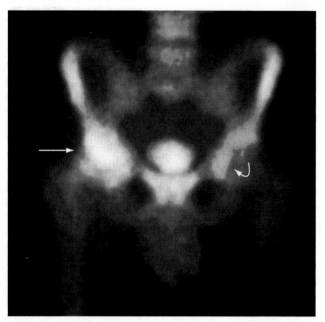

Figure 94-5 Bone scintigraphy of osteonecrosis of both femoral heads using Tc 99m MDP shows moderate uptake of radiopharmaceutical at the site of the osteonecrotic segment in the right femoral head and markedly increased uptake at the site of bone repair *(straight arrow)*. The left femoral head *(curved arrow)* exhibits early-stage disease.

and coworkers in 1984,[103] and it is defined by appearance of abnormal signals on T1-weighted images. The degree of head involvement was classified into three categories: less than 15%, 15% to 30%, and greater than 30%. The second method used is the index of necrotic extent, which is determined by measuring the angle created by the extent of subchondral involvement. Lesion size was estimated using a "necrotic arc angle," defined as the angle of the arc of the necrotic segment from the center of the femoral head. Two angles were obtained: "A," representing the necrotic arc angle seen on midcoronal images, and "B," representing the necrotic arc angle seen on midsagittal images. The index is a compilation of these two angles. A third method is a variation of the second, in which the angle is identified not on midcoronal or midsagittal images, but on the image that shows the maximum lesion size in the sagittal and coronal images. It was thought that this method would correct for the underestimation that may be inherent in the second method.

Table 94-6 shows a comparison of various radiographic techniques used in the diagnosis and staging of osteonecrosis. Hip arthroscopy also is used in the staging of osteonecrosis. In a study comparing radiography, MRI, and arthroscopy, there was only moderate correlation among the three methods. Arthroscopy was able to detect osteochondral degeneration, not detected by radiography or MRI in 36% of postcollapse femoral heads.[104,105] Recently, the measurement of serum and urine carboxy-terminal cross-linking telopeptide of type I collagen (CTX-1), a marker of bone resorption, has been proposed as a method of evaluating the risk of osteonecrosis of the jaw secondary to bisphosphonate usage.[105a]

BONE MARROW EDEMA

Bone marrow edema is a common observation in osteonecrosis and frequently is accompanied by vascular congestion. Bone marrow edema is not specific for osteonecrosis and

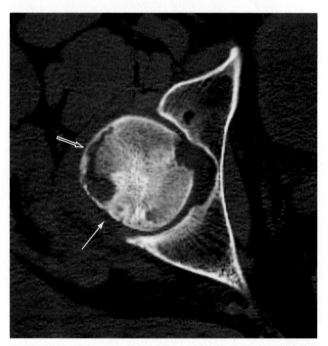

Figure 94-6 CT shows advanced osteonecrosis of the femoral head. Note increased sclerosis posteriorly *(solid arrow)* and subchondral collapse of necrotic bone anterolaterally *(open arrow)*.

may be seen in many musculoskeletal disorders, including osteomyelitis, osteoarthritis, occult intraosseous fracture, stress fracture, osteoporosis, and sickle cell crisis.

A specific syndrome known as bone marrow edema syndrome has been described and was initially thought to be a precursor to osteonecrosis, but it is now believed to be a separate entity. Bone marrow edema syndrome is a transitory,

Table 94-5 Magnetic Resonance Imaging (MRI) Changes and Their Correlation with Histology in Osteonecrosis

Type of Appearance	Category of Observations	Histology	MRI Appearance
A	Fatlike	Premature fatty marrow development in the femoral neck or intertrochanteric region	Normal fat signal; sclerotic margin may be seen circumscribing lesion
B	Bloodlike	Bone resorption; replacement by vascular granulation tissue	High signal intensity of inner border; low signal intensity of surrounding rim
C	Fluid-like	Presence of edema	Diffusely decreased signal on T1-weighted images; high signal on T2-weighted images
D	Fibrotic	Sclerosis owing to reinforcement of existing trabeculae at margin of live bone (repair tissue interface)	Decreased signal on T1-weighted and T2-weighted images

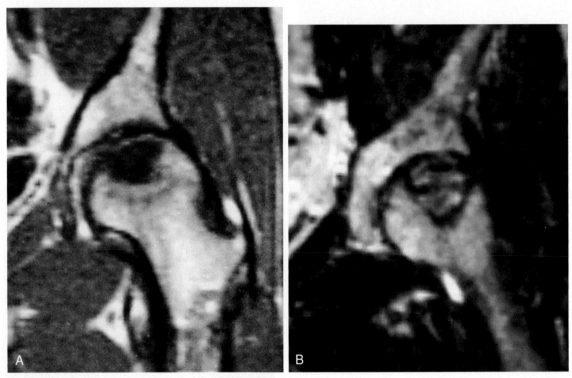

Figure 94-7 A, On T1-weighted coronal MR image of the left hip, the osteonecrotic segment in the subchondral portion of the femoral head shows low signal intensity. **B,** On T2-weighted coronal image, the necrotic bone exhibits high signal intensity, surrounded by a sclerotic low-signal rim.

self-limiting condition, typically seen in middle-aged men and in women in their third trimester of pregnancy. Patients complain of pain, limited range of motion, and an abnormal gait. Osteopenia is detected on conventional radiographs and MRI (low signal on T1-weighted images and high signal on T2-weighted images). The three phases of bone marrow edema syndrome include an initial phase lasting about 1 month, followed by a plateau phase lasting 1 or 2 months, and finally a regression phase lasting for an additional 4 to 6 months.[106] Subchondral fractures do not occur. Biopsy specimens obtained in the initial phase show diffuse interstitial edema, fragmentation of fatty marrow cells, and increased new bone formation.[107]

A study of 24 cases of bone marrow edema syndrome of the knee showed that although migrating bone marrow edema occurred in a third of patients at a 5-year follow-up, the patients were asymptomatic, and MRI signal alterations

had resolved. Biopsy specimens of the affected bone were obtained using arthroscopic surgery and core decompression, and histology revealed areas of bone marrow edema and vital trabeculae covered by osteoblasts and osteoid seams. None of the cases progressed to osteonecrosis.[108]

TREATMENT

The key to the successful treatment of osteonecrosis is early detection. The choice of conservative nonsurgical versus more aggressive surgical options depends on the clinical and pathologic staging of the disease.

Surgical management of femoral head osteonecrosis includes core decompression, structural bone grafting, vascularized fibula grafting, osteotomy, resurfacing arthroplasty, hemiarthroplasty, and total hip replacement.[109] Arthroscopy has been used as a tool to treat osteonecrosis.

It has been used to determine the position of the core decompression tract to the necrotic part of the femoral head,[110] and arthroscopic débridement has been used in treatment of osteonecrosis of the capitellum of the humerus in adolescents,[111] Kienböck's disease,[112] and osteonecrosis of the scaphoid.[113]

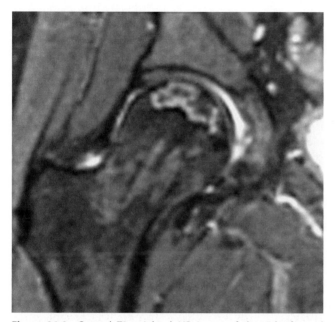

Figure 94-8 Coronal T2-weighted MR image of the right femoral head shows the double-line sign, characteristic for osteonecrosis: low signal line at periphery of the lesion, and high signal band located more centrally.

Core decompression involves the removal of a core of bone from the femoral neck and head. The core acts as a vent to reduce intraosseous pressure and intramedullary pressure, reversing ischemia and improving symptoms. Other changes that may occur include stimulation of angiogenesis, leading to improved vascularization during the repair process. It is generally used in less advanced stages of osteonecrosis. Core decompression in the treatment of nontraumatic osteonecrosis of the femoral head was done in 34 patients with 54 affected hips.[114] The average age at presentation was 38 years. The patients were monitored for a mean duration of 120 months. Success was defined as absence of symptoms, no progression of disease, and no further surgery. Clinical success was established in 26 hips (48%), and radiographic success was established in 20 hips (37%). The later the stage at which core decompression was performed, the greater the failure rate.[115] Core decompression also has been used in the treatment of humeral head osteonecrosis with good outcome.[116]

More recently, computer-assisted core decompression has been used to provide greater precision in directing the core into the ischemic area, and to minimize the radiation exposure time to patients.[117] Because early diagnosis improves outcome, and because there is a high incidence of developing osteonecrosis in a contralateral hip, core decompression is frequently done on both hips simultaneously. This approach has been shown to have little added risk over unilateral core decompression with the added benefit of better outcomes secondary to early surgical treatment of the contralateral hip.[118]

In structural bone grafting, or bone impaction grafting, the bone graft is inserted into the necrotic segment through the core tract. The bone graft acts in similar fashion to a stent, providing support to overlying subchondral

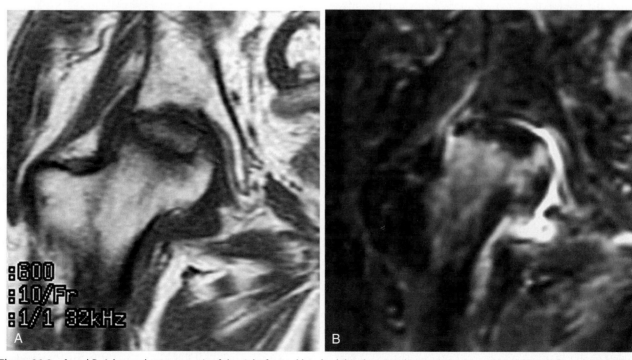

Figure 94-9 **A** and **B,** Advanced osteonecrosis of the right femoral head exhibits low signal intensity on T1-weighted (**A**) and T2-weighted (**B**) MR images.

Table 94-6 Comparative Sensitivity and Specificity of Diagnostic Radiologic Imaging Modalities in Osteonecrosis

Radiologic Imaging	Earliest Sign Seen	Earliest Seen (Stage)	Degree of Specificity
Radiography	Crescent sign	Sclerotic rim of reactive bone (stage 2)	High
CT	Asterisk sign	Sclerotic rim surrounding a mottled area of osteolysis and sclerosis (stage 2)	High
MRI	Low signal intensity on T1-weighted images; high signal intensity on T2-weighted images	Bone marrow edema (stage 1)	High
Skeletal scintigraphy	Decreased uptake in subchondral distribution	"Cold spot" (stage 1)	Low
	Increased uptake in subchondral distribution	"Hot spot" (stage 2)	Low

CT, computed tomography; MRI, magnetic resonance imaging.

bone. The goal is to prevent collapse. This combination of procedures is frequently used in treating stage I or II osteonecrotic femoral heads. Allogeneic and autologous bone grafts, mostly harvested from the tibia or fibula, are used. When this technique was attempted in patients with stages III and IV lesions, the outcome was generally poor (100% failure after 2 to 4 years), with progression to collapse and further surgical procedures.[119]

Vascularized structural bone grafting also uses the core tract to insert a corticocancellous bone graft into the femoral neck and head along with its vascular pedicle. The vascular pedicle is anastomosed to a nearby vessel, adding a source of blood to the graft. The results of vascularized fibular grafting in the treatment of hips with osteonecrosis showed a survival of 61% of hips at 5-year follow-up, and 42% at a median time of 8 years.[120] In another study, 197 patients with 226 osteonecrotic hips were treated with a combination of autologous cancellous bone impaction and pedicled iliac bone block transfer. The anastomosis was to the ascending branch of the lateral femoral circumflex artery. Fourteen hips required conversion to total hip arthroplasty because of collapse or severe pain or both. Of the remaining 212 hips, 92% were considered a clinical success, and 76% were considered radiographically successful. The success rate declined from stage II to stage IV hips (96% for stage II hips, 90% for stage III hips, and 57% for stage IV hips).[121]

Osteotomy of the femur involves shifting the position of the osteonecrotic segment by making a cut in the proximal femur so that the osteonecrotic segment is rotated or flexed out of the weight-bearing region of the acetabulum, and replacing the weight-bearing region with viable bone. Healing of the necrotic region can proceed without the stress of weight bearing. Several different osteotomy techniques have been attempted to salvage hips in stage II or III osteonecrosis.

Resurfacing arthroplasty uses a metallic or ceramic shell placed over a femoral head that has been débrided of the necrotic area. The potential advantages of resurfacing arthroplasty include preservation of joint mechanics, bone conservation,[122] more physiologic loading of the bone, a lower incidence of perioperative complications, and easier conversion to total hip arthroplasty in case of failure.[123] Complications of this procedure include femoral neck fractures, a secondary osteonecrosis when

the procedure is done for other reasons,[124] and increased metal ion levels.[125] Resurfacing arthroplasty has been recommended for patients with later stage osteonecrosis, including patients with femoral head collapse.[126] A retrospective study compared the results of limited femoral head resurfacing and total hip arthroplasty in 30 consecutive patients with Steinberg stage III or IV disease. The survival rate at a 7-year mean follow-up period for the resurfacing group was 90%, whereas the survival rate at an 8-year mean follow-up for the total hip arthroplasty group was 93%.[127]

In hemiarthroplasty, only part of the hip joint is replaced. The original acetabulum is preserved, but the femoral head is replaced with a prosthesis. Two kinds of prostheses are used—a unipolar prosthesis and a bipolar prosthesis. In a unipolar prosthesis, the articulation is between the artificial femoral head and the acetabulum. In the bipolar prosthesis, presently the most frequently used, the articulation is within the prosthesis itself. Failure rates for hemiarthroplasties in osteonecrosis are 50% to 60% at 3 years for unipolar prostheses and 44% for bipolar prostheses.[128] Another study evaluated the success rate of Charnley/Bicentric hemiarthroplasty in the treatment of Ficat and Arlet stage III osteonecrosis of the femoral head. Failures included three hips that needed to be revised to cementless total hip replacement, two hips with radiographic changes of loosening and imminent failure, and one hip with progressive loss of joint space and secondary degenerative changes. The success rate was 84.2% after a mean of 56 months.[129]

Total hip arthroplasty is complete replacement of the hip joint with a prosthesis including the femoral head and the acetabulum. In a study of 55 consecutive hip arthroplasty procedures, cementless total hip arthroplasty was shown to provide favorable results in advanced-stage osteonecrosis of the femoral head. Although 10 of the 48 hips available for follow-up after a minimum of 5 years required revision, all of these patients had Ficat and Arlet stage III or IV disease.[130] A study of 53 hips in 41 patients treated with cemented total hip replacement showed that at a minimum of 10 years of follow-up, 17.4% required revision. Compared with cemented total hip replacements done for other conditions, osteonecrosis had a greater risk for loosening of acetabular and femoral components.[131] A survivorship analysis of cemented total hip replacements in renal transplant patients with osteonecrosis of the femoral head showed that there was excellent survival after 10 years (98.8%). After 20 years, the survival decreased to 63.8%.

Nonsurgical treatment of osteonecrosis of the femoral head consists of refraining from weight bearing on the affected joint, analgesic and anti-inflammatory medications, and physiotherapy. Conservative medical treatment is effective only in the early stages for symptomatic relief. Nonsurgical management does not seem to change the natural course of the disease.[132]

Electric stimulation has been used in the treatment of osteonecrosis, frequently in conjunction with core decompression. Electric stimulation enhances osteogenesis and neovascularization. It also alters the balance between osteoblast and osteoclast activity so that more bone is produced, and less is resorbed, leading to an increase in bone substance. The three methods for delivery of electric stimulation include direct current, pulsed electromagnetic field, and capacitance coupling. Core decompression with placement of an electric stimulating coil in the anterosuperior segment of the femoral head was done in 11 hips in eight patients who had Ficat stage II osteonecrosis. Results were poor, with 5 of 11 hips requiring reoperation after an average of 13 months after initial placement of the electric coil, and the other 6 having progressive deterioration in function. There was minimal evidence of new bone formation around the coil under histologic examination.[133]

A study compared the effectiveness of nonsurgical treatment with core decompression with and without direct current electric stimulation. The clinical symptoms scores and progression to arthroplasty rates were worst in the nonoperative treatment group, whereas the results were best in the patients treated with core decompression and DC stimulation.[134]

Capacitive coupling is a noninvasive method of providing electric stimulation that can be administered with or without core decompression and grafting. Core decompression and grafting were done on 40 patients with stage I to III osteonecrosis; half of the patients wore active capacitive coupling units with electrodes over the femoral head for 6 months. The control group was 55 patients with osteonecrosis who were treated conservatively. Two-year to 4-year follow-up showed that core decompression with or without capacitive coupling provided better clinical and radiologic outcome than conservative treatment, but that capacitive coupling did not improve the results further when used with core decompression and grafting.[135]

Extracorporeal shock wave therapy has been used in the treatment of osteonecrosis of the femoral head. A study of 48 patients and 57 hips compared extracorporeal shock wave therapy with core decompression and bone grafting. Twenty-three patients with 29 affected hips were assigned to the shock wave group, and the remaining patients and hips received surgical treatment. The patients in the shock wave group were given one treatment of 6000 pulses of shock waves at 28 kV to the affected hip. The patients were evaluated by their reports of symptoms (pain), by Harris hip scores, by quality of life (daily work and activity assessment), and radiographically. Shock wave therapy produced better results than the nonvascularized bone grafting procedure, with comparatively less progression of disease.[136]

Conservative treatment of osteonecrosis of the talus is not promising, and the affected ankles generally continue to progress, requiring either core decompression or arthrodesis.[60] Conservative treatment of bisphosphonate-induced osteonecrosis of the jaw includes cessation of bisphosphonate usage or surgical débridement.[17] Good oral hygiene, regular dental assessment, and avoidance of dental procedures during bisphosphonate usage can prevent onset of osteonecrosis. Figure 94-10 is an algorithm for the treatment of osteonecrosis.

NEW MODALITIES OF TREATMENT OF OSTEONECROSIS

Mesenchymal stem cells are thought to play a role in the development of osteonecrosis. Corticosteroids seem to cause enhanced adipogenesis and decreased osteogenesis by mesenchymal cells in vitro, and they cause a decrease in a potent angiogenic factor, vascular endothelial growth factor. This activity suggests that steroids shunt uncommitted osteoprogenitor cells in marrow from osteoblastic differentiation to the adipocytic pathway, leading to diminished vascularization and eventual osteonecrosis.[137] Alcohol also seems to have a similar effect on the differentiation of stem cells.[76] Consequently, more recent studies on the use of mesenchymal stem cells in the treatment of osteonecrosis have been performed. Multipotential mesenchymal stem cells from femoral bone marrow near osteonecrosis sites are able to express mRNA for aggrecan and collagen type II. They also can deposit immunoreactive collagen type II and sulfated proteoglycans into the bone matrix. These features are characteristics of chondrogenic differentiation. The mesenchymal stem cells can be differentiated into osteocytic lineage in vitro.[138]

A pilot study evaluating the effectiveness of implantation of autologous bone marrow cells in the treatment of osteonecrosis used core decompression to implant stem cells into the necrotic lesions of the femoral head.[139,140] The patients were divided into two groups—one that received core decompression alone as treatment for osteonecrosis (the control group), and one that received autologous bone marrow cell implantation along with core decompression (the treatment group). The patients were followed for 24 months, and at that time, 5 of 8 hips in the control group, but only 1 of 10 in the treatment group advanced to stage III osteonecrosis. In addition, there was greater improvement in pain and joint symptoms in the treatment group, and the treatment seemed to be safe. Because of the small number of patients involved, further studies need to be done to confirm these results.

More recently, 28 patients with 44 necrotic hips were treated with percutaneous decompression and autologous bone marrow mononuclear cell infusion. Patients were followed for a minimum of 2 years and evaluated for clinical and radiographic progression of the disease. There seemed to be overall slowing in the progression of disease stage. The mean Harris hip score improved from 58 to 86.[141]

OUTCOME AND PROGNOSIS

The natural history of osteonecrosis depends on the size of the infarcted segment, the site of occurrence, and the clinical and radiologic staging of the disease. At the onset of the disease, range of motion may be well preserved, but gradually

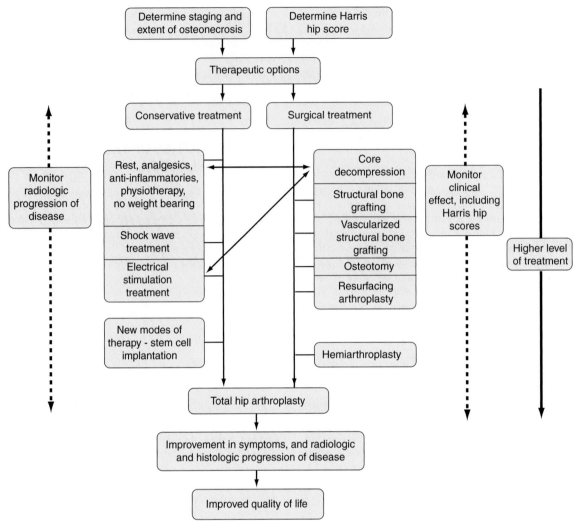

Figure 94-10 Algorithm for treatment of osteonecrosis.

deteriorates over time. Patients are frequently asymptomatic initially. By the time they present, many patients already may have later stage disease. Although spontaneous resolution of osteonecrosis of the femoral head can occur, it is rare and occurs only when lesion size is small.[142] A study of the prognosis of osteonecrosis of the femoral head as a function of symptoms (pain) and radiographic findings showed that in patients who were asymptomatic and had normal radiographs, progression of the disease was slow, with only 1 of 23 hips progressing to pain and radiographic changes after 5 years. If radiographic changes are already present, disease progresses to pain in 14 of 19 patients after 5 years.[143] In a study of stage I osteonecrotic lesions of the hip diagnosed with MRI, 40 patients were followed for an average of 11 years. All patients had a stage I lesion on the contralateral hip. Overall, 35 of the 40 stage I hips became symptomatic, and 29 hips showed collapse. The mean interval between diagnosis and collapse was 92 months, whereas the mean interval between symptoms and diagnosis was 80 months.[144] Most stage I hips eventually progress to a more advanced stage, requiring surgery, so these hips should be monitored closely.

Future Directions

The recent recognition of the role of cellular mediators or regulatory factors of inflammation in the pathogenesis of bone diseases may provide greater insight into completely novel modes of prevention and treatment of osteonecrosis in the future.

REFERENCES

1. McCarthy EF: Aseptic necrosis of bone: An historic perspective. Clin Orthop 168:216-221, 1982.
2. Nixon JE: Avascular necrosis of bone: A review. J R Soc Med 76: 681-692, 1983.
3. Axhausen G: Archiv fur klinische Chirurgie 151:72-98, 1928.
4. Hutter CD: Dysbaric osteonecrosis: A reassessment and hypothesis. Med Hypotheses 54:585-590, 2000.
5. **Assouline-Dayan Y, Chang C, Greenspan A, et al: Pathogenesis and natural history of osteonecrosis. Semin Arthritis Rheum 32:94-124, 2002.**
6. **Chang CC, Greenspan A, Gershwin ME: Osteonecrosis: Current perspectives on pathogenesis and treatment. Semin Arthritis Rheum 23:47-69, 1993.**

7. Sevitt S: Avascular necrosis and revascularisation of the femoral head after intracapsular fractures: A combined arteriographic and histological necropsy study. J Bone Joint Surg Br 46:270-296, 1964.

8. Mankin HJ: Nontraumatic necrosis of bone (osteonecrosis). N Engl J Med 326:1473-1479, 1992.

9. D'Aubigne RM, Frain PG: [Theory of osteotomies]. Rev Chir Orthop Reparatrice Appar Mot 58:159-167, 1972.

10. Peitrogrando V, Mastromarino R: Osteopatia de prolongato trattamento cortisono. Ortop Traumatol 25:793, 1957.

11. Koo KH, Kim R, Kim YS, et al: Risk period for developing osteonecrosis of the femoral head in patients on steroid treatment. Clin Rheumatol 21:299-303, 2002.

12. Hurel SJ, Kendall-Taylor P: Avascular necrosis secondary to postoperative steroid therapy. Br J Neurosurg 11:356-358, 1997.

13. Gogas H, Fennelly D: Avascular necrosis following extensive chemotherapy and dexamethasone treatment in a patient with advanced ovarian cancer: Case report and review of the literature. Gynecol Oncol 63:379-381, 1996.

14. Vreden SG, Hermus AR, van Liessum PA, et al: Aseptic bone necrosis in patients on glucocorticoid replacement therapy. Neth J Med 39 (3-4):153-157, 1991.

15. Haajanen J, Saarinen O, Laasonen L, et al: Steroid treatment and aseptic necrosis of the femoral head in renal transplant recipients. Transplant Proc 16:1316-1319, 1984.

16. Chandler GN, Jones DT, Wright V, et al: Charcot's arthropathy following intra-articular hydrocortisone. BMJ 1:952-953, 1959.

17. Farrugia MC, Summerlin DJ, Krowiak E, et al: Osteonecrosis of the mandible or maxilla associated with the use of new generation bisphosphonates. [Laryngoscope 116:115-120, 2006.

18. Axhausen G: Die nekrose des proximaler Bruchstuecks beim Schenkelhals bruch und ihre Bedentung Fuer das Heuft gelenk. Langebachs Arch Klin Chir 120:325-346, 1922.

19. Matsuo K, Hirohata T, Sugioka Y, et al: Influence of alcohol intake, cigarette smoking, and occupational status on idiopathic osteonecrosis of the femoral head. Clin Orthop 234:115-123, 1988.

20. Antti-Poika I, Karaharju E, Vankka E, et al: Alcohol-associated femoral head necrosis. Ann Chir Gynaecol 76:318-322, 1987.

21. Orlic D, Jovanovic S, Anticevic D, et al: Frequency of idiopathic aseptic necrosis in medically treated alcoholics. Int Orthop 14:383-386, 1990.

22. Hirota Y, Hirohata T, Fukuda K, et al: Association of alcohol intake, cigarette smoking, and occupational status with the risk of idiopathic osteonecrosis of the femoral head. Am J Epidemiol 137:530-538, 1993.

23. Mont MA, Glueck CJ, Pacheco IH, et al: Risk factors for osteonecrosis in systemic lupus erythematosus. J Rheumatol 24:654-662, 1997.

24. Calvé J: Sur une forme particuliere de pseudocoxalgie greffee sur des deformations caracteristiques de l'extremite superieure du femur. Rev Chir 30:54-58, 1910.

25. Legg A: An obscure affection of the hip joint. Boston Med Surg J 162:202-204, 1910.

26. Perthes G: Ueber Arthritis deformans juvenilis. Deutsche Zeitschr Chir 107:111-159, 1910.

27. Bentzon P: Experimental studies on the pathogenesis of coxa plana (Calvé-Legg-Perthes-Waldenstrom's disease) and other manifestations of "local dyschondroplasia." Acta Radiol 6:155-172, 1926.

28. Ryder C, LeBouvier J, Kane R: Coxa plana. Pediatrics 19:979-992, 1957.

29. Goff CW: Legg-Calvé-Perthes syndrome (LCPS): An up-to-date critical review. Clin Orthop 22:93-107, 1962.

30. Landin LA, Danielsson LG, Wattsgard C: Transient synovitis of the hip: Its incidence, epidemiology and relation to Perthes' disease. J Bone Joint Surg Br 69:238-242, 1987.

31. Burwell RG: Perthes' disease: Growth and aetiology. Arch Dis Child 63:1408-1412, 1988.

32. Burwell RG, Dangerfield PH, Hall DJ, et al: Perthes' disease: An anthropometric study revealing impaired and disproportionate growth. J Bone Joint Surg Br 60:461-477, 1978.

33. Kristmundsdottir F, Burwell RG, Harrison MH: Delayed skeletal maturation in Perthes' disease. Acta Orthop Scand 58:277-279, 1987.

34. Hall DJ, Harrison MH, Burwell RG: Congenital abnormalities and Perthes' disease: Clinical evidence that children with Perthes' disease may have a major congenital defect. J Bone Joint Surg Br 61:18-25, 1979.

35. Burwell RG, Vernon CL, Dangerfield PH, et al: Raised somatomedin activity in the serum of young boys with Perthes' disease revealed by bioassay: A disease of growth transition? Clin Orthop 209:129-138, 1986.

36. Rayner PH, Schwalbe SL, Hall DJ: An assessment of endocrine function in boys with Perthes' disease. Clin Orthop 209:124-128, 1986.

37. Montella BJ, Nunley JA, Urbaniak JR: Osteonecrosis of the femoral head associated with pregnancy: A preliminary report. J Bone Joint Surg Am 81:790-798, 1999.

38. Hernigou P, Allain J, Bachir D, et al: Abnormalities of the adult shoulder due to sickle cell osteonecrosis during childhood. Rev Rhum Engl Ed 65:27-32, 1998.

39. Hernigou P, Galacteros F, Bachir D, et al: Deformities of the hip in adults who have sickle-cell disease and had avascular necrosis in childhood: A natural history of fifty-two patients. J Bone Joint Surg Am 73:81-92, 1991.

40. Kandzierski G, Gregosiewicz A, Malek U, et al: [Femur head necrosis in haemophilia and after prolonged steroid therapy—description of two cases]. Chir Narzadow Ruchu Ortop Pol 69:269-271, 2004.

41. Kemnitz S, Moens P, Peerlinck K, et al: Avascular necrosis of the talus in children with haemophilia. J Pediatr Orthop B 11:73-78, 2002.

42. Kilcoyne RF, Nuss R: Femoral head osteonecrosis in a child with hemophilia. Arthritis Rheum 42:1550-1551, 1999.

43. MacNicol MF, Ludlam CA: Does avascular necrosis cause collapse of the dome of the talus in severe haemophilia? Haemophilia 5:139-142, 1999.

44. Paton RW, Evans DI: Silent avascular necrosis of the femoral head in haemophilia. J Bone Joint Surg Br 70:737-739, 1988.

45. Perri G, Giordano V: [Aseptic necrosis of the femur head in hemophiliacs]. Radiol Med (Torino) 68:137-140, 1982.

46. Twynham G: A case of Caisson disease. BM J 1:190-191, 1888.

47. Davidson JK: Dysbaric disorders: Aseptic bone necrosis in tunnel workers and divers. Baillieres Clin Rheumatol 3:1-23, 1989.

48. Cushner MA, Friedman RJ: Osteonecrosis of the humeral head. J Am Acad Orthop Surg 5:339-346, 1997.

49. Hasan SS, Romeo AA: Nontraumatic osteonecrosis of the humeral head. J Shoulder Elbow Surg 11:281-298, 2002.

50. Hattrup SJ, Cofield RH: Osteonecrosis of the humeral head: Relationship of disease stage, extent, and cause to natural history. J Shoulder Elbow Surg 8:559-564, 1999.

51. L'Insalata JC, Pagnani MJ, Warren RF, et al: Humeral head osteonecrosis: Clinical course and radiographic predictors of outcome. J Shoulder Elbow Surg 5:355-361, 1996.

52. Baumgarten KM, Mont MA, Rifai A, et al: Atraumatic osteonecrosis of the patella. Clin Orthop 383:191-196, 2001.

53. Berger CE, Kroner A, Kristen KH, et al: Spontaneous osteonecrosis of the knee: Biochemical markers of bone turnover and pathohistology. Osteoarthritis Cartilage 13:716-721, 2005.

54. Mont MA, Baumgarten KM, Rifai A, et al: Atraumatic osteonecrosis of the knee. J Bone Joint Surg Am 82:1279-1290, 2000.

55. Barnes R, Brown JT, Garden RS, et al: Subcapital fractures of the femur: A prospective review. J Bone Joint Surg 58:2-24, 1976.

56. Kusayama T: Idiopathic osteonecrosis of the femoral condyle after meniscectomy. Tokai J Exp Clin Med 28:145-150, 2003.

57. Murakami H, Soejima T, Inoue T, et al: A long-term follow-up study of four cases who underwent curettage and autogenous bone grafting for steroid-related osteonecrosis of the femoral condyle. Kurume Med J 51(3-4):277-281, 2004.

58. Muscolo DL, Costa-Paz M, Ayerza M, et al: Medial meniscal tears and spontaneous osteonecrosis of the knee. Arthroscopy 22:457-460, 2006.

59. Radke S, Wollmerstedt N, Bischoff A, et al: Knee arthroplasty for spontaneous osteonecrosis of the knee: Unicompartimental vs bicompartimental knee arthroplasty. Knee Surg Sports Traumatol Arthrosc 13:158-162, 2005.

60. Delanois RE, Mont MA, Yoon TR, et al: Atraumatic osteonecrosis of the talus. J Bone Joint Surg Am 80:529-536, 1998.

61. Hirohata S, Ito K: Aseptic necrosis of unilateral scaphoid bone in systemic lupus erythematosus. Intern Med 31:794-797, 1992.

62. Allen BL Jr, Jinkins WJ 3rd: Vertebral osteonecrosis associated with pancreatitis in a child: A case report. J Bone Joint Surg Am 60:985-987, 1978.

63. Ito M, Motomiya M, Abumi K, et al: Vertebral osteonecrosis associated with sarcoidosis: Case report. J Neurosurg Spine 2:222-225, 2005.

64. Sigmundsson FG, Andersen PB, Schroeder HD, et al: Vertebral osteonecrosis associated with pancreatitis in a woman with pancreas divisum: A case report. J Bone Joint Surg Am 86:2504-2508, 2004.

65. Chowdhury S, Pickering LM, Ellis PA: Adjuvant aromatase inhibitors and bone health. J Br Menopause Soc 12:97-103, 2006.

66. Van Poznak C, Estilo C: Osteonecrosis of the jaw in cancer patients receiving IV bisphosphonates. Oncology (Williston Park) 20:1053-1062; discussion 1065-1066, 2006.

67. Pathak I, Bryce G: Temporal bone necrosis: Diagnosis, classification, and management. Otolaryngol Head Neck Surg 123:252-257, 2000.

68. Gardeniers J: ARCO international classification of osteonecrosis. ARCO Newsletter 5:79, 1993.

69. Glimcher MJ, Kenzora JE: The biology of osteonecrosis of the human femoral head and its clinical implications, III: Discussion of the etiology and genesis of the pathological sequelae; commments on treatment. Clin Orthop 140:273-312, 1979.

70. Cui Q, Wang GJ, Balian G: Steroid-induced adipogenesis in a pluripotential cell line from bone marrow. J Bone Joint Surg Am 79:1054-1063, 1997.

71. Cui Q, Wang GJ, Su CC, et al: The Otto Aufranc Award. Lovastatin prevents steroid induced adipogenesis and osteonecrosis. Clin Orthop 344:8-19, 1997.

72. Wang GJ, Cui Q, Balian G: The Nicolas Andry award. The pathogenesis and prevention of steroid-induced osteonecrosis. Clin Orthop 370:295-310, 2000.

73. Wang Y, Li Y, Mao K, et al: Alcohol-induced adipogenesis in bone and marrow: A possible mechanism for osteonecrosis. Clin Orthop 410:213-224, 2003.

74. Yin L, Li YB, Wang YS: Dexamethasone-induced adipogenesis in primary marrow stromal cell cultures: Mechanism of steroid-induced osteonecrosis. Chin Med J (Engl) 119:581-588, 2006.

75. Preedy VR, Patel VB, Reilly ME, et al: Oxidants, antioxidants and alcohol: Implications for skeletal and cardiac muscle. Front Biosci 4:e58-e66, 1999.

76. Suh KT, Kim SW, Roh HL, et al: Decreased osteogenic differentiation of mesenchymal stem cells in alcohol-induced osteonecrosis. Clin Orthop 431:220-225, 2005.

77. Lee JS, Lee JS, Roh HL, et al: Alterations in the differentiation ability of mesenchymal stem cells in patients with nontraumatic osteonecrosis of the femoral head: Comparative analysis according to the risk factor. J Orthop Res 24:604-609, 2006.

78. Miyanishi K, Yamamoto T, Irisa T, et al: Bone marrow fat cell enlargement and a rise in intraosseous pressure in steroid-treated rabbits with osteonecrosis. Bone 30:185-190, 2002.

79. Kim YH, Kim JS: Histologic analysis of acetabular and proximal femoral bone in patients with osteonecrosis of the femoral head. J Bone Joint Surg Am 86:2471-2474, 2004.

80. Laogun AA, Ajayi NO, Osamo NO, et al: Plasma viscosity in sickle-cell anemia. Clin Phys Physiol Meas 1:145, 1980.

81. Kleinman RG, Bleck EE: Increased blood viscosity in patients with Legg-Perthes disease: A preliminary report. J Pediatr Orthop 1:131-136, 1981.

82. Migliorati CA, Casiglia J, Epstein J, et al: Managing the care of patients with bisphosphonate-associated osteonecrosis: An American Academy of Oral Medicine position paper. J Am Dent Assoc 136:1658-1668, 2005.

83. Koo KH, Lee JS, Lee YJ, et al: Endothelial nitric oxide synthase gene polymorphisms in patients with nontraumatic femoral head osteonecrosis. J Orthop Res 24:1722-1728, 2006.

84. Glueck CJ, Fontaine RN, Gruppo R, et al: The plasminogen activator inhibitor-1 gene, hypofibrinolysis, and osteonecrosis. Clin Orthop Relat Res 366:133-146, 1999.

85. Jones JP Jr: Intravascular coagulation and osteonecrosis. Clin Orthop 277:41-53, 1992.

86. Jones LC, Mont MA, Le TB, et al: Procoagulants and osteonecrosis. J Rheumatol 30:783-791, 2003.

87. Saito S, Ohzono K, Ono K: Early arteriopathy and postulated pathogenesis of osteonecrosis of the femoral head: The intracapital arterioles. Clin Orthop 277:98-110, 1992.

88. Ohzono K, Takaoka K, Saito S, et al: Intraosseous arterial architecture in nontraumatic avascular necrosis of the femoral head: Microangiographic and histologic study. Clin Orthop 277:79-88, 1992.

89. Heikkinen ES, Puranen J, Suramo I: The effect of intertrochanteric osteotomy on the venous drainage of the femoral neck in Perthes' disease. Acta Orthop Scand 47:89-95, 1976.

90. Liu SL, Ho TC: The role of venous hypertension in the pathogenesis of Legg-Perthes disease: A clinical and experimental study. J Bone Joint Surg Am 73:194-200, 1991.

91. Thompson GH, Salter RB: Legg-Calvé-Perthes disease: Current concepts and controversies. Orthop Clin North Am 18:617-635, 1987.

92. Chryssanthou CP: Dysbaric osteonecrosis: Etiological and pathogenetic concepts. Clin Orthop 130:94-106, 1978.

93. Lehner CE, Adams WM, Dubielzig RR, et al: Dysbaric osteonecrosis in divers and caisson workers: An animal model. Clin Orthop 344:320-332, 1997.

94. Gangji V, Hauzeur JP, Schoutens A, et al: Abnormalities in the replicative capacity of osteoblastic cells in the proximal femur of patients with osteonecrosis of the femoral head. J Rheumatol 30:348-351, 2003.

95. Sato M, Sugano N, Ohzono K, et al: Apoptosis and expression of stress protein (ORP150, HO1) during development of ischaemic osteonecrosis in the rat. J Bone Joint Surg Br 83:751-759, 2001.

96. Kenzora JE, Glimcher MJ: Accumulative cell stress: The multifactorial etiology of idiopathic osteonecrosis. Orthop Clin North Am 16:669-679, 1985.

97. Zizic TM, Marcoux C, Hungerford DS, et al: Corticosteroid therapy associated with ischemic necrosis of bone in systemic lupus erythematosus. Am J Med 79:596-604, 1985.

98. Chiandussi S, Biasotto M, Dore F, et al: Clinical and diagnostic imaging of bisphosphonate-associated osteonecrosis of the jaws. Dentomaxillofac Radiol 35:236-243, 2006.

99. Dihlmann W: CT analysis of the upper end of the femur: The asterisk sign and ischaemic bone necrosis of the femoral head. Skeletal Radiol 8:251-258, 1982.

100. Dihlmann W, Heller M: [The asterisk sign and adult ischemic femur head necrosis]. Rofo 142:430-435, 1985.

101. Specchiulli F, Mele M, Capocasale N, et al: The early diagnosis of idiopathic femoral osteonecrosis. Ital J Orthop Traumatol 14:519-526, 1988.

102. Mitchell DG, Steinberg ME, Dalinka MK, et al: Magnetic resonance imaging of the ischemic hip: Alterations within the osteonecrotic, viable, and reactive zones. Clin Orthop 244:60-77, 1989.

103. Steinberg ME, Hayken GD, Steinberg DR: A new method for evaluation and staging of avascular necrosis of the femoral head. In Arlet J, Ficat RP, Hungerford DS (eds): Bone Circulation. Baltimore, Williams & Wilkins, 1984, pp 398-403.

104. Ruch DS, Sekiya J, Dickson Schaefer W, et al: The role of hip arthroscopy in the evaluation of avascular necrosis. Orthopedics 24:339-343, 2001.

105. Sekiya JK, Ruch DS, Hunter DM, et al: Hip arthroscopy in staging avascular necrosis of the femoral head. J South Orthop Assoc 9:254-261, 2000.

105a. Marx RE, Cillo JE, Ulloa JJ: Oral bisphosphonate-induced osteonecrosis: Risk factors, prediction of risk using serum CTX testing, prevention and treatment. J Oral Maxillofacial Surgery 65:2397-2410, 2007.

106. Schapira D: Transient osteoporosis of the hip. Semin Arthritis Rheum 22:98-105, 1992.

107. Plenk H Jr, Hofmann S, Eschberger J, et al: Histomorphology and bone morphometry of the bone marrow edema syndrome of the hip. Clin Orthop 334:73-84, 1997.

108. Berger CE, Kroner AH, Kristen KH, et al: Transient bone marrow edema syndrome of the knee: Clinical and magnetic resonance imaging results at 5 years after core decompression. Arthroscopy 22:866-871, 2006.

109. Mont MA, Ragland PS, Parvizi J: Surgical treatment of osteonecrosis of the hip. Instr Course Lect 55:167-172, 2006.

110. Ruch DS, Satterfield W: The use of arthroscopy to document accurate position of core decompression of the hip. Arthroscopy 14:617-619, 1998.

111. Ruch DS, Cory JW, Poehling GG: The arthroscopic management of osteochondritis dissecans of the adolescent elbow. Arthroscopy 14:797-803, 1998.

112. Menth-Chiari WA, Poehling GG, Wiesler ER, et al: Arthroscopic debridement for the treatment of Kienbock's disease. Arthroscopy 15:12-19, 1999.

113. Ruch DS, Chang DS, Poehling GG: The arthroscopic treatment of avascular necrosis of the proximal pole following scaphoid nonunion. Arthroscopy 14:747-752, 1998.

114. Bozic KJ, Zurakowski D, Thornhill TS: Survivorship analysis of hips treated with core decompression for nontraumatic osteonecrosis of the femoral head. J Bone Joint Surg Am 81:200-209, 1999.

115. Rodriguez-Merchan EC: Osteonecrosis of the femoral head after traumatic hip dislocation in the adult. Clin Orthop 377:68-77, 2000.
116. Mont MA, Payman RK, Laporte DM, et al: Atraumatic osteonecrosis of the humeral head. J Rheumatol 27:1766-1773, 2000.
117. Beckmann J, Goetz J, Baethis H, et al: Precision of computer-assisted core decompression drilling of the femoral head. Arch Orthop Trauma Surg 126:374-379, 2006.
118. Israelite C, Nelson CL, Ziarani CF, et al: Bilateral core decompression for osteonecrosis of the femoral head. Clin Orthop 441:285-290, 2005.
119. Marcus ND, Enneking WF, Massam RA: The silent hip in idiopathic aseptic necrosis: Treatment by bone-grafting. J Bone Joint Surg Am 55:1351-1366, 1973.
120. Marciniak D, Furey C, Shaffer JW: Osteonecrosis of the femoral head: A study of 101 hips treated with vascularized fibular grafting. J Bone Joint Surg Am 87:742-747, 2005.
121. Zhao D, Xu D, Wang W, et al: Iliac graft vascularization for femoral head osteonecrosis. Clin Orthop 442:171-179, 2006.
122. Vendittoli PA, Lavigne M, Girard J, et al: A randomised study comparing resection of acetabular bone at resurfacing and total hip replacement. J Bone Joint Surg Br 88:997-1002, 2006.
123. Grecula MJ: Resurfacing arthroplasty in osteonecrosis of the hip. Orthop Clin North Am 36:231-242, x, 2005.
124. Little CP, Ruiz AL, Harding IJ, et al: Osteonecrosis in retrieved femoral heads after failed resurfacing arthroplasty of the hip. J Bone Joint Surg Br 87:320-323, 2005.
125. Shimmin AJ, Bare J, Back DL: Complications associated with hip resurfacing arthroplasty. Orthop Clin North Am 36:187-193, ix, 2005.
126. Hungerford MW, Mont MA, Scott R, et al: Surface replacement hemiarthroplasty for the treatment of osteonecrosis of the femoral head. J Bone Joint Surg Am 80:1656-1664, 1998.
127. Mont MA, Rajadhyaksha AD, Hungerford DS: Outcomes of limited femoral resurfacing arthroplasty compared with total hip arthroplasty for osteonecrosis of the femoral head. J Arthroplasty 16(8 Suppl 1):134-139, 2001.
128. Cabanela ME: Bipolar versus total hip arthroplasty for avascular necrosis of the femoral head: A comparison. Clin Orthop 261:59-62, 1990.
129. Learmonth ID, Opitz M: Treatment of grade III osteonecrosis of the femoral head with a Charnley/Bicentric hemiarthroplasty. J R Coll Surg Edinb 38:311-314, 1993.
130. Hartley WT, McAuley JP, Culpepper WJ, et al: Osteonecrosis of the femoral head treated with cementless total hip arthroplasty. J Bone Joint Surg Am 82A:1408-1413, 2000.
131. Fyda TM, Callaghan JJ, Olejniczak J, et al: Minimum ten-year follow-up of cemented total hip replacement in patients with osteonecrosis of the femoral head. Iowa Orthop J 22:8-19, 2002.
132. Musso ES, Mitchell SN, Schink-Ascani M, et al: Results of conservative management of osteonecrosis of the femoral head: A retrospective review. Clin Orthop 207:209-215, 1986.
133. Trancik T, Lunceford E, Strum D: The effect of electrical stimulation on osteonecrosis of the femoral head. Clin Orthop 256:120-124, 1990.
134. Steinberg ME, Brighton CT, Corces A, et al: Osteonecrosis of the femoral head: Results of core decompression and grafting with and without electrical stimulation. Clin Orthop 249:199-208, 1989.
135. Steinberg ME, Brighton CT, Bands RE, et al: Capacitive coupling as an adjunctive treatment for avascular necrosis. Clin Orthop 261:11-18, 1990.
136. Wang CJ, Wang FS, Huang CC, et al: Treatment for osteonecrosis of the femoral head: Comparison of extracorporeal shock waves with core decompression and bone-grafting. J Bone Joint Surg Am 87:2380-2387, 2005.
137. Li X, Jin L, Cui Q, et al: Steroid effects on osteogenesis through mesenchymal cell gene expression. Osteoporos Int 16:101-108, 2005.
138. Lee HS, Huang GT, Chiang H, et al: Multipotential mesenchymal stem cells from femoral bone marrow near the site of osteonecrosis. Stem Cells 21:190-199, 2003.
139. Gangji V, Hauzeur JP: Treatment of osteonecrosis of the femoral head with implantation of autologous bone-marrow cells: Surgical technique. J Bone Joint Surg Am 87(Suppl 1[Pt 1]):106-112, 2005.
140. Gangji V, Hauzeur JP, Matos C, et al: Treatment of osteonecrosis of the femoral head with implantation of autologous bone-marrow cells: A pilot study. J Bone Joint Surg Am 86:1153-1160, 2004.
141. Yan ZQ, Chen YS, Li WJ, et al: Treatment of osteonecrosis of the femoral head by percutaneous decompression and autologous bone marrow mononuclear cell infusion. Chin J Traumatol 9:3-7, 2006.
142. Cheng EY, Thongtrangan I, Laorr A, et al: Spontaneous resolution of osteonecrosis of the femoral head. J Bone Joint Surg Am 86:2594-2599, 2004.
143. Jergesen HE, Khan AS: The natural history of untreated asymptomatic hips in patients who have non-traumatic osteonecrosis. J Bone Joint Surg Am 79:359-363, 1997.
144. Hernigou P, Poignard A, Nogier A, et al: Fate of very small asymptomatic stage-I osteonecrotic lesions of the hip. J Bone Joint Surg Am 86:2589-2593, 2004.
145. Cruess RL: Steroid-induced avascular necrosis of the head of the humerus: Natural history and management. J Bone Joint Surg Br 58:313-317, 1976.
146. Cruess RL: Steroid-induced osteonecrosis: A review. Can J Surg 24:567-571, 1981.
147. Scotter E, Moody A: Dysbaric osteonecrosis (caisson disease). Radiogr Today 54:41-43, 1988.
148. Hungerford DS, Zizic TM: Alcoholism associated ischemic necrosis of the femoral head: Early diagnosis and treatment. Clin Orthop 130:144-153, 1978.
149. Abylaev ZhA, Bukhman AI: [Possible mechanisms of the development of osteopathies in patients with chronic lead poisoning]. Gig Tr Prof Zabol 2:31-35, 1990.
150. Kazakos K, Chatzipapas C, Xarchas KC, et al: Knee osteonecrosis due to lead poisoning: Case report and review of the literature. Med Sci Monit 12:CS85-CS89, 2006.
151. Graziani F, Cei S, La Ferla F, et al: Association between osteonecrosis of the jaws and chronic high-dosage intravenous bisphosphonates therapy. J Craniofac Surg 17:876-879, 2006.
152. Rubinstein RA Jr, Beals RK: The results of treatment of posttraumatic avascular necrosis of the femoral head in young adults: Report of 31 patients. Contemp Orthop 27:527-532, 1993.
153. Burwell RG: Perthes' disease. J Bone Joint Surg Br 60:1-3, 1978.
154. Herold HZ: Avascular necrosis of the femoral head in children under the age of three. Clin Orthop 126:193-195, 1977.
155. Morcuende JA, Meyer MD, Dolan LA, et al: Long-term outcome after open reduction through an anteromedial approach for congenital dislocation of the hip. J Bone Joint Surg Am 79:810-817, 1997.
156. Narayanan UG: Reduction increasing osteonecrosis risk in slipped capital femoral epiphysis. J Bone Joint Surg Am 86:437; author reply, 2004.
157. Yamasaki T, Yasunaga Y, Hisatome T, et al: Bone remodeling of a femoral head after transtrochanteric rotational osteotomy for osteonecrosis associated with slipped capital femoral epiphysis: A case report. Arch Orthop Trauma Surg 125:486-489, 2005.
158. Sellman DC, Froimson AI: Long-term follow-up of a total articular resurfacing arthroplasty and a cup arthroplasty in Gaucher's disease. Orthop Rev 21:1099-1101, 1104, 1107, 1992.
159. Irisa T, Yamamoto T, Miyanishi K, et al: Osteonecrosis induced by a single administration of low-dose lipopolysaccharide in rabbits. Bone 28:641-649, 2001.
160. Jones JP Jr: Fat embolism and osteonecrosis. Orthop Clin North Am 16:595-633, 1985.
161. Barbezat GO, Miles T, Bank S, et al: Necrosis of the femoral head in a black patient with pancreatitis. S Afr Med J 50:160, 1976 (letter).
162. Chao YC, Wang SJ, Chu HC, et al: Investigation of alcohol metabolizing enzyme genes in Chinese alcoholics with avascular necrosis of hip joint, pancreatitis and cirrhosis of the liver. Alcohol Alcohol 38:431-436, 2003.
163. Pais MJ: Disease states affecting both liver and bone. Radiol Clin North Am 18:253-267, 1980.
164. Watson RM, Roach NA, Dalinka MK: Avascular necrosis and bone marrow edema syndrome. Radiol Clin North Am 42:207-219, 2004.
165. Horiuchi H, Saito N, Kobayashi S, et al: Avascular necrosis of the femoral head in a patient with Fabry's disease: Identification of ceramide trihexoside in the bone by delayed-extraction matrix-assisted laser desorption ionization-time-of-flight mass spectrometry. Arthritis Rheum 46:1922-1925, 2002.
166. Ross G, Kuwamura F, Goral A: Association of Fabry's disease with femoral head avascular necrosis. Orthopedics 16:471-473, 1993.
167. Mielants H, Veys EM, DeBussere A, et al: Avascular necrosis and its relation to lipid and purine metabolism. J Rheumatol 2:430-436, 1975.
168. Heaf JG: Bone disease after renal transplantation. Transplantation 75:315-325, 2003.

169. Kjaergaard GH, Laursen JO: [Osteonecrosis of a knee joint in a young man with IDDM]. Ugeskr Laeger 162:4663-4664, 2000.

170. Hernigou P, Bachir D, Galacteros F: The natural history of symptomatic osteonecrosis in adults with sickle-cell disease. J Bone Joint Surg Am 85:500-504, 2003.

171. Onuba O: Bone disorders in sickle-cell disease. Int Orthop 17:397-399, 1993.

172. Mahachoklertwattana P: Zoledronic acid for the treatment of thalassemia-induced osteonecrosis. Haematologica 91:1155A, 2006.

173. Campbell WN, Joshi M, Sileo D: Osteonecrosis following meningococcemia and disseminated intravascular coagulation in an adult: Case report and review. Clin Infect Dis 24:452-455, 1997.

174. **Jones JP Jr: Fat embolism, intravascular coagulation, and osteonecrosis. Clin Orthop 292:294-308, 1993.**

175. Jones JP Jr: Coagulopathies and osteonecrosis. Acta Orthop Belg 65(Suppl 1):5-8, 1999.

176. Seipolt B, Dinger J, Rupprecht E: Osteonecrosis after meningococcemia and disseminated intravascular coagulation. Pediatr Infect Dis J 22:1021-1022, 2003.

177. Glueck CJ, Freiberg RA, Fontaine RN, et al: Hypofibrinolysis, thrombophilia, osteonecrosis. Clin Orthop 386:19-33, 2001.

178. Glueck CJ, Freiberg R, Glueck HI, et al: Hypofibrinolysis: A common, major cause of osteonecrosis. Am J Hematol 45:156-166, 1994.

179. Strau G, Kainz L, Kienzer H: [Spontaneous osteonecrosis of the knee joint in clinically suspected thrombosis of the leg veins]. Rontgenblatter 41:122-124, 1988.

180. Tektonidou MG, Malagari K, Vlachoyiannopoulos PG, et al: Asymptomatic avascular necrosis in patients with primary antiphospholipid syndrome in the absence of corticosteroid use: A prospective study by magnetic resonance imaging. Arthritis Rheum 48:732-736, 2003.

181. Neidel J, Boehnke M, Kuster RM: The efficacy and safety of intraarticular corticosteroid therapy for coxitis in juvenile rheumatoid arthritis. Arthritis Rheum 46:1620-1628, 2002.

182. Abu-Shakra M, Buskila D, Shoenfeld Y: Osteonecrosis in patients with SLE. Clin Rev Allergy Immunol 25:13-24, 2003.

183. Nagasawa K, Ishii Y, Mayumi T, et al: Avascular necrosis of bone in systemic lupus erythematosus: Possible role of haemostatic abnormalities. Ann Rheum Dis 48:672-676, 1989.

184. Rascu A, Manger K, Kraetsch HG, et al: Osteonecrosis in systemic lupus erythematosus, steroid-induced or a lupus-dependent manifestation? Lupus 5:323-327, 1996.

185. Freeman HJ, Freeman KJ: Prevalence rates and an evaluation of reported risk factors for osteonecrosis (avascular necrosis) in Crohn's disease. Can J Gastroenterol 14:138-143, 2000.

186. Stiles RG, Carpenter WA, Tigges S: Osteonecrosis of the femoral heads in inflammatory bowel disease. N Engl J Med 330:791; author reply 792, 1994.

187. Wang TY, Avlonitis EG, Relkin R: Systemic necrotizing vasculitis causing bone necrosis. Am J Med 84:1085-1086, 1988.

188. Yanagitani Y, Fujita M: Avascular necrosis of the femoral head associated with mucocutaneous lymph node syndrome. J Pediatr Orthop 6:107-109, 1986.

189. Clarke AE, Bloch DA, Medsger TA Jr, et al: A longitudinal study of functional disability in a national cohort of patients with polymyositis/dermatomyositis. Arthritis Rheum 38:1218-1224, 1995.

190. **Scribner AN, Troia-Cancio PV, Cox BA, et al: Osteonecrosis in HIV: A case-control study. J Acquir Immune Defic Syndr 25:19-25, 2000.**

191. Chaudhuri R, McKeown B, Harrington D, et al: Mucormycosis osteomyelitis causing avascular necrosis of the cuboid bone: MR imaging findings. AJR Am J Roentgenol 159:1035-1037, 1992.

192. Appel M, Pauleto AC, Cunha LA: Osteochondral sequelae of meningococcemia: Radiographic aspects. J Pediatr Orthop 22:511-516, 2002.

193. Bradford DS, Szalapski EW Jr, Sutherland DE, et al: Osteonecrosis in the transplant recipient. Surg Gynecol Obstet 159:328-334, 1984.

194. Danzig LA, Coutis RD, Resnick D: Avascular necrosis of the femoral head following cardiac transplantation: Report of a case. Clin Orthop 117:217-220, 1976.

195. Fink JC, Leisenring WM, Sullivan KM, et al: Avascular necrosis following bone marrow transplantation: A case-control study. Bone 22:67-71, 1998.

196. Helenius I, Jalanko H, Remes V, et al: Avascular bone necrosis of the hip joint after solid organ transplantation in childhood: A clinical and MRI analysis. Transplantation 81:1621-1627, 2006.

197. Lieberman JR, Scaduto AA, Wellmeyer E: Symptomatic osteonecrosis of the hip after orthotopic liver transplantation. J Arthroplasty 15:767-771, 2000.

198. Marston SB, Gillingham K, Bailey RF, et al: Osteonecrosis of the femoral head after solid organ transplantation: A prospective study. J Bone Joint Surg Am 84:2145-2151, 2002.

199. Dzik-Jurasz AS, Brooker S, Husband JE, et al: What is the prevalence of symptomatic or asymptomatic femoral head osteonecrosis in patients previously treated with chemoradiation? A magnetic resonance study of anal cancer patients. Clin Oncol (R Coll Radiol) 13:130-134, 2001.

200. Curtis MA, Tung GA, Dawamneh MF: Radiation osteonecrosis of the clavicle. Acad Radiol 3:971-974, 1996.

201. Epstein J, van der Meij E, McKenzie M, et al: Postradiation osteonecrosis of the mandible: A long-term follow-up study. Oral Surg Oral Med Oral Pathol Oral Radiol Endod 83:657-662, 1997.

202. Holler U, Petersein A, Golder W, et al: [Radiation-induced osteonecrosis of the pelvic bones vs. bone metastases—a difficult differential diagnosis]. Aktuelle Radiol 8:196-197, 1998.

203. Niewald M, Barbie O, Schnabel K, et al: Risk factors and dose-effect relationship for osteoradionecrosis after hyperfractionated and conventionally fractionated radiotherapy for oral cancer. Br J Radiol 69:847-851, 1996.

204. Stebbings JH: Dose-response analyses of osteonecrosis in New Jersey radium workers point to roles for other alpha emitters. Health Phys 74:602-607, 1998.

205. Balzer S, Schneider DT, Bernbeck MB, et al: Avascular osteonecrosis after hyperthermia in children and adolescents with pelvic malignancies: A retrospective analysis of potential risk factors. Int J Hyperthermia 22:451-461, 2006.

206. Gurkan E, Yildiz I, Ocal F: Avascular necrosis of the femoral head as the first manifestation of acute lymphoblastic leukemia. Leuk Lymphoma 47:365-367, 2006.

207. Wei SY, Esmail AN, Bunin N, et al: Avascular necrosis in children with acute lymphoblastic leukemia. J Pediatr Orthop 20:331-335, 2000.

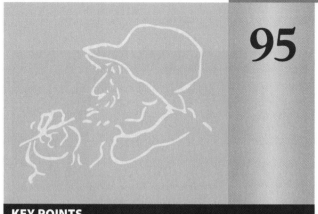

95 Relapsing Polychondritis

JEAN-CHARLES PIETTE • PHILIPPE VINCENEUX

Inflammation associated with relapsing polychondritis involves the auricles (sparing the soft earlobe), the skin, and occasionally the vasculature.

Relapsing polychondritis is associated occasionally with antibodies to type II collagen and with HLA-DR4.

Relapsing polychondritis occasionally may extend to inflammation of cartilage of the larynx and trachea, and peripheral arthritis.

Differential diagnosis includes Wegener's granulomatosis, Behçet's syndrome, Cogan's syndrome, and cellulitis.

Relapsing polychondritis may be seen with myelodysplasia syndromes.

DEFINITION AND CRITERIA

Relapsing polychondritis is a rare, long-lasting, and potentially life-threatening disorder characterized by recurrent inflammatory episodes affecting the cartilaginous structures of the external ears, nose, larynx, and tracheobronchial tree, sometimes leading to their destruction.[1-5] Systemic manifestations involving the auricles, eyes, skin, inner ears, and vessels are frequently associated. Several sets of clinical diagnostic criteria are available[1-3]; Table 95-1 lists the most commonly used criteria. Biopsy confirmation is not required for diagnosis except for atypical cases.

EPIDEMIOLOGY

Since its first description by Jaksch-Wartenhorst in 1923, less than 800 cases of polychondritis have been published, with two series of 100 or more.[3,6] Epidemiologic data are scarce. Most reported patients are white, but the disease has been found in all ethnic groups. Although polychondritis may develop at any age,[5,7] it usually occurs in mid-adulthood, with a mean age at onset of 43 years (slightly older in men). Sex distribution is usually reported as equal, but a female predominance has been reported in more recent series,[4,6] leading to a female-to-male ratio of 1:2 based on 600 patients. Familial cases are extremely rare.[8] Maternofetal transmission of polychondritis, reported only once,[9] has never occurred in our experience.[10]

PATHOPHYSIOLOGY

The etiology of polychondritis is unknown. A history of mechanical insult to cartilage is infrequent. Cartilage destruction by degradative enzymes is supported by peculiar animal models[8] and by electron microscopic studies.[11]

The release of degradative enzymes is thought to result from autoimmune reactions. The pathogenetic role of the immune system is suggested by the presence of a lymphocytic infiltrate and of immune deposits in tissue lesions,[1,8,12] by humoral[13-17] and cell-mediated[18,19] responses to cartilage components, by frequent overlaps with various autoimmune disorders, and principally by more recent advances in animal models. Polychondritis has been induced in rats and mice by immunization with type II collagen[20,21] or with matrilin-1, a noncollagenous cartilage matrix protein.[22] The importance of the genetic background is shown by a murine model, using a mouse doubly transgenic for human HLA-DQ6 and HLA-DQ8 after immunization with type II collagen,[21] and by the association of human polychondritis with HLA-DR4.[23] Finally, a two-step process has been suggested in which the initiator is considered to be possibly matrilin-1 or type II collagen, among other proteins.[20,24]

CLINICAL FEATURES

The onset is usually abrupt, with highly variable presenting manifestations including isolated general symptoms.[1,18] The occurrence of chondritis may be delayed months to years.[4] Table 95-2 lists the main cumulative clinical features.

CHONDRITIS

Auricular chondritis is a key manifestation, rarely absent in the course of the disease. Acute episodes manifest with pain, tenderness, swelling, warmth, and marked redness affecting the helix, antihelix, and sometimes tragus on one or both sides, but, importantly for the differential diagnosis, sparing the soft earlobe, which lacks cartilage. Attacks resolve spontaneously or with treatment within days, but relapses invariably occur sooner or later, their features being attenuated by steroids. Recurrent inflammation may lead to permanent sequelae, either a drooping "cauliflower" ear or more frequently an induration of the pinna (Fig. 95-1). A prior history of inflammatory episodes is necessary to confirm the diagnosis of chondritis in patients with a "flat" auricle, devoid of its normal relief.

Nasal chondritis is far less obvious than auricular chondritis during acute episodes. Symptoms are restricted to nose pain, tenderness, mild swelling, and infrequent redness, sometimes accompanied by fullness, crusting, rhinorrhea, and rare epistaxis. A suggestive saddle-nose deformity resulting from cartilage collapse (Fig. 95-2) may develop progressively in the absence of apparent prior acute attacks, especially in women.[3,25]

Laryngeal, tracheal, or bronchial chondritis, which may extend to the subsegmental level, is frequently associated

Table 95-1 Empiric Diagnostic Criteria for Relapsing Polychondritis

Major Criteria
Proven inflammatory episodes involving auricular cartilage
Proven inflammatory episodes involving nasal cartilage
Proven inflammatory episodes involving laryngotracheal cartilage

Minor Criteria
Ocular inflammation (conjunctivitis, keratitis, episcleritis, uveitis)
Hearing loss
Vestibular dysfunction
Seronegative inflammatory arthritis
Diagnosis is made by two major criteria or one major plus two minor criteria
Histologic examination of affected cartilage is not required

From Michet CJ Jr, McKenna CH, Luthra HS, et al: Relapsing polychondritis: Survival and predictive role of early disease manifestations. Ann Intern Med 104:74-78, 1986.

Table 95-2 Main Cumulative Clinical Features of Relapsing Polychondritis*

Clinical Feature	Frequency (%)
Auricular chondritis	85
Nasal chondritis	65
Laryngotracheobronchial chondritis	48
Costal chondritis	38
Arthropathy	78
Ocular inflammation	60
Fever ≥38°C	38
Hearing loss	33
Dermatologic manifestations	33
Cardiovascular manifestations	30
Vestibular dysfunction	22
Renal involvement	13

*Compiled from published series and personal experience, totaling >500 patients. Data should be regarded as approximations.

and worsens prognosis.[1,5,25-28] Laryngeal chondritis is responsible for hoarseness or aphonia, tenderness over the thyroid cartilage, and inspiratory dyspnea with stridor. Subglottic stenosis mainly occurs in women[3] and may require emergency tracheostomy. Tracheobronchial manifestations (i.e., cough, chest pain, expiratory dyspnea, wheezing, and frequent infections owing to inability to clear secretions) are nonspecific. When polychondritis manifests with isolated lower respiratory tract involvement, the diagnosis may be delayed by months.[29] Severe respiratory failure resulting from permanent stenoses or expiratory collapse secondary to tracheobronchomalacia or both may lead to death.

Costal chondritis provokes localized parietal pain and costochondral tumefactions. This chondritis rarely results in depression of the anterior chest wall.[30]

OTHER MANIFESTATIONS

In addition to chondritis, diverse symptoms may occur as a presenting feature or later in the disease course. Joint manifestations vary from arthralgias to an oligoarthritis or polyarthritis, either acute or episodic and migratory or, less frequently, chronic, nonerosive, nondeforming, and not accompanied by nodules.[31-33] Peripheral arthropathy is usually asymmetric and mainly affects the wrists, metacarpophalangeal and proximal interphalangeal joints, elbows, knees, ankles, and parasternal joints. Synovial fluid may be paucicellular. Tenosynovitis and other para-articular manifestations are common, such as cervical or lumbar inflammatory pain.[31] The presence of radiographic abnormalities in peripheral joints or in the spine is infrequent and suggestive of an overlap with another condition, mainly with spondyloarthropathies[34] or rheumatoid arthritis.[23,35]

Eye involvement results from polychondritis itself or from associated Sjögren's syndrome.[36,37] Recurrent episcleritis/scleritis or conjunctivitis is more frequent than keratitis or uveitis. Vision is rarely threatened by retinal vasculitis, optic neuropathy, or necrotizing scleritis. Frank proptosis obligates one to rule out Wegener's granulomatosis and lymphoma.[38]

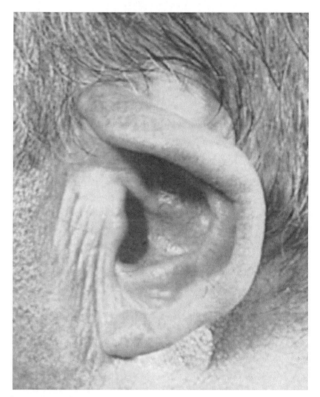

Figure 95-1 Distortion and collapse of the external ear in a patient with relapsing polychondritis.

Audiovestibular manifestations are frequent.[2] Hearing impairment may result from stenosis of the external auditory meatus, otitis media caused by eustachian tube chondritis, or more specifically from neurosensory lesions owing to vasculitis of the internal auditory artery. In the last-mentioned condition, deafness is abrupt, unilateral or bilateral, of variable magnitude, and accompanied by buzzing, and inconsistently reverses with prompt high-dose steroids. Transient vertigo may be associated or occur independently.

Vascular involvement is uncommon, extremely diverse, and frequently multifocal. It carries a negative prognosis.

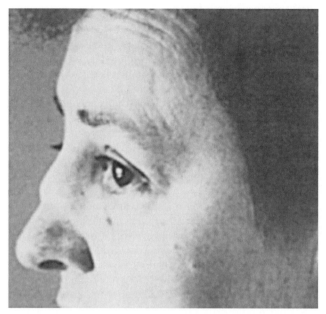

Figure 95-2 Destruction of the nasal cartilage in a patient with relapsing polychondritis, creating the characteristic saddle-nose deformity. *(From McKay DAR, Watson PG, Lyne AJ, et al: Relapsing polychondritis and eye disease. Br J Ophthalmol 58:600, 1974.)*

Acquired inflammatory aneurysms usually affecting the ascending thoracic aorta may progressively develop late in the course of polychondritis.[39-43] Large arteries at various sites also may be affected by aneurysms, stenosis, or both.[44] A microvasculitic process sometimes involves the skin or organs such as kidney, brain, sclera, inner ear, or testes.[3,39,45] Its implication in most cases of polychondritis remains disputed. Thrombophlebitis occasionally is related to antiphospholipid antibodies.[46] Cardiac lesions include aortic failure resulting from dilated aortic anulus associated with ascending aortic aneurysms, mitral valve failure sometimes resulting from active inflammation, steroid-sensitive conduction disturbances, myocarditis, pericarditis, and coronary aneurysms.[1,3,41,43,47-49]

Dermatologic manifestations consist of oral or complex aphthosis, nodules, purpura, papules, sterile pustules, superficial phlebitis, livedo, ulcerations, and distal necrosis.[6] Histologic findings include leukocytoclastic vasculitis, neutrophil infiltrates, and thrombosis. These lesions frequently occur in association with myelodysplasia,[6] and sometimes resemble those of Behçet's syndrome. The acronym MAGIC syndrome (mouth and genital ulcers with inflamed cartilage) has been proposed for this overlap.[50,51]

Kidney involvement, shown by microscopic hematuria, proteinuria, and sometimes severe loss of renal function, is usually attributed by biopsy to a crescentric pauci-immune glomerulonephritis within an accompanying micropolyangiitis.[45] Less frequently, immune complex nephritis is related to overlapping systemic lupus or cryoglobulinemia.

Neurologic manifestations consist of peripheral or cranial neuropathies, hemiplegia, seizures, rhombencephalitis, and lymphocytic or aseptic neutrophilic meningitis.[52,53]

Flares are accompanied by fever, asthenia, weight loss, and sometimes liver or lymph node enlargement.[1] The clinical picture may be modified by various associated conditions, such as thyroiditis or ulcerative colitis.[4]

LABORATORY FINDINGS

To date, the contribution of laboratory findings to diagnosis is limited. A major elevation of acute-phase reactants and erythrocyte sedimentation rate is observed during flares, with a few exceptions associated with mild-to-moderate anemia of chronic disease, leukocytosis, and thrombocytosis.[1,5] Polyclonal elevation of serum IgA, IgG, or IgM is common. Tests for rheumatoid factors or antinuclear antibodies may be positive, but high titers suggest an overlap with rheumatoid arthritis, Sjögren's syndrome, or systemic lupus erythematosus.[4,23,54,55] Antineutrophil cytoplasmic antibodies devoid of proteinase-3 specificity are present in some patients.[56] Antibodies to cartilage detected by indirect fluorescence staining are not routinely determined.[13] Although initially claimed to be sensitive and specific,[14] tests for antibodies to type II collagen have limited clinical significance.[20] Preliminary data on antibodies to matrilin-1 seem promising, but require confirmation.[16,17]

Histologic examination of an affected cartilage, mainly auricular, is considered suggestive when it shows the association of degenerative changes with the presence of an inflammatory infiltrate (Fig. 95-3). The infiltrate, containing CD4+ lymphocytes, macrophages, neutrophils, and capillaries, penetrates the cartilage from its outer surface to its depth.[1,8,12] Loss of basophilic staining of the matrix reflects

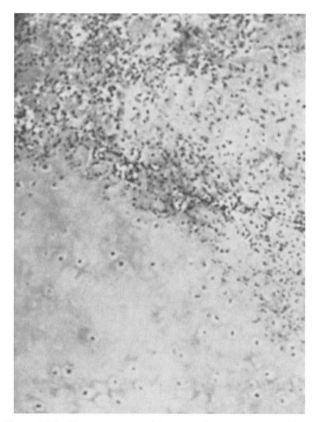

Figure 95-3 Biopsy specimen of the external ear in a patient with relapsing polychondritis. The specimen shows necrotizing chondritis with inflammatory cell infiltrate, depletion of matrix proteoglycans, chondrocyte degeneration, and fibrosis. (Original magnification, ×400.) *(From Herman JH, Dennis MV: Immunopathologic studies in relapsing polychondritis. J Clin Invest 52:549, 1973; by copyright permission of the American Society for Clinical Investigation.)*

proteoglycan depletion. Chondrocytes become vacuolated and die. The destroyed cartilage is replaced by fibrous tissue where calcification or even ossification may occur. Because degenerative changes are commonly found in normal subjects age 40 or older, the biopsy specimen must be obtained during an acute flare to evaluate the infiltrate best.

Acquired myelodysplasia frequently occurs in men with late-onset polychondritis.[6,57,58] Chronic macrocytic nonregenerative anemia requiring regular transfusions is sometimes accompanied by leukopenia and thrombocytopenia. Myeloproliferative disorders and other forms of hematologic malignancies also have been reported.[3,38]

DIFFERENTIAL DIAGNOSIS

Auricular chondritis is frequently misdiagnosed as infectious perichondritis, although infection does not spare the lobule and occurs in peculiar circumstances.[2,8] Confusing aspects of the auricle may be observed in cellulitis, leprosy, leishmaniasis, frostbite, and after repeated trauma, such as with rugby players. Another consideration in this area would be external otitis, frequently caused by *Pseudomonas aeruginosa* or *Staphylococcus aureus*.

A saddle-nose deformity may result from congenital syphilis, direct trauma, nasal septal perforation, and mainly Wegener's granulomatosis. Rare differential diagnoses of nasal chondritis include the recessive genetic defect affecting expression of the transporter associated with antigen presentation (TAP) genes,[59] and two pediatric disorders, chronic infantile neurologic cutaneous and articular syndrome[60] and an autosomal dominant degenerative chondropathy.[61] Early symptoms may mimic acute sinusitis.

Lower respiratory tract involvement may be confused with asthma or chronic bronchitis. Stenoses occur in amyloidosis, sarcoidosis, inflammatory bowel disorders, tracheobronchopathia osteochondroplastica, rhinoscleroma in endemic areas, and mainly Wegener's granulomatosis.[62,63] Arterial involvement shares similarities with closely related Takayasu's arteritis, Behçet's disease, and Cogan's syndrome.[40,50] Involvement of the aortic root also occurs in Marfan syndrome, Ehlers-Danlos syndrome, syphilis, medial cystic necrosis, and spondyloarthropathies.[49]

Taken together, Wegener's granulomatosis remains the main differential diagnosis of polychondritis. Both disorders share acquired saddle-nose deformity, subglottic stenosis, scleritis, and sometimes audiovestibular involvement or pauci-immune glomerulopathy. Auricular chondritis has been described in Wegener's granulomatosis,[45] and proptosis or nasal septum perforation has been described in polychondritis.[44] Key features that suggest Wegener's granulomatosis are pansinusitis, parenchymal lung involvement, mononeuritis multiplex, granulomatous vasculitis, and antineutrophil cytoplasmic antibodies directed to proteinase-3. Conversely, diffuse tracheomalacia is a distinctive feature of polychondritis. Although these disorders are distinct entities, overlaps probably exist.[39,64,65]

EVALUATION, COURSE, AND PROGNOSIS

Evaluation of airway disease is crucial. Pulmonary function tests using forced inspiratory and expiratory flow volume loop studies quantify the deficit and localize the structures involved.[26,28] Tracheobronchoscopy may worsen hypoxia and lead to death.[26,28] In most cases, it should be replaced by computed tomography or magnetic resonance imaging.[26,27,66,67] Reconstruction techniques, including virtual endoscopy, and dynamic studies easily visualize the respiratory tree without the hazards of real endoscopy.

Routine echocardiograms check the valves and ascending aorta. Repeated vascular imaging is needed in patients with large artery involvement because lesions are frequently multiple and tend to recur.[40,43] The use of nontraumatic methods, such as magnetic resonance angiograms, prevents the development of false aneurysms induced by arterial puncture.[50]

The course of polychondritis varies. Disease remains smoldering in a few patients, whereas most experience flares affecting independently cartilage, joints,[33] or vessels.[40] Very few patients undergo a progressive downhill course refractory to therapy. Although durable remissions may occur, polychondritis rarely evolves to extinction. Pregnancy has no influence on disease activity.[10] The discrimination between tracheobronchial flare and superimposed infection may be difficult because both may coexist. Functional impairment, related to the disease itself or to treatment, frequently develops with time.

The severity of prognosis reflects the frequent requirement for high-dose steroids and the extreme duration of polychondritis. The 5-year and 10-year probabilities of survival after diagnosis were 74% and 55% in the Mayo Clinic series.[3] More recent data[4] and our experience are much more encouraging. The leading causes of death are airway obstruction and pneumonia in women and specific cardiovascular involvement in men.[3,5] In patients younger than 51 years old, saddle-nose deformity and systemic vasculitis were the worst prognostic factors.[3] For older patients, only anemia predicted outcome. Survival is limited when repeated transfusions are required for myelodysplasia.[57]

TREATMENT

Systemic treatment is empiric and should be adapted to disease activity and severity.[4] Minor cases may respond to nonsteroidal anti-inflammatory drugs, colchicine, or dapsone.[4,5,68] Prednisone remains the cornerstone of treatment for most patients. Initial doses are 0.5 to 1 mg/kg/day. Methylprednisolone pulses (1 g/day for 3 days) are used in frank respiratory flares, recent neurosensorial hearing loss, or systemic microvasculitis.[69] Progressive tapering frequently is limited by the requirement for substantial maintenance doses.

Combined immunosuppression is indicated initially in severe respiratory or vasculitic involvement or secondarily to improve disease control and allow steroid tapering. Methotrexate (0.3 mg/kg/wk) is frequently effective[4,70] and carries no risk of secondary myelodysplasia. Cyclophosphamide, azathioprine, chlorambucil, and mycophenolate mofetil also have been used, and cyclosporine in case of preexisting cytopenias.[1,4,5,44,45,71] In our experience, cyclophosphamide is the most potent. Infliximab has been reported to be effective in two cases,[72] but our results in six patients with refractory polychondritis were disappointing. Such patients, who do not respond to plasmapheresis or high-dose immunoglobulins, might be candidates for experimental regimens, such as tolerance induction with oral collagen[7] or autologous stem cell transplantation.[73]

Focal steroid treatment includes eye drops, intra-articular injections, and inhaled steroids sometimes combined with ephedrine.[74] Propranolol is used empirically to limit aortic dilation. Airway obstruction may require tracheostomy, mechanical ventilation, tracheal surgery, or stenting.[26,29,75,76] Sustained disease control allows successful nasal reconstruction. The initial medium-term results of heart or arterial surgery are frequently jeopardized in the long-term by valve disinsertion or relapsing aneurysms occurring despite immunosuppression.[39-41,49,50] A careful preoperative anesthesia evaluation is mandatory.[77]

CONCLUSION

Although early recognition and conventional management have improved the prognosis of relapsing polychondritis, a better comprehension of its pathophysiology is needed to elaborate targeted intervention.

REFERENCES

1. **McAdam LP, O'Hanlan MA, Bluestone R, et al: Relapsing polychondritis: Prospective study of 23 patients and a review of the literature. Medicine (Balt) 55:193-215, 1976.**
2. Damiani JM, Levine HL: Relapsing polychondritis: Report of ten cases. Laryngoscope (St Louis) 89:929-946, 1979.
3. **Michet CJ Jr, McKenna CH, Luthra HS, et al: Relapsing polychondritis: Survival and predictive role of early disease manifestations. Ann Intern Med 104:74-78, 1986.**
4. Trentham DE, Le CH: Relapsing polychondritis. Ann Intern Med 129:114-122, 1998.
5. Vinceneux P, Pouchot J, Piette JC: Polychondrite atrophiante. In Kahn MF, Peltier AP, Meyer O (eds): Maladies et Syndromes Systémiques. Paris, Flammarion Médecine-Sciences, 2000, pp 623-649.
6. Francès C, el Rassi R, Laporte JL, et al: Dermatologic manifestations of relapsing polychondritis: A study of 200 cases at a single center. Medicine (Balt) 80:173-179, 2001.
7. Navarro MJ, Higgins GC, Lohr KM, et al: Amelioration of relapsing polychondritis in a child treated with oral collagen. Am J Med Sci 324:101-103, 2002.
8. Arkin CR, Masi AF: Relapsing polychondritis: Review of current status and case report. Semin Arthritis Rheum 5:41-61, 1975.
9. Arundell FW, Haserick JR: Familial chronic atrophic polychondritis. Arch Dermatol 82:439-440, 1960.
10. Papo T, Wechsler B, Bletry O, et al: Pregnancy in relapsing polychondritis: Twenty-five pregnancies in eleven patients. Arthritis Rheum 40:1245-1249, 1997.
11. Giroux L, Paquin F, Guerard-Desjardins MJ, et al: Relapsing polychondritis: An autoimmune disease. Semin Arthritis Rheum 13:182-187, 1983.
12. Riccieri V, Spadaro A, Taccari E, et al: A case of relapsing polychondritis: Pathogenetic considerations. Clin Exp Rheumatol 6:95-96, 1988.
13. Ebringer R, Rook G, Swana GT, et al: Autoantibodies to cartilage and type II collagen in relapsing polychondritis and other rheumatic diseases. Ann Rheum Dis 40:473-479, 1981.
14. **Foidart JM, Abe S, Martin GR, et al: Antibodies to type II collagen in relapsing polychondritis. N Engl J Med 299:1203-1207, 1978.**
15. Yang CL, Brinckmann J, Rui HF, et al: Autoantibodies to cartilage collagens in relapsing polychondritis. Arch Dermatol Res 285:245-249, 1993.
16. Buckner JH, Wu JJ, Reife RA, et al: Autoreactivity against matrilin-1 in a patient with relapsing polychondritis. Arthritis Rheum 43:939-943, 2000.
17. Hansson AS, Heinegard D, Piette JC, et al: The occurrence of autoantibodies to matrilin 1 reflects a tissue-specific response to cartilage of the respiratory tract in patients with relapsing polychondritis. Arthritis Rheum 44:2402-2412, 2001.
18. Alsalameh S, Mollenhauer J, Scheuplein F, et al: Preferential cellular and humoral immune reactivities to native and denatured collagen types IX and XI in a patient with fatal relapsing polychondritis. J Rheumatol 20:1419-1424, 1993.
19. Buckner JH, Van Landeghen M, Kwok WW, et al: Identification of type II collagen peptide 261-273-specific T cell clones in a patient with relapsing polychondritis. Arthritis Rheum 46:238-244, 2002.
20. Cremer MA, Rosloniec EF, Kang AH: The cartilage collagens: A review of their structure, organization, and role in the pathogenesis of experimental arthritis in animals and in human rheumatic disease. J Mol Med 76:275-288, 1998.
21. **Bradley DS, Das P, Griffiths MM, et al: HLA-DQ6/8 double transgenic mice develop auricular chondritis following type II collagen immunization: A model for human relapsing polychondritis. J Immunol 161:5046-5053, 1998.**
22. Hansson AS, Heinegard D, Holmdahl R: A new animal model for relapsing polychondritis, induced by cartilage matrix protein (matrilin-1). J Clin Invest 104:589-598, 1999.
23. Zeuner M, Straub RH, Rauh G, et al: Relapsing polychondritis: Clinical and immunogenetic analysis of 62 patients. J Rheumatol 24:96-101, 1997.
24. **Hansson AS, Holmdahl R: Cartilage-specific autoimmunity in animal models and clinical aspects in patients—focus on relapsing polychondritis. Arthritis Res 4:296-301, 2002.**
25. McCaffrey TV, McDonald TJ, McCaffrey LA: Head and neck manifestations of relapsing polychondritis: Review of 29 cases. Otolaryngology 86:473-478, 1978.
26. **Eng J, Sabanathan S: Airway complications in relapsing polychondritis. Ann Thorac Surg 51:686-692, 1991.**
27. Davis SD, Berkmen YM, King T: Peripheral bronchial involvement in relapsing polychondritis: Demonstration by thin-section CT. AJR Am J Roentgenol 153:953-954, 1989.
28. Tillie-Leblond I, Wallaert B, Leblond D, et al: Respiratory involvement in relapsing polychondritis: Clinical, functional, endoscopic, and radiographic evaluations. Medicine (Balt) 77:168-176, 1998.
29. Sarodia BD, Dasgupta A, Mehta AC: Management of airway manifestations of relapsing polychondritis: Case reports and review of literature. Chest 116:1669-1675, 1999.
30. Lim MC, Chan HL: Relapsing polychondritis—a report on two Chinese patients with severe costal chondritis. Ann Acad Med Singapore 19:396-403, 1990.
31. **O'Hanlan M, McAdam LP, Bluestone R, et al: The arthropathy of relapsing polychondritis. Arthritis Rheum 19:191-194, 1976.**
32. Balsa A, Espinosa A, Cuesta M, et al: Joint symptoms in relapsing polychondritis. Clin Exp Rheumatol 13:425-430, 1995.
33. Gunaydin I, Daikeler T, Jacki S, et al: Articular involvement in patients with relapsing polychondritis. Rheumatol Int 18:93-96, 1998.
34. Pazirandeh M, Ziran BH, Khandelwal BK, et al: Relapsing polychondritis and spondylarthropathies. J Rheumatol 15:630-632, 1988.
35. Rajaee A, Voossoghi AA: Classical rheumatoid arthritis associated with relapsing polychondritis. J Rheumatol 16:1263-1265, 1989.
36. Isaak BL, Liesegang TJ, Michet CJ Jr: Ocular and systemic findings in relapsing polychondritis. Ophthalmology 93:681-689, 1986.
37. Letko E, Zafirakis P, Baltatzis S, et al: Relapsing polychondritis: A clinical review. Semin Arthritis Rheum 31:384-395, 2002.
38. Lichauco JJ, Lauer S, Shigemitsu HH, et al: Orbital mucosa-associated lymphoid tissue (MALT)-type lymphoma in a patient with relapsing polychondritis. Arthritis Rheum 44:1713-1715, 2001.
39. Michet CJ Jr: Vasculitis and relapsing polychondritis. Rheum Dis Clin N Am 16:441-444, 1990.
40. Piette JC, Vinceneux P, Francès C: Vascular manifestations in relapsing polychondritis. In Asherson RA, Cervera R, Abramson S, et al (eds): Vascular Manifestations of Systemic Autoimmune Diseases. Boca Raton, CRC Press, 2001, pp 351-359.
41. **Del Rosso A, Petix NR, Pratesi M, et al: Cardiovascular involvement in relapsing polychondritis. Semin Arthritis Rheum 26:840-844, 1997.**
42. Selim AG, Fulford LG, Mohiaddin RH, et al: Active aortitis in relapsing polychondritis. J Clin Pathol 54:890-892, 2001.
43. Barretto SN, Oliveira GH, Michet CJ Jr, et al: Multiple cardiovascular complications in a patient with relapsing polychondritis. Mayo Clin Proc 77:971-974, 2002.
44. Esdaile J, Hawkins D, Gold P, et al: Vascular involvement in relapsing polychondritis. Can Med Assoc J 116:1019-1022, 1977.

45. Chang-Miller A, Okamura M, Torres VE, et al: Renal involvement in relapsing polychondritis. Medicine (Balt) 66:202-217, 1987.

46. Empson M, Adelstein S, Garsia R, et al: Relapsing polychondritis presenting with recurrent venous thrombosis in association with anticardiolipin antibody. Lupus 7:132-134, 1998.

47. Bowness P, Hawley IC, Dearden A, et al: Complete heart block and severe aortic incompetence in relapsing polychondritis: Clinicopathologic findings. Arthritis Rheum 34:97-100, 1991.

48. Buckley LM, Ades PA: Progressive aortic valve inflammation occurring despite apparent remission of relapsing polychondritis. Arthritis Rheum 35:812-814, 1992.

49. Lang-Lazdunski L, Hvass U, Paillole C, et al: Cardiac valve replacement in relapsing polychondritis: A review. J Heart Valve Dis 4:227-235, 1995.

50. Le Thi Huong D, Wechsler B, Piette JC, et al: Aortic insufficiency and recurrent valve prosthesis dehiscence in MAGIC syndrome. J Rheumatol 20:397-398, 1993.

51. Imai H, Motegi M, Mizuki N, et al: Mouth and genital ulcers with inflamed cartilage (MAGIC syndrome): A case report and literature review. Am J Med Sci 314:330-332, 1997.

52. Hanslik T, Wechsler B, Piette J-C, et al: Central nervous system involvement in relapsing polychondritis. Clin Exp Rheumatol 12:539-541, 1994.

53. Kothare SV, Chu CC, VanLandingham K, et al: Migratory leptomeningeal inflammation with relapsing polychondritis. Neurology 51:614-617, 1998.

54. Kitridou RC, Wittmann AL, Quismorio FP: Chondritis in systemic lupus erythematosus: Clinical and immuno-pathologic studies. Clin Exp Rheumatol 5:349-353, 1987.

55. Piette JC, El-Rassi R, Amoura Z: Antinuclear antibodies in relapsing polychondritis. Ann Rheum Dis 58:656-657, 1999.

56. Papo T, Piette JC, Le Thi Huong D, et al: Antineutrophil cytoplasmic antibodies in polychondritis. Ann Rheum Dis 52:384-385, 1993.

57. **Piette JC, Papo T, Chavanon P, et al: Myelodysplasia and relapsing polychondritis. J Rheumatol 22:1208-1209, 1995.**

58. Diebold J, Rauh G, Jäger K, et al: Bone marrow pathology in relapsing polychondritis: High frequency of myelodysplastic syndromes. Br J Haematol 89:820-830, 1995.

59. Moins-Teisserenc HT, Gadola SD, Cella M, et al: Association of a syndrome resembling Wegener's granulomatosis with low surface expression of HLA class-I molecules. Lancet 354:1598-1603, 1999 (erratum in Lancet 356:170, 2000).

60. Prieur AM, Griscelli C, Lampert F, et al: A chronic, infantile, neurological, cutaneous and articular (CINCA) syndrome: A specific entity analysed in 30 patients. Scand J Rheumatol 66(suppl):57-68, 1987.

61. Kurien M, Seshadri MS, Zacharia A: Inherited degenerative chondropathy—an autosomal dominant new clinical entity: Report on two cases and follow-up of four cases. J Laryngol Otol 109:433-436, 1995.

62. Loehrl TA, Smith TL: Inflammatory and granulomatous lesions of the larynx and pharynx. Am J Med 111(Suppl 8A):113S-117S, 2001.

63. Prince JS, Duhamel DR, Levin DL, et al: Nonneoplastic lesions of the tracheobronchial wall: Radiologic findings with bronchoscopic correlation. RadioGraphics 22(Spec No):S215-S30, 2002 (erratum in RadioGraphics 23:191, 2003).

64. Case Records of the Massachusetts General Hospital (case 26-1985). N Engl J Med 312:1695-1703, 1985.

65. Cauhape P, Aumaitre O, Papo T, et al: A diagnostic dilemna: Wegener's granulomatosis, relapsing polychondritis or both? Eur J Med 2:497-498, 1993.

66. Behar JV, Choi YW, Hartman TA, et al: Relapsing polychondritis affecting the lower respiratory tract. AJR Am J Roentgenol 178:173-177, 2002.

67. Heman-Ackah YD, Remley KB, Goding GS Jr: A new role for magnetic resonance imaging in the diagnosis of laryngeal relapsing polychondritis. Head Neck 21:484-489, 1999.

68. Barranco VP, Minor DB, Solomon M: Treatment of relapsing polychondritis with dapsone. Arch Dermatol 112:1286-1288, 1976.

69. Lipnick RN, Fink CW: Acute airway obstruction in relapsing polychondritis: Treatment with pulse methylprednisolone. J Rheumatol 18:98-99, 1991.

70. **Park J, Gowin KM, Schumacher HR Jr: Steroid sparing effect of methotrexate in relapsing polychondritis. J Rheumatol 23:937-938, 1996.**

71. Svenson KLG, Holmdahl R, Klareskog L, et al: Cyclosporin A treatment in a case of relapsing polychondritis. Scand J Rheumatol 13:329-333, 1984.

72. Saadoun D, Deslandre CJ, Allanore Y, et al: Sustained response to infliximab in 2 patients with refractory relapsing polychondritis. J Rheumatol 30:1394-1395, 2003.

73. Rosen O, Thiel A, Massenkeil G, et al: Autologous stem-cell transplantation in refractory autoimmune diseases after in vivo immunoablation and ex vivo depletion of mononuclear cells. Arthritis Res 2:327-336, 2000.

74. Gaffney RJ, Harrison M, Blayney AW: Nebulized racemic ephedrine in the treatment of acute exacerbations of laryngeal relapsing polychondritis. J Laryngol Otol 106:63-64, 1992.

75. Adliff M, Ngato D, Keshavjee S, et al: Treatment of diffuse tracheomalacia secondary to relapsing polychondritis with continuous positive airway pressure. Chest 112:1701-1704, 1997.

76. Dunne JA, Sabanathan S: Use of metallic stents in relapsing polychondritis. Chest 105:864-867, 1994.

77. Biro P, Rohling R, Schmid S, et al: Anesthesia in a patient with acute respiratory insufficiency due to relapsing polychondritis. J Clin Anesth 6:59-62, 1994.

Websites

http://www.emedicine.com/derm/topic375.htm
http://www.orpha.net/data/patho/GB/uk-RP.html
http://www.polychondritis.org/
http://rpolychondritis.tripod.com/

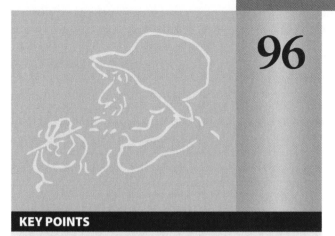

96

Heritable Diseases of Connective Tissue

DEBORAH KRAKOW

KEY POINTS

Heritable disorders of connective tissues are a diverse group of disorders and can be associated with extreme variation in height ranging from very short (dwarfs) to tall stature.

The osteochondrodysplasias or skeletal dysplasias are a heterogeneous group of more than 300 disorders frequently associated with profound short stature and orthopaedic complications.

These disorders are diagnosed based on radiographic, morphologic, clinical, and molecular criteria.

The molecular mechanisms have been elucidated in many of these disorders providing for improved clinical diagnosis and reproductive choices for affected individuals and their families.

Treatment options have been offered in osteogenesis imperfecta and Marfan syndrome that may improve the quality of life and life span in affected individuals.

Heritable disorders of connective tissues are a heterogeneous group of disorders characterized by abnormalities in skeletal tissues including cartilage, bone, tendon, ligament, muscle, and skin. These disorders, originally defined by McKusick,[1] have been classified based on clinical findings and molecular criteria. They are subclassified into disorders that primarily affect cartilage and bone (the skeletal dysplasias), and disorders that have a more profound effect on connective tissue, including Ehlers-Danlos syndrome (EDS), Marfan syndrome, and other disorders manifested by abnormal extracellular matrix molecules.

The skeletal dysplasias are associated with abnormalities in the size and shape of the appendicular and axial skeleton and frequently result in disproportionate short stature. Until the early 1960s, most individuals with short stature were considered to have pituitary dwarfism, achondroplasia (short-limb dwarfism), or Morquio disease (short-trunked dwarfism). Presently, there are more than 300 well-characterized disorders that are classified primarily on the basis of clinical, radiographic, and molecular criteria.[2] Disorders of connective tissue are genetic defects that result from mutations in genes that encode extracellular matrix proteins, transcription factors, tumor suppressors, signal transducers, enzymes, chaperones, intracellular binding proteins, RNA processing molecules, and genes of unknown function.

SKELETAL DYSPLASIAS

The skeletal dysplasias, or osteochondrodysplasias, are defined as disorders that are associated with a generalized abnormality in the skeleton. Although each skeletal dysplasia is relatively rare, collectively, the birth incidence of these disorders is almost 1 in 5000.[3] These disorders range in severity from "precocious" arthropathy to perinatal lethality owing to pulmonary insufficiency. Individuals with these disorders can have significant orthopaedic, neurologic, and psychological complications. Many of these individuals seek medical attention for orthopaedic complaints owing to ongoing pain, arthritic complaints in large joints, and back pain primarily caused by ongoing abnormalities in bone and cartilage.

EMBRYOLOGY

The human skeleton (from the Greek, *skeletos*, "dried up") is a complex organ consisting of 206 bones (126 appendicular bones, 74 axial bones, and 6 ossicles). The skeleton, including tendons, ligaments, and muscles in addition to cartilage and bone, has multiple embryonic origins and serves many key functions throughout life, including linear growth, mechanical support for movement, a blood and mineral reservoir, and protection of vital organs.

The patterning and architecture of the skeleton occurs during fetal development (see Chapter 4). During that period, the number, size, and shape of the future skeletal elements are determined, a process that is under complex genetic control.[4] Uncondensed mesenchyme undergoes cellular condensations (cartilage anlagen) at sites of future bones, and this occurs by two mechanisms.[5] In the process of endochondral ossification, mesenchyme first differentiates into a cartilage model (anlagen), and then the center of the anlagen degrades, mineralizes, and is removed by osteoclast-like cells. This process spreads up and down the bones and allows for vascular invasion and influx of osteoprogenitor cells. The periosteum in the midshaft region of the bone produces osteoblasts, which synthesize the cortex; this is known as the primary ossification center.

At the ends of the cartilage anlagen, a similar process leading to the removal of cartilage occurs (secondary center of ossification) leaving a portion of cartilage model "trapped" between the expanding primary and secondary ossification centers. This area is referred to as a cartilage growth plate or epiphysis. There are four chondrocyte cell types in the growth plate: reserve, resting, proliferative, and hypertrophic. These growth plate chondrocytes undergo a tightly regulated program of proliferation, hypertrophy, degradation, and replacement by bone (primary spongiosa). This is the major mechanism of skeletogenesis and is the mechanism by which bones increase in length, and the articular surfaces increase in diameter. In contrast, the flat bones of the cranial vault and part of the clavicles and pubis form by intramembranous ossification, whereby fibrous tissue, derived from mesenchymal cells, differentiates directly into osteoblasts, which directly lay down bone.[5] These processes are under specific and direct genetic control, and abnormalities in the genes that encode these pathways frequently lead to skeletal dysplasias.[6-9]

CARTILAGE STRUCTURE

Collagen accounts for two thirds of the adult weight of adult articular cartilage and provides significant strength and structure to the tissue (Chapter 3). Collagens are a family of proteins that consist of single molecules (monomers) that combine into three polypeptide chains to form a triple helix structure. In the triple helix, every third amino acid is a glycine residue, and the general chain structure is denoted as Gly-X-Y, where X and Y are commonly proline and hydroxyproline. The collagen helix can be composed of identical chains (homotrimeric), as in type II collagen, or can consist of different collagen chains (heterotrimeric), as seen in collagen type XI.[10]

Collagens are widely distributed throughout the body, and 33 collagen gene products are expressed in a tissue-specific manner, leading to 19 triple helical collagens. Collagens are classified further by the structures they form in the extracellular matrix. The most abundant collagens are the fibrillar types (I, II, III, V, and XI), and their extensive cross-linking provides mechanical strength that is necessary for high stress tissue, such as cartilage, bone, and skin.[11] Another collagen species is the fibril-associated collagens with interrupted triple helices, which include collagen types IX, XII, XIV, and XVI. These collagens interact with fibrillar collagens and other extracellular molecules, including aggrecan, cartilage oligomeric matrix protein, and other sulfated proteoglycans.[11] Collagen types VIII and X are nonfibrillar, short-chain collagens, and type X collagen is the most abundant extracellular matrix molecule expressed by hypertrophic chondrocytes during endochondral ossification.[12] The major collagens of articular cartilage are fibrillar collagen types II, IX, XI, and X. In developing cartilage, the core fibrillar network is a cross-linked copolymer of collagens II, IX, and XI.[13] Mutations in genes that encode these collagens result in various skeletal dysplasias and highlight the importance of these molecules in skeletal development.

CLASSIFICATION AND NOMENCLATURE

As mentioned earlier, in the 1970s, there was recognition of the genetic and clinical heterogeneity of heritable disorders of connective tissue and a new awareness of the complexity of these disorders. As a result, there have been multiple attempts to classify these disorders in a manner that clinicians and scientists could use effectively to diagnose and determine their pathogenicity (International Nomenclature of Constitutional Diseases of Bone, 1970, 1977, 1983, 1992, 2001, and 2005). The initial categories were purely descriptive and clinically based. With the more recent explosion in determining the genetic basis of these diseases, the classification has evolved into one that combines the older clinical one (including the eponyms and Greek terms) and blends these disorders into families that share a molecular basis or pathway. The most recent updated classification can be found at www.isds.ch; some of the chondrodysplasia families are listed in Table 96-1.

The most widely used method for differentiating the skeletal disorders has been through the detection of skeletal radiographic abnormalities. Radiographic classifications are based on the different parts of the long bones that are abnormal (epiphyses, metaphyses, and diaphyses) (Fig. 96-1). These epiphyseal, metaphyseal, and diaphyseal disorders can be differentiated further depending on whether or not the spine is involved (spondyloepiphyseal, spondylometaphyseal, or spondyloepimetaphyseal dysplasias). Each of these classes of these disorders can be differentiated further into distinct disorders based on other clinical and radiographic findings.

CLINICAL EVALUATION AND FEATURES

The skeletal dysplasias are generalized disorders of the skeleton and usually result in disproportionate short stature. Affected individuals usually present because they are disproportionately short. This finding needs to be documented on the appropriate growth curves for gender and ethnicity if possible. Most individuals with disproportionate short stature have skeletal dysplasias, and individuals with proportionate short stature have endocrine, nutritional, or prenatal-onset growth deficiency, or other nonskeletal dysplasia disorders. There are exceptions to the rule, such as congenital hypothyroidism, which is associated with disproportionate short stature, and disorders such as osteogenesis imperfecta (OI) and hypophosphatasia can be associated with normal body proportions.

A disproportionate body habitus may not be immediately visible on physical examination. Anthropometric dimensions, such as upper-to-lower segment (U/L) ratio, sitting height, and arm span, must be measured when considering the possibility of a skeletal dysplasia and should be measured in centimeters. Sitting height is an accurate measurement of head and trunk length, but it requires special equipment for precise measurements. U/L ratios are easy to obtain and provide an accurate measurement of proportion. The lower segment is measured from the symphysis pubis to the floor at the inside of the heel. The upper segment is measured by subtracting the lower segment measurement from the total height. McKusick[14] has published standard U/L segment ratios for whites and African-Americans across ages. A white child 8 to 10 years old has a U/L segment ratio of approximately 1 and as an adult has a U/L segment ratio of 0.95. Individuals presenting with disproportionate short stature have altered U/L segment ratios depending on whether they have short limbs, short trunk, or both. An individual with short limbs and normal trunk has an increased U/L segment ratio, and an individual with normal limbs but short trunk has a diminished U/L segment ratio (Fig. 96-2). Another means of determining if there is disproportion is based on arm span measurements, which are very close to total height in an average-proportioned individual. A short-limbed individual has an arm span considerably shorter than the height.

As in any disorder that has a genetic basis, it is crucial to obtain an accurate family history, and this should include any history of previously affected children or parental consanguinity. The skeletal dysplasias are genetically

Table 96-1   Classification of the Chondrodysplasias

Dysplasia	Mode of Inheritance	Chromosomal Location	Gene
Achondroplasia Group			
Achondroplasia	AD	4p16.3	FGFR3
Thanatophoric dysplasia, type I	AD	4p16.3	FGFR
Thanatophoric dysplasia, type II	AD	4p16.3	FGFR3
Achondroplasia	AD	4p16.3	FGFR3
Hypochondroplasia	AD	4p16.3	FGFR3
SADDAN*	AD	4p16.3	FGFR3
Osteoglophonic dysplasia	AD	8p11	FGFR1
Severe Spondylodysplastic Dysplasias			
Achondrogenesis IA	AR		
Opsismodysplasia	AR		
Spondylometaphyseal dysplasia, type Sedaghatian	AR		
Metatropic Dysplasia Group			
Fibrochondrogenesis	AR		
Schneckenbecken dysplasia	AR		
Metatropic dysplasia	AD/AR (more than one form)		
Short Rib Dysplasia (Polydactyly) Group			
Short-rib polydactyly type I/III	AR		
Short-rib polydactyly type II/IV	AR		
Asphyxiating thoracic dysplasia	AR		
Chondroectodermal dysplasia	AR	4p16	EVC1, EVC2
Thoracolaryngopelvic dysplasia	AD		
Omodysplasia Group			
Omodysplasia I	AD		
Omodysplasia II	AR		
Filamin-Related Disorders			
Atelosteogenesis I	AD	3p14.3	FLNB
Atelosteogenesis III	AD	3p14.3	FLNB
Larsen syndrome	AD	3p14.3	FLNB
Otopalatodigital syndrome type II	XLR	Xq28	FLNA
Osteodysplasty of Melnick and Needles	XLD	Xq28	FLNA
Diastrophic Dysplasia Group			
Achondrogenesis IB	AR	5q31-q34	DTDST
Achondrogenesis II	AR	5q31-q34	DTDST
Diastrophic dysplasia	AR	5q31-q34	DTDST
Recessive multiple epiphyseal dysplasia	AR	5q31-q34	DTDST
Dyssegmental Dysplasia Group			
Dyssegmental dysplasia, Silverman-Handmaker type	AR		HSPG2
Dyssegmental dysplasia, Rolland-Desbuquois type	AR		
Type II Collagenopathies			
Achondrogenesis II	AD	12q13	COL2A1
Kniest dysplasia	AD	12q13	COL2A1
Spondyloepiphyseal dysplasia, congenital	AD	12q13	COL2A1
Spondyloepiphyseal dysplasia, Strudwick type	AD	12q13	COL2A1
Spondyloperipheral dysplasia	AD	12q13	COL2A1
Arthro-ophthalmopathy (Stickler syndrome)	AD	12q13	COL2A1
Type XI Collagenopathies			
Stickler dysplasia	AD	1p21	COL11A1
Otospondylometaepiphyseal dysplasia	AR	6p21.3	COL11A2
Weissenbacher-Zweymuller syndrome	AD	6p21.3	COL11A2
Other Spondyloepi-(meta)-physeal Dysplasias			
Spondyloepimetaphyseal dysplasia, Pakistani type	AR	10q23-q24	ATPSK2
Spondyloepiphyseal dysplasia tarda	XLR	Xp22	SEDL
Progressive pseudorheumatoid dysplasia	AR	6q22-q23	WISP3
Dyggve-Melchior-Clausen dysplasia	AR	18q12-q21.1	FLJ90130
Wolcott-Rallison dysplasia	AR	2p12	EIF2AK3
Acrocapitofemoral dysplasia	AR	2q35-q36	IHH
Schimke immuno-osseous dysplasia	AR	2q34-q36	SMARCAL1
Sponastrime	AR		
Spondyloepimetaphsyseal dysplasia, with joint laxity	AR		

*Severe achondroplasia with developmental delay and acanthosis nigricans.
 AD, autosomal dominant; AR, autosomal recessive; SP, sporadic; XLD, X-linked dominant; XLR, X-linked recessive.

Continued

Table 96-1 Classification of the Chondrodysplasias—cont'd

Dysplasia	Mode of Inheritance	Chromosomal Location	Gene
Multiple Epiphyseal Dysplasia and Pseudoachondroplasia			
Multiple epiphyseal dysplasia, types Fairbanks and Ribbing	AD	6q12-q14	COL9A1
		1p33-q32	COL9A2
		20q13.3	COL9A
		2q24-q23	MATN
		19p13.1	COMP
Pseudoachondroplasia	AD	19p13.1	COMP
Chondrodysplasia Punctata			
Chondrodysplasia punctata, rhizomelic type	AR	6q22-q24	PEX7
		1q42	DHAPAT
		2q31	AGPS
Chondrodysplasia punctata, Conradi-Hünermann type	XLD	Xp11.2	EBP
Hydrops-ectopic-calcifications-moth-eaten bones	AR	1q42.1	LBR
Chondrodysplasia punctata, brachytelephalangic type	XLR	Xp22-p32	ARSE
Chondrodysplasia punctata, tibial-metacarpal type	SP		
Metaphyseal Dysplasias			
Metaphyseal chondrodysplasia, Jansen type	AD	3p21-p22	PTHrP
Eiken dysplasia	AR	3p21-p22	PTHrP
Bloomstrand dysplasia	AR	3p21-p22	PTHrP
Metaphyseal chondrodysplasia, Schmidt type	AD	6q21-q22	COL10A1
Metaphyseal chondrodysplasia, McKusik type	AR	9p21-p13	RMRP
Metaphyseal chondrodysplasia, with pancreatic insufficiency, and cyclin neutropenia	AR	7q11	SBDS
Adenosine deaminase deficiency	AR	20q13.11	ADA
Spondylometaphyseal dysplasias			
Spondylometaphyseal dysplasia, Koslowski type	AD		
Spondylometaphyseal dysplasia, corner fracture type	AD		
Brachyolmia Spondylodysplasias			
Brachyolmia (Hobek type; Toledo type)	AR		
Brachyolmia (Maroteaux type)	AR		
Brachyolmia (AD)	AD		
Mesomelic Dysplasias			
Dyschondrosteosis	XLD	Xp22.3	SHOX
Mesomelic dysplasia, Langer type	XLR	Xp22.3	SHOX
Mesomelic dysplasia, Nievergelt type	AD		
Mesomelic dysplasia, Robinow type	AD		
	AR	9q22	ROR2
Mesomelic dysplasia, Reinhardt type	AD		
Mesomelic dysplasia, Werner type	AD		
Mesomelic dysplasia, Kantapura type	AD	2q24-32	
Acromelic and Acromesomelic Dysplasias			
Acromicric dysplasia	SP		
Geleophysic dysplasia	AR		
Trichorhinophalangeal dysplasia, type I	AD	8q24.12	TRPS1
Trichorhinophalangeal dysplasia, type II	AD	del8q24.11-q13	TRPS2
Acrodysplasia with retinitis pigmentosa and nephropathy	AR		
Acrodysostosis	AD		
Grebe dysplasia	AR	20q11.2	CDMP1
Acromesomelic dysplasia, Hunter-Thompson	AR	20q11.2	CDMP1
Angel-shaped phalangoepiphyseal dysplasia			
Acromesomelic dysplasia, Maroteaux type	AR	9p21-12	NPRB
Dysplasia with Prominent Membranous Bone Involvement			
Cleidocranial dysplasia	AD	6p21	CBFA1
Bent Bone Dysplasias			
Campomelic dysplasia	AD	17q24.1-q25.1	SOX9
Stuve-Wiedemann dysplasia	AR	5p13.1	LIFR
Multiple Dislocations with Dysplasias			
Desbuquois syndrome	AR		
Pseudodiastrophic dysplasia	AR		
Spondyloepimetaphyseal dysplasia with joint laxity	AR		

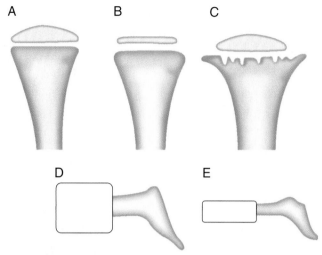

Figure 96-1 **A-E,** Classification of chondrodysplasias based on radiographic involvement of the long bones (**A-C**) and vertebrae (**D** and **E**). **A** and **D** are normal, **B** is an epiphyseal abnormality, **C** is a metaphyseal abnormality, and **E** is a "spondylo-" abnormality.

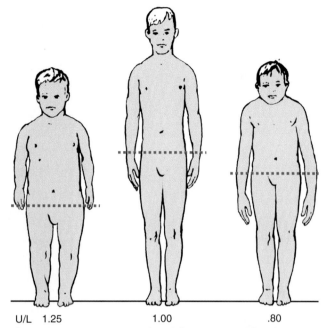

Figure 96-2 Upper segment length/lower segment length (U/L) in 8- to 10-year-old individuals with short limb and short trunk dwarfism. The child on the left has short limbs and an increased U/L ratio; the child on the right has a short trunk and reduced U/L ratio.

heterogeneous and can be inherited as autosomal dominant, autosomal recessive, X-linked recessive, and X-linked dominant disorders, and rarer genetic mechanisms of disease, including germline mosaicism and uniparental disomy, have been seen.[15-18] For many patients and families, accurate diagnosis and recurrence risk can have a significant impact on their reproductive decisions. Another consideration for patients with short stature is that there is increased nonrandom mating, which leads to reproductive outcomes that have been previously unknown.[19] Homozygous achondroplasia is lethal, and many newborns who inherit two dominant mutations (compound heterozygotes) die early with severe abnormalities of the skeleton.[20]

It also is important to obtain an accurate history relative to the onset of short stature, and whether it developed immediately in the postnatal period or was noticed at age 2 or 3. Of the 300 skeletal dysplasias, approximately 100 of them have onset in the prenatal period, but many affected individuals do not develop disproportionate short stature and joint discomfort until childhood.[21]

A detailed physical examination may reveal a diagnosis or help differentiate the most likely group of possible diagnoses. It is crucial when disproportion and short stature have been established and the limbs are involved to determine which segment is involved: upper segment (rhizomelic—humerus and femur), middle segment (mesomelic—radius, ulna, tibia, and fibula), and distal segment (acromelic—hands and feet). Numerous head and facial dysmorphisms are seen in the skeletal disorders. Affected individuals frequently have disproportionately large heads. Frontal bossing and flattened nasal bridge is characteristic of achondroplasia, one of the most common skeletal dysplasias.[22] Cleft palate and micrognathia are commonly found in the type II collagen abnormalities, abnormally flattened midface with a turned-up nose is frequently found in the chondrodysplasia punctata disorders,[23] and abnormal swollen pinnae are seen in diastrophic dysplasia.[24] Individuals with skeletal dysplasias should be screened for ophthalmologic and hearing abnormalities because some of these disorders are associated with eye abnormalities and hearing loss.

Further evaluation of the hands and feet can lead to further differentiation of these disorders. Postaxial polydactyly is characteristically found in chondroectodermal dysplasia and the short-rib polydactyly disorders (see Table 96-1). Short, hypermobile, radially displaced thumbs are seen in diastrophic dysplasia. Nails can be abnormally hypoplastic in chondroectodermal dysplasia and short and broad in cartilage hair hypoplasia. Clubfeet may be seen in many disorders, including Kneist dysplasia, spondyloepiphyseal dysplasia congenita, Larsen syndrome, OI types II and III, and diastrophic dysplasia. Bone fractures occur most commonly in two types of disorders—those that result from undermineralized bone (OI, hypophosphatasia, achondrogenesis IA), or those that result from overmineralized bone (osteopetrosis syndromes and dysosteosclerosis).

Organ systems other than the skeleton can be involved, although rarely. Congenital cardiac defects are seen in chondroectodermal dysplasia (atrial septal defects), the short-rib polydactyly disorders (complex outlet defects including isolated ventricular septal defects), and Larsen syndrome (ventricular septal defects). Gastrointestinal anomalies are rare among the skeletal disorders, but congenital megacolon can be seen in cartilage hair hypoplasia, malabsorption syndrome in Schwachmann-Diamond syndrome, and omphaloceles in otopalatodigital syndrome and atelosteogenesis I.

DIAGNOSIS AND TESTING

After obtaining a thorough family history and physical examination, the next step is to obtain a full set of skeletal radiographs. A full series of skeletal views includes anterior, lateral, and Towne views of the skull; anterior and lateral views of the entire spine; and anteroposterior views of the pelvis and extremities, with separate views of the hands and

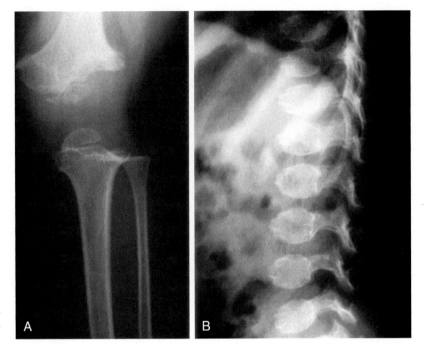

Figure 96-3 Radiographs showing abnormalities in the chondrodysplasias, specifically pseudoachondroplasia. **A,** Irregular metaphyses and small epiphyses. **B,** Small, rounded vertebrae with anterior beaking.

feet, especially after the newborn period. Most of the important clues to diagnosis are in skeletal radiographs that are obtained before puberty. When the epiphyses have fused to the metaphyses, determining the precise diagnosis can be extremely challenging. If an adult is evaluated, all attempts should be made to obtain any available childhood radiographs. Many subtle clues in these skeletal radiographs can lead to precise diagnosis. Punctate calcifications in the areas of the epiphyses in the chondrodysplasia punctata disorders, multiple ossification centers of the calcaneus in more than 20 disorders,[25] and the type of hand shortening can aid in differentiating many disorders.

After obtaining radiographs, close attention should be paid to the specific parts of the skeleton (spine, limbs, pelvis, skull) involved and to the location of the lesions (epiphyses, metaphyses, and vertebrae) (Fig. 96-3). As mentioned earlier, these radiographic abnormalities can change with age, and if available, radiographs across a few years or

decades aid in diagnosis. Fractures can be seen in OI (all types) (Fig. 96-4; see Table 96-1) and severe hypophosphatasia. In older individuals, fractures may be seen in disorders associated with increased mineralization, such as the osteopetrosis syndromes and dysosteosclerosis. When a thorough evaluation of the radiographs reveals abnormalities, but a diagnosis still cannot be made, resources are available. The International Skeletal Dysplasia Registry (http://www.csmc.edu/3805.html) is available to provide diagnosis for these rare disorders.

Morphologic studies of chondro-osseous tissue have revealed specific abnormalities in many of the skeletal dysplasias.[26-28] In these disorders, histologic evaluation of chondro-osseous morphology can aid in making an accurate diagnosis, and absence of histopathologic alterations can rule out diagnoses. These studies need to be done on cartilage growth plate, and although commonly performed on perinatal lethal skeletal disorders at autopsy, obtaining

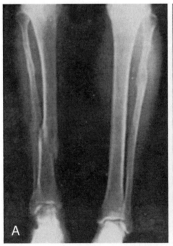
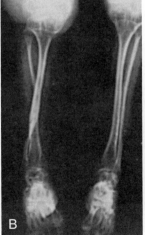
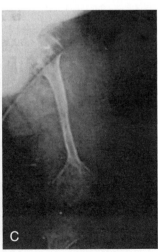

Figure 96-4 Radiographs illustrating skeletal differences among variants of osteogenesis imperfecta (OI). **A,** Dominant OI—mild, with minimal deformity. **B,** Moderate OI—mild epiphyseal dysplasia. **C,** Severe OI—marked diaphyseal narrowing and widening of the metaphysis with severe epiphyseal dysplasia. Lethal OI is not illustrated.

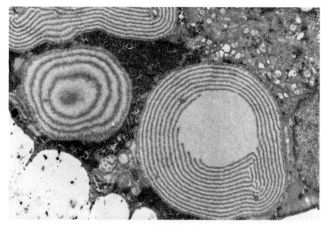

Figure 96-5 Electron micrograph of a chondrocyte from an individual with pseudoachondroplasia. Note the characteristic lamellar pattern in the rough endoplasmic reticulum.

growth plate histology on individuals with nonlethal disorders is difficult. If affected individuals (children) are undergoing surgery, an iliac crest biopsy specimen can be evaluated.

Histomorphology studies done on these disorders have led to important insights on the pathogenesis of these disorders. On morphologic grounds, the chondrodysplasias can be broadly classified into disorders (1) that have a qualitative abnormality in endochondral ossification, (2) that have abnormalities in cellular morphology, (3) that have abnormalities in matrix morphology, and (4) in which the abnormality is primarily localized to the area of chondro-osseous transformation. In thanatophoric dysplasia, there is a defect in endochondral ossification with a very short, almost hypertrophic zone, shortened proliferative zone, and overgrowth of the periosteum; in pseudoachondroplasia, there is a distinct lamellar pattern (alternating electron-dense and electron-lucent lamellae) in the rough endoplasmic reticulum of chondrocytes (Fig. 96-5) and a grossly abnormal matrix in diastrophic dysplasia, which leads to a characteristic ring around the chondrocytes. All of these findings are characteristic and diagnostic for these disorders and illustrate how morphology studies can have an integral part in the investigation of these disorders.

There has been significant progress in gene identification in these disorders, which has impact for affected individuals. As illustrated in Table 96-1, for disorders in which the gene is identified, molecular diagnostic testing is potentially available. Molecular diagnosis can be used to confirm a clinical and radiographic diagnosis, predict carrier status in families at risk for a recessive disorder, and, for some individuals, allow for prenatal diagnosis of at-risk fetuses. Because these are rare disorders, commercial testing is not always readily available; however, GeneTests (www.genetests.org) is a publically funded medical genetics website developed for physicians that provides information on diseases and available genetic testing.

MANAGEMENT AND TREATMENT

The optimal management of this diverse set of disorders requires an understanding of the medical, skeletal, and psychosocial consequences. This is often best accomplished by centers that have a multidisciplinary approach, which includes adult and pediatric physicians, orthopaedists, rheumatologists, otolaryngologists, neurologists, neurosurgeons, and ophthalmologists who are committed to the care of these patients.

Most medical complications in these disorders result from orthopaedic complications, and they vary depending on the specific disorder. In disorders associated with significant odontoid hypoplasia, such as Morquio disease, type II collagenopathies, metatropic dysplasia, and Larsen syndrome, flexion-extension films should be monitored at regular intervals to assess for C1-C2 subluxation. If there is evidence for subluxation, surgery for C1-C2 fixation is indicated. Genu varum—lateral curvature of the lower extremity—is common in many skeletal disorders caused by overgrowth of the fibula; this causes knee or ankle pain in many individuals, especially children, and correction by osteotomy should be considered. Children and adults with skeletal dysplasias should have regular eye and hearing examinations because they are at increased risk for myopia, retinal degeneration, glaucoma, and hearing loss depending on the disorder.

Frequently, patients with these disorders have significant joint pain and in some cases joint limitations. Because most of these disorders result from mutations in genes crucial to cartilage function, the cartilage at the joint surfaces may not provide adequate support and cushioning function. Many of these patients seek attention for joint pain. Evaluation should include radiographs and magnetic resonance imaging (MRI), when appropriate, to determine the etiology of the pain. In some disorders, such as the type II collagenopathies, pseudoachondroplasia, multiple epiphyseal dysplasia, and cartilage hair hypoplasia, by adulthood, so little cartilage remains at the knee or hips that joint replacement is indicated for pain relief. Lastly, overweight in adults with short stature is an ongoing issue and contributes to inactivity, loss of function, adult-onset diabetes, hypertension, and coronary disease.[29]

Achondroplasia

Achondroplasia is the most common of the nonlethal skeletal dysplasias (approximately 1 in 20,000) and serves as an example on how to approach these disorders. Most affected individuals are of normal intelligence, have a normal life span, and lead independent and productive lives. The mean final height in achondroplasia is 130 cm for men and 125 cm for women; specific growth charts have been developed to document and track linear growth, head circumference, and weight in these individuals.[30,31]

In early infancy, there is potentially serious compression of the cervicomedullary spinal cord secondary to a narrow foramen magnum, cervical canal, or both. Clinically, these infants have central apnea, sleep apnea, profound hypotonia, motor delay, or excessive sweating. MRI with flow studies is necessary to document the obstruction; if present, obstruction requires decompressive surgery.[32] Other complications include nasal obstruction, thoracolumbar kyphosis, and hydrocephalus in a few individuals.[32]

From early childhood, and as children begin to walk, they develop several orthopaedic manifestations, which include progressive bowing of the legs owing to fibular overgrowth, lumbar lordosis, and hip flexion contractures. Recurrent ear infections can lead to chronic serous otitis media and deafness. Tympanic membrane tube placement is indicated in many of these patients. Craniofacial abnormalities lead to dental malocclusion, and appropriate treatment is necessary.

In adults, the main potential medical complication is impingement of the spinal root canals. This complication can be manifested by lower limb paresthesias, claudication, clonus, or bladder or bowel dysfunction. It is crucial that these complaints are addressed because without appropriate decompression surgery, paralysis of the spinal cord can result.[32]

Growth hormone has not been effective in increasing height in this disorder.[33] Surgical limb lengthening has been employed successfully to increase limb length by 12 inches,[34] but this technique needs to be done during the teen years and is performed over a 2-year period and is associated with complications. Throughout their lives, individuals with achondroplasia and other skeletal dysplasias and their families experience various psychosocial challenges.[35] These challenges can be addressed by specialized medical and social support systems. Interactions with advocacy groups such as Little People of America (http://www.lpaonline.org) can provide emotional support and medical information.

BIOCHEMICAL AND MOLECULAR ABNORMALITIES

Similarities in clinical and radiographic findings and histomorphology have placed bone dysplasia into families.[36] These families share common pathophysiologic or pathway mechanisms. In recent years, there has been an explosion in understanding of the basic biology of these disorders. This explosion has resulted from the successful human genome project, which improved various methodologies, including candidate gene approach, linkage analysis, positional cloning, and human/mouse synteny allowing for identification of the disease genes (see Table 96-1). With gene discovery in more than 100 of these osteochondrodysplasias, these genes can be placed into several categories designed to understand their pathogenesis: (1) defects in extracellular proteins; (2) defects in metabolic pathways (enzymes, ion channels, and transporters); (3) defects in folding and degradation of macromolecules; (4) defects in hormones and signal transduction; (5) defects in nuclear proteins; (6) defects in oncogenes and tumor-suppressor genes; (7) defects in RNA and DNA processing molecules; (8) defects in intracellular structural proteins; and (9) genes of unknown function. There are still many skeletal dysplasias for which the chromosomal location and gene are unknown. Following are descriptions of some of the molecular mechanisms involved in the skeletal dysplasias.

DEFECTS IN EXTRACELLULAR STRUCTURAL PROTEINS

TYPE II COLLAGEN AND TYPE XI COLLAGEN

Because type II collagen was found primarily in cartilage, the nucleus pulposus, and the vitreous of the eye, it was hypothesized that skeletal disorders with significant spine and eye abnormalities would result from defects in type II collagen.

Type II collagen defects have been identified in a spectrum of disorders ranging from lethal to mild arthropathy, which include achondrogenesis II, hypochondrogenesis, spondyloepiphyseal dysplasia congenita, spondyloepimetaphyseal dysplasia, Strudwick type, Kniest dysplasia, Stickler syndrome, and "precocious" familial arthopathy. These disorders are referred to as type II collagenopathies, and they all result from heterozygosity for mutations in COL2A1.[37,38] Biochemical analysis of cartilage derived from these individuals shows electrophoretically detectable abnormal type II collagen. Type I collagen is not normally present in cartilage, but in the presence of abnormal type II collagen, there is increased type I collagen in the growth plate.

Mutations that result in a substitution for a triple helical glycine residue seem to be the most common type of mutation.[39-41] There are some correlations between the location of the mutation and the disease phenotype. In spondyloepiphyseal dysplasia, the glycine substitutions are scattered throughout the molecule; however, in Kniest dysplasia, the mutations are in the more amino-terminal end of the molecule.[42-44] Stickler syndrome (see Table 96-1) is genetically heterogeneous and results from mutations in COL2A1 and COL11A1, and nonocular forms result from mutations in COL11A2.[45,46] In Stickler syndrome, the COL2A1 and COL11A1 mutations tend to be nonsense mutations resulting in premature translation stop codons; however, patients with COL11A1 mutations tend to have a more severe eye phenotype and hearing loss than patients with COL2A1 mutations.

Individuals heterozygous for various COL11A2 mutations[47] have a nonocular form of Stickler syndrome, consistent with the absent expression of COL11A2 in the vitreous humor. Otospondylomegaepiphyseal dysplasia is a rare autosomal recessive disorder caused by loss of function mutations in COL11A2.[47] This disorder has radiographic similarities to Kniest dysplasia, but is associated with profound sensorineural hearing loss and lack of ocular involvement.

CARTILAGE OLIGOMERIC MATRIX PROTEIN

Heterozygosity for mutations in cartilage oligomeric matrix protein leads to pseudoachondroplasia and multiple epiphyseal dysplasia.[48] Cartilage oligomeric matrix protein is a member of the thrombospondin family of proteins and consists of an epidermal growth factor domain and calcium binding, calmodulin domain.[49] In pseudoachondroplasia and multiple epiphyseal dysplasia, disease-producing mutations occur in the calmodulin domain, with a few in the globular carboxy-terminal domain (Fig. 96-6).

DEFECTS IN METABOLIC PATHWAYS

Defects in metabolic pathways comprise defects in enzymes, ion channels, and transporters essential for cartilage metabolism and homeostasis. An example is the diastrophic dysplasia group (see Table 96-1), a spectrum of disorders (lethal to mild short stature) resulting from mutations in the DTDST gene. These disorders result from a varying defect in the degree of sulfate uptake or transport into chondrocytes.[50] Lack of adequate intracellular sulfate affects the normal post-translational modification of proteoglycans and leads to abnormal chondrogenesis that is proportional to the degree of transporter compromise.[50]

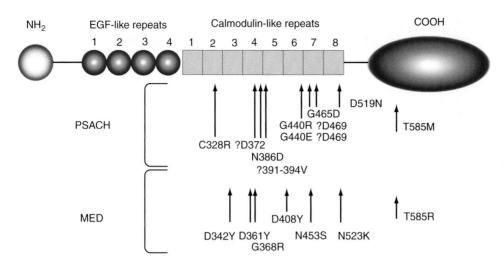

Figure 96-6 Diagram of the cartilage oligomeric matrix protein (COMP) delineating the domains— NH$_2$ amino terminus, EGF-like (epidermal growth factor-like), calmodulin-like, COOH (carboxy-terminus), PSACH (pseudoachondroplasia), and MED (multiple epiphyseal dysplasia). Amino acid substitutions are listed below the molecule.

DEFECTS IN INTRACELLULAR STRUCTURAL PROTEINS

Intracellular proteins are ubiquitously expressed proteins; the finding that mutations in the genes encoding filamin A and filamin B produced primarily skeletal disorders was surprising.[51-53] The filamins are cytoskeleton proteins involved in multicellular processes, including providing structure to the cell, facilitating signal transduction and transport of small solutes, allowing communication between the intracellular and extracellular environment, and participating in cell division and motility. Defects in these genes have a profound effect on the skeleton ranging from absence of bone formation to significant joint dislocations. The mechanisms by which these mutations produce disease are unclear.

SUMMARY

Although these osteochondrodysplasias are rare disorders, affected individuals have significant skeletal complications throughout their lives, first owing to patterning defects, then effects on linear growth, and finally loss of normal structural cartilage as a cushion later in life. The explosion in delineating the molecular defects has shown the complexity of cartilage as a tissue and the large number of cellular processes necessary for a normal skeleton.

OSTEOGENESIS IMPERFECTA

OI is a heritable disorder of bone and was one of the first disorders hypothesized to be a defect in collagen by McKusick.[1] Although an osteochondrodysplasia, OI is discussed separately from the chondrodysplasias delineated previously. OI is a generalized disorder of connective tissue that predominantly affects the skeletal system[54] and affects numerous individuals (estimates at about 1 in 20,000 individuals).

Initially, there were four types of recognized OI in the clinical classification of Sillence.[55] There are now seven types of recognized OI, and because there is enormous clinical variability in these types, the subtypes are discussed separately (Table 96-2). These disorders all share the same phenotypic finding of hypomineralization of the skeleton.

MILD OSTEOGENESIS IMPERFECTA (TYPE I)

Affected individuals with OI type I disease have mild disease in terms of clinical course, the extent of skeletal deformity, and the radiologic appearance of the skeleton (see Fig. 96-4A and Table 96-2). They also account for most individuals with OI. Individuals are usually short for their age or their unaffected family members. Many of these individuals experience numerous fractures, especially in childhood; children with OI type I may have 20 fractures by the age of 5.

The disorder is autosomal dominant, and in many cases the individual is the first affected in the family. There is mild facial dysmorphism in OI type I with a mild triangular facial shape. The sclerae are blue that become gray-to-pale blue in adulthood. Arcus senilis not related to lipid abnormalities may occur in some patients. Other reported ocular defects include scleromalacia, keratoconus, and retinal detachment.[56] The teeth frequently show dentinogenesis imperfecta owing to the effects of mutation on the tooth dentin. The deciduous and permanent teeth have an opalescent and translucent appearance, which tends to darken with age. The enamel is normal, but the dentin is dysplastic; chipping of enamel occurs, and the teeth are subjected to erosion and breakage. Teeth of affected individuals appear discolored or gray. This finding varies in the disorder, but does cosegregate in families with OI. Dentinogenesis imperfecta can be seen in all forms of OI. During the second and third decades of life, a characteristic high-frequency sensorineural or mixed hearing loss can be detected.[57] The incidence of mitral valve prolapse is not increased in these patients compared with the population at large, but individual kindreds with increased diameter of the aortic root or patients with aortic regurgitation have been reported.[58] Many patients complain of easy bruising, and this may result from the effects of mutation on skin and the vessels below.

Mildly affected patients may not have fractures at birth, although occasionally a fracture of a clavicle or extremity occurs during delivery. Radiographically, affected newborns have wormian bones seen on lateral views of the skull, with significant osteopenia seen through the skeleton, especially the spine. After birth, the frequency of fracture depends on the child's activity, the need for

Table 96-2 Characteristics of Osteogenesis Imperfecta

Type	Clinical Features	Inheritance	Biochemical Abnormality	Gene
I	Normal stature; little or no deformity; blue sclerae; hearing loss; dentinogenesis imperfecta	AD (new mutations are common)	50% reduction in type I collagen synthesis	COL1A1
II	Lethal; minimal calvarial mineralization; beaded ribs; compressed femurs; long bone deformity	AD (new mutations; mosaicism)	Structural alterations of type I collagen chains—overmodification of type I collagen	COL1A1
		AR (rare)		COL1A2 CRTAP P3H1
III	Progressively deforming bones; dentinogenesis imperfecta; hearing loss; very short stature	AD	Structural alterations of type I collagen chains—overmodification of type I collagen	COL1A1
		AR		COL1A2 CRTAP P3H1
IV	Normal sclerae in adult; mild-to-moderate deformity; variable short stature; dentinogenesis imperfecta; some hearing loss	AD	Structural alterations of type I collagen chains—overmodification of type I collagen	COL1A1 COL1A2
V	Similar to type IV plus calcification of interosseous membrane of forearm; hyperplastic callus formation	AD	None described	Unknown
VI	Similar to type IV with vertebral compression; mineralization defect	Unknown	None described	Unknown
VII	Moderate-to-severe; fractures at birth; early deformity and rhizomelia	AR	None described	CRTAP

AD, autosomal dominant; AR, autosomal recessive; CRTAP, cartilage-associated protein; P3H1, prolyl-3-hydroxylase 1.

immobilization after lower extremity fractures, and the attitude of the family toward independent activity. Generally, these patients may experience 5 to 15 major fractures before puberty and several minor traumatic fractures of the digits or the small bones of the feet. Characteristically, the fracture rate declines dramatically after puberty, only to increase during later life. Mild scoliosis approximating 20 degrees is common. Osteopenia is observed in vertebral bodies and the peripheral skeleton and progresses with age. In OI type I, the long bones usually heal with no significant deformity. Compared with more severe phenotypes, children with OI type I only infrequently require the insertion of intramedullary rods and almost never experience nonunion at a fracture site.

Although osteopenia with rarefaction of the medullary space and cortical thinning are observed in radiographs, many OI type I cases are so mild as to be missed on routine radiographic examination. Measurement of bone mineral density by dual-energy x-ray absorptiometry at any age discloses a significant decrease in bone mass.[59] T scores (i.e., standard deviation from the young-adult mean bone mineral density) are frequently in the range of −2.5 to −4.0 at the lumbar spine or proximal femur, consistent with the diagnosis of osteoporosis as defined by the World Health Organization. Low bone mineral density in children with recurrent fractures may assist in identifying children with OI.

Molecular Pathology

As in other phenotypes, OI type I is the result of mutations affecting the COL1A1(I) and COL1A2(I) polypeptide chains of type I collagen. Cultured fibroblasts from individuals with mild OI synthesize low amounts (approximately one half) of the expected amounts of type I collagen. The molecular basis for the low production of type I collagen seems to be diminished activity of one of the COL1A1(I) or COL1A2(I) collagen alleles. Many of the reported mutations in OI type I are nonsense and frameshift mutations and are predicted to lead to premature termination codons, although there are some exceptions.[60,61]

LETHAL OSTEOGENESIS IMPERFECTA (TYPE II)

Approximately 10% of OI patients have the severe neonatal form of the disease, lethal OI. Most cases result from sporadic mutations; however, more recently, a recessive form of the disease has been documented.[62-64] These infants present with severe bone fragility, multiple intrauterine fractures at various stages of healing, deformed extremities, and occasionally hydrops fetalis (Fig. 96-7). Radiographic features include wormian bones, multiple fractures, crumbled bones, and characteristic beading of the ribs owing to healing callus formation. There is a subtype of the lethal form, OI type IIC, which is autosomal recessive and is differentiated by the absence of beaded ribs (thin ribs).

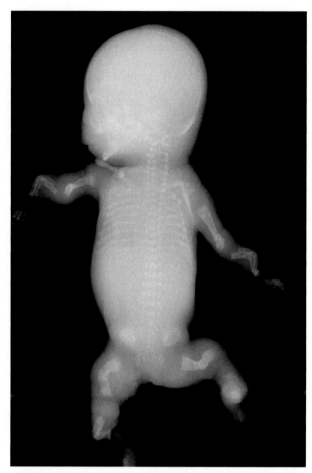

Figure 96-7 Radiograph of lethal osteogenesis imperfecta (type II) showing poorly mineralized calvaria, bent, crumbled bones, and ribs with fractures and callus formation.

Molecular Pathology

Most cases occur de novo, as new dominant mutations; however, an autosomal recessive form has been established, as has recurrence based on germline mosaicism.[62-65] The biochemical abnormality in lethal OI is the inability to synthesize and secrete normal type I collagen.[66] As a result, the amount of type I collagen in bone is low, much of the secreted collagen is abnormally overmodified, and the quantity of the minor collagen types III and V is high. Bone collagen fibers are thinner than normal, and at the intracellular level, type I collagen is retained within dilated endoplasmic reticulum.

Similar to other forms of OI, mutations in the genes encoding COL1A1 and COL1A2A lead to the dominant form or de novo form of lethal OI.[67] Single glycine substitutions with the Gly-X-Y triplet of either COL1A1 or COL1A2 lead to this form of OI, as do some small deletions, all producing severe effects on the triple helix. The recessive form accounts for a few of these cases and results from mutations in the genes encoding either CRTAP (cartilage associated protein) or P3H1 (prolyl-3-hydroxylase 1).[64] These molecules form a complex that hydroxylates (add an -OH group) to a third position residue at proline 986 (Pro986). This modification of a single residue stabilizes the collagen helix.[64] Nonsense or frameshift mutations predicted to lead to premature termination codons and absent function of CRTAP or P3H1 produce this form of OI.

SEVERELY DEFORMING OSTEOGENESIS IMPERFECTA (TYPE III)

The deforming variant of OI is the classic form of OI. Similar to lethal OI (OI type II), most cases are inherited as autosomal dominant (or a de novo mutation), although recurrent cases based on autosomal recessive inheritance owing to CRTAP or P3H1 mutations have been described more recently.[62-64] This variant is characterized by severe deformity of the limbs and marked kyphoscoliosis, thorax deformity, and significant short stature. The extent of growth retardation is remarkable, and in many adults the height may not surpass 3 feet (90 to 100 cm). Abnormal cranial molding occurs in utero and during infancy, producing frontal bossing and a characteristic triangular-shaped facies. Radiographically, wormian bones and delayed closure of the fontanelles may be observed well into the first decade.

Pulmonary function can be diminished because of distortion of the spine and thorax, and this can progress over time and lead to restrictive lung disease and sleep apnea. Because of diminished vital capacity, pulmonary insufficiency is a leading cause of death in patients with OI type III. Many patients with scoliosis greater than 60 degrees develop respiratory compromise and need pulmonary investigations. Many of these individuals need supplemental oxygen.

Platybasia secondary to soft bone at the base of the skull may cause the external ear canals to slant upward as the base of the skull sinks on the cervical vertebrae; this may lead to communicating or obstructive hydrocephalus, cranial nerve palsies, and upper and lower motor neuron lesions. Headache, diplopia, nystagmus, cranial nerve neuralgia, decline in motor function, urinary dysfunction, and respiratory compromise are complications of basilar invagination.[68] As opposed to OI type I, most affected OI type III patients have white sclerae as adults. Approximately 25% of patients with type III OI have dentinogenesis imperfecta, necessitating constant dental care throughout childhood. Severe hearing impairment occurs in 10% of patients, although milder degrees of hearing loss are more common.

The skeleton in these patients has significant osteopenia, leading to multiple fractures in the upper and lower extremities and vertebral bodies, particularly before puberty. In contrast to OI type I, in which fractures tend to heal without deformity, fractures in OI type III frequently lead to skeletal deformity. Radiographs of the skeleton reveal marked osteopenia, thinning of cortical bone, narrowing of the diaphysis, and widening of the metaphysis, which merges into a dysplastic epiphyseal zone filled with whorls of partially calcified cartilage (i.e., popcorn deformity) (see Fig. 96-4C).[81] Osteoporosis leads to collapse of vertebral end plates contributing to worsening kyphoscoliosis. Pectus excavatum or pectus carinatum adds to thoracic deformity. In addition, lack of weight bearing increases the severity of osteoporosis and increases the risk of fracture. Many individuals become wheelchair bound at an early age or walk with mechanical assistance.

Molecular Pathology

The molecular basis of OI type III is very similar to OI type II. Most cases result from heterozygosity for mutations in COL1A1(I) and COL1A2.[1] These mutations are glycine substitutions scattered throughout the triple helix and in-frame deletions.[69] As in OI type II, familial recurrences result from mutations in *CRTAP* and *P3H1* and rare cases of germline mosaicism.

OSTEOGENESIS IMPERFECTA OF MODERATE SEVERITY (TYPE IV)

Clinically, the phenotype of patients with moderately severe OI (OI type IV) falls between the milder OI type I and OI type III. In most cases, OI type IV is inherited in an autosomal dominant fashion. Fractures occur rarely at birth, and some patients may not have an initial fracture until later in the first decade. The extent of skeletal deformity involving the spine, thorax, and extremities is usually intermediate between that of OI types I and III, and these patients have short stature and frequently have scoliosis. Patients may have some mild facial dysmorphisms, but not as severe as OI type III. Hearing loss occurs, but less than in OI types I and III.

Most fractures occur during childhood and may reoccur during the postmenopausal period in women or in men older than age 50 years. Long bone deformity tends to develop after fractures, which may lead to a difficulty in ambulation. Radiographs of the long bones and vertebral bodies show marked osteopenia with vertebral collapse. Although there is marked cortical thinning, bowing, and coarsening of trabeculae, the overall architecture of the bone is normal (see Fig. 96-4B).

Molecular Pathology

The molecular mechanisms for OI type IV are similar to the other forms. The mutations are in *COL1A1*(I) and *COL1A2*(I) and include glycine substitution and in-frame deletions.[69,70] At present, there is no evidence for an autosomal recessive form of OI type IV.

OSTEOGENESIS IMPERFECTA TYPE V

OI type V was reported in 2000 as a variant within the heterogeneous group classified under OI type IV.[71] In the initial report of seven OI patients, the phenotype was distinguished by the following criteria: moderate fracture history, hyperplastic callus formation, limitation in forearm pronation and supination as a result of intramembraneous bone formation at the joint, normal sclerae, and no dentinogenesis imperfecta. Bone biopsy specimens showed a meshlike appearance of irregularly spaced lamellae, different from the woven bone seen in OI types II, III, and IV. The etiology of this rare form has not been established, but it does not result from mutations in *COL1A1*(I) or *COL1A2*(I).

OSTEOGENESIS IMPERFECTA TYPE VI

The brittle bone phenotype OI type VI also was reported among the heterogeneous OI type IV group of patients. Characteristic among the eight subjects was the occurrence of a first fracture at an early age (4 to 18 months old).[72] The bone is severely brittle, and affected patients have white sclerae. All patients had vertebral compression fractures, and patients showed elevated serum alkaline phosphatase levels. No type I collagen mutations were identified in this cohort.

OSTEOGENESIS IMPERFECTA TYPE VII

In addition to OI types V and VI, Glorieux reported on an autosomal recessive form of OI and used the designation OI type VII.[72a] This form occurred with a small genetic isolate among the First Nations community in northern Quebec, Canada (S89). The phenotype includes fractures at birth, blue sclerae, osteopenia, rhizomelia, and deformities of the lower extremities. The disorder has been localized to chromosome 3p22-24 and has been shown to result from a hypomorphic allele in *CRTAP*.[64]

HISTOPATHOLOGY OF BONE IN OSTEOGENESIS IMPERFECTA

The range of histologic appearances of bone in the different OI phenotypes is as variable as the clinical phenotypes. Undermineralization and overmineralization of bone have been recognized within the same specimen.[73] Bone histomorphology appears relatively normal in OI type I, but osteopenia secondary to thin lamellar plates and diminished cortical width is evident. Immature woven bone and lamellar disarray are characteristic of more severe OI phenotypes.[73]

TREATMENT

Over the years, there have been multiple attempts to treat OI with a variety of vitamins, hormones, and drugs, none of which has been successful. The list includes administration of mineral supplements, fluoride, androgenic steroids, ascorbic acid, and vitamin D. During the last decade, bisphosphonates administered parenterally or orally to children and adults have shown favorable results. The bisphosphonate pamidronate administered intravenously increased bone mass, decreased skeletal pain, and decreased fracture incidence in children with severe OI.[74] Similar results involving cyclic administration of pamidronate have been reported by other investigators.[75] Dosage regimens in different series for children and adults range from 1 to 3 mg/kg, administered intravenously at 2- to 4-month intervals; lower dosage regimens also have been reported.[76] Generally, reports indicate a significant increase in bone mass in children and a decrease in fracture rate. The effect is most marked in the spine, where vertebral remodeling may improve vertebral height. Metabolic studies have shown a decrease in serum ionized calcium and increase in serum parathyroid hormone.

Urinary excretion of N-telopeptide as an index of bone resorption decreased from 61% to 73%. The major side effects of intravenous bisphosphonate treatment include the acute-phase response (24 hours after infusion) and the occurrence of otitis and vestibular imbalance in a few patients. The currently recommended treatment regimen includes the use of a bisphosphonate, with adequate calcium and vitamin D supplementation to avoid the occurrence of hypercalciuria and to maintain normal serum vitamin D levels.

The use of surgery to correct deformities and to facilitate weight bearing has been the subject of several reviews.[77] Multiple osteotomies and realignment of a deformed bone over intramedullary rods is an option for many children with severe bowing.[78] Indications include frequent fractures at the apex of the bow, impaired standing, and limb-length inequality owing to bowing.[79] Expanding (telescoping) rods are best for growing children because they require fewer revisions. Spinal deformities are common and usually progressive. Surgical stabilization is most advisable in the teen years or early adulthood when patients are best able to tolerate these complex reconstructions.[80,81] Early basilar invagination may be halted with prophylactic posterior fusion of the occipital-cervical junction with plate fixation.[82] Patients with severe brainstem compression may require anterior transoral decompression and posterior instrumented fusion. Patients with various types of OI seem to be at increased risk of premature osteoarthritis, and the reasons for this are unclear. Total joint arthroplasty is usually successful in these patients, and referral is appropriate if arthroplasty is indicated.[83]

Every child with OI benefits from appropriate rehabilitative therapy.[84,85] Bracing with lightweight plastics as the child begins to walk can minimize microfracture and bowing of the upper femurs. Muscle strengthening exercises are essential as primary care and after immobilization for fracture. Perhaps the most beneficial programs have been developed around swimming, preferably in heated pools, and as part of continuous rehabilitative medical care.

EHLERS-DANLOS SYNDROME

The heterogeneous group of disorders grouped together as EDS illustrates the genetic and clinical variability characteristic of the heritable disorders of connective tissue. The most cardinal feature of these disorders is the presence of joint hypermobility, associated with an increase in skin elasticity and skin fragility. In 1997, a simplified classification was proposed dividing EDS into six major clinical types. The classification includes the classic, hypermobility, vascular, kyphoscoliosis, arthrochalasia, and dermatosparaxis types, and several rarer EDS types grouped into "other forms."[86] Clinically, EDS can be difficult to separate, however, because of considerable overlap in phenotype findings.

CLASSIC TYPE

The classic type of EDS accounts for about 80% of reported cases[87] and is inherited as an autosomal dominant trait. Originally, EDS was classified as types I and II, and now these types are classified as the classic form, although these subclassifications are still in use. Previously, types I and II EDS were distinguished from each other based on joint laxity and skin fragility, which are less severe in type I than in type II EDS. Most prototypic forms of EDS (Fig. 96-8) are characterized by various degrees of hyperextensibility of large and small joints, which are classic findings in EDS. It is crucial that hyperextensibility be defined, and differentiating mild "normal" laxity from hyperextensibility can be challenging. Beighton and colleagues[86] have presented a clinically useful classification of joint laxity (Fig. 96-9), as follows:

1. Passive dorsiflexion of the fifth digit beyond 90 degrees = 1 point for each hand
2. Passive apposition of the thumbs to the flexor surface of the radius = 1 point for each hand
3. Hyperextension of the elbows beyond 10 degrees = 1 point for each side

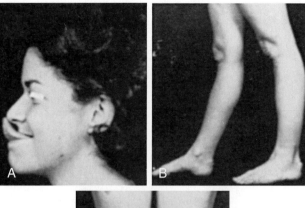
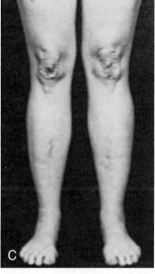

Figure 96-8 Ehlers-Danlos syndrome type I. **A-C,** Tissue elasticity, joint hypermobility, and tissue fragility are shown by the patient's ability to extend her tongue to the tip of the nose (Gorlin's sign) **(A)**, by hyperextensibility at the knee (genu recurvatum) **(B)**, and by characteristic "cigarette paper" or papyraceous scars of the knees and tibial skin **(C)**. *(Courtesy of V. McKusick, MD.)*

4. Hyperextension of the knees beyond 10 degrees = 1 point for each knee
5. Flexion of the trunk forward so that the palms can be placed flat on the ground = 1 point

A score of 5 or more points is defined as joint hypermobility.

Large joint hyperextensibility is seen in varying degrees in the classic form and decreases with age. Recurrent joint dislocations, periodic joint effusion related to trauma, and the eventual appearance of osteoarthritis pose significant management problems. Bilateral synovial thickening has been observed in EDS, along with the accumulation of small masses of crystalline material in synovial villi. It has been observed that EDS patients constituted 5% of cases in a pediatric arthritis clinic population.[88] There is debate about whether affected infants may be born prematurely to affected mothers because of early rupture of amniotic membranes. Patients with EDS have characteristic facies, with a broad nasal root and epicanthal folds. They may have large, lax ears, and traction on the ears or elbows reveals skin hyperextensibility. Another sign of hypermobility is the ability to touch the tip of the tongue to the nose (Gorlin's sign). In addition, absence of the lingual frenulum is characteristic for this disorder.

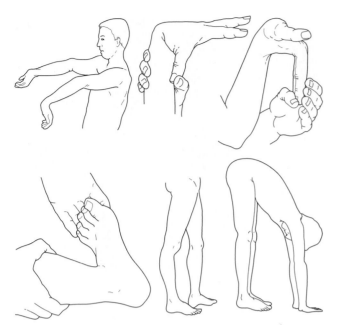

Figure 96-9 Maneuvers that may be used to establish the presence of clinically significant joint laxity found in Ehlers-Danlos syndrome. It is not unusual to find extreme laxity of the small joints and less laxity in large joints. Laxity decreases with age, so the dominant nature of most of these syndromes may not be appreciated when examining older family members. (*Redrawn and modified from Wynne-Davies R: Acetabular dysplasia and familial joint laxity: Two etiological factors in congenital dislocation of the hip—a review of 589 patients and their families. J Bone Joint Surg Br 52:704, 1970.*)

In EDS, the skin has a characteristically pleasant soft or "velvety" feel that can be appreciated by stroking the forearms. Thin, atrophic corrugated and hyperpigmented scars are found on the forehead, under the chin, and on the lower extremities (known as cigarette paper or papyraceous scars), although this is not a uniform finding. Typically, skin lesions heal slowly after injury or surgery. Molluscoid pseudotumors (violaceous subcutaneous tumors ranging in size from 0.5 to 3 cm) may be palpated in tissue over pressure points on the forearms and lower extremities and may be seen on radiographs. Although many patients claim to bruise easily, ecchymoses distributed on the extremities are found only in patients with the more severe forms of the disorder. Severe bilateral varicose veins are a common problem.

Associated pulmonary complications of EDS include spontaneous pneumothorax, pneumomediastinum, and subpleural blebs.[89] Mitral valve prolapse and tricuspid valve insufficiency may complicate classic EDS, and aortic root dilation has been reported, although the rate of progression is unknown.[90,91] Skeletal abnormalities include thoracolumbar kyphoscoliosis; a long, giraffe-like neck; downward sloping of the ribs of the upper part of the thorax; and a tendency toward reversal of the normal cervical, thoracic, and lumbar curves. Anterior wedging of thoracic vertebral bodies occasionally is seen.[92]

HYPERMOBILITY TYPE

The hypermobile type of EDS is a dominantly inherited disorder that manifests as marked joint and spine hypermobility, recurrent joint dislocations, and the typical soft skin that is neither hyperextensible nor velvety. Individuals with

EDS type III may have virtually normal skin. Because of the extent of joint laxity affecting large and small joints, these patients experience multiple dislocations and may require surgical repair. The shoulders, patellae, and temporomandibular joints are frequently sites of dislocation. Musculoskeletal pain may mimic that of fibromyalgia syndrome, and patients frequently seek medical attention for symptoms consistent with chronic pain.

One difficulty in this subtype is differentiating it from benign hypermobility syndrome. Benign hypermobility syndrome is used to describe patients with generalized joint laxity, associated musculoskeletal complaints, but normal skin.[93] They do not have the classic stigmata of either EDS or Marfan syndrome. Many of these patients present in their 20s and 30s with rheumatologic symptoms that can pose problems in diagnosis and treatment. The precise approach and treatment for these patients are unclear.

Structural and Molecular Pathology of the Classic and Hypermobile Types of Ehlers-Danlos Syndrome

Abnormally large, small, or frayed dermal collagen fibrils and disordered elastic fibers have been observed in the classic and hypermobile forms of EDS by electron microscopy.[94] Type V collagen is a heterotrimeric collagen composed of the products of three genes, *COL5A1(V)*, *COL5A2(V)*, and *COL5A3(V)*. Type V collagen may stabilize type I collagen by coassembling with that protein. Initially, linkage analysis was used to show that some families with the classic form of EDS (originally types I and II) were linked to *COL5A1*. Subsequently, it has been established that about 50% of patients with either the classic or the hypermobility type of EDS have mutations in *COL5A1(V)* or *COL5A2(V)*. There seems to be no genotype-phenotype correlation in these disorders, and no mutations have been identified in *COL5A3(V)*. In some cases of EDS classic type, heterozyosity for mutations in *COL1A1(I)* have been shown.[94a]

VASCULAR TYPE

The vascular type of EDS is an autosomal dominant disorder and one of the most severe forms of EDS and was formerly referred to as EDS type IV. It is associated with arterial rupture, commonly involving iliac, splenic, or renal arteries or the aorta and resulting in either massive hematomas or death.[95] Arterial rupture may lead to stroke or intracompartmental bleeding in a limb. Patients with vascular EDS also are susceptible to rupture of internal viscera and may experience repeated rupture of diverticula on the antimesenteric border of the large bowel. Problems with pregnancy vary from preterm delivery to uterine or vascular rupture, although delivery is uneventful in many instances.[96,97] Typical causes of death in EDS families have included gastrointestinal rupture, peripartum uterine rupture, rupture of the hepatic artery, and vascular ruptures.

In contrast to the other forms of EDS, EDS type IV is not associated with hyperextensiblity of large joints, although small joints may be minimally hypermobile. These patients have thin, soft, transparent skin, through which a prominent venous pattern is seen, especially on their chest walls. Their skin is not velvety as in the classic form. Excessive bruisability may occur. Vascular EDS includes, as a subgroup, patients who have been described as acrogyric—having characteristically thin faces, prominent eyes, and extremities that lack subcutaneous fat, giving the appearance of premature aging. Peripheral joint contractures and acro-osteolysis have been described.

Spontaneous hemopneumothorax associated with hemoptysis and mitral valve prolapse occurs frequently. Surgical repair of ruptured vessels or internal viscera is extremely difficult because of friable tissues. Anesthetic and surgical difficulties related to intubation, spontaneous arterial bleeding during surgery, and ligation of vessels that tear under pressure complicate surgical maneuvers. Similarly, arteriography may be dangerous in these individuals. These patients can be quite difficult to manage. Imaging studies may reveal normal-appearing aorta or other large vessels that rupture shortly after a "normal study."

Molecular Pathology

Although EDS type IV was clinically recognized as a disorder distinct from the other forms of EDS, the finding that tissues from these individuals were deficient in type III collagen clearly distinguished this as a separate form of EDS. Type III collagen is a homotrimer [1(III)3] found in skin, blood vessels, and the walls of hollow viscera. Heterozygosity for mutations in the gene encoding COL3A1 leads to EDS vascular type and affects the synthesis and secretion of type III collagen.[98,99] Various types of mutations have been identified, including missense, nonsense, and deletions, and there is no correlation between the clinical phenotype and type III collagen mutation.[98,99] In this disorder, the biochemical abnormalities include decreased or absent type III collagen or production of an abnormal homotrimer that is retained in the endoplasmic reticulum and if secreted contributes to abnormal matrix. Biochemical and mutational analysis for this disorder is available (GeneTests) and should be considered because this is dominantly inherited.

THERAPY IN CLASSIC, HYPERMOBILITY, AND VASCULAR TYPES OF EHLERS-DANLOS SYNDROME

There are no specific treatments for the classic, hypermobility, and vascular forms of EDS. Supportive therapy is essential, however, for preservation of normal joint function and alleviation of joint pain. Planned exercise programs and muscle strengthening exercises are useful and do much to maintain a positive outlook in these individuals, who may have a poor prognosis if joint stability and articular surfaces are compromised by excessive activity or chronic trauma. Many children and young adults with large joint hypermobility are attracted to activities such as gymnastics and dance, and these activities promote hypermobility and joint damage. The presence of multiple ecchymoses raises concern about a bleeding diathesis, particularly at the time of elective surgery. Although there is no consistent basis for the hemorrhagic tendency in the classic and hyperextensibility forms of EDS, anecdotally, these patients tend to have greater blood losses than expected at surgery. In our center, we discourage pregnancy in patients with the vascular form because the mortality rate is increased.

ARTHROCHALASIA TYPE

Formerly known as EDS types VIIA and VIIB, the arthrochalasia type of EDS is another autosomal dominant form resulting from mutations that cause faulty processing of type I collagen at the N-terminus. The arthrochalasia type of EDS is characterized by pronounced and generalized joint hypermobility, moderate cutaneous elasticity, moderate bruising, a characteristic round facies with midface hypoplasia, and significant short stature. The skin has a doughy feel and is fragile and hyperelastic. Kyphoscoliosis and muscle hypotonia are frequently present. These patients experience multiple dislocations, particularly involving large joints, including the hips, knees, and ankles. These dislocations manifest in the newborn period, especially hip and ankle dislocations. Patients frequently need orthopaedic surgery for joint dislocation, and their tissues are highly friable, which complicates orthopaedic procedures.

Molecular Pathology

The two disorders EDS types VIIA and VIIB, now termed arthrochalasia type, result from mutations involving the N-terminal propeptide cleavage site of type I collagen.[100] The arthrochalasia type of EDS has provided insight into the process of normal type I collagen fiber formation. The initial observation was of an accumulation of unprocessed procollagen within the dermis of affected individuals. With subsequent recognition that procollagen had N-terminal and C-terminal extension propeptides, and that separate enzymes were responsible for their removal, the syndrome became more sharply defined as an accumulation of procollagen with the N-terminal peptides still attached (pN collagen).[101] Of the two distinctly different genetic abnormalities resulting in procollagen accumulation, the more frequent form is the mutational resistance of a procollagen cleavage site to the action of the N-terminal procollagen peptidase. The resistance results from an amino acid substitution or deletion in the proCOL1A1[1] (EDS type VIIA) or pro2COL2A1 (EDS type VIIB) chain, leading to a portion of the collagen chains containing an abnormal N-terminal extension; this results from mutations in COL1A1[1] or COL1A2[2] in exon 6 of the molecule, which alters the proteinase cleavage site.[100] Individuals with mutations in exon 6 of COL1A1[1] are more severely affected than individuals with similar mutations in COL1A2.[102]

DERMATOSPARAXIS TYPE

The dermatosparaxis type of EDS was formerly known as EDS type VIIC and is an autosomal recessive form of EDS. In this type, the skin is extremely fragile, soft, and doughy with easy bruising. The phenotype includes blue sclerae, marked joint hypermobility, micrognathia, large umbilical hernia, epiphyseal delay, and mild hirsutism.[103] The dermatosparaxis type results from a deficiency of the procollagen N-propeptidase, in contrast to the arthrochalasia form, which involves the enzyme cleavage site, and individuals have been identified who are homozygous for mutations in the gene.[104] This defect is homologous to the dermatosparaxis defect in sheep and cattle.[105]

KYPHOSCOLIOSIS TYPE

The kyphoscoliosis type of EDS, formerly known as EDS type VI, is inherited as an autosomal recessive disease. The findings in this disorder include severe kyphoscoliosis noted at birth, recurrent joint dislocations, hyperextensible skin and joints, poor tone, and reduced muscle mass.[106] The skin is grossly abnormal and has been described as pale, translucent, and velvety; on trauma, the skin shows gaping wounds that heal poorly. One difference in this form of EDS is that there is significant ocular involvement. Affected individuals have microcornea, retinal detachment, and glaucoma leading to blindness in some individuals. In addition, patients with severe kyphoscoliosis may develop respiratory and cardiac compromise and ultimately cardiorespiratory failure.

Molecular Pathology

The kyphoscoliosis type of EDS results from lysyl hydroxylase deficiency.[107] A variety of mutations within the lysyl hydroxylase gene have been defined and include premature stop codons, amino acid substitutions, internal deletions, and compound heterozygotes.[107] Defective lysyl hydroxylase impairs the conversion of lysyl residues to hydroxylysine on procollagen peptides. The consequence of deficient hydroxylysine content of collagen is the effect it has on cross-linking, which helps stabilize the mature collagen molecule.

OTHER EHLERS-DANLOS SYNDROME TYPES

Numerous other rare forms of EDS have some overlap with other disorders or have been reported only in a small cohort of individuals, and these are not discussed in this chapter.

MARFAN SYNDROME

One of the most common inherited disorders of connective tissue, Marfan syndrome is an autosomal dominant disorder with a reported incidence of 1 in 10,000 to 20,000 individuals.[108] Clinical presentations range from the severe infantile form to individuals who are only mildly affected. Although the most impressive findings in Marfan syndrome are relative to the musculoskeletal, cardiac, and ocular findings, affected individuals also have pulmonary, neurologic, and psychological complications. Marfan syndrome also has become one of the few genetic disorders for which there has been advocacy for treatment to slow the progression of the disease, and physicians need to recognize the phenotype because many affected individuals present with life-threatening emergencies.

CLINICAL FEATURES

Marfan syndrome can be difficult to diagnose in some individuals and families, and it has been recognized that it also has been overdiagnosed. Stringent criteria for this diagnosis were proposed in 1996.[108] The 1996 criteria rely on the recognition of "major" and "minor" clinical manifestations involving the skeletal, cardiovascular, dura, and ocular systems. Major criteria include four of eight typical skeletal manifestations, ectopia lentis, aortic root dilation involving the sinuses of Valsalva or aortic dissection, and lumbosacral

dural ectasia by computed tomography or MRI. Major criteria for establishing the diagnosis in a family member include having a parent, child, or sibling who meets major criteria independently, the presence of a *fibrillin-1* mutation known to cause the syndrome, or a haplotype around *fibrillin-1* inherited by descent and identified in a familial Marfan syndrome patient.

Establishing the diagnosis unequivocally in the absence of a family history requires a major manifestation from two systems and involvement of a third system. If a mutation known to cause Marfan syndrome is identified, the diagnosis requires one major criterion and involvement of a second organ system. The reason is that there is a great deal of intrafamilial variability in this disorder, and there are individuals who harbor heterozygosity for mutations, but do not meet criteria for Marfan syndrome and may have different prognoses.[109] Similar to other connective tissue disorders, there is wide variability in phenotypic expression.

Aortic disease leading to the formation of aneurysmal dilation and dissection is the main cause of morbidity and mortality in Marfan syndrome.[110] Dilation of the aorta is found in 50% of children and progresses over time. Echocardiography shows that 60% to 80% of adult patients have dilation of the aortic root that may involve other segments of the thoracic aorta, the abdominal aorta, or even the carotid and intracranial arteries. Dissection usually begins above the coronary ostia and extends the entire length of the aorta. Of Marfan syndrome patients, 60% to 70% have mitral valve prolapse with regurgitation. Heart failure and myocardial infarction may complicate the course of Marfan syndrome patients. Pregnant women are at particular risk for aortic dissection, particularly women who already have aortic root dilation, and this should be taken into consideration when treating a woman of reproductive age with Marfan syndrome.[111]

Arachnodactyly occurs in 90% of patients. Following are techniques that aid in determining arachnodactyly (Fig. 96-10):

1. The thumb: The Steinberg test is positive when the thumb, enclosed in the clenched fist, extends beyond the hypothenar border.
2. The wrist: The Walker-Murdoch sign is positive when there is overlap of the thumb and fifth digit as they encircle the opposite wrist.
3. The metacarpal: The metacarpal index is done by radiographic determination and is the mean value of the lengths divided by the midpoint widths of the second, third, and fourth metacarpals. In normal subjects, the metacarpal index ranges from 5.4 to 7.9, whereas this range is 8.4 to 10.4 in patients with Marfan syndrome.

Thoracic kyphosis may be associated with reduced lung capacity and residual volume that may lead to pulmonary insufficiency. Dural ectasia, which may occur in 40% of patients, results from enlargement of the spinal canal owing to progressive ectasia of the dura and neural foramina and erosion of vertebral bone; this usually involves the lower spine.[112] Diminished bone mineral density has been reported in several patients with Marfan syndrome.[113] Ectopia lentis occurs in 50% to 80% of patients with Marfan syndrome. Subluxation of the lens is usually bilateral and appears by age 5 years. Although the lens is typically displaced upward, displacement into any quadrant may occur. Visual acuity is diminished in many patients because of lens subluxation

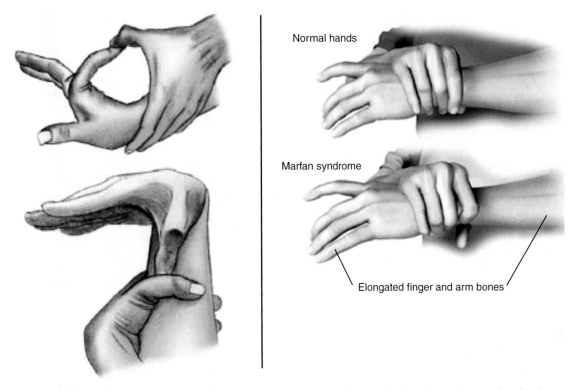

Normal hands

Marfan syndrome

Elongated finger and arm bones

Figure 96-10   Marfan syndrome. The Steinberg test (thumb) and the Walker-Murdoch test (wrist) show arachnodactyly.

or secondary acute glaucoma. Secondary myopia, retinal detachment, and iritis with loss of vision contribute to most of the ocular related morbidity.[114]

Marfan syndrome patients have been found to develop large epidural venous plexuses in the lumbar and cervical regions, a major diagnostic criterion for the syndrome. These engorged venous plexuses, which are visualized by MRI myelography, have been associated with the syndrome of spontaneous intracranial hypotension, which also is associated with dural tears. Clinical signs are severe headache, back and leg pain, radiculopathies, and incontinence secondary to cerebral displacement.[115] Spinal abnormalities in Marfan syndrome include increased interpedicle distance of nonrotated vertebrae, vertebral inversion (flattening of the normal kyphosis at the dorsal level and kyphosis or disappearance of the physiologic lordosis at the lumbar level), and vertebral dysplasia (dolichospondylic, elongated vertebral bodies with increased concavity). Scoliosis constitutes one of the major management problems in Marfan syndrome. In one series, the average age of onset was 10.5 years (range 3 to 15 years), with rapid progression during adolescence.[116] If mechanical bracing or physical therapy fails to halt progression, spinal fusion should be considered, particularly when the curvature exceeds 45 to 50 degrees.

DIFFERENTIAL DIAGNOSIS: HOMOCYSTINURIA

Homocystinuria, which shares several skeletal and ocular features with Marfan syndrome, is the prime diagnostic consideration. Homocystinuria is an autosomal recessive disease. The characteristic features of this metabolic disorder of sulfur metabolism are marfanoid phenotype with joint laxity,

scoliosis, lens dislocation, early-onset osteoporosis, vascular thrombosis affecting arteries and veins owing to increased clotting activity and the cytotoxic effect of homocysteine on vascular endothelial cells, and mild mental retardation.[117]

Cystathionine β-synthase deficiency is the most common cause of homocystinuria.[118] Affected individuals have elevated levels of homocystine and methionine levels, whereas cystathionine and cysteine levels in blood are decreased. This disorder is differentiated from Marfan syndrome because the direction of ectopia lentis is different than in Marfan syndrome, and there is no progressive aortic root dilation.

MOLECULAR BIOLOGY OF MARFAN SYNDROME

Fibrillin-1 protein is an important component of elastic and nonelastic connective tissues throughout the body.[119] It is the main protein of a group of connective tissue microfibrils that are essential for normal elastic fibrillogenesis. In nonelastic tissues, the fibrillin-1-containing microfibril functions as an anchoring fiber. *FBN-1* is a large gene (65 exons) located at chromosome 15q21.1.

Since the first report of an *FBN-1* mutation in Marfan syndrome in 1991, more than 500 different *FBN-1* mutations have been described in Marfan syndrome and related disorders.[120] *FBN-1* mutations occur across a wide range of milder phenotypes that overlap the classic Marfan phenotype, including dominantly inherited ectopia lentis, Shprintzen-Goldberg syndrome, and familial or isolated forms of aortic aneurysms.[121,122] Most of these are private mutations (occur genetically independent with no "hot spot" in the molecule). The one exception are the rare infantile Marfan syndrome mutations that cluster between exons 24 and

26 and exon 32.[123] Heterozygosity for missense, frameshifts, deletions and insertions, splice site alterations, and nonsense mutations all have been seen.[124] Robinson and associates[125] stated that at least 337 mainly unique mutations in the *FBN-1* gene had been reported in Marfan syndrome up to that time. The clinical presentation of the fibrillinopathies caused by *FBN-1* mutations ranged from isolated ectopia lentis to neonatal Marfan syndrome, which generally leads to death within the first 2 years of life.

TREATMENT

In 1972, the life span of untreated patients with classic Marfan syndrome was about 32 years. The early mortality in Marfan syndrome results primarily from complications associated with aortic dilation. This symmetric dilation of the sinuses of Valsalva is progressive throughout life and is often detectable in infancy. In the early 1970s, McKusick suggested that he might reduce the risk of aortic dissection in patients with Marfan syndrome.[125a] Shores and coworkers[126] reported on a 10-year open-label trial of propranolol in 70 patients with Marfan syndrome. When compared with the control group, the treated individuals had a significantly slower rate of dilation of the aortic root, improved survival, and fewer treated patients reaching a clinical end point (death, congestive heart failure, aortic regurgitation, aortic dissection, or cardiovascular surgery).

More recent data generated from a mouse model of Marfan syndrome suggest excessive signaling by the transforming growth factor (TGF)-β family of cytokines.[127] There is evidence that aortic aneurysm in the mouse model of Marfan syndrome is associated with increased TGF-β signaling and TGF-β antagonists such as TGF-β–neutralizing antibody or the angiotensin II type 1 receptor blocker, losartan. In this mouse model, losartan (angiotensin II type 1 blockade) fully corrected the abnormalities in the aortic wall. There was some evidence that alveolar septation, which contributes to pulmonary problems in Marfan syndrome, was partially reversed with losartan treatment. The authors concluded that because this drug is in clinical use for hypertension, it merits further investigation as a preventive treatment in Marfan syndrome.

Electrocardiogram monitoring is done yearly until the aortic root diameter exceeds 45 mm, at which time monitoring is done every 6 months. Elective repair of aortic root disease before enlargement to 6 cm has occurred is preferable to emergency repair required for marked dilation or dissection. Surgical intervention is considered when the aortic root diameter approaches twice the upper limit of normal for body surface area, or the absolute measurement exceeds 50 to 55 mm. Total aortic root replacement with a composite valve graft (Bentall procedure) and coronary artery implantation have become the surgical procedures of choice and are associated with an 81% 10-year survival rate and a 75% 20-year survival rate.[128,129] Mitral valve replacement and coronary artery implantation may be accomplished during the same procedure. Most importantly, repeated trials have shown that patients who undergo elective repair, as opposed to emergent repair, do substantially better.

Correction of scoliosis may be attempted with bracing; however, surgical repair should be considered when the curve exceeds 40 degrees. Progressive scoliosis in Marfan syndrome may require fixation with rods, and complications of joint laxity may require orthopaedic correction. Arthropathy associated with excessive joint mobility may require orthopaedic intervention. Dislocated lenses should not be removed surgically, unless more conventional means of correcting vision are ineffective.

LOEYS-DIETZ SYNDROME

In 2005, Loeys and colleagues[130] described individuals with a previously undescribed autosomal dominant aortic aneurysm syndrome. This disorder, now referred to as Loeys-Dietz syndrome, also is characterized by hypertelorism, bifid uvula or cleft palate or both, and generalized arterial tortuosity with ascending aortic aneurysm and dissection. Other abnormal findings include craniosynostosis, structural brain abnormalities, mental retardation, congenital heart disease, and aneurysms with dissection throughout the arterial tree.

Some individuals with Loeys-Dietz syndrome had a clinical phenotype that overlapped with Marfan syndrome, but none met diagnostic criteria set forth in 1996.[108] Although Marfan syndrome is associated with progressive arterial disease, in Loeys-Dietz syndrome the aneurysms tended to be particularly aggressive and rupture at an earlier stage and size than seen in Marfan syndrome. Heterozygosity for mutations in *TGFBR1* and *TGFBR* have been identified.[130] From a management perspective, it is important to recognize these individuals because they are managed more aggressively than patients with Marfan syndrome. Aortic aneurysms are corrected at smaller sizes (4 cm), and complaints such as abdominal pain and headache should be thoroughly investigated because they may be associated with aneurysms.

CONGENITAL CONTRACTURAL ARACHNODACTYLY

Congenital contractural arachnodactyly is an autosomal dominant condition that includes tall stature, arachnodactyly, dolichostenomelia, and multiple contractures involving large joints.[131] There is a characteristic "crumpled ear" deformity as a result of a flattened helix with partial obliteration of the concha. Marked deformity of the chest cage also occurs, and scoliosis may be progressive and severe. For unknown reasons, the contractures tend to become less severe with age. Radiographically, osteopenia can be seen. The ocular and typical cardiac lesions of classic Marfan syndrome are absent. This disorder results from heterozygosity for mutation in *fibrillin-2* (*FNB-2*).[132]

There are many other extremely rare disorders of connective tissue, especially with profound effects on the skin, including the group of disorders termed *cutis laxa* and *pseudoxanthoma elasticum*.[133,134]

SUMMARY

Heritable disorders of connective tissues are a heterogeneous group of disorders characterized by abnormalities in skeletal tissues including cartilage, bone, tendon, ligament, muscle, and skin. The clinical spectrum ranges from extreme short stature to excessively tall individuals, and the types of altered genes span all of the numerous gene families and pathways. Affected individuals usually need medical attention their entire lives and have been victims of appearing different because they cannot mask their abnormalities. Understanding and appreciation for the unique set of medical issues in each disorder would improve these individuals' quality of life and their life span.

REFERENCES

1. McKusick VA: Heritable Disorders of Connective Tissue. St Louis, CV Mosby, 1956.
2. Superti-Furga A, Unger S: Nosology and classification of genetic skeletal disorders: 2006 revision. Am J Med Genet A 143:1-18, 2007.
3. Orioli IM, Castilla EE, Barbosa-Neto JG: The birth prevalence rates for the skeletal dysplasias. J Med Genet 23:328-332, 1986.
4. Kornak U, Mundlos S: Genetic disorders of the skeleton: A developmental approach. Am J Hum Genet 73:447-474, 2003.
5. Rosenberg A: Bones and joints and soft tissue tumors. In Contran RS, Kumar V, Collins T (eds): Robbins Pathologic Basis of Disease, 6th ed. Philadelphia, WB Saunders, 1999, pp 1215-1221.
6. **Karsenty G: Genetics of skeletogenesis. Dev Genet 22:301-313, 1998.**
7. Dreyer SD, Zhou G, Lee B: The long and the short of it: Developmental genetics of the skeletal dysplasias. Clin Genet 54:464-473, 1998.
8. Shum L, Nuckolls G: The life cycle of chondrocytes in the developing skeleton. Arthritis Res 4:94-106, 2002.
9. Zelzer E, Olsen BR: The genetic basis for skeletal diseases. Nature 423:343-348, 2003.
10. Kuivaniemi H, Tromp G, Prockop DJ: Mutations in fibrillar collagens (types I, II, III, and XI), fibril-associated collagen (type IX), and network-forming collagen (type X) cause a spectrum of diseases of bone, cartilage, and blood vessels. Hum Mutat 9:300-315, 1997.
11. Eyre DR: Collagens and cartilage matrix homeostasis. Clin Orthop 427(Suppl):S118-S122, 2004.
12. Chan D, Ho MS, Cheah KS: Aberrant signal peptide cleavage of collagen X in Schmid metaphyseal chondrodysplasia: Implications for the molecular basis of the disease. J Biol Chem 276:7992-7997, 2001.
13. Eyre D: Collagen of articular cartilage. Arthritis Res 4:30-35, 2002.
14. McKusick VA: Heritable Disorders of Connective Tissue, 4th ed. St Louis, CV Mosby, 1972.
15. Rimion DL: Molecular defects in the skeletal chondrodysplasias. J Med Genet 63:106-110, 1996.
16. Superti-Furga A, Bonafe L, Rimoin DL: Molecular-pathogenetic classification of the skeleton. Am J Med Genet 106:282-293, 2001.
17. Edwards MJ, Wenstrup RJ, Byers PH, et al: Recurrence of lethal osteogenesis imperfecta due to parental mosaicism for a mutation in the COL1A2 gene of type I collagen: The mosaic parent exhibits phenotypic features of a mild form of the disease. Hum Mutat 1:47-54, 1992.
18. Stevenson DA, Brothman AR, Chen Z, et al: Paternal uniparental disomy of chromosome 14: Confirmation of a clinically-recognizable phenotype. Am J Med Genet A 130:88-91, 2004.
19. Unger S, Korkko J, Krakow D, et al: Double heterozygosity for pseudoachondroplasia and spondyloepiphyseal dysplasia congenita. Am J Med Genet 101:140-146, 2001.
20. Pauli RM, Conroy MM, Langer LO, et al: Homozygous achondroplasia with survival beyond infancy. Am J Med Genet 16:459-473, 1983.
21. Lachman RS: Radiology of Syndromes, Skeletal and Metabolic Disorders, 4th ed. Chicago, Year Book Medical Publishers, 2007.
22. Hunter AG, Bankier A, Rogers JG, et al: Medical complications of achondroplasia: A multicentre patient review. J Med Genet 35:705-712, 1998.
23. Sheffield LJ, Danks DM, Mayne V, et al: Chondrodysplasia punctata—23 cases of a mild and relatively common variety. J Pediatr 89:916-923, 1976.
24. Lamy M, Maroteaux P: Le nanisme diastrophique. Presse Med 68:1977-1980, 1960.
25. Cormier-Daire V, Savarirayan R, Unger S, et al: "Duplicate calcaneus": A rare developmental defect observed in several skeletal dysplasias. Pediatr Radiol 31:38-42, 2001.
26. Rimoin DL: The chondrodystrophies. Adv Hum Genet 5:1-118, 1975.
27. Sillence DO, Horton WA, Rimoin DL: Morphologic studies in the skeletal dysplasias. Am J Pathol 96:813-870, 1979.
28. Rimoin DL, Sillence DO: Chondro-osseous morphology and biochemistry in the skeletal dysplasias. Birth Defects Orig Artic Ser 17:249-265, 1981.
29. Hecht JT, Hood OJ, Schwartz RJ, et al: Obesity in achondroplasia. Am J Med Genet 31:597-602, 1988.
30. Horton WA, Rotter JI, Rimoin DL, et al: Standard growth curves for achondroplasia. J Pediatr 93:435-438, 1978.
31. Hunter AG, Hecht JT, Scott CI Jr: Standard weight for height curves in achondroplasia. Am J Med Genet 62:255-261, 1996.
32. Gordon N: The neurological complications of achondroplasia. Brain Dev 22:3-7, 2000.
33. Kanaka-Gantenbein C: Present status of the use of growth hormone in short children with bone diseases (diseases of the skeleton). J Pediatr Endocrinol Metab 14:17-26, 2001.
34. Yasui N, Kawabata H, Kojimoto H, et al: Lengthening of the lower limbs in patients with achondroplasia and hypochondroplasia. Clin Orthop 344:298-306, 1997.
35. Hill V, Sahhar M, Aitken M, et al: Experiences at the time of diagnosis of parents who have a child with a bone dysplasia resulting in short stature. Am J Med Genet A 122:100-107, 2003.
36. Spranger J: Pattern Recognition in Bone Dysplasias: Endocrine and Genetics. New York, Wiley, 1985, pp 315-342.
37. **Horton WA: Molecular genetic basis of the human chondrodysplasias. Endocrinol Metab Clin North Am 3:683-697, 1996.**
38. Francomano CA, McIntosh I, Wilkin DJ: Bone dysplasias in man: Molecular insights. Curr Opin Genet Dev 3:301-308, 1996.
39. Korkko J, Cohn DH, Ala-Kokko L, et al: Widely distributed mutations in the COL2A1 gene produce achondrogenesis type II/hypochondrogenesis. Am J Med Genet 92:95-100, 2000.
40. Lee B, Vissing H, Ramirez F, et al: Identification of the molecular defect in a family with spondyloepiphyseal dysplasia. Science 244:978-980, 1998.
41. Nishimura G, Haga N, Kitoh H, et al: The phenotypic spectrum of COL2A1 mutations. Hum Mutat 26:36-43, 2005.
42. Wilkin DJ, Artz AS, South S, et al: Small deletions in the type II collagen triple helix produce Kniest dysplasia. Am J Med Genet 85:105-112, 1999.
43. Wilkin DJ, Bogaert R, Lachman RS, et al: A single amino acid substitution (G103D) in the type II collagen triple helix produces Kniest dysplasia. Hum Mol Genet 3:1999-2003, 1994.
44. Winterpacht A, Hilbert M, Schwarze U, et al: Kniest and Stickler dysplasia phenotypes caused by collagen type II gene (COL2A1) defect. Nat Genet 3:323-326, 1994.
45. Williams CJ, Ganguly A, Considine E, et al: A(-2)-to-G transition at the 3-prime acceptor splice site of IVS17 characterizes the COL2A1 gene mutation in the original Stickler syndrome kindred. Am J Med Genet 63:461-467, 1996.
46. Annunen S, Korkko J, Czarny M, et al: Splicing mutations of 54-bp exons in the COL11A1 gene cause Marshall syndrome, but other mutations cause overlapping Marshall/Stickler phenotypes. Am J Hum Genet 65:974-983, 1999.
47. Vikkula M, Mariman ECM, Lui VCH, et al: Autosomal dominant and recessive osteochondrodysplasias associated with the COL11A2 locus. Cell 80:431-437, 1995.
48. **Briggs MD, Hoffman SMG, King LM, et al: Pseudoachondroplasia and multiple epiphyseal dysplasia due to mutations in the cartilage oligomeric matrix protein gene. Nat Genet 10:330-336, 1995.**
49. Newton G, Weremowicz S, Morton CC, et al: Characterization of human and mouse cartilage oligomeric matrix protein. Genomics 24:435-439, 1994.
50. Karniski LP: Mutations in the diastrophic dysplasia sulfate transporter (DTDST) gene: Correlation between sulfate transport activity and chondrodysplasia phenotype. Hum Mol Genet 14:1485-1490, 2001.
51. Robertson SP, Twigg SRF, Sutherland-Smith AJ, et al: Localized mutations in the gene encoding the cytoskeletal protein filamin A cause diverse malformations in humans. Nat Genet 33:487-491, 2003.
52. Krakow D, Robertson SP, King LM, et al: Mutations in the gene encoding filamin B disrupt vertebral segmentation, joint formation and skeletogenesis. Nat Genet 36:405-410, 2004.
53. Farrington-Rock C, Firestein MH, Bicknell LS, et al: Mutations in two regions of FLNB result in atelosteogenesis I and III. Hum Mutat 27:705-710, 2006.

54. Rowe D, Shapiro J: Osteogenesis imperfecta. In Avioli I, Krane S (eds): Metabolic Bone Disease. Philadelphia, WB Saunders, 1990.

55. Sillence D: Osteogenesis imperfecta: An expanding panorama of variants. Clin Orthop 159:11-25, 1981.

56. Madigan WP, Wertz D, Cockerham GC, et al: Retinal detachment in osteogenesis imperfecta. J Pediatr Ophthalmol Strabismus 4:268-269, 1994.

57. Pedersen U: Osteogenesis imperfecta clinical features, hearing loss and stapedectomy: Biochemical, osteodensitometric, corneometric and histological aspects in comparison with otosclerosis. Acta Otolaryngol Suppl 415:1-36, 1985.

58. Hortop J, Tsipouras P, Hanley JA, et al: Cardiovascular involvement in osteogenesis imperfecta. Circulation 73:54-61, 1986.

59. Davie MW, Haddaway MJ: Bone mineral content and density in healthy subjects and in osteogenesis imperfecta. Arch Dis Child 70:331-334, 1994.

60. Willing MC, Cohn DH, Byers PH: Frameshift mutation near the 3′ end of the COL1A1 gene of type I collagen predicts an elongated Pro alpha 1(I) chain and results in osteogenesis imperfecta type I. J Clin Invest 85:282-290, 1990.

61. Mundlos S, Chan D, Weng YM, et al: Multiexon deletions in the type I collagen COL1A2 gene in osteogenesis imperfecta type IB: Molecules containing the shortened alpha2(I) chains show differential incorporation into the bone and skin extracellular matrix. J Biol Chem 271:21068-21074, 1996.

62. Cabral WA, Chang W, Barnes AM, et al: Prolyl 3-hydroxylase 1 deficiency causes a recessive metabolic bone disorder resembling lethal/severe osteogenesis imperfecta. Nat Genet 39:359-365, 2007.

63. Barnes AM, Chang W, Morello R, et al: Deficiency of cartilage-associated protein in recessive lethal osteogenesis imperfecta. N Engl J Med 355:2757-2764, 2006.

64. Morello R, Bertin TK, Chen Y, et al: CRTAP is required for prolyl 3-hydroxylation and mutations cause recessive osteogenesis imperfecta. Cell 127:291-304, 2006.

65. Edwards MJ, Wenstrup RJ, Byers PH, et al: Recurrence of lethal osteogenesis imperfecta due to parental mosaicism for a mutation in the COL1A2 gene of type I collagen: The mosaic parent exhibits phenotypic features of a mild form of the disease. Hum Mutat 1: 47-54, 1992.

66. Byers PH: Brittle bones—fragile molecules: Disorders of collagen gene structure and expression. Trends Genet 9:293-300, 1990.

67. Marini JC, Forlino A, Cabral WA, et al: Consortium for osteogenesis imperfecta mutations in the helical domain of type I collagen: Regions rich in lethal mutations align with collagen binding sites for integrins and proteoglycans. Hum Mutat 28:209-221, 2007.

68. Charnas LR, Marini JC: Communicating hydrocephalus, basilar invagination, and other neurologic features in osteogenesis imperfecta. Neurology 3:2603-2608, 1993.

69. Cohen-Solal L, Bonaventure J, Maroteaux P: Dominant mutations in familial lethal and severe osteogenesis imperfecta. Hum Genet 87:297-301, 1991.

70. Molyneux K, Starman BJ, Byers PH, et al: A single amino acid deletion in the alpha-2(I) chain of type I collagen produces osteogenesis imperfecta type III. Hum Genet 90:621-628, 1993.

71. Glorieux FH, Rauch F, Plotkin H: Type V osteogenesis imperfecta: A new form of brittle bone disease. J Bone Miner Res 15:1650-1658, 2000.

72. Glorieux FH, Ward LM, Rauch F: Osteogenesis imperfecta type VI: A form of brittle bone disease with a mineralization defect. J Bone Miner Res 17:30-38, 2002.

72a. Ward LM, Rauch F, Travers R, et al: Osteogenesis imperfecta type VII: an autosomal recessive form of brittle bone disease. Bone 31: 12-18, 2002.

73. Traub W, Arad T, Vetter U, et al: Ultrastructural studies of bones from patients with osteogenesis imperfecta. Matrix Biol 14:337-345, 1994.

74. Glorieux FH: Experience with bisphosphonates in osteogenesis imperfecta. Pediatrics 119:S163-S165, 2007.

75. Plotkin H, Rauch F, Bishop NJ, et al: Pamidronate treatment of severe osteogenesis imperfecta in children under 3 years of age. J Clin Endocrinol Metab 85:1846-1850, 2000.

76. Gonzalez E, Pavia C, Ros J, et al: Efficacy of low dose schedule pamidronate infusion in children with osteogenesis imperfecta. J Pediatr Endocrinol Metab 14:529-533, 2001.

77. Wilkinson JM, Scott BW, Clarke AM, et al: Surgical stabilisation of the lower limb in osteogenesis imperfecta using the Sheffield Telescopic Intramedullary Rod System. J Bone Joint Surg Br 80: 999-1004, 1998.

78. Zeitlin L, Fassier F, Glorieux FH: Modern approach to children with osteogenesis imperfecta. J Pediatr Orthop B 12:77-87, 2003.

79. Naudie D, Hamdy RC, Fassier F, et al: Complications of limb-lengthening in children who have an underlying bone disorder. J Bone Joint Surg Am 80:18-24, 1998.

80. Widmann RF, Laplaza FJ, Bitan FD, et al: Quality of life in osteogenesis imperfecta. Int Orthop 26:3-6, 2002.

81. Widmann RF, Bitan FD, Laplaza FJ, et al: Spinal deformity, pulmonary compromise, and quality of life in osteogenesis imperfecta. Spine 24:1673-1678, 1999.

82. Sawin PD, Menezes AH: Basilar invagination in osteogenesis imperfecta and related osteochondrodysplasias: Medical and surgical management. J Neurosurg 86:950-960, 1997.

83. Papagelopoulos PJ, Morrey BF: Hip and knee replacement in osteogenesis imperfecta. J Bone Joint Surg Am 75:572-580, 1993.

84. Binder H, Conway A, Gerber LH: Rehabilitation approaches to children with osteogenesis imperfecta: A ten-year experience. Arch Phys Med Rehabil 74:386-390, 1993.

85. Binder H, Conway A, Hason S, et al: Comprehensive rehabilitation of the child with osteogenesis imperfecta. Am J Med Genet 45: 265-269, 1993.

86. Beighton P, De Paepe A, Steinmann B, et al: Ehlers-Danlos syndromes: Revised nosology, Villefranche, 1997. Ehlers-Danlos National Foundation (USA) and Ehlers-Danlos Support Group (UK). Am J Med Genet 77:31-37, 1998.

87. Hollister DW: Heritable disorders of connective tissue: Ehlers-Danlos syndrome. Pediatr Clin North Am 3:575-591, 1978.

88. Osborn TG, Lichtenstein JR, Moore TL, et al: Ehlers-Danlos syndrome presenting as rheumatic manifestations in the child. J Rheumatol 8:79-85, 1981.

89. Ayres JG, Pope FM, Reidy JF, et al: Abnormalities of the lungs and thoracic cage in the Ehlers-Danlos syndrome. Thorax 40:300-305, 1985.

90. Leier CV, Call TD, Fulkerson PK, et al: The spectrum of cardiac defects in the Ehlers-Danlos syndrome, types I and III. Ann Intern Med 92:171-178, 1980.

91. Tiller GE, Cassidy SB, Wensel C, et al: Aortic root dilatation in Ehlers-Danlos syndrome types I, II and III: A report of five cases. Clin Genet 53:460-465, 1998.

92. Coventry MB: Some skeletal changes in the Ehlers-Danlos syndrome: A report of two cases. J Bone Joint Surg Am 43A:855-860, 1961.

93. Kirk JA, Ansell BM, Bywaters EG: The hypermobility syndrome: Musculoskeletal complaints associated with generalized joint hypermobility. Ann Rheum Dis 26:419-425, 1967.

94. Holbrook KA, Byers PH: Skin is a window on heritable disorders of connective tissue. Am J Med Genet 34:105-121, 1989.

94a. Malfait F, Symoens S, DeBacker J, et al: Three arginine to cysteine substitutions in the pro-alpha (I)-collagen chain cause Ehlers-Danlos syndrome with a propensity to arterial rupture in early adulthood. Hum Mutat 28(4):387-395, 2007.

95. Hamel BC, Pals G, Engels CH, et al: Ehlers-Danlos syndrome and type III collagen abnormalities: A variable clinical spectrum. Clin Genet 53:440-446, 1998.

96. Gilchrist D, Schwarze U, Shields K, et al: Large kindred with Ehlers-Danlos syndrome type IV due to a point mutation (G571S) in the COL3A1 gene of type III procollagen: Low risk of pregnancy complications and unexpected longevity in some affected relatives. Am J Med Genet 82:305-311, 1999.

97. Rudd NL, Nimrod C, Holbrook KA, et al: Pregnancy complications in type IV Ehlers-Danlos syndrome. Lancet 1:50-53, 1983.

98. Anderson DW, Thakker-Varia S, Tromp G, et al: A glycine (415)-to-serine substitution results in impaired secretion and decreased thermal stability of type III procollagen in a patient with Ehlers-Danlos syndrome type IV. Hum Mutat 9:62-63, 1997.

99. Thakker-Varia S, Anderson DW, Kuivaniemi H, et al: Aberrant splicing of the type III procollagen mRNA leads to intracellular degradation of the protein in a patient with Ehlers-Danlos type IV. Hum Mutat 6:116-125, 1995.

100. Lichtenstein JR, Martin GR, Kohn LD, et al: Defect in conversion of procollagen to collagen in a form of Ehlers-Danlos syndrome. Science 182:298-299, 1973.

101. Byers PH, Duvic M, Atkinson M, et al: Ehlers-Danlos syndrome type VIIA and VIIB result from splice-junction mutations or genomic deletions that involve exon 6 in the COL1A1 and COL1A2 genes of type I collagen. Am J Med Genet 72:94-105, 1997.

102. D'Alessio M, Ramirez F, Blumberg BD, et al: Characterization of a COL1A1 splicing defect in a case of Ehlers-Danlos syndrome type VII: Further evidence of molecular homogeneity. Am J Hum Genet 49:400-406, 1991.

103. Wertelecki W, Smith LT, Byers PH: Initial observations of human dermatosparaxis: Ehlers-Danlos syndrome type VIIC. J Pediat 121:558-564, 1992.

104. Colige A, Sieron AL, Li SW, et al: Human Ehlers-Danlos syndrome type VII C and bovine dermatosparaxis are caused by mutations in the procollagen I N-proteinase gene. Am J Hum Genet 65:308-317, 1999.

105. Nusgens BV, Verellen-Dumoulin C, Hermanns-Le T, et al: Evidence for a relationship between Ehlers-Danlos type VII C in humans and bovine dermatosparaxis. Nat Genet 1:214-217, 1992.

106. Heim P, Raghunath M, Meiss L, et al: Ehlers-Danlos syndrome type VI (EDS VI): Problems of diagnosis and management. Acta Paediatr 87:708-710, 1998.

107. Yeowell HN, Walker LC: Mutations in the lysyl hydroxylase 1 gene that result in enzyme deficiency and the clinical phenotype of Ehlers-Danlos syndrome type VI. Mol Genet Metab 71:212-220, 2000.

108. De Paepe A, Devereux RB, Dietz HC, et al: Revised diagnostic criteria for the Marfan syndrome. Am J Med Genet 62:417-426, 1996.

109. Montgomery RA, Geraghty MT, Bull E, et al: Multiple molecular mechanisms underlying subdiagnostic variants of Marfan syndrome. Am J Hum Genet 63:1703-1711, 1998.

110. Adams JN, Trent RJ: Aortic complications of Marfan's syndrome. Lancet 352:1722-1723, 1998.

111. Elkayam U, Ostrzega E, Shotan A, et al: Cardiovascular problems in pregnant women with the Marfan syndrome. Ann Intern Med 123:117-122, 1995.

112. Ahn NU, Sponseller PD, Ahn UM, et al: Dural ectasia in the Marfan syndrome: MR and CT findings and criteria. Genet Med 2:173-179, 2000.

113. Kohlmeier L, Gasner C, Bachrach LK, et al: The bone mineral status of patients with Marfan syndrome. Bone Miner Res 10:1550-1555, 1995.

114. Maumenee IH: The eye in the Marfan syndrome. Trans Am Ophthalmol Soc 79:684-733, 1981.

115. Nallamshetty L, Ahn NU, Ahn UM, et al: Plain radiography of the lumbosacral spine in Marfan syndrome. Spine J 2:327-333, 2002.

116. Savini R, Cervellati S, Beroaldo E: Spinal deformities in Marfan's syndrome. Ital J Orthop Traumatol 6:19-40, 1980.

117. Mudd SH, Skovby F, Levy HL, et al: The natural history of homocystinuria due to cystathionine beta-synthase deficiency. Am J Hum Genet 37:1-31, 1985.

118. Mudd SH, Edwards WA, Loeb PM, et al: Homocystinuria due to cystathionine synthase deficiency: The effect of pyridoxine. J Clin Invest 49:1762-1773, 1970.

119. Sakai LY, Keene DR, Engvall E: Fibrillin, a new 350kD glycoprotein, is a component of extracellular microfibrils. J Cell Biol 103:2499-2509, 1986.

120. Collod-Beroud G, Beroud C, Ades L, et al: Marfan database (third edition): New mutations and new routines for the software. Nucleic Acids Res 26:229-233, 1998.

121. Collod-Beroud G, Boileau C: Marfan syndrome in the third millennium. Eur J Hum Genet 10:673-681, 2002.

122. Stoll C: Shprintzen-Goldberg marfanoid syndrome: A case followed up for 24 years. Clin Dysmorphol 11:1-7, 2002.

123. Wang M, Wang JY, Cisler J, et al: Three novel fibrillin mutations in exons 25 and 27: Classic versus neonatal Marfan syndrome. Hum Mutat 9:359-362, 1997.

124. Dietz HC, Pyeritz RE: Mutations in the human gene for fibrillin-1 (FBN1) in the Marfan syndrome and related disorders. Hum Mol Genet 4:1799-1809, 1995.

125. Robinson PN, Booms P, Katzke S, et al: Mutations of FBN1 and genotype-phenotype correlations in Marfan syndrome and related fibrillinopathies. Hum Mutat 20:153-161, 2002.

125a. Halpern BL, Char F, Murdoch JL, et al: A prospectus on the prevention of aortic rupture in the Marfan syndrome with data on survivorship without treatment. Johns Hopkins Med J 129:123-129, 1971.

126. Shores J, Berger KR, Murphy EA, et al: Progression of aortic dilatation and the benefit of long-term beta-adrenergic blockade in Marfan's syndrome. N Engl J Med 330:1335-1341, 1994.

127. Habashi JP, Judge DP, Holm TM, et al: Losartan, an AT1 antagonist, prevents aortic aneurysm in a mouse model of Marfan syndrome. Science 312:117-121, 2006.

128. Gott VL, Greene PS, Alejo DE, et al: Replacement of the aortic root in patients with Marfan's syndrome. N Engl J Med 340:1307-1313, 1999.

129. Gott VL, Cameron DE, Alejo DE, et al: Aortic root replacement in 271 Marfan patients: A 24-year experience. Ann Thorac Surg 73:438-443, 2002.

130. Loeys BL, Chen J, Neptune ER, et al: A syndrome of altered cardiovascular, craniofacial, neurocognitive and skeletal development caused by mutations in TGFBR1 or TGFBR2. Nat Genet 37:275-281, 2005.

131. Beals RK, Hecht F: Congenital contractural arachnodactyly: A heritable disorder of connective tissue. J Bone Joint Surg Am 53:987-993, 1971.

132. Putnam EA, Zhang H, Ramirez F, et al: Fibrillin-2 (FBN2) mutations result in the Marfan-like disorder, congenital contractural arachnodactyly. Nat Genet 11:456-458, 1995.

133. Ringpfeil F: Selected disorders of connective tissue: Pseudoxanthoma elasticum, cutis laxa, and lipoid proteinosis. Clin Dermatol 23:41-46, 2005.

134. Milewicz DM, Urban Z, Boyd C: Genetic disorders of the elastic fiber system. Matrix Biol 19:471-480, 2000.

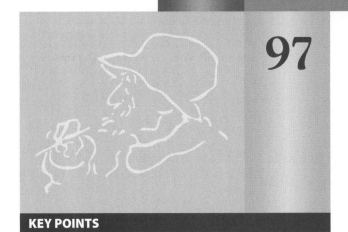

97

Juvenile Idiopathic Arthritis ◘

KIRAN NISTALA • PATRICIA WOO •
LUCY R. WEDDERBURN

KEY POINTS

Juvenile idiopathic arthritis (JIA) is an umbrella term for childhood arthritis of unknown cause.

JIA affects 1 in 1000 children.

Many of the subtypes of JIA have particular features, but some complications are common to several subtypes.

JIA is clearly distinct from adult rheumatoid arthritis.

Progress in the understanding of the genetics and pathogenesis of JIA has revealed subtype-specific associations and some common mechanisms of disease.

The principles of treating JIA are common to all subtypes because they involve a multidisciplinary approach, aiming to suppress inflammation early and maintain function.

DEFINITION AND CLASSIFICATION

It has been more than a century since Still eloquently described the differences between forms of childhood arthritis and adult rheumatoid arthritis.[1] Despite many advances in understanding of genetic, pathologic, and molecular influences on the disease, the cause or causes of juvenile arthritis are unknown, and it remains a leading cause of acquired disability in childhood. In more recent years, *juvenile idiopathic arthritis* (JIA) has become widely accepted as an umbrella term to cover this heterogeneous group of conditions.[2,3] The classification of JIA (Table 97-1), proposed and subsequently revised by the International League of Associations for Rheumatology (ILAR), has now replaced previous nomenclature, including the European term, *juvenile chronic arthritis*, and the American term, *juvenile rheumatoid arthritis*.[4]

JIA is defined as arthritis in one or more joints persisting for 6 weeks or more, which begins before the 16th birthday and has no other known cause.[2,3] Each category has a list of possible exclusions (see Table 97-1). A primary goal of such a system is to define mutually exclusive categories of idiopathic childhood arthritis based on predominant clinical and laboratory features, with the aim of improving therapy and management.[4,5] Although the classification of JIA is based primarily on clinical features of the disease, with emphasis on presenting features, it is widely accepted that improved knowledge should lead to a more precise definition of the types of JIA, perhaps based on genetic, pathologic, or mechanistic information, and that such a classification would need to evolve or change, as understanding of the subtypes of juvenile arthritis and their pathophysiology improves. The increasing use of one system of classification would facilitate ready comparison of data and information from many studies and clinical trials.

Table 97-2 provides an overview of the main features of each type of JIA. Many of the types of childhood arthritis have distinct clinical features, and some of these features are rare in adult inflammatory arthritis. In JIA, in contrast to adult rheumatoid arthritis, large joints, such as the knees, wrists, and ankles, are typically more prominently involved than small joints. Subcutaneous nodules and rheumatoid factor (RF) seropositivity are unusual, but antinuclear antibody (ANA) seropositivity is frequent in some JIA subtypes. Some JIA subtypes have a majority onset in young childhood, although as yet there is no clear biologic explanation for why this is so. Examples include the systemic-onset and oligoarticular subtypes of JIA. In contrast, some JIA subtypes have an adult counterpart, such as psoriatic arthritis and RF-positive polyarticular JIA; these subtypes tend to have a slightly older onset in children. Some complications of JIA, such as osteoporosis or uveitis, can occur in many subtypes; others are more restricted to particular subtypes.

Long-term studies have shown that, as a whole, JIA is not as benign as previously thought, with rates of complete remission off medication still low in many subtypes,[6] evidence for loss of quality of life in childhood,[7] and 30% to 50% of patients experiencing ongoing inflammation or disability into adulthood.[8,9] The imperative to investigate mechanisms of disease pathogenesis and search for new therapeutic avenues remains as strong as ever. A further drive to continue to aim for complete remission in JIA is the observation that when inflammation is fully controlled, juvenile tissues, including synovium, cartilage, and bone, can undergo remarkable "healing" with restoration of function, in sharp contrast to adult arthritis.

◘ Supplemental images available on the Expert Consult Premium Edition website.

Table 97-1 International League of Associations for Rheumatology Classification of Juvenile Idiopathic Arthritis (JIA)

Category	Definition	Exclusions
Systemic onset JIA	Arthritis in ≥1 joints with, or preceded by, fever of at least 2 wk duration that is documented to be daily ("quotidian"*) for at least 3 days and accompanied by ≥1 of the following: 1. Evanescent (nonfixed) erythematous rash 2. Generalized lymph node enlargement 3. Hepatomegaly or splenomegaly or both 4. Serositis†	A. Psoriasis or a history of psoriasis in the patient or a first-degree relative B. Arthritis in an HLA-B27+ male beginning after the 6th birthday C. Ankylosing spondylitis, enthesitis-related arthritis, sacroiliitis with inflammatory bowel disease, Reiter's syndrome, or acute anterior uveitis, or a history of one of these disorders in a first-degree relative D. Presence of IgM RF on at least 2 occasions at least 3 mo apart
Oligoarticular JIA	Arthritis affecting 1-4 joints during the first 6 mo of disease. Two subcategories are recognized: 1. Persistent oligoarthritis—affecting ≤4 joints throughout the disease course 2. Extended oligoarthritis—affecting >4 joints after the first 6 mo of disease	A, B, C, D above, plus E. Presence of systemic JIA in the patient
Polyarthritis (RF negative)	Arthritis affecting ≥5 joints during the first 6 mo of disease; a test for RF is negative	A, B, C, D, E
Polyarthritis (RF positive)	Arthritis affecting ≥5 joints during the first 6 mo of disease; ≥2 tests for RF at least 3 mo apart during the first 6 mo of disease are positive	A, B, C, E
Psoriatic arthritis	Arthritis and psoriasis, or arthritis and at least 2 of the following: 1. Dactylitis‡ 2. Nail pitting§ and onycholysis 3. Psoriasis in a first-degree relative	B, C, D, E
Enthesitis-related arthritis	Arthritis and enthesitis,‖ or arthritis or enthesitis with at least 2 of the following: 1. Presence of or a history of sacroiliac joint tenderness or inflammatory lumbosacral pain or both¶ 2. Presence of HLA-B27 antigen 3. Onset of arthritis in a male >6 yr old 4. Acute (symptomatic) anterior uveitis 5. History of ankylosing spondylitis, enthesitis-related arthritis, sacroiliitis with inflammatory bowel disease, Reiter's syndrome, or acute anterior uveitis in a first-degree relative	A, D, E
Undifferentiated arthritis	Arthritis that fulfills criteria in no category or in ≥2 of the above categories	

*Quotidian fever is defined as a fever that rises to 39°C once a day and returns to 37°C between fever peaks.
†Serositis refers to pericarditis, pleuritis, or peritonitis, or some combination of the three.
‡Dactylitis is swelling of ≥1 digits, usually in an asymmetric distribution, which extends beyond the joint margin.
§A minimum of 2 pits on any one or more nails at any time.
‖Enthesitis is defined as tenderness at the insertion of a tendon, ligament, joint capsule, or fascia to bone.
¶Inflammatory lumbosacral pain refers to lumbosacral pain at rest with morning stiffness that improves on movement.
RF, rheumatoid factor.

EPIDEMIOLOGY

By definition, JIA begins before age 16 years. Young children 1 to 3 years old are most commonly affected, a pattern most noticeable in girls, in whom the disease is twice as common. Boys have a wider distribution of age at onset, with a small peak in incidence at 8 to 10 years.[10,11] Systemic-onset JIA is an exception with a 1:1 female-to-male ratio.[12] Studies of the incidence of childhood arthritis using either juvenile rheumatoid arthritis or juvenile chronic arthritis classifications have documented rates of 3.5 to 13.9 (confidence limits 9.9 to 18.8) per 100,000 children/yr in population-based cohorts,[13-16] and a population-based study using ILAR JIA criteria suggested a rate of 15/100,000 children/yr.[11] Prevalence of chronic arthritis in childhood has been estimated as 148/100,000 children in a Norwegian study, and 400/100,000 children in a survey of 12-year-old schoolchildren.[17,18] In the latter study, all children were examined by a pediatric rheumatologist, which may explain the higher prevalence estimate. Most quoted studies are from populations of northern European descent, but some reports suggest arthritis may be less common in Japanese,[19] black,[20] and Asian children.[20]

ETIOLOGY

GENETICS

Despite significant advances in genetics and molecular immunology, understanding of the etiology of JIA is piecemeal. Genetic factors and environmental triggers are thought to play a part ultimately leading to abnormalities in the cellular, humoral, and innate arms of the immune system. The evidence for a genetic contribution to JIA comes from several sources. Twin studies show a high concordance

Table 97-2 Overview of the Main Features of the Subtypes of Juvenile Idiopathic Arthritis (JIA)

ILAR Subtype	Peak Age of Onset (yr)	Female: Male; % of All JIA	Arthritis Pattern	Extra-articular Features	Investigations	Notes on Therapy
Systemic arthritis	2-4	1:1; ~10% of JIA cases	Polyarticular, often knees, wrists, and ankles; also fingers, neck, and hips	Daily fever; evanescent rash; pericarditis; pleuritis	Anemia; WBC ↑↑; ESR ↑↑; CRP ↑↑; ferritin ↑; platelets ↑↑ (normal or ↓ in MAS)	Less responsive to standard treatment with MTX and anti-TNF agents; consider IL-1Ra in resistant cases
Oligoarthritis	<6	4:1; 50-60% of JIA (but ethnic variation)	Knees ++; ankles, fingers +	Uveitis in ~30%	ANA positive in ~60%; other tests usually normal; may have mildly ↑ ESR/CRP	NSAIDS and intra-articular steroids; occasionally require MTX
Polyarthritis, RF negative	6-7	3:1; 30% of JIA cases	Symmetric or asymmetric; small and large joints; cervical spine; TMJ	Uveitis in ~10%	ANA positive in 40%; RF negative; ESR ↑ or ↑↑; CRP ↑/normal; mild anemia	Standard therapy with MTX and NSAIDs, then if nonresponsive, anti-TNF agents or other biologics
Polyarthritis, RF positive	9-12	9:1; <10% of JIA cases	Aggressive symmetric polyarthritis	Rheumatoid nodules in 10%; low-grade fever	RF positive; ESR ↑↑; CRP ↑/normal; mild anemia	Long-term remission unlikely; early aggressive therapy is warranted
Psoriatic arthritis	7-10	2:1; <10% of JIA cases	Asymmetric arthritis of small or medium sized joints	Uveitis in 10%; psoriasis in 50%	ANA positive in 50%; ESR ↑; CRP ↑/normal; mild anemia	NSAIDS and intra-articular steroids; second-line agents less commonly
Enthesitis-related arthritis	9-12	1:7; 10% of JIA cases	Predominantly lower limb joints affected; sometimes axial skeleton (but less than adult AS)	Acute anterior uveitis; association with reactive arthritis and IBD	80% HLA-B27+	NSAIDS and intra-articular steroids; consider sulfasalazine as alternative to MTX

ANA, antinuclear antibody; AS, ankylosing spondylitis; CRP, C-reactive protein; ESR, erythrocyte sedimentation rate; IBD, inflammatory bowel disease; ILAR, International League of Associations for Rheumatology; IL-1Ra, interleukin-1 receptor antagonist; MAS, macrophage activation syndrome; MTX, methotrexate; NSAID, nonsteroidal anti-inflammatory drug; RF, rheumatoid factor; TMJ, temporomandibular joint; TNF, tumor necrosis factor; WBC, white blood cell count.

of disease in monozygotic twins.[21,22] A study of 164 affected sibling pairs with JIA showed a 70% concordance for gender, 73% for disease onset, and 66% for disease course, considerably higher than in a non–affected sibling pair cohort.[23] First-degree relatives of children with JIA have a higher rate of autoimmune disease than controls.[24] Genetic influences on JIA susceptibility and phenotype are polygenic,[25] and a more recent genome-wide scan in JIA affected sibling pair families has supported the idea that multiple genetic loci contribute to JIA susceptibility.[26]

The strong associations of specific alleles with JIA are within the major histocompatibility complex (MHC) system and were the first to be documented.[27,28] Among the MHC class I loci, HLA-B27 is strongly associated with spondyloarthropathy, which in children is now termed *enthesitis-related arthritis* (ERA), whereas HLA-A*0201 is increased in oligoarthritis.[29] Multiple studies have revealed an increase in HLA-DR alleles, of which the strongest are DRB1*0801 and DRB1*1101 with oligoarticular JIA and DRB1*1301, in particular in ANA-positive cases.[30-32] Several haplotypes across the MHC confer an increased risk for all types of JIA, such as DRB1*08-DQA1*0401-DQB1*0402, which confers an odds ratio of 6.1 for persistent oligoarticular

JIA and 10.3 for extended oligoarticular JIA. Frequency of the DRB1*1301-DQA1*01-DQB1*06 haplotype distinguishes persistent from extended oligoarticular JIA, whereas DRB1*0801 and DRB1*1401 are associated with polyarticular JIA.[29]

Together these effects may be large; in one study, the presence of the combination of the HLA-DRB1*0801, HLA-DRB1*1101, and HLA-DPB1*0201 alleles conferred a relative risk of 236.[33] Some associations closely mirror the associations of the corresponding adult disease, such as the strong association of the HLA-B27 allele with ERA and the HLA-DRB1*0401 with RF-positive polyarticular JIA. Some of these allele/subtype associations show an age-specific effect, in that they confer risk over a specific age range only.[34] Although systemic JIA shows weaker associations with HLA alleles, even in this subtype, specific haplotypes (e.g., DRB1*11-DQA1*05-DQB1*03) are increased compared with control subjects.[29]

Inflammatory cytokines have been an important target for drug development in JIA, and similarly their gene polymorphisms have been a key area of scrutiny. Several HLA-independent tumor necrosis factor (TNF) haplotypes are significantly associated with JIA, but the functional consequences of these alleles are unclear.[35] Some of the best characterized non-HLA genetic associations in JIA have been established in systemic JIA. The hypothesis suggesting a link between systemic JIA and interleukin (IL)-6 was proposed in 1993,[36] with many of the clinical features in systemic JIA resembling the phenotype of IL-6 overexpression (e.g., fevers, stunted growth, anemia).[37] A polymorphism (−174G/C) in the regulatory region of the IL-6 gene alters transcription of IL-6 in response to IL-1 and lipopolysaccharide; patients with systemic JIA have significantly lower frequency of the protective CC genotype,[38] and the IL-6 −174G allele was confirmed as a susceptibility gene for systemic JIA.[39]

More recent haplotype analysis of the IL-6 gene has confirmed a haplotype association with systemic JIA.[40] A polymorphism in the promoter region of the macrophage inhibitory factor (MIF) gene is associated with JIA.[41] This polymorphism (MIF −173*C) results in higher MIF production in the serum and synovium of JIA patients and has been shown to be predictive of outcome of intra-articular steroid injections in systemic JIA.[42]

The anti-inflammatory gene IL-10 was first studied in oligoarticular JIA. The "ATA" haplotype of three single nucleotide polymorphisms at the 5′ flanking end of the gene is associated with lower production of IL-10 by peripheral blood mononuclear cells, and was found more frequently in the more severe subtype of JIA, extended oligoarticular JIA, than the milder persistent oligoarticular JIA.[43] IL-10 and its family member IL-20 were found to be associated with systemic JIA.[44] The gene *PTPN22*, a negative regulator of T cell responses, has been suggested to be associated with JIA also, but current evidence is conflicting.[45,46] In contrast to studies using the candidate gene approach, future novel genetic associations will be elucidated through whole-genome scanning, requiring large multicenter case-control cohorts.

ENVIRONMENT

A study of socioeconomic factors in the etiology of JIA suggested that high parental income and being an only child may be associated with a higher risk of disease,[47] and in a Finnish study of more than 58,000 births, fetal exposure to smoking has been suggested to increase the risk of JIA in girls.[48] The evidence that genetic risk alleles, such as those associated with HLA antigens, confer different risk of JIA across different ages, strongly suggests that crucial environmental triggers, which change with age, may be involved in the initiation of JIA.[34]

Microbial triggers for JIA remain elusive. *Borrelia burgdoferi*, the infectious agent responsible for Lyme disease; *Mycoplasma pneumoniae*; and several viruses, such as rubella and parvovirus, can cause a clinical picture similar to JIA, leading to the hypothesis that JIA represents an immunologic response to an infectious trigger.[49] Bacterial or viral DNA can be isolated from the joints or serum of JIA patients,[50,51] but no single agent has been identified as a cause of JIA, and in most cases of JIA no persisting infectious agent can be shown. Epidemiologic studies searching for infectious "outbreaks" or seasonal variation in incident JIA cases, or in pregnant mothers whose children subsequently develop JIA, have provided conflicting results.[47,52-54]

An alternative role for microbial pathogens in the pathogenesis of JIA has been suggested through molecular mimicry. Heat shock proteins are proteins expressed by microbial and human cells in response to stress. Bacterial heat shock proteins are strong immunogens and may generate cross-reactive immune responses to self–heat shock proteins in humans. In oligoarticular JIA, reactivity to self–heat shock proteins correlates with disease remission,[55] and synovial T cells generate a regulatory cell phenotype in response to self–heat shock protein 60, which was not detectable in the more severe polyarthritis subgroup.[56]

PATHOGENESIS

The pathologic hallmark of juvenile inflammatory arthritis is the inflamed synovium. Histology of this tissue shows thickened synovium that is highly vascular and shows marked hyperplasia of synoviocytes in the lining layer and a dense infiltrate of inflammatory cells, comprising T cells, macrophages, and in some cases B cells and natural killer cells (Fig. 97-1).[57-61] The hypertrophied synovial layer is highly vascular, with endothelium expressing markers of activation such as HLA-DR and intracellular adhesion molecule 1. The vascularity is likely related to the increased production of proangiogenic factors, such as vascular endothelial growth factor, and the angiogenic chemokines.[62,63] Recruitment of this inflammatory infiltrate is likely mediated by multiple chemokines shown to be increased in JIA, including CCL3, CCL5, and CXCL10; IL-8; and monocyte chemotactic protein-1.[64-68]

The strong association of many JIA subtypes with genetic variants at HLA loci, the central role of HLA class I and II proteins in T cell function, and the predominance of T cells in pathologic JIA synovial tissue and fluid led to intense investigation of the role of T cells in the pathology of JIA. T cells within the JIA joint are highly activated memory cells, expressing rapidly upregulated (CD69) and persistent (DR) activation markers.[59,69,70] These T cells express a restricted set of T cell receptors:[71,72] The clonotypes are large and long-lived, and the same hierarchy of clones re-expands during a relapse or flare of disease.[71] The finding that this oligoclonality in the intra-articular T cell population is more marked in CD4[+] T cells in oligoarthritis (which is associated with class II HLA-DR genes), and yet more marked in CD8[+] T cells in ERA (which is associated with the class I allele HLA-B27), supports the concept that recognition of MHC-peptide complexes by T cells plays a role in the pathogenesis of JIA.[72]

Early work on inflammatory cytokines produced by synovial T cells suggested that these were heavily skewed toward a T helper type 1 (Th1) CCR5[+]CXCR3[+] interferon-γ-producing lineage.[59,73,74] More recent evidence suggests, however, that another proinflammatory T cell cytokine, IL-17, produced by Th17 cells, has an important role in JIA. Th17 cells are enriched in the joint in JIA, and their numbers are higher in children with the more severe extended oligoarticular JIA compared with children with milder, persistent oligoarticular disease.[75]

Many inflammatory cytokines and chemokines are abnormally increased in JIA and found at the site of destructive synovitis. Subtype differences have emerged, which may allow a "subtype-specific" profiling of serum or synovial fluid

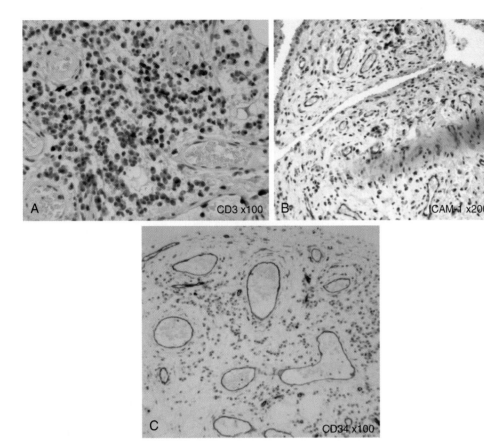

Figure 97-1 Sections of synovium from the knee of a child with oligoarticular juvenile idiopathic arthritis showing intense inflammatory infiltrate and highly vascular hypertrophied tissue. **A,** Stained for CD3 (surface protein expressed on T lymphocytes) (magnification, ×100). **B,** Stained for intracellular adhesion molecule 1, which is expressed on the endothelium and a proportion of the infiltrating cells (magnification, ×200). **C,** Stained for CD34, expressed on vascular endothelium (and hematopoietic stem cells) (magnification, ×100).

in the future, although such measurements have to take into account circadian rhythms and the short half-lives of these mediators.[67,76,77] Systemic JIA is associated with high levels of TNF, IL-1, IL-6, MIF, and IL-18. In cases of classic systemic JIA, the levels of IL-6 and IL-1 receptor antagonist increase and decrease in parallel with the fever and rash.[78] IL-6 and MIF levels are each associated with disease activity in systemic JIA, and high synovial MIF levels predict poor response to intra-articular steroid injection.[79] IL-1 has been suggested to have a major role in the pathogenesis of systemic JIA,[80] although results in this field are conflicting.

In addition to the proinflammatory, destructive process within the joint, there is strong evidence for ongoing immunoregulation in JIA. The existence of a mild form of arthritis in which full-blown immunopathology can resolve and disease can enter full remission (known as persistent oligoarticular JIA) provides a unique model in autoimmunity: a mild self-remitting autoimmune pathology, which can be compared with more severe clinical subtypes. Children with persistent oligoarticular JIA have evidence of immunoregulation as shown by high numbers of CD25+ foxp3+ regulatory T cells in the joint,[81] and these cells correlate with clinical phenotype and outcome. In addition, T cells specific for the conserved self-antigen heat shock proteins have been shown to be present at significantly higher numbers in children destined to have a mild disease course, and these self-antigen heat shock protein–specific cells are thought to play a regulatory role.[55,56] The crucial role of dendritic cells in the control of this immunoregulation of JIA is a field of intense investigation.

In addition to cells of the adaptive immune system, many other parts of the immune system are abnormally activated in JIA, including synovial macrophages,[79] dendritic cells,[82,83] and neutrophils.[84,85] Modern high-throughput methods of gene expression profiling and proteomics have shown differences between JIA clinical subtypes in several cell populations and between JIA patients before and after treatment and compared with controls.[63,86-89] Ultimately, the understanding of pathologic mechanisms and alterations in the balance between immune activation and regulation, during disease and in response to treatment, should lead to a new set of molecular tools with which to separate clinical subtypes, predict disease course, and select tailored therapies for every child more accurately.

PRINCIPLES OF TREATMENT

JIA is a disease with great diversity, with patients ranging from a child with arthritis affecting one joint to an acutely sick child with systemic arthritis. Successfully caring for these children and their families as they progress from infancy to adulthood requires myriad skills that cannot be provided by one clinician alone. The essential principle of managing JIA is to deliver care as a multidisciplinary team, including pediatric rheumatologists, physical therapists, occupational therapists, podiatrists or orthotists, specialist nurses, psychologists, social workers, school liaison workers, family support groups, general practitioners, ophthalmologists, dentists or orthodontists, orthopaedic surgeons, and pain management teams. The long-term goal is to achieve early and *complete* suppression of inflammation without treatment toxicity, while maintaining muscle power, joint range of movement, and function, through active physical therapy and occupational therapy input, and maximize the child's potential for normal growth and development and educational and vocational success.

A persistent block to good outcome in many areas of the world is a delay in recognition or diagnosis of JIA.[90] When recognized, most children with JIA now have a good outcome, however, in terms of functional ability. Despite these good functional outcomes and educational achievements, studies of adults who had JIA as children show that JIA may still have a profound effect on quality of life and vocational achievements.[9,91]

ISSUES SPECIFIC TO MANAGEMENT OF CHILDHOOD ARTHRITIS

The challenges of assessing and treating children with arthritis are quite distinct from managing patients with rheumatoid arthritis. The child's symptoms are often filtered through the parents' preconceptions and fears. A skilled pediatric rheumatologist needs to listen to the child and the parent and address the concerns of both, communicating in language that is appropriate for the parents and the developmental stage of the child. The wishes of the patient may not always mirror that of their parents, particularly with adolescents.

In children, arthritis more commonly manifests with reduced function or deformity, rather than pain or swelling. The assessment of pain can be difficult in young children; pain may manifest as altered mood or restricted play, rather than localizing symptoms. The wider rheumatology team plays a vital role, which includes assessing an apprehensive child. Therapists can achieve a detailed examination by "simply" observing and interacting with the child in a natural state of play. With an older child, therapists, specialist nurses, and social workers have key roles in communicating with schools and acting as child advocates, such as requesting computer laptops to help with writing difficulties, or helping parents to engage with school authorities if their child's educational needs are not being met. Table 97-3 provides an overview of the role of physical therapists and occupational therapists during the course of managing a long-term patient with JIA.

For an adolescent who has been under the long-term care of the pediatric rheumatology team, moving to adult care is stressful and can precipitate poor adherence and disease flares. Transition is the process that builds up to the successful transfer of care. This is a "multifaceted active process that attends to the medical, psychosocial and educational-vocational needs of the adolescent as they move from child to adult-orientated care."[92] The aim is to equip an adolescent with a range of skills that gives him or her a sense of control over his or her healthcare and enables the adolescent to function independently (Table 97-4). Ideally, this transition service would be provided in a dedicated adolescent rheumatology clinic. This service may not be feasible outside large pediatric rheumatology centers, but many of the principles still can be adopted regardless of the size of the service.

Table 97-3 Overview of the Role of Physical Therapy and Occupational Therapy in Juvenile Idiopathic Arthritis

Treatment Goals of Early Disease
Identify and control pain (e.g., splinting)
Improve function (e.g., progressive home exercise program)
Educate child and family
Input in Established Arthritis
Limit/reverse impairments (e.g., serial casting)
Teach self-management and problem-solving skills (e.g., pacing)
Advocate for child (e.g., ergonomic assessment at school)
Plan for the Future
Support adolescent healthy living goals
Vocational counseling
Teach independent living skills
Surgical intervention planning

Adapted from Kachta G, Davidson I: Physiotherapy and occupational therapy. In Szer IS, Kimura Y, Malleson PN, Southwood TR (eds): Arthritis in Children and Adolescents. Oxford, UK, Oxford University Press, 2006, pp 381-391.

Table 97-4 Essentials of a Transitional Care Service

Policy on timing of transition and transfer that agrees with adult services
Preparation period
Disease education program
Address needs of the adolescent and parent or guardian
Transfer process that is coordinated with other medical specialties
Committed adult rheumatology service with key liaison personnel
Administrative support
Primary care involvement
Involvement of adolescent Developing his or her own individualized transition plans As advisor to adolescent rheumatology service development As educator of peers and health professionals
Regular evaluation and audit

From McDonagh JE, White P: Adolescent rheumatology services. In Szer IS, Kimura Y, Malleson PN, Southwood TR (eds): Arthritis in Children and Adolescents. Oxford, UK, Oxford University Press, 2006, pp 315-329.

GENERAL PRINCIPLES OF MEDICAL MANAGEMENT OF JUVENILE IDIOPATHIC ARTHRITIS

Algorithms of suggested treatment decision routes are shown in Figures 97-2 and 97-3. Nonsteroidal anti-inflammatory drugs (NSAIDs) should be given from the time of diagnosis, and at adequate doses (Table 97-5). When there are only a few joints involved (e.g., oligoarticular JIA and some cases of psoriatic or ERA JIA), initial management should include intra-articular steroid injection with triamcinolone hexacetonide, given under sedation or general anesthetic for children. Triamcinolone hexacetonide has been found to be superior to triamcinolone acetonide, betamethasone, and methylprednisolone acetate in randomized controlled trials,[93,94] and early treatment is associated with better outcome.[95]

When intra-articular steroid injection is inadequate to control synovitis, or arthritis involves three or more joints, methotrexate is the second-line agent of choice. Its efficacy has been confirmed in two randomized trials, with maximum benefit at an intermediate dose of 15 mg/m^2 administered subcutaneously.[96,97] The main side effects that limit use of methotrexate are nausea, vomiting, and deranged liver

MEDICAL MANAGEMENT OF OLIGOARTHRITIS
(PERSISTENT OLIGOARTHRITIS JIA,
PSORIATIC JIA AND MILD ERA)

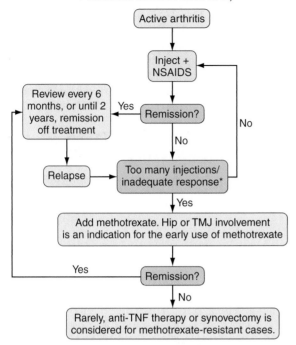

Figure 97-2 Algorithm to outline the treatment principles for persistent oligoarticular juvenile idiopathic arthritis (JIA), psoriatic JIA, and enthesitis-related arthritis JIA. *There is no evidence to support a limit on the number of steroid injections per joint, and some centers have injected more than 10 times without adverse effects. NSAIDs, nonsteroidal anti-inflammatory drugs; TMJ, temporomandibular joint; TNF, tumor necrosis factor.

MEDICAL MANAGEMENT OF POLYARTHRITIS
(EXTENDED OLIGOARTICULAR JIA, RF+/RF–
POLYARTICULAR JIA AND SOME ERA PATIENTS)

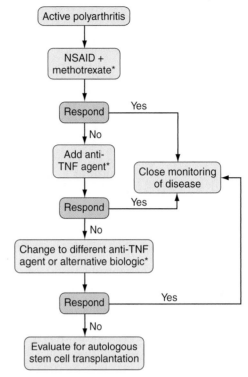

Figure 97-3 Algorithm to outline the treatment principles for extended oligoarticular juvenile idiopathic arthritis (JIA), and rheumatoid factor–negative and rheumatoid factor–positive polyarticular JIA. *Consider joint injections or pulsed intravenous steroid and short-course oral steroid. NSAIDs, nonsteroidal anti-inflammatory drugs; TNF, tumor necrosis factor.

function tests. Folic acid usually is recommended to ameliorate these effects, but there is limited evidence from pediatric studies to substantiate this practice.[98] The more toxic effects of methotrexate seen in adults, such as liver cirrhosis and lung fibrosis, are extremely rare in children.

Alternatives to methotrexate to consider include leflunomide, an oral inhibitor of pyrimidine synthesis, which seems to be less efficacious than methotrexate in JIA.[99] Sulfasalazine is shown to be of sustained benefit in oligoarticular and polyarticular JIA, but at the cost of gastrointestinal and skin side effects.[100,101] In recent years, biologic therapies have revolutionized the treatment of rheumatoid arthritis. In children, only one agent, etanercept (recombinant soluble TNF receptor), is currently licensed for use in the United Kingdom; criteria for approval include a failure of or intolerance to methotrexate, in the presence of active synovitis.

In 2000, etanercept was tested in JIA using a unique placebo-controlled withdrawal design and was shown to be efficacious in patients resistant to methotrexate therapy,[102] although the benefits are not equal for all subtypes.[103] Long-term follow-up has confirmed its benefits and good safety record.[104] A trial of infliximab showed a good response to treatment, but was not adequately powered to establish superiority to methotrexate alone.[105] Treatment with 6 mg/kg of infliximab was recommended because this dose was associated with significantly fewer antibodies to the drug

and infusion-related adverse events than the smaller 3 mg/kg dose. Preliminary data from trials with CTLA4-Ig (abatacept) and adalimumab show promising results in methotrexate-naive and treated JIA patients.[106,107]

Patients with systemic arthritis fare less well with anti-TNF-α therapy compared with other subtypes, which likely reflects the distinct etiopathogenesis of systemic JIA (see section on systemic arthritis). Early-phase trials of IL-1 receptor antagonist (anakinra)[80] and IL-6 blockade[108,109] offer future hope for this recalcitrant group of patients, who pose one of the greatest challenges to pediatric rheumatology. The long-term safety of immune blockade of specific mediators such as TNF-α or IL-1 is unknown; however, despite concerns about infections (e.g., tuberculosis) or malignancy, to date the available data are reassuring.[103] In patients who achieve remission on methotrexate or biologic treatments it is not clear when treatment should be stopped. Without definitive clinical or biologic markers to predict relapse off treatment, most centers continue treatment for 1 to 2 years of continuous remission. MRP8 and MRP14 may be useful biomarkers to predict long-term remission off methotrexate, and a recent randomized trial comparing withdrawal at 6 versus 12 months hopes to answer this question.[109a]

In situations where current drug therapies fail, the option of autologous stem cell transplantation has been widely used in Europe for children with severe resistant JIA. The

Table 97-5 Doses of Common Nonsteroidal Anti-inflammatory Drugs (NSAIDs) Used for Juvenile Idiopathic Arthritis (JIA)

NSAID	Dose	Comments
Ibuprofen (from 6 mo of age)	30-40 mg/kg/day in 3-4 divided doses	Up to 60 mg/kg/day in sJIA in divided doses
Naproxen (>2 yrs)	20-30 mg/kg/day in 2 divided doses	Maximum, 1 g/day
Piroxicam	<15 kg, 5 mg; 16-25 kg, 10 mg; 26-45 kg, 15 mg; >46 kg, 20 mg once a day	
Diclofenac	1-3 mg/kg/day in 2-3 divided doses	SR preparation available; maximum 150 mg/day
Indomethacin (>1 mo of age)	1-2 mg/kg/day in 2 divided doses	SR preparations useful to alleviate morning stiffness; maximum, 50 mg/day

SR, sustained release.

restoration of "immune balance" by autologous stem cell transplantation has been successfully carried out in more than 65 children with severe JIA; 53% of these children have achieved remission,[110,111] with good long-term disease-free survival rates.[112] Children who relapse may show a milder disease phenotype, which is more easily controlled with standard therapy. Guidelines for the consideration of autologous stem cell transplantation are updated on a regular basis to include available biologic therapies.[113]

GROWTH DISTURBANCES IN JUVENILE IDIOPATHIC ARTHRITIS

In a growing child, uncontrolled arthritis leads to secondary systemic and localized growth disturbances. Generalized growth failure is most marked in systemic JIA and is related to high levels of IL-6 and corticosteroid toxicity. Sick children are often anorexic despite their catabolic state, and dietary advice is needed to avoid compounding their existing growth failure. In older children, poor growth is associated with pubertal delay and osteoporosis. Osteoporosis should be considered in all children with prolonged active disease and is most marked in children with systemic JIA (see section on systemic arthritis). Bisphosphonates and calcium and vitamin D supplements have been used,[114,115] but evidence for the optimal combination is lacking; a large multicenter trial is currently in progress to determine this (BSPAR arc website available at http://www.arc.org.uk/news/pressreleases/15936.asp).

Local growth disturbances vary according the anatomic site involved. Unrecognized arthritis affecting large joints can cause bony overgrowth, most commonly affecting the knee. Leg-length abnormalities greater than 2 cm are an indication for orthoses to prevent mechanical back pain. Muscle atrophy around affected joints is common and requires intensive physical therapy.

Overgrowth of the medial tibial epiphyses leads to a valgus deformity of the knees, which may require epiphyseal stapling or osteotomy for correction. Arthritis of the temporomandibular joint is often asymptomatic, manifesting late with growth failure of the jaw, micrognathia,

retrognathia, and overbite. Arthritis of the facet joints in the cervical spine causes bony ankylosis with major functional consequences from the limited extension and rotational movements. Hip involvement is common in systemic JIA and polyarticular JIA, and the most frequent cause of reduced mobility. In early-onset hip disease, overgrowth of the femoral head coupled with a short broad femoral neck leads to anteversion and bowing of the femoral shaft. With disease onset after about age 11 years, the architecture is often normal, but protrusio acetabuli may develop.

CLINICAL FEATURES OF SUBTYPES OF JUVENILE IDIOPATHIC ARTHRITIS

Table 97-2 provides a summary of the epidemiology and clinical features of the subtypes of JIA.

SYSTEMIC ARTHRITIS

Systemic JIA is defined as arthritis associated with systemic features, typically quotidian spiking fevers of 39°C or greater for more than 2 weeks, accompanied by at least one of the following: an evanescent rash, lymphadenopathy, serositis, or hepatosplenomegaly.[3] This clinical subtype was previously known as Still's disease and has a recognized adult-equivalent condition, adult-onset Still's disease.[116] Systemic JIA occurs in young children with a peak age in most series of 2 to 4 years.[16] The incidence is the same in both sexes in whites, in contrast to the other types of JIA. The prevalence of systemic JIA approximates to 10 cases per 100,000, representing about 10% of JIA as a whole, although some surveys have suggested that it may be more frequent in Japan and India.[12]

There is only a weak association between the HLA region and systemic JIA in whites, but there is good evidence that genetic predisposition constitutes at least part of the cause of systemic JIA. Non-HLA genes, such as those coding for macrophage MIF, have been shown to be associated with JIA as a whole, and a variant of the IL-6 gene confers susceptibility.[39,41] These genes are thought to predispose the patient to a vigorous inflammatory response to stimuli, such as infectious agents, and the net effect of the interaction between proinflammatory and anti-inflammatory proteins is probably the key to the clinical features in this subtype of JIA. IL-6 and IL-1 may play a role in the pathogenesis of systemic JIA[80] and have been proposed as therapeutic targets. Several monocyte-derived and neutrophil-derived proinflammatory factors also are abnormal in systemic JIA, including the myeloid-related proteins S100A8 and S100A9, and neutrophil-derived S100A12.[84] Abnormalities of the adaptive immune system in systemic JIA may include a defect in perforin. Low levels are associated with severe disease, but can reverse when disease is controlled.[117,118]

Clinical Manifestations

The fever is typically spiking in character with a peak of at least 39°C (Fig. 97-4A). It occurs once or twice a day and recurs each day (quotidian). This quotidian fever is accompanied by an evanescent salmon pink macular/urticarial rash, which can be itchy (Fig. 97-4B). The child is usually

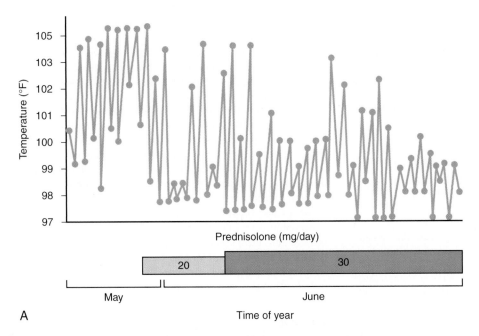

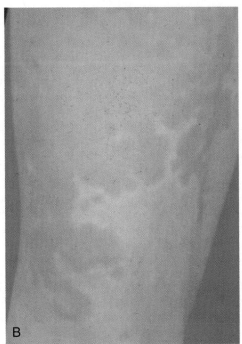

Figure 97-4 **A,** Regular spiking fever typical of systemic juvenile idiopathic arthritis (JIA). **B,** Evanescent rash of systemic JIA.

unwell and irritable during the fever, but often recovers in between. Other accompanying symptoms are headaches (sometimes with signs of meningism), arthralgia or arthritis, myalgia, abdominal pains from serositis that can mimic an acute abdomen, breathlessness and chest pains on lying flat indicating pericarditis, and acute chest pains from pleuritis. The severity of symptoms varies widely, ranging from fever and rash for 2 to 3 weeks followed by mild arthritis, to simultaneous onset of all the above-described symptoms. In the most severe cases, children also may present with features of secondary hemophagocytic lymphohistiocytosis (also known as macrophage activation syndrome),[119] with signs of anemia, jaundice, and purpura in later stages.

Laboratory Features

There are no specific tests for systemic JIA, but there are characteristic patterns of laboratory abnormalities. There is typically a very high C-reactive protein and erythrocyte sedimentation rate, leukocytosis with neutrophilia, thrombocytosis, and anemia, which may be profound. Liver enzymes, ferritin, and coagulation screen may be abnormal in severe cases, and polyclonal hypergammaglobulinemia is frequent. There are no specific autoantibodies, but RF and complement levels are normal or high (as acute-phase reactants). Investigative tests that may be required to exclude other conditions include urinary vanillylmandelic acid and bone marrow aspiration (see later).

Table 97-6 Differential Diagnosis of Systemic Juvenile Idiopathic Arthritis (JIA)

Condition	Differentiating Features from Systemic JIA
Infection	Positive cultures, PCR, or specific antibodies; continuous or irregular fever, nonquotidian; various rashes (not typical systemic JIA rash)
Leukemia	Nonquotidian fevers; bone pain; systemically unwell constantly
Neuroblastoma	Nonquotidian fevers; systemically unwell constantly
CINCA or NOMID	Fixed rash; undulating fevers; neurologic complications
Kawasaki disease	Fixed rash; mucocutaneous symptoms; coronary artery dilation
Other primary vasculitis	Undulating fevers; fixed, painful rashes or purpura; systemically ill constantly; renal involvement
SLE	Constant or nonquotidian fevers; positive ANA and dsDNA antibodies; cytopenias; other organs involved

ANA, antinuclear antibody; CINCA, chronic infantile neurologic cutaneous and articular syndrome; dsDNA, double-stranded DNA; NOMID, neonatal-onset multisystem inflammatory disease; PCR, polymerase chain reaction; SLE, systemic lupus erythematosus.

Differential Diagnosis

Many illnesses can mimic systemic JIA (Table 97-6). Apart from arthritis, fever is classic, and a careful fever chart often helps eliminate some of the differential diagnoses. The rash is similar to a viral exanthema, but the difference is that it is evanescent. If these criteria are not fulfilled unequivocally, it is necessary to screen for infectious agents, measure urinary vanillylmandelic acid, and obtain a bone marrow aspirate to exclude infection, neuroblastoma, and leukemia. Some physicians do these tests routinely because malignancies are often close mimics in the early stages of systemic JIA. The recurrent fever syndromes are often mistaken for systemic JIA, but the character of the fevers and the fixed rashes associated with these syndromes should alert the clinician to a different diagnosis. Between the subtypes of JIA, polyarticular disease also can manifest with an unwell child and arthritis, but an absence of systemic features (see Tables 97-1 and 97-2).

Treatment

Mild systemic JIA often needs nothing more than NSAIDs given to cover the whole 24-hour period (see Table 97-5). Indomethacin is helpful for fever and pericarditis. In more severe cases, steroids are needed, usually given as pulsed intravenous high-dose methylprednisolone (30 mg/kg bolus), up to a maximum dose of 1000 mg (1g), followed by tapering doses of oral prednisolone.[120] Disease-modifying drugs, such as methotrexate and cyclosporine, are often used, but there is evidence that these are less effective than in polyarthritis.[97] Some disease-modifying antirheumatic drugs are associated with macrophage activation syndrome in patients with systemic JIA (e.g., sulfasalazine, methotrexate).[119] Etanercept is less effective in systemic JIA compared with polyarticular JIA.[103,121] Newer biologics to block IL-6 and IL-1 signaling

are more promising,[80,108,109,122] and the results of phase II/III trials are awaited. The restoration of "immune balance" by autologous stem cell transplantation has been successfully carried out in more than 60 children with severe JIA, many of these systemic JIA (see section on general principles of medical management of JIA).

The complications of systemic JIA require special consideration. Osteoporosis and growth retardation may be severe owing to disease activity itself[123] and steroid use,[124] and the use of growth hormone may be warranted.[125] Evidence to establish a role for bisphosphonates and calcium and vitamin D supplements is currently being sought in a multicenter trial (see Growth Disturbances in JIA, earlier). Amyloidosis, previously a major cause of death in systemic JIA, is now less common, presumably as a result of better control of inflammatory activity, but still may affect severe refractory cases. There is evidence for the use of chlorambucil for this complication,[126] but concerns about risk of malignancy remain. Amyloidosis is a relative contraindication to autologous stem cell transplantation.[113]

Outcome

Systemic JIA is heterogeneous in severity, disease course, and outcome. It can be monocyclic, with remission within 2 to 4 years; relapsing, characterized by flares of systemic features with mild arthritis; or continuing with persistent destructive arthritis, usually more prominent after the regression of systemic features.[12] Patients with severe disease can have flares of extra-articular features at any time and may have active arthritis into adult life despite standard therapies. An Italian study of 80 patients suggested a remission rate of only 33% 10 years after disease onset,[127] whereas a retrospective analysis of active/inactive disease, including 59 patients with systemic JIA, suggested that children had only 30% of time with inactive disease (median follow-up 7 years).[6]

Overall, outcome in this subtype is poor with more children having long-term functional disability.[127] Predictors of poor outcome include the presence of systemic features 6 months after onset, thrombocytosis, and the presence of polyarthritis with hip involvement.[128,129] The mortality rate for systemic JIA is still perceived to be higher than the mortality rate associated with other subtypes of JIA in clinical practice now, although no formal figures are available. As a result of the inadequate control of the disease with the available therapies, growth failure and osteoporosis are serious and lasting complications. Social isolation and unemployment also have been described as more prevalent in this group.[8]

OLIGOARTHRITIS

Oligoarticular arthritis is the most common form of JIA and preferentially affects girls (female-to-male ratio of 4:1), with a peak onset before 6 years of age. It affects about 60 per 100,000 white children, but rates vary in different ethnic groups.[130] Oligoarticular JIA affects four or fewer joints in the first 6 months of disease. If more than four joints become involved after 6 months, it is defined as extended oligoarthritis; otherwise, it is known as persistent oligoarthritis.[3] There are several exclusion factors (see Table 97-1), including psoriasis in the patient or a first-degree relative, systemic features, a positive IgM RF on more than one occasion 3 months apart, or a positive HLA-B27 test when in a boy in whom arthritis starts at 6 years or older.

These details are crucial to consider if the ILAR criteria are to be used correctly; many studies are likely to include patients of other subtypes (e.g., ERA and psoriatic JIA) in the oligoarticular group inadvertently, where these exclusions are overlooked. There is a strong genetic association with the HLA alleles at class I (HLA A2) and class II (DRB1*0801, DRB1*1104, DRB1*1301) loci.[29,131] The rate of extension to the extended oligoarthritis subtype has been reported as 30% to 50%.[132,133] Increasing evidence for real differences between the persistent and extended subtypes include genetic[29,43] and pathologic[75,81] data. Currently, there is no single reliable predictor of extension,[132,134] but much work is in progress to establish such predictors.

Clinical Manifestations

Children with oligoarthritis present with involvement of one to four joints, most commonly the knees and ankles (Fig. 97-5). Small joints of the hand are the third most commonly affected, but this pattern may portend the later

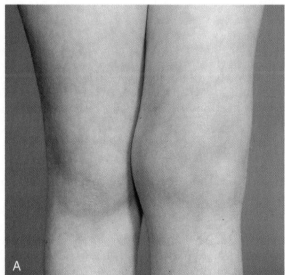

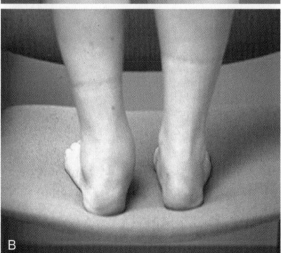

Figure 97-5 Oligoarticular juvenile idiopathic arthritis. **A,** Unilateral arthritis of the left knee showing swelling, flexion, and muscle atrophy. **B,** Unilateral arthritis of the left ankle showing valgus deformity of the hind foot. (**A** courtesy of Professor T. Southwood; **B** from Woo et al: Paediatr Rheumatol Clin Pract, 2007.)

onset of psoriatic arthritis.[135] Temporomandibular joint arthritis is common, but is often detected late in the course of the disease because symptoms are uncommon. Initial wrist involvement is rare and may indicate progression to extended oligoarthritis, or polyarticular disease. Shoulders are rarely involved. Cervical spine disease may be manifest by torticollis. Most children complain of pain, morning stiffness, and gelling, and a parent may notice a limp and joint swelling, or in a young child, a reluctance to walk and return to crawling. Twenty-five percent of cases seem to be painless, however, and only swelling is observed.

The most common extra-articular manifestation is iridocyclitis, also known as chronic anterior uveitis. Twenty percent to 30% of children with oligoarticular JIA develop uveitis, which is generally asymptomatic.[136] The eye is neither red nor photophobic. Uveitis is more prevalent in children who are ANA positive.[137] All children with oligoarticular JIA should have a mandatory slit lamp examination of the eyes by an experienced ophthalmologist at presentation and every 3 to 4 months for the first year and then for several years, with recommended screening times depending on age at onset.[138,139] Some physicians decrease the surveillance to every 6 months if the ANA is negative because a positive ANA test is a predictor of uveitis.[140]

Laboratory Features

Of children with oligoarthritis, 50% to 70% have a positive ANA test, typically 1:40 to 1:320 depending on the test system, and the rate is even higher in girls with an early onset.[140,141] In some cases, a child has mildly or moderately elevated acute-phase reactants, such as erythrocyte sedimentation rate or C-reactive protein, and in a few cases a mild anemia is present. A high erythrocyte sedimentation rate may predict progression to the extended subtype.[132] Elevated acute-phase reactants may suggest other conditions, such as subclinical inflammatory bowel disease with associated arthropathy.

Differential Diagnosis

The differential diagnosis of oligoarticular JIA includes other JIA subtypes, such as ERA and psoriatic JIA (see Table 97-1), and septic arthritis, reactive arthritis, foreign body synovitis, pigmented villonodular synovitis, arteriovenous malformation, bleeding disorders (e.g., hemophilia), or severe trauma, including nonaccidental injury. Mild trauma, such as from a fall, does not cause persistent joint swelling, and trauma is rarely a cause of joint swelling, unless there is an internal derangement seen in older, but not younger, children. Children with hypermobility can develop transient joint effusions after exercise.[142] Lyme disease (in an endemic area) frequently causes knee swelling usually for less than 6 weeks, although it is frequently recurrent. Leukemia may manifest with joint swelling, commonly a monarthritis, but usually is associated with systemic manifestations, high erythrocyte sedimentation rate or lactate dehydrogenase, and more pain than in children with JIA.[143]

Treatment

Figure 97-2 is an algorithm showing the principles of treatment. Initial treatment should be with intra-articular injection with triamcinolone hexacetonide, 1 mg/kg large joints such as the knee and 0.5 mg/kg in smaller joints such as the ankle, given under sedation or general anesthetic for young children. Triamcinolone hexacetonide has been found to be superior to triamcinolone acetonide, beta-methasone, and methylprednisolone acetate in randomized controlled trials,[93,94] and early treatment is associated with better outcome.[95] Levels of proinflammatory factors, such as MIF, may predict response to intra-articular steroids.[79] If the arthritis recurs, joint injections can be repeated three times in a 12-month period. The response to a second joint injection is not predicted by the response of the first. NSAIDs should be given at adequate doses (see Table 97-2)[120] and may help control symptoms, but do not alter the natural history. There is little evidence base for differences between NSAIDs, and choice is usually made according to preferred dosing schedules, availability of liquid preparations, and patient preference.

When oligoarthritis is resistant to injections, a disease-modifying agent, such as methotrexate or an anti-TNF-α agent, should be used, especially when extended disease develops. Some physicians add a disease-modifying agent at the time of an injection of a hip or the temporomandibular joint because these are particularly prone to destruction. In addition, the hip and the temporomandibular joint are important for function and are hard to evaluate clinically when disease has been established. Rarely, synovectomy is required.

Physical therapy is required for all children with JIA, for stretches, muscle building, and consequent joint protection. Children who present late in the course of oligoarthritis already may have flexion contractures. Besides exercise and stretching, night splints and serial casting may be required. Serial casting is done two or three times a week for 1 month if needed, and is probably most effective when started just after joint injection. Some children with marked leg-length discrepancy (resulting from overgrowth of the affected knee) may require a shoe lift/raise. Screening for uveitis is compulsory for all cases of JIA. Uveitis is generally controlled with topical medications (glucocorticoids and mydriatics) and may require control of glaucoma. Where uveitis is resistant to topical therapy or side effects develop, methotrexate and anti-TNF-α agents can be effective.[137,144] Newer biologics, such as adalimumab, have been used when other agents have failed.[145] There are no data from randomized controlled trials of uveitis of JIA.

Outcome

Most children with oligoarthritis do well, and the disease remits in 68% in the persistent oligoarthritis subgroup.[6,132] About 30% to 50% of cases become extended oligoarthritis, and the outcome of this subtype is not as good; these patients have high cumulative times of active arthritis.[6] This picture has improved, however, since the introduction of methotrexate as the treatment of choice. Partial or complete remission is induced in 60% to 70% of patients on methotrexate in the extended oligoarticular group.[96,97,146] Anti-TNF-α agents are effective in many patients who fail to respond fully to methotrexate,[102] especially if given in combination with methotrexate. A continuing morbidity with poor outcome is visual loss, which is more frequent in children with significant eye involvement at the time of the first ophthalmologic visit. Other sequelae include leg-length discrepancy, especially in patients with knee arthritis, and muscle atrophy. Later morbidity can include other joint involvement, such as the temporomandibular joint. Long-term studies of adults treated before the use of biologic agents have shown that 50% of adults who had oligoarticular-onset JIA may have ongoing active disease, or functional problems, in adulthood.[8]

POLYARTHRITIS, RHEUMATOID FACTOR NEGATIVE

RF-negative polyarthritis is defined as arthritis affecting five or more joints in the first 6 months of disease, with a negative RF test.[3] Patients who meet the criteria for systemic arthritis, ERA, and psoriatic arthritis are excluded. Extended oligoarthritis, another subgroup with a polyarticular course, is distinguished from RF-negative polyarthritis by having five or more affected joints after only 6 months of disease. There is a risk of misclassifying these two groups if a patient's presentation is delayed, or progression of arthritis occurs around the time point of 6 months.

RF-negative polyarthritis constitutes 20% to 30% of new cases.[147] The British Paediatric Rheumatology National Diagnostic Register of 311 patients recorded a mean age of onset of 6.5 years for this subtype, with girls outnumbering boys by 3:1.[16] Age-related analysis reveals a bimodal distribution of onset, however, with one peak around 3.5 years and the other around 10 to 11 years.

Clinical Manifestations

Arthritis is usually insidious and can be symmetric or asymmetric, affecting large and small joints. Typically, small joint synovitis is distinct from adult rheumatoid arthritis (as noted by Still[1]) because it frequently involves proximal interphalangeal joints, but spares metacarpophalangeal joints at onset. The cervical spine and temporomandibular joint are often involved.[148,149] Some authors distinguish two clinical subgroups on the basis of ANA: (1) an ANA-positive group consisting of young girls (<6 years old) with an asymmetric-onset arthritis and at a high risk of uveitis, and (2) a slightly older group (7 to 9 years old) of ANA-negative patients having symmetric involvement of large and small joints.[150] Uveitis occurs in 5% to 20% of patients in the RF-negative polyarthritis JIA subtype, generally patients with few affected joints.[151]

Laboratory Features

Polyarthritis may be associated with elevated acute-phase reactants and mild anemia. The ANA test is positive in 40%, and the RF is negative by definition.

Differential Diagnosis

The differential diagnosis of RF-negative polyarthritis JIA includes other JIA subtypes, such as extended oligoarticular JIA, ERA, and psoriatic JIA. Other major diagnostic considerations include autoimmune connective tissue diseases such as systemic lupus erythematosus, particularly in older girls who are ANA positive, and lymphoma and leukemia. Septic polyarthritis is unusual, but *Neisseria gonorrhoeae* and Lyme disease can present in this way. ERA should be considered in particular in older boys (>6 years old; HLA-B27 testing is mandatory) (see later).

Treatment

Figure 97-3 is an algorithm showing the principles of treatment. Children with polyarthritis require a disease-modifying agent as soon as practically possible after the diagnosis has been confirmed. Methotrexate is typically the first agent of choice, but its slow onset of action may necessitate a short course of oral steroids, intravenous methylprednisolone, or multiple joint injections to control inflammation quickly and help reduce pain and stiffness. This initial rapid response to steroids also serves to gain the parents, and patient's confidence.

Most patients respond to methotrexate within 6 months, and nonresponders should be considered for the use of anti-TNF-α agents by this time.[96,102] If anti-TNF-α therapy is begun, methotrexate can be continued because half of methotrexate nonresponders show a late response. The combination of methotrexate and etanercept has been shown more recently to be the only combination that prevents bony erosion in adults with RA (see Chapter 67).[152] Sulfasalazine and leflunomide are still used in some centers before starting an anti-TNF-α agent in mild disease, although evidence suggests that leflunomide may be slightly less effective than methotrexate.[99] As described in the section on principles of treatment of JIA, JIA with a polyarticular course of any type that does not respond well to methotrexate or etanercept is now increasingly being treated with a range of newer biologics. Physical therapy is required, as for all children with JIA, for stretches, muscle building, and consequent joint protection. Children with hand involvement need occupational therapy assessment and input.

Outcome

Approximately 30% of children go into long-term remission; the chance of remission is highest in the first 5 years of disease.[6,53] Symmetric arthritis and early hand involvement predicted future disability and poorer overall well-being.[153] Final height maybe reduced, but usually much less than in patients with systemic arthritis.

POLYARTHRITIS, RHEUMATOID FACTOR POSITIVE

RF-positive polyarticular JIA is defined as arthritis affecting five or more joints in the first 6 months of disease and a positive RF test on two occasions at least 3 months apart. RF-positive polyarthritis constitutes 5% to 10% of cases under the juvenile rheumatoid arthritis or juvenile chronic arthritis classifications.[154] In the JIA classification, RF testing is crucial to avoid large numbers of children with polyarthritis being unclassifiable.[11] RF-positive polyarthritis is more common in girls, with reported female-to-male ratios of 5.7 to 12.8,[16,155] and can be considered as part of the spectrum of rheumatoid arthritis, sharing immunogenetic and serologic factors. HLA-DRB1*0401 is strongly associated,

and the HLA-DRB1*0401 DQA1*03 DQB1*03 haplotype carries an increased odds ratio of 3.9 for this subtype, yet is protective for other subtypes of JIA.[29] Anti–cyclic citrullinated peptide antibodies have been reported in 57% to 73% of this JIA subtype.[156,157] Disease expression differs from adults, perhaps because of the effects of environmental factors, the effects of arthritis on a growing body, and the psychosocial impact of chronic disease during adolescence, which is itself a period of significant change in an individual's independence and self-identity.

Clinical Manifestations

The arthritis is typically an aggressive, symmetric polyarthritis affecting the small joints of the hands, typically the proximal interphalangeal joints, metacarpophalangeal joints, and wrists, and with a large joint involvement in a pattern that resembles rheumatoid arthritis. Children frequently have more than 30 joints with arthritis. At onset, low-grade fever may be present, but it is distinctly different from systemic JIA. Felty's syndrome (splenomegaly and leukopenia) (see Chapter 66) can occur in childhood RF-positive polyarthritis. Rheumatoid nodules occur in 10% of cases, most frequently around the elbow. Other extra-articular manifestations are reported less often than in adults. Uveitis is an unusual feature of this subtype.

Laboratory Features

Polyarthritis may be associated with elevated acute-phase reactants and anemia (normocytic, normochromic). The ANA test is positive in a few cases, and the RF is by definition positive on two occasions 3 months apart. Similar to adult rheumatoid arthritis, RF testing typically detects IgM-anti-IgG. In these patients, anti–cyclic citrullinated peptide antibodies may be more specific and as in adults are associated with erosive arthritis.[157]

Differential Diagnosis

The differential diagnosis of RF-positive polyarthritis JIA includes other JIA subtypes, especially when there is no confirmed RF-positive test on two occasions. Such cases are frequently unclassified in the JIA system; however, management and therapy are unaffected.

Treatment

Figure 97-3 is an algorithm showing the principles of treatment. Children with RF-positive polyarthritis are at high risk of prolonged erosive arthritis and require a disease-modifying agent at the time of diagnosis. Methotrexate has proven efficacy and should be given at 10 to 15 mg/m²/wk, if possible by the parenteral route.[96] In view of the now well-established evidence in rheumatoid arthritis (see Chapter 67), clinicians need to consider the use of combination therapy of an anti-TNF-α agent with methotrexate because this has been shown to be superior to methotrexate alone in the prevention of bony erosions.[152] Although most data exist for etanercept, a more recent randomized controlled trial of infliximab plus methotrexate suggested benefit from this combination.[105] Data from children treated with anti-TNF-α and methotrexate are beginning to emerge from postmarketing surveillance registries.[158] Some children benefit from multiple joint injections to maintain control of the arthritis, and all require physical and occupational therapy.

Outcome

Children with RF-positive polyarthritis have a poor long-term prognosis compared with the other JIA subgroups. In a study of 437 children with JIA with at least 4 years of follow-up, 65% of RF-positive polyarthritis patients achieved clinical remission on treatment, but only 5% maintained remission 12 months after cessation of medications, an outlook that was markedly worse than other subgroups.[6] In long-term follow-up studies, patients with RF-positive polyarthritis were more likely to have a poorer Steinbrocker functional class health assessment questionnaire score, major arthritis-related surgery, and active erosive disease; patients with RF-negative polyarthritis had a similar functional outcome to systemic patients, which was better than the outcome of patients with RF-positive polyarthritis, but significantly worse than persistent oligoarthritis patients.[9,159,160]

PSORIATIC ARTHRITIS

Psoriatic JIA is defined as the combination of arthritis and psoriasis, or arthritis and at least two of the following: dactylitis, nail abnormalities (two or more nail pits, or onycholysis), or family history of psoriasis in a first-degree relative. The earlier proposed ILAR classification[2] included second-degree relatives with psoriasis, but this was believed to classify too many cases incorrectly.[161,162] A full family history is crucial, and without this children may be misclassified.[161]

Psoriatic JIA represents 2% to 15% of all JIA.[11,15] In the United States, it is more common in whites than other racial groups; approximately 90% of patients are white. Girls are slightly more affected than boys, and the typical age of onset is 7 to 10 years, with psoriasis typically occurring within 2 years of the onset of arthritis, although it can follow arthritis by many years. The specific etiology is unknown, but there is a strong genetic component with 40% of patients with psoriasis having an affected relative, and several candidate HLA and non-HLA genes have been identified (see Chapter 72).[29] More recent data from adults have implicated the newly identified IL-17-secreting T cells (Th17) and related cytokine IL-22 in the pathogenesis of psoriasis.[163]

Clinical Manifestations

Arthritis is typically asymmetric and can involve large joints (commonly knees and ankles) and small joints, classically dactylitis, more commonly in the feet than in the hands, and distal interphalangeal joints. The total number of joints generally is limited, and children frequently follow an oligoarticular course. Psoriatic JIA is associated with uveitis in 15% of children. These features are typical of oligoarthritis, and many children are first classified as having oligoarticular JIA before psoriasis is manifest in the child or relative. A more recent study of childhood psoriatic arthritis argued for two distinct subpopulations. Using cluster analysis, the authors identified a younger group, median age 2.7 years, ANA-positive with a female preponderance, all of whom had dactylitis.

The older group, median age 9.5 years, were more likely to have oligoarthritis and had higher remission rates.[164] Although many adults with psoriatic arthritis have features of a spondyloarthropathy, such as sacroiliitis or enthesitis, in the JIA classification these children are classified as having ERA (see later), or, if they have psoriasis, are unclassified.

Laboratory Features

Children with psoriatic arthritis may have mild elevation of the erythrocyte sedimentation rate, C-reactive protein, and platelets, and a mild anemia of chronic disease. The ANA test is positive in half of children with psoriatic arthritis. RF is negative by definition.

Differential Diagnosis

Children with psoriatic arthritis are frequently misdiagnosed as having oligoarticular JIA if the history of psoriasis in the child or first-degree relatives is not sought. Exclusions include a positive IgM RF on more than one occasion 3 months apart, HLA-B27 if in a boy with onset after the 6th birthday, and any of the following: ERA, sacroiliitis with inflammatory bowel disease, Reiter's syndrome, or acute anterior uveitis, or a history of one of these disorders in a first-degree relative, or systemic features.

Treatment

The treatment is similar to oligoarthritis (see Fig. 97-2); intra-articular corticosteroid injections are beneficial for patients with limited arthritis (see section on general principles of medical management of JIA). NSAIDs help with symptoms, such as morning stiffness, but do not alter the long-term outcome. Methotrexate is beneficial for the skin psoriasis and arthritis and, when used in children, is recommended as a single weekly dose rather than split doses more commonly used by dermatologists for psoriasis alone.[165] In children with more aggressive disease, anti-TNF-α therapy is indicated and may limit bony destruction significantly. Oral corticosteroids are rarely needed. Regular screening for uveitis is compulsory, and management is as for oligoarticular JIA (see section on oligoarthritis).

Outcome

There are few long-term outcome data of psoriatic JIA defined by the ILAR criteria. In a retrospective review of 63 patients with juvenile psoriatic arthritis diagnosed using the Vancouver criteria (i.e., including HLA-B27-associated disease and accepting psoriatic-like skin rash instead of physician-diagnosed psoriasis), 40% had ongoing active disease, and 8% had severe functional limitations after a mean follow-up of 7 years.[166] The uveitis of psoriatic arthritis, similar to that of oligoarticular disease, is insidious and painless and can lead to blindness if untreated, so close monitoring is indicated.

ENTHESITIS-RELATED ARTHRITIS

ERA is a subtype that has replaced, but is not exactly overlapping with, previous definitions in children such as juvenile ankylosing spondylitis or syndrome of seronegative enthesitis arthritis.[167] ERA is defined as arthritis and enthesitis, or arthritis or enthesitis with at least two of the following: (1) sacroiliac joint tenderness, or inflammatory lumbosacral pain; (2) positive HLA-B27; (3) onset of arthritis in a boy 6 years old or older; (4) acute anterior symptomatic uveitis; or (5) history of ankylosing spondylitis, ERA, sacroiliitis with inflammatory bowel disease, Reiter's syndrome, or acute anterior uveitis in a first-degree relative. Exclusions include psoriasis in a first-degree relative, systemic features, and a positive IgM RF on more than one occasion 3 months apart.

This form of JIA is more frequent in boys (male-to-female ratio of syndrome of seronegative enthesitis arthritis 7:1), although in some geographic areas it may be underrecognized in symptomatic girls, who can have milder disease with less axial skeleton involvement.[168] The onset is typically in boys older than 6 years (commonly preteen or teenage) with peripheral arthritis affecting large joints, and there is a familial predilection. ERA is generally thought to be a form of spondyloarthropathy and has a strong association with HLA-B27. In patients who have the HLA-B27 gene, mechanisms may parallel those in adults with ankylosing spondylitis (see Chapter 70). There is overlap in terms of genetic factors and putative causative factors with reactive arthritis, although children with reactive arthritis are excluded from the ILAR criteria for JIA.

Clinical Manifestations

A typical feature of ERA is the presence of enthesitis (i.e., inflammation of the tendons and ligaments where they attach to bone [the enthesis]). The typical sites are the inferior pole of the patella, Achilles' tendon, and plantar fascia insertions into the calcaneus. Not all entheses are equally significant in ERA, and some are prone to mechanical damage in other pediatric conditions, such as in Osgood-Schlatter disease. Metatarsalgia is common in children and should not count as enthesitis. The arthritis of ERA typically affects the hips, knees, or ankles, and may be symmetric or asymmetric. Joints are painful and stiff, sometimes with night pain. At onset, spinal symptoms are rare, but in a subgroup of children with ERA progress to features more typical of adult ankylosing spondylitis with sacroiliac joint and spinal inflammation. This progression is more likely in boys, who are HLA-B27 positive and have spinal or sacroiliac joint pain within 1 year of diagnosis.[169] ERA is associated with an acute anterior uveitis, which typically presents as an acutely red, painful eye and needs immediate medical attention because if untreated it may lead to blindness (see Chapter 46).

Laboratory Features

There is no defining laboratory test, although HLA-B27 is present in 80% to 90% of cases and helps establish this diagnosis. The erythrocyte sedimentation rate may be mildly or markedly increased, and there may be a mild anemia, but these also should raise the suspicion that the patient may have subclinical inflammatory bowel disease. RF is negative by definition; ANA may be positive. Ultrasound can distinguish enthesitis.

Differential Diagnosis

Some children with prolonged reactive arthritis, or arthritis associated with inflammatory bowel disease, have enthesitis and would be classified as having ERA if the infective agent were not identified, or until inflammatory bowel disease is discovered. Other conditions that may mimic ERA include reactive arthritis in children and pain syndromes; children with widespread amplified musculoskeletal pain may have very tender entheses that can be mistaken for enthesitis.

Treatment

Treatment of ERA is similar to that for oligoarthritis and polyarthritis (see Figs. 97-2 and 97-3). Most patients respond to intra-articular corticosteroid injections, but many need a disease-modifying antirheumatic drug and respond well to sulfasalazine or methotrexate, although there has been no comparison of the two agents in children.[170] If disease is severe, a course of intravenous pulse methylprednisolone is often helpful. Children with enthesitis require an NSAID for symptomatic relief. Many physicians empirically favor certain NSAIDs for enthesitis, specifically diclofenac and indomethacin. Occasionally, corticosteroid injection of the plantar fascial insertion on the calcaneus is helpful or, for a limited time, oral steroids. Physical therapy is central to management (as for all JIA), and orthotics and shoe modification can help greatly. These measures have not proved to modify the course of disease significantly, in particular, axial and spinal inflammation.

In open label studies, the anti-TNF-α agents infliximab and etanercept have been shown to be effective agents for axial disease.[171,172] Anti-TNF-α agents should be used early in the course of axial disease, before irreversible damage from spinal erosion and fusion occurs. Anti-TNF-α agents also are associated with improvement in peripheral arthritis and enthesitis.[172]

Outcome

Long-term outcome of ERA is unknown, but a proportion of these children progress to the adult form of ankylosing spondylitis. Enthesitis can be more symptomatic in teens and young adults and improves with age. Spinal and sacroiliac joint involvement in teenagers, if left untreated, can lead to ankylosis, as in adults. Boys with HLA-B27 and hip arthritis are at higher risk of developing progressive spinal involvement.

UNCLASSIFIED JUVENILE IDIOPATHIC ARTHRITIS

Because of the exclusion criteria within the ILAR classification, strict adherence to the ILAR system leads to some children being defined as unclassifiable[173,174]; this is distinct from the previous European League Against Rheumatism or American College of Rheumatology criteria for juvenile arthritis, which did not include an unclassified group. The unclassified cases are patients who are defined as not having fulfilled sufficient inclusion criteria for any category or are excluded by fulfilling criteria for more than one category. A child in the oligoarthritis subgroup would be excluded if he or she had a family history of psoriasis in a first-degree relative. Although this system caused considerable controversy when proposed, it is based on the premise that classification is primarily a research tool, and so the provision of an undifferentiated category would offer greater homogeneity for the remaining subgroups.

For clinical purposes, treatment of such children follows the same guidelines as outlined earlier. Ultimately, the system for classifying JIA reflects current understanding of the disease's pathophysiology. As this knowledge improves, future revisions would be increasingly useful in a clinical setting because patient categorization would offer accurate predictions of clinical response and prognosis.

CONCLUSION

The modern treatment of JIA involves a range of specialists. Early use of one of numerous disease-modifying agents can suppress disease activity in many cases. Pediatric rheumatologists have in their favor the remarkable capacity for childhood growth and development to allow repair and restoration of function, in contrast to adults with inflammatory arthritis. A persistent block to good outcome in many areas of the world is a delay in recognition or diagnosis of JIA. When JIA is recognized, children who receive active treatment through a multidisciplinary approach should have an improving prognosis in the years to come. The advent of new biologic therapies and rapid translation of basic research into therapeutic strategies and an increased willingness on the part of regulatory bodies to make new therapies available to children should combine to continue to improve the outlook for children with arthritis.

REFERENCES

1. Still GF: On a form of arthritis in children. Med Chir Trans 80:47, 1897. Reprinted in Arch Dis Child 16:156-165, 1941.
2. Petty RE, Southwood TR, Baum J, et al: Revision of the proposed classification criteria for juvenile idiopathic arthritis: Durban, 1997. J Rheumatol 25:1991-1994, 1998.
3. **Petty RE, Southwood TR, Manners P, et al: International League of Associations for Rheumatology classification of juvenile idiopathic arthritis: Second revision, Edmonton, 2001. J Rheumatol 31:390-392, 2004.**
4. Southwood TR: Classification of childhood arthritis. In Szer IS, Kimura Y, Malleson PN, Southwood TR (eds): Arthritis in Children and Adolescents. 2006, pp 205-209.
5. Petty RE: Growing pains: The ILAR classification of juvenile idiopathic arthritis. J Rheumatol 28:927-928, 2001.
6. Wallace CA, Huang B, Bandeira M, et al: Patterns of clinical remission in select categories of juvenile idiopathic arthritis. Arthritis Rheum 52:3554-3562, 2005.
7. Gutierrez-Suarez R, Pistorio A, Cespedes Cruz A, et al: Health-related quality of life of patients with juvenile idiopathic arthritis coming from 3 different geographic areas: The PRINTO multinational quality of life cohort study. Rheumatology 46:314-320, 2007.
8. Packham JC, Hall MA: Long-term follow-up of 246 adults with juvenile idiopathic arthritis: Functional outcome. Rheumatology 41:1428-1435, 2002.
9. Foster HE, Marshall N, Myers A, et al: Outcome in adults with juvenile idiopathic arthritis: A quality of life study. Arthritis Rheum 48:767-775, 2003.
10. Cassidy JT: Juvenile rheumatoid arthritis. In: Kelley's Textbook of Rheumatology 7th ed. Philadelphia, WB Saunders, pp 1579-1596.
11. **Berntson L, Andersson Gare B, Fasth A, et al: Incidence of juvenile idiopathic arthritis in the Nordic countries: A population based study with special reference to the validity of the ILAR and EULAR criteria. J Rheumatol 30:2275-2282, 2003.**
12. Woo P: Systemic juvenile idiopathic arthritis: Diagnosis, management, and outcome. Nat Clin Pract Rheumatol 2:28-34, 2006.
13. Towner SR, Michet CJ Jr, O'Fallon WM, et al: The epidemiology of juvenile arthritis in Rochester, Minnesota 1960-1979. Arthritis Rheum 26:1208-1213, 1983.
14. Denardo BA, Tucker LB, Miller LC, et al: Demography of a regional pediatric rheumatology patient population. Affiliated Children's Arthritis Centers of New England. J Rheumatol 21:1553-1561, 1994.
15. Malleson PN, Fung MY, Rosenberg AM: The incidence of pediatric rheumatic diseases: results from the Canadian Pediatric Rheumatology Association Disease Registry. J Rheumatol 23:1981-1987, 1996.
16. Symmons DP, Jones M, Osborne J, et al: Pediatric rheumatology in the United Kingdom: Data from the British Paediatric Rheumatology Group National Diagnostic Register. J Rheumatol 23:1975-1980, 1996.
17. Moe N, Rygg M: Epidemiology of juvenile chronic arthritis in northern Norway: A ten-year retrospective study. Clin Exp Rheumatol 16:99-101, 1998.
18. Manners PJ, Diepeveen DA: Prevalence of juvenile chronic arthritis in a population of 12-year-old children in urban Australia. Pediatrics 98:84-90, 1996.
19. Fujikawa S, Okuni M: A nationwide surveillance study of rheumatic diseases among Japanese children. Acta Paediatr Jpn 39:242-244, 1997.
20. Saurenmann RK, Rose JB, Tyrrell P, et al: Epidemiology of juvenile idiopathic arthritis in a multiethnic cohort: Ethnicity as a risk factor. Arthritis Rheum 56:1974-1984, 2007.
21. Ansell BM, Bywaters EG, Lawrence JS: Familial aggregation and twin studies in Still's disease: Juvenile chronic polyarthritis. Rheumatology 2:37–61, 1969.
22. Prahalad S, Ryan MH, Shear ES, et al: Twins concordant for juvenile rheumatoid arthritis. Arthritis Rheum 43:2611-2612, 2000.
23. Moroldo MB, Chaudhari M, Shear E, et al: Juvenile rheumatoid arthritis affected sibpairs: Extent of clinical phenotype concordance. Arthritis Rheum 50:1928-1934, 2004.
24. Prahalad S, Shear ES, Thompson SD, et al: Increased prevalence of familial autoimmunity in simplex and multiplex families with juvenile rheumatoid arthritis. Arthritis Rheum 46:1851-1856, 2002.
25. Prahalad S: Genetics of juvenile idiopathic arthritis: An update. Curr Opin Rheumatol 16:588-594, 2004.
26. Thompson SD, Moroldo MB, Guyer L, et al: A genome-wide scan for juvenile rheumatoid arthritis in affected sibpair families provides evidence of linkage. Arthritis Rheum 50:2920-2930, 2004.
27. Edmonds J, Metzger A, Terasaki P, et al: Proceedings: HL-A antigen W27 in juvenile chronic polyarthritis. Ann Rheum Dis 33:576, 1974.
28. Brunner HI, Ivaskova E, Haas JP, et al: Class I associations and frequencies of class II HLA-DRB alleles by RFLP analysis in children with rheumatoid-factor-negative juvenile chronic arthritis. Rheumatol Int 13:83-88, 1993.
29. **Thomson W, Barrett JH, Donn R, et al: Juvenile idiopathic arthritis classified by the ILAR criteria: HLA associations in UK patients. Rheumatology 41:1183-1189, 2002.**
30. Donn RP, Ollier WE: Juvenile chronic arthritis—a time for change? Eur J Immunogenet 23:245-260, 1996.
31. Prahalad S, Glass DN: Is juvenile rheumatoid arthritis/juvenile idiopathic arthritis different from rheumatoid arthritis? Arthritis Res Ther 4(Suppl 3):303-310, 2002.
32. Donn RP, Thomson W, Pepper L, et al: Antinuclear antibodies in early onset pauciarticular juvenile chronic arthritis (JCA) are associated with HLA-DQB1*0603: A possible JCA-associated human leucocyte antigen haplotype. Br J Rheumatol 34:461-465, 1995.
33. Paul C, Schoenwald U, Truckenbrodt H, et al: HLA-DP/DR interaction in early onset pauciarticular juvenile chronic arthritis. Immunogenetics 37:442-448, 1993.
34. Murray KJ, Moroldo MB, Donnelly P, et al: Age specific (susceptibility and protection) for JRA-associated HLA alleles. Arthritis Rheum 42:1843-1853, 1999.
35. Zeggini E, Thomson W, Kwiatkowski D, et al: Linkage and association studies of single-nucleotide polymorphism-tagged tumor necrosis factor haplotypes in juvenile oligoarthritis. Arthritis Rheum 46:3304-3311, 2002.
36. Woo P: Cytokines in childhood rheumatic diseases. Arch Dis Child 69:547-549, 1993.
37. De Benedetti F, Martini A: Is systemic juvenile rheumatoid arthritis an interleukin 6 mediated disease? J Rheumatol 25:203-207, 1998.

38. Fishman D, Faulds G, Jeffery R, et al: The effect of novel polymorphisms in the interleukin-6 (IL-6) gene on IL-6 transcription and plasma IL-6 levels, and an association with systemic-onset juvenile chronic arthritis. J Clin Invest 102:1369-1376, 1998.

39. Ogilvie EM, Fife MS, Thompson SD, et al: The −174G allele of the interleukin-6 gene confers susceptibility to systemic arthritis in children: A multicenter study using simplex and multiplex juvenile idiopathic arthritis families. Arthritis Rheum 48:3202-3206, 2003.

40. Fife MS, Ogilvie EM, Kelberman D, et al: Novel IL-6 haplotypes and disease association. Genes Immun 6:367-370, 2005.

41. Donn R, Alourfi Z, Zeggini E, et al: A functional promoter haplotype of macrophage migration inhibitory factor is linked and associated with juvenile idiopathic arthritis. Arthritis Rheum 50:1604-1610, 2004.

42. De Benedetti F, Meazza C, Vivarelli M, et al: Functional and prognostic relevance of the −173 polymorphism of the macrophage migration inhibitory factor gene in systemic-onset juvenile idiopathic arthritis. Arthritis Rheum 48:1398-1407, 2003.

43. Crawley E, Kay R, Sillibourne J, et al: Polymorphic haplotypes of the interleukin-10 5′ flanking region determine variable interleukin-10 transcription and are associated with particular phenotypes of juvenile rheumatoid arthritis. Arthritis Rheum 42:1101-1118, 1999.

44. Fife MS, Gutierrez A, Ogilvie EM, et al: Novel IL10 gene family associations with systemic juvenile idiopathic arthritis. Arthritis Res Ther 8:R148, 2006.

45. Hinks A, Barton A, John S, et al: Association between the PTPN22 gene and rheumatoid arthritis and juvenile idiopathic arthritis in a UK population: Further support that PTPN22 is an autoimmunity gene. Arthritis Rheum 52:1694-1699, 2005.

46. Seldin MF, Shigeta R, Laiho K, et al: Finnish case-control and family studies support PTPN22 R620W polymorphism as a risk factor in rheumatoid arthritis, but suggest only minimal or no effect in juvenile idiopathic arthritis. Genes Immun 6:720-722, 2005.

47. Nielsen HE, Dorup J, Herlin T, et al: Epidemiology of juvenile chronic arthritis: Risk dependent on sibship, parental income, and housing. J Rheumatol 26:1600-1605, 1999.

48. Jaakkola JJ, Gissler M: Maternal smoking in pregnancy as a determinant of rheumatoid arthritis and other inflammatory polyarthropathies during the first 7 years of life. Int J Epidemiol 34:664-671, 2005.

49. Pugh MT, Southwood TR, Gaston JS: The role of infection in juvenile chronic arthritis. Br J Rheumatol 32:838-844, 1993.

50. Hokynar K, Brunstein J, Soderlund-Venermo M, et al: Integrity and full coding sequence of B19 virus DNA persisting in human synovial tissue. J Gen Virol 81:1017-1025, 2000.

51. Gonzalez B, Larranaga C, Leon O, et al: Parvovirus B19 may have a role in the pathogenesis of juvenile idiopathic arthritis. J Rheumatol 34:1336-1340, 2007.

52. Pritchard MH, Matthews N, Munro J: Antibodies to influenza A in a cluster of children with juvenile chronic arthritis. Br J Rheumatol 27:176-180, 1988.

53. Oen K, Fast M, Postl B: Epidemiology of juvenile rheumatoid arthritis in Manitoba, Canada, 1975-92: Cycles in incidence. J Rheumatol 22:745-750, 1995.

54. Uziel Y, Pomeranz A, Brik R, et al: Seasonal variation in systemic onset juvenile rheumatoid arthritis in Israel. J Rheumatol 26:1187-1189, 1999.

55. Prakken AB, van Hoeij MJ, Kuis W, et al: T-cell reactivity to human HSP60 in oligo-articular juvenile chronic arthritis is associated with a favorable prognosis and the generation of regulatory cytokines in the inflamed joint. Immunol Lett 57:139-142, 1997.

56. de Kleer IM, Kamphuis SM, Rijkers GT, et al: The spontaneous remission of juvenile idiopathic arthritis is characterized by CD30+ T cells directed to human heat-shock protein 60 capable of producing the regulatory cytokine interleukin-10. Arthritis Rheum 48:2001-2010, 2003.

57. Bywaters EG: Pathologic aspects of juvenile chronic polyarthritis. Arthritis Rheum 20:271-276, 1977.

58. Murray KJ, Luyrink L, Grom AA, et al: Immunohistological characteristics of T cell infiltrates in different forms of childhood onset chronic arthritis. J Rheumatol 23:2116-2124, 1996.

59. Wedderburn LR, Robinson N, Patel A, et al: Selective recruitment of polarized T cells expressing CCR5 and CXCR3 to the inflamed joints of children with juvenile idiopathic arthritis. Arthritis Rheum 43:765-774, 2000.

60. Chan AT, Kollnberger SD, Wedderburn LR, et al: Expansion and enhanced survival of natural killer cells expressing the killer immunoglobulin-like receptor KIR3DL2 in spondylarthritis. Arthritis Rheum 52:3586-3595, 2005.

61. Gregorio A, Gambini C, Gerloni V, et al: Lymphoid neogenesis in juvenile idiopathic arthritis correlates with ANA positivity and plasma cells infiltration. Rheumatology 46:308-313, 2007.

62. Vignola S, Picco P, Falcini F, et al: Serum and synovial fluid concentration of vascular endothelial growth factor in juvenile idiopathic arthritides. Rheumatology 41:691-696, 2002.

63. Barnes MG, Aronow BJ, Luyrink LK, et al: Gene expression in juvenile arthritis and spondyloarthropathy: Pro-angiogenic ELR+ chemokine genes relate to course of arthritis. Rheumatology 43:973-979, 2004.

64. De Benedetti F, Pignatti P, Bernasconi S, et al: Interleukin 8 and monocyte chemoattractant protein-1 in patients with juvenile rheumatoid arthritis: Relation to onset types, disease activity, and synovial fluid leukocytes. J Rheumatol 26:425-431, 1999.

65. Pharoah DS, Varsani H, Tatham RW, et al: Expression of the inflammatory chemokines CCL5, CCL3 and CXCL10 in juvenile idiopathic arthritis, and demonstration of CCL5 production by an atypical subset of CD8+ T cells. Arthritis Res Ther 8:R50-R60, 2006.

66. Yao TC, Kuo ML, See LC, et al: RANTES and monocyte chemoattractant protein 1 as sensitive markers of disease activity in patients with juvenile rheumatoid arthritis: A six-year longitudinal study. Arthritis Rheum 54:2585-2593, 2006.

67. de Jager W, Hoppenreijs EP, Wulffraat NM, et al: Blood and synovial fluid cytokine signatures in patients with juvenile idiopathic arthritis: A cross-sectional study. Ann Rheum Dis 66:589-598, 2007.

68. Aggarwal A, Agarwal S, Misra R: Chemokine and chemokine receptor analysis reveals elevated interferon-inducible protein-10 (IP)-10/CXCL10 levels and increased number of CCR5+ and CXCR3+ CD4 T cells in synovial fluid of patients with enthesitis-related arthritis (ERA). Clin Exp Immunol 148:515-519, 2007.

69. Black AP, Bhayani H, Ryder CA, et al: T-cell activation without proliferation in juvenile idiopathic arthritis. Arthritis Res 4:177-183, 2002.

70. Gattorno M, Prigione I, Morandi F, et al: Phenotypic and functional characterisation of CCR7+ and CCR7− CD4+ memory T cells homing to the joints in juvenile idiopathic arthritis. Arthritis Res Ther 7:R256-R267, 2005.

71. Wedderburn LR, Maini MK, Patel A, et al: Molecular fingerprinting reveals non-overlapping T cell oligoclonality between an inflamed site and peripheral blood. Int Immunol 11:535-543, 1999.

72. Wedderburn LR, Patel A, Varsani H, et al: Divergence in the degree of clonal expansions in inflammatory T cell subpopulations mirrors HLA-associated risk alleles in genetically and clinically distinct subtypes of childhood arthritis. Int Immunol 13:1541-1550, 2001.

73. Gattorno M, Facchetti P, Ghiotto F, et al: Synovial fluid T cell clones from oligoarticular juvenile arthritis patients display a prevalent Th1/Th0 pattern of cytokine secretion irrespective of immunophenotype. Clin Exp Immunol 109:4-11, 1997.

74. Scola MP, Thompson SD, Brunner HI, et al: Interferon-gamma:interleukin 4 ratios and associated type 1 cytokine expression in juvenile rheumatoid arthritis synovial tissue. J Rheumatol 29:369-378, 2002.

75. Nistala K, Moncrieffe H, Newton KR, et al: IL-17-producing T cells are enriched in the joints of children with arthritis, but have a reciprocal relationship to regulatory T cells numbers. Arthritis Rheum 58:875-887, 2008.

76. De Benedetti F, Pignatti P, Gerloni V, et al: Differences in synovial fluid cytokine levels between juvenile and adult rheumatoid arthritis. J Rheumatol 24:1403-1409, 1997.

77. Woo P: Cytokines and juvenile idiopathic arthritis. Curr Rheumatol Rep 4:452-457, 2002.

78. Rooney M, David J, Symons J, et al: Inflammatory cytokine responses in juvenile chronic arthritis. Br J Rheumatol 34:454-460, 1995.

79. Meazza C, Travaglino P, Pignatti P, et al: Macrophage migration inhibitory factor in patients with juvenile idiopathic arthritis. Arthritis Rheum 46:232-237, 2002.

80. Pascual V, Allantaz F, Arce E, et al: Role of interleukin-1 (IL-1) in the pathogenesis of systemic onset juvenile idiopathic arthritis and clinical response to IL-1 blockade. J Exp Med 201:1479-1486, 2005.

81. **de Kleer IM, Wedderburn LR, Taams LS, et al: CD4+CD25(bright) regulatory T cells actively regulate inflammation in the joints of patients with the remitting form of juvenile idiopathic arthritis. J Immunol 172:6435-6443, 2004.**

82. Varsani H, Patel A, van Kooyk Y, et al: Synovial dendritic cells in juvenile idiopathic arthritis (JIA) express receptor activator of NF-kappaB (RANK). Rheumatology 42:583-590, 2003.

83. Gattorno M, Chicha L, Gregorio A, et al: Enrichment of plasmacytoid dendritic cells in synovial fluid of juvenile idiopathic arthritis. Arthritis Rheum 48:S101, 2003.

84. Foell D, Wittkowski H, Hammerschmidt I, et al: Monitoring neutrophil activation in juvenile rheumatoid arthritis by S100A12 serum concentrations. Arthritis Rheum 50:1286-1295, 2004.

85. Jarvis JN, Petty HR, Tang Y, et al: Evidence for chronic, peripheral activation of neutrophils in polyarticular juvenile rheumatoid arthritis. Arthritis Res Ther 8:R154, 2006.

86. Jarvis JN, Dozmorov I, Jiang K, et al: Novel approaches to gene expression analysis of active polyarticular juvenile rheumatoid arthritis. Arthritis Res Ther 6:R15-R32, 2004.

87. Ogilvie EM, Khan A, Hubank M, et al: Specific gene expression profiles in systemic juvenile idiopathic arthritis. Arthritis Rheum 56:1954-1965, 2007.

88. Allantaz F, Chaussabel D, Stichweh D, et al: Blood leukocyte microarrays to diagnose systemic onset juvenile idiopathic arthritis and follow the response to IL-1 blockade. J Exp Med 204:2131-2144, 2007.

89. Gibson DS, Blelock S, Brockbank S, et al: Proteomic analysis of recurrent joint inflammation in juvenile idiopathic arthritis. J Proteome Res 5:1988-1995, 2006.

90. Foster HE, Eltringham MS, Kay LJ, et al: Delay in access to appropriate care for children presenting with musculoskeletal symptoms and ultimately diagnosed with juvenile idiopathic arthritis. Arthritis Rheum 57:921-927, 2007.

91. Peterson LS, Mason T, Nelson AM, et al: Psychosocial outcomes and health status of adults who have had juvenile rheumatoid arthritis: A controlled, population-based study. Arthritis Rheum 40:2235-2240, 1997.

92. Blum RW, Garell D, Hodgman CH, et al: Transition from child-centered to adult health-care systems for adolescents with chronic conditions. A position paper of the Society for Adolescent Medicine. J Adolesc Health 14:570-576, 1993.

93. Balogh Z, Ruzsonyi E: Triamcinolone hexacetonide versus betamethasone: A double-blind comparative study of the long-term effects of intra-articular steroids in patients with juvenile chronic arthritis. Scand J Rheumatol Suppl 67:80-82, 1987.

94. **Zulian F, Martini G, Gobber D, et al: Triamcinolone acetonide and hexacetonide intra-articular treatment of symmetrical joints in juvenile idiopathic arthritis: A double-blind trial. Rheumatology 43:1288-1291, 2004.**

95. Lepore L, Del Santo M, Malorgio C, et al: Treatment of juvenile idiopathic arthritis with intra-articular triamcinolone hexacetonide: Evaluation of clinical effectiveness correlated with circulating ANA and T gamma/delta + and B CD5+ lymphocyte populations of synovial fluid. Clin Exp Rheumatol 20:719-722, 2002.

96. **Ruperto N, Murray KJ, Gerloni V, et al: A randomized trial of parenteral methotrexate comparing an intermediate dose with a higher dose in children with juvenile idiopathic arthritis who failed to respond to standard doses of methotrexate. Arthritis Rheum 50:2191-2201, 2004.**

97. **Woo P, Southwood TR, Prieur AM, et al: Randomized, placebo-controlled, crossover trial of low-dose oral methotrexate in children with extended oligoarticular or systemic arthritis. Arthritis Rheum 43:1849-1857, 2000.**

98. Ramanan AV, Whitworth P, Baildam EM: Use of methotrexate in juvenile idiopathic arthritis. Arch Dis Child 88:197-200, 2003.

99. Silverman E, Mouy R, Spiegel L, et al: Leflunomide or methotrexate for juvenile rheumatoid arthritis. N Engl J Med 352:1655-1666, 2005.

100. van Rossum MA, Fiselier TJ, Franssen MJ, et al: Sulfasalazine in the treatment of juvenile chronic arthritis: A randomized, double-blind, placebo-controlled, multicenter study. Dutch Juvenile Chronic Arthritis Study Group. Arthritis Rheum 41:808-816, 1998.

101. van Rossum MA, van Soesbergen RM, Boers M, et al: Long-term outcome of juvenile idiopathic arthritis following a placebo-controlled trial: Sustained benefits of early sulfasalazine treatment. Ann Rheum Dis 66:1518-1524, 2007.

102. **Lovell DJ, Giannini EH, Reiff A, et al: Etanercept in children with polyarticular juvenile rheumatoid arthritis. Pediatric Rheumatology Collaborative Study Group. N Engl J Med 342:763-769, 2000.**

103. Quartier P, Taupin P, Bourdeaut F, et al: Efficacy of etanercept for the treatment of juvenile idiopathic arthritis according to the onset type. Arthritis Rheum 48:1093-1101, 2003.

104. Lovell DJ, Giannini EH, Reiff A, et al: Long-term efficacy and safety of etanercept in children with polyarticular-course juvenile rheumatoid arthritis: Interim results from an ongoing multicenter, open-label, extended-treatment trial. Arthritis Rheum 48:218-226, 2003.

105. **Ruperto N, Lovell DJ, Cuttica R, et al: A randomized, placebo-controlled trial of infliximab plus methotrexate for the treatment of polyarticular-course juvenile rheumatoid arthritis. Arthritis Rheum 56:3096-3106, 2007.**

106. Giannini E, Ruperto N, Prieur AM, et al: Efficacy of abatacept in different sub-populations of JIA: Results of a randomized withdrawal study. Arthritis Rheum 56:s291, 2007.

107. Lovell DJ, Ruperto N, Goodman S, et al: Adalimumab is safe and effective during long term treatment of patients with juvenile rheumatoid arthritis: Results from a 2 year study. Arthritis Rheum 56:s292, 2007.

108. Woo P, Wilkinson N, Prieur AM, et al: Open label phase II trial of single, ascending doses of MRA in Caucasian children with severe systemic juvenile idiopathic arthritis: Proof of principle of the efficacy of IL-6 receptor blockade in this type of arthritis and demonstration of prolonged clinical improvement. Arthritis Res Ther 7:R1281-R1288, 2005.

109. Yokota S, Miyamae T, Imagawa T, et al: Therapeutic efficacy of humanized recombinant anti-interleukin-6 receptor antibody in children with systemic-onset juvenile idiopathic arthritis. Arthritis Rheum 52:818-825, 2005.

109a. Foell D, Frosch M, Schulze zur Wiesch A, et al: Methotrexate treatment in juvenile idiopathic arthritis: When is the right time to stop? Ann Rheum Dis 63:206-208, 2004.

110. **De Kleer IM, Brinkman DM, Ferster A, et al: Autologous stem cell transplantation for refractory juvenile idiopathic arthritis: Analysis of clinical effects, mortality, and transplant related morbidity. Ann Rheum Dis 63:1318-1326, 2004.**

111. Wedderburn LR, Abinun M, Palmer P, et al: Autologous haematopoietic stem cell transplantation in juvenile idiopathic arthritis. Arch Dis Child 88:201-205, 2003.

112. Brinkman DM, de Kleer IM, ten Cate R, et al: Autologous stem cell transplantation in children with severe progressive systemic or polyarticular juvenile idiopathic arthritis: Long-term follow-up of a prospective clinical trial. Arthritis Rheum 56:2410-2421, 2007.

113. Foster H, Davidson J, Baildam E, et al: Autologous haematopoietic stem cell rescue (AHSCR) for severe rheumatic disease in children: Guidance for BSPAR members—executive summary. Rheumatology 45:1570-1571, 2006.

114. Cimaz R: Osteoporosis in childhood rheumatic diseases: Prevention and therapy. Best Pract Res Clin Rheumatol 16:397-409, 2002.

115. Lovell DJ, Glass D, Ranz J, et al: A randomized controlled trial of calcium supplementation to increase bone mineral density in children with juvenile rheumatoid arthritis. Arthritis Rheum 54:2235-2242, 2006.

116. Yamaguchi M, Ohta A, Tsunematsu T, et al: Preliminary criteria for classification of adult Still's disease. J Rheumatol 19:424-430, 1992.

117. Wulffraat NM, Rijkers GT, Elst E, et al: Reduced perforin expression in systemic juvenile idiopathic arthritis is restored by autologous stem-cell transplantation. Rheumatology 42:375-379, 2003.

118. Grom AA, Villanueva J, Lee S, et al: Natural killer cell dysfunction in patients with systemic-onset juvenile rheumatoid arthritis and macrophage activation syndrome. J Pediatr 142:292-296, 2003.

119. Sawhney S, Woo P, Murray KJ: Macrophage activation syndrome: A potentially fatal complication of rheumatic disorders. Arch Dis Child 85:421-426, 2001.

120. McCann L, Wedderburn LR, Hasson N: Juvenile idiopathic arthritis: Best practice. Arch Dis Child 91:29-36, 2006.

121. Kimura Y, Pinho P, Walco G, et al: Etanercept treatment in patients with refractory systemic onset juvenile rheumatoid arthritis. J Rheumatol 32:935-942, 2005.

122. Lequerre T, Quartier P, Rosellini D, et al: Interleukin-1 receptor antagonist (anakinra) treatment in patients with systemic-onset juvenile idiopathic arthritis or adult onset Still's disease: Preliminary experience in France. Ann Rheum Dis 67:302-308, 2008.

123. Cassidy JT, Hillman LS: Abnormalities in skeletal growth in children with juvenile rheumatoid arthritis. Rheum Dis Clin N Am 23:499-522, 1997.

124. Simon D, Lucidarme N, Prieur AM, et al: Effects on growth and body composition of growth hormone treatment in children with juvenile idiopathic arthritis requiring steroid therapy. J Rheumatol 30:2492-2499, 2003.

125. Davies UM, Rooney M, Preece MA, et al: Treatment of growth retardation in juvenile chronic arthritis with recombinant human growth hormone. J Rheumatol 21:153-158, 1994.

126. David J, Vouyiouka O, Ansell BM, et al: Amyloidosis in juvenile chronic arthritis: A morbidity and mortality study. Clin Exp Rheumatol 11:85-90, 1993.

127. Lomater C, Gerloni V, Gattinara M, et al: Systemic onset juvenile idiopathic arthritis: A retrospective study of 80 consecutive patients followed for 10 years. J Rheumatol 27:491-496, 2000.

128. Spiegel LR, Schneider R, Lang BA, et al: Early predictors of poor functional outcome in systemic-onset juvenile rheumatoid arthritis: A multicenter cohort study. Arthritis Rheum 43:2402-2409, 2000.

129. Modesto C, Woo P, Garcia-Consuegra J, et al: Systemic onset juvenile chronic arthritis, polyarticular pattern and hip involvement as markers for a bad prognosis. Clin Exp Rheumatol 19:211-217, 2001.

130. Graham TB, Glass DN: Juvenile rheumatoid arthritis: Ethnic differences in diagnostic types. J Rheumatol 24:1677-1679, 1997.

131. Thomas E, Barrett JH, Donn RP, et al: Subtyping of juvenile idiopathic arthritis using latent class analysis. British Paediatric Rheumatology Group. Arthritis Rheum 43:1496-1503, 2000.

132. Guillaume S, Prieur AM, Coste J, et al: Long-term outcome and prognosis in oligoarticular-onset juvenile idiopathic arthritis. Arthritis Rheum 43:1858-1865, 2000.

133. Hofer MF, Mouy R, Prieur AM: Juvenile idiopathic arthritides evaluated prospectively in a single center according to the Durban criteria. J Rheumatol 28:1083-1090, 2001.

134. Al-Matar MJ, Petty RE, Tucker LB, et al: The early pattern of joint involvement predicts disease progression in children with oligoarticular (pauciarticular) juvenile rheumatoid arthritis. Arthritis Rheum 46:2708-2715, 2002.

135. Huemer C, Malleson PN, Cabral DA, et al: Patterns of joint involvement at onset differentiate oligoarticular juvenile psoriatic arthritis from pauciarticular juvenile rheumatoid arthritis. J Rheumatol 29:1531-1535, 2002.

136. Petty RE, Smith JR, Rosenbaum JT: Arthritis and uveitis in children: A pediatric rheumatology perspective. Am J Ophthalmol 135:879-884, 2003.

137. Saurenmann RK, Levin AV, Feldman BM, et al: Prevalence, risk factors, and outcome of uveitis in juvenile idiopathic arthritis: A long-term followup study. Arthritis Rheum 56:647-657, 2007.

138. Edelsten C, Lee V, Bentley CR, et al: An evaluation of baseline risk factors predicting severity in juvenile idiopathic arthritis, associated uveitis, and other chronic anterior uveitis in early childhood. Br J Ophthalmol 86:51-56, 2002.

139. BSPAR Guidelines. Available at: http://bspar.org.uk/pages/clinical_guidelines.asp. Accessed 2008.

140. Petty RE, Cassidy JT, Sullivan DB: Clinical correlates of antinuclear antibodies in juvenile rheumatoid arthritis. J Pediatr 83:386-389, 1973.

141. Schaller JG, Johnson GD, Holborow EJ, et al: The association of antinuclear antibodies with the chronic iridocyclitis of juvenile rheumatoid arthritis (Still's disease). Arthritis Rheum 17:409-416, 1974.

142. Adib N, Davies K, Grahame R, et al: Joint hypermobility syndrome in childhood: A not so benign multisystem disorder? Rheumatology 44:744-750, 2005.

143. Trapani S, Grisolia F, Simonini G, et al: Incidence of occult cancer in children presenting with musculoskeletal symptoms: A 10-year survey in a pediatric rheumatology unit. Semin Arthritis Rheum 29:348-359, 2000.

144. Foeldvari I, Nielsen S, Kummerle-Deschner J, et al: Tumor necrosis factor-alpha blocker in treatment of juvenile idiopathic arthritis-associated uveitis refractory to second-line agents: Results of a multinational survey. J Rheumatol 34:1146-1150, 2007.

145. Biester S, Deuter C, Michels H, et al: Adalimumab in the therapy of uveitis in childhood. Br J Ophthalmol 91:319-324, 2007.

146. Ravelli A, Viola S, Migliavacca D, et al: The extended oligoarticular subtype is the best predictor of methotrexate efficacy in juvenile idiopathic arthritis. J Pediatr 135:316-320, 1999.

147. Andersson Gare B, Fasth A, Andersson J, et al: Incidence and prevalence of juvenile chronic arthritis: A population survey. Ann Rheum Dis 46:277-281, 1987.

148. Laiho K, Savolainen A, Kautiainen H, et al: The cervical spine in juvenile chronic arthritis. Spine J 2:89-94, 2002.

149. Twilt M, Mobers SM, Arends LR, et al: Temporomandibular involvement in juvenile idiopathic arthritis. J Rheumatol 31:1418-1422, 2004.

150. Ravelli A, Felici E, Magni-Manzoni S, et al: Patients with antinuclear antibody-positive juvenile idiopathic arthritis constitute a homogeneous subgroup irrespective of the course of joint disease. Arthritis Rheum 52:826-832, 2005.

151. Chalom EC, Goldsmith DP, Koehler MA, et al: Prevalence and outcome of uveitis in a regional cohort of patients with juvenile rheumatoid arthritis. J Rheumatol 24:2031-2034, 1997.

152. van der Heijde D, Klareskog L, Rodriguez-Valverde V, et al: Comparison of etanercept and methotrexate, alone and combined, in the treatment of rheumatoid arthritis: Two-year clinical and radiographic results from the TEMPO study, a double-blind, randomized trial. Arthritis Rheum 54:1063-1074, 2006.

153. Deleted in press.

154. Gare BA, Fasth A: Epidemiology of juvenile chronic arthritis in southwestern Sweden: A 5-year prospective population study. Pediatrics 90:950-958, 1992.

155. Bowyer S, Roettcher P: Pediatric rheumatology clinic populations in the United States: results of a 3 year survey. Pediatric Rheumatology Database Research Group. J Rheumatol 23:1968-1974, 1996.

156. van Rossum M, van Soesbergen R, de Kort S, et al: Anti-cyclic citrullinated peptide (anti-CCP) antibodies in children with juvenile idiopathic arthritis. J Rheumatol 30:825-828, 2003.

157. Ferucci ED, Majka DS, Parrish LA, et al: Antibodies against cyclic citrullinated peptide are associated with HLA-DR4 in simplex and multiplex polyarticular-onset juvenile rheumatoid arthritis. Arthritis Rheum 52:239-246, 2005.

158. Horneff G, Schmeling H, Biedermann T, et al: The German etanercept registry for treatment of juvenile idiopathic arthritis. Ann Rheum Dis 63:1638-1644, 2004.

159. Oen K, Malleson PN, Cabral DA, et al: Disease course and outcome of juvenile rheumatoid arthritis in a multicenter cohort. J Rheumatol 29:1989-1999, 2002.

160. Zak M, Pedersen FK: Juvenile chronic arthritis into adulthood: A long-term follow-up study. Rheumatology 39:198-204, 2000.

161. Ramsey SE, Bolaria RK, Cabral DA, et al: Comparison of criteria for the classification of childhood arthritis. J Rheumatol 27:1283-1286, 2000.

162. Berntson L, Fasth A, Andersson-Gare B, et al: The influence of heredity for psoriasis on the ILAR classification of juvenile idiopathic arthritis. J Rheumatol 29:2454-2458, 2002.

163. Zheng Y, Danilenko DM, Valdez P, et al: Interleukin-22, a T(H)17 cytokine, mediates IL-23-induced dermal inflammation and acanthosis. Nature 445:648-651, 2007.

164. Stoll ML, Zurakowski D, Nigrovic LE, et al: Patients with juvenile psoriatic arthritis comprise two distinct populations. Arthritis Rheum 54:3564-3572, 2006.

165. Lewkowicz D, Gottlieb AB: Pediatric psoriasis and psoriatic arthritis. Dermatol Ther 17:364-375, 2004.

166. Roberton DM, Cabral DA, Malleson PN, et al: Juvenile psoriatic arthritis: Followup and evaluation of diagnostic criteria. J Rheumatol 23:166-170, 1996.

167. Rosenberg AM, Petty RE: A syndrome of seronegative enthesopathy and arthropathy in children. Arthritis Rheum 25:1041-1047, 1982.

168. Burgos-Vargas R, Pacheco-Tena C, Vazquez-Mellado J: Juvenile-onset spondyloarthropathies. Rheum Dis Clin N Am 23:569-598, 1997.

169. Burgos-Vargas R, Vazquez-Mellado J, Cassis N, et al: Genuine ankylosing spondylitis in children: A case-control study of patients with early definite disease according to adult onset criteria. J Rheumatol 23:2140-2147, 1996.

170. Burgos-Vargas R, Vazquez-Mellado J, Pacheco-Tena C, et al: A 26 week randomised, double blind, placebo controlled exploratory study of sulfasalazine in juvenile onset spondyloarthropathies. Ann Rheum Dis 61:941-942, 2002.

171. Henrickson M, Reiff A: Prolonged efficacy of etanercept in refractory enthesitis-related arthritis. J Rheumatol 31:2055-2061, 2004.

172. Tse SM, Burgos-Vargas R, Laxer RM: Anti-tumor necrosis factor alpha blockade in the treatment of juvenile spondylarthropathy. Arthritis Rheum 52:2103-2108, 2005.

173. Berntson L, Fasth A, Andersson-Gare B, et al: Construct validity of ILAR and EULAR criteria in juvenile idiopathic arthritis: A population based incidence study from the Nordic countries. International League of Associations for Rheumatology. European League Against Rheumatism. J Rheumatol 28:2737-2743, 2001.

174. Merino R, De Inocencio J, Garcia-Consuegra J: Evaluation of ILAR classification criteria for juvenile idiopathic arthritis in Spanish children. J Rheumatol 28:2731-2736, 2001.

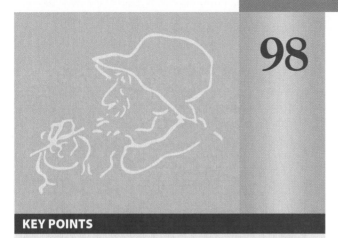

98

Systemic Lupus Erythematosus, Juvenile Dermatomyositis, Scleroderma, and Vasculitis ▪

JAMES T. CASSIDY

KEY POINTS

Pediatric systemic lupus erythematosus (SLE) accounts for 11% of patients referred to pediatric rheumatology clinics and approximately 20% of all cases of SLE.

Children with SLE appear to have more severe disease than adults, with an especially high incidence of renal involvement.

Thrombocytopenic purpura and autoimmune hemolytic anemia may be presenting manifestations of SLE in children.

With the use of aggressive treatment regimens, including intravenous cyclophosphamide and (presumably) mycophenolate mofetil, the prognosis for children with lupus nephritis has improved considerably, with greater than 90% survival and good renal function at 5 years.

Neonatal lupus, characterized by rash, fever, and other systemic manifestations, with or without congenital complete heart block, is caused by maternal anti-Ro antibodies in association with other factors, one of which is maternal HLA-DR3.

Inflammatory muscle disease in children almost always takes the form of juvenile dermatomyositis, with childhood polymyositis being very rare. Unlike in adults with dermatomyositis, an immune complex vasculitis is often present in childhood dermatomyositis and may be a major cause of morbidity and mortality. It has a predilection to involve the skin and the gastrointestinal tract.

Myositis is present in as many as 25% of children with systemic sclerosis and may be the presenting manifestation.

Localized scleroderma, including linear scleroderma and morphea, is three times more common than diffuse systemic sclerosis in children. In most cases, the disease remains localized and does not progress to diffuse disease.

Although the cause of Kawasaki's disease is still unknown, treatment with intravenous immunoglobulin (Ig) G has been shown to improve mortality results by decreasing the number and severity of coronary artery aneurysms.

Henoch-Schönlein purpura, an IgA-mediated vasculitis, is the most common cause of vasculitis in children. It usually has a good prognosis, even in children with nephritis.

This chapter covers four of the major connective tissue diseases of children—systemic lupus erythematosus (SLE), juvenile dermatomyositis (JDM), scleroderma, and vasculitis—and their variants. The discussion is limited to aspects of these disorders important or unique to children,[1] to avoid the repetition of data presented elsewhere in this text. Studies on the incidence and prevalence of these diseases are not as complete as those for juvenile rheumatoid arthritis (JRA).

However, data are available from a number of referral clinics in North America that provide reasonable estimates of the relative frequency of these disorders (Table 98-1).

SYSTEMIC LUPUS ERYTHEMATOSUS

DEFINITION AND CLASSIFICATION

SLE is an episodic multisystem disorder characterized by persistent antinuclear antibody (ANA) seropositivity, widespread inflammation, and immune complex deposition in key target organs. It is a prototype of autoimmune diseases in humans that results from a genetic predisposition and altered immunologic reactivity.

EPIDEMIOLOGY

SLE accounts for 11% of children referred to pediatric rheumatology clinics, and 20% of all cases of lupus are in children (see Table 98-1). The incidence of SLE in children has been estimated at 0.6 per 100,000.[2] The incidence in a Canadian study was 0.36 per 100,000 (confidence interval [CI] 0.23 to 0.61).[3] The disease is probably more frequent in Asians, Polynesians, Native Americans, and African Americans than in whites in the United States. The disease is generally regarded as more serious in children than in adults.[4] SLE is unusual in a child younger than 4 years and becomes increasingly more common from age 9 through the teenage years. The female-to-male ratio is approximately 4.1:1 to 5:1, depending on age; in younger children, relatively more boys are affected.

CAUSE AND PATHOGENESIS

The pathogenesis of SLE is complex, consisting of abnormal homeostatic control of immunologic reactivity to nuclear and cytoplasmic antigens, which may be antigen driven; cytokine polymorphisms; and other immunologic perturbations. Defective antigen presentation, immune complex clearance, and Fas-mediated apoptotic cell death may also be involved. An environmental trigger such as sun exposure, drug reaction, or a slow virus infection may precipitate the onset of disease in a genetically susceptible host. Female hormones (estrogen, prolactin) are associated with the development of SLE in the F_1 hybrid NZB/NZW mouse and potentially in humans.

▪ Supplemental images available on the Expert Consult Premium Edition website.

1677

Table 98-1 Frequency of the Major Pediatric Connective Tissue Diseases

Disease	Number	Percentage
Juvenile rheumatoid arthritis	7368	65.2
Systemic lupus erythematosus	1214	10.7
Juvenile dermatomyositis	658	5.8
Systemic scleroderma	90	0.8
Localized scleroderma	340	3.0
Polyarteritis nodosa	42	0.4
Kawasaki's disease	259	2.3
Henoch-Schönlein purpura	838	7.4
Other vasculitides	491	4.3

Data based on 57,729 diagnoses from 48,934 consecutive patients entered into the Pediatric Rheumatic Disease Registry of the Pediatric Rheumatology Database Research Group, 1992-2002. Courtesy of Suzanne Bowyer, MD.

Genetics

In approximately 1 in 10 families in which a person is afflicted with SLE, another connective tissue disease is identified. This observation emphasizes the heritability of this disorder; however, susceptibility is complex and polygenic. Lupus has been described in identical twins with a concordance rate of 24%, compared with 2% in dizygotic twins.[5] It is also associated with selective immunoglobulin A (IgA) deficiency and inherited deficiencies of complement components such as C2, C1q, C1r, and C1 esterase inhibitor. The C4A null allele is strongly associated with SLE; human leukocyte antigen (HLA)-DR3 is increased in frequency in whites, and HLA-DR2 is increased in African Americans.

Drug-Induced Lupus

Acute SLE is precipitated by a drug reaction in some children. Implicated medications include anticonvulsant drugs, hydralazine, D-penicillamine, isoniazid, penicillin, minocycline, and the sulfonamides. Most of these disorders are self-limited and abate on withdrawal of the offending agent. The most frequent clinical manifestations are fever, dermatitis, and pleuropericardial disease. Antibodies to double-stranded DNA (dsDNA) are usually not present; however, ANA reactivity specific for histones is characteristic (but is also found in children with idiopathic SLE). The serum complement concentration remains normal; central nervous system (CNS) disease and nephritis are uncharacteristic.

Pathology

The basic inflammatory lesion is an immune complex vasculitis with fibrinoid necrosis, inflammatory cell infiltrates, and sclerosis of collagen. Vascular deposition of immune complexes affects both arterioles and venules and is widespread throughout the parenchymal organs, in supporting tissues underlying the dermis and panniculus, and in mucosal and serosal surfaces. In the kidney, immune complexes are deposited in the mesangium and in subendothelial spaces beneath the glomerular basement membrane. Diffuse proliferative glomerulonephritis may represent a more severe form of focal proliferative nephritis, and progression from

Table 98-2 Clinical Manifestations of Systemic Lupus Erythematosus in Childhood

Manifestation	Occurrence (%)
Skin	15-80
Malar erythema	55
Photosensitivity	40
Raynaud's phenomenon	25
Alopecia	20
Kidneys	85-100
Hypertension	30
Renal failure	10
Musculoskeletal system	20-95
Arthritis	75
Myositis	20
Cardiopulmonary system	30-50
Pericarditis	45
Pleuritis	35
Pulmonary hemorrhage	5
Gastrointestinal tract	5-20
Oral or nasopharyngeal ulcerations	15
Mesenteric thrombosis	10
Sterile peritonitis	5
Hepatosplenomegaly	45
Nervous system	30-40
Central	30
Peripheral	5

one to the other has been identified in sequential biopsies. In membranous glomerulonephritis, which is uncommon in children, immune complexes form along the subepithelial surface of the glomerular basement membrane and obliterate the foot processes.

CLINICAL FEATURES

Clinically, SLE is an extremely variable and diverse disease and may develop with any degree of severity, ranging from an acute, rapidly fatal illness to an insidious, chronic disability with repeated exacerbations (Table 98-2).[6] Constitutional symptoms such as fever, malaise, and weight loss are common. Mucocutaneous involvement and a malar erythematous rash in a butterfly distribution are characteristic of acute disease. Hepatomegaly and splenomegaly are common. Lupus hepatitis is an infrequent complication.

Arthritis affects most children with SLE and involves both large and small joints. Characteristics of this arthritis are its transient nature and the fact that it may be migratory. Pain is often more severe than expected based on objective signs of inflammation. The arthritis of SLE seldom results in permanent deformity; however, SLE may evolve from JRA in a few children. Raynaud's phenomenon, with digital vasculitic ulcerations, is a common finding and is often present at disease onset. Ischemic necrosis of bone, particularly of the femoral heads and tibial plateaus, is frequent in long-standing disease, especially after treatment with glucocorticoids.

Pericarditis is the most common manifestation of cardiac involvement, although asymptomatic abnormalities of myocardial perfusion or dysfunction may be more common than generally suspected.[7] Valvular insufficiency may occur; Libman-Sacks verrucous endocarditis is characteristic and, based on echocardiographic studies, is more common than was previously thought. Abnormalities of pulmonary function and pleuritis, along with a basilar pneumonitis, are frequent. Pulmonary hemorrhage, mesenteric thrombosis, and acute pancreatitis are often life-threatening events. Autoimmune endocrinopathies occur with increased frequency in affected children.

The two affected systems most closely correlated with survival are the CNS and the kidneys. Disease of the CNS and the peripheral nervous system is a common cause of morbidity in children.[8] Severe recurrent headaches, seizures, chorea closely resembling that of acute rheumatic fever, and neuropsychiatric manifestations ranging from disordered personality to frank psychosis occur in a majority of children. A labile, inappropriate affect is particularly characteristic in older children and adolescents. Intracranial hemorrhage and cerebral vein thrombosis may result from hypertension, thrombocytopenia, or the presence of antiphospholipid antibodies. Pseudotumor cerebri may be a complication of SLE or of glucocorticoid therapy. Magnetic resonance imaging (MRI) and single photon emission computed tomography (SPECT) aid in differentiating functional and potentially reversible lesions from organic defects. Systemic polyneuropathy, Guillain-Barré syndrome, transverse myelopathy, and involvement of the cranial nerves have all been reported. The so-called cytoid body of retinal vasculitis is often associated with CNS vasculitis or a lupus crisis that may also present as optic neuropathy or a visual field defect.

Lupus nephritis is present to some degree in virtually all children with SLE. Nephritis may not be reflected initially in changes in creatinine clearance, proteinuria, or abnormal urinary sediment. Clinically evident nephritis, if it is going to develop, usually manifests within a few years of disease onset. Continuing evidence of immune complex disease, such as increased levels of anti-dsDNA antibodies or hypocomplementemia, correlates with active nephritis in most children. It is generally agreed that prognostically important renal lesions are more common in young patients than in adults, and the prognosis in children with renal disease is more guarded.

DIAGNOSIS AND DIAGNOSTIC TESTS

The 11 criteria developed by the American College of Rheumatology (ACR) for the classification of SLE, as modified in 1994, are applicable to children.[9,10] The presence of four criteria has a sensitivity of 90% and a specificity of 98%. A skin biopsy is occasionally helpful diagnostically because soluble immune complexes containing IgG and C3 are deposited in the vascular endothelium and along the dermoepidermal junction in both involved and uninvolved skin. This finding is known as the lupus band test.

Persistent leukopenia is particularly characteristic of SLE. Most children are leukopenic at onset, with a predominance of neutrophils in the peripheral white blood cell count. Leukocytosis may not develop to an appropriate degree, however, even with severe infection. Thrombocytopenia is common (30% to 50% of cases). SLE may present as thrombocytopenic purpura with or without hemolytic anemia; Coombs' antibodies are often present in these children. Thrombotic thrombocytopenic purpura is a rare diagnosis of exclusion. Other causes of anemia include posthemorrhagic conditions, septicemia, and gastrointestinal bleeding.

ANAs are a hallmark of the immunologic abnormalities of SLE and are present in nearly all children with the disease. They generally occur in high titers in a homogeneous or peripheral immunofluorescent pattern on indirect immunofluorescent testing. The peripheral nuclear pattern is diagnostic of the presence of anti-dsDNA antibodies, which are associated with active systemic disease, and especially with nephritis. Antigen-antibody complex deposition leads to widespread vasculopathy and lupus nephritis.

Serum antibodies in children with SLE also include those that are tissue specific (e.g., antiplatelet antibodies) and result in specific manifestations of the disease, such as thrombocytopenia. Other antibodies may be associated with an acute hemolytic anemia and leukopenia. An elevated partial thromboplastin time may signal the presence of a lupus anticoagulant. Anticardiolipin antibodies lead to recurrent thromboses (in about 10% of cases) and are associated with the development of neuropsychiatric lupus, chorea,[11,12] epilepsy,[13] and the catastrophic antiphospholipid syndrome.[14] This antibody, a specificity of B_2 glycoprotein I–dependent anticardiolipin antibodies, is also directed against cardiolipin substrate in the serologic reaction for syphilis. Both these specificities are more common in children than in adults. A young person with a false-positive result on these tests for syphilis is at risk for the development of SLE. Antiribosomal P and antineuronal antibodies are also characteristics of children with CNS disease and psychosis. Rheumatoid factors are often present in high titer. Cold agglutinins and cryoglobulins may also be present, resulting in peripheral anoxic phenomena and gangrene.

Both the classic and alternative complement pathways are activated in the immune complex vasculitis of SLE. A depressed whole hemolytic complement determination (CH50 assay) reflects the status of the total complement cascade; a low concentration of C3 or C4 is usually a reliable indicator of active disease, if persistent. Dyslipoproteinemia is characteristic of active disease and is also a consequence of glucocorticoid therapy.

A number of other diseases should be considered in the differential diagnosis of a child with suspected SLE. Among these are polyarticular or systemic-onset JRA, acute poststreptococcal glomerulonephritis, idiopathic hemolytic anemia, immune thrombocytopenic purpura, leukemia, allergic or contact dermatitis, idiopathic seizure disorder, mononucleosis, acute rheumatic fever, septicemia, and infectious endocarditis. Sjögren's syndrome is a multisystem disorder that may be misdiagnosed as SLE, particularly in the presence of high titers of multiple autoantibodies, including anti-Ro/La. It is often insidious in onset and slowly progressive. Primary Sjögren's syndrome is rare in children and may present as recurrent parotid and lacrimal swelling, dry mouth, and persistent keratoconjunctivitis.

TREATMENT

Because SLE is an extremely serious and complex disease, most children benefit from management by the same multidisciplinary medical team over the course of their illness. Long-term supportive care includes adequate nutrition, prompt treatment of infections, and control of hypertension, if present. Unnecessary restraints on a child's general level of activity and psychosocial peer group interactions are undesirable. The prophylactic measures of avoiding unnecessary drug exposure, transfusion, and excessive sunlight should be emphasized. Appropriate clothing and sunscreens are prescribed to minimize exposure to ultraviolet radiation.

Nonsteroidal anti-inflammatory drugs (NSAIDs), except for ibuprofen, are helpful in treating minor manifestations of SLE such as arthralgia and myalgia. Aspirin or anticoagulation may be indicated for the antiphospholipid antibody syndrome (see Chapter 76). Hydroxychloroquine is used as an adjunctive medication to control dermatitis or to moderate the glucocorticoid dosage.[15] Glucocorticoids are, however, the mainstay of treatment. Prednisone is the preferred analogue for oral administration. The lowest dose that achieves the objectives of the treatment program should be prescribed. Initial therapy usually requires a split dosage regimen. Low-dose therapy, defined as 0.5 mg/kg per day, is used to treat persistent fever, dermatitis, arthritis, or serositis. These manifestations are often suppressed promptly. A period of weeks is usually required to control anemia and achieve a serologic remission, with suppression of anti-dsDNA antibodies and return of serum complement levels toward normal. A low-dose program is often sufficient to control clinical disease in children with mesangial or focal glomerulonephritis. Treatment of children with active SLE is monitored by the clinical course and periodic assessments of anti-dsDNA antibodies and serum complement levels. Exacerbation of the disease during steroid tapering may be signaled by a deterioration in the serologic indices and clinical measures of disease activity.

High-dose prednisone therapy, defined as 1 to 2 mg/kg per day in divided doses, is indicated for lupus crisis, CNS disease, acute hemolytic anemia, and the more severe forms of nephritis. Intravenous (IV) pulse therapy with methylprednisolone is preferred for acute exacerbations in a variety of protocols at a dose of 10 to 30 mg/kg. Although the approach to the diagnosis and therapy of nephritis is controversial, the precise glucocorticoid regimen and the decision whether to add immunosuppressive drugs must be based on the degree and type of kidney involvement. Renal biopsy is warranted in most children with SLE to establish the type, activity, and chronicity of the disease, unless there is no clinical or serologic evidence of kidney involvement.

In addition to glucocorticoids, immunosuppressive agents are required in some children. Although azathioprine has been employed extensively, and methotrexate more recently, clinical experience suggests that IV cyclophosphamide pulse therapy (500 to 750 mg/m² every 4 weeks for 6 months, followed by maintenance therapy) is preferable in patients with severe nephritis.[16,17] Data on the use of mycophenolate mofetil in children are limited, but studies in adults indicate that it is superior to cyclophosphamide in patients with active nephritis.[18] Dialysis and kidney transplantation have been used in end-stage renal disease.[19] Stem cell transplantation is currently being evaluated. Resistant cutaneous disease may respond to topical tacrolimus. Clinical measures of therapeutic responsiveness[20] and preliminary core measures of disease activity and severity have been developed for clinical assessment and response to therapy.[21]

OUTCOME

SLE is characterized by repeated exacerbations and remissions; active disease usually lasts for many years. Predicting the outcome for a specific child is difficult, and generalizations about outcome are especially unreliable during the first 1 to 2 years after disease onset. Later, a more realistic determination can be made, depending on the degree of systemic activity and the observed response to therapy. Outcome is poorest in children with diffuse proliferative nephritis or an organic brain syndrome; it is best in children with minimal or controlled systemic disease or mesangial nephritis or in those who respond promptly to steroid therapy. Morbidity is often underestimated, however.[22] There was no definite association between poor outcome and male sex or nonwhite ethnicity in one study,[23] but in others, nonwhite children were at increased risk of nephritis and a poor outcome.[24,25]

Although the course of the disease and its severity are highly variable, prognosis has improved dramatically during the past 3 decades.[105] Life-table analysis in a study from Minnesota indicated that survival in 21 children with diffuse proliferative glomerulonephritis was only 70% at 10 years.[26] In more recent studies, the survival rate was 91% at 5 years and 94% among children followed for at least 11 years.[24,27] Although nephritis and CNS disease continue to be leading causes of death, infection has replaced them in some series as the most common preterminal event. Functional asplenia may predispose children to an increased risk of septicemia. Accelerated atherosclerosis of the coronary arteries may be a late complication and cause of death in approximately one fourth of cases. Cumulative organ damage occurs in many children.[28] Duration of disease, hypertension, total glucocorticoid dose, and use of cyclophosphamide were associated with evidence of organ damage in 61% of 71 children followed until a mean age of approximately 26 ± 10 years.[29] Osteopenia is common and is related to disease severity and duration and to medication (glucocorticoids).[30]

NEONATAL LUPUS SYNDROMES

Children of mothers who have active SLE or are at risk of developing it may present with lupus-like syndromes in the neonatal period related to transplacental passage of maternal IgG autoantibodies.[31] Neonatal lupus is divided into two types: a transient syndrome and congenital complete heart block.[32] In a study of 128 infants born to mothers with anti-Ro antibodies, 16% developed cutaneous neonatal lupus and 1.6% developed complete heart block.[33]

Transient neonatal lupus syndrome results from the transplacental transport of maternal anti-Ro/La ribonucleoprotein antibodies in the presence of specific HLA-DR and DQ genes. In some infants, malar erythema develops in conjunction with discoid or annular lesions either immediately after birth or within a few months (Fig. 98-1). In most babies, there is no associated systemic disease, and serologic abnormalities abate in the first few months of life with the metabolic decay of maternal immunoglobulin. Thrombocytopenia may be present along with mild hemolytic anemia or leukopenia. CNS involvement may occur.[34] Usually, this form of the syndrome requires no specific treatment. Occasionally, glucocorticoids are indicated for severe dermatologic disease or gastrointestinal bleeding. An autoimmune disease may develop in young adults who have had neonatal lupus,[35] although there is apparently no increased risk of SLE.[36]

Congenital complete heart block, alone or associated with other cardiac defects such as myocarditis, septal and endocardial cushion defects, and endomyocardial fibroelastosis, is a distinct and permanent neonatal lupus syndrome. Congenital complete heart block can be diagnosed in utero by fetal echocardiography. Extreme bradycardia results in fetal hydrops. The correct obstetric approach is unclear, but it includes treating the mother with glucocorticoids (dexamethasone), plasmapheresis, and intrauterine pacing. The neonatal death rate is approximately 15%, and survival at 3 years is only 20%. Most of the remaining children require pacemakers.

Approximately one third of affected babies are born to mothers who have or are at risk for the development of SLE or an associated autoimmune disease.[37,38] More than 90% of these mothers are HLA-DR3-positive. Anti-Ro (SSA) antibodies directed against a small cytoplasmic RNA protein complex and, in most cases, antibodies to the La (SSB) ribonucleoprotein complex have been found in virtually every child and mother with this syndrome who have been studied. The predominant anti-Ro specificity is for the 52-kD peptide. These antibodies result in the absence or degeneration and fibrosis of the atrioventricular node, which results in heart block during maturation of the fetal heart at approximately 16 to 18 weeks.

JUVENILE DERMATOMYOSITIS

DEFINITION AND CRITERIA

JDM is a multisystem disease characterized by nonsuppurative inflammation of striated muscle, skin, and the gastrointestinal tract.[39] It is characterized early in its course by an immune complex vasculitis of varying severity and later by the development of calcinosis.

An acute onset of proximal muscle weakness accompanied by the characteristic dermatitis is pathognomonic for JDM. The 25% of children who do not have the classic rash almost invariably have an atypical rash that still suggests this diagnosis. Polymyositis—that is, inflammatory myositis without dermatitis—is an unusual presentation in children. Serum "muscle" enzymes are elevated in 98% of affected children, and sequential measurements are important for diagnosis and to monitor the effectiveness of therapy. Atrophy, fatty infiltration, or signal abnormalities indicative of active disease can be demonstrated by MRI. A muscle biopsy is sometimes indicated during the initial evaluation to determine prognosis and provide support for the institution of long-term glucocorticoid therapy or immunosuppressive drugs. The muscle undergoing biopsy should be clinically involved but not atrophied. The best site is generally the deltoid or quadriceps.

Diagnostic histopathologic changes involve striated muscles, skin, and the gastrointestinal tract. The initial lesion is an acute patchy, inflammatory lymphocytic infiltration (Fig. 98-2). Concomitant degeneration and regeneration of striated muscle fibers follow, resulting in a moderate variation in fiber size. Areas of focal necrosis are replaced during the healing phase by an interstitial proliferation of connective tissue and fat. An immune complex necrotizing vasculitis occurs in arterioles, capillaries, and venules and is especially characteristic in children with this disorder.

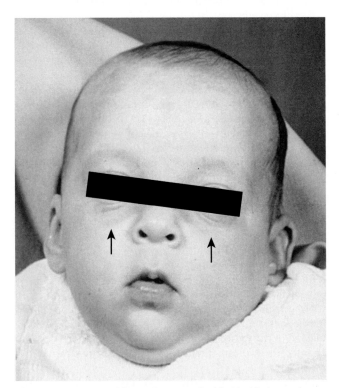

Figure 98-1 Neonatal lupus. Four-month-old girl with the erythematous rash of neonatal lupus across the bridge of the nose, lower eyelids, and superior forehead. This baby was born at 33 weeks' gestation with complete congenital heart block. Her mother had high titers of anti-Ro antibody.

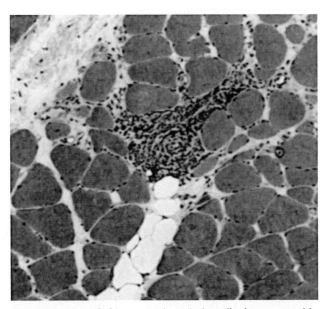

Figure 98-2 Muscle biopsy specimen in juvenile dermatomyositis. In the center is a perivascular, mononuclear cell inflammatory infiltrate, with arterial thickening and prominent endothelial cells (hematoxylin and eosin, ×100).

Diffuse linear and occasionally granular deposits of IgM, C3d, and fibrin are present in the areas of noninflammatory vasculopathy. Electromyography is often not attempted in children because of difficulty in obtaining cooperation during the painful procedure. Notable electromyographic changes include myopathy and denervation.

EPIDEMIOLOGY

JDM is relatively uncommon and accounts for approximately 6% of children with major connective tissue diseases in pediatric rheumatology clinics (see Table 98-1). Incidence in a study from the United Kingdom and Ireland was 0.19 per 100,000 (95% CI 0.14 to 0.26).[40] In the United States, it was 2.5 to 4.1 cases per 1 million (4-year average, 3.2; 95% CI 2.9 to 3.4) in children 2 to 17 years of age.[41] The disease is more frequent in girls. Onset is especially common between ages 5 and 14 years.

CAUSE AND PATHOGENESIS

Although the cause of JDM remains unknown, data support a dynamic model of autoimmune disease involving muscle, the vascular system, and immune regulation in a genetically susceptible child.[42] Immune complex vasculitis may be an important initiating or perpetuating event,[43] with immunoglobulins and complement deposited in the walls of small blood vessels in skeletal muscle. Shared epitopes between skeletal muscle and *Streptococcus pyogenes* M5 protein may be targets of immune responses.[44] HLA-DQA1*0501 is increased in frequency in white children[45] and is associated with an increase in the TNFα-308A allele.[46] JDM has occurred after a history of respiratory infections or gastrointestinal complaints, vaccinations, hypersensitivity reactions to drugs, and sunburn. Acute transient inflammatory myositis has been reported after viral and parasitic infections (e.g., coxsackievirus B, influenza, toxoplasmosis) in otherwise normal children. A fatal myositis has been described in children with agammaglobulinemia in association with echovirus infection. JDM has been reported in patients with selective IgA deficiency and C2 complement component deficiency.

Maternal cell chimerism has been identified in mononuclear cells in the vascular compartment and in muscle in 80% to 90% of children with JDM.[47-49] It was present in 25% of siblings and 15% of controls in these reports. Reed and colleagues[49] found chimeric cells in 60 of 72 children with JDM, in 11 of 48 unaffected siblings, and in 5 of 29 healthy controls. In all groups, microchimerism was associated with the maternal HLA-DQA1*0501 allele.[50]

CLINICAL FEATURES

Proximal muscle weakness, dermatitis, fever, and constitutional symptoms such as fatigue, malaise, weight loss, and anorexia are presenting features of this disorder (Table 98-3).[51] The limb girdle muscles of the lower extremities are affected initially, followed by the shoulder girdle and proximal arm muscles. Affected muscles are occasionally edematous and indurated. A child may also complain of muscle pain, tenderness, or stiffness or may stop walking or be unable to climb stairs or dress. An inability to get up off the floor without the classic Gower's maneuver or to get out of bed is common.

Table 98-3 Clinical Manifestations of Juvenile Dermatomyositis

Manifestation	Occurrence (%)
Musculoskeletal system	100
Muscle weakness	
Proximal pelvic girdle	95
Proximal shoulder girdle	75
Neck flexors	60
Pharyngeal muscles	45
Distal muscles of the extremities	30
Facial and extraocular muscles	5
Arthritis	25
Skin	85-100
Periungual and articular rash (Gottron's papules)	80
Heliotrope rash of eyelids and periorbital edema	15
Malar rash	40
Photosensitivity	40
Ulcerations	25
Raynaud's phenomenon	15
Calcinosis	40
Gastrointestinal tract	10-60
Pharyngitis	40
Dysphagia	10
Hemorrhage	5
Lungs	15-80
Restrictive disease	80
Fibrosis	<1

It has been proposed that the course of JDM in most children can be divided into four clinical phases:[52]
1. A prodromal period of weeks to months with nonspecific symptoms
2. Progressive muscle weakness and dermatitis that lasts days to weeks
3. Persistent myositis and dermatitis of 1 to 2 years' duration
4. Recovery with residual muscle atrophy and contractures with or without calcinosis

Although muscle weakness may be impressive, deep tendon reflexes are preserved. Weakness of the anterior neck flexors and back leads to an inability to hold the head upright or maintain a sitting posture. Facial and extraocular muscles are uncommonly involved. Ten percent of children develop pharyngeal, hypopharyngeal, or palatal muscle weakness. Dysphonia results along with dysphagia, which may be related to esophageal hypomotility. These children are at risk for sudden and often fatal aspiration. Palatal speech and nasal regurgitation of liquids are early warning signs of potential respiratory compromise. Profound involvement of the thoracic and respiratory muscles occurs in a few children. Later in the disease, or in children with an acute onset, the distal muscles of the extremities may be affected. Rarely, there is generalized acute inflammation of the entire striated musculature; this may be more characteristic of an infantile onset. CNS involvement is rare.

Most children have the classic rash of JDM over the malar area, the upper eyelids (with periorbital edema), and the dorsal surfaces of the knuckles (Fig. 98-3), elbows, and knees. The basic lesion is angiitis on a background of cutaneous photosensitivity. At onset, indurative edema of the

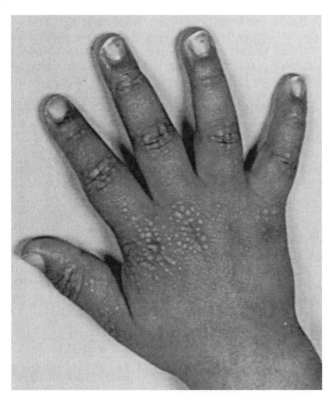

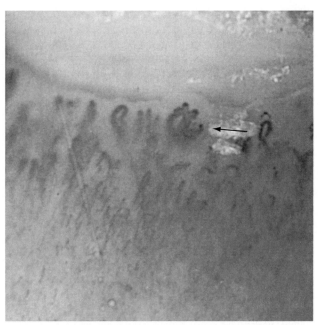

Figure 98-4 **Abnormal nail-fold capillary pattern of juvenile derma-tomyositis (×100).** The vessels are thickened and tortuous and show a peripheral pattern of arborization (*arrow*). There are clear areas of capillary dropout. *(Courtesy of Dr. Jay Kenik.)*

Figure 98-3 Gottron's papules present since the age of 18 months in a 4-year-old girl with juvenile dermatomyositis. Raised hypopigmented papules are present on an erythematous base over the dorsum of the hand, with accentuation over the metacarpophalangeal, proximal interphalangeal, and distal phalangeal joints.

skin and subcutaneous tissues is often present. Later there is epidermal thinning and atrophy of the accessory structures, with loss of hair and telangiectases. Vasculitic ulcers at the corners of the eyes, around the axillae, and in "stretch marks" may be difficult to treat. Although a few children have calcinosis at disease onset, the development of calcification and dystrophic mineralization with hydroxyapatite is more characteristic of the healing phase. Nail-fold capillary loop abnormalities are identifiable through the +40 lens of an ophthalmoscope in half the children and have prognostic importance.[53] The nail folds show simultaneous dilation of isolated loops, dropout of surrounding vessels, and an arborized cluster of capillary loops—all distinctive features of JDM (Fig. 98-4).

Dermatomyositis sine myositis or amyopathic dermatomyositis is rare in children, although the classic rash may occur before clinical muscle involvement. However, in a review of established dermatomyositis sine myositis by Plamondon and Dent,[54] none of their 27 patients developed clinical myopathy at a mean follow-up of 32.8 months. Polymyositis is rare in childhood.

The association of lipodystrophy with JDM may be more common than previously recognized (20% to 50%).[41,55] The disorder may be generalized, localized, or unilateral. It is characterized by a slow and progressive loss of subcutaneous and visceral fat, often most noticeable over the upper body and face, accompanied by hirsutism, acanthosis nigricans, clitoral enlargement, hepatic steatosis, insulin resistance, abnormal glucose tolerance, and hypertriglyceridemia.

DIAGNOSIS AND DIAGNOSTIC TESTS

Serum concentrations of the muscle enzymes creatine kinase, aldolase, aspartate aminotransferase, and alanine aminotransferase are elevated in active disease. The extent of the increase is variable, but levels can range from 20 to 40 times normal for creatine kinase or aspartate aminotransferase. Detection of MB bands on the creatine kinase isozyme pattern is usually evidence of regeneration of striated muscle, not cardiac damage. Nonspecific tests of inflammation tend to correlate with the degree of clinical activity. Leukocytosis and anemia are uncommon at disease onset, except in children with associated gastrointestinal bleeding. The occurrence of rheumatoid factors and ANAs is variable. Myositis-specific and myositis-associated antibodies have been described in only a minority of children.[39,56] Half of the affected children had circulating immune complexes. The serum concentration of von Willebrand's factor VIII antigen is elevated in active disease (evidence of vasculitis), as is the serum neopterin concentration.

Considerations in the differential diagnosis include the other multisystem connective tissue diseases. JDM that presents predominantly with arthritis may be confused with either an acute systemic onset of JRA or SLE. Scleroderma poses unique diagnostic problems, in that approximately 25% of children with the disorder have a primary myositis. Although early cutaneous abnormalities of scleroderma and JDM are different, the skin changes tend to merge and become more similar later in the course of the two diseases.

In children with muscular dystrophy, there is a selective pattern of muscle weakness, an insidious onset of progressive or remitting illness, and a positive family history. Dermatitis is absent. The serum creatine kinase concentration is elevated in first-degree relatives, especially in the mothers of children with X-linked disease. Congenital myopathies, myotonias, hypotonic syndromes, and the metabolic and endocrine myopathies, especially hypothyroidism, must also be considered. Paroxysmal myoglobulinuria and thyrotoxic myopathy may occasionally be encountered. Myasthenia gravis is rare in children.

Rhabdomyolysis may be a complication of an acute infection, trauma, or extreme muscular exertion. Onset is abrupt and is characterized by profound weakness, myoglobinuria, and occasionally oliguria and renal failure. Trichinosis and toxoplasmosis cause myositis of varying severity, and severe pustular acne may occasionally be associated with inflammatory disease of muscle. Influenza B, coxsackievirus B infection, poliomyelitis, and Guillain-Barré syndrome are other diagnostic considerations.

TREATMENT

The presence of a noninflammatory vasculopathy is associated with a poorer outcome and is an important prognostic factor in survival. Zonal loss of the capillary bed, areas of focal infarction of muscle, lymphocytic non-necrotizing vasculopathy, and a noninflammatory endarteropathy have been associated with progressive infarction of muscle and the gastrointestinal tract and with cutaneous ulcerations. Smooth muscle is not affected, except for isolated vasculitis. The heart is generally not involved in the primary pathologic process. A few children with cardiac disease have been described with focal myocardial fibrosis and contraction band necrosis.

General supportive care and a coordinated team approach are vital and should include scheduled, individualized rest and positioning. Muscle strengthening should be added only when clinical evidence of acute inflammation has subsided. During the convalescent phase, physical therapy is focused on normalizing function as much as possible and minimizing the development of contractures secondary to muscle weakness or atrophy. The Childhood Health Assessment Questionnaire is a valid measure to assess physical function.[57] Preliminary core measures of disease activity and damage assessment have been developed.[58] Osteopenia is almost universally present.[30,59]

The introduction of glucocorticoids dramatically improved the prognosis of JDM. For initial treatment of acute disease, it is generally necessary to use 2 mg/kg per day of prednisone in four divided doses for at least the first month; then, if indicated by clinical response and a decrease in the serum muscle enzyme concentrations, a lower dose in the range of 1 mg/kg per day can be prescribed. Thereafter, the daily steroid dose is slowly tapered in amount and frequency of administration, as determined by improvement in clinical status, degree of muscle weakness (repeated testing on a 0 to 5 scale), and level of serum muscle enzymes. Satisfactory control is not achieved until enzyme levels have returned to normal or nearly normal and remain there during tapering of the steroid dose and as the child's level of physical activity increases. IV methylprednisolone pulse therapy is indicated for acute exacerbations and should be considered as initial treatment to minimize the daily steroid dose. Alternate-day steroid therapy may be useful only late in the recovery phase. Addition of hydroxychloroquine aids in controlling the dermatitis and appears to be steroid sparing.

Acute complications (e.g., cutaneous ulcerations) and failure to respond to steroids may be indications for the use of immunosuppressive agents or alternative therapeutic regimens, which include methotrexate, IV cyclophosphamide, IV immunoglobulin (IVIG),[60] cyclosporine, mycophenolate mofetil, hydroxychloroquine, plasmapheresis, extracorporeal photochemotherapy, and potentially monoclonal antibody to tumor necrosis factor-α (TNFα). Experience with stem cell transplantation is limited. Cutaneous disease can be approached with emollients and agents such as tacrolimus. Many approaches to the therapy of calcinosis have been advocated, including colchicine, probenecid, aluminum salts, warfarin, and bisphosphonates. None of these has been uniformly successful in studies with adequate numbers of patients. Surgical excision of calcific tumors in areas of ulceration or pressure remains an option. Chronicity of disease and pathologic calcifications have been associated with the presence of the TNFα-308A allele.[46] Hypercalcemia has been described during resolution of the calcinosis.

OUTCOME

The basic nature of the inflammatory disease, its initial response to treatment, and the presence or absence of vasculitis or progressive involvement of other organ systems, such as the gastrointestinal tract and lungs, are major factors that influence outcome. Children with varying degrees of disease activity have decreased aerobic and work capacity.[61] A duration of active myositis as short as 8 months has been reported. In up to 60% of children, the disease course lasts approximately 2 years and consists of only one or two exacerbations. The remaining 40% continue to have acute exacerbations and remissions; a disease that is more typical of systemic vasculitis eventually develops in a few. In a small number of children, sclerodactyly and cutaneous atrophy or areas of lipoatrophy associated with insulin resistance may develop late in the course. New data emphasize the potential role of leptin deficiency in the abnormalities characteristic of lipodystrophy.[62] Acanthosis nigricans or a recurrence of arthritis may occur. Even years after onset, some children have persistent elevations of serum muscle enzymes, especially creatine kinase, and characteristic histopathologic features of the disease may be noted on repeat biopsy.

The course of the dermatitis often does not follow that of the myositis. Many clinicians are convinced that children who have a generalized rash and cutaneous ulcerations have the worst prognosis. The characteristic nail-fold capillary loop abnormalities of thickening and arborization, along with a noninflammatory vasculopathy, correlate with more severe disease. During the healing phase of the myositis, calcium salts (hydroxyapatite or fluorapatite) are deposited in skin and subcutaneous tissues, around the joints, and within interfascial planes of the muscles in up to half of children. Later, calcification may be slowly resorbed spontaneously (Figs. 98-5 and 98-6). It has been proposed that early use of IV pulse steroid therapy may minimize the later development of calcinosis.[39]

Despite these findings, the average child progressively improves to achieve functional recovery (Table 98-4). The

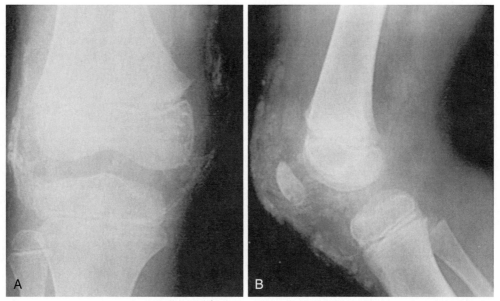

Figure 98-5 Massive deposits of calcium salts in the subcutaneous tissue and fascia about the right knee in an 11-year-old boy. Calcinosis followed the acute phase of juvenile dermatomyositis by 3 years. **A,** Anteroposterior view. **B,** Lateral view.

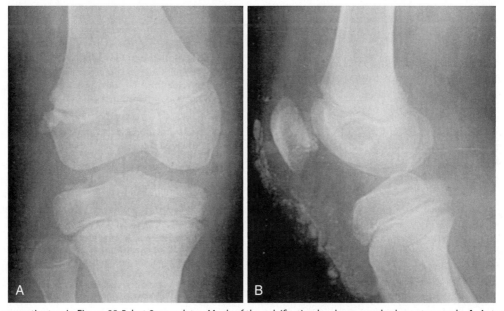

Figure 98-6 Same patient as in Figure 98-5, but 2 years later. Much of the calcification has been resorbed spontaneously. **A,** Anteroposterior view, **B,** Lateral view.

outcome is best in children who are diagnosed early and receive vigorous treatment. Most children should be able to function independently as adults, although some have residual atrophy of skin or muscle groups. Difficulties during pregnancy have been described in women who have had JDM. In the preglucocorticoid era, JDM was associated with a mortality rate that approached 50%. Surviving children often had devastating residual problems, including contractures, muscle atrophy, and widespread calcinosis. At present, the long-term survival rate approaches 90%, and functional outcome has been greatly improved. The greatest risk of death is within the first 2 years after onset. An acute gastrointestinal complication or respiratory insufficiency

leading to hypoxia with or without aspiration is a serious, often preterminal event.

SCLERODERMA

The sclerodermas are systemic or localized connective tissue diseases of unknown cause. Often, their development is unrecognized initially because these disorders are so rare. A classification is presented in Table 98-5. Systemic disease is divided into diffuse cutaneous scleroderma and limited cutaneous scleroderma. The localized forms of the disease, such as morphea or linear scleroderma,[63] are often regarded as more dermatologic than rheumatic in nature. Some

Table 98-4 Outcome for Children with Juvenile Dermatomyositis

Outcome	Occurrence (%)
Complete functional recovery	65
Minimal disease (atrophy or contracture)	25
Calcinosis	20-40
Significant disability or dependence	5
Death	7

Table 98-5 Classification of Scleroderma

Systemic Disease
Scleroderma
Diffuse
Limited
Overlap syndromes
Sclerodermatomyositis or other connective tissue diseases
Mixed connective tissue disease
Localized Disease
Morphea
Generalized morphea
Linear scleroderma
Eosinophilic fasciitis

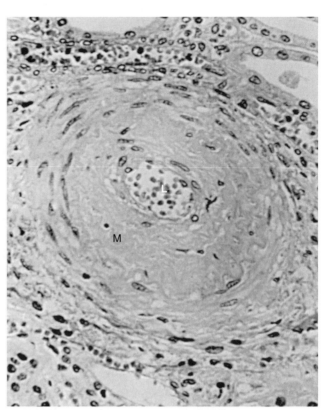

Figure 98-7 Renal arteriole from a patient who died of scleroderma and hypertensive crisis. There is virtual obliteration of the vessel lumen (L) by intimal proliferation and medial mucoid hyperplasia (M).

rheumatologists also include mixed connective tissue disease and eosinophilic fasciitis in this category.

DIFFUSE CUTANEOUS SYSTEMIC SCLERODERMA

The early clinical presentation of diffuse cutaneous systemic scleroderma (DCSS) is often subtle. Although not validated in children, the ACR classification criteria seem to be applicable to this age group.[64]

Epidemiology

DCSS is rare and accounts for about 1% of major connective tissue disorders in pediatric rheumatology clinics (see Table 98-1).[65] Girls are affected more frequently than boys in a ratio of 3:1, except in the youngest age group.[1] There is no peak age at onset during childhood and no racial predilection. Familial clustering has been demonstrated.[66]

Cause and Pathogenesis

Scleroderma-like disease occurs in children with insulin-dependent (type 1) diabetes mellitus, phenylketonuria, and progeria and has developed after exposure to vinyl chloride, bleomycin, and pentazocine. It occurred in an epidemic in Spain related to a toxin in adulterated rapeseed oil.

The pathogenesis is basically unknown. There is an increased number of high collagen-producing fibroblasts in the skin. Endothelial perturbation is present, with accelerated endothelial cell apoptosis and anti–endothelial cell antibodies. The similarities between scleroderma and graft-versus-host disease in bone marrow transplant recipients has led to the hypothesis that a persistence of fetal progenitor cells and microchimerism may be involved in

the pathogenesis.[67,68] Although not uncommon in healthy adults, microchimerism is increased in scleroderma but may be detected only in bone marrow or affected tissues.[69]

Angiitis is regarded as the basic initial lesion. The skin and gastrointestinal tract are involved early, along with the lungs, heart, and kidneys. Perivascular infiltrates of mononuclear cells are often present and have been identified in some studies to consist predominantly of T lymphocytes. Arterioles eventually undergo hyalinization and fibrosis (Fig. 98-7). In the skin, there is thinning of the epidermis, loss of the rete pegs, and atrophy of the dermal appendages. In the deeper layers, homogenization of the collagen fibers, with loss of structural detail; increased density and thickness of collagen deposition; and predominance of embryonal fibers are characteristic.

Clinical Features

Clinical manifestations of DCSS are summarized in Table 98-6. The onset is often marked by the appearance of Raynaud's phenomenon; tightening, thinning, and atrophy of the skin of the hands and face; or the appearance of cutaneous telangiectases about the face, upper trunk, and hands. There is often a diagnostic delay of years because of the subtle, insidious nature of the presentation of this disease.

Raynaud's phenomenon occurs in most children with DCSS and often antedates the onset of cutaneous abnormalities. It is characterized by obstructive digital arterial disease and sympathetic hyperactivity. Vascular spasm within

Table 98-6 Clinical Manifestations of Systemic Scleroderma in Childhood

Manifestation	Occurrence (%)
Skin	100
Raynaud's phenomenon	75
Digital ulcerations	60
Telangiectases	30
Subcutaneous calcification	25
Pigmentary changes	20
Gastrointestinal tract	75-100
Abnormal esophageal motility	75
Dysphagia	20
Colonic sacculations	20
Duodenal dilation	5
Lungs	75-100
Dyspnea	20
Abnormal diffusion	75
Decreased vital capacity	70
Musculoskeletal system	25-75
Joint contractures	75
Resorption of digital tufts	75
Muscle weakness and pain	40
Heart	15-30
Electrocardiographic abnormalities and arrhythmias	30
Cardiomegaly	15
Congestive failure	15

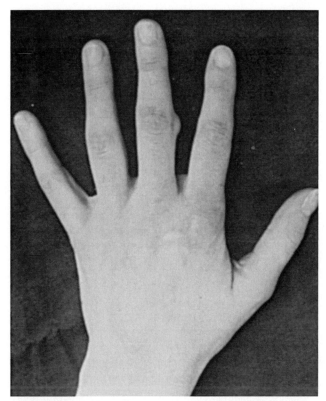

Figure 98-8 Subcutaneous nodule of periarticular calcification in a teenage girl with acrosclerosis.

viscera such as the esophagus may accompany the peripheral anoxia. Digital gangrene may supervene, with the development of small atrophic pits on the fingertips.

Characteristic abnormalities of the nail-fold capillaries have been identified. There is a reduction in the number of vessels and a marked tortuosity and "puddling" of the remaining capillaries. Scattered white fibrotic areas are prominent. Skin tightening is virtually universal and tends to become more generalized with time. Hypopigmentation and hyperpigmentation are characteristic, as are subcutaneous calcification and deposition of calcium salts around joints (Fig. 98-8). Erythema and ulcerations may develop over the elbows, knees, and malleoli.

Many children have contractures about joints, and a few have objective evidence of arthritis. A crepitant tenosynovitis develops in others. Muscle pain and tenderness are present in approximately 20%. Elevation of the serum muscle enzymes tends to be mild to moderate and not as striking as in JDM. Dyspnea on exertion may be related to skin tightness, muscle weakness, or interstitial pulmonary fibrosis. Myocarditis and cardiomyopathy also lead to dyspnea, arrhythmia, and signs of heart failure. Although widespread gastrointestinal involvement occurs in most children, symptomatic disease is often confined to the esophagus, with complaints of dysphagia or reflux esophagitis. Esophageal ulceration and constriction may develop. Malabsorption may become severe and lead to a fatal outcome.

Renal blood flow is characteristically decreased, especially in the cortex, although normal glomerular filtration may be preserved by intrarenal shifts in blood flow. Plasma renin levels correlate with the degree of histologic abnormality of the renal arteries and arterioles. Renal arteriography may document arterial narrowing, tortuosity of the interlobular and arcuate arterioles, cortical hypoperfusion,

and other changes that accompany malignant hypertension. Kidney size is small to normal.

Diagnosis and Diagnostic Tests

High-titer ANAs with speckled patterns are present in the serum in most children. Distinct antigenic specificity may be present, with anticentromere in limited disease, anti-Scl 70 (topoisomerase 1) in diffuse disease, or antinucleolar antibodies. Pulmonary diffusion testing and spirometry are sensitive measures of involvement of the respiratory tract and document a decrease in the timed vital capacity and forced expiratory flow, an early decrease in diffusion, and an increase in functional residual volume. High-resolution CT may confirm the presence of pulmonary disease despite a normal chest radiograph.

Even in early asymptomatic disease, upper gastrointestinal fluoroscopy often documents disordered peristalsis of the distal esophagus. Esophageal motility studies by manometry, however, are more sensitive indicators of functional abnormalities, and a 24-hour pH probe study for potential reflux is helpful. Dilation of the second portion of the duodenum and pseudosacculations of the colon may also be present. Acro-osteolysis of the digits, accompanied by focal areas of soft tissue calcification, may be present on radiographs of the hands (Fig. 98-9).

Plethysmography confirms abnormal vascular responses in affected digits in children with Raynaud's phenomenon and documents both obstructive vascular disease and overactivity of the sympathetic nervous system. Arteriography should be performed with care, if at all, because it may exacerbate digital anoxia.

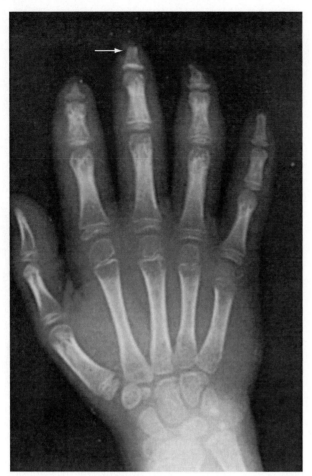

Figure 98-9 Hand of a girl with complaints of Raynaud's phenomenon for 2 years. *Arrow* points to early resorption of the tuft of a distal phalanx (acro-osteolysis).

Considerations in the differential diagnosis include JDM, SLE, and, less frequently, JRA. Patients with limited disease may have features of the previously designated CREST syndrome (calcinosis, Raynaud's phenomenon, esophageal dysmotility, sclerodactyly, and telangiectases), now referred to as limited cutaneous systemic scleroderma. Other overlap syndromes, mixed connective tissue disease, and eosinophilic fasciitis should also be considered.

Treatment

No uniformly effective therapy is available.[1] NSAIDs may relieve some of the musculoskeletal symptoms. Vigorous physical therapy is important in most patients to prevent or minimize joint contractures. D-penicillamine or colchicine may be useful in the management of cutaneous manifestations, if prescribed early; cyclosporine, methotrexate, and cyclophosphamide have been suggested. Because of its apparent safety and tolerability, mycophenolate mofetil has been advocated as a potential immunomodulatory agent for maintenance. Glucocorticoid drugs are contraindicated in most children, because these agents may exacerbate small blood vessel disease and renal involvement with hypertension. Malignant hypertension demands immediate lowering of the blood pressure to normal and merits expert intensive care. Angiotensin-converting enzyme inhibitors are effective in the treatment of hypertension and may have some long-term beneficial effect on abnormalities of the skin and subcutaneous tissues. Autologous stem cell transplantation is being evaluated.[70,71]

Raynaud's phenomenon is best managed with calcium channel blockers such as nifedipine, α-adrenergic blocking agents such as phenoxybenzamine or prazosin, and potentially new agents such as sidenofil. Prostacyclin analogues appear to be safe and effective for the treatment of severe vaso-occlusive disease.[72] Biofeedback has been advocated for the management of less threatening vasospasm. Children with Raynaud's phenomenon must also dress appropriately for the season and avoid cold liquids and objects that exacerbate peripheral arteriolar constriction.

Outcome

The prognosis for pediatric patients with diffuse scleroderma is poor, especially for those with DCSS.[73] Death is often related to cardiopulmonary failure or gastrointestinal complications, including severe inanition. Cardiac arrhythmias may develop during the course of the disease secondary to myocardial fibrosis, and congestive heart failure is often a terminal event. Pulmonary interstitial disease and vascular lesions are probably universal. Renal failure or acute hypertensive encephalopathy supervenes as a potentially fatal outcome in a few children; in adults, these complications are more likely to occur early in the course of the disease. A child may live decades after the onset of systemic scleroderma; therefore, an optimistic but realistic attitude should prevail in discussions with parents. Patients with limited disease were originally thought to have a more favorable prognosis, but evidence is lacking because of the rarity of this subtype.

LOCALIZED SCLERODERMA

The localized sclerodermas are three times as common as systemic disease in children and adolescents (accounting for about 3% of referrals; see Table 98-1). Linear scleroderma is approximately twice as frequent as morphea, which has an estimated incidence of 2.7 per 100,000 children.[63,74] Linear scleroderma develops primarily in the first 2 decades of life. Laboratory abnormalities are few, with the exception of ANAs in almost half the children.[75] Antibodies to centromere or Scl 70 are generally not present. In the localized syndromes, fibrosis of the connective tissues most commonly affects the dermis, subdermis, and superficial striated muscle. However, in a multinational review of 750 children, extracutaneous disease developed in approximately one fourth.[76] Trauma often precedes the onset of cutaneous disease.

It has been proposed that morphea be subdivided into five types: (1) single or multiple plaques, (2) smaller lesions in a more generalized distribution (guttate morphea), (3) bullous, (4) linear, and (5) deep.[77] All these subtypes demonstrate homogenization of collagen bundles. In early disease, acute inflammatory erythema and edema are present in one or more circumscribed lesions, followed by hypopigmentation and induration surrounded by areas of hyperpigmentation (Fig. 98-10). Lesions may be located anywhere on the trunk or extremities and may coalesce or enlarge centrifugally to involve larger areas of the body. Paresthesia or pain may be present over these lesions.

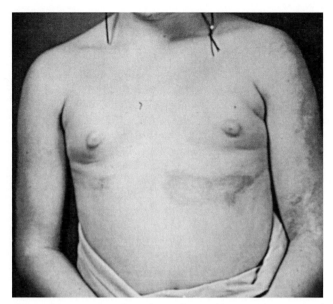

Figure 98-10 Lesions of morphea with central hypopigmentation and active borders on the thorax of a young girl. Another extensive lesion is present on the outer left arm.

Linear scleroderma is the most common subtype in children and is characterized by the presence of one or more areas of linear involvement of the skin of the head, trunk, or extremities. Underlying bone is often affected, with resultant abnormalities of growth or joint contractures. Linear scleroderma often affects only one side of the body, producing hemiatrophy of involved areas. Indeed, it is this lack of normal development, such as in hemifacial atrophy and failure of an extremity to grow in proportion to its opposite member, that causes the most severe disabilities (Fig. 98-11). Linear scleroderma is also associated with syndromes of progressive facial hemiatrophy (Parry-Romberg syndrome) or uveitis.[78] Because linear lesions of the face or scalp may have the appearance of dueling scars, the term *scleroderma en coup de sabre* has been used.

D-penicillamine may be effective in the more generalized form of morphea if used early. Hydroxychloroquine has been recommended by some experts, and ultraviolet A$_1$ phototherapy is advocated by others. Glucocorticoids, as well as methotrexate, may be indicated in clinically active disease. Local emollients and steroid ointments and, more recently, imiquimod may also result in cutaneous improvement. Localized scleroderma may regress spontaneously without treatment, or fibrosis of the involved skin and subcutaneous tissues may progress to produce "hide binding" and marked contractures of an extremity. Active disease is often characterized by exacerbations and remissions occurring over many months to a few years. Prognosis is generally satisfactory in the absence of severe deformity or systemic involvement. Occasionally, visceral disease or a seizure disorder develops late in the course of linear scleroderma. In a few children, the disease may evolve into an overlap syndrome with another connective tissue disease, such as SLE.

EOSINOPHILIC FASCIITIS

Controversy continues over whether eosinophilic fasciitis is a distinct clinicopathologic entity or an unusual variant of deep morphea.[79] It is also associated with plaque

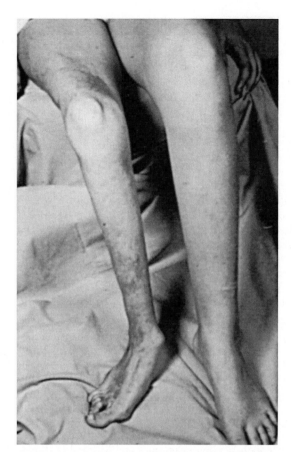

Figure 98-11 Linear scleroderma affecting the right leg of a 14-year-old girl. The disease began at age 6 years and resulted in severe atrophy and shortening of the extremity.

morphea in some children. This disorder is exceptionally rare in the pediatric population. Affected children present with marked induration of cutaneous and subcutaneous tissues of the upper or lower extremities and occasionally the trunk or face. Unusual physical exertion may precede the onset of disease. Raynaud's phenomenon, nail-fold capillary abnormalities, and visceral disease are absent.

Diagnosis is confirmed by a full-thickness biopsy of skin, fascia, and muscle. Inflammation is present in all layers, but the most characteristic features are thickened fascia, with infiltration of histiocytes and often eosinophils, and a prominent perivascular infiltrate of lymphocytes and plasma cells. IgG, IgM, and C3 may be deposited in areas of inflammation. Associated laboratory findings include hypergammaglobulinemia and a remarkable peripheral eosinophilia of 40% to 60%. Eosinophilic fasciitis must be differentiated from the eosinophilia-myalgia syndrome.

As originally reported, eosinophilic fasciitis was self-limited, with spontaneous resolution after months to years. There was often marked relief with the administration of low-dose glucocorticoids. Occasionally, a more severe form of the disease with hematologic abnormalities evolved. These complications may be more common with childhood-onset disease.

MIXED CONNECTIVE TISSUE DISEASE

Mixed connective tissue disease was initially reported as a disorder associated with a favorable prognosis and an excellent initial response to relatively low-dose glucocorticoid therapy. It had a frequency of 0.3% in the U.S. Pediatric Rheumatology Data Base. Children present with arthritis, myositis, and cutaneous disease characteristic of scleroderma, SLE, or JDM.[80] Progression to a more scleroderma-like disease has occurred, with sclerodactyly and gastrointestinal involvement, or an SLE-like disease may evolve.[81,82] Nephritis may be more frequent and more severe in children than in adults. Children often have less pulmonary disease (hypertension) and more hematologic complications (thrombocytopenia) than adults. ANAs are present in very high titers, often in a speckled pattern, to an extractable nuclear antigen and ribonucleoprotein (RNP). Epitope specificity is to U_1RNP and the associated 70-kD A and C polypeptides and, in some instances, to U_1RNA.[83] The predominant HLA associations in these patients are to DR2 and DR4. Other ANAs delineate a subset of children with an overlap syndrome who have the immune complex characteristics of SLE. Antibodies to dsDNA and to the Sm nuclear antigen are present in this latter group.

VASCULITIS

Inflammatory vasculitis is a prominent component of virtually all the systemic connective tissue diseases. The current classification of idiopathic vasculitis is somewhat unsatisfactory,[84] but it is based on the size of the vessels predominantly involved, the type of visceral involvement, and whether the predominant histopathologic feature is vessel wall necrosis or a granulomatous response.[1] All forms of vasculitis, except for Henoch-Schönlein purpura and Kawasaki's disease, are rare in children (Table 98-7). In national diagnostic registries, the various forms of vasculitis account for 1% to 6% of the pediatric rheumatic diseases.[3,85,86] A major study of classification criteria for the vasculitic diseases (predominantly in adults) has been published by a committee of the ACR,[87] with modification by a consensus conference.[88]

NECROTIZING VASCULITIS OF MEDIUM AND SMALL ARTERIES

Medium-sized muscular arteries are involved in necrotizing vasculitis; the predominant histopathologic change is fibrinoid necrosis of the entire thickness of the vessel wall.[89] Lesions tend to be segmental, with a predilection for bifurcations of the vessels. Biopsy specimens usually demonstrate vasculitis in all stages of development from acute to chronic.

Polyarteritis Nodosa

Polyarteritis nodosa (PAN) was initially described more than a century ago, and small numbers of patients have periodically been reported in the pediatric literature. The classic disease remains rare and accounts for approximately 0.4% of referrals to pediatric rheumatology clinics (see Table 98-1). The course and progression of this disease are highly variable, and multisystem involvement leads to diagnostic confusion with numerous other disorders. Early diagnosis and correct classification are often difficult (Table 98-8).[90]

Clinical Features. Although the onset of PAN is frequently insidious, constitutional symptoms of fever and weight loss are often the presenting complaints. The renal, gastrointestinal, and cardiovascular systems are prominently involved, as are both the central and peripheral nervous systems (Table 98-9). The initial clinical diagnosis may be renovascular hypertension or a surgical abdomen. Severe sensorimotor peripheral neuropathy that is often asymmetric in distribution—so-called

Table 98-8 Proposed Criteria for the Diagnosis of Polyarteritis Nodosa in Childhood*

Major Criteria
Renal disease
Musculoskeletal findings

Minor Criteria
Cutaneous findings
Gastrointestinal involvement
Peripheral neuropathy
Central nervous system disease
Hypertension
Cardiac disease
Lung disease
Constitutional symptoms
Increased acute-phase reactants
Presence of hepatitis B surface antigen

*Diagnosis requires the presence of five criteria, including at least one major criterion. Antinuclear antibody and anti–double-stranded DNA must be absent.

From Ozen S, Besbas N, Saatci U, et al: Diagnostic criteria for polyarteritis nodosa in childhood. J Pediatr 120:206-209, 1992.

Table 98-7 Relative Frequencies of Vasculitides in Childhood

Disease	U.S. Registry No. of Patients (N = 434)	Percentage
Kawasaki's disease	97	22.4
Henoch-Schönlein purpura	213	49.1
Wegener's granulomatosis	6	1.4
Polyarteritis nodosa	14	3.2
Takayasu's arteritis	8	1.8
Unclassified	96	22.1

Data from Bowyer S, Roettcher P: Pediatric rheumatology clinic populations in the United States: Results of a 3 year survey. J Rheumatol 23:1968-1974, 1996.

Table 98-9 Clinical Manifestations of Polyarteritis Nodosa in Childhood

Manifestation	Occurrence (%)
Hypertension	80
Gastrointestinal tract	68
Musculoskeletal system	74
Skin	69
Nervous system	45
Central nervous system	16
Peripheral neuropathy	10
Heart	21
Kidneys	25
Lungs	7

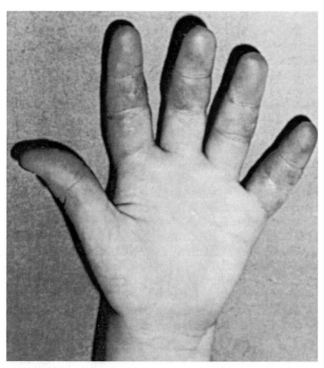

Figure 98-12 Marked digital cyanosis and swelling in a young boy with polyarteritis nodosa. The digital anoxia was accompanied by chronic pain that was exacerbated during acute vasospastic episodes.

Table 98-10 Criteria for the Diagnosis of Kawasaki's Disease

Criterion*	Occurrence (%)
1. Fever lasting 5 days or more	100

2. Changes in lips and oral cavity
   a. Dry, red, vertically fissured lips
   b. Strawberry tongue
   c. Diffuse erythema of mucous membranes
	90

3. Bilateral nonsuppurative bulbar conjunctivitis	85
4. Polymorphous rash (primarily on trunk)	80

5. Changes in peripheral extremities
   a. Erythema of palms and soles
   b. Indurative edema of hands and feet
   c. Desquamation from digital tips
	70

6. Acute nonpurulent enlargement of cervical lymph node to >1.5 cm in diameter	70

*Five criteria are required for diagnosis, or four criteria plus coronary aneurysms on echocardiography. For criteria 2 and 5, any one of the three findings will suffice.

Modified from Sakaguchi M, Taka A, Endo M, et al: On the mucocutaneous lymph node syndrome or Kawasaki disease. In Yu PN, Goodwin JF (eds): Progress in Cardiology 13. Philadelphia, Lea & Febiger, 1985, p 97.

study to study. Death is most commonly secondary to renal failure, myocardial infarction, or hypertensive encephalopathy.

Kawasaki's Disease

Definition and Classification Criteria. An acute febrile illness associated with systemic vasculitis that primarily affects infants and young children was initially reported in 1967 by Kawasaki in Japan.[92] The first descriptions in the English literature appeared in 1974 under the designation "mucocutaneous lymph node syndrome." Previously, a number of infants with a febrile illness that lasted a few weeks to months and was often fatal were described with a syndrome referred to as "infantile polyarteritis nodosa," which probably represented undiagnosed Kawasaki's disease. Clinical criteria were established by Japanese investigators in 1974 to aid in diagnosis. The revised criteria are listed in Table 98-10, but they remain imperfect guidelines with less than optimal sensitivity or specificity.[93] Atypical or incomplete disease may be common in a number of geographic areas.[94]

Epidemiology. Kawasaki's disease has occurred sporadically and in mini-epidemics in the United States, with an incidence of 6 to 7.6 per 100,000 children younger than 5 years.[95] It is currently the leading cause of acquired heart disease in children in developed countries. The disease accounts for approximately 3% of referrals to U.S. pediatric rheumatology clinics (see Table 98-1) and has not changed in incidence during the last decade.[96] The disease is distinctly more common among the Japanese. In Japan, an incidence of 90 per 100,000 was recorded.[97] In the United States, the risk of developing Kawasaki's disease is 17 times greater among children of Japanese ancestry than among white children. In North America, a seasonal variation is often present, with most cases occurring in the spring.[98] The mean age at onset is around 1.5 years, and the male-to-female ratio is 1.5:1. Kawasaki's disease is more common in very young boys, and the single most important complication, coronary aneurysm, is also most frequent

mononeuritis multiplex—may be present. Cutaneous lesions are frequent and include purpura, peripheral gangrene, and nodular vasculitis (Fig. 98-12).

The degree and extent of multisystem involvement are often reflected in anemia, leukocytosis, marked elevation of the erythrocyte sedimentation rate, urinary sediment changes, and abnormalities in serum immunoglobulin concentrations. Rheumatoid factor and ANA seropositivity are unusual. Increased levels of von Willebrand's factor and β-thromboglobulin are associated with activity of the vascular disease. Immune complexes may be present. A few children (<5%) demonstrate seropositivity for hepatitis B– or C–associated antigens. Diagnosis depends on confirmation by biopsy of an involved, accessible site (skin, muscle, nerve) or an angiogram that demonstrates aneurysms in the celiac or renal vasculature.[89,91]

Treatment. Glucocorticoid therapy is the mainstay of treatment. Suppressive amounts of prednisone are indicated, in the range of 1 to 2 mg/kg per day in divided doses. The aggressiveness of the therapeutic program must be closely monitored, according to the extent of cardiac and renal involvement and the presence of hypertension. A child may not respond adequately to oral prednisone alone or to IV steroid pulse therapy. Extensive systemic involvement, particularly of the abdominal vasculature with aneurysms and thrombosis, is generally accepted as an indication for the use of intermittent IV pulse therapy with cyclophosphamide in conjunction with glucocorticoids.

Outcome. PAN is characterized by a chronic relapsing course of many years' duration, with eventual remission possible in some children. Mortality varies widely from in these children. This disease rarely occurs after the age of 11 years. A diagnosis of Kawasaki's disease in adults has been problematic: patients may have this disease or another similar disorder, such as toxic shock syndrome or severe scarlet fever.

Cause and Pathogenesis. The seasonality and temporal clustering of Kawasaki's disease suggest an infectious vector that is currently unidentified; however, secondary cases in a home are unusual. Many causative factors have been suggested but none have been proved, despite 40 years of research. A relationship to heat shock proteins, mycobacterial superantigens, staphylococcal toxins, or Epstein-Barr virus has been postulated. A recent study demonstrated IgA-secreting plasma cells in the vasculature of children who died of Kawasaki's disease, suggesting that a pathogenic organism or antigen had gained entry through mucosal surfaces.[99] Numerous immunologic abnormalities have been reported.[100] The pathogenesis probably represents, in part, a generalized stimulation of the inflammatory response, with increased production of cytokines resulting in cytokine-mediated endothelial damage.[101] A family-based study suggested that genetic variation in the IL-4 gene or linked regions was involved in susceptibility and pathogenesis[102] or in the receptor-ligand pair CCR5 and CCL3L1.[103] The extreme thrombocytosis (550,000 to 1 million/mm^3) observed may contribute to thrombus formation on damaged vascular endothelium. Von Willebrand's factor concentrations are elevated in children with active vasculitis. There is no simple relation to antigens of the major histocompatibility complex in North American white children. A similar disease can be induced in mice by intraperitoneal injection of *Lactobacillus casei*.[104]

Clinical Features. The usual monocyclic course has been divided into three phases that aid in diagnosis and approach to treatment. The acute febrile onset of the disease has already been described. The subacute period begins with return of the temperature to normal and elevation of the platelet count. The convalescent phase follows, with a return of the platelet count to normal. Recurrences are unusual.[106] In rare instances, systemic involvement continues in a pattern indistinguishable from that of undifferentiated vasculitis.

Fever is universal at onset and is usually sustained and remittent. Temperatures of 40°C are common and may be higher. The febrile phase lasts 5 to 25 days, with a mean of about 10 days. Young children may present with a febrile seizure, although other causes of CNS involvement must be carefully excluded. Cerebrospinal fluid protein may be elevated, and pleocytosis is common. Extreme irritability is common.

Mucocutaneous changes are also prominent. Nonsuppurative conjunctival injection may persist for several weeks. Erythema of the lips, with cracking, peeling, and bleeding, is present in most children. Pharyngeal erythema and a strawberry tongue often accompany these changes. A polymorphous rash develops in most children and represents a small vessel vasculitis and perivasculitis of the dermis and subcutaneous tissues. This rash accompanies the fever throughout the acute phase of the disease and then gradually fades. Pruritus is frequently present; vesiculation and purpura do not occur. Painful erythema and edema of the hands, fingers, feet, and toes occur within a few days after onset, and the child may refuse to walk. During recovery, desquamation of the hands and feet occurs, with peeling of the skin beginning underneath the

tips of the nails. This feature is most common during the third week after onset and persists for 1 to 2 weeks. Desquamation and indurative edema can also occur elsewhere, including the perineal area, early in the course (a valuable diagnostic clue). Beau's lines of the nails develop 1 to 2 months after onset.

Although lymphadenopathy occurs in about half the children, it is often not prominent and resolves rapidly toward the end of the febrile period. Involvement of the cervical nodes is common and may be unilateral; a sentinel cervical node 1 to 2 cm in diameter is the most characteristic physical finding. Involvement of almost any system can occur. Relatively common at presentation and during the initial course are pneumonitis, with the development of nodules in some children; tympanitis; meningitis; photophobia and uveitis; diarrhea; meatitis; and sterile pyuria. Arthritis or arthralgia occurs in more than one third of children. Relatively uncommon clinical findings are pleural effusions, severe abdominal colic, hydrops of the gallbladder, intestinal pseudo-obstruction, jaundice, and tonsillar exudate. The kidneys are not involved.

The most serious manifestations are myocarditis and coronary vasculitis. It is assumed that a panmyocarditis is universal during the acute febrile phase of the disease. In a variable number of children, the disease progresses to coronary vasculitis with vessel wall necrosis, aneurysm formation, or thrombosis. Coronary artery aneurysms are often present at onset or as early as the second week of the illness. Development of these aneurysms reaches a peak during the subacute period; they are usually multiple and are identified in approximately 20% of children with Kawasaki's disease in the United States. In children with risk factors for coronary artery aneurysms (i.e., male, age at onset of 18 months or younger or older than 6 years, Japanese ancestry, prolonged febrile course with early clinical myocarditis), their frequency increases to greater than 50%. Aneurysms also occur in arteries other than the coronaries, such as the brachial, subclavian, and axillary vessels.

Diagnosis and Diagnostic Tests. Acute-phase indices are elevated early in the course. Abnormalities of the transaminase enzymes and sterile pyuria may be present. Two-dimensional echocardiography is the most sensitive technique for delineating proximal coronary vasculitis and aneurysms (Fig. 98-13). This study should be performed immediately in a child with fever and rash in whom there is a high index of suspicion of Kawasaki's disease. Echocardiography should also be repeated during the course of the disease—for example, at 1 week, 6 weeks, and 3 months—with the timing and frequency dependent on the course of disease and whether aneurysms were initially detected. A committee of the American Heart Association has issued general recommendations based on disease severity.[107] These recommendations have recently been reviewed.[93,108] Angiography in selected children may demonstrate multiple lesions of the proximal or peripheral cardiac vessels. Abnormal lipoprotein patterns have been described,[109] as well as elevated levels of osteoprotegerin.[110]

Treatment. The current approach to treatment is divided into two parts: (1) aspirin in anti-inflammatory doses and then as an antiplatelet agent and (2) IVIG.[93,111,112] In the presence of developing, progressive, or unstable cardiac disease, close observation in the hospital with cardiac monitoring is extremely

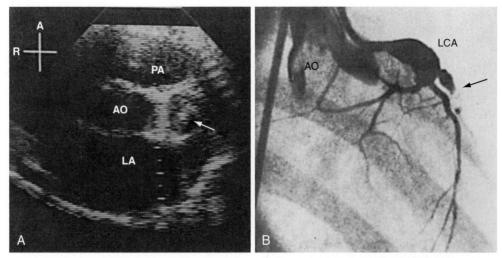

Figure 98-13 A, Echocardiographic demonstration of an aneurysm of the left coronary artery *(arrow)* in a young boy with Kawasaki's disease. **B,** Angiogram of this giant aneurysm *(arrow)*. AO, aorta; LA, left atrium, LCA, left coronary artery; PA, pulmonary artery.

important. Only by detecting the initial signs of cardiac de-compensation or arrhythmia can appropriate emergency measures be taken in a severely affected child. High-dose aspirin (e.g., 100 mg/kg per day in divided doses) is traditionally instituted during the acute phase of the illness, although this practice has been questioned.[113-115] During the subacute period (resolution of fever and development of thrombocytosis), antiplatelet dosages are prescribed (e.g., 5 mg/kg per day in a single dose). This dosage is continued for months to years in children with or at risk for coronary artery involvement.

Controlled studies have demonstrated that a single high dose of IVIG (2000 mg/kg) is efficacious.[111,116,117] This therapy is probably most effective if given within the first 10 days of the illness. Children often have a dramatic response to IVIG in terms of fever, constitutional symptoms, and general well-being. In addition, IVIG therapy reduces the frequency, size, and severity of coronary aneurysms and improves the outcome compared with control groups. Glucocorticoids are generally contraindicated because of early studies that reported an increased frequency of coronary aneurysms in children who received steroids compared with those receiving no therapy or aspirin alone. Use of these agents may be considered, however, in a subgroup of children with recurrent disease or severe active myocarditis[118] or in IVIG-resistant disease.[119-121] Additional recommendations include the use of infliximab.[122] Thrombolytic therapy with tissue plasminogen activator or urokinase should be considered in cases of acute coronary thrombosis. Coronary abnormalities may require prolonged medication, interventional catheterization, or cardiac surgery.

Outcome. Long-term damage to the coronary arteries occurs in approximately one fourth of children.[123] Almost all early deaths and most cases of long-term disability are related to cardiac involvement.[95,97,124] Myocardial infarction has been described in approximately 2.5% of reported cases and occurs most commonly in the subacute phase. Death may be due to infarction, coronary thrombosis, or rupture of an aneurysm. Giant aneurysms (>8 mm) represent an especially serious development.[125] Late death several years after onset has occurred as a result of aneurysm rupture or premature atherosclerosis

with calcification and occlusion.[126,127] Extensive scarring, arterial calcification, multiple areas of stenosis, or recanalization may develop in children who survive an initial severe coronary insult and result in progressive myocardial dysfunction.[124,128] Selected children may be candidates for coronary bypass surgery and revascularization.[129-131]

A careful history to uncover previous Kawasaki's disease is indicated in all older children and young adolescents who present for pre-sports physical examinations, because there may be long-term persistence of vascular abnormalities.[124,132,133] If the history includes a febrile illness accompanied by features suggestive of the disorder, clinical evaluation must include specific measures of cardiac function (e.g., stress testing, echocardiography).

NECROTIZING VASCULITIS OF SMALL VESSELS

Necrotizing vasculitis that affects smaller vessels, including postcapillary venules, is referred to as *leukocytoclastic vasculitis*.[89] In these disorders, the vessel wall undergoes necrosis and is infiltrated with polymorphonuclear leukocytes, and nuclear debris is scattered around the lesions. Fibrinoid necrosis is present, and deposition of immunoglobulin and complement can often be demonstrated by fluorescent microscopy. This form of vasculitis may be encountered as a sequela to drug hypersensitivity, infectious endocarditis, or hematologic malignancy. Cryoglobulinemia, either essential or secondary to another disease, causes an immune complex vasculitis that mimics various forms of vasculopathy.

Henoch-Schönlein Purpura

Definition and Criteria. Henoch-Schönlein purpura (HSP) is common in children and adolescents[89,134,135] between 3 and 15 years of age and is more frequent in boys than in girls (1.5:1). It is recognized as a putative IgA-mediated immune vasculitis. Diagnosis is based on the clinical tetrad of arthritis, abdominal pain, hematuria, and nonthrombocytopenic purpura.[136] The classic purpuric skin rash (palpable purpura) is generally regarded as essential for diagnosis (Fig. 98-14). HSP is relatively uncommon in adults and often more severe.[137,138]

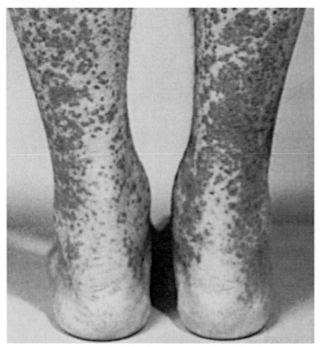

Figure 98-14 Petechial and papular rash over the lower extremities of a teenage boy with Henoch-Schönlein purpura.

Epidemiology. An incidence of 13.5 per 100,000 children was reported from Belfast, Northern Ireland.[139] HSP accounts for about 8% of new patient referrals (see Table 98-1). It commonly occurs after an upper respiratory tract infection, often in the spring. Streptococcal disease has been implicated in some cases, and others have been related to vaccination, varicella, hepatitis B infection, insect bites, dietary allergens, malignancy, or mycoplasma infection. Occasionally, a familial occurrence is reported, but no definite HLA association has been demonstrated. HSP occurs more frequently in children with C2 complement component deficiency. It is more frequent in the Middle East in children who also have familial Mediterranean fever.

Clinical Features. Disease onset is often acute, with sequential manifestations appearing over a few days to weeks. A leukocytoclastic vasculitis with deposition of IgA, IgG, fibrin, C3, and properdin occurs in all affected organs,[89] although the skin, gastrointestinal tract, joints, and kidneys are the primary structures affected. Vasculitic involvement may lead to an acute scrotal syndrome. The universal vascular deposition of IgA suggests that HSP is an IgA-mediated immune response and may operate through the alternative complement pathway. The CNS may be involved, and an isolated cerebral vasculitis has been described. Pulmonary disease with hemorrhage can occur.

Purpura is the first sign in more than half the children. The buttocks and lower extremities are most often affected; the trunk is usually spared. The lesions often appear in crops; some may have central hemorrhage or ulceration, and others mimic urticaria. Individual purpuric lesions often coalesce to form larger areas of involvement interspersed with petechiae. Subcutaneous edema is observed in 25% of children. It commonly involves the dorsa of the hands and feet and, less commonly, the scalp, forehead, periorbital areas, perineum, and scrotum. Extensive edema is most common in children younger than 2 years. Acute hemorrhagic edema of infancy may be a variant of HSP.

More than 85% of affected children have gastrointestinal signs and symptoms. These include colicky abdominal pain, melena, ileus, vomiting, and hematemesis. Extensive submucosal and mucosal edema, hemorrhage, perforation, and intussusception occur in less than 5% of children and are more common in children older than 4 years. Clinical evidence of glomerulitis is found in up to 50% of cases.[139-141] The degree of renal involvement varies from mild endocapillary glomerulitis to extensive crescentic disease. Mesangial involvement is prominent at onset and is similar to Berger's (IgA) nephropathy in adults.[142]

Arthritis that is symmetric or asymmetric and predominantly involves the larger joints is a prominent finding in about 75% of children. Although often initially painful, with limitation of motion, it may be less dramatic and is usually not migratory. The knees and ankles are most commonly affected, but wrists, elbows, and fingers may also be involved with prominent periarticular swelling and tenderness, usually without erythema or warmth. Joint effusions per se are unusual. The arthritis is transient, often resolves within a few days, and leaves no residual damage.

A moderate leukocytosis occurs, along with a normocytic, normochromic anemia that may be related in part to gastrointestinal blood loss. The platelet count is normal. Activated C3d is present in the circulation, and concentrations of properdin and factor B are decreased in half the children during the acute illness. Serum IgA and IgM concentrations are elevated in half the patients. Fibrin split products are increased in the circulation and urine, providing evidence of involvement of the fibrinolytic system.

Diagnosis and Diagnostic Tests. HSP must be differentiated from a wide variety of other illnesses of childhood, including poststreptococcal glomerulonephritis, rheumatic fever, SLE, septicemia, and disseminated intravascular coagulation. Other causes of an acute surgical abdomen or gastrointestinal bleeding must be considered, along with intussusception and pancreatitis. CT in HSP may delineate multifocal areas of bowel wall thickening, mesenteric edema, vascular engorgement, or intussusception. Although the presence of purpura is traditionally required for a diagnosis of HSP, there are undoubtedly children who either do not develop purpura or do not have it at disease onset. Biopsy of a cutaneous lesion may be diagnostic in difficult cases if it demonstrates a leukocytoclastic vasculitis characterized by deposition of IgA and C3.

Treatment. General supportive measures are critical in seriously ill children with HSP. In general, glucocorticoids have potential therapeutic value only for the management of gastrointestinal vasculitis and hemorrhage or in severe symptomatic disease in a carefully selected group of patients. The response to their use in these cases may be dramatic. Prednisone, 1 to 2 mg/kg per day in divided doses, is used for at least a week and is then gradually tapered, based on clinical improvement and extent of bleeding. There is no concrete evidence that prednisone otherwise modifies the clinical expression of the disease, shortens its course, or has any direct effect on the frequency or severity of renal involvement.[143] Clinical studies have not thoroughly evaluated the efficacy of steroids administered early to children with nephritis; however, in children with progressive renal disease, consideration should be given to their use and to cytotoxic agents and antiplatelet drugs.

Kidney biopsy is generally not indicated, except to clarify the extent and nature of renal disease in children who are severely affected. Azathioprine, cyclosporine, and IVIG have also been recommended for severe nephritis. Renal transplantation has been successfully performed in children, and nephritis does not generally recur in the allografts.[144]

Outcome. HSP is usually a self-limited disease and often consists of a single episode of clinical involvement. In most children, the disease runs its course in 4 to 6 weeks. Although approximately 30% of young children have a second or third exacerbation, an increasing percentage of older children have recurrences: the younger the child and the shorter the course, the fewer recurrences that are expected. Exacerbations usually occur within the initial 6-week period, but an occasional child may develop recurrences for as long as 2 years after onset. The prognosis is generally excellent and depends on the extent of systemic involvement and the age of the child, being better in younger children. Morbidity and mortality are predominantly related to involvement of the gastrointestinal tract or kidneys.[140] Nephrotic syndrome, decreased creatinine clearance, severe histopathology, and persistence of urinary abnormalities are ominous signs.[145] Pregnancy may exacerbate occult renal disease. Mortality was less than 1% in the Belfast study, and the morbidity rate was 1.1%.[139]

Other Forms of Leukocytoclastic Vasculitis

Smaller blood vessels, including arterioles, capillaries, and venules, are typically involved in hypersensitivity angiitis.[89,134] A form of this disease, serum sickness, was once more common than at present; it occurred secondary to the therapeutic use of heterologous antisera and the introduction of sulfa drugs and penicillin. In addition to these medications, many other drugs have been implicated in the pathogenesis. Cutaneous disease is common and consists of painful, palpable purpura or hemorrhagic infarcts. The vascular inflammatory lesions are at similar stages of evolution in all vessels; the cellular infiltrate often contains many eosinophils. Immune complexes can often be demonstrated in the circulation. Arthritis is usually a prominent component of the clinical presentation; Cogan's syndrome is rare. Hypersensitivity angiitis is characterized by a variable course whose outcome is often determined by the presence and severity of cardiac, pulmonary, or renal abnormalities. Prednisone is usually effective in suppressing this disorder and in preventing severe complications or death. The disease generally runs its course in approximately 6 weeks.

Isolated cutaneous polyarteritis, usually without systemic or constitutional symptoms, is occasionally encountered in a child who presents with palpable purpura, painful nodules, or inflammatory ridges that develop along the course of medium and small vessels of the dermis and panniculus.[146] The clinical course is variable but is characterized by benign remissions and recurrences, often over many years. Few children develop systemic involvement. Although each exacerbation may respond to glucocorticoids or occasionally to aspirin, this disease is frequently of such long duration that it is difficult to treat a growing child with prednisone during its entire course. Alternate-day dosing may offer a more rational approach to therapy.

Hypocomplementemic urticarial vasculitis, although occurring primarily in young women, has also been described in children.[147] The eruption affects principally the face, upper extremities, and trunk but also occurs on the palms and soles. The urticarial lesions last 2 to 4 days with each exacerbation and then fade without scarring. Systemic features of variable severity (arthritis, myositis, uveitis, serositis, involvement of the lungs or kidneys) accompany the cutaneous disease. The degree of hypocomplementemia parallels the severity of the illness. In some patients, the condition warrants treatment with glucocorticoid drugs.

Microscopic polyarteritis is a rare form of vasculitis and glomerulonephritis in childhood. It is associated with perinuclear antineutrophil cytoplasmic and antimyeloperoxidase antibodies. Many children progress to end-stage renal disease.[148] Therapy generally includes glucocorticoids and cyclophosphamide.

GIANT CELL ARTERITIS

Characteristic features of giant cell arteritis are involvement of the aorta and its major branches, disruption of the internal elastic lamina, intimal proliferation, and infiltration of vessel walls with mononuclear cells and giant cells. Systemic giant cell arteritis is rare and involves major branches or segments of the aorta at single or multiple locations. The child may present with constitutional symptoms, fever of unknown origin, or hypertension. A diagnosis is established by angiography combined with biopsy of a vessel, if accessible (Fig. 98-15). Vascular occlusion leads to peripheral anoxia, cyanosis, and gangrene. Recanalization may occur spontaneously or during treatment with glucocorticoid drugs.

Cranial or temporal arteritis is generally a disease of older adults, but it has been described in children and is characterized by a persistent, severe headache and localized pain and tenderness over a cranial or temporal vessel. The erythrocyte sedimentation rate is dramatically elevated. The threat of blindness from involvement of the ophthalmic and central retinal arteries is an important consideration and an indication for the prompt initiation of glucocorticoid therapy. Diagnosis is established by biopsy of an affected vessel, with care taken to secure a generous specimen. CNS vasculitis occurs secondary to a variety of conditions.[149]

Takayasu's Arteritis

Takayasu's arteritis is a giant cell arteritis that occurs predominantly in children and adolescents, especially teenage girls (female-to-male ratio 8:1), and involves the aorta and its major branches and the pulmonary arteries.[150] Features of the disease include stenosis, occlusion, dilation, and aneurysms. Takayasu's arteritis has been referred to as "pulseless disease" or "reverse coarctation" because of the characteristic obliteration of the radial pulses. These signs of peripheral vascular insufficiency often direct attention to the correct diagnosis, which is confirmed by angiography,[151] ultrasonography, MRI, or magnetic resonance angiography.[152] Criteria for diagnosis have been developed by the ACR.[153]

This disorder is more common in Asians, Hispanics, Sephardic Jews, and African Americans. It occasionally occurs in the families of children with other connective tissue diseases or in conjunction with other rheumatic disorders and

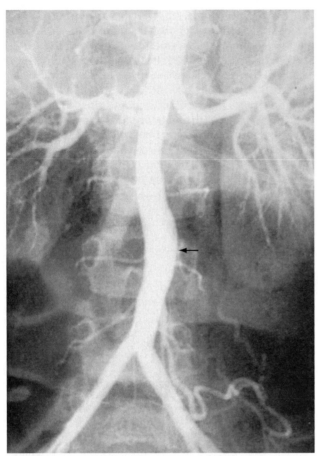

Figure 98-15 Angiogram demonstrating tortuosity and dilation of the lower aorta *(arrow)* in a 6-year-old girl with giant cell arteritis of the abdominal vessels. Note involvement of the right renal artery.

has been reported in monozygotic twin sisters. Hypertension is frequent during the course of the disease and is related in part to stenosis of the renal arteries. Calcification is sometimes identified in affected vessels on plain films.

The course of the disease may be as short as 3 to 6 months or as long as many years. Survival rates in one study were 93% at 5 years and 87% at 10 years.[154] It is generally believed that glucocorticoids are effective if used early, before stenosis and thrombosis develop (after a negative cutaneous purified protein derivative test, because of a putative association with tuberculosis in some areas of the world), but there have been insufficient clinical studies to confirm the efficacy of either this therapeutic approach or the use of cyclophosphamide, azathioprine, or methotrexate. NSAIDs are useful to relieve symptoms during the early phases of the illness. Anticoagulants and antiplatelet agents may be indicated if there is widespread chronic occlusion of vessels. Vessel grafts have been successful late in the course of the disease for vascular occlusion,[155] which is the most common indication for surgical intervention.[156]

Granulomatous Arteritis

Wegener's granulomatosis is a rare example of granulomatous arteritis in children and is characterized by the clinical triad of upper and lower respiratory involvement and renal

disease.[89,157-159] Onset of the disease has been described as early as 3 months of age. Constitutional symptoms are prominent. Unexplained pain, rhinorrhea, mucosal ulceration, or bleeding from the upper respiratory tract is characteristic. Destruction of nasal cartilage may result in a saddle nose. Hemoptysis and pleuritic pain are frequent. Chest radiographs demonstrate multiform pulmonary infiltrates; pulmonary disease may progress to hemorrhage, obstruction, atelectasis, or repeated episodes of infection. More than 80% of affected children have renal disease, which may become rapidly progressive, although hypertension is less common than in other types of nephritis. Necrotizing granulomas also occur in the skin, heart, CNS, gastrointestinal tract, and synovia. Limited forms of Wegener's granulomatosis have been described, possibly including midline granuloma, which is exceedingly rare in children.

The differential diagnosis includes berylliosis, Löffler's syndrome, tuberculosis, syphilis, and lymphoma. Goodpasture's syndrome, lymphomatoid granulomatosis, relapsing polychondritis, and other forms of vasculitis are sometimes confused with Wegener's granulomatosis. Sarcoidosis can occur in children with systemic necrotizing vasculitis, cutaneous vasculitis, or granulomatous arteritis.

Biopsy of an affected site, generally nasal mucosa or lung, is essential to an early diagnosis. Necrotizing granulomas with leukocytic, lymphocytic, and giant cell infiltration are present.[89] Overt vasculitis may not be evident. Antineutrophil cytoplasmic antibodies directed against serine protease 3 are characteristic of Wegener's granulomatosis.[160] The perinuclear pattern of staining, usually associated with antibodies to myeloperoxidase, is less specific and has been described in other forms of vasculitis and connective tissue diseases.

In untreated children, death from renal or pulmonary complications usually occurs in a matter of months, but long-term survival in the absence of specific therapy has been reported. Glucocorticoid drugs and trimethoprim-sulfamethoxazole may be useful early in the disease, but studies confirm that cyclophosphamide is the most effective treatment.[158] The use of methotrexate as an alternative immunosuppressive agent has been proposed to avoid the long-term morbidity associated with cyclophosphamide.[161]

Allergic granulomatosis (Churg-Strauss syndrome) is a systemic vasculitis that occurs predominantly in males on a background of chronic asthma and peripheral eosinophilia.[89] Other manifestations are similar to those characteristic of PAN, especially in the gastrointestinal tract, CNS, and musculoskeletal system. Renal disease is, however, less frequent. Pulmonary involvement is often the single most important manifestation. The histopathologic pattern in biopsy specimens is that of a necrotizing vasculitis with an eosinophilic infiltrate and extravascular necrotizing granulomas. Administration of glucocorticoid drugs is the main approach to treatment, occasionally in combination with cyclophosphamide. Prognosis is variable; death often results from cardiopulmonary failure.

REFERENCES

1. Cassidy JT, Petty RE, Laxer RM, et al: Textbook of Pediatric Rheumatology, 5th ed. Philadelphia, Elsevier Saunders, 2005.
2. Fessel WJ: Epidemiology of systemic lupus erythematosus. Rheum Dis Clin North Am 14:15-23, 1988.

3. Malleson PN, Fung MY, Rosenberg AM: The incidence of pediatric rheumatic diseases: Results from the Canadian Pediatric Rheumatology Association Disease Registry. J Rheumatol 23:1981-1987, 1996.

4. Tucker LB, Menon S, Schaller JG, et al: Adult- and childhood-onset systemic lupus erythematosus: A comparison of onset, clinical features, serology, and outcome. Br J Rheumatol 34:866-872, 1995.

5. Deapen D, Escalante A, Weinrib L, et al: A revised estimate of twin concordance in systemic lupus erythematosus. Arthritis Rheum 35:311-318, 1992.

6. Bader-Meunier B, Armengaud JB, Haddad E, et al: Initial presentation of childhood-onset systemic lupus erythematosus: A French multicenter study. J Pediatr 146:648-653, 2005.

7. Gazarian M, Feldman BM, Benson LN, et al: Assessment of myocardial perfusion and function in childhood systemic lupus erythematosus. J Pediatr 132:109-116, 1998.

8. Sibbitt WL Jr, Brandt JR, Johnson CR, et al: The incidence and prevalence of neuropsychiatric syndromes in pediatric onset systemic lupus erythematosus. J Rheumatol 29:1536-1542, 2002.

9. Tan EM, Cohen AS, Fries JF, et al: The 1982 revised criteria for the classification of systemic lupus erythematosus. Arthritis Rheum 25:1271-1277, 1982.

10. Ferraz MB, Goldenberg J, Hilario MO, et al: Evaluation of the 1982 ARA lupus criteria data set in pediatric patients. Committees of Pediatric Rheumatology of the Brazilian Society of Pediatrics and the Brazilian Society of Rheumatology. Clin Exp Rheumatol 12:83-87, 1994.

11. Ravelli A, Martini A: Antiphospholipid antibody syndrome in pediatric patients. Rheum Dis Clin North Am 23:657-676, 1997.

12. **Cimaz R, Descloux E: Pediatric antiphospholipid syndrome. Rheum Dis Clin North Am 32:553-573, 2006.**

13. Cimaz R, Romeo A, Scarano A, et al: Prevalence of anti-cardiolipin, anti-beta2 glycoprotein I, and anti-prothrombin antibodies in young patients with epilepsy. Epilepsia 43:52-59, 2002.

14. Armenti VT, Radomski JS, Moritz MJ, et al: Report from the National Transplantation Pregnancy Registry (NTPR): Outcomes of pregnancy after transplantation. Clin Transpl 121-130, 2002.

15. Canadian Hydroxychloroquine Study Group: A randomized study of the effect of withdrawing hydroxychloroquine sulfate in systemic lupus erythematosus. N Engl J Med 324:150-154, 1991.

16. Steinberg AD, Steinberg SC: Long-term preservation of renal function in patients with lupus nephritis receiving treatment that includes cyclophosphamide versus those treated with prednisone only. Arthritis Rheum 34:945-950, 1991.

17. Lehman TJ: A practical guide to systemic lupus erythematosus. Pediatr Clin North Am 42:1223-1238, 1995.

18. **Ginzler EM, Dooley MA, Aranow C, et al: Mycophenolate mofetil or intravenous cyclophosphamide for lupus nephritis. N Engl J Med 353:2219-2228, 2005.**

19. Gipson DS, Ferris ME, Dooley MA, et al: Renal transplantation in children with lupus nephritis. Am J Kidney Dis 41:455-463, 2003.

20. Brunner HI, Silverman ED, Bombardier C, et al: European consensus lupus activity measurement is sensitive to change in disease activity in childhood-onset systemic lupus erythematosus. Arthritis Rheum 49:335-341, 2003.

21. **Ruperto N, Ravelli A, Oliveira S, et al: The Pediatric Rheumatology International Trials Organization/American College of Rheumatology provisional criteria for the evaluation of response to therapy in juvenile systemic lupus erythematosus: Prospective validation of the definition of improvement. Arthritis Rheum 55:355-363, 2006.**

22. Lacks S, White P: Morbidity associated with childhood systemic lupus erythematosus. J Rheumatol 17:941-945, 1990.

23. Miettunen PM, Ortiz-Alvarez O, Petty RE, et al: Gender and ethnic origin have no effect on long term outcome of childhood-onset systemic lupus erythematosus. J Rheumatol 31:1650-1654, 2004.

24. Hagelberg S, Lee Y, Bargman J, et al: Long term followup of childhood lupus nephritis. J Rheumatol 29:2635-2642, 2002.

25. **Bernatsky S, Boivin JF, Joseph L, et al: Mortality in systemic lupus erythematosus. Arthritis Rheum 54:2550-2557, 2006.**

26. Platt JL, Burke BA, Fish AJ, et al: Systemic lupus erythematosus in the first two decades of life. Am J Kidney Dis 2:212-222, 1982.

27. Yang LY, Chen WP, Lin CY: Lupus nephritis in children—a review of 167 patients. Pediatrics 94:335-340, 1994.

28. Ravelli A, Duarte-Salazar C, Buratti S, et al: Assessment of damage in juvenile-onset systemic lupus erythematosus: A multicenter cohort study. Arthritis Rheum 49:501-507, 2003.

29. Lilleby V, Flato B, Forre O: Disease duration, hypertension and medication requirements are associated with organ damage in childhood-onset systemic lupus erythematosus. Clin Exp Rheumatol 23:261-269, 2005.

30. Alsufyani KA, Ortiz-Alvarez O, Cabral DA, et al: Bone mineral density in children and adolescents with systemic lupus erythematosus, juvenile dermatomyositis, and systemic vasculitis: Relationship to disease duration, cumulative corticosteroid dose, calcium intake, and exercise. J Rheumatol 32:729-733, 2005.

31. Silverman ED, Laxer RM: Neonatal lupus erythematosus. Rheum Dis Clin North Am 23:599-618, 1997.

32. **Buyon JP, Clancy RM: Neonatal lupus: Review of proposed pathogenesis and clinical data from the US-based Research Registry for Neonatal Lupus. Autoimmunity 36:41-50, 2003.**

33. Cimaz R, Spence DL, Hornberger L, et al: Incidence and spectrum of neonatal lupus erythematosus: A prospective study of infants born to mothers with anti-Ro autoantibodies. J Pediatr 142:678-683, 2003.

34. Prendiville JS, Cabral DA, Poskitt KJ, et al: Central nervous system involvement in neonatal lupus erythematosus. Pediatr Dermatol 20:60-67, 2003.

35. Neiman AR, Lee LA, Weston WL, et al: Cutaneous manifestations of neonatal lupus without heart block: Characteristics of mothers and children enrolled in a national registry. J Pediatr 137:674-680, 2000.

36. **Martin V, Lee LA, Askanase AD, et al: Long-term followup of children with neonatal lupus and their unaffected siblings. Arthritis Rheum 46:2377-2383, 2002.**

37. Waltuck J, Buyon JP: Autoantibody-associated congenital heart block: Outcome in mothers and children. Ann Intern Med 120:544-551, 1994.

38. Press J, Uziel Y, Laxer RM, et al: Long-term outcome of mothers of children with complete congenital heart block. Am J Med 100:328-332, 1996.

39. **Rider LG, Miller FW: Classification and treatment of the juvenile idiopathic inflammatory myopathies. Rheum Dis Clin North Am 23:619-655, 1997.**

40. Symmons DP, Sills JA, Davis SM: The incidence of juvenile dermatomyositis: Results from a nation-wide study. Br J Rheumatol 34:732-736, 1995.

41. **Mendez EP, Lipton R, Ramsey-Goldman R, et al: US incidence of juvenile dermatomyositis, 1995-1998: Results from the National Institute of Arthritis and Musculoskeletal and Skin Diseases Registry. Arthritis Rheum 49:300-305, 2003.**

42. Tezak Z, Hoffman EP, Lutz JL, et al: Gene expression profiling in DQA1*0501+ children with untreated dermatomyositis: A novel model of pathogenesis. J Immunol 168:4154-4163, 2002.

43. Pachman LM: Juvenile dermatomyositis: Immunogenetics, pathophysiology, and disease expression. Rheum Dis Clin North Am 28:579-602, 2002.

44. **Massa M, Costouros N, Mazzoli F, et al: Self epitopes shared between human skeletal myosin and Streptococcus pyogenes M5 protein are targets of immune responses in active juvenile dermatomyositis. Arthritis Rheum 46:3015-3025, 2002.**

45. Reed AM, Pachman LM, Hayford J, et al: Immunogenetic studies in families of children with juvenile dermatomyositis. J Rheumatol 25:1000-1002, 1998.

46. **Pachman LM, Fedczyna TO, Lechman TS, et al: Juvenile dermatomyositis: The association of the TNF alpha-308A allele and disease chronicity. Curr Rheumatol Rep 3:379-386, 2001.**

47. Artlett CM, Ramos R, Jiminez SA, et al: Chimeric cells of maternal origin in juvenile idiopathic inflammatory myopathies. Childhood Myositis Heterogeneity Collaborative Group. Lancet 356:2155-2156, 2000.

48. Reed AM, Picornell YJ, Harwood A, et al: Chimerism in children with juvenile dermatomyositis. Lancet 356:2156-2157, 2000.

49. **Reed AM, McNallan K, Wettstein P, et al: Does HLA-dependent chimerism underlie the pathogenesis of juvenile dermatomyositis? J Immunol 172:5041-5046, 2004.**

50. Artlett CM, O'Hanlon TP, Lopez AM, et al: HLA-DQA1 is not an apparent risk factor for microchimerism in patients with various autoimmune diseases and in healthy individuals. Arthritis Rheum 48:2567-2572, 2003.

51. Pachman LM: Juvenile dermatomyositis. Pathophysiology and disease expression. Pediatr Clin North Am 42:1071-1098, 1995.

52. Spencer CH, Hanson V, Singsen BH, et al: Course of treated juvenile dermatomyositis. J Pediatr 105:399-408, 1984.

53. Dolezalova P, Young SP, Bacon PA, et al: Nailfold capillary microscopy in healthy children and in childhood rheumatic diseases: A prospective single blind observational study. Ann Rheum Dis 62:444-449, 2003.

54. Plamondon S, Dent PB: Juvenile amyopathic dermatomyositis: Results of a case finding descriptive survey. J Rheumatol 27:2031-2034, 2000.

55. Huang JL: Juvenile dermatomyositis associated with partial lipodystrophy. Br J Clin Pract 50:112-113, 1996.

56. Feldman BM, Reichlin M, Laxer RM, et al: Clinical significance of specific autoantibodies in juvenile dermatomyositis. J Rheumatol 23:1794-1797, 1996.

57. **Huber AM, Hicks JE, Lachenbruch PA, et al: Validation of the Childhood Health Assessment Questionnaire in the juvenile idiopathic myopathies. Juvenile Dermatomyositis Disease Activity Collaborative Study Group. J Rheumatol 28:1106-1111, 2001.**

58. Ruperto N, Ravelli A, Murray KJ, et al: Preliminary core sets of measures for disease activity and damage assessment in juvenile systemic lupus erythematosus and juvenile dermatomyositis. Rheumatology (Oxford) 42:1452-1459, 2003.

59. Falcini F, Bindi G, Simonini G, et al: Bone status evaluation with calcaneal ultrasound in children with chronic rheumatic diseases: A one year followup study. J Rheumatol 30:179-184, 2003.

60. Lang BA, Laxer RM, Murphy G, et al: Treatment of dermatomyositis with intravenous gammaglobulin. Am J Med 91:169-172, 1991.

61. Hicks JE, Drinkard B, Summers RM, et al: Decreased aerobic capacity in children with juvenile dermatomyositis. Arthritis Rheum 47:118-123, 2002.

62. **Oral EA, Simha V, Ruiz E, et al: Leptin-replacement therapy for lipodystrophy. N Engl J Med 346:570-578, 2002.**

63. Nelson AM: Localized scleroderma including morphea, linear scleroderma, and eosinophilic fasciitis. Curr Probl Pediatr 26:318-324, 1996.

64. LeRoy EC, Medsger TA Jr: Criteria for the classification of early systemic sclerosis. J Rheumatol 28:1573-1576, 2001.

65. Uziel Y, Miller ML, Laxer RM: Scleroderma in children. Pediatr Clin North Am 42:1171-1203, 1995.

66. Mayes MD: Scleroderma epidemiology. Rheum Dis Clin North Am 29:239-254, 2003.

67. Nelson JL, Furst DE, Maloney S, et al: Microchimerism and HLA-compatible relationships of pregnancy in scleroderma. Lancet 351:559-562, 1998.

68. **Johnson KL, Nelson JL, Furst DE, et al: Fetal cell microchimerism in tissue from multiple sites in women with systemic sclerosis. Arthritis Rheum 44:1848-1854, 2001.**

69. Lemaire R, Farina G, Kissin E, et al: Mutant fibrillin 1 from tight skin mice increases extracellular matrix incorporation of microfibril-associated glycoprotein 2 and type I collagen. Arthritis Rheum 50:915-926, 2004.

70. **Wulffraat NM, Sanders LA, Kuis W: Autologous hemopoietic stem-cell transplantation for children with refractory autoimmune disease. Curr Rheumatol Rep 2:316-323, 2000.**

71. Farge D, Marolleau JP, Zohar S, et al: Autologous bone marrow transplantation in the treatment of refractory systemic sclerosis: Early results from a French multicentre phase I-II study. Br J Haematol 119:726-739, 2002.

72. Zulian F, Corona F, Gerloni V, et al: Safety and efficacy of iloprost for the treatment of ischaemic digits in paediatric connective tissue diseases. Rheumatology (Oxford) 43:229-233, 2004.

73. Scalapino K, Arkachaisri T, Lucas M, et al: Childhood onset systemic sclerosis: Classification, clinical and serologic features, and survival in comparison with adult onset disease. J Rheumatol 33:1004-1013, 2006.

74. Peterson LS, Nelson AM, Su WP, et al: The epidemiology of morphea (localized scleroderma) in Olmsted County 1960-1993. J Rheumatol 24:73-80, 1997.

75. Rosenberg AM, Uziel Y, Krafchik BR, et al: Antinuclear antibodies in children with localized scleroderma. J Rheumatol 22:2337-2343, 1995.

76. **Zulian F, Vallongo C, Woo P, et al: Localized scleroderma in childhood is not just a skin disease. Arthritis Rheum 52:2873-2881, 2005.**

77. **Peterson LS, Nelson AM, Su WP: Classification of morphea (localized scleroderma). Mayo Clin Proc 70:1068-1076, 1995.**

78. Lehman TJ: The Parry Romberg syndrome of progressive facial hemiatrophy and linear scleroderma en coup de sabre: Mistaken diagnosis or overlapping conditions? J Rheumatol 19:844-845, 1992.

79. Grisanti MW, Moore TL, Osborn TG, et al: Eosinophilic fasciitis in children. Semin Arthritis Rheum 19:151-157, 1989.

80. Mier RJ, Shishov M, Higgins GC, et al: Pediatric-onset mixed connective tissue disease. Rheum Dis Clin North Am 31:483-496, 2005.

81. Michels H: Course of mixed connective tissue disease in children. Ann Med 29:359-364, 1997.

82. Yokota S, Imagawa T, Katakura S, et al: Mixed connective tissue disease in childhood: A nationwide retrospective study in Japan. Acta Paediatr Jpn 39:273-276, 1997.

83. Hoffman RW, Cassidy JT, Takeda Y, et al: U1-70-kd autoantibody-positive mixed connective tissue disease in children: A longitudinal clinical and serologic analysis. Arthritis Rheum 36:1599-1602, 1993.

84. Ozen S: Problems in classifying vasculitis in children. Pediatr Nephrol 20:1214-1218, 2005.

85. Bowyer S, Roettcher P: Pediatric rheumatology clinic populations in the United States: Results of a 3 year survey. Pediatric Rheumatology Database Research Group. J Rheumatol 23:1968-1974, 1996.

86. Symmons DP, Jones M, Osborne J, et al: Pediatric rheumatology in the United Kingdom: Data from the British Pediatric Rheumatology Group National Diagnostic Register. J Rheumatol 23:1975-1980, 1996.

87. Hunder GG, Arend WP, Bloch DA, et al: The American College of Rheumatology 1990 criteria for the classification of vasculitis: Introduction. Arthritis Rheum 33:1065-1067, 1990.

88. Jennette JC, Falk RJ, Andrassy K, et al: Nomenclature of systemic vasculitides: Proposal of an international consensus conference. Arthritis Rheum 37:187-192, 1994.

89. Lie JT: American College of Rheumatology Subcommittee on Classification of Vasculitis: Illustrated histopathologic classification criteria for selected vasculitis syndromes. Arthritis Rheum 33:1074-1087, 1990.

90. **Ozen S, Anton J, Arisoy N, et al: Juvenile polyarteritis: Results of a multicenter survey of 110 children. J Pediatr 145:517-522, 2004.**

91. Brogan PA, Davies R, Gordon I, et al: Renal angiography in children with polyarteritis nodosa. Pediatr Nephrol 17:277-283, 2002.

92. Kawasaki T: Acute febrile mucocutaneous syndrome with lymphoid involvement with specific desquamation of the fingers and toes in children. Jpn J Allergy 16:178-222, 1967.

93. **Newburger JW, Takahashi M, Gerber MA, et al: Diagnosis, treatment, and long-term management of Kawasaki disease: A statement for health professionals from the Committee on Rheumatic Fever, Endocarditis, and Kawasaki Disease, Council on Cardiovascular Disease in the Young, American Heart Association. Pediatrics 114:1708-1733, 2004.**

94. **Falcini F, Cimaz R, Calabri GB, et al: Kawasaki's disease in northern Italy: A multicenter retrospective study of 250 patients. Clin Exp Rheumatol 20:421-426, 2002.**

95. Taubert KA, Rowley AH, Shulman ST: Nationwide survey of Kawasaki disease and acute rheumatic fever. J Pediatr 119:279-282, 1991.

96. Holman RC, Curns AT, Belay ED, et al: Kawasaki syndrome hospitalizations in the United States, 1997 and 2000. Pediatrics 112:495-501, 2003.

97. Nakamura Y, Yanagawa H, Kato H, et al: Mortality rates for patients with a history of Kawasaki disease in Japan. Kawasaki Disease Follow-up Group. J Pediatr 128:75-81, 1996.

98. Chang RK: Hospitalizations for Kawasaki disease among children in the United States, 1988-1997. Pediatrics 109:e87, 2002.

99. **Rowley AH, Eckerley CA, Jack HM, et al: IgA plasma cells in vascular tissue of patients with Kawasaki syndrome. J Immunol 159:5946-5955, 1997.**

100. Falcini F, Trapani S, Turchini S, et al: Immunological findings in Kawasaki disease: An evaluation in a cohort of Italian children. Clin Exp Rheumatol 15:685-689, 1997.

101. Nakatani K, Takeshita S, Tsujimoto H, et al: Circulating endothelial cells in Kawasaki disease. Clin Exp Immunol 131:536-540, 2003.

102. Burns JC, Shimizu C, Shike H, et al: Family-based association analysis implicates IL-4 in susceptibility to Kawasaki disease. Genes Immun 6:438-444, 2005.

103. Burns JC, Shimizu C, Gonzalez E, et al: Genetic variations in the receptor-ligand pair CCR5 and CCL3L1 are important determinants of susceptibility to Kawasaki disease. J Infect Dis 192:344-349, 2005.

104. Lehman TJ, Walker SM, Mahnovski V, et al: Coronary arteritis in mice following the systemic injection of group B *Lactobacillus casei* cell walls in aqueous suspension. Arthritis Rheum 28:652-659, 1985.

105. Urowitz MB, Gladman DD, Abu-Shakra M, et al: Mortality studies in systemic lupus erythematosus: Results from a single center. III. Improved survival over 24 years. J Rheumatol 24:1061-1065, 1997.

106. Nakamura Y, Yanagawa H, Ojima T, et al: Cardiac sequelae of Kawasaki disease among recurrent cases. Arch Dis Child 78:163-165, 1998.

107. Dajani AS, Taubert KA, Takahashi M, et al: Guidelines for long-term management of patients with Kawasaki disease: Report from the Committee on Rheumatic Fever, Endocarditis, and Kawasaki Disease, Council on Cardiovascular Disease in the Young, American Heart Association. Circulation 89:916-922, 1994.

108. Kushner HI, Bastian JF, Turner CH, et al: Rethinking the boundaries of Kawasaki disease: Toward a revised case definition. Perspect Biol Med 46:216-233, 2003.

109. Weng KP, Hsieh KS, Huang SH, et al: Serum HDL level at acute stage of Kawasaki disease. Chung Hua Min Kuo Hsiao Erh Ko I Hsueh Hui Tsa Chih 39:28-32, 1998.

110. Simonini G, Masi L, Giani T, et al: Osteoprotegerin serum levels in Kawasaki disease: An additional potential marker in predicting children with coronary artery involvement. J Rheumatol 32:2233-2238, 2005.

111. Newburger JW, Takahashi M, Beiser AS, et al: A single intravenous infusion of gamma globulin as compared with four infusions in the treatment of acute Kawasaki syndrome. N Engl J Med 324:1633-1639, 1991.

112. American Academy of Pediatrics: Kawasaki syndrome. In Pickering LK (ed): Red Book: 2003 Report of the Committee on Infectious Diseases. Elk Grove Village, Ill, American Academy of Pediatrics, 2003, pp 392-395.

113. Sundel RP, Baker AL, Fulton DR, et al: Corticosteroids in the initial treatment of Kawasaki disease: Report of a randomized trial. J Pediatr 142:611-616, 2003.

114. Hsieh KS, Weng KP, Lin CC, et al: Treatment of acute Kawasaki disease: Aspirin's role in the febrile stage revisited. Pediatrics 114:e689-e693, 2004.

115. Wooditch AC, Aronoff SC: Effect of initial corticosteroid therapy on coronary artery aneurysm formation in Kawasaki disease: A meta-analysis of 862 children. Pediatrics 116:989-995, 2005.

116. Yanagawa H, Nakamura Y, Sakata K, et al: Use of intravenous gamma-globulin for Kawasaki disease: Effects on cardiac sequelae. Pediatr Cardiol 18:19-23, 1997.

117. Oates-Whitehead RM, Baumer JH, Haines L, et al: Intravenous immunoglobulin for the treatment of Kawasaki disease in children. Cochrane Database Syst Rev CD004000, 2003.

118. Lang BA, Yeung RS, Oen KG, et al: Corticosteroid treatment of refractory Kawasaki disease. J Rheumatol 33:803-809, 2006.

119. Hashino K, Ishii M, Iemura M, et al: Re-treatment for immune globulin-resistant Kawasaki disease: A comparative study of additional immune globulin and steroid pulse therapy. Pediatr Int 43:211-217, 2001.

120. Takeshita S, Kawamura Y, Nakatani K, et al: Standard-dose and short-term corticosteroid therapy in immunoglobulin-resistant Kawasaki disease. Clin Pediatr (Phila) 44:423-426, 2005.

121. Tsai MH, Huang YC, Yen MH, et al: Clinical responses of patients with Kawasaki disease to different brands of intravenous immunoglobulin. J Pediatr 148:38-43, 2006.

122. Burns JC, Mason WH, Hauger SB, et al: Infliximab treatment for refractory Kawasaki syndrome. J Pediatr 146:662-667, 2005.

123. Burns JC: Kawasaki disease: The mystery continues. Minerva Pediatr 54:287-294, 2002.

124. Kato H, Sugimura T, Akagi T, et al: Long-term consequences of Kawasaki disease: A 10- to 21-year follow-up study of 594 patients. Circulation 94:1379-1385, 1996.

125. Levy DM, Silverman ED, Massicotte MP, et al: Longterm outcomes in patients with giant aneurysms secondary to Kawasaki disease. J Rheumatol 32:928-934, 2005.

126. Fukushige J, Takahashi N, Ueda K, et al: Long-term outcome of coronary abnormalities in patients after Kawasaki disease. Pediatr Cardiol 17:71-76, 1996.

127. Dadlani GH, Gingell RL, Orie JD, et al: Coronary artery calcifications in the long-term follow-up of Kawasaki disease. Am Heart J 150:1016, 2005.

128. Burns JC, Shike H, Gordon JB, et al: Sequelae of Kawasaki disease in adolescents and young adults. J Am Coll Cardiol 28:253-257, 1996.

129. Kitamura S: The role of coronary bypass operation on children with Kawasaki disease. Coron Artery Dis 13:437-447, 2002.

130. Tsuda E, Kitamura S: National survey of coronary artery bypass grafting for coronary stenosis caused by Kawasaki disease in Japan. Circulation 110:II61-II66, 2004.

131. Wong D, Harder J, Jadavji T: Kawasaki disease, myocardial infarction and coronary artery revascularization. Can J Cardiol 21:601-604, 2005.

132. Hirata S, Nakamura Y, Matsumoto K, et al: Long-term consequences of Kawasaki disease among first-year junior high school students. Arch Pediatr Adolesc Med 156:77-80, 2002.

133. Cimaz R, Falcini F: An update on Kawasaki disease. Autoimmun Rev 2:258-263, 2003.

134. Michel BA, Hunder GG, Bloch DA, et al: Hypersensitivity vasculitis and Henoch-Schönlein purpura: A comparison between the 2 disorders. J Rheumatol 19:721-728, 1992.

135. Fukuda T, Ishibashi M, Shinohara T, et al: Follow-up assessment of the collateral circulation in patients with Kawasaki disease who underwent dipyridamole stress technetium-99m tetrofosmin scintigraphy. Pediatr Cardiol 26:558-564, 2005.

136. Mills JA, Michel BA, Bloch DA, et al: The American College of Rheumatology 1990 criteria for the classification of Henoch-Schönlein purpura. Arthritis Rheum 33:1114-1121, 1990.

137. Garcia-Porrua C, Calvino MC, Llorca J, et al: Henoch-Schönlein purpura in children and adults: Clinical differences in a defined population. Semin Arthritis Rheum 32:149-156, 2002.

138. Uppal SS, Hussain MA, Al Raqum HA, et al: Henoch-Schönlein's purpura in adults versus children/adolescents: A comparative study. Clin Exp Rheumatol 24:S26-S30, 2006.

139. Stewart M, Savage JM, Bell B, et al: Long term renal prognosis of Henoch-Schönlein purpura in an unselected childhood population. Eur J Pediatr 147:113-115, 1988.

140. Goldstein AR, White RH, Akuse R, et al: Long-term follow-up of childhood Henoch-Schönlein nephritis. Lancet 339:280-282, 1992.

141. Chang WL, Yang YH, Wang LC, et al: Renal manifestations in Henoch-Schönlein purpura: A 10-year clinical study. Pediatr Nephrol 20:1269-1272, 2005.

142. Blanco R, Martinez-Taboada VM, Rodriguez-Valverde V, et al: Henoch-Schönlein purpura in adulthood and childhood: Two different expressions of the same syndrome. Arthritis Rheum 40:859-864, 1997.

143. Huber AM, King J, McLaine P, et al: A randomized, placebo-controlled trial of prednisone in early Henoch-Schönlein purpura [ISRCTN85109383]. BMC Med 2:7, 2004.

144. Hasegawa A, Kawamura T, Ito H, et al: Fate of renal grafts with recurrent Henoch-Schönlein purpura nephritis in children. Transplant Proc 21:2130-2133, 1989.

145. Tarshish P, Bernstein J, Edelmann CM Jr: Henoch-Schönlein purpura nephritis: Course of disease and efficacy of cyclophosphamide. Pediatr Nephrol 19:51-56, 2004.

146. Sheth AP, Olson JC, Esterly NB: Cutaneous polyarteritis nodosa of childhood. J Am Acad Dermatol 31:561-566, 1994.

147. Martini A, Ravelli A, Albani S, et al: Hypocomplementemic urticarial vasculitis syndrome with severe systemic manifestations. J Pediatr 124:742-744, 1994.

148. Valentini RP, Smoyer WE, Sedman AB, et al: Outcome of antineutrophil cytoplasmic autoantibodies-positive glomerulonephritis and vasculitis in children: A single-center experience. J Pediatr 132:325-328, 1998.

149. Lanthier S, Lortie A, Michaud J, et al: Isolated angiitis of the CNS in children. Neurology 56:837-842, 2001.

150. Mwipatayi BP, Jeffery PC, Beningfield SJ, et al: Takayasu arteritis: Clinical features and management: report of 272 cases. Aust N Z J Surg 75:110-117, 2005.

151. McCulloch M, Andronikou S, Goddard E, et al: Angiographic features of 26 children with Takayasu's arteritis. Pediatr Radiol 33:230-235, 2003.

152. Saltoglu N, Tasova Y, Midikli D, et al: Fever of unknown origin in Turkey: Evaluation of 87 cases during a nine-year-period of study. J Infect 48:81-85, 2004.

153. Arend WP, Michel BA, Bloch DA, et al: The American College of Rheumatology 1990 criteria for the classification of Takayasu arteritis. Arthritis Rheum 33:1129-1134, 1990.

154. Park MC, Lee SW, Park YB, et al: Clinical characteristics and outcomes of Takayasu's arteritis: Analysis of 108 patients using standardized criteria for diagnosis, activity assessment, and angiographic classification. Scand J Rheumatol 34:284-292, 2005.

155. Miyata T, Sato O, Koyama H, et al: Long-term survival after surgical treatment of patients with Takayasu's arteritis. Circulation 108:1474-1480, 2003.

156. Fields CE, Bower TC, Cooper LT, et al: Takayasu's arteritis: Operative results and influence of disease activity. J Vasc Surg 43:64-71, 2006.

157. Leavitt RY, Fauci AS, Bloch DA, et al: The American College of Rheumatology 1990 criteria for the classification of Wegener's granulomatosis. Arthritis Rheum 33:1101-1107, 1990.

158. Rottem M, Fauci AS, Hallahan CW, et al: Wegener granulomatosis in children and adolescents: Clinical presentation and outcome. J Pediatr 122:26-31, 1993.

159. **Belostotsky VM, Shah V, Dillon MJ: Clinical features in 17 paediatric patients with Wegener granulomatosis. Pediatr Nephrol 17:754-761, 2002.**

160. Hoffman GS: Classification of the systemic vasculitides: Antineutrophil cytoplasmic antibodies, consensus and controversy. Clin Exp Rheumatol 16:111-115, 1998.

161. Gottlieb BS, Miller LC, Ilowite NT: Methotrexate treatment of Wegener granulomatosis in children. J Pediatr 129:604-607, 1996.

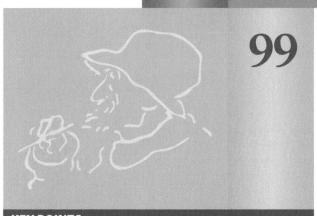

99 Bacterial Arthritis

GEORGE HO, JR. • DAWD S. SIRAJ •
PAUL P. COOK

KEY POINTS

Acute bacterial arthritis is a medical emergency that warrants rapid, accurate diagnosis and immediate treatment.

Most instances of native joint infection are the result of bacteremic seeding.

Staphylococcus aureus is the most frequent microorganism in adult nongonococcal septic arthritis.

The initial selection of an antibiotic regimen should be broad enough to take into account host factors, clinical characteristics, likely causative microorganisms, and regional antibiotic sensitivity data pending confirmation of bacteria by culture and sensitivities.

An infected joint must be adequately drained, and an antibiotic course that is sufficiently long to cure the infection must be instituted. Surgical drainage must be considered without delay if needle aspirations are unsuccessful.

Poor prognostic factors in bacterial joint infection include old age, underlying rheumatoid arthritis, and infection in a prosthetic joint.

To optimize the outcome, prompt aggressive treatment must be instituted, and consultations with orthopaedic surgery, rheumatology, infectious diseases, and physical medicine and rehabilitation should be sought.

Late prosthetic joint infections require antibiotic treatment directed at the isolated microorganism and the complete removal of the infected prosthesis before reimplantation of a new prosthesis in a one-stage or two-stage operation.

Reducing the risk of a prosthetic joint infection involves a thorough preoperative evaluation, perioperative use of antibiotics, and the careful use of antibiotic prophylaxis when a patient with a prosthesis is exposed to transient bacteremia during an invasive dental procedure.

EPIDEMIOLOGY

Bacterial infections of the joint are usually curable with treatment, but morbidity and mortality are still significant in patients with underlying rheumatoid arthritis (RA), patients with prosthetic joints, elderly patients, and patients who have severe and multiple comorbidities. Goldenberg[1]

wrote in 1994, "Treatment and outcome (of septic arthritis) have not improved substantially over the past 20 years." This statement is probably still true today. Incremental knowledge of the pathogenesis of septic arthritis caused by two common organisms, *Neisseria gonorrhoeae* and *Staphylococcus aureus*, and understanding of the pathobiology of prosthetic devices may lead to innovations in the management and prevention of bacterial joint infections, however.

The normal diarthrodial joint is very resistant to bacterial infection because of local and systemic host defenses. Bacteria can reach the synovial-lined joint, however, via the hematogenous route and result in septic arthritis. The large joints are affected more commonly than the small joints, and monarticular infection is the rule, with polyarticular infection (more than one joint involved) in less than 20% of cases. A prospective series from a community-based population in the Netherlands reflected a representative distribution of joint involvement: knee 55%, ankle 10%, wrist 9%, shoulder 7%, hip 5%, elbow 5%, sternoclavicular joint 5%, sacroiliac joint 2%, and foot joint 2%.[2]

The incidence of septic arthritis ranges from 2 to 5/100,000/yr in the general population, 5.5 to 12/100,000/yr in children, 28 to 38/100,000/yr in patients with RA, and 40 to 68/100,000/yr in patients with joint prostheses.[3,4] The organisms causing bacterial arthritis depend on the epidemiologic circumstances (Table 99-1).[5] Monarthritis of a prosthetic joint in an elderly man is likely due to *Staphylococcus*, whereas a migratory arthritis in a sexually active woman with skin lesions is likely due to disseminated gonococcal infection.

ETIOLOGY AND PATHOGENESIS

Most cases of septic arthritis result from hematogenous seeding of the synovial membrane. The abundant vascular supply of the synovium and the lack of a limiting basement membrane allow organisms to target joints during bacteremia. Less common causes of septic arthritis include direct inoculation after joint aspiration or corticosteroid injection of a joint[6]; animal or human bites; nail puncture wounds or plant thorn injury[7]; joint surgery, especially hip and knee arthroplasties; and spread by contiguous osteomyelitis, cellulitis, or septic

Table 99-1 Etiologic Organisms Causing Joint Infection in Various Hosts

Adults	Children ≤5 yr old	Children >5 yr old	Neonates	Prosthetic
Common	**Common**	**Common**	**Common**	**Common**
Staphylococcus aureus	*S. aureus*	*S. aureus*	*S. aureus*	Coagulase-negative staphylococci
Streptococcus pneumoniae	*Haemophilus influenzae**	Group A streptococci	Group B streptococci	*S. aureus*
β-Hemolytic streptococci (mainly Lancefield groups A, G, and B)	Group A streptococci		Enterobacteriaceae	
Neisseria gonorrhoeae (adult and sexually active adolescent)	*S. pneumoniae*			
Enterobacteriaceae (age >60 or predisposing condition)				
Salmonella				
Rare	**Rare**	**Rare**	**Rare**	**Less Common**
Pseudomonas	*Salmonella*		*Pseudomonas*	*Corynebacterium*
Mycobacterium tuberculosis	*H. influenzae*		*H. influenzae*	Enterococci and streptococci
H. influenzae	*N. meningitidis*	*N. meningitidis*	*N. gonorrhoeae*	*Pseudomonas aeruginosa*
Neisseria meningitidis	*N. gonorrhoeae*	*N. gonorrhoeae*		Enterobacteriaceae
Pasteurella	*Kingella kingae*	*Kingella kingae*		*Propionibacterium*
Anaerobes	*M. tuberculosis*	*M. tuberculosis*		Other anaerobes
Mycoplasma/Ureaplasma	*B. burgdorferi*	*B. burgdorferi*		*Candida*
Fungi (*Sporothrix*, dimorphic fungi, *Cryptococcus*)				*M. tuberculosis*
Borrelia burgdorferi				

*Rare in children immunized with Hib vaccine.
Adapted from Atkins BL, Bowler IC: The diagnosis of large joint sepsis. J Hosp Infect 40:263-274, 1998.

bursitis. Arthrocentesis is a common procedure frequently used in conjunction with corticosteroid administration in patients with various forms of joint diseases. Septic arthritis after joint aspiration and injection is extremely rare, occurring in 0.0002% of patients.[8] Arthroscopic surgery also is a common procedure that is complicated by a very low incidence of septic arthritis (<0.5% of procedures).[9,10] Coagulase-positive and coagulase-negative staphylococci account for more than 87% of these infections. In rare cases of septic arthritis of the knee related to anterior cruciate ligament repair, the tissue allografts were identified as the source of the infection.[11] Cultures yielded gram-negative organisms, such as *Pseudomonas aeruginosa*, *Citrobacter*, *Klebsiella oxytoca*, and mixed infection with *S. aureus*, *Enterococcus faecalis*, and *P. aeruginosa*.

Acute bacterial arthritis usually is designated gonococcal or nongonococcal. In the case of gonococcal arthritis, *N. gonorrhoeae* possesses a variety of virulence factors on the cell surface. *N. gonorrhoeae* is able to attach to cell surfaces via filamentous outer-membrane appendages, or pili. Another outer membrane protein, protein I, has forms IA and IB. Protein IA binds the host factor H and inactivates complement component, C3b, circumventing the host's complement system.[12] Protein IA also prevents phagolysosomal fusion in neutrophils, enabling survival of the organism within the phagocytes. Lipo-oligosaccharide is a gonococcal molecule similar to lipopolysaccharide of other gram-negative bacteria and possesses endotoxin activity, which contributes to the joint damage seen in gonococcal arthritis.[13]

S. aureus is the most common organism that causes nongonococcal arthritis. The virulence of *S. aureus* is associated with its ability to attach to host tissue within the joint, evade host defenses, and cause damage to the joint. Table 99-2 lists some of these virulence factors and their mechanisms of action. The attachment of *S. aureus* to the joint tissues is facilitated by microbial surface components recognizing adhesive matrix molecules (MSCRAMMs). MSCRAMMs are embedded in the cell wall peptidoglycan of *S. aureus* (Fig. 99-1).[14,15] They bind to host matrix proteins, including collagen, fibrinogen, elastin, vitronectin, laminin, and fibronectin. Knockout gene experiments in animal models showed that the gene coding for the protein that binds collagen is an important virulence factor for *S. aureus* joint infections.[16] Most *S. aureus* isolates also express the fibronectin-binding proteins, FnbpA and FnbpB. Disruption of the respective genes, *fnbpA* and *fnbpB*, by knockout gene experiments completely obliterates adherence of *S. aureus* to fibronectin-coated surfaces (e.g., prosthetic joints).[17]

The genes of several *S. aureus* cell surface proteins (e.g., protein A, fibronectin-binding proteins, coagulase) and exotoxins (e.g., toxic shock syndrome toxin-1 [TSST-1], enterotoxin B, proteases, and hemolysins) are regulated by the accessory gene regulator *agr*.[18,19] At low cell numbers, such as at the time of infection, production of cell surface proteins for attachment to host tissues is facilitated by the *agr* gene. When the cells have attached to tissue or an orthopaedic device and have passed from exponential to stationary phase of growth, *agr* represses the expression of genes coding for cell surface proteins and activates genes coding for exotoxins and tissue-destroying exoenzymes. Because of this complex effect on the different stages of infection, inhibitors of *agr* may reduce tissue destruction, but enhance tissue colonization. This effect could have implications for chronic infections such as occur with prosthetic joints.

Adherence receptors may allow for the intracellular movement of *S. aureus* into host cells (e.g., osteoblasts, endothelial cells, and neutrophils).[20] When internalized, the organism is protected from the host's immune system and from antimicrobial agents. After adherence to the joint tissue, the bacteria activate the host immune response. Opsonization and phagocytosis are key defenses to eradicate the organism. *S. aureus* possesses two virulence factors,

Table 99-2 Virulence Factors of *Staphylococcus aureus* and Their Mechanisms of Action

Virulence Factor	Mechanism of Action
Collagen-binding protein	Binds collagen
Clumping factor A and B	Binds fibrinogen
Fibronectin-binding protein A and B	Binds fibronectin
Capsular polysaccharide	Antiphagocytic
Protein A	Binds fragment crystallizable portion of IgG
Toxic shock syndrome toxin-1	Superantigen
Enterotoxins	Superantigens

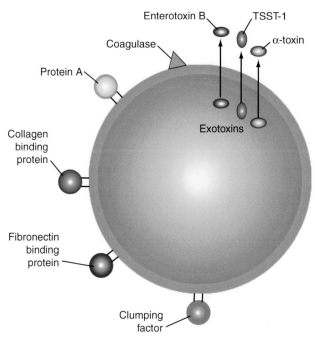

Figure 99-1 Schematic diagram of *Staphylococcus aureus*. Many of the cell-surface proteins are regulated by the *agr* locus (see text). At low cell concentrations, *agr* facilitates the production of the cell-surface proteins, which facilitate attachment to tissue. At higher cell concentrations, as occurs with establishment of infection, *agr* downregulates production of the cell-surface proteins and activates genes coding for exotoxins.

protein A and capsular polysaccharide, which interfere with these defenses. Protein A interferes with binding of complement by binding to the fragment crystallizable (Fc) portion of IgG. Protein A has been termed a *superantigen* for B cells because 30% of human B cells show Fab-mediated binding of the protein A molecule.[21] Binding of protein A by B cells leads to activation and subsequently to depletion of B cells through apoptosis.[22] This process may have implications regarding the ability of the immune system to control infection with *S. aureus*. The gene coding for protein A had been experimentally disrupted, and joint infection caused by the altered strain in a mouse model resulted in less joint destruction than infection caused by the wild-type strain.[23]

Capsular polysaccharide interferes with opsonization and phagocytosis. Of the 11 reported capsule serotypes of *S. aureus*, types 5 and 8 account for 85% of clinical infections.[24] The capsule of these two serotypes is thinner,

which facilitates the attachment to host fibronectin and fibrin.[25] When attached to these host proteins, capsule production is upregulated to form a thicker capsule, which makes the bacteria more resistant to opsonization and phagocytosis. The thicker capsule also is able to conceal the highly immunogenic adherence proteins (MSCRAMMs).[26] A mutant of the type 5 capsule in a murine model had a lower rate of infection and resulted in less severe arthritis compared with mice infected with the wild-type strain.[27] A vaccine consisting of types 5 and 8 polysaccharide reduced *S. aureus* bacteremia by more than half in hemodialysis patients.[28] The duration of protection was approximately 40 weeks after a single vaccination.

S. aureus exotoxins (e.g., TSST-1 and enterotoxins) act as superantigens that bind to host major histocompatibility complex (MHC) class II molecules and T cell receptors, resulting in clonal expansion and activation of some T cells. This activation triggers the release of numerous cytokines, including interleukin (IL)-2, interferon-γ, and tumor necrosis factor (TNF)-α.[29] Induction of these cytokines results in systemic toxicity and joint damage. The stimulated T cells initially proliferate, but later disappear, likely owing to apoptosis, and result in immunosuppression.[30] Internalized organisms that had been protected from this inflammatory response may cause fulminant or persistent infection. Mice injected with strains of *S. aureus* lacking TSST-1 and enterotoxins rarely develop arthritis; when arthritis is induced, it is much milder compared with arthritis in animals injected with the wild-type strain.[29] Vaccination of mice with a mutated, recombinant form of enterotoxin A devoid of superantigen function was associated with a significant reduction in mortality.[31]

In response to bacterial infection of the joint space, the host releases a variety of cytokines and inflammatory mediators. Initially, IL-1β and IL-6 are released into the joint space, leading to an influx of inflammatory cells. These neutrophils and macrophages engulf invading bacteria and release additional cytokines, including TNF-α, IL-1, IL-6, and IL-8. Blocking TNF-α with a monoclonal antibody and IL-1 with an IL-1 receptor antagonist inhibited leukocyte infiltration into the joint by 80% in a rabbit model of *S. aureus*–induced arthritis when the cytokine inhibitors were given simultaneously with *S. aureus*.[32] When the same inhibitors were given 24 hours after infection, however, there was no effect on leukocyte infiltration, suggesting the crucial roles of TNF-α and IL-1 in the early stages of *S. aureus*–induced arthritis. Release of interferon-γ is associated with the influx of T cells, which occurs a few days after infection. In a mouse model of *S. aureus* septic arthritis, interferon-γ has been associated with a worsening of the severity of arthritis, while protecting the animals from septicemia.[33] The host's early cytokine response may aid the clearance of organisms and limit infection in the host. A late cytokine response may amplify the destructiveness of an established infection.

CLINICAL FEATURES

Acute bacterial arthritis is most commonly monarticular. Polyarticular infection occurs in 5% to 8% of pediatric cases and in 10% to 19% of adult nongonococcal cases.[34,35] The differential diagnosis of acute monarthritis overlaps with many causes of polyarthritis because virtually any arthritic disorder can initially manifest as a single swollen joint. The three main etiologies to consider when a patient presents with acute monarticular arthritis are trauma, infection, and crystal-induced synovitis such as gout or pseudogout. Polyarticular septic arthritis is usually seen in patients with systemic inflammatory disorders such as the spondyloarthropathies, RA, systemic lupus erythematosus, and other connective tissue diseases or patients with overwhelming sepsis.[36]

Disseminated gonococcal infection occurs in 1% to 3% of patients infected with *N. gonorrhoeae*. Gonococcal arthritis is the most common cause of acute monarthritis in sexually active young adults. In the preantibiotic era, gonococcal arthritis was a well-recognized illness in neonates. Disseminated gonococcal infection is three times more common in women than men. Women are more commonly affected because they are more likely to have asymptomatic and untreated primary infections. Bacterial dissemination has been associated with intrauterine devices and has occurred during menstruation, pregnancy, and pelvic operation.[37-39]

Patients with gonococcal joint disease typically present with one of two forms. The first form is characterized by fever, shaking chills, vesiculopustular skin lesions, tenosynovitis, and polyarthralgias. Blood cultures are frequently positive, whereas synovial fluid cultures are rarely positive. *N. gonorrhoeae* can be cultured from genital, rectal, and pharyngeal sites. Tenosynovitis of multiple tendons of the wrist, fingers, ankle, and toes is a unique feature of this form of disseminated gonococcal infection and distinguishes it from other forms of infectious arthritis. In the second form of gonococcal infection, patients have purulent arthritis, most commonly of the knee, wrist, or ankle, and more than one joint can be infected simultaneously. *N. gonorrhoeae* frequently can be cultured from the synovial fluid.[40]

The classic presentation of nongonococcal septic arthritis is the acute onset of pain and swelling in a single joint. Large joints are affected most commonly. In adults, the knee is involved in more than 50% of cases; hip, ankle, and shoulder infections are less common.[41] In infants and small children, the hip is more often involved.[42] Patients with septic arthritis often have underlying illnesses and predispositions to infections. Many are immunocompromised; are intravenous drug abusers; have prosthetic joints; and have diseases such as neoplasia, renal failure, and RA. Table 99-3 lists the risk factors that predispose to septic arthritis.[3,6,43-45]

Most patients with bacterial arthritis are febrile, although chills are unusual. Fever may be absent in elderly patients. In children, septic arthritis usually is accompanied by fever, malaise, poor appetite, irritability, and progressive reluctance to use the affected limb. Physical examination typically reveals warmth and tenderness of the affected joint, joint effusion, and limited active and passive range of motion. Septic arthritis among patients with RA has been a special challenge to clinicians because of the high incidence of infection and the poor outcome. Septic arthritis in patients with RA is associated with poor joint outcome and high mortality.[34,46-50] In many cases, it is difficult to differentiate septic arthritis in a joint already affected by RA from rheumatoid flare. Whenever bacterial arthritis is suspected, the most important diagnostic procedure is arthrocentesis and examination of the synovial fluid. For joints that are

Table 99-3 Risk Factors for the Development of Septic Arthritis

Age >80 years[3]
Diabetes mellitus[3]
Presence of a prosthetic joint in the knee or the hip[3]
Recent joint surgery[3]
Skin infection[3]
Previous septic arthritis[43]
Recent intra-articular injection[6]
HIV or AIDS
Intravenous drug abuse
End-stage renal disease on hemodialysis
Advanced hepatic disease
Hemophilia with or without AIDS
Sickle cell disease
Underlying malignancy
Hypogammaglobulinemia (susceptible to *Mycoplasma* infections)[45]
Late complement-component deficiency (susceptible to *Neisseria* infections)[44]
Low socioeconomic status with high rate of comorbidities[43]

AIDS, acquired immunodeficiency syndrome; HIV, human immunodeficiency virus.

deep and more difficult to aspirate, ultrasound-guided or fluoroscopy-guided needle aspiration should be done.

DIAGNOSIS AND DIAGNOSTIC TESTS

Arthrocentesis and synovial fluid analysis should be done for all patients who present with an inflamed joint. Normal joints contain a small amount of synovial fluid that is clear, is highly viscous, and has very few white blood cells (WBCs). The protein concentration is approximately one third that of plasma, and the glucose concentration is similar to that of plasma. Infected synovial fluid is usually purulent with an elevated leukocyte count typically greater than 50,000 WBC/mm^3 and often exceeding 100,000 WBC/mm^3 with polymorphonuclear cell predominance. Synovial fluid levels of glucose, lactate dehydrogenase, and total protein have limited value in the diagnosis of septic arthritis. Although a low synovial fluid glucose (<40 mg/dL or less than half the serum glucose concentration) and an elevated lactate dehydrogenase suggest bacterial infection, they are not sufficiently sensitive or specific for the diagnosis.[51] Figure 99-2 is an algorithm for synovial fluid analysis; Table 99-4 lists the differential diagnoses of septic arthritis and the known causes of pseudoseptic arthritis.[6,52,53]

A definite diagnosis of bacterial arthritis can be made only by visualizing bacteria on a Gram-stained smear or by culturing bacteria from the synovial fluid. In patients not previously treated with antibiotics, synovial fluid cultures are positive in 70% to 90% of cases of nongonococcal bacterial arthritis.[54,55] Blood cultures are positive in 40% to 50% of cases of septic arthritis and are the only method of identifying the pathogen in about 10% of cases. An extra-articular site of infection offers a clue to the etiologic organism infecting the joint. Examples include septic arthritis in

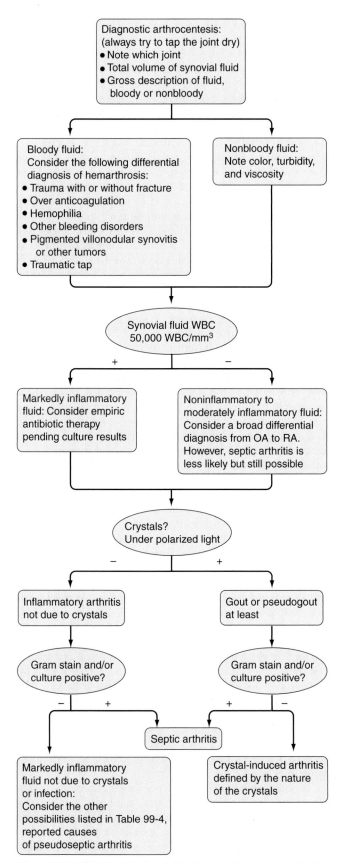

Figure 99-2 Algorithm for synovial fluid analysis in septic arthritis. OA, osteoarthritis; RA, rheumatoid arthritis; WBC, white blood cells.

Table 99-4 Differential Diagnosis of Septic Arthritis or Reported Causes of Pseudoseptic Arthritis*

Partially treated septic arthritis
Rheumatoid arthritis
Juvenile rheumatoid arthritis
Gout
Pseudogout
Apatite-related arthropathy
Reactive arthritis
Psoriatic arthritis
Systemic lupus erythematosus
Sickle cell disease
Dialysis-related amyloidosis
Transient synovitis of the hip
Plant thorn synovitis
Metastatic carcinoma
Pigmented villonodular synovitis
Hemarthrosis
Neuropathic arthropathy
Synovitis after injection of hylan

*Extremely inflammatory synovitis with negative culture is referred to as pseudoseptic arthritis. Typically, synovial fluid analysis shows ≥50,000 white blood cells (WBC)/mm³. Often the WBC count is >100,000 WBC/mm³.
Data from references 6, 52, and 53.

association with pneumococcal pneumonia, *Escherichia coli* urinary tract infection, and cellulitis caused by staphylococci or streptococci. Gram-positive cocci are identified in 50% to 75% of synovial fluid Gram-stained smears, but gram-negative bacilli are identified less than 50% of the time in culture-proven cases.[55]

Culture for *N. gonorrhoeae* is almost always negative in skin lesions and is positive in less than 50% of synovial fluids and in less than one third of blood cultures; this may be the result of the fastidious growth requirements of *N. gonorrhoeae*. The organism can be easily recovered from other sites (i.e., the genitourinary tract). Alternatively, immune response to the organism or its components may be responsible for some of the clinical manifestations of disseminated gonococcal infection. The tenosynovitis and dermatitis associated with disseminated gonococcal infection may not yield viable organisms. Polymerase chain reaction techniques can detect gonococcal DNA in the synovial fluid of some culture-negative cases of suspected gonococcal arthritis, but the technique is not standardized and is not widely avilable.[56,57]

When culturing the synovial fluid, it should be brought directly to the laboratory and placed on conventional broth and solid media or into aerobic and anaerobic blood culture bottles. Inoculating blood culture bottles with 5 to 10 mL of joint fluid or smaller volumes into isolator tubes may increase the yield of positive cultures beyond that of standard techniques.[58,59] Synovial fluid culture using the BACTEC Peds Plus/F bottle and the BACTEC 9240 instrument (Becton Dickinson Diagnostic Systems, Sparks, Md) detected significantly more pathogens and fewer contaminants than culture by the agar-plate method.[60]

Table 99-1 lists the common organisms that cause joint infections according to the age of the patient and whether the joint is native or prosthetic.[5] Overall, S. aureus is the most common etiologic agent among children of all age groups, followed by group A streptococci and Streptococcus pneumoniae. Neonates and infants younger than 2 months old are more susceptible to group B streptococci and gram-negative enteric bacilli than older children. Rarely, Pseudomonas, N. gonorrhoeae, and Candida albicans may be responsible in very young children. Since the introduction of the Haemophilus influenzae type b vaccine, the incidence of septic arthritis caused by H. influenzae has declined dramatically.[61,62] In sexually active adolescents, N. gonorrhoeae must be considered.[63] P. aeruginosa and Candida are potential pathogens in adolescent intravenous drug abusers. Patients with sickle cell anemia are prone to develop Salmonella arthritis, and immunocompromised children are at higher risk for infection with gram-negative bacilli. Other unusual joint pathogens in children include Neisseria meningitidis, anaerobes, Brucella, and Kingella kingae.

The organisms causing nongonococcal septic arthritis in adults are 75% to 80% gram-positive cocci and 15% to 20% gram-negative bacilli.[64] S. aureus is the most common organism in native and prosthetic joint infections. Staphylococcus epidermidis is common in prosthetic joint infections, but is a rare cause of native joint infections. The streptococci, including S. pneumoniae, are the next most common group of gram-positive aerobes. Streptococcus pyogenes is followed by groups B, G, C, and F in frequency. Patients with non–group A streptococcal disease often have comorbidities, such as immunosuppression, diabetes mellitus, malignancy, and severe genitourinary or gastrointestinal infections.[65] Group B streptococcal arthritis in adults is uncommon, but it can be a serious infection in adult diabetics and patients with late prosthetic hip infections.[66] Aggressive polyarthritis caused by group B streptococci resulted in serious functional damage and permanent morbidity.[67,68] Patients predisposed to gram-negative bacillary infections include patients with a history of intravenous drug abuse, very young and very old patients, and immunocompromised patients.[69] The most common gram-negative organisms are E. coli and P. aeruginosa.

Anaerobes account for 5% to 7% of septic arthritis.[2,3,54] Common anaerobes include Bacteroides, Propionibacterium acnes, and various anaerobic gram-positive cocci. Predisposing factors include wound infections, joint arthroplasty, and immunocompromised hosts. Foul-smelling synovial fluid or air in the joint space should raise the suspicion of anaerobic infection, and appropriate cultures should be obtained and held for at least 2 weeks. Anaerobes and coagulase-negative staphylococci are more common in prosthetic joint infections.

Polyarticular septic arthritis is much less common than monarticular infection.[34,36] Many of the patients have one or more comorbidities, and some have been intravenous drug abusers. Occurrence of polyarticular septic arthritis is high in patients with RA and averages 25% (range 18% to 35%).[70] Although S. aureus is the most common pathogen, group G streptococci, H. influenzae, S. pneumoniae, or mixed aerobic and anaerobic bacteria have been responsible for polyarticular infections. Involvement of more than one joint also can occur in certain patient populations, such as neonates and patients with sickle cell anemia, or with certain organisms, such as N. gonorrhoeae, N. meningitidis, and Salmonella.[71]

Polymicrobial (two or more bacterial species), polyarticular (two or more joints) septic arthritis is a rare clinical entity. Large joints are usually affected. Among five reported cases, the knee was affected in four cases (bilaterally in two); the elbow and wrist were affected in three cases, and the shoulder was affected in two cases. The mean number of joints infected was three. Bacteremia was present in all but one case (80%) and always involved the same organisms that were in the synovial fluids. Most bacterial species isolated were the usual organisms seen in septic arthritis. Combinations of gram-positive aerobic and anaerobic organisms were common. A characteristic of most cases (80%) was the extension of locally destructive processes as a result of the contiguous spread of infection from the affected joints, such as osteomyelitis, fasciitis with compartment syndrome, and abscess or sinus tract formation. Systemic complications, including septic shock, multiorgan failure, and toxic shock syndrome, were noted in 60% of cases. The mortality rate of polymicrobial, polyarticular septic arthritis in this small series was 60%.[72]

Plain radiographs in septic arthritis are usually normal early in the course of the infection, but baseline films should be obtained to look for evidence of other disease and contiguous osteomyelitis. Radiographs often show nonspecific changes of inflammatory arthritis, including periarticular osteopenia, joint effusion, soft tissue swelling, and joint space loss. In more advanced infection, periosteal reaction, marginal or central erosions, and destruction of subchondral bone may be seen. Bony ankylosis is a late sequela of septic arthritis. Dislocation or subluxation of the femoral head is unique to hip infection of neonates.[42]

Ultrasound of the hip is the modality of choice to detect fluid collections in this deep joint and can serve as a guide in its aspiration. Ultrasound can be similarly used in other joints, such as the popliteal cyst of the knee, shoulder, acromioclavicular, or sternoclavicular joints. Triple-phase bone scan using technetium 99m is often done in children to identify an associated metaphyseal osteomyelitis or avascular necrosis of the femoral head. Whole-body bone scan is preferred in young children because, despite focal symptoms, septic arthritis and osteomyelitis may be multifocal in this age group.[73] In septic arthritis of all age groups, the periarticular distribution of increased uptake is seen on the early "blood-pool" phase and the delayed images of the joint. Bone scans provide only nonspecific information, however, and cannot differentiate septic from noninfectious causes of joint inflammation. A suggestive bone scan must be interpreted in the proper clinical context and supported by microbiologic data for a definitive diagnosis of joint or bone infection.

In joints that are difficult to evaluate otherwise or that have complex anatomic structures, computed tomography (CT) and magnetic resonance imaging (MRI) can provide useful images to delineate the extent of the infection.[74] MRI is highly sensitive in early detection of joint fluid and is superior to CT in the delineation of soft tissue structures. These images can show early bone erosion; reveal soft tissue extension; and facilitate arthrocentesis of joints such as shoulders, hips, acromioclavicular,[75] sternoclavicular, sacroiliac, and facet joints of the spine.

TREATMENT

Treatment of septic arthritis must begin immediately after the clinical evaluation is complete and all appropriate cultures are taken. A serious clinical suspicion of a joint infection warrants the initiation of antibiotic therapy before culture confirmation is available. Delays in treatment allow the infection to become more established in the joint and damage permanently the articular cartilage. Untreated, there is the opportunity for the joint infection to spread to other body sites via the hematogenous route and become more widespread and more difficult to cure.

The principles of treatment of an infected joint, whether natural or prosthetic, follow those of treatment of an infected body cavity in which antibiotics must be used in conjunction with adequate drainage of the infected closed space. The clinical circumstances and the preliminary laboratory data aid the selection of antibiotic agents. Host factors, any extra-articular sites of infection, and the Gram-stained smear of the synovial fluid are the best early guides for the antibiotic agents with which to start. Table 99-5 lists antibiotic agents for adults,[76-80] and Table 99-6 lists agents for children.[71]

Narrow antibiotic coverage is indicated if gram-positive cocci are found in the synovial fluid, and the clinician suspects a primary source of staphylococcal infection from the skin. Appropriate monotherapy in this case may be a penicillinase-resistant penicillin or vancomycin if methicillin resistance is likely. If gram-negative bacilli are noted in the synovial fluid, and the patient has a kidney infection, specific agents (e.g., ampicillin or a cephalosporin) against *E. coli* and other common urinary tract pathogens may be used. In healthy, sexually active individuals with community-acquired septic arthritis and a negative synovial fluid Gram-stained smear, a reasonable initial empiric therapy to cover gonococci, *S. aureus*, and streptococci can be ceftriaxone or cefotaxime pending final culture results. In elderly debilitated patients with an acute monarthritis, if the Gram-stained smear of synovial fluid is nonrevealing, and no clue is found after searching for an extra-articular source of infection, broad antibiotic coverage against a wide variety of organisms should be given initially. A typical regimen includes an antistaphylococcal agent, an aminoglycoside against gram-negative bacilli, and an antipseudomonal penicillin or a third-generation cephalosporin.

When the identity and the sensitivities of the organism are known, antibiotic therapy should continue with the most efficacious agent that has the best safety profile and the lowest cost. The parenteral route of antibiotic administration is the preferred initial treatment. Continued antibiotic therapy may be switched to oral agents if adequate blood levels can be achieved and maintained by this route. There is no evidence that the direct intra-articular instillation of drugs is necessary or preferable in septic arthritis because there is no barrier against the free diffusion of antibiotic agents from the blood to the synovial fluid. In cases in which uncertainty exists, serum and synovial fluid levels of antibiotic drugs can be measured to ensure that therapeutic levels are reached.

Most individuals with septic arthritis respond adequately to appropriate antimicrobial agents after initial joint aspiration for fluid analysis. In experimental infectious arthritis cases, early antibiotic therapy was shown to reduce the loss of collagen and erosion of articular surface, which should minimize the need for open surgical drainage.[81] It is generally accepted that prompt and adequate drainage of the septic joint is essential to decrease the risks of substantial loss of articular function; however, the best approach to drain the joint remains controversial.[82]

From retrospective studies, daily aspiration of an infected joint showed better functional outcome than open surgical drainage, although the former had higher overall mortality.[83-85] An explanation for higher mortality could be the higher comorbid conditions of patients who had daily aspirations than the ones who were more fit and underwent open surgical drainage.[83] If the synovial fluid cell count and polymorphonuclear percentage decrease with successive aspiration, the antimicrobial therapy is probably effective.[54,86] If needle aspiration is technically difficult (as in the hip or the shoulder) or does not provide thorough drainage of the joint, if the joint effusion does not resolve promptly, if sterilization of the joint fluid is delayed, if the infected joint is already damaged by preexisting rheumatoid disease, or if infected synovial tissue or bone needs débridement, surgical drainage should be considered sooner rather than later.[54,55,87] Arthroscopy is emerging as an alternative to arthrotomy with the advantage of reduced surgical morbidity. Wound healing is faster, and rehabilitation time is shortened.[88]

During the first few days of management, immobilization of the infected joint by external splinting and adequate analgesic administration ensure patient comfort. Physical therapy, starting with passive then graduating to active motion, should be instituted as soon as the patient can tolerate mobilization of the inflamed joint because early active range-of-motion exercises are beneficial for ultimate functional recovery. Involving the orthopaedic surgeon and the physical therapist early on in the course of treatment facilitates the best choice of drainage procedure and results in the best functional outcome.[89]

The optimal duration of antibiotic treatment has not been prospectively studied. For native joint infections, antibiotic administration can be 2 weeks for uncomplicated infection by susceptible microorganisms or 4 to 6 weeks for more extensive infection in an immunocompromised host. For septic arthritis caused by *H. influenzae*, streptococci, or gram-negative cocci, 2 weeks of antibiotic therapy is usually adequate. Staphylococcal septic arthritis usually requires 3 to 4 weeks of therapy, and for pneumococcal or gram-negative bacillary infections, therapy should be continued for at least 4 weeks.[87,90]

PROSTHETIC JOINT INFECTIONS

Total joint replacement for advanced arthritis is one of the major advances in medicine in the 20th century and continues to improve in the 21st century. Infection of prosthetic joints is an uncommon, but devastating complication of joint replacement surgery. Approximately 600,000 joint replacements are done each year in the United States, with an infection rate of 1% to 3%.[91] The infection rate is higher for knee arthroplasty (1% to 2%) compared with hip and shoulder arthroplasty (0.3% to 1.3%) and is much higher in patients undergoing reimplantation because of infection

Table 99-5 Antibiotic Agents Used in Adults

Synovial Fluid Gram Stain	Organism	Antibiotic	Dose
Gram-positive cocci (clusters)	Staphylococcus aureus (methicillin-sensitive)	Nafcillin/oxacillin	2 g IV q4h
		or	
		Cefazolin	1-2 g IV q8h
	S. aureus (methicillin-resistant)	Vancomycin	1 g IV q12h
		or	
		Clindamycin	900 mg IV q8h
		or	
		Linezolid	600 mg IV q12h
Gram-positive cocci (chains)	Streptococcus	Nafcillin	2 g IV q4h
		or	
		Penicillin	2 million U IV q4h
		or	
		Cefazolin	1-2 g IV q8h
Gram-negative diplococci	Neisseria gonorrhoeae	Ceftriaxone	2 g IV q24h
		or	
		Cefotaxime	1 g IV q8h
		or	
		Ciprofloxacin	400 mg IV q12h
Gram-negative bacilli	Enterobacteriaceae (E. coli, Proteus, Serratia)	Ceftriaxone	2 g IV q24h
		or	
		Cefotaxime	2 g IV q8h
	Pseudomonas	Cefepime	2 g IV q12h
		or	
		Piperacillin	3 g IV q6h
		or	
		Imipenem	500 mg IV q6h
		plus	
		Gentamicin	7 mg/kg IV q24h
Polymicrobial infection	S. aureus, Streptococcus, gram-negative bacilli	Nafcillin/oxacillin*	2 g IV q4h
		plus	
		Ceftriaxone	2 g IV q24h
		or	
		Cefotaxime	2 g IV q8h
		or	
		Ciprofloxacin	400 mg IV q12h

*If penicillin allergic, vancomycin plus third-generation cephalosporin or ciprofloxacin.
IV, intravenously; q4h, every 4 hours; q6h, every 6 hours; q8h, every 8 hours; q12h, every 12 hours; q24h, every 24 hours.
Data from references 76-80.

of the initial prosthesis (3% for hips and 6% for knees).[92-94] The risk of infection is about twofold higher in patients with RA compared with patients with osteoarthritis.[95]

The risk of infection is related to many factors. In a retrospective study of 462 infected orthopaedic implants, the most important risks for infection included (1) a surgical site infection at a site other than the prosthesis (odds ratio 35.9), (2) a score of 2 on the National Nosocomial Infections Surveillance System surgical patient risk index (odds ratio 3.9), (3) the presence of a malignancy (odds ratio 3.1), and (4) a history of joint arthroplasty (odds ratio 2.0).[96] Certain patient populations are at increased risk of infection because of comorbid conditions (e.g., diabetes mellitus and RA).

Orthopaedic implants adversely affect host defenses. Prosthetic devices impair opsonic activity and diminish the ability of neutrophils to kill bacteria.[97] Polymorphonuclear leukocytes release lysosomal enzymes and superoxide into the area surrounding the prosthesis, resulting in tissue damage and local devascularization.[98] Phagocytes may be focused on removal of the foreign body such that fewer cells are available to fight infection.[99] Finally, polymethyl methacrylate bone cement can inhibit neutrophil and complement functions,

and the heat produced by the polymerization of polymethyl methacrylate can damage adjacent cortical bone and result in a devascularized necrotic area, which is ideal for bacterial growth. After implantation, prosthetic joints are immediately coated by host proteins, including albumin, fibrinogen, and fibronectin. S. aureus, which possesses numerous host protein binding receptors (MSCRAMMs), is a common pathogen in infection of prosthetic joints. Patients with a prosthetic joint who develop S. aureus bacteremia have an approximate one in three chance of developing an infection of the implant.[100]

Another phenomenon crucial to development of infection is the ability of organisms to form biofilms on the surface of the prosthetic device. A biofilm is defined as "an assemblage of microbial cells that is irreversibly associated with a surface and enclosed in a matrix of primarily polysaccharide material."[101] Biofilm formation is a natural process. Organisms grow on indwelling medical devices, potable water system pipes, and living tissues. S. epidermidis is particularly adept at attaching to and forming biofilms on foreign bodies, such as prosthetic joints. Small numbers of these organisms from the patient's skin or mucous membranes, or from the hands of the surgeons or clinical staff, contaminate and

Table 99-6 Antibiotic Agents Used in Children

Age	Likely Pathogen	Antibiotic	Dosage (mg/kg/day)	Doses/day
Neonate	Staphylococcus aureus; group B streptococci; gram-negative bacilli	Nafcillin plus Cefotaxime or Gentamicin	100 150 5-7.5	4 3 3
Child <5 yr old	S. aureus; Haemophilus influenzae*; group A streptococci; Streptococcus pneumoniae	Nafcillin† plus Cefotaxime or Ceftriaxone or Cefuroxime	150 100-150 50 150-200	4 3-4 1-2 3-4
Child >5 yr old	S. aureus; group A streptococci	Nafcillin† or Cefazolin	150 50	4 3-4
Adolescent (sexually active)	Previous organisms; Neisseria gonorrhoeae	Ceftriaxone	50	1-2

*Decreased incidence in children fully immunized with Hib vaccine.
†If patient is penicillin allergic, alternatives include vancomycin (40 mg/kg/day divided into four doses) or clindamycin (20-40 mg/kg/day divided into four doses).
Adapted from Gutierrez KM: Infectious and inflammatory arthritis. In Long SS, Pickering LK, Prober CG (eds): Principles and Practice of Pediatric Infectious Diseases, 2nd ed. New York, Churchill Livingstone, 2002, pp 475-481.

colonize the orthopaedic device at the time of implantation. Staphylococcal surface proteins, SSP-1 and SSP-2, are fimbria-like polymers that facilitate adherence of S. epidermidis to polystyrene.[102] S. epidermidis produces a polysaccharide/adhesin substance crucial to the formation of this extracellular matrix known as slime. Polysaccharide/adhesin mutants have been shown to be less virulent than the wild-type strain in a rabbit model of endocarditis.[103]

Prosthetic joint infections are divided into early onset (<3 months after placement), delayed (3 to 24 months postsurgery), and late onset (>24 months after placement).[104] Early and delayed infections usually are related to surgical contamination at the time of the implantation, whereas late infections usually result from hematogenous seeding of the joint. Owing to its high virulence, S. aureus accounts for most early and late infections (see Table 99-1). Delayed infections usually are caused by less virulent microorganisms, such as coagulase-negative staphylococci and P. acnes. Because these low-virulence organisms are common skin contaminants, it is important to interpret culture results carefully.

Clinically, the most common symptom in patients with prosthetic joint infection is pain of the affected joint. Differentiating pain from mechanical loosening of the prosthesis from pain related to infection can be difficult. Typically, a patient with mechanical loosening but no infection has pain only with motion, whereas a patient with infection experiences pain at rest and with motion. Warmth at the implant site, effusion, erythema, and fever frequently are associated with early and late, but not delayed, infections. This difference in clinical presentation likely represents the virulence of the most common organisms associated with the three categories of infection. The presence of a sinus tract with purulent discharge suggests involvement of the implant and is an indication for removal of the prosthesis.

Laboratory tests are not useful in the diagnosis because an elevated C-reactive protein or erythrocyte sedimentation rate may be part of the underlying disease process, such as RA. Serial plain radiographs may be helpful; the presence of subperiosteal bone growth and transcortical sinus tracts is specific for infection.[105] Bone scans using technetium 99m–labeled methylene diphosphonate are very sensitive, but lack specificity because the bone scan is typically positive for 6 to 12 months after the original implantation.[106] Bone scans may be a useful screening test for patients with suspected late prosthetic joint infection. CT has limitations because of the imaging artifacts caused by the metal implant. MRI can be performed only in patients with titanium or tantalum implants.

Aspiration of the joint may be helpful in differentiating infection from noninfectious causes of joint pain, particularly in patients without RA. In one study, a synovial fluid leukocyte count of greater than 1700/mm³ had a sensitivity of 94% for determining infection, whereas a differential count of greater than 65% neutrophils had a sensitivity of 97%.[107] The specificities of these two measurements were 88% and 98% in patients without underlying inflammatory diseases such as RA. Gram-stained smear of the synovial fluid has a low sensitivity (<20%), but a high specificity (>97%).[108,109] Cultures of drainage from a sinus tract are not helpful, unless the culture grows S. aureus.[110]

Generally, at least three tissue specimens should be taken at the time of surgery, including tissue from the joint capsule, synovial lining, bone-cement interface, and samples from purulent material or sequestrum.[109,111] Swabs of the joint have a low sensitivity and should be avoided. Unless the patient is septic or otherwise systemically ill, antimicrobial therapy should be discontinued a minimum of 2 weeks before the revision surgery, and perioperative antibiotics should not be administered until all of the tissue cultures have been obtained. Using this methodical approach, there is a direct correlation of the number of tissue specimens positive for a particular microorganism and the probabiltiy of infection. The probability of infection has been estimated to be less than 5% if all tissue specimens are negative, and greater than 94% if three or more tissue specimens are positive for growth.[109] Finally, the location of the prosthesis is helpful in the interpretation of the positive culture. The isolation of *P. acnes* from a single tissue culture from a knee prosthesis is more likely to be a contaminant than if the same organism is obtained from a shoulder prosthesis.[112]

Medical therapy of patients with prosthetic joint infections is challenging. Organisms existing in biofilms are much more resistant to antimicrobial agents for several reasons. First, the drugs have difficulty penetrating the biofilm layer. The biofilm-associated organisms also grow much more slowly than organisms in suspension. As a result, antimicrobial agents such as vancomycin, penicillins, and cephalosporins, which act on rapidly dividing organisms, are not effective in treating device-related infections.[113] Rifampin and fluoroquinolones may be more effective because they are active against organisms in the stationary phase of growth.[114,115] The role of newer antibiotics, such as linezolid, daptomycin, and tigecycline, is unclear at this time.[116,117] In a rabbit experimental model of *S. aureus* osteomyelitis, the combination of tigecycline and rifampin eradicated infection in 100% of 14 rabbits.[118]

Treatment of late prosthetic joint infections is complex. In most patients, effective therapy requires a combination of antibiotics with the removal of the orthopaedic device. Failure to remove the infected prosthesis is frequently associated with an unacceptably high rate of relapse, probably related to biofilm formation on the orthopaedic implant. Removal of the joint prosthesis, débridement of infected bone, and placement of a new prosthesis during the same operation has been associated with a high rate of recurrence of infection,[119,120] but studies indicate that single-stage revision or débridement with retention of the prosthesis may be effective in certain situations.[121-124] Patients whose symptoms of pain and swelling of the joint have been less than 8 days[124] or less than 3 weeks,[125] and who have a stable prosthesis with little soft tissue damage and no sinus tract are candidates for débridement with retention of the prosthesis if the preoperative synovial fluid cultures are negative, or if the cultures grow an easily treatable organism (Fig. 99-3). The treatment of choice for most patients is a two-stage process involving removal of the infected prosthesis and débridement of infected bone, stabilization of the joint using an antibiotic-impregnated methyl methacrylate spacer, and 6 weeks of intravenous antibiotics (first stage), followed by reimplantation of a second orthopaedic implant (second stage).[126] Using this approach, the success rate is approximately 80% to 90%. Rarely, antibiotic treatment is continued indefinitely in a patient in whom the risk of removing the infected prosthesis is too great, the prosthesis is not loose, and the organism responsible for the infection can be reasonably suppressed by the use of an oral antibiotic agent.[127]

The pathogenesis of bacterial infection in prosthetic joints is complex. Anatomic, virulence, and host factors affect prognosis and approach to therapy. An understanding of these interactions may lead to novel therapeutic and preventive strategies, such as vaccines against capsule antigens or surface adhesins in patients undergoing elective joint replacements.

PREVENTION OF PROSTHETIC JOINT INFECTIONS

There is consensus that preoperative evaluation of a patient for occult infection, such as periodontal disease or bacteriuria, is warranted, and corrective steps to eradicate any

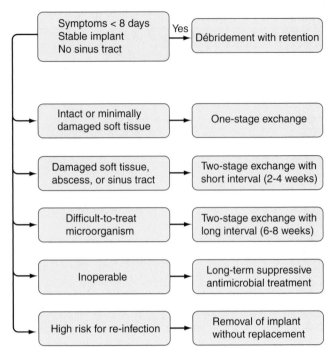

Figure 99-3 Algorithm for the management of an infected joint prosthesis. *(Adapted from Trampuz A, Zimmerli W: Prosthetic joint infections: Update in diagnosis and treatment. Swiss Med Wkly 135:243-251, 2005.)*

infection are essential before joint replacement. There also is consensus that perioperative antibiotic prophylaxis significantly reduces the rate of early postoperative infection, and this practice is routine. The role of antibiotic prophylaxis to prevent late prosthetic joint infection before diagnostic or therapeutic procedures that lead to transient bacteremia, especially dental treatment, is controversial.

In 2003, the American Dental Association and the American Academy of Orthopedic Surgeons jointly updated an advisory on antibiotic prophylaxis for dental patients with total joint replacements.[128] The advisory stated that antibiotic prophylaxis is not routinely indicated for most dental patients with total joint replacements. All patients with a total joint replacement within 2 years of the implant procedure, and some immunocompromised patients with total joint replacements who may be at higher risk for hematogenous infections, should be considered, however, to receive antibiotic prophylaxis before undergoing dental procedures with a higher bacteremic risk. Other orthopaedic and oral and maxillofacial surgeons have argued that there is "no scientific evidence to support the view that patients with arthroplasties, even in the high-risk groups, require antibiotic prophylaxis during dental treatment."[129]

Professional societies take opposing positions citing evidence from clinical experience, descriptive studies, and reports of expert committees.[130-132] Surveys of physicians and dentists have shown that most are in favor of the use of antibiotic prophylaxis before bacteremia-producing procedures to prevent prosthetic joint infection.[133-135] Proponents believe the prevention of prosthetic joint infection is analogous to the prevention of bacterial endocarditis.[136] Other reasons are fear of litigation and previous experience of dealing with the catastrophe of a late prosthetic joint infection. Opponents to prophylactic antibiotic use cite the lack of data to support a clear-cut relationship between transient bacteremia and infection of a prosthetic joint. Others object because of the concern for antibiotic resistance in bacteria from the excessive use of antibiotics, and the cost and consequences of unnecessary drug use. There are no data from randomized controlled trials, cohort or case-control studies, or multiple time series with or without the intervention.

In the absence of good evidence-based data, opting for antibiotic for the purpose of prophylaxis is a reasonable choice of the well-informed clinician.[137] The incidence of late infection of a prosthetic joint as a result of procedure-related bacteremia is extremely low—10 to 100 cases per 100,000 patients with total joint replacement per year. The cost of providing antibiotic prophylaxis to all patients with prosthetic joints before all procedures that are associated with transient bacteremia is substantial. The efficacy of such antibiotic prophylaxis is unknown. Cost-effective analyses have shown mixed results.[138-141] These discrepancies are due to the lack of reliable data and the different assumptions used in the calculations. In the patient with the greatest risk of infection, an invasive procedure that leads to bacteremia sometimes can result in an infected total joint replacement. Counseling these patients on the risks and benefits of antibiotic prophylaxis would lead to an informed decision on which the patient and the physician can agree.[52]

As we gain experience since 1999 with the use of biologic agents in the management of RA and other inflammatory arthritides, there remains the conundrum of whether the increased risk of infection from TNF inhibitor and methotrexate warrants holding them before an elective orthopaedic procedure. A retrospective analysis of 10 cases of postoperative infections showed the use of a TNF inhibitor was significantly associated with the development of a serious infection (OR 4.4).[142] A meta-analysis of the clinical literature on TNF inhibitors through December 2005 found an increased risk of serious infection and dose-related increased risk of malignancy in RA patients treated with TNF inhibitors.[143] The risks and benefits must be weighed carefully, and the patients must be fully informed on how these agents should be used on a case-by-case basis.

OUTCOME AND PROGNOSIS

In the 21st century, patients with septic arthritis as a group are becoming older, with more risk factors for infection and more comorbidities. The number of patients with prosthetic joints is increasing as the population of older patients grows and people live longer. It is not surprising to see more cases of infection in total joint replacements. The organisms have not changed significantly, however. Staphylococci (44% to 66%) are still the dominant organism followed by streptococci (18% to 28%) and gram-negative bacilli (9% to 19%).[144] The emerging challenges in the treatment of septic arthritis are how to improve outcome, how to deal with resistant organisms, and how to overcome host factors that portend a poor prognosis.

The outcome of the treatment of septic arthritis can be measured as mortality, as the functional outcome of the infected joint, or as short-term and long-term outcomes. Among the survivors, loss of articular cartilage, loss of

Table 99-7 Factors That May Portend a Poor Outcome in Septic Arthritis

Older age
Preexisting arthritis, especially rheumatoid arthritis, but also osteoarthritis and tophaceous gout
Presence of synthetic material (e.g., total joint replacement)
Delay in diagnosis or long duration of symptoms before seeking medical attention
Polyarticular infection, especially if >3 joints and small hand joints are affected
Presence of bacteremia
Infection caused by virulent or difficult-to-treat organisms (e.g., *Staphylococcus aureus, Pseudomonas aeruginosa,* or some gram-negative bacilli)
Patients receiving immunosuppressive therapy
Serious underlying comorbidities (e.g., liver, kidney, or heart diseases)
Peripheral leukocytosis at presentation
Worsening renal function

Data from references 36, 43, 49, 145-147.

motion, or increase in pain in the affected joint would be considered poor functional outcomes. Loss of the limb to infection and need for surgery to fuse the joint or restore function also are poor outcomes. Most studies report the outcome at the time of hospital discharge, and long-term data on adults with septic arthritis are unavailable. The rate of development of degenerative joint disease, the rate of relapse or recurrence of infection, and the rate of progression of functional impairment in the affected joint over time have not been well studied.

Many retrospective studies have characterized features that may increase the chance of a poor outcome at the time of hospital discharge (Table 99-7).[36,43,49,145-147] One prospective community-based study of adults and children found poor joint outcome in 33% of survivors among 154 patients with bacterial arthritis and noted older age, preexisting joint disease, and an infected joint containing synthetic material as negative prognostic factors by univariate analysis.[147] These investigators noted no association between poor outcome and young age, comorbidity, immunosuppressive medication, functional class, multiple infected joints, type of organism, or treatment delay. In a large retrospective study from the United Kingdom on the outcome of 243 patients, 11.5% died secondary to septic arthritis, and additional morbidity was noted in 31.6% of patients. Multivariate analysis suggests that important predictors of death are confusion at presentation, age 65 years or older, multiple joint sepsis, and involvement of the elbow joint. Predictors of morbidity were age 65 years or older, diabetes mellitus, open surgical drainage, and gram-positive infections other than *S. aureus.*[84]

REFERENCES

1. Goldenberg DL: Bacterial arthritis. Curr Opin Rheumatol 6:394-400, 1994.
2. Kaandorp CJE, Dinant HJ, van de Laar MAFJ, et al: Incidence and sources of native and prosthetic joint infection: A community based prospective survey. Ann Rheum Dis 56:470-475, 1997.

3. Kaandorp CJ, Van Schaardenburg D, Krijnen P, et al: Risk factors for septic arthritis in patients with joint disease: A prospective study. Arthritis Rheum 38:1819-1825, 1995.
4. Gillespie WJ: Epidemiology in bone and joint infection. Infect Dis Clin North Am 4:361-376, 1990.
5. Atkins BL, Bowler IC: The diagnosis of large joint sepsis. J Hosp Infect 40:263-274, 1998.
6. Roberts WN Jr, Hauptman HW: Joint aspiration or injection: Complications. In Rose BD (ed): UpToDate. Wellesley, Mass, UpToDate, 2002.
7. Ho G Jr: Bacterial arthritis. Curr Opin Rheumatol 13:310-314, 2001.
8. Esterhai JL Jr, Gelb I: Adult septic arthritis. Orthop Clin North Am 22:503-514, 1991.
9. Armstrong RW, Bolding F, Joseph R: Septic arthritis following arthroscopy: Clinical syndromes and analysis of risk factors. Arthroscopy 8:213-223, 1992.
10. Babcock HM, Matava MJ, Fraser V: Postarthroscopy surgical site infections: Review of the literature. Clin Infect Dis 34:65-71, 2002.
11. Centers for Disease Control and Prevention: Septic arthritis following anterior cruciate ligament reconstruction using tendon allografts—Florida and Louisiana, 2000. MMWR Morb Mortal Wkly Rep 50:1081-1083, 2001.
12. Ram S, Mackinnon FG, Gulati S, et al: The contrasting mechanisms of serum resistance of *Neisseria gonorrhoeae* and group B *Neisseria meningitidis*. Mol Immunol 36:915-928, 1999.
13. Goldenberg DL, Reed JI, Rice PA: Arthritis in rabbits induced by killed *Neisseria gonorrhoeae* and gonococcal lipopolysaccharide. J Rheumatol 11:3-8, 1984.
14. Herrmann, M, Vaudaux PE, Pittet D, et al: Fibronectin, fibrinogen, and laminin act as mediators of adherence of clinical staphylococcal isolates to foreign material. J Infect Dis 158:693-701, 1988.
15. Patti JM, Allen BL, McGavin MJ, et al: MSCRAMM-mediated adherence of microorganisms to host tissues. Annu Rev Microbiol 48:585-617, 1994.
16. Patti JM, Bremell T, Krajewska-Pietrasik D, et al: The *Staphylococcus aureus* collagen adhesin is a virulence determinant in experimental septic arthritis. Infect Immun 62:152-161, 1994.
17. Greene C, McDevitt D, Francois P, et al: Adhesion properties of mutants of *Staphylococcus aureus* defective in fibronectin-binding proteins and studies on the expression of fnb genes. Mol Microbiol 17:1143-1152, 1995.
18. Novick RP, Muir TW: Virulence gene regulation by peptides in staphylococci and other gram-positive bacteria. Curr Opin Microbiol 2:40-45, 1999.
19. Winzer K, Williams P: Quorum sensing and the regulation of virulence gene expression in pathogenic bacteria. Int J Med Microbiol 291:131-143, 2001.
20. Hudson MC, Ramp WK, Nicholson NC, et al: Internalization of *Staphylococcus aureus* by cultured osteoblasts. Microb Pathog 19:409-419, 1995.
21. Silverman GJ, Sasano M, Wormsley SB: Age-associated changes in binding of human B lymphocytes to a VH3-restricted unconventional bacterial antigen. J Immunol 151:5840-5855, 1993.
22. Palmqvist N, Silverman GJ, Josefsson E, et al: Bacterial cell wall-expressed protein A triggers supraclonal B-cell responses upon in vivo infection with *Staphylococcus aureus*. Microb Infect 7:1501-1511, 2005.
23. Gemmell CG, Goutcher SC, Reid R, et al: Role of certain virulence factors in a murine model of *Staphylococcus aureus* arthritis. J Med Microbiol 46:208-213, 1997.
24. Albus A, Arbeit RD, Lee JC: Virulence of *Staphylococcus aureus* mutants altered in type 5 capsule production. Infect Immun 59:1008-1014, 1991.
25. Buxton TB, Rissing JP, Horner JA, et al: Binding of a *Staphylococcus aureus* bone pathogen to type I collagen. Microb Pathog 8:441-448, 1990.
26. Vandenesch F, Projan SJ, Kreiswirth B, et al: Agr-related sequences in *Staphylococcus lugdunensis*. FEMS Microbiol Lett 111:115-122, 1993.
27. Nilsson IM, Lee JC, Bremell T, et al: The role of staphylococcal polysaccharide microcapsule expression in septicemia and septic arthritis. Infect Immun 65:4216-4221, 1997.
28. Shinefield H, Black S, Fattom A, et al: Use of a *Staphylococcus aureus* conjugate vaccine in patients receiving hemodialysis. N Engl J Med 346:491-496, 2002.
29. Bremell T, Tarkowski A: Preferential induction of septic arthritis and mortality by superantigen-producing staphylococci. Infect Immun 63:4185-4187, 1995.
30. Renno T, Hahne M, MacDonald HR: Proliferation is a prerequisite for bacterial superantigen-induced T cell apoptosis in vivo. J Exp Med 181:2283-2287, 1995.
31. Nilsson IM, Verdrengh M, Ulrich RG, et al: Protection against *Staphylococcus aureus* sepsis by vaccination with recombinant staphylococcal enterotoxin A devoid of superantigenicity. J Infect Dis 180:1370-1373, 1999.
32. Kimura M, Matsukawa A, Ohkawara S, et al: Blocking of TNF-alpha and IL-1 inhibits leukocyte infiltration at early, but not at late stage of *S. aureus*-induced arthritis and the concomitant cartilage destruction in rabbits. Clin Immunol Immunopathol 82:18-25, 1997.
33. Zhao YX, Nilsson IM, Tarkowski A: The dual role of interferon-gamma in experimental *Staphylococcus aureus* septicemia versus arthritis. Immunology 93:80-85, 1998.
34. Epstein JH, Zimmermann B III, Ho G Jr: Polyarticular septic arthritis. J Rheumatol 13:1105-1107, 1986.
35. Smith JW: Infectious arthritis. In Mandell GL, Douglas RG Jr, Bennett JE (eds): Principles and Practice of Infectious Diseases, 3rd ed. New York, Churchill Livingstone, 1990, pp 911-918.
36. Dubost J, Fis I, Denis P, et al: Polyarticular septic arthritis. Medicine 72:296-310, 1993.
37. Brown TJ, Yen-Moore A, Tyring SK: An overview of sexually transmitted diseases, Part I. J Am Acad Dermatol 41:511-532, 1999.
38. Cucurull E, Espinoza LR: Gonococcal arthritis. Rheum Dis Clin N Am 24:305-322, 1998.
39. Al-Suleiman SA, Grimes EM, Jonas HS: Disseminated gonococcal infections. Obstet Gynecol 61:48-51, 1983.
40. O'Brien JP, Goldenberg DL, Rice PA: Disseminated gonococcal infection: A prospective analysis of 49 patients and a review of pathophysiology and immune mechanisms. Medicine 62:395-406, 1983.
41. Goldenberg DL: Septic arthritis and other infections of rheumatologic significance. Rheum Dis Clin N Am 17:149-156, 1991.
42. Bennett OM, Namnyak SS: Acute septic arthritis of the hip joint in infancy and childhood. Clin Orthop 281:123-132, 1992.
43. Gupta MN, Sturrock RD, Field M: A prospective 2-year study of 75 patients with adult-onset septic arthritis. Rheumatology (Oxf) 40:24-30, 2001.
44. Petersen BH, Lee TJ, Snyderman R, et al: *Neisseria meningitidis* and *Neisseria gonorrhoeae* bacteremia associated with C6, C7, or C8 deficiency. Ann Intern Med 90:917-920, 1979.
45. Franz A, Webster AD, Furr PM, et al: Mycoplasmal arthritis in patients with primary immunoglobulin deficiency: Clinical features and outcome in 18 patients. Br J Rheumatol 36:661-668, 1997.
46. Nolla JM, Gomez-Vaquero C, Fiter J, et al: Pyarthrosis in patients with rheumatoid arthritis: A detailed analysis of 10 cases and literature review. Semin Arthritis Rheum 30:121-126, 2000.
47. Gardner GC, Weisman MH: Pyarthrosis in patients with rheumatoid arthritis: A report of 13 cases and a review of the literature from the past 40 years. Am J Med 88:503-511, 1990.
48. Goldenberg DL: Infectious arthritis complicating rheumatoid arthritis and other chronic rheumatic disorders. Arthritis Rheum 32:496-502, 1989.
49. Mateo Soria L, Miquel Nolla Sole J, Rozadilla Sacanell A, et al: Infectious arthritis in patients with rheumatoid arthritis. Ann Rheum Dis 51:402-403, 1992.
50. Ostensson A, Geborek P: Septic arthritis as a non-surgical complication in rheumatoid arthritis: Relation to disease severity and therapy. Br J Rheumatol 30:35-38, 1991.
51. Shmerling RH, Delbanco TL, Tosteson ANA, et al: Synovial fluid tests: What should be ordered? JAMA 264:1009-1014, 1990.
52. Ho G Jr: Septic arthritis. In Klippel JH (ed): Primer on the Rheumatic Diseases, 12th ed. Atlanta, Arthritis Foundation, 2001, pp 259-264.
53. Perez-Ruiz F, Testillano M, Gastaca MA, et al: Pseudoseptic pseudogout associated with hypomagnesemia in liver transplant patients. Transplantation 71:696-698, 2001.
54. Pioro MH, Mandell BF: Septic arthritis. Rheum Dis Clin N Am 23:239-258, 1997.
55. Goldenberg DL: Septic arthritis. Lancet 351:197-202, 1998.
56. Liebling MR, Arkfeld DG, Michelini GA, et al: Identification of *Neisseria gonorrhoeae* in synovial fluid using the polymerase chain reaction. Arthritis Rheum 37:702-709, 1994.
57. Muralidhar B, Rumore PM, Steinman CR: Use of the polymerase chain reaction to study arthritis due to *Neisseria gonorrhoeae*. Arthritis Rheum 37:710-717, 1994.

58. von Essen R: Culture of joint specimens in bacterial arthritis: Impact of blood culture bottle utilization. Scand J Rheumatol 26:293-300, 1997.

59. Yagupsky P, Press J: Use of the isolator 1.5 microbial tube for culture of synovial fluid from patients with septic arthritis. J Clin Microbiol 35:2410-2412, 1997.

60. Hughes JG, Vetter EA, Patel R, et al: Culture with BACTEC Peds Plus/F bottle compared with conventional methods for detection of bacteria in synovial fluid. J Clin Microbiol 39:4468-4471, 2001.

61. Adams WG, Deaver KA, Cochi SL, et al: Decline of childhood *Haemophilus influenzae* type b Hib disease in the Hib vaccine era. JAMA 269:221-226, 1993.

62. Broadhurst LE, Erickson RL, Kelley PW: Decreases in invasive *Haemophilus influenzae* disease in US Army children, 1984-1991. JAMA 269:227-231, 1993.

63. Brewer GF, Davis JR, Grossman M: Gonococcal arthritis in an adolescent girl. Am J Dis Child 122:253-254, 1971.

64. Goldenberg DL, Cohen AS: Acute infectious arthritis. Am J Med 60:369-377, 1976.

65. Schattner A, Vosti KL: Bacterial arthritis due to beta-hemolytic streptococci of serogroups A, B, C, F, and G: Analysis of 23 cases and review of the literature. Medicine 77:122-139, 1998.

66. Duggan JM, Georgiadis G, VanGorp C, et al: Group B streptococcal prosthetic joint infections. J South Orthop Assoc 10:209-214, 2001.

67. Straus C, Caplanne D, Bergemer AM, et al: Destructive polyarthritis due to a group B streptococcus. Rev Rhum Engl Educ 64:339-341, 1997.

68. **Pischel KD, Weisman MH, Cone RO: Unique features of group B streptococcal arthritis in adults. Arch Intern Med 145:97-102, 1985.**

69. Goldenberg DL, Brandt K, Cathcart E, et al: Acute arthritis caused by gram-negative bacilli: A clinical characterization. Medicine 53:197-208, 1974.

70. Ho G Jr: Bacterial arthritis. In McCarty DJ, Koopman WJ (eds): Arthritis and Allied Conditions, 12th ed. Philadelphia, Lea & Febiger, 1993, pp 2003-2023.

71. Gutierrez KM: Infectious and inflammatory arthritis. In Long SS, Pickering LK, Prober CG (eds): Principles and Practice of Pediatric Infectious Diseases, 2nd ed. New York, Churchill Livingstone, 2002, pp 475-481.

72. Gilad J, Borer A, Riesenberg K, et al: Polymicrobial polyarticular septic arthritis: A rare clinical entity. Scand J Infect Dis 33:381-383, 2001.

73. Mandell GA: Imaging in the diagnosis of musculoskeletal infections in children. Curr Probl Pediatr 26:218-237, 1996.

74. Sanchez RB, Quinn SF: MRI of inflammatory synovial processes. Magn Reson Imaging 7:529-540, 1989.

75. Widman DS, Craig JG, Van Holsbeeck MT: Sonographic detection, evaluation and aspiration of infected acromioclavicular joints. Skeletal Radiol 30:388-392, 2001.

76. Espinoza LR: Infectious arthritis. In Goldman L, Bennett JC (eds): Cecil Textbook of Medicine, 21st ed. Philadelphia, WB Saunders, 2000, pp 1507-1509.

77. Gilbert DN, Moellering RC, Sande MA (eds): The Sanford Guide. Hyde Park, Vermont, Antimicrobial Therapy, Inc, 2002.

78. Goldenberg DL, Sexton DJ: Bacterial (nongonococcal) arthritis. In Rose BD (ed): UpToDate. Wellsley, Mass, UpToDate, 2002.

79. Nicolau DP, Freeman CD, Belliveau PP, et al: Experience with a once-daily aminoglycoside program administered to 2184 adult patients. Antimicrob Agents Chemother 39:650-655, 1995.

80. Smith JW, Hasan MS: Infectious arthritis. In Mandell GL, Bennett JE, Dolin R (eds): Principles and Practice of Infectious Diseases, 5th ed. Philadelphia, Churchill Livingstone, 2000, pp 1175-1182.

81. Smith RL, Schurman DJ, Kajiyama G, et al: The effect of antibiotics on the destruction of cartilage in experimental infectious arthritis. J Bone Joint Surg Am 69:1063-1068, 1987.

82. Manadan AM, Block JA: Daily needle aspiration versus surgical lavage for the treatment of bacterial septic arthritis in adults. Am J Therap 11:412-415, 2004.

83. **Goldenberg D, Brandt K, Cohen A, et al: Treatment of septic arthritis: Comparison of needle aspiration and surgery as initial modes of joint drainage. Arthritis Rheum 18:83-90, 1975.**

84. Weston VC, Jones AC, Bradbury N, et al: Clinical features and outcome of septic arthritis in a single UK Health District 1982-1991. Ann Rheum Dis 58:214-219, 1999.

85. Broy S, Schmid F: A comparison of medical drainage (needle aspiration) and surgical drainage in the initial treatment of infected joints. Clin Rheum Dis 12:501-521, 1986.

86. Goldenberg DL, Reed JI: Bacterial arthritis. N Engl J Med 312:764-771, 1985.

87. Smith JW, Piercy EA: Infectious arthritis. Clin Infect Dis 20:225-231, 1995.

88. Parisien JS, Shafer B: Arthroscopic management of pyoarthrosis. Clin Orthop 275:243-247, 1992.

89. Ho G Jr: How best to drain an infected joint: Will we ever know for certain? J Rheumatol 20:2001-2003, 1993.

90. Ross JJ, Saltzman CL, Carling P, et al: Pneumococcal septic arthritis: Review of 190 cases. Clin Infect Dis 36:319-327, 2003.

91. Darouiche RO: Device-associated infections: A macroproblem that starts with microadherence. Clin Infect Dis 33:1567-1572, 2001.

92. Lidgren L, Knutson K, Stefansdottir A: Infection and arthritis: Infection of prosthetic joints. Best Pract Res Clin Rheumatol 17:209-218, 2003.

93. Hanssen AD, Rand JA: Evaluation and treatment of infection at the site of a total hip or knee arthroplasty. Instr Course Lect 48:111-122, 1999.

94. Sperling JW, Kozak TK, Hanssen AD, et al: Infection after shoulder arthroplasty. Clin Orthop 382:206-216, 2001.

95. Robertsson O, Knutson K, Lewold S, et al: The Swedish Knee Arthroplasty Register 1975-1997: An update with special emphasis on 41,223 knees operated on in 1988-1997. Acta Orthop Scand 72:503-513, 2001.

96. Berbari EF, Hanssen AD, Duffy MC, et al: Risk factors for prosthetic joint infection: Case-control study. Clin Infect Dis 27:1247-1254, 1998.

97. Zimmerli W, Waldvogel FA, Vaudaux P, et al: Pathogenesis of foreign body infection: Description and characteristics of an animal model. J Infect Dis 146:487-497, 1982.

98. Roisman FR, Walz DT, Finkelstein AE: Superoxide radical production by human leukocytes exposed to immune complexes: Inhibitory action of gold compounds. Inflammation 7:355-362, 1983.

99. Wang JY, Wicklund BH, Gustilo RB, et al: Prosthetic metals impair murine immune response and cytokine release in vivo and in vitro. J Orthop Res 15:688-697, 1997.

100. Murdoch DR, Roberts SA, Fowler VG, et al: Infection of orthopedic prostheses after *Staphylococcus aureus* bacteremia. Clin Infect Dis 32:647-649, 2001.

101. Donlan RM: Biofilms: Microbial life on surfaces. Emerg Infect Dis 8:881-890, 2002.

102. Veenstra GJ, Cremers FF, van Dijk H, et al: Ultrastructural organization and regulation of a biomaterial adhesin in *Staphylococcus epidermidis*. J Bacteriol 178:537-541, 1996.

103. Shiro H, Muller E, Gutierrez N, et al: Transposon mutants of *Staphylococcus epidermidis* deficient in elaboration of capsular polysaccharide/adhesin and slime are avirulent in a rabbit model of endocarditis. J Infect Dis 169:1042-1049, 1994.

104. **Zimmerli W, Trampuz A, Ochsner PE: Prosthetic-joint infections. N Engl J Med 351:1645-1654, 2004.**

105. Tigges S, Stiles RG, Roberson JR: Appearance of septic hip prosthesis on plain radiographs. AJR Am J Roentgenol 163:377-380, 1994.

106. Smith SL, Wastie ML, Forster I: Radionuclide bone scintigraphy in the detection of significant complications after total knee joint replacement. Clin Radiol 56:221-224, 2001.

107. Trampuz A, Hanssen AD, Osmon DR, et al: Synovial fluid leukocyte count and differential for the diagnosis of prosthetic knee infection. Am J Med 117:556-562, 2004.

108. Spangehl MJ, Masri BA, O'Connell JX, et al: Prospective analysis of preoperative and intraoperative investigations for the diagnosis of infection at the sites of two hundred and two revision total hip arthroplasties. J Bone Joint Surg Am 81:672-683, 1999.

109. Atkins BL, Athanasou N, Deeks JJ, et al: Prospective evaluation of criteria for microbiological diagnosis of prosthetic-joint infection at revision arthroplasty. The OSIRIS Collaborative Study Group. J Clin Microbiol 36:2932-2939, 1998.

110. Mackowiak PA, Jones SR, Smith JW: Diagnostic value of sinus-tract cultures in chronic osteomyelitis. JAMA 239:2772-2775, 1978.

111. Kamme C, Lindberg L: Aerobic and anaerobic bacteria in deep infections after total hip arthroplasty: Differential diagnosis between infectious and non-infectious loosening. Clin Orthop 154:201-207, 1981.

112. Steckelberg J, Osmon D: Prosthetic joint infections. In Waldvogel F, Bisno A (eds): Infections Associated with Indwelling Medical Devices, 3rd edition. Washington, DC, American Society for Microbiology Press, 2000.

113. Stewart PS, Costerton JW: Antibiotic resistance of bacteria in biofilms. Lancet 358:135-138, 2001.

114. Widmer AF, Frei R, Rajacic Z, et al: Correlation between in vivo and in vitro efficacy of antimicrobial agents against foreign body infections. J Infect Dis 162:96-102, 1990.

115. Widmer AF, Wiestner A, Frei R, et al: Killing of nongrowing and adherent *Escherichia coli* determines drug efficacy in device-related infections. Antimicrob Agents Chemother 35:741-746, 1991.

116. Trampuz A, Widmer AF: Infections associated with orthopedic implants. Curr Opin Infect Dis 19:349-356, 2006.

117. Razonable RR, Osmon DR, Steckelberg JM: Linezolid therapy for orthopedic infections. Mayo Clin Proc 79:1137-1144, 2004.

118. Yin LY, Lazzarini L, Fan L, et al: Comparative evaluation of tigecycline and vancomycin, with and without rifampicin, in the treatment of methicillin-resistant *Staphylococcus aureus* experimental osteomyelitis in a rabbit model. J Antimicrob Chemother 55:995-1002, 2005.

119. Brandt CM, Sistrunk WW, Duffy MC, et al: *Staphylococcus aureus* prosthetic joint infection treated with debridement and prosthesis retention. Clin Infect Dis 24:914-919, 1997.

120. Raut VV, Siney PD, Wroblewski BM: One-stage revision of total hip arthroplasty for deep infection: Long term followup. Clin Orthop 321:202-207, 1995.

121. Giulieri SG, Graber P, Ochsner PE, et al: Management of infection associated with total hip arthroplasty according to a treatment algorithm. Infection 32:222-228, 2004.

122. Callaghan JJ, Katz RP, Johnston RC: One-stage revision surgery of the infected hip: A minimum 10-year followup study. Clin Orthop 369:139-143, 1999.

123. Ure KJ, Amstutz HC, Nasser S, et al: Direct-exchange arthroplasty for the treatment of infection after total hip replacement: An average ten-year follow-up. J Bone Joint Surg Am 80:961-968, 1998.

124. Marculescu CE, Berberi EF, Hanssen AD, et al: Outcome of prosthetic joint infections treated with debridement and retention of components. Clin Infect Dis 42:471-478, 2006.

125. Trampuz A, Zimmerli W: Prosthetic joint infections: Update in diagnosis and treatment. Swiss Med Wkly 135:243-251, 2005.

126. Brandt CM, Duffy MCT, Berbari EF, et al: *Staphylococcus aureus* prosthetic joint infection treated with prosthesis removed and delayed reimplantation arthroplasty. Mayo Clin Proc 74:553-558, 1999.

127. Stein A, Bataille JF, Drancourt M, et al: Ambulatory treatment of multi-drug resistant *Staphylococcus*-infected orthopedic implants with high-dose oral co-trimoxazole. Antimicrob Agents Chemother 42:3086-3091, 1998.

128. American Dental Association, American Academy of Orthopedic Surgeons Advisory statement: Antibiotic prophylaxis for dental patients with total joint replacements. J Am Dent Assoc 134:895-899, 2003.

129. Sandhu SS, Lowry JC, Morton ME, et al: Antibiotic prophylaxis, dental treatment and arthroplasty: Time to explode a myth. J Bone Joint Surg Br 79:521-522, 1997.

130. American Society for Gastrointestinal Endoscopy: Antibiotic prophylaxis for gastrointestinal endoscopy. Gastrointest Endosc 58:475-482, 2003.

131. American Society of Colon and Rectal Surgeons: Practice parameters for antibiotic prophylaxis to prevent infective endocarditis or infected prosthesis during colon and rectal endoscopy. Dis Colon Rectum 44:899, 2001.

132. Working Party of the British Society for Antimicrobial Chemotherapy: Case against antibiotic prophylaxis for dental treatment of patients with joint prostheses. Lancet 339:301, 1992.

133. Howell RM, Green JG: Prophylactic antibiotic coverage in dentistry: A survey of need for prosthetic joints. Gen Dent 33:320-323, 1985.

134. Meyer GW, Artis AL: Antibiotic prophylaxis for orthopedic prostheses and GI procedures: Report of a survey. Am J Gastroenterol 92:989-991, 1997.

135. Shrout MK, Scarbrough F, Powell BL: Dental care and the prosthetic joint patient: A survey of orthopedic surgeons and general dentists. J Am Dent Assoc 125:429-436, 1994.

136. Dajani AS, Taubert KA, Wilson W, et al: Prevention of bacterial endocarditis: Recommendations by the American Heart Association. JAMA 277:1794-1801, 1997.

137. Mason JC, Dollery CT, So A, et al: An infected prosthetic hip: Is there a role for prophylactic antibiotics? BMJ 305:300-302, 1992.

138. Jacobson JJ, Schweitzer SO, Kowalski CJ: Chemoprophylaxis of prosthetic joint patients during dental treatment: A decision-utility analysis. Oral Surg Oral Med Oral Pathol 72:167-177, 1991.

139. Jaspers MT, Little JW: Prophylactic antibiotic coverage in patients with total arthroplasty: Current practice. J Am Dent Assoc 111:943-948, 1985.

140. Krijnen P, Kaandorp CJE, Steyerberg EW, et al: Antibiotic prophylaxis for haematogenous bacterial arthritis in patients with joint disease: A cost effective analysis. Ann Rheum Dis 60:359-366, 2001.

141. Tsevat J, Durand-Zaleski I, Pauker SG: Cost-effectiveness of antibiotic prophylaxis for dental procedures in patients with artificial joints. Am J Public Health 79:739-743, 1989.

142. Giles JT, Bartlett SJ, Gelber AC, et al: Tumor necrosis factor inhibitor therapy and risk of serious postoperative orthopedic infection in rheumatoid arthritis. Arthritis Care Res 55:333-337, 2006.

143. Bongartz T, Sutton AJ, Sweeting MJ, et al: Anti-TNF antibody therapy in rheumatoid arthritis and the risk of serious infections and malignancies: Systematic review and meta-analysis of rare harmful effects in randomized controlled trials. JAMA 295:2275-2285, 2006.

144. Dubost JJ, Soubrier M, De Champs C, et al: No change in the distribution of organisms responsible for septic arthritis over a 20 year period. Ann Rheum Dis 61:267-269, 2002.

145. Ho G Jr, Su EY: Therapy for septic arthritis. JAMA 247:797-800, 1982.

146. Yu LP, Bradley JD, Hugenberg ST, et al: Predictors of mortality in non-post-operative patients with septic arthritis. Scand J Rheumatol 21:142-144, 1992.

147. Kaandorp CJE, Krijnen P, Moens HJB, et al: The outcome of bacterial arthritis: A prospective community-based study. Arthritis Rheum 40:884-892, 1997.

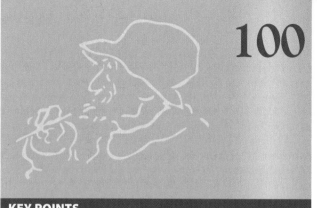

100 Lyme Disease

LINDA K. BOCKENSTEDT

KEY POINTS

Lyme disease is due to infection with tick-transmitted spirochetes of the genus *Borrelia burgdorferi sensu lato*, and has a worldwide distribution. Variation in genospecies may account for differences in the clinical expression of Lyme disease, with neurologic and late skin disease more common in Europe and arthritis more common in North America.

Lyme disease has a characteristic pattern of signs and symptoms (see Table 100-1) and usually begins with the hallmark skin lesion erythema migrans. Earlier recognition and treatment has led to a decline in the incidence of carditis and acute neurologic and late disease manifestations.

Musculoskeletal manifestations occur in more than 50% of patients and at all stages of infection, but frank arthritis is now considered a sign of late disease and is uncommon (<10% of patients).

The diagnosis of Lyme disease should be suspected when a patient who lives, works, or vacations in an endemic area presents with signs and symptoms of *B. burgdorferi* infection. Two-tiered (enzyme-linked immunosorbent assay and immunoblot) serologic tests can be negative with early infection, but become positive in most patients with disease of greater than 1 month's duration.

Most patients are cured with 2 to 4 weeks of antibiotic therapy, although the time to disease resolution may extend beyond the duration of therapy, and irreversible tissue damage may occur.

Coinfection with other tick-borne pathogens (*Babesia microti* or *Anaplasma phagocytophilum*) can lead to more severe symptoms and should be suspected in patients who have a poor response to treatment for Lyme disease.

Antibiotic-refractory arthritis occurs in less than 10% of patients who develop arthritis secondary to Lyme disease and may be due to persistent foreign antigen, abnormal regulation of the inflammatory response, or infection-induced autoimmunity. These patients respond to nonsteroidal anti-inflammatory drugs and hydroxychloroquine, and arthritis typically resolves over 4 to 5 years.

A minority of patients have persistent debilitating complaints of fatigue, mild cognitive dysfunction, and musculoskeletal pain after antibiotic treatment for Lyme disease. Viable *B. burgdorferi* cannot be detected in these individuals, and controlled treatment trials show no benefit of prolonged antibiotic therapy over placebo.

Although maternal-fetal transmission of *B. burgdorferi* can occur, there is no evidence that the organism causes a congenital syndrome. *B. burgdorferi* infection in the mother should not cause harm to the fetus if pregnant patients with Lyme disease are treated with recommended antibiotic regimens.

Lyme disease is a multisystem disorder caused by the tick-borne spirochete *Borrelia burgdorferi*.[1] The disease first came to medical attention in the late 1970s with the investigation of a clustering of cases of juvenile arthritis in the region of Lyme, Connecticut.[2] A characteristic skin rash described as single or multiple expanding red macules often heralded the onset of arthritis.[2] This rash, termed *erythema migrans* (EM), had been linked in Europe to the bite of *Ixodes* ticks and the subsequent development of neurologic abnormalities.[3] Further investigation revealed that arthritis was one manifestation of a systemic disorder affecting the skin, heart, joints, and nervous system. In 1982, Burgdorfer[4] isolated the causative agent, the spirochete *B. burgdorferi*, from *Ixodes* ticks. Demonstration that Lyme disease patients developed antibodies to this organism and its eventual culture from skin, cerebrospinal fluid (CSF), and synovial tissue confirmed the infectious etiology of the disorder.[5] It is now the most common vector-borne disease in the United States.[1]

ECOLOGY AND EPIDEMIOLOGY OF LYME DISEASE

Lyme disease has a worldwide distribution, with most cases reported in North America, Europe, and Asia.[6] On each of these continents, hard-shelled ticks of the *Ixodes* family serve as vectors for the disease. The incidence of Lyme disease varies geographically and is determined by the prevalence of *B. burgdorferi*–infected ticks. In the United States, cases of Lyme disease have been reported in 49 states and the District of Columbia, but most are clustered in the Northeast and mid-Atlantic region, upper Midwest, and northern California. In 2005, 23,305 cases were reported to the Centers for Disease Control and Prevention, with 93% originating from eight states: New York, Pennsylvania, New Jersey, Massachusetts, Connecticut, Maryland, Minnesota, and Delaware.[7]

The spirochetes associated with Lyme disease reside within the genus *B. burgdorferi sensu lato* (sl) and include *B. burgdorferi sensu stricto* (ss), *Borrelia garinii*, and *Borrelia afzelii*.[6] All three genospecies can be found in Europe, whereas only *B. burgdorferi* ss is found in North America. Variation among the genospecies may account for the differences in clinical expression of Lyme disease between the two continents, with *B. garinii* associated with neurologic disease, *B. afzelii* associated with late skin involvement, and *B. burgdorferi* ss associated with arthritis. Because of the prominence of musculoskeletal manifestations with *B. burgdorferi* ss infection, the only genospecies in North America, this chapter focuses on Lyme disease in the United States.

TICKS AND LYME DISEASE

Lyme disease is found primarily in temperate climates where humans can have incidental exposure to questing ticks. *Ixodes* ticks have a 2-year life span in which they pass through three developmental stages—larva, nymph, and adult—feeding only once per stage.[8,9] *B. burgdorferi* is not passed transovarially and is maintained by passage between a reservoir host and ticks. Small rodents are the main reservoirs for *B. burgdorferi* ss and *B. afzelii*, whereas birds are the principal haven for *B. garinii* in Europe.[6] In the southern United States, ticks feed preferentially on lizards, which are not competent reservoirs for *B. burgdorferi*; this may explain in part the rarity of Lyme disease in this region.

Larvae acquire *B. burgdorferi* after feeding on an infected reservoir host in early spring, then molt to nymphs, which lay dormant until the following late spring and summer. The peak incidence of Lyme disease is in the summer months when humans come in contact with questing nymphs, which have more promiscuous feeding patterns.[8] Engorged nymphs molt into adult ticks, which feed almost exclusively on deer. *B. burgdorferi* does not persist in deer, which serve to maintain and propagate the tick population.

PATHOGENESIS

BORRELIA BURGDORFERI INVASION OF THE MAMMALIAN HOST

During tick feeding, *B. burgdorferi* migrates from the tick midgut to the salivary glands for egress into the blood meal host.[9] Migration takes about 24 hours, during which time spirochetes multiply and undergo phenotypic changes that permit the survival of *B. burgdorferi* in the new host. Spirochetes multiply first at the tick bite site in the skin, and if not dealt with by the innate immune system, they can disseminate through tissues and the bloodstream to infect any organ system at least transiently. The degree to which *B. burgdorferi* causes disease in tissues depends on spirochete virulence, growth conditions that allow it to persist at a particular site, and host factors that modulate the inflammatory response.

Analysis of the *B. burgdorferi* genome has revealed no known virulence factors common to other bacterial pathogens to help explain the pathogenesis of Lyme disease.[10] Instead the genome is remarkably rich in genes encoding putative lipoproteins, only a handful of which have been studied in detail. Outer surface protein (Osp) A is a midgut adhesin required for spirochete infection of ticks.[11] Osp C is essential for initial infection of the mammal, but is dispensable after spirochetes have disseminated and colonized other tissue.[12] To do so, *B. burgdorferi* harnesses host plasmin to move through tissues and expresses adhesins, including decorin binding proteins A and B, BBK32, and p66, which allow it to bind to extracellular matrix proteins and integrins on cells.

PATHOLOGY OF LYME DISEASE

Because intact spirochetes are seen only rarely in tissue specimens, the inflammatory response to *B. burgdorferi* components rather than tissue destruction by the spirochete itself is believed to underlie the pathology of Lyme disease. Histopathologic studies of EM lesions, cardiac tissue, synovial biopsy specimens, and limited nervous system tissue (meninges, spinal cord, and nerve roots) reveal varying degrees of monocytic and lymphoplasmacytic infiltrates, especially perivascular, that stain positively for cell surface markers for macrophages, T cells, and B cells.[13] The joint effusions of patients with Lyme arthritis reveal acute inflammation with elevated leukocyte counts, whereas the synovium resembles that of rheumatoid arthritis, with chronic inflammation mediated by mononuclear cell infiltration and pseudolymphoid follicles formed by T cells, B cells, and plasma cells. In the synovium and less commonly the epineural area, perivascular infiltrates can be associated with endarteritis obliterans, but *B. burgdorferi* infection does not typically cause a true vasculitis.

IMMUNE RESPONSE TO *BORRELIA BURGDORFERI*

Innate immune cells respond to *B. burgdorferi* through engagement of the Toll-like receptor (TLR) family of pattern recognition receptors, especially TLR2 (lipoproteins), TLR5 (flagellin), and TLR9 (spirochete DNA).[14] As a consequence, proinflammatory cytokines (including interleukin-1β and tumor necrosis factor-α), chemokines (interleukin-8), nitric oxide, and prostaglandins are produced that recruit inflammatory cells to the site of infection.[14,15] *B. burgdorferi* also induces matrix metalloproteinase expression in tissues through TLR-dependent and non–TLR-dependent pathways that contribute to pathology.[16]

Humoral immunity is a key host defense against *B. burgdorferi* infection. *B. burgdorferi* lipoproteins are B cell mitogens, and antibodies that arise in the absence of T cell help are sufficient to resolve inflammation and prevent challenge infection in the mouse model of Lyme borreliosis.[17,18] With the induction of adaptive immunity, IgG-containing immune complexes and cryoglobulins can be found in the serum of patients with Lyme disease and are concentrated in the joints of patients who develop Lyme arthritis.[19] Evidence of pathogen-specific intrathecal antibody production can be found in patients with neuroborreliosis[20]; some of these antibodies also can bind neural glycolipid antigens.[21,22]

B. burgdorferi infection primes CD4+ and CD8+ T cells, and the predominance of T helper type 1 responses correlates with more severe arthritis and neuroborreliosis.[23,24] There is an association between T cell and B cell responses to Osp A and the development of antibiotic-refractory Lyme arthritis.[25,26] Although evidence has been presented to suggest an autoimmune etiology (see later section on antibiotic-refractory arthritis), the self-limited nature of Lyme arthritis also raises the possibility that the immune responses detected are appropriate and directed toward eliminating persisting antigens rather than viable organisms. Alternatively, prolonged arthritis may be due to abnormal or delayed regulation of the host immune response when the pathogen and its inflammatory products have been eliminated. Deficiency in CD25+ T regulatory cells prolongs murine Lyme arthritis,[27] and synovial fluid γδ T cells isolated from patients with Lyme arthritis can modulate *B. burgdorferi*–specific CD4+ T cell responses by inducing apoptosis in a Fas-dependent fashion.[28]

MECHANISMS OF SPIROCHETE PERSISTENCE

When visualized in vivo, *B. burgdorferi* resides primarily in the extracellular matrix in connective tissue.[13] Despite occasional sightings of spirochetes inside cells,[29] an intracellular phase of the *B. burgdorferi* life cycle has not been shown. *B. burgdorferi* employs immune evasion strategies of an extracellular pathogen, which are directed toward deterring phagocyte ingestion and antibody and complement-mediated lysis.[14] *B. burgdorferi* expresses Erp and complement regulator–acquiring surface proteins that bind host factor H to prevent complement-mediated lysis. To impede antibody-mediated clearance, *B. burgdorferi* undergoes antigenic variation[30] and reduces expression of lipoproteins as infection progresses.[31] The *vlsE* gene undergoes random rearrangement of its expression locus, producing antigenically distinct variants of VlsE, a protein essential for spirochete survival in vivo. In the chronic phase of *B. burgdorferi* infection in mice, spirochetes can be visualized in the extracellular matrix of connective tissue, especially the skin, without an associated inflammatory response.[32]

CLINICAL FEATURES OF LYME DISEASE

Lyme disease occurs in stages that reflect the immune response to the spirochete as it establishes infection in the skin and later disseminates to distant organ sites (Table 100-1). Presenting clinical manifestations depend on the stage of the illness in which patients first seek medical attention. A characteristic feature of Lyme disease is that clinical signs can resolve without specific therapy, and patients may present in later stages of the illness without exhibiting signs of early disease.

EARLY LOCALIZED INFECTION

The hallmark of Lyme disease is the skin lesion EM, which is present in 80% to 90% of patients (Fig. 100-1).[33] The lesion arises within 1 month (median 7-10 days) at the tick bite site, especially in skin folds or where clothes bind in adults and around the hairline in children. EM begins as a red macule that expands at the rate of 2 to 3 cm/day, enlarging to more than 70 cm in diameter. Characteristic lesions greater than 5 cm in diameter in an appropriate clinical setting are sufficient for establishing the diagnosis of Lyme disease.[34] EM most often manifests with uniform erythema, but central clearing can occur in larger lesions, producing a classic "bull's eye" appearance (see Fig. 100-1D). Vesicular or necrotic centers are rarer, but even these EM lesions have relatively few symptoms other than a tingling or burning sensation. Intense pruritus or pain is unusual and should raise concern for alternative diagnoses.

EM may be accompanied by systemic flulike symptoms, including low-grade fever, malaise, neck pain or stiffness, arthralgias, and myalgias.[8] Particularly severe systemic symptoms should alert the physician to possible coinfection with another tick-borne pathogen, such as *Babesia microti* or *Anaplasma phagocytophilum* (the agent of human granulocytic anaplasmosis, formerly known as human granulocytic erhlichiosis). Lyme disease also can manifest with systemic symptoms alone in the absence of EM.[35,36] Absence of upper respiratory or gastrointestinal symptoms may help distinguish Lyme disease from common viral infections.

Table 100-1 Clinical Manifestations of Lyme Disease

Early Localized Infection
Occurs 3±30 days after tick bite
Erythema migrans (EM) in 80%-90% of patients; single lesion, occasionally associated with fever, malaise, neck pain or stiffness, arthralgias and myalgias
Systemic symptoms noted above in the absence of EM during summer months
Borrelial lymphocytoma (rare, seen primarily in Europe)
Early Disseminated Infection
Occurs weeks to months after tick bite
Profound malaise and fatigue common
Multiple EM lesions with systemic symptoms similar to early localized infection
Musculoskeletal   Migratory polyarthralgias and myalgias

Carditis (<3% of untreated patients)
   Varying degrees of atrioventricular nodal block
   Mild myopericarditis

Neurologic (<10% of untreated patients)
   Cranial neuropathies (especially facial nerve palsy)
   Lymphocytic meningitis
   Radiculoneuropathies
   Encephalomyelitis

Late Disease
Occurs months to years after tick bite

Arthritis (<10% of patients)
   Acute monarticular or migratory pauciarticular inflammatory arthritis, usually involving the knee
   Chronic antibiotic-refractory arthritis (<10% of patients with arthritis)

Neurologic (rare)
   Peripheral neuropathies
   Mild encephalopathy
   Encephalomyelitis (primarily seen in Europe)

Skin   Acrodermatitis chronica atrophicans (primarily seen in Europe)

Musculoskeletal complaints and debilitating fatigue associated with Lyme disease should be distinguished from fibromyalgia and chronic fatigue syndrome, which typically are more insidious in onset and are not associated with objective findings or laboratory abnormalities.

A newly recognized southern tick–associated rash illness (STARI) can produce a skin lesion similar to the bull's eye form of EM.[37] The rash is associated with the bite of the Lone Star tick, *Amblyomma americanum*, which is endemic to the southeastern and south-central states, but which also can be found as far north as Maine or west as central Texas and Oklahoma. Similar to EM, systemic symptoms can accompany the rash of STARI, but disease in organs other than the skin does not occur. The etiology of STARI is unknown. Although a noncultivatable spirochete named *Borrelia lonestari* has been found in *A. americanum*, STARI patients do not develop positive Lyme serologies, and the organism has not been found in skin biopsy specimens of the STARI lesions. Antibiotics resolve EM and STARI, but STARI patients recover more quickly from systemic symptoms than do patients with EM.

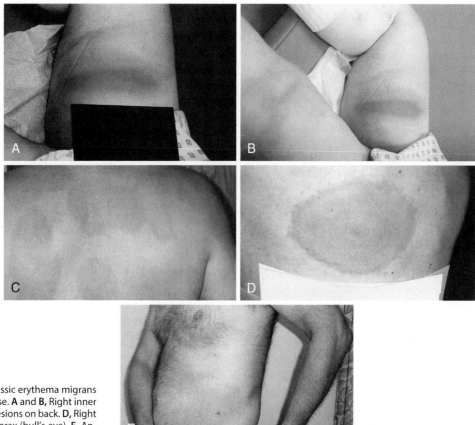

Figure 100-1 Classic erythema migrans rash of Lyme disease. **A** and **B**, Right inner thigh. **C**, Multiple lesions on back. **D**, Right lateral posterior thorax (bull's eye). **E**, Anterior side.

EARLY DISSEMINATED INFECTION

Within weeks of the onset of infection, *B. burgdorferi* can disseminate through the skin, blood, and lymphatics to infect multiple tissues. Clinically apparent disease at this stage is usually seen, however, in the skin, heart, or nervous system. Patients with disseminated infection have debilitating fatigue and appear ill. Specific localizing signs and symptoms may fluctuate, but profound fatigue is a consistent complaint.

SKIN DISEASE

Fifty percent of patients with untreated Lyme disease develop multiple EM lesions, a sign of disseminated infection (see Fig. 100-1C).[33] Secondary lesions are typically smaller and can occur anywhere on the body, but are most noticeable on the trunk. The lesions usually appear as flat macules and can develop partial central clearing. EM lesions may be accompanied by migratory muscle, joint, and periarticular pain that lasts hours to days, but frank arthritis is now considered a late manifestation.

CARDIAC DISEASE

The incidence of cardiac involvement has declined to 1% to 3% in recent years, possibly owing to earlier recognition and treatment of *B. burgdorferi* infection. It most often occurs within the first 2 months of infection and manifests as varying degrees of atrioventricular block, occasionally accompanied by mild myopericarditis.[38] Electrophysiologic studies have mapped the conduction defect to the area above the bundle of His and involving the atrioventricular node, although multiple levels can be affected. Overt congestive heart failure is rare, and chronic cardiomyopathy, reported in Europe, has not been documented to occur in the United States.[39] Patients with Lyme carditis often have a history of EM and may have concomitant arthralgia and myalgia at the time of presentation. Absence of valvular heart disease helps distinguish Lyme carditis from acute rheumatic fever, and prominent myocardial dysfunction or pericardial involvement should suggest other infectious etiologies.

NERVOUS SYSTEM INVOLVEMENT

Acute neurologic Lyme disease occurs in less than 10% of patients and most commonly manifests as cranial nerve palsy or meningitis, although radiculopathy and encephalomyelitis also are occasionally seen.[40-42] Cranial palsy usually affects the seventh nerve, resulting in unilateral or bilateral facial palsy. Even in endemic areas, however, onset of seventh nerve palsy in the nonwinter months is due to *B. burgdorferi* infection in only 25% of cases. Bilateral facial palsy is seen in only a few other conditions—Guillain-Barré syndrome, human immunodeficiency virus infection, sarcoidosis, and other causes of chronic meningitis—all of which are readily distinguished from Lyme disease. Rarely, other cranial nerves (III, IV, V, VI, or VIII) may be involved. Lyme meningitis manifests with fever, headache, and stiff neck similar to viral meningitis, along with a CSF lymphocytosis and elevated protein.[43] In children, meningitis may occur with EM, cranial nerve involvement, and increased intracranial pressure (papilledema), which is rare in adults.[42,44] Lyme radiculopathy typically manifests as pain, weakness, numbness, and reflex loss in a dermatomal distribution, resembling mechanical radiculopathies.[42] Lyme disease should be considered when there is no obvious precipitating factor for disk-related symptoms, and imaging studies do not delineate pathology at the appropriate root level. Untreated Lyme radiculopathy can progress to become bilateral, which helps distinguish it from mechanical disease. When truncal involvement causes unilateral chest or abdominal pain, Lyme radiculopathy is often mistaken for visceral disease or early herpes zoster before the development of vesicular lesions.

OTHER ORGAN SYSTEM INVOLVEMENT

A variety of other organs can exhibit pathology with disseminated *B. burgdorferi* infection, including the eye (keratitis), the ear (sensorineural hearing loss), the liver (hepatitis), the spleen (necrosis), skeletal muscle (myositis), and subcutaneous tissue (panniculitis).[45] In general, other, more classic manifestations of Lyme disease are present concurrently or have been present in the recent past to suggest the diagnosis.

LATE DISEASE

Months after the onset of infection, untreated patients can develop late manifestations of Lyme disease, usually involving the joints (discussed separately later), nervous system, and the skin. At this stage of infection, two-tier (enzyme-linked immunosorbent assay [ELISA] and IgG immunoblot) serologic testing for *B. burgdorferi* should be positive.

Late Neurologic Disease

Late neurologic Lyme disease is now rare; patients may present with encephalomyelitis, peripheral neuropathy, or encephalopathy.[46,47] Encephalomyelitis, seen predominantly in Europe with *B. garinii* infection, is a slowly progressive, unifocal or multifocal inflammatory disease of the central nervous system, with increased T2 signals in the white matter on MRI. CSF examination often reveals a lymphocytic pleocytosis, elevated protein, and normal glucose, and serum IgG to *B. burgdorferi* and intrathecal antibody production can be found. These findings help distinguish Lyme encephalomyelitis from multiple sclerosis, which may rarely be associated with positive IgG reactivity to *B. burgdorferi* in serum and CSF samples, but there is no intrathecal antibody production.[48] Multiple sclerosis patients with positive Lyme serologies do not respond to antibiotics used for neurologic Lyme disease.

Late peripheral nervous system involvement manifests as a mild sensorimotor neuropathy in a "stocking and glove" distribution, with evidence of a mild confluent mononeuritis multiplex on electrophysiologic studies.[49] Patients may have intermittent limb paresthesias and occasionally radicular pain. The most common finding on physical examination is reduced vibratory sensation in the lower extremities. Serum IgG to *B. burgdorferi* should be present, but CSF examination is normal, consistent with disease confined to the peripheral nervous system. Patients with this form of neuropathy should

be evaluated for other infectious diseases (syphilis, human immunodeficiency virus, and hepatitis C virus), metabolic disorders (especially vitamin B_{12} deficiency, diabetes mellitus, and thyroid disease), and autoimmune diseases (antinuclear antibody [ANA] or rheumatoid factor associated).

Patients with Lyme encephalopathy complain of memory impairment and cognitive dysfunction that is best shown by formal neuropsychologic testing.[50,51] Occasionally, patients may have CSF abnormalities with elevated protein, lymphocytic pleocytosis, and intrathecal antibody to *B. burgdorferi*, but CSF examination also can be normal. Serum IgG to *B. burgdorferi* should be present, however, to consider the diagnosis. The mild cognitive dysfunction seen in patients with Lyme encephalopathy must be distinguished from neurocognitive deficits secondary to chronic stress, sleep deprivation, fibromyalgia, chronic fatigue syndrome, or aging. As for any chronic encephalopathy, toxic-metabolic causes should be excluded. Brain imaging studies generally are normal or show only nonspecific abnormalities and are not useful in establishing a diagnosis of encephalopathy associated with Lyme disease.

Late Skin Disease

The late skin lesion acrodermatitis chronica atrophicans is found mainly in Europe because of its association with *B. afzelii* infection, although any *B. burgdorferi* species can cause the lesion. Acrodermatitis chronica atrophicans develops insidiously over years and most often is found on the dorsum of the hands or feet.[52] It begins as a unilateral bluish red discoloration and swelling, which evolves to atrophic, cellophane-like skin with prominent appearance of the blood vessels. About 60% of patients also have a peripheral sensory neuropathy affecting the involved extremity. A prominent lymphoplasmacytic infiltrate is shown on the skin biopsy specimen. Antibiotics can lead to improvement in pain and swelling, but atrophic skin remains.

LYME ARTHRITIS AND OTHER MUSCULOSKELETAL MANIFESTATIONS OF LYME DISEASE

Musculoskeletal symptoms are common in all stages of Lyme disease and include migratory pain in joints, tendons, bursae, and muscles.[53] Typically, musculoskeletal pain affects one or two sites at a time, lasts only hours to a few days at any one location, and is associated with significant fatigue. The incidence of frank arthritis has declined from 50% in early studies to less than 10% in more recent years.[15] ELISA and IgG immunoblot for *B. burgdorferi* are positive when arthritis appears, and *B. burgdorferi* DNA can be detected by polymerase chain reaction (PCR) in synovium and synovial fluid even though cultures are usually negative. Although Lyme arthritis can resemble pauciarticular juvenile arthritis or reactive arthritis, patients generally test negative for ANA, rheumatoid factor, and anti–cyclic citrullinated peptide antibodies, and do not have an increased frequency of HLA-B27 alleles. Joint fluid analysis and synovial histopathology cannot distinguish these entities. Axial and sacroiliac joint involvement is not a feature of Lyme disease, but enthesitis can be seen. Most patients with Lyme arthritis have positive two-tier serologic tests for *B. burgdorferi* infection.

Arthritis usually begins months or years after *B. burgdorferi* infection and is predated by migratory arthralgias in half of patients.[53] The most typical pattern is a monarticular or oligoarticular arthritis involving one or a few large joints (fewer than five total), with the knee affected in 80% of cases. Joints are warm with large effusions, often greater than 100 mL in the knee, but comparatively little pain. Synovial fluid is inflammatory with white blood cell counts ranging from approximately 2000 to 70,000/mm[3] (median approximately 24,000/mm[3]), with a predominance of neutrophils.[54] Depending on the chronicity of the arthritis, synovial biopsy specimens reveal only mononuclear cell infiltration or more advanced changes consistent with rheumatoid synovium.[13] Large effusions can lead to Baker cyst formation and rupture. The temporomandibular joint also is frequently involved and in one study was the first joint to be affected in 25% of patients with arthritis.[53] Other joints commonly affected include the shoulder, ankle, elbow, wrist, and hip. Lyme arthritis is often intermittent, with episodes lasting a few weeks to months. Recurrent episodes are notable for smaller effusions and progressive synovial hypertrophy, bony erosion, and cartilage destruction. A small percentage (<10%) of patients with intermittent arthritis settle into a pattern of chronic arthritis, generally affecting only a single joint, often the knee. Inflammation of a single joint that persists for more than 12 months would be an unusual presenting manifestation of Lyme arthritis, as is the prominent involvement of small joints.

The natural history of Lyme arthritis suggests that it is a self-limited disorder. In the late 1970s, before the use of antibiotics for Lyme disease, 21 patients who presented with EM and later developed Lyme arthritis were followed for 1 to 8 years without antimicrobial therapy.[53] Six patients had only a single episode of arthritis, and the remaining 15 had recurrent episodes that decreased in frequency over the study period. On average, the number of patients who continued to experience episodes of arthritis decreased by 10% to 20% each year. Similar results were found in children in whom antibiotic treatment for arthritis was delayed 4 years.[55]

ANTIBIOTIC-REFRACTORY LYME ARTHRITIS

A few patients treated with standard antibiotic regimens for Lyme arthritis have persistent joint inflammation and proliferative synovitis that does not respond to further antimicrobial therapy.[15,56] The pathogenesis of "antibiotic-refractory" Lyme arthritis is unknown, but may be due to persistent spirochetes or their antigens, infection-induced autoimmunity, or inadequate regulation of the inflammatory response.[15] Patients with antibiotic-refractory Lyme arthritis no longer have PCR evidence for spirochete DNA in tissues[56] and have an increased frequency of the rheumatoid arthritis–related alleles HLA DRB1*0401, HLA DRB1*0101, and HLA DRB1*0404, suggesting a genetic predisposition to joint inflammation.[57] Because of the high prevalence of B cell and T cell responses to *B. burgdorferi* Osp A in patients with antibiotic-refractory arthritis, it has been proposed that immune responses to Osp A triggered by infection may be perpetuated by a self-antigen after the pathogen has been eliminated.[15] An Osp A peptide corresponding to amino acids 163 through 175 (Osp A$_{163-175}$) was found to share an epitope with human leukocyte function–associated antigen 1α, an adhesion molecule expressed on inflamed tissues.[58] The leukocyte function–associated antigen 1α peptide stimulated Osp A$_{163-175}$-specific T cells only weakly, however, and did not promote production of the T helper type 1 cytokine interferon-γ normally found in antibiotic-refractory arthritis.[59] Antibodies to cytokeratin 10, a constituent of synovial capillaries, have been found in the blood and synovial tissue of patients with antibiotic-refractory Lyme arthritis.[60] These antibodies also react with Osp A and may contribute to ongoing inflammation when infection is cleared. If autoimmunity is responsible for antibiotic-refractory Lyme arthritis, it must eventually succumb to immune regulation because even this form of Lyme arthritis generally resolves within 4 to 5 years.[53,56]

DIAGNOSIS

The diagnosis of Lyme disease should be considered in individuals who present with an appropriate clinical history, and who have a reasonable risk of exposure to *B. burgdorferi*–infected ticks (Fig. 100-2).[20] Supporting serologic evidence is necessary to secure the diagnosis for all stages of infection except for early localized disease in which EM can be recognized by morphologic features alone. Routine laboratory tests are nonspecific, with some patients exhibiting mildly elevated white blood cell (neutrophil) counts, erythrocyte sedimentation rates, and liver function tests. Culture or microscopic visualization of spirochetes in clinical samples is not sensitive enough for routine use in diagnosis. Culture of a skin biopsy specimen taken from the leading margin of an EM lesion is an exception, with *B. burgdorferi* detected in more than 40% of samples, but is rarely necessary to identify EM.

SEROLOGIC TESTING

Detection of antibodies to *B. burgdorferi* is the mainstay of laboratory testing for Lyme disease.[20] Presence of antibodies to *B. burgdorferi* at best indicates previous exposure to the organism, however, and should not be considered evidence of active infection. In nonendemic areas, about 5% of normal human serum samples yield positive results on serologic tests for Lyme disease. In endemic areas, asymptomatic IgG seroconversion to *B. burgdorferi* has been found in about 7% of subjects.[61]

A two-tiered approach is recommended for detection of *B. burgdorferi*–specific antibodies.[62] An ELISA or an indirect immunofluorescence assay to detect IgM and IgG reactivity to *B. burgdorferi* should be used as an initial screening test, followed by an immunoblot (Western blot) to confirm that positive or equivocal results are due to antibodies that bind *B. burgdorferi* antigens. ELISA and immunofluorescence assay are highly sensitive tests, but lack specificity because of cross-reactivity of *B. burgdorferi* antigens with other bacterial pathogens.[20] A positive or equivocal ELISA or immunofluorescence assay should be confirmed by immunoblot analysis of *B. burgdorferi* proteins (Table 100-2). Banding patterns characteristic of early infection include antibodies to the 41-kD flagellin protein and Osp C, which has a molecular weight ranging from 21 to 24 kD depending on the *B. burgdorferi* strain used

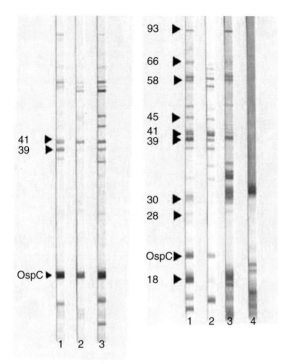

Figure 100-2 *Left,* Selected IgM immunoblot reactivities. *Lane 1,* Serum band locator control showing several bands, including the significant 41-kD protein, 39-kD protein, and OspC *(arrows). Lane 2,* Serum sample from a patient with early Lyme borreliosis with erythema migrans. *Lane 3,* Serum sample from a patient with early disseminated Lyme borreliosis with multiple erythema migrans lesions. Note the larger number of bands observed in a serum sample of the patient with early disseminated Lyme borreliosis. *Right,* Selected IgG immunoblot reactivities. *Lane 1,* Serum band locator control showing several immunoreactive bands, including those considered significant in the IgG blot criteria *(arrows). Lane 2,* Serum sample from a patient with early disseminated Lyme borreliosis with neurologic involvement. *Lane 3,* Serum sample from a patient with Lyme arthritis. *Lane 4,* Serum sample from an individual who received three doses of OspA vaccine; note the strong reactivity with OspA (31 kD) and other antigens below OspC. *(From Aguero-Rosenfeld ME, Wang G, Schwartz I, et al: Diagnosis of Lyme borreliosis. Clin Microbiol Rev 18:484, 2005.)*

(Fig. 100-3). With disseminated infection and especially with late Lyme disease, IgG reactivity to an expanding array of *B. burgdorferi* proteins can be seen (see Fig. 100-3).

Some commercial laboratories have developed assays using recombinant antigens or employ criteria for the interpretation of immunoblots that have not been validated and published in peer-reviewed literature.[63] For this reason, the Centers for Disease Control and Prevention advises using only validated tests approved by the Food and Drug Administration (FDA) for serologic diagnosis of Lyme disease. Two-tier testing for IgM and IgG should be performed for individuals with suspected Lyme disease and signs and symptoms of less than 1 month's duration, whereas only IgG results should be considered for illnesses of longer duration.[62] Positive IgM serologies alone after 1 month of illness are most often false-positive tests, which arise in the setting of other infectious diseases (especially infectious mononucleosis and other spirochetal and tick-borne infections), rheumatoid arthritis (with or without rheumatoid factor), and conditions associated with a positive ANA (systemic lupus erythematosus).[64] No further testing is recommended if ELISA or immunofluorescence assay results are negative. Two-tier testing has overall sensitivities of 29% to 40% in

Table 100-2 Criteria for Western Blot Interpretation in the Serologic Confirmation of Lyme Disease

Duration of Disease	Isotype Tested	Criteria for Positive Test
First month of infection	IgM	Two of the following 3 bands are present: 23 kDa (OspC), 39 kDa (BmpA), and 41 kDa (Fla)
After first month of infection	IgG	Five out of 10 bands are present: 18 kDA, 21 kDa, 28 kDa, 39 kDa, 41 kDa, 45 kDa, 58 kDa (not GroEL), 66 kDa, and 93 kDa

Adapted from Centers for Disease Control and Prevention: Recommendations for Test Performance and Interpretation from the Second National Conference on Serologic Diagnosis of Lyme Disease. Morb Mort Wkly Rept MMWR 44:590-591, 1995.

EM during the acute phase; 29% to 78% for EM in the convalescent phase; and greater than 95% in neurologic, arthritis, and other manifestations of late disease.[20]

A new peptide-based immunoassay that uses a highly conserved invariant region of the VlsE protein, termed C6 (IR6), is now commercially available.[65,66] Although the C6 peptide ELISA measures only IgG reactivity, it has a high degree of sensitivity and specificity in all stages of Lyme disease and may be particularly useful in early Lyme disease.[66]

After antibiotic therapy, IgM and IgG titers to *B. burgdorferi* measured by either whole cell ELISA or the C6 peptide ELISA (IgG only) generally decrease slowly, but can remain positive for years.[67,68] Repeat serologic testing is not recommended as a means for assessing response to treatment.

DETECTION OF ANTIBODIES TO *BORRELIA BURGDORFERI* IN CEREBROSPINAL FLUID

In suspected cases of neuroborreliosis, intrathecal antibody production usually is assessed by measuring the ratio of IgG to *B. burgdorferi* in CSF and serum.[20,69] Intrathecal antibody production is more commonly found in European neuroborreliosis than in North American Lyme disease, which may be due to the higher prevalence of *B. garinii* in central nervous system infection than *B. burgdorferi ss.* Antibodies to *B. burgdorferi* may persist in CSF after treatment for Lyme disease and should not be used to assess efficacy of therapy.

POLYMERASE CHAIN REACTION

PCR has been used to detect *B. burgdorferi* DNA in a variety of clinical specimens with variable success.[70] The greatest utility of PCR clinically is in Lyme arthritis, in which the sensitivity of PCR for detection of *B. burgdorferi* DNA is 85%. In contrast, the sensitivity of PCR for detecting *B. burgdorferi* DNA in CSF is low (<40%) and most often positive in patients with a CSF pleocytosis. PCR of urine specimens is not recommended because of inconsistent sensitivity and documented nonspecific amplification of non–*B. burgdorferi* DNA targets.[20] Although certain commercial laboratories currently offer PCR tests for *B. burgdorferi* DNA in blood or urine specimens, these have not been validated.[63] There are no FDA-approved tests for PCR-based molecular techniques for detecting *B. burgdorferi* DNA in patient specimens.

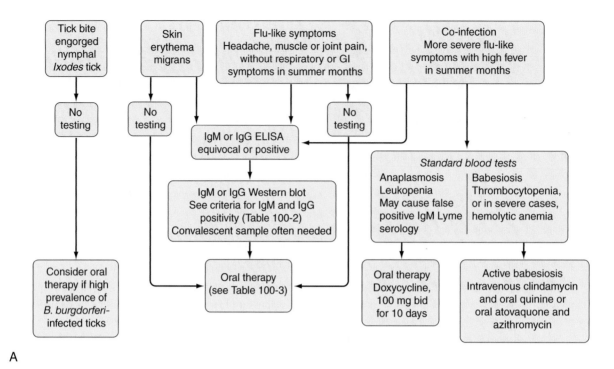

A

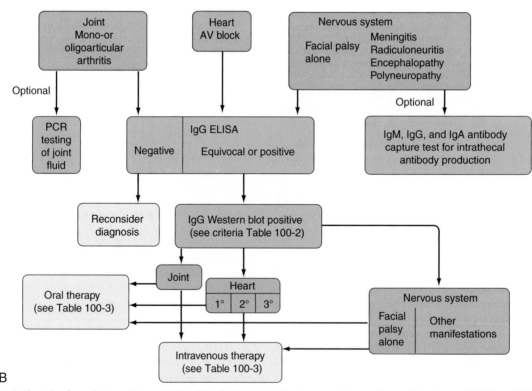

B

Figure 100-3 **A,** Algorithm for early Lyme disease. **B,** Algorithm for later organ involvement in Lyme disease. *(From Steere AC, Coburn J, Glickstein L: The emergence of Lyme disease. J Clin Invest 113:1093-1101, 2004.)*

OTHER TESTS FOR LYME DISEASE

A urine antigen test, immunofluorescent staining for cell wall–deficient forms of *B. burgdorferi*, and lymphocyte transformation assays are offered by some commercial laboratories to aid in the diagnosis of Lyme disease. These tests have not been adequately validated for accuracy or clinical usefulness, and the Centers for Disease Control and Prevention cautions against their use.[63]

DIAGNOSTIC IMAGING

Imaging studies have a limited role in the evaluation of patients with Lyme disease because no feature is sufficiently distinctive to confirm the diagnosis. Plain radiographs of arthritic joints show changes consistent with an inflammatory arthropathy, including joint effusions, synovial hypertrophy, periarticular osteoporosis, cartilage loss, bony erosions, and calcified entheses.[71] MRI of arthritic joints can confirm the radiographic findings and reveal associated myositis and adenopathy, which may be useful in distinguishing Lyme arthritis from septic arthritis in children.[72]

Cranial and spinal MRI findings in neuroborreliosis can reveal focal nodular lesions or patchy white matter lesions on T2-weighted images, consistent with inflammatory or demyelinating processes.[73,74] These lesions typically resolve after treatment for Lyme disease,[74] in some cases only after several years.[75] In patients with post–Lyme disease syndrome, cerebral MRI and the more sensitive technique of fluid-attenuated inversion recovery are normal in about 50% of cases or show nonspecific findings of small white matter lesions.[76] Positron emission tomography and single-photon emission computed tomography studies are often normal or show only nonspecific changes with subcortical and cortical hypoperfusion.[77,78]

TREATMENT AND PROGNOSIS

Updated guidelines for the clinical assessment and treatment of Lyme disease have been published (Table 100-3).[79] Because many of the manifestations of Lyme disease resolve without specific therapy, the goal of antibiotic treatment is to hasten resolution of signs and symptoms and to prevent later clinical manifestations. Generally, oral antibiotics are sufficient therapy for EM, disseminated EM, uncomplicated facial palsy, mild carditis (first-degree atrioventricular block), and arthritis. Disseminated infection and late manifestations of Lyme disease may require longer courses of antibiotics, and there is often a greater lag time to symptom resolution compared with early disease. Doxycycline is the antibiotic of choice in nonpregnant adults and children 8 years old and older because it is also effective against *A. phagocytophilum*, which may occur with early Lyme disease.[79] Amoxicillin and cefuroxime axetil are acceptable alternatives for the treatment of EM, facial palsy, and other non-neurologic manifestations of Lyme disease. Macrolide antibiotics are less effective than other antimicrobials and should be used only in individuals who cannot take doxycycline, amoxicillin, or cefuroxime axetil. First-generation cephalosporins are not effective therapy for Lyme disease.

Documented nervous system involvement (other than isolated facial palsy) and symptomatic cardiac involvement are the two main indications for intravenous antibiotic therapy.[79] Ceftriaxone administered intravenously for 2 to 4 weeks is the preferred antimicrobial, with parenteral cefotaxime or penicillin G acceptable alternatives. There is increasing evidence, however, that oral doxycycline, which is well absorbed and has a high central nervous system penetration, may be effective for meningitis or radiculopathy. Lumbar puncture is recommended in individuals with cranial nerve palsies who have symptoms of meningeal irritation because a CSF pleocytosis would be an indication to treat with intravenous therapy. Asymptomatic CSF pleocytosis can occur in the setting of facial palsy and is not an indication for intravenous therapy. Repeat treatment is not recommended for chronic neurologic abnormalities, unless objective signs of relapse are present.

Patients with symptomatic cardiac involvement (chest pain, shortness of breath, syncope) or with significant conduction system disease (first-degree atrioventricular block with P-R intervals ≥0.3 msec, or second-degree or third-degree block) should be hospitalized for cardiac monitoring and intravenous antibiotic therapy. Consultation with a cardiologist is recommended and placement of a temporary pacemaker may be necessary. Oral antibiotics can be substituted for intravenous antibiotics at the time of hospital discharge to complete the course of therapy.[79]

For arthritis, a 1-month course of oral doxycycline or amoxicillin is recommended, with a repeat course of oral therapy if inflammation does not resolve within 3 months of treatment.[79] For patients with moderate-to-severe joint swelling after a 1-month course of oral antibiotics, intravenous ceftriaxone for 2 to 4 weeks can be used[80]; when inflammation is mild, an additional 1-month course of oral antibiotics can be considered, although arthritis usually resolves without additional therapy. Longer courses of antibiotics provide no additional benefit when PCR for *B. burgdorferi* in joint fluid is negative.[56] In this situation, nonsteroidal anti-inflammatory drugs and hydroxychloroquine are recommended for treatment of antibiotic-refractory Lyme arthritis. In rare patients who fail to respond to these disease-modifying antirheumatic drugs, methotrexate, and tumor necrosis factor-α inhibitors have been anecdotally used with success. Arthroscopic synovectomy is curative in most patients who fail to respond to medical management.[81] Intra-articular corticosteroids may be associated with a higher rate of antibiotic unresponsiveness and are rarely used.[56]

PREGNANCY AND LYME DISEASE

Pregnant and lactating women with Lyme disease can be treated with the same antibiotic regimens recommended for nonpregnant patients except that doxycycline should be avoided.[79] Maternal-fetal transmission of *B. burgdorferi* does occur,[82] but in contrast to syphilis in pregnancy, there is no evidence that the organism causes a congenital syndrome.[83,84] Pregnant patients should be reassured that with recommended therapy for Lyme disease, *B. burgdorferi* infection in the mother should not cause harm to the fetus.[84]

EXPECTED OUTCOMES

Most patients treated for Lyme disease with recommended courses of antibiotics experience resolution of all signs and symptoms of the disorder.[43,85,86] About 15% of patients treated for Lyme disease may experience a Jarisch-Herxheimer reaction, a self-limited worsening of symptoms within 24 to 48 hours of initiation of antibiotic therapy.[14] Within the first week of treatment, patients may rarely show evolution of disease, such as the development of new EM lesions or facial nerve palsy, but these signs should improve as therapy progresses. Most patients with Lyme arthritis experience resolution of joint inflammation after a 1-month

Table 100-3 Recommended Treatment of Lyme Disease[a]

Manifestation	Drug	Adult Dosage	Pediatric Dosage	Duration (days) (Range)
Erythema migrans (Recommended)	Doxycycline[b]	100 mg PO bid	<8 years: not recommended ≥8 years: 4 mg/kg/day in 2 divided doses (max 100 mg/dose)	14 days (10-21)
	Amoxicillin	500 mg PO tid	50 mg/kg/day in 3 divided doses	14 days (10-21)
	Cefuroxime axetil	500 mg PO bid	30 mg/kg/day in 2 divided doses	14 days (10-21)
Erythema migrans (Alternative)[c]	Azithromycin	500 mg PO qd	10 mg/kg qd (max 500 mg/day)	7-10 days
	Clarithromycin	500 mg PO bid	7.5 mg/kg bid	14-21 days
	Erythromycin	500 mg PO qid	12.5 mg/kg qid (max 500 mg/dose)	14-21 days
Acute neurologic disease Cranial nerve palsy[d] Meningitis or radiculopathy[e] (Alternative IV)	Same as oral regimens for erythema migrans Ceftriaxone	2 g IV qd	50-75 mg/kg IV qd in single dose (max 2 g/day)	14 days (10-21) 14 days (10-28)
	Cefotaxime	2 g IV q8h	150-200 mg/kg/day IV in 3-4 divided doses (max 6 g/day)	
	Penicillin G	18-24 million units	200,000-400,000 U/kg/day divided q4h (max 18-24 million U/day)	
Cardiac disease[f]	Same as for erythema migrans *or* IV regimen as for neurologic disease			14 days (10-21) 14 days (10-21)
Late disease Arthritis without neurologic involvement	Same as for erythema migrans			28 days (28)
Recurrent arthritis after oral regimen	Repeat oral regimen *or* IV regimen as for neurologic disease			14 days (14-28)
Central or peripheral nervous system disease	IV regimen as for acute neurologic disease			14 days (14-28)

[a]Complete response to treatment may be delayed beyond the treatment period, regardless of the clinical manifestation, and relapse may recur. Patients with objective signs of relapse may need a second course of treatment.

[b]Tetracyclines are relatively contraindicated in pregnant or lactating women and in children < 8 years of age.

[c]Due to their lower efficacy, macrolides are reserved for patients who are unable to take or who are intolerant of tetracyclines, penicillins, and cephalosporins.

[d]Patients without clinical evidence of meningitis may be treated with an oral regimen. The recommendation is based on experience with seventh cranial nerve palsy. Whether oral therapy would be as effective for patients with other cranial neuropathies is unknown; the decision between oral and parenteral therapy should be individualized.

[e]For nonpregnant adult patients intolerant of β-lactam agents, doxycycline 200-400 mg/day orally (or IV if unable to take oral medications) in two divided doses may be adequate. For children ≥ 8 years of age, the dosage of doxycycline for this indication is 4-8 mg/kg/day in two divided doses (maximum daily dosage of 200-400 mg).

[f]A parenteral antibiotic regimen is recommended at the start of therapy for patients who have been hospitalized for cardiac monitoring; an oral regimen may be substituted to complete a course of therapy or to treat outpatients. A temporary pacemaker may be required for patients with advanced heart block.

course of oral antibiotics, and less than 10% of patients progress to antibiotic-refractory arthritis, which nevertheless resolves within 4 years.[56]

Subjective complaints of fatigue and musculoskeletal pain may persist for months after treatment for Lyme disease.[87] When patients complain of persistent pain and fatigue, evaluation for coinfection with *B. microti* or *A. phagocytophilum* should be performed.[88] Patients with coinfection tend to be more symptomatic at presentation and can have a delayed resolution of symptoms compared with patients with Lyme disease alone. Objective, nonprogressive signs, such as mild facial weakness after facial palsy, likely are due to irreversible tissue damage, and further antibiotic therapy does not seem to be beneficial.[89,90]

POST–LYME DISEASE SYNDROMES

There is a great deal of controversy over the potential for Lyme disease to cause life-altering chronic morbidity in patients. As noted earlier, it is unusual to have objective signs after recommended antibiotic regimens, and when such signs (e.g., Lyme arthritis) are present, further antibiotic therapy does not alter outcome.[56] Even when objective signs are present, they usually are nonprogressive (e.g., residual facial weakness after facial palsy) or resolve over time (as is the case for Lyme arthritis). The term *chronic Lyme disease*, which implies ongoing infection, is invalid.

A few patients treated for Lyme disease may have fatigue, musculoskeletal pain, and complaints of memory impairment despite conventional or prolonged courses of antibiotic therapy.[89,91] In several controlled, population-based cohort studies that used validated standardized measures of outcomes (e.g., SF-36), patients with Lyme disease had more joint pain, symptoms of memory impairment, and worse functional status because of pain compared with controls.[86,92,93] These complaints could not be documented by abnormalities on physical examination or by neurocognitive testing, however, and a follow-up study showed that quality-of-life measures improved with time.[94] Children are less likely than adults to have persistent complaints after treatment for Lyme disease.[93]

Two randomized, double-blind, placebo-controlled trials of antibiotic therapy were conducted on seropositive and seronegative patients with chronic symptoms (>6 months) after treatment for Lyme disease.[90] Patients were randomly assigned to receive either intravenous ceftriaxone for 1 month followed by 2 months of oral doxycycline or matched intravenous and oral placebos. An interim analysis of the first 129 subjects enrolled (78 seropositive, 51 seronegative) resulted in termination of the study because no differences in outcome between groups receiving antibiotics or placebo were found, and evidence of ongoing infection could not be documented. Another trial of antibiotics for post-treatment Lyme disease symptoms found that fatigue, as assessed by the Fatigue Severity Scale–11, improved in the group receiving intravenous ceftriaxone, but cognitive dysfunction did not.[95] Individuals who had positive IgG immunoblots for Lyme disease and who had not received prior treatment with intravenous antibiotics were more likely to have improvement in fatigue. An open pilot study provided evidence that gabapentin may be effective in the treatment of chronic pain syndromes after Lyme disease.[96]

A growing number of patients with similar subjective complaints are being treated for months or years with antibiotics for presumed *B. burgdorferi* infection.[97-100] Often these patients have no serologic evidence of *B. burgdorferi* exposure despite years of not feeling well, and they experience only partial resolution of their symptoms owing to antibiotics. Occasionally, patients may have other conditions, such as rheumatoid arthritis or fibromyalgia, for which therapy has been delayed because of a misdiagnosis of Lyme disease.[97] Musculoskeletal pain is common in the general population; 20% to 30% of adults complain of chronic fatigue.[101] In the absence of a clinical history with objective manifestations of Lyme disease or positive two-tiered serologic tests, definitive attribution of symptoms to *B. burgdorferi* infection cannot be made. Caution should be exercised when attributing the response of symptoms to the antimicrobial effects of antibiotics because ceftriaxone and other β-lactam antibiotics can modulate neurotransmitter activity,[102] and tetracyclines inhibit matrix metalloproteinases.[103] Prolonged antibiotic use is not without risk. Minor side effects are common, and serious adverse events, such as biliary complications from ceftriaxone therapy or indwelling catheter–related infections, occur at high enough rates to warrant only judicious use of antibiotics.[90,99]

PREVENTION

The most effective way to prevent Lyme disease is to reduce exposure risk to *B. burgdorferi*–infected ticks through personal protective measures and environmental controls.[104]

These measures include avoidance of tick habitats such as wooded areas, stone fences, woodpiles, and tall grass; wearing protective clothing; and performing daily surveillance and prompt removal of ticks (within 24 hours of feeding). Other effective measures include use of DEET-containing insecticide sprays, yearly application of acaricides to property to kill ticks, construction of four-poster bait stations that apply acaricides onto deer as they feed, and tall fences to prevent deer from incidentally transporting ticks to an area.

A single 200-mg dose of doxycycline (or 4 mg/kg up to 200 mg for children ≥8 years old) has been shown to reduce the incidence of Lyme disease after a recognized tick bite,[105] but is not routinely recommended because of the low rate of infection.[79] An FDA-approved recombinant Osp A–based vaccine to prevent Lyme disease was withdrawn because of low market demand and concern for potential vaccine-related side effects.[106,107]

SUMMARY

Lyme disease is a localized or systemic infection that usually manifests with skin and musculoskeletal signs and symptoms, but it can involve other organ systems, especially the heart and nervous system. The diagnosis should be based on objective clinical findings consistent with Lyme disease and supporting serologic tests. Most patients are cured with 2 to 4 weeks of antibiotic therapy, although the time to disease resolution may be prolonged, especially for individuals in whom therapy was delayed; irreversible tissue damage may occur. A poor response to antibiotic therapy should raise concern for alternative diagnoses or coinfection with other tick-borne pathogens. Antibiotic-refractory Lyme arthritis occurs in less than 10% of patients. Treatment with nonsteroidal anti-inflammatory drugs and hydroxychloroquine usually resolves arthritis within 4 to 5 years. Some patients treated for Lyme disease develop a post–Lyme disease syndrome of fatigue, headaches, mild memory impairment, and musculoskeletal pain. Ongoing infection cannot be shown and controlled treatment trials show no benefit of prolonged antibiotic therapy over placebo. Referral to an academic medical center with experience in the diagnosis and treatment of Lyme disease should be considered when patients do not respond as expected to therapy.

REFERENCES

1. Bockenstedt LK, Malawista SE: Lyme disease. In Cecil RL, Goldman L, Bennett JC (eds): The Cecil Textbook of Medicine, 23rd ed. Philadelphia, WB Saunders, 2008, pp 2289-2294.
2. **Steere AC, Malawista SE, Snydman DR, et al: Lyme arthritis: An epidemic of oligoarticular arthritis in children and adults in three Connecticut communities. Arthritis Rheum 20:7-17, 1977.**
3. Weber K, Pfister HW: History of Lyme borreliosis in Europe. In Weber K, Burgdorfer W (eds): Aspects of Lyme borreliosis. Berlin, Springer-Verlag, 1993, pp 1-20.
4. Burgdorfer W, Barbour AG, Hayes SF, et al: Lyme disease—a tick-borne spirochetosis? Science 216:1317-1319, 1982.
5. **Steere AC, Grodzicki RL, Kornblatt AN, et al: The spirochetal etiology of Lyme disease. N Engl J Med 308:733-740, 1983.**
6. Piesman J, Gern L: Lyme borreliosis in Europe and North America. Parasitology 129(Suppl):S191-S220, 2004.
7. Centers for Disease Control and Prevention: Reported Lyme disease cases by state, 1993-2005. Available at: http://www.cdc.gov/ncidod/dvbid/lyme/Id_rptdLymeCasesbyState.htm. Accessed 2006.

8. Steere AC, Coburn J, Glickstein L: The emergence of Lyme disease. J Clin Invest 113:1093-1101, 2004.

9. De Silva AM, Fikrig E: *Borrelia burgdorferi* genes selectively expressed in ticks and mammals. Parasitol Today 13:267-270, 1997.

10. Fraser CM, Casjens S, Huang WM, et al: Genomic sequence of a Lyme disease spirochaete, *Borrelia burgdorferi*. Nature 390:580-586, 1997.

11. Pal U, de Silva AM, Montgomery RR, et al: Attachment of *Borrelia burgdorferi* within *Ixodes scapularis* mediated by outer surface protein A. J Clin Invest 106:561-569, 2000.

12. Tilly K, Krum JG, Bestor A, et al: *Borrelia burgdorferi* OspC protein required exclusively in a crucial early stage of mammalian infection. Infect Immun 74:3554-3564, 2006.

13. Duray PH: Histopathology of clinical phases of human Lyme disease. Rheum Dis Clin N Am 15:691-710, 1989.

14. Bockenstedt LK: Lyme disease. In Stone JH, Crofford LJ, White PH (eds): Primer on the Rheumatic Diseases, 13th ed. Springer Science+Business Media, 2008, pp 282-289.

15. Steere AC, Glickstein L: Elucidation of Lyme arthritis. Nat Rev Immunol 4:143-152, 2004.

16. Behera AK, Hildebrand E, Uematsu S, et al: Identification of a TLR-independent pathway for *Borrelia burgdorferi*-induced expression of matrix metalloproteinases and inflammatory mediators through binding to integrin alpha 3 beta 1. J Immunol 177:657-664, 2006.

17. Fikrig E, Barthold SW, Chen M, et al: Protective antibodies in murine Lyme disease arise independently of CD40 ligand. J Immunol 157:1-3, 1996.

18. McKisic MD, Barthold SW: T-cell-independent responses to *Borrelia burgdorferi* are critical for protective immunity and resolution of Lyme disease. Infect Immun 68:5190-5197, 2000.

19. Hardin JA, Steere AC, Malawista SE: Immune complexes and the evolution of Lyme arthritis: Dissemination and localization of abnormal C1q binding activity. N Engl J Med 301:1358-1363, 1979.

20. Aguero-Rosenfeld ME, Wang G, Schwartz I, et al: Diagnosis of Lyme borreliosis. Clin Microbiol Rev 18:484-509, 2005.

21. Dai Z, Lackland H, Stein S, et al: Molecular mimicry in Lyme disease: Monoclonal antibody H9724 to *B. burgdorferi* flagellin specifically detects chaperonin-HSP60. Biochim Biophys Acta 1181:97-100, 1993.

22. Aberer E, Brunner C, Suchanek G, et al: Molecular mimicry and Lyme borreliosis: A shared antigenic determinant between *Borrelia burgdorferi* and human tissue. Ann Neurol 26:732-737, 1989.

23. Gross DM, Steere AC, Huber BT: T helper 1 response is dominant and localized to the synovial fluid in patients with Lyme arthritis. J Immunol 160:1022-1028, 1998.

24. Widhe M, Jarefors S, Ekerfelt C, et al: *Borrelia*-specific interferon-gamma and interleukin-4 secretion in cerebrospinal fluid and blood during Lyme borreliosis in humans: Association with clinical outcome. J Infect Dis 189:1881-1891, 2004.

25. Kalish RA, Leong JM, Steere AC: Association of treatment-resistant chronic Lyme arthritis with HLA-DR4 and antibody reactivity to OspA and OspB of *Borrelia burgdorferi*. Infect Immun 61:2774-2779, 1993.

26. Lengl-Janssen B, Strauss AF, Steere AC, et al: The T helper cell response in Lyme arthritis: Differential recognition of *Borrelia burgdorferi* outer surface protein A in patients with treatment-resistant or treatment-responsive Lyme arthritis. J Exp Med 180:2069-2078, 1994.

27. Iliopoulou BP, Alroy J, Huber BT: CD28 deficiency exacerbated joint inflammation upon *Borrelia burgdorferi* infection, resulting in the development of chronic Lyme arthritis. J Immunol 179:8076-8082, 2007.

28. Vincent MS, Roessner K, Lynch D, et al: Apoptosis of Fas(high) CD4+ synovial T cells by borrelia-reactive Fas-ligand(high) gamma delta T cells in Lyme arthritis. J Exp Med 184:2109-2117, 1996.

29. Chary-Valckenaere I, Jaulhac B, Champigneulle J, et al: Ultrastructural demonstration of intracellular localization of *Borrelia burgdorferi* in Lyme arthritis. Br J Rheumatol 37:468-470, 1998.

30. Norris SJ: Antigenic variation with a twist—the *Borrelia* story. Mol Microbiol 60:1319-1322, 2006.

31. Liang FT, Nelson FK, Fikrig E: Molecular adaptation of *Borrelia burgdorferi* in the murine host. J Exp Med 196:275-280, 2002.

32. Barthold SW, de Souza MS, Janotka JL, et al: Chronic Lyme borreliosis in the laboratory mouse. Am J Pathol 143:959-971, 1993.

33. Edlow JA: Erythema migrans. Med Clin North Am 86:239-260, 2002.

34. Centers for Disease Control and Prevention: Case definitions for infectious conditions under public health surveillance: Lyme disease (revised 9/96). MMWR Morb Mortal Wkly Rep 46:1-51, 1997.

35. Feder HM Jr, Gerber MA, Krause PJ, et al: Early Lyme disease: A flu-like illness without erythema migrans. Pediatrics 91:456-459, 1993.

36. Steere AC, Dhar A, Hernandez J, et al: Systemic symptoms without erythema migrans as the presenting picture of early Lyme disease. Am J Med 114:58-62, 2003.

37. Centers for Disease Control and Prevention: Southern tick-associated rash illness. Available at: http://www.cdc.gov/ncidod/dvbid/stari/

38. Steere AC, Batsford WP, Weinberg M, et al: Lyme carditis: Cardiac abnormalities of Lyme disease. Ann Intern Med 93:8-16, 1980.

39. Sangha O, Phillips CB, Fleischmann KE, et al: Lack of cardiac manifestations among patients with previously treated Lyme disease. Ann Intern Med 128:346-353, 1998.

40. Reik L, Steere AC, Bartenhagen NH, et al: Neurologic abnormalities of Lyme disease. Medicine (Balt) 58:281-294, 1979.

41. **Halperin JJ, Pass HL, Anand AK, et al: Nervous system abnormalities in Lyme disease. Ann N Y Acad Sci 539:24-34, 1988.**

42. Halperin JJ: Lyme disease and the peripheral nervous system. Muscle Nerve 28:133-143, 2003.

43. Nachman SA, Pontrelli L: Central nervous system Lyme disease. Semin Pediatr Infect Dis 14:123-130, 2003.

44. Eppes SC, Nelson DK, Lewis LL, et al: Characterization of Lyme meningitis and comparison with viral meningitis in children. Pediatrics 103:957-960, 1999.

45. Steere AC: Lyme disease. N Engl J Med 321:586-596, 1989.

46. Logigian EL, Kaplan RF, Steere AC: Chronic neurologic manifestations of Lyme disease. N Engl J Med 323:1438-1444, 1990.

47. Halperin JJ: Central nervous system Lyme disease. Curr Neurol Neurosci Rep 5:446-452, 2005.

48. Coyle PK, Krupp LB, Doscher C: Significance of reactive Lyme serology in multiple sclerosis. Ann Neurol 34:745-747, 1993.

49. Halperin JJ, Little BW, Coyle PK, et al: Lyme disease: Cause of a treatable peripheral neuropathy. Neurology 37:1700-1706, 1987.

50. Halperin JJ, Krupp LB, Golightly MG, et al: Lyme borreliosis-associated encephalopathy. Neurology 40:1340-1343, 1990.

51. Logigian EL, Kaplan RF, Steere AC: Successful treatment of Lyme encephalopathy with intravenous ceftriaxone. J Infect Dis 180:377-383, 1999.

52. Asbrink E, Hovmark A, Olsson I: Clinical manifestations of acrodermatitis chronica atrophicans in 50 Swedish patients. Zentralbl Bakteriol Mikrobiol Hyg [A] 263:253-261, 1986.

53. **Steere AC, Schoen RT, Taylor E: The clinical evolution of Lyme arthritis. Ann Intern Med 107:725-731, 1987.**

54. Steere AC, Malawista SE, Hardin JA, et al: Erythema chronicum migrans and Lyme arthritis: The enlarging clinical spectrum. Ann Intern Med 86:685-698, 1977.

55. Szer IS, Taylor E, Steere AC: The long-term course of Lyme arthritis in children. N Engl J Med 325:159-163, 1991.

56. **Steere AC, Angelis SM: Therapy for Lyme arthritis: Strategies for the treatment of antibiotic-refractory arthritis. Arthritis Rheum 54: 3079-3086, 2006.**

57. Steere AC, Klitz W, Drouin EE, et al: Antibiotic-refractory Lyme arthritis is associated with HLA-DR molecules that bind a *Borrelia burgdorferi* peptide. J Exp Med 203:961-971, 2006.

58. Gross DM, Forsthuber T, Tary-Lehmann M, et al: Identification of LFA-1 as a candidate autoantigen in treatment-resistant Lyme arthritis. Science 281:703-706, 1998.

59. Trollmo C, Meyer AL, Steere AC, et al: Molecular mimicry in Lyme arthritis demonstrated at the single cell level: LFA-1 alpha L is a partial agonist for outer surface protein A-reactive T cells. J Immunol 166:5286-5291, 2001.

60. Ghosh S, Seward R, Costello CE, et al: Autoantibodies from synovial lesions in chronic, antibiotic treatment-resistant Lyme arthritis bind cytokeratin-10. J Immunol 177:2486-2494, 2006.

61. Steere AC, Sikand VK, Schoen RT, et al: Asymptomatic infection with *Borrelia burgdorferi*. Clin Infect Dis 37:528-532, 2003.

62. Centers for Disease Control and Prevention: Recommendations for test performance and interpretation from the Second National Conference on Serologic Diagnosis of Lyme Disease. MMWR Morb Mortal Wkly Rep 44:590-591, 1995.

63. Centers for Disease Control and Prevention: Notice to readers: Caution regarding testing for Lyme disease. MMWR Morb Mortal Wkly Rep 54:125, 2005.

64. Aguero-Rosenfeld ME, Nowakowski J, Bittker S, et al: Evolution of the serologic response to *Borrelia burgdorferi* in treated patients with culture-confirmed erythema migrans. J Clin Microbiol 34:1-9, 1996.

65. Bacon RM, Biggerstaff BJ, Schriefer ME, et al: Serodiagnosis of Lyme disease by kinetic enzyme-linked immunosorbent assay using recombinant VlsE1 or peptide antigens of *Borrelia burgdorferi* compared with 2-tiered testing using whole-cell lysates. J Infect Dis 187:1187-1199, 2003.

66. Liang FT, Steere AC, Marques AR, et al: Sensitive and specific serodiagnosis of Lyme disease by enzyme-linked immunosorbent assay with a peptide based on an immunodominant conserved region of *Borrelia burgdorferi* vlsE. J Clin Microbiol 37:3990-3996, 1999.

67. Kalish RA, McHugh G, Granquist J, et al: Persistence of immunoglobulin M or immunoglobulin G antibody responses to *Borrelia burgdorferi* 10-20 years after active Lyme disease. Clin Infect Dis 33:780-785, 2001.

68. Peltomaa M, McHugh G, Steere AC: Persistence of the antibody response to the VlsE sixth invariant region (IR6) peptide of *Borrelia burgdorferi* after successful antibiotic treatment of Lyme disease. J Infect Dis 187:1178-1186, 2003.

69. Wilske B, Schierz G, Preac-Mursic V, et al: Intrathecal production of specific antibodies against *Borrelia burgdorferi* in patients with lymphocytic meningoradiculitis (Bannwarth's syndrome). J Infect Dis 153:304-314, 1986.

70. Schmidt BL: PCR in laboratory diagnosis of human *Borrelia burgdorferi* infections. Clin Microbiol Rev 10:185-201, 1997.

71. Lawson JP, Steere AC: Lyme arthritis: Radiologic findings. Radiology 154:37-43, 1985.

72. Ecklund K, Vargas S, Zurakowski D, et al: MRI features of Lyme arthritis in children. AJR Am J Roentgenol 184:1904-1909, 2005.

73. Kalina P, Decker A, Kornel E, et al: Lyme disease of the brainstem. Neuroradiology 47:903-907, 2005.

74. Agosta F, Rocca MA, Benedetti B, et al: MR imaging assessment of brain and cervical cord damage in patients with neuroborreliosis. AJNR Am J Neuroradiol 27:892-894, 2006.

75. Steinbach JP, Melms A, Skalej M, et al: Delayed resolution of white matter changes following therapy of B *burgdorferi* encephalitis. Neurology 64:758-759, 2005.

76. Morgen K, Martin R, Stone RD, et al: FLAIR and magnetization transfer imaging of patients with post-treatment Lyme disease syndrome. Neurology 57:1980-1985, 2001.

77. Logigian EL, Johnson KA, Kijewski MF, et al: Reversible cerebral hypoperfusion in Lyme encephalopathy. Neurology 49:1661-1670, 1997.

78. Fallon BA, Keilp J, Prohovnik I, et al: Regional cerebral blood flow and cognitive deficits in chronic Lyme disease. J Neuropsychiatry Clin Neurosci 15:326-332, 2003.

79. **Wormser GP, Dattwyler RJ, Shapiro ED, et al: The clinical assessment, treatment, and prevention of Lyme disease, human granulocytic anaplasmosis, and babesiosis: Clinical practice guidelines by the Infectious Diseases Society of America. Clin Infect Dis 43: 1089-1134, 2006.**

80. Dattwyler RJ, Wormser GP, Rush TJ, et al: A comparison of two treatment regimens of ceftriaxone in late Lyme disease. Wien Klin Wochenschr 117:393-397, 2005.

81. Schoen RT, Aversa JM, Rahn DW, et al: Treatment of refractory chronic Lyme arthritis with arthroscopic synovectomy. Arthritis Rheum 34:1056-1060, 1991.

82. Schlesinger PA, Duray PH, Burke BA, et al: Maternal-fetal transmission of the Lyme disease spirochete, *Borrelia burgdorferi*. Ann Intern Med 103:67-68, 1985.

83. **Williams CL, Strobino B, Weinstein A, et al: Maternal Lyme disease and congenital malformations: A cord blood serosurvey in endemic and control areas. Paediatr Perinat Epidemiol 9:320-330, 1995.**

84. Strobino BA, Williams CL, Abid S, et al: Lyme disease and pregnancy outcome: A prospective study of two thousand prenatal patients. Am J Obstet Gynecol 169:367-374, 1993.

85. Shapiro ED: Long-term outcomes of persons with Lyme disease. Vector Borne Zoonotic Dis 2:279-281, 2002.

86. Shadick NA, Phillips CB, Sangha O, et al: Musculoskeletal and neurologic outcomes in patients with previously treated Lyme disease. Ann Intern Med 131:919-926, 1999.

87. Wormser GP, Ramanathan R, Nowakowski J, et al: Duration of antibiotic therapy for early Lyme disease: A randomized, double-blind, placebo-controlled trial. Ann Intern Med 138:697-704, 2003.

88. Krause PJ, McKay K, Thompson CA, et al: Disease-specific diagnosis of coinfecting tickborne zoonoses: Babesiosis, human granulocytic ehrlichiosis, and Lyme disease. Clin Infect Dis 34:1184-1191, 2002.

89. Asch ES, Bujak DI, Weiss M, et al: Lyme disease: An infectious and postinfectious syndrome. J Rheumatol 21:454-461, 1994.

90. **Klempner MS, Hu LT, Evans J, et al: Two controlled trials of antibiotic treatment in patients with persistent symptoms and a history of Lyme disease. N Engl J Med 345:85-92, 2001.**

91. Bujak DI, Weinstein A, Dornbush RL: Clinical and neurocognitive features of the post Lyme syndrome. J Rheumatol 23:1392-1397, 1996.

92. Shadick NA, Phillips CB, Logigian EL, et al: The long-term clinical outcomes of Lyme disease. A population-based retrospective cohort study. Ann Intern Med 121:560-567, 1994.

93. Seltzer EG, Gerber MA, Cartter ML, et al: Long-term outcomes of persons with Lyme disease. JAMA 283:609-616, 2000.

94. Shadick NA, Phillips CB, Sangha O, et al: Diminished health-related quality-of-life improves over time in Lyme disease: The 12 yr followup from the Nantucket Lyme disease cohort study. IX International Conference on Lyme Borreliosis and Other Tick-borne Diseases, New York, 2002, O-36.

95. Krupp LB, Hyman LG, Grimson R, et al: Study and treatment of post Lyme disease (STOP-LD): A randomized double masked clinical trial. Neurology 60:1923-1930, 2003.

96. Weissenbacher S, Ring J, Hofmann H: Gabapentin for the symptomatic treatment of chronic neuropathic pain in patients with late-stage Lyme borreliosis: A pilot study. Dermatology 211:123-127, 2005.

97. Sigal LH: Summary of the first 100 patients seen at a Lyme disease referral center. Am J Med 88:577-581, 1990.

98. Steere AC, Taylor E, McHugh GL, et al: The overdiagnosis of Lyme disease. JAMA 269:1812-1816, 1993.

99. **Reid MC, Schoen RT, Evans J, et al: The consequences of overdiagnosis and overtreatment of Lyme disease: An observational study. Ann Intern Med 128:354-362, 1998.**

100. Qureshi MZ, New D, Zulqarni NJ, et al: Overdiagnosis and overtreatment of Lyme disease in children. Pediatr Infect Dis J 21:12-14, 2002.

101. Wessely S: Chronic fatigue: Symptom and syndrome. Ann Intern Med 134:838-843, 2001.

102. Rothstein JD, Patel S, Regan MR, et al: Beta-lactam antibiotics offer neuroprotection by increasing glutamate transporter expression. Nature 433:73-77, 2005.

103. Sadowski T, Steinmeyer J: Effects of tetracyclines on the production of matrix metalloproteinases and plasminogen activators as well as of their natural inhibitors, tissue inhibitor of metalloproteinase-1 and plasminogen activator inhibitor-1. Inflamm Res 50:175-182, 2001.

104. **Hayes EB, Piesman J: How can we prevent Lyme disease? N Engl J Med 348:2424-2430, 2003.**

105. Nadelman RB, Nowakowski J, Fish D, et al: Prophylaxis with single-dose doxycycline for the prevention of Lyme disease after an *Ixodes scapularis* tick bite. N Engl J Med 345:79-84, 2001.

106. Steere AC, Sikand VK, Meurice F, et al: Vaccination against Lyme disease with recombinant *Borrelia burgdorferi* outer-surface lipoprotein A with adjuvant. Lyme Disease Vaccine Study Group. N Engl J Med 339:209-215, 1998.

107. Hanson MS, Edelman R: Progress and controversy surrounding vaccines against Lyme disease. Expert Rev Vaccines 2:683-703, 2003.

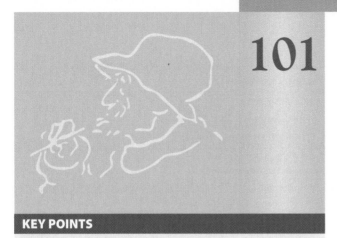

101 Mycobacterial Infections of Bones and Joints

WALTER G. BARR •
J. TIMOTHY HARRINGTON •
JOHN P. FLAHERTY

KEY POINTS

Global rates of tuberculosis disease have been increasing as a result of the expanding HIV pandemic and the growing problem of antituberculous drug resistance; rheumatologists have seen an increase in tuberculosis disease in response to the expanded use of anti-TNF agents.

Musculoskeletal tuberculosis typically presents as a chronic localized infection, most commonly involving the spine, less often the hip or knee.

Diagnosis may be very difficult and requires biopsy for histopathology and culture of the bone or synovium; rapid diagnostic test techniques have not yet proven reliable in bone and joint specimens.

The tuberculin skin test can be helpful in identifying latent tuberculosis prior to treatment with anti-TNF agents, but it is limited by false-positive and false-negative results; the availability of interferon-gamma release assays might improve test specificity.

Treatment requires multiple agents selected on the basis of susceptibility testing for 6 to 9 months and has been complicated by the increasing incidence of drug resistance.

The recognition of tuberculosis (TB) and other mycobacterial infections of the musculoskeletal system has become a major challenge for rheumatologists in the United States and other developed countries. Before 1999, most rheumatologists could easily go an entire year without seeing a single case of mycobacterial infection. Such cases were rare even at academic centers, where they would likely be presented as unusual teaching cases at clinical conferences.

However, 1999 introduced the routine clinical use of anti–tumor necrosis factor (TNF) therapy in the United States, and with it came an unexpected increase in TB cases. These infections have been notably extrapulmonary in their proclivity, with 5% to 7% of TB cases emerging after the initiation of anti-TNF therapy reported to occur in bone, joint, or tendon. Fortunately, routine screening with tuberculin skin test (TSTs) led to a sharp decline in the number of new cases. However, the limitations of TSTs in assessing for latent TB and the expanding indications for anti-TNF therapy mandate continued vigilance in these patients.

Another major force driving the increase in mycobacterial infections is the human immunodefiency virus (HIV) epidemic that continues to be a worldwide problem. By 1991, 21% of extrapulmonary TB cases in the United States were associated with acquired immunodeficiency syndrome (AIDS). In developing countries, the HIV pandemic has led to marked increases in osteoarticular TB coinfection.[1] These cases are distinguished by disseminated multifocal disease suggestive of hematogenous spread, rapid progression, and more common coexistence with pulmonary infection.[2,3] HIV testing should be a routine part of the workup of any patient presenting with a musculoskeletal infection secondary to *Mycobacterium tuberculosis*. The good news is that since the introduction of effective antiretroviral therapy, the incidence of TB and nontuberculous mycobacteria in HIV/AIDS patients has sharply declined in the United States.

Although TB is uncommon among the non–HIV-infected population in the developed world (in the United States, TB is steadily declining among the general population), it remains a major problem in developing countries. There, TB continues to ravage the population, with 9 million new cases of active disease and 1.6 million deaths each year.[4] Worldwide, it is the number two infectious disease killer after HIV/AIDS. Someone in the world is newly infected with TB bacilli every second. About one third of the world's population is infected with TB, providing a reservoir that will continue to complicate its global control.[5] More alarming is the emergence of extremely drug-resistant TB (XDR-TB).[6] These strains fail to respond to all first-line and most second-line TB agents. An outbreak of XDR-TB in South Africa was associated with a mortality rate of 100%, with a median survival of only 16 days after diagnosis. Globalization of the world economy is encouraging increased contact between populations of the developed and developing worlds. Recent immigrants to the United States from endemic areas constitute an expanding reservoir of patients with latent TB.

The challenge of diagnosing musculoskeletal mycobacterial infection reaches beyond the rarity of the disease. Such infections are often indolent and lack the pain, fevers, chills, and other prominent symptoms that typically accompany bacterial infections of the musculoskeletal system. In addition, unless the diagnosis of TB is a consideration from the outset, routine culture techniques will not isolate the organism. Delay in the diagnosis of mycobacterial infections of the musculoskeletal system is often measured in extended periods of 6 to 9 months. Unless we lower our threshold of suspicion for mycobacterial infection, it is unlikely that such delays will be substantially shortened.

For all these reasons, 21st-century rheumatologists need to be well informed about a set of diseases they have had little or no experience with during their formal medical training.

CLINICAL SCENARIOS

To appreciate the entire spectrum of clinical problems a rheumatologist may encounter in dealing with mycobacterial infections, it is useful to think in terms of several distinct categories. Franco-Paredes and colleagues[7] provided a clinically useful division of mycobacterial infections into four major categories. The following sections reflect that division.

DIRECT INVOLVEMENT OF THE MUSCULOSKELETAL SYSTEM

Musculoskeletal infections caused by mycobacteria typically manifest with chronic, indolent, localized involvement of the bones, spine, peripheral joints, or soft tissues that produces a focus of nonspecific pain and, less often, swelling. In infections initiated by direct tissue inoculation, the traumatic event is often trivial or remote in time from the onset of clinical disease. Diagnosis may be delayed for months to years, in part because of minimal early symptoms and attribution of those symptoms to a noninfectious disorder until disease progression and disability prompt a more aggressive diagnostic investigation.

Constitutional symptoms are typically subtle or absent, and laboratory indicators of inflammation are often normal. Synovial effusion is frequently minimal, and the fluid, if it is obtainable, shows nonspecific inflammation. Radiographic abnormalities may be delayed, although newer imaging techniques have allowed the earlier detection of abnormalities and the distinction of TB from other infections and neoplasm.[8,9] Characteristic pulmonary or extrapulmonary findings are not always present; for example, more than 50% of osteoarticular TB manifests without evidence of past or present pulmonary disease. Tuberculin and other skin tests may provide useful clues to the cause, but results are not invariably positive, especially in debilitated or immunosuppressed patients. Correct diagnosis is highly dependent, in most cases, on demonstration of the infectious agent by microscopic examination and culture of affected tissue.

In HIV-infected patients, mycobacterial infections are often diagnosed before the patients' HIV-positive status is known, sometimes leading to its recognition.[10] Atypical pulmonary TB and extrapulmonary (often multifocal) infection are common; extrapulmonary infection occurs in 60% to 70% of such cases, compared with 16% of all TB patients.

The clinical patterns of musculoskeletal TB include spondylitis, osteomyelitis, peripheral joint infection, and soft tissue abscess. In a series of 230 consecutive cases of TB from the preantibiotic era, 5.2% had skeletal involvement; the spine was affected in 60% of cases.[11] The incidence of extrapulmonary and osteoarticular disease has risen during the last decade at a rate exceeding that of lung involvement. TB of the bones and joints is spread hematogenously. The sites most commonly affected are the spine and hips, followed by the knees and wrists; other joint involvement is rare. Constitutional symptoms are unusual in musculoskeletal TB and, when present, suggest TB in other organs. Vertebral collapse due to spinal TB may initially be attributed to the more common osteoporosis-caused spinal compression fracture. TB only rarely involves skeletal muscle but must be considered in the differential diagnosis of an enlarging muscle lesion.[12-16] Isolated cases involving tendons,[17] trochanteric bursa,[18] and fascia lata[19] illustrate the variety of possibilities. Biopsy and culture are required for diagnosis. Imaging studies do not distinguish TB from neoplasm.

Table 101-1 Causes of False-Negative Purified Protein Derivative Test

Old age (>70 yr)
Steroid use (prednisone ≥15 mg/day)
Hypoalbuminemia (<2 g/dL)
Azotemia
Impaired cellular immunity
HIV infection

In nonendemic areas, skeletal TB usually occurs in elderly, debilitated patients, most often in the form of solitary osteolytic lesions in the axial skeleton. The development of skeletal disease is often remote from the initial infection, which strongly implies reactivation of previous subclinical disease. Patients may have false-negative tuberculin tests for several reasons, including long-term corticosteroid use or coexisting debilitating diseases, such as rheumatoid arthritis or chronic renal failure, that compromise resistance (Table 101-1).[20,21] The occurrence of spinal disease in children has largely been eliminated by effective medical therapy of pulmonary infection.

In contrast, in endemic areas with high infectivity rates, those infected are more commonly children and young to middle-aged adults. These individuals have a higher incidence of multifocal skeletal involvement in the ribs, pelvis, vertebral appendages, cervical spine, feet, and long bone diaphyses, and they show positive TST reactivity.[22] Bone seeding occurs through hematogenous spread, sometimes secondarily from another extrapulmonary site. When pulmonary findings are present, a miliary pattern is typical. Spread to bone may also occur from infected nodes, either by direct extension or through draining lymph channels.[23]

Spondylitis

The spine is the dominant site of involvement in skeletal TB, accounting for 50% to 60% of cases.[24] Between 48% and 67% of lesions occur in the lower thoracic and thoracolumbar spine in HIV-negative patients, whereas the lumbar spine is most commonly involved in HIV-positive patients.[2] The cervical spine is less often involved. Unilateral sacroiliac involvement is not uncommon. Infection usually begins in the anterior subchondral bone of a single vertebra adjacent to the intervertebral disk (Figs. 101-1 and 101-2). Progression to bone changes takes 2 to 5 months and begins with extension from cancellous to cortical bone, and then across the disk space to adjacent vertebrae (Fig. 101-3). Bone destruction may lead to vertebral collapse. Isolated neural arch involvement and intraspinal abscess may also occur.

Paravertebral abscess begins with the extension of infection under the anterior longitudinal ligament. In the thoracic spine, this may extend into the pleural space and lung parenchyma. In the cervical region, it may present in the posterior cervical triangle or retropharyngeal space. In the lumbar spine, a cold abscess characteristically produces lateral displacement of the psoas muscle and may dissect along its length to present as a mass in the inguinal triangle, gluteal muscle, or upper thigh. In isolated cases, a cold abscess occurs with inapparent bone involvement.

A particular variant of this presentation is subligamentous TB, in which infection spreads up and down the spine beneath the longitudinal ligament, producing scalloping of multiple anterior vertebral bodies without disk involvement. This pattern is more common in the cervical spine.[25]

The clinical presentation of spinal TB usually consists of localized pain, often accompanied by low-grade fever, weight loss, chills, and nonspecific constitutional symptoms. Patients may also present initially with abscess formation or kyphosis, or there may be symptoms of spinal cord or nerve root involvement. Paraparesis and paraplegia have been reported in 1% to 27% of patients in various series. In comparison to pyogenic and brucellar vertebral osteomyelitis, spinal TB more often presents with a prolonged clinical course, thoracic segment involvement, absence of fever, spinal deformity, neurologic deficit, and paravertebral or epidural masses.[25] On occasion, tuberculous spondylitis may present with chronic inflammatory-type back pain more typical of the spondyloarthropathies.[26]

Mycobacterial colony counts in bone biopsy specimens are relatively low. Only 40% of smears and cultures from psoas abscesses are positive. Among patients meeting strict clinical and radiographic criteria in one series, between 73% and 82% had compatible histologic features on biopsy; of these, 80% to 95% had positive culture results.[23] The differential diagnosis, which is extensive, includes pyogenic and fungal osteomyelitis, primary and metastatic tumors, sarcoidosis, multiple myeloma, and eosinophilic granuloma.

Cervical spine involvement is relatively rare, accounting for only 0.4% to 1.2% of cases of extrapulmonary TB in the United States.[27] The most common presenting symptoms are neck pain and stiffness, although hoarseness, dysphagia, torticollis, fever, anorexia, and neurologic disorders may also occur. Spinal involvement can progress to myelopathy because of delays in diagnosis. Radiographs may show characteristic osteolysis of the anterior vertebral body with sparing of the posterior portion, gibbus deformity, disk involvement, and a partially calcified paraspinous mass. Computed tomography (CT) or magnetic resonance imaging (MRI) is useful for assessing compromise of the spinal canal. Retropharyngeal infection may extend into the craniocervical junction and, if not promptly recognized, may cause atlantoaxial dislocation and neurologic complications.[28,29]

The sacroiliac joint is involved in up to 10% of cases of skeletal TB, often without other evidence of disease.[30] Infection, and TB in particular, should be suspected in all cases of unilateral sacroiliitis. Emigration from an endemic area and a past history of TB increase the likelihood of this cause. Buttock pain on the involved side is the presenting symptom and is often accompanied by proximal leg or radicular pain. Examination reveals sacroiliac tenderness to palpation and stress maneuvers. Sacroiliac films show joint widening and erosion in all cases. An elevated erythrocyte sedimentation rate (ESR) and anemia are common, and a

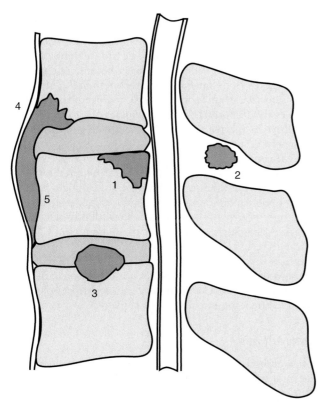

Figure 101-1   Tuberculous spondylitis: sites of involvement. Tuberculous lesions can localize in the vertebral body (1) or, more rarely, the posterior osseous or ligamentous structures (2). Extension to the intervertebral disk (3) or prevertebral tissues (4) is not infrequent. Subligamentous spread (5) can lead to erosion of the anterior vertebral surface. *(From Resnick D: Diagnosis of Bone and Joint Disorders, 3rd ed. Philadelphia, WB Saunders, 1995, p 2464.)*

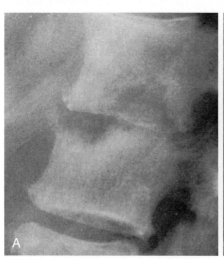 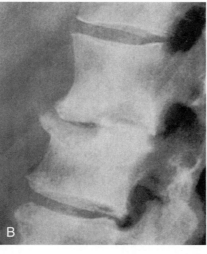

Figure 101-2   Tuberculous spondylitis: diskovertebral lesion. A, The initial radiograph reveals subchondral destruction of two vertebral bodies, with mild surrounding eburnation and loss of intervertebral disk height. The appearance is identical to that in pyogenic spondylitis. **B,** Several months later, an osseous response is evident. Note the increased sclerosis. Osteophytosis and improved definition of the osseous margins can be seen. *(From Resnick D: Diagnosis of Bone and Joint Disorders, 3rd ed. Philadelphia, WB Saunders, 1995, p 2465.)*

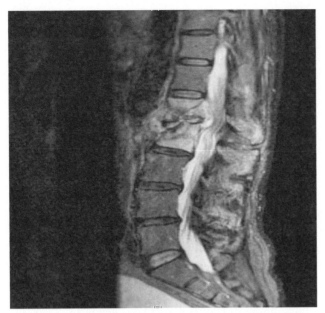

Figure 101-3 Tuberculous spondylitis: spinal cord compression. Magnetic resonance image of the lumbar spine shows destruction of contiguous vertebral bodies and an inflammatory mass pressing on the spinal cord. This patient was successfully treated with medical therapy alone.

positive tuberculin reaction is typical. Biopsy of the sacroiliac joint shows granulomatous histologic features or nonspecific inflammation and a positive culture in most cases.

Atypical spinal lesions, which occur in about 10% of cases, may lead to delayed diagnosis and treatment. Atypical radiographic presentations in single vertebra include concentric collapse, sclerotic foci, and selective involvement of the vertebral arches and costotransverse joints. Multiple vertebrae may be involved either in continuity or as skipped lesions. Atypical clinical presentations may suggest a herniated intervertebral disk, failed back syndrome, spinal tumor, meningeal granuloma, or cold abscess without vertebral destruction.[24,31]

Tuberculous Osteomyelitis

Bone lesions begin with hematogenous implantation of organisms in the medullary area. Metaphyseal involvement is most common, and lesions may spread through the growth plate to involve the adjacent joint, usually late in the disease course. Lesions are typically destructive. Lytic lesions in unusual areas, such as the pubic symphysis, sacroiliac joint, and elbow, can be misdiagnosed as malignancy.[32] Osteomyelitis may develop in a bone or joint that has been previously exposed to trauma. Sternal osteomyelitis due to M. tuberculosis has been described following coronary artery bypass surgery.

Tuberculous osteomyelitis occurs in both children and adults.[33] Although any bone can be involved, the femur and tibia are most commonly affected. Dactylitis may also occur in children. In one large series from an endemic area,[34] such cases represented 19% of bone and joint TB and 15% of cases of osteomyelitis of hematogenous origin. Bone pain was the most common presentation; a draining sinus, abscess formation, and local swelling and tenderness were also common. The average delay before diagnosis was 28 months.

Multifocal osteoarticular TB is a less common variant of the disease,[35] but TB should be considered in all patients from endemic areas who present with multiple destructive skeletal lesions.

For a definitive diagnosis of osteoarticular TB, a biopsy specimen of an affected site must be obtained.[19] Soft tissue lesions characteristically demonstrate rim enhancement on CT examination. CT may also facilitate percutaneous needle biopsy or abscess drainage.[36] Histologic examination generally reveals granulomatous inflammation. In one series of 121 cases, biopsy showed a positive culture in 33%, granulomatous histologic features in 46% and both in 21%.[37]

Radiographic findings include cavity formation with a thin adjacent layer of sclerosis in about 50% of cases, sometimes containing a sequestrum. The true extent of bone involvement may be difficult to detect because of clinically silent lesions. Bone imaging with technetium 99, although more sensitive than conventional radiographs, provides false-negative information in some cases of early, indolent, or highly destructive disease. Tuberculin test reactions are positive in 92% of cases.

Treatment with chemotherapy is generally effective. In a minority of cases, surgical débridement is required for healing. Initiation of therapy on the basis of histologic findings is appropriate pending culture results. Sinus cultures are commonly positive for pyogenic bacteria both before and after antituberculous therapy, but these are presumed to be contaminants. Healing is associated with sclerosis at the margin of lesions. Misdiagnosis of the condition as pyogenic osteomyelitis may lead to unnecessary surgery or to delayed antituberculous treatment, resulting in extension of infection into the joint and chronic disability.

Septic Arthritis

Tuberculous joint involvement is second in frequency to vertebral infection.[24] The typical pattern is a monarticular arthritis involving the large and medium joints, most commonly the hip and knee (Figs. 101-4 and 101-5).[38,39] Other joints less commonly involved include the sacroiliac, shoulder, elbow, ankle, carpal, and tarsal joints. Infection begins in the synovium, with progression of destructive changes being slower than in pyogenic septic arthritis.

The diagnosis of tuberculous arthritis is often missed. A consecutive series spanning the years 1970 to 1984 emphasized typical features.[40] Of 23 cases of musculoskeletal TB, 9 involved the spine, 1 the hip, and the remaining 13 the peripheral joints. Most patients were men older than 50 years. The history of TB or exposure was generally forgotten. In all cases, presenting symptoms were joint pain and swelling. Four patients had evidence of active pulmonary TB, and in two patients with sterile pyuria, M. tuberculosis grew from the urine. Only 5 of 10 patients tested had a positive tuberculin reaction. Radiographs showed changes of erosive arthritis in 7 and no changes in 4 of 11 joints studied. The median delay in diagnosis was 8 months.

Arriving at a correct diagnosis requires vigorous pursuit and usually a synovial biopsy and culture. Initial studies are often misleading and may contribute to delayed diagnosis or misdiagnosis. Synovial fluid findings are variable and do not distinguish this arthropathy from other inflammatory or septic arthritides.[41] Cell counts more often suggest inflammatory

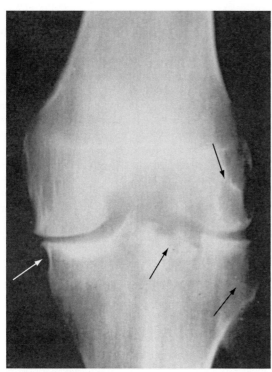

Figure 101-4 Tuberculous arthritis of the knee. On conventional computed tomography, typical marginal and central osseous erosions *(arrows)* accompany tuberculous arthritis. Osteoporosis is not prominent. *(From Resnick D: Diagnosis of Bone and Joint Disorders, 3rd ed. Philadelphia, WB Saunders, 1995, p 2480.)*

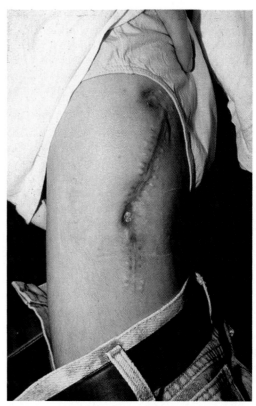

Figure 101-5 Tuberculous arthritis following total hip replacement. A sinus tract emerges from the scar following total hip arthroplasty for childhood destructive arthritis of unknown cause. The young man was originally from Vietnam.

rather than septic arthritis and may contain a preponderance of neutrophils. Synovial fluid glucose tends to be low and more than 10 mg/dL below fasting serum levels, but nonfasting determinations are often misleading. The diagnosis may be facilitated if the organism is observed on an acid-fast smear of synovial fluid, but only 10% to 20% of reported cases are positive. In contrast, 79% of synovial fluid cultures are positive. Radiographic changes are similar to those seen in other septic arthritides, beginning with juxta-articular bone demineralization and progressing to marginal bone erosion and articular cartilage destruction (see Fig. 101-4).

With the open biopsy technique, granulomatous histologic features and positive cultures are present in 94% of cases. No data are available for direct amplification tests in mycobacterial arthritis, but their use can be considered in suspected cases to provide an earlier diagnosis. The histologic examination alone may be confusing, because granulomatous synovitis can also be found in nontuberculous mycobacterial infection, sarcoidosis, erythema nodosum, brucellosis, Crohn's disease, and foreign body reaction. As noted earlier, synovial acid-fast smear is of limited value. Tuberculous arthritis is also reported in children, sometimes early in the disease course; synovial biopsy and culture are recommended in patients with monarthritis and a positive tuberculin reaction.[42]

TB must be considered among the possible causes of septic arthritis occurring in patients with preexisting rheumatoid arthritis,[43] although it is not widely seen in developed countries.[43,44] Conversely, rheumatoid factor may be present in TB, leading to diagnostic confusion in the presence of chronic monarthritis.[44]

EMERGENCE OF TUBERCULOSIS DURING THE TREATMENT OF RHEUMATIC DISEASES

Many patients with systemic rheumatic disease have dysregulated immune systems that are treated with immunosuppressive drugs. Such an impaired immune response may permit the reactivation of latent TB. TNF-α plays a key role in granuloma formation and stabilization, which promotes the containment of M. *tuberculosis*. The rate of TB among patients with rheumatoid arthritis before the widespread use of anti-TNF drugs was approximately 6 cases per 100,000. In one large patient registry, the estimated incidence of TB associated with infliximab in rheumatoid arthritis patients was in excess of 1000 per 100,000 person-years of exposure during the years 2000–2001.[45] Etanercept may be associated with a lower risk for TB reactivation than infliximab: 10 cases per 100,000 person-years of exposure with etanercept, versus 41 per 100,000 person-years with infliximab, according to an analysis of Food and Drug Administration data.[46] Early experience with adalimumab (13 cases in 2400 treated patients) suggests that it may be associated with a relatively high risk for TB reactivation. Monoclonal antibodies to TNF may play a greater role in destabilizing granulomas than TNF receptors. Nonetheless, similar precautions should be taken with any TNF antagonist.

These reactivations in the face of anti-TNF therapy typically occur within 6 to 12 months of treatment and often present as extrapulmonary disease. The institution of a TB screening protocol in rheumatoid arthritis patients, and treatment of latent TB before infliximab administration, resulted in a 78% decrease in active TB.[47] Strategies to treat latent TB infection that are tailored to the at-risk population can effectively and safely lessen the likelihood of active TB in patients treated with TNF antagonists. Although screening for latent TB infection has reduced the incidence of active disease, false-negative TSTs can undermine such good intentions (see Table 101-1).

The approach to a patient with latent TB who needs anti-TNF therapy has not been determined. Patients with positive TSTs and normal chest radiographs who have never been treated for TB should probably receive at least 1 to 2 months of therapy before beginning an anti-TNF drug. Patients discovered to have active TB should receive a complete course of a standard antituberculous regimen before any consideration is given to using an anti-TNF drug. Other biologic agents, including abatacept and rituximab, may pose a lower risk for reactivation of TB because the mechanisms of action are not intimately involved with host defense related to intracellular organisms. Patients treated with abatacept in clinical trials were prescreened with a TST and excluded if positive, thus making a direct comparison difficult. There is little or no evidence that B cells play a major role in containing TB, and no recommendation for TST screening is included in the labeling for rituximab.

Glucocorticoid use also poses a significant hazard for patients with latent TB. Many mechanisms account for this effect, including impairment of cellular immune responses and monocyte chemotaxis and function, including the monocyte's production of TNF-α. The use of glucocorticoids has recently been associated with a five times increased risk for the development of TB in a case-control study based on a large general practice database in the United Kingdom.[48] The risk appeared to be dose related but was seen even at the physiologic dose of prednisone 7.5 mg/day. Just as with anti-TNF therapy, the risk for TB is greatest early in the course of treatment.

Although anti-TNF therapy and steroids stand out as particular risk factors for the development of TB, all rheumatic disease patients treated with immunosuppressives that impair cellular immunity should be considered at risk. This is especially true in the elderly, the malnourished, and immigrants from countries with high endemic rates of TB.

RHEUMATIC DISORDERS PRECIPITATED BY THE TREATMENT OF TUBERCULOSIS

A variety of rheumatic conditions may be precipitated by drugs used in the treatment of TB. These include drug-induced lupus caused by isoniazid (INH) and rifampin. As with other cases of drug-induced lupus, they are associated with positive antinuclear antibodies and the presence of antihistone antibodies. Typically, these patients follow a benign course, with reversal of disease after the drug is discontinued.

Arthropathy and tendinopathy have been described with the use of fluoroquinolones, especially ciprofloxacin and levofloxacin. The risk of tendon rupture (usually the Achilles tendon) is greatest in patients older than 50 years and increases with the concomitant use of corticosteroids.

Pyrazinamide interferes with the renal tubular excretion of uric acid and has been associated with the development of hyperuricemia and gout in adults.

Some patients develop a paradoxical worsening of their condition upon the initiation of antituberculous therapy. Such a development may raise questions about a flare of the underlying disease, especially if immunosuppressive therapy has been withdrawn in the face of infection. Symptoms include fever, malaise, weight loss, and increasing respiratory symptoms. The mechanism for such reactions is not completely understood but has been categorized within the spectrum of immune reconstitution inflammatory syndromes. Such reactions are more common in HIV patients and have also been seen in patients treated with infliximab following cessation of the anti-TNF therapy.[49]

All these drug-induced syndromes occur rarely but should be recalled in appropriate circumstances.

REACTIVE IMMUNOLOGIC PHENOMENON IN THE SETTING OF TUBERCULOSIS

A variety of reactive immunologic phenomena have been associated with M. tuberculosis infection. These are uncommonly found in clinical practice.

Poncet's disease is an aseptic inflammatory polyarthritis that occurs in the presence of active TB. Although any joints can be involved, the most commonly affected are the knees, ankles, and elbows.[50] The mechanism is thought to be similar to other forms of reactive arthritis secondary to remote infection. Most cases resolve after satisfactory treatment of the TB. A reactive arthritis has been described following the intravesicular instillation of bacille Calmette-Guérin (BCG) vaccine for bladder cancer.[51]

Other seldom-encountered immune reaction patterns described with M. tuberculosis include erythema nodosum, erythema induratum, and amyloidosis (AA type).

DIAGNOSIS

TUBERCULIN SKIN TEST

The TST—also called the purified protein derivative (PPD)—has been in use for nearly a century and remains the most widely used screening test for TB. It is routinely administered in rheumatology offices that prescribe anti-TNF therapy. The test represents a crude mix of antigens from M. tuberculosis and is plagued by both false-positive and false-negative results. It is unable to distinguish latent infection from active disease and may be negative in the face of severe active TB. Corticosteroids (≥15 mg/day prednisone) may render the PPD negative in the face of latent TB. Elderly and malnourished patients may not exhibit a positive TST. Table 101-1 provides a partial list of causes for a false-negative TST that are of special interest to rheumatologists.

False-positive results may likewise occur in the case of infection with nontuberculous mycobacteria or previous BCG vaccine. PPD positivity degrades over time in BCG-vaccinated patients, at a variable rate. The degree of positivity is influenced by a number of factors, including the number of BCG vaccinations and the number of subsequent PPD tests performed. Some patients may retain a response as long as 15 years after BCG vaccine. However, a PPD result of

20 mm or greater is rarely due to BCG. In addition, if faced with a high-risk situation, such as the initiation of anti-TNF therapy, one should probably make a presumption of latent TB even if the induration measures as little as 5 mm.

The important message for rheumatologists is that the TST is an important but imperfect screening tool for M. tuberculosis, with a sensitivity and specificity in the range of 70%. A negative TST should not eliminate the clinician's vigilance in monitoring patients being treated with anti-TNF therapy for reactivated or new-onset TB, especially in high-risk populations.

IMAGING

Although imaging patterns suggestive of TB have been discussed, there are no pathognomonic skeletal radiographic features that can establish the diagnosis. Early features on radiographs may be equivocal or nonexistent. Chest radiographs are often normal or fail to show features characteristic of TB.

Conventional radiography is generally a useful approach for defining bone destruction, the extent of disease, and adjacent soft tissue lesions.[52] MRI is more effective in identifying early disease; it may help distinguish TB from other infections and neoplasm and can aid in evaluating the extent of disease.[8,53] Scintiscans with technetium and gallium may also be helpful in localizing bone and soft tissue lesions, but early false-negative findings are not uncommon.[54] CT can be helpful in guiding diagnostic needle biopsy. Fine-needle biopsy is an acceptable alternative to core-needle biopsy and open biopsy for the diagnosis of osteoarticular TB in both the axial and peripheral skeleton, and it has the advantage of obviating general anesthesia.[55,56] Both CT and MRI may also be helpful in monitoring therapy.[57]

CULTURE

Nearly all species of Mycobacteria are slow growing, with M. tuberculosis being the slowest. Other bacteria may rapidly outgrow mycobacteria if the specimen is not inoculated on special isolation media. The small number of mycobacteria found in clinically infected areas further challenges the ability to confirm mycobacterial infection and accounts for the dismally low yield of positive Ziehl-Neelsen staining (10% to 20%) in synovial fluid and other biologic fluids.

Synovial fluid and other bodily fluids are less likely than tissue to yield a positive culture. If a joint is suspected of harboring TB, a synovial biopsy should be obtained. Arthroscopically derived tissue yields higher positive cultures than needle biopsies do. CT-guided needle aspiration and biopsy can provide invaluable information in the case of spinal involvement. Characteristic features on tissue pathology, including caseating and noncaseating granulomas, may allow an early presumptive diagnosis of TB pending culture results, which may take 4 to 6 weeks to be finalized.

ADVANCED DIAGNOSTIC TESTING

Interferon-γ Release Assays

The limitations of the traditional PPD skin test in terms of specificity and sensitivity in identifying latent TB have led to the development of new T cell–based testing. These assays measure the production of interferon-γ by whole-blood mononuclear cells stimulated by specific M. tuberculosis antigens. The interferon-γ release assays (IGRAs) appear to be promising as a test for latent TB and have good sensitivity and specificity for latent TB infection.[58] These assays may prove particularly helpful in distinguishing TB from nontuberculous mycobacteria and in patients who have had recent BCG vaccines. They also offer the opportunity to circumvent operator error with TST administration and do not require patients to return for a reading. IGRAs have replaced the TST in some centers for routine screening for latent TB infection.

Nucleic Acid Amplification

Molecular diagnostics using nucleic acid amplification may be helpful in patients with low mycobacterial loads. The presence of polymerase chain reaction inhibitors, especially in extrapulmonary specimens, can lead to false-negative results. Despite more than a decade of experience, the role of nucleic acid amplification tests in diagnosing TB infection is still being defined. These assays must be interpreted with caution in extrapulmonary tissue specimens and when the clinical suspicion of infection is low.[59-61] Although the specificity is quite good, the sensitivity is actually lower than with traditional cultures.

TREATMENT

The appropriate management of tuberculous infections of bones and joints is a complex and evolving process. Proper selection of antibiotic regimens and ongoing disease monitoring should involve comanagement with an infectious disease consultant. Nonetheless, rheumatologists should be familiar with the basic treatment principles.

Treatment of M. tuberculosis infections that involve the musculoskeletal system consists of the same combination chemotherapy regimens that are effective in pulmonary TB. Treatment regimens for infections of the bone and spine traditionally involved 12- to 18-month courses of antibiotics, even when much shorter courses were recommended for lung disease and other extrapulmonary sites. The longer courses for musculoskeletal disease were based on poor tissue penetration into osseous tissues and high rates of relapse. Experience with regimens that include rifampin indicate that a 9-month course of therapy is effective in musculoskeletal disease. In some cases, 6 months may be adequate.

Current guidelines on the treatment of TB published jointly by the Centers for Disease Control, American Thoracic Society, and Infectious Diseases Society of America recommend a 6-month course of therapy for all sites except the bone (6 to 9 months) and the central nervous system (9 to 12 months).[62] Rifampin is the critical component that allows shorter-course therapy.

The standard approach to TB therapy (both pulmonary and extrapulmonary) in the United States currently includes four drugs to start: isoniazid, rifampin, ethambutol, and pyrazinamide—known as IREZ therapy. Once the bacillus is confirmed to be sensitive to INH, the ethambutol can be discontinued. Pyrazinamide is administered for 2 months, and rifampin and INH are continued for the duration of therapy.

Longer courses of therapy are required for patients who are slow to respond. Radiographic features of mycobacterial disease may not change much after 6 months of treatment, and response to treatment is based mainly on clinical features, including reduction in pain, resolution of constitutional symptoms, and emergence of increased mobility. Longer courses are also advised for cases of relapse and resistant organisms.

Surgical intervention is seldom indicated for the initial management of osteoarticular TB. Possible exceptions at presentation include patients with advanced or progressive disease or spinal kyphosis of 40 degrees or greater. Patients who have extensive joint destruction and immobility after an adequate course of chemotherapy may also be candidates for surgery.

Following successful antibiotic therapy, arthroplasty of the hip and knee may be undertaken and is usually successful. Recurrence of disease in the prosthetic joint is less likely if the surgery is performed years after the infection and the tissue obtained at surgery is culture negative. This may be impractical, however, when a patient is unable to ambulate following an adequate course of therapy. In such cases, the TB therapy is continued through surgery and for at least 3 months postoperatively. If TB recurs in the prosthetic joint, it can sometimes be managed with antibiotic therapy alone. However, in many cases, removal of the prosthesis is necessary for complete resolution of the infection.

The increasing incidence of drug-resistant TB complicates the selection of appropriate drugs.[63-65] Primary monoresistance to isoniazid occurs in about 7% of TB isolates in the United States. When identified, this does not substantially impact the treatment outcome. Multidrug-resistant TB (MDR-TB) refers to isolates that are resistant to isoniazid and rifampin. The rate of MDR-TB in the United States has been relatively stable for the past decade, at less than 1%. In other parts of the world, MDR-TB rates may exceed 6% for new cases and 30% in previously treated individuals. The treatment of MDR-TB is complex and often requires the use of multiple (often toxic) second-line agents for 18 to 24 months or longer. XDR-TB—that is, strains resistant to all first-line TB drugs and at least three second-line agents—has been reported in at least 17 countries, with particularly high rates in Kazakhstan, Iran, and South Africa.[66] The options for treatment of XDR-TB are very limited, and treatment failure and death are the likely outcome.

Incomplete adherence with treatment is a particularly important risk factor for secondary drug resistance, and the likelihood of drug resistance increases following relapse after treatment. Directly observed therapy is strongly advocated to reduce the spread of infection and the frequency of drug-resistant TB.[67]

OSTEOARTICULAR INFECTIONS CAUSED BY NONTUBERCULOUS (ATYPICAL) MYCOBACTERIA

Nontuberculous mycobacteria have a ubiquitous presence in the environment, including soil, water, and animal reservoirs. They are not typically spread from human to human. In normal hosts, they usually result in localized infections of the skin. Some infections are the result of aspiration and may spread hematogenously to other sites.[68]

Immunosuppressed hosts may develop nontuberculous mycobacterial infections of the musculoskeletal system, but these infections are much less common than TB. In contrast to TB, nontuberculous infection is more likely to cause tenosynovitis, synovitis, or osteomyelitis and less likely to cause spinal infection. Although there are some 50 species of nontuberculous mycobacteria, the majority of musculoskeletal infections are caused by *Mycobacterium marinum*, *Mycobacterium kansasii*, and *Mycobacterium avium-intracellulare* (also called M. *avium* complex, or MAC).

Three distinct patterns of musculoskeletal involvement are reported: tenosynovitis, synovitis, and osteomyelitis.[69,70] Tenosynovitis typically presents as chronic unilateral hand and wrist swelling (Figs. 101-6 to 101-8).[71] Synovitis typically presents as chronic indolent asymmetric swelling in a knee, hand, or wrist. A number of species have been associated with these syndromes, and the number isolated from immunosuppressed patients is growing.[10] Predisposing factors, in addition to immunosuppression and direct inoculation, include environmental exposure and preexisting joint disease.[72]

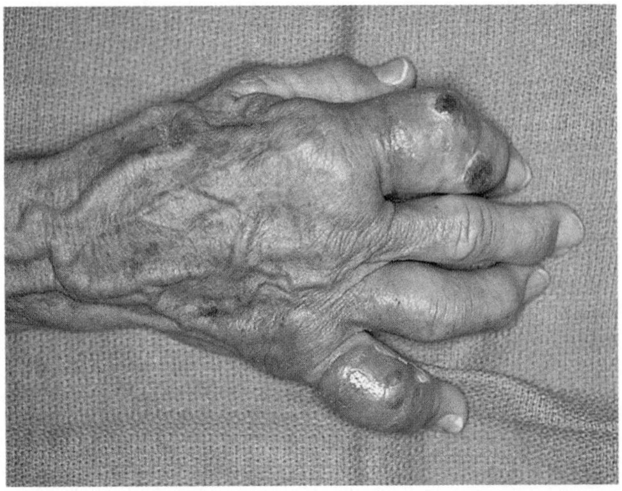

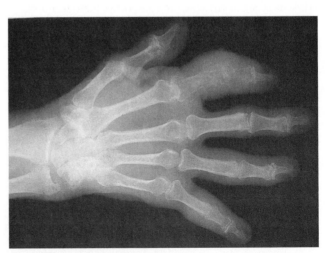

Figure 101-6 Hand demonstrating tenosynovitis and synovitis secondary to *M. marinum*.

Figure 101-7 Radiograph of the hand in Figure 101-6 demonstrates joint destruction secondary to *M. marinum*.

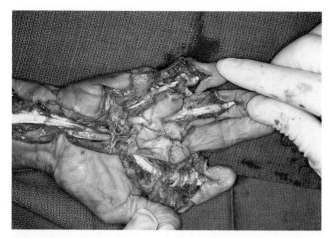

Figure 101-8 The hand depicted in Figures 101-6 and 101-7, infected with *M. marinum,* shows extensive tenosynovitis at the time of synovectomy.

Correct diagnosis usually requires tissue biopsy and culture. Synovial fluid, when it is obtainable, is typically inflammatory, and a culture may be helpful only if mycobacterial techniques are requested. Identification of acid-fast bacilli on smear and granulomatous inflammation from a tissue biopsy specimen often provides direction for an appropriate microbiologic investigation, but histologic features do not consistently demonstrate granuloma formation. With a compatible clinical presentation and histologic findings, mycobacterial culture, including special techniques for M. marinum, should be requested. Direct amplification testing may be useful for more rapid identification of mycobacterial species in tissue specimens, but data from musculoskeletal cases are limited.[59,73] In addition to mycobacteria, other causes of granulomatous synovitis include fungi, brucellosis, sarcoidosis, inflammatory bowel disease, and nonmetallic foreign bodies. Mycobacteria other than M. *tuberculosis* are responsible for a significant proportion of these cases.[74]

MAC has become the most common mycobacterial infectious agent affecting patients with HIV/AIDS, in whom it has a greater tendency to cause disseminated disease.[10] Fortunately, there has been a sharp decline in the incidence of MAC following the introduction of effective antiretroviral therapy and MAC prophylaxis.

When dealing with TB, isolation of the organism is always clinically significant. In contrast, when dealing with a nontuberculous mycobacterial isolate, the clinician must judge whether it is a contaminant, represents insignificant colonization, or is the cause of disease. Certain guidelines have proved useful in this respect[72,75-77]:

- The illness should be consistent with one or more syndromes associated with mycobacterial infection.
- Other causes of disease, such as TB and fungi, should be excluded.
- A mycobacterial species should be isolated that is associated with human disease, the most significant being those that are not common environmental contaminants (M. *kansasii,* M. *marinum,* M. *simiae,* M. *szulgai,* and M. *ulcerans*).
- The site of isolation of the organism should favor true infection over contamination or colonization.

- Heavier growth suggests significant infection.
- With significant disease, multiple isolations of the responsible organism are the rule.

Because laboratory identification of the organism and sensitivities may take weeks to months, initial therapy often includes multiple drugs to cover both TB and other mycobacteria. One common approach to initial empiric therapy is to link standard IREZ therapy for TB with clarithromycin until cultures return. The latest American Thoracic Society guidelines for the treatment of nontuberculous mycobacteria were published in 2007.[78] Surgical débridement of infected tissue may play an important role in the treatment of selected patients, especially for resistant organisms. The most efficacious drugs remain controversial, prolonged treatment is often necessary, and relapses are not uncommon. As with TB, therapy customized to the individual patient is crucial with nontuberculous mycobacteria infection. The key to effective therapy lies in the unique characteristics of the culture and sensitivity of the particular isolate.

REFERENCES

1. Shafer RW, Kim DS, Weiss JP, et al: Extrapulmonary tuberculosis in patients with human immunodeficiency virus infection. Medicine (Baltimore) 70:384, 1991.
2. Jellis JE: Human immunodeficiency virus and osteoarticular tuberculosis. Clin Orthop 398:27, 2002.
3. Havlir DV, Barnes PF: Tuberculosis in patients with human immunodeficiency virus infection. N Engl J Med 340:367, 1999.
4. Global Tuberculosis Control: Surveillance, Planning, Financing. WHO Report WHO/HTM/TB/2007.376. Geneva, World Health Organization, 2007.
5. **Bloom BR: Tuberculosis—the global view. N Engl J Med 346:1434, 2002.**
6. **Gandhi NR, Moll A, Sturm AW, et al: Extensively drug-resistant tuberculosis as a cause of death in patients co-infected with tuberculosis and HIV in a rural area of South Africa. Lancet 638:1575, 2006.**
7. **Franco-Paredes C, Diaz-Borjon A, Senger M, et al: The everexpanding association between rheumatologic diseases and tuberculosis. Am J Med 119:470, 2006.**
8. Moore SL, Rafii M: Imaging of musculoskeletal and spinal infections: Imaging of musculoskeletal and spinal tuberculosis. Radiol Clin North Am 39:329, 2001.
9. Griffith JF, Kumta SM, Leung PC, et al: Imaging of musculoskeletal tuberculosis: A new look at an old disease. Clin Orthop 398:32, 2002.
10. American Thoracic Society and the Centers for Disease Control: Mycobacterioses and the acquired immunodeficiency syndrome. Am Rev Respir Dis 136:492, 1987.
11. La Fond EM: An analysis of adult skeletal tuberculosis. J Bone Joint Surg Am 40:346, 1958.
12. Ashworth MJ, Meadows TH: Isolated tuberculosis of a skeletal muscle. J Hand Surg Br 17:235, 1992.
13. Hasan N, Baithun S, Swash M, Wagg A: Tuberculosis of striated muscle. Muscle Nerve 16:984, 1993.
14. Indudhara R, Singh SK, Minz M, et al: Tuberculous pyomyositis in a renal transplant recipient. Tuber Lung Dis 73:239, 1992.
15. George JC, Buckwalter KA, Braunstein EM: Tuberculosis presenting as a soft tissue forearm mass in a patient with a negative tuberculin skin test. Skeletal Radiol 23:79, 1994.
16. Abdelwahab IF, Kenan S, Hermann G, et al: Tuberculous gluteal abscess without bone involvement. Skeletal Radiol 27:36, 1998.
17. Albornoz MA, Mezgarzedeh M, Neumann CH, et al: Granulomatous tenosynovitis: A rare musculoskeletal manifestation of tuberculosis. Clin Rheumatol 17:166, 1998.
18. King AD, Griffith J, Rushton A, et al: Tuberculosis of the greater trochanter and the trochanteric bursa. J Rheumatol 25:391, 1998.
19. Chen W-S: Tuberculosis of the fascia lata. Clin Rheumatol 17:77, 1998.

20. Alvarez S, McCabe WR: Extrapulmonary tuberculosis revisited: A review of experience at Boston City and other hospitals. Medicine (Baltimore) 63:25, 1984.

21. el-Shahawy MA, Gadallah MF, Campese VM: Tuberculosis of the spine (Pott's disease) in patients with end-stage renal disease. Am J Nephrol 14:55, 1994.

22. Jacobs P: Osteo-articular tuberculosis in coloured immigrants: A radiologic study. Clin Radiol 15:59, 1964.

23. **Gorse GJ, Pais MJ, Kusske JA, Cesario TC: Tuberculous spondylitis. Medicine (Baltimore) 62:178, 1983.**

24. Chapman M, Murray RD, Stoker DJ: Tuberculosis of bones and joints. Semin Roentgenol 14:266, 1985.

25. Colmenero JD, Jimenez-Mejias ME, Sanchez-Lora FJ, et al: Pyogenic, tuberculous, and brucellar vertebral osteomyelitis: A descriptive and comparative study of 219 cases. Ann Rheum Dis 56:709, 1997.

26. Cantini F, Salvarani C, Olivieri I, et al: Tuberculous spondylitis as a cause of inflammatory spinal pain: A report of 4 cases. Clin Exp Rheumatol 16:305, 1998.

27. Slater RR Jr, Beale RW, Bullitt E: Pott's disease of the cervical spine. South Med J 84:521, 1991.

28. Krishnan A, Patkar D, Patankar T, et al: Craniovertebral junction tuberculosis: A review of 29 cases. J Comput Assist Tomogr 25:171, 2001.

29. Bhojraj SY, Shetty N, Shah PJ: Tuberculosis of the craniocervical junction. J Bone Joint Surg Br 83:222, 2001.

30. Pouchot J, Vinceneus P, Barge J, et al: Tuberculosis of the sacroiliac joint: Clinical features, outcome, and evaluation of closed needle biopsy in 11 consecutive cases. Am J Med 84:622, 1988.

31. Pande KC, Babhulkar SS: Atypical spinal tuberculosis. Clin Orthop 398:64, 2002.

32. Tsay MH, Chen MC, Jaung GY, et al: Atypical skeletal tuberculosis mimicking tumor metastasis: Report of a case. J Formos Med Assoc 94:428, 1995.

33. Shih HN, Hsu RW, Lin TY: Tuberculosis of the long bone in children. Clin Orthop 335:246, 1997.

34. Babhulkar SS, Pande SK: Unusual manifestations of osteoarticular tuberculosis. Clin Orthop 398:114, 2002.

35. Muradali D, Gold WL, Vellend H, Becker E: Multifocal osteoarticular tuberculosis: Report of four cases and review of management. Clin Infect Dis 17:204, 1993.

36. Coppola J, Muller NL, Connell DG: Computed tomography of musculoskeletal tuberculosis. J Can Assoc Radiol 38:199, 1987.

37. **Martini M, Adjrad A, Boudjemaa A: Tuberculous osteomyelitis: A review of 125 cases. Int Orthop 10:201, 1986.**

38. Babhulkar S, Pande S: Tuberculosis of the hip. Clin Orthop 398:93, 2002.

39. Hoffman EB, Allin J, Campbell JAB, Leisegang FM: Tuberculosis of the knee. Clin Orthop 398:100, 2002.

40. Evanchick CC, Davis DE, Harrington TM: Tuberculosis of peripheral joints: An often missed diagnosis. J Rheumatol 13:187, 1986.

41. Wallace R, Cohen AS: Tuberculous arthritis: A report of two cases with a review of biopsy and synovial fluid findings. Am J Med 61:277, 1976.

42. Jacobs JC, Li SC, Ruzal-Shapiro C, et al: Tuberculous arthritis in children: Diagnosis by needle biopsy of the synovium. Clin Pediatr 33:344, 1994.

43. Sorio LM, Sole JMN, Sacanell AR, et al: Infectious arthritis in patients with rheumatoid arthritis. Ann Rheum Dis 51:402, 1992.

44. Davidson PT, Horowitz I: Skeletal tuberculosis: A review with patient presentations and discussion. Am J Med 48:77, 1970.

45. **Gomez-Reino JJ, Carmona L, Rodriquez Valverde V, et al: Treatment of rheumatoid arthritis with tumor necrosis factor inhibitors may predispose to a significant increase in tuberculosis risk: A multicenter active surveillance report. Arthritis Rheum 48:2122, 2003.**

46. Mohan AK, Cote TR, Block JA, et al: Tuberculosis following the use of etanercept, a tumor necrosis factor inhibitor. Clin Infect Dis 39:295, 2004.

47. **Carmona L, Gomez-Reino JJ, Rodriquez Valverde V, et al: Effectiveness of recommendations to prevent reactivation of latent TB infection in patients treated with tumor necrosis antagonists. Arthritis Rheum 52:1766, 2005.**

48. Jick SS, Lieberman ES, Rahman MU, et al: Glucocorticoid use, other associated factors, and the risk of tuberculosis. Arthritis Rheum (Arthritis Care Res) 55:19, 2006.

49. Garcia Vidal C, Rodriquez Fernandez S, Martinez Lacasa J, et al: Paradoxical response to antituberculous therapy in infliximab-treated patients with disseminated tuberculosis. Clin Infect Dis 40:756, 2005.

50. Dall L, Long L, Standford J: Poncet's disease: Tuberculous rheumatism. Rev Infect Dis 11:105, 1989.

51. Pancaldi P, Van Linthoudt D, Aborino S, et al: Reiter's syndrome after intravesical bacillus Calmette-Guerin treatment for superficial bladder carcinoma. Br J Rheumatol 32:1096, 1993.

52. Resnick D: Osteomyelitis, septic arthritis, and soft tissue infection. In Resnick D (ed): Diagnosis of Bone and Joint Disorders, 4th ed. Philadelphia, WB Saunders, 2002, pp 2510-2624.

53. Gupta RK, Gupta S, Kumar S, et al: MRI in intraspinal tuberculosis. Neuroradiology 36:39, 1994.

54. Lifeso RM, Weaver P, Harder EH: Tuberculous spondylitis in adults. J Bone Joint Surg Am 67:1405, 1985.

55. Mondal A: Cytological diagnosis of vertebral tuberculosis with fine-needle aspiration biopsy. J Bone Joint Surg Am 76:181, 1994.

56. Masood S: Diagnosis of tuberculosis of bone and soft tissue by fine-needle aspiration biopsy. Diagn Cytopathol 8:451, 1992.

57. Omari B, Robertson JM, Nelson RJ, Chiu LC: Pott's disease: A resurgent challenge to the thoracic surgeon. Chest 95:145, 1989.

58. **Menzies D, Madhakur PA, Comstock G: Meta-analysis: New tests for the diagnosis of latent tuberculosis infection: Areas of uncertainty and recommendations for research. Ann Intern Med 146:340, 2007.**

59. Harrington JT: The evolving role of direct amplification tests in diagnosing osteoarticular infections caused by mycobacteria and fungi. Curr Opin Rheumatol 11:289, 1999.

60. Catanzaro A, Perry S, Clarridge JE, et al: The role of clinical suspicion in evaluating a new diagnostic test for active tuberculosis: Results of a multicenter prospective trial. JAMA 283:639, 2000.

61. Woods GL: Molecular techniques in mycobacterial detection. Arch Pathol Lab Med 125:122, 2001.

62. **Recommendations for the treatment of tuberculosis. MMWR 52:1-77, 2003.**

63. Hannachi MR, Martini M, Boulahal F, et al: A comparison of three daily short-course regimens in osteoarticular tuberculosis in Algiers. Bull Int Union Tuberc 57:46, 1982.

64. Parsons LM, Driscoll JR, Taber HW, et al: Antimicrobial resistance: Drug resistance in tuberculosis. Infect Dis Clin North Am 11:906, 1997.

65. Bradford WZ, Daley CL: Emerging infectious diseases: Multiple drug-resistant tuberculosis. Infect Dis Clin North Am 12:157, 1998.

66. Raviglione MC, Smith IM: XDR tuberculosis: Implications for global health. N Engl J Med 356:656, 2007.

67. Chaulk CP, Kazandjian VA: Directly observed therapy for treatment completion of pulmonary tuberculosis: Consensus statement of the Public Health Tuberculosis Guidelines Panel. JAMA 279:943, 1998.

68. Brown-Elliot BA, Wallace RJ: Infections caused by nontuberculous mycobacteria. In Mandell GL, Bennett JE, Dolin R (eds): Mandell, Douglas, and Bennett's Principles and Practice of Infectious Diseases, 6th ed. Philadelphia, Churchill Livingstone, 2005, pp 2909-2916.

69. Kelly PJ, Karlson AG, Weed LA, et al: Infection of synovial tissues by mycobacteria other than Mycobacterium tuberculosis. J Bone Joint Surg Am 49:1521, 1967.

70. Marchevsky AM, Damsker B, Green S, Tepper S: The clinicopathological spectrum of non-tuberculous mycobacterial osteoarticular infections. J Bone Joint Surg Am 67:925, 1985.

71. Zenone T, Boibieux A, Tigaud S, et al: Non-tuberculous mycobacterial tenosynovitis: A review. Scand J Infect Dis 31:221, 1999.

72. Glickstein SL, Nashel DJ: Mycobacterium kansasii septic arthritis complicating rheumatic disease: Case report and review of the literature. Semin Arthritis Rheum 16:231, 1987.

73. Weigl JAI, Haas WH: Postoperative Mycobacterium avium osteomyelitis confirmed by polymerase chain reaction. Eur J Pediatr 159:64, 2000.

74. Sutker WL, Lankford LL, Tompsett R: Granulomatous synovitis: The role of atypical mycobacteria. Rev Infect Dis 1:729, 1979.

75. Wolinsky E: When is an infection disease? Rev Infect Dis 3:1025, 1981.

76. Wallace RJ Jr, O'Brien R, Glassroth J, et al: Diagnosis and treatment of disease caused by nontuberculous mycobacteria. Am Rev Respir Dis 142:940, 1990.

77. Ahn CH, McLarty JW, Ahn SS, et al: Diagnostic criteria for pulmonary disease caused by Mycobacterium kansasii and Mycobacterium intracellulare. Am Rev Respir Dis 125:388, 1992.

78. **Griffith DE, Aksamit T, Brown-Elliot BA, et al: An official ATS-IDSA statement: Diagnosis, treatment, and prevention of nontuberculous mycobacterial diseases. Am J Resp Crit Care Med 175:367-416, 2007.**

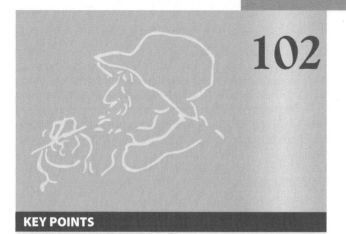

102 Fungal Infections of the Bones and Joints

J. TIMOTHY HARRINGTON •
JOHN P. FLAHERTY •
WALTER G. BARR

KEY POINTS

Fungi are an infrequent but clinically important cause of osteoarticular infections.

A high index of suspicion is required to diagnose and correctly treat these infections, because they are often indolent in onset and masquerade as other disorders.

Travel and immigration have affected the geographic localization of several important fungal infections.

Immunocompromise, including antirheumatic biologic therapies, predisposes to fungal infections, often resulting in more acute and widely disseminated disease.

Although diagnosis may be assisted by clinical presentation and serologic testing, examination and culture of infected tissue are critical.

New antifungal therapies have broadened the effective options, but choice of drugs, duration of treatment, and combined surgical débridement must be carefully considered to achieve optimal outcomes.

Fungal infection is a relatively infrequent but important cause of osteomyelitis and arthritis. Fungal diseases that commonly cause osteomyelitis include coccidioidomycosis, blastomycosis, cryptococcosis, candidiasis, and sporotrichosis (Table 102-1). Fungal arthritis is less common and is most often associated with sporotrichosis, coccidioidomycosis, blastomycosis, candidiasis, and, occasionally, other species. The epidemiology of these fungal infections, their musculoskeletal presentations, and their treatment are considered in this chapter. Additional information may be accessed by electronic search at UpToDate.

The epidemiology and clinical features of individual deep mycoses may suggest the diagnosis in some cases, but their indolent presentation, which often resembles that of other noninfectious diseases, may be misleading. Travel and immigration have blurred their geographic localization. Infection may be acute and overwhelming in immunocompromised patients, for whom disseminated fungal infections are a major risk. Anticytokine treatments for rheumatic diseases are associated with disseminated fungal infection,[1] as are acquired immunodeficiency syndrome (AIDS), pregnancy, and treatments for transplantation and malignancies,[2] in some cases. For rheumatologists, disseminated fungal infections are an important diagnostic consideration in some patients and must be considered before starting biologic treatments in those at risk; they may also complicate the clinical course of other arthritides.

Fungal infections are generally diagnosed by histologic examination or culture of involved tissues. Improved biopsy techniques facilitate the diagnosis, provided the possibility of fungal infection is considered and proper studies are requested. Synovial fluid leukocyte counts and culture results vary among fungal infections and in individual cases and may be misleading. Serologic testing may also assist in diagnosing and staging several fungal infections. Detecting fungal antigens and DNA in blood and tissue is now possible in some cases, but the clinical use of these methods is still under investigation.[3]

COCCIDIOIDOMYCOSIS

Coccidioides immitis, a soil fungus, generally causes a primary respiratory illness after spores are inhaled. A self-limited acute pneumonia may result, associated with systemic manifestations such as arthralgia and erythema nodosum (valley fever), but infection is often inapparent and only infrequently becomes chronic or disseminated.[4] Coccidioidomycosis is endemic to the southwestern United States and areas of Central and South America, but cases are increasingly diagnosed in nonendemic areas because of travel, infection from fomites, and reactivation of remote infection. Cases increase when soil is disturbed and in windy conditions. Direct human-to-human transmission is rare. Extrapulmonary infection is almost always caused by hematogenous spread from an initial pulmonary focus. The bones and joints are frequent sites of dissemination, particularly in immunocompromised hosts.

Septic arthritis of the knee is common, generally arising from direct infection of the synovium. Other joint infections are caused by spread from a contiguous osteomyelitis involving the vertebrae, wrists, hands, ankles, feet, pelvis, and long bones.[5] The onset is characterized by gradually increasing pain and joint stiffness, with little swelling but early radiographic changes. In one series, arthritis was the only manifestation of disseminated coccidioidomycosis in 51 of 57 patients and was an aspect of more generalized disease in the remaining 6 patients.[6]

Diagnostic confusion is common in osteoarticular coccidioidomycosis because of the delayed dissemination (months to years) after primary infection and because of atypical clinical presentations. The criteria for diagnosis include compatible clinical features, serologic studies, histologic examination, and culture. Early infections, often before systemic spread, are associated with a positive antibody precipitin test that detects immunoglobulin (Ig) M antibody. Complement fixation serologic values detecting IgG antibodies are in a range indicative of disseminated disease in a majority of patients and show a significant decrease with

Table 102-1 Fungi Causing Osteoarticular Infections

Infection	Geographic Distribution	Infection Site
Coccidioidomycosis	Southwestern US, Central and South America, elsewhere	Bones and joints, especially knee
Blastomycosis	North-central and southern US	Bones and joints
Cryptococcosis	Ubiquitous	Bones; rarely joints
Candidiasis	Ubiquitous	Bones; rarely joints
Sporotrichosis	Ubiquitous	Bones and joints
Aspergillosis	Ubiquitous	Spine, ribs; rarely joints
Histoplasmosis	Midwestern and southeastern US	Rarely bones and joints; hypersensitivity arthritis
Scedosporiosis	Undefined	Bones and joints

effective treatment. The definitive diagnosis is most commonly made by the demonstration of granulomatous synovitis and typical spherules in a biopsy specimen, confirmed in some cases by positive culture and direct amplification testing. Synovial fluid, when it is obtainable, does not necessarily demonstrate septic leukocyte counts, and it is culture positive in less than 5% of cases. Radioisotope bone scans may be helpful to identify areas of infection.[7]

With early diagnosis of effusive synovitis, antifungal treatment alone is appropriate. With more widely disseminated infection or involvement of critical areas such as the spine, and in high-risk hosts, the choice and duration of treatments are often complicated.[8] Indications for combined medical and surgical treatment include (1) chronic joint inflammation with pannus formation and progressive disease during medical treatment, (2) involvement of contiguous bone, (3) rising complement fixation titers, and (4) extra-articular dissemination. Combined antifungal and surgical treatment is superior to either medical or surgical treatment alone.[6,9] A high priority for combined treatment is identified by a complement fixation titer at or above 1:128. For skeletal infections, itraconazole is more effective than fluconazole and has been successful in some patients who relapsed after previous treatment with amphotericin or ketoconazole.[10,11] New antifungal agents such as voriconazole and posaconazole are under investigation.[8]

Coccidioidal synovitis may also occur in a noninfectious inflammatory variety that complicates either primary pulmonary or disseminated disease and is typically a polyarthritis. It is accompanied by fever, erythema nodosum or multiforme, eosinophilia, and hilar adenopathy. It abates in 2 to 4 weeks.[4,12]

BLASTOMYCOSIS

Blastomycosis, caused by *Blastomyces dermatitidis*, is endemic in the north-central and southern United States. Infection most commonly produces sporadic or clustered cases of pulmonary disease and is induced by exposure to soil or dust containing decomposed wood and, presumably, contaminated with the organism.[13] Affected individuals

do not appear to have any distinguishing or predisposing characteristics except for exposure to the organism during work or recreation. Clinical presentation includes high fever and other constitutional symptoms, pulmonary and skin involvement, and a significant mortality rate. Hematogenous dissemination is common; skin disease and osteoarticular disease occur most frequently. Bone involvement occurs in 25% to 60% of disseminated cases, and arthritis is estimated to occur in 3% to 5%.[14] The skeletal areas most commonly affected are the long bones, vertebrae, and ribs (Fig. 102-1).[15-17]

Arthritis is usually monarticular in the knee, ankle, or elbow but may rarely be polyarticular.[14,18] Joint infection is an isolated skeletal disorder in only a few cases; joint radiographs more commonly show punched-out bone lesions (Fig. 102-2A). Synovial fluid is commonly purulent, and organisms are evident on microscopic examination as well as by culture. The synovial histologic examination shows epithelioid granulomas with budding yeast forms (Fig. 102-2B). The diagnosis is also commonly made from involved nonarticular sites. Urinary antigen testing appears to be very sensitive. The therapeutic response to amphotericin B or itraconazole is generally favorable.[13,19,20]

CRYPTOCOCCOSIS

Cryptococcus neoformans, the fungus causing cryptococcosis, is geographically ubiquitous and is found in pigeon feces; a related species, *Cryptococcus gattii*, is associated with certain types of eucalyptus trees in tropical climates. It is a common pathogen only in association with defects in cell-mediated host defense, including human immunodeficiency virus (HIV) infection,[21] transplantation, lymphoreticular malignant neoplasms, tumor necrosis factor-α (TNF-α) antagonist treatment,[22] and corticosteroid therapy.

Cryptococcosis varies in acuteness, usually affecting the lungs in its primary form, but it sometimes disseminates hematogenously to a wide variety of sites, including the central nervous system and skin. Although bone infection is common, causing osteolytic lesions in 5% to 10% of cases, articular involvement is rarely reported.[23] Bone lesions may be confused with metastatic neoplasm (Fig. 102-3).

Cryptococcal arthritis is an indolent monarticular arthritis in about 60% of reported cases and a polyarthritis in the remainder.[24,25] The knee is most commonly involved. A single case of tenosynovitis with carpal tunnel syndrome has been recognized. The majority of cases reported from the pre-AIDS era also demonstrated radiographic evidence of periarticular osteomyelitis. These patients were young adults, did not have debilitating disease or other evidence of dissemination, and had pulmonary involvement in only 50% of cases. Synovial tissue showed acute and chronic synovitis, multinucleate giant cells, prominent granuloma formation, and large numbers of budding cryptococci with special stains. Most recently reported cases are associated with immunosuppression and disseminated infection. Myositis and fasciitis have also been reported.[26,27] Serum cryptococcal antigen testing appears to be very sensitive, in part because osteoarticular infection results from hematogenous dissemination. The choice of treatment for cryptococcal disease depends on both the anatomic sites of involvement and the host's immune status, with amphotericin B and

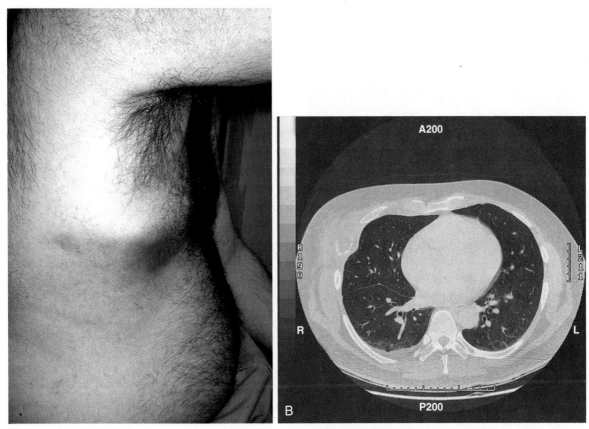

Figure 102-1 **A,** Blastomycosis osteomyelitis of a rib and chest wall. **B,** Computed tomography scan appearance. Primary infection in the blood may spread to the skeleton. *(Courtesy of John Flaherty, MD, Feinberg School of Medicine, Northwestern University.)*

fluconazole being considered most effective.[25,28] 5-Flucytosine is often added to amphotericin B or fluconazole in cases of severe cryptococcal infections.[29]

CANDIDIASIS

Candida species are widely distributed yeasts. *Candida albicans* is a normal commensal of humans, and other species can probably live in nonanimal environments such as soil. Since the advent of antibiotic therapy in the 1940s, and related to the common use of immunosuppression and parenteral lines, candidiasis has been responsible for an increasing incidence of mucocutaneous and deep-organ infections.[29]

Osteomyelitis, though rarely reported, is a potentially serious complication of hematogenous dissemination in both adults and children.[30,31] It may also occur from direct tissue inoculation during surgery or by injection of contaminated heroin,[32] and bone infection may emerge after successful amphotericin B treatment of other sites. Infection is commonly located in two adjacent vertebrae[33] or in a single long bone. Surgical inoculation has occurred in the sternum, spine, and mandible. A few patients have had multiple sites of involvement.

The clinical presentation is localized pain. Other symptoms and laboratory abnormalities vary. Bone changes of osteomyelitis are commonly demonstrated by radiographs of the symptomatic site. The diagnosis is established when culture of involved bone obtained by either open or needle biopsy has identified a variety of *Candida* species. Use of direct amplification testing has been reported.[34] Treatment

with ketoconazole, itraconazole, or amphotericin B is effective.[35,36] The use of surgical débridement must be individualized. With vertebral involvement but no neurologic complications, medication alone has been effective.

Candidiasis is an uncommon cause of monarticular arthritis.[37-41] Reported cases commonly involve a knee, occur in the context of multifocal extra-articular *Candida* infection, and are accompanied by constitutional symptoms. Both children and adults have been affected. Predisposing conditions include gastrointestinal and pulmonary disorders, narcotic addiction, intravenous catheters, leukopenia, immunosuppressive treatment, broad-spectrum antibiotics, and corticosteroids. Some involved joints were previously affected by arthritis, and infection has followed arthrocentesis in isolated cases. In most cases, radiographs reveal coincident osteomyelitis. Synovial fluid leukocyte counts may vary; *Candida* species have been cultured from synovial fluid in all cases but are not commonly identified on smear. Histologic studies of synovium show nonspecific chronic inflammation rather than granulomas. Muscle infection by *Candida* has also been reported in neutropenic patients, in the form of either diffuse myositis or localized abscess.[42-44]

SPOROTRICHOSIS

Sporotrichosis is caused by *Sporothrix schenckii*, a saprophyte found widely in soil and plants. Infection in humans occurs through inoculation of the skin or, rarely, inhalation into the respiratory tract; it is a source of infection among agricultural

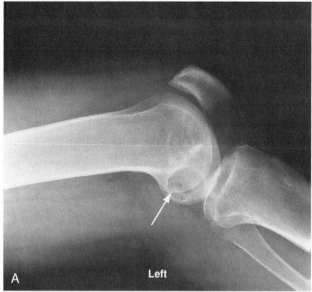

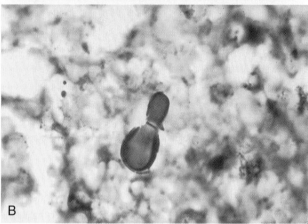

Figure 102-2   **Blastomycosis joint infection. A,** Radiographs commonly show punched-out bone lesions. **B,** Synovial histology shows epithelioid granulomas with budding yeast forms. *(Courtesy of John Flaherty, MD, Feinberg School of Medicine, Northwestern University.)*

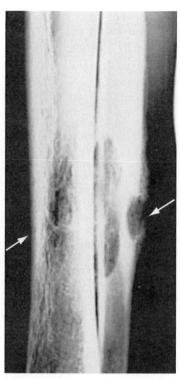

Figure 102-3   **Cryptococcosis (torulosis).** Discrete osteolytic foci with surrounding sclerosis and, in some places, periosteal reaction are seen *(arrows).* This involvement of bone protuberances, such as the calcaneus, is not unexpected in this disease. The resulting appearance simulates that of other fungal diseases, especially coccidioidomycosis, as well as neoplastic disorders. *(From Resnick D: Diagnosis of Bone and Joint Disorders, 3rd ed. Philadelphia, WB Saunders, 1995, p 2507.)*

workers in tropical and subtropical areas. It most commonly involves the skin and lymphatics but may disseminate from the lungs to the central nervous system, eyes, bones, and joints.[45] In immunocompetent hosts, a single site is typically involved; in immunocompromised hosts, including patients on anticytokine therapy, multifocal disease may occur.[46]

In contrast to the relatively common occurrence of skin infection, articular sporotrichosis is a rare disorder.[47,48] In 84% of patients in one series, there was no accompanying skin involvement, suggesting entry through the lungs. Sporotrichosis most often occurs in individuals with a chronic illness that alters host defense, such as alcoholism or a myeloproliferative disorder. Sporotrichosis arthritis is most often indolent and infects a single joint or multiple joints in equal proportions. The knee, hand, wrist, elbow, and shoulder are most frequently involved; hand and wrist involvement distinguishes this from other fungal arthritides. Articular infection shows a propensity to spread to adjacent soft tissues, forming draining sinuses. Constitutional symptoms are unusual.

Radiographic changes vary from juxta-articular osteopenia to the commonly observed punched-out bone lesions.

When it is obtainable, synovial fluid is inflammatory. Synovitis is characterized on gross evaluation by destructive pannus and on microscopic examination by granulomatous histologic features or, less frequently, by nonspecific inflammation. Organisms are difficult to identify in tissue, and the diagnosis is often made by positive culture of joint fluid or involved tissue. Serologies may aid in the diagnosis of disseminated infection. In a small number of cases, sporotrichosis may disseminate to cause a potentially fatal infection characterized by low-grade fever, weight loss, anemia, osteolytic bone lesions, arthritis, skin lesions, and involvement of the eyes and central nervous system.[49-52] These infections occur in immunosuppressed patients with either hematologic malignant neoplasias or HIV infection.

In 44 cases reported in 1979, treatment was optimal with combined joint débridement and high-dose intravenous amphotericin B (11 of 11 cured) and slightly less effective with amphotericin alone (14 of 19 cured).[47] Oral potassium iodide (5 of 15 cured) and other forms of treatment were not adequate. More recently, itraconazole has proved effective for initial therapy of most patients, with amphotericin B being reserved for those with extensive involvement and for itraconazole failures. In contrast, fluconazole has demonstrated only modest success in osteoarticular sporotrichosis.[53,54]

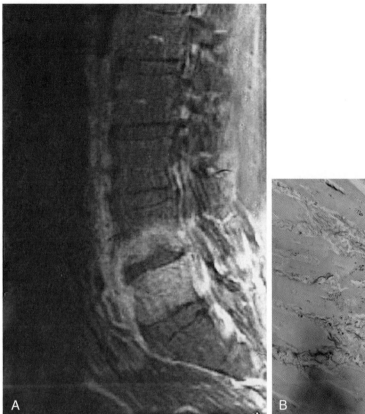
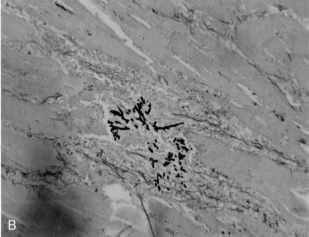

Figure 102-4 **Aspergillosis vertebral osteomyelitis and diskitis. A,** *Aspergillus* may spread directly from the lung to adjacent vertebrae, disk spaces, and ribs (more often in children) or through the bloodstream. **B,** Infected tissue may show characteristic organisms. *(Courtesy of John Flaherty, MD, Feinberg School of Medicine, Northwestern University.)*

ASPERGILLOSIS

Aspergillus species are ubiquitous, but infection occurs only rarely in normal individuals. In contrast, invasive infection is an important life-threatening complication in immunocompromised adults and children.[55-57] It may spread directly from the lung to adjacent vertebrae, disk spaces, and ribs (more often in children) or through the bloodstream (Fig. 102-4).[58-60] Rare cases of monarthritis with adjacent osteomyelitis are also reported.[61] The organism may be observed in infected tissue (see Fig. 102-4B). Treatment with combined surgical débridement and antifungal therapy is an ongoing challenge.[57,60] Voriconazole is superior to amphotericin in invasive pulmonary aspergillosis and appears to be the treatment of choice for all cases of invasive aspergillosis.[62,63]

HISTOPLASMOSIS

Histoplasma capsulatum is a soil fungus that causes endemic disease in the midwestern and southeastern United States.[24,64] Bone and joint involvement is rare but has been reported in the knee, wrist, and ankle. Immunosuppression, including the use of TNF antagonists, predisposes to disseminated histoplasmosis in adults and children, which may be confused clinically with sarcoidosis, tuberculosis, and reactive inflammatory conditions.[65-67] Diagnosis depends on appropriate use of fungal staining and culture methods, antigen detection, and serologic antibody testing.[68] A case report emphasizes the rare occurrence of fungal prosthetic joint arthritis.[69] The more common osteoarticular involvement with histoplasmosis is a hypersensitivity syndrome accompanying acute pulmonary infection; it is characterized by self-limited polyarthritis, erythema nodosum, and erythema multiforme. Amphotericin B is the preferred treatment for severe infection and itraconazole for less severe cases.[70,71]

SCEDOSPORIOSIS

Scedosporium species are environmental molds that have recently been identified as fungal pathogens in both immunocompetent and immunocompromised hosts. They may cause focally invasive and disseminated infection after cutaneous inoculation. *Scedosporium prolificans* has a predilection for bone and cartilage, leading to both septic arthritis and osteomyelitis. Infections are difficult to eradicate with surgery and antifungal agents.[72,73] Case reports suggest improved infection control with voriconazole.[74,75]

TREATMENT OF FUNGAL INFECTION

Antifungal chemotherapy has improved over the past several decades, first with the introduction of amphotericin B and then with the oral antifungal agents flucytosine, ketoconazole, fluconazole, and itraconazole. More recent advances include the development of less toxic formulations

Table 102-2 Drug Treatment of Osteoarticular Mycotic Infections

Infection	Drug Recommended	Infection-Specific References
Coccidioidomycosis	Itraconazole*	6, 9–11
Blastomycosis	Itraconazole*	19, 20
Cryptococcosis	Fluconazole†	25, 28
Candidiasis	Fluconazole‡	35–41
Sporotrichosis	Itraconazole*	47, 53, 54
Aspergillosis	Voriconazole	56, 59
Histoplasmosis	Itraconazole	70, 71
Scedosporiosis	Voriconazole	72-75

*Amphotericin B is indicated for severe infections.
†Amphotericin B plus 5-flucytosine is indicated for severe infections.
‡Caspofungin is indicated for infections due to *Candida krusei* and *Candida glabrata*.

of amphotericin B, liposomal amphotericin B, and amphotericin B lipid complex. Voriconazole and posaconazole, which are broad-spectrum antifungals, have demonstrated improved activity against aspergillosis and mucormycosis, respectively. The echinocandin antifungal agents caspofungin, micafungin, and anidulafungin have emerged as alternative therapies for aspergillosis and as the treatments of choice for some *Candida* infections. For detailed treatment guidelines, several excellent reviews are available.[76-85] In choosing an appropriate drug (Table 102-2) and course of treatment, the clinician must consider the infecting agent, clinical manifestations of the disease, immune status of the host, antimicrobial resistance, drug side effect profile, and direct and indirect costs of treatment. Treatment has become more complex because of immune system compromise in infected patients being treated for transplant rejection, autoimmune disorders, malignant disease, and AIDS. In AIDS-related cases, after the initial control of infection, lifelong oral suppressive therapy is mandated by the high frequency of recurrence, although successful antiretroviral therapy may modify this risk.[86]

Itraconazole has become the first choice for treatment of the endemic mycoses—blastomycosis, histoplasmosis, and sporotrichosis. The initial dose is 200 mg/day, which should be increased to twice daily if a clinical response is not obtained in 2 to 3 weeks. At least 6 months of treatment is required, and some patients may need up to a year of therapy. For cryptococcosis, fluconazole is the recommended azole.[25,28] Amphotericin B is the preferred drug for meningeal and life-threatening infections. Specific treatment protocols and detailed side effect profiles are presented in reviews[76-84] and infection-specific references (see Table 102-2).

REFERENCES

1. Giles JT, Bathon JM: Serious infections associated with anticytokine therapies in the rheumatic diseases. J Intensive Care Med 19:320-334, 2004.
2. Blair JE, Smilack JD, Caples SM: Coccidioidomycosis in patients with hematologic malignancies. Arch Intern Med 165:113-117, 2005.
3. Bialek R, Gonzalez GM, Begerow D, Zelck UE: Coccidioidomycosis and blastomycosis: Advances in molecular diagnosis. FEMS Immunol Med Microbiol 45:355-360, 2005.
4. Chiller TM, Galgiani JN, Stevens DA: Coccidioidomycosis. Infect Dis Clin North Am 17:41-57, 2003.
5. Holley K, Muldoon M, Taskar S: *Coccidioides immitis* osteomyelitis: A case series review. Orthopedics 25:827-831, 2002.
6. Bayer AS, Guze LB: Fungal arthritis. II. Coccidioidal synovitis: Clinical, diagnostic, therapeutic, and prognostic considerations. Semin Arthritis Rheum 8:200-211, 1979.
7. Stadalnik RC, Goldstein E, Hoeprich PD, et al: Diagnostic value of gallium and bone scans in evaluation of extrapulmonary coccidioidal lesions. Am Rev Respir Dis 121:673-676, 1980.
8. Galgiani JN, Ampel NM, Blair JE, et al: Treatment guidelines for coccidioidomycosis. Clin Infect Dis 41:1217-1223, 2005.
9. Bried JM, Galgiani JN: *Coccidioides immitis* infections in bones and joints. Clin Orthop Relat Res 211:235-243, 1986.
10. **Galgiani JN, Catanzaro A, Cloud GA, et al: Comparison of oral fluconazole and itraconazole for progressive, nonmeningeal coccidioidomycosis: A randomized, double-blind trial. Ann Intern Med 133:676-686, 2000.**
11. Graybill JR, Stevens DA, Galgiani JN, et al: Itraconazole treatment of coccidioidomycosis. Am J Med 89:282-290, 1990.
12. Smith CE: Coccidioidomycosis. Pediatr Clin North Am 62:109-125, 1955.
13. Bradsher RW, Chapman SW, Pappas PG: Blastomycosis. Infect Dis Clin North Am 17:21-40, 2003.
14. Bayer AS, Scott VJ, Guze LB: Fungal arthritis. IV. Blastomycotic arthritis. Semin Arthritis Rheum 9:145-151, 1979.
15. MacDonald PB, Black GB, MacKenzie R: Orthopaedic manifestations of blastomycosis. J Bone Joint Surg Am 72:860-864, 1990.
16. Pritchard DJ: Granulomatous infections of the bones and joints. Orthop Clin North Am 6:1029-1047, 1975.
17. Saccente M, Abernathy RS, Pappas PG, et al: Vertebral blastomycosis with paravertebral abscess: Report of eight cases and review of the literature. Clin Infect Dis 26:413-418, 1998.
18. Abril A, Campbell MD, Cotten VR, et al: Polyarticular blastomycotic arthritis. J Rheumatol 25:1019-1021, 1998.
19. Bradsher RW: Therapy of blastomycosis. Semin Respir Infect 12:263-267, 1997.
20. **Chapman SW, Bradsher RW Jr, Campbell DG, et al: Practice guidelines for the management of patients with blastomycosis. Clin Infect Dis 30:679-683, 2000.**
21. Levitz SM: The ecology of *Cryptococcus neoformans* and the epidemiology of cryptococcosis. J Infect Dis 13:1163-1169, 1991.
22. True DG, Penmetcha M, Peckham SJ: Disseminated cryptococcal infection in rheumatoid arthritis treated with methotrexate and infliximab. J Rheumatol 29:1561-1563, 2002.
23. Behrman RE, Masci JR, Nicholas P: Cryptococcal skeletal infections: Case report and review. Rev Infect Dis 12:181-190, 1900.
24. Bayer AS, Choi C, Tillman DB, Guze LB: Fungal arthritis. V. Cryptococcal and histoplasmal arthritis. Semin Arthritis Rheum 9:218-227, 1980.
25. Bruno KM, Farhoomand L, Libman BS, et al: Cryptococcal arthritis, tendonitis, tenosynovitis, and carpal tunnel syndrome: Report of a case and review of the literature. Arthritis Rheum 47:104-108, 2002
26. Gave AA, Torres R, Kaplan L: Cryptococcal myositis and vasculitis: An unusual necrotizing soft tissue infection. Surg Infect 5:309-313, 2004.
27. Basaran O, Emiroglu R, Arikan U, et al: Cryptococcal necrotizing fasciitis with multiple sites of involvement in the lower extremities. Dermatol Surg 29:1158-1160, 2003.
28. **Saag MS, Graybill RJ, Larsen RA, et al: Practice guidelines for the management of cryptococcal disease. Infectious Diseases Society of America. Clin Infect Dis 30:710-718, 2000.**
29. Edwards JE Jr: *Candida* species. In Mandell GL, Bennett JE, Dolin R (eds): Mandell, Douglas, and Bennett's Principles and Practice of Infectious Diseases. Philadelphia, Churchill Livingstone, 2000, pp 2656-2674.
30. McCullers JA, Flynn PM: *Candida tropicalis* osteomyelitis: Case report and review. Clin Infect Dis 26:1000-1001, 1998.
31. Arias F, Mata-Essayag S, Landaeta ME, et al: *Candida albicans* osteomyelitis: Case report and literature review. Int J Infect Dis 8:307-314, 2004.
32. Lafont A, Olive A, Gelman M, et al: *Candida albicans* spondylodiscitis and vertebral osteomyelitis in patients with intravenous heroin drug addiction: Report of 3 new cases. J Rheumatol 21:953-956, 1994.

33. Chia SL, Tan BH, Tan CT, Tan SB: Candida spondylodiscitis and epidural abscess: Management with shorter courses of anti-fungal therapy in combination with surgical debridement. J Infect 51:17-23, 2005.

34. Harrington JT: The evolving role of direct amplification tests in diagnosing osteoarticular infections caused by mycobacteria and fungi. Curr Opin Rheumatol 11:289-292, 1999.

35. Martin MV: The use of fluconazole and itraconazole in the treatment of Candida albicans infections: A review. J Antimicrob Chemother 44:429-437, 1999.

36. **Pappas PG, Rex JH, Sobel JD, et al: Guidelines for treatment of candidiasis. Clin Infect Dis 38:161-189, 2004.**

37. Bayer AS, Guze LB: Fungal arthritis. I. Candida arthritis: Diagnostic and prognostic implications and therapeutic considerations. Semin Arthritis Rheum 8:142-150, 1978.

38. Barson WJ, Marcon MJ: Successful therapy of Candida albicans arthritis with a sequential intravenous amphotericin B and oral fluconazole regimen. Pediatr Infect Dis J 15:1119-1122, 1996.

39. Weers-Pothoff G, Havermans JF, Kamphuis J, et al: Candida tropicalis arthritis in a patient with acute myeloid leukemia successfully treated with fluconazole: Case report and review of the literature. Infection 25:109-111, 1997.

40. Evdoridou J, Roilides E, Bibashi G, et al: Multifocal osteoarthritis due to Candida albicans in a neonate: Serum level monitoring of liposomal amphotericin B and literature review. Infection 25:112-116, 1997.

41. Fraucher J-F, Thiebaut M-M, Reynes J, et al: Unusual outcome of disseminated candidiasis treated with fluconazole: A matter of pharmacodynamics. Clin Infect Dis 26:197-198, 1998.

42. Arena FP, Perlin M, Brahman H: Fever, rash, and myalgias of disseminated candidiasis during antifungal therapy. Arch Intern Med 141:1233, 1981.

43. Fornadley JA, Parker GS, Rickman LS, et al: Candida myositis manifesting as a discrete neck mass. Otolaryngol Head Neck Surg 102:74-76, 1990.

44. Behar SM, Chertow GM: Olecranon bursitis caused by infection with Candida lusitaniae. J Rheumatol 25:598-600, 1998.

45. Morris-Jones R: Sporotrichosis. Clin Exp Dermatol 27:427-431, 2002.

46. Gottlieb GS, Lesser CF, Holmes KK, Wald A: Disseminated sporotrichosis associated with treatment with immunosuppressants and tumor necrosis factor-α antagonists. Clin Infect Dis 37:838-840, 2003.

47. Bayer AS, Scott VJ, Guze LB: Fungal arthritis. III. Sporotrichal arthritis. Semin Arthritis Rheum 9:66-74, 1979.

48. Crout JE, Brewer NS, Tompkins RB: Sporotrichosis arthritis: Clinical features in seven patients. Ann Intern Med 86:294-297, 1977.

49. Wilson DE, Mann JJ, Bennett JE, Utz JP: Clinical features of extracutaneous sporotrichosis. Medicine (Baltimore) 46:265-279, 1967.

50. Lynch PJ, Voorhees JJ, Harrell ER: Systemic sporotrichosis. Ann Intern Med 73:23-30, 1970.

51. Oscherwitz SL, Rinaldi MG: Disseminated sporotrichosis in a patient infected with human immunodeficiency virus. Clin Infect Dis 15:568-569, 1992.

52. al-Tawfiq JA, Wools KK: Disseminated sporotrichosis and Sporothrix schenckii fungemia as the initial presentation of immunodeficiency infection. Clin Infect Dis 26:1403-1406, 1998.

53. Sharkey-Mathis PK, Kauffman CA, Graybill JR, Stevens DA: Treatment of sporotrichosis with itraconazole: Am J Med 95:279-285, 1993.

54. **Kauffman CA, Hajjeh R, Chapman SW: Practice guidelines for management of patients with sporotrichosis. For the Mycoses Study Group, Infectious Diseases Society of America. Clin Infect Dis 30:684-687, 2000.**

55. Cuellar ML, Silveira LH, Espinoza LR: Fungal arthritis. Ann Rheum Dis 51:690-697, 1992.

56. Kontoyiannis DP, Bodey GP: Invasive aspergillosis in 2002: An update. Eur J Microbiol Infect Dis 21:161-172, 2002.

57. Dotis J, Roilides E: Osteomyelitis due to Aspergillus spp. in patients with chronic granulomatous disease: Comparison of Aspergillus nidulans and Aspergillus fumigatus. Int J Infect Dis 8:103-110, 2004.

58. Pasic S, Abinun M, Pistignjat B, et al: Aspergillus osteomyelitis in chronic granulomatous disease: Treatment with recombinant gamma-interferon and itraconazole. Pediatr Infect Dis J 15:833-834, 1996.

59. Vinas FC, King PK, Diaz FG: Spinal aspergillus osteomyelitis. Clin Infect Dis 28:1223-1229, 1999.

60. Paterson DL: New clinical presentations of invasive aspergillosis in non-conventional hosts. Clin Microbiol Infect 10(Suppl 1):24-30, 2004.

61. Steinfeld S, Durez P, Hauzeur J-P, et al: Articular aspergillosis: Two case reports and review of the literature. Br J Rheumatol 36:1331-1334, 1997.

62. **Perfect JR, Marr KA, Walsh TJ, et al: Voriconazole treatment for less-common, emerging, or refractory fungal infections. Clin Infect Dis 36:1122-1131, 2003.**

63. Stratov I, Korman TM, Johnson PD: Management of aspergillus osteomyelitis: Report of failure of liposomal amphotericin B and response to voriconazole in an immunocompetent host and literature review. Eur Clin Microbiol Infect Dis 22:277-283, 2003.

64. Wheat J: Histoplasmosis: Recognition and treatment. Clin Infect Dis 19(Suppl 1):S19-S27, 1994.

65. Weinberg JM, Ali R, Badve S, Pelker RR: Musculoskeletal histoplasmosis: A case report and review of the literature. J Bone Joint Surg Am 83:1718-1722, 2001.

66. Lee JH, Slifman NR, Gershon SK, et al: Life-threatening histoplasmosis complicating immunotherapy with tumor necrosis factor alpha antagonists infliximab and etanercept. Arthritis Rheum 46:2565-2570, 2002.

67. Wood KL, Hage C, Knox KS, et al: Histoplasmosis after treatment with anti-tumor necrosis factor-α therapy. Am J Respir Crit Care Med 167:1279-1282, 2003.

68. Wheat LJ: Laboratory diagnosis of histoplasmosis: Update 2000. Semin Respir Infect 16:131, 2001.

69. Fowler VG, Nacinovich FM, Alspaugh JA, et al: Prosthetic joint infection due to Histoplasma capsulatum: Case report and review. Clin Infect Dis 26:1017, 1998.

70. **Wheat J, Sarosi G, McKinsey D, et al: Practice guidelines for management of patients with histoplasmosis. Infectious Diseases Society of America. Clin Infect Dis 30:688-695, 2000.**

71. Mocherla S, Wheat JL: Treatment of histoplasmosis. Semin Respir Infect 16:141-148, 2001.

72. Wilson CM, O'Rourke EJ, McGinnis MR, Salkin IF: Scedosporium inflatum: Clinical spectrum of a newly recognized pathogen. J Infect Dis 161:102-107, 1990.

73. Levine NB, Kurokawa R, Fichtenbaum CJ, et al: An immunocompetent patient with primary Scedosporium apiospermum vertebral osteomyelitis. J Spinal Disord Tech 15:425-430, 2002.

74. Steinbach WJ, Schell WA, Miller JL, Perfect JR: Scedosporium prolificans osteomyelitis in an immunocompetent child treated with voriconazole and caspofungin, as well as locally applied polyhexamethylene biguanide. J Clin Microbiol 41:3981-3985, 2003.

75. Studahl M, Backteman T, Staulhammar F, et al: Bone and joint infection after traumatic implantation of Scedosporium prolificans treated with voriconazole and surgery. Acta Paediatr 92:980-982, 2003.

76. Terrell CL, Hughes CE: Antifungal agents used for deep-seated mycotic infections. Mayo Clin Proc 67:69-91, 1992.

77. Sarosi GA, Davies SF: Therapy for fungal infections. Mayo Clin Proc 69:1111-1117, 1994.

78. Meier JL: Mycobacterial and fungal infections of the bones and joints. Curr Opin Rheumatol 6:408-414, 1994.

79. Martino P, Girmenia C: Are we making progress in antifungal therapy? Curr Opin Oncol 9:314-320, 1997.

80. Perez-Gomez A, Prieto A, Torresano M, et al: Role of the new azoles in the treatment of fungal osteoarticular infections. Semin Arthritis Rheum 27:226-244, 1998.

81. Rapp RP, Gubbins PO, Evans ME: Amphotericin B lipid complex. Ann Pharmacother 31:1174-1186, 1997.

82. Alexander BD, Perfect JR: Antifungal resistance trends toward the year 2000: Implications for therapy and new approaches. Drugs 54:657-678, 1997.

83. Espinel-Ingroff A: Clinical relevance of antifungal resistance. Infect Dis Clin North Am 11:929-944, 1997.

84. Summers KK, Hardin TC, Gore SJ, Graybill JR: Therapeutic drug monitoring of systemic antifungal therapy. J Antimicrob Chemother 40:753-764, 1997.

85. Mora-Duarte J, Bettis R, Rotstein C, et al: Comparison of caspofungin and amphotericin B for invasive candidiasis. N Engl J Med 347:2020-2029, 2002.

86. Currier JS, Williams PL, Koletar SL, et al: Discontinuation of Mycobacterium avium complex prophylaxis in patients with anti-retroviral therapy-induced increases in CD4+ cell count: A randomized double-blind, placebo-controlled trial. AIDS Clinical Trials Study Group 362 Study Team. Ann Intern Med 133:493-503, 2000.

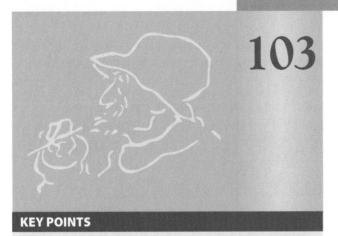

103

Rheumatic Manifestations of Human Immunodeficiency Virus Infection

JOHN D. REVEILLE • RASHMI M. MAGANTI

KEY POINTS

With patients with human immunodeficiency virus (HIV) living longer as a result of more effective and available treatments, the challenges of HIV-associated rheumatic manifestations are growing.

Certain diseases seem to be particular to HIV infection (i.e., HIV-associated arthritis, diffuse infiltrative lymphocytosis syndrome [DILS], HIV-associated polymyositis).

Other diseases, specifically CD4-mediated diseases such as rheumatoid arthritis and systemic lupus erythematosus, tend to go into remission with disease activity and flare with antiretroviral treatment.

Effective antiretroviral therapy has resulted in certain diseases (i.e., DILS, late opportunistic infections) decreasing in prevalence, but also is associated with new side effects (e.g., osteonecrosis, myopathy, rhabdomyolysis).

With immune reconstitution after antiretroviral therapy, a new spectrum of autoimmune and autoinflammatory disease has emerged requiring special attention.

In the years since acquired immunodeficiency syndrome (AIDS) was initially described in 1981, the human immunodeficiency virus (HIV) pandemic has become one of the leading global health crises. According to new data in the UNAIDS 2006 report, the AIDS epidemic seems to be slowing down globally, but new cases are continuing to increase at alarming rates in certain regions, such as southern Africa, Eastern Europe, and central and eastern Asia. An estimated 39 million people are living with HIV worldwide (Fig. 103-1). Approximately 4.1 million people became newly infected with HIV in 2005, and 2.8 million people died. More than 92% of new cases occur in developing countries.

Progress in dealing with the HIV epidemic, including in education and public health awareness, has undoubtedly influenced the decrease in prevalence seen among young people in some countries in recent years. As availability of newer treatment strategies and better access to health care result in increased life expectancy in the next decade, it is expected that HIV infection increasingly will be managed as a chronic illness, and complications such as musculoskeletal and rheumatic conditions associated with HIV infection and its treatment are expected to increase (Table 103-1).

Among the rheumatologic disorders, clinicians face the challenge of treating potentially disabling inflammatory disorders with immunosuppressive therapy in the face of ongoing viral-induced immunocompromise. Diagnosing infection is especially important in an immunocompromised patient because the probability of an opportunistic infection as a cause for a musculoskeletal complaint increases with advancing stages of the patient's HIV disease. At early stages (CD4+ count >300/μL), opportunistic infections are unlikely, although bacterial infections (especially tuberculosis) still can occur. There should be a very high threshold to using immunosuppressive drugs in this population.

HUMAN IMMUNODEFICIENCY VIRUS–ASSOCIATED BONE AND JOINT DISEASE

HUMAN IMMUNODEFICIENCY VIRUS–ASSOCIATED ARTHRALGIA

Forty-five percent of HIV-positive patients may have otherwise unexplained arthralgia (Table 103-2); arthralgias and myalgias also form a part of the constitutional symptoms of HIV seroconversion. Whether the arthralgia can be attributed to circulating viral and host immune complexes owing to HIV infection per se or to other infections (e.g., hepatitis C) has not been determined. The pathogenesis is unclear, but may involve cytokines or transient bone ischemia.[1] Patients presenting with arthralgia alone rarely progress to inflammatory joint disease, however. The most appropriate treatment is non-narcotic analgesics and reassurance.

PAINFUL ARTICULAR SYNDROME

Painful articular syndrome is a self-limited syndrome lasting less than 24 hours, associated with few objective clinical findings, and characterized by severe bone and joint pain.[2] It occurs predominantly in the late stages of HIV infection. Its etiology is unknown, and there is no evidence of synovitis in these patients. The knee is most commonly affected, but the elbow and shoulders also can be involved. Radiographic features are nonspecific; occasionally, periarticular osteopenia is seen. Treatment is symptomatic.

HUMAN IMMUNODEFICIENCY VIRUS–ASSOCIATED ARTHRITIS

The first reports of a seronegative arthritis associated with HIV infection appeared in 1988, with frequencies of 12% (Table 103-3). HIV-associated arthritis seems to be most common in sub-Saharan Africa, where HIV infection is pandemic. In the Congo, where the seroprevalence of HIV infection is 7% to 8%, AIDS is the leading cause of aseptic arthritis (60% of cases).[3] This is usually an oligoarthritis,

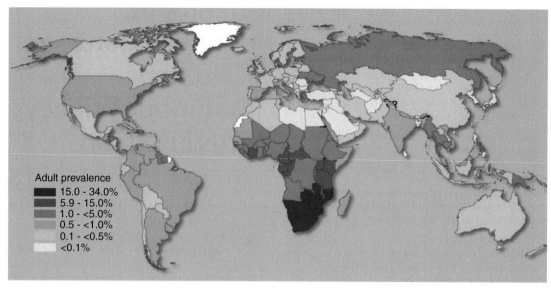

Figure 103-1 A global view of human immunodeficiency virus (HIV) infection—39 million living with HIV in 2005. *(Extracted from 2006 Report on the Global AIDS Epidemic. UNAIDS, 2006.)*

predominantly involving the lower extremities, and tends to be self-limited, lasting less than 6 weeks.[2,4] Most commonly involved are the knees (84%), ankles (59%), and metatarsophalangeal joints (23%) in the lower limbs and the wrists (41%), elbows (29%), and metacarpophalangeal and interphalangeal joints (25%) in the upper limbs, similar to other viral arthritides. Some patients have been reported as having a longer course, however, with joint destruction.[5,6]

The etiology is unclear; there is no association with HLA-B27 or any other known genetic factor. Synovial fluid cultures are typically sterile, although one report described the presence of tubuloreticular inclusions, suggesting a viral etiology, possibly HIV itself.[2,4] Radiographs of the affected joints are usually normal except in uncommon cases with prolonged symptoms, in which joint space narrowing and destruction can occur. Treatment includes nonsteroidal

Table 103-1 Rheumatic Diseases Associated with or Occurring in Patients with Human Immunodeficiency Virus (HIV) Infection

Unique to HIV Infection	Encountered in HIV-Infected Patients	Ameliorated by HIV Infection but Worsening or Reappearing with IRIS
Diffuse infiltrative leukocytosis syndrome	HIV-associated Reiter's syndrome	Rheumatoid arthritis
HIV-associated arthritis	Polymyositis	Systemic lupus erythematosus
Zidovudine-associated myopathy	Psoriatic arthritis	
Painful articular syndrome	Polyarteritis nodosa	
	Giant cell arteritis	
	Hypersensitivity angiitis	
	Wegener's granulomatosis	
	Henoch-Schönlein purpura	
	Behçet's syndrome	
	Infectious arthritis (bacterial, fungal)	

IRIS, immune reconstitution inflammatory syndrome.

Table 103-2 Distribution of Various Rheumatic Diseases from Various Sites

Feature	Cincinnati, Ohio	Houston, Texas	Madrid, Spain
No. patients	1100	4467	556
HIV-associated arthralgia	NA	0.7%	1.6%
Myalgia	0.7%	0.6%	4.5%
PsA/Reiter's syndrome	0.5%	0.6%	0.5%
HIV-associated arthritis	0%	0.47%	0.4%
DILS/Sjögren's syndrome	NR	3%-4%	NR

DILS, diffuse infiltrative lymphocytosis syndrome; HIV, human immunodeficiency virus; NA, not applicable; NR, not reported; PsA, psoriatic arthritis.

Table 103-3 Contrasting Features of Human Immunodeficiency Virus (HIV)–Associated Arthritis and Reiter's Syndrome

Feature	HIV-Associated Arthritis	HIV-Associated Reactive Arthritis
Joint involvement	Asymmetric oligoarthritis/polyarthritis	Asymmetric oligoarthritis/polyarthritis
Mucocutaneous involvement	Absent	Present
Enthesopathy	Absent	Frequent
Synovial fluid white blood cell count	500-2000/μL	2000-10,000/μL
Synovial fluid cultures	Negative	Negative
Microorganisms in synovial membranes	HIV-1 virus (?)	*Chlamydia**
HLA-B27 association	Absent	70%-90%†

*Shown in non–HIV-associated Reiter's syndrome. Reports of such infections in patients with HIV-associated Reiter's syndrome are lacking.
†In whites.

anti-inflammatory drugs (NSAIDs) and, in more severe cases, low-dose glucocorticoids. Hydroxychloroquine and sulfasalazine also have been used.[7]

REACTIVE ARTHRITIS OCCURRING IN HUMAN IMMUNODEFICIENCY VIRUS INFECTION

Early reports in the United States suggested that reactive arthritis occurred more commonly in the setting of HIV infection; however, later studies showed that this may be reflective of the sexually active nature of the population at highest risk for HIV infection.[8] This contention is not borne out in studies from sub-Saharan Africa, where HLA-B27 is rare, as were reports of spondyloarthritis before the HIV epidemic. With the arrival of AIDS, a dramatic upsurge in the prevalence of reactive arthritis and undifferentiated spondyloarthritis, and less often psoriatic arthritis,[6,9] was seen, suggesting a pathogenic role of HIV infection.

The typical presentation is a seronegative lower extremity peripheral arthritis, usually accompanied by enthesitis (sausaging of toes or fingers, Achilles tendinitis, and plantar fasciitis). Mucocutaneous features are common, especially keratoderma blennorrhagicum (Fig. 103-2) and circinate balanitis. Extensive psoriaform skin rashes can occur. The clinical overlap makes it difficult sometimes to distinguish HIV-associated reactive arthritis from psoriatic arthritis.[10] Urethritis occurs in similar frequency as in HIV-negative reactive arthritis. Axial involvement and uveitis seem to be less common, but do occur. Longitudinal studies from Africa have described an aggressive course with a poor prognosis.[11,12]

HLA-B27 is found in 80% to 90% of patients with HIV-associated reactive arthritis, at least in whites.[10] Studies from Africa have found most to be HLA-B27 negative, however.[6,9] Some studies suggest the presence of HLA-B27 antigen may slow the progression to AIDS.[11,12] In asymptomatic HIV-infected, HLA-B27–positive individuals, cytotoxic T lymphocyte response is dominated by recognition of a gag-encoded p24 protein epitope that is not seen in HIV-positive, HLA-B27–negative individuals.[13,14] Other HLA class I antigens that have been associated with a better outcome in HIV infection also have been implicated in psoriasis and psoriatic arthritis and include HLA-B13 and HLA-B17 (B57, B58).[12,13] HLA-B*2703 was protective against HIV progression in a Zambian population.[15]

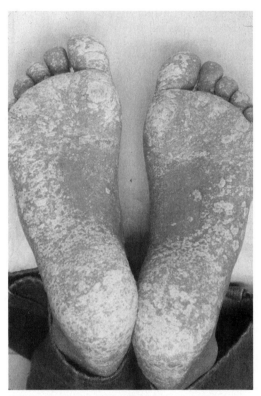

Figure 103-2 Keratoderma blennorrhagicum in a patient with Reiter's syndrome and human immunodeficiency virus infection.

Treatment

The treatment is similar to that for HIV-negative patients with reactive arthritis. NSAIDs are the mainstay; in particular, indomethacin is recommended, not only for its efficacy, but also for its inhibition of HIV replication that has been observed in vitro, which seems to be unique to this NSAID.[16] Patients frequently have an inadequate response to NSAIDs alone. Sulfasalazine has been shown to be effective in some studies at doses of 2 g/day, and one study suggested that it ameliorated HIV infection.[17,18] Methotrexate was initially believed to be contraindicated because of its immunosuppressive effect, but with careful monitoring of HIV viral loads, CD4+ counts, and the patient's clinical status, more recent studies have suggested a place for methotrexate in the treatment of reactive arthritis and psoriatic arthritis occurring in HIV infection.[19]

Hydroxychloroquine also has been reported to be efficacious not only in treating HIV-associated reactive arthritis, but also in reducing HIV replication in vitro and in reducing HIV viral loads in vivo.[20] The arthritis and the cutaneous lesions of HIV-associated reactive arthritis and psoriatic arthritis have been found to respond to etretinate (0.5 to 1 mg/kg/day),[21] although because of the side effects of this drug, its use should be reserved for patients unresponsive to other treatments. Tumor necrosis factor blockers also have been used,[22,23] although these agents should be used with extreme caution and only in patients with CD4+ counts greater than 200 mm[3] and HIV viral load less than 60,000 copies/mm[3].[24,25]

PSORIASIS AND PSORIATIC ARTHRITIS

The psoriatic rash can be extensive (Fig. 103-3) in HIV-positive patients, especially in patients not on antiretroviral treatment.[26] A report from Zambia found 27 of 28 African patients with psoriatic arthritis to be HIV positive.[27] The arthritis was predominantly polyarticular, lower limb, and progressive. Psoriasis was commonly an extensive guttate-plaque admixture and, in contrast to the articular disease, was nonremittive with onset of AIDS.[28] Antiretroviral treatment has been shown to be effective in treating HIV-associated psoriasis and its associated arthritis.[29] Phototherapy may improve the skin rash, but also may enhance viral replication and worsen HIV disease. Other agents reported to be efficacious include cyclosporine (although renal function must be monitored carefully) and etretinate. Methotrexate also can be used, albeit with caution.[19] Tumor necrosis factor blockers may be used in patients with refractory disease,

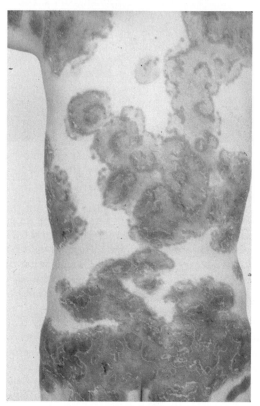

Figure 103-3 Disseminated psoriasis vulgaris in a patient with human immunodeficiency virus–associated psoriasis.

although with the usual cautions (see earlier) because frequent polymicrobial infections while on the drug resulted in its discontinuation in some patients.[30]

UNDIFFERENTIATED SPONDYLOARTHRITIS

Symptoms of reactive arthritis or psoriatic arthritis are found in patients who do not otherwise develop full-blown disease, such as enthesopathy (plantar fasciitis, Achilles tendinitis).[31] The treatment is symptomatic (NSAIDs, intralesional corticosteroid injections), although sulfasalazine should be considered in patients with more extensive disease.

AVASCULAR NECROSIS OF BONE

Most cases of osteonecrosis have occurred after the introduction of highly active antiretroviral therapy (HAART).[32] Dyslipidemia associated with protease inhibitors has been implicated most frequently, although there have been no controlled studies to establish if antiretroviral drugs per se predispose to this.[33] Other contributing factors include alcohol abuse and use of corticosteroids, megestrol acetate, and antiphospholipid antibodies.[34] The most common presenting symptom of osteonecrosis is pain on weight bearing and activity.[35] Some patients may be asymptomatic, and the diagnosis is made based on incidental findings in radiologic studies. Most patients tend to present when subchondral collapse already has occurred. Radiographs, computed tomography (CT), magnetic resonance imaging (MRI), and nuclear medicine studies have been used successfully to diagnose osteonecrosis, as in HIV-negative patients.

HYPERTROPHIC PULMONARY OSTEOARTHROPATHY

Hypertrophic pulmonary osteoarthropathy affects bones, joints, and soft tissues and can develop in HIV-infected patients with *Pneumocystis carinii* pneumonia. It is characterized by severe pain in the lower extremity; digital clubbing; arthralgia; nonpitting edema; and periarticular soft tissue involvement of the ankle, knees, and elbows. The skin over the affected areas is glistening, edematous, and warm. Radiography reveals extensive periosteal reaction and subperiosteal proliferative changes in the long bones of the lower extremity. A bone scan shows increased uptake along the cortical surfaces. Treatment of *P. carinii* pneumonia usually alleviates this condition.[36]

OSTEOPENIA AND OSTEOPOROSIS

Osteopenia and osteoporosis occur more than three times as commonly in HIV-infected patients regardless of antiretroviral treatment[37] and can result in pathologic fractures. Abnormal bone metabolism was attributed to the HIV infection itself by some authors.[38] Risk factors for the development of osteopenia are use of protease inhibitors, longer duration of HIV infection, high viral load, high lactate levels, low bicarbonate levels, increased alkaline phosphatase level, and lower body weight before antiretroviral therapy.[39] Bisphosphonates and, in patients with HIV wasting syndrome, testosterone have been used to preserve bone density.[40]

HUMAN IMMUNODEFICIENCY VIRUS–ASSOCIATED MUSCLE DISEASE

Muscle involvement in HIV infection varies from uncomplicated myalgias or asymptomatic creatine kinase elevation to severe, disabling, HIV-associated polymyositis or pyomyositis. HIV seroconversion also can coincide with myoglobinuria and acute myalgia, suggesting that myotropism for HIV may be present early in the infection.

MYALGIA AND FIBROMYALGIA

One third of HIV-positive outpatients complain of myalgias,[41] and 11% complain of fibromyalgia.[42] Fibromyalgia is associated with longer disease duration and a history of depression. Treatment is similar to that for fibromyalgia in the non-HIV setting.

NONINFLAMMATORY NECROTIZING MYOPATHY AND HUMAN IMMUNODEFICIENCY VIRUS–RELATED WASTING SYNDROME

Severe wasting from chronic infections, malignancy, malabsorption, and nutritional deficiency often accounts for weakness and disability in patients with AIDS. This wasting leads to loss of lean body and muscle mass. Cachexia and muscle wasting associated with HIV is called "slim's disease" in Africa. A noninflammatory necrotizing myopathy of unclear pathogenesis has been described, accounting for 42% of patients diagnosed with myopathy.[43] Even in patients without significant wasting, muscle biopsy specimens have shown diffuse atrophy, mild neurogenic atrophy, or thick filament loss without conspicuous inflammation. Whether this condition is immune mediated, as some have suggested,[44] or due to metabolic or nutritional factors is unclear. Corticosteroids have been reported to restore muscle strength and mass.[45]

NEMALINE MYOPATHY

Nemaline myopathy is a rare disorder that has been described in some HIV-positive patients, in addition to occurring as a congenital disorder. Nemaline myopathy represents a nonspecific myofibril alteration resulting from Z band disruption.[46] Muscle biopsy specimens disclose prominent, randomly distributed atrophic type 1 fibers with numerous intracytoplasmic rod bodies in the centers of the fibers, corresponding to nemaline rods at electron microscopy. Necrotic fibers and inflammatory infiltrates usually are not found. Some patients have been described to have associated monoclonal gammopathy.[47] Although there is no inflammation, corticosteroids may be useful.

HUMAN IMMUNODEFICIENCY VIRUS–ASSOCIATED POLYMYOSITIS

HIV-associated polymyositis most typically manifests early in the course of HIV infection and may be the presenting feature. In one large series of HIV-positive outpatients from a county clinic in Texas, the frequency was 2.2/1000.[48] The pathogenesis of HIV-associated polymyositis is unclear—possibly stemming from direct viral invasion (leading to a cytopathic effect and subsequent muscle necrosis), as

suggested in one pathologic study,[49] or from an autoimmune response of the HIV host, as suggested by another study.[50]

The most common manifestation is a subacute, progressive proximal muscle weakness occurring in the setting of an elevated creatine kinase. Myalgia is not a prominent presenting feature. Skin involvement is unusual, as is involvement of extraocular muscles and facial muscles.[51]

On MRI, T2-weighted studies with or without fat saturation show high signal intensity without rim enhancement, in contrast to in pyomyositis, in which rim enhancement is seen.[52] MRI also is helpful in guiding muscle biopsy, the definitive diagnostic test. Electromyographic studies reveal myopathic motor unit potentials with early recruitment and full interference patterns and fibrillation potentials, positive sharp waves, and complex repetitive discharges indicative of an irritative process. Light microscopy of muscle biopsy specimens shows interstitial inflammatory infiltrates of variable intensity accompanied by degenerating and regenerating myofibrils, similar to those seen in polymyositis without HIV-1 (Fig. 103-4). Concomitant vasculitis rarely occurs. In specimens from HIV-positive and HIV-negative patients with myositis, the predominant cell populations were CD8+ T cells and macrophages invading or surrounding healthy muscle fibers that express major histocompatibility complex (MHC) class I antigens on their cell surfaces.[53] The endomysial infiltrates in specimens from HIV-positive patients differed from patients with polymyositis without HIV infection only by a significant reduction of CD4+ cells.[50]

Treatment is similar to that for other inflammatory myopathies. The creatine kinase elevation and the muscle weakness respond to moderate-dose glucocorticoids.[48] Refractory cases may require immunosuppressive agents, such as methotrexate, azathioprine, or mycophenolate mofetil. Intravenous immunoglobulin has been used with some success. These agents should be used with caution, however, with careful monitoring of the patient's clinical status, CD4+ counts, and HIV mRNA levels (Table 103-4).

Creatine kinase elevation is commonly encountered in outpatients with HIV infection, secondary to HIV per se, behaviors associated with higher risk for HIV infection (e.g., cocaine use), or HIV treatment.[48] In most patients, these elevations are transient and of little consequence, but they require careful follow-up for any sign of clinical deterioration before electrodiagnostic and biopsy studies are undertaken.

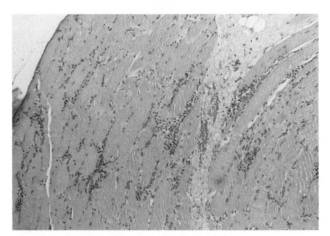

Figure 103-4 Muscle biopsy specimen from a patient with human immunodeficiency virus–associated polymyositis.

Table 103-4 Myopathies Associated with Human Immunodeficiency Virus (HIV) Infection

HIV-Associated Myopathies	Myopathies Secondary to Antiretrovirals	Others
HIV polymyositis	Zidovudine myopathy	Opportunistic infections involving muscle
Inclusion-body myositis	Toxic mitochondrial myopathies related to other NRTIs	Tumor infiltrations of skeletal muscle
Nemaline myopathy	HIV-associated lipodystrophy syndrome	Rhabdomyolysis
Diffuse infiltrative lymphocytosis syndrome	Immune restoration syndrome related to HAART	
HIV-wasting syndrome		
Vasculitic processes		
Myasthenia gravis and other myasthenic syndromes		
Chronic fatigue and fibromyalgia		

HAART, highly active antiretroviral therapy; NRTIs, nucleoside-analogue reverse-transcriptase inhibitors.

INCLUSION BODY MYOSITIS

Inclusion body myositis has been recognized as a complication of HIV infection.[54] This condition is clinically, histologically, and immunologically identical to sporadic inclusion body myositis. Muscle biopsy specimens suggest two concurrently ongoing processes—an autoimmune-mediated process by cytotoxic T cells and a degenerative process manifested by the vacuolated muscle fibers and deposits of amyloid-related proteins. Of particular interest has been the finding of elevated mRNA levels and constitutive expression of Toll-like receptor 3, which is known to mediate inflammatory stimuli from pathogens and endogenous danger signals and to link the innate and adaptive immune system, in muscle fibers of patients with HIV-associated inclusion body myositis in close proximity of infiltrating mononuclear cells.[55]

MYOPATHY ASSOCIATED WITH TREATMENT

A reversible toxic mitochondrial myopathy occurring in patients who received high doses of zidovudine has been described, which manifests as myalgias, muscle tenderness, and proximal muscle weakness mimicking HIV polymyositis.[56] Histologically, it is characterized by the presence of *ragged red fibers*, a term coined to designate atrophic ragged red fibers with marked myofibril alterations, including thick myofilament loss and cytoplasmic body formation,[57] and minimal inflammatory infiltrates. The symptoms tend to improve as the drug is discontinued, with creatine kinase levels returning to normal within 4 weeks of discontinuing the drug, and muscle strength returning within 8 weeks. In any HIV-infected patient presenting with an elevated creatine kinase, especially when symptoms of myalgia or muscle weakness are present, zidovudine should be discontinued for 4 weeks and the patient re-evaluated before electromyography or muscle biopsies are undertaken.

RHABDOMYOLYSIS

Rhabdomyolysis can occur at all stages of HIV infection and may be separated into three groups: (1) HIV-associated rhabdomyolysis, including rhabdomyolysis in primary HIV infection, recurrent rhabdomyolysis, and isolated rhabdomyolysis; (2) drug-induced rhabdomyolysis; and (3) rhabdomyolysis at the end stage of AIDS, associated or not with opportunistic infections of muscle. Drugs implicated in rhabdomyolysis in HIV patients include didanosine, lamivudine, trimethoprim-sulfamethoxazole, ritonavir, and indinavir.[58]

DIFFUSE INFILTRATIVE LYMPHOCYTOSIS SYNDROME

Diffuse infiltrative lymphocytosis syndrome (DILS), found exclusively in HIV-positive patients, is characterized by salivary gland enlargement and peripheral CD8 lymphocytosis often accompanied by sicca symptoms and other extraglandular features. The prevalence of DILS is declining since the introduction of HAART.[59] Using parotid enlargement as a criterion, the prevalence in Houston, Texas, was 4% in the pre-HAART era, declining to 0.8% after the introduction of aggressive HIV therapy.[59,60] In another study from Greece, using xerophthalmia and xerostomia as the defining criteria (and requiring confirmatory minor salivary gland biopsy specimen and technetium scintigraphy),[61] the prevalence of DILS was 7.8% and decreased dramatically after the introduction of HAART.

The primary immunogenetic association has been with HLA-DRB1 alleles expressing the ILEDE amino acid sequence in the third diversity region—usually HLA-DRB1*1102, DRB1*1301, and DRB1*1302.[59,62] The delayed progression to AIDS in patients with DILS has been attributed to delay in the evolution of the HIV-1 virus from the less aggressive M-tropic strain to the more rapidly replicating T-tropic strain by a more effective CD8 lymphocyte response.[62] This response has been attributed in part to the finding of sequence homology of a six-residue epitope shared by HLA-DRB1 alleles associated with DILS with a V3 loop on M-tropic HIV strains. Studies of immunophenotypes of circulating and tissue-infiltrating lymphocytes and salivary gland T cell receptor sequence analysis suggested that DILS represents an MHC-restricted, antigen-driven, oligoclonal selection of CD8+, CD29− lymphocytes that express selective homing receptors and infiltrate the salivary glands, lungs, and other organs, where they are postulated to suppress HIV-1 replication.[63]

Minor salivary gland biopsy specimens show a focal sialadenitis, similar to that observed in Sjögren's syndrome, although there tends to be less destruction of the salivary glands (Fig. 103-5). CD8+ lymphocytes constitute most of

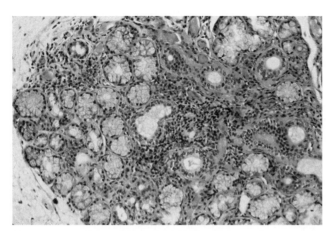

Figure 103-5 Minor salivary gland biopsy specimen from a patient with diffuse infiltrative lymphocytosis syndrome. Note the relative preservation of the glandular architecture, even with significant interstitial inflammation.

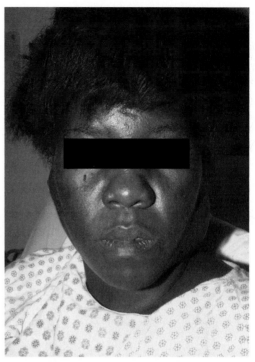

Figure 103-6 Massive bilateral asymmetric salivary gland enlargement in a patient with diffuse infiltrative lymphocytosis syndrome. This was the presenting feature of human immunodeficiency virus infection in this patient. CT revealed this to be a solid mass. At follow-up 2 years after this photograph was taken, the gland had not changed in size.

the inflammatory infiltrate,[64,65] in contrast to that seen in primary (non–HIV-associated) Sjögren's syndrome. Lymphoepithelial cysts are seen frequently in the parotid glands of patients with DILS, leading to inspissated salivary secretions that may be painful.

The characteristic, if not defining, presentation of DILS is painless parotid enlargement, often massive (Fig. 103-6). This enlargement is accompanied by sicca symptoms in greater than 60% of patients. Although parotid and submandibular enlargement is nearly universal in this disorder, certain extraglandular features also are prominent (Table 103-5). DILS and Sjögren's syndrome share some similarities and differences (Table 103-6).

Diagnostic criteria have been proposed for DILS as follows[66]:

1. HIV seropositive by enzyme-linked immunosorbent assay and Western blot analysis
2. Bilateral salivary gland enlargement or xerostomia persisting for more than 6 months
3. Histologic confirmation or salivary or lacrimal gland lymphocytic infiltration in the absence of granulomatous or neoplastic enlargement

Minor salivary gland biopsy specimens are usually positive (see Fig. 103-5). Gallium-67 scintigraphy (Fig. 103-7) of the salivary glands has been used when lip biopsy was not feasible or equivocal. Tc 99m pertechnetate scanning offers little diagnostic help. Scintigraphy is being used as a primary diagnostic aid in patients on protease inhibitors because minor salivary gland biopsy specimens are rarely positive in patients on these drugs. CT also has been used to determine the extent of glandular swelling and in the evaluation of parotid cysts and possible salivary glandular malignancy (Table 103-7).

Patients with asymptomatic glandular swelling and mild, if any, sicca symptoms can be observed over time. Antiretroviral treatment is effective in treating the glandular swelling and sicca symptoms associated with DILS and complications such as neuropathy.[59] We have found also that moderate doses of corticosteroids (30 to 40 mg/day of prednisone) are effective in treating the glandular swelling and sicca symptoms of DILS without adversely affecting the frequency of opportunistic infections, increasing the viral

Table 103-5 Extraglandular Features of Diffuse Infiltrative Lymphocytosis Syndrome

Pulmonary
Lymphocytic interstitial pneumonitis*
Neurologic
Cranial nerve VII palsy†
Aseptic lymphocytic meningitis
Peripheral neuropathy
Gastrointestinal
Lymphocytic hepatitis
Renal
Renal tubular acidosis
Interstitial nephritis
Musculoskeletal
Peripheral arthritis
Polymyositis
Hematologic
Lymphoma‡

*25% to 50%, but decreasing.
†Owing to mechanical compression by inflamed parotid tissue.
‡Poor prognostic indicator.

loads, or depressing the CD4+ counts, although the effect is transient. Lymphocytic interstitial pneumonitis may require higher doses of corticosteroids (60 mg/day of prednisone), sometimes for extended periods. Radiation therapy should be avoided. Cranial nerve VII palsy tends to respond poorly to any treatment. Combination antiretroviral therapy also

Table 103-6 Similarities and Differences between Diffuse Infiltrative Lymphocytosis Syndrome (DILS) and Sjögren's Syndrome

Feature	DILS	Sjögren's Syndrome
Parotid swelling	Ubiquitous	Uncommon
Sicca symptoms	Common	Very common
Extraglandular symptoms	Common	Uncommon
Autoantibodies (antinuclear antibodies, anti-Ro/La)	Rare	Common
HLA class II association	DRB1*1102, DRB1*1301, DRB1*1302	DRB1*0301, DQA1*0501, DQB1*0201

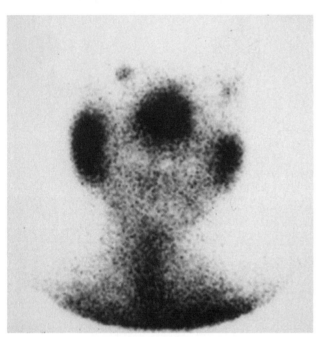

Figure 103-7 The "snowman" sign. Gallium-67 scintigraphy of the parotid glands of a patient with diffuse infiltrative lymphocytosis syndrome occurring in the setting of hemophilia.

Table 103-7 Treatment of Diffuse Infiltrative Lymphocytosis Syndrome

Reassurance and education
Regular dental care
No specific treatment for asymptomatic individuals
Effective antiretroviral treatment
Pilocarpine (5-10 mg) or cevimeline (30 mg orally 3 times daily) for sicca symptoms
Systemic glucocorticoids
Drainage and instillation of corticosteroids into parotid lymphoepithelial cysts
Radiation of parotid cysts

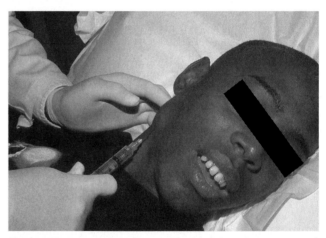

Figure 103-8 Aspiration of a parotid epithelial cyst in a patient with diffuse infiltrative lymphocytosis syndrome.

has been reported to be effective in resolving parotid epithelial cysts, although when refractory the cysts can be managed by aspiration and instillation of 1 mL of a depot steroid into the cyst (Fig. 103-8). Frequent recurrence may necessitate surgical excision.

VASCULITIS ASSOCIATED WITH HUMAN IMMUNODEFICIENCY VIRUS INFECTION

A wide spectrum of vasculitis has been described in patients with HIV infection.[66] Fevers, malaise, weakness, rashes, headaches, and neurologic symptoms are common in HIV-positive patients, and the triggers of vasculitis range from specific infective agents and drugs to idiopathic vasculitis. Among infective causes, cytomegalovirus and tuberculosis are probably the most common. Inflammatory vasculitides are less common rheumatologic diseases that occur in less than 1% of HIV patients.

One series found 34 (23%) of 148 "symptomatic" HIV-positive patients to have vasculitis.[67] Of these patients, 11 met American College of Rheumatology criteria for a

distinct category of vasculitis, including hypersensitivity vasculitis in 6, polyarteritis nodosa in 4, and Henoch-Schönlein purpura in 1. Wegener's granulomatosis and pulmonary microscopic polyangiitis can occur in patients with high CD4+ counts and during immune reconstitution. Behçet's syndrome and relapsing polychondritis occur in HIV infection[68] and respond to HAART.[69] A rapidly progressive focal necrotizing vasculitis of the aorta and large arteries with aneurysm formation and rupture has been described in Africans with HIV infection.[70] Giant cell arteritis likewise has been described in patients with HIV infection with aortic root dilation.[71] Kawasaki disease has been reported in HIV-positive children and adults. Cryoglobulinemic vasculitis with associated lymphocytic interstitial pneumonia occurs with and without hepatitis C coinfection.[66,67]

Patients with isolated central nervous system angiitis usually present with organic brain syndromes and neurologic deficit.[72] In children and in one case report in an adult, HIV-associated cerebral aneurysmal arteriopathy was described causing multiple fusiform aneurysms in the circle of Willis.[73] Central nervous system vasculitis may manifest as recurrent strokes. Although imaging studies (MRI, angiography) may be helpful, brain biopsy may be necessary to establish the diagnosis. Although this syndrome is rarely encountered clinically, perivascular mononuclear cell infiltrates have been described in brain tissue specimens collected at autopsy from five of six children with AIDS.[74] Necrotizing granulomatous vasculitis not limited to the central nervous system has been reported in patients with low CD4+ counts that responds to antiretroviral therapy.[71] More recently, there has been a case report of leukocytoclastic cerebral vasculitis treated with anti-CD25 antibody.[75]

Diagnosis is based on a high degree of suspicion and angiography and biopsy of specific organ beds. Similar to in immunocompetent patients, perinuclear antineutrophil cytoplasmic antigen (pANCA) and cytoplasmic antineutrophil cytoplasmic antigen (cANCA) may be useful with Wegener's granulomatosis or microscopic polyangiitis. Biopsy with cultures is important to rule out infectious mimics, however.

Corticosteroids are the mainstay of treatment of HIV-associated vasculitis, although cytotoxic agents such as cyclophosphamide, intravenous immunoglobulin, and plasmapheresis have been used in refractory cases. Painful neuropathy secondary to vasculitis responds well to high-dose glucocorticoids, in contrast to HIV-associated peripheral neuropathy.[76]

PRIMARY PULMONARY HYPERTENSION

Pulmonary hypertension is a severe life-limiting disease, often affecting younger patients. Patients with AIDS and primary pulmonary hypertension present with a higher degree of pulmonary hypertension than non-AIDS patients.[77,78] The predominant histopathologic finding has been a plexogenic pulmonary arteriopathy, although thromboembolic changes also have been reported. One group found an association with HLA-DRB1*1301 and HLA-DRB1*1302 and with the linked allele HLA-DRB3*0301.[79] A potential role of human herpes virus-8 and occult Kaposi's sarcoma has been postulated.[85]

Symptoms are progressive shortness of breath, pedal edema, nonproductive cough, fatigue, syncope or near-syncope, and chest pain. Pulmonary function tests show mild restrictive patterns with variably reduced diffusing capacities. In a review of 131 reviewed cases of pulmonary hypertension associated with HIV infection, the interval between the diagnosis of HIV disease and the diagnosis of pulmonary hypertension was 33 months. The median length of time from diagnosis to death was 6 months.[80] The responses to vasodilator agents—calcium channel blockers, sildenafil, intravenous and inhaled prostanoids, and endothelin antagonists—and HAART vary, with some studies showing improved mortality.[81]

HUMAN IMMUNODEFICIENCY VIRUS–ASSOCIATED MUSCULOSKELETAL INFECTIONS

PYOMYOSITIS

Pyomyositis is a primary infection of skeletal muscle not arising from contiguous infection, presumably hematogenous in origin, and often associated with abscess formation. Rarely seen in developed countries, infectious myositis nonetheless is an important complication of HIV infection in areas most endemic for HIV, such as Africa and India. It tends to occur in later stages of the infection with CD4+ counts less than 200/μL. *Staphylococcus aureus* is the most common pathogen.[82] Other organisms that have been implicated include *Streptococcus pyogenes, Cryptococcus neoformans, Mycobacterium tuberculosis, Mycobacterium avium-intracellulare, Nocardia asteroides, Salmonella enteritidis, Escherichia coli, Citrobacter freundii, Morganella morganii, Pseudomonas aeruginosa,* and group A streptococci.

The clinical course of pyomyositis can be roughly divided into three stages—invasive, suppurative, and late. The first stage, which typically lasts 1 to 3 weeks, is characterized by localized cramplike pain and induration in conjunction with a low-grade fever. Large muscle groups, particularly those of the lower extremities, are most often affected. The degrees of pain and fever increase in the second stage, which is characterized further by the development of edema and pus in the affected muscle. Untreated, the disease progresses to the third stage; within 3 weeks of onset, sepsis and death can occur.[83] The mortality rate associated with pyomyositis has been estimated to range from 1% to 20%. Ultrasound and MRI with contrast enhancement are effective in localizing infection, although sometimes tagged white blood cell scans may be needed. Oral and intravenous antibiotics in conjunction with surgical drainage are often required.[52]

BACTERIAL ARTHRITIS AND OSTEOMYELITIS

There are no data to suggest that bacterial infections of bones or joints occur more frequently in patients with HIV infection. *S. aureus* is the most common infectious agent encountered, but parenteral drug use and not HIV infection per se may account for this. Many other organisms have been reported to cause osteomyelitis in HIV-infected patients, including *Salmonella, N. asteroides, Streptococcus pneumoniae, Neisseria gonorrhoeae,* cytomegalovirus, invasive *Aspergillus, Toxoplasma gondii, Torulopsis glabrata, C. neoformans,* and *Coccidioides immitis.* Osteomyelitis is associated with mortality rates of greater than 20% in HIV-infected patients. The most frequently involved bones are the wrist, tibia, femoral heads, and thoracic cage, but other rare sites, such as the patella and the mandible, have been reported.[52]

MUSCULOSKELETAL TUBERCULOSIS

Musculoskeletal involvement, the fourth most common extrapulmonary manifestation of tuberculosis, is found in about 1% to 5% of patients with tuberculosis. It can mimic many skeletal diseases and can manifest in various locations. Less than 50% of reported patients with musculoskeletal tuberculosis have radiographic evidence of pulmonary tuberculosis. M. *tuberculosis* disseminates hematogenously after an acute or reactivated pulmonary infection. Usually the skeletal tuberculosis lesions in immunocompetent patients are solitary, but in AIDS patients they may have a multicentric distribution in about 30% of cases.[84] The vertebrae are the most common site involved, mostly the lower thoracic or upper lumbar segments. The frequency of tuberculous spondylitis is 50% to 66%; peripheral arthritis, 20% to 30%; osteomyelitis, 10% to 20%; and tenosynovitis and bursitis, about 1% to 3%. Treatment includes four-drug antitubercular therapy and often surgical intervention.

ATYPICAL MYCOBACTERIAL INFECTIONS

Musculoskeletal infections caused by atypical mycobacterial species are unusual in immunocompetent individuals. Atypical mycobacterial species most commonly implicated in causing septic arthritis or osteomyelitis in HIV include M. *avium-intracellulare* complex, *Mycobacterium kansasii*, *Mycobacterium haemophilum*, *Mycobacterium terrae,* and *Mycobacterium fortuitum*. M. *haemophilum* has been most frequently implicated in skeletal infection, accounting for more than half of cases, and M. *kansasii* is second, accounting for an additional 25%. These are systemic infections that have involved several joints or skeletal sites. Cutaneous lesions, such as nodules, ulcers, and draining sinus tracts, occur in approximately 50% of patients.[85] These infections tend to occur late in the course of HIV, usually when the CD4+ T lymphocyte count is less than 100/μL. Along with standard antituberculosis therapy, clarithromycin is effective.

BACILLARY ANGIOMATOSIS OSTEOMYELITIS

Bacillary angiomatosis is a multisystem infectious disease caused by two closely related organisms—*Bartonella henselae* and *Bartonella quintana*—initially described in patients with AIDS by Stoler and colleagues in 1983.[85a] It seems to be a disease unique to HIV-infected patients and to a lesser degree to other immunocompromised patients.[1]

The name *bacillary angiomatosis* came from the descriptions of the vascular proliferation, seen on histologic examination of clinical specimens, and from the bacilli identified on Warthin-Starry silver stain. The bacterial infection results in a vascular proliferative response ensuing in lesions in the skin (resembling Kaposi's sarcoma), lymph nodes (adenitis), central nervous system (aseptic meningitis or intracranial masses), bone (osteomyelitis), and liver (peliosis hepatis). Osteomyelitis is found in about one third of the patients in association with skin disease. These lesions usually are characterized by extensive destruction of the cortical bone, periostitis, medullary invasion, and an overlying soft tissue mass that might resemble cellulitis. A complete remission of bacillary angiomatosis after doxycycline or erythromycin therapy occurs, although bone lesions may need surgical drainage.

FUNGAL INFECTIONS

In addition to bacterial infections, patients with advanced HIV infection (CD4+ T lymphocyte count <100/μL) are at high risk for fungal musculoskeletal infections, particularly infections caused by *Candida albicans*[86] and *Sporothrix schenckii*.[87] S. *schenckii* can manifest with oligoarticular or even polyarticular involvement, with tendon sheath effusions (Fig. 103-9), and can be particularly difficult to eradicate, requiring long-term suppressive antifungal therapy. Various disseminated fungal infections, such as histoplasmosis, cryptococcosis, and blastomycosis, occur in HIV and often cause osteomyelitis.

PARASITIC INFECTIONS

Muscle toxoplasmosis is found in profoundly immunodepressed patients, typically presenting with a painful subacute myopathy and concurrent multivisceral toxoplasmosis.[88] *Toxoplasma* cysts are observed mainly in muscle fibers in muscle biopsy specimens, and identification of cysts as *Toxoplasma* may be easier by using specific antibodies or electron microscopy. Muscle weakness such as in polymyositis

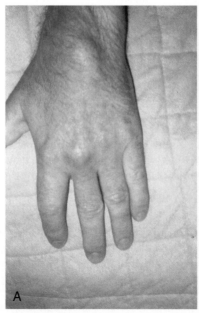 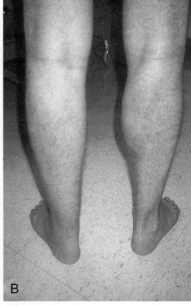

Figure 103-9 **A,** Third metacarpophalangeal synovitis and common extensor digitorum longus tendon sheath effusion at the dorsal surface of the wrist. **B,** Dissecting a Baker's cyst in the same patient with disseminated *Sporotrichum schenckii* infection (organism cultured from synovial fluid obtained from both sites).

can occur in muscle toxoplasmosis. Treatment is based on a combination of drugs acting synergistically against *T. gondii*, including pyrimethamine and sulfadiazine or trisulfapyrimidines.

RESPONSE OF OTHER RHEUMATIC DISEASES TO HUMAN IMMUNODEFICIENCY VIRUS INFECTION

Early reports suggested that rheumatoid arthritis went into remission in the face of HIV infection. Early reports likewise suggested that HIV infection might reduce activity of systemic lupus erythematosus, particularly at times of low CD4+ T cell counts. With the emergence of the newly described immune reconstitution syndrome, most autoimmune diseases appear de novo or recur with institution of HAART and increase in CD4+ counts.[10]

HIGHLY ACTIVE ANTIRETROVIRAL THERAPY–RELATED IMMUNE RECONSTITUTION SYNDROME

The coverage of antiretroviral therapy has increased from 7% in 2003 to 20% in 2005. Immune reconstitution inflammatory syndrome is a paradoxical clinical deterioration in patients with HIV who receive HAART, as a result of improvement in cellular immunity. It was initially described with the recrudescence of infections, but more recently autoinflammatory and autoimmune phenomena are being described.

Shelburne and coworkers[89] put forth four criteria required for the diagnosis of immune reconstitution inflammatory syndrome, as follows:
1. Patient has been diagnosed with AIDS.
2. Treatment with anti-HIV therapy results in increased CD4+ counts and decreased HIV-1 viral load.
3. Infectious and inflammatory symptoms appear during therapy.
4. Symptoms cannot be explained by a new etiology.

More recent understanding of the immunology of immune reconstitution inflammatory syndrome has helped elucidate how atypical, hyperaccentuated inflammatory host responses to preexisting or coexisting infections can occur in HIV patients taking HAART. HIV infection causes a relentless decline in CD4+ memory and naive cells, an increase in activated T cells in the peripheral blood, and thymic dysfunction. HAART can lead to sustained suppression of HIV and a concomitant repopulation of T cell counts in a biphasic mode.[90] The first phase represents the release of predominantly memory CD4+ cells and lasts a few weeks to months. The second phase, from approximately 6 months on, represents the main phase of naive T cell proliferation and is accompanied by changes in T helper cytokine production profiles.[91,92] Immune reconstitution inflammatory syndrome can occur during both phases of immune recovery, and different infections and autoimmune phenomena occur in phase 1 compared with phase 2.

Organ-specific autoimmune phenomena have been described more often than generalized systemic autoimmune disease and tend to occur later during reconstitution. These phenomena may be a manifestation of naive T cell release as opposed to memory T cell reconstitution. Graves' thyroiditis occurring about 21 months after initiation of HAART has been described in about 17 cases.[93] Terminal ileitis, alopecia universalis, cerebral CD8 lymphocytosis, and Guillain-Barré syndrome[90,94] have been reported. Polymyositis,[95] rheumatoid arthritis,[102] systemic lupus erythematosus,[96] Kawasaki-like febrile illness, and sarcoidosis[97,98] newly developing after initiation of HAART also have been described. These conditions tend to occur earlier during reconstitution compared with the organ-specific autoimmunity.

If a diagnosis of immune reconstitution inflammatory syndrome is made, HAART is continued, and most symptoms resolve with little or no therapy. If the inflammatory symptoms involve areas where significant damage secondary to uncontrolled inflammation is likely to occur, such as in the central nervous system or eye, HAART should be stopped, and careful use of corticosteroids should be considered. Immune reconstitution inflammatory syndrome is less likely to occur if the CD4+ count is greater than $200/\mu L$ when HAART is initiated. More systematic analysis is needed, however, and guidelines need to be established for defining the autoimmunity associated with immune reconstitution. The prognosis for most immune reconstitution inflammatory syndrome cases is favorable because a robust inflammatory response may predict an excellent response to HAART in terms of immune reconstitution and, perhaps, improved survival.

RHEUMATOLOGIC COMPLICATIONS OF HUMAN IMMUNODEFICIENCY VIRUS TREATMENT

The myopathy associated with nucleoside transcriptase inhibitors such as zidovudine and osteonecrosis and parotid lipomatosis associated with the use of protease inhibitors have been discussed previously. In addition to these conditions, cases of adhesive capsulitis, Dupuytren's contractures, tenosynovitis, and temporomandibular joint dysfunction have been reported as a consequence of indinavir treatment.[99]

LABORATORY ABNORMALITIES ASSOCIATED WITH HUMAN IMMUNODEFICIENCY VIRUS INFECTION

Humoral immunologic abnormalities are frequent in patients with HIV, but are rarely associated with severe clinical signs. The most common laboratory abnormality is polyclonal hyperglobulinemia, found in 45% of HIV-positive individuals.[100] Hypocomplementemia is rare. Rheumatoid factor and antinuclear antibodies, usually in low titer, have been described in 17% of patients with HIV infection in some series.[100] IgG anticardiolipin antibodies are found in 95% of patients with AIDS, particularly in patients with advanced disease, and in 20% to 30% overall of HIV-positive individuals.[101] Cryoglobulinemia is decreasing in this population since the introduction of HAART.[102] cANCA and pANCA have been described in the serum of HIV-positive individuals, in frequencies of 43% by enzyme-linked immunosorbent assay and 18% by indirect immunofluorescence.[103]

CONCLUSION

The impact of the global HIV pandemic continues to grow, and rheumatologists need to keep aware of the wide spectrum of rheumatic diseases that occur in HIV-positive patients. HAART has changed the natural history of HIV infection: It has modified the frequency and expression of some HIV-related clinical syndromes and has been associated directly (toxicity) and indirectly (immune reconstitution) with the development of new ones. With longer survival and newer refinements in treatment, the spectrum of rheumatic disease seen in HIV-positive patients is very much a "moving target" for rheumatologists that is likely to continue to evolve.

REFERENCES

1. Biviji AA, Paiement GD, Steinbach LS: Musculoskeletal manifestations of human immunodeficiency virus infection. J Am Acad Orthop Surg 10:312-320, 2002.
2. **Rynes RI, Goldenberg DL, DiGiacomo R, et al: Acquired immunodeficiency syndrome-associated arthritis. Am J Med 84:810-816, 1988.**
3. Bileckot R, Mouaya A, Makuwa M: Prevalence and clinical presentations of arthritis in HIV-positive patients seen at a rheumatology department in Congo-Brazzaville. Rev Rhum Engl Ed 65:549-554, 1998.
4. Berman A, Cahn P, Perez H, et al: Human immunodeficiency virus infection associated arthritis: Clinical characteristics. J Rheumatol 26:1158-1162, 1999.
5. Reveille JD: The changing spectrum of rheumatic disease in human immunodeficiency virus infection. Semin Arthritis Rheum 30:147-166, 2000.
6. Mody GM, Parke FA, Reveille JD: Articular manifestations of human immunodeficiency virus infection. Best Pract Res Clin Rheumatol 17:265-287, 2003.
7. Ornstein MH, Sperber K: The antiinflammatory and antiviral effects of hydroxychloroquine in two patients with acquired immunodeficiency syndrome and active inflammatory arthritis. Arthritis Rheum 39:157-161, 1996.
8. Clark MR, Solinger AM, Hochberg MC: Human immunodeficiency virus infection is not associated with Reiter's syndrome: Data from three large cohort studies. Rheum Dis Clin N Am 18:267-276, 1992.
9. Njobvu P, McGill P: Human immunodeficiency virus related reactive arthritis in Zambia. J Rheumatol 32:1299-1304, 2005.
10. **Reveille JD, Conant MA, Duvic M: Human immunodeficiency virus-associated psoriasis, psoriatic arthritis, and Reiter's syndrome: A disease continuum? Arthritis Rheum 33:1574-1578, 1990.**
11. Kaslow RA, Carrington M, Apple R, et al: Influence of combinations of human major histocompatibility complex genes on the course of HIV-1 infection. Nat Med 2:405-411, 1996.
12. Carrington M, O'Brien SJ: The influence of HLA genotype on AIDS. Annu Rev Med 54:535-551, 2003.
13. Altfeld M, Kalife ET, Qi Y, et al: HLA alleles associated with delayed progression to AIDS contribute strongly to the initial CD8(+) T cell response against HIV-1. PLoS Med 3:e403, 2006.
14. Frahm N, Kiepiela P, Adams S, et al: Control of human immunodeficiency virus replication by cytotoxic T lymphocytes targeting subdominant epitopes. Nat Immunol 7:173-178, 2006.
15. Lopez-Larrea C, Njobvu PD, Gonzalez S, et al: The HLA-B*5703 allele confers susceptibility to the development of spondylarthropathies in Zambian human immunodeficiency virus-infected patients with slow progression to acquired immunodeficiency syndrome. Arthritis Rheum 52:275-279, 2005.
16. Bourinbaiar AS, Lee-Huang S: The non-steroidal anti-inflammatory drug, indomethacin, as an inhibitor of HIV replication. FEBS Lett 360:85-88, 1995.
17. Njobvu PD, McGill PE: Sulphasalazine in the treatment of HIV-related spondyloarthropathy. Br J Rheumatol 36:403-404, 1997.
18. Disla E, Rhim HR, Reddy A, et al: Improvement in CD4 lymphocyte count in HIV-Reiter's syndrome after treatment with sulfasalazine. J Rheumatol 21:662-664, 1994.
19. Maurer TA, Zackheim HS, Tuffanelli L, et al: The use of methotrexate for treatment of psoriasis in patients with HIV infection. J Am Acad Dermatol 31:372-375, 1994.
20. Chiang G, Sassaroli M, Louie M, et al: Inhibition of HIV-1 replication by hydroxychloroquine: Mechanism of action and comparison with zidovudine. Clin Ther 18:1080-1092, 1996.
21. Louthrenoo W: Successful treatment of severe Reiter's syndrome associated with human immunodeficiency virus infection with etretinate: Report of 2 cases. J Rheumatol 20:1243-1246, 1993.
22. Gaylis N: Infliximab in the treatment of an HIV positive patient with Reiter's syndrome. J Rheumatol 30:407-411, 2003.
23. Ting PT, Koo JY: Use of etanercept in human immunodeficiency virus (HIV) and acquired immunodeficiency syndrome (AIDS) patients. Int J Dermatol 45:689-692, 2006.
24. Filippi J, Roger PM, Schneider SM, et al: Infliximab and human immunodeficiency virus infection: Viral load reduction and CD4+ T-cell loss related to apoptosis. Arch Intern Med 166:1783-1784, 2006.
25. Beltran B, Nos P, Bastida G, et al: Safe and effective application of anti-TNF-alpha in a patient infected with HIV and concomitant Crohn's disease. Gut 55:1670-1671, 2006.
26. Arnett FC, Reveille JD, Duvic M: Psoriasis and psoriatic arthritis associated with human immunodeficiency virus infection. Rheum Dis Clin N Am 17:59-78, 1991.
27. Njobvu P, McGill P: Psoriatic arthritis and human immunodeficiency virus infection in Zambia. J Rheumatol 27:1699-1702, 2000.
28. **Espinoza LR, Berman A, Vasey FB, et al: Psoriatic arthritis and acquired immunodeficiency syndrome. Arthritis Rheum 31:1034-1040, 1988.**
29. Duvic M, Crane MM, Conant M, et al: Zidovudine improves psoriasis in human immunodeficiency virus-positive males. Arch Dermatol 130:447-451, 1994.
30. Bartke U, Venten I, Kreuter A, et al: Human immunodeficiency virus-associated psoriasis and psoriatic arthritis treated with infliximab. Br J Dermatol 150:784-786, 2004.
31. McGonagle D, Reade S, Marzo-Ortega H, et al: Human immunodeficiency virus associated spondyloarthropathy: Pathogenic insights based on imaging findings and response to highly active antiretroviral treatment. Ann Rheum Dis 60:696-698, 2001.
32. Gerster JC, Camus JP, Chave JP, et al: Multiple site avascular necrosis in HIV infected patients. J Rheumatol 18:300-302, 1991.
33. Allison GT, Bostrom MP, Glesby MJ: Osteonecrosis in HIV disease: Epidemiology, etiologies, and clinical management. AIDS 17:1-9, 2003.
34. **Gutierrez F, Padilla S, Masia M, et al: Osteonecrosis in patients infected with HIV: Clinical epidemiology and natural history in a large case series from Spain. J Acquir Immune Defic Syndr 42:286-292, 2006.**
35. Morse CG, Mican JM, Jones EC, et al: The incidence and natural history of osteonecrosis in HIV-infected adults. Clin Infect Dis 44:739-748, 2007.
36. Gunnarsson G, Karchmer AW: Hypertrophic osteoarthropathy associated with Pneumocystis carinii pneumonia and human immunodeficiency virus infection. Clin Infect Dis 22:590-591, 1996.
37. Brown TT, Qaqish RB: Antiretroviral therapy and the prevalence of osteopenia and osteoporosis: A meta-analytic review. AIDS 20:2165-2174, 2006.
38. Pan G, Yang Z, Ballinger SW, et al: Pathogenesis of osteopenia/osteoporosis induced by highly active anti-retroviral therapy for AIDS. Ann N Y Acad Sci 1068:297-308, 2006.
39. Amorosa V, Tebas P: Bone disease and HIV infection. Clin Infect Dis 42:108-114, 2006.
40. Lin D, Rieder M: Interventions for the treatment of decreased bone mineral density associated with HIV infection. Cochrane Database Syst Rev CD005645, 2007.
41. Buskila D, Gladman D: Musculoskeletal manifestations of infection with human immunodeficiency virus. Rev Infect Dis 12:223-235, 1990.
42. Simms RW, Zerbini CA, Ferrante N, et al: Fibromyalgia syndrome in patients infected with human immunodeficiency virus. The Boston City Hospital Clinical AIDS Team. Am J Med 92:368-374, 1992.
43. Miro O, Pedrol E, Cebrian M, et al: Skeletal muscle studies in patients with HIV-related wasting syndrome. J Neurol Sci 150:153-159, 1997.

44. Gherardi R, Chariot P, Authier FJ: [Muscular involvement in HIV infection]. Rev Neurol (Paris) 151:603-607, 1995.

45. Simpson DM, Bender AN, Farraye J, et al: Human immunodeficiency virus wasting syndrome may represent a treatable myopathy. Neurology 40:535-538, 1990.

46. Miro O, Masanes F, Pedrol E, et al: [A comparative study of the clinical and histological characteristics between classic nemaline myopathy and that associated with the human immunodeficiency virus]. Med Clin (Barc) 105:500-503, 1995.

47. Nakagawa M, Hirata K: [Adult onset nemaline myopathy and monoclonal gammopathy]. Ryoikibetsu Shokogun Shirizu 35:406-413, 2001.

48. **Johnson RW, Williams FM, Kazi S, et al: Human immunodeficiency virus-associated polymyositis: A longitudinal study of outcome. Arthritis Rheum 49:172-178, 2003.**

49. Seidman R, Peress NS, Nuovo GJ: In situ detection of polymerase chain reaction-amplified HIV-1 nucleic acids in skeletal muscle in patients with myopathy. Mod Pathol 7:369-375, 1994.

50. Leon-Monzon M, Lamperth L, Dalakas MC: Search for HIV proviral DNA and amplified sequences in the muscle biopsies of patients with HIV polymyositis. Muscle Nerve 16:408-413, 1993.

51. Reveille JD: The changing spectrum of rheumatic disease in human immunodeficiency virus infection. Semin Arthritis Rheum 30: 147-166, 2000.

52. Tehranzadeh J, Ter-Oganesyan RR, Steinbach LS: Musculoskeletal disorders associated with HIV infection and AIDS, Part I: Infectious musculoskeletal conditions. Skeletal Radiol 33:249-259, 2004.

53. Illa I, Nath A, Dalakas M: Immunocytochemical and virological characteristics of HIV-associated inflammatory myopathies: Similarities with seronegative polymyositis. Ann Neurol 29:474-481, 1991.

54. Cupler EJ, Leon-Monzon M, Miller J, et al: Inclusion body myositis in HIV-1 and HTLV-1 infected patients. Brain 119(Pt 6):1887-1893, 1996.

55. Schreiner B, Voss J, Wischhusen J, et al: Expression of toll-like receptors by human muscle cells in vitro and in vivo: TLR3 is highly expressed in inflammatory and HIV myopathies, mediates IL-8 release and up-regulation of NKG2D-ligands. FASEB J 20:118-120, 2006.

56. Walsh K, Kaye K, Demaerschalk B, et al: AZT myopathy and HIV-1 polymyositis: One disease or two? Can J Neurol Sci 29:390-393, 2002.

57. Dalakas MC, Illa I, Pezeshkpour GH, et al: Mitochondrial myopathy caused by long-term zidovudine therapy. N Engl J Med 322: 1098-1105, 1990.

58. Authier FJ, Gherardi RK: [Muscular complications of human immunodeficiency virus (HIV) infection in the era of effective anti-retroviral therapy]. Rev Neurol (Paris) 162:71-81, 2006.

59. **Basu D, Williams FM, Ahn CW, et al: Changing spectrum of the diffuse infiltrative lymphocytosis syndrome. Arthritis Rheum 55: 466-472, 2006.**

60. Williams FM, Cohen PR, Jumshyd J, et al: Prevalence of the diffuse infiltrative lymphocytosis syndrome among human immunodeficiency virus type 1-positive outpatients. Arthritis Rheum 41:863-868, 1998.

61. Kordossis T, Paikos S, Aroni K, et al: Prevalence of Sjogren's-like syndrome in a cohort of HIV-1-positive patients: Descriptive pathology and immunopathology. Br J Rheumatol 37:691-695, 1998.

62. **Itescu S, Rose S, Dwyer E, et al: Certain HLA-DR5 and -DR6 major histocompatibility complex class II alleles are associated with a CD8 lymphocytic host response to human immunodeficiency virus type 1 characterized by low lymphocyte viral strain heterogeneity and slow disease progression. Proc Natl Acad Sci U S A 91:11472-11476, 1994.**

63. Itescu S, Dalton J, Zhang HZ, et al: Tissue infiltration in a CD8 lymphocytosis syndrome associated with human immunodeficiency virus-1 infection has the phenotypic appearance of an antigenically driven response. J Clin Invest 91:2216-2225, 1993.

64. Kazi S, Cohen PR, Williams F, et al: The diffuse infiltrative lymphocytosis syndrome: Clinical and immunogenetic features in 35 patients. AIDS 10:385-391, 1996.

65. Itescu S, Winchester R: Diffuse infiltrative lymphocytosis syndrome: A disorder occurring in human immunodeficiency virus-1 infection that may present as a sicca syndrome. Rheum Dis Clin N Am 18: 683-697, 1992.

66. Garcia-Garcia JA, Macias J, Castellanos V, et al: Necrotizing granulomatous vasculitis in advanced HIV infection. J Infect 47:333-335, 2003.

67. **Gherardi R, Belec L, Mhiri C, et al: The spectrum of vasculitis in human immunodeficiency virus-infected patients: A clinicopathologic evaluation. Arthritis Rheum 36:1164-1174, 1993.**

68. Belzunegui J, Cancio J, Pego JM, et al: Relapsing polychondritis and Behcet's syndrome in a patient with HIV infection. Ann Rheum Dis 54:780, 1995.

69. Cicalini S, Gigli B, Palmieri F, et al: Remission of Behcet's disease and keratoconjunctivitis sicca in an HIV-infected patient treated with HAART. Int J STD AIDS 15:139-140, 2004.

70. Chetty R, Batitang S, Nair R: Large artery vasculopathy in HIV-positive patients: Another vasculitic enigma. Hum Pathol 31:374-379, 2000.

71. Javed MA, Sheppard MN, Pepper J: Aortic root dilation secondary to giant cell aortitis in a human immunodeficiency virus-positive patient. Eur J Cardiothorac Surg 30:400-401, 2006.

72. Brannagan TH III: Retroviral-associated vasculitis of the nervous system. Neurol Clin 15:927-944, 1997.

73. Ake JA, Erickson JC, Lowry KJ: Cerebral aneurysmal arteriopathy associated with HIV infection in an adult. Clin Infect Dis 43: e46-e50, 2006.

74. Katsetos CD, Fincke JE, Legido A, et al: Angiocentric CD3(+) T-cell infiltrates in human immunodeficiency virus type 1-associated central nervous system disease in children. Clin Diagn Lab Immunol 6: 105-114, 1999.

75. Nieuwhof CM, Damoiseaux J, Cohen Tervaert JW: Successful treatment of cerebral vasculitis in an HIV-positive patient with anti-CD25 treatment. Ann Rheum Dis 65:1677-1678, 2006.

76. Bradley WG, Verma A: Painful vasculitic neuropathy in HIV-1 infection: Relief of pain with prednisone therapy. Neurology 47: 1446-1451, 1996.

77. Coplan NL, Shimony RY, Ioachim HL, et al: Primary pulmonary hypertension associated with human immunodeficiency viral infection. Am J Med 89:96-99, 1990.

78. Morse JH, Barst RJ, Itescu S, et al: Primary pulmonary hypertension in HIV infection: An outcome determined by particular HLA class II alleles. Am J Respir Crit Care Med 153:1299-1301, 1996.

79. Gutierrez F, Masia M, Padilla S, et al: Occult lymphadenopathic Kaposi's sarcoma associated with severe pulmonary hypertension: A clinical hint about the potential role of HHV-8 in HIV-related pulmonary hypertension? J Clin Virol 37:79-82, 2006.

80. Mehta NJ, Khan IA, Mehta RN, et al: HIV-related pulmonary hypertension: Analytic review of 131 cases. Chest 118:1133-1141, 2000.

81. Nunes H, Humbert M, Sitbon O, et al: Prognostic factors for survival in human immunodeficiency virus-associated pulmonary arterial hypertension. Am J Respir Crit Care Med 167:1433-1439, 2003.

82. Ansaloni L: Tropical pyomyositis. World J Surg 20:613-617, 1996.

83. Scharschmidt TJ, Weiner SD, Myers JP: Bacterial pyomyositis. Curr Infect Dis Rep 6:393-396, 2004.

84. Jellis JE: Human immunodeficiency virus and osteoarticular tuberculosis. Clin Orthop 398:27-31, 2002.

85. Hirsch R, Miller SM, Kazi S, et al: Human immunodeficiency virus-associated atypical mycobacterial skeletal infections. Semin Arthritis Rheum 25:347-356, 1996.

85a. Stoler MH, Bonfiglio TA, Steigbigel RT, et al: An atypical subcutaneous infection associated with acquired immune deficiency syndrome. Am J Clin Pathol 80:714-718, 1983.

86. Edelstein H, McCabe R: *Candida albicans* septic arthritis and osteomyelitis of the sternoclavicular joint in a patient with human immunodeficiency virus infection. J Rheumatol 18:110-111, 1991.

87. Heller HM, Fuhrer J: Disseminated sporotrichosis in patients with AIDS: Case report and review of the literature. AIDS 5:1243-1246, 1991.

88. Gherardi R, Baudrimont M, Lionnet F, et al: Skeletal muscle toxoplasmosis in patients with acquired immunodeficiency syndrome: A clinical and pathological study. Ann Neurol 32:535-542, 1992.

89. **Shelburne SA III, Hamill RJ, Rodriguez-Barradas MC, et al: Immune reconstitution inflammatory syndrome: Emergence of a unique syndrome during highly active antiretroviral therapy. Medicine (Balt) 81:213-227, 2002.**

90. DeSimone JA, Pomerantz RJ, Babinchak TJ: Inflammatory reactions in HIV-1-infected persons after initiation of highly active antiretroviral therapy. Ann Intern Med 133:447-454, 2000.

91. Hardy G, Worrell S, Hayes P, et al: Evidence of thymic reconstitution after highly active antiretroviral therapy in HIV-1 infection. HIV Med 5:67-73, 2004.

92. Lederman MM, Connick E, Landay A, et al: Immunologic responses associated with 12 weeks of combination antiretroviral therapy consisting of zidovudine, lamivudine, and ritonavir: Results of AIDS Clinical Trials Group Protocol 315. J Infect Dis 178:70-79, 1998.

93. Chen F, Day SL, Metcalfe RA, et al: Characteristics of autoimmune thyroid disease occurring as a late complication of immune reconstitution in patients with advanced human immunodeficiency virus (HIV) disease. Medicine (Balt) 84:98-106, 2005.

94. Gray F, Bazille C, dle-Biassette H, et al: Central nervous system immune reconstitution disease in acquired immunodeficiency syndrome patients receiving highly active antiretroviral treatment. J Neurovirol 11(Suppl 3):16-22, 2005.

95. Calza L, Manfredi R, Colangeli V, et al: Polymyositis associated with HIV infection during immune restoration induced by highly active anti-retroviral therapy. Clin Exp Rheumatol 22:651-652, 2004.

96. Calabrese LH, Kirchner E, Shrestha R: Rheumatic complications of human immunodeficiency virus infection in the era of highly active antiretroviral therapy: Emergence of a new syndrome of immune reconstitution and changing patterns of disease. Semin Arthritis Rheum 35:166-174, 2005.

97. Schneider J, Zatarain E: IRIS and SLE. Clin Immunol 118:152-153, 2006.

98. Ferrand RA, Cartledge JD, Connolly J, et al: Immune reconstitution sarcoidosis presenting with hypercalcaemia and renal failure in HIV infection. Int J STD AIDS 18:138-139, 2007.

99. Florence E, Schrooten W, Verdonck K, et al: Rheumatological complications associated with the use of indinavir and other protease inhibitors. Ann Rheum Dis 61:82-84, 2002.

100. **Kaye BR: Rheumatologic manifestations of infection with human immunodeficiency virus (HIV). Ann Intern Med 111:158-167, 1989.**

101. Petrovas C, Vlachoyiannopoulos PG, Kordossis T, et al: Anti-phospholipid antibodies in HIV infection and SLE with or without antiphospholipid syndrome: Comparisons of phospholipid specificity, avidity and reactivity with beta2-GPI. J Autoimmun 13:347-355, 1999.

102. Bonnet F, Pineau JJ, Taupin JL, et al: Prevalence of cryoglobulinemia and serological markers of autoimmunity in human immunodeficiency virus infected individuals: A cross-sectional study of 97 patients. J Rheumatol 30:2005-2010, 2003.

103. de Habegger SA, Motta P, Iliovich E, et al: [Anti-neutrophil cytoplasmic antibodies (ANCA) in patients with symptomatic and asymptomatic HIV infection]. Medicina (B Aires) 57:294-298, 1997.

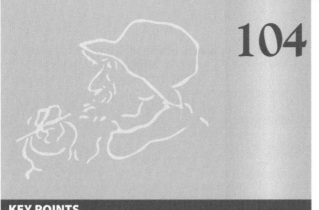

104 Viral Arthritis

STANLEY J. NAIDES

KEY POINTS

Acute-onset, symmetric polyarthritis suggests viral infection, especially when accompanied by rash.

Always take exposure, travel, occupation, and vaccination histories.

Parvovirus B19 is the most common viral arthritis in the United States.

In adults with parvovirus B19 infection, rash may be subtle or absent.

Rubella arthritis occurs in young adults. Rubella vaccination has reduced the overall incidence of rubella infection but has shifted the peak age to young adults.

Arthralgia, arthritis, or neuropathic pain may occur after rubella vaccination; these conditions are usually self-limited in duration.

Alphaviruses are mosquito-borne causes of arthritis and rash. Outbreaks occur in endemic areas associated with rising mosquito populations and should be considered in travelers entering the United States.

Hepatitis B virus infection presents as an arthritis-urticaria syndrome.

Hepatitis C virus infection causes cryoglobulinemia and vasculitis. Cryoglobulinemic vasculitis often presents as palpable purpura of the lower legs.

The history of risk behaviors associated with hepatitis C virus infection may be remote.

Viruses are candidate causative agents for various rheumatic diseases in part because arthralgia and arthritis are prominent features of certain viral infections. Understanding how viruses cause arthritis and the nature of virus-host cell interactions may suggest how viruses precipitate, establish, or maintain chronic inflammatory arthritis such as rheumatoid arthritis.

Viral effects in a given host may depend on host factors such as age, gender, genetic background, infection history, and immune response. The ability of a given virus to infect a host may also depend on the viral mode of host entry, tissue tropism, replication strategy, cytopathologic effects, ability to establish persistent infection, viral expression of hostlike antigens, and ability to alter host antigens. Viral modification of the regulation of cellular gene expression may contribute to autoimmunity. Infected cells may die by classic cell necrosis, programmed cell death (apoptosis), or autophagy. Initiation of an immune response to virally encoded antigens on the cell surface may target that cell for destruction and alter cell-cell interactions. The antibody response may generate immune complexes that are deposited locally at the site of viral infection or systemically in synovium. Alternatively, cells may survive, but their behavior may be altered by the expression of viral genes. Transactivation of cellular genes by viral gene products may induce the cell cycle or cytokines that elicit or perpetuate an immune response targeting host cells. Molecular mimicry of host autoantigens by viral proteins may break immune tolerance. Viral components may elicit "danger signals" that trigger an immune response.[1,2]

PARVOVIRUS B19

Human parvovirus B19 is a member of the family Parvoviridae, subfamily Parvovirinae, genus *Erythrovirus*. It consists of the small, single-stranded DNA viruses that autonomously replicate in erythroid precursors (hence the genus name). B19 has no envelope and is approximately 23 nm in diameter. Productive infection occurs in erythroid precursors; infection of nonerythroid tissues occurs but is restricted, which means that if assembly of virions occurs, it is inefficient, or that nonstructural but not capsid structural viral genes are expressed, preventing virion assembly. Parvoviruses are species specific and not known to readily cross species barriers. The common canine parvovirus does not infect humans.

EPIDEMIOLOGY

B19 infection is common and occurs worldwide. B19 is typically transmitted by respiratory secretions but may also be transmitted via pooled blood products. Outbreaks commonly occur in late winter and spring, when close contact is most common, although epidemics may also occur in summer and fall. Most B19 infections, especially in children, remain asymptomatic or are diagnosed as nonspecific viral illnesses. Outbreaks tend to occur in 3- to 5-year cycles, representing the time required for a new cohort of susceptible children to enter school. Up to 60% of adults have serologic evidence of past B19 infection.[3,4] Susceptible adults in occupations with multiple exposures to children, such as schoolteachers and pediatric nurses, are at greatest risk (up to 50%) of acquiring infection during outbreaks.[4,5] Sporadic cases do occur during nonepidemic periods. The diagnosis should be entertained even in the absence of surveillance data suggesting an outbreak.

PATHOGENESIS

The onset of joint symptoms and rash is associated temporally with appearance of serum anti-B19 immunoglobulin (Ig) M antibody, suggesting a role for circulating immune complexes during the acute phase of the illness.[6] Although there is little evidence of circulating virus in patients who have chronic joint symptoms, B19 DNA may be found in the bone marrow and synovium of patients with chronic B19 arthropathy. Persistence in chronic B19 arthropathy may be facilitated by failure to develop IgG antibodies to the N-terminal region of the minor capsid protein VP1, known to encode neutralizing epitopes.[6] The presence of antibody to the B19 nonstructural protein NS1 in some cases of chronic B19 arthropathy probably reflects immune response to NS1 on the surface of B19 virions or NS1 spilled during cell death.[7] NS1 protein itself, however, may play a pathogenic role in perpetuating chronic B19 arthropathy through its interaction with cellular genes.[8] NS1 protein upregulates in vitro transcription from the interleukin-6 (IL-6) promoter and from human immunodeficiency virus (HIV) long terminal repeats in the presence of *tat* and an intact *tar* element.[9,10] A high prevalence of B19 DNA and proteins in synovium from rheumatoid arthritis patients was reported in association with enhanced synovial production of IL-6 and tumor necrosis factor-α.[8] These findings remain controversial.[11] B19 may induce apoptosis through NS1, which is known to be toxic to cells.[12,13] Production of NS1 in nonpermissive synoviocytes could theoretically induce autoimmunity by disrupting normal patterns of cell interactions and intercellular regulation.

DIAGNOSIS

Clinical Features

The incubation period from B19 infection to symptom onset is 7 to 18 days. B19 causes transient aplastic crisis in the setting of chronic hemolytic anemia.[6] In otherwise healthy children, B19 causes erythema infectiosum, or fifth disease, characterized by bright red "slapped cheeks" and a macular or maculopapular eruption on the torso and extremities. Up to 70% of infected children may be asymptomatic; others may have mild flulike symptoms including fever, headache, sore throat, cough, anorexia, vomiting, diarrhea, and arthralgia. In adults, the rash tends to be subtler, and the slapped-cheek rash is usually absent. Uncommon dermatologic manifestations include vesicular or hemorrhagic vesiculopustular eruptions, purpura with or without thrombocytopenia, Henoch-Schönlein purpura, and a "socks and gloves" acral erythema. B19 infection may be associated with paresthesias in the fingers and, rarely, with numbness of the toes. Progressive arm weakness has been associated with mild nerve conduction slowing and decreased motor and sensory potential amplitudes. B19 may cross the placenta to infect the fetus, which may develop hydrops fetalis on the basis of B19-induced anemia or viral cardiomyopathy. Less commonly, B19 may cause pancytopenia, isolated anemia, thrombocytopenia, leukopenia, myocarditis, neuropathy, or hepatitis.[14] Reports suggest that B19 may be associated with vasculitis, including giant cell arteritis.[15,16]

Patients with congenital or acquired immunodeficiencies, including prior chemotherapy or acquired immunodeficiency syndrome (AIDS) due to HIV infection, may develop persistent B19 infection with chronic or recurrent anemia, thrombocytopenia, or leukopenia. B19 infection is the leading cause of pure red cell aplasia in patients with AIDS.[17,18]

Table 104-1 Prevalence of Joint Symptoms in Fifth Disease by Age: Port Angeles, Washington, 1961-1962

Symptom	Prevalence (%) by Age		
	0-9 Years	10-19 Years	>20 Years
Pain	5.1	11.5	77.2
Swelling	2.8	5.3	59.6

Data from Ager EA, Chin TDY, Poland JD: Epidemic erythema infectiosum. N Engl J Med 275:1326, 1966.

In a study of an erythema infectiosum outbreak in Port Angeles, Washington, in which subjects were identified on the basis of rash, the incidence of arthralgia and joint swelling increased with age (Table 104-1).[19] In adults, a severe flulike illness consisting of fever, chills, malaise, and myalgias may precede or accompany sudden-onset, moderately severe, symmetric polyarthritis in a rheumatoid-like distribution. The arthritis is characterized by prominent involvement of the finger proximal interphalangeal, metacarpophalangeal, wrist, knee, and ankle joints. Within 24 to 48 hours of onset, all affected joints become involved. Axial skeleton involvement is uncommon. Joint symptoms are usually self-limited.

After the initial infection, objective joint swelling, heat, and erythema, when present, tend to resolve over several weeks. A minority of patients have prolonged symptoms that fall into one of two patterns. Approximately two thirds have continuous morning stiffness and arthralgias with intermittent flares. The other third are symptom free between flares. Chronic B19 arthropathy may last months to years. Pain remains a prominent feature during flares; patients commonly report morning stiffness. Approximately 12% of patients presenting with "early synovitis" have B19 infection, most of whom are women.[6]

Laboratory Tests

Viremia lasts 5 to 6 days and is associated with an absence of reticulocytosis and, in otherwise normal individuals, a minimal decrease in the concentrations of hemoglobin, neutrophils, and lymphocytes. Flulike symptoms may occur during viremia. An IgM antibody response follows the initial viremia in 4 to 6 days and is associated with clearing of viremia and cessation of nasal shedding of virus.

The antibody response is associated with the second phase of clinical illness, characterized by rash and joint symptoms. Onset of the anti-B19 IgG antibody response occurs almost concurrently with the IgM response. The two clinical phases of illness often overlap. Low to moderate titers of rheumatoid factor and anti-DNA, antilymphocyte, antinuclear, and antiphospholipid antibodies may be present initially.[20-24]

During viremia, immune electron microscopy may detect virions in serum. However, this method is not readily available to clinicians. B19 DNA may be detected during viremia. However, because adult patients usually present after the onset of joint symptoms, the most useful diagnostic test is anti-B19 IgM serology. Radioimmunoassays and enzyme-linked immunosorbent assays have been used to detect B19 antigen and specific antibody to B19 capsid.[6,25,26] The anti-B19 IgM antibody response is usually positive for 2 months after the acute illness and may wane shortly thereafter. In some patients, anti-B19 IgM may be detected for 6 months or longer. A positive anti-B19 IgG antibody test in the absence of anti-B19 IgM is usually not diagnostically helpful because of the high seroprevalence of anti-B19 IgG in the adult population. Reports of B19 DNA in normal synovium suggest that testing for B19 DNA in these tissues is of little clinical utility in the absence of anti-B19 IgM.[27]

Differential Diagnosis

Many patients with B19 arthropathy meet the American Rheumatism Association criteria for a diagnosis of rheumatoid arthritis: morning stiffness lasting more than an hour; symmetric involvement; involvement of at least three joints; and involvement of the finger proximal interphalangeal, metacarpophalangeal, and wrist joints. Rheumatoid factor may be present at low to moderate titers. Absence of rheumatoid nodules and joint destruction differentiates B19 arthropathy from classic, erosive rheumatoid arthritis.

Occasionally, B19 infection may present with features of systemic lupus erythematosus (SLE). Whether this represents a clinical mimic or indicates that B19 plays a role in initiating or precipitating SLE in these patients remains to be determined.[6]

Rubella in adults may present with rash and symmetric polyarthralgia or polyarthritis that is clinically indistinguishable from B19 infection. A history of prenatal rubella testing, prior rubella vaccination, or rubella exposure may aid in choosing the appropriate diagnostic serologies.

TREATMENT AND PROGNOSIS

There is no specific treatment or vaccine for B19 infection. Treatment is therefore symptomatic, with nonsteroidal anti-inflammatory drugs. Intravenous immunoglobulin has been successful in the treatment of bone marrow suppression and B19 persistence in immunocompromised patients,[18] but initial studies suggest that this is not applicable to chronic arthropathy patients. Long-term prognosis is good. Although subjective arthralgias and morning stiffness may be prolonged, joint destruction is not a feature of chronic B19 arthropathy. B19's role as a cofactor in the development of classic erosive rheumatoid arthritis has not been confirmed.

TOGAVIRUSES

The family Togaviridae includes the *Rubivirus* and *Alphavirus* genera.

RUBELLA VIRUS

Rubella virus is the sole member of the genus *Rubivirus*. It consists of enveloped, single-stranded RNA viruses. The rubella virion is spherical and measures 50 to 70 nm in diameter, with a 30-nm dense core. Envelope glycoproteins form 5- to 6-nm spikelike projections that contain hemagglutination activity.[28]

Epidemiology

Transmission is by nasopharyngeal secretions, with a peak incidence in late winter and spring. Vaccination has reduced the incidence of rubella outbreaks and shifted the demographic profile from children to college students and adults. The incubation period from infection to rash is 14 to 21 days. Viremia precedes rash by 6 to 7 days, peaks just before the onset of rash, and clears within 48 hours after the onset of rash. Nasopharyngeal shedding of virus is detectable from 7 days before the appearance of rash until 14 days afterward, but it is maximal from just before the rash until 5 to 6 days later.[29]

Pathogenesis

Rubella virus can persistently infect synoviocytes and chondrocytes in vitro. An inadequate humoral immune response to specific rubella envelope glycoprotein epitopes may allow rubella virus to persistently infect synovium and lymphocytes in chronic rubella arthritis patients. The onset of rash and arthritis is concurrent with antibody production, suggesting a role for antibody or immune complexes.[29] Concentrations of rubella antibody are higher in synovial fluid than in serum. Synovial lymphocytes from infected individuals spontaneously secrete rubella antibody in vitro, suggesting that there is also an immune response to rubella infection in the joint.[30]

Diagnosis

Clinical Features. Asymptomatic infection occurs in children and adults. Low-grade fever, malaise, coryza, and prominent lymphadenopathy involving posterior cervical, postauricular, and occipital nodes may precede rash by 5 days. A morbilliform rash may initially appear on the face and then spread to the torso, upper extremities, and lower extremities over 2 to 3 days. The facial rash may coalesce and clear as the extremities become involved. In some cases, the rash is only a transient blush.

Joint symptoms commonly occur in women beginning 1 week before or 1 week after the appearance of the rash. Symmetric or migratory arthralgias are more common than synovitis. Morning stiffness is prominent. Joint symptoms usually resolve over a few days to 2 weeks. Proximal interphalangeal, metacarpophalangeal, wrist, elbow, ankle, and knee joints are most frequently affected. Periarthritis, tenosynovitis, and carpal tunnel syndrome may be seen. In some patients, symptoms may persist for months to years.[31,32]

Live attenuated rubella vaccines have caused a high frequency of postvaccination myalgia, arthralgia, arthritis, and paresthesia—symptoms similar to those in natural infection—beginning 2 weeks after inoculation and lasting less than a week. However, in some patients, symptoms may persist for more than a year. RA27/3, the vaccine strain in current use, may cause postvaccination joint symptoms in 15% or more of recipients.[31,32]

Two rheumatologic syndromes may complicate natural infection or vaccination in children. In the catcher's crouch syndrome, a lumbar radiculoneuropathy causes popliteal fossa pain on arising in the morning. Exacerbation of the pain by knee extension encourages the assumption of a baseball catcher's crouch position (Fig. 104-1). The pain gradually subsides through the day but recurs the next morning. In the arm syndrome, brachial neuropathy causes arm and hand pain and dysesthesias that are worse at night. Both syndromes may occur beginning 1 to 2 months after infection or vaccination, with the initial episode lasting up to 2 months. Episodes recur for up to 1 year but eventually resolve without long-term sequelae.[33]

Laboratory Tests. Although rubella may be cultured from tissues and body fluids, including throat swabs, detecting antirubella IgM antibody usually establishes the diagnosis of acute rubella infection. Diagnosis by anti-IgG antibody seroconversion requires paired acute and convalescent sera. IgM and IgG are usually present at the onset of joint symptoms. IgM antibody levels peak 8 to 21 days after symptom onset and wane by 5 weeks. Antirubella IgG rises rapidly over a period of 1 to 3 weeks and is long lived. A single positive IgG serum sample or a set of untitered IgG-positive screens only documents immunity.[29]

Differential Diagnosis. Rubella arthritis needs to be differentiated from other viral arthritides and from inflammatory arthritides, including rheumatoid arthritis. It may be confused with parvovirus B19 infection.

Treatment and Prognosis

Nonsteroidal anti-inflammatory drugs are useful to control symptoms. Some investigators have suggested the use of low to moderate doses of steroids to control symptoms and viremia.[34] Long-term prognosis is good.

ALPHAVIRUSES

The members of the genus *Alphavirus* are enveloped, single-stranded RNA viruses transmitted by mosquitoes.[35] Several cause acute febrile arthropathy, and their names reflect local appreciation of their clinical impact. For example, *chikungunya* means 'that which twists or bends up' (Tanzania). The related *o'nyong-nyong* virus means 'joint breaker' in the Acholi (Uganda) dialect. *Igbo-ora* is 'the disease that breaks your wings."

Epidemiology

Chikungunya, o'nyong-nyong, and igbo-ora viruses form a serologically related group. Chikungunya virus was isolated during an epidemic of febrile arthritis in Tanzania between 1952 and 1953. Similar epidemics probably occurred in Africa, Asia, India, Indonesia, and possibly the southern United States as early as 1779.[35] Mosquitoes responsible for transmission to humans define its geographic distribution (Table 104-2). A feared consequence of global warming is spread of the geographic range of infected mosquitoes.[36-39]

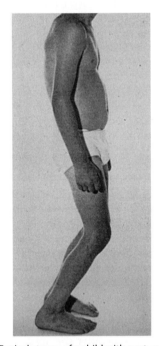

Figure 104-1 Typical stance of a child with post–rubella vaccination "catcher's crouch" syndrome. *(From Schaffner W, Fleet WF, Kilroy AW, et al: Polyneuropathy following rubella immunization: A follow-up study and review of the problem. Am J Dis Child 127:684, 1974.)*

Table 104-2 Mosquito Vectors and Reservoirs of Alphaviruses

Virus	Mosquito	Reservoir	Region
Chikungunya virus	*Aedes* species *Mansonia africana*	Baboons, monkeys, *Scotophilis* bat species	Africa, Asia
O'nyong-nyong virus	*Anopheles funestus* *Anopheles gambiae*	Unknown	Africa
Igbo-ora virus	*Anopheles funestus* *Anopheles gambiae*	Unknown	Ivory Coast
Ross River virus	*Aedes vigilax* *Aedes camptorbynchus* *Culex annulirostris* *Mansonia uniformus* *Aedes polynesiensis* *Aedes aegypti*	Rodents, marsupials, domestic animals	Australia, New Zealand, Papua New Guinea, Pacific islands
Barmah forest virus	*Aedes* species *Anopheles* species *Culex* species	Unknown	Australia
Sindbis virus	*Aedes* species *Culex* species *Culiseta* species	Unknown	Sweden, Finland, Karelian isthmus of Russia
Mayaro virus	*Haemagogus janthinomys*	Marmosets	Bolivia, Brazil, Peru

Chikungunya fever occurs endemically and in epidemics.[40] Outbreaks have been described in the Indian Ocean islands, Malaysia, and Hong Kong.[41-44] An outbreak occurred in Italy in 2007. A large-scale outbreak of the serologically related o'nyong-nyong virus occurred in the Acholi province of northwestern Uganda in February 1959; this outbreak spread through Uganda and the surrounding region at a rate of 2 to 3 kilometers daily, affecting more than 2 million people within 2 years.[45] After the initial o'nyong-nyong epidemic, clinical disease was not detected again until it re-emerged in the Acholi region in 1996.[46] Despite the absence of outbreaks in the intervening years, serologic surveys have demonstrated that o'nyong-nyong virus is endemic.[47]

Weber's line is a hypothetical demarcation separating the Australian and Asiatic geographic zones. Antibodies to chikungunya virus are found west of Weber's line, and Ross River virus antibodies are found only east of it. Ross River virus causes epidemics of fever and rash in Australia, New Zealand, and the western Pacific islands.[48] In the Fiji Islands from 1979 to 1980, Ross River virus caused febrile polyarthritis in more than 40,000 individuals.[49] In Australia, endemic cases and epidemics occur in tropical and temperate regions annually.[50] Most cases occur in Queensland and New South Wales territories, where high rainfall and subsequent increases in mosquito populations usually precede epidemic periods. Infection rates in Australia range from 0.2% to 3.5% per year. Male and female infection rates are similar, but there is a female predominance in presenting cases. Most infected adults are symptomatic; the case rate for children is lower. Barmah Forest virus, another alphavirus with an increasing incidence in Australia, may manifest in a fashion similar to Ross River virus.[51-56]

Individuals involved in outdoor activities or occupations in forested areas in Sweden, Finland, and the neighboring Karelian isthmus of Russia are at greatest risk for infection with Sindbis virus; in those regions, it is known as Okelbo disease, Pogosta disease, and Karelian fever, respectively. Birds are the intermediate host.[57] It has also been reported in central Africa, Zimbabwe, South Africa, and Australia in sporadic cases or small outbreaks.[35]

Mayaro virus, first recognized in Trinidad in 1954, is endemic in the tropical rain forests of Bolivia, Brazil, and Peru. Cases have been imported into the United States in individuals traveling from endemic areas.[58]

Diagnosis

Clinical Features. Chikungunya fever presents with an explosive onset of high fever and severe arthralgia after a 1- to 12-day incubation period. The fever lasts 1 to 7 days. Typically, a macular or maculopapular, sometimes pruritic rash on the torso, extremities, and occasionally the face, palms, and soles occurs on day 2 to 5 of illness as the patient defervesces. The rash may last 1 to 5 days and may recur with fever. Isolated petechiae and mucosal bleeding may occur. In some patients, involved skin desquamates.[59,60] Chemosis is prominent. Headache, photophobia, retro-orbital pain, pharyngitis, anorexia, nausea, vomiting, and abdominal pain may be present. Diffuse myalgia and back and shoulder pain are common. Migratory polyarthralgia, stiffness, and swelling affect predominantly the small joints of the hands, wrists, feet, and ankles. Large joints are less severely affected. Previously injured joints may be disproportionately affected. Large effusions are uncommon. Symptoms in children tend to be milder. Low-titer rheumatoid factor may be found in those with long-standing symptoms.

O'nyong-nyong fever is clinically similar to chikungunya fever.[61,62] In 1984, igbo-ora caused an epidemic of fever, myalgias, arthralgias, and rash in four Ivory Coast villages. Sequencing the isolates from the 1996 outbreak of o'nyong-nyong fever suggested that igbo-ora virus is a variant of o'nyong-nyong virus.[46]

Ross River virus polyarthralgia is severe, incapacitating, and often migratory and asymmetric.[63] Symptoms follow a 7- to 11-day incubation period. Finger interphalangeal and metacarpophalangeal joints, wrists, knees, ankles, shoulders, elbows, and toes are often involved. Polyarticular swelling and tenosynovitis are common. Arthralgias are worse in the morning and after inactivity. Rash is macular, papular, or maculopapular and may be pruritic. Vesicles, papules, or petechiae are typically seen on the trunk and extremities. The palms, soles, and face may be involved. Rash typically appears 1 to 2 days before joint symptoms, but it may occur anywhere from 11 days before to 15 days after the onset of arthralgias, and it resolves by fading to a brownish discoloration or by desquamation. Half of patients have no fever, and those who do may have only modest fevers lasting 1 to 3 days. Nausea, headache, and myalgia are common. Respiratory symptoms, mild photophobia, and lymphadenopathy may occur. Up to a third of patients have paresthesias and palm or sole pain. Carpal tunnel syndrome may be seen. Arthritis is less common and less prominent in Barmah Forest virus infection than in Ross River virus infection, but the rash is more common and florid.[64,65]

Rash and arthralgia are the presenting symptoms in Sindbis virus infection, although one may precede the other by a few days. Constitutional symptoms are usually mild and include low-grade fever, headache, fatigue, malaise, nausea, vomiting, pharyngitis, and paresthesias. A macular rash typically begins on the torso and then spreads to the arms and legs, palms, soles, and occasionally head. Macules evolve to form papules that tend to vesiculate. Vesiculation is prominent on pressure points, including the palms and soles. As the rash fades, a brownish discoloration is left. Vesicles on the palms and soles may become hemorrhagic. The rash may recur during convalescence.[66]

A Mayaro virus outbreak in Belterra, Brazil, in 1988 was characterized by sudden onset of fever, headache, dizziness, chills, and arthralgias in the wrists, fingers, ankles, and toes. The clinical attack rate was 80%. Joint swelling, unilateral inguinal lymphadenopathy, and leukopenia may be present. A maculopapular rash on the trunk and extremities lasts about 3 days.[67]

Laboratory Tests. The diagnosis of alphavirus infection requires laboratory confirmation. Any febrile patient residing in or returning from an endemic area should have a laboratory investigation. Chikungunya virus may be isolated from serum on days 2 through 4 of illness.[68] Neutralizing antibody, hemagglutination inhibition activity, and complement fixation tests may be used to detect antibodies. Chikungunya virus–specific IgM antibodies may be found for

6 months or longer.[69] O'nyong-nyong virus may be isolated by intracerebral injection into suckling mice, in which it produces alopecia, rash, and runting. Hemagglutination inhibition or complement fixation tests identify o'nyong-nyong virus.[70,71] Because chikungunya and o'nyong-nyong viruses are closely related serologically, mouse antisera raised to chikungunya virus or o'nyong-nyong virus react equally well with o'nyong-nyong virus, but o'nyong-nyong antisera does not react well with chikungunya virus. Molecular detection methods have improved diagnostic specificity.[72-75] Specific reverse-transcriptase polymerase chain reaction–based assays for viral RNA detection have been developed.[73,76]

In chikungunya fever, synovial fluid shows decreased viscosity, poor mucin clot, and 2000 to 5000 white blood cells/mm³. Ross River virus has been isolated only from antibody-negative sera. In the Australian epidemics before 1979, patients were antibody positive at the time of presentation. In contrast, patients in the Pacific island epidemics of 1979 to 1980 remained viremic and seronegative for up to 1 week after the onset of the symptoms. Synovial fluid cell counts range from 1500 to 13,800 cells/mm³, predominantly monocytes and vacuolated macrophages.[77] Barmah Forest virus infection is confirmed by rising titers of specific IgG.[64] Diagnosis of Sindbis virus infection is confirmed by specific serology.

Pathogenesis

Little is known about the pathogenesis of chikungunya fever or arthritis. Involved skin shows erythrocyte extravasation from superficial capillaries and perivascular cuffing. The virus adsorbs to human platelets, causing aggregation, suggesting a mechanism for bleeding. Synovitis probably results from direct viral infection of synovium. In one patient with chronic arthropathy, the synovium appeared atrophic on arthroscopy and was histologically normal.[78] The mechanisms of o'nyong-nyong virus pathogenesis are unknown. However, the virus was isolated from peripheral blood mononuclear cells in a patient in Chad.[79]

Ross River virus antigen may be detected early in monocytes and macrophages by immunofluorescence, but intact virus is not identifiable by electron microscopy or cell culture.[80] Erythematous and purpuric rashes show mild dermal perivascular mononuclear cell infiltrates, mostly T lymphocytes. Purpuric areas also show erythrocyte extravasation. Viral antigen may be detected in epithelial cells in erythematous and purpuric skin lesions and in perivascular zones in erythematous lesions.[81]

Sindbis virus has been isolated from a skin vesicle in the absence of viremia. Skin lesions show perivascular edema, hemorrhage, lymphocytic infiltrates, and areas of necrosis. Anti–Sindbis virus IgM may persist for years, raising the possibility that Sindbis virus arthritis is associated with viral persistence.[82]

Treatment and Prognosis

Management is supportive. Nonsteroidal anti-inflammatory agents are useful, but aspirin should be avoided in view of the tendency for alphavirus rashes to develop a hemorrhagic component. Chloroquine has been used in chikungunya fever when nonsteroidal anti-inflammatory agents failed.[83]

During the acute attack, range-of-motion exercises may decrease stiffness. In general, the management of alphavirus infection is symptomatic; patients recover without sequelae. After acute chikungunya fever, symptoms may persist for months before resolution. Approximately 10% of patients still have joint symptoms 1 year after infection.[78] A few patients may develop chronic arthralgia. Case reports suggest that a few patients with chronic arthropathy develop destructive joint lesions, but a second process cannot be ruled out.

For persons with Ross River virus arthritis, mild exercise tends to improve joint symptoms. Half of all patients are able to resume their daily activities within 4 weeks, although residual polyarthralgia may be present. Joint symptoms may recur.[84] Arthralgia, myalgia, and lethargy may continue for at least 6 months in up to half of patients.[64] Relapsing episodes gradually resolve, but joint symptoms have been reported in a few patients for up to 3 years.[63,85]

Nonerosive chronic arthropathy is common after Sindbis virus infection, with up to one third of patients having arthropathy 2 years or longer after onset. A smaller number have symptoms as long as 5 to 6 years.[82] Mayaro virus–infected patients have persistent arthralgias for months.

HEPATITIS B VIRUS

Hepatitis B virus (HBV), a member of the family Hepadnaviridae, genus *Orthohepadnavirus*, is an enveloped, double-stranded, icosahedral DNA virus measuring 42 nm in diameter.[86,87]

EPIDEMIOLOGY

HBV occurs worldwide and is transmitted by parenteral and sexual routes. Prevalence is highest in Asia, the Middle East, and sub-Saharan Africa. In China, the prevalence is as high as 10%, compared with 0.01% in the United States. In endemic regions, infection occurs at an early age, frequently perinatally. Early HBV infection is usually asymptomatic. Rates of HBV carriage and specific antibody positivity decline with age. In the West, most infections are acquired during adulthood through sexual or needle exposures, leading to acute hepatitis. Of those with hepatitis, 5% to 10% develop persistent infection. In endemic regions, HBV is a common cause of chronic liver disease and a leading cause of hepatocellular carcinoma.[86]

CLINICAL FEATURES

The time from infection to clinical hepatitis is usually 45 to 120 days. A preicteric prodromal period lasts several days to a month and may be associated with fever, myalgia, malaise, anorexia, nausea, and vomiting. Joint involvement is usually sudden in onset and often severe, with symmetric and simultaneous involvement of several joints. Alternatively, arthritis may be migratory or additive.[88,89] The joints of the hand and knee are most often affected, but wrists, ankles, elbows, shoulders, and other large joints may be involved as well. Fusiform swelling occurs in the small joints of the hand. Morning stiffness is common. Arthritis and urticaria may precede jaundice by days to weeks and persist for several weeks, but they usually subside soon after the onset of clinical jaundice. Arthritis is usually limited to the preicteric prodrome. Those who develop chronic active hepatitis or chronic HBV viremia may have recurrent polyarthralgia or polyarthritis.[90] Polyarteritis nodosa may be associated with chronic hepatitis B viremia.[91]

DIAGNOSIS

Urticaria in the presence of polyarthritis should suggest the possibility of HBV infection. Acute hepatitis may be asymptomatic, but elevated bilirubin and transaminases are usually present when arthritis appears. At the onset of arthritis, peak levels of serum hepatitis B surface antigen (HBsAg) are detectable. Virions, viral DNA, polymerase, and hepatitis B antigen may be detectable in serum. Anti–hepatitis B core antigen IgM antibodies indicate acute HBV infection rather than past or chronic infection.[92]

PATHOGENESIS

Significant viremia occurs early in infection. Soluble immune complexes with circulating HBsAg form as anti-HBsAg antibodies are produced. An immune complex–mediated arthritis usually results, with immune complex deposition in synovium. Immune complexes containing HBsAg, antibody, and complement components may be detected.

HEPATITIS C VIRUS

Hepatitis C virus (HCV), a member of the family Flaviviridae, is an enveloped, single-stranded, spherical RNA virus measuring 38 to 50 nm in diameter.[93,94]

EPIDEMIOLOGY

HCV infection occurs worldwide. Like HBV infection, seroprevalence is higher in Africa and Asia, where it may cause one fourth of acute and chronic hepatitis cases. In Japan, up to 50% of hepatitides may be caused by HCV.[95] In the United States, an estimated 2.7 million individuals are infected.[96,97]

HCV is transmitted by the parenteral route. Sexual transmission may occur but is uncommon.[98] More than half of all cases of non-A, non-B hepatitis are attributable to HCV infection.[99] Multiple HCV genotypes and quasi-species are organized into six major groups. They differ in pathogenicity, severity of disease, and response to interferon.[99-103]

CLINICAL FEATURES

Acute HCV infection is usually benign. Up to 80% of posttransfusion infections are anicteric and asymptomatic. Liver enzyme elevations, when present, are usually minimal. Normal transaminase levels do not exclude HCV infection. Community-acquired cases may present more symptomatically and with significant transaminase elevations. Acute fulminant HCV hepatitis is rare. Acute HCV infection may be accompanied by acute-onset polyarthritis in a rheumatoid distribution, including the small joints of the hand, wrists, shoulders, knees, and hips.[104]

HCV is often associated with mixed (type II and III) cryoglobulinemia. Essential mixed cryoglobulinemia—a triad of arthritis, palpable purpura, and cryoglobulinemia—is associated with HCV infection in most cases. Cryoglobulinemia in HCV infection is also seen in the absence of arthritis and purpura.[105] Cryoglobulinemia may be associated with necrotizing vasculitis. The presence of anti-HCV antibodies in essential mixed cryoglobulinemia is associated with more severe cutaneous involvement, such as Raynaud's phenomena, purpura, livedo, distal ulcers, and gangrene.[106] HCV RNA may be found in 75% of cryoprecipitates from patients with essential mixed cryoglobulinemia and anti-HCV antibodies.[107]

DIAGNOSIS

Serologic tests use an array of antigens in an enzyme immunoassay. A recombinant antigen strip immunoblot assay is confirmatory.[108] Polymerase chain reaction–based diagnostics allow confirmation of HCV viremia, viral load, and genotype.[100,101] A minority of patients may have HCV RNA detectable by polymerase chain reaction amplification methods in the absence of positive serologic findings.[108-113] A liver biopsy for staging of liver disease is usually indicated in patients who have serum anti-HCV antibody or RNA, even in the setting of normal liver enzymes, because liver enzymes do not reflect liver histology. A number of algorithms based on blood measures of liver involvement have been proposed to aid in staging.[114-118]

PATHOGENESIS

HCV infection persists despite antibody response to viral epitopes. Increased $CD4^+CD25^+$ regulatory T lymphocytes may blunt the immune response to HCV.[118] A high rate of mutation in the envelope protein is responsible for the emergence of neutralization-escape mutants and quasi-species.[119] HCV may contain an IgG Fc binding region on its surface; humoral immune response to HCV would, by epitope spreading, also target bound immunoglobulin Fc structures.[120] Chronic HCV infection leads to cirrhosis, end-stage liver failure, and hepatocellular carcinoma after a period of up to 20 years, but the frequency of these sequelae is debated and the mechanisms by which they occur are unknown.[121]

TREATMENT

Interferon-α2b at a dose of 3 million units or higher three times weekly for 6 months suppresses viral titers and ameliorates HCV liver disease in about half of patients and may benefit HCV-associated cryoglobulinemia.[122] Relapse after completion of the initial course of therapy is common. The use of pegylated interferons to increase drug half-life and decrease clearance and the addition of ribavirin have improved outcomes.[123] There is controversy whether interferon therapy precipitates autoimmune diseases such as autoimmune thyroiditis.[124,125] Those with cryoglobulinemia who fail interferon therapy require immunosuppressive therapy when vasculitis is present.

HUMAN T-LYMPHOTROPIC VIRUS TYPE 1

Human T-lymphotropic virus type 1 (HTLV-1), a retrovirus, is endemic in southern Japan, where it has been associated with oligoarthritis and a nodular rash (Fig. 104-2).

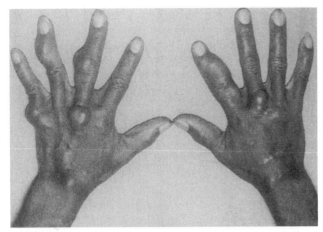

Figure 104-2 Nodular synovitis associated with human T-lymphotropic virus type 1 infection. *(From Yancey WB Jr, Dolson LH, Oblon D, et al: HTLV-I-associated adult T-cell leukemia/lymphoma presenting with nodular synovial masses. Am J Med 89:676, 1990.)*

Anti-HTLV serology is positive. Type C viral particles are found in skin nodules. Synovial tissue is infiltrated by leukemic T lymphocytes with lobulated nuclei.[126-128]

OTHER VIRUSES

There are numerous other commonly encountered viral syndromes in which joint involvement occasionally occurs. Children with varicella rarely develop brief monarticular or pauciarticular arthritis.[129] Mumps in adults is occasionally associated with small or large joint synovitis preceding or following the onset of parotitis by up to 4 weeks. Mumps arthritis may last several weeks.[130] Infection with adenovirus and coxsackieviruses A9, B2, B3, B4, and B6 has been associated with recurrent episodes of polyarthritis, pleuritis, myalgia, rash, pharyngitis, myocarditis, and leukocytosis.[131] Epstein-Barr virus–induced mononucleosis is frequently accompanied by polyarthralgia, but monarticular knee arthritis sometimes occurs. A few cases of polyarthritis, fever, and myalgias due to echovirus 9 infection have been reported.[132] Arthritis associated with herpes simplex virus or cytomegalovirus infection is rare, but a severe cytomegalovirus polyarthritis has been described in several immunocompromised bone marrow transplant recipients.[133] *Herpes hominis* occasionally causes arthritis of the knee in wrestlers, a condition referred to as herpes gladiatorum.[134] Knee arthritis after vaccinia inoculation has been reported as a rare complication.[135]

REFERENCES

1. Pennisi E: Teetering on the brink of danger. Science 271:1665, 1996.
2. Albert LJ, Inman RD: Molecular mimicry and autoimmunity. N Engl J Med 341:2068, 1999.
3. Gillespie SM, Cartter ML, Asch S, et al: Occupational risk of human parvovirus B19 infection for school and day-care personnel during an outbreak of erythema infectiosum. JAMA 263:2061, 1990.
4. **Bell LM, Naides SJ, Stoffman P, et al: Human parvovirus B19 infection among hospital staff members after contact with infected patients. N Engl J Med 321:485, 1989.**
5. Anderson MJ, Higgins PG, Davis LR, et al: Experimental parvoviral infection in humans. J Infect Dis 152:257, 1985.
6. **Naides SJ: Rheumatic manifestations of parvovirus B19 infection. Rheum Dis Clin North Am 24:375, 1998.**
7. Von Poblotzki A, Hemauer A, Gigler A, et al: Antibodies to the nonstructural protein of parvovirus B19 in persistently infected patients: Implications for pathogenesis. J Infect Dis 172:1356, 1995.
8. Takahashi Y, Murai C, Shibata S, et al: Human parvovirus B19 as a causative agent for rheumatoid arthritis. Proc Natl Acad Sci U S A 95:8227, 1998.
9. Hsu TC, Tzang BS, Huang CN, et al: Increased expression and secretion of interleukin-6 in human parvovirus B19 non-structural protein (NS1) transfected COS-7 epithelial cells. Clin Exp Immunol 144:152, 2006.
10. Sol N, Morinet F, Alizon M, et al: Trans-activation of the long terminal repeat of human immunodeficiency virus type 1 by the parvovirus B19 NS1 gene product. J Gen Virol 74:2011, 1993.
11. Peterlana D, Puccetti A, Beri R, et al: The presence of parvovirus B19 VP and NS1 genes in the synovium is not correlated with rheumatoid arthritis. J Rheumatol 30:1907, 2003.
12. Poole BD, Karetnyi YV, Naides SJ: Parvovirus B19-induced apoptosis of hepatocytes. J Virol 78:7775, 2004.
13. Poole BD, Zhou J, Grote A, et al: Apoptosis of liver-derived cells induced by parvovirus B19 nonstructural protein. J Virol 80:4114, 2006.
14. Karetnyi YV, Beck PR, Markin RS, et al: Human parvovirus B19 infection in acute fulminant liver failure. Arch Virol 144:1713, 1999.
15. Gabriel SE, Espy M, Erdman DD, et al: The role of parvovirus B19 in the pathogenesis of giant cell arteritis: A preliminary evaluation. Arthritis Rheum 42:1255, 1999.
16. Veraldi S, Mancuso R, Rizzitelli E, et al: Henoch-Schönlein syndrome associated with human parvovirus B19 primary infection. Eur J Dermatol 9:232, 1999.
17. Heegaard ED, Rosthoj S, Petersen B, et al: Role of parvovirus B19 infection in childhood idiopathic thrombocytopenic purpura. Acta Paediatr 88:614, 1999.
18. Frickhofen N, Abkowitz JL, Safford M, et al: Persistent B19 parvovirus infection in patients infected with human immunodeficiency virus type 1 (HIV-1): A treatable cause of anemia in AIDS. Ann Intern Med 113:926, 1990.
19. Ager EA, Chin TDY, Poland JD: Epidemic erythema infectiosum. N Engl J Med 275:1326, 1966.
20. Naides SJ, Field EH: Transient rheumatoid factor positivity in acute parvovirus B19 infection. Arch Intern Med 148:2587, 1988.
21. Kerr JR, Boyd N: Autoantibodies following parvovirus B19 infection. J Infect 32:41, 1996.
22. Lunardi C, Tiso M, Borgato L, et al: Chronic parvovirus B19 infection induces the production of anti-virus antibodies with autoantigen binding properties. Euro J Immunol 28:936, 1998.
23. Meyer O: Parvovirus B19 and autoimmune diseases. Joint Bone Spine 70:6, 2003.
24. von Landenberg P, et al: Antiphospholipid antibodies in pediatric and adult patients with rheumatic disease are associated with parvovirus B19 infection. Arthritis Rheum 48:1939, 2003.
25. Anderson LJ, Tsou C, Parker RA, et al: Detection of antibodies and antigens of human parvovirus B19 by enzyme-linked immunosorbent assay. J Clin Microbiol 24:522, 1986.
26. Cohen BJ: Detection of parvovirus B19-specific IgM by antibody capture radioimmunoassay. J Virol Methods 66:1, 1997.
27. Soderlund M, von Essen R, Haapasaari J, et al: Persistence of parvovirus B19 DNA in synovial membranes of young patients with and without chronic arthropathy. Lancet 349:1063, 1997.
28. Frey TK: Molecular biology of rubella virus. Adv Virus Res 44:69, 1994.
29. Chantler J, Wolinsky JS, Tingle A: Rubella. In Knipe DM, Howley PM, et al (eds): Fields Virology, 4th ed. Philadelphia, Lippincott Williams & Wilkins, 2001, pp 963-990.
30. Mims CA, Stokes A, Grahame R: Synthesis of antibodies, including antiviral antibodies, in the knee joints of patients with arthritis. Ann Rheum Dis 44:734, 1985.
31. **Tingle AJ, Allen M, Petty RE, et al: Rubella-associated arthritis. I. Comparative study of joint manifestations associated with natural rubella infection and RA 27/3 rubella immunization. Ann Rheum Dis 45:110, 1986.**
32. Howson CP, Katz M, Johnston RB Jr, et al: Chronic arthritis after rubella vaccination. Clin Infect Dis 15:307, 1992.

33. Schaffner W, Fleet WF, Kilroy AW, et al: Polyneuropathy following rubella immunization: A follow-up study and review of the problem. Am J Dis Child 127:684, 1974.

34. Mitchell LA, Tingle AJ, Shukin R, et al: Chronic rubella vaccine-associated arthropathy. Arch Intern Med 153:2268, 1993.

35. Griffin DE: Alphaviruses. In Knipe DM, Howley PM, et al (eds): Fields Virology, 4th ed. Philadelphia, Lippincott Williams & Wilkins, 2001, pp 917-962.

36. Bryan JH, Foley DH, Sutherst RW: Malaria transmission and climate change in Australia. Med J Aust 164:345, 1996.

37. Jetten TH, Focks DA: Potential changes in the distribution of dengue transmission under climate warming. Am J Trop Med Hyg 57:285, 1997.

38. Reiter P: Climate change and mosquito-borne disease. Environ Health Perspect 109(Suppl 1):141, 2001.

39. Rydzanicz K, Kiewra D, Lonc E: Changes in range of mosquito-borne diseases affected by global climatic fluctuations. Wiad Parazytol 52:73, 2006.

40. Halstead SB, Nimmannitya S, Margiotta MR: Dengue and chikungunya virus infection in man in Thailand, 1962-1964. II. Observations on disease in outpatients. Am J Trop Med Hyg 18:972, 1969.

41. Sam IC, AbuBakar S: Chikungunya virus infection. Med J Malaysia 61:264, 2006.

42. Schuffenecker I, Iteman I, Michault A, et al: Genome microevolution of chikungunya viruses causing the Indian Ocean outbreak. Plo S Med 3:e263, 2006.

43. Lee N, Wong CK, Lam WY, et al: Chikungunya fever, Hong Kong. Emerg Infect Dis 12:1790, 2006.

44. AbuBakar S, Sam JC, Wong PF, et al: Reemergence of endemic Chikungunya, Malaysia. Emerg Infect Dis 13:147, 2007.

45. Williams MC, Woodall JP, Gillett JD: O'nyong-nyong fever: An epidemic in East Africa. VII. Virus isolations from man and serological studies up to July 1961. Trans R Soc Trop Med Hyg 59:186, 1965.

46. Lanciotti RS, Ludwig ML, Rwaguma EB, et al: Emergence of epidemic o'nyong-nyong fever in Uganda, after a 35 year absence. Virology 252:258, 1998.

47. Marshall TF, Keenlyside RA, Johnson BK, et al: The epidemiology of o'nyong-nyong in the Kano Plain, Kenya. Ann Trop Med Parasitol 76:153, 1982.

48. Harley D, Sleigh A, Ritchie S: Ross River virus transmission, infection, and disease: A cross-disciplinary review. Clin Microbiol Rev 14:909, 2001.

49. Bennett NM, Cunningham AL, Fraser JR, et al: Epidemic polyarthritis acquired in Fiji. Med J Aust 1:316, 1980.

50. Mudge PR, Aaskov JG: Epidemic polyarthritis in Australia, 1980-1981. Med J Aust 2:269, 1983.

51. Lindsay MDA, Johansen CA, Broom AK, et al: Emergence of Barmah Forest virus in western Australia. Emerg Infect Dis 1:22, 1995.

52. Harvey L, Dwyer D: Recent increases in the notification of Barmah Forest virus infections in New South Wales. N S W Public Health Bull 15:199, 2004.

53. Liu C, Broom AK, Kurcz N, et al: Communicable Diseases Network Australia: National Arbovirus and Malaria Advisory Committee annual report 2004-05. Commun Dis Intell 29:341, 2005.

54. Quinn HE, Gatton ML, Hall G, et al: Analysis of Barmah Forest virus disease activity in Queensland, Australia, 1993-2003: Identification of a large, isolated outbreak of disease. J Med Entomol 42:882, 2005.

55. Liu C, Johansen C, Kurucz N, et al: Communicable Diseases Network Australia: National Arbovirus and Malaria Advisory Committee annual report, 2005-06. Commun Dis Intell 30:411, 2006.

56. Kelly-Hope LA, Kay BH, Purdie DM, et al: The risk of Ross River and Barmah Forest virus disease in Queensland: Implications for New Zealand. Aust N Z J Public Health 26:69, 2002.

57. Brummer-Korvenkontio M, Vapalahti O, Kuusisto P, et al: Epidemiology of Sindbis virus infections in Finland 1981-96: Possible factors explaining a peculiar disease pattern. Epidemiol Infect 129:335, 2002.

58. Tesh RB, Watts DM, Russell KL, et al: Mayaro virus disease: An emerging mosquito-borne zoonosis in tropical South America. Clin Infect Dis 28:67, 1999.

59. Moore CG: *Aedes albopictus* in the United States: Current status and prospects for further spread. J Am Mosq Control Assoc 15:221, 1999.

60. **Halstead SB, Udomsakdi S, Singharaj P, et al: Dengue and chikungunya virus infection in man in Thailand, 1962-1964. III. Clinical, epidemiologic, and virologic observations on disease in non-indigenous white persons. Am J Trop Med Hyg 18:984, 1969.**

61. Sanders EJ, Rwaguma EB, Kawamata J, et al: O'nyong-nyong fever in south-central Uganda, 1996-1997: Description of the epidemic and results of a household-based seroprevalence survey. J Infect Dis 180:1436, 1999.

62. **Kiwanuka N, Sanders EJ, Rwaguma EB, et al: O'nyong-nyong fever in south-central Uganda, 1996-1997: Clinical features and validation of a clinical case definition for surveillance purposes. Clin Infect Dis 29:1243, 1999.**

63. Fraser JRE: Epidemic polyarthritis and Ross River virus disease. Clin Rheum Dis 12:369, 1986.

64. Flexman JP, Smith DW, Mackenzie JS, et al: A comparison of the diseases caused by Ross River virus and Barmah Forest virus. Med J Aust 169:159, 1998.

65. Passmore J, O'Grady KA, Moran R, et al: An outbreak of Barmah Forest virus disease in Victoria. Commun Dis Intell 26:600, 2002.

66. Julkunen I, Brummer-Korvenkontio M, Hautanen A, et al: Elevated serum immune complex levels in Pogosta disease, an acute alphavirus infection with rash and arthritis. J Clin Lab Immunol 21:77, 1986.

67. **Pinheiro FP, Freitas RB, Travassos da Rosa JF, et al: An outbreak of Mayaro virus disease in Belterra, Brazil. I. Clinical and virological findings. Am J Trop Med Hyg 30:674, 1981.**

68. Nimmannitya S, Halstead SB, Cohen SN, et al: Dengue and chikungunya virus infection in man in Thailand, 1962-1964. I. Observations on hospitalized patients with hemorrhagic fever. Am J Trop Med Hyg 18:954, 1969.

69. Nakitare GW, Bundo K, Igarashi A: Enzyme-linked immunosorbent assay (ELISA) for antibody titers against chikungunya virus of human serum from Kenya. Trop Med 25:119, 1983.

70. Williams MC, Woodall JP, Porterfield JS: O'nyong-nyong fever: An epidemic virus disease in East Africa. V. Human antibody studies by plaque inhibition and other serological tests. Trans R Soc Trop Med Hyg 56:166, 1962.

71. Williams MC, Woodall JP, Porterfield JS: O'nyong-nyong fever: An epidemic virus disease in East Africa. Trans R Soc Trop Med Hyg 59:186, 1965.

72. Hasebe F, Parquet MC, Pandey BD, et al: Combined detection and genotyping of chikungunya virus by a specific reverse transcription-polymerase chain reaction. J Med Virol 67:370, 2002.

73. Pfeffer M, Linssen B, Parke MD, et al: Specific detection of chikungunya virus using a RT-PCR/nested PCR combination. J Vet Med B Infect Dis Vet Public Health 49:49, 2002.

74. Corwin A, Simanjuntak CH, Ansari A: Emerging disease surveillance in Southeast Asia. Ann Acad Med Singapore 26:628, 1997.

75. Junt T, Heraud JM, Lelarge J, et al: Determination of natural versus laboratory human infection with Mayaro virus by molecular analysis. Epidemiol Infect 123:511, 1999.

76. Pastorino B, Bessaud M, Grandadam M, et al: Development of a TaqMan RT-PCR assay without RNA extraction step for the detection and quantification of African chikungunya viruses. J Virol Methods 124:65, 2005.

77. **Aaskov JG, Mataika JU, Lawrence GW, et al: An epidemic of Ross River virus infection in Fiji, 1979. Am J Trop Med Hyg 30:1053, 1981.**

78. Brighton SW, Prozesky OW, De la Harpe AL: Chikungunya virus infection: A retrospective study of 107 cases. S Afr Med J 63:313, 1983.

79. Bessaud M, Peyrefitte CN, Pastorino BA, et al: O'nyong-nyong virus, Chad. Emerg Infect Dis 12:1248, 2006.

80. Fraser JR, Cunningham AL, Clarris BJ, et al: Cytology of synovial effusions in epidemic polyarthritis. Aust N Z J Med 11:168, 1981.

81. Fraser JR, Ratnamohan VM, Dowling JP, et al: The exanthem of Ross River virus infection: Histology, location of virus antigen and nature of inflammatory infiltrate. J Clin Pathol 36:1256, 1983.

82. Niklasson B, Espmark A, Lundstrom J: Occurrence of arthralgia and specific IgM antibodies three to four years after Ockelbo disease. J Infect Dis 157:832, 1988.

83. Brighton SW: Chloroquine phosphate treatment of chronic chikungunya arthritis: An open pilot study. S Afr Med J 66:217, 1984.

84. Mylonas AD, Brown AM, Carthew TL, et al: Natural history of Ross River virus-induced epidemic polyarthritis. Med J Aust 177:356, 2002.

85. Laine M, Luukkainen R, Jalava J, et al: Prolonged arthritis associated with Sindbis-related (Pogosta) virus infection. Rheumatology (Oxford) 41:829, 2002.

86. Robinson WS: Hepatitis B viruses: General features (human). In Webster RG, Granoff A (eds): Encyclopedia of Virology. San Diego, Academic Press, 1994, pp 554-559.

87. Bendinelli M, Pistello M, Maggi F, et al: Blood-borne hepatitis viruses: Hepatitis B, C, D, and G viruses and TT virus. In Specter S, Hodinka RL, Young SA (eds): Clinical Virology Manual. Washington, DC, ASM Press, 2000, pp 306-337.

88. Hollinger FB, Liang TJ: Hepatitis B virus. In Knipe DM, Howley PM, Griffin DE, et al (eds): Fields Virology, Philadelphia, Lippincott Williams & Wilkins, 2001, pp 2971-3036.

89. **Alarcon GS, Townes AS: Arthritis in viral hepatitis: Report of two cases and review of the literature. Johns Hopkins Med J 132:1, 1973.**

90. Csepregi A, Rojkovich B, Nemesanszky E, et al: Chronic seropositive polyarthritis associated with hepatitis B virus-induced chronic liver disease: A sequel of virus persistence. Arthritis Rheum 43:232, 2000.

91. Guillevin L, Lhote F, Cohen P, et al: Polyarteritis nodosa related to hepatitis B virus: A prospective study with long-term observation of 41 patients. Medicine (Baltimore) 74:238, 1995.

92. Hoofnagle JH: Serologic markers of hepatitis B virus infection. Annu Rev Med 32:1, 1981.

93. Gronboek KE, Jensen OJ, Krarup HB, et al: Biochemical, virological and histopathological changes in Danish blood donors with antibodies to hepatitis C virus. Dan Med Bull 43:186, 1996.

94. Lindebach BD, Rice CM: Flaviviridae: The viruses and their replication. In Knipe DM, Howley PM, Griffin DE, et al (eds): Fields Virology. Philadelphia, Lippincott Williams & Wilkins, 2001, pp 991-1041.

95. Kuboki M, Shinzawa H, Shao L, et al: A cohort study of hepatitis C virus (HCV) infection in an HCV epidemic area of Japan: Age and sex-related seroprevalence of anti-HCV antibody, frequency of viremia, biochemical abnormality and histological changes. Liver 19:88, 1999.

96. Alter MJ, Mast EE: The epidemiology of viral hepatitis in the United States. Gastroenterol Clin North Am 23:437, 1994.

97. Williams I: Epidemiology of hepatitis C in the United States. Am J Med 107:2S, 1999.

98. Neumayr G, Propst A, Schwaighofer H, et al: Lack of evidence for the heterosexual transmission of hepatitis C. QJM 92:505, 1999.

99. Bhandari BN, Wright TL: Hepatitis C: An overview. Annu Rev Med 46:309, 1995.

100. Pawlotsky JM: Hepatitis C virus genetic variability: Pathogenic and clinical implications. Clin Liver Dis 7:45, 2003.

101. Pawlotsky JM: Use and interpretation of hepatitis C virus diagnostic assays. Clin Liver Dis 7:127, 2003.

102. Davis GL: Hepatitis C virus genotypes and quasispecies. Am J Med 107:21S, 1999.

103. Simmonds P, Bukh J, Combet C, et al: Consensus proposals for a unified system of nomenclature of hepatitis C virus genotypes. Hepatology 42:962, 2005.

104. **Siegel LB, Cohn L, Nashel D: Rheumatic manifestations of hepatitis C infection. Semin Arthritis Rheum 23:149, 1993.**

105. Arranz FR, Diaz RD, Diez LI, et al: Cryoglobulinemic vasculitis associated with hepatitis C virus infection: A report of eight cases. Acta Derm Venereol (Stockh) 75:234, 1995.

106. Sansonno D, Cornacchiulo V, Iacobelli AR, et al: Localization of hepatitis C virus antigens in liver and skin tissues of chronic hepatitis C virus-infected patients with mixed cryoglobulinemia. Hepatology 21:305, 1995.

107. Munoz-Fernandez S, Barbado FJ, Martin Mola E, et al: Evidence of hepatitis C virus antibodies in the cryoprecipitate of patients with mixed cryoglobulinemia. J Rheumatol 21:229, 1994.

108. van der Poel CL: Hepatitis C virus: Into the fourth generation. Vox Sang 67(Suppl 3):95, 1994.

109. Schmidt WN, Klinzman D, LaBrecque DR, et al: Direct detection of hepatitis C virus (HCV) RNA from whole blood, and comparison with HCV RNA in plasma and peripheral blood mononuclear cells. J Med Virol 47:153, 1995.

110. Schmidt WN, Wu P, Cederna J, et al: Surreptitious hepatitis C virus (HCV) infection detected in the majority of patients with cryptogenic chronic hepatitis and negative HCV antibody tests. J Infect Dis 176:27, 1997.

111. Stapleton JT, Klinzman D, Schmidt WN, et al: Prospective comparison of whole-blood- and plasma-based hepatitis C virus RNA detection systems: Improved detection using whole blood as the source of viral RNA. J Clin Microbiol 37:484, 1999.

112. Schmidt W, Stapleton JT: Whole-blood hepatitis C virus RNA extraction methods. J Clin Microbiol 39:3812, 2001.

113. George SL, Gebhardt J, Klinzman D, et al: Hepatitis C virus viremia in HIV-infected individuals with negative HCV antibody tests. J Acquir Immune Defic Syndr 31:154, 2002.

114. Colletta C, Smirne C, Fabris C, et al: Value of two noninvasive methods to detect progression of fibrosis among HCV carriers with normal aminotransferases. Hepatology 42:838, 2005.

115. Wilson LE, Torbenson M, Astemborski J, et al: Progression of liver fibrosis among injection drug users with chronic hepatitis C. Hepatology 43:788, 2006.

116. Zaman A, Rosen HR, Ingram K, et al: Assessment of FIBROSpect II to detect hepatic fibrosis in chronic hepatitis C patients. Am J Med 120:e9, 2007.

117. Adams LA, Bulsara M, Rossi E, et al: Hepascore: An accurate validated predictor of liver fibrosis in chronic hepatitis C infection. Clin Chem 51:1867, 2005.

118. Bolacchi F, Sinistro A, Ciaprini C, et al: Increased hepatitis C virus (HCV)-specific CD4+CD25+ regulatory T lymphocytes and reduced HCV-specific CD4+ T cell response in HCV-infected patients with normal versus abnormal alanine aminotransferase levels. Clin Exp Immunol 144:188, 2006.

119. Shimizu YK, Hijikata M, Iwamoto A, et al: Neutralizing antibodies against hepatitis C virus and the emergence of neutralization escape mutant viruses. J Virol 68:1494, 1994.

120. Wunschmann S, Medh JD, Klinzmann D, et al: Characterization of hepatitis C virus (HCV) and HCV E2 interaction with CD81 and the low density lipoprotein receptor. J Virol 74:10055, 2000.

121. Seeff LB: Natural history of hepatitis C. In Liang TJ, Hoofnagle JH (eds): Hepatitis C. San Diego, Academic Press, 2000, pp 85-105.

122. Gish RG: Standards of treatment in chronic hepatitis C. Semin Liver Dis 19(Suppl 1):35, 1999.

123. Baker DE: Pegylated interferon plus ribavirin for the treatment of chronic hepatitis C. Rev Gastroenterol Disord 3:93, 2003.

124. Morisco F, Mazziotti G, Rotondi M, et al: Interferon-related thyroid autoimmunity and long-term clinical outcome of chronic hepatitis C. Dig Liver Dis 33:247, 2001.

125. Rocco A, Gargano S, Provenzano A, et al: Incidence of autoimmune thyroiditis in interferon-alpha treated and untreated patients with chronic hepatitis C virus infection. Neuroendocrinol Lett 22:39, 2001.

126. Yancey WB Jr, Dolson LH, Oblon D, et al: HTLV-I-associated adult T-cell leukemia/lymphoma presenting with nodular synovial masses. Am J Med 89:676, 1990.

127. **Masuko-Hongo K, Nishioka K: HTLV-I associated arthropathy (HAAP)—a review. Ryoikibetsu Shokogun Shirizu 32:525, 2000.**

128. Nishioka K, Nakajima T, Hasunuma T, et al: Rheumatic manifestation of human leukemia virus infection. Rheum Dis Clin North Am 19:489, 1993.

129. Chen MK, Wang CC, Lu JJ, et al: Varicella arthritis diagnosed by polymerase chain reaction. J Formos Med Assoc 98:519, 1999.

130. Gordon SC, Lauter CB: Mumps arthritis: A review of the literature. Rev Infect Dis 6:338, 1984.

131. Bayer AS: Arthritis associated with common viral infections: Mumps, coxsackievirus, and adenovirus. Postgrad Med 68:55, 1980.

132. Blotzer JW, Myers AR: Echovirus-associated polyarthritis: Report of a case with synovial fluid and synovial histologic characterization. Arthritis Rheum 21:978, 1978.

133. Burns LJ, Gingrich RD: Cytomegalovirus infection presenting as polyarticular arthritis following autologous BMT. Bone Marrow Transplant 11:77, 1993.

134. Shelley WB: Herpetic arthritis associated with disseminated herpes simplex in a wrestler. Br J Dermatol 103:209, 1980.

135. Silby HM, Farber R, O'Connell CJ, et al: Acute monarticular arthritis after vaccination: Report of a case with isolation of vaccinia virus from synovial fluid. Ann Intern Med 62:347, 1965.

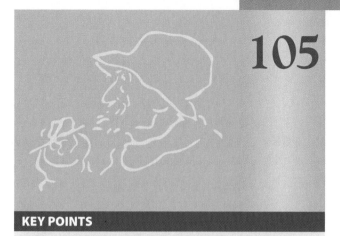

105

Poststreptoccocal Arthritis and Rheumatic Fever

ALLAN GIBOFSKY •
JOHN B. ZABRISKIE

KEY POINTS

Acute rheumatic fever (ARF) is a delayed, nonsuppurative sequela of a pharyngeal infection with group A streptococci. Although there has been a dramatic decline in the severity and the mortality of the disease, there have been reports of its resurgence in the United States.

Adequate treatment of documented streptococcal pharyngitis markedly reduces the incidence of subsequent ARF. Appropriate antimicrobial prophylaxis prevents recurrences of disease in known patients with ARF.

The clinical presentation of ARF varies. The lack of a single pathognomonic feature has resulted in the development of the revised Jones criteria, which should be used to establish a diagnosis.

The terms *migrating* and *migratory* are often used to describe the polyarthritis of ARF, but these designations are not meant to signify that the inflammation disappears in one joint when it appears in another. Rather, the various localizations usually overlap in time, and the onset, as opposed to the full course of the arthritis, "migrates" from joint to joint.

Many investigators have suggested that poststreptococcal migratory arthritis (in adults and children) in the absence of carditis might be a entity distinct from ARF. Although these features may be seen (admittedly rarely), migratory arthritis without evidence of other major Jones criteria but supported by two minor manifestations still should be considered ARF, especially in children.

Antibiotic prophylaxis with penicillin should be started immediately after the resolution of the acute episode. The optimal regimen consists of oral penicillin VK, 250,000 U twice a day, or parenteral penicillin G, 1.2 million U intramuscularly every 4 weeks.

Acute rheumatic fever (ARF) is a delayed, nonsuppurative sequela of pharyngeal infection with group A streptococci. After the initial streptococcal pharyngitis, there is a latent period of 2 to 3 weeks. The onset of disease usually is characterized by an acute febrile illness, which may manifest itself in one of three classic ways: (1) The patient may present with migratory arthritis predominantly involving the large joints of the body. (2) There may be concomitant clinical and laboratory signs of carditis and valvulitis. (3) There may be involvement of the central nervous system, manifesting as Sydenham's chorea. The clinical episodes are self-limiting, but damage to the valves may be chronic and progressive, resulting in cardiac decompensation and death.

Although there has been a dramatic decline in the severity and the mortality of the disease since the turn of the 20th century, there have been reports in recent years of its resurgence in the United States[1] and in many military installations throughout the world, a reminder that the disease remains a public health problem even in developed countries. In addition, the disease continues essentially unabated in many developing countries. Estimates suggest there will be 10 to 20 million new cases per year in countries where two thirds of the world population lives.

EPIDEMIOLOGY

The incidence of ARF began to decline long before the introduction of antibiotics into clinical practice, decreasing from 250 to 100 patients/100,000 population from 1862 to 1962 in Denmark.[2] The introduction of antibiotics in 1950 rapidly accelerated this decline, until by 1980 the incidence ranged from 0.23 to 1.88 patients/100,000, with disease occurring primarily in children and teenagers. A notable exception has been in the native Hawaiian and Maori populations (both of Polynesian ancestry), where the incidence continues to be 13.4/100,000 hospitalized children/year.[3]

Only a few M serotypes (types 5, 14, 18, and 24) have been identified with outbreaks of ARF, suggesting that certain strains of group A streptococci may be more "rheumatogenic" than others.[4] In Trinidad, types 41 and 11 have been the most common strains isolated from the oropharynx of patients with ARF, however. In our own series, gathered over a 20-year period (Table 105-1), many different M serotypes were isolated, including six strains that could not be typed. Kaplan and colleagues[5] isolated several M types from patients seen during an outbreak of ARF in Utah, and these strains were mucoid and nonmucoid in character. Whether or not certain strains are more "rheumatogenic" than others remains unresolved. What is true, however, is that a streptococcal strain capable of causing well-documented pharyngitis is generally capable of causing ARF, although some notable exceptions have been recorded.[6]

PATHOGENESIS

Although there is little evidence for the direct involvement of group A streptococci in the affected tissues of ARF patients, there is a large body of epidemiologic and immunologic evidence indirectly implicating group A streptococci in the initiation of the disease process: (1) It is well known that outbreaks of ARF closely follow epidemics of either streptococcal sore throat or scarlet fever.[6] (2) Adequate treatment of documented streptococcal pharyngitis markedly reduces the incidence of subsequent ARF.[7] (3) Appropriate antimicrobial prophylaxis prevents recurrence of disease in known patients with ARF.[8] (4) If one tests the sera of most ARF patients for three antistreptococcal

Table 105-1 Positive Throat Cultures for Group A
β-Hemolytic Streptococci among Rockefeller
University Hospital Rheumatic Fever
Patients (*N*=87)

M Type	RHD	No RHD	Total
Nontypable	1	5	6
1	1	1	2
2	0	1	1
5	1	1	2
6	1	1	2
12	0	2	2
18	2	2	4
19	2	1	3
28	1	0	1
Total	9	11	23

RHD, patients with rheumatic heart disease; No RHD, patients without rheumatic heart disease.

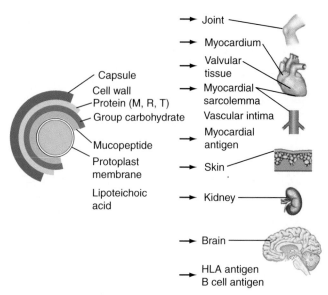

Figure 105-1 Schematic representation of the various structures of group A streptococci. Note the wide variety of cross-reactions between its antigens and mammalian tissues.

antibodies (streptolysin O, hyaluronidase, and streptokinase), most ARF patients (whether or not they recall an antecedent streptococcal sore throat) have elevated antibody titers to these antigens.[9]

A note of caution is necessary concerning documentation (either clinical or microbiologic) of an antecedent streptococcal infection. The frequency of isolation of group A streptococci from the oropharynx is extremely low even in populations with limited access to antibiotics. There seems to be an age-related discrepancy in the clinical documentation of an antecedent sore throat. In older children and young adults, the recollection of a streptococcal sore throat approaches 70%; in younger children, this rate approaches only 20%.[1] It is important to have a high index of suspicion of ARF in children or young adults presenting with signs of arthritis or carditis or both even in the absence of a clinically documented sore throat.

Another intriguing, and as yet unexplained, observation has been the invariable association of ARF only with streptococcal pharyngitis. Although there have been many outbreaks of impetigo, ARF almost never occurs after infection with these strains. In Trinidad, where impetigo and ARF are common infections, the strains colonizing the skin are different from the strains associated with ARF, and did not influence the incidence of ARF.[10] The explanation for these observations remains obscure.

Group A streptococci fall into two main classes based on differences in the C repeat regions of the M protein.[11] One class is associated with streptococcal pharyngeal infection, and the other (with some exceptions) is commonly associated with impetigo. The particular strain of streptococci may be crucial in initiating the disease process. The pharyngeal site of infection with its large repository of lymphoid tissue also may be important in the initiation of the abnormal humoral response by the host to the antigens cross-reactive with target organs. Finally, although impetigo strains do colonize the pharynx, they do not seem to elicit as strong an immunologic response to the M protein moiety as do the pharyngeal strains.[12,13] This may prove to be an important factor, especially in light of the known cross-reactions between various streptococcal structures and mammalian proteins.

GROUP A STREPTOCOCCI

Figure 105-1 is a schematic cross-section of group A streptococci. The capsule is composed of equimolar concentrations of *N*-acetyl glucosamine and glucuronic acid and is structurally identical to hyaluronic acid of mammalian tissues.[14] Although numerous attempts to produce antibodies to this capsule have been unsuccessful,[15,16] Fillet and colleagues[17] were able to show high antibody titers to hyaluronic acid using techniques designed to detect nonprecipitating antibodies in the sera of immunized animals. Similar antibodies have been noted in humans.[18] The data establishing the importance of this capsule in human infections have been almost nonexistent, although Stollerman[19] commented on the presence of a large mucoid capsule as being one of the more important characteristics of certain "rheumatogenic" strains.

With respect to the M protein moiety, investigations by Lancefield and others spanning almost 70 years[20] have established that the M protein molecule (at least 80 distinct serologic types) is perhaps the most important virulence factor in group A streptococcal infections of humans. The protein is a helical, coiled-coil structure and bears a striking structural homology to the cardiac cytoskeletal proteins, tropomyosin and myosin, and to many other coil-coiled structures, including keratin, DNA, lamin, and vimentin. When the amino acid sequence of many M proteins was delineated, it was possible to localize specifically the cross-reactive areas of the molecules. The studies of Dale and Beachey[21] showed that the segment of the M protein involved in the opsonic reaction also cross-reacted with human sarcolemma antigens. Sargent and coworkers[22] more precisely localized this cross-reaction to the M protein amino acid residues 164-197.

The evidence implicating these cross-reactions in the pathogenesis of ARF remains scant. Antibodies to myosin have been detected in the sera of ARF patients, but they also are present in a high percentage of the sera obtained from individuals who had a streptococcal infection, but did

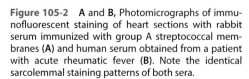

Figure 105-2 **A** and **B,** Photomicrographs of immunofluorescent staining of heart sections with rabbit serum immunized with group A streptococcal membranes (**A**) and human serum obtained from a patient with acute rheumatic fever (**B**). Note the identical sarcolemmal staining patterns of both sera.

not subsequently develop ARF.[23] The significance of this observation is unclear because myosin is an internal protein of cardiac muscle cells and not easily exposed to M protein cross-reacting antibodies. The group-specific carbohydrate of the streptococcus is a polysaccharide chain consisting of repeating units of rhamnose capped by N-acetyl glucosamine molecules. The N-acetyl glucosamine is immunodominant and gives rise to the serologic group specificity of group A streptococci.[24]

Goldstein and associates[25] first described the cross-reaction between group A carbohydrate and valvular glycoproteins, and the reactivity was related to the N-acetyl glucosamine moiety present in both structures. Goldstein and Caravano[26] noted that rheumatic fever (RF) sera reacted to the heart valve glycoprotein. Fillet (unpublished data) observed strong reactivity of RF sera with purified proteoglycan material. These cross-reactions could involve the sugar moiety present in the proteoglycan portion of the glycoprotein and the carbohydrate.

It generally has been assumed that group A anticarbohydrate antibodies do not play a role in phagocytosis of group A streptococci. Salvadori and coworkers[27] showed, however, that human sera containing high titers of anti–group A carbohydrate antibody promoted opsonization and phagocytosis of many different M protein–specific strains, and the opsonophagocytic antibodies were directed to the N-acetyl glucosamine moiety of the group A carbohydrate. The mucopeptide portion of the cell wall is the "backbone" of the organism and quite rigid in structure. It is composed of repeating units of muramic acid and N-acetyl glucosamine, cross-linked by peptide bridges.[28] It is particularly difficult to degrade and induces a wide variety of lesions when injected into various species, including arthritis in rats[29] and myocardial granulomas in mice resembling (but not identical to) RF Aschoff lesions.[30]

The relationship of cell wall mucopeptides to the pathogenesis of ARF remains obscure. Elevated levels of antimucopeptide antibody not only have been detected in the sera of patients with ARF, but also in the sera of patients with

rheumatoid arthritis and juvenile rheumatoid arthritis[31]; however, its pathogenetic relationship to clinical disease has been difficult to establish. There is no evidence that cell wall antigens are present either in the Aschoff lesion or in the myocardial tissue obtained from patients with ARF. Perhaps the most significant cross-reactions lie in the streptococcal membrane structure. We have shown that immunization with membrane material[32] elicited antibodies that bound to heart sections in a pattern similar to that observed with acute RF sera (Fig. 105-2).

Kingston and Glynn[33] were the first to show that animals immunized with streptococcal antigens developed antibodies in their sera that stained astrocytes. Husby and associates[34] showed that sera from ARF patients with chorea exhibited antibodies that were specific for caudate cells. Absorption of the sera with streptococcal membrane antigens eliminated the reactivity with caudate cells. Numerous other cross-reactions between streptococcal membranes and other organs also have been reported (e.g., renal basement membranes, basement membrane proteoglycans, and skin, particularly keratin). In the context of this chapter, space does not permit an exhaustive discussion of these cross-reactions, and the reader is referred to a previous review[35] for a more detailed discussion. Whether or not these cross-reactions (especially the cross-reactions seen with basement membranes and skin) play a role in the disease awaits further study.

GENETICS

The concept that ARF might be the result of a host genetic predisposition has intrigued investigators for more than a century.[36] It has been variously suggested that the disease gene is transmitted in an autosomal dominant fashion,[37] or autosomal recessive fashion with limited penetrance,[38] or that it is possibly related to the genes conferring blood group secretor status.[39] Renewed interest in the genetics of ARF occurred with the recognition that gene products of the human major histocompatibility complex (MHC) were associated with certain clinical disease states. Using an alloserum from a multiparous donor, an increased frequency of a B cell alloantigen was reported in several genetically distinct and ethnically diverse populations of ARF patients and was not MHC related.[40]

More recently, a monoclonal antibody (D8/17) was prepared by immunizing mice with B cells from an ARF patient.[41] A B cell antigen identified by this antibody was found to be expressed on increased numbers of B cells in 100% of rheumatic patients of diverse ethnic origins, and only in 10% of normal individuals. The antigen defined by this monoclonal antibody showed no association with or linkage to any of the known MHC haplotypes, and it did not seem to be related to B cell activation antigens. Studies with D8/17 have been expanded to a larger number of patients with RF (see Table 105-1) of diverse ethnic origins with essentially the same results. As discussed subsequently, the presence or absence of elevated levels of D8/17+ B cells in cases of questionable RF has been helpful in establishing or ruling out the diagnosis.

These studies are in contrast to other reports in which an increased frequency of HLA-DR4 and HLA-DR2 has been seen in white and black patients with rheumatic heart disease (RHD).[42] Other studies have implicated HLA-DR1 and HLA-DRW6 as susceptibility factors in South African black patients with RHD.[43] More recently, Guilherme and associates[44] have reported an increased frequency of HLA-DR7 and HLA-DW53 in RF patients in Brazil.

These seemingly conflicting results concerning HLA antigens and RF susceptibility prompt speculation that these reported associations might be of class II genes close to (or in linkage disequilibrium with), but not identical to the putative RF susceptibility gene. Alternatively, and more likely, susceptibility to ARF is polygenic, and the D8/17 antigen might be associated with only one of the genes (i.e., genes of the MHC complex encoding for DR antigens) conferring susceptibility. Although the explanation remains to be determined, the presence of the D8/17 antigen does seem to identify a population at special risk of contracting ARF (Table 105-2).

ETIOLOGIC CONSIDERATIONS

Although a large body of immunologic and epidemiologic evidence has implicated group A streptococci in the induction of the disease process, the precise pathologic mechanisms involved remain obscure. At least three main theories have been proposed. The first theory is concerned with the question of whether persistence of the organism is important. Despite several controversial reports, no investigators have been able to show consistently and reproducibly live organisms in RF cardiac tissues or valves.[45]

The second theory revolves around the question of whether deposition of toxic products is required. Although an attractive hypothesis, little or no experimental evidence has been obtained to support this concept. Halbert and colleagues[46] have suggested that streptolysin O (an extracellular product of group A streptococci) is cardiotoxic and might be carried to the site by circulating complexes containing streptolysin O and antibody. Despite an intensive search for these products, no such complexes in situ have been identified, however.[47,48] Renewed interest in these extracellular toxins has emerged more recently with

Table 105-2 Frequency of the D8/17 Marker in Patients with Rheumatic Fever, Patients with Other Diseases, and Controls in Various Geographic Populations

	No.	% Positive
Rheumatic Fever Patients		
New York	43/45	93
New Mexico	30/31	97
Utah*	18/18	100
Russia (Georgian)	27/30	90
Russia (Moscow)	50/52	96
Mexico	35/39	89
Chile	45/50	90
Normals		
Russia	4/78	5
New York	6/68	8
Chile	8/50	16
Mexico	6/72	8
Other Diseases		
Rheumatoid arthritis	2/42	4
Ischemic heart disease	0/10	0
Multiple sclerosis	1/25	4
Systemic lupus erythematosus	1/12	9

*Acute patients.

the observation by Schlievert and coworkers[49] that certain streptococcal pyrogenic toxins (A and C) may act as superantigens. These antigens may stimulate large numbers of T cells through their unique bridging interaction with T cell receptors of specific Vβ types and class II MHC molecules. This interaction is distinct from conventional antigen presentation in the context of the MHC complex. When activated, these cells elaborate tumor necrosis factor, interferon-γ, and numerous interleukin moieties, contributing to the initiation of pathologic damage. It has been suggested[50] that in certain disease states, such as rheumatoid arthritis, autoreactive cells of specific Vβ lineage may "home" to the target organ.

Although an attractive hypothesis, no data concerning the role of these superantigens in ARF have yet been forthcoming. Perhaps the best evidence to date favors a third theory of an abnormal host immune response (humoral and cellular) in a genetically susceptible individual to the streptococcal antigens cross-reactive with mammalian tissues. The evidence supporting this theory may be divided into three broad categories.

(1) Employing a wide variety of methods, numerous investigators have documented the presence of heart-reactive antibodies in ARF sera. The prevalence of these antibodies has ranged from 33% to 85% in various series. Although these antibodies are seen in other individuals (notably individuals with uncomplicated streptococcal infections that do not progress to RF and patients with poststreptococcal glomerulonephritis), the titers are always lower than the titers seen in RF and decrease with time during the convalescent period (Table 105-3). An important point in terms of diagnosis and prognosis has been the observation by Zabriskie and associates[51] that these heart-reactive antibody titers decline over time. By the end of 3 years, these titers are essentially undetectable in patients

Table 105-3   Heart-Reactive Antibody Titers in Sera of Patients with Acute Rheumatic Fever Compared with Uncomplicated Streptococcal Infections and Other Arthritic Infections

Clinical Disorder	No. Patients	Serum Dilutions			Average ASO Titer
		1:5	1:10	1:20	
Acute rheumatic fever (grade I)	34	4+	2+	+*	700
Uncomplicated streptococcal infections (grade II)	40	1+	0	0	561
APSGN	20	+/−	0	0	520
Rheumatoid arthritis	10	0	0	0†	ND
Systemic lupus erythematosus	10	0	0	0	ND

*Serum samples obtained at onset of rheumatic fever and at a comparable time in the group with uncomplicated scarlet fever.
†Serum samples obtained during active disease.
APSGN, acute poststreptococcal glomerulonephritis; ASO, antistreptolysin O; ND, not determined.

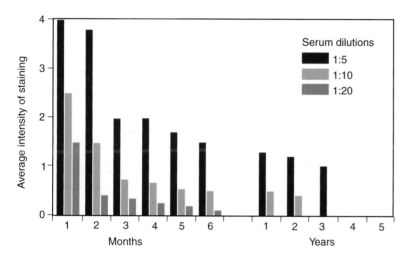

Figure 105-3 Serial heart-reactive antibody titers in 40 patients with documented acute rheumatic fever. Note the slow decline of these titers over the first 2 years after the initial episode and the absence of these antibodies 5 years after the initial attack.

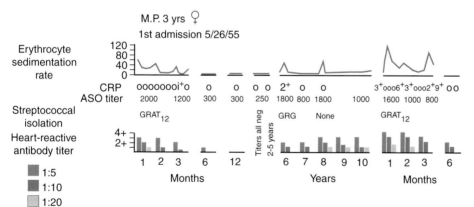

Figure 105-4 Heart-reactive antibody titers and laboratory data obtained from a patient with rheumatic fever who had two well-documented acute attacks 11 years apart. Note absence of the heart-reactive antibody during years 2 to 5 and its reappearance during years 6 to 10 after evidence of two intercurrent streptococcal infections secondary to breaks in penicillin prophylaxis (see antistreptolysin O [ASO] titers). High titers of heart-reactive antibody appeared with the second attack. CRP, C-reactive protein.

who had only a single attack (Fig. 105-3). This pattern is consistent with the well-known clinical observations that recurrences of RF most often occur within the first 2 to 3 years after the initial attack and become rarer 5 years after an initial episode.

As illustrated in Figure 105-4, this pattern of titers also has prognostic value. During the 2- to 5-year period after the initial attack, a patient's titers decreased to undetectable levels. With a known break in prophylaxis starting in year 6, at least two streptococcal infections occurred, as evidenced by an increase in antistreptolysin O (ASO) titers during that period. The concomitant increase in heart-reactive antibody titers was notable. The final infection was followed by a clinical recurrence of classic rheumatic carditis complete with isolation of the organism, elevated heart-reactive antibodies, and acute-phase reactants 11 years after the initial attack.

(2) Sera from patients with ARF also contain increased levels of antibodies to myosin and tropomyosin compared with sera from patients with pharyngeal streptococcal infections that do not progress to ARF. These myosin affinity purified antibodies also cross-react with M protein moieties, suggesting this molecule could be the antigenic stimulus for the production of myosin antibodies in these sera.[23,52]

Table 105-4   Composition of Mononuclear Cellular Infiltrates in Acute and Chronic Active Rheumatic Valvulitis

Patient	Type of Valve	Type of Valvulitis*	Composition of Infiltrate (%)						CD4/CD8 Ratio
			HLA-DR+	CD1+†	CD20+‡	CD3+§	CD4+¶	CD8+‖	
Acute Valvulitis									
1	Mitral	Acute	58.9	42.6	5.1	49.5	75.6	23.9	3.1
2	Mitral	Acute	49.8	43.1	6.9	43.1	58.7	34.3	1.9
	Aortic	Acute	52.7	51	3.9	38.1	65.9	26.5	2.3
3	Mitral	Acute	63.9	42	5.5	52.4	75.4	18.9	4
4	Aortic	Acute	68.1	56	7.4	33.7	71.6	22	1.9
Chronic Valvulitis									
4	Mitral	Chronic active	49.4	47.4	7.4	44.3	53.7	38.8	1.4
5	Mitral	Chronic active	48.8	39.1	1.4	53.9	45.2	51.5	0.9
	Aortic	Chronic active	67.8	35	4	36.8	47.5	49.1	1
6	Mitral	Chronic active	41.8	23.4	8	65.9	57.3	33.3	1.7
	Aortic	Chronic active	69.6	48.7	6.2	30.1	58.2	32.6	1.8
7	Mitral	Chronic active	55.4	24.2	8.1	59.8	64.9	24.7	2.6
8	Mitral	Chronic active	80.4	34.1	13.4	44.4	44.8	50.9	0.9
9	Mitral	Chronic active	46.1	29.6	0.8	65.6	61.6	33.3	1.8

*Determined in the frozen valve samples studied.
†(63D3) monocytes/macrophages.
‡(Leu 16) B cells.
§Pan T cells.
¶Helper T cells.
‖Suppressor cells.

(3) Finally, as indicated earlier, autoimmune antibodies are a prominent finding in chorea, another major clinical manifestation of ARF, and these antibodies are directed against the cells of the caudate nucleus. The titer of this antibody corresponds with clinical disease activity.[34] Although not autoimmune in nature, the presence of elevated levels of immune complexes in ARF has been well documented in the sera and in the joints of ARF patients.[53] Elevated levels of immune complexes, which may be as high as the levels seen in classic poststreptococcal glomerulonephritis, may be responsible for the immune complex vasculitis seen in ARF tissues and may provide the initial impetus for vascular damage, followed by the secondary penetration of autoreactive antibodies. Support for this concept is the close clinical similarity of RF arthritis to experimentally induced serum sickness in animals or the arthritis seen secondary to drug hypersensitivity.

Deposition of host immunoglobulin and complement also is seen in the cardiac tissues of ARF patients, suggesting autoimmune deposition of immunoglobulins in or near the Aschoff lesions. At a cellular level, there is now ample evidence for the presence of lymphocytes and macrophages at the site of pathologic damage in the heart in patients with ARF.[54] The cells are predominantly CD4+ helper lymphocytes during acute stages of the disease (4:1). The ratio of CD4+ to CD8+ lymphocytes (2:1) more closely approximates the normal ratio in chronic valvular specimens. Most of these cells express DR antigens. A potentially important finding has been the observation that macrophage-like fibroblasts present in the diseased valves express DR antigens[55] and might be the antigen-presenting cells for the CD4+ lymphocytes. Increased cellular reactivity to streptococcal antigens also has been noted in the peripheral blood mononuclear cell preparations of ARF patients compared with these cells isolated from nephritis patients.[56]

This abnormal reactivity peaks at 6 months after the attack, but may persist for 2 years after the initial episode.

The reactivity was specific only for the strains associated with ARF, suggesting an abnormal humoral and cellular response to streptococcal antigens unique to RF-associated streptococci. Support for the potential pathologic importance of these T cells is strengthened further by the observation that lymphocytes obtained from experimental animals sensitized to cell membranes, but not cell walls, are specifically cytotoxic for syngeneic embryonic cardiac myofibers in vitro.[57] In humans, normal mononuclear cells primed in vitro by M protein molecules from an RF-associated strain also are cytotoxic for myofibers, but specificity solely for cardiac cells was lacking in the human studies.[58] Similar studies have not been performed yet using lymphocytes from active ARF patients (Table 105-4).

CLINICAL FEATURES

The clinical presentation of ARF varies, and the lack of a single pathognomonic feature has resulted in the development of the revised Jones criteria (Table 105-5),[59] which are used to establish a diagnosis. These criteria were established only as guidelines for the diagnosis and were never intended to be "etched in stone." Depending on the age, geographic location, and ethnic population, emphasis on one criterion for the diagnosis of ARF may be more important than others. Manifestations of RF that are not clearly expressed pose a dilemma because of the importance of identifying a first rheumatic attack definitively to establish the need for prophylaxis of recurrences (see later). Some of the isolated manifestations, particularly polyarthritis, may be difficult or impossible to distinguish from other diseases, especially at their onset. The diagnosis can be made, however, when "pure" chorea is the sole manifestation because of the rarity with which this syndrome is due to any other cause. More recently, the World Health Organization updated the Jones criteria to allow for the diagnosis of recurrent ARF in patients with established RHD and chronic RHD (Table 105-6).

Table 105-5 Revised Jones Criteria for Diagnosis of Acute Rheumatic Fever

Major Manifestations	Minor Manifestations
Carditis	Fever
Polyarthritis	Arthralgia
Chorea	Previous RF or RHD
Erythema marginatum	
Subcutaneous nodules	
Laboratory Findings	
Elevated acute-phase reactants	
C-reactive protein	
Erythrocyte sedimentation rate	
Prolonged P-R interval rate	
Supporting evidence of preceding streptococcal infection	
Increased ASO or other streptococcal antibodies	
Positive throat culture for group A β-hemolytic streptococci	
Recent scarlet fever	

ASO, antistreptolysin O; RF, rheumatic fever; RHD, rheumatic heart disease.
From Jones Criteria 1992 update: Guidelines for diagnosis of rheumatic fever. JAMA 268:2069-2070, 1992.

ARTHRITIS

In classic, untreated cases, the arthritis of ARF affects several joints in quick succession, each for a short time. The legs usually are affected first, and the arms are affected later. The terms *migrating* and *migratory* are often used to describe the polyarthritis of ARF, but these designations are not meant to signify that the inflammation disappears in one joint when it appears in another. Rather, the various localizations usually overlap in time, and the onset, as opposed to the full course of the arthritis, "migrates" from joint to joint.

Joint involvement is more common, and also more severe, in teenagers and young adults than in children. Arthritis is usually the earliest symptomatic manifestation of the disease, although asymptomatic carditis may precede it. Rheumatic polyarthritis may be excruciatingly painful, but is almost always transient. The pain is usually more prominent than the objective signs of inflammation. When the disease is allowed to express itself fully, unmodified by anti-inflammatory treatment, more than half of patients studied show a true polyarthritis, with inflammation in 6 to 16 joints. Classically, each joint is maximally inflamed for only a few days, or a week at the most; the inflammation decreases, perhaps lingering for another week or so, and then disappears completely. Radiographs at this point may show a slight effusion, but most likely are unremarkable.

In routine practice, many patients with arthritis or arthralgias are treated empirically with salicylates or other nonsteroidal anti-inflammatory drugs, and arthritis subsides quickly in the joints already affected and does not migrate to new joints. Therapy may deprive the diagnostician of a useful sign. In a large series of patients with ARF and associated arthritis, most of whom had been treated, involvement of only a single large joint was common (25%). One or both knees were affected in 76%, and one or both ankles were affected in 50%. Elbows, wrists, hips, or small joints of the feet were involved in 12% to 15% of patients, and shoulders or small joints of the hand were affected in 7% to 8%. Rarely affected joints included the lumbosacral (2%), cervical (1%), sternoclavicular (0.5%), and temporomandibular

Table 105-6 Summary of 2002 World Health Organization Criteria for the Diagnosis of Rheumatic Fever and Rheumatic Heart Disease

Diagnostic Categories	Criteria
Primary episode of RF	Two major or one major and two minor manifestations plus evidence of a preceding group A streptococcal infection
Recurrent attack of RF in patients without established RHD	Two major or one major and two minor manifestations plus evidence of a preceding group A streptococcal infection
Recurrent attack of RF in patients with established RHD	Two minor manifestations plus evidence of a preceding group A streptococcal infection
Rheumatic chorea, insidious onset of rheumatic carditis	One major manifestation or evidence of a preceding group A streptococcal infection
Chronic valve lesions of RHD (i.e., patients presenting for the first time with pure mitral stenosis, mixed mitral valve disease, and aortic valve disease)	Do not require any other criteria to be diagnosed as having RHD

RF, rheumatic fever; RHD, rheumatic heart disease.
From Rheumatic Fever and Rheumatic Heart Diseases. Report of a WHO expert consultation. WHO technical report series no. 923. World Health Organization, 2004.

(0.5%). Involvement of the small joints of the hands or feet alone occurred in only 1% of these patients.[60] Analysis of the synovial fluid in well-documented cases of ARF with arthritis generally reveals a sterile, inflammatory fluid. There may be a decrease of the complement components C1q, C3, and C4, indicating their consumption by immune complexes in the joint fluid.[9]

POSTSTREPTOCOCCAL REACTIVE ARTHRITIS

Numerous investigators[61-63] have suggested that poststreptococcal migratory arthritis (in adults and children) in the absence of carditis might be a distinct entity from ARF for the following reasons: (1) The latent period between the antecedent streptococcal infection and the onset of poststreptococcal reactive arthritis is shorter (1 to 2 weeks) than the 3 to 4 weeks usually seen in classic ARF. (2) The response of the poststreptococcal reactive arthritis to aspirin and other nonsteroidal medications is poor compared with the dramatic response seen in classic ARF. (3) Evidence of carditis is not usually seen in these patients; the severity of the arthritis is marked. (4) Extra-articular manifestations (e.g., tenosynovitis and renal abnormalities) are often seen in these patients.

Although these features may be seen (admittedly rarely), migratory arthritis without evidence of other major Jones criteria, if supported by two minor manifestations (see Table 105-5), still must be considered ARF, especially in children. Variations in the response to aspirin in these children often are not documented with serum salicylate levels, and an unusual clinical course is insufficient to exclude the diagnosis of ARF. Appropriate prophylactic measures should be taken.[64] Support for this concept may be found in the work of Crea and Mortimer.[65] In their series of patients with ARF, 50% of the children who presented solely with signs of migratory arthritis went on to develop significant valvular damage. RF in adults also occurs. Although migratory arthritis is a common presenting symptom, an outbreak in San Diego Naval Training Camp[66] revealed a 30% incidence of valvular damage in these patients. The importance of clearly defining this reactive arthritis as an RF variant has obvious implications for secondary prophylactic treatment. As suggested by some investigators, poststreptococcal reactive arthritis is a benign condition without need for prophylaxsis. Because these patients largely do fulfill the Jones criteria (one major, two minor), they should be considered as having RF and in our opinion treated as such.

CARDITIS

Cardiac valvular and muscle damage can manifest in a variety of signs or symptoms. These manifestations include organic heart murmurs, cardiomegaly, congestive heart failure, and pericarditis. Mild-to-moderate chest discomfort, pleuritic chest pain, and a pericardial friction rub are indications of pericarditis. On clinical examination, the patient can have new or changing organic murmurs, most commonly mitral regurgitant murmurs and occasionally aortic regurgitant murmurs and systolic ejection murmurs, caused by acute valvular inflammation and deformity. Rarely, a Carey Coombs mid-diastolic murmur caused by rapid flow over the mitral valve is heard. If the valvular damage is severe, and there is concurrent cardiac dysfunction, congestive heart failure can occur. Congestive heart failure is the most life-threatening clinical syndrome of ARF and must be treated aggressively and early with a combination of anti-inflammatory drugs, diuretics, and, occasionally, steroids to decrease cardiac inflammation acutely.

Electrocardiogram abnormalities may include all degrees of heart block, including atrtioventricular dissociation, but first-degree heart block is not associated with a poor prognosis. Second-degree or third-degree heart block occasionally can be symptomatic. If heart block is associated with congestive heart failure, temporary pacemaker placement may be required. The most common manifestation of carditis is cardiomegaly, as seen on radiograph. Among patients at the Rockefeller University Hospital who were diagnosed with ARF between 1950 and 1970 with an average of 20 years of follow-up, 90% had evidence of carditis at diagnosis (Table 105-7). In Bland and Jones'[67] classic review of 1000 patients with ARF, only 65% of the patients were diagnosed with carditis. When Doppler sonography was employed in the clinical evaluation of patients during the Utah outbreak, 91% of patients had carditis,[1] however, indicating that, with more sensitive measurements of cardiac dysfunction, almost all ARF patients have signs of acute carditis.

RHEUMATIC HEART DISEASE

RHD is the most severe sequela of ARF. Usually occurring 10 to 20 years after the original attack, it is the major cause of acquired valvular disease in the world. The mitral valve is mainly involved, and aortic valve involvement occurs less often. Mitral stenosis is a classic RHD finding and can manifest as a combination of mitral insufficiency and stenosis, secondary to severe calcification of the mitral valve. When symptoms of left atrial enlargement are present, mitral valve replacement may become necessary.

In various studies, the incidence of RHD in patients with a history of ARF has varied. In Bland and Jones'[67] classic follow-up study of patients with ARF, after 20 years, one third of patients had no murmur, another one third died, and the remaining one third were alive with RHD. Most of the patients who died had RHD. Although the classic dogma is that patients with RHD invariably had more than one attack of ARF, more recent analysis of our patients at the Rockefeller University Hospital disproves this notion. The population studied was 87 patients who had only one documented attack of ARF, without any evidence (clinical or laboratory) of a recurrence during a 20-year follow-up under close supervision. Greater than 80% had carditis at admission, and approximately 50% now have organic murmurs (see Table 105-7). Valvular damage manifesting as organic murmurs later in life is still likely to occur in 50% of the patients, particularly if they presented with evidence of carditis at initial diagnosis. All of the patients in our population who ended up with RHD had carditis at diagnosis.

CHOREA

Sydenham's chorea (chorea minor or St. Vitus' dance) is a neurologic disorder consisting of abrupt, purposeless, nonrhythmic involuntary movements, muscular weakness, and emotional disturbances. Involuntary movements disappear during sleep, but may occur at rest and may interfere with voluntary activity. Initially, it may be possible to suppress these movements, which may affect all voluntary muscles, with the hands and face usually the most obvious. Grimaces and inappropriate smiles are common. Handwriting usually

Table 105-7 Physical Signs and Symptoms of Acute Rheumatic Fever: Rockefeller University Hospital, 1950 to 1970

	RHD (n = 40) (%)	No RHD (n = 47) (%)	Total (N = 87) (%)	Bland and Jones (%)
Carditis	100	83	90.1	65.3
Arthritis	67.5	68.1	67.8	41
Epistaxis	0	10.6	5.7	27.4
Chorea	5	2.1	3.4	51.8
Pericarditis	2.5	4.3	3.4	13
Subcutaneous nodules	7.5	0	3.4	8.8
Erythema marginatum	0	4.3	2.3	7.1

becomes clumsy and provides a convenient way of following the patient's course. Speech is often slurred.

The movements are commonly more marked on one side and occasionally are completely unilateral (hemichorea). The muscular weakness is best revealed by asking the patient to squeeze the examiner's hands: The pressure of the patient's grip increases and decreases continuously and capriciously, a phenomenon known as relapsing grip, or milking sign. The emotional changes manifest in outbursts of inappropriate behavior, including crying and restlessness. In rare cases, psychological manifestions may be severe and may result in transient psychosis. The neurologic examination fails to reveal sensory losses or pyramidal tract involvement. Diffuse hypotonia may be present.

Chorea may follow streptococcal infections after a latent period, which is longer, on the average, than the latent period of other rheumatic manifestations. Some patients with chorea have no other symptoms, but other patients develop chorea weeks or months after arthritis. In both cases, examination of the heart may reveal murmurs.

It has been known for years that often the early symptoms of chorea may manifest as emotional or behavioral changes in the patient,[68] and only later do the choreiform motor symptoms appear. It also was noted that many chorea patients years after the choreiform symptoms had subsided would present with behavioral disorders, such as tics or obsessive-compulsive disorders. These earlier observations combined with the known presence of antibrain antibodies in the sera of Sydenham's chorea patients raised the question of whether a prior streptococcal infection (or infection with other microbes) might induce antibodies cross-reactive with brain antigen involved in neural pathways associated with behavior. Two more recent articles[69,70] indicate there is a strong association of the D8/17 B cell marker (described earlier) with children with obsessive-compulsive disorder (see Table 105-6). Although Swedo and coworkers[69] selected patients on the basis of a strong history of prior streptococcal infections, Murphy and colleagues[70] noted a strong association of the marker in patients with obsessive-compulsive disorder without a history of streptococcal infections. These preliminary studies suggest that streptococci and probably other microbes may induce antibodies that functionally disrupt the basal ganglia pathways leading not only to classic chorea, but also to behavioral disorders in these children without evidence of classic chorea.

SUBCUTANEOUS NODULES

The subcutaneous nodules of ARF are firm and painless. The overlying skin is not inflamed and usually can be moved over the nodules. The diameter of these round lesions varies from a few millimeters to 1 or 2 cm. They are located over bony surfaces or prominences or near tendons. Their number varies from a single nodule to a few dozen and averages three or four; when numerous, they are usually symmetric. Nodules are rarely present for more than 1 month. They are smaller and more short-lived than the nodules of rheumatoid arthritis. Although in both diseases the elbows are most frequently involved, the rheumatic nodules are more common on the olecranon, whereas nodules of rheumatoid arthritis are usually found 3 or 4 cm distal to it. Rheumatic subcutaneous nodules generally

appear only after the first few weeks of illness, usually only in patients with carditis.

ERYTHEMA MARGINATUM

Erythema marginatum is an evanescent, nonpruritic skin rash, pink or faintly red, affecting usually the trunk, sometimes the proximal parts or the limbs, but not the face. This lesion extends centrifugally, while the skin in the center returns gradually to normal—hence the name *erythema marginatum*. The outer edge of the lesion is sharp, whereas the inner edge is diffuse. Because the margin of the lesion is usually continuous, making a ring, it is also termed *erythema annulare*. The individual lesions may appear and disappear in a matter of hours, usually to return. A hot bath or shower may make them more evident or may reveal them for the first time. Erythema marginatum usually occurs in the early phase of the disease. It often persists or recurs, even when all other manifestations of disease have disappeared. Occasionally, the lesions appear for the first time, or, more likely, are noticed for the first time, late in the course of the illness or even during convalescence. This disorder usually occurs only in patients with carditis.

MINOR MANIFESTATIONS

Fever

Temperature is increased in almost all ARF attacks and ranges from 38.4°C to 40°C. Usually fever decreases in approximately 1 week without antipyretic treatment and may become low grade for another 1 or 2 weeks. Fever rarely lasts for more than 3 to 4 weeks.

Abdominal Pain

The abdominal pain of RF resembles that of other conditions associated with acute microvascular mesenteric inflammation and is nonspecific. It usually occurs at or near the onset of the RF attack so that other manifestations may not yet be present to clarify the diagnosis. In many cases, abdominal pain may mimic acute appendicitis.

Epistaxis

In the past, epistaxis occurred most prominently and severely in patients with severe and protracted rheumatic carditis. Early clinical studies reported a frequency of 48%, but it probably occurs even less frequently now (see Table 105-6). Although epistaxis has been correlated in the past with the severity of rheumatic inflammation, it is difficult to assess retrospectively the possible thrombasthenic effect of large doses of salicylates, administered for prolonged periods in protracted attacks.

Rheumatic Pneumonia

Pneumonia may appear during the course of severe rheumatic carditis. This inflammatory process is difficult or impossible to distinguish from pulmonary edema or the alveolitis associated with respiratory distress syndromes owing to a variety of pathophysiologic states.

LABORATORY FINDINGS

The diagnosis of ARF cannot readily be established by laboratory tests. Nevertheless, such tests may be helpful in two ways: first, in showing that an antecedent streptococcal infection has occurred and, second, in documenting the presence or persistence of an inflammatory process. Serial chest radiographs may be helpful in following the course of carditis, and an electrocardiogram may reflect the inflammatory process on the conduction system. Throat cultures are usually negative by the time ARF appears, but an attempt should be made to isolate the organism. It is our practice to take three throat cultures during the first 24 hours, before administration of antibiotics. Streptococcal antibodies are more useful because (1) they reach a peak titer at about the time of onset of ARF; (2) they indicate true infection, rather than transient carriage; and (3) by performing several tests for different antibodies, any significant recent streptococcal infection can be detected.

To show a rising titer, it is useful to take a serum specimen when the patient is first seen and to take another 2 weeks later for comparison. The specific antibody tests that have been used to diagnose streptococcal infections most frequently are those directed against extracellular products, including ASO, anti-DNAse B, antihyaluronidase (anti–diphosphopyridine nucleotide [anti-DPNase]), and antistreptokinase. ASO has been the most widely used test and is generally available in U.S. hospitals. ASO titers vary with age, season, and geography. They reach peak levels in elementary school–age children; titers of 200 to 300 Todd units/mL are common in healthy children. After streptococcal pharyngitis, the antibody response peaks at about 4 to 5 weeks, which is usually during the second or third week of ARF (depending on how early it is detected). Thereafter, antibody titers decrease rapidly in the next several months, and after 6 months, they decline more slowly.

Because only 80% of cases of documented ARF exhibit an increase in the ASO titer, it is recommended that other antistreptococcal antibody tests be done in the absence of a positive ASO titer. These include anti-DNAse B, antihyaluronidase, or anti-Streptozyme (which is a combination of various streptococcal antigens). Streptococcal antibodies, when increased, support, but do not prove the diagnosis of ARF, and they are not a measure of rheumatic activity. Even in the absence of intercurrent streptococcal infection, titers decline during the rheumatic attack despite the persistence or severity of rheumatic activity.

ACUTE-PHASE REACTANTS

Acute-phase reactants are elevated during ARF, just as they are during other inflammatory conditions. C-reactive protein and erythrocyte sedimentation rate are almost invariably elevated during the active rheumatic process, if they are not suppressed by antirheumatic drugs. These values may be normal, however, during episodes of pure chorea or persistent erythema marginatum. Particularly when treatment has been discontinued or is being tapered off, C-reactive protein and erythrocyte sedimentation rate are useful in monitoring "rebounds" of rheumatic inflammation, which indicate that the rheumatic process is still active. If either C-reactive protein or erythrocyte sedimentation rate remains normal a few weeks after discontinuing antirheumatic therapy, the

attack may be considered ended unless chorea appears. Usually, there is no exacerbation of the systemic inflammation, and chorea is present as an isolated manifestation.

ANEMIA

A mild, normochromic, normocytic anemia of chronic infection or inflammation may be seen during ARF. Suppressing the inflammation usually improves the anemia; hematinic therapy usually is not indicated.

OTHER SUPPORTING FINDINGS

As noted in Figures 105-3 and 105-4 and Table 105-2, two other tests have been helpful in our experience in confirming the diagnosis of ARF, especially when the diagnosis is in doubt. First, one can detect elevated titers of heart-reactive antibodies directed against sarcolemmal antigens in most ARF patients. Elevated levels of these antibodies are not seen in either uncomplicated streptococcal infections or acute poststreptococcal glomerulonephritis. Using enzyme-linked immunosorbent assay, antibodies directed against cytoskeletal constituents such as myosin and tropomyosin also are elevated in ARF patients and might be helpful in determining whether or not cross-reactive antibodies unique to ARF exist.[50] Second, the use of the D8/17 monoclonal antibody mentioned earlier also has proved helpful in the differential diagnosis of ARF from other disorders. In our hands, all RF patients express abnormal levels of D8/17+ B cells, especially during the acute attack. In cases in which the diagnosis of ARF has been doubtful, the presence of elevated levels of D8/17+ B cells has proved to be very helpful in establishing the correct diagnosis.[40]

CLINICAL COURSE AND TREATMENT

The mainstay of treatment for ARF has always been anti-inflammatory agents, most commonly aspirin. Dramatic improvement in symptoms usually is seen after the initiation of therapy. Usually 80 to 100 mg/kg/day in children and 4 to 8 g/day in adults is required for an effect to be seen. Aspirin levels can be measured; 20 to 30 mg/dL is the therapeutic range. Duration of anti-inflammatory therapy can vary, but needs to be maintained until all symptoms are absent, and laboratory values are normal. If severe carditis also is present (as indicated by significant cardiomegaly, congestive heart failure, or third-degree heart block), steroid therapy can be instituted. The usual dosage is 2 mg/kg/day of oral prednisone during the first 1 to 2 weeks. Depending on clinical and laboratory improvement, the dosage is tapered over the next 2 weeks, and during the last week, aspirin may be added in the above-recommended dose, sufficient to achieve 20 to 30 mg/dL.

As noted by Cillers[71] in a clinical review, studies have shown no difference in the risk of cardiac disease at 1 year in groups treated with either aspirin or corticosteroids. Similarly, although nonsteroidal anti-inflammatory drugs also have been used to treat the acute inflammation, none have been the subject of randomized controlled trials. Whether or not signs of pharyngitis are present at the time of diagnosis, antibiotic therapy with penicillin should be started and maintained for at least 10 days, given in doses recommended for the eradication of streptococcal pharyngitis. Additionally, all family contacts should be cultured and treated for streptococcal infection if positive. If compliance is an issue, depot penicillins (i.e., benzathine penicillin G, 600,000 U in children and 1.2 million U in adults) should be given. Recurrences of ARF are most common within 2 years of the original attack, but can occur at any time. The risk of recurrence decreases with age. Recurrence rates have been decreasing, from 20% in past years to 2% to 4% in more recent outbreaks. This decrease might be due to better surveillance and treatment.

PROPHYLAXIS

Antibiotic prophylaxis with penicillin should be started immediately after the resolution of the acute episode. The optimal regimen consists of oral penicillin V potassium, 250,000 U twice a day, or parenteral penicillin G, 1.2 million U intramuscularly every 4 weeks. One study suggests, however, that injections every 3 weeks are more effective than every-4-week injections at preventing ARF recurrences.[72] If the patient is allergic to penicillin, erythromycin, 250 mg/day, can be substituted.

The end point of prophylaxis is unclear; most authors believe it should continue at least until the patient is a young adult, which is usually 10 years from an acute attack with no recurrence. In our opinion, individuals with documented evidence of RHD should be on continuous prophylaxis indefinitely because our experience has been that ARF recurrences can occur even in the fifth or sixth decade. A potential problem for ARF recurrences are young children in the household who could transmit new group A streptococcal infections to RF-susceptible individuals. The alternative to long-term prophylaxis in an individual with ARF would be the introduction of streptococcal vaccines designed not only to prevent recurrent infections in susceptible individuals with previous ARF, but also to prevent streptococcal disease in general.

STREPTOCOCCAL VACCINES

The difficulties in developing a streptococcal vaccine have been related mainly to the numerous reports that streptococcal antigens are known to cross-react with mammalian tissues.[64] Despite these caveats, more recent work indicates progress in this area. Perhaps the most advanced has been the work of Dale and colleagues,[73] in which they synthesized short peptides (20 to 30 amino acids) of many different M proteins and linked them together and showed that they can develop type-specific antibodies that also are opsonic. Little toxicity or cross-reactivity to human tissues has been noted with the antigen or the antibodies. Phase II trials are now in progress.

A second approach revolves around the C-repeat region of the M protein moiety, which is common to all group A streptococci. Bessen and Fischetti[74] used a commensural organism commonly found in the oral mucosa of humans in which by genetic engineering they inserted the C-repeat of the M protein, which is preferentially displayed on the surface of the organism. This induces IgA antibodies, preventing oral colonization of mice by live group A streptococci. Others[75] have confirmed these results using a different

M-type organism. Good and colleagues[76] used similar methods except that they added additional amino acids making their antibodies opsonic.

Based on the observation by Lancefield[77] that human sera rarely, if ever, contained more than one type-specific M protein antibody, Salvadori and coworkers[27] examined other possible streptococcal antigens that might explain the broad-based immunity to streptococcal infections that occurs with increasing age. Their studies indicated that the streptococcal group A carbohydrate (GRA-CHO) might be a good immunogen for the following reasons. Antibodies to GRA-CHO are present in human sera, increase with age, and are opsonic for several distinct M⁺-type strains. Active and passive immunization with GRA-CHO in mice exhibited protection against a live lethal challenge in mice. No cross-reactive antibodies have been detected.

Two other candidates also are under consideration. Ji and associates[78] described a surface antigen present on group A streptococci called C5a peptidase. This enzyme specifically cleaves the human serum chemotoxin C5a at the polymorphonuclear binding site. These observations led to experiments in which intranasal inoculation with C5a peptidase resulted in the appearance of antibodies that clearly reduced the potential of several different M⁺ strains to colonize mice.[78] Finally, Lukomski and colleagues[79] showed that the presence of *SPEB* markedly increases the virulence of a given group A streptococcal strain. Inactivation of the *SPEB* gene markedly decreases the lethality (IP challenge) of at least two strains—type 49 and S43 type 6. The mechanism whereby SPEB⁻ strains decrease the lethality of the strain seems to be related to the fact that polymorphonuclear neutrophils were able to clear the mutant strain from the circulation and tissues much more rapidly than the wild-type strain.[79]

CONCLUSION

Despite its disappearance in many areas of the world, ARF continues to be a serious problem in the geographic areas where two thirds of the population live. Even in developed countries with full access to medical care, better nutrition, and housing, the resurgence of the disease in these areas emphasizes the need for continued vigilance of physicians and other health officials in diagnosing and treating ARF. Whether this resurgence represents a change in the virulence of the organism or failure to recognize the importance and adequate treatment of an antecedent streptococcal infection remains an area of intense debate and requires careful and controlled epidemiologic surveillance.

The importance of early diagnosis and therapy cannot be overemphasized. Although the joint manifestations are transient and self-limiting, the cardiac sequelae are chronic and life-threatening. Nevertheless, ARF remains one of the few autoimmune disorders known to occur as a result of infection with a specific organism. The confirmed observation of an increased frequency of a B cell alloantigen in several populations of rheumatic patients suggests that it might be possible to identify susceptible individuals to ARF at birth. If so, from a public health standpoint, (1) these individuals would be prime candidates for immunization with any streptococcal vaccine that might be developed in the future; (2) careful monitoring of streptococcal disease in the susceptible population could lead to early and effective antibiotic strategies, resulting in disease prevention; and (3) in individuals previously infected, who later present with subtle or nonspecific manifestations of the disease, the presence or absence of the marker could be valuable in arriving at a diagnosis.

The continued study of ARF as a paradigm for microbial-host interactions also has important implications for the study of autoimmune diseases in general and rheumatic diseases in particular. Further insights into this intriguing host-parasite relationship may shed additional light into diseases where the infection is presumed, but has not been identified yet.

REFERENCES

1. Veasy LG, Orsmond GS, et al: Resurgence of acute rheumatic fever in the intermountain area of the United States. N Engl J Med 316:421-427, 1987.
2. **Gordis L: The virtual diappearance of rheumatic fever in the United States: Lessons in the rise and fall of disease. Circulation 72: 1155-1162, 1985.**
3. Pope RM: Rheumatic fever in the 1980s. Bull Rheum Dis Arthritis Foundation 38:1-8, 1989.
4. Markowitz M, Gordis L: Rheumatic Fever, 2nd ed. Philadelphia, WB Saunders, 1972.
5. Kaplan EL, Anthony BF, Chapman SS, et al: The influence of the site of infection on the immune response to group A streptococci. J Clin Invest 49:1405-1414, 1970.
6. Whitnack E, Bisno AL: Rheumatic fever and other immunologically mediated cardiac diseases. In Parker C (ed): Clinical Immunology, vol II. Philadelphia, WB Saunders, 1980, pp 894-929.
7. **Denny FW Jr, Wannamaker LW, Brink WR, et al: Prevention of rheumatic fever: Treatment of the preceeding streptococcal infection. JAMA 143:151-153, 1950.**
8. Markowitz M: Rheumatic fever: Recent outbreaks of an old disease. Conn Med 51:229-233, 1987.
9. Stollerman GH, Lewis AJ, Schultz I, et al: Relationship of the immune response to group A streptococci to the cause of acute, chronic and recurrent rheumatic fever. Am J Med 20:163-169, 1956.
10. Potter EV, Svartman M, Mohammed I, et al: Tropical acute rheumatic fever and associated streptococcal infections compared with concurrent acute glomerulonephritis. J Pediatr 92:325-333, 1978.
11. Bessen D, Jones KF, Fischetti VA: Evidence for the distinct classes of streptococcal M protein and their relationship to rheumatic fever. J Exp Med 169:269-283, 1989.
12. Kaplan EL, Johnson DR, Cleary PP: Group A streptococcal serotypes isolated from patients and sibling contacts during the resurgence of rheumatic fever in the United States in the mid 1980's. J Infect Dis 159:101-103, 1989.
13. Bisno AL, Nelson KE: Type-specific opsonic antibodies in streptococcal pyoderma. Infect Immun 10:1356-1361, 1975.
14. Kendall F, Heidelberger M, Dawson M: A serologically inactive polysaccharide elaborated by mucoid strains of group A hemolytic streptococcus. J Biol Chem 118:61-82, 1937.
15. Seastone CV: The virulence of group C hemolytic streptococci of animal origin. J Exp Med 70:361-378, 1939.
16. Quinn RW, Singh KP: Antigenicity of hyaluronic acid. Biochem J 95:290-301, 1957.
17. Fillet HM, McCarty M, Blake M: Induction of antibodies to hyaluronic acid by immunization of rabbits with encapsulated streptococci. J Exp Med 164:762-776, 1986.
18. Faarber P, Capel PJ, Rigke PM, et al: Cross reactivity of anti DNA antibodies with proteoglycans. Clin Exp Immunol 55:402-412, 1984.
19. **Stollerman GH: In Rheumatic Fever and Streptococcal Infection. New York, Grune & Stratton, 1975, p 70.**
20. Fischetti VA: Streptococcal M protein: Molecular design and biological behavior. Clin Microbiol Rev 2:285-314, 1989.
21. Dale JB, Beachey EH: Multiple cross reactive epitopes of streptococcal M proteins. J Exp Med 161:113-122, 1985.
22. Sargent SJ, Beachey EH, Corbett CE, et al: Sequence of protective epitopes of streptococcal M proteins shared with cardiac sarcolemmal membranes. J Immunol 139:1285-1290, 1987.
23. Cunningham MW, McCormack JM, Talaber LR, et al: Human monoclonal antibodies reactive with antigens of the group A streptococcus and human heart. J Immunol 141:2760-2766, 1988.
24. **McCarty M: The streptococcal cell wall. The Harvey Lectures Series 65:73-96, 1970.**
25. Goldstein I, Rebeyrotte P, Parlebas J, et al: Isolation from heart valves of glycopeptides which share immunological properties with streptococcus haemolyticus group A polysaccharides. Nature 219:866-868, 1968.
26. Goldstein I, Caravano R: Determination of anti group A streptococcal polysaccharide antibodies in human sera by an hemagglutination technique. Proc Soc Exp Biol Med 124:1209-1212, 1967.
27. Salvadori LG, Blake MS, McCarty M, et al: Group A streptococcus-liposome ELISA antibody titers to group A polysaccharide and opsonophagocytic capabilities of the antibodies. J Infect Dis 171:593-600, 1995.
28. Chetty C, Schwab JH: Chemistry of endotoxins. In Rietschel ET (ed): Handbook of Endotoxin, vol 1. Amsterdam, Elsevier Science, 1984, pp 376-410.
29. Cromartie WJ, Craddock JB, Schwab JH, et al: Arthritis in rats after systemic injection of streptococcal cells or cell walls. J Exp Med 146:1585-1602, 1977.
30. Cromartie WJ, Craddock JB: Rheumatic-like cardiac lesions in mice. Science 154:285-287, 1966.
31. Heymer B, Schleifer KH, Read SE, et al: Detection of antibodies to bacterial cell wall peptidoglycan in human sera. J Immunol 117:23-26, 1976.
32. **Zabriskie JB: Rheumatic fever: The interplay between host genetics and microbe. Circulation 71:1077-1086, 1985.**
33. Kingston D, Glynn LE: A cross-reaction between *Streptococcus pyogenes* and human fibroblasts, endothelial cells and astrocytes. Immunology 21:1003-1016, 1971.
34. **Husby G, van de Rijn I, Zabriskie JB, et al: Antibodies reacting with cytoplasm of subthalamic and caudate nuclei neurons in chorea and acute rheumatic fever. J Exp Med 144:1094-1110, 1976.**
35. Froude J, Gibofsky A, Buskirk DR, et al: Cross reactivity between streptococcus and human tissue: A model of molecular mimicry and autoimmunity. Curr Top Microbiol Immunol 145:5-26, 1989.
36. Cheadle WB: Harvean lectures on the various manifestations of the rheumatic state as exemplified in childhood and early life. Lancet 1:821-832, 1889.
37. **Wilson MG, Schweitzr MD, Lubschez R: The familial epidemiology of rheumatic fever. J Pediatr 22:468-482, 1943.**
38. Taranta A, Torosdag S, Metrakos JD, et al: Rheumatic fever in monozygotic and dizygotic twins. Circulation 20:778-792, 1959.
39. Glynn LE, Halborrow EJ: Relationship between blood groups, secretion status and susceptibility to rheumatic fever. Arthritis Rheum 4:203, 1961.
40. **Patarroyo ME, Winchester RJ, Vejerano A, et al: Association of a B cell alloantigen with susceptibility to rheumatic fever. Nature 278: 173-174, 1979.**
41. Khanna AK, Buskirk DR, Williams RC Jr, et al: Presence of a non-HLA B cell antigen in rheumatic fever patients and their families as defined by a monoclonal antibody. J Clin Invest 83:1710-1716, 1989.
42. Ayoub EA, Barrett DJ, Maclaren NK, et al: Association of class II human histocompatibility leucocyte antigens with rheumatic fever. J Clin Invest 77:2019-2026, 1986.
43. Maharaj B, Hammond MG, Appadoo B, et al: HLA-A, B, DR and DQ antigens in black patients with severe chronic rheumatic heart disease. Circulation 765:259-261, 1987.
44. Guilherme L, Weidenbach W, Kiss MH, et al: Association of human leucocyte class II antigens with rheumatic fever or rheumatic heart disease in a Brazilian population. Circulation 83: 1995-1998, 1991.
45. Watson RF, Hirst GK, Lancefield RC: Bacteriological studies of cardiac tissues obtained at autopsy from eleven patients dying with rheumatic fever. Arthritis Rheum 4:74-85, 1961.
46. Halbert SP, Bircher R, Dahle E: The analysis of streptococcal infections, V: Cardiotoxicity of streptolysin O for rabbits in vivo. J Exp Med 113:759-784, 1961.

47. Wagner BM: Studies in rheumatic fever, III: Histochemical reactivity of the Aschoff body. Ann N Y Acad Sci 86:992-1008, 1960.
48. Zabriskie JB: Unpublished data, 1959.
49. Schlievert PM, Johnson LP, Tomai MA, et al: Characterization and genetics of group A streptococcal pyrogenic exotoxins. In Ferretti J, Curtis R (eds): Streptococcal Genetics. Washington, DC, ASM, 1987, pp 136-142.
50. Paliard X, West SG, Lafferty JA, et al: Evidence for the effects of superantigen in rheumatoid arthritis. Science 253:325-329, 1991.
51. Zabriskie JB, Hsu KC, Seegal BC: Heart-reactive antibody associated with rheumatic fever: Characterization and diagnostic significance. Clin Exp Immunol 7:147-159, 1970.
52. Khanna AK, Nomura Y, Fischetti VA, et al: Antibodies in the sera of acute rheumatic fever patients bind to human cardiac tropomyosin. J Autoimmun 10:99-106, 1997.
53. van de Rijn I, Fillit H, Brandis WE, et al: Serial studies on circulating immune complexes in post-streptococcal sequelae. Clin Exp Immunol 34:318-325, 1978.
54. Kemeny E, Grieve T, Marcus R, et al: Identification of mononuclear cells and T cell subsets in rheumatic valvulitis. Clin Immunol Immunopathol 52:225-237, 1989.
55. Amoils B, Morrison RC, et al: Aberrant expression of HLA-DR antigen on valvular fibroblasts from patients with acute rheumatic carditis. Clin Exp Immunol 66:84-94, 1986.
56. Read SE, Reid HFM, Fischetti V, et al: Serial studies on the cellular immune response to streptococcal antigens in acute and convalescent rheumatic fever patients in Trinidad. J Clin Immunol 6:433-441, 1986.
57. Yang LC, Soprey PR, Wittner MK, et al: Streptococcal induced cell mediated immune destruction of cardiac myofibers in vitro. J Exp Med 146:344-360, 1977.
58. Dale JB, Beachey EH: Human cytotoxic T lymphocytes evoked by group A streptococcal M proteins. J Exp Med 166:1825-1835, 1987.
59. Jones Criteria 1992 update: Guidelines for diagnosis of rheumatic fever. JAMA 268:2069-2070, 1992.
60. Feinstein AR, Spagnulo M: The clinical patterns of rheumatic fever: A reappraisal. Medicine 41:279-305, 1962.
61. Goldsmith DP, Long SS: Poststreptococcal disease of chlidhood—a changing syndrome. Arthritis Rheum 25:S18, 1982 (abstract).
62. Arnold MH, Tyndall A: Post-streptococcal reactive arthritis. Ann Rheum Dis 48:681-688, 1989.
63. Fink CW: The role of streptococcus in post streptococcal reactive arthritis and childhood polyarteritis nodosa. J Rheumatol 18:14-20, 1991.
64. Gibofsky A, Zabriskie JB: Rheumatic fever: New insights into an old disease. Bull Rheum Dis Arthritis Foundation 42:5-7, 1994.
65. Crea MA, Mortimer EA: The nature of scarlatinal arthritis. Pediatrics 23:879-884, 1959.
66. Wallace MR, Garst PD, Papadimos TJ, et al: The return of acute rheumatic fever in young adults. JAMA 262:2557-2561, 1989.
67. Bland EF, Jones TD: Rheumatic fever and rheumatic heart disease: A twenty year report on 1,000 patients followed since childhood. Circulation 4:836-843, 1951.
68. Osler W: On Chorea and Choreiform Movements. HK Lewis & Co, 1894.
69. Swedo SE, Leonard HL, Mittleman BB, et al: Children with PANDAS (pediatric autoimmune neuropsychiatric disorders associated with strep. infections) are identified by a marker associated with rheumatic fever. Am J Psychiatry 154:110-112, 1997.
70. Murphy T, Goodman W: D8/17 reactivity as an immunologic marker of susceptibility to nonpsychiatric disorders. J Am Acad Child Adolesc Psychiatry 41:98-100, 2002.
71. Cillers AM: Rheumatic fever and its management. BMJ 333:1153-1156, 2006.
72. Lue HC, Mil-Wham W, Hsieh KH, et al: Rheumatic fever recurrences: Controlled study of 3 week verus 4 week benzathine penicillin prevention programs. J Pediatr 108:299-304, 1986.
73. Dale JB, Simmons M, Chiang EC, et al: Recombinant, octavalent group A streptococcal M protein vaccine. Vaccine 14:944-948, 1996.
74. Bessen D, Fischetti VA: Influence of intranasal immunization with synthetic peptides corresponding to conserved epitopes of M protein on mucosal colonization by group A streptococci. Infect Immun 56:2666-2672, 1988.
75. Bronze MS, Courtney HS, Dale JB: Epitopes of group A streptococcal M protein that evoke cross protection local immune responses. J Immunol 148:888-893, 1992.
76. Good MF, Brandt ER, Currie B, et al: Strategies for developing a group A streptococoal vaccine based on the M protein. Presented at the XIV Lancefield International Symposium on Streptococci and Streptococcal Diseases, Auckland, New Zealand, 1999.
77. Lancefield RC: Persistence of type specific antibodies in man following infection with group A streptococci. J Exp Med 110:271-292, 1959.
78. Ji Y, Carlson B, Kondagunta A, et al: Intranasal immunization with C5a peptidase prevents nasopharyngeal colonization of mice by the group A streptococcus. Infect Immun 65:2080-2087, 1997.
79. Lukomski S, Burns EH, Wyde PR, et al: Genetic inactivation of an extracellular cysteine protease (SPEB) expression by *Streptococcus pyogenes* decreases resistance to phagocytosis and dissemination to organs. Infect Immun 66: 771-776, 1998.

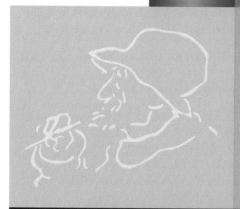

106 Amyloidosis

DAVID C. SELDIN • MARTHA SKINNER

KEY POINTS

Amyloidosis is a term for systemic diseases in which aggregated proteins deposit in tissues of the body, eventually leading to organ failure and death if not effectively treated.

Patients with amyloidosis can present with joint symptoms and soft tissue deposits that mimic rheumatologic disorders, and chronic inflammation or infection can lead to secondary AA amyloidosis.

The diagnosis of amyloidosis requires a tissue biopsy that demonstrates green birefringence of deposits on polarization microscopy after staining with Congo red.

Appropriate treatment depends upon the accurate biochemical or immunochemical identification of amyloid type, distinguishing hereditary genetic from acquired forms of amyloidosis.

The term *amyloidosis* comprises diseases that have in common the extracellular deposition of insoluble fibrillar proteins in tissues and organs. These diseases are a subset of a growing group of disorders recognized to be caused by misfolding of proteins; these disorders include Alzheimer's and other neurodegenerative diseases, prion diseases, serpinopathies, some of the cystic fibroses, and others. A unifying feature of amyloidoses is that the deposits share a common β-pleated sheet structural conformation that confers unique staining properties. The name "amyloid" is attributed to the pathologist Virchow, who in 1854 thought such deposits in autopsy livers were cellulose because of their peculiar staining reaction with iodine and sulfuric acid.[1] In the 20th century, "amyloid" was found to be a proteinaceous fibrillar deposit in tissues.[2] Biochemical characterization of the fibril proteins from clinical cases proved the "amyloidoses" to be a spectrum of diseases, many with a fatal outcome owing to progressive deposition of amyloid fibrils in major organs. A growing number of treatments are available to target the source of the abnormal protein and, for some types, to inhibit the amyloidogenic protein misfolding process.

CLASSIFICATION AND EPIDEMIOLOGY

Amyloid diseases are defined by the biochemical nature of the protein in the deposited fibril. The proteins are diverse and unrelated in primary amino acid sequence, resulting in amyloid diseases being classified according to whether they are systemic or localized, whether they are acquired or inherited, and their recognized clinical patterns (Table 106-1).[3] Each amyloid disease has a shorthand nomenclature, expressed asA for amyloidosis and an abbreviation for the biochemical nature of the fibrils: for example, *AL* is amyloid of immunoglobulin light chain origin. The discussion in this chapter is limited to the systemic amyloidoses because these are the diseases that can involve the joints and are potentially confused with autoimmune rheumatologic disorders.

The acquired systemic amyloidoses are AL (immunoglobulin light chain, or primary), AA (reactive, secondary), and $A\beta_2M$ (β_2-microglobulin, dialysis-associated) types. The AL type is most common, although epidemiologic data are limited. One study based on National Center for Health Statistics data estimated the incidence as 4.5 per 100,000.[4] AL amyloidosis usually manifests after age 40 years and is associated with rapid progression, multisystem involvement, and a short survival. AA amyloidosis is rare, occurring in less than 1% of patients with chronic inflammatory diseases in the United States and Europe, but it is more common in Turkey and the Middle East, where it occurs in association with familial Mediterranean fever.[5-7] It may begin within 1 year after onset of the underlying inflammatory disease or many years later. It is the only type of amyloidosis that occurs in children. $A\beta_2M$ amyloidosis is a chronic rheumatologic complication that occurs in a few patients on long-term dialysis and is related to a high concentration of β_2-microglobulin.[8]

The inherited amyloidoses are rare, with an estimated incidence of less than 1 per 100,000.[9] They are autosomal dominant diseases in which a variant plasma protein forms amyloid deposits beginning in midlife. The most common form is caused by variant transthyretin (TTR), of which there are nearly 100 known to be associated with amyloidosis.[10] One variant, Val-122-Ile, has a carrier frequency that may be 4% of the black population and is associated with late-onset cardiac amyloidosis.[11] Even wild-type TTR can form fibrils, leading to senile systemic amyloidosis, which

Table 106-1   Classification of Amyloidosis

Term	Fibril Composition	Systemic (S) or Localized (L)	Clinical Syndrome
AL	Immunoglobulin light chains (κ or λ)	S, L	Primary; myeloma-associated; systemic or localized in skin, lymph nodes, bladder, tracheobronchial tree
AA	Amyloid A protein	S	Secondary; reactive; familial Mediterranean fever
Aβ₂M	β₂-microglobulin	S	Long-term hemodialysis or ambulatory peritoneal dialysis
ATTR	Transthyretin (92 familial variants); wild-type TTR in senile systemic amyloidosis	S	Familial amyloidotic polyneuropathy and cardiomyopathy; senile systemic amyloidosis
AApoA	Apolipoprotein A-I (11 familial variants) or apolipoprotein A-II (4 familial variants)	S	Familial polyneuropathy with nephropathy
AGel	Gelsolin (variant Asn 187, Tyr 187)	S	Familial polyneuropathy with lattice corneal dystrophy, cranial neuropathy, nephropathy
AFib	Fibrinogen A alpha (3 familial variants)	S	Familial amyloidosis with nephropathy
ALys	Lysozyme (4 familial variants)	S	Familial amyloidosis with nephropathy
Aβ	Amyloid β protein	L	Alzheimer's disease; Down syndrome; cerebral amyloid angiopathy (Dutch)
ACys	Cystatin C (variant with N-terminal deletion and Glu 68)	S	Cerebral amyloid angiopathy (Icelandic)
AIAPP	Islet amyloid polypeptide	L	Type 2 diabetes mellitus; insulinoma
ACal	Calcitonin	L	Medullary carcinoma of the thyroid
AANF	Atrial natriuretic factor	L	Atrial amyloid, localized

predominantly affects the heart, in older patients.[12,13] Other familial amyloidoses, caused by variant apolipoprotein A-I, A-II, gelsolin, fibrinogen Aα, or lysozyme, are reported in only a few families worldwide.

PATHOLOGY AND PATHOGENESIS OF AMYLOID FIBRIL FORMATION

PATHOLOGIC FEATURES

Amyloid deposits are widespread in AL amyloidosis and can be present in the extracellular spaces and the blood vessels of all organs. Deposits in AA amyloidosis usually develop in the kidneys, liver, and spleen, although widespread deposits can be found late in the course of the disease. In Aβ₂M amyloidosis, deposits tend to occur in synovial membrane, cartilage, and bone, but visceral organs are sometimes affected. In ATTR amyloidosis, the nervous system, heart, and thyroid are frequently affected organs, with only small deposits found elsewhere.

All amyloid deposits stain with Congo red dye and exhibit a unique green birefringence by polarized light microscopy,[14] although the deposits also can be recognized on routine hematoxylin and eosin–stained sections. By electron microscopy, amyloid fibrils are 8 to 10 nm wide and of varying lengths, with a 2.5- to 3.5-nm filamentous subunit arranged along the long axis of the fibril in a slow twist.[15] Typing of amyloid deposits can be done with conventional immunohistochemical staining. False-positive results can occur, however, owing to the presence of nonamyloid serum proteins, and immunoelectron microscopy can provide more definitive immunologic identification of the protein in the fibril itself.[16] Fibrils can be extracted from tissues, and their composition can be analyzed by mass spectrometry, providing a definitive identification; however, this is not available yet as a routine clinical test.

PATHOGENESIS OF AMYLOID FIBRIL FORMATION

The exact mechanism of fibril formation is unknown and may differ among the various types of amyloid.[17,18] Studies suggest there may be a common underlying mechanism, however, in which a partially unfolded protein intermediate forms multimers and then higher order polymers. Factors that contribute to fibrillogenesis include variant or unstable protein structure, extensive β-conformation of the precursor protein, proteolytic processing of the precursor protein, association with components of the serum or extracellular matrix (e.g., amyloid P-component, amyloid enhancing factor, apolipoprotein E, or glycosaminoglycans), and physical properties including pH of the tissue site.

AL amyloidosis is a plasma cell dyscrasia with an excess of clonal plasma cells in the bone marrow; it can occur in isolation or along with multiple myeloma. Similar cytogenetic changes have been identified in both plasma cell diseases, suggesting they may have a common molecular pathogenesis.[19] By two-dimensional gel electrophoresis and mass spectrometry, it can be seen that the amyloid fibril deposits are composed of intact 23-kD monoclonal immunoglobulin light chains and C-terminal truncated fragments.[20] Although all κ and λ light chain subtypes have been identified in amyloid fibrils, λ subtypes predominate, and the λ VI subtype seems to have unique structural properties that predispose it to fibril formation,[21] often in the kidney.[22] AL amyloidosis is usually a rapidly progressive disease with amyloid deposits in multiple tissue sites.

The AA type of amyloidosis is a complication of severe, long-standing inflammation, as occurs in rheumatic diseases or infection. The AA amyloid fibrils usually are composed of an 8-kD, 76-amino acid amino-terminal portion of the 12-kD precursor, serum amyloid A (SAA).[23] SAA is a polymorphic protein encoded by a family of SAA genes, which are acute-phase apoproteins synthesized in the liver and transported by a high-density lipoprotein, HDL3, in the plasma.[24] An underlying inflammatory disease of several years' duration causing an elevated SAA usually precedes fibril formation, although infections can produce AA deposition more quickly. AA fibril formation can be accelerated by an amyloid enhancing factor present in high concentration in the spleen (which may be early SAA aggregates or deposits), by basement membrane heparan sulfate proteoglycan, or by seeding with AA or heterologous fibrils.[25,26]

Factors related to β_2-microglobulin fibril formation are under investigation. The high prevalence of Aβ_2M disease in patients undergoing long-term dialysis argues against an amyloidogenic variant β_2-microglobulin molecule. Permeability of dialysis membranes may be a factor because the molecular weight of β_2-microglobulin is 11.8 kD, above the porosity of standard membranes. It has been hypothesized that dialysis membranes may be bioincompatible and induce proinflammatory mediators that stimulate β_2-microglobulin and contribute to fibril formation.[27]

In ATTR (also called familial amyloidotic polyneuropathy), and all other forms of familial amyloidosis, inherited mutations or polymorphisms in the genes encoding large serum proteins produce amyloid-prone variants. The process of fibrillogenesis has been best studied for TTR, in which variant TTR molecules seem to be prone to dissociation from stable tetramers and to unfolding, leading to misfolding, polymerization, and fibril formation.[28] The role of aging is intriguing because patients with the variant proteins do not have clinically apparent disease until midlife or later, despite the lifelong presence of the abnormal protein.[29] Further evidence of an age-related trigger is that senile cardiac amyloidosis, caused by the deposition of fibrils derived from normal TTR, is exclusively a disease of elderly individuals.[13]

DIAGNOSIS

A tissue biopsy specimen showing amyloid fibrils is necessary for the diagnosis of amyloidosis (Fig. 106-1). The least invasive biopsy is the abdominal fat aspirate, which is positive in 80% to 90% of patients with either AL or ATTR amyloidosis and in 60% to 70% of patients with AA amyloidosis.[30,31] It is easy to perform after local injection of anesthetic and has a low rate of infectious or hemorrhagic complications (Fig. 106-2). If the aspirate is negative, but clinical suspicion for disease persists, a more invasive tissue biopsy should be done. Although a biopsy specimen of a clinically involved organ is recommended, almost any tissue biopsy specimen is likely to be positive if the patient has systemic amyloidosis: In a series of 100 patients with AL amyloidosis, 85% of 249 tissue biopsy specimens were positive, including all samples from the kidney, heart, and liver.[32] When the diagnosis of amyloidosis is made, a careful evaluation of the entire

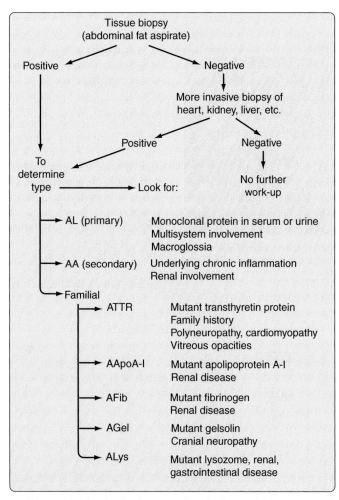

Figure 106-1 Algorithm for the diagnosis of amyloidosis and determination of type.

clinical picture, including manner of presentation, organ system involvement, underlying diseases, and family history should provide a clue to the type of amyloid.

Identification of a plasma cell dycrasia distinguishes AL from other types of amyloidosis (Fig. 106-3). More than 90% of patients have a serum or urine monoclonal immunoglobulin protein or a free light chain on testing by immunofixation electrophoresis or by a recently available nephelometric assay for free light chains.[33,34] In addition, there is often an increased percentage of plasma cells in the bone marrow, which are monoclonal on immunohistochemical staining (Fig. 106-4).[35] A monoclonal serum protein by itself is not diagnostic of amyloidosis because monoclonal gammopathy of uncertain significance is common in older patients. When "monoclonal gammopathy of uncertain significance" is present in a patient with biopsy-proven amyloidosis, however, the AL type is strongly suspected. Immunohistochemical

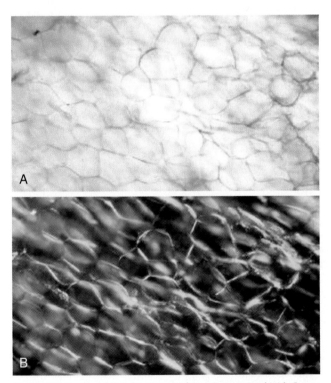

Figure 106-2 **A** and **B,** Subcutaneous fat aspirate stained with Congo red viewed by light microscopy (**A**) and viewed under polarized light (**B**) (×200). The staining and birefringence is evident in the walls and connective tissue surrounding the adipose cells.

staining by light or electron microscopy should be done by a laboratory familiar with the techniques and able to perform appropriate controls.[16] Mass spectrometry–based microsequencing of small amounts of protein extracted from fibril deposits ultimately may be the most reliable way to identify the components of the fibrils.[36]

AA amyloidosis is suspected in patients with renal amyloidosis and a chronic inflammatory condition or infection. AL and ATTR amyloidosis must be ruled out. AA amyloidosis must be confirmed by immunohistochemical staining for AA protein.

Familial amyloidosis must be excluded in every patient who does not have a plasma cell dyscrasia or the AA type of amyloidosis. Although the disease has a dominant inheritance, family history may not be apparent when the disease occurs later in life; also, some cases occur through new mutations. Variant TTR proteins usually can be detected by isoelectric focusing (Fig. 106-5).[37] Abnormal isoelectric focusing should prompt genetic testing to determine the precise TTR mutation. Genetic testing should be employed when screening tests fail to identify the fibril protein. Using polymerase chain reaction–based sequencing, abnormal fibrinogens and apolipoproteins and variant TTRs can be detected.[38]

CLINICAL FEATURES AND TREATMENT OF SYSTEMIC AMYLOIDOSES

AL AMYLOIDOSIS

AL amyloidosis usually occurs in middle-aged or older individuals, but also can occur in the third or fourth decade of life. It has a wide spectrum of organ system involvement, and presenting features reflect the organs most prominently affected.[39,40] Initial symptoms of fatigue and weight loss are frequent, but the diagnosis is rarely made until symptoms referable to a specific organ appear.

The kidneys are commonly affected; renal amyloidosis is manifested by proteinuria, sometimes massive with edema and hypoalbuminemia. Mild renal dysfunction is frequent, but rapidly progressing renal failure is rare. Cardiac involvement, often with congestive heart failure, is a common presentation.[41] The electrocardiogram may show low voltage with a pattern of myocardial infarction. The echocardiogram frequently shows concentrically thickened ventricles and a normal or mildly reduced ejection fraction. Nervous system features include peripheral sensory neuropathy, carpal tunnel syndrome, and autonomic dysfunction with

Figure 106-3 **A,** Pretreatment serum immunofixation electrophoresis shows an IgG κ monoclonal protein. **B,** Post-treatment serum immunofixation electrophoresis shows absence of the monoclonal protein.

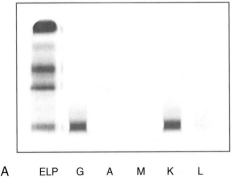

A   ELP   G   A   M   K   L

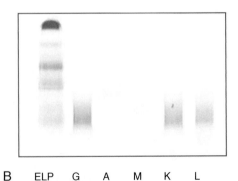

B   ELP   G   A   M   K   L

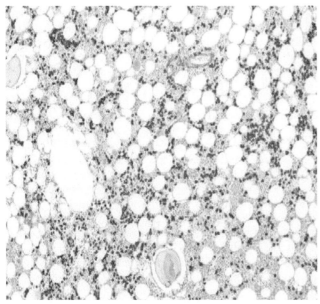

Figure 106-4 Bone marrow biopsy specimen stained with antibody to λ light chain shows preferential staining of plasma cells and staining of amyloid deposit around a blood vessel (×400).

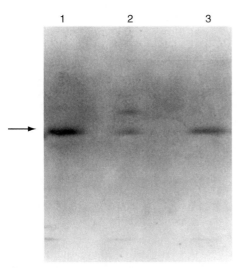

Figure 106-5 Isoelectric focusing of serum samples shows bands of variant and wild-type TTR protein *(arrow)* from a patient with ATTR *(lane 2)* and a single band of wild-type TTR in normal subjects *(lanes 1 and 3)*.

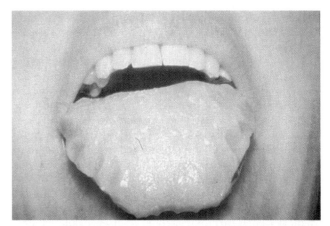

Figure 106-6 Enlarged tongue of a patient with AL amyloidosis.

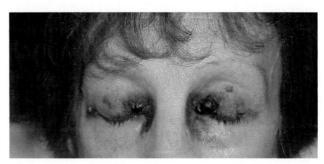

Figure 106-7 Periorbital ecchymoses in a patient with AL amyloidosis.

series of almost 200 patients.[42] Symptoms and signs mimicking rheumatologic diseases, with arthropathy, subcutaneous tissue deposits, muscle pseudohypertrophy, adenopathy, carpal tunnel syndrome, submandibular gland enlargement, and macroglossia occur in more than 40% of patients with AL amyloidosis, particularly in patients with light chain deposits.

Timely diagnosis of AL amyloidosis is crucial. Patients with any of these clinical syndromes should have immunofixation electrophoresis performed. The sensitivity of serum or urine protein electrophoresis without immunofixation is inadequate for diagnosis.

gastrointestinal motility disturbances (early satiety, diarrhea, constipation) and orthostatic hypotension. Macroglossia, a classic feature pathognomonic of AL amyloidosis, is found in 10% of patients (Fig. 106-6). Hepatomegaly may be massive with mild cholestatic abnormalities of liver function, although liver failure is uncommon, even when hepatomegaly is massive. The spleen is frequently involved, and there may be functional hyposplenism even in the absence of significant splenomegaly. Cutaneous ecchymoses are common, particularly around the eyes, giving the "raccoon-eyes" sign, and appear spontaneously or when provoked by minor trauma (Fig. 106-7). Other findings include nail dystrophy (Fig. 106-8), alopecia, and amyloid arthropathy with thickening of synovial membranes. We have reviewed the soft tissue and joint manifestations of AL amyloidosis in a

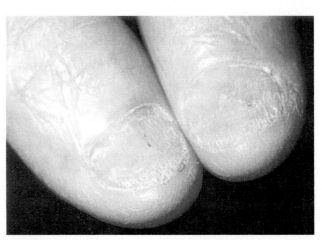

Figure 106-8 Fingernail dystrophy in a patient with AL amyloidosis.

Extensive multisystem involvement typifies AL amyloidosis, and median survival with no treatment is usually only about 1 year from diagnosis. Current therapies target the clonal bone marrow plasma cells using chemotherapy approaches employed for multiple myeloma (Table 106-2). Cyclic oral melphalan and prednisone can decrease the plasma cell burden, but produce complete hematologic remission in only a small percentage of patients, and modestly increase median survival.[32,43] Substitution of high-dose dexamethasone for prednisone seems to increase response rates markedly.[44]

High-dose intravenous melphalan followed by autologous stem cell transplantation is highly effective. Of more than 300 patients treated on such protocols at Boston Medical Center, approximately 40% of evaluable patients achieve a hematologic complete response, and most of these experience significant improvement or stabilization of organ function.[45] Median survival in the treated patients exceeds 4.5 years. Other centers have replicated these results.[46-48] Patients with amyloidosis and organ impairment have a high rate of treatment-related morbidity and mortality with aggressive treatment, however, particularly at centers without extensive multidisciplinary experience in the management of the disease. Factors that contribute to mortality are amyloid cardiomyopathy, nutritional status as measured by weight loss, performance status, and, in some studies, number of involved organs. The bleeding diathesis resulting from absorption of clotting factor X to amyloid fibrils also confers high mortality during myelosuppressive therapy. Age alone[49] or renal failure[50] should not exclude patients from such treatment, however.

For patients with impaired cardiac function or arrhythmias owing to amyloid involvement of the myocardium, median survival is only about 6 months without treatment, and stem cell mobilization and high-dose chemotherapy are associated with great morbidity. In a few such patients, cardiac transplantation has been performed followed by treatment with intravenous melphalan and stem cell rescue to prevent fibrillogenesis in the transplanted heart or other organs.

New agents that are efficacious in reducing the plasma cell burden in multiple myeloma are being tested for AL amyloidosis. The immunomodulators thalidomide and lenalidomide have activity in AL amyloidosis,[51,52] although the former is not well tolerated. Excellent responses have been seen with lenalidomide and dexamethasone, even in heavily pretreated patients. The proteasome inhibitor bortezomib is being tested in a multicenter trial.

Innovative approaches target the amyloid fibrils themselves or accessory binding proteins. The anthracycline derivative 4'-iodo-4'-deoxydoxorubicin (IDOX) was serendipitously noted to cause resorption of amyloid deposits in model systems, but preliminary trials with single-agent IDOX have not produced clinically significant responses.[53,54] The agent R-1-[6-[R-2-carboxy-pyrrolidin-1-yl]-6-oxo-hexanoyl]pyrrolidine-2-carboxylic acid (CPHPC) binds serum amyloid P protein and accelerates clearance from the circulation and from amyloid fibrils.[55] The efficacy of CPHPC in promoting fibril resorption and reducing amyloid disease has so far not been shown.

Supportive treatment is recommended for patients with all types of amyloidosis (Table 106-3). At times, supportive treatments are lifesaving (e.g., heart or kidney transplantation, renal dialysis, cardiac pacemaker, and nutritional support). Digitalis, calcium channel blockers, and β-blockers are relatively contraindicated because toxicity has been observed at therapeutic levels.

AA AMYLOIDOSIS

AA amyloidosis can occur at any age. The primary clinical manifestation is proteinuria or renal insufficiency or both.[5] A study from Finland found AA amyloidosis to be the most common cause of nephrotic syndrome in patients with rheumatoid arthritis.[56] Hepatomegaly, splenomegaly, and autonomic neuropathy frequently occur as the disease progresses; cardiomyopathy occurs rarely. With chronic inflammatory diseases, amyloid progression is slow, and survival is often more than 10 years, particularly with treatment for end-stage renal disease. In contrast, untreated infections, such as osteomyelitis, tuberculosis, or leprosy, can produce a more rapidly progressive amyloid syndrome, which remits with effective medical or surgical treatment of the infection.

The major therapy in AA amyloidosis is treatment of the underlying inflammatory or infectious disease. Treatment that suppresses or eliminates the inflammation or infection also decreases the serum amyloid A (SAA) protein. For familial Mediterranean fever, colchicine, 1.2 to 1.8 mg/day, is the appropriate treatment. Colchicine has not been helpful for AA amyloidosis of other causes or for other amyloidoses. A multicenter trial using a new antiamyloid drug, eprodisate, has been completed, and the drug was found to delay significantly worsening of renal function in patients with AA amyloidosis.[57] Eprodisate interferes with the interaction of AA amyloid protein and glycosaminoglycans in tissues and prevents fibril formation and deposition.

Table 106-2 Major Treatment Options for Amyloidosis

AL Amyloidosis

Intravenous melphalan with autologous stem cell rescue
  Granulocyte colony-stimulating factor mobilized peripheral blood stem cell collection
  Intravenous melphalan 100-200 mg/m²
  Autologous stem cell reinfusion
Cyclic oral melphalan and dexamethasone
  Melphalan 0.22 mg/kg/day × 4 days
  Dexamethasone 20-40 mg/day × 4 days
  Repeat administration every 4 wk
Immunomodulators
  Thalidomide 50-200 mg/day or lenalidomide 5-15 mg/day × 21 days
  Dexamethasone 20-40 mg/day × 4 days
  Repeat administration every 4 wk
Proteasome inhibitors
  Intravenous bortezomib, in clinical trials

AA Amyloidosis

Aggressive treatment of underlying inflammatory disease
Medical or surgical treatment of underlying infection
Colchicine 1.2-1.8 mg/day for AA amyloidosis secondary to familial Mediterranean fever
Antifibril drug, eprosidate (FDA approval pending)

ATTR Amyloidosis

Orthotopic liver transplantation
Diflunisal in clinical trials

Table 106-3 Supportive Treatment for All Types of Amyloidosis

Organ System	Symptom	Treatment Options
Cardiac	Congestive failure	Salt restriction of 1-2 g/day Diuretics: furosemide, spironolactone, metolazone
	Arrhythmia	Pacemaker Automatic implantable cardiac defibrillator Antiarrhythmics
Renal	Nephrotic syndrome	Salt restriction of 1-2 g/day Elastic stockings, leg elevation Maintain dietary protein Angiotensin-converting enzyme inhibitor, if blood pressure tolerates
	Renal failure	Dialysis (long-term ambulatory peritoneal dialysis or hemodialysis)
Autonomic nervous	Orthostatic hypotension	Midodrine Increase dietary salt or add fludrocortisone, depending on edema Elastic stockings
	Gastric atony or ileus	Small frequent feedings (6/day) low in fat Oral nutritional supplements Jejunostomy tube feeding Parenteral nutrition
Gastrointestinal	Diarrhea	Low-fat diet (≤40 g) Psyllium hydrophilic muciloid (Metamucil) Loperamide hydrochloride (Imodium) Tincture of opium Parenteral nutrition
	Macroglossia	Soft solid diet Partial glossectomy (rarely effective)
Peripheral nervous	Sensory neuropathy	Avoid trauma Gabapentin (Neurontin) 100-300 mg 3 times daily Amitriptyline, 25-50 mg at bedtime Carbamazepine (Tegretol)
	Motor neuropathy	Ankle/foot orthotics for footdrop Physical therapy
Hematologic	Intracutaneous bleeding	Avoid trauma, antiplatelet agents
	Factor X deficiency	Factor replacement (recombinant factor VIIa, prothrombin complex concentrates) Splenectomy if massively enlarged spleen

Aβ₂M AMYLOIDOSIS

Several distinct rheumatologic conditions are observed in Aβ₂M amyloidosis, including carpal tunnel syndrome, persistent joint effusions, spondyloarthropathy, and cystic bone lesions. Carpal tunnel syndrome is usually the first symptom of disease. Persistent joint effusions accompanied by mild discomfort occur in 50% of patients on dialysis for more than 12 years. Involvement is bilateral, and large joints (shoulders, knees, wrists, and hips) are more frequently affected. The synovial fluid is noninflammatory and β₂-microglobulin amyloid deposits can be found if the sediment is examined with Congo red staining. Spondyloarthropathy with destructive changes of the intervertebral disks and paravertebral erosions have occurred in association with β₂-microglobulin amyloid deposits. Cystic bone lesions sometimes leading to pathologic fractures have been described in the femoral head, acetabulum, humerus, tibial plateau, vertebral bodies, and carpal bones. Although less common, visceral β₂-microglobulin amyloid deposits occasionally occur in the gastrointestinal tract, heart, tendons, and subcutaneous tissues of the buttocks.

The treatment for Aβ₂M amyloidosis is difficult because the 11-kD β₂-microglobulin molecule is too large to pass through a dialysis membrane. Consistent with a postulated role of copper in initiating Aβ₂M fibrillogenesis,[58] copper-free dialysis membranes seem to reduce the incidence of disease. Patients on continuous ambulatory peritoneal dialysis

usually have lower plasma levels of β₂-microglobulin than patients on hemodialysis and may not develop amyloid deposits as quickly. Symptoms of arthropathy are common, and prevalence may approach 100% of individuals on dialysis for more than 15 years. Patients who have received kidney transplants after developing Aβ₂M report an improvement in symptoms.

ATTR FAMILIAL AMYLOIDOSIS

The clinical features of ATTR amyloidosis overlap AL amyloidosis such that the diseases cannot be reliably distinguished on clinical grounds alone. A family history makes ATTR more likely, but many patients seem to present sporadically with new mutations. Within each family, disease begins at nearly the same age, and symptoms usually include neuropathy or cardiomyopathy or both. Peripheral neuropathy begins as a lower extremity sensory and motor neuropathy and progresses to the upper extremities. Autonomic neuropathy is manifest by gastrointestinal symptoms of diarrhea with weight loss and orthostatic hypotension. Patients with TTR Val-30-Met, the most common mutation, have normal echocardiograms, but may have conduction system defects and require a pacemaker. Patients with TTR Thr-60-Ala and several other mutations have myocardial thickening similar to that caused by AL amyloidosis, although heart failure is less common, and the prognosis is better.

Vitreous opacities caused by amyloid deposits are pathognomonic of ATTR amyloidosis.

The TTR variant, Val 122 Ile, is a common allele in African-Americans and seems to be associated with cardiomyopathy. In a large referral population, 25% of African-American patients with amyloidosis had this TTR variant.[59] This disease likely is underdiagnosed because of a lack of physician awareness and the difficulty of distinguishing amyloid and hypertensive cardiomyopathy without an endomyocardial biopsy.[11]

Without intervention, survival after ATTR disease onset is 5 to 15 years. Orthotopic liver transplantation, which removes the major source of variant TTR production and replaces it with normal TTR, is the major treatment for ATTR amyloidosis.[60,61] Liver transplantation arrests disease progression, and some improvement in autonomic and peripheral neuropathy can occur.[62] Cardiomyopathy does not improve, and in some patients seems to worsen, after liver transplantation.[63] Long-term outcome and the timing of transplantation are being evaluated.[64] An international multicenter randomized placebo-controlled clinical trial is under way to test the efficacy of the nonsteroidal anti-inflammatory drug, diflunisal, for the treatment of TTR amyloidosis (www.bu.edu/amyloid/doctors/trials/html). Laboratory studies have suggested that diflunisal stabilizes variant TTRs and prevents unfolding and aggregation.[65]

SUMMARY

Treatment of the amyloidoses begins with recognition of the clinical amyloid syndromes and obtaining appropriate biopsy specimens and screening tests to rule in or out AL amyloidosis. For difficult cases and for identification of variant serum proteins, amyloid referral centers can provide specialized diagnostic techniques. Effective therapy is now available for AL, AA, and ATTR amyloidosis. An understanding of the biophysical properties of amyloid proteins and of the mechanisms of protein misfolding in a wide variety of diseases would enable the further development of more specific and less toxic antifibril drugs.

Acknowledgments

This chapter was supported by grants from the National Institutes of Health (HL 68705), the Gerry Foundation, the Young Family Amyloid Research Fund, and the Amyloid Research Fund at Boston University.

REFERENCES

1. Virchow VR: Ueber einem Gehirn and Rueckenmark des Menchen auf gefundene Substanz mit chemischen reaction der Cellulose. Virchows Arch Pathol Anat 6:135-138, 1854.
2. Cohen AS, Calkins E: Electron microscopic observations on a fibrous component in amyloid of diverse origins. Nature 183:1202-1203, 1959.
3. Westermark P, Benson MD, Buxbaum JN, et al: Amyloid: Towards terminology clarification. Report from the Nomenclature Committee of the International Society of Amyloidosis. Amyloid J Protein Folding Disorders 12:1-4, 2005.
4. Simms RW, Prout MN, Cohen AS: The epidemiology of AL and AA amyloidosis. Baillieres Clin Rheumatol 8:627-634, 1994.
5. Gertz MA, Kyle RA: Secondary systemic amyloidosis: Response and survival in 64 patients. Medicine 70:246-256, 1991.
6. David J, Vouyiouka O, Ansell BM, et al: Amyloidosis in juvenile chronic arthritis: A morbidity and mortality study. Clin Exp Rheumatol 11:85-90, 1993.
7. Livneh A, Langevitz P, Shinar Y, et al: MEFV mutation analysis in patients suffering from amyloidosis of familial Mediterranean fever. Amyloid 6:1-6, 1999.
8. Drueke TB: Beta 2-microglobulin and amyloidosis. Nephrol Dial Transplant 15(Suppl 1):17-24, 2000.
9. Benson MD: Amyloidosis. In Scriver CR, Beaudet AL, Sly WS, et al (eds): The Metabolic and Molecular Bases of Inherited Disease, 8th ed, Vol IV. New York, McGraw Hill, 2001, pp 5345-5378.
10. **Connors LH, Lim A, Prokaeva T, et al: Tabulation of human transthyretin (TTR) variants, 2003. Amyloid J Protein Folding Disorders 10:160-184, 2003.**
11. Jacobson DR, Pastore RD, Yaghoubian R, et al: Variant-sequence transthyretin (isoleucine 122) in late-onset cardiac amyloidosis in black Americans. N Engl J Med 336:466-473, 1997.
12. Kyle RA, Spittell PC, Gertz MA, et al: The premortem recognition of systemic senile amyloidosis with cardiac involvement. Am J Med 101:395-400, 1996.
13. Ng B, Connors LH, Davidoff R, et al: Senile systemic amyloidosis presenting with heart failure: A comparison with light chain-associated amyloidosis. Arch Intern Med 165:1425-1429, 2005.
14. **Bennhold H: Eine spezifische Amyloidfarbung mit Kongorot. Munch Med Wochenschr 69:1537-1538, 1922.**
15. **Shirahama T, Cohen AS: High-resolution electron microscopic analysis of the amyloid fibril. J Cell Biol 33:679-708, 1967.**
16. Arbustini E, Morbini P, Verga L, et al: Light and electrom microscopy immunohistochemical characterization of amyloid deposits. Amyloid Int J Exp Clin Invest 4:157-170, 1997.
17. Bellotti V, Mangione P, Merlini G: Review: Immunoglogulin light chain amyloidosis—the archetype of structural and pathologic variability. J Struct Biol 130:280-289, 2000.
18. Lansbury PT: Evolution of amyloid: What normal protein folding may tell us about fibrillogenesis and disease. Proc Natl Acad Sci U S A 96:3342-3344, 1999.
19. Hayman SR, Bailey RJ, Jalal SM, et al: Translocations involving the immunoglobulin heavy-chain locus are possibly early genetic events in patients with primary systemic amyloidosis. Blood 98:2266-2268, 2001.
20. Lavatelli F, Perlman DH, Spencer B, et al: A proteomic approach to the study of systemic amyloidosis. In Skinner M, Berk JL, Connors LH, et al (eds): XIth International Symposium on Amyloidosis. Boca Raton, CRC Press, 2007, pp 360-362.
21. **Solomon A, Frangione B, Franklin EC: Bence Jones proteins and light chains of immunoglobulins: Preferential association of the V lambda VI subgroup of human light chains with amyloidosis AL (lambda). J Clin Invest 70:453-460, 1982.**
22. Teng J, Russell WJ, Gu X, et al: Different types of glomerulopathic light chains interact with mesangial cells using a common receptor but exhibit different intracellular trafficking patterns. Lab Invest 84:440-451, 2004.
23. Husby G, Marhung G, Dowton B, et al: Serum amyloid A (SAA): Biochemistry, genetics, and the pathogenesis of AA amyloidosis. Amyloid Int J Exp Clin Invest 1:119-137, 1994.
24. Kluve-Beckerman B, Dwulet FE, Benson MD: Human serum amyloid A. J Clin Invest 82:1670-1675, 1988.
25. Johan K, Westermark G, Engstrom U, et al: Acceleration of amyloid protein A amyloidosis by amyloid-like synthetic fibrils. Proc Natl Acad Sci U S A 95:2558-2563, 1998.
26. Kluve-Beckerman B, Manaloor J, Liepnieks J: A pulse-chase study tracking the conversion of macrophage-endocytosed serum amyloid A into extracellular amyloid. Arthritis Rheum 46:1905-1913, 2002.
27. Zingraff J, Drueke T: Beta2-microglobulin amyloidosis: Past and future. Artif Organs 22:581-584, 1998.
28. Hammarstrom P, Wiseman RL, Powers ET, et al: Prevention of transthyretin amyloid disease by changing protein misfolding energetics. Science 299:713-716, 2003.
29. Suhr OE, Svendsen IH, Ohlsson P, et al: Impact of age and amyloidosis on thiol conjugation of transthyretin in hereditaty transthyretin amyloidosis. Amyloid Int J Exp Clin Invest 6:187-191, 1999.
30. **Libbey CA, Skinner M, Cohen AS: Use of abdominal fat tissue aspirate in the diagnosis of systemic amyloidosis. Arch Intern Med 143:1549-1552, 1983.**
31. Duston MA, Skinner M, Shirahama T, et al: Diagnosis of amyloidosis by abdominal fat aspiration: Analysis of four years' experience. Am J Med 82:412-414, 1987.
32. Skinner M, Anderson J, Simms R, et al: Treatment of 100 patients with primary amyloidosis: A randomized trial of melphalan, prednisone, and colchicine versus colchicine only. Am J Med 100:290-298, 1996.

33. Abraham RS, Clark RJ, Bryant SC, et al: Correlation of serum immunoglobulin free light chain quantification with urinary Bence Jones protein in light chain myeloma. Clin Chem 48:655-657, 2002.

34. Akar H, Seldin DC, Magnani B, et al: Quantitative serum free light-chain assay in the diagnostic evaluation of AL amyloidosis. Amyloid J Protein Folding Disorders 12:210-215, 2005.

35. Swan N, Skinner M, O'Hara C: Bone marrow core biopsy specimens in AL (primary) amyloidosis: A morphologic and immunohistochemical study of 100 cases. Am J Clin Pathol 120:610-616, 2003.

36. Lim A, Wally J, Walsh MT, et al: Identification and localization of a cysteinyl posttranslational modification in an amyloidogenic kappa 1 light chain protein by electrospray ionization and matrix-assisted laser deposition/ionization mass spectrometry. Anal Biochem 295:45-56, 2001.

37. Connors LH, Ericsson T, Skare J, et al: A simple screening test for variant transthyretins associated with familial transthyretin amyloidosis using isoelectric focusing. Biochim Biophys Acta 1407:185-192, 1998.

38. Benson MD: Amyloidosis. In Scriver CR, Beaudet AL, Sly WS, et al (eds): The Metabolic and Molecular Bases of Inherited Disease, 7th ed. New York, McGraw-Hill, 1999, pp 4159-4191.

39. Falk RH, Comenzo RL, Skinner M: The systemic amyloidoses. N Engl J Med 337:898-909, 1997.

40. Merlini G, Bellotti V: Molecular mechanisms of amyloidosis. N Engl J Med 349:583-596, 2003.

41. Dubrey SW, Cha K, Anderson J, et al: The clinical features of immunoglobulin light-chain (AL) amyloidosis with heart involvement. QJM 91:141-157, 1998.

42. Prokaeva T, Spencer B, Kaut M, et al: Soft tissue, joint, and bone manifestations of AL amyloidosis: Clinical presentation, molecular features, and survival. Arthritis Rheum 56:3858-3868, 2007.

43. Kyle RA, Gertz MA, Greipp PR, et al: A trial of three regimens for primary amyloidosis: Colchicine alone, melphalan and prednisone, and melphalan, prednisone, and colchicine. N Engl J Med 336:1202-1207, 1997.

44. Pallidini G, Perfetti V, Obici L, et al: Association of melphalan and high-dose dexamethasone is effective and well tolerated in patients with AL (primary) amyloidosis who are ineligible for stem cell transplantation. Blood 103:2936-2938, 2004.

45. Skinner M, Sanchorawala V, Seldin DC, et al: High-dose melphalan and autologous stem-cell transplantation in patients with AL amyloidosis: An 8-year study. Ann Intern Med 140:85-93, 2004.

46. Dispenzieri A, Kyle RA, Lacy MQ, et al: Superior survival in primary systemic amyloidosis patients undergoing peripheral blood stem cell transplantation: A case-control study. Blood 103:3960-3963, 2004.

47. Schonland SO, Lokhorst H, Buzyn A, et al: Allogeneic and syngeneic hematopoietic cell transplantation in patients with amyloid light-chain amyloidosis: A report from the European Group for Blood and Marrow Transplantation. Blood 107:2578-2584, 2006.

48. Perfetti V, Siena S, Palladini G, et al: Long-term results of a risk-adapted approach to melphalan conditioning in autologous peripheral blood stem cell transplantation for primary (AL) amyloidosis. Haematologica 91:1635-1643, 2006.

49. Seldin DC, Anderson JJ, Skinner M, et al: Successful treatment of AL amyloidosis with high-dose melphalan and autologous stem cell transplantation in patients over age 65. Blood 108:3945-3947, 2006.

50. Casserly LF, Fadia A, Sanchorawala V, et al: High-dose intravenous melphalan with autologous stem cell transplantation in AL amyloidosis-associated end-stage renal disease. Kidney Int 63:1051-1057, 2003.

51. Seldin DC, Choufani EB, Dember LM, et al: Tolerability and efficacy of thalidomide for the treatment of patients with light chain-associated (AL) amyloidosis. Clin Lymphoma 3:241-246, 2003.

52. Sanchorawala V, Wright DG, Rosenzweig M, et al: Lenalidomide and dexamethasone in the treatment of AL amyloidosis: Results of a phase II trial. Blood 109:492-496, 2007.

53. Gianni L, Bellotti V, Gianni AM, et al: New drug therapy of amyloidoses: resorption of AL-type deposits with 4'-iodo-4'-deoxydoxorubicin. Blood 86:855-861, 1995.

54. Gertz MA, Lacy MQ, Dispenzieri A, et al: A multicenter phase II trial of 4'-iodo-4'-deoxydoxorubicin (IDOX) in primary amyloidosis (AL). Amyloid J Protein Folding Disorders 9:24-30, 2002.

55. Pepys MB, Herbert J, Hutchinson WL, et al: Targeted pharmacological depletion of serum amyloid P component (SAP) for treatment of human amyloidosis. Nature 417:254-259, 2002.

56. Helin HJ, Korpela MM, Mustonen JT, et al: Renal biopsy findings and clinicopathologic correlations in rheumatoid arthritis. Arthritis Rheum 38:242-247, 1995.

57. Dember LM, Hawkins PN, Hazenberg BPC, et al: Eprodisate for the treatment of AA amyloidosis. N Engl J Med 356:2349-2360, 2007.

58. Morgan CJ, Gelfand M, Atreya C, et al: Kidney dialysis-associated amyloidosis: A molecular role for copper in fiber formation. J Mol Biol 309:339-345, 2001.

59. Berg A, Falk RH, Connors LH, et al: Transthyretin ILE-122 in a series of black patients with amyloidosis. In Kyle RA, Gertz MA (eds): Amyloid and Amyloidosis 1998. New York, Parthenon Publishing Group, 1999.

60. Holmgren G, Steen L, Ekstedt J, et al: Biochemical effect of liver transplantation in two Swedish patients with familial amyloidotic polyneuropathy (FAP-met30). Clin Genet 40:242-246, 1991.

61. Lewis WD, Skinner M, Simms RW, et al: Orthotopic liver transplantation for familial amyloidotic polyneuropathy. Clin Transplant 8:107-110, 1994.

62. Bergethon P, Sabin T, Lewis D, et al: Improvement in the polyneuropathy associated with familial amyloid polyneuropathy after liver transplantation. Neurology 47:944-951, 1996.

63. Dubrey SW, Davidoff R, Skinner M, et al: Progression of ventricular wall thickening after liver transplantation for familial amyloidosis. Transplantation 64:74-80, 1997.

64. de Carvalho M, Conceicao I, Bentes C, et al: Long-term quantitative evaluation of liver transplantation in familial amyloid polyneuropathy (Portuguese V30M). Amyloid J Protein Folding Disorders 9:126-133, 2002.

65. Sekijima Y, Dendle MA, Kelly JW: Orally administered diflunisal stabilizes transthyretin against dissociation required for amyloidogenesis. Amyloid J Protein Folding Disorders 13:236-249, 2006.

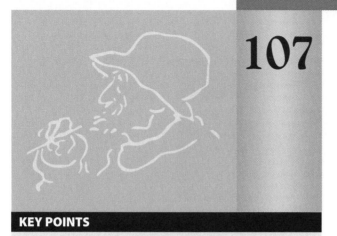

107 Sarcoidosis

LEE S. NEWMAN • HOLLY M. SACKETT

KEY POINTS

Sarcoidosis is a multisystem inflammatory disease of unknown cause.

Sarcoidosis occurs worldwide and affects people of all racial and ethnic backgrounds.

No single infectious agent or antigen has consistently been linked to sarcoidosis.

Some clinical subtypes, especially Löfgren's syndrome and acute resolving sarcoidosis, have an immunologic and genetic basis that is distinct from other forms of sarcoidosis.

Rheumatologic manifestations are common in sarcoidosis and are often overlooked or misdiagnosed.

Magnetic resonance imaging has improved the detection of musculoskeletal involvement in sarcoidosis.

New treatment modalities, including tumor necrosis factor-α inhibitors, appear to be promising for the treatment of extrathoracic sarcoidosis based on case series, although randomized controlled trials have shown limited benefit in cases of pulmonary involvement.

Sarcoidosis is a multisystem immunologic disorder that preferentially involves the lungs. Characterized by non-caseating granulomas in virtually any organ, sarcoidosis is the consequence of an antigen-specific immune and inflammatory response to unidentified triggering agents. Clinically, sarcoidosis often presents with hilar lymphadenopathy, pulmonary infiltration, and ocular and skin lesions. With protean clinical manifestations, this disease can mimic many inflammatory and infectious disorders.[1] Particular targets include the lungs, lymphatics, eyes, skin, liver, bones, and neurologic system. This chapter emphasizes the rheumatologic and immunologic aspects of this condition.

The American Thoracic Society (ATS), European Respiratory Society (ERS), and World Association of Sarcoidosis and Other Granulomatous Disorders (WASOG) criteria for the diagnosis of sarcoidosis include (1) the presence of a consistent clinical and radiographic picture; (2) the demonstration of noncaseating granulomatous disease (Fig. 107-1), often in more than one affected organ; and (3) the exclusion of other conditions that can produce similar pathology, including a panoply of infections, autoimmune disorders, and inhalation diseases, as discussed in the differential diagnosis section.[2]

EPIDEMIOLOGY

Sarcoidosis occurs worldwide and affects people of all racial and ethnic backgrounds, both genders, and all ages.[1] Most patients are diagnosed in early adulthood, before age 40 years; there is a slight female predominance and a peak incidence in the 20 to 29 age group. Estimated prevalence rates vary from 1 to 80 per 100,000 population. Similarly, there is a range of age-adjusted annual incidence rates, from 10.9 per 100,000 for whites to 35.5 per 100,000 for African Americans in the United States. Similar rates have been reported in many countries; however, the published rates, including those for the United States, are likely underestimates, because many cases go undiagnosed or are misdiagnosed. Familial and twin studies demonstrate much higher prevalence of disease in first-generation relatives of those with sarcoidosis.[3] The highest risk for familial sarcoidosis occurs in African Americans (although familial risk has also been demonstrated in whites), women, and patients with active disease. Interestingly, when sarcoidosis occurs in siblings, the clinical pattern of illness often differs between the siblings.[4]

CAUSE AND PATHOGENESIS

The cause of sarcoidosis remains unknown. However, available evidence strongly supports the hypothesis that the disease develops when a specific environmental exposure with antigenic properties occurs in a genetically susceptible individual. Spatial and temporal clustering of cases, reports of community outbreaks, and reports of work-related risks for health care workers suggest either shared environmental exposure or possibly person-to-person transmission. Environmental investigation of new cases has uncovered clusters of disease among nurses, firefighters, and military personnel. A case-control study of a sarcoidosis cluster on the Isle of Mann demonstrated that a greater percentage of cases than controls reported previous contact with a sarcoidosis patient, although this study has been criticized for its information and recall biases. A recent case-control study identified exposure to industrial organic dust as an occupational risk factor, as well as occupations in the building material, hardware, gardening supplies, and education trades.[5] No single infective agent or antigen has been consistently linked to sarcoidosis. Numerous studies have investigated the possibility that mycobacteria and viruses cause sarcoidosis, but to date, no infectious agent evaluated has fulfilled Koch's postulates. However, recent studies strongly suggest a role of mycobacteria antigens in a sizable proportion of cases.[6-9] This is compatible with immunologic evidence of oligoclonal T cells, presumably due to antigen-driven accumulation of T cells in sarcoidosis patients' affected organs, as reflected

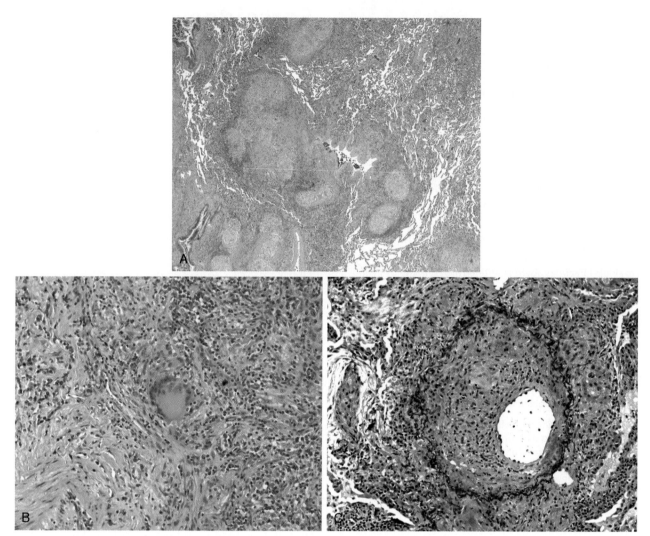

Figure 107-1 **A,** The typical pathologic appearance of sarcoidosis consists of non-necrotizing granulomas, which are mononuclear cell infiltrates with varying degrees of adjacent collagen deposition. Shown here is tissue from the lung, the most commonly affected organ, infiltrated by multiple noncaseating granulomas adjacent to vessels and bronchioles (hematoxylin and eosin, ×100). **B,** This photomicrograph (×400) demonstrates the classic, but not pathognomonic, features of noncaseating granulomas, including multinucleated giant cell (center), abundant lymphocytes, macrophages, epithelioid cells, mast cells, plasma cells, and fibroblasts. **C,** Although uncommon, sarcoidosis can cause a non-necrotizing granulomatous vasculitis in virtually any organ. Shown here is a pulmonary artery using an elastic tissue Verhoeff-van Gieson stain (×200). The elastic lamina (dark stain) is intact. Within the intima is a large area of non-necrotizing granulomatous inflammation, producing a narrowing of the vessel lumen. Efforts must be made to exclude other causes of vasculitis, as discussed in the text. Prognosis is generally poor for this form of sarcoidosis.

by bronchoalveolar lavage. Evidence of an upregulated T helper type 1 (Th1) pattern of cytokine production, along with tumor necrosis factor-α (TNF-α) release, suggests that regardless of whether the granulomatous inflammation of sarcoidosis is initiated by a microbe-related antigen, the pathologic consequence is due to enhanced immune reactivity, as discussed later.

A case-control etiologic study of sarcoidosis (ACCESS) examined 706 affected and unaffected pairs but did not identify a single proximate cause of sarcoidosis by questionnaire.[10] Questionnaire results suggested a possible role for exposure in the work environment, including environments rich in microbial bioaerosols and occupational exposure to insecticides. A previous case-control study evaluated the rural predominance of the disease and identified exposure to wood stoves or fireplaces as potential risk factors.[11] A more recent study found that these inhalational exposures are principally associated with pulmonary

sarcoidosis,[12] providing little insight into the triggering exposure for nonpulmonary forms of the disease. Similarly, seasonal and geographic variations in sarcoidosis risk raise questions about cause. In one study, the incidence of sarcoidosis varied by season, with symptoms presenting more often in spring and less often in winter.[13] Available lines of immunologic evidence suggest that sarcoidal granulomas form as a result of antigen exposure, an antigen-specific cell-mediated immune response, and inflammatory or innate immune responses that amplify and perpetuate the antigen-specific immunologic reaction.

The disease is mediated primarily through CD4+ T helper cells and cells derived from mononuclear phagocytes.[14] These cells accumulate within affected tissue, where they organize into noncaseating granulomas.[1,2,15] The earliest manifestation of sarcoidosis is a mononuclear infiltration of the target organ, thought to be mediated primarily by CD4+ T lymphocytes and a host of other inflammatory cells (e.g., macrophages, mast cells, fibroblasts), as well as epithelial and endothelial cells, which promotes the nonspecific inflammatory response and leads to increased tissue permeability and cell migration. Mononuclear cell recruitment is enhanced by the production of chemokines, as well as adhesion molecules and selectins, which are chemoattractants and promote cell binding.

In the early stages of disease, an elevated lymphocyte count and a marked increase in the CD4/CD8 T lymphocyte ratio is observed in affected organs, such as the lungs. Antigen presenting cells, such as dendritic cells and macrophages, present antigen to T cells and drive the production of proinflammatory cytokines such as interleukin (IL)-12 and IL-15, resulting in a Th1 pattern of cytokine production, including the release of interferon-γ and IL-2. IL-15 may act synergistically with IL-2 and TNF-α to stimulate further T cell proliferation.

Naive T cells become activated, undergo clonal expansion, and differentiate into effector and central memory T cells. In sarcoidosis, it appears that most T cells have been previously stimulated, likely in regional lymph nodes, and have migrated back to the affected organ. Studies of the T lymphocyte antigen receptor (TCR) repertoire in sarcoidosis demonstrate that the disorder is initiated by an antigen-specific immune response, based on observed oligoclonal expansion of T lymphocyte subsets bearing particular, restricted αβ TCRs. Notably, in patients with Löfgren's syndrome and in those with acute, remitting sarcoidosis, there is a strong association between a lung-restricted expansion of AV2.3 CD4+ T cells and the expression of one of two specific class II major histocompatibility complex (MHC) molecules (HLA-DRB3*0101 and *0301),[16,17] suggesting that the combination of a specific TCR and a particular MHC class II molecule interacts with the putative sarcoidosis antigen to trigger the acute form of disease.

The release of inflammatory cytokines serves to recruit additional peripheral blood monocytes to the affected organ, where they differentiate into exudate macrophages that show enhanced antigen-presenting capacity and release many cytokines, particularly TNF-α and IL-1β. Notably, from a therapeutic perspective, TNF-α upregulates endothelial cell adhesion molecule expression, drives the acute-phase response via IL-6, promotes downstream cytokine release in tissues, and can promote systemic features of disease, including fatigue and altered cognitive function. The net result of cytokine cascade is an amplification loop involving antigen recognition, proinflammatory cytokine release, cell activation, cell recruitment, and granuloma formation.

Progression from granulomatous inflammation to increasing amounts of fibrosis may be a prognostically bad sign in sarcoidosis. Factors leading from granuloma to fibrosis are poorly understood but probably involve changes in local cytokine production toward a Th2 pattern.

Substantial evidence suggests that genetic susceptibility is important to disease development and that multiple genes account for this genetic predisposition. Both German and U.S. genome-wide sibling pair analyses have been performed. In the United States, African Americans with sarcoidosis show linkage on chromosome 1p22, 2p25, 5p15-13, 5q11, 5q35, 9q34, 11p15, and 20q13.[18] Disease is two to four times more common among monozygotic than dizygotic twins. Up to 19% of affected African American

families and 5% of affected white families have more than one member with sarcoidosis.[19] An analysis of nearly 11,000 first-degree relatives and more than 17,000 second-degree relatives of the 706 ACCESS case-control pairs yielded an adjusted familial relative risk of developing sarcoidosis of 4.7 (95% confidence interval 2.3 to 9.7). White cases had a much higher familial relative risk than did African American cases (18.0 versus 2.8; P = .098).[20] The distribution of human leukocyte antigen (HLA) and angiotensin-converting enzyme (ACE) polymorphic alleles in German families suggests an excess of specific alleles among affected first-degree relatives.[21-23] Further analysis of ACE gene polymorphisms in a population study found differences between the natural history of disease (acute versus chronic) and presentation (Löfgren's syndrome versus non-Löfgren's).[24] Interestingly, Biller and colleagues[25] provided evidence that the ACE genotype should be taken into account when examining the clinical significance of sarcoidosis patients' ACE activity levels in serum.

Using a candidate gene approach, and based on our understanding of immune mechanisms, both case-control studies and microsatellite linkage analysis in familial sarcoidosis strongly support the existence of a susceptibility locus for sarcoidosis on chromosome 6 in the HLA region. Studies of Löfgren's syndrome and other acute, resolving forms of sarcoidosis in Sweden, Holland, and England have largely elucidated the genetic basis of this particular clinical phenotype. HLA-DR17 (DRB1*03) was found nearly four times as often in patients with these forms of disease as in normal controls.[26] In a large population of British and Dutch cases and controls, HLA-DQB1*0201 was strongly associated with reversible disease.[27] A more recent Polish study showed a combined effect of HLA-DRB1*03 and interferon-γ 3,3 homozygosity in increasing the risk of Löfgren's syndrome, suggesting a complex gene-gene interaction.[28] Within racial groups, HLA-DRB1*1101 is a significant susceptibility risk factor for both black and white Americans, with population-attributable risks of 16% and 9%, respectively. However, different clinical patterns, such as specific organ involvement[29] and chronic, severe disease, are also associated with particular genetic patterns in HLA.[30] In patients with small fiber neuropathy, there is an association with HLA-DQB1 alleles.[31]

Investigation of other genes in the MHC region has yielded significant associations with antigen transporter protein TAP1 and 2 polymorphisms and with polymorphic alleles in the TNF-α gene promoter.[32] Recently, a variant of the butyrophilin-like 2 (BTNL2) gene, which resides in the MHC class II region and probably encodes for a protein that functions as a T cell costimulatory molecule, has been associated with sarcoidosis susceptibility in both Caucasian German and U.S. populations. Haplotypes for this gene show a significantly weaker association with sarcoidosis risk in African Americans.[33,34] Other candidate gene studies have yielded negative or confounding results, with a few notable exceptions. Various C-C chemokine receptor genes are of particular interest, because studies in three distinct populations (Japanese, Czech, and Dutch) identified both strong positive and negative associations between specific polymorphic alleles and sarcoidosis. In one study, a particular haplotype of the C-C chemokine receptor A was strongly associated with Löfgren's syndrome, even after adjusting for other known risk factors for this sarcoidosis variant, such as HLA haplotype and female sex.[35] However, data from a recent family-based study suggest that the gene of interest might not be the C-C chemokine receptor itself but rather other genes in the surrounding area.[36]

CLINICAL FEATURES

The clinical presentation of sarcoidosis is diverse, ranging from asymptomatic disease captured on an incidental chest radiograph to acute febrile illness to chronic insidious organ failure. Although the disease appears typically between the ages of 20 and 50 years, both childhood and geriatric cases occur with some regularity. The vast majority of patients (>90%) have evidence of pulmonary involvement. However, sarcoidosis can affect any organ and thus can present with symptoms referable to any organ. Some patients present with nonspecific but debilitating symptoms, including fatigue, fever, anorexia, and weight loss.

A distinct subgroup of sarcoidosis patients is characterized by an acute presentation, classically with Löfgren's syndrome. This presentation consists of acute erythema nodosum or other skin lesions, such as vesicles or maculopapular rash; bilateral hilar lymphadenopathy; uveitis; fever; and polyarthritis. Acute iritis, conjunctivitis, and even conjunctival nodules are common. Bell's palsy may occur prior to or concomitant with the acute symptoms. In a study of 55 patients with acute sarcoidosis arthritis, Visser and colleagues[17] found that four clinical features—symmetric ankle arthritis, symptoms for less than 2 months, age younger than 40 years, and erythema nodosum—provided a high degree of diagnostic certainty in an outpatient rheumatology practice in the Netherlands. In acute disease, bone cysts are rare; however, hypercalcemia and hypercalciuria may be found in approximately 20% of patients. Chest radiographs are typically normal or show significant hilar and mediastinal lymphadenopathy without pulmonary infiltrates. Arrhythmias may occur due to acute granulomatous cardiac involvement. The acute form of disease has a higher probability of spontaneous resolution. Although relapse may occur, it is thought to be less common than in those patients with a more chronic presentation. Prognosis is generally good.

Although a true dividing line between chronic and acute forms of the disease does not exist, certain features of sarcoidosis enhance the likelihood that the disease will persist. Chronic disease is usually insidious in onset and occurs in older patients. Skin lesions in chronic disease are more typically plaques, keloids, nodules within surgical incision lines and scars, or lupus pernio, which is a persistent, disfiguring, violaceous rash over the nose, cheeks, and ears. Chronic eye involvement includes chronic uveitis, cataracts, glaucoma, or keratoconjunctivitis sicca, which can be confused with Sjögren's syndrome. Bone involvement is much more common in chronic than acute cases, as are pulmonary infiltrates, nephrocalcinosis, and cardiac involvement with cor pulmonale. Persistence of disease and recurrence after treatment are common in the chronic form. The remainder of this section focuses specifically on the rheumatologic manifestations of sarcoidosis.

BONE

Sarcoidal changes in bone are most commonly found in the hands or feet. Bone lesions are reported in approximately 3% to 13% of cases. This is likely an underestimation because osseous lesions are typically asymptomatic, and imaging procedures not performed routinely.[37] There is a higher prevalence of radiographically evident osseous disease in the progressive, chronic form of sarcoidosis; in patients with pulmonary involvement; among African American patients; and in those who have granulomatous skin lesions, especially lupus pernio. Asymptomatic bone cysts are more common in females and in patients with lupus pernio.[38] Bone involvement is usually bilateral and asymptomatic; however, it may present as localized pain, swelling, and stiffness. Lesions are most commonly lytic, sometimes with associated expansion of the shaft, pathologic fractures, and cavitation. Lesions also may be sclerotic, starting with progressive cortical tunneling and remodeling, and they are sometimes associated with rapid destruction, periosteal reaction, and secondary involvement of joint surfaces.[39,40] Involvement of the metacarpals, metatarsals, and phalanges of the hands and feet are typical, although any bone can be affected; case reports and case series have described vertebral, iliac, scapular, and even skull sarcoidosis.[37,41-47]

The classic lacy, reticular (lytic) radiographic appearance of sarcoidosis usually produces little disturbance of adjacent soft tissues, although subchondral lesions sometimes extend into the joint space.[37] Figure 107-2 illustrates the range of radiographic findings in osseous sarcoidosis, from early disease to the more typical abnormalities found in untreated, advanced disease. Bone cysts have also been observed, sometimes large enough to result in pathologic fractures.[40] Periostitis is rare. Recent reports suggest that bone scans using either technetium 99m methylene diphosphonate or gallium 67 citrate may detect bone changes not seen on plain radiographic films. However, abnormalities on these scans are not specific for sarcoidosis and may represent other pathology, even in a patient with biopsy-proven sarcoidosis elsewhere.[48,49] Magnetic resonance imaging (MRI) is more sensitive than plain radiographs for the detection of osseous sarcoidosis. On MRI, the lesions may appear hypointense on T1-weighted images and hyperintense on T2-weighted images.[50] Scintigraphy may be superior in detecting multiple bone involvement or osteonecrosis associated with glucocorticoid therapy. MRI offers the greater precision needed if biopsies are to be performed or if osteonecrosis is suspected.[51] When diagnostic biopsies are performed, they can demonstrate noncaseating granulomas in both the bone marrow and the bone cortex.[40]

Sarcoid dactylitis is characterized by diffuse soft tissue swelling of the affected digit; when the terminal phalanx is involved, the proximal nail becomes distorted, thickened, and dystrophic. Dactylitis is often associated with painful stiffness of the adjacent joints and tenderness. The overlying skin may be erythematous. There is marked angular deformity or ankylosis due to bone loss or joint damage in severe cases. Bone involvement may also be associated with tenosynovitis, as has been reported in several cases involving the wrists.[52-54] Osteopenia and osteoporosis occur in up to two thirds of patients with sarcoidosis, partly as a consequence of dysregulated calcium metabolism.[55,56] Case series data support the existence of bone loss in untreated sarcoidosis; some authors suggest that this occurs independent of dysregulated calcium and vitamin D metabolism and is instead related to osteoclast activation by granulomas.[40]

Because of the common use of corticosteroids to treat the disease, patients are also at risk for glucocorticoid-related bone loss. This is particularly true of postmenopausal women, whose loss of bone mineral density is significantly greater than that of other sarcoidosis patients on prednisone therapy.[57] Although there is no standardized approach to the management of this problem in sarcoidosis, a few small studies have attempted to address the issue. One trial randomized 30 sarcoidosis patients who were being started on prednisone therapy to receive either alendronate or placebo. After 1 year of follow-up, the alendronate group demonstrated a slight increase in bone mineral density, whereas the placebo group demonstrated a statistically significant decrease (4.5%) in bone mineral density.[58] In a nonrandomized study, a group of glucocorticoid-treated sarcoidosis patients was followed, and a subset was treated with salmon calcitonin for 15 months. This additional

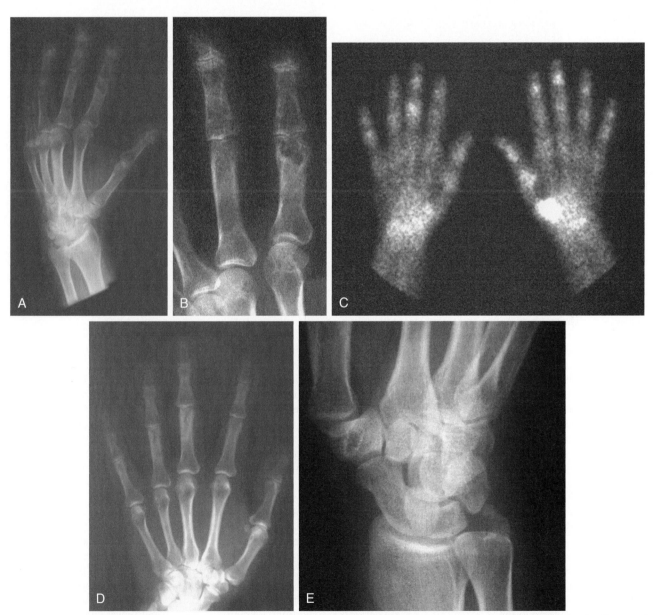

Figure 107-2   A, This plain film demonstrates multiple areas of radiolucency, including cystic changes in the small finger metacarpal and proximal phalanx and the index finger proximal and middle phalanges. A destructive process can also be seen in the ulnar styloid, whereas the joint space is well maintained. **B,** A closer view of the same hand reveals large cystic lesions involving the subchondral bone adjacent to the proximal interphalangeal joint of the index finger. Similar lesions involve the middle phalanx of the long finger, with a reticular pattern of radiolucency. Unrelated osteoarthritis changes can be noted at the proximal and distal interphalangeal joints. **C,** This bone scan demonstrates increased uptake of technetium 99m methylene diphosphonate in the left long finger proximal to the interphalangeal joint region. This corresponds to a subtle lesion visible on the plain film (see **D**). **D,** The subtle lesion is seen as an increase in radiolucency in the distal portion of the long finger proximal phalanx, as well as associated fusiform soft tissue swelling. **E,** This plain film demonstrates an unusual destructive lesion at the ulnar styloid and a sharply demarcated cyst in the trapezium in a patient with sarcoidosis arthritis.

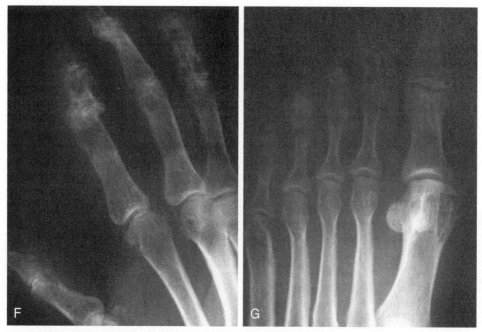

Figure 107-2 Cont'd **F,** This radiograph highlights advanced destructive sarcoidosis arthritis involving all the proximal and distal interphalangeal joints. A cystic lesion is present in the head of the long finger metacarpal bone, and a destructive lesion can be noted in the head of the index finger metacarpal bone, with preservation of the joint space. **G,** In this study, a cystic region of radiolucency with a reticular pattern on the head of the metatarsal bone of the great toe is associated with destruction of the cortical margin. It is important to note the absence of periarticular osteopenia or uniform joint space loss, which would be observed in rheumatoid arthritis.

treatment resulted in significant benefit in terms of maintenance of bone mineral density. The efficacy of salmon calcitonin is supported by at least one other nonrandomized trial.[59,60] In practice, most sarcoidosis clinics apply the same primary and secondary treatment strategies advocated for the management of other patients with glucocorticoid-induced osteoporosis. However, it is particularly important to monitor serum and urinary calcium levels more frequently when introducing therapy with cholecalciferol or bisphosphonates. Calcitriol should be avoided owing to the risk of inducing hypercalcemia in sarcoidosis patients receiving corticosteroids, especially because pretreatment serum calcitriol levels are usually elevated in this disease.

JOINT

Sarcoidal joint involvement produces symmetric arthralgia or arthritis, often with accompanying erythema nodosum. Sarcoidosis most commonly affects the larger joints (ankles, knees, wrists, elbows), although any joint can be involved. Joint pain and stiffness may be the presenting symptoms of the disease. In the acute form of disease presentation, the arthropathy is symmetric, peripheral, and most often associated with erythema nodosum. The majority of these patients report bilateral ankle arthralgias.[17] Within a few weeks to a few months, the arthralgias tend to subside, without recurrence or joint deformity. If the joint disease persists, it can result in joint destruction. In such cases, the arthritis is usually accompanied by chronic skin lesions. Arthralgias without erythema nodosum are more common in white males with hilar adenopathy, whereas arthralgias associated with

erythema nodosum are more frequent in women. Chronic polyarthritis without involvement of the adjacent bone has been reported mostly in African American patients. The prevalence of spondyloarthropathy in sarcoidosis patients is estimated at 6.6%,[61] with a number of cases well described in the literature.[62,63]

Acute sarcoid arthritis is diagnosed mainly on clinical grounds. When performed, synovial fluid analysis typically demonstrates a sterile lymphocytosis and elevated protein.[40] Synovial biopsies of involved joints tend to be indeterminate, demonstrating a mild inflammatory synovitis, but often without granulomas.[64-66] Chronic destructive joint disease occurs in a minority of patients. It is often associated with other manifestations of more severe disease, such as lupus pernio and chronic uveitis.[40] Synovial biopsies in this form of arthritis show inflammatory infiltrates of lymphocytes and plasma cells, proliferation of fibroblasts, and noncaseating granulomas.[40]

Löfgren's syndrome, or acute erythema nodosum with bilateral hilar lymphadenopathy, may be accompanied by fever, arthralgias or arthritis, anterior uveitis, and lung involvement. In a retrospective review of 187 cases, Mana and colleagues[67] reported a significant seasonal clustering in spring and winter for erythema nodosum and Löfgren's syndrome. Asymptomatic myopathy was common. This disease was self-limited in most cases. In a review of sequential clinical cases of erythema nodosum, Garcia-Porrua and coworkers[68] found that approximately one third were due to sarcoidosis. They emphasize that other causes must be excluded, including nonstreptococcal upper respiratory tract infection and pharmaceutical use, particularly oral contraceptives.

MUSCLE

Muscle involvement is usually subclinical. Symptomatic muscle involvement occurs in less than 0.5% of cases.[40] When it does occur, it is often in concert with osseous disease. In systemic sarcoidosis without clinical manifestations of muscle disease, 50% to 80% of patients are found to have granulomas on muscle biopsy. Gastrocnemius muscle biopsy has been evaluated as a diagnostic tool in patients presenting with hilar adenopathy but no muscle symptoms. In one series of 22 patients, this procedure was 100% sensitive and specific for diagnosing sarcoidosis.[69] Other studies have found that muscle biopsy is not useful in asymptomatic patients, and it is not routinely performed to establish a diagnosis in this patient population.[40]

When clinically evident, sarcoidosis muscle involvement takes one of three major forms: chronic myopathy, nodular, and granulomatous myositis. The most common form is a chronic, progressive myopathy of gradual onset. It is associated with proximal muscle wasting in the extremities, trunk, and neck. It must be distinguished from glucocorticoid-induced myopathy. Of note, cardiac muscle involvement is often found concurrently with this form of sarcoid muscle disease.[40] Electromyography is often normal, but it can sometimes help distinguish between myopathic and neuropathic disorders.

The nodular form of muscular sarcoidosis is the next most common form and may present as small nodules or as a frank soft tissue mass, which is often mistaken for a soft tissue neoplasm.[70] Some characteristic findings of this presentation on MRI include the "dark star" sign on axial images, which consists of a star-shaped central structure of decreased signal intensity, and the "three stripes" sign seen on coronal and sagittal images, which consists of an inner stripe of decreased signal intensity and outer stripes of increased signal intensity. Gallium 67 scanning can sometimes help distinguish between a sarcoidosis nodule (significantly greater uptake) and a soft tissue mass.[40]

The rarest form of muscle involvement is granulomatous myositis, which typically presents with an acute to subacute onset of proximal muscle weakness, muscle pain or tenderness, and weight loss. The majority of these patients are female and African American, have an elevated creatine phosphokinase level and erythrocyte sedimentation rate, and demonstrate a myopathic pattern on electromyography.[40] Even rarer clinical presentations include respiratory muscle weakness and painful ophthalmoplegia due to enlargement of the extraocular muscles.[71-73]

The diagnosis of myositis or myopathy may be suggested by MRI and gallium or technetium scanning; however, the increased uptake during scintigraphy is nonspecific.[74] As noted previously, MRI findings may be more characteristic in the nodular form of the disease. The "gold standard" for diagnosis in all forms of muscle involvement is muscle biopsy. Biopsies may demonstrate typical noncaseating granulomas, muscle fiber degeneration and regeneration, perivascular inflammation, and occasional vasculitis. Neurogenic atrophy and granulomatous infiltration of nerves are also common in sarcoidal myositis.[75] Fine-needle aspiration biopsies can be strongly suggestive of the diagnosis, demonstrating multinucleated giant cells, epithelioid histiocytes, or both.[70,76] MRI of sarcoidosis patients with musculoskeletal symptoms shows nonspecific marrow and soft tissue lesions that often go undetected on plain radiographs.[77] Myelopathy, cranial neuropathies, and encephalopathy may also be detected more readily on MRI.

VASCULITIS

Systemic vasculitis is a rare but serious form of sarcoidal involvement. Either large or small vessels may be affected in virtually any organ. Biopsies may demonstrate vasculitis associated with noncaseating granulomas[78] (see Fig. 107-1C) or frank necrotizing sarcoidal granulomas. Although the relationship between sarcoidosis and vasculitis is unclear in some cases, associations have been reported between sarcoidosis and such diverse vasculitic processes as Takayasu's arteritis,[79,80] hypersensitivity vasculitis, polyarteritis nodosa, microscopic polyangiitis,[81] and Churg-Strauss syndrome.[82] Significant morbidity and relapse despite corticosteroid therapy are common. Discovery of vasculitis in one organ generally implies involvement elsewhere.

DIAGNOSIS AND DIAGNOSTIC TESTS

Diagnosis of sarcoidosis is a two-step process: (1) identifying clinical and pathologic features consistent with the disease, and (2) excluding other conditions that have clinical overlap. Diagnostic considerations for pulmonary granulomatous inflammation include infections with mycobacteria, bacteria, fungi, spirochetes, and protozoa (Table 107-1). Diseases caused by occupational and environmental inhaled agents must also be considered, including hypersensitivity pneumonitis due to inhaled organic and inorganic antigens and metal-induced disorders such as chronic beryllium disease[83] and silicosis.[84] Tissue biopsy is recommended to diagnose multiorgan sarcoidosis, depending on the clinical presentation.[85] Neoplasms can be associated with granulomatous inflammation. Local sarcoidal reactions can occur, especially in skin, but they are not associated with systemic symptoms and lack multiorgan distribution.[1,2]

Sarcoidosis must be distinguished from inflammatory conditions of unknown cause, especially the autoimmune disorders, as discussed later. Sarcoidosis has been associated with the elevation of various autoantibodies in serum, including nonspecific elevations of rheumatoid factor and antinuclear antibody (ANA). In a recent retrospective study of 34 patients with sarcoidosis, ANA positivity was observed in one third of patients, two of whom had antibodies to double-stranded DNA. None of these antibody-positive patients developed systemic lupus erythematosus during the 10- to 15-year follow-up.[86] Several researchers have suggested an association between autoimmune endocrinopathies and sarcoidosis. One series demonstrated significantly higher levels of antibodies against thyroid peroxidase and purified thyroglobulin, as well as Hashimoto's thyroiditis, in sarcoidosis patients compared with diseased and nondiseased controls.[87] Similarly, in another series of 78 sarcoidosis patients, nearly 20% had evidence of autoimmune endocrine disease such as polyglandular autoimmune syndromes, Graves' disease, and autoimmune thyroiditis.[88] Finally, a Japanese group found an association between antiphospholipid antibodies and sarcoidosis, with 21 of 55 sarcoidosis patients having either immunoglobulin (Ig) G or IgM antiphospholipid antibodies. The antibody-positive subset was found to have significantly more

Table 107-1 Differential Diagnosis of Granulomatous Disease

Cause	Disease Examples
Infectious agents	
Mycobacteria	Tuberculosis, atypical mycobacterial infections
Fungi	Histoplasmosis, coccidioidomycosis
Bacteria	Brucellosis
Spirochetes	Syphilis
Metazoa	Schistosomiasis
Parasites	Leishmaniasis, toxoplasmosis
Neoplasms	Carcinoma, sarcoma, malignant nasal granuloma
Hypersensitivity pneumonitis	Farmer's lung, bird fancier's lung, suberosis, bagassosis
Metals	Chronic beryllium disease, zirconium granuloma, aluminum granuloma
Silicates	Silicosis with granulomatous inflammation
Vasculitic granulomatoses and autoimmune disorders	Wegener's granulomatosis, Churg-Strauss, lymphomatoid granulomatosis, polyarteritis nodosa, bronchocentric granulomatosis, systemic lupus erythematosus, primary biliary cirrhosis, juvenile rheumatoid arthritis
Other conditions	Chronic granulomatous disease (children), Whipple's disease, lymphocytic infiltration after cancer chemotherapy, Blau's syndrome, local sarcoidal reactions

Table 107-2 Recommended Baseline and Follow-up Clinical Evaluation for Sarcoidosis

Baseline

Occupational and environmental history
Medication history
Examination emphasizing lungs, lymphatics, skin, eyes, liver, heart, joints
Biopsy of an affected organ, with special stains and cultures
Chest radiography
Pulmonary function tests, including gas exchange
Electrocardiogram
Slit-lamp examination
Liver function tests, renal function tests
Serum calcium
24-hour urinary calcium excretion
Other tests, depending on clinical presentation and organ systems involved

Follow-up

Monitoring for resolution or progression.
Tracking of organs previously involved using least invasive method.
Monitoring for new involvement of common disease target organs.

expected major organs targeted by sarcoidosis. Other tests may be appropriate, depending on which other organs are affected.

As a general principle, because there is no single specific diagnostic test for sarcoidosis, the diagnosis depends on establishing the compatible clinicopathologic picture and excluding other granulomatous diseases. Ideally, the evaluation should provide histologic confirmation of disease and negative cultures and special stains for organisms.

The clinical impact of sarcoidosis depends on the extent of granulomatous inflammation and the particular organs affected. In determining the extent and severity of disease, clinicians should use noninvasive tools whenever possible to assess which organs are clinically involved and to assess the extent and severity of organ injury. Asymptomatic organ involvement may be missed, but it is usually of little or no clinical significance, with two significant exceptions. A slit-lamp examination is recommended for all patients with suspected sarcoidosis, to look for clinically undetected uveitis. Subclinical hypercalciuria, even in the absence of hypercalcemia, is associated with nephrolithiasis; therefore, a baseline 24-hour urine calcium measurement is advisable. Additionally, periodic electrocardiograms should be obtained to screen for rare but potentially life-threatening cardiac arrhythmias and conduction abnormalities.

A baseline complete blood count is recommended to evaluate for anemia, leukopenia, and thrombocytopenia. Serum calcium and liver enzymes may reflect organ involvement meriting treatment. Serum ACE activity is frequently elevated in sarcoidosis. It is not specific but can be useful to monitor disease progression and response to therapy. As discussed earlier, in the future, ACE activity may be more useful when interpreted in the context of a person's ACE genotype. Tests for cutaneous anergy may suggest a diagnosis of sarcoidosis and help rule out tuberculosis, but the anergy panel is neither sensitive nor specific.

In patients who present with arthritic or bone symptoms, a chest radiograph or, in some cases, a high-resolution computed tomography scan of the thorax can detect evidence of hilar or mediastinal lymphadenopathy. In the proper clinical

extrathoracic organ involvement and a longer persistence of abnormal chest radiographs.[89]

The putative link between sarcoidosis and autoimmunity is supported by cases of concurrent diagnoses, as well as by some of the obvious similarities between sarcoidosis and the autoimmune diseases. Although sarcoidosis is rare in children, when it does occur in preschool children, it may mimic the manifestations of juvenile rheumatoid arthritis, with skin, eye, and joint involvement without lung disease. Distinction between the two entities usually requires biopsy of skin, synovium, lymph node, or liver.[90-93] In contrast, the clinical presentations of rheumatoid arthritis and sarcoidosis in adults are quite distinct. Interestingly, the coexistence of the two diseases, with biopsy verification of both, has been demonstrated in numerous case reports, suggesting a possible etiologic similarity.[94-97] Sjögren's syndrome also occurs concurrently with or is difficult to distinguish from sarcoidosis, particularly when there is lung involvement. Both diseases can present with keratoconjunctivitis sicca, parotid swelling, lung involvement, and cutaneous anergy. Some authors suggest that labial minor salivary gland biopsy or lung biopsy can distinguish between the two diseases, but even biopsy findings are sometimes inconclusive.[98-104]

Table 107-2 summarizes the recommended baseline and follow-up tests used in the evaluation and management of sarcoidosis.[1] These recommendations are based on the setting, this can help make the diagnosis of sarcoidosis and also point to a logical site for biopsy, because the majority of patients with hilar adenopathy are found to have pulmonary granulomas when transbronchial lung biopsies are performed by bronchoscopy.

Kveim-Siltzbach skin testing—using a preparation of sarcoidosis spleen that is intradermally injected—has been used in the past to establish a diagnosis of sarcoidosis in patients with unexplained erythema nodosum, uveitis, liver granulomas, or hypercalciuria. However, this is not approved for general use in the United States and is not recommended.

Gallium 67 citrate scanning adds no specificity to the diagnosis of sarcoidosis, except in the case of patients with lacrimal and salivary gland involvement, in which case the so-called panda sign is observed due to increased uptake in those sites.[105]

Monitoring for disease progress, regression, or response to therapy should be customized, relying on the least invasive markers of disease activity and vital organ involvement. The clinician must remain vigilant, given the tendency of this disorder to relapse and emerge in new organs.

TREATMENT

In the majority of patients with sarcoidosis, the disease resolves spontaneously. However, the natural history and prognosis of sarcoidosis are highly variable. It is not known why some sarcoidosis patients recover and others progress, although some clues are coming from the emerging genetics literature discussed earlier. Although general rules can be applied, there are many exceptions. Acute-onset sarcoidosis is more likely to resolve spontaneously than is chronic, insidious disease. The presence of multiorgan involvement at the time of initial presentation portends a more protracted and clinically severe illness. Even after apparent recovery, a proportion of patients may relapse months or years later. Factors associated with worse prognosis include older age at diagnosis, African American race, duration of illness longer than 6 months, pulmonary infiltrates, splenomegaly, lupus pernio, and greater number of organs involved. A more favorable prognosis has been found in patients with acute disease who expressed HLA-DR3 and -DQ2, regardless of whether erythema nodosum was present.[17,106,107]

Because sarcoidosis can resolve spontaneously without treatment, most treatment protocols incorporate a period of observation whenever possible. A detailed summary of current pharmacotherapy in sarcoidosis has been the subject of several recent reviews.[8,108,109] This section addresses the general treatment of sarcoidosis, with an emphasis on rheumatologic manifestations when data are available. Oral corticosteroids remain the first-line therapy in most cases; however, there is no consensus about when corticosteroids should be initiated.[109] Further, there is evidence that corticosteroids may actually be detrimental in some cases. Their use is aimed at the relief of symptoms and the modulation of disease activity in vital organs. It is debatable whether all these goals can be achieved, especially in light of corticosteroid side effects. In a synthesis of data from eight randomized trials of oral or inhaled corticosteroids in pulmonary sarcoidosis that included control groups, Paramothayan and Jones[109] concluded that oral corticosteroids improved chest radiographs after 6 to 24 months of treatment and produced

a small improvement in lung function and gas exchange. They found no evidence of sustained improvement after the withdrawal of corticosteroids.[109] Only two of the eight trials examined the efficacy of inhaled corticosteroid therapy. In these trials, there was no effect on chest radiograph abnormalities, no consistent effects on lung function, and only a small improvement in symptoms in one of the studies. In another review, Reich[110] suggested that patients with a recent diagnosis of stage II or III sarcoidosis might experience more long-term harm than benefit from systemic steroids; that the effect on those with disease of intermediate duration is neutral; and that patients with chronic, progressive pulmonary disease respond favorably, at least in the intermediate term.[111-115] A review of oral corticosteroid use in sarcoidosis patients in Japanese hospitals reported that eye involvement, followed by lung and heart involvement, was the main reason for steroid treatment. Doses ranged from 30 to 60 mg/day. Approximately 70% to 80% of those treated responded well to oral corticosteroids in an unblinded case series.[116]

The ATS-ERS-WASOG consensus statement suggests that patients with acute pulmonary sarcoidosis should not be treated. The lack of randomized, controlled clinical trials, especially for all the various forms of organ involvement, limits the conclusions that can be drawn. Studies examining outcomes at greater than 2 years suggest no significant benefit from corticosteroid therapy in asymptomatic sarcoidosis patients with more advanced forms of pulmonary involvement. In a British Thoracic Society study,[117] patients not meeting the criteria for immediate therapy were observed for 6 months. At that point, participants were assigned to receive either long-term corticosteroid therapy or corticosteroids based on symptoms. After 2 years, the long-term therapy group showed modest improvements in pulmonary function compared with the symptom-based treatment group. Based on the available literature and a survey of clinical practice in the United States and abroad, it is our general recommendation that corticosteroids should not be initiated until after a period of clinical observation, unless there is a life- or sight-threatening reason to treat, such as cardiac, neurologic, or eye disease that failed topical therapy. There is no consensus regarding the optimal initial dosage of corticosteroids. The ATS consensus statement suggests a starting dose of 20 to 40 mg of prednisone or its equivalent, either daily or on alternate days. The British Thoracic Society similarly used prednisolone 30 mg/day as a starting dose. After an initial period of treatment lasting approximately 8 to 18 weeks, those who objectively improve on corticosteroids can start tapering to as low a dose as tolerated without a return of symptoms or organ dysfunction, usually 5 to 10 mg daily or on alternate days. The ATS statement recommends that for those who respond to steroids, treatment should be continued for at least 1 year. If intolerable side effects occur or if the disease does not respond to steroid therapy, patients are considered candidates for the addition of a second-line immunosuppressive agent. If patients suffer relapse on maintenance therapy, there are many options, none of which has been substantiated by rigorous clinical research. In many practices, such patients are placed back on higher-dose prednisone, and a second-line agent is considered. Patients who have evidence of a clinical response to corticosteroids are reevaluated using objective measures before attempts to completely withdraw immunosuppressive medication. Even patients who are believed to have entered remission should be followed periodically, given the tendency for sarcoidosis to relapse. The use of other immunosuppressive agents in sarcoidosis should be reserved for those patients who experience symptomatic disease progression despite the use of systemic corticosteroids or who require therapy but cannot tolerate steroid side effects.

Methotrexate (MTX) has emerged as one of the preferred second-line drugs. One randomized clinical trial of MTX in sarcoidosis indicated steroid-sparing benefits.[118] The largest published experience comes from Lower and Baughman,[119] who reported improvement in 33 of 50 patients treated with MTX for a minimum of 2 years. A follow-up report of 209 patients showed that 52% on MTX entered remission and 16% remained stable, with or without low-dose prednisone.[120] Other reports confirm the beneficial effects of MTX in cutaneous and musculoskeletal sarcoidosis.[121,122] In a study by Kaye and colleagues,[121] low-dose MTX (average 10 mg/wk; range, 7.5 to 15 mg) used for an average of 30 months controlled clinical symptoms in patients with musculoskeletal involvement and helped reduce the corticosteroid dose. In most studies, treatment doses of MTX range from 5 to 15 mg/week, usually taken as a single or divided oral dose one day per week. MTX may take up to 6 months to become fully effective in sarcoidosis. During this period, patients are usually maintained on corticosteroids.

Case reports on the benefits of cyclosporine A in sarcoidosis have not been supported by larger cohort studies.[123-125] The first study to examine cyclosporine in a more rigorous fashion found that when administered at doses that achieved blood levels between 150 and 250 ng/mL, cyclosporine failed to produce clinical improvement in 20 patients who had pulmonary involvement, despite 6 months of therapy.[124] Cyclosporine was undetectable in bronchoalveolar lavage fluid, suggesting poor penetration into the lung as a possible reason for its failure. A more recent study, using a standardized treatment protocol, found the combination of prednisone and cyclosporine to be no better and possibly worse than prednisone alone in treating pulmonary sarcoidosis.[125]

Azathioprine may be an effective second-line agent in a subset of sarcoidosis patients. It is frequently used in titrated oral doses up to 100 to 150 mg/day, despite a paucity of published studies examining the drug's efficacy in sarcoidosis.[126] Some data suggest that it may be efficacious for extrapulmonary disease. Two more recent case series evaluated combined therapy with azathioprine and corticosteroids in patients with chronic pulmonary sarcoidosis. A retrospective review of 10 patients demonstrated sustained improvement in lung function in only 2 patients, but a prospective evaluation of 11 patients demonstrated symptomatic relief and improvement in lung physiology and radiographic abnormalities in 9 after an average of 20 months of therapy. Thus, azathioprine may be an effective second-line agent in a subset of sarcoidosis patients.[127,128]

Chloroquine has proved effective in treating cutaneous manifestations of sarcoidosis,[129] hypercalcemia and hypercalciuria associated with sarcoidosis, and steroid-refractory neurosarcoidosis.[130,131] Generally, chloroquine therapy is initiated at a dosage of 500 mg/day and may be titrated up to a maximum of 1000 mg/day and decreased to a low of 250 mg/day. Hydroxychloroquine may be used instead, at a dosage

of 200 to 400 mg/day, because of the lower risk of ophthalmic toxicity. In one study of chronic pulmonary sarcoidosis, after an average of 19.7 months of treatment, subjects who received maintenance therapy with low-dose (250 mg/day) chloroquine demonstrated a significantly slower decline in lung function and a trend toward fewer relapses compared with those who were simply observed.

Cyclophosphamide is employed in selected cases of corticosteroid-refractory sarcoidosis.[132,133] It appears to be beneficial for both cardiac and neurosarcoidosis. Oral cyclophosphamide is given at a dose of 1 to 2 mg/kg per day, up to a maximum dose of 150 mg/day. Therapy is maintained for several months before tapering. Intravenous monthly pulse cyclophosphamide has been used for the treatment of neurosarcoidosis at a dosage of 0.75 to 1.5 g/month.[133]

Based on our present understanding of cytokine expression in sarcoidosis, it is logical to expect that anti–TNF-α therapies such as etanercept, infliximab, and adalimumab, and surrogates for this mode of action such as thalidomide and pentoxifylline, should be effective. There are individual published cases and small case series supporting the use of thalidomide in patients with cutaneous sarcoidosis, including lupus pernio.[134-138] High doses of pentoxifylline improved lung function in a group of patients with mild pulmonary sarcoidosis.[139] A prospective, open-label study with etanercept was terminated before full enrollment owing to excessive treatment failures; however, design flaws limit the extent to which conclusions can be drawn. Case reports and case series support the use of infliximab in the treatment of lupus pernio, neurosarcoidosis, and progressive cutaneous sarcoidosis.[140-142] Results of a recent major clinical trial demonstrated that at 24 weeks, patients with chronic, steroid-treated pulmonary sarcoidosis who received infliximab showed a small but statistically significant improvement in forced vital capacity compared with those who received placebo. A more sizable improvement was seen in the subgroup of patients who entered the study with more severe pulmonary impairment. No differences in the frequency of adverse events were seen between placebo-treated and infliximab-treated subjects at week 24. In light of these studies, infliximab has joined the armamentarium of second-line treatments for patients with refractory, debilitating, or life-threatening sarcoidosis, but it must be recognized that the benefit for mild or moderate pulmonary involvement may be small.[143] Tuberculosis should be carefully excluded in these patients before and during treatment, although it is a rare complication. Combined regimens are increasingly being used to treat sarcoidosis, although there have been few trials. Most of these regimens include corticosteroids and one or more second-line agents.

Future Directions

Larger, better-controlled studies of diagnostic tests used in the detection of musculoskeletal sarcoidosis are needed.

Attention must be paid to the clinical subtypes of sarcoidosis when applying current literature to the treatment of patients.

Controlled clinical trials that examine nonpulmonary outcomes in patients with extrathoracic sarcoidosis are needed.

SUMMARY

Sarcoidosis should be considered in any patient presenting with systemic and multiorgan symptoms or whenever granulomatous inflammation is discovered on histology. Therapeutic advances based on an understanding of immune mechanisms will likely improve our approaches to the medical management of this enigmatic condition.

REFERENCES

1. **Newman LS, Rose CS, Maier LA: Sarcoidosis. N Engl J Med 336: 1224-1234, 1997.**
2. **Statement on sarcoidosis. Joint statement of the American Thoracic Society (ATS), the European Respiratory Society (ERS) and the World Association of Sarcoidosis and Other Granulomatous Disorders (WASOG) adopted by the ATS Board of Directors and by the ERS Executive Committee, February 1999. Am J Respir Crit Care Med 160:736-755, 1999.**
3. Baughman RP, et al: Clinical characteristics of patients in a case control study of sarcoidosis. Am J Respir Crit Care Med 164:1885-1889, 2001.
4. Judson MA, et al: Comparison of sarcoidosis phenotypes among affected African-American siblings. Chest 130:855-862, 2006.
5. Barnard J, et al: Job and industry classifications associated with sarcoidosis in a case-control etiologic study of sarcoidosis (ACCESS). J Occup Environ Med 47:226-234, 2005.
6. Drake WP, et al: Molecular analysis of sarcoidosis tissues for mycobacterium species DNA. Emerg Infect Dis 8:1334-1341, 2002.
7. Song Z, et al: Mycobacterial catalase-peroxidase is a tissue antigen and target of the adaptive immune response in systemic sarcoidosis. J Exp Med 201:755-767, 2005.
8. Moller DR: Treatment of sarcoidosis—from a basic science point of view. J Intern Med 253:31-40, 2003.
9. Drake WP, Newman LS: Mycobacterial antigens may be important in sarcoidosis pathogenesis. Curr Opin Pulm Med 12:359-363, 2006.
10. **Newman LS, et al: A case control etiologic study of sarcoidosis: Environmental and occupational risk factors. Am J Respir Crit Care Med 170:1324-1330, 2004.**
11. Kajdasz DK, et al: A current assessment of rurally linked exposures as potential risk factors for sarcoidosis. Ann Epidemiol 11:111-117, 2001.
12. Kreider ME, et al: Relationship of environmental exposures to the clinical phenotype of sarcoidosis. Chest 128:207-215, 2005.
13. Sipahi Demirkok S, et al: Analysis of 87 patients with Lofgren's syndrome and the pattern of seasonality of subacute sarcoidosis. Respirology 11:456-461, 2006.
14. **Hunninghake GW, et al: Inflammatory and immune processes in the human lung in health and disease: Evaluation by bronchoalveolar lavage. Am J Pathol 97:149-206, 1979.**
15. Moller DR, Chen ES: Genetic basis of remitting sarcoidosis: Triumph of the trimolecular complex? Am J Respir Cell Mol Biol 27:391-395, 2002.
16. **Grunewald J, et al: Lung restricted T cell receptor AV2S3+ CD4+ T cell expansions in sarcoidosis patients with a shared HLA-DRbeta chain conformation. Thorax 57:348-352, 2002.**
17. Visser H, et al: Sarcoid arthritis: Clinical characteristics, diagnostic aspects, and risk factors. Ann Rheum Dis 61:499-504, 2002.
18. Iannuzzi MC, et al: Genome-wide search for sarcoidosis susceptibility genes in African Americans. Genes Immun 6:509-518, 2005.
19. Rybicki BA, et al: Genetics of sarcoidosis. Clin Chest Med 18: 707-717, 1997.
20. Rybicki BA, et al: Familial aggregation of sarcoidosis: A case-control etiologic study of sarcoidosis (ACCESS). Am J Respir Crit Care Med 164:2085-2091, 2001.
21. Schurmann M, et al: HLA-DQB1 and HLA-DPB1 genotypes in familial sarcoidosis. Respir Med 92:649-652, 1998.
22. Schurmann M, et al: Familial sarcoidosis is linked to the major histocompatibility complex region. Am J Respir Crit Care Med 162: 861-864, 2000.
23. Schurmann M, et al: Angiotensin-converting enzyme (ACE) gene polymorphisms and familial occurrence of sarcoidosis. J Intern Med 249:77-83, 2001.
24. Alia P, et al: Association between ACE gene I/D polymorphism and clinical presentation and prognosis of sarcoidosis. Scand J Clin Lab Invest 65:691-697, 2005.
25. Biller H, et al: Genotype-corrected reference values for serum angiotensin-converting enzyme. Eur Respir J 28:1085-1091, 2006.
26. Berlin M, et al: HLA-DR predicts the prognosis in Scandinavian patients with pulmonary sarcoidosis. Am J Respir Crit Care Med 156:1601-1605, 1997.
27. Sato H, et al: HLA-DQB1*0201: A marker for good prognosis in British and Dutch patients with sarcoidosis. Am J Respir Cell Mol Biol 27:406-412, 2002.
28. Wysoczanska B, et al: Combined association between IFN-gamma 3,3 homozygosity and DRB1*03 in Lofgren's syndrome patients. Immunol Lett 91:127-131, 2004.
29. Rossman MD, et al: HLA-DRB1*1101: A significant risk factor for sarcoidosis in blacks and whites. Am J Hum Genet 73:720-735, 2003.
30. Pabst S, et al: Toll-like receptor (TLR) 4 polymorphisms are associated with a chronic course of sarcoidosis. Clin Exp Immunol 143:420-426, 2006.
31. Voorter CE, et al: Association of HLA DQB1 0602 in sarcoidosis patients with small fiber neuropathy. Sarcoidosis Vasc Diffuse Lung Dis 22:129-132, 2005.
32. Grutters JC, et al: Increased frequency of the uncommon tumor necrosis factor-857T allele in British and Dutch patients with sarcoidosis. Am J Respir Crit Care Med 165:1119-1124, 2002.
33. Rybicki BA, et al: The BTNL2 gene and sarcoidosis susceptibility in African Americans and whites. Am J Hum Genet 77:491-499, 2005.
34. Valentonyte R, et al: Sarcoidosis is associated with a truncating splice site mutation in BTNL2. Nat Genet 37:357-364, 2005.
35. Spagnolo P, et al: C-C chemokine receptor 2 and sarcoidosis: Association with Lofgren's syndrome. Am J Respir Crit Care Med 168: 1162-1166, 2003.
36. Valentonyte R, et al: Study of C-C chemokine receptor 2 alleles in sarcoidosis, with emphasis on family-based analysis. Am J Respir Crit Care Med 171:1136-1141, 2005.
37. Wilcox A, Bharadwaj P, Sharma OP: Bone sarcoidosis. Curr Opin Rheumatol 12:321-330, 2000.
38. Yanardag H, Pamuk ON: Bone cysts in sarcoidosis: What is their clinical significance? Rheumatol Int 24:294-296, 2004.
39. Atanes A, et al: [The bone manifestations in 94 cases of sarcoidosis]. An Med Interna 8:481-486, 1991.
40. Zisman DA, Shorr AF, Lynch JP 3rd: Sarcoidosis involving the musculoskeletal system. Semin Respir Crit Care Med 23:555-570, 2002.
41. Rua-Figueroa I, et al: Vertebral sarcoidosis: Clinical and imaging findings. Semin Arthritis Rheum 31:346-352, 2002.
42. Cohen NP, et al: Vertebral sarcoidosis of the spine in a football player. Am J Orthop 30:875-877, 2001.
43. Andres E, et al: Iliac bone defects revealing systemic sarcoidosis. Joint Bone Spine 68:74-75, 2001.
44. Sundaram M, et al: Progressive destructive vertebral sarcoid leading to surgical fusion. Skeletal Radiol 28:717-722, 1999.
45. Franco M, et al: Long-term radiographic follow-up in a patient with osteosclerotic sarcoidosis of the spine and pelvis. Rev Rhum Engl Ed 65:586-590, 1998.
46. Finelli DA, et al: Leptomeningeal and calvarial sarcoidosis: CT and MR appearance. J Comput Assist Tomogr 19:639-642, 1995.
47. Marymont JV, Murphy DA: Sarcoidosis of the axial skeleton. Clin Nucl Med 19:1060-1062, 1994.
48. Matsuoka S, et al: Positivity of extrapulmonary Ga-67 uptake in sarcoidosis: Thyroid uptake due to chronic thyroiditis and bone uptake due to fibrous dysplasia. Ann Nucl Med 15:537-539, 2001.
49. Milman N, et al: Diagnostic value of routine radioisotope bone scanning in a series of 63 patients with pulmonary sarcoidosis. Sarcoidosis Vasc Diffuse Lung Dis 17:67-70, 2000.
50. Fisher AJ, et al: MR imaging changes of lumbar vertebral sarcoidosis. AJR Am J Roentgenol 173:354-356, 1999.
51. Shorr AF, et al: Osseous disease in patients with pulmonary sarcoidosis and musculoskeletal symptoms. Respir Med 94:228-232, 2000.
52. Gonzalez del Pino J, et al: Sarcoidosis of the hand and wrist: A report of two cases. J Hand Surg (Am) 22:942-945, 1997.
53. Katzman BM, et al: Sarcoid flexor tenosynovitis of the wrist: A case report. J Hand Surg (Am) 22:336-337, 1997.
54. Larsen TK: Tenosynovitis as initial diagnosis of sarcoidosis: Case report. Scand J Plast Reconstr Surg Hand Surg 30:157-159, 1996.

55. Rizzato G, et al: Multi-element follow up in biological specimens of hard metal pneumoconiosis. Sarcoidosis 9:104-117, 1992.

56. Conron M, Young C, Beynon HL: Calcium metabolism in sarcoidosis and its clinical implications. Rheumatology (Oxford) 39:707-713, 2000.

57. Montemurro L, et al: Bone loss in prednisone treated sarcoidosis: A two-year follow-up. Ann Ital Med Int 5:164-168, 1990.

58. Gonnelli S, et al: Prevention of corticosteroid-induced osteoporosis with alendronate in sarcoid patients. Calcif Tissue Int 61:382-385, 1997.

59. Rizzato G, et al: Bone protection with salmon calcitonin (sCT) in the long-term steroid therapy of chronic sarcoidosis. Sarcoidosis 5:99-103, 1988.

60. Montemurro L, et al: Prevention of corticosteroid-induced osteoporosis with salmon calcitonin in sarcoid patients. Calcif Tissue Int 49:71-76, 1991.

61. Erb N, et al: An assessment of back pain and the prevalence of sacroiliitis in sarcoidosis. Chest 127:192-196, 2005.

62. Kremer P, et al: Sarcoidosis and spondylarthropathy: Three case-reports. Rev Rhum Engl Ed 63:405-411, 1996.

63. Kotter I, Durk H, Saal JG: Sacroiliitis in sarcoidosis: Case reports and review of the literature. Clin Rheumatol 14:695-700, 1995.

64. Kremer JM: Histologic findings in siblings with acute sarcoid arthritis: Association with the B8,DR3 phenotype. J Rheumatol 13:593-597, 1986.

65. Palmer DG, Schumacher HR: Synovitis with non-specific histological changes in synovium in chronic sarcoidosis. Ann Rheum Dis 43:778-782, 1984.

66. Scott DG, et al: Chronic sarcoid synovitis in the Caucasian: An arthroscopic and histological study. Ann Rheum Dis 40:121-123, 1981.

67. **Mana J, et al: Lofgren's syndrome revisited: A study of 186 patients. Am J Med 107:240-245, 1999.**

68. Garcia-Porrua C, et al: Erythema nodosum: Etiologic and predictive factors in a defined population. Arthritis Rheum 43:584-592, 2000.

69. Andonopoulos AP, et al: Asymptomatic gastrocnemius muscle biopsy: An extremely sensitive and specific test in the pathologic confirmation of sarcoidosis presenting with hilar adenopathy. Clin Exp Rheumatol 19:569-572, 2001.

70. Yamamoto T, et al: Aspiration biopsy of nodular sarcoidosis of the muscle. Diagn Cytopathol 26:109-112, 2002.

71. Ost D, Yeldandi A, Cugell D: Acute sarcoid myositis with respiratory muscle involvement: Case report and review of the literature. Chest 107:879-882, 1995.

72. Dewberry RG, et al: Sarcoid myopathy presenting with diaphragm weakness. Muscle Nerve 16:832-835, 1993.

73. Cornblath WT, Elner V, Rolfe M: Extraocular muscle involvement in sarcoidosis. Ophthalmology 100:501-505, 1993.

74. Otake S, Ishigaki T: Muscular sarcoidosis. Semin Musculoskelet Radiol 5:167-170, 2001.

75. Prayson RA: Granulomatous myositis: Clinicopathologic study of 12 cases. Am J Clin Pathol 112:63-68, 1999.

76. Guo M, Lemos L, Baliga M: Nodular sarcoid myositis of skeletal muscle diagnosed by fine needle aspiration biopsy: A case report. Acta Cytol 43:1171-1176, 1999.

77. **Moore SL, Teirstein AE: Musculoskeletal sarcoidosis: Spectrum of appearances at MR imaging. Radiographics 23:1389-1399, 2003.**

78. Diri E, Espinoza CG, Espinoza LR: Spinal cord granulomatous vasculitis: An unusual clinical presentation of sarcoidosis. J Rheumatol 26:1408-1410, 1999.

79. Weiler V, et al: Concurrence of sarcoidosis and aortitis: Case report and review of the literature. Ann Rheum Dis 59:850-853, 2000.

80. Schapiro JM, et al: Sarcoidosis as the initial manifestation of Takayasu's arteritis. J Med 25:121-128, 1994.

81. Fernandes SR, Singsen BH, Hoffman GS: Sarcoidosis and systemic vasculitis. Semin Arthritis Rheum 30:33-46, 2000.

82. Ohori N, Arita K, Ohta M: [A case of Churg-Strauss syndrome overlapping with sarcoidosis]. Rinsho Shinkeigaku 38:631-636, 1998.

83. Newman LS: Metals that cause sarcoidosis. Semin Respir Infect 13:212-220, 1998.

84. Safirstein BH, et al: Granulomatous pneumonitis following exposure to the World Trade Center collapse. Chest 123:301-304, 2003.

85. Teirstein AS, et al: The spectrum of biopsy sites for the diagnosis of sarcoidosis. Sarcoidosis Vasc Diffuse Lung Dis 22:139-146, 2005.

86. Weinberg I, Vasiliev L, Gotsman I: Anti-dsDNA antibodies in sarcoidosis. Semin Arthritis Rheum 29:328-331, 2000.

87. Nakamura H, et al: High incidence of positive autoantibodies against thyroid peroxidase and thyroglobulin in patients with sarcoidosis. Clin Endocrinol (Oxf) 46:467-472, 1997.

88. Papadopoulos KI, et al: High frequency of endocrine autoimmunity in patients with sarcoidosis. Eur J Endocrinol 134:331-336, 1996.

89. Ina Y, et al: Antiphospholipid antibodies: A prognostic factor in sarcoidosis? Chest 105:1179-1183, 1994.

90. Sarigol SS, Hay MH, Wyllie R: Sarcoidosis in preschool children with hepatic involvement mimicking juvenile rheumatoid arthritis. J Pediatr Gastroenterol Nutr 28:510-512, 1999.

91. Sahn EE, et al: Preschool sarcoidosis masquerading as juvenile rheumatoid arthritis: Two case reports and a review of the literature. Pediatr Dermatol 7:208-213, 1990.

92. Ukae S, et al: Preschool sarcoidosis manifesting as juvenile rheumatoid arthritis: A case report and a review of the literature of Japanese cases. Acta Paediatr Jpn 36:515-518, 1994.

93. Sakurai Y, et al: Preschool sarcoidosis mimicking juvenile rheumatoid arthritis: The significance of gallium scintigraphy and skin biopsy in the differential diagnosis. Acta Paediatr Jpn 39:74-78, 1997.

94. Fallahi S, et al: Coexistence of rheumatoid arthritis and sarcoidosis: Difficulties encountered in the differential diagnosis of common manifestations. J Rheumatol 11:526-529, 1984.

95. Kucera RF: A possible association of rheumatoid arthritis and sarcoidosis. Chest 95:604-606, 1989.

96. Menard O, et al: Association of histologically proven rheumatoid arthritis with pulmonary sarcoidosis. Eur Respir J 8:472-473, 1995.

97. Yutani Y, et al: A rare case of sarcoidosis with rheumatoid arthritis. Osaka City Med J 41:85-89, 1995.

98. Justiniani FR: Sarcoidosis complicating primary Sjogren's syndrome. Mt Sinai J Med 56:59-61, 1989.

99. Radenne F, et al: [Sjogren's syndrome and necrotizing sarcoid-like granulomatosis]. Rev Mal Respir 16:554-557, 1999.

100. Giotaki H, et al: Labial minor salivary gland biopsy: A highly discriminatory diagnostic method between sarcoidosis and Sjogren's syndrome. Respiration 50:102-107, 1986.

101. Miyata M, et al: Primary Sjogren's syndrome complicated by sarcoidosis. Intern Med 37:174-178, 1998.

102. Lois M, et al: Coexisting Sjogren's syndrome and sarcoidosis in the lung. Semin Arthritis Rheum 28:31-40, 1998.

103. Drosos AA, et al: Sicca syndrome in patients with sarcoidosis. Rheumatol Int 18:177-180, 1999.

104. Gal I, Kovacs J, Zeher M: Case series: Coexistence of Sjogren's syndrome and sarcoidosis. J Rheumatol 27:2507-2510, 2000.

105. Oates E, Metherall J: Images in clinical medicine: Sarcoidosis. N Engl J Med 329:1394, 1993.

106. Grunewald J, et al: T-cell receptor variable region gene usage by CD4+ and CD8+ T cells in bronchoalveolar lavage fluid and peripheral blood of sarcoidosis patients. Proc Natl Acad Sci U S A 91:4965-4969, 1994.

107. Grunewald J, et al: Restricted V alpha 2.3 gene usage by CD4+ T lymphocytes in bronchoalveolar lavage fluid from sarcoidosis patients correlates with HLA-DR3. Eur J Immunol 22:129-135, 1992.

108. Vourlekis JS, Sawyer RT, Newman LS: Sarcoidosis: Developments in etiology, immunology, and therapeutics. Adv Intern Med 45:209-257, 2000.

109. Paramothayan S, Jones PW: Corticosteroid therapy in pulmonary sarcoidosis: A systematic review. JAMA 287:1301-1307, 2002.

110. Reich JM: Adverse long-term effect of corticosteroid therapy in recent-onset sarcoidosis. Sarcoidosis Vasc Diffuse Lung Dis 20:227-234, 2003.

111. Young RL, et al: Pulmonary sarcoidosis: A prospective evaluation of glucocorticoid therapy. Ann Intern Med 73:207-212, 1970.

112. Harkleroad LE, et al: Pulmonary sarcoidosis: Long-term follow-up of the effects of steroid therapy. Chest 82:84-87, 1982.

113. Israel HL, Fouts DW, Beggs RA: A controlled trial of prednisone treatment of sarcoidosis. Am Rev Respir Dis 107:609-614, 1973.

114. Eule H, et al: The possible influence of corticosteroid therapy on the natural course of pulmonary sarcoidosis: Late results of a continuing clinical study. Ann N Y Acad Sci 465:695-701, 1986.

115. Zaki MH, et al: Corticosteroid therapy in sarcoidosis: A five-year, controlled follow-up study. N Y State J Med 87:496-499, 1987.

116. Sugisaki K, et al: Clinical characteristics of 195 Japanese sarcoidosis patients treated with oral corticosteroids. Sarcoidosis Vasc Diffuse Lung Dis 20:222-226, 2003.

117. Gibson GJ, et al: British Thoracic Society sarcoidosis study: Effects of long term corticosteroid treatment. Thorax 51:238-247, 1996.

118. Baughman RP, Winget DB, Lower EE: Methotrexate is steroid sparing in acute sarcoidosis: Results of a double blind, randomized trial. Sarcoidosis Vasc Diffuse Lung Dis 17:60-66, 2000.

119. Lower EE, Baughman RP: Prolonged use of methotrexate for sarcoidosis. Arch Intern Med 155:846-851, 1995.

120. Baughman RP, Lower EE: Alternatives to corticosteroids in the treatment of sarcoidosis. Sarcoidosis Vasc Diffuse Lung Dis 14:121-130, 1997.

121. Kaye O, et al: Low-dose methotrexate: An effective corticosteroid-sparing agent in the musculoskeletal manifestations of sarcoidosis. Br J Rheumatol 34:642-644, 1995.

122. Webster GF, et al: Weekly low-dose methotrexate therapy for cutaneous sarcoidosis. J Am Acad Dermatol 24:451-454, 1991.

123. Rebuck AS, et al: Cyclosporin for pulmonary sarcoidosis. Lancet 1:1174, 1984.

124. Martinet Y, et al: Evaluation of the in vitro and in vivo effects of cyclosporine on the lung T-lymphocyte alveolitis of active pulmonary sarcoidosis. Am Rev Respir Dis 138:1242-1248, 1988.

125. Wyser CP, et al: Treatment of progressive pulmonary sarcoidosis with cyclosporin A: A randomized controlled trial. Am J Respir Crit Care Med 156:1371-1376, 1997.

126. Pacheco Y, et al: Azathioprine treatment of chronic pulmonary sarcoidosis. Sarcoidosis 2:107-113, 1985.

127. Lewis SJ, Ainslie GM, Bateman ED: Efficacy of azathioprine as second-line treatment in pulmonary sarcoidosis. Sarcoidosis Vasc Diffuse Lung Dis 16:87-92, 1999.

128. Muller-Quernheim J, et al: Treatment of chronic sarcoidosis with an azathioprine/prednisolone regimen. Eur Respir J 14:1117-1122, 1999.

129. Zic JA, et al: Treatment of cutaneous sarcoidosis with chloroquine: Review of the literature. Arch Dermatol 127:1034-1040, 1991.

130. O'Leary TJ, et al: The effects of chloroquine on serum 1,25-dihydroxyvitamin D and calcium metabolism in sarcoidosis. N Engl J Med 315:727-730, 1986.

131. Sharma OP: Effectiveness of chloroquine and hydroxychloroquine in treating selected patients with sarcoidosis with neurological involvement. Arch Neurol 55:1248-1254, 1998.

132. Demeter SL: Myocardial sarcoidosis unresponsive to steroids: Treatment with cyclophosphamide. Chest 94:202-203, 1988.

133. Lower EE, et al: Diagnosis and management of neurological sarcoidosis. Arch Intern Med 157:1864-1868, 1997.

134. Carlesimo M, et al: Treatment of cutaneous and pulmonary sarcoidosis with thalidomide. J Am Acad Dermatol 32:866-869, 1995.

135. Rousseau L, et al: Cutaneous sarcoidosis successfully treated with low doses of thalidomide. Arch Dermatol 134:1045-1046, 1998.

136. Lee JB, Koblenzer PS: Disfiguring cutaneous manifestation of sarcoidosis treated with thalidomide: A case report. J Am Acad Dermatol 39:835-838, 1998.

137. Oliver SJ, et al: Thalidomide induces granuloma differentiation in sarcoid skin lesions associated with disease improvement. Clin Immunol 102:225-236, 2002.

138. Baughman RP, et al: Thalidomide for chronic sarcoidosis. Chest 122:227-232, 2002.

139. Zabel P, et al: Pentoxifylline in treatment of sarcoidosis. Am J Respir Crit Care Med 155:1665-1669, 1997.

140. Baughman RP, Lower EE: Infliximab for refractory sarcoidosis. Sarcoidosis Vasc Diffuse Lung Dis 18:70-74, 2001.

141. Pettersen JA, et al: Refractory neurosarcoidosis responding to infliximab. Neurology 59:1660-1661, 2002.

142. Mallbris L, et al: Progressive cutaneous sarcoidosis responding to anti-tumor necrosis factor-alpha therapy. J Am Acad Dermatol 48:290-293, 2003.

143. Baughman RP, et al: Infliximab therapy in patients with chronic sarcoidosis and pulmonary involvement. Am J Respir Crit Care Med 174:795-802, 2006.

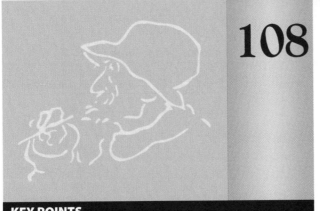

108 Hemochromatosis

GAYE CUNNANE

KEY POINTS

Elevated ferritin (>200 µg/L) and transferrin saturation (>45%) in the absence of other causes are useful screening measures for hereditary hemochromatosis (HHC).

Genetic testing should be reserved for patients with suggestive biochemical abnormalities or a positive family history of HHC or both.

Disease phenotype varies greatly among individuals with similar genetic mutations.

Diet, alcohol intake, and other risk factors for chronic liver disease all influence the clinical expression of HHC.

Phlebotomy is effective treatment for decreasing iron stores.

Some clinical manifestations of disease improve with treatment (constitutional symptoms, diabetes mellitus, liver enzyme abnormalities), whereas others are unaltered (arthritis, hypogonadism, cirrhosis).

Atypical osteoarthritis or chondrocalcinosis should trigger a search for an underlying metabolic disorder.

The earlier the diagnosis, the better the prognosis.

Hemochromatosis refers to the presence of excess iron in body tissues because of increased iron absorption. Primary or hereditary hemochromatosis (HHC) is an autosomal recessive disease, whereas secondary hemochromatosis refers to iron overload as a result of increased iron availability, ineffective erythropoiesis, or inherited abnormalities of iron metabolism (Table 108-1).

Hemochromatosis was first recognized in the 1880s in a series of case reports that described "bronze diabetes" and "pigmented cirrhosis," but von Recklinghausen is credited with the first use of the term in 1889.[1] In 1935, the familial pattern of HHC was described by Sheldon,[2] who suggested that the disease was due to an inborn error of metabolism. Finch and Finch in 1955[3] showed that HHC was caused by abnormal iron absorption in the presence of a normal diet. At that time, premorbid recognition of the problem was uncommon, however, and most cases were diagnosed at autopsy. In 1972, serum ferritin became available as a measure of iron stores. Three years later, Simon and colleagues[4] discovered that the HHC gene was present on chromosome 6, close to the HLA-A locus. It took 21 more years for the mutated gene, *HFE*, to be described, and in the last decade it has been recognized that other gene mutations also can cause iron overload.[5] Genetic testing has revolutionized the diagnosis of HHC, although the phenotype of any given mutation may vary greatly.[6] Nevertheless, the detection of such genes has greatly improved the overall prognosis of this condition by allowing the disease to be diagnosed at a preclinical stage in high-risk individuals. This discovery has helped many patients with HHC achieve a normal life expectancy.

NORMAL IRON METABOLISM

The average total body iron content in adults is 3 to 4 g, mostly contained within hemoglobin, but also present in myoglobin and cytochromes in addition to the storage proteins ferritin and hemosiderin. Of a typical daily Western diet of 10 to 20 mg of iron, 1 to 2 mg is absorbed by duodenal enterocytes each day.[7,8] Heme dietary sources from fish and meat have a higher bioavailability than nonheme sources, such as vegetables. The addition of ascorbic acid to the meal increases absorption of nonheme iron, whereas tannins, bran, and phytates inhibit iron absorption.[9,10] The rate of iron absorption is thought to be controlled by numerous mechanisms, including recent dietary iron intake, the extent of iron stores in the body, and a putative erythroid regulator that signals the state of bone marrow erythropoiesis to the intestine.[7] When there is poor dietary iron intake or body iron stores are low, or in the presence of increased or ineffective erythropoiesis, iron absorption is increased. When iron stores are normal, however, iron is retained in the intestinal cells by the protein mobilferritin and is subsequently excreted when these cells are shed. Iron homeostasis is regulated at the level of intestinal absorption.[7,11] There is no effective control mechanism, however, if the absorption process becomes disturbed.

When body iron stores reach an adequate level, ferritin production is increased to facilitate storage, and the transferrin receptor is downregulated to minimize the entry of iron into the cells. The iron responsive element binding protein mediates this process by detaching from ferritin mRNA so that more ferritin can be produced.[12] With increasing iron stores, circulating transferrin becomes saturated, and iron is preferentially offloaded to tissue sites that contain cells with high levels of transferrin receptors, such as liver, heart, thyroid, gonads, and pancreatic islet cells.[13]

IRON OVERLOAD SYNDROMES OTHER THAN HEREDITARY HEMOCHROMATOSIS

Because there is no physiologic mechanism to increase iron excretion, the inevitable result of increased iron entry into the body is iron overload. This iron overload may occur because of ineffective erythropoiesis or excessive intake of iron by oral or parenteral means. Chronic liver disease also is associated with increased iron deposition in hepatic parenchymal cells, accompanied by high ferritin, but normal serum iron concentrations. Transferrin saturation levels

Table 108-1   Definitions of Terms Used in Iron Metabolism

Ferritin	Major iron storage protein ↑ in iron storage diseases and inflammation Preferentially ↑ in adult-onset Still's disease Plasma levels reflect iron stores (e.g., 1 ng/mL ferritin = 10 mg iron)
Transferrin	Transporter protein for iron in plasma Synthesized in liver Increased in iron deficiency states
Transferrin saturation	Serum iron (µg/dL) ÷ TIBC (µg/dL) × 100 ↓ in iron deficiency/anemia of chronic disease/ferroportin mutation ↑ in hemochromatosis/ineffective erythropoiesis/iron overload states/severe liver failure
Iron regulatory proteins	Maintain iron homeostasis by modulating synthesis of transferrin receptors/ferritin/duodenal iron transporter
HFE protein	Identified in cells of deep crypts of duodenum and in Kupffer cells Modulates uptake of transferrin-bound iron into duodenal crypt cells
Iron exporter proteins	Ferroportin/Hephaestin/divalent metal transporter 1 (DMT1)
Hepcidin	Acute-phase reactant produced by liver Intrinsic antimicrobial activity Negative regulator of iron absorption Reduces iron release from macrophages Thought to interact with and inactivate ferroportin Hepcidin mutations found in some families with juvenile HHC
Hemojuvelin	Modulates hepcidin expression
Hemosiderin	Histologic identification of iron stain in tissues

HCC, hereditary hemochromatosis; TIBC, total iron-binding capacity.

Table 108-2   Hereditary Hemochromatosis

Name	Gene	Gene Product	Pattern of Inheritance
HFE-related HHC Type 1	HFE, 6p21.3	HFE	Autosomal recessive
Juvenile type HHC Type 2a	HJV, 1q21	Hemojuvelin	Autosomal recessive
Type 2b	HAMP, 19q13.1	Hepcidin	
TfR2-related HHC Type 3	TfR2, 7q22	Transferrin receptor 2	Autosomal recessive
Ferroportin-related HHC Type 4	SLC40A1, 2q32	Ferroportin	Autosomal dominant

HHC, hereditary hemochromatosis.

are usually within the high-normal range in chronic liver disease, in contrast to long-standing HHC, in which such levels are typically very high.

GENETICS OF HEMOCHROMATOSIS

Four types of HHC have now been described, all linked to gene mutations (Table 108-2).[14] Classic HHC (type 1) is an autosomal recessive disorder, with a mutation of the HFE gene, located on chromosome 6. Although numerous such mutations have been described, the most common is a single amino acid substitution of tyrosine for cysteine at position 282 (C282Y). This particular mutation is thought to have arisen in a Celtic/Viking ancestor more than 2000 years ago and is now one of the most common genetic defects in individuals of Northern European origin. This anomaly had no reproductive implications, but may have had survival advantages by protecting against iron deficiency in a susceptible population. Homozygosity for this mutation is a risk factor for organ damage secondary to iron deposition, although phenotypic expression varies widely. Other mutations of the HFE gene include the replacement of histidine with aspartic acid at position 63 (H63D) and the substitution of serine for cysteine at position 65 (S65C). The clinical manifestations of the latter mutations seem to be less serious, although compound heterozygosity of such defects may be associated with evidence of iron overload.

Mutations of the HFE gene cause adult HHC that becomes clinically obvious in middle age. In contrast, hemojuvelin or hepcidin mutations result in juvenile HHC (type 2), which may manifest in the teens or twenties. The rate of iron accumulation seems to be greater than in adult HHC and is often associated with widespread organ involvement and early mortality.[15] In contrast to the Northern European inheritance of HFE mutations, juvenile HHC has been most commonly reported in Italy.[16] The clinical manifestations of transferrin receptor mutations (type 3) seem to resemble the manifestations of the classic HFE-related HHC. Such mutations are rare, and few cases have been described.[17,18]

Ferroportin is an iron regulatory protein that helps in the export of iron from enterocytes, macrophages, and hepatocytes. Ferroportin mutations are inherited in an autosomal dominant fashion and have been described in European and Australian families.[19,20] Phenotypic expression varies, with some patients having the effects of iron overload in a similar manner to classic HHC, and others showing minimal evidence of organ damage.[21]

Many other inherited iron overload syndromes have been identified. The African iron overload syndrome occurs in a few Africans who drink locally brewed beer containing extremely high levels of iron (80 mg/L). Not all Africans who drink this beer develop hemochromatosis, leading to suggestions that additional genetic factors contribute to the development of disease. It is thought that a polymorphism of the ferroportin 1 gene is involved.[22] Separately, there is a familial association with a syndrome of very high ferritin levels (>1000 ng/mL) and bilateral congenital cataracts. This "hereditary hyperferrinemia-cataract syndrome" involves several mutations in the iron responsive element of L-ferritin and is inherited in an autosomal dominant fashion. The cataracts are thought to be due to excessive ferritin production within the lens fibers.[23]

EPIDEMIOLOGY

Although HHC previously was thought to be a rare condition, the availability of genetic testing has revealed that it is one of the most common inheritable disorders. Although 5 out of every 1000 individuals of Northern European origin is homozygous for the *HFE* mutation, phenotypic expression varies, and clinical cases are much fewer in number. In study of nearly 100,000 individuals from primary care practices in the United States, the prevalence for C282Y homozygosity was as follows: white, 0.44%; Native American, 0.11%; Hispanic, 0.027%; African-American, 0.014%; Pacific Islander, 0.012%; and Asian, 0.0004%.[24] Peak age at time of diagnosis is 40 to 60 years for classic HHC. Clinical manifestations vary widely between individuals with the same mutation, however, suggesting that the disease may be influenced by other factors, including diet, alcohol intake, smoking, and comorbid features such as chronic liver disease.[25] Gender is an obvious influencing factor because premenopausal women are likely to have lower iron stores secondary to menstrual blood loss.

PATHOGENESIS

Inappropriate absorption of iron by cells of the gastrointestinal tract is the hallmark of HHC. The duodenal cells seem to be iron deficient with abnormally low ferritin levels, which may be due to a local defect of the enterocytes or an aberration of a regulatory signal elsewhere.[14,26] Two theories have been suggested to explain the pathophysiology of iron overload in HHC. The crypt-programming model, first mooted in 1997, proposes that anomalous iron absorption by duodenal crypt cells is associated with the perception of iron deficiency despite adequate iron stores.[27] The mutated HFE protein cannot interact normally with transferrin receptor-1. Upregulation of an iron transporter protein (divalent metal transporter 1) has been shown in these cells allowing continued absorption of iron from the intestinal lumen, regardless of the extent of iron stores. Macrophages in HHC also have been found to reflect an iron-deficient state, suggesting that they share the same defect as the enterocytes in this condition.[14,28]

The second theory, called the hepcidin model, proposes that the abnormal HFE protein is unable to influence levels of hepcidin, an iron inhibitory protein. Normally, when plasma iron levels are adequate, hepcidin manufacture increases, slowing down release of iron from enterocytes and macrophages by interacting with iron transport proteins. In HHC, it is thought that hepcidin levels are inappropriately low, allowing excessive iron absorption to occur.[29] Absence of hepcidin results in early severe iron loading, whereas overexpression of this protein can improve iron deposition significantly in a mouse model of HHC.[30]

If the genetic subtypes of HHC have been identified, why does the phenotypic expression vary so greatly? The answer to this question is unknown, but it is postulated that the presence of modifier genes may affect disease manifestations. Abnormalities of the genes associated with hepcidin, hemojuvelin, or transferrin receptor in addition to abnormalities involved in fibrogenesis and antioxidation all may influence the age and extent of disease onset in patients with *HFE*-related HHC.[31-33] Other factors include lifestyle risk factors, such as smoking, alcohol intake, and diet. The presence of chronic liver conditions, such as chronic hepatitis, hepatic porphyrias, and thalassemias, may accelerate the development of cirrhosis in patients with HHC.[34-37]

Chronic iron overload is thought to cause organ damage via several mechanisms, including weakening of lysosomal membranes and consequent discharge of enzymes into the cytoplasm. Increased free radical formation contributes to lipid peroxidation of cell membranes. There is accelerated fibrogenesis and a reduction in the stores of vitamins C and E that are essential for tissue viability.[38,39] Iron deposition in HHC occurs first in parenchymal cells, with reticuloendothelial involvement a late feature, in contrast to transfusional iron overload, in which the reticuloendothelial cells are primarily involved.[36]

CLINICAL FEATURES

EXTRA-ARTICULAR MANIFESTATIONS

HHC is more common in men than women and typically manifests in middle-aged adults as iron stores gradually accumulate, often reaching 20 to 30 g. Organ involvement varies and is unpredictable, although the liver, as the major site of iron storage, is typically affected. Commonly, abnormalities of the liver enzymes, checked as part of a routine health screen, are the initial indication of disease. The degree of iron overload has a direct impact on the life expectancy of the affected individual. Without an early diagnosis, progressive fibrosis leading to cirrhosis may occur.[36,40] The risk of hepatocellular carcinoma is greatly increased in patients with established cirrhosis.[41]

Glucose intolerance tends to be a late finding in HHC and is due to progressive iron accumulation in pancreatic beta cells causing low C-peptide and insulin levels. Alpha cell function is usually preserved, however, and serum glucagon levels are normal or increased.[42] The risk of diabetes mellitus also is higher in C282Y heterozygotes with no clinical evidence of HHC compared with controls.[43]

Iron deposition in the heart can result in conduction system abnormalities and heart failure.[44] It is unclear whether or not HHC is associated with an increased risk of atherosclerosis, with different studies showing conflicting results.[45]

Pituitary involvement in HHC is due to iron deposition resulting in reduced serum levels of secreted hormones from this gland. Low levels of gonadotropic hormone cause loss of libido and erectile dysfunction.[36,46] Hypothyroidism in HHC is thought to be due to a direct toxic effect of iron on thyroid cells and is associated with low thyroxine and elevated thyroid-stimulating hormone.[47] Such endocrine abnormalities may contribute to the development of osteoporosis in these individuals.

Skin discoloration occurs as a result of extra melanin and iron in the epidermis. It is a late finding, and the development of "bronze diabetes" represents the end stage of years of iron accumulation in the tissues.

Patients with HHC have increased susceptibility to certain infections. High serum iron concentrations may increase bacterial virulence, whereas excess iron in macrophages is thought to reduce phagocytosis.[48] Particular caution is advised with uncooked seafood because of the risk of septicemia from *Vibrio vulnificus*. In addition, *Yersinia enterocolitica*, *Listeria monocytogenes*, *Salmonella enteritidis* serotype *typhimurium*, *Klebsiella pneumoniae*, *Escherichia coli*, *Rhizopus arrhizus*, and *Mucor* species all have been reported to cause severe illness in patients with iron overload.[7]

ARTICULAR FEATURES

Arthritis is a common symptom in HHC, affecting 50% to 80% of patients and significantly interfering with quality of life.[49-54] Although it tends to be a late feature, joint pain may nevertheless be the presenting symptom of HHC, alerting a diligent physician to the presence of an underlying metabolic disorder. Articular involvement may be widespread, but changes to the second and third metacarpophalangeal joints are most characteristic.[55] Arthritis also may be present in the proximal interphalangeal joints, wrists, shoulders, hips, knees, and ankles.[49-56] Patients notice pain and stiffness of the involved joints, but evidence of synovitis is usually absent. Hip damage develops in approximately 25% of individuals with HHC, and after hip arthroplasty, there is an increased risk of aseptic loosening of the prosthesis.[57,58] The differential diagnosis of HHC-related arthropathy includes severe osteoarthritis, rheumatoid arthritis, other forms of inflammatory arthritis, and crystal arthritis. Rheumatoid factor is typically negative, however, and the radiographs, in established cases, show distinctive findings, such as joint space narrowing of the second and third metacarpophalangeal joints, hooklike osteophytes on the radial aspect of the metacarpal heads, and chondrocalcinosis particularly of the triangular fibrocartilage adjacent to the ulnar styloid.

The pathogenetic mechanism underlying HHC-related arthritis is unknown, and the prevalence of joint pains in this condition has not been found to correlate with body iron stores. Toxic effects from local iron deposition, the acceleration of cartilage defects, and immunologic mechanisms all have been implicated.[52,53,59] Using light microscopy, the involved synovium shows iron deposits, particularly in the lining cells, but inflammatory cell infiltration is not typical.[60,61] Apatite and calcium pyrophosphate dihydrate crystals may be observed, but why they are preferentially expressed in HHC is unknown. In association with the increased incidence of calcium pyrophosphate dihydrate deposition disease in HHC, a putative role for a parathyroid hormone fragment (PTH 44-68) also has been suggested.[62]

INVESTIGATIONS

A high index of suspicion is helpful when a patient presents with joint pains and abnormal liver enzymes. Although the differential diagnosis is wide, the presence of elevated ferritin and transferrin saturation levels (serum iron × 100/total iron-binding capacity) strongly points to the answer. Serum iron should be measured with the patient fasting because concentrations may be increased after a meal.[36] High ferritin levels also may be caused by systemic inflammation or malignancy, but these conditions tend to be associated with a reduced transferrin saturation. Other causes of elevated transferrin saturation include high serum iron secondary to hepatic cytolysis or low transferrin levels secondary to liver failure, and these possibilities should be excluded. If ferritin measures greater than 200 µg/L, and transferrin saturation is greater than 45%, genetic screening is recommended.[14,24] The finding of homozygosity for the C282Y mutation or compound heterozygosity for C282Y/H63D confirms the diagnosis.

Liver biopsy may be considered for prognostic purposes in established cases.[6,13,36,63] HHC can be distinguished histologically from alcoholic cirrhosis by the preferential distribution of iron in the hepatocytes in the former and in the Kuffper cells in the latter.[36] Magnetic resonance imaging of the abdomen also can be used to determine iron overload in the internal organs. Gradient T2-weighted sequences show decreased signal intensity and correlate highly with liver iron concentrations. This imaging method also can identify other locations of iron deposition (e.g., in the spleen, pancreas, lymph nodes, and heart).[36]

Because HHC is a systemic condition, other investigations should include a search for diabetes, thyroid disease, hypogonadism, osteoporosis, and cardiomyopathy. Disease mimickers, such as porphyria cutanea tarda, ineffective erythropoiesis, and chronic alcohol excess, should be excluded.

SCREENING

Greater disease awareness and the availability of genetic screening have meant that HHC is increasingly likely to be diagnosed before the classic triad of cirrhosis, diabetes, and skin hyperpigmentation develops. Late presentation with evidence of end-organ damage does occur, however, particularly in patients with additional risk factors for iron overload or liver disease.

HHC is an attractive clinical target for population screening because of its high prevalence, potential disease severity, availability of effective treatment, and impact of early diagnosis on the morbidity and mortality of affected individuals. Certain groups are more at risk than others, however, and the disease prevalence is higher in white than nonwhite individuals.[6,24,64] Biochemical measures, such as transferrin saturation, may be a cost-effective method of screening in whites during routine health checks and in individuals who complain of nonspecific symptoms, such as excessive fatigue and arthralgias. Levels of transferrin saturation greater than 45% in men and greater than 35% in premenopausal women, in the absence of other causes, warrant further investigation.[13,14]

Genetic testing should be reserved for patients with suggestive biochemical abnormalities or a family history of HHC. Routine population screening for C282Y or H63D mutations is not recommended because of the variable clinical penetrance of these genes and the potential negative consequences of a positive result in asymptomatic patients, such as financial, legal, insurance, and psychological implications.[14] When a case of HHC is diagnosed, however, and two gene mutations are identified (i.e., C282Y/C282Y or C282Y/H63D), siblings also should be tested for these mutations. H63D/H63D homozygotes are not thought to be at risk of clinical disease. Children of a patient with HHC or of an individual with C282Y/H63D heterozygosity are at risk only if the other parent also carries hemochromatosis gene mutations.

For individuals in whom genetic testing has identified a risk of HHC, but with no clinical evidence of disease, yearly biochemical screening should be done, with measures of ferritin, transferrin saturation, and liver enzymes. Such monitoring allows early detection of organ compromise and timely initiation of treatment (Fig. 108-1).

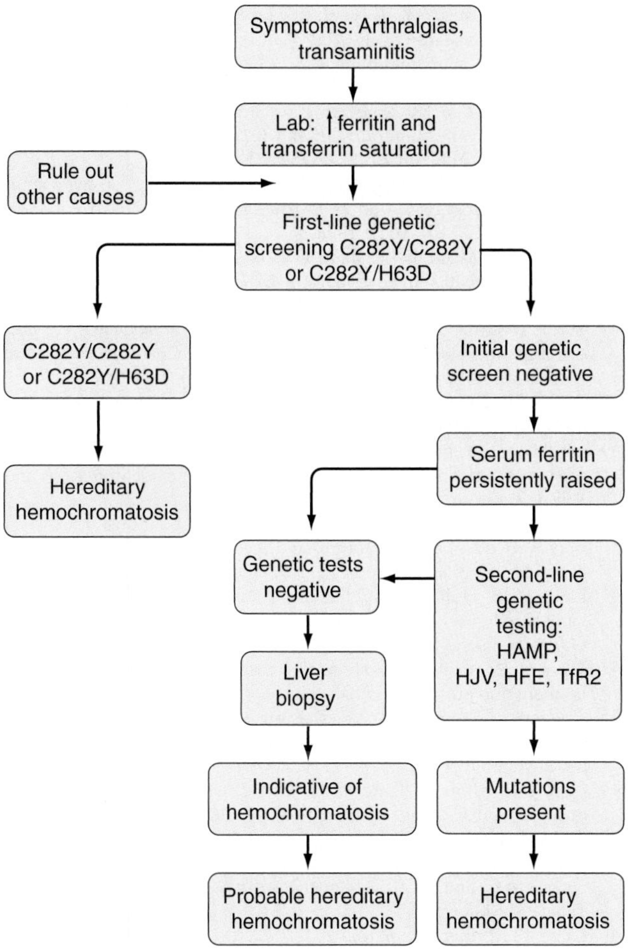

Figure 108-1   Algorithm for the diagnosis of hereditary hemochromatosis.

MANAGEMENT

Removing excess iron before the development of organ damage significantly abrogates the adverse consequences of HHC. Target groups for treatment include asymptomatic individuals with biochemical evidence of high iron stores, in addition to patients with overt clinical disease. Some features of HHC improve with bloodletting, including constitutional symptoms, diabetes, and liver enzyme abnormalities. Phlebotomy has no effect, however, on arthritis, hypogonadism, and liver fibrosis.[13] When cirrhosis is established, the risk of hepatocellular carcinoma is greatly increased, even after a satisfactory reduction in iron stores.[13,65]

Phlebotomy is an effective method of removing excess iron. The use of chelating agents is rarely necessary. Every 500 mL of whole blood contains 200 to 250 mg of iron, depending on the hematocrit. Phlebotomy can be arranged once or twice weekly, as tolerated by the patient, aiming for a serum ferritin of 50 ng/mL and a transferrin saturation of less than 45%. It can take more than 1 year for iron stores to normalize with this regimen. Iron deficiency anemia should always be avoided, and when ferritin levels reach their target, the frequency of bloodletting may be reduced. Phlebotomy continues for life, and the maintenance schedule depends on the patient's ability to sustain the ferritin level in the low-normal range. Blood removal in HHC is not without risks. In particular, life-threatening cardiac arrhythmias may develop during rapid mobilization of iron stores. Vitamin C supplementation may precipitate such problems by facilitating iron release and increasing pro-oxidant and free radical activity.[13] Patients undergoing phlebotomy for HHC should not take extra vitamin C, but can continue to eat fresh produce containing this vitamin.

Other dietary recommendations include a reduction or avoidance of food containing high doses of iron, such as red meat and internal organs. Uncooked shellfish is a particular hazard because of the risk of contamination with *V. vulnificus*. Some alcoholic drinks contain iron, and all are potentially hepatotoxic. Alcohol should be consumed only occasionally because it seems to have a synergistic effect in the presence of iron overload on the development of cirrhosis and hepatocellular carcinoma.[37]

Just as the pathogenesis of joint pain in HHC is unclear, the treatment of arthritis in this condition is unsatisfactory. The arthritis may continue to progress despite effective phlebotomy. Nonsteroidal anti-inflammatory drugs, colchicine, and intra-articular corticosteroids may be helpful in some cases. It is important to recognize osteoporosis as a potential disease complication, particularly in the setting of hypogonadism or reduced thyroid function. Hormone replacement, if indicated, should be instituted, although some patients may require additional treatment with calcium and bisphosphonates.

PROGNOSIS

The earlier HHC is diagnosed, the better the prognosis because morbidity and mortality are directly related to the extent of iron overload and consequent organ damage. The development of cirrhosis is a serious indicator of reduced longevity. For patients with HHC-related hepatic failure who undergo liver transplantation, survival rates are lower compared with individuals who receive liver transplants for other reasons. Postoperative death in these circumstances is typically due to cardiac complications or infection.[13,66]

In the absence of cirrhosis or diabetes, patients with HHC have a normal life expectancy. Given the importance of timely recognition of this common metabolic problem, a vigilant physician can make an enormous difference to the lives of patients who present with early symptoms of this disease. In this context, the rheumatologist has a particularly relevant role in keeping a high index of suspicion for the diagnosis of HHC in patients with atypical osteoarthritis or chondrocalcinosis.

REFERENCES

1. von Recklinghausen FD: Uber Haemochromatose. Tageblatt Versammlung Dtsche Naturforscher Artzte Heidelberg 62:324-325, 1889.
2. Sheldon JH: Haemochromatosis. London, Oxford University Press, 1935.
3. Finch SC, Finch CA: Idiopathic hemochromatosis, an iron storage disease. Medicine (Balt) 34:381-430, 1955.
4. Simon M, Pawlotsky Y, Bourel M, et al: Hémochromatose idiopathique maladie associée à l'antigene tissulaire HLA-3. Nouv Presse Med 4:1432, 1975.
5. Feder JN, Gnirke A, Thomas W, et al: A novel MHC class 1-like gene is mutated in patients with hereditary hemochromatosis. Nat Genet 13:399-408, 1996.

6. Olynyk JK, Cullen DJ, Sina Aquilia BA, et al: A population based study of the clinical expression of the hemochromatosis gene. N Engl J Med 341:718-724, 1999.

7. **Andrews NC: Disorders of iron metabolism. N Engl J Med 341:1986-1995, 1999.**

8. Finch CA, Huebers H: Perspectives in iron metabolism. N Engl J Med 306:1520-1528, 1982.

9. Hallberg L, Brune M, Rossander L: The role of vitamin C in iron absorption. Int J Vitam Nutr Res Suppl 30:103-108, 1989.

10. Hallberg L, Rossander L, Skanberg AB: Phytates and the inhibitory effect of bran on iron absorption in man. Am J Clin Nutr 45:988-996, 1987.

11. Fleming RE, Bacon BR: Orchestration of iron homeostasis. N Engl J Med 352:1741-1744, 2005.

12. Dix DJ, Lin PN, Kimata Y, et al: The iron regulatory region of ferritin mRNA is also a positive control element for iron-dependent translation. Biochemistry 31:2818-2822, 1992.

13. **Tavill AS: Diagnosis and management of hemochromatosis. Hepatology 33:1321-1328, 2001.**

14. **Pietrangelo A: Hereditary hemochromatosis—a new look at an old disease. N Engl J Med 350:2383-2397, 2004.**

15. Cazzola M, Cerani P, Rovati A, et al: Juvenile genetic hemochromatosis is clinically and genetically distinct from the classical HLA-related disorder. Blood 92:2979-2981, 1998.

16. Lanzara C, Roetto A, Daraio F, et al: Spectrum of hemojuvelin gene mutations in 1q-linked juvenile hemochromatosis. Blood 103: 4317-4321, 2004.

17. Roetto A, Totaro A, Piperno A, et al: New mutations inactivating transferrin receptor 2 in hemochromatosis type 3. Blood 97: 2555-2560, 2001.

18. Girelli D, Bozzini C, Roetto A, et al: Clinical and pathologic findings in hemochromatosis type 3 due to a novel mutation in transferrin receptor 2 gene. Gastroenterology 122:1295-1302, 2002.

19. Njajou OT, Vaessen N, Joosse M, et al: A mutation in SLC11A3 is associated with autosomal dominant hemochromatosis. Nat Genet 28:213-214, 2001.

20. Montosi G, Donovan A, Totaro A, et al: Autosomal dominant hemochromatosis is associated with a mutation in the ferroportin (SLC11A3) gene. J Clin Invest 108:619-623, 2001.

21. Cremonesi L, Forni GL, Soriani N, et al: Genetic and clinical heterogeneity of ferroportin disease. Br J Haematol 131:663-670, 2005.

22. Gordeuk VR, Caleffi A, Corradini E, et al: Iron overload in Africans and African-Americans and a common mutation in the SLC40A1 (ferroportin 1) gene. Blood Cells Mol Dis 31:299-304, 2003.

23. Cazzola M: Role of ferritin and ferroportin genes in unexplained hyperferritinaemia. Best Pract Res Clin Haematol 18:251-263, 2005.

24. **Adams PC, Reboussin DM, Barton JC, et al: Hemochromatosis and iron-overload screening in a racially diverse population. N Engl J Med 352:1769-1778, 2005.**

25. Waalen J, Nordestgaard BG, Beutler E: The penetrance of hereditary hemochromatosis. Best Pract Res Clin Haematol 18:203-220, 2005.

26. Pietrangelo A, Rocchi E, Casalgrandi G, et al: Regulation of transferrin, transferrin receptor and ferritin genes in human duodenum. Gastroenterology 102:802-809, 1992.

27. Parkkila S, Waheed A, Britton RS, et al: Immunohistochemistry of HLA-H, the protein defective in patients with hereditary hemochromatosis, reveals unique pattern of expression in gastrointestinal tract. Proc Natl Acad Sci U S A 94:2534-2539, 1997.

28. Cairo G, Recalcati S, Montosi G, et al: Inappropriately high iron regulatory protein activity in monocytes of patients with genetic hemochromatosis. Blood 89:2546-2553, 1997.

29. **Bridle KR, Frazer DM, Wilkins SJ, et al: Disrupted hepcidin regulation in HFE-associated haemochromatosis and the liver as a regulator of body iron homeostasis. Lancet 361:669-673, 2003.**

30. Nicolas G, Viatte L, Lou DQ, et al: Constitutive hepcidin expression prevents iron overload in a mouse model of hemochromatosis. Nat Genet 34:97-101, 2003.

31. Pietrangelo A, Caleffi A, Henrion J, et al: Juvenile hemochromatosis associated with pathogenic mutations of adult hemochromatosis genes. Gastroenterology 128:470-479, 2005.

32. Jacolot S, Le Gac G, Scotet V, et al: HAMP as a modifier gene that increases the phenotypic expression of the HFE pC282Y homozygous genotype. Blood 103:2835-2840, 2004.

33. Le Gac G, Scotet V, Ka C, et al: The recently identified type 2A juvenile hemochromatosis gene (HJV), a second candidate modifier of the C282Y homozygous phenotype. Hum Mol Genet 13:1913-1918, 2004.

34. Thorburn D, Curry G, Spooner R, et al: The role of iron and hemochromatosis gene mutations in the progression of liver disease in chronic hepatitis C. Gut 50:248-252, 2002.

35. Bonkovsky HL, Poh Fitzpatrick M, Pimstone N, et al: Porphyria cutanea tarda, hepatitis C and HFE gene mutations in North America. Hepatology 27:1661-1669, 1998.

36. **Chung RT, Misdraji J, Sahani DV: Case 33-2006: A 43-year-old man with diabetes, hypogonadism, cirrhosis, arthralgias and fatigue. N Engl J Med 355:1812-1819, 2006.**

37. Stal P, Olsson J, Svoboda P, et al: Studies on genotoxic effects of iron overload and alcohol in an animal model of hepatocarcinogenesis. J Hepatol 27:562-571, 1997.

38. Bacon BR, Britton RS: Hereditary hemochromatosis and alcohol: A fibrogenic cocktail. Gastroenterology 122:563-565, 2002.

39. von Herbay A, DeGroot H, Hegi U, et al: Low vitamin E content in plasma of patients with alcoholic liver disease, hemochromatosis and Wilson's disease. J Hepatol 20:41-46, 1994.

40. Adams PC, Deugnier Y, Moirand R, et al: The relationship between iron overload, clinical symptoms and age in 410 patients with genetic hemochromatosis. Hepatology 25:162-166, 1997.

41. Elmberg M, Hultcrantz R, Ekbom A, et al: Cancer risk in patients with hereditary hemochromatosis and in their first-degree relatives. Gastroenterology 125:1733-1741, 2003.

42. Yaouanq JM: Diabetes and hemochromatosis: Current concepts, management and prevention. Diabetes Metab 21:319-329, 1995.

43. Salonen JT, Tuomainen TP, Kontula K: Role of C282Y mutation in haemochromatosis gene in the development of type 2 diabetes in healthy men. BMJ 320:1706-1707, 2000.

44. Gore JM, Fallon JT: Case 31-1994: A 25 year old man with recent onset of diabetes and congestive heart failure. N Engl J Med 331: 460-466, 1994.

45. Ellervik C, Tybjaerg-Hansen A, Grande P, et al: Hereditary hemochromatosis and risk of ischemic heart disease. Circulation 112: 185-193, 2005.

46. Cundy T, Butler J, Bomford A, et al: Reversibility of hypogonadotropic hypogonadism associated with genetic haemochromatosis. Clin Endocrinol 38:617-620, 1993.

47. Edwards CQ, Kelly TM, Ellwein G, et al: Thyroid disease in hemochromatosis. Arch Intern Med 143:1890-1893, 1983.

48. van Asbeck BS, Verbrugh HA, van Oost VA, et al: *Listeria monocytogenes* meningitis and decreased phagocytosis associated with iron overload. BMJ 284:542-544, 1982.

49. Bulaj ZJ, Ajioka RS, Phillips JD, et al: Disease-related conditions in relatives of patients with hemochromatosis. N Engl J Med 343: 1529-1535, 2000.

50. Ross JM, Kowalchuk RM, Shaulinsky J, et al: Association of heterozygous hemochromatosis C282Y gene mutation with hand osteoarthritis. J Rheumatol 30:121-125, 2000.

51. von Kempis J: Arthropathy in hereditary hemochromatosis. Curr Opin Rheumatol 13:80-83, 2001.

52. **Schumacher HR: Haemochromatosis. Bailliere's Best Pract Clin Res Rheumatol 14:277-284, 2000.**

53. Ines LS, da Silva JA, Malcata AB, et al: Arthropathy of genetic hemochromatosis: A major and distinctive manifestation of disease. Clin Exp Rheumatol 19:98-102, 2001.

54. Adams PC, Speechley M: The effect of arthritis on the quality of life in hereditary hemochromatosis. J Rheumatol 23:707-710, 1996.

55. Cunnane G, O'Duffy JD: The iron salute sign of haemochromatosis. Arthritis Rheum 38:558, 1995.

56. Carroll GJ: Primary osteoarthritis in the ankle joint is associated with finger metacarpophalangeal osteoarthritis and the H63D mutation in the HFE gene. J Clin Rheumatol 12:109-113, 2006.

57. Axford JS, Bomford A, Revell P, et al: Hip arthropathy in genetic hemochromatosis: Radiographic and histologic features. Arthritis Rheum 34:357-361, 1991.

58. Lunn JV, Gallagher PM, Hegarty S, et al: The role of hereditary hemochromatosis in aseptic loosening following primary total hip arthroplasty. J Orthop Res 23:542-548, 2005.

59. Arosa FA, Oliveira L, Porto G, et al: Anomalies of the CD8+ T cell pool in haemochromatosis. Clin Exp Immunol 107:548-554, 1997.

60. Schumacher HR: Ultrastructural characteristics of the synovial membrane in idiopathic hemochromatosis. Ann Rheum Dis 31:465-473, 1972.
61. Walker RJ, Dymock IW, Ansell ID, et al: Synovial biopsy in hemochromatosis arthropathy. Ann Rheum Dis 31:98-102, 1972.
62. Pawlotsky Y, Le Dantec P, Moirand R, et al: Elevated parathyroid hormone 44-68 and osteoarticular changes in patients with genetic hemochromatosis. Arthritis Rheum 42:799-806, 1999.
63. Tavill AS, Adams PC: A diagnostic approach to hemochromatosis. Can J Gastroenterol 20:535-540, 2006.
64. Tavill AS: Clinical implications of the hemochromatosis gene. N Engl J Med 341:755-757, 1999.
65. Niederau C, Fischer R, Purschel A, et al: Long term survival in patients with hereditary hemochromatosis. Gastroenterology 110:1107-1119, 1996.
66. Kowdley KV, Brandhagen DJ, Gish RG, et al: Survival after liver transplantation in patients with hepatic iron overload: The national hemochromatosis transplant registry. Gastroenterology 129:494-503, 2005.

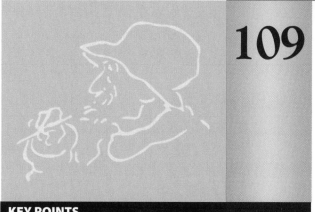

109

Hemophilic Arthropathy

KATHERINE S. UPCHURCH •
DOREEN B. BRETTLER

KEY POINTS

Severe hemophilia, if not aggressively treated, is most often complicated by recurrent hemarthrosis.

Recurrent hemarthrosis causes chronic arthropathy with overlapping clinical and pathologic features of osteoarthritis and rheumatoid arthritis.

Septic arthritis should be considered in hemophilic patients with risk factors (previous arthrocentesis, intravenous drug use, human immunodeficiency virus infection), and acute monarticular arthritis.

Soft tissue and muscle hemorrhage are frequent complications of hemophilia.

With continuous factor infusion, surgical procedures, including total joint replacements, can be done safely in hemophilic patients.

The best treatment for hemophilic arthropathy is prevention of recurrent hemarthrosis through regular prophylactic factor replacement.

Although spontaneous joint hemorrhage has been described in a variety of inherited disorders of coagulation,[1-3] and in the setting of anticoagulation therapy,[4] it occurs most frequently in hemophilia. Bleeding into the joints is the complication of hemophilia that most often requires therapeutic intervention and, when it is recurrent, can lead to chronic, deforming arthritis that is independent of bleeding episodes.

Hemophilia refers to a group of inherited diseases in which there is a functional deficiency of a specific clotting factor. The most common are hemophilia A (classic hemophilia) and hemophilia B (Christmas disease); the deficient factors are factor VIII (hemophilia A) and factor IX (hemophilia B). The incidence and severity of hemorrhagic complications of hemophilia are directly related to the severity of the underlying coagulation defect.

Although the intrinsic pathway of coagulation is severely impaired in hemophilia, the extrinsic tissue-dependent pathway remains intact and is probably the major hemostatic regulatory system. Normal synovial tissue and cultures of synovial fibroblasts have been found to be deficient in tissue factor,[5] which suggests that in synovium-lined joints, hemophiliacs have functional inactivity of intrinsic and extrinsic coagulation pathways. This situation may explain the marked propensity toward hemorrhage in joints compared with other tissue sites in these patients.

CLINICAL FEATURES

The spectrum of articular disease in hemophiliacs has been the subject of numerous comprehensive reviews[6-10] and includes acute hemarthrosis, subacute or chronic arthritis, and end-stage hemophilic arthropathy. The usual distribution of joint involvement is shown in Figure 109-1. Involvement of the small joints of the hands and feet also may occur, although infrequently.

ACUTE HEMARTHROSIS

Nearly all patients with severe hemophilia A or B (<1% activity of the deficient factor) and half of patients with moderate disease activity experience hemarthrosis. Acute hemarthroses generally first occur when a child begins to walk and continue, usually cyclically, into adulthood, when the frequency diminishes. Patients frequently have premonitory symptoms, such as stiffness or warmth in the affected joint, followed by intense pain, which may be due partly to rapid joint capsule distention.

Pain is accompanied by objective clinical findings of warmth, a tense effusion, tenderness, limitation of motion, and a joint that is often held in a flexed position. Joint pain responds rapidly to replacement of the deficient clotting factor. If hemostasis is achieved early after onset of hemarthrosis, full joint function may be regained within 12 to 24 hours. If the hemorrhage is more advanced, however, blood is resorbed slowly over 5 to 7 days, and full joint function is regained within 10 to 14 days.

SUBACUTE OR CHRONIC ARTHRITIS

Recurrent hemarthroses, particularly in patients with severe factor deficiency, may lead to a self-perpetuating condition in which joint abnormalities persist in intervals between bleeding episodes. The involved joint is chronically swollen, although painless and only slightly warm. Chronic synovitis, including prominent synovial proliferation with or without effusion, may be present. There may be mild limitation of motion, often with a flexion deformity. Factor replacement does not modify these findings.

END-STAGE HEMOPHILIC ARTHROPATHY

Long-standing end-stage hemophilic arthropathy has features in common with degenerative joint disease and advanced rheumatoid arthritis. The joint appears enlarged and "knobby," owing to osteophytic bone overgrowth. Synovial thickening and effusion are not prominent, however. Range of motion is severely restricted, and fibrous ankylosis

Percentage joints with:

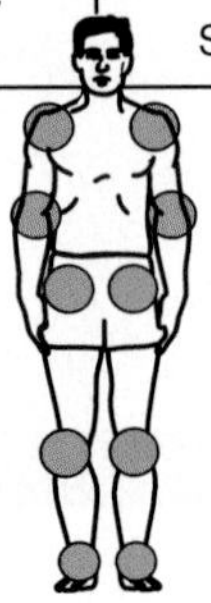

Any hemarthrosis	Many hemarthroses	Chronic pain	Synovitis	Limitation of motion	Any radiologic abnormality
34.5	13.3	13.9	—	16.9	21.6
54.0	38.5	13.8	9.8	27.0	52.6
28.6	8.0	5.4	—	19.8	18.8
63.1	50.9	26.8	11.6	27.0	50.2
60.8	42.8	15.2	2.2	34.2	52.4

Figure 109-1 Distribution of acute hemarthrosis based on a study of 139 patients with hemophilia. Clinical and radiologic features of chronic arthritis in hemophilia. *(Adapted from Steven MM, Yogarojah S, Madhok R, et al: Haemophilic arthritis. QJM 58:181, 1986.)*

is common. Subluxation, joint laxity, and malalignment are frequently present. Hemarthroses decrease in frequency, however.

SEPTIC ARTHRITIS

Until the early 1980s, septic arthritis rarely occurred in hemophiliac patients. With the widespread occurrence of human immunodeficiency virus (HIV) infection as a result of contaminated factor concentrates, the incidence of this complication has increased significantly.[11,12] Septic arthritis is seen more often in adult than in pediatric hemophiliacs and is most commonly monarticular, usually involving the knee. In contrast to spontaneous hemarthrosis, septic arthritis is significantly associated with a temperature greater than 38°C within 12 hours of presentation and articular pain that does not improve with replacement therapy.[11] Peripheral leukocyte count may not be elevated, particularly in HIV-positive patients.[13] A predisposing factor other than hemophilic arthropathy is often identifiable, including previous arthrocentesis or arthroplasty, intravenous drug use, and infected indwelling venous access catheters. *Staphylococcus aureus* is the most frequently identified organism even in HIV-infected patients, followed by *Streptococcus pneumoniae*.[13]

MUSCLE AND SOFT TISSUE HEMORRHAGE

Bleeding into muscles and soft tissue is common in hemophiliacs and may be more insidious than hemarthrosis because of the lack of premonitory symptoms. Bleeding into the iliopsoas and gastrocnemius muscles and the forearm results in well-described syndromes with which the rheumatologist should be familiar. Iliopsoas hemorrhage produces acute groin pain with marked pain on hip extension and a hip flexion contracture. Rotation is preserved, in contrast to intra-articular hemorrhage. If untreated, the expanding soft tissue mass may compress the femoral nerve, causing signs and symptoms of femoral neuropathy.[6,14] Bleeding into the gastrocnemius muscle can cause an equinus deformity from heel cord contracture.[6] Finally, hemorrhage into closed compartments can cause acute muscle necrosis and nerve compression.[15] Of particular importance is bleeding into the volar compartment of the forearm, which can cause flexion deformities of the wrist and fingers. If a

compartment syndrome is suspected, compartment pressures should be measured to confirm the diagnosis.

A large intramuscular hemorrhage uncommonly results in the formation of a simple muscle cyst, which clinically appears to be an encapsulated soft tissue area of swelling overlying muscle. Cyst formation in this setting is confined by the muscular fascial plane and most likely results from inadequate resorption of blood and clot. Subperiosteal or intraosseous hemorrhage, in contrast, may lead to a pseudotumor, a rare skeletal complication of hemophilia. Hemophilic pseudotumors are of two types: the adult type, which occurs proximally, usually in the pelvis or femur; and the childhood type, which occurs distal to the elbows or knees and carries a better prognosis.[16,17]

Conservative early management of muscle cysts and childhood-type pseudotumors is indicated, including immobilization and factor replacement. In adult-type pseudotumors, which are usually refractory to conservative therapy, and in progressive childhood pseudotumors, surgical removal is indicated[16] to prevent serious complications, such as spontaneous rupture, fistula formation, neurologic or vascular entrapment, and fracture of adjacent bone. Aspiration of a pseudotumor or cyst is contraindicated.

DIAGNOSTIC IMAGING

RADIOGRAPHS

The earliest radiographic changes in hemophilic arthropathy are confined to the soft tissue and reflect acute hemarthrosis. The joint capsule is distended with displacement of fat pads, and there is an increased hazy density caused by intra-articular blood. Hemarthrosis before epiphyseal plate closure may result in epiphyseal overgrowth and irregularity. Occasionally, premature epiphyseal closure is seen.

With the progression of chronic proliferative synovitis, irreversible radiologic changes appear.[18] These changes reflect the inflammatory and the degenerative nature of chronic hemophilic arthropathy (Table 109-1 and Fig. 109-2A). Certain changes unique to hemophilic arthropathy occur as well (Table 109-1 and Fig. 109-2B). A study of serial radiographs of symptomatic joints in hemophilic patients suggests that serial scoring with conventionally accepted techniques may be a cost-effective alternative to magnetic resonance imaging (MRI) in predicting progressive synovial hypertrophy.[19]

OTHER IMAGING METHODS

MRI is now routinely used to stage hemophilic arthritis accurately to determine optimal treatment and to follow response to therapy.[20] A scoring system based on MRI has been proposed.[21] Additionally, MRI and ultrasonography are useful in the detection and the quantitation of soft tissue bleeding, cysts, and pseudotumors.[22,23]

Table 109-1 Radiologic Manifestations of Chronic Hemophilic Arthropathy

Characteristic	Also Seen in
Periarticular soft tissue swelling	RA
Periarticular demineralization	RA
Marginal erosions	RA
Subchondral irregularity and cyst formation	RA, OA
Decreased joint space	OA
Osteophyte formation	CPPD*
Chondrocalcinosis	

Specific
  Femoral intercondylar notch widening
  Squaring of distal patellar margin (lateral view)
  Proximal radial enlargement (see Fig. 109-2B)
  Talar flattening ± ankle ankylosis†	

CPPD, calcium pyrophosphate deposition disease; OA, osteoarthritis; RA, rheumatoid arthritis.
*From Jensen PS, Putnam CE: Chondrocalcinosis and hemophilia. Clin Radiol 28:401, 1977.
†From Schreiber RR: Musculoskeletal system: Radiologic findings. In Brinkhous KM, Hemker HC (eds): Handbook of Hemophilia, I. New York, American Elsevier, 1975.

PATHOLOGIC FEATURES AND PATHOGENESIS

Pathologic studies of human hemophilic arthropathy have been limited to synovial specimens obtained at surgery[24,25] or at postmortem examination and reflect changes of advanced disease only. Studies of experimentally produced hemarthrosis in animals,[26,27] post-traumatic hemarthrosis in nonhemophilic humans,[28] and canine and murine models of hemophilia A[29-31] have provided an understanding of the earliest changes induced by acute hemarthrosis and their evolution to chronic arthritis.

As reviewed more recently,[32] the process most likely includes catabolic activation of synovial cells by exposure to blood components with subsequent cartilage destruction and a direct destructive effect of intra-articular blood on cartilage. A single synovial hemorrhage induces serial changes in the synovial membrane, including early focal villous synovial proliferation and subsynovial diapedesis of erythrocytes, followed by the appearance of perivascular inflammatory cells, patchy subsynovial fibrosis, and intracellular iron accumulation in synovial cells and subsynovial macrophages. With repeated hemarthroses, the synovium becomes grossly hypertrophied and hyperpigmented, with eventual organization into a pannus that invades and erodes marginal cartilage. On histologic examination, villous hypertrophy and subsynovial fibrosis progress, but inflammatory cells are scarce (Fig. 109-3).[25] Seventy-five percent of synoviocytes contain siderosomes (electron-dense, iron-filled deposits within lysosomes), in contrast to 10% in normal synovium and 25% in rheumatoid synovium.[33] Iron deposits are associated with the production of proinflammatory cytokines and synovial inhibition of the formation of human cartilage matrix. Although the inflammatory synovial changes are mild, the synovial production of proinflammatory mediators, including interleukin-1 and interleukin-6 and tumor necrosis factor-α, approaches that of rheumatoid synovium.[32] The articular cartilage is grossly and microscopically abnormal in the setting of recurrent hemarthrosis.[26] There are areas of cartilaginous fissuring and rarefaction

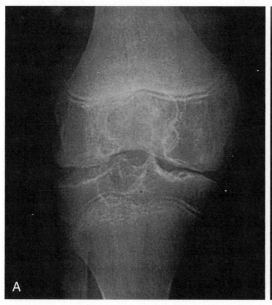 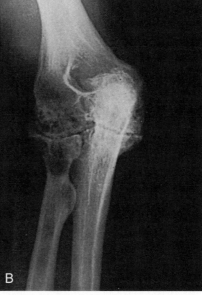

Figure 109-2 Radiographic changes of hemophilic arthropathy. **A,** Early arthritis of the knee, showing soft tissue swelling, widening of the femoral condyles and tibial plateau, irregularity of the distal femoral epiphysis, and a few subchondral bone cysts. **B,** More advanced arthritis involving the elbow, showing almost complete loss of joint space and extensive subchondral cyst formation. The widening of the proximal radius is characteristic of hemophilic arthropathy.

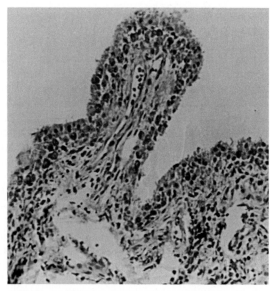

Figure 109-3   Proliferative synovitis of hemophilia. Villous hypertrophy of synovium with pigment deposition in superficial cells. The reaction is mainly synovial cell hyperplasia. Infiltrating inflammatory cells are scarce (Hematoxylin and eosin, ×2500).

exposing sclerotic bone. The remaining cartilage is thin and unevenly distributed, often freely protruding into the joint cavity. Bone erosions appear at weight-bearing surfaces. There is loss of matrix glycosaminoglycan, which also is seen in degenerative arthritis.[25,34]

Current studies suggest that recurrent hemarthrosis induces joint destruction in hemophilic arthropathy through direct and indirect effects of iron on the synovium[33,35] and cartilage,[34,36] by the degradative effect of the proliferative synovium,[37] and through an alteration in cartilage biochemical composition similar to that seen in degenerative arthritis. There may be a relationship between hemarthrosis-induced overexpression of oncogenes (e.g., *c-myc* and *mdm-2*) and the dysregulated, tumor-like proliferation of hemophilic synovium.[38,39]

DIAGNOSIS

In most cases of congenital coagulopathy, the diagnosis has been made before presentation to a rheumatologist. In the case of hemophilia, if there is an affected family member, prenatal diagnosis is possible. Because the spontaneous mutation rate in hemophilia is significant, the diagnosis may not be suspected until infancy, when recurrent, large ecchymoses or sustained oral hemorrhages commonly develop in most affected patients. In the case of hemophilia A or hemophilia B, hemarthrosis is usually a later manifestation, but it may be the initial symptom of other, less severe coagulopathies, even in adulthood. When a coagulopathy is suspected, baseline screening tests, including prothrombin time, activated partial thromboplastin time, and platelet count, should be performed. In patients with hemophilia, the prothrombin time and platelet count are normal, and the activated partial thromboplastin time is prolonged, denoting a defect in the intrinsic clotting cascade. Referral to a hematologist, who obtains the appropriate factor assays, is the next step.

Individuals with factor VIII or IX levels of 1% or less of the normal level have joint and muscle hemorrhages requiring therapy an average four or five times per month. Such patients are classified as having severe hemophilia. Individuals with factor VIII or IX levels greater than 5% of normal are considered to have mild hemophilia and usually bleed only with trauma or at surgery. Occasional "spontaneous" hemarthrosis may occur in such patients, especially in joints damaged by previously undertreated hemorrhage.

Patients whose factor VIII or IX levels fall between these two ranges are considered to have moderately severe hemophilia, and their clinical picture falls somewhere between the extremes. If such patients have had multiple untreated or suboptimally treated hemarthroses with subsequent joint damage, the anatomic instability of these joints would cause frequent and severe bleeding, and the condition would appear clinically more severe than the factor VIII or IX assay might suggest.

TREATMENT OF HEMOPHILIA

Until recent years, in most hemophilia centers factor replacement therapy has been given on demand; that is, factor concentrate has been infused at the earliest sign of a hemorrhage. With the introduction of highly purified, safe concentrates, prophylactic treatment is now much more common in countries where this product is available, especially in pediatric patients.[40,41] Instead of being infused when a hemorrhage has occurred, factor concentrate is given regularly three times per week to prevent bleeds. Prophylaxis is started before any joint damage has occurred, usually at approximately 2 years of age, with the goal of minimizing bleeding episodes to no more than four to six per year. Indwelling catheters, such as Port-A-Cath and Hickman lines, are required for factor administration because frequent venipunctures are painful and cumbersome. More recent data suggest that the institution of prophylactic factor infusion would significantly decrease the long-term joint sequelae of hemophilia and decrease lifetime disability.[42-44]

With adequate factor replacement, all types of surgery, including joint replacements, can be done. Surgical intervention in a patient with hemophilia should be done, however, only at specialized centers with blood bank and coagulation laboratory support and with the participation of a hematologist who specializes in clotting disorders. A surgeon who feels comfortable operating on patients with clotting disorders also is essential. Constant-infusion techniques for administering factor concentrate during and after surgery have made adequate factor levels easier to maintain and have decreased overall perioperative use of factor concentrates.[45] Many types of commercial factor VIII concentrate are available, most of which are manufactured with recombinant technology.

FACTOR VIII REPLACEMENT

All plasma-derived factor concentrates are virally inactivated by various methods, including exposure to solvent detergent, heat, and pasteurization. Recombinant factor VIII concentrates, manufactured by inserting the human factor VIII gene into a mammalian cell line, are widely available and used almost exclusively, especially in developed countiries.[46,47] Because human plasma is not used in their production, transfusion-transmitted diseases, such as hepatitis and HIV-1, are no longer a risk. Recombinant concentrates at doses similar to those of plasma-derived concentrates have been efficacious in the treatment of hemorrhages. Half-life and recovery times for the infused factor VIII are similar to those for plasma-derived concentrates. Current prices range from $0.35 to $0.90 per unit for factor VIII plasma-derived concentrates and from $1.00 to $1.20 per unit for recombinant factor VIII. In most hemophilia centers in the United States, recombinant factor concentrates are the only concentrates used, although high-purity, plasma-derived concentrates are still available. Because these concentrates have made early and intensive home therapy possible, overall costs of health care have greatly declined for patients treated with these materials.

Arginine vasopressin (desmopressin), a vasopressin analogue, can be used in the treatment of mild hemophilia A to increase the endogenous factor VIII level. Desmopressin increases the baseline factor VIII level about threefold, so a baseline level of at least 10% is required for efficacy.[48] Because this is not a blood product, it poses no danger of transmitting blood-borne viruses. Although cryoprecipitate contains factor VIII, its use has been discouraged because it is not virally inactivated. It is less safe than concentrates.

FACTOR IX REPLACEMENT

Factor IX is not found in either cryoprecipitate or factor VIII concentrate; these two materials are totally ineffective for the treatment of hemophilia B. Fresh-frozen plasma does contain factor IX and has been used in the past. Most fresh-frozen plasma products are not virally inactivated, however, and are less safe than factor IX concentrates.

The principles of treatment are similar to those for factor VIII replacement. Because the half-life of factor IX is longer, however, it can be given less frequently. Demand therapy is still commonly used; as for factor VIII deficiency, however, prophylaxis is beginning to be used in pediatric patients. Several plasma-derived factor IX concentrates are available, all virally inactivated. In the past, all such concentrates also contained factors II, VII, and X (prothrombin complex concentrates). Currently, only pure factor IX concentrates are used to treat factor IX deficiency. As with factor VIII concentrates, a recombinant factor IX concentrate is available and is widely used. Recovery is less than that of its plasma-derived counterpart, however, and higher doses (approximately 1.5 times calculated levels) must be infused to reach appropriate levels.

COMPLICATIONS OF FACTOR REPLACEMENT THERAPY

Inhibitor Antibodies

Inhibitor antibodies may develop after exposure to factor concentrate. They occur most often in patients with severe hemophilia after 9 to 30 exposures of replacement therapy, usually before the age of 5 years. There may be a familial predisposition to the development of this complication. Because bleeding cannot be reliably controlled in patients with inhibitor antibodies, elective surgery in these patients should be done only after careful deliberation.

Inhibitor antibodies in factor VIII–deficient hemophiliacs are IgG antibodies (usually IgG4) and may have an unpredictable natural history. Low titer and clinically weak antibodies sometimes are easily neutralized by factor VIII and do not undergo anamnestic increases in titer after multiple factor VIII challenges. Such antibodies may rarely become high in titer. In other patients, antibody titers increase after each exposure to factor VIII. Still other patients seem to lose antibody spontaneously despite multiple subsequent factor VIII challenges. The type of antibody response to factor VIII infusion and the patient's clinical response dictate therapy.

Therapy for patients with inhibitor antibodies has been reviewed more recently.[49] Induction of immune tolerance through frequent administration of factor VIII successfully eliminates inhibitors in 80% of patients. In patients in whom immune tolerance therapy is unsuccessful, there are several approaches for management of acute bleeding episodes, including the administration of activated prothrombin complex concentrate or, more recently, recombinant activated factor VIIa (rVIIa, Novo-Seven; Novo Nordisk, Bagsvaerd, Denmark). rVIIa is thought to function directly at the site of injury, causing activation of factor IX and the extrinsic clotting system locally. Porcine factor VIII, which has limited cross-reactivity with the human antibody, was used previously, but has been removed from the market because of contamination with porcine parvovirus. A recombinant form of this protein is being investigated.

The use of immunosuppressives or glucocorticoids has been abandoned in most centers owing to lack of efficacy in this condition and serious side effects. Regimens of regular factor VIII infusions for induction of tolerance have been successful in eliminating the antibody. It has been suggested by some groups that an immune tolerance regimen be started as early as possible after an inhibitor develops. Rituximab may be useful to suppress inhibitor titers in refractory patients.[50]

Inhibitor antibodies against factor IX are exceedingly rare. There is no generally accepted efficacious therapy. Treatment usually includes large and frequent doses of factor IX concentrate. Induction of immune tolerance with elimination of the antibody also has been used, but with less success than with antibodies to factor VIII. Using large doses of purified factor IX concentrate in some patients with inhibitor antibodies to factor IX has resulted in anaphylactic reactions and nephrotic syndrome secondary to immune complex formation and deposition in the kidney.[51,52]

Human Immunodeficiency Virus

HIV was introduced into the U.S. blood supply in the 1970s. By the late 1970s, factor concentrate was widely contaminated. By 1982, approximately 50% of patients with hemophilia were infected with HIV.[53] Currently, approximately 10% to 20% of American hemophiliacs are infected with HIV. As with other infected individuals, CD4+ lymphocyte counts and HIV titers are used to guide treatment regimens. Since 1985, in the manufacture of plasma-derived concentrates a triple barrier to viral contamination of plasma-derived concentrates has been employed: (1) self exclusion for donors, (2) donor screening with serologic tests for HIV, and (3) viral inactivation during concentrate production. Recombinant concentrates also are now widely available. Acquisition of HIV-1 through factor concentrate in patients with hemophilia has been virtually nonexistent since 1985.

Viral Hepatitis

A second infectious side effect of either cryoprecipitate or factor concentrate is hepatitis, which may be a result of parenterally transmitted hepatitis A, B, C, or G virus; cytomegalovirus; or other as yet unidentified pathogens. In most series, most patients with hemophilia treated before the 1980s have plasma levels of hepatitis B virus surface antibody, and a few (2% to 5%) carry hepatitis B virus surface antigen. Approximately 80% of hemophiliacs transfused before 1990 have antibody to hepatitis C virus,[54] which, in contrast to hepatitis B virus antibody, is a marker for ongoing infection. Virucidal concentrate treatment methods have reduced, but not eliminated, parenteral transmission of hepatitis B and C viruses. Transmission of hepatitis A and G viruses also has been reported with the use of plasma-derived concentrates. Vaccination against hepatitis B and hepatitis A is now recommended for infants born in the United States, and vaccination against hepatitis A is recommended for infants with hemophilia. Transmission of hepatitis has decreased dramatically because almost all pediatric patients are treated with recombinant products.

THERAPY FOR MUSCULOSKELETAL COMPLICATIONS OF HEMOPHILIA

Acute Hemarthrosis

The most important measure in therapy for acute hemarthrosis is prompt correction of the clotting abnormality by administration of the deficient factor. Arthrocentesis, if it is accomplished within 24 hours of the onset of symptoms (but after factor replacement), may be symptomatically beneficial in advanced acute hemarthrosis; however, for diagnostic and potentially therapeutic purposes, it should be considered mandatory at any time if suspicion of infection is high.[12,14] Analgesia and brief joint immobilization for no more than 2 days often aid in pain control. Subsequently, passive range-of-motion isometric exercise should be initiated to reduce the likelihood of joint contracture (Fig. 109-4).

Chronic Hemophilic Arthropathy

Conservative. A variety of conservative measures can bring remarkable benefit in the setting of chronic hemophilic arthropathy,[55-58] including the following:
   Prophylactic factor infusions
   Intensive physical therapy for muscle building and increased joint stability
   Periods of avoidance of weight bearing to allow regression of synovitis
   Correction of flexion contractures by wedging casts, night splints, or the judicious use of traction
   Training in sports to allow future maintenance of muscle mass

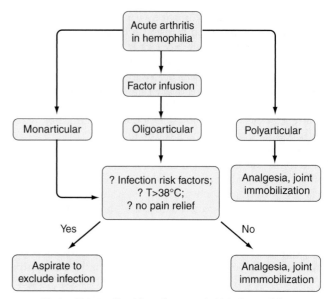

Figure 109-4   Algorithm of acute arthritis in hemophilia.

In modern treatment programs, aspiration of joints with chronic synovial effusions is rarely necessary or of lasting benefit. Failure of these conservative modalities to relieve symptoms or produce regression of synovitis should prompt consideration of other options, including local corticosteroid injections (which have been described as useful more recently),[59] the use of nonsteroidal anti-inflammatory drugs (NSAIDs), synovectomy, and joint replacement in the end stage.

Despite the obvious theoretical contraindications to the use of NSAIDs in hemophilia (i.e., the antiplatelet effects), several NSAIDs may be used safely for short periods as adjuncts to the conservative regimen. Ibuprofen, salsalate, and magnesium salicylate have been shown in a few patients to be safe and efficacious in reducing joint pain and analgesic dependence,[60,61] although long-term regression of synovitis and modification of the course of chronic hemophilic arthropathy have not been shown with any NSAID. The selective cyclooxygenase-2 inhibitors class of NSAIDs do not have significant antiplatelet effects and theoretically should be safer than conventional NSAIDs in patients with hemophilia. Rofecoxib and valdecoxib have been withdrawn from the market because of a causative link to increased risk of cardiovascular events. Although others are in development, celecoxib, the only remaining cyclooxygenase-2 inhibitor on the market, has not been specifically tested in hemophilic patients and, similar to other NSAIDs, should be used with caution.

Synovectomy. Synovectomy in the setting of hemophilic arthritis has been shown to reduce the incidence of recurrent hemarthrosis and the severity of synovitis. This procedure can be accomplished surgically, arthroscopically, or through intra-articular injections of radioactive colloids. Patients should be considered for synovectomy if, despite aggressive conservative measures as outlined previously, persistent hemarthroses continue with ongoing chronic synovitis. In our center, specific indications for synovectomy include persistence of at least two hemarthroses per month in the same joint accompanied by symptoms and signs of chronic synovitis despite at least 4 months of conservative therapy, including intensive factor replacement. The major drawback to surgical synovectomy remains the observation, confirmed in most series,[62,63] that joint motion is reduced postoperatively compared with preoperative baseline joint motion, despite intensive rehabilitation.

To overcome this finding and the high cost of hospitalization and factor replacement therapy attendant with surgical synovectomy, arthroscopic synovectomy has been employed in chronic hemophilic arthritis in recent years. Most follow-up series report that this technique is as successful as surgical synovectomy and results in less loss of motion,[64-66] particularly when continuous passive motion is used in the postoperative period.[67] The total cost of the procedure is less than that of surgical synovectomy, as is the rehabilitation period. Postoperative bleeding after arthroscopic synovectomy has been associated with poor results.

An alternative to surgical or arthroscopic synovectomy is ablation of the synovium using either radioisotopic or chemical agents, as reviewed more recently.[41,68,69] Such a nonoperative approach has been successful in reducing bleeding episodes by 70% to 80% in patients with hemophilia[70] and is especially useful in patients with circulating factor inhibitors, in whom surgery is relatively contraindicated. Commonly used radioisotopes in the United States include colloidal ^{32}P chromic phosphate, yttrium 90, and radioactive colloidal gold (^{198}Au). Theoretical long-term carcinogenic and teratogenic effects remain the major concerns associated with this technique in patients who may have long life expectancies and are still of reproductive age; these effects have limited the use of radioisotopes in the United States, but less so in Europe. Chemical synovectomies using osmic acid, rifampicin, and hyaluronic acid have been attempted in some European centers with modest success, especially in children.[68] The short-term results of radioactive and chemical synovectomies are similar, although long-term outcomes may be superior in radioisotopic synovectomy.[41] Radioactive and chemical synovectomies remain experimental in the United States. Both have the advantages of being minimally invasive, requiring little factor replacement, and resulting in little morbidity, and both are much less expensive than operative procedures.

Total Joint Replacement. Major orthopaedic procedures, including total joint replacements,[71-74] have been employed safely and successfully in end-stage hemophilic arthropathy, including in patients with inhibitor antibodies.[75] The primary indication for total joint replacement is pain in an involved joint that is refractory to all conservative measures. Careful preoperative planning is imperative, including assessment for the presence of inhibitors, planning for factor replacement, and planning for a multidisciplinary rehabilitative program.[76] It is concerning, however, that most hemophilic patients in need of total joint replacement are young and may, if they are not infected with HIV, have a long life expectancy. If the procedure is performed at a young age, this virtually ensures the need for one or more revisions during the patient's lifetime. In addition, patients are at increased risk for complications of surgery because of their underlying coagulopathy, and loosening is observed more commonly than

in nonhemophilic patients in long-term follow-up. These findings suggest that total joint replacement should be reserved for the most severe cases of hemophilic arthropathy and deferred as long as possible. A comprehensive recent review details the many orthopaedic procedures that are now available for alleviating the pain and deformity resulting from hemophilic arthropathy.[77]

CONCLUSION

Gene therapy or repair to cure hemophilia may someday be a reality, although this approach currently is still fraught with serious safety concerns.[78,79] Until then, the best therapy for hemophilic arthropathy remains its prevention, and prevention is now achievable in many patients. With improvement in the safety and availability of factor concentrates, prophylactic infusion is now feasible. Through a combination of prevention of hemarthrosis or correction of the hemostatic defect at the earliest symptom of joint hemorrhage, education of the patient, application of comprehensive care, and emphasis on the importance of physical activity to maintain muscle mass, the incidence of new or progressive arthropathy can be significantly reduced.

REFERENCES

1. Roberts HR, Escobar M, White GC: Hemophilia A and hemophilia B. In Lichtman MA, Beutler E, Kaushansky K, et al (eds): Williams Hematology, 7th ed. New York, McGraw-Hill, 2005, pp 1867-1886.
2. Larrieu MJ, Caen JP, Meyer DO, et al: Congenital bleeding disorders with long bleeding time and normal platelet count, II: Von Willebrand's disease (report of thirty-seven patients). Am J Med 45:354-372, 1968.
3. Ahlberg A, Silwer J: Arthropathy in von Willebrand's disease. Acta Orthop Scand 41:539-544, 1970.
4. Wild JH, Zvaifler NJ: Hemarthrosis associated with sodium warfarin therapy. Arthritis Rheum 19:98-102, 1976.
5. Green D, Ryan C, Malandruccuolo N, et al: Characterization of the coagulant activity of cultured human fibroblasts. Blood 37:47-51, 1971.
6. **Hilgartner MW: Hemophilic arthropathy. Adv Pediatr 21:165-193, 1975.**
7. **Arnold WD, Hilgartner MW: Hemophilic arthropathy: Current concepts of pathogenesis and management. J Bone Joint Surg Am 59:287-305, 1977.**
8. **Gilbert MS: Musculoskeletal manifestations of hemophilia. Mt Sinai J Med 44:339-358, 1977.**
9. Steven MM, Yogarajah S, Madhok SY, et al: Hemophilic arthritis. QJM 58:181-197, 1986.
10. Rodriguez-Merchan EC: Pathogenesis, early diagnosis, and prophylaxis for chronic hemophilic synovitis. Clin Orthop 343:6-11, 1997.
11. Ellison RT, Reller LB: Differentiating pyogenic arthritis from spontaneous hemarthrosis in patients with hemophilia. West J Med 144:42-45, 1986.
12. Gilbert MS, Aledort LM, Seremetis S, et al: Long term evaluation of septic arthritis in hemophilic patients. Clin Orthop 328:54-59, 1996.
13. Merchan EC, Magallon M, Manso F, et al: Septic arthritis in HIV positive haemophiliacs. Int Orthop 16:302-306, 1992.
14. Helm M, Horoszowski H, Seligsohn U, et al: Iliopsoas hematoma: Its detection and treatment with special reference to hemophilia. Arch Orthop Trauma Surg 99:195-197, 1982.
15. Madigan RP, Hanna WT, Wallace SL: Acute compartment syndrome in hemophilia. J Bone Joint Surg Am 63:1327-1329, 1981.
16. Gilbert MS, Kreel I, Hermann G: The hemophilic pseudotumor. In Hilgartner MW, Pochedly C. (eds): Hemophilia in the Child and Adult. New York, Raven Press, 1989.
17. Magallon M, Monteagudo J, Altisent C, et al: Hemophilic pseudotumor: Multicenter experience over a 25-year period. Am J Hematol 45:103-108, 1994.

18. Kilcoyne RF, Nuss R: Radiological evaluation of hemophilic arthropathy. Semin Thromb Hemost 29:43-48, 2003.

19. Ng WH, Chu WCW, Shing MK, et al: Role of imaging in management of hemophilic patients. AJR Am J Roentgenol 184:1619-1623, 2005.

20. **Kilcoyne RF, Nuss R: Radiological assessment of haemophilic arthropathy with emphasis on MRI findings. Haemophilia 9(Suppl 1): 57-64, 2003.**

21. Soler R, Lopez-Fernandez F, Rodriguez E, et al: Hemophilic arthropathy: A scoring system for magnetic resonance imaging. Eur Radiol 12:836-843, 2002.

22. Wilson DA, Prince JR: MR imaging of hemophilic pseudotumors. AJR Am J Roentgenol 150:349-350, 1988.

23. Wilson DJ, McLardy-Smith PD, Woodham CH, et al: Diagnostic ultrasound in haemophilia. J Bone Joint Surg Br 69:103-107, 1987.

24. Ghadially FN, Ailsby RL, Yong NK: Ultrastructure of the hemophilic synovial membrane and electron-probe x-ray analysis of hemosiderin. J Pathol 120:201-208, 1976.

25. Roosendaal G, Mauser-Bunschoten EP, De Kleijn P, et al: Synovium in hemophilic arthropathy. Haemophilia 4:502-505, 1998.

26. Roy S, Ghadially FN: Pathology of experimental hemarthrosis. Ann Rheum Dis 25:402-415, 1966.

27. **Hoaglund FT: Experimental hemarthrosis. J Bone Joint Surg Am 49:285-298, 1967.**

28. Roy S, Ghadially FN: Ultrastructure of synovial membrane in human hemarthrosis. J Bone Joint Surg Am 49:1636-1646, 1967.

29. Swanton MC, Wysocki GP: Pathology of joints in canine hemophilia A. In Brinkhous KM, Hemker HC (eds): Handbook of Hemophilia. Part I. New York, American Elsevier, 1975.

30. Bi L, Lawler AM, Antonarakis SE, et al: Targeted disruption of the mouse factor VIII gene produces a model of haemophilia A. Nat Genet 10:119-121, 1995.

31. Valentino LA, Hakobyan N, Kazarian T, et al: Experimental synovitis in a murine model of human haemophilia. Haemophilia 10:280-287, 2004.

32. **Hoots WK: Pathogenesis of hemophilic arthropathy. Semin Hematol 43(1 Suppl 1):S18-S22, 2006.**

33. Morris CJ, Blake DR, Wainwright AC, et al: Relationship between iron deposits and tissue damage in the synovium: An ultrastructural study. Ann Rheum Dis 45:21-26, 1986.

34. Hough AJ, Banfield WG, Sokoloff L: Cartilage in hemophilic arthropathy. Arch Pathol Lab Med 100:91-96, 1976.

35. Okazaki I, Brinckerhoff CE, Sinclair JF, et al: Iron increases collagenase production by rabbit synovial fibroblasts. J Lab Clin Med 97:396-402, 1981.

36. Choi YC, Hough AJ, Morris GM, et al: Experimental siderosis of articular chondrocytes cultured in vitro. Arthritis Rheum 24:809-823, 1981.

37. Mainardi CL, Levine PH, Werb Z, et al: Proliferative synovitis in hemophilia: Biochemical and morphologic observations. Arthritis Rheum 21:137-144, 1978.

38. Wen FQ, Jabbar AA, Chen YX, et al: c-myc protooncogene expression in hemophilic synovitis: In vitro studies of the effects of iron and ceramide. Blood 100:912-916, 2002.

39. Hakobyan N, Kazarian T, Jabbar AA, et al: Pathobiology of hemophilic synovitis I: Overexpression of mdm2 oncogene. Blood 104:2060-2064, 2004.

40. Berntorp E, Michiels J: A healthy hemophilic patient without arthropathy: From concept to clinical reality. Semin Thromb Hemost 29:5-10, 2003.

41. **Hilgartner MW: Current treatment of hemophilic arthropathy. Curr Opin Pediatr 14:46-49, 2002.**

42. Nilsson IM, Berntorp E, Lofqvist T, et al: Twenty-five years' experience of prophylactic treatment in severe haemophilia A and B. J Intern Med 232:25-32, 1992.

43. Astermark J, Petrini P, Tengborn L, et al: Primary prophylaxis in severe haemophilia should be started at an early age but can be individualized. Br J Haematol 105:1109-1113, 1999.

44. Fischer K, van der Bom J, Mauser-Bunschoten EP, et al: The effects of postponing prophylactic treatment on long-term outcome in patients with severe hemophilia. Blood 99:2337-2341, 2002.

45. Varon D, Martinowitz U: Continuous infusion therapy in hemophilia. Haemophilia 4:431-435, 1998.

46. **White GC, MacMillan CW, Kingdon HS, et al: Use of recombinant hemophilic factor in the treatment of two patients with classic hemophilia. N Engl J Med 320:166-170, 1989.**

47. **Schwartz RS, Agilgaard CF, Aledort LM, et al: Human recombinant DNA derived antihemophilic factor (factor VIII) in the treatment of hemophilia A. N Engl J Med 323:1800-1805, 1990.**

48. Mannucci PM, Ruggeri ZM, Pareti FI, et al: DDAVP in haemophilia. Lancet 2:1171-1172, 1977.

49. Young G: New approaches in the management of inhibitor patients. Acta Haematol 115:172-179, 2006.

50. Mathias M, Khair K, Hann I, et al: Rituximab in the treatment of alloimmune factor VIII and IX antibodies in two children with severe haemophilia. Br J Haematol 125:366-368, 2004.

51. Warrier I: Factor IX antibody and immune tolerance. Vox Sang 77(Suppl 1):70-71, 1999.

52. Ewenstein B, Takemoto C, Warrier I, et al: Nephrotic syndrome as a complication of immune tolerance in hemophilia B. Blood 89:1115-1116, 1997 (letter).

53. Levine PH: The acquired immune deficiency syndrome in persons with hemophilia. Ann Intern Med 103:723-726, 1985.

54. Brettler DB, Alter, Dienstag JL, et al: Prevalence of hepatitis C virus antibody in a cohort of hemophilia patients. Blood 76:254-256, 1990.

55. Miser AW, Miser JS, Newton WA: Intensive factor replacement for management of chronic synovitis in hemophilic children. Am J Pediatr Hematol Oncol 8:66-69, 1986.

56. Buzzard BM: Physiotherapy for prevention and treatment of chronic hemophilic synovitis. Clin Orthop 343:42-46, 1997.

57. Schumacher P: Discussion paper: Orthotic management in hemophilia. Ann N Y Acad Sci 240:344, 1975.

58. Atkins RM, Henderson NJ, Duthie RB: Joint contractures in the hemophilias. Clin Orthop 219:97-106, 1987.

59. Fernandez-Palazzi F, Caviglia HA, Salazar JR, et al: Intraarticular dexamethasone in advanced chronic synovitis in hemophilia. Clin Orthop 343:25-29, 1997.

60. Thomas P, Hepburn B, Kim HC, et al: Non-steroidal anti-inflammatory drugs in the treatment of haemophilic arthropathy. Am J Hematol 12:131-137, 1982.

61. Inwood MJ, Killackey B, Startup SJ: The use and safety of ibuprofen in the haemophiliac. Blood 61:709-711, 1983.

62. Montane I, McCollough NC, Lian EC-Y: Synovectomy of the knee for hemophilic arthropathy. J Bone Joint Surg Am 68:210-216, 1986.

63. Post M, Watts G, Telfer M: Synovectomy in hemophilic arthropathy: A retrospective review of 17 cases. Clin Orthop 202:139-146, 1986.

64. Weidel JD: Arthroscopic synovectomy for chronic hemophilic synovitis of the knee. Arthroscopy 1:205-209, 1985.

65. **Weidel JD: Arthroscopic synovectomy of the knee in hemophilia: 10- to 15-year follow-up. Clin Orthop 328:46-53, 1996.**

66. Klein KS, Aland CM, Kin HC, et al: Long-term follow-up of arthroscopic synovectomy for chronic hemophilic synovitis. Arthroscopy 3:231-236, 1987.

67. Limbird TJ, Dennis SC: Synovectomy and continuous passive motion (CPM) in hemophiliac patients. Arthroscopy 3:74-79, 1987.

68. Heim M: The treatment of intra-articular synovitis by the use of chemical and radioactive substances. Haemophilia 8:369-371, 2002.

69. Schneider P, Farahati J, Reiners C: Radiosynovectomy in rheumatology, orthopedics and hemophilia. J Nucl Med 46(Suppl 1):48S-54S, 2005.

70. Siegel HJ, Luck JV. Jr, Siegel ME, et al: Phosphate-32 colloid radiosynovectomy in hemophilia: Outcome in 125 patients. Clin Orthop 392:409-417, 2001.

71. Birch NC, Ribbans WJ, Goldman E, et al: Knee replacement in haemophilia. J Bone Joint Surg Br 76:165-166, 1994.

72. Kelley SS, Lachiewicz PF, Gilbert MS, et al: Hip arthroplasty in hemophilic arthropathy. J Bone Joint Surg Am 77:828-834, 1995.

73. Thomason HC, Wilson FC, Lachiewicz PF, et al: Knee arthroplasty in hemophilic arthropathy. Clin Orthop 360:169-173, 1999.

74. Norian JM, Ries MD, Karp S, et al: Total knee arthroplasty in hemophilic arthopathy. J Bone Joint Surg Am 84:1138-1141, 2002.

75. Rodriguez-Merchan EC, Wiedel JD, Wallny T, et al: Elective orthopedic procedures for hemophilia patients with inhibitors. Semin Hematol 41(Suppl 1):109-116, 2004.

76. Ingerslev J, Hvid I: Surgery in hemophilia: The general view: Patient selection, timing, and preoperative assessment. Semin Hematol 43(Suppl 1):S23-S26, 2006.
77. Rodriguez-Merchan EC: Orthopedic surgery of haemophilia in the 21st century: An overview. Haemophilia 8:360-368, 2002.
78. Lozier J: Gene therapy of the hemophilias. Semin Hematol 41:287-296, 2004.
79. Gan SU, Kon OL, Calne RY: Genetic engineering for haemophilia A. Exp Opin Biol Ther 6:1023-1030, 2006.

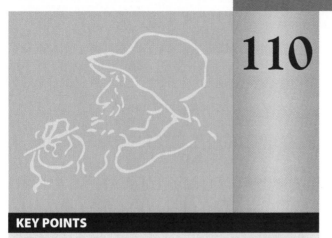

110 Rheumatic Manifestations of Hemoglobinopathies

KENNETH C. KALUNIAN •
BOB SUN

KEY POINTS

Rheumatic manifestations are common in various hemoglobinopathies owing to the profound intravascular effects of these diseases.

Sickle cell disease is associated with arthritis, dactylitis, osteomyelitis, septic arthritis, avascular necrosis (AVN), hyperuricemia, and gout.

Recent studies using magnetic resonance imaging suggest that the prevalence of AVN in sickle cell disease is more than 40%.

Prevalence rates of hyperuricemia in sickle cell disease approach 50%, but gout is rare.

Because of functional asplenia, abnormal opsonization and complement function, and poor antibody responses to polysaccharide components of bacterial capsules, patients with sickle cell disease are predisposed to osteomyelitis with encapsulated organisms.

Precipitation of α-globin chains occurs in the thalassemias, accounting for a variety of bone and joint problems.

Because the maintenance and survival of bone and joint structures are dependent on the proper circulation of blood, rheumatic manifestations are common in various hemoglobinopathies such as sickle cell disease and thalassemias, diseases that have profound intravascular effects. Common bone and joint complications from sickle cell disease include an associated arthritis, dactylitis, osteomyelitis, septic arthritis, avascular necrosis (AVN), hyperuricemia, and gout. In thalassemias, precipitation of α-globin chains occurs, and a variety of clinical manifestations, including bone and joint problems, can arise. Treatment for iron overload, which is common in ß-thalassemia, can also lead to arthropathy.

CAUSE

Sickle cell diseases are an inherited group of disorders that cause production of abnormal hemoglobin. The most widely recognized disorder is sickle cell anemia (HbSS). Other hemoglobinopathies that are common variants of this disease include sickle cell trait (HbSA), sickle cell–hemoglobin C disease (HbSC), and sickle cell–α thalassemia (HbS-αThal). HbSS is a result of the substitution of a valine for glutamic acid as the sixth amino acid of the β-globin chain, which produces a hemoglobin tetramer that is poorly soluble when deoxygenated.[1] HbSC is less common and is caused by the substitution of lysine for glutamine acid in the β-globin chains. Sickling of erythrocytes in small vessels is thought to be responsible for the painful vaso-occlusive crises, with important interactions between erythrocytes and vascular endothelium. Hemolysis and pain caused by vaso-occlusive crises are clinical hallmarks of this disease.[2]

Complications from sickle cell disease can range from pulmonary disorders such as acute chest syndrome to rare hematologic disorders such as hemophagocytic syndrome. Acute chest syndrome is thought to arise from vasoconstriction, which eventually results in chest pain, a new infiltrate on chest radiographs, and fever, usually without bacteremia.[2] It is the most frequently reported cause of death in adults with sickle cell disease. There has been one case report of a patient with sickle cell disease who developed thrombocytopenia, microcytic anemia, elevated ferritin, and hemophagocytic syndrome on biopsy.[3] Complex interactions of sickled cells with endothelium can induce red cell binding to the endothelial cell–receptor complex of glycoproteins Ib, Ix, and V; endothelial CD36; and vascular cell adhesion molecule-1 (VCAM-1), providing potential targets for therapy.[4] Repeated vaso-occlusive crises are thought to significantly contribute to some of these manifestations through decreased blood flow, which can lead to impaired nourishment of critical structures such as the femoral head and vertebral bodies (Fig. 110-1).[5]

ß-Thalassemia is a result of the impaired production of ß-globin chains, which leads to a relative excess of α-globin chains.[6] The degree of impaired ß-globin production leads to various phenotypes of this disease, including ß-thalassemia major, intermedia, and minor. Among the clinical features of patients with ß-thalassemia are hemolytic anemia, which is usually severe and often causes transfusion dependence in homozygotes; splenomegaly; and hyperplastic bone marrow, with changes apparent on skeletal radiographs. These excess α-globin chains are unstable and incapable of forming soluble tetramers on their own.[7]

EPIDEMIOLOGY

Prevalence studies of the various rheumatic manifestations of the hemoglobinopathies are generally limited to reports from small case series. Arthritis associated with HbSS has been studied in a prospective series of 70 patients followed over a 6- to 18-month period; 32 patients developed arthritis that affected primarily the knees and, less commonly, the elbows, hands, and lumbar and sacral spine.[8] In another series, it appeared that by 2 years of age, as many as 45% of all children with HbSS developed dactylitis.[9] The prevalence of osteomyelitis was 12% in a French study of a cohort of 299 patients.[10] The estimated risk of *Salmonella* osteomyelitis in HbSS patients appears to be 100 times greater than

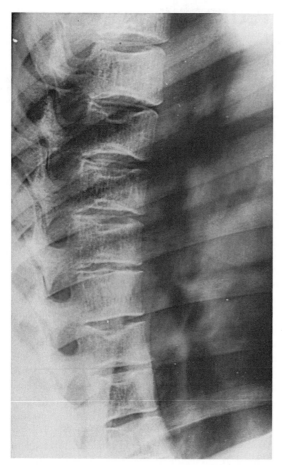

Figure 110-1 Cuplike indentation of vertebral bodies in a radiograph of a patient with sickle cell disease.

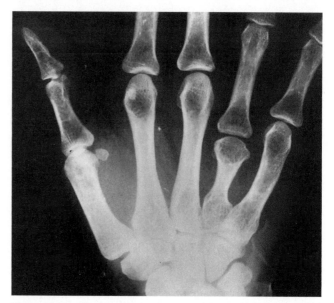

Figure 110-2 Shortened metacarpal in an adult with hemoglobin SC disease. Longitudinal growth of the fourth metacarpal was arrested in childhood as a result of infarction of the growth plate and subsequent premature epiphyseal fusion. *(Courtesy of Richard H. Gold, MD.)*

in the normal population.[11] In some case series, *Staphylococcus aureus* is the most common pathogen responsible for HbSS-related osteomyelitis.[12] AVN of the femoral head is found in individuals of all ages, including children as young as 5 years.[13] The true prevalence of AVN is difficult to estimate because of the lack of sensitive methods for detection. In a study of 2590 patients with HbSS, plain radiographic evidence of AVN of the femoral head was found in 9.8% of patients.[13] In contrast, recent studies using magnetic resonance imaging (MRI) found that the prevalence of AVN was as high as 41% in adults with HbSS.[14] Among adults with HbSS, the prevalence of hyperuricemia appears to be about 50%[15]; however, gout rarely occurs.

Arthritis has been described in patients with ß-thalassemia major. In one case series, 24 of 50 patients from 5 to 23 years of age had ankle joint pain.[16] Up to 52% of patients with ß-thalassemia minor had arthralgias in one case series.[17] In studies of ß-thalassemia patients from the United Kingdom and India treated with deferiprone, the frequency of arthralgias was 33% and 38%, respectively.[18]

PATHOGENESIS

The pathogenesis of some hemoglobinopathy-related rheumatic manifestations is a direct result of the vaso-occlusion caused by the sickling of red blood cells. Hand-foot syndrome, also known as dactylitis, results from repeated vaso-occlusive crises involving the small bones of the hands and feet; it classically presents at about 6 months of age, when hemoglobin S reaches pathologic levels.[19] AVN in HbSS occurs when vaso-occlusion results in infarction of the articular surfaces and heads of the long bones (Fig. 110-2).[20] Progressive occlusion of the microcirculation within the femoral head leads to increased intraosseous pressure and subsequent cell death.[21] Patients with HbSS have functional asplenia, abnormal opsonization and complement function, and poor antibody responses to the polysaccharide components of bacterial capsules.[22] As a result, these patients are predisposed to osteomyelitis with encapsulated organisms such as *Salmonella* and *S. aureus*.[23]

Hyperuricemia and uric acid overproduction are often present and are thought to be due to the high turnover in red blood cells associated with HbSS. The pathogeneses of the arthritis associated with HbSS and thalassemias are unknown, as is the pathogenesis of deferiprone-associated arthralgias.

CLINICAL FEATURES

Episodes of sickle cell crisis are the most common type of vaso-occlusive event. Acute pain is the first symptom of disease in more than 25% of patients and is the most frequent symptom after the age of 2 years.[2] The episodes can affect any area of the body, with the back, chest, abdomen, and extremities being most commonly affected.

Arthritis associated with HbSS involves primarily the knees but can also involve elbows, hands, and the lumbar and sacral spine.[8] Episodes of arthritis correlate temporally with episodes of sickle cell crisis. In one series of 70 patients with HbSS, 32 had arthritis that was thought to be associated with hemoglobinopathy.[8] Of these 32 patients, 13 had synovial fluid studies performed; 8 patients had fluid of an inflammatory type, and 5 five had noninflammatory fluid. The synovial white cell count varied from 600 to 270,000 cells/mm³. None of the patients had synovial evidence of crystals or infection. Most patients had recurrent episodes of arthritis that were transient in nature, with each episode lasting an average of 5 days. However, chronic synovitis with destruction of hyaline articular cartilage has been reported in two patients with sickle cell anemia.[24]

Patients with dactylitis typically experience an acute onset of symmetric swelling of the hands and feet, with mild erythema and a low-grade fever (Fig. 110-3) . In addition, severe anemia and leukocytosis may be present. Radiographic changes are seen an average of 10 days after the onset of symptoms; these consist of subperiosteal new bone formation in the hands and feet. Cortical thinning, multiple irregular intramedullary deposits, and areas of spotty destruction and formation of periosteal new bone may be seen later.[25] These changes can lead to a "moth-eaten" appearance.[25]

In osteomyelitis, many sites can be involved, and the process can be symmetric. The diaphysis is most commonly affected, with occasional epiphyseal involvement and progression to pyarthrosis.[26] Clinically, patients present with persistently high fever, leukocytosis, and severe local pain in the affected bones. Seeding of the bone is usually hematogenous, although infection occasionally spreads locally from a septic joint.

AVN typically affects the femoral heads and, less commonly, the heads of the humeri, knees, and small joints of the hands and feet. Pain and limited motion of the affected joint are usually the first symptoms noted. Pain is constant and increases with weight bearing on the limb when the lower extremities are involved.

Gouty attacks in patients with HbSS, though very rare despite the high frequency of hyperuricemia, are similar to attacks in patients with primary gout. Patients with HbSS are generally younger than patients with primary gout, and urate clearance is greater in younger individuals; this may account for the low frequency of secondary gout in HbSS.[27]

There are descriptions of patients with ß-thalassemia major developing arthritis. One case series reported that 24 of 50 patients from 5 to 23 years of age had ankle joint pain.[16] Two of these patients had effusions that were not inflammatory. Radiographic changes included marked reduction in trabecular and cortical bone, consistent with severe osteoporosis, and the presence of microfractures.[16] Sporadic case reports and series have described the arthropathy of ß-thalassemia minor as an oligoarticular or monarticular process. Gerster and colleagues[28] reported that over a 10-year period, 4 of 32 patients developed acute-onset oligoarticular pain that lasted 2 to 10 days and occurred approximately 2 to 10 times per year. The erythrocyte sedimentation rate was consistently low in all these patients, and joint effusions were found in two of the four patients. Dorwart and Schumacher[29] reported a case of a woman with ß-thalassemia and persistent nonerosive seronegative knee arthritis; synovial fluid analyses in this patient revealed that the fluid was noninflammatory.

Regular blood transfusions are often required for ß-thalassemia; these transfusions often lead to iron overload that requires subsequent treatment with deferiprone to chelate iron and prevent iron-related visceral and cardiac toxicity.[30] A common side effect of deferiprone therapy is arthropathy of the knees. One case series of ß-thalassemia patients treated with deferiprone found that 3 of 16 patients developed bilateral knee pain on exertion, morning stiffness, and joint warmth and swelling.[31] In studies of ß-thalassemia patients treated with deferiprone in the United Kingdom and India, the frequency of arthralgias was 33% and 38%, respectively.[18] Radiography of affected joints revealed joint effusion, subchondral bone irregularity, and patellar beaks. MRI revealed thickening and enhancement of the synovium and irregularly thickened epiphyseal and articular cartilage overlying subchondral bone defects.[18]

DIAGNOSIS AND DIAGNOSTIC TESTS

The histopathology of sickle cell arthropathy has been evaluated using needle synovial biopsies in patients with HbSS-related joint disease.[32] Focal intimal lining cell proliferation and scattered chronic inflammatory cells were identified in most patients. Small vessel congestion, evidence of microvascular thrombosis, and electron microscopic confirmation of occluded vessels was also observed, suggesting that red cells can sickle in the hypoxic environment of the joint.

When considering the diagnosis of a rheumatic manifestation related to hemoglobinopathies, a high index of suspicion for infection is essential. For example, dactylitis and other types of painful vaso-occlusive crises are difficult to distinguish from osteomyelitis. Recent studies have attempted to address the difficulty of distinguishing these entities, focusing on newer imaging modalities. In one study that retrospectively assessed the use of sequential radionuclide bone marrow and bone scans, bone infarction during a vaso-occlusive crisis appeared to be associated with reduced activity of radionuclide on bone marrow scans and corresponding abnormal activity on bone scans.[33] In contrast, acute osteomyelitis resulted in normal activity on bone marrow scans and abnormal activity on bone scans.[33] MRI can also be useful for the diagnosis of acute osteomyelitis. A small study demonstrated that contrast-enhanced MRI might allow one to differentiate between acute infarction and osteomyelitis.[34] Despite advances in imaging modalities, sensitivity and specificity can be limited, and a

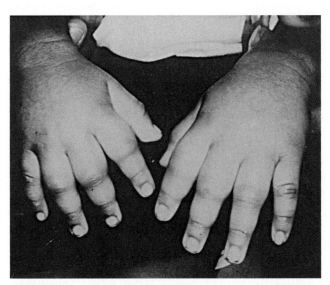

Figure 110-3 Diffusely swollen hands are seen in the hand-foot syndrome of young children with sickle cell disease.

definitive diagnosis of osteomyelitis still depends on clinical assessment combined with positive cultures from blood or bone obtained by aspiration or biopsy.

The diagnosis of AVN is obtained through clinical assessment combined with typical radiographic findings. Initially, radiographs demonstrate local sclerosis near the joint margin. Patchy lucencies then develop and may include a lucency between sclerotic and intact bone. Flattening, separation of the necrotic fragment, and secondary osteoarthritis may be seen later. MRI can detect AVN earlier than plain radiographs and can potentially distinguish it from other causes of acute pain, such as osteomyelitis.

The diagnosis of gout in the setting of hemoglobinopathies is similar to that of idiopathic gout. There are no specific diagnostic tests for arthritis associated with HbSS, ß-thalassemia–related arthritis, or deferiprone-related arthropathy; these diagnoses should be considered when other causes of arthritis, such as septic arthritis, have been excluded.

TREATMENT

For most patients with transient arthritis associated with HbSS crises, treatment usually involves analgesics and hydration. Intra-articular corticosteroids are not useful. There are no data on treatment strategies to prevent or treat chronic synovitis associated with HbSS. Transfusion therapy can improve the oxygen carrying capacity during aplastic or splenic sequestration crisis and can provide protection during acute chest syndrome, but it has not been helpful in treating arthritis associated with HbSS crises. It can, however, decrease the frequency of painful crises. Treatment of dactylitis typically consists of hydration and analgesic and anti-inflammatory medications. Recurrent episodes may warrant the use of hydroxyurea. Antibiotics directed toward the involved pathogen are the optimal treatment for osteomyelitis. *Salmonella* infections respond well to antibiotics, and surgical drainage is generally not required. The treatment of hemoglobinopathy-related gout is the same as the treatment of primary gout. There are no proven treatment approaches for AVN; conservative methods, such as avoidance of weight bearing with crutches and bed rest, have been used; however, these approaches have a drastic impact on quality of life, and their success rates are low.[35] Core decompression is a common procedure used to treat early stages of AVN; however, failure rates in some studies of HbSS-related AVN are as high as 50% at 5 years.[36] Joint replacement is usually required in later stages of AVN.

Evidence of effective treatment strategies for ß-thalassemia–related arthritis is scarce. Nonsteroidal anti-inflammatory drugs and intra-articular corticosteroids appear to be ineffective.[28,29] Arthropathy from deferiprone therapy is usually self-limited; however, if the arthropathy persists, a few case series have reported some success with intra-articular corticosteroid injections.

PROGNOSIS

The prognosis of the various rheumatic manifestations of hemoglobinopathies has not been well defined. However, studies have attempted to identify predictors of adverse outcomes in patients with HbSS. The presence of dactylitis

in a patient with HbSS may suggest a poorer outcome. In an observational study of children with HbSS, dactylitis along with a hemoglobin of less than 7 g/dL and leukocytosis correlated significantly with adverse outcomes later in childhood.[37] Another longitudinal study demonstrated that children diagnosed with dactylitis before the age of 6 months are more likely to have severe events later in life, such as cerebrovascular accident and acute chest syndrome (defined as the presence of a new pulmonary infiltrate, a defect on radionuclide imaging of the chest, or both, in association with an acute respiratory tract illness).[38] Surgical treatment of AVN in HbSS patients can lead to a higher incidence of perioperative complications such as excessive blood loss, acute chest syndrome, and prosthesis failure.[39]

REFERENCES

1. **Bunn HF: Pathogenesis and treatment of sickle cell disease. N Engl J Med 11:762-769, 1997.**
2. Bainbridge R, Higgs DR, Maude GH, et al: Clinical presentation of homozygous sickle cell disease. J Pediatr 106:881-885, 1985.
3. Kio E, Onitilo A, Lazarchick J, et al: Sickle cell crisis associated with hemophagocytic lymphohistiocytosis. Am J Hematol 77:229-232, 2004.
4. Hebbel RP: Blockade of adhesion of sickle cells to endothelium by monoclonal antibodies. N Engl J Med 342:1911, 2000.
5. Smith JA: Bone disorders in sickle cell disease. Hematol Oncol Clin North Am 10:1345-1356, 1996.
6. Adams JG, Coleman MB: Structural hemoglobin variants that produce the phenotype of thalassemia. Semin Hematol 27:229-238, 1990.
7. **Rund D, Rachmilewitz E: ß-Thalassemia. N Engl J Med 353: 1135-1146, 2005.**
8. Espinoza LR, Spilberg I, Osterland CK, et al: Joint manifestations of sickle cell disease. Medicine 53:295-305, 1971.
9. Stevens MC, Padwick M, Serjeant GR: Observations on the natural history of dactylitis in homozygous sickle cell disease. Clin Pediatr 20:311-317, 1981.
10. Neonato MG, Guilloud-Bataille M, Beauvais P, et al: Acute clinical events in 299 homozygous sickle cell patients living in France. French Study Group on Sickle Cell Disease. Eur J Haematol 65:155-164, 2000.
11. Chambers JB, Forsythe DA, Bertrand SL, et al: Retrospective review of osteoarticular infections in a pediatric sickle cell age group. J Pediatr Orthop 20:682-685, 2000.
12. Okorama EO, Agbo DC: Childhood osteomyelitis. Clin Pediatr 23:411-413, 1984.
13. **Milner PF, Kraus AP, Sebeds JI, et al: Sickle cell disease as a cause of osteonecrosis of the femoral head. N Engl J Med 21:1476-1481, 1991.**
14. **Cordner S, De Ceulaer K: Musculoskeletal manifestations of hemoglobinopathies. Curr Opin Rheumatol 15:44-47, 2003.**
15. Reynolds MD: Gout and hyperuricemia associated with sickle cell anemia. Semin Arthritis Rheum 12:404-413, 1983.
16. Gratwick GM, Bullough PG, Bohne WH, et al: Thalassemic osteoarthropathy. Ann Intern Med 88:494-501, 1978.
17. Arman MI, Butun B, Doseyen A, et al: Frequency and features of rheumatic findings in thalassemia minor: A blind controlled study. Br J Rheumatol 31:197, 1992.
18. **Kellenberger CJ, Schmugge M, Saurenmann T: Radiographic and MRI features of deferiprone-related arthropathy of the knees in patients with ß-thalassemia. Am J Radiol 183:989-994, 2004.**
19. Gill FM, Sleeper LA, Weiner SJ, et al: Clinical events in the first decade in a cohort of infants with sickle cell disease. Cooperative Study of Sickle Cell Disease. Blood 86:776-783, 1995.
20. Mukisi-Mukaza M, Elbaz A, Samuel-Leborgne Y, et al: Prevalence, clinical features, and risk factors of osteonecrosis of the femoral head among adults with sickle cell disease. Orthopedics 23:357-363, 2000.
21. Hawker H, Neilson H, Hayes RJ, et al: Haematological factors associated with avascular necrosis of the femoral head in homozygous sickle cell disease. Br J Haematol 50:29-34, 1982.
22. **Aguilar C, Vichinsky E, Neumayr L: Bone and joint disease in sickle cell disease. Hematol Oncol Clin North Am 19:929-941, 2005.**

23. Burnett MW, Bass JW, Cook BA: Etiology of osteomyelitis complicating sickle cell disease. Pediatrics 101:296-297, 1998.
24. Schumacher HR, Dorwart BB, Bond J, et al: Chronic synovitis with early cartilage destruction in sickle cell disease. Ann Rheum Dis 36:413-419, 1977.
25. Babhulkar SS, Pande K, Babhulkar B: The hand-foot syndrome in sickle-cell haemoglobinopathy. J Bone Joint Surg 77:310-312, 1995.
26. Anand AJ, Glatt AI: Salmonella osteomyelitis and arthritis in sickle cell disease. Semin Arthritis Rheum 24:211-221, 1994.
27. Diamond HS, Meisel A, Sharon E, et al: Hyperuricosuria and increased tubular secretion of urate in sickle cell anemia. Am J Med 59:796-802, 1975.
28. Gerster JC, Dardel R, Guggi S: Recurrent episodes of arthritis in thalassemia minor. J Rheumatol 11:352-354, 1984.
29. Dorwart BB, Schumacher HR: Arthritis in β thalassaemia trait: Clinical and pathological features. Ann Rheum Dis 40:185-189, 1981.
30. **Kontoghiorghes GJ, Pattichi K, Hadjigavriel M, et al: Transfusional iron overload and chelation therapy with deferoxamine and deferiprone (L1). Transfus Sci 23:211-223, 2000.**
31. **Berkovitch M, Laxer RM, Inman R, et al: Arthropathy in thalassaemia patients receiving deferiprone. Lancet 343:1471-1472, 1994.**
32. Schumacher HR, Andrews R: McLaughin G: Arthropathy in sickle cell disease. Ann Intern Med 78:203, 1973.
33. Skaggs DL, Kim SK, Greene NW, et al: Differentiation between bone infarction and acute osteomyelitis in children with sickle-cell disease with use of sequential radionuclide bone-marrow and bone scans. J Bone Joint Surg 83:1810-1813, 2001.
34. Umans H, Haramati N, Flusser G: The diagnostic role of gadolinium enhanced MRI in distinguishing between acute medullary bone infarct and osteomyelitis. Magn Reson Imaging 18:255-262, 2000.
35. Garino JP, Steinberg ME: Total hip arthroplasty in patients with avascular necrosis of the femoral head: A 2- to 10-year follow-up. Clin Orthop Relat Res 334:108-115, 1997.
36. Bishop AR, Roberson JR, Eckman JR, et al: Total hip arthroplasty in patients who have sickle-cell hemoglobinopathy. J Bone Joint Surg 70:853-855, 1988.
37. **Miller ST, Sleeper LA, Pegelow CH, et al: Prediction of adverse outcomes in children with sickle cell disease. N Engl J Med 342:83-89, 2000.**
38. **Foucan L, Ekouevi D, Etienne-Julan M, et al: Early onset dactylitis associated with the occurrence of severe events in children with sickle cell anaemia. The Paediatric Cohort of Guadeloupe. Paediatr Perinat Epidemiol 20:59-66, 2006.**
39. Vichinsky EP, Neumayr LD, Haberkern C, et al: The perioperative complication rate of orthopedic surgery in sickle cell disease: Report of the National Sickle Cell Surgery Study Group. Am J Hematol 62:129-138, 1999.

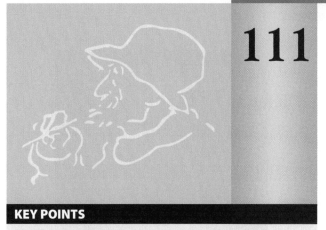

111 Arthritis Accompanying Endocrine and Metabolic Disorders

JOHN S. SERGENT

KEY POINTS

The diabetic stiff hand syndrome (cheirarthropathy) is related to both the duration of disease and the degree of hyperglycemia. It is predictive of other end-organ complications of diabetes.

Other important complications of diabetes affecting the musculoskeletal system include frozen shoulder, Charcot joints, especially in the feet, Dupuytren's contractures, trigger fingers, and diabetic amyotrophy, also known as diabetic muscle infarction.

Patients with mild primary hyperparathyroidism may present with fractures due to osteoporosis as their initial symptom, and patients with unexplained osteoporosis should also be screened for hyperparathyroidism.

Renal osteodystrophy is largely a complication of secondary hyperparathyroidism due to phosphate retention, among other factors.

Proximal weakness, which can be profound and intermittent, is commonplace in hyperthyroidism from any cause, and patients with unexplained weakness should also be screened for hyperthyroidism.

Hyperthyroidism can cause myopathy as well, and may be associated with elevated creatine kinase levels, but the degree of weakness is usually mild to moderate.

Hypothyroid arthropathy is associated with viscous joint effusion, usually in joints previously affected by osteoarthritis. It resolves quickly with correction of the hypothyroidism.

Carpal tunnel syndrome can be the first symptom of several endocrine disorders, including diabetes mellitus, acromegaly, and hypothyroidism.

Complications of exogenous corticosteroid therapy include osteoporosis, avascular necrosis, and steroid myopathy.

Untreated acromegaly is virtually always associated with severe osteoarthritis and degenerative disk disease.

A rheumatologist or primary care physician must always be cognizant of the many ways that systemic diseases affect muscles and joints. These may be manifest in numerous ways, as follows:

1. A primary endocrine or metabolic disorder may occur with important musculoskeletal problems (e.g., proximal muscle weakness in Cushing's syndrome, carpal tunnel syndrome in diabetes mellitus, and acromegaly).
2. A patient with long-standing endocrine or metabolic disease may develop musculoskeletal complications (e.g., diabetic stiff-hand syndrome).
3. A patient with a well-established rheumatic disease may develop an endocrine disorder (e.g., hypothyroidism in scleroderma).
4. An endocrine or metabolic disorder may develop as a result of therapy for a rheumatic disease (e.g., iatrogenic Cushing's syndrome).

Many of these disorders can be subtle when occurring in previously normal individuals. When they occur in association with preexisting rheumatic disease, or when their manifestations are atypical, considerable skill is often necessary to establish the diagnosis.

DIABETES MELLITUS

Diabetes mellitus is associated with a wide variety of complications involving joints. In many of these complications, there is a direct cause; in others, there is a reported epidemiologic association, although the actual cause-and-effect relationship is unproven (Table 111-1).

The hand is an important target for diabetic complications. The diabetic stiff-hand syndrome, also known as diabetic cheirarthropathy and the limited joint-mobility syndrome, is a common complication of type 1 and type 2 diabetes mellitus (Fig. 111-1).[1] The condition is believed to be due to excessive glycosylation of collagen in the skin, blood vessels, and periarticular structures[2] and to decreased collagen degeneration and removal,[3] resulting in thick, inelastic tissues. In its advanced stages, the fingers remain permanently contracted at the metacarpophalangeal and proximal interphalangeal joints, and the thick, shiny skin may resemble that of scleroderma.[4] This complication, usually only bothersome and not disabling, increases in association with the duration of the disease.[5] As might be expected, it is predictive of renal, retinal, and other diabetic complications[6,7] and occurs in 30% of patients with long-standing diabetes.[8] Therapy with aldose reductase inhibitors has been reported to be beneficial for the stiff-hand syndrome[9] and has improved nerve conduction in diabetic neuropathy,[10] but further use has been limited by side effects.

Dupuytren's contractures may be seen in patients with diabetic stiff-hand syndrome, or they may occur independently. It is thought that the pathogenesis is similar to stiff-hand syndrome, with glycosylation and increased collagen deposition playing a role. In contrast to most cases of stiff-hand syndrome, Dupuytren's contractures may be seen early in the course of the disease. The prevalence of Dupuytren's contractures in adult diabetics is about 30%.[8]

Trigger fingers, a catching and snapping of the fingers, occasionally painful, also is frequent in diabetic patients. This complication is due to flexor tenosynovitis and believed to have the same pathogenesis as stiff-hand syndrome.[11]

Table 111-1 Joint Complications of Diabetes Mellitus

Manifestation	Typical Joint Involved
Diabetic stiff-hand syndrome	Metacarpophalangeal, proximal interphalangeal joints
Dupuytren's contractures	Fourth (and other) flexion tendons
Trigger fingers	Flexor tendons
Adhesive capsulitis	Shoulders
Reflex sympathetic dystrophy	Shoulders, hands
Carpal tunnel syndrome	First 4 fingers
Charcot's arthropathy	Foot, ankle
Diffuse idiopathic skeletal hyperostosis	Spine
Osteomyelitis	Foot
Diabetic angiotrophy	Shoulder, back, thighs

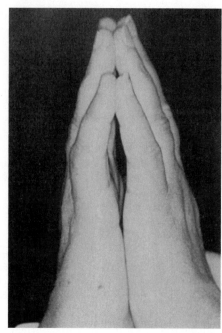

Figure 111-1 The prayer sign in the diabetic stiff-hand syndrome. As a result of progressive thickening of tendons, joint capsules, and subcutaneous tissues, progressive stiffness and flexion contractures develop in these patients.

Adhesive capsulitis of the shoulders, with or without calcific tendinitis, is well established as a complication of diabetes.[12,13] It can be associated with reflex sympathetic dystrophy.[14] Although sometimes associated with recurrent painful tendinitis and bursitis, the loss of motion can be painless and insidious.

Carpal tunnel syndrome occurs in about 25% of individuals with diabetes mellitus[8] and can be subtle, especially in patients with preexisting peripheral neuropathy. Because nocturnal paresthesias are common in both, the clinician must be alert to the possibility of carpal tunnel syndrome to intervene early in disease to prevent thenar muscle atrophy.

Charcot's arthropathy in diabetes usually involves the ankle or midfoot and invariably occurs in individuals with sensory neuropathy.[15] The onset can be sudden,[16] occasionally in association with minor trauma. The abrupt onset, with swelling and radiographs showing the bone fragments and disorganization, can lead an unwary clinician on an unnecessary search for infection. As with Charcot joints of other causes, treatment is generally unsatisfactory, with little more to offer than splinting and bracing.

Diffuse idiopathic skeletal hyperostosis (see Chapter 93) is associated with diabetes, although it is unclear whether the relationship is to diabetes per se, relative insulin resistance, or other factors that make up the metabolic syndrome. This complication is seen most prominently in obese patients with type 2 diabetes. It also has been seen in nondiabetic individuals with abnormal insulin responses to hyperglycemia.[17] It is manifest by proliferative new bone formation at joint margins, particularly in the axial skeleton. Clinically, patients may have diminished mobility similar to that seen in ankylosing spondylitis. There is no evidence to date that diabetic control improves the condition or delays diffuse idiopathic skeletal hyperostosis, although no careful studies have yet been done to evaluate the relationship. The pathophysiologic mechanism of the condition also has not yet been elucidated, although it may be related more to hyperlipidemia and other metabolic factors than to diabetes itself.[18,19]

Osteomyelitis in the foot is a major problem in long-standing diabetics. Because of the peripheral sensory neuropathy, foot injuries and pressure ulcers tend to be underappreciated, and patients may not realize anything is seriously wrong until advanced osteomyelitis has developed. In addition, subcutaneous foreign bodies, such as needles and splinters, can be present for weeks or months before a diabetic patient is aware of them. There is good evidence that infections and other complications of these problems can be markedly diminished by meticulous foot care.[20,21]

Diabetic amyotrophy, also known as diabetic muscle infarction, is a rare condition associated with the abrupt onset of pain and rapid atrophy in large muscle groups, usually the thighs, the perispinous muscles, and the shoulder girdle.[22,23] Fasciculations are often prominent, and electromyography reveals a neuropathic picture. Severe pain is the most frequent complaint, although profound weakness of the affected muscles also is a problem. This problem slowly resolves in most cases.

PARATHYROID DISORDERS

Hyperparathyroidism has major effects on the skeleton, the most important of which is osteopenia (see Chapter 92). The most important joint manifestation of primary hyperparathyroidism is chondrocalcinosis with associated calcium pyrophosphate dihydrate deposition disease (see Chapter 88).[24] Although the most common arthritic manifestation is acute pseudogout, the entire spectrum of arthropathies associated with calcium pyrophosphate dihydrate may be seen in this disorder, including a crippling and slowly progressive polyarthritis.[25]

Most patients with long-standing hyperparathyroidism have proximal muscle weakness, a condition rapidly reversed by removal of the parathyroid adenoma.[26,27] In these patients, the muscle enzymes are normal, and electromyography and muscle biopsy show a picture most consistent with denervation.

Patients with secondary hyperparathyroidism associated with advanced renal disease have numerous abnormalities in the bones and joints. The changes of renal osteodystrophy resulting from secondary hyperparathyroidism include an erosive arthritis in the hands,[28] resorption of the distal clavicle,[29] and erosions in the axial skeleton.[30] In children, the widespread bone deformities of osteitis fibrosa cystica can be crippling.[31] Other musculoskeletal manifestations of advanced renal failure include aluminum-induced osteomalacia[32] and β_2-microglobulin amyloidosis (see Chapter 92).

Hypoparathyroidism, usually secondary to surgical removal of the parathyroid glands, most commonly causes proximal muscle weakness related to the degree of hypocalcemia. This condition responds dramatically to treatment with vitamin D and calcium. Idiopathic hypoparathyroidism is a rare disorder, usually seen as part of the DiGeorge syndrome with thymic hypoplasia.

Pseudohypoparathyroidism, known as Albright's hereditary osteodystrophy, is due to end-organ resistance to the effect of parathyroid hormone. These patients have persistent hypocalcemia and hyperphosphatemia, but parathyroid hormone levels are consistently elevated.

Type Ia pseudohypoparathyroidism, which is autosomal dominant, is associated with short stature, calcification of the perispinal ligaments, and, usually, mental retardation. Most patients have an impressive shortening of the fourth metacarpal and metatarsal bones that can be seen by having the patient clench the fist. Instead of the usual knuckle appearance over the fourth metacarpal head, these individuals have a dimple. Patients with type Ib pseudohypoparathyroidism also have resistance to parathyroid hormone, but have normal phenotype.

Patients with pseudohypoparathyroidism have a defect in the genes encoding the alpha subunit of the cell membrane–associated guanine nucleotide stimulating unit of adenyl cyclase.[33] Type Ia pseudohypoparathyroidism is almost always inherited maternally,[34] and type Ib is inherited paternally.[35] The musculoskeletal manifestations of osteomalacia and rickets are covered in Chapter 92.

THYROID DISORDERS

Hyperthyroidism (Graves' disease) may affect the musculoskeletal system in several ways. The most common complication is osteopenia and frank osteoporosis, which can be a major problem in patients with idiopathic Graves' disease or in patients with iatrogenic hyperthyroidism.[36] Failure to recognize the declining need for thyroid replacement with age is an important cause of iatrogenic hyperthyroidism in older women. For that reason, patients with hypothyroidism who are on thyroid hormone and estrogen therapy should have thyroid-stimulating hormone levels monitored and the dose readjusted to keep the thyroid-stimulating hormone level within the normal range.[37,38] Bone density has been shown to increase after correction of the hyperthyroid state.[39]

Pretibial myxedema is a syndrome of painless nodules that occur over the pretibial areas. Virtually all affected patients have concomitant Graves' ophthalmopathy.[40] The lesions vary in size, ranging from nodules of 1-cm diameter to very large lesions covering most of the pretibial surface. They are variably colored, ranging from pink to a light purple hue, and can mimic erythema nodosum. In contrast to erythema nodosum, these lesions are painless. They are caused by the accumulation of hyaluronic acid in the skin,[41] and in some cases they have a shiny appearance resembling scleroderma or morphea.

Hyperthyroidism also can be associated with numerous changes in the nails,[42] including onycholysis, or elevation of the nail from the nail bed, and clubbing. Clubbing is usually part of the condition known as thyroid acropachy, a rare manifestation of hyperthyroidism also associated with periostitis around the metacarpal joints and distal soft tissue swelling of the digits. The condition is not clearly related to the levels of thyroid hormone because it may be seen after the patient has reverted to the euthyroid state.

Proximal muscle weakness is a common complication of hyperthyroidism and is present in most patients. Most of these patients have lost weight and have other evidence of loss of muscle mass. The proximal muscle weakness corrects rapidly with correction of the hyperthyroid state.[43] Perhaps related to the proximal myopathy, adhesive capsulitis of the shoulder seems to be increased in patients with hyperthyroidism. In these patients, the condition can be insidious and difficult to treat, with frozen-shoulder syndrome often the initial manifestation.

There are strong relationships between Graves' disease and Hashimoto's disease and other rheumatic diseases. Seventy-five percent to 90% of patients with Graves' disease[44] and a smaller percentage of patients with Hashimoto's thyroiditis have antinuclear antibodies, and many have anti-DNA antibodies as well, despite the fact that overt systemic lupus erythematosus (SLE) is uncommon. There is a true increased incidence of hypothyroidism in patients with scleroderma, and there is some evidence that other rheumatic diseases also are associated with an increased incidence, including SLE, rheumatoid arthritis (RA), mixed connective tissue disease, Sjögren's syndrome, and polymyositis.

Graves' disease is associated with HLA-B8, HLA-A1, HLA-Cw7, and HLA-DR3, and combinations of these antigens correlate with persistent disease.[45] Hashimoto's disease is associated with HLA-B8, HLA-DR3, HLA-Aw30, and HLA-DR5. These diseases occur with increased frequency in individuals with other autoimmune diseases that are associated with these HLA antigens.[46]

Hypothyroidism in its idiopathic form is almost always caused by Hashimoto's thyroiditis and can be associated with an unusual arthropathy. Patients present with swelling and stiffness in large joints, usually the knees. The hands also may be involved, and this is often very impressive in joints previously involved with osteoarthritis. Examination of the swollen joint reveals a thick, gelatinous sensation that causes a very slow fluid wave (bulge sign). Synovial thickening on palpation can be impressive. Aspiration of the fluid from patients with the arthropathy of myxedema reveals noninflammatory fluid that is extremely viscous with very high hyaluronic acid levels. Calcium pyrophosphate dihydrate crystals may be present, but inflammation is not.[47] This arthropathy resolves quickly with correction of the hypothyroid state.

The myopathy of hypothyroidism can be confusing. Many patients have proximal muscle weakness; however, some complain only of generalized lassitude and fatigue. In one study, 25% of hypothyroid patients had muscle symptoms, although creatine kinase levels were usually normal.[48] Occasionally, levels can be quite elevated, and rhabdomyolysis has been reported.[49] Muscle biopsy specimens are usually normal, although moderate inflammatory changes are sometimes present.[50] This condition can resemble either polymyalgia rheumatica or polymyositis, depending on the predominance of stiffness versus weakness.

Carpal tunnel syndrome is increased in patients with hypothyroidism, and in one study hypothyroidism was present in 7% of patients with carpal tunnel syndrome.[51] It is frequent enough that most patients with idiopathic carpal tunnel syndrome should be screened for early myxedema.

Because of all these considerations, the clinician encountering patients with musculoskeletal complications must always keep thyroid disorders in mind. Many of these conditions can be subtle, and the musculoskeletal manifestations—ranging from myopathy to pretibial myxedema to frank arthropathies—can be the presenting manifestation of thyroid disorders.

ADRENAL DISORDERS

Iatrogenic Cushing's syndrome secondary to exogenous glucocorticoid therapy of an underlying inflammatory disease is the most common condition involving adrenal hormones seen in patients with rheumatic diseases (see Chapter 55). A few complications of iatrogenic Cushing's syndrome warrant special comment.

Osteonecrosis is a common late complication of glucocorticoid therapy[52] and may first become evident months or years after glucocorticoid therapy has been discontinued. It also can be seen following short courses of therapy, however, or after intermittent high-dose intravenous therapy.[53] Because many patients receiving glucocorticoid therapy have diseases associated with joint pain, the clinician must be alert to this condition. When it affects the hip, which is the most common joint involved, the pain is usually dull, located in the groin, increased by weight bearing, and progressive. An increased incidence of osteonecrosis has been seen in patients on replacement glucocorticoid therapy, pointing out the need to treat with the lowest acceptable dose of the drug.[54]

Steroid myopathy can be particularly perplexing in patients being treated for primary or secondary inflammatory myopathies. Steroid myopathy is characteristically more severe in the pelvic girdle and can be so severe that patients are bedridden. It may come on gradually or abruptly, heralded by weakness and muscle aching. Biopsy specimens show type II fiber atrophy, and muscle enzymes are normal. There is evidence that longer acting and fluorinated compounds are more likely to cause myopathy.[55] When myopathy has developed, it usually requires nearly total discontinuation of the glucocorticoids before any improvement is seen, and even then it may be weeks or months before strength begins to return.

Osteopenia (see Chapters 55 and 92) is related to the dose and the duration of glucocorticoid therapy. No "safe" dose has yet been established. Because osteoporosis can develop rapidly after beginning glucocorticoid therapy, prophylaxis is recommended in most patients. Regimens shown to be effective at preventing or treating glucocorticoid-induced osteoporosis include calcium and vitamin D_3,[56] calcitonin,[57] and bisphosphonates.[58,59]

Idiopathic Cushing's syndrome may be confused with primary musculoskeletal disease. More than 50% of patients have muscle weakness, and a similar percentage have back pain, often secondary to osteoporotic fractures. In patients with Cushing's syndrome secondary to ectopic adrenocorticotropic hormone production, glucocorticoid levels may be extremely high, resulting in profound myopathy and other features such as steroid psychosis. Because weight loss, rather than typical centripetal obesity, is often present in these patients, the appearance may not be typical of idiopathic Cushing's syndrome of pituitary origin.

Other effects of glucocorticoids on the musculoskeletal system are less well understood. Some patients complain of intense joint pain, usually most severe in the knees, when high doses of glucocorticoids are first administered. This pain typically resolves even if the dose is left unchanged.

The so-called steroid withdrawal syndrome consists of widespread arthralgias, myalgias, malaise, and sometimes low-grade fever.[60] It may be seen when glucocorticoids have been used for nonrheumatic conditions, such as asthma or inflammatory bowel disease, and does not require suppression of the pituitary-adrenal axis. Finally, the abrupt reduction of the dose of a glucocorticoid can cause a severe rebound flare in the underlying disease. This may be seen even though the dose of the glucocorticoid remains in the pharmacologic range.

Patients with idiopathic Addison's disease present with weakness, weight loss, abdominal pain, hyperpigmentation, nausea, and hypotension. Iatrogenic Addison's disease can be much more subtle. Because mineralocorticoids are still being produced, salt wasting, hyperkalemia, and postural hypotension are usually less impressive, and hyperpigmentation is not seen because the pituitary is suppressed. As in idiopathic Addison's disease, the features may not be impressive unless the individual undergoes a second exogenous stress, such as surgery or an infection. In that setting, addisonian crisis has been seen even in individuals still receiving physiologic or "replacement" doses of glucocorticoids. It should be assumed that individuals taking glucocorticoids at more than the equivalent of 5 mg/day of prednisone have a pituitary-adrenal axis unable to respond to severe stress, and appropriate increases in the glucocorticoid dose should be considered. In addition, the development of idiopathic Addison's disease in individuals receiving low-dose glucocorticoids can result in similar diagnostic difficulty.[61]

ACROMEGALY

Growth hormone levels tend to decline with age, and there is evidence that treatment of the elderly with growth hormone increases muscle mass[62] and, in some cases, increases bone density as well. At this time, the most important musculoskeletal manifestations related to growth hormone are those seen in acromegaly.

Growth hormone is secreted primarily in nocturnal pulses, and it stimulates hepatocytes to produce somatomedin C, or insulin-like growth factor. Somatomedin C has variable effects on adult tissues, but osteocytes, chondrocytes, and fibroblasts all are responsive in adults. Acromegaly, caused by an adenoma in the anterior pituitary gland, is an insidious disease, and often years have passed before the diagnosis is made. During those years, a variety of musculoskeletal consequences have usually developed.

Carpal tunnel syndrome occurs in about half of patients with acromegaly and is one of the few musculoskeletal manifestations that may develop early in the disease course.[63] It is due to enlargement of the nerve and to expansion of the transverse carpal ligament and other soft tissues. Raynaud's phenomenon owing to compression of the distal arteries by soft tissues occurs in about one third of patients with acromegaly.

If the diagnosis is not made early, and it rarely is, premature osteoarthritis almost inevitably develops. The knee is the most frequently involved joint, followed by the hip and the spine. The hypertrophied cartilage tends to fissure and ulcerate, and the ligaments of the knee become elongated and lax. This combination of instability and abnormal cartilage can lead to severe disability.[64] Other areas affected include the temporomandibular joints and the small joints of the hands and feet. The reason that glove size increases in acromegalics is not because bones grow; it is because cartilage in each joint increases in thickness, and the soft tissues proliferate.

The early radiographic picture of acromegalic joints shows joint space widening as a result of cartilage hypertrophy. In the spine, disk spaces also may be widened. Later, as the inevitable degeneration occurs, the changes are indistinguishable from those of idiopathic osteoarthritis.

Back pain is a particularly troubling feature of acromegaly. Most patients complain of dull, diffuse pain in the lumbar spine. The pain does not radiate into the legs and is often present at rest and with activity. These changes are caused by several factors, including disk space enlargement, osteophyte production, and ligamentous calcifications. Some patients improve when growth hormone levels are reduced after surgery, radiation, or treatment with a somatostatin analogue.[65]

Most acromegalic patients develop proximal muscle weakness, which is occasionally an early symptom. Muscle enzymes are normal. Biopsy specimens show no inflammation, but do reveal abnormal variations in fiber size.

PREGNANCY

The pregnant state produces a complex series of musculoskeletal changes in normal individuals. Probably the most common is the near-universal problem of low back pain, especially during the third trimester. This pain is believed to be primarily mechanical in nature and is due to the increased lumbar lordosis. In addition, the increased mobility of the sacroiliac and other joints of the pelvic girdle, under the influence of the hormone relaxin, may be a factor in many women.

Carpal tunnel syndrome is common in the last trimester, resulting primarily from increased fluid retention. It is usually mild and responsive to wrist splints. It resolves quickly after delivery.

Pregnancy has impressive effects in patients with inflammatory rheumatic diseases. Virtually all the rheumatic diseases, especially RA and SLE, have been reported to develop in the early postpartum period.

There is evidence that rheumatoid factor positivity during pregnancy predicts subsequent RA.[66] This finding could be interpreted in several ways, but a likely interpretation is that the pregnant state itself has delayed the clinical onset of the disease until the postpartum period. In other words, the true incidence of RA may be unaffected by pregnancy, but the time of its onset is. This observation would be compatible with the well-known improvement in the course of RA in about three fourths of patients when they become pregnant. This improvement usually begins in the first trimester, but virtually all patients relapse in the first 3 or 4 months postpartum. Many investigators have attempted to explain this amelioration of the disease during the pregnant state. HLA incompatibilities in DRB1, DQA1, and DQB1 all have been associated with a greater likelihood of disease improvement during pregnancy.[67] In addition, cytokines are affected by the pregnant state. Interleukin-2 production is decreased, and production of soluble tumor necrosis factor receptors is increased.[68]

In other rheumatic diseases, the situation during pregnancy is more complex. In SLE, fetal wastage is increased, and there is some evidence that the disease is more apt to flare during the postpartum period. The relationship between SLE and pregnancy is discussed in detail in Chapter 75.

The use of hormone therapy to treat rheumatic diseases has had a stormy history. Based partly on murine studies showing that SLE can be made worse by estrogen and improved by androgen,[69] SLE has been the subject of extensive study. Patients with SLE metabolize the active metabolite of estrogen (i.e., estrone) preferentially to the feminizing metabolites 16-hydroxyestrone and estriol.[70] In addition, there is some evidence that testosterone levels are lower and that inactive forms predominate.[71] This has led to some interest in using dehydroepiandrosterone, which also has been reported to be low in patients with SLE, in treatment of fatigue and other manifestations of the disease.[72]

The role of birth control pills also has been investigated. Studies have suggested that oral contraceptive use diminishes the lifetime risk of RA.[73] In contrast, SLE may flare more often in women taking birth control pills containing estrogen.[74] If progesterone-only birth control pills are used, however, SLE activity may be decreased. At this time, the decision to use oral contraceptives in patients with SLE requires careful considerations of the risks, which are probably small, versus the benefits. If an oral contraceptive is chosen, the lowest effective dose of estrogen or a progesterone-only preparation should be used.[75] There is no evidence to suggest that postmenopausal hormone replacement therapy with estrogen adversely affects the course of SLE.

REFERENCES

1. Kapoor A, Sibbitt WL Jr: Contractures in diabetes mellitus: The syndrome of limited joint mobility. Semin Arthritis Rheum 18:168, 1989.
2. Sheetz MJ, King GL: Molecular understanding of hyperglycemia adverse effects for diabetic complications. JAMA 288:2579, 2002.
3. Seibold JR, Uitto J, Dorwart BB, et al: Collagen synthesis and collagenase activity in dermal fibroblasts from patients with diabetes and digital sclerosis. J Lab Clin Med 105:664, 1985.
4. Iwasaki T, Kohama T, Houjou S, et al: Diabetic scleroderma and scleroderma-like changes in a patient with maturity onset type diabetes of young people. Dermatology 188:228, 1994.

5. Gamstedt A, Holm-Glad J, Ohlson CG, et al: Hand abnormalities are strongly associated with the duration of diabetes mellitus. J Intern Med 234:189, 1993.

6. Lawson PM, Maneschi F, Kohner EM: The relationship of hand abnormalities to diabetes and diabetic retinopathy. Diabetes Care 6:140, 1983.

7. Rosenbloom AL, Silverstein JH, Lezotte DC, et al: Limited joint mobility in diabetes mellitus indicating increased risk for microvascular disease. N Engl J Med 305:191, 1981.

8. Chammas M, Bousquet P, Renard E, et al: Dupuytren's disease, carpal tunnel syndrome, trigger finger, and diabetes mellitus. J Hand Surg Am 20:109, 1995.

9. Eaton P, Sibbitt WL Jr, Harsh A: The effect of an aldose reductase inhibiting agent on limited joint mobility in diabetic patients. JAMA 253:1437, 1985.

10. Goto Y, Hotta N, Shigeta Y, et al: Effects of an aldose reductase inhibitor, Epalrestat, on diabetic neuropathy. Biomed Pharmacother 49:296, 1995.

11. Benedetti A, Noacco C, Simonatti M, et al: Diabetic trigger finger. N Engl J Med 306:1552, 1982.

12. Arkkila PE, Kantola IM, Viikari JS, et al: Shoulder capsulitis in type I and II diabetic patients: Association with diabetic complications and related diseases. Ann Rheum Dis 55:907, 1996.

13. Boyle-Walker KL, Gabard DL, Bietsch E, et al: A profile of patients with adhesive capsulitis. J Hand Ther 10:222, 1997.

14. Lequesne M, Dang N, Benasson M, et al: Increased association of diabetes mellitus with capsulitis of the shoulder and shoulder-hand syndrome. Scand J Rheumatol 6:53, 1997.

15. Serra F, Mancini L, Ghirlanda G, et al: Charcot's foot. RAYS 22:524, 1997.

16. Armstrong DG, Lavery LA: Acute Charcot's arthropathy of the foot and ankle. Phys Ther 78:74, 1998.

17. Julkunen H, Heinonen OP, Pyorala K: Hyperostosis of the spine in an adult population: Its relationship to hyperglycemia and obesity. Ann Rheum Dis 30:605, 1971.

18. Daragon A, Mejjad O, Czernichow P, et al: Vertebral hyperostosis and diabetes mellitus: A case-control study. Ann Rheum Dis 54:375, 1995.

19. Vezyroglou G, Mitropoulos A, Antoniadis C: A metabolic syndrome in diffuse idiopathic skeletal hyperostosis: A controlled study. J Rheumatol 23:672, 1996.

20. Suico JG, Marriott DJ, Vinicor F, et al: Behaviors predicting foot lesions in patients with non-insulin-dependent diabetes mellitus. J Gen Intern Med 13:482, 1998.

21. Rith-Najarian S, Branchaud C, Beulieu O, et al: Reducing lower-extremity amputations due to diabetes: Application of the staged diabetes management approach in a primary care setting. J Family Pract 47:127, 1998.

22. Thomas PK: Classification, differential diagnosis, and staging of diabetic peripheral neuropathy. Diabetes 46(Suppl 2):S54, 1997.

23. Naftulin S, Fast A, Thomas M: Diabetic lumbar radiculopathy: Sciatica without disc herniation. Spine 18:2419, 1993.

24. Rynes RI, Merzig EG: Calcium pyrophosphate crystal deposition disease and hyperparathyroidism: A controlled, prospective study. J Rheumatol 5:460, 1978.

25. Resnick DL: Erosive arthritis of the hand and wrist in hyperparathyroidism. Radiology 110:263, 1974.

26. Frame B, Heinze EG, Block M, et al: Myopathy in primary hyperparathyroidism: Observations in 3 patients. Ann Intern Med 68:1022, 1968.

27. Nudelman I, Deutsch AA, Reiss R: Surgical treatment of primary hyperparathyroidism in the elderly patient. Isr J Med Sci 19:150, 1983.

28. Rubin LA, Fam AG, Rubenstein J, et al: Erosive azotemic osteoarthropathy. Arthritis Rheum 27:1086, 1984.

29. Pecovnik-Balon B, Kramberger S: Tumoral calcinosis in patients on hemodialysis: Care report and review of the literature. Am J Nephrol 17:93, 1997.

30. Kuntz D, Navean B, Bardin T, et al: Destructive spondyloarthropathy in hemodialyzed patients. Arthritis Rheum 27:369, 1984.

31. Dabbagh S: Renal osteodystrophy. Curr Opin Pediatr 10:190, 1998.

32. Pei Y, Hercz G, Greenwood C, et al: Risk factors for renal osteodystrophy: A multivariant analysis. J Bone Miner Res 10:149, 1995.

33. Ringel MD, Schwindinger WF, Levine MA: Clinical implications of genetic defects in G proteins: The molecular basis of McCune-Albright syndrome and Albright hereditary osteodystrophy. Medicine 75:171, 1996.

34. Hayward BE, Kamiya M, Strain L, et al: The human GNAS1 gene is imprinted and encodes distinct paternally and biallelically expressed G proteins. Proc Natl Acad Sci U S A 95:10038, 1998.

35. Juppner H, Schipani E, Bastepe M, et al: The gene responsible for pseudohypoparathyroidism type Ib is paternally imprinted and maps in four unrelated kindreds of chromosome 20Q13.3. Proc Natl Acad Sci U S A 95:11798, 1998.

36. Jodar E, Munoz-Torres M, Escobar-Jimenez F, et al: Bone loss in hyperthyroid patients and in former hyperthyroid patients controlled on medical therapy: Influence of etiology and menopause. Clin Endocrinol 47:279, 1997.

37. Chiovato L, Mariotti S, Pinchera A: Thyroid diseases in the elderly. Baillieres Clin Endocrinol Metab 11:251, 1997.

38. Shetty KR, Duthie EH Jr: Thyroid disease and associated illness in the elderly. Clin Geriatr Med 11:311, 1995.

39. Rosen CJ, Alder RA: Longitudinal changes in lumbar bone density among thyrotoxic patients after attainment of euthyroidism. J Clin Endocrinol Metab 75:1531, 1992.

40. Fatourechi V, Pajouhi M, Fransway AF: Dermopathy of Graves disease (pretibial myxedema): Review of 150 cases. Medicine 73:1, 1994.

41. Kriss JP: Pathogenesis and treatment of pretibial myxedema. Endocrinol Metab Clin N Am 16:409, 1987.

42. Nixon DW, Samols E: Acral changes associated with thyroid diseases. JAMA 212:1175, 1970.

43. Ramsey ID: Muscle dysfunction in hyperthyroidism. Lancet 2:931, 1966.

44. Katakura M, Yamada T, Aizawa T, et al: Presence of antideoxyribonucleic acid antibody in patients with hyperthyroidism of Graves' disease. J Clin Endocrinol Metab 64:405, 1987.

45. Baldini M, Pappalettera M, Lecchi L, et al: Human lymphocyte antigens in Graves' disease: Correlation with persistent course of disease. Am J Med Sci 309:43, 1995.

46. Torfs CP, King M, Huey B, et al: Genetic interrelationship between insulin-dependent diabetes mellitus, the autoimmune thyroid diseases, and rheumatoid arthritis. Am J Hum Genet 38:170, 1986.

47. Dorwart BB, Schumacher HR: Joint effusions, chondrocalcinosis and rheumatic manifestations of hypothyroidism. Am J Med 59:780, 1975.

48. Hartl E, Finsterer J, Grossegger C, et al: Relationship between thyroid function and skeletal muscle involvement in subclinical and overt hypothyroidism. Endocrinologist 11:217, 2001.

49. Bhansazi A, Chandran V, Ranesh J, et al: Acute myoedema: An unusual presenting manifestation of hypothyroid myopathy. Postgrad Med J 76:99, 2000.

50. Mastaglia FL, Ojeda VJ, Sarnat HB, et al: Myopathies associated with hypothyroidism: A review based upon 13 cases. Aust N Z J Med 18:799, 1988.

51. Katz JN, Larson MG, Sabra A: The carpal tunnel syndrome: Diagnostic utility of the history and physical examination findings. Ann Intern Med 112:321, 1990.

52. Weiner ES, Abeles M: Aseptic necrosis and glucocorticosteroids in systemic lupus erythematosus: A reevaluation. J Rheumatol 16:604, 1989.

53. Wollheim FA: Acute and long-term complications of corticosteroid pulse therapy. Scand J Rheumatol Suppl 54:27, 1984.

54. Vreden SG, Hermus AR, van Liessum PA, et al: Aseptic bone necrosis in patients on glucocorticoid replacement therapy. Neth J Med 39:153, 1991.

55. Lane RJ, Mastaglia FL: Drug-induced myopathies in man. Lancet 2:562, 1978.

56. Buckley LM, Leib ES, Cartularo KS, et al: Calcium and vitamin D_3 supplementation prevents bone loss in the spine secondary to low dose corticosteroids in patients with rheumatoid arthritis. Ann Intern Med 125:961, 1996.

57. Adachi JD, Bensen WG, Bell MJ, et al: Salmon calcitonin nasal spray in the prevention of corticosteroid-induced osteoporosis. Br J Rheumatol 36:255, 1997.

58. Saag KG, Emkey R, Schnitzer TJ, et al: Alendronate for the prevention and treatment of glucocorticoid-induced osteoporosis. N Engl J Med 339:292, 1998.

59. Adachi JD, Bensen WG, Brown J, et al: Intermittent etidronate therapy to prevent corticosteroid-induced osteoporosis. N Engl J Med 337:382, 1997.

60. Dixon RB, Nicholas PC: On the various forms of corticosteroid withdrawal syndrome. Am J Med 68:224, 1980.

61. Cronin CC, Callaghan N, Kearney PJ, et al: Addison disease in patients treated with glucocorticoid therapy. Arch Intern Med 157:456, 1997.

62. Schwartz RS: Trophic factor supplementation: Effect on the age-associated changes in body composition. J Gerontol Series A 50(Spec. No.):151, 1995.

63. Baum H, Ludecke DK, Herrmann HD: Carpal tunnel syndrome and acromegaly. Acta Neurochirurg 83:54, 1986.

64. Bluestone R, Bywaters EG, Hartog M, et al: Acromegalic arthropathy. Ann Rheum Dis 30:243, 1971.

65. **Layton MW, Fudman EJ, Barkan A, et al: Acromegalic arthropathy: Characteristics and response to therapy. Arthritis Rheum 31:1, 1990.**

66. Iijima T, Tada H, Hidaka Y, et al: Prediction of postpartum onset of rheumatoid arthritis. Ann Rheum Dis 57:460, 1998.

67. Van der Horst-Bruinsma IE, de Vries RR, de Buck PD, et al: Influence of HLA-class II incompatibility between mother and fetus on the development and course of rheumatoid arthritis of the mother. Ann Rheum Dis 57:286, 1998.

68. **Russell AS, Johnston C, Chew C, et al: Evidence for reduced Th1 function in normal pregnancy: A hypothesis for the remission of rheumatoid arthritis. J Rheumatol 24:1045, 1997.**

69. Van Vollenhoven RF, McGuire JL: Estrogen, progesterone, and testosterone: Can they be used to treat autoimmune diseases? Cleve Clin J Med 61:276, 1994.

70. Lahita RG: The role of sex hormones in systemic lupus erythematosus. Curr Opin Rheumatol 11:352, 1999.

71. Lahita RG, Bradlow HL, Ginzler E, et al: Low plasma androgens in women with systemic lupus erythematosus. Arthritis Rheum 30:241, 1987.

72. Van Vollenhoven RF, Morabito LM, Engleman EG, et al: Treatment of systemic lupus erythematosus with dehydroepiandrosterone: 50 patients tested up to 12 months. J Rheumatol 25:285, 1998.

73. Hazes JM, Dijkmans BA, Vandenbroucke JP, et al: Reduction of the risk of rheumatoid arthritis among women who take oral contraceptives. Arthritis Rheum 33:173, 1990.

74. Julkunen HA: Oral contraceptives in systemic lupus erythematosus: Side effects and influence on the activity of SLE. Scand J Rheumatol 20:427, 1991.

75. Buyon JP: Oral contraceptives in women with systemic lupus erythematosus. Ann Intern Med 147:259, 1996.

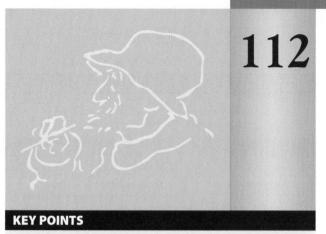

112 Musculoskeletal Syndromes in Malignancy

ELIZA F. CHAKRAVARTY

KEY POINTS

Musculoskeletal and rheumatic syndromes can occasionally be the first presentation of an underlying malignancy. Older age of onset, prominent constitutional symptoms, atypical features of rheumatic disease, and absence of response to glucocorticoids or other conventional therapy may be suggestive of a paraneoplastic process.

Data from numerous cohorts have confirmed an elevated (> threefold) incidence of malignancy associated with dermatomyositis. Solid organ tumors, including lung, colon, and ovarian in European populations and nasopharyngeal tumors in Asian populations, are among the most common tumors found in dermatomyositis patients; most malignancies are diagnosed within 1 year of diagnosis of myopathy.

Although to a lesser magnitude than dermatomyositis, polymyositis has been associated with an increased incidence of malignancies in several large population-based studies.

Chronic autoimmune conditions including Sjögren's syndrome, rheumatoid arthritis, and systemic lupus erythematosus are associated with an increased risk for the development of lymphoid malignancies compared to the general population. This is felt to be, at least in part, due to chronic inflammation and immune stimulation.

Commonly used immunosuppressive medications have been associated with later development of malignancies, some of which may be related to reactivation of latent Epstein-Barr virus.

Possible associations between anti-TNF-α therapy and increased risk of development of lymphoma are confounded by increased disease activity and previous DMARD use in patients who receive biologic therapy.

Patients with systemic sclerosis are at increased risk for the development of solid organ tumors primarily involving tissues affected by the fibrotic process.

Musculoskeletal syndromes seem to be associated with malignancy in a variety of ways. Cause and effect are difficult to define clearly in many situations, however. Certain rheumatic diseases have been associated with an increased risk of the subsequent development of malignancy; one example is the development of lymphoma in an individual with primary Sjögren's syndrome. The converse situation also exists, in that certain rheumatic diseases are seen more frequently in the presence of an underlying malignancy, such as dermatomyositis. Little is understood regarding the pathogenesis of connective tissue disease in association with neoplastic disease. Other factors can contribute to the association of musculoskeletal syndromes and malignancy. Many of the medications used to treat rheumatic diseases modulate the immune system and may be associated directly or indirectly with an increased risk for the subsequent development of malignancy. In unusual circumstances, musculoskeletal involvement occurs as a paraneoplastic process, defined as a hormonal, neurologic, hematologic, or biochemical disturbance associated with malignancy, but not directly related to invasion by the neoplasm or its metastases.[1]

PARANEOPLASTIC SYNDROMES

Musculoskeletal syndromes can develop as a manifestation of a paraneoplastic process and occasionally can be the first presentation of an underlying malignancy. Hematologic malignancies, lymphoproliferative disorders, and solid tumors are associated with a wide variety of paraneoplastic rheumatic syndromes. Older age of onset, atypical features of rheumatic disease, and absence of response to glucocorticoids or other conventional therapy may suggest a paraneoplastic process. Knowledge of the associations with rheumatic syndromes and underlying malignancy is crucial when caring for these patients. Hypertrophic osteoarthropathy, amyloidosis, and secondary gout are reviewed in Chapters 93, 106, and 87. Table 112-1 lists common paraneoplastic associations.

CARCINOMATOUS POLYARTHRITIS

The term *carcinomatous polyarthritis* is used to describe the development of arthritis in association with malignancy, but it is distinct from arthritis associated with metastasis or direct tumor invasion. Table 112-2 lists common features of carcinomatous polyarthritis. It generally occurs in patients who are older in age, has an explosive onset, and often develops in close temporal correlation with the discovery of the malignancy. Although it can have various presentations and may mimic the appearance of rheumatoid arthritis (RA),[2] carcinomatous polyarthritis is more often a seronegative asymmetric disease with predominant involvement of the lower extremities and some sparing of the small joints of the hands. There is no evidence of direct tumor extension or metastasis and no specific identifying histologic or radiographic appearance. Carcinomatous polyarthritis can occur in association with many types of malignancy, but has been reported in the greatest frequency in association with breast, colon, lung, and ovarian cancers and with lymphoproliferative disorders.[3] The underlying pathogenesis of

Table 112-1 Paraneoplastic Syndromes

Connective Tissue Disease	Malignancy	Clinical Setting	Clinical Alert
Carcinomatous polyarthritis	Multiple types of solid tumors, including breast; lymphoproliferative disorders	See Table 112-2	See Table 112-2
Vasculitis	Lymphopoietic and hematopoietic malignancies	Cutaneous vasculitis most common; systemic vasculitis rare	Vasculitis not related to infections, medications, or autoimmune disease
Mixed cryoglobulinemia	Non-Hodgkin's lymphoma	Immune complex–mediated disease with cutaneous vasculitis, neuropathy, fatigue, and visceral organ involvement	Usually appears 5-10 yr after diagnosis of cryoglobulinemia
Panniculitis	Hematologic malignancies; pancreatic, breast, and prostate cancers	Induration of skin and deeper tissues; eosinophilia often present	Usually refractory to prednisone
Fasciitis	Ovarian, breast, gastric, and pancreatic cancers	Palmar fasciitis with inflammatory polyarthritis; similar in presentation to reflex sympathetic dystrophy	Bilateral presentation; severe fibrosis and contractures; aggressive course
Reflex sympathetic dystrophy syndrome	Multiple cancer types; Pancoast tumors	Tumors may invade stellate ganglion or brachial plexus on affected side	Absence of typical antecedent factors; failure to respond to conventional therapies
Erythromelalgia	Myeloproliferative disorders	Often seen in setting of thrombocytosis	—
Atypical polymyalgia rheumatica	Renal, lung, and colon cancer; multiple myeloma	—	Age <50 yr; asymmetric involvement; poor response to prednisone
Digital necrosis	Gastrointestinal and pulmonary tumors	Severe Raynaud's phenomenon with onset >50 yr old	Asymmetric features; digital necrosis
Remitting seronegative symmetric synovitis with pitting edema	Several tumor types	Abrupt onset of arthritis and edema surrounding wrists and small joints of hands	Presence of fever, weight loss; poor response to prednisone
Multicentric reticulohistiocytosis	Lung, stomach, breast, cervix, colon, and ovarian carcinomas	—	—
Lupus-like syndromes	Variety of solid tumors and lymphoproliferative disorders	—	Rare associations with malignancy limited to case reports
Antiphospholipid antibodies	Multiple cancer types	Association between antibodies, cancer, and risk of thrombosis unclear	Higher presence of antibodies found in patients with malignancy
Osteogenic osteomalacia	Solid tumors and tumors of mesenchymal origin	Bone pain and muscle weakness	Diligent search is indicated in all patients with late-onset apparent idiopathic osteomalacia
Sarcoidosis	Cervical, bladder, gastric, lung, breast, and renal cancers and cutaneous and pulmonary squamous cell carcinomas	Highest incidence of "malignancy" during first 4 yr after detection of granulomas	Malignant tumors can cause sarcoid-like tissue reactions leading to mistaken diagnosis of sarcoidosis before recognition of malignancy
Lymphomatoid granulomatosis	Lymphoma	Unusual granulomatous form of vasculitis with angiodestructive infiltration of various tissues	—

this process has not been elucidated; however, the arthritic symptoms may be improved with successful treatment of the malignancy.[4]

VASCULITIS

Vasculitis in association with malignancy is uncommon and has a reported prevalence of only 8% of patients with malignancy.[5] The association seems to be significantly higher with lymphoproliferative and myeloproliferative disorders than with solid tumors, and vasculitis commonly predates the identification of malignancy. The vasculitic process is most often small vessel and cutaneous and only rarely involves significant organs. Treatment often requires the use of glucocorticoids and therapy directed against the underlying malignancy, although it seems this is often ineffective. Table 112-1 shows malignancies associated with vasculitis. In the setting of malignancy, it is believed that the persistent antigen stimulation from the tumor results in T cell activation or immune complex formation and deposition.

Table 112-2 Features of Carcinomatous Polyarthritis

Close temporal relationship between onset of arthritis and discovery of malignancy
Late age of onset of arthritis
Asymmetric joint involvement
Explosive onset
Predominant lower extremity involvement with sparing of wrists and small joints of hands
Absence of rheumatoid nodules
Absence of rheumatoid factor
No family history of rheumatoid disease
Nonspecific histopathologic appearance of synovial lining
No periosteal reaction

The development of small vessel vasculitis has been reported to antedate and postdate the development of lymphoproliferative and myeloproliferative diseases. One group looked at 222 patients with vasculitis retrospectively and identified 11 who had developed an associated malignancy. Of these 11 patients, 7 had hematologic neoplasia, and 4 had malignant solid tumors. Nine of the patients manifested cutaneous vasculitis, and the remaining two had vasculitic involvement in the bowel. In four of the patients, the development of vasculitis antedated the diagnosis of malignancy.[6] Similar findings were reported by investigators who found an underlying malignancy in 8 of 192 patients with cutaneous vasculitis. Most malignancies were hematologic (six of eight) and predated (five of eight) the diagnosis of cancer.[7] In a retrospective analysis of 23 patients with cutaneous vasculitis and hematologic malignancies, the authors were able to attribute the presence of vasculitis to the malignancy itself in 61% of cases.[8]

Systemic vasculitis is much less commonly associated with underlying malignancy. Case reports and small series have found antineutrophil cytoplasmic antibody (ANCA)–negative and ANCA-positive vasculitis associated with hematologic malignancies.[9-11] Wegener's granulomatosis has likewise been associated with the development of several types of malignancies, including lymphoproliferative disorders, bladder cancer, and renal cell carcinoma.[12,13] In some cases, the malignancy was diagnosed within months of the diagnosis of Wegener's granulomatosis,[12] and in other reports, cancer developed many years after diagnosis and treatment of vasculitis,[13] making it unclear whether the malignancies were a result of the vasculitis or possibly the treatment. A group from the Cleveland Clinic did a retrospective study to assess directly the temporal relationship between vasculitis and cancer.[14] During an 18-year study period, the authors found only 12 cases of vasculitis and cancer diagnosed within the same 12-month period: Six patients had lymphoproliferative disorders, and six had solid tumors. In most cases, the vasculitis responded partially to immunosuppressive therapy, but the investigators observed a more impressive improvement of vasculitis with definitive treatment for the underlying malignancy. A more recent study found 20 cases of malignancy among 200 patients with ANCA-positive vasculitis; 6 were diagnosed concurrently with diagnosis of vasculitis, and 14 predated vasculitis by a median of 96 months.[15] Only 4 of 20 malignancies in this series were lymphoproliferative; the remaining malignancies were solid organ tumors.

Vasculitis associated with underlying malignancy is often poorly responsive to conventional therapy directed against the vasculitis. In one series of 13 patients with cutaneous vasculitis and lymphoproliferative or myeloproliferative disorders, symptoms of vasculitis were poorly responsive to therapy with nonsteroidal anti-inflammatory drugs (NSAIDs), glucocorticoids, antihistamines, and antiserotonin agents. Although the investigators reported a lessening of the severity of the vasculitis after chemotherapy directed against the malignancy, they generally found chemotherapy to be ineffective. Of the 13 patients identified, 10 died as a direct result of the malignancy.[16] Similarly, Hutson and Hoffman[14] found a general concurrence between improvement in vasculitic syndrome with definitive treatment for the associated underlying malignancy.

CRYOGLOBULINEMA

Cryoglobulins are immunoglobulins that precipitate at reduced temperature. Cryoglobulinemia can be characterized by hyperviscosity symptoms or by vasculitis. Patients often have fatigue, arthralgia or arthritis, cutaneous vasculitis or purpura, neuropathy, digital ischemia, and visceral organ involvement (renal or pulmonary). There are three types of cryoglobulins, as follows:

Type I: Monoclonal immunoglobulin, either IgG or IgM; this type is associated with lymphoproliferative disorders.

Type II: Monoclonal IgM directed against polyclonal IgG; type II cryoglobulins were initially thought to be idiopathic and were known as mixed essential cryoglobulinemia. With the identification of hepatitis C virus (HCV), it has been discovered that most of these patients have HCV infection that is directly involved in the pathogenesis of the cryoglobulins. Specific epitopes of HCV antigens are recognized by IgG components of immune complexes, and viral particles are found in the cryoprecipitate.[17] One study found clonal B cell populations in the peripheral blood of 48% of HCV-positive patients with type II cryoglobulemia, many of whom were eventually diagnosed with a B cell malignancy.[18] Overall, it is estimated that approximately 5% to 8% of patients with mixed cryoglobulinemia may go on to develop non-Hodgkin's lymphoma, usually after 5 to 10 years of cryoglobulinemia.[19,20] The risk of developing non-Hodgkin's lymphoma among HCV-positive cryoglobulinemic patients may be 35 times higher than that in the general population.[21] Other data suggest that HCV infection may be associated with other hematologic malignancies.[22,23] At this time, the subset of patients with mixed cryoglobulinemia who will develop lymphoma cannot be predicted.

Type III: Mixed polyclonal IgG and IgM; type III cryoglobulins are commonly seen with a variety of illnesses, including connective tissue diseases (systemic lupus erythematosus [SLE] and RA) and infections. In one study of 607 patients diagnosed with mixed cryoglobulinemia, 27 cases of hematologic malignancies were identified. Of these, systemic autoimmune diseases were detected in 56% of the cases of non-Hodgkin's lymphoma.[23]

PANNICULITIS

The fasciitis-panniculitis syndrome, which includes eosinophilic fasciitis, is characterized by swelling and induration of the skin that extends into deeper subcutaneous tissues and is associated with fibrosis and chronic inflammation. Patients may develop arthritis and subcutaneous nodules similar to those seen in erythema nodosum. The arthropathy seems to be secondary to periarticular fat necrosis, can be monarticular or polyarticular,[24] and may mimic RA or juvenile RA.[25] Blood and tissue eosinophilia is commonly, but not always, present.[26] This syndrome can be idiopathic and have a benign course, or it can be secondary to a variety of infectious, vascular, or traumatic etiologies. In a few patients, the fasciitis-panniculitis syndrome is associated with an underlying malignancy. Hematologic malignancies are most often associated with this syndrome and are usually diagnosed concurrently or within the first year.[27,28] Pancreatic cancer and pancreatitis also can be associated with this syndrome.[24,25] Patients with cancer-associated fasciitis-panniculitis syndrome are predominantly female and are generally refractory to prednisone.[27]

PALMAR FASCIITIS

Palmar fasciitis and arthritis is a syndrome characterized by progressive bilateral contractures of the digits, fibrosis of palmar fascia, and inflammatory polyarthritis.[29,30] The metacarpophalangeal and proximal interphalangeal joints are most commonly affected; other affected joints include the elbows, wrists, knees, ankles, and feet. Palmar fasciitis is almost uniformly associated with the presence of an underlying malignancy, most often ovarian, breast, gastric, and pancreatic tumors.[30-32] Although initially thought to be an atypical variant of reflex sympathetic dystrophy, the severity of manifestations, bilateral presentation, and strong association with occult malignancy suggest that, in these cases, palmar fasciitis is a distinct entity that behaves as a paraneoplastic syndrome. Glucocorticoids, chemotherapy, or both do not seem to result in improvement, although fasciitis occasionally regresses with treatment of the underlying malignancy.[29]

REFLEX SYMPATHETIC DYSTROPHY SYNDROME

Reflex sympathetic dystrophy and a variant, shoulder-hand syndrome, are characterized by regional pain, swelling, vasomotor instability, and focal osteoporosis in a given limb; this condition is thought to be caused by sympathetic dysfunction. The absence of associated antecedent factors, such as stroke, myocardial infarction, or trauma, and failure to respond to conventional therapy warrant a search for an underlying malignancy. A variety of malignancies have been associated with the development of reflex sympathetic dystrophy or its variants.[33,34] Pancoast tumor of the lung apices or other malignancies that infiltrate the stellate ganglion or brachial plexus have been described in patients with reflex sympathetic dystrophy.[35-37] Therapy directed against the underlying malignancy may lead to some amelioration of symptoms associated with reflex sympathetic dystrophy.

ERYTHROMELALGIA

Erythromelalgia is an enigmatic condition characterized by attacks of severe burning, erythema, and warmth of the extremities with symptoms predominantly involving the feet.[38,39] Symptoms are often exacerbated when the extremities are placed in a dependent position, during ambulation, or during exposure to increased temperatures. Partial relief can be obtained through elevation or cooling of the extremity. This disorder can occur idiopathically (60%) or secondary to another disease (40%).[38,40] Myeloproliferative disorders, including polycythemia vera and essential thrombocytosis, are common primary causes and have been found to precede the diagnosis of erythromelalgia by several years.[39,41] The underlying pathophysiology of this disease is unknown; however, it is often associated with thrombocythemia. In the largest published retrospective cohort, 168 patients at the Mayo Clinic were identified with this diagnosis between 1970 and 1994.[42] The authors found that after a mean follow-up of 8.7 years, 31.9% of patients reported worsening of disease, 26.6% reported no change, 30.9% reported improvement, and 10.6% reported complete resolution of symptoms. Kaplan-Meier survival curves revealed a significant decrease in survival compared with controls. A history of myeloproliferative disease was found in 15 of 168 patients. The exact cause of the symptoms is unclear, but microvascular arteriovenous shunting has been hypothesized.[43] The most effective therapy seems to be the use of daily aspirin, leading to a significant relief of symptoms, which is believed to be related to inhibition of cyclooxygenase-1. A host of other therapies have been tried with varying success.[44] Because of the association with myeloproliferative diseases, routine monitoring with complete blood counts is prudent.

POLYMYALGIA RHEUMATICA

Polymyalgia rheumatica is a disorder affecting older adults that manifests with discomfort and stiffness in the shoulder and hip girdle, fatigue, anemia of chronic disease, and elevated erythrocyte sedimentation rate (ESR). Classically, this condition responds to moderate doses of prednisone within 48 hours. A variety of other conditions can have presentations that mimic polymyalgia rheumatica, including other rheumatic disorders, systemic infections, and malignancy.[45] Although the association between polymyalgia rheumatica and malignancy has been controversial, atypical features of polymyalgia rheumatica may suggest the presence of occult malignancy, including age younger than 50 years, limited or asymmetric involvement of typical sites, ESR less than 40 mm/hr or greater than 100 mm/hr, severe anemia, proteinuria, and poor or delayed response to 20 mg daily of prednisone. Kidney, lung, and colon cancer and multiple myeloma are most often found in patients presenting with atypical polymyalgia rheumatica.[46-48] One study of patients undergoing evaluation for possible polymyalgia rheumatica found 10% to have a diagnosis of malignant neoplasms.[49] In contrast, several prospective studies have shown that patients who present with classic polymyalgia rheumatica or temporal arteritis do not seem to have an increased risk of developing malignancy over age-matched controls.[50-52]

DIGITAL NECROSIS

The development of digital necrosis or profound Raynaud's phenomenon may suggest the presence of infection, inflammatory disease, or an underlying malignancy. In patients older than age 50 years, the development of Raynaud's phenomenon, particularly in an asymmetric fashion or in association with digital necrosis, should raise the possibility that this is a paraneoplastic process. These features often antedate the diagnosis of the malignancy by an average of 7 to 9 months.[53,54] A variety of solid tumors and lymphoproliferative disorders have been associated with this syndrome.[53-59] Mechanisms proposed include cryoglobulinemia, immune complex–induced vasospasm, hypercoagulability, marantic endocarditis with emboli, and necrotizing vasculitis.[59] Therapy with interferon-α also has been reported in association with the development of Raynaud's phenomenon and digital necrosis.[60-62]

REMITTING SERONEGATIVE SYMMETRIC SYNOVITIS WITH PITTING EDEMA

Remitting seronegative symmetric synovitis with pitting edema is an uncommon disorder primarily affecting the metacarpophalangeal joints and the wrists. Although the underlying etiology and pathogenesis of this illness are unclear, lymphoma, myelodysplastic syndrome, and several solid tumors, mostly adenocarcinoma, all have been reported in association with it.[63-67] Characteristics that suggest possible underlying malignancy include the presence of systemic features, such as fever or weight loss, and a poor response to glucocorticoids.[65,66]

MULTICENTRIC RETICULOHISTIOCYTOSIS

Multicentric reticulohistiocytosis is a rare condition characterized by the presence of cutaneous papules; it is often associated with a destructive arthritis. The papules are flesh-colored to brown-yellow and are classically present in the periungual region and on the dorsal hands and face. Arthritis mutilans may develop in 50% of cases. The characteristic histologic appearance of tissue infiltration with histiocytes and multinucleated giant cells can be found in affected skin, joints, and occasionally internal organs.[68] Multicentric reticulohistiocytosis has been reported in association with hyperlipidemia, malignancies, and autoimmune diseases. Malignancy has been associated in 25% to 31% of cases.[69] The most frequently seen malignancies include carcinoma of the lung, stomach, breast, cervix, colon, and ovary.[68]

LUPUS-LIKE SYNDROMES

Lupus-like syndromes are rarely associated with underlying malignancy. Isolated case reports have described lupus-like syndromes with ovarian carcinoma[70,71] and hairy cell leukemia[72]; subacute cutaneous lupus was reported in a patient with breast carcinoma.[73] Studies on the presence of antinuclear antibodies (ANAs) in patients with cancer have yielded mixed results. Two studies were unable to find a significantly increased prevalence of ANAs in patients with solid tumors or lymphomas compared with healthy controls.[74,75] In contrast, one smaller study found an increased prevalence in patients with non-Hodgkin's lymphoma compared with controls (21% versus 0),[76] and another study found a prevalence of ANAs in 274 patients with various malignancies of 27.7% compared with 6.45% of 140 healthy controls.[77] There do not seem to be any predictive features that suggest occult malignancy in patients presenting with lupus-like syndromes or positive ANAs.

ANTIPHOSPHOLIPID ANTIBODIES

Antiphospholipid antibodies and their association with thromboses have been described as a primary syndrome and a secondary phenomenon in autoimmune diseases, primarily SLE. More recently, antiphospholipid antibodies have been associated with a variety of malignancies. Correlations between antiphospholipid antibodies in cancer patients and thromboembolic events have been less clear, however.

Several studies have shown the presence of antiphospholipid antibodies in patients with solid tumors and lymphoproliferative disorders at a higher frequency than the 1% to 5% seen in the general population.[78,79] An early study of 216 consecutive patients with cancer found 22% positive for anticardiolipin antibodies compared with 3.4% in controls. This study found a twofold increase in the development of thromboembolism in patients with positive antibodies compared with patients with negative serologies; it also indicated that most thromboembolic events occurred in patients with higher antibody titers.[80] Other studies have confirmed the association between malignancy and antiphospholipid antibodies (12.5% to 68%), but have been unable to show a correlation with thromboembolic events.[76,78,81-85] A correlation between antibody titer and disease activity has been shown in some studies,[81,83] and decreased survival in others.[85] A review of the literature concluded that antiphospholipid antibodies resolve in one third of cancer patients after treatment for the underlying malignancy.[86]

Studies of the prevalence of antiphospholipid antibodies in unselected patient populations have shown an association with underlying malignancy. A prospective study in France found that 7% of 1014 consecutive patients admitted to a medical ward had antiphospholipid antibodies.[87] In antibody-positive patients, cancer was the most frequently associated disease. A more recent study in patients presenting with a first ischemic stroke found a significantly higher rate of development of cancer within 12 months in patients who had anticardiolipin antibodies (19% versus 5%).[88]

OSTEOMALACIA

Osteomalacia is the softening of bones often associated with the failure of adequate calcification secondary to renal dysfunction or a lack of vitamin D. Osteomalacia has been associated with benign and malignant solid tissue and mesenchymal tumors.[89] Tumors causing oncogenic osteomalacia have been shown to overproduce fibroblast growth factor 23 (FGF-23), and elevated serum levels of FGF-23 can be detected in patients with this paraneoplastic condition.[90] Octreotide scintigraphy may be a useful tool for identifying occult tumors.[91] With removal of the tumor, there often seems to be resolution of the osteomalacia and normalization of serum FGF-23 levels.[90]

SARCOIDOSIS

Noncaseating granulomas can occur in numerous settings and are not pathognomonic for sarcoidosis. Granulomas resembling those of sarcoidosis may be found in lymph nodes that drain sites of malignancy. These tumor-related tissue reactions resulting in granuloma formation have been described with many types of malignant lesions, including solid tumors and lymphomas.[92,93] The clinical and radiographic presentation of sarcoidosis and cancer can be virtually indistinguishable, making it important to pursue aggressive evaluation in a patient with sarcoidosis.[94]

The risk of malignancy developing in patients with established diagnoses of sarcoidosis is controversial. Some studies have shown an increased risk of developing lung cancer and lymphoma,[95,96] whereas others have shown no increased risk of cancer over the general population.[94,97]

LYMPHOMATOID GRANULOMATOSIS

Lymphomatoid granulomatosis is a rare disorder with angiodestructive and lymphoproliferative features involving the lung and, less often, the skin and central nervous system. Although lymphocytic infiltration of vessels is a hallmark of the disease, lymphomatoid granulomatosis now seems to fall within the spectrum of lymphoproliferative disorders. Despite the predominance of T cells within inflammatory infiltrates, studies have suggested that an Epstein-Barr virus (EBV)–associated B cell proliferation may underlie the pathogenesis of the disease.[98,99] Prognosis is generally poor with a median survival from diagnosis of 14 months,[100] although more recent reports suggest some response to rituximab therapy.[101,102] Frank lymphomas evolve in 25% of cases.[103]

INFLAMMATORY MYOPATHIES

The inflammatory myopathies in adult populations encompass a group of illnesses characterized by an idiopathic immune-mediated attack on skeletal muscle that results in muscle weakness. There have been many associations between the inflammatory myopathies and the presence of malignancy, but the etiology of the association is controversial.[104] Dermatomyositis has classically been associated with occult malignancies, whereas the associations between polymyositis and inclusion body myositis are less clear. A further issue is whether the inflammatory myopathy predates the malignancy and can be considered a primary rheumatic disease with known risks of developing malignancy, or whether it simply represents a manifestation of a paraneoplastic process.

On average, the prevalence of malignancy in association with the inflammatory myopathies has been approximately 25%. The frequency of malignancy has ranged, however, from 6% to 60% in patients with dermatomyositis and from 0 to 28% in patients with polymyositis.[104] Other estimates have placed the incidence of cancer in patients with inflammatory myopathies at five to seven times that of the general population.[104]

Dermatomyositis has been associated with a wide range of malignancies. Most common are ovarian, lung, and gastric tumors in European populations, and nasopharyngeal malignancies in Asian populations. Studies have confirmed a strong association between dermatomyositis and malignancy. Hill and colleagues[105] studied a pooled cohort of patients from Sweden, Denmark, and Finland and found 198 cases of cancer in 618 patients with dermatomyositis. The standardized incidence ratio (SIR) for malignancy with dermatomyositis was 3. Similar results were found in a Scottish cohort of 286 patients with dermatomyositis.[106] Of patients, 77 were found to have underlying malignancies, with an SIR of 3.3 to 7.7. Buchbinder and coworkers[107] used strict histopathologic criteria to classify myositis in patients from Victoria, Australia. This group found 36 cases of cancer in 85 patients diagnosed with dermatomyositis and an SIR of 4.3 to 6.2.

In contrast to the previous work, studies of Asian populations have shown a higher association of nasopharyngeal carcinomas with dermatomyositis. In a Taiwanese study, 18% of 91 patients with dermatomyositis were found to have an underlying malignancy, the most common of which was nasopharyngeal cancer, followed by lung cancer.[108] In a smaller study, 66.6% of 15 dermatomyositis patients in Singapore had malignancies, most of which were nasopharyngeal carcinoma.[109] Eight white patients with nasopharyngeal carcinoma within 1 year of diagnosis of dermatomyositis were reported more recently in Tunisia.[110]

In polymyositis, the relative risk for developing internal malignancies seems to be lower than that for dermatomyositis, but it is consistently increased over that expected in the general population. Studies have found a 14% to 30% prevalence of cancer among patients with polymyositis with SIRs increased to 1.2 to 2.1.[105-108] Small numbers of many types of cancers were found in these studies.

These more recent studies confirm results found in previous large studies of Swedish and Finnish populations and a 1994 meta-analysis of all published case-control and cohort studies of malignancy and myositis that identified an odds ratio for the association of cancer with dermatomyositis of 4.4 and of cancer with polymyositis of 2.1.[111]

In amyopathic dermatomyositis, a variant of dermatomyositis in which typical cutaneous manifestations are present with subclinical or no identifiable muscle disease, the association with underlying malignancy is controversial, and published reports are limited to small groups of patients.[109,112-114] A systematic review of the amyopathic dermatomyositis literature has suggested similar associations between amyopathic dermatomyositis and internal malignancies.[115]

Far less is known about the association of inclusion body myositis and underlying malignancy. In Buchbinder's study from Northern Europe, 52 patients were identified with inclusion body myositis. Of the patients, 12 were found to have internal malignancies, with an SIR of 2.4. The numbers of each type of cancer seen were too small to find specific associations.[107]

Not all studies concur regarding the association between the inflammatory myopathies and malignancy.[116,117] In a study done at the Mayo Clinic, patients with myositis did not seem to be at a statistically significant risk for the development of malignancy. No clinical differences were seen between patients who developed a malignancy and patients who did not.[117]

Despite the negative results of some studies, it seems that most work supports the notion of an increased risk of malignancy in association with dermatomyositis and polymyositis. For patients in whom an inflammatory myopathy has been diagnosed, a workup for the presence of malignancy should be done. The extent of this workup has been debated, however, because extensive undirected searches often result in a very low yield. It is probably rare for an undirected workup to yield evidence of malignancy in polymyositis and dermatomyositis patients[118]; any workup should be tailored to the individual patient's age, symptoms, and signs. Studies have suggested that imaging of the chest, abdomen, and pelvis may increase the potential for discovery of underlying malignancy.[119,120] Other studies have suggested the use of serum tumor markers (CA125 and CA19-9) to augment detection of patients with dermatomyositis or polymyositis at highest risk for associated malignancy.[121] Malignancies associated with inflammatory myopathies have been known to develop many years after the diagnosis of muscle disease, so continued vigilance and repeated screening for malignancy are warranted.

There are certain cohorts in whom the risk of malignancy may be higher, including patients who have active dermatomyositis but exhibit a normal creatine kinase level,[122] patients with evidence of distal extremity weakness,[123] and patients with prominent pharyngeal and diaphragmatic involvement.[123] Patients with myositis-associated autoantibodies may be at less risk for the development of malignancy.[123,124] More recent work has suggested that

the presence of leukocytoclastic vasculitis[125] or cutaneous ulceration[123] increases further the risk of underlying malignancy.

Although the pathogenesis is unknown, the types of malignancy associated with the inflammatory myopathies have been varied, including adenocarcinomas of the breast, ovaries, and stomach. Most cases of dermatomyositis and malignancy seem to occur within 1 year of each other, with myositis diagnosed first in most cases.[104] When identified, removal of the malignancy may result in improvement of the myopathic process, which further supports the paraneoplastic nature of myositis in some cases.[126]

RISKS OF DEVELOPING LYMPHOPROLIFERATIVE DISORDERS IN RHEUMATIC DISEASES

Since the 1960s, there have been increasing reports of the association between rheumatic diseases and the development of malignancies, particularly lymphoproliferative disorders. Table 112-3 shows preexisting connective tissue

Table 112-3 Preexisting Connective Tissue Diseases Associated with Malignancy

Connective Tissue Disease	Malignancy	Associated Factors	Clinical Alert
Sjögren's syndrome	Lymphoproliferative disorders	Glandular features—lymphadenopathy, parotid or salivary enlargement Extraglandular features—purpura, vasculitis, splenomegaly, lymphopenia, low C4 cryoglobulins	Clues to progression from pseudolymphoma to lymphoma include worsening of clinical features, disappearance of rheumatoid factor, and decline of IgM
Rheumatoid arthritis	Lymphoproliferative disorders	Presence of paraproteinemia, greater disease severity, longer disease duration, immunosuppression, Felty's syndrome	Rapidly progressive, refractory flare in long-standing rheumatoid disease may suggest an underlying malignancy
SLE	Lymphoproliferative disorders	—	Non-Hodgkin's lymphoma should be considered in SLE patients who develop adenopathy or masses; lymphoma of the spleen is another cause of splenic enlargement in SLE
Discoid lupus erythematosus	Squamous cell epithelioma	Found in oldest plaques, ≥20 yr after onset of discoid lesion, primarily in men 30-60 yr old	Poorly healing skin lesion within discoid plaques should be evaluated
Systemic sclerosis (scleroderma)	Alveolar cell carcinoma Nonmelanoma skin cancer Adenocarcinoma of the esophagus	Pulmonary fibrosis, interstitial lung disease Areas of scleroderma and fibrosis in the skin Barrett's metaplasia	Annual chest radiograph after fibrosis is detected Change in skin features or poorly healing lesions should be evaluated Esophagoscopy and biopsy, if indicated, of distal esophageal constricting lesions
Paget's disease of bone	Osteogenic sarcoma	Development of severe pain; increasing incidence with age	Swelling and bone destruction in preexisting Paget's disease may be sarcoma; diagnosis may require biopsy
Dermatomyositis	Ovarian, lung, and gastric cancer in Western populations; nasopharyngeal carcinoma in Asian populations	Older in age, normal creatinine kinase levels, presence of cutaneous vasculitis; less likely in setting of myositis-specific antibodies	Malignancy evaluation needs to be tailored to individual patient's age, symptoms, and signs

SLE, systemic lupus erythematosus.

diseases that have been associated with malignancy. Much of what is known about associations between rheumatic disease and malignancy is drawn from retrospective and prospective cohort studies, registry-linkage studies, small series, and case reports. In addition, certain confounding factors need to be considered when assessing the risk of the development of malignancy, including the potential oncogenic properties of many of the immunosuppressive and cytotoxic medications prescribed to treat autoimmune diseases. Lymphoproliferative disorders have developed in patients with rheumatic diseases and in recipients of solid organ transplantations treated with immunosuppressive agents. EBV has been implicated in the development of lymphoid neoplasia in immunosuppressed patients. In the following sections, many of the rheumatic diseases and the therapies used to treat them are discussed.

SJÖGREN'S SYNDROME

Sjögren's syndrome, an autoimmune exocrinopathy, is characterized by a benign lymphocytic infiltrate of salivary and lacrimal glands that leads to the development of sicca syndrome (keratoconjunctivitis and xerostomia). The development of lymphoproliferative disorders in the setting of Sjögren's syndrome is perhaps the prototypic example of chronic autoimmune disease and an increased risk of malignancy. In 1964, investigators first reported the development of four cases of lymphoproliferative disorders in a cohort of 58 patients with Sjögren's syndrome.[127] In 1978, 7 of 136 patients with sicca syndrome were identified as having developed non-Hodgkin's lymphoma. Compared with the expected incidence of cancer among women of the same age range, there was a 44-fold increased risk of developing non-Hodgkin's lymphoma.[128] These findings have been reproduced numerous times in other cohorts. Lymphoproliferative disorders complicate approximately 4% to 10% of cases of primary Sjögren's syndrome.[129-133] The relative risk for development of lymphoproliferative disorders in patients with primary Sjögren's syndrome ranges from 6 to 44,[128,134-139] and a meta-analysis of cohort studies has found a pooled SIR of 18.8.[136] Most lymphoproliferative disorders were non-Hodgkin's lymphoma, specifically low-grade B cell lymphoma, diffuse large B cell lymphoma, and lymphoma of mucosa-associated lymphoid tissue. Waldenström's macroglobulinemia, chronic lymphocytic leukemia, and multiple myeloma were more rarely reported.[128,132,133,135]

Generally, the development of lymphoma is a late manifestation of Sjögren's syndrome, often seen after 6.5 years of disease.[130,131,140] Several clinical and laboratory features seem to be associated with or predictive of development of lymphoproliferative disorders, including palpable purpura,[127,132,133,139] cutaneous ulcerations,[129] cryoglobulinemia,[133] low serum complement levels[132,133,139,141] monoclonal gammopathies,[142,143] cytopenias,[127,139] splenomegaly,[127] and adenopathy.[129] Progression to high-grade lymphoma portends a poor prognosis.[130,132,133,140] In contrast, the incidence of other malignancies or all-cause mortality was not increased in patients with Sjögren's syndrome compared with the general population.[135,139,144] It is believed that chronic B cell stimulation may lead to the malignant transformation of clonal lines characteristic of Sjögren's syndrome. The presence of a viral trigger accounting for malignant transformation is one possible theory. EBV, among other viruses, has been implicated, but studies have failed to find EBV or other viral particles in lymphoma specimens associated with Sjögren's syndrome.[145]

There also have been reports of chromosomal translocations being present with increased frequency in patients with Sjögren's syndrome who have developed lymphoma. One group of investigators identified the presence of translocations of the proto-oncogene *bcl-2*[146] in five of seven patients with Sjögren's syndrome and lymphoma by the use of polymerase chain reaction. Such translocations were found in peripheral blood or bone marrow in 5% of unselected patients with Sjögren's syndrome without evidence of lymphoma in another study.[147] Conversely, no evidence of *bcl-2* translocations was present in 50 salivary gland biopsy specimens of patients with Sjögren's syndrome without evidence of lymphoma.[148] Analysis of biopsy specimens taken before the development of lymphoma from the seven patients previously mentioned showed no evidence of *bcl-2* translocation. Translocation seemed to correlate with the development of lymphoma in at least a subset of patients with Sjögren's syndrome, and the use of polymerase chain reaction technology may allow for early detection of malignant transformation.[147-149]

RHEUMATOID ARTHRITIS

Data from numerous studies since the 1970s are persuasive that RA is associated with a twofold to threefold increased risk for the development of lymphoproliferative disorders, the magnitude of which has remained constant despite dramatic changes in therapy. Many factors, including chronic inflammation and immune dysregulation, in addition to potential oncogenic properties of immunosuppressive therapies for the treatment of RA, must be considered when evaluating the risk of the development of hematologic malignancies. It is often difficult to separate the effects of medication use from the underlying severity of inflammation that makes medication use necessary or indicated, a concept termed *confounding by indication*.[150] This association has been highlighted further with widespread use of tumor necrosis factor (TNF)-α inhibitors for patients with refractory disease and the potential for these medications to interfere with innate immune tumor surveillance.

In 1978, an SIR of 2.7 for lymphoma was reported in a group of 46,101 Finnish RA patients compared with the general population.[151] A similarly increased risk of 2.4 for lymphoma was seen later in a group of 20,699 Danish patients[152]; an SIR of 1.9 to 2 was reported in a large cohort of 76,527 Swedish patients.[153,154] In the United States, an increased risk of 1.9 was found in a cohort of 18,527 patients,[155] and an SIR of 2.2 was found in a separate cohort of 8458 patients 65 years old and older.[156] Similar results were seen in the United Kingdom: A SIR of 2 to 2.4 for lymphoma was observed in an inception cohort of 2015 patients with inflammatory arthritis in England compared with the general population,[157] and an SIR of 2.04 to 2.39 was seen for non-Hodgkin's lymphoma in a cohort of 26,623 RA patients in Scotland.[158] A meta-analysis of nine cohort studies of RA patients found a pooled SIR of 3.9 for lymphoma using a random effects model.[137] Canadian investigators found an increased risk of leukemia (SIR 2.47) among RA patients, but were unable to confirm elevated rates of lymphomas compared with the general population.[159] Data from case-control studies of patients with non-Hodgkin's lymphoma have shown similar results: Odds ratios of 1.3 to 1.5 were found for underlying RA.[136,138] In general, lymphomas in patients with RA do not seem to be different with respect to grade, histology, or immunophenotype from the lymphomas seen in the general population.[160] Lymphoma patients with underlying RA, although having similar overall survival, seemed in one study to have a lower risk of progression, relapse, or death from lymphoma.[161]

Most studies have suggested that the risk for the development of lymphoma is related to the degree of inflammation. The Swedish group identified high inflammatory activity (defined by ESR, swollen and tender joint counts, and the physician's global assessment of disease activity) as a significant risk factor, with an odds ratio of 25.8 compared with low disease activity.[162] No association between any specific drug and the development of lymphoma was identified; however, the cohort examined was treated between 1965 and 1983, and few of these patients were apparently treated with immunosuppressive drugs, making the lack of association less certain.[162] In a follow-up case-control study of 378 lymphomas in a Swedish group of RA patients published more recently, a 71-fold increased risk of lymphoma in patients with high cumulative disease activity compared with low disease activity was seen.[163] Immunosuppressive therapy did not seem to modify risk for lymphoma in this study.

Patients with active RA often exhibit elevated immunoglobulin levels. In most cases, this is polyclonal in origin and may reflect the presence of rheumatoid factor. The possibility exists, however, that the paraprotein may be of monoclonal B cell origin and may reflect early development of a lymphoproliferative disorder. The incidence of monoclonal gammopathy in patients with RA has been estimated to be 1% to 2%,[164] which is comparable to the incidence of monoclonal gammopathy of unknown significance in the general population.[165] Other factors, such as the presence of secondary Sjögren's syndrome or the presence of urinary free light chains, seem to be of less prognostic significance for the development of a lymphoproliferative disorder.[164] Patients with Felty's syndrome (a variant of RA associated with neutropenia and splenomegaly) were found in a Veterans Affairs study of 906 men to have a 2-fold increase in total cancer incidence, but a 12-fold increase in risk of non-Hodgkin's lymphoma.[166]

Traditional Disease-Modifying Antirheumatic Drug Therapy

Several studies have looked at the contribution of disease-modifying antirheumatic drug (DMARD) therapy to the elevated risk of malignancies in RA patients. A prospective, observational study was performed in a group of Canadian RA patients enrolled in a DMARD registry.[167] Although this study found an increased rate of lymphoproliferative disorders in this cohort compared with the general Canadian population (SIR 8.05), there were no significant differences in DMARD exposure between patients who developed malignancy and patients who did not. A second group of Canadian investigators similarly identified an increased risk for the development of lymphoma and myeloma in RA patients overall compared with control groups.[168] In this study, the risk of lymphoma and myeloma seemed to be 4-fold greater

in the RA group when DMARD use was not controlled for and 3.4-fold greater when individual DMARD use was controlled for. Despite the low level of DMARD exposure in this population, no strong effect of DMARD use was seen.

Similar effects of DMARD use were seen in the study of Swedish patients with RA and lymphoma: Treatment with any DMARD (odds ratio 0.9), or specific use of methotrexate (odds ratio 0.8), did not seem to be associated with increased risk of lymphoma compared with DMARD-naive RA patients; however, no patients had been treated with TNF inhibition.[166] In contrast, a European cohort of RA patients enrolled in a DMARD registry was evaluated longitudinally for the development of malignancies.[169] These investigators found an increased risk of lymphoproliferative disorders in patients with the highest cumulative exposure to DMARDs compared with patients with less than 1 year of exposure (SIR 4.82).

Although inconclusive, data from these studies when taken together suggest a possible increased risk for the development of lymphoproliferative disorders in RA patients treated with DMARDs. More recent studies have suggested, however, that this increased risk may be due to the duration and severity of the underlying disorder, rather than to specific medication use.

Methotrexate

The recognition that erosion and joint destruction begin early has increased the use of DMARDs earlier in the course of disease, and methotrexate has become the most commonly used DMARD for the treatment of RA. Numerous long-term clinical studies have shown mixed data regarding the risk of lymphoproliferative diseases specifically related to treatment with methotrexate in patients with RA.[138,155,166,170] More than 50 cases of non-Hodgkin's lymphoma in RA patients treated with methotrexate have been cited in the literature[170]; most patients are reported to have B cell lymphoma, and extranodal involvement is common. Only 17 of these cases were assayed for the presence of EBV, of which 7 (41%) were positive.[170] This rate is less than that seen in post-transplantation patients or in patients with acquired immunodeficiency syndrome (AIDS) who develop lymphoma, but it is still significantly higher than that for lymphoma in the general population.[171] It has been postulated that, although methotrexate may carry a small risk of EBV-associated lymphoma in patients with RA, its ability to reduce disease activity of RA (which is an established risk factor for development of lymphoproliferative disorders) may lead in time to an overall reduction in the rate of malignancies seen in the RA population.[172]

Of the 50 original cases of B cell lymphoma cited in the literature, 8 patients have been reported to experience spontaneous remission after stopping methotrexate; of these, 4 patients were positive for EBV.[170] Of the patients who developed Hodgkin's disease in the French study, none treated with withdrawal of methotrexate alone achieved remission.[171] This finding suggests that, in at least a few methotrexate-treated patients with non-Hodgkin's lymphoma, the lymphoma might go into remission spontaneously, and that a brief period of observation without immunosuppressive therapy might be considered, particularly in patients found to be EBV positive.[170,172] The mechanisms by which lymphoma may develop in RA patients and be potentiated by methotrexate include persistent immunologic stimulation, which might lead to clonal selection and malignant transformation of CD5[+] B cells; reactivation of latent EBV[173]; direct oncogenic action; decreased apoptosis of infected B cells; and decreased natural killer cell activity.[170]

Tumor Necrosis Factor Inhibitors

The advent and widespread use of TNF-α inhibitors has dramatically changed the treatment options for patients with RA. Because of the role of TNF in innate immune tumor surveillance and cytotoxic response to B cell lymphomas, long-term use of such inhibitors brings concerns regarding further increases in risk for lymphoma development in RA patients.[174] After an initial report to the U.S. Food and Drug Administration of 26 cases of lymphoma in patients treated with etanercept and infliximab for RA or Crohn's disease,[175] numerous additional studies have examined the roles played by these agents with conflicting results.

Wolfe and Michaud[155] found an SIR of 2.9 in U.S. RA patients (10,012 patient-years) receiving anti-TNF therapy compared with 1.9 for all participating RA patients (29,314 patient-years), regardless of therapy. A larger Swedish study evaluated 4160 RA patients receiving TNF inhibitors and found an SIR of 2.9 for lymphoma compared with the general population.[181] Further analysis found a nonsignificant adjusted relative risk of lymphoma in the anti-TNF–treated group of 1.1 compared with 56,770 TNF-naive RA patients.[176] This study was followed by an analysis of pooled administrative databases in North America, which found a nonsignificant hazard ratio (1.1) for the development of lymphoma among RA patients 65 years old and older using biologic agents, primarily TNF inhibitors (N = 1152), compared with patients receiving methotrexate (N = 7306).[156] In contrast, a population-based study from Sweden evaluating 757 anti-TNF–treated patients (1603 patient-years) found an extremely high SIR of 11.5 compared with an SIR of 1.3 for TNF-naive patients (3948 patient-years).[177]

A meta-analysis specifically evaluating harmful events occurring during nine randomized, clinical trials of infliximab and adalimumab (data on etanercept were not included) has been published.[178] The authors found an odds ratio of developing any malignancy of 3.3 for patients receiving infliximab or adalimumab compared with patients receiving placebo. The odds ratio remained elevated after malignancies occurring within 6 weeks of initiating anti-TNF therapy and all nonmelanoma skin cancers were excluded. Of the 29 malignancies found in anti-TNF–treated patients, 4 were lymphomas. Criticisms of this study include heterogeneity of patient populations, concomitant medications, and comorbidities among clinical trials[179]; differential follow-up between placebo and treated groups; and an unusually low rate of malignancy seen in the placebo-treated patients.[180]

Overall, these data raise the possibility that TNF inhibition further increases risks of lymphoproliferative disorders in patients with RA. Several factors make these possible associations far from conclusive: Patients with RA already seem to be at an increased risk for the development of lymphoproliferative disorders; patients with the highest disease activity may be at the highest risk; and these patients also are more likely to have received previous immunomodulatory agents, to be on multiple agents in combination, and

to be receiving anti-TNF therapy. Separating the impact of disease activity, other DMARD therapy including prior or concomitant methotrexate, and the role of TNF inhibition on the risk of lymphoma is impossible; these confounders will always be present to some degree in studies of malignancy in relation to RA and its treatment.

Risk of Solid Tumors in Patients with Rheumatoid Arthritis

Despite persuasive evidence of increased risks of lymphoproliferative disorders associated with underlying RA, rates of overall all-site malignancies do not seem to be higher compared with the general population.[151-153,158,159] The overall "null" result of all malignancies is due to the combination of an increased risk of lymphoproliferative disorders offset by an apparent decreased risk of colorectal malignancies.[151-153,158,159,181] The decreased risk of colorectal cancer has been attributed to long-term use of NSAIDs among RA patients.[182]

Aside from lymphoproliferative disorders, only a few solid tumors have been associated with RA, including lung cancer and nonmelanoma skin cancer. An increased risk of lung cancer in RA patients has been seen in multiple studies.[151-153,158,159,181] A study evaluating three separate RA cohorts (an inpatient registry of 53,067 prevalent cases of RA, an inception cohort of 3703 incident RA cases, and a registry of 4160 RA patients treated with TNF inhibitors) found a consistently increased risk of lung cancer in all cohorts (SIR 1.48 to 2.4) compared with the general population.[181] This association may be related to tobacco use, which seems to be a common risk factor for the development of RA in addition to its well-known association with lung cancer,[183] although the particular association of lung cancer among RA patients who smoke is unknown. A slightly increased risk for the development of nonmelanoma skin cancer has been noted in several studies,[151,152,181,184] although the significance of these tumors, which carry a low probability of metastasis, is unclear.

SYSTEMIC LUPUS ERYTHEMATOSUS

The risks of developing malignancy in association with SLE have been difficult to estimate in the past. Small series and cohort studies have noted that patients with SLE might be at increased risk for malignancy, including non-Hodgkin's lymphomas, sarcomas, and breast carcinoma.[185-189] Other small series have not found differences,[190] however, or have found infrequent associations[191] in numbers or types of malignancy between patients with lupus and the general population.[190] Conflicting results also are seen in case-control studies of larger groups of patients, with some cohorts showing an increased overall risk of malignancy,[192-194] whereas others have failed to do so.[195-198] Some studies that did not find an increased risk of overall malignancies in patients with SLE have shown an increased risk of lymphoproliferative disorders, however.[136,138,196-198] Confounding factors complicating interpretation of these studies include possible incomplete ascertainment of malignancies, inclusion of nonrepresentative cohorts of patients with SLE, and selection of inappropriate control populations.[199]

To determine more adequately whether individuals with SLE are at an increased risk, systematic reviews and meta-analyses of pooled data are necessary. The SIR of individual studies has ranged from 1.1 to 2.6.[200] A meta-analysis of six of the clinical cohort studies found a slightly increased risk of overall malignancies in cohorts of patients with SLE, with an SIR of 1.58.[201] This analysis showed an increased risk of lymphomas in these cohorts, with an SIR of 3.57 for non-Hodgkin's lymphoma and 2.35 for Hodgkin's disease. A separately performed meta-analysis of the incidence of lymphoma in patients with SLE found an SIR of 7.4.[137] Individual hospital discharge database studies have shown a consistently higher risk of non-Hodgkin's lymphoma (SIR 3.72 to 6.7), but these studies examined only hospitalized patients with SLE.[200] Pooled analysis showed a slightly elevated risk for the development of breast cancer, with an SIR of 1.53, but they did not find an increased risk of lung or colorectal cancers in these patients.[201] The same confounding factors influencing the individual studies are a factor in interpreting these pooled data. A more recent series of studies analyzing nearly 9500 lupus patients (approximately 77,000 patient-years of observation) in a multinational cohort study has helped to define better potential associations with malignancy.[202,203]

The authors of these studies have found a slightly increased risk of malignancies overall (SIR 1.15) and higher risks for the development of hematologic malignancies (SIR 2.75), particularly non-Hodgkin's lymphoma (SIR 3.64).[202] Forty-two cases of non-Hodgkin's lymphomas were identified, most of which were of aggressive histologic subtypes.[204] The elevated risk of non-Hodgkin's lymphoma seemed to be independent of race or ethnicity in this cohort, although white patients seemed to have higher rates of malignancy in general compared with patients of other ethnicities.[205]

Several studies have additionally raised concerns about an increased risk of gynecologic malignancies among women with SLE.[192,201,203] Data supporting an increased risk of developing breast cancer have been mixed; however, increased risks may have been masked by differential rates of known risk factors for breast cancer compared with women in the general population.[203] Women with SLE have been shown to have less exposure to oral contraceptives and greater prevalence of nulliparity, obesity, and tobacco use, all of which may mitigate the numbers of breast or other hormonal malignancies seen in this population.[206] The number of breast cancers seen in large cohorts of women with SLE well exceeds what would be expected based on traditional Gail model risk factors, including age, parity, family history, reproductive history, and use of exogenous estrogens (SIR 2.1).[207,208] Breast cancers in women with SLE do not seem to be diagnosed at earlier stages than in the general population, making surveillance bias an unlikely explanation for the associations seen.[209] One study suggested that women with SLE receive age-appropriate screening mammography less frequently than do healthy women.[210]

The relative prevalence of cervical cancer in SLE patients is more difficult to estimate because national cancer registries often do not record malignancies in situ. In the large multinational study performed more recently, the SIR for invasive cervical cancer was found to be elevated at 1.26,

albeit with confidence intervals that cross the null.[202] Other studies have confirmed an increased risk of abnormal Pap smears and cervical dysplasia in women with SLE.[211-214] Different studies have implicated increased prevalence of human papillomavirus infection and other sexually transmitted diseases,[213,215] oral contraceptive use,[215] and immunosuppression[212,215] that may partly explain this association. Similarly to mammography, women with SLE seem less likely to undergo routine Pap testing than women in the general population.[210]

Although the exact etiology of the association is unknown, several theories have arisen to explain the possible connection between SLE and malignancy, especially B cell lymphoma. Some authors have postulated that certain immunologic defects may predispose patients to SLE and B cell lymphoma, including apoptosis dysfunction, chronic antigenic stimulation, and overexpression of *bcl-2* oncogene.[200,216] Viruses, EBV in particular, also have been postulated as part of the development of SLE and lymphoma.[200,216] Studies have not conclusively validated any of these theories to date, however.

Overall, the presence of SLE seems to carry a small increased risk for the development of lymphoproliferative disorders, particularly non-Hodgkin's lymphoma. The underlying cause of this association is unknown. The association does not seem to be related to the use of immunosuppressive or cytotoxic agents.[185,196,198,200] Data also suggest that lupus patients may be less likely to receive recommended cancer screening.[210]

SYSTEMIC SCLEROSIS

Although data are conflicting, most evidence suggests that individuals with systemic sclerosis seem to have an increased risk of developing malignancy.[217] The malignancies that have been implicated are often in organs affected by inflammation and fibrosis, including the lung, breast, esophagus, and skin. The SIR of malignancy in the scleroderma population is 1.5 to 5.1 compared with that of the general population.[218-223] There is an apparent increase in the observed number of cases of lung cancers that occur in the setting of pulmonary fibrosis but not in association with tobacco use.[222,224] There also seems to be a temporal correlation between the onset of systemic sclerosis and the development of breast cancer, although not an increased incidence of breast cancer.[218] Older age at the time of diagnosis with systemic sclerosis seems to be a significant risk factor for the development of cancer.[219] Data are mixed regarding associations between systemic sclerosis–specific autoantibodies and the development of cancer: Selected studies support potential associations,[221,225] whereas others do not.[222,226]

Although the SIR for all malignancies is 1.5 to 2.4, the incidence ratio for lung cancer can be as high as 7.8 and for non-Hodgkin's lymphoma 9.6. Cases of non-Hodgkin's lymphoma seem to be more likely to occur within the first year of the diagnosis of systemic sclerosis.[220] Elevations in incidence also were found for other specific cancers, including nonmelanoma skin cancers (4.2), primary liver cancers (3.3), and hematopoietic cancers (2.3)—all having a higher incidence than that in the general population. The greatest risk seems to correspond to areas commonly affected by fibrosis, particularly the lung and skin. Esophageal involvement, common to limited and diffuse systemic sclerosis, is the likely etiology for an increased incidence of Barrett's esophagus (12.7%)[227] and development of esophageal cancer (SIR 9.6).[223] Potential biologic explanations for a possible increased incidence of carcinoma of the tongue seen in one cohort of systemic sclerosis patients are less clear.[228] In contrast to the above-mentioned data, one study found no increase in overall or specific malignancies in patients with systemic sclerosis (SIR 0.91 overall).[226] Localized scleroderma, including morphea or linear scleroderma, does not seem to convey an increased risk of malignancy.[229] Several reports have described the development of postirradiation morphea in patients treated for breast cancer.[230]

PRIMARY TUMORS AND METASTATIC DISEASE

PRIMARY MUSCULOSKELETAL TUMORS

This section does not provide in-depth knowledge of the primary tumors of the musculoskeletal system. Rather, it provides a reference to the most common primary malignant musculoskeletal tumors and symptoms that may arise in association with them. The primary tumors of bone, including benign and malignant tumors, are discussed in more detail in Chapter 114.

A primary malignant bone cancer is any neoplasm that develops from the tissues or cells found within bone that has the ability to metastasize. Neoplasms may develop or arise from any of the types of cells present within the bone—osteoblasts, chondrocytes, adipose and fibrous tissue, vascular cells, hematopoietic cells, and neural tissue.[231] A neoplasm developing from any of these tissues is called a sarcoma, which signifies that it is derived from mesenchymal tissue. The bone sarcomas are named for the predominant differentiated tissue type, such as osteosarcomas, chondrosarcomas, liposarcomas, and angiosarcomas.[231]

The most common manifestation of these tumors is the development of pain in the area of the lesion, which may be accompanied by a sympathetic effusion or stiffness in the surrounding joint. This discomfort does not seem to be activity related and is often worse at night. These tumors can manifest, however, as painless masses or as pathologic fractures. Systemic features, such as fatigue, malaise, weight loss, fevers, and night sweats, are rare with all of these tumors except for Ewing's sarcoma.[231] Primary malignant bone tumors are uncommon, particularly compared with other types of cancer. They have their highest incidence in childhood and adolescence and constitute 3.2% of childhood malignancies that occur before age 15 years. The incidence has been reported in this age group as 3 per 100,000 individuals.[232] These tumors commonly arise out of areas of rapid growth, with the most common site of primary bone sarcomas being the metaphysis near the growth plate.[232]

Table 112-4 lists the most common types of primary malignant bone tumors. Osteosarcoma is the most common of the tumors and generally occurs in individuals in the second decade of life or in elderly individuals.[233] Osteosarcoma also can occur secondary to radiation therapy delivered as treatment for other malignancies. Paget's disease of bone can rarely (<1% of cases) proceed to malignant transformation.[234] Severe pain in the setting of Paget's disease may signal transformation to

Table 112-4 Primary Bone Tumors

Nonosseous Tumors	Osseous Tumors
Multiple myeloma	Osteosarcoma
Round cell tumors	Chondrosarcoma
	Giant cell tumors
	Fibrosarcoma

osteogenic sarcoma. Tumors most frequently affect the femur, humerus, skull, and pelvis and can result in pathologic fractures. Survival is usually less than 1 year. Differentiating malignancy from Paget's disease may require a biopsy.[235,236]

Chondrosarcoma has been reported as the second most common of the malignant bone tumors. This tumor may occur as a primary tumor or as a malignant transformation in the setting of benign lesions, such as an enchondroma or osteochondroma.[237] Fibrosarcoma is significantly less common than the previously mentioned tumors and accounts for less than 4% of primary malignant bone tumors.[238]

As a group, round cell tumors include primary lymphomas of bone, Ewing's sarcoma, and metastatic neuroblastoma. Ewing's sarcoma is a common primary bone tumor of childhood. Giant cell tumors as a group account for 4.5% of bone tumors. They usually arise from the metaphysis or epiphysis of long bones, generally around the knee. Most are benign, but a few are malignant lesions, usually arising out of a previously irradiated benign giant cell tumor.[231]

In addition to the primary malignancies of bone, there are a plethora of malignant tumors that can arise from mesenchymal connective tissue; these are also known as sarcomas.[238,239] They can result in joint complaints, but more often result in soft tissue complaints. They are very rare. Rhabdomyosarcoma is a malignant tumor arising from muscle tissue. It is the fourth most common solid tumor in children and is responsible for more than half of all soft tissue sarcomas in children. Rhabdomyosarcoma rarely occurs in adults. It can appear at any site, and the symptoms are most often referable to the site involved. Most commonly, rhabdomyosarcoma affects the orbits, genitourinary tract, limbs, head and neck, and parameningeal areas. It commonly metastasizes to the lymph nodes, lungs, and bone.[232,240]

METASTATIC DISEASE

When bone lesions are identified, primary tumors need to be considered, although most malignant lesions in bone are metastatic. Metastasis rarely affects muscles, joints, or adjacent connective tissue. More commonly, it affects bone. The most common sites of metastasis are the spine and pelvis. It is uncommon to find metastatic lesions distal to the elbow, and, although rare, metastasis to the foot is more common than to the hand.[241] When distal or acral metastasis is identified, it is often associated with lung cancer.[242] Primary tumors generally associated with metastases to bone include tumors in the prostate, thyroid, lung, breast, and kidney.[243] Although most skeletal metastases do not produce pain, one of the most common causes of cancer pain is the infiltration of bone. The pain can be intense and stabbing or dull. It is often constant rather than intermittent, is worse at night, and often is worse with weight bearing and movement.[244] Rheumatic or arthritic complaints often can occur before lesions are easily identified on radiographs. Arthritis associated with metastatic carcinoma

Table 112-5 Frequent Features of Arthritis Resulting from Metastatic Carcinoma

Presence of constitutional symptoms
Prior history of malignancy
Protracted clinical course
Negative culture results, negative crystal analysis
Medical therapeutic failure
Rapid reaccumulation of hemorrhagic noninflammatory effusion
Radiologic evidence of destructive process

is most commonly monarticular and most commonly affects the knee. Metastases to the hip, ankle, wrist, hand, and foot have been reported, but occur less frequently. Breast and lung carcinomas are present in most patients.[245] Metastases to the extremities can simulate gout, osteomyelitis, tenosynovitis, or acro-osteolysis. The development of joint involvement can be related to direct synovial implantation or involvement of the juxta-articular or subchondral bone.[246] Table 112-5 presents the clinical features suggestive of underlying metastases.

Radiographic features of bone tumors can be significant when interpreting the duration of disease and the type of malignancy. Lesions may be lytic or blastic, and patterns of destruction often reflect the aggressiveness of tumors. Well-circumscribed lesions may be more indicative of slower growth, whereas a "moth-eaten" pattern with evidence of cortical destruction typically signifies a more rapid rate of growth. What has been described as a permeative pattern suggests an extremely rapid rate of destruction and is often associated with an extraosseous soft tissue mass.[231] Computed tomography, magnetic resonance imaging, and radionucleotide imaging also can provide significant information for diagnosis, staging, prognosis, and therapy.

POSTCHEMOTHERAPY RHEUMATISM

Several rheumatic or musculoskeletal manifestations can develop in patients after administration of chemotherapy for the treatment of malignancy. Postchemotherapy rheumatism has been best described in patients treated for breast cancer, but also has been described in other malignancies, including ovarian cancer and non-Hodgkin's lymphoma.[247-249] The phenomenon has been described as a noninflammatory, self-limited, migratory arthropathy. Typically, symptoms develop several weeks to several months after the completion of chemotherapy and often include myalgia, stiffness, arthralgia, and arthritis involving the small joints of the hands, ankles, and knees.[248] It can be mistaken for RA based on its symptoms; however, most patients have little or no evidence of synovial thickening and have no radiographic or serologic evidence to suggest RA. The pathogenesis of this process is unknown; however, it is self-limited, usually lasting less than 1 year, and is best treated in a conservative fashion. Evaluation should be performed to exclude recurrent carcinoma or another inflammatory condition. The medications most frequently implicated in this phenomenon include cyclophosphamide, 5-fluorouracil, methotrexate, and tamoxifen.[249-251]

Other immunomodulatory agents also have been linked to the development of musculoskeletal findings. Tamoxifen use has been associated with the development of an acute inflammatory arthritis similar to RA.[251] Use of interleukin-2 can

result in spondyloarthritis or inflammatory arthritis. Interferon-α administration can result in seropositive nodular RA and myalgia and arthralgia.[252,253] The use of interferon also can result in autoantibody formation and features suggestive of SLE and autoimmune thyroid disease.[253-255]

LYMPHOPROLIFERATIVE AND MYELOPROLIFERATIVE DISEASES

LEUKEMIA

Leukemia can result in the development of musculoskeletal complaints. Bone pain is the most common musculoskeletal manifestation, and it has been reported to occur in 50% of adults with leukemia.[256] Long bone pain is more common in children, whereas axial pain is more common in adults. Generally, the bone pain is more common in the lower than the upper extremities.[257] Overt synovitis can develop in association with acute and chronic leukemia and can result in the development of monarticular or polyarticular arthritis.[258] The pathogenesis seems to be leukemic infiltration of the synovium and subperiosteal tissue. Bleeding or hemorrhage in the joint also may be associated with the process. Most cases of arthritis associated with leukemia are seen in children— 14% to 50% compared with 4% to 16.5% in adults.[259-261]

In a series of adult patients with acute leukemia studied over a 10-year period, 5.8% (8 of 139) of the patients presented with rheumatic manifestations. On average, symptoms of arthritis preceded the diagnosis of leukemia by 3.25 months.[262] The most common patterns of presentation were an asymmetric large joint involvement in association with low back pain, followed by symmetric polyarthritis mimicking early RA. Rheumatic manifestations included morning stiffness, low back pain, nonarticular bone pain, pain out of proportion to objective findings, low-grade fever, and elevation of the ESR. The response to NSAIDs, glucocorticoids, and conventional antirheumatic therapy was reportedly poor, but tumor-directed chemotherapy resulted in substantial improvement of the rheumatic manifestations. Patients with these manifestations also were more likely to exhibit early osteopenia or lytic bone lesions. Ultimately, prognosis and mortality rates were no different between patients presenting with or without rheumatic manifestations.[262]

In contrast, a large retrospective study of children with leukemia found 21.4% (36 of 168) with acute lymphoblastic leukemia and 10.5% (6 of 57) with acute nonlymphoblastic leukemia developed symptoms associated with bones and joints. Thirteen of these patients with acute lymphoblastic leukemia had evidence of bony lesions on radiographs.[263] Many of these children had been incorrectly treated for juvenile RA or osteomyelitis before the diagnosis of leukemia. The group with bone lesions seemed to do very well, and their condition might fall into a subgroup of childhood leukemia that has a better prognosis.[258,263] A more recent study found that the presence of subtle blood count changes and nighttime pain may help distinguish leukemia from juvenile RA.[261]

MULTIPLE MYELOMA

Multiple myeloma is a neoplastic proliferation of plasma cells, a nonosseous malignant tumor arising in the marrow. In contrast to the other primary tumors of bone, which have their highest incidence in children and adolescents, myeloma is a tumor of adults, occurring most commonly in the fifth and sixth decades of life. The most common musculoskeletal feature of this disease is the development of bone pain. Other hallmark features are diffuse pain and stiffness. Patients characteristically develop osteopenia, and osteolytic lesions are seen on radiographs. The lytic lesions, which can occur in any area of the skeleton, are produced by focal accumulations of plasma cells. Osteosclerotic lesions also have been reported.[264] True arthritis is rare, but cases of arthritis secondary to articular and periarticular invasion with malignant cells have been reported in multiple myeloma and in Waldenström's macroglobulinemia.[265] A secondary feature of the disease, which can often lead to additional musculoskeletal complaints, is the development of hyperuricemia and secondary gout. Sjögren's syndrome and other autoimmune phenomena also have been described in association with multiple myeloma.[266]

LYMPHOMA

Musculoskeletal symptoms have been reported in 25% of cases of non-Hodgkin's lymphoma.[267] The most common musculoskeletal problem associated with lymphoma is the development of bone pain associated with metastases or lymphoma in the bone. By report, more than 50% of patients have evidence of bone lesions at autopsy; however, few patients actually present with arthritis or bone pain.[258,268] Nonetheless, non-Hodgkin's lymphoma has been reported to manifest as a seronegative arthritis with or without other features, such as lymphadenopathy and hepatomegaly, typically seen with this disease. Monarticular and polyarticular involvement can occur. Cases have been reported of polyarthritis simulating RA in the setting of non-Hodgkin's lymphoma.[269] Although it is unusual to see direct involvement of the synovium, this also has been reported. There have been cases with radiographic evidence of bone destruction associated with non-Hodgkin's lymphomatous arthropathy.[270] Suspicion of lymphoma should be heightened in patients in whom severe constitutional symptoms seem out of proportion to the degree of arthritis, especially in patients who are negative for rheumatoid factor.[267]

ANGIOIMMUNOBLASTIC LYMPHADENOPATHY

Angioimmunoblastic lymphadenopathy is a rare lymphoproliferative disorder marked by the clinical features of lymphadenopathy, hepatosplenomegaly, rash, and hypergammaglobulinemia. Patients can develop a nonerosive, symmetric, seronegative polyarthritis concurrent with other features or as an initial complaint of the disease.[271-273] Similar features have been reported with intravascular lymphoma, with a report of a patient presenting with a symmetric polyarthritis accompanied by fever.[274] Table 112-6 lists musculoskeletal complaints found with hematologic malignancy.

GRAFT-VERSUS-HOST DISEASE

Graft-versus-host disease is a complication of bone marrow transplantation and a major cause of morbidity and mortality in the transplant population. Numerous musculoskeletal

Table 112-6 Musculoskeletal Manifestations of Hematologic Malignancy

Malignancy	Pathogenesis
Leukemia	Infiltration of synovium
Lymphoma	Metastases or invasion of bone, rarely joint
Angioblastic lymphadenopathy	Vasculitis, cryoglobulinemia
Multiple myeloma	Metastasis or invasion of bone, hyperuricemia

complaints arise in the setting of acute graft-versus-host disease (lasting 0 to 3 months) and in chronic graft-versus-host disease (lasting >3 months after transplantation). The most frequent manifestation is the involvement of the skin, which in many cases can progress to resemble the changes of systemic sclerosis. Skin changes consistent with eosinophilic fasciitis also have been reported.[257] Graft-versus-host disease can lead to symptoms of keratoconjunctivitis sicca and xerostomia resembling Sjögren's syndrome. Other features including arthralgias, arthritis, myositis, Raynaud's phenomenon, and serositis also have been reported.[257,275]

ASSOCIATION OF IMMUNOMODULATORY AGENTS WITH MALIGNANCY

Many of the medications used to treat rheumatic diseases are modulators of the immune system. As such, they may be associated directly or indirectly with an increased risk of the subsequent development of malignancy associated with the underlying disorder. An individual agent may confer this risk through direct mutagenesis of DNA, through generalized immunosuppression with the risk of developing an EBV-associated lymphoproliferative disorder, or through injury to an unintended organ system, such as the bladder with the use of cyclophosphamide. Longer duration of use of these agents has been associated with increasing risk of developing subsequent malignancies.[276] It is often difficult, however, to differentiate adequately the individual risk of an agent, particularly in the background of an autoimmune disease that itself can convey an increased risk for the development of malignancy. Table 112-7 provides an overview of the potential oncologic risks of various immunomodulatory therapies.

CYCLOPHOSPHAMIDE

Cyclophosphamide is an alkylating agent that kills resting and cycling cells and has cytotoxic, mutagenic, and carcinogenic potential. It is used predominantly for the treatment of vasculitis, glomerulonephritis, and other life-threatening or organ-threatening manifestations of rheumatic disease. The use of cyclophosphamide in RA seems to result in an increased risk of the development of bladder cancer, skin cancer, and hematologic malignancies including non-Hodgkin's lymphoma and leukemia.[277,278] Risk factors for the development of neoplasia include higher total dosage, longer duration of therapy, and tobacco use.[279] The overall relative risk of developing malignancy seems to be 1.5 to 4.1 for those treated compared with controls, and the increased

Table 112-7 Immunomodulatory Agents and Risk of Malignancy

DMARD	Risk of Malignancy
Cyclophosphamide	Non-Hodgkin's lymphoma, leukemia, bladder cancer, skin cancer
Azathioprine	Non-Hodgkin's lymphoma
Cyclosporine	Immunosuppression-associated lymphoma
Methotrexate	Immunosuppression-associated lymphoma
Gold salts	None known
Hydroxychloroquine	None known
Penicillamine	None known
Sulfasalazine	None known
Leflunomide	None known
Biologic response modifiers	Unknown, possible lymphoma

DMARD, disease-modifying antirheumatic drug.

risk of bladder cancer continues more than 17 years after cyclophosphamide therapy.[278,279]

The increased incidence of bladder cancer and other malignancies in patients with Wegener's granulomatosis treated with cyclophosphamide has been shown in a series of studies from Sweden.[280,281] Patients with Wegener's granulomatosis treated with cyclophosphamide had a twofold increased risk for cancer overall, with higher risks for specific tumors: bladder cancer (SIR 4.8), leukemia (SIR 5.7), and lymphoma (SIR 4.2).[280] As with RA patients, higher cumulative doses of cyclophosphamide were associated with higher risks of developing bladder cancer.[281] The increased risk for the development of bladder cancer is believed to be a direct result of high concentrations of active metabolites in the bladder, such as acrolein. The overall risks of bladder cancer may be less with pulsed, intravenous treatment than with daily oral cyclophosphamide. The use of cyclophosphamide generally is restricted to life-threatening or organ-threatening disease in which the risks associated with treatment are outweighed by the serious effects of untreated rheumatic disease.

METHOTREXATE

Methotrexate is one of the most commonly used agents in the treatment of rheumatic diseases and generally has a favorable side-effect profile. Similar to many other immunomodulatory agents, questions have been raised regarding the oncogenic potential of methotrexate when used to treat autoimmune or inflammatory disorders. There has been no strong evidence to suggest that methotrexate conveys an increased risk for the development of solid tumors. There have been reports, however, of a relationship between methotrexate use and the development of lymphomas, as previously discussed in the section on RA-associated malignancies. Despite this possible association, methotrexate has been shown to reduce all-cause, cardiovascular, and noncardiovascular mortality in patients with RA compared with RA patients treated with other agents.[282] Although this work may not directly address questions regarding the use of methotrexate in RA and the risk of developing malignancy,

it helps to answer the overall question of whether this agent's benefits outweigh its risks.

Studies have been published regarding the possible association of methotrexate use in the treatment of RA and the development of lymphoproliferative disorders associated with EBV, as was previously mentioned in the section on RA-associated malignancies. EBV has been reported in non-Hodgkin's lymphoma, Hodgkin's disease, and T cell lymphomas in RA patients treated with methotrexate.[171,172,283,284]

One set of investigators reviewed all reported cases of lymphoproliferative disorders in RA patients treated with methotrexate.[285] They subsequently identified most of the cases as non-Hodgkin's B cell lymphomas, either large cell or diffuse mixed type. In many of the cases, there was extranodal involvement. In patients tested, 46% showed evidence of EBV infection, and in 14 patients treated solely by withdrawal of methotrexate, 8 achieved full remission. The rate of EBV association is less than that seen in posttransplantation patients or in patients with AIDS who develop lymphoma, but it is nevertheless higher than that for lymphoma in the general population.[285]

Further investigation into the association of immunomodulatory agents for the treatment of rheumatic diseases and the development of lymphoproliferative disorders also has shown an association with EBV. After analyzing 10 EBV-associated lymphoid neoplasms in patients with RA or dermatomyositis using polymerase chain reaction, investigators found that these lymphoproliferative disorders can harbor EBV strain type A or B, with type A being the most prevalent; this is similar to what has been reported in post–solid organ transplantation, immunosuppression-associated lymphoproliferative disorders. EBV-latent membrane protein-1 deletions seem to occur in one third of the cases, but are not required for the neoplasm to develop.[286]

It is possible that, although not increasing the overall risk for the development of lymphoproliferative disorders, treatment with methotrexate may carry a small risk for the development of EBV-associated lymphoid malignancies similar to malignancies seen in other immunosuppressed individuals. A subset of these patients may respond with regression of the tumor after discontinuation of methotrexate.

AZATHIOPRINE

Azathioprine is a purine analogue that leads to inhibition of purine synthesis and direct cytotoxic effects. The use of azathioprine is associated with an increased risk of lymphoma and nonlymphoproliferative cancers.[278,287-289] Compared with the risk to the general population, azathioprine treatment can result in a 10-fold increased risk for the development of lymphoproliferative disorders[289]; this amounts to 1 case of lymphoma per 1000 patient-years of azathioprine treatment.[288] A correlation between the cumulative dose of azathioprine used and the incidence of cancer has been seen.[278,289] Leukemia also has been reported in association with azathioprine use.[290,291] In contrast, one study reported outcomes of 148 SLE patients treated with azathioprine compared with 210 unexposed SLE patients.[292] In this 24-year longitudinal study, only 5.4% of azathioprine-treated patients developed malignancies (none were lymphoma) compared with 6.7% of azathioprine-naive patients (three with lymphoma).

CYCLOSPORINE

Cyclosporine is currently used for the treatment of RA and SLE, particularly for lupus nephritis. Based on experience with solid organ transplantation in which post-transplantation lymphoproliferative disorders are well recognized as complications arising in allograft recipients treated with immunosuppressive drugs, there has been a concern for an increased risk of the development of malignancy, especially lymphoproliferative disorders, with cyclosporine treatment of rheumatic diseases. Although cyclosporine has been used formally in the treatment of RA since the 1980s, there have not been sufficient numbers of patients followed longitudinally for sufficient time to determine whether the drug may convey an increased risk for the development of malignancy. Cyclosporine has been associated with the development of EBV-associated lymphomas in some patients with RA[293]; however, a retrospective study looked at more than 1000 RA patients treated with cyclosporine in clinical trials and concluded that the use of cyclosporine did not increase the potential risk for the development of malignancy or the type of malignancy beyond that seen with the use of other DMARDs.[294] A second retrospective and case-control study found that cyclosporine treatment in RA patients does not increase the risk of malignancies in general or the risk of malignant lymphoproliferative disorders.[295] This finding may be due partly to the lower doses generally used for the treatment of rheumatic diseases compared with allograft recipients.[278]

LEFLUNOMIDE

Leflunomide is a selective inhibitor of de novo pyrimidine synthesis and leads to cell cycle arrest in rapidly replicating cell lines, such as activated T cells in RA. Currently, there does not seem to be evidence that leflunomide conveys an increased risk for the development of malignancy. As is so important with the introduction of any new medication, long-term safety studies and postmarketing surveillance are necessary to ascertain whether there is increased risk at 10 and 20 years.

BIOLOGIC RESPONSE MODIFIERS

As a group, commercially available biologic response modifiers include TNF inhibitors and interleukin-1 antagonists. Risk of developing malignancies in association with TNF inhibitors in patients with RA is discussed in detail in the section on RA-associated malignancies. A study examined the incidence of malignancies developing in 180 patients with Wegener's granulomatosis participating in a randomized controlled multicenter clinical trial of etanercept or placebo in addition to conventional therapy for induction of remission followed by monotherapy for maintenance.[296] No hematologic malignancies were seen during the study. All solid malignancies found during the trial were in subjects receiving etanercept in addition to cyclophosphamide during the trial. There is a suggestion that etanercept may increase the risk of solid tumors above that expected from treatment with cyclophosphamide alone; however, patients randomly assigned to etanercept were nearly 5 years older than the patients in the placebo group and were less likely to have newly diagnosed Wegener's granulomatosis.[296]

RADIATION

Radiation therapy is no longer used for the treatment of inflammatory arthritis. Its use in ankylosing spondylitis in the early part of the 20th century resulted in significant increases in malignancies, including leukemia; lymphoma; myeloma; and esophageal, colon, pancreas, lung, bone, soft tissue, prostate, bladder, and kidney cancers. It also resulted in an increased relative risk of mortality of 1.3 compared with expected deaths. There were clear dose-response relationships between the amount of radiation and the development of individual cancers.[210,211]

CONCLUSION

A plethora of factors contribute to the development of musculoskeletal syndromes in the setting of autoimmune disease and malignancy. There are a great many autoimmune disorders, and for most, the underlying etiology and pathogenesis have not been elucidated. This incredible diversity often makes understanding the relationship between associated symptoms difficult. To make any generalizations regarding association between an autoimmune disorder and the subsequent development of malignancy, large numbers of patients must be studied longitudinally for exceptionally long periods. Other confounders complicate the picture. Many of the agents used in the treatment of connective tissue and autoimmune disorders modulate the immune system. These agents may have direct carcinogenic potential, whereas others may affect the immune system in a way that may decrease tumor surveillance and subsequently lead to the development of a neoplasm. Intricately entwined are the unique differences of individual immune systems not only in healthy individuals, but also in individuals whose immune systems are already altered based on an underlying autoimmune disorder. Although uncommon, it is plausible that virtually any of the autoimmune-based diseases and the agents used to treat them might be associated with malignancy in certain circumstances. Most important, when musculoskeletal symptoms arise, malignancy or paraneoplastic syndromes should be considered in the differential diagnosis, especially when patients present with atypical features of autoimmune disease or are refractory to conventional treatment. In addition, the potential for any agent to induce a neoplastic process must be weighed against its proposed benefits before initiating it as therapy.

REFERENCES

1. Stedman's Medical Dictionary, 26th ed. Baltimore, Williams & Wilkins, 1995.
2. Caldwell DS: Carcinoma polyarthritis: Manifestations and differential diagnosis. Med Grand Rounds 1:378, 1982.
3. Chan MK, Hendrickson CS, Taylor KE: Polyarthritis associated with breast carcinoma. West J Med 137:132, 1982.
4. Stummvoll GH, Aringer M, Machold KP, et al: Cancer polyarthritis resembling rheumatoid arthritis as a first sign of hidden neoplasms. Scand J Rheumatol 30:40, 2001.
5. Gonzalez-Gay MA, Garcia-Porrua C, Salvarani C, et al: Cutaneous vasculitis and cancer: A clinical approach. Clin Exp Rheumatol 18:305, 2000.

6. Sanchez-Guerrero J, Gutierrez-Urena S, Vidaller A, et al: Vasculitis as a paraneoplastic syndrome: Report of 11 cases and review of the literature. J Rheumatol 17:1458, 1990.
7. Garcia-Porrua C, Gonzalez-Gay MA: Cutaneous vasculitis as a paraneoplastic syndrome in adults. Arthritis Rheum 41:1133, 1998.
8. Bachmeyer C, Wetterwald E, Aractingi S: Cutaneous vasculitis in the course of hematologic malignancies. Dermatology 210:8, 2005.
9. Hamidou MA, Derenne S, Audrain MAP, et al: Prevalence of rheumatic manifestations and antineutrophil cytoplasmic antibodies in haematological malignancies: A prospective study. Rheumatology 39:417, 2000.
10. Hamidou MA, Boumalassa A, Larroche C, et al: Systemic medium-sized vessel vasculitis associated with chronic myelomonocytic leukemia. Semin Arthritis Rheum 31:119, 2001.
11. Hamidou MA, El Kouri D, Audrain M, et al: Systemic antineutrophil cytoplasmic antibody vasculitis associated with lymphoid neoplasia. Ann Rheum Dis 60:295, 2001.
12. Tatsis E, Reinhold-Keller E, Steindorf K, et al: Wegener's granulomatosis associated with renal cell carcinoma. Arthritis Rheum 42:751, 1999.
13. Knight AM, Ekbom A, Askling J: Cancer risk in a population based cohort of patients with Wegener's granulomatosis. Arthritis Rheum 44:S332, 2001 (abstract 1677).
14. Hutson TE, Hoffman GS: Temporal concurrence of vasculitis and cancer: A report of 12 cases. Arthritis Care Res 13:417, 2000.
15. Pankhurst T, Savage COS, Gordon C, et al: Malignancy is increased in ANCA-associated vasculitis. Rheumatology (Oxf) 43:1532, 2004.
16. Greer JM, Longley S, Edwards NL, et al: Vasculitis associated with malignancy: Experience with 13 patients and literature review. Medicine (Balt) 67:220, 1988.
17. Dammacco F, Sansonno D, Piccoli C, et al: The cryoglobulins: An overview. Eur J Clin Invest 31:628, 2001.
18. Vallat L, Benhamou Y, Gutierrez M, et al: Clonal B cell populations in the blood and liver of patients with chronic hepatitis C virus infection. Arthritis Rheum 50:3668, 2004.
19. La Civita L, Zignego AL, Monti M, et al: Mixed cryoglobulinemia as a possible preneoplastic disorder. Arthritis Rheum 38:1859, 1995.
20. Ramos-Casals M, Garcia-Carrasco M, Trejo O, et al: Lymphoproliferative diseases in patients with cryoglobulinemia: Clinical description of 27 cases. Arthritis Rheum 44:S58, 2001.
21. Monti G, Pioltelli P, Saccardo F, et al: Incidence and characteristics of non-Hodgkin lymphomas in a multicenter case file of patients with hepatitis C virus-related symptomatic mixed cryoglobulinemias. Arch Intern Med 165:101, 2005.
22. Bianco E, Marcucci F, Mele A, et al: Prevalence of hepatitis C virus infection in lymphoproliferative diseases other than B-cell non-Hodgkin's lymphoma, and in myeloproliferatives diseases: An Italian multi-center case-control study. Haematologica 89:70, 2004.
23. Trejo O, Ramos-Casals M, Lopez-Guillermo A, et al: Hematologic malignancies in patients with cryoglobulinemia: Association with autoimmune and chronic viral diseases. Semin Arthritis Rheum 33:19, 2003.
24. Virshup AM, Sliwinski AJ: Polyarthritis and subcutaneous nodules associated with carcinoma of the pancreas. Arthritis Rheum 16:388, 1973.
25. Marhaug G, Hvidsten D: Arthritis complicating acute pancreatitis: A rare but important condition to be distinguished from juvenile rheumatoid arthritis. Scand J Rheumatol 12:397, 1988.
26. Naschitz JE, Boss JH, Misselevich I, et al: The fasciitis-panniculitis syndromes: Clinical and pathologic features. Medicine (Balt) 75:6, 1996.
27. Naschitz JE, Yeshurun D, Zucherman E, et al: Cancer-associated fasciitis panniculitis. Cancer 73:231, 1994.
28. Masuoka H, Kikuchi K, Takahashi S, et al: Eosinophilic fasciitis associated with low-grade T-cell lymphoma. Br J Dermatol 139:928, 1998.
29. Pfinsgraff J, Buckingham RB, Killian PJ, et al: Palmar fasciitis and arthritis with malignant neoplasms: A paraneoplastic syndrome. Semin Arthritis Rheum 16:118, 1986.
30. Enomoto M, Takemura H, Suzuki M, et al: Palmar fasciitis and polyarthritis associated with gastric carcinoma: Complete resolution after total gastrectomy. Intern Med 39:754, 2000.
31. Saxman SB, Seitz D: Breast cancer associated with palmar fasciitis and arthritis. J Clin Oncol 15:3515, 1997.
32. Martorell EA, Murray PM, Peterson JJ, et al: Palmar fasciitis and arthritis syndrome associated with metastatic ovarian carcinoma: A report of 4 cases. J Hand Surg 29A:4, 2004.
33. Mekhail N, Kapural L: Complex regional pain syndrome type I in cancer patients. Current Rev Pain 4:227, 2000.
34. Michaels RM, Sorber JA: Reflex sympathetic dystrophy as a probable paraneoplastic syndrome: Case report and literature review. Arthritis Rheum 27:1183, 1984.
35. Olson WL: Reflex sympathetic dystrophy associated with tumour infiltration of the stellate ganglion. J R Soc Med 86:482, 1993.
36. Derbekyan V, Novales-Diaz J, Lisbona R: Pancoast tumor as a cause of reflex sympathetic dystrophy. J Nucl Med 34:1993, 1992.
37. Ku A, Lachmann E, Tunkel R, et al: Upper limb reflex sympathetic dystrophy associated with occult malignancy. Arch Phys Med Rehabil 77:726, 1996.
38. Kalgaard OM, Seem E, Kvernebo K: Erythromelalgia: A clinical study of 87 cases. J Intern Med 242:191, 1997.
39. Kurzrock R, Cohen PR: Erythromelalgia and myeloproliferative disorders. Arch Intern Med 149:105, 1989.
40. Kraus A, Alarcon-Segovia D: Erythermalgia, erythromelalgia, or both? Conditions neglected by rheumatologists. J Rheumatol 20:1, 1993.
41. Babb RR, Alarcon-Segovia D, Fairbairn JF II: Erythermalgia. Circulation 19:136, 1964.
42. Davis MD, O'Fallon WM, Rogers RS III, et al: Natural history of erythromelalgia: Presentation and outcome in 168 patients. Arch Dermatol 136:330, 2000.
43. Mork C, Asker CL, Salerud EG, et al: Microvascular arteriovenous shunting is a probable pathogenic mechanism in erythromelalgia. J Invest Dermatol 43:841, 2000.
44. Cohen JS: Erythromelalgia: New theories and new therapies. J Am Acad Dermatol 43(5 Pt 1):841, 2000.
45. Gonzalez-Gay MA, Garcia-Porrua C, Salvarani C, et al: Polymyalgia manifestations in different conditions mimicking polymyalgia rheumatica. Clin Exp Rheum 18:755, 2000.
46. Kohli M, Bennett RM: An association of polymyalgia rheumatica with myelodysplastic syndromes. J Rheumatol 21:1357, 1994.
47. Naschitz JE, Slobodin G, Yeshurun D, et al: Atypical polymyalgia rheumatica as a presentation of metastatic cancer. Arch Intern Med 157:2381, 1997.
48. Gonzalez-Gay MA, Garcia-Porrua C, Calvarani C, et al: The spectrum of conditions mimicking polymyalgia rheumatica in northwestern Spain. J Rheumatol 27:2179, 2000.
49. Haugeberg G, Dovland H, Johnsen V: Increased frequency of malignancy found in patients presenting with new-onset polymyalgic symptoms suggested to have polymyalgia rheumatica. Arthritis Rheum 47:346, 2002.
50. Myklebust G, Wilsgaard T, Jacobsen BK, et al: No increased frequency of malignancy neoplasms in polymyalgia rheumatica and temporal arteritis: A prospective longitudinal study of 398 cases and matched population controls. J Rheumatol 29:2143, 2002.
51. Liozon E, Loustaud V, Fauchais AL, et al: Concurrent temporal (giant cell) arteritis and malignancy: Report of 20 patients with review of the literature. J Rheumatol 33:1606, 2006.
52. Haga HJ, Eide GE, Brun J, et al: Cancer in association with polymyalgia rheumatica and temporal arteritis. J Rheumatol 20:1335, 1993.
53. DeCross AJ, Sahasrabudhe DM: Paraneoplastic Raynaud's phenomenon. Am J Med 92:571, 1992.
54. Chow SF, McKenna CH: Ovarian cancer and gangrene of the digits: Case report and review of the literature. Mayo Clin Proc 71:253, 1996.
55. Petri M, Fye KH: Digital necrosis: A paraneoplastic syndrome. J Rheumatol 12:800, 1985.
56. Ohtsuka T, Yamakage A, Yamazaki S: Digital ulcers and necroses: Novel manifestations of angiocentric lymphoma. Br J Dermatol 142:1013, 2000.
57. D'Hondt L, Guillaume T, Humblet Y, et al: Digital necrosis associated with chronic myeloid leukemia: a rare paraneoplastic phenomenon … and not a toxicity of recombinant interferon. Acta Clin Belg 52:49, 1997.
58. Courtney PA, Sandhu S, Gardiner PV, et al: Resolution of digital necrosis following treatment of multiple myeloma. Rheumatology (Oxf) 39:1163, 2000.
59. Hebbar S, Thomas GAO: Digital ischemia associated with squamous cell carcinoma of the esophagus. Dig Dis Sci 50:691, 2005.

60. Bachmeyer C, Farge D, Gluckman E, et al: Raynaud's phenomenon and digital necrosis induced by interferon-alpha. Br J Dermatol 135:481, 1996.

61. Reid TJ III, Lombardo FA, Redmond J III, et al: Digital vasculitis associated with interferon therapy. Am J Med 92:702, 1992.

62. Al-Zahrani H, Gupta V, Minded MD, et al: Vascular events associated with alpha interferon therapy. Leuk Lymphoma 44:471, 2003.

63. Sibilia J, Friess S, Schaeverbeke T, et al: Remitting seronegative symmetrical synovitis with pitting edema (RS3PE): A form of paraneoplastic polyarthritis? J Rheumatol 26:115, 1999.

64. Cantini F, Salvarani C, Olivieri I: Paraneoplastic remitting seronegative symmetrical synovitis with pitting edema. Clin Exp Rheumatol 17:741, 1999.

65. Olivieri I, Salvarani C, Cantini F: RS3PE syndrome: An overview. Clin Exp Rheumatol 18(4 Suppl 20):S53, 2000.

66. Paira S, Graf C, Roverano S, et al: Remitting seronegative symmetrical synovitis with pitting oedema: A study of 12 cases. Clin Rheumatol 21:146, 2002.

67. Russell EB: Remitting seronegative symmetrical synovitis with pitting edema syndrome: Followup for neoplasia. J Rheumatol 32:1760, 2005.

68. Trotta F, Castellino G, Lo Monaco A: Multicentric reticulohistiocytosis. Best Pract Res Clin Rheumatol 18:759, 2004.

69. Snow JL, Muller SA: Malignancy-associated multicentric reticulohistiocytosis: A clinical, histological, and immunophenotypic study. Br J Dermatol 133:71, 1995.

70. Freundlich B, Makover D, Maul GG: A novel antinuclear antibody associated with a lupus-like paraneoplastic syndrome. Ann Intern Med 109:295, 1988.

71. Chtourou M, Aubin F, Savariault I, et al: Digital necrosis and lupus-like syndrome preceding ovarian carcinoma. Dermatology 196:348, 1998.

72. Strickland RW, Limmani A, Wall JG, et al: Hairy cell leukemia presenting as a lupus-like syndrome. Arthritis Rheum 31:566, 1988.

73. Schewach-Millet M, Shpiro D, Ziv R, et al: Subacute cutaneous lupus erythematosus associated with breast carcinoma. J Am Acad Dermatol 19:406, 1988.

74. Swissa M, Amital-Teplizki H, Haim N, et al: Autoantibodies in neoplasia: an unresolved enigma. Cancer 65:2554, 1990.

75. Armas JB, Dantas J, Mendonca D, et al: Anticardiolipin and antinuclear antibodies in cancer patients: A case control study. Clin Exp Rheumatol 18:227, 2000.

76. Timuragaoglu A, Duman A, Ongut G, et al: The significance of autoantibodies in non-Hodgkin's lymphoma. Leuk Lymphoma 40:119, 2000.

77. Solans-Laque R, Perez-Bocanegra C, Salud-Salvia A, et al: Clinical significance of antinuclear antibodies in malignant diseases: Association with rheumatic and connective tissue paraneoplastic syndromes. Lupus 13:159, 2004.

78. Petri M: Epidemiology of the antiphospholipid antibody syndrome. J Autoimmun 15:145, 2000.

79. Asherson RA: Antiphospholipid antibodies, malignancy and paraproteinemias. J Autoimmun 15:117, 2000.

80. Zuckerman E, Toubi E, Dov Golan T, et al: Increased thromboembolic incidence in anti-cardiolipin-positive patients with malignancy. Br J Cancer 72:447, 1995.

81. Ozguroglu M, Arun B, Erzin Y, et al: Serum cardiolipin antibodies in cancer patients with thromboembolic events. Clin Appl Thromb Hemost 5:181, 1999.

82. Stasi R, Stipa E, Masi M, et al: Antiphospholipid antibodies: Prevalence, clinical significance and correlation to cytokine levels in acute myeloid leukemia and non-Hodgkin's lymphoma. Thromb Haemost 70:568, 1993.

83. Lossos IS, Bogomolski-Yahalom V, Matzner Y: Anticardiolipin antibodies in acute myeloid leukemia: Prevalence and clinical significance. Am J Hematol 57:139, 1998.

84. Genvresse I, Luftner D, Spath-Schwalbe E, et al: Prevalence and clinical significance of anticardiolipin and anti-β2-glycoprotein-I antibodies in patients with non-Hodgkin's lymphoma. Br J Haematol 68:84, 2002.

85. Bairey O, Blickstein D, Monselise Y, et al: Antiphospholipid antibodies may be a new prognostic parameter in aggressive non-Hodgkin's lymphoma. Br J Haematol 76:384, 2006.

86. Gomez-Puerta JA, Cervera R, Espinosa G, et al: Antiphospholipid antibodies associated with malignancies: Clinical and pathological characteristics of 120 patients. Semin Arthritis Rheum 35:322, 2006.

87. Schved JF, Dupuy-Fons C, Biron C, et al: A prospective epidemiological study on the occurrence of antiphospholipid antibody: The Montpellier Antiphospholipid (MAP) study. Haemostasis 24:175, 1994.

88. Tanne D, D'Olhaberriague L, Trivedi AM, et al: Anticardiolipin antibodies and mortality in patients with ischemic stroke: A perspective follow-up study. Neuroepidemiology 21:93, 2002.

89. Jan de Beur SM: Tumor-induced osteomalacia. JAMA 294:1260, 2005.

90. Jonsson KB, Zahradruk R, Larsson T, et al: Fibroblast growth factor 23 in oncogenic osteomalacia and X-linked hypophosphatemia. N Engl J Med 348:1656, 2003.

91. Seufert J, Ebert K, Muller J, et al: Octreotide therapy for tumor induced osteomalacia. N Engl J Med 345:1883, 2001.

92. Moder KG, Litin SC, Gaffey TA: Renal cell carcinoma associated with sarcoid-like tissue reaction. Mayo Clin Proc 65:1498, 1990.

93. Rawlings DJ, Bernstein B, Rowland JM, et al: Prolonged course of illness in a child with malignant lymphoma mimicking sarcoidosis. J Rheumatol 20:1583, 1993.

94. Bouros D, Hatzakis K, Labrakis H, et al: Association of malignancy with diseases causing interstitial pulmonary changes. Chest 121:1278, 2002.

95. Reich JM, Mullooly JP, Johnson RE: Linkage analysis of malignancy-associated sarcoidosis. Chest 107:605, 1995.

96. Caras WE, Dillard T, Baker T, et al: Coexistence of sarcoidosis and malignancy. South Med J 96:918, 2003.

97. Seersholm N, Vestbo J, Viskum K: Risk of malignant neoplasms in patients with pulmonary sarcoidosis. Thorax 52:892, 1997.

98. Nicholson AG, Wotherspoon AC, Diss TC, et al: Lymphomatoid granulomatosis: Evidence that some cases represent EBV-associated B-cell lymphoma. Histopathology 29:317, 1996.

99. Jaffe ES, Wilson WH: Lymphomatoid granulomatosis: Pathogenesis, pathology and clinical implications. Cancer Surv 30:233, 1997.

100. Katzenstein AA, Carrington CB, Liebow AA: Lymphomatoid granulomatosis: A clinicopathologic study of 152 cases. Cancer 43:360, 1979.

101. Zaidi A, Kampalath B, Peltier WL, et al: Successful treatmetns of systemic and central nervous system lymphomatoid granulomatosis with rituximab. Leuk Lymphoma 45:777, 2004.

102. Jordan K, Grothey A, Grothe W, et al: Successful treatment of mediastinal lymphomatoid granulomatosis with rituximab monotherapy. Eur J Haematol 74:263, 2005.

103. Carson S: The association of malignancy with rheumatic and connective tissue diseases. Semin Oncol 24:360, 1997.

104. Barnes B: Dermatomyositis and malignancy: A review of the literature. Ann Intern Med 84:68, 1976.

105. Hill CL, Zhang Y, Sigurgeirsson B, et al: Frequency of specific cancer types in dermatomyositis and polymyositis: A population based study. Lancet 357:96, 2001.

106. Stockton D, Doherty VR, Brewster DH: Risk of cancer in patients with dermatomyositis or polymyositis, and follow-up implications: A Scottish population-based cohort study. Br J Cancer 85:41, 2001.

107. Buchbinder F, Forbes A, Hall S, et al: Incidence of malignant disease in biopsy-proven inflammatory myopathy. Ann Intern Med 134:1087, 2001.

108. Chen YJ, Wu CY, Shen JL: Predicting factors of malignancy in dermatomyositis and polymyositis: A case-control study. Br J Dermatol 144:825, 2001.

109. Ang P, Sugeng MW, Chua SH: Classical and amyopathic dermatomyositis seen at the National Skin Centre of Singapore: A 3-year retrospective review of their clinical characteristics and association with malignancy. Ann Acad Med Singapore 29:219, 2000.

110. Boussen H, Megazaa A, Nasr C, et al: Dermatomyositis and nasopharyngeal carcinoma: Report of 8 cases. Arch Dermatol 142:112, 2006.

111. Zantos D, Zhang Y, Felson D: The overall and temporal association of cancer with polymyositis and dermatomyositis. J Rheumatol 21:1855, 1994.

112. Jorizzo JL: Dermatomyositis: Practical aspects. Arch Dermatol 138:114, 2002.

113. Caproni M, Cardinali C, Parodi A, et al: Amyopathic dermatomyositis: A review by the Italian Group of Immunodermatology. Arch Dermatol 138:23, 2002.

114. el-Azhari RA, Pakzad SY: Amyopathic dermatomyositis: Retrospective review of 37 cases. J Am Acad Dermatol 46:560, 2002.
115. Gerami P, Schope JM, McDonald L, et al: A systematic review of adult-onset clinically amyopathic dermatomyositis (dermatomyositis sine myositis): A missing link within the spectrum of the idiopathic inflammatory myopathies. J Am Acad Dermatol 54:597, 2006.
116. Medsger TA Jr, Dawson WN Jr, Masi AT: The epidemiology of polymyositis. Am J Med 48:715, 1970.
117. Lakhanpal S, Bunch TW, Ilstrup DM, et al: Polymyositis-dermatomyositis and malignant lesions: Does an association exist? Mayo Clin Proc 61:645, 1986.
118. Callen JP: Relationship of cancer to inflammatory muscle diseases: Dermatomyositis, polymyositis and inclusion body myositis. Rheum Dis Clin N Am 20:943, 1994.
119. Callen JP: When and how should the patient with dermatomyositis or amyopathic dermatomyositis be assessed for possible cancer? Arch Dermatol 138:969, 2002.
120. Sparsa A, Liozon E, Herrmann F, et al: Routine versus extensive malignancy search for adult dermatomyositis and polymyositis: A study of 40 patients. Arch Dermatol 138:885, 2002.
121. Amoura Z, Duhaut P, Huong DLT, et al: Tumor antigen markers for the detection of solid cancers in inflammatory myopathies. Cancer Epidemiol Biomarkers Prev 14:1279, 2005.
122. Fudman EJ, Schnitzer TJ: Dermatomyositis without creatine kinase elevation: A poor prognostic sign. Am J Med 80:329, 1986.
123. Ponyi A, Constantin T, Garami M, et al: Cancer-associated myositis: Clinical features and prognostic signs. Ann N Y Acad Sci 1051:64, 2005.
124. Love LA, Leff RL, Fraser DD, et al: A new approach to the classification of idiopathic inflammatory myopathy: Myositis-specific autoantibodies define useful homogeneous patient groups. Medicine (Balt) 70:360, 1991.
125. Hunger RE, Durr C, Brand CU: Cutaneous leukocytoclastic vasculitis in dermatomyositis suggests malignancy. Dermatology 202:123, 2001.
126. Hidano A, Kaneko K, Arai Y, et al: Survey of the prognosis for dermatomyositis with special reference to its association with malignancy and pulmonary fibrosis. J Dermatol 13:233, 1986.
127. Talal N, Bunim J: The development of malignant lymphoma in the course of Sjögren's syndrome. Am J Med 36:529, 1964.
128. Kassan SS, Thomas TL, Moutsopoulos HM, et al: Increased risk of lymphoma in sicca syndrome. Ann Intern Med 89:888, 1978.
129. Sutcliffe N, Inanc M, Speight P, et al: Predictors of lymphoma development in primary Sjögren's syndrome. Semin Arthritis Rheum 28:80, 1998.
130. Zufferey P, Meyer OC, Grossin M, et al: Primary Sjögren's syndrome (SS) and malignant lymphoma: A retrospective cohort study of 55 patients with SS. Scand J Rheumatol 24:342, 1995.
131. Voulgarelis M, Dafni RG, Isenberg DA, et al: Malignant lymphoma in primary Sjögren's syndrome: A multicenter, retrospective, clinical study by the European concerted action on Sjögren's syndrome. Arthritis Rheum 42:1765, 1999.
132. Skopouli FN, Dafni U, Ioannidis JPA, et al: Clinical evolution, and morbidity and mortality of primary Sjögren's syndrome. Semin Arthritis Rheum 29:296, 2000.
133. Ioannidis JPA, Vassiliou VA, Moutsopoulos HM: Long-term risk of mortality and lymphoproliferative disease and predictive classification of primary Sjögren's syndrome. Arthritis Rheum 46:741, 2002.
134. Valesini G, Priori R, Bavoillot D, et al: Differential risk of non-Hodgkin's lymphoma in Italian patients with primary Sjögren's syndrome. J Rheumatol 24:2376, 1997.
135. Pertovaara M, Pukkala E, Laippala P, et al: A longitudinal cohort study of Finnish patients with primary Sjögren's syndrome: Clinical, immunological, and epidemiological aspects. Ann Rheum Dis 60:467, 2001.
136. Smedby KE, Hjalgrim H, Askling J, et al: Autoimmune and chronic inflammatory disorders and risk of non-Hodgkin lymphoma by subtype. J Natl Cancer Inst 98:51, 2006.
137. Zintzaras E, Voulgarelis M, Moutsopoulos HM: The risk of lymphoma development in autoimmune diseases. Arch Intern Med 165:2337, 2005.
138. Engels EA, Cerhan JR, Linet MS, et al: Immune-related conditions and immune-modulating medications as risk factors for non-Hodgkin's lymphoma: A case-control study. Am J Epidemiol 162:1153, 2005.

139. Theander E, Henriksson G, Ljungbery O, et al: Lymphoma and other malignancies in primary Sjögren's syndrome. Ann Rheum Dis 65:796, 2006.
140. Biasi D, Caramaschi P, Ambrosetti A, et al: Mucosa-associated lymphoid tissue lymphoma of the salivary glands occurring in patients affected by Sjögren's syndrome: Report of 6 cases. Acta Haematol 105:83, 2001.
141. Ramos-Casals M, Brito-Zeron P, Yague J, et al: Hypocomplementaemia as an immunological marker of morbidity and mortality in patients with primary Sjögren's syndrome. Rheumatology 44:89, 2005.
142. Moutsopoulos HM, Costello R, Drosos AA, et al: Demonstration and identification of monoclonal proteins in the urine of patients with Sjögren's syndrome. Ann Rheum Dis 44:109, 1985.
143. Brito-Zeron P, Ramos-Casals M, Nardi N, et al: Circulating monoclonal immunoglobulins in Sjögren syndrome: Prevalence and clinical significance in 237 patients. Medicine (Balt) 84:90, 2005.
144. Theander E, Manthorpe R, Jacobsson LTH: Mortality and causes of death in primary Sjögren's syndrome: A prospective cohort study. Arthritis Rheum 50:1262, 2004.
145. Mariette X: Lymphomas in patients with Sjögren's syndrome: Review of the literature and physiopathologic hypothesis. Leuk Lymphoma 33:93, 1999.
146. Banks PM, Witrak GA, Conn DL: Lymphoid neoplasia developing after connective tissue disease. Mayo Clin Proc 54:104, 1979.
147. Takacs I, Zeher M, Urban L, et al: Frequency and evaluation of t(14; 18) translocations in Sjögren's syndrome. Ann Hematol 79:444, 2000.
148. Pisa EK, Pisa P, Kang HI, et al: High frequency of t(14; 18) translocation in salivary gland lymphomas from Sjögren's syndrome patients. J Exp Med 174:1245, 1991.
149. De Vita S, Ferraccioli G, De Re V, et al: The polymerase chain reaction detects B cell clonalities in patients with Sjögren's syndrome and suspected malignant lymphoma. J Rheumatol 21:1497, 1994.
150. Chakravarty EF: Associations between rheumatoid arthritis, TNF inhibition, and risk of lymphoma. Curr Med Literature Leuk Lymphoma 13:85, 2005.
151. Isomaki HA, Hakulinen T, Joutsenlathi U: Excess risk of lymphomas, leukemia and myeloma in patients with rheumatoid arthritis. J Chronic Dis 31:691, 1978.
152. Mellemkjaer L, Linet MS, Gridley G, et al: Rheumatoid arthritis and cancer risk. Eur J Cancer 32A:1753, 1996.
153. Gridley G, McLaughlin JK, Ekbom A, et al: Incidence of cancer among patients with rheumatoid arthritis. J Natl Cancer Inst 85:307, 1993.
154. Ekström K, Hjalgrim H, Brandt L, et al: Risk of malignant lymphomas in patients with rheumatoid arthritis and in their first-degree relatives. Arthritis Rheum 48:963, 2003.
155. Wolfe F, Michaud K: Lymphoma in rheumatoid arthritis: The effect of methotrexate and anti-tumor necrosis factor therapy in 18,572 patients. Arthritis Rheum 50:1740, 2004.
156. Setoguchi S, Solomon DH, Weinblatt ME, et al: Tumor necrosis factor α antagonist use and cancer in patients with rheumatoid arthritis. Arthritis Rheum 54:2757, 2006.
157. Franklin J, Lunt M, Bunn D, et al: Incidence of lymphoma in a large primary-care derived cohort of inflammatory polyarthritis. Ann Rheum Dis 65:617, 2006.
158. Thomas E, Brewster DH, Black RJ: Risk of malignancy among patients with rheumatic conditions. Int J Cancer 88:497, 2000.
159. Cibere J, Sibley J, Haga M: Rheumatoid arthritis and the risk of malignancy. Arthritis Rheum 40:1580, 1997.
160. Kamel OW, Holly EA, van de Rijn M, et al: A population based, case control study of non-Hodgkin's lymphoma in patients with rheumatoid arthritis. J Rheumatol 26:1676, 1999.
161. Mikuls TR, Endo JO, Puumala SE, et al: Prospective study of survival outcomes in non-Hodgkin's lymphoma patients with rheumatoid arthritis. J Clin Oncol 24:1597, 2006.
162. Baecklund E, Ekbom A, Sparen P, et al: Disease activity and risk of lymphoma in patients with rheumatoid arthritis: Nested case-control study. BMJ 317:180, 1998.
163. Baecklund E, Iliadou A, Askling J, et al: Association of chronic inflammation, not its treatment, with increased lymphoma risk in rheumatoid arthritis. Arthritis Rheum 54:692, 2006.
164. Kelly C, Sykes H: Rheumatoid arthritis, malignancy, and paraproteins. Ann Rheum Dis 49:657, 1990.

165. Kyle RA, Therneau TM, Rajkumar SV, et al: Prevalence of monoclonal gammopathy of undetermined significance. N Engl J Med 354:1362, 2006.

166. Gridley G, Klippel JH, Hoover RN, et al: Incidence of cancer among men with the Felty syndrome. Ann Intern Med 120:35, 1994.

167. Matteson EL, Hickey AR, Maguire L, et al: Occurrence of neoplasia in patients with rheumatoid arthritis enrolled in a DMARD Registry: Rheumatoid Arthritis Azathioprine Registry Steering Committee. J Rheumatol 18:809, 1991.

168. Tennis P, Andrews E, Bombardier C, et al: Record linkage to conduct an epidemiologic study on the association of rheumatoid arthritis and lymphoma in the province of Saskatchewan, Canada. J Clin Epidemiol 46:685, 1993.

169. Asten P, Barrett J, Symmons D: Risk of developing certain malignancies is related to duration of immunosuppressive drug exposure in patients with rheumatic diseases. J Rheumatol 26:1705, 1999.

170. Georgescu L, Quinn GC, Schwartzman S, et al: Lymphoma in patients with rheumatoid arthritis: Association with the disease state or methotrexate treatment. Semin Arthritis Rheum 26:794, 1997.

171. Mariette X, Cazals-Hatem D, Warszawki J, et al: Lymphomas in rheumatoid arthritis patients treated with methotrexate: A 3-year prospective study in France. Blood 99:3909, 2002.

172. Starkebaum G: Rheumatoid arthritis, methotrexate, and lymphoma: Risk substitution, or cat and mouse with Epstein-Barr virus? J Rheumatol 28:2573, 2001.

173. Feng WH, Cohen JI, Fischer S, et al: Reactivation of latent Epstein-Barr virus by methotrexate: A potential contributor to methotrexate associated lymphomas. J Natl Cancer Inst 96:1691, 2004.

174. Franklin JP, Symmons DPM, Silman AJ: Risk of lymphoma in patients with RA treated with anti-TNFα agents. Ann Rheum Dis 64:657, 2005.

175. Brown SL, Greene MH, Gershon SK, et al: Tumor necrosis factor antagonist therapy and lymphoma development: Twenty-six cases reported to the Food and Drug Administration. Arthritis Rheum 46:3151, 2002.

176. Askling J, Fored CM, Baecklund E, et al: Haematopoietic malignancies in rheumatoid arthritis: Lymphoma risk and characteristics after exposure to tumor necrosis factor antagonists. Ann Rheum Dis 64:1414, 2005.

177. Geborek P, Bladstrom A, Turesson C, et al: Tumour necrosis factor blockers do not increase overall tumour risk in patients with rheumatoid arthritis, but they may be associated with an increased risk of lymphomas. Ann Rheum Dis 64:699, 2005.

178. Bongartz T, Sutton AJ, Sweeting MJ, et al: Anti-TNF antibody therapy in rheumatoid arthritis and the risk of serious infections and malignancies: Systematic review and meta-analysis of rare harmful effects in randomized controlled trials. JAMA 295:2275, 2006.

179. American College of Rheumatology Hotline: Update on safety issues concerning TNF inhibitors. 2006. Available at: http://www.rheumatology.org/publications/hotline/0506JAMATNF.asp.

180. Dixon W, Silman A: Is there an association between anti-TNF monoclonal antibody therapy in rheumatoid arthritis and risk of malignancy and serious infection? Commentary on the meta-analysis by Bongartz et al. Arthritis Res Ther 8:111, 2006.

181. Askling J, Fored CM, Brandt L, et al: Risks of solid cancers in patients with rheumatoid arthritis and after treatment with tumour necrosis factor antagonists. Ann Rheum Dis 64:1421, 2005.

182. Berkel H, Holcombe RF, Middlebrooks M, et al: Nonsteroidal anti-inflammatory drugs and colorectal cancer. Epidemiol Rev 18:205, 1996.

183. Gorman JD: Smoking and rheumatoid arthritis: Another reason to just say no. Arthritis Rheum 54:10, 2006.

184. Chakravarty EF, Michaud K, Wolfe F: Skin cancer, rheumatoid arthritis, and tumor necrosis factor inhibitors. J Rheumatol 32:2130, 2005.

185. Pettersson T, Pukkala E, Teppo L, et al: Increased risk of cancer in patients with systemic lupus erythematosus. Ann Rheum Dis 51:437, 1992.

186. Canoso JJ, Cohen AS: Malignancy in a series of 70 patients with systemic lupus erythematosus. Arthritis Rheum 17:383, 1974.

187. Lewis RB, Castor CW, Knisley RE, et al: Frequency of neoplasia in systemic lupus erythematosus and rheumatoid arthritis. Arthritis Rheum 19:1256, 1976.

188. Green JA, Dawson AA, Walker W: Systemic lupus erythematosus and lymphoma. Lancet 2:753, 1978.

189. Menon S, Snaith ML, Isenberg DA: The association of malignancy with SLE: An analysis of 150 patients under long-term review. Lupus 2:177, 1993.

190. Lopez Dupla M, Khamashta M, Pintado Garcia V, et al: Malignancy in systemic lupus erythematosus: A report of five cases in a series of 96 patients. Lupus 2:377, 1993.

191. Sulkes A, Naparstek Y: The infrequent association of systemic lupus erythematosus and solid tumors. Cancer 68:1389, 1991.

192. Ramsey-Goldman R, Mattai SA, Schilling E, et al: Increased risk of malignancy in patients with systemic lupus erythematosus. J Invest Med 46:217, 1998.

193. Mellemkjaer L, Andersen V, Linet MS, et al: Non-Hodgkin's lymphoma and other cancers among a cohort of patients with systemic lupus erythematosus. Arthritis Rheum 40:761, 1997.

194. Bjornadal L, Lofstrom B, Yin L, et al: Increased cancer incidence in a Swedish cohort of patients with systemic lupus erythematosus. Scand J Rheumatol 31:66, 2002.

195. Sweeney DM, Manzi S, Janosky J, et al: Risk of malignancy in women with systemic lupus erythematosus. J Rheumatol 22:1478, 1995.

196. Abu-Shakra M, Gladman DD, Urowitz MB: Malignancy in systemic lupus erythematosus. Arthritis Rheum 39:1050, 1996.

197. Nived O, Bengtsson A, Jonsen A, et al: Malignancies during follow-up in an epidemiologically defined systemic lupus erythematosus inception cohort in southern Sweden. Lupus 10:500, 2001.

198. Sultan SM, Ioannou Y, Isenberg A: Is there an association of malignancy with systemic lupus erythematosus? An analysis of 276 patients under long-term review. Rheumatology 39:1147, 2000.

199. Ramsey-Goldman R, Clarke AE: Double trouble: Are lupus and malignancy associated? Lupus 10:388, 2001.

200. Bernatsky S, Clarke A: Ramsey-Goldman R: Malignancy and systemic lupus erythematosus. Curr Rheum Rep 4:351, 2002.

201. Bernatsky S, Boivin J, Clarke A, et al: Cancer risk in SLE: A meta-analysis. Arthritis Rheum 44:S244, 2001.

202. Bernatsky S, Boivin JF, Joseph L, et al: An international cohort study of cancer in systemic lupus erythematosus. Arthritis Rheum 52:1481, 2005.

203. Bernatsky S, Ramsey-Goldman R, Clarke A: Exploring the links between systemic lupus erythematosus and cancer. Rheum Dis Clin N Am 31:387, 2005.

204. Bernatsky S, Ramsey-Goldman R, Rajan R, et al: Non-Hodgkin's lymphoma in systemic lupus erythematosus. Ann Rheum Dis 64:1507, 2005.

205. Bernatsky S, Boivin JF, Joseph L, et al: Race/ethnicity and cancer occurrence in systemic lupus erythematosus. Arthritis Rheum 53:781, 2005.

206. Bernatsky S, Boivin JF, Joseph L, et al: Prevalence of factors influencing cancer risk in women with lupus: Social habits, reproductive issues, and obesity. J Rheumatol 29:2551, 2002.

207. Bernatsky S, Ramsey-Goldman R, Boivin JF, et al: Do traditional Gail model risk factors account for increased breast cancer in women with lupus? J Rheumatol 30:1505, 2003.

208. Bernatsky S, Clarke A, Ramsey-Goldman R, et al: Hormonal exposures and breast cancer in a sample of women with systemic lupus erythematosus. Rheumatology (Oxf) 43:1178, 2004.

209. Bernatsky S, Clarke A, Ramsey-Goldman R, et al: Breast cancer stage at time of detection in women with systemic lupus erythematosus. Lupus 13:469, 2004.

210. Bernatsky SR, Cooper GS, Mill C, et al: Cancer screening in patients with systemic lupus erythematosus. J Rheumatol 33:45, 2006.

211. Dhar JP, Kmak D, Bhan R, et al: Abnormal cervicovaginal cytology in women with lupus: A retrospective cohort study. Gynecol Oncol 82:4, 2001.

212. Ognenovski VM, Marder W, Somers EC, et al: Increased incidence of cervical intraepithelial neoplasia in women with systemic sclerosis treated with intravenous cyclophosphamide. J Rheumatol 31:1763, 2004.

213. Lai-Shan T, Chan AYK, Chan PKS: Increased prevalence of squamous intraepithelial lesions in systemic lupus erythematosus. Arthritis Rheum 50:3619, 2004.

214. Tam LS, Chan AYK, Chan PKS, et al: Increased prevalence of squamous intraepithelial lesions in systemic lupus erythematosus. Arthritis Rheum 50:3619, 2004.

215. Bernatsky S, Ramsey-Goldman R, Gordon C, et al: Factors associated with abnormal Pap results in systemic lupus erythematosus. Rheumatology (Oxf) 43:1386, 2004.

216. Xu Y, Wiernik PH: Systemic lupus erythematosus and B-cell hematologic neoplasm. Lupus 10:841, 2001.

217. Pearson JE, Silman AJ: Risk of cancer in patients with scleroderma. Ann Rheum Dis 62:697, 2003.

218. Roumm AD, Medsger TA Jr: Cancer and systemic sclerosis: An epidemiologic study. Arthritis Rheum 28:1336, 1985.

219. Abu-Shakra M, Guillemin F, Lee P: Cancer in systemic sclerosis. Arthritis Rheum 36:460, 1993.

220. Rosenthal AK, McLaughlin JK, Linet MS, et al: Scleroderma and malignancy: An epidemiological study. Ann Rheum Dis 52:531, 1993.

221. Higuchi M, Horiuchi T, Ishibashi N, et al: Anticentromere antibody as a risk factor for cancer in patients with systemic sclerosis. Clin Rheumatol 19:123, 2000.

222. Hill CL, Nguyen AM, Roder D, et al: Risk of cancer in patients with scleroderma: A population based cohort study. Ann Rheum Dis 62:728, 2003.

223. Derk CT, Rasheed M, Artlett CM, et al: A cohort study of cancer incidence in systemic sclerosis. J Rheumatol 33:1123, 2006.

224. Hesselstrand R, Scheja A, Akesson A: Mortality and causes of death in a Swedish series of systemic sclerosis patients. Ann Rheum Dis 57:682, 1998.

225. Rothfield N, Kurtzman S, Vazques-Abad D, et al: Association of anti-topoisomerase I with cancer. Arthritis Rheum 35:724, 1992.

226. **Chatterjee S, Dombi GW, Severson RK, et al: Risk of malignancy in scleroderma: A population-based cohort study. Arthritis Rheum 52:2415, 2005.**

227. Wipff J, Allanore Y, Soussi F, et al: Prevalence of Barrett's esophagus in systemic sclerosis. Arthritis Rheum 52:2882, 2005.

228. Derk CT, Rasheed M, Spiegel JR, et al: Increased incidence of carcinoma of the tongue in patients with systemic sclerosis. J Rheumatol 32:637, 2005.

229. Rosenthal AK, McLaughlin JK, Gridley G, et al: Incidence of cancer among patients with systemic sclerosis. Cancer 76:910, 1995.

230. Reddy SM, Pui JC, Gold LI, et al: Postirradiation morphea and subcutaneous polyarteritis nodosa: Case report and literature review. Semin Arthritis Rheum 34:728, 2005.

231. Rosier RN, Konski A, Boros L: Bone tumors. In Rubin P (ed): Clinical Oncology: A Multidisciplinary Approach for Physicians and Students, 7th ed. Philadelphia, WB Saunders, 1993, pp 509-530.

232. Arndt CA, Crist WM: Common musculoskeletal tumors of childhood and adolescence. N Engl J Med 341:342, 1999.

233. Hayden JB, Hoang BH: Osteosarcoma: Basic science and clinical implications. Orthop Clin North Am 37:1, 2006.

234. Weber KL: What's new in musculoskeletal oncology. J Bone Joint Surg Am 87:1400, 2005.

235. Hadjipavlou A, Lander P, Srolovitz H, et al: Malignant transformation in Paget's disease of bone. Cancer 70:2802, 1992.

236. Mankin HJ, Hornicek FJ: Paget's sarcoma: A historical and outcome review. Clin Orthop 438:97, 2005.

237. Terek RM: Recent advances in the basic science of chondrosarcoma. Orthop Clin North Am 37:9, 2006.

238. Rosier RN, Constine LS III: Soft tissue sarcoma. In Rubin P (ed): Clinical Oncology: A Multidisciplinary Approach for Physicians and Students, 7th ed. Philadelphia, WB Saunders, 1993, pp 487-507.

239. Mankin HJ, Hornicek FJ: Diagnosis, classification, and management of soft tissue sarcomas. Cancer Control 12:5, 2005.

240. Breitfeld PP, Meyer WH: Rhabdomyosarcoma: New windows of opportunity. Oncologist 10:518, 2005.

241. Spjut HJ, Dorfman HD, Fechner RE, et al: Tumors of Bone and Cartilage. Washington, DC, Armed Forces Institute of Pathology, 1983.

242. Mirra JM: Bone Tumors: Diagnosis and Treatment. Philadelphia, JB Lippincott, 1989.

243. Stummvol GH, Aringer M, Machold KP, et al: Cancer polyarthritis resembling rheumatoid arthritis as a first sign of hidden neoplasms. Scand J Rheumatol 30:40, 2001.

244. Patt RB: Basic and advanced methods of pain control. In Rubin P (ed): Clinical Oncology: A Multidisciplinary Approach for Physicians and Students, 7th ed. Philadelphia, WB Saunders, 1993, pp 709-733.

245. Murray GC, Persellin RH: Metastatic carcinoma presenting as monarticular arthritis: A case report and review of the literature. Arthritis Rheum 23:95, 1980.

246. Dunne C, Illidge T: Arthritis and carcinoma. Ann Rheum Dis 52:86, 1993.

247. Raderer M, Scheithauer W: Postchemotherapy rheumatism following adjuvant therapy for ovarian cancer. Scand J Rheumatol 23: 291-292, 1994.

248. Loprinzi CL, Duffy J, Ingle JN: Postchemotherapy rheumatism. J Clin Oncol 11:768-770, 1993.

249. Kim MJ, Ye YM, Park HS: Chemotherapy-related arthropathy. J Rheumatol 33:1364, 2006.

250. Creamer P, Lim K, George E, et al: Acute inflammatory polyarthritis in association with tamoxifen. Br J Rheumatol 33:583-585, 1994.

251. Warner E, al Keshavjee N, Shupak R, et al: Rheumatic symptoms following adjuvant therapy for breast cancer. Am J Clin Oncol 20:322, 1997.

252. Passos de Souza E, Evangelista Segundo PT, Jose FF, et al: Rheumatoid arthritis induced by alpha-interferon therapy. Clin Rheumatol 20:297, 2001.

253. Raanani P, Ben-Bassat I: Immune-mediated complications during interferon therapy in hematological patients. Acta Haematol 107:133, 2002.

254. Wandl UB, Nagel-Hiemke M, May D, et al: Lupus like autoimmune disease induced by interferon therapy for myeloproliferative disorders. Clin Immunol Immunopathol 65:70, 1992.

255. Ronnblom LE, Alm GV, Oberg KE: Autoimmunity after alpha-interferon therapy for malignant carcinoid. Ann Intern Med 115:178, 1991.

256. Thomas LB, Forkner CE, Frei E III, et al: The skeletal lesions of acute leukemia. Cancer 14:608, 1961.

257. Rennie JAN, Auchterlonie IA: Leukaemias and GVH disease. Baillieres Clin Rheumatol 5:231, 1991.

258. Ehrenfeld M, Gur H, Shoenfeld Y: Rheumatologic features of hematologic disorders. Curr Opin Rheumatol 11:62, 1999.

259. Silverstein MN, Kelly P: Leukemia with osteoarticular symptoms and signs. Ann Intern Med 59:637, 1963.

260. Spilberg I, Meyer GJ: The arthritis of leukemia. Arthritis Rheum 15:630, 1972.

261. Jones OY, Spencer CH, Bowyer SL: A multicenter case-control study on predictive factors distinguishing leukemia from juvenile rheumatoid arthritis. Pediatrics 117:840, 2006.

262. Gur H, Koren V, Ehrenfeld M, et al: Rheumatic manifestations preceding adult acute leukemia: Characteristics and implication on course and prognosis. Acta Haematol 101:1, 1999.

263. Kai T, Ishii E, Matsuzaki A, et al: Clinical and prognostic implications of bone lesions in childhood leukemia at diagnosis. Leuk Lymphoma 23:119, 1996.

264. Lacy MZ, Gertz MA, Hanson CA, et al: Multiple myeloma associated with diffuse osteosclerotic bone lesions: A clinical entity distinct from osteosclerotic myeloma (POEMS syndrome). Am J Hematol 56:288, 1997.

265. Roux S, Fermand JP, Brechignac S, et al: Tumoral joint involvement in multiple myeloma and Waldenström's macroglobulinemia: Report of 4 cases. J Rheumatol 23:2175, 1996.

266. Terpos E, Angelopoulou MK, Variami E, et al: Sjögren's syndrome associated with multiple myeloma. Ann Hematol 79:449, 2000.

267. Hermaszewski RA, Ratnavel RC, Denman DJ, et al: Immunodeficiency and lymphoproliferative disorders. Baillieres Clin Rheumatol 5:277, 1991.

268. Falcini F, Bardare M, Cimaz R, et al: Arthritis as a presenting feature of non-Hodgkin's lymphoma. Arch Dis Child 78:367, 1998.

269. Nishiya K, Tanaka Y: Co-existence of non-Hodgkin's lymphoma in the leukemic phase and polyarthritis simulating rheumatoid arthritis. Intern Med 36:227, 1997.

270. Dorfman HD, Siegel HL, Perry MC, et al: Non-Hodgkin's lymphoma of the synovium simulating rheumatoid arthritis. Arthritis Rheum 30:155, 1987.

271. Davies PG, Fordham JN: Arthritis and angioimmunoblastic lymphadenopathy. Ann Rheum Dis 42:516, 1983.

272. Layton MA, Musgrove C, Dawes PT: Polyarthritis, rash and lymphadenopathy: Case reports of two patients with angioimmunoblastic lymphadenopathy presenting to a rheumatology clinic. Clin Rheumatol 17:148, 1998.

273. Tsochatzis E, Vassilopoulos D, Deutsch M: Antioblastic T-cell lymphoma-associated arthritis: Case report and literature review. J Clin Rheumatol 11:326, 2005.

274. von Kempis J, Kohler G, Herbst EW, et al: Intravascular lymphoma presenting as symmetric polyarthritis. Arthritis Rheum 41:1126, 1998.

275. Tichelli A, Duell T, Weill M, et al: Late-onset keratoconjunctivitis sicca syndrome after bone marrow transplantation: Incidence and risk factors—European Group or Blood and Marrow Transplantation (EBMT) Working Party on Late Effects. Bone Marrow Transplant 17:1105, 1996.

276. Asten P, Barrett J, Symmons D: Risk of developing certain malignancies is related to duration of immunosuppressive drug exposure in patients with rheumatic diseases. J Rheumatol 26:1705, 1999.

277. Baltus JA, Boersma JW, Hartman AP, et al: The occurrence of malignancies in patients with rheumatoid arthritis treated with cyclophosphamide: A controlled retrospective follow-up. Ann Rheum Dis 42:368, 1983.

278. Kinlen LJ: Incidence of cancer in rheumatoid arthritis and other disorders after immunosuppressive treatment. Am J Med 21:44, 1985.

279. Radis CD, Kahl LE, Baker GL, et al: Effects of cyclophosphamide on the development of malignancy and on long-term survival of patients with rheumatoid arthritis: A 20-year follow-up study. Arthritis Rheum 38:1120, 1995.

280. Knight A, Askling J, Ekbom A: Cancer incidence in a population-based cohort of patients with Wegener's granulomatosis. Int J Cancer 100:82, 2002.

281. Knight A, Askling J, Granath F, et al: Urinary bladder cancer in Wegener's granulomatosis, risks and relation to cyclophosphamide. Ann Rheum Dis 63:1307, 2004.

282. Choi HK, Hernan MA, Seeger JD, et al: Methotrexate and mortality in patients with rheumatoid arthritis: A prospective study. Lancet 359:1173, 2002.

283. Liote F, Pertuiset E, Cochand-Priollet B, et al: Methotrexate-related B lymphoproliferative disease in a patient with rheumatoid arthritis: Role of Epstein-Barr virus infection. J Rheumatol 22:1174, 1995.

284. Bachman TR, Sawitzke AD, Perkins SL, et al: Methotrexate-associated lymphoma in patients with rheumatoid arthritis: Report of two cases. Arthritis Rheum 39:325, 1996.

285. Sibilia J, Liote F, Mariette X: Lymphoproliferative disorders in rheumatoid arthritis patients on low-dose methotrexate. Rev Rhum Engl Ed 65:267, 1998.

286. Natkunam Y, Elenitoba-Johnson KS, Kingma DW, et al: Epstein-Barr virus strain type and latent membrane protein 1 gene deletions in lymphomas in patients with rheumatic diseases. Arthritis Rheum 40:1152, 1997.

287. van Wanghe P, Dequeker J: Compliance and long-term effect of azathioprine in 65 rheumatoid arthritis cases. Ann Rheum Dis 41(Suppl 1):40, 1982.

288. Silman AJ, Petrie J, Hazleman B, et al: Lymphoproliferative cancer and other malignancy in patients with rheumatoid arthritis treated with azathioprine: A 20-year follow-up study. Ann Rheum Dis 47:988, 1988.

289. Pitt PI, Sultan AH, Malone M, et al: Association between azathioprine therapy and lymphoma in rheumatoid disease. J R Soc Med 80:428, 1987.

290. Vasquez S, Kavanaugh AF, Schneider NR, et al: Acute nonlymphocytic leukemia after treatment of systemic lupus erythematosus with immunosuppressive agents. J Rheumatol 19:1625, 1992.

291. Seidenfeld AM, Smythe HA, Ogryzlo MA, et al: Acute leukemia in rheumatoid arthritis treated with cytotoxic agents. J Rheumatol 11:586, 1984.

292. Nero P, Rahman A, Isenberg DA: Does long term treatment with azathioprine predispose to malignancy and death in patients with systemic lupus erythematosus? Ann Rheum Dis 63:325, 2004.

293. Zijlmans JM, van Rijthoven AW, Kluin PM, et al: Epstein-Barr virus-associated lymphoma in a patient with rheumatoid arthritis treated with cyclosporine. N Engl J Med 326:1363, 1992.

294. Arellano F, Krupp P: Malignancies in rheumatoid arthritis patients treated with cyclosporin A. Br J Rheumatol 32(Suppl 1):72, 1993.

295. van den Borne BE, Landewe RB, Houkes I, et al: No increased risk of malignancies and mortality in cyclosporin A-treated patients with rheumatoid arthritis. Arthritis Rheum 41:1930, 1998.

296. Stone JH, Holbrook JT, Marriott MA: Solid malignancies among patients in the Wegener's Granulomatosus Etanercept Trial. Arthritis Rheum 54:1608, 2006.

297. Darby SC, Doll R, Gill SK, et al: Long-term mortality after a single course with x-rays in patients treated for ankylosing spondylitis. Br J Cancer 55:179, 1987.

298. Weiss HA, Darby SC, Doll R: Cancer mortality following x-ray treatment for ankylosing spondylitis. Int J Cancer 59:327, 1994.

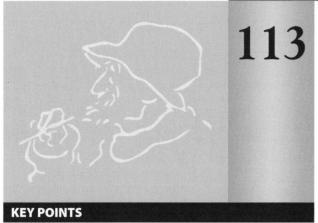

113 Familial Autoinflammatory Syndromes

ANNA SIMON •
JOS W. M. VAN DER MEER •
JOOST P. H. DRENTH

KEY POINTS

Autoinflammatory disorders are characterized by recurrent or chronic inflammation without signs of infection or autoimmune phenomena.

Dysregulation of the interleukin-1β pathway is central to many familial autoinflammatory syndromes, especially the cryopyrin-associated periodic syndromes and familial Mediterranean fever.

The need for a definite diagnosis in the familial autoinflammatory syndromes has increased because of advances in treatment options.

A severe complication of these disorders is type AA amyloidosis, which often leads to renal failure; the risk of this complication is greatly reduced when patients receive adequate treatment.

In a substantial portion of patients presenting with a clear phenotype of recurrent inflammation, with or without family history, the diagnosis can remain elusive, which indicates that other disorders remain to be discovered.

DEFINITION

The familial autoinflammatory syndromes, often referred to as hereditary periodic fever syndromes, comprise rare disorders with a common phenotype of lifelong, recurrent inflammatory episodes, with fever and usually accompanied by other inflammatory symptoms, such as abdominal pain, diarrhea, rash, or arthralgia.[1] Between the fever episodes, patients generally feel healthy and function normally. Routine laboratory investigations during a fever attack invariably reveal a severe acute-phase response with a high erythrocyte sedimentation rate, leukocytosis, and high concentrations of acute-phase proteins such as C-reactive protein (CRP), serum amyloid A (SAA), and several proinflammatory cytokines. The episodes of fever occur without an obvious trigger, although some patients note a relationship to physical stimuli (e.g., exposure to cold), emotional stress, or the menstrual cycle. The episodes resolve spontaneously in days or weeks. Patients with periodic fever occur go undiagnosed for years, generating a high level of discouragement and frustration for patients and physicians when no diagnosis is made.[2,3] The term *autoinflammatory*, coined by McDermott and colleagues in 1999,[4] adequately describes the phenotype of recurrent, acute inflammatory responses. It is preferable to the term *autoimmune* in these cases because typical autoimmune phenomena are not found.

Several distinct types of hereditary autoinflammatory syndromes are recognized. Despite the common phenotype described previously, these genetically distinct types often can be differentiated clinically by numerous specific characteristics, in particular by the mode of inheritance, age of onset, average duration of the fever episodes and the fever-free interval, geographic region of origin of the patient's family, and occurrence of long-term complications such as amyloidosis or deafness (Table 113-1 and Fig. 113-1). A significant number of patients with a periodic fever phenotype still do not fit into this genetically based classification, probably representing additional (genetic) defects that can lead to periodic fevers. This chapter describes six different types of familial autoinflammatory syndromes that have been characterized at this time.

DIFFERENTIAL DIAGNOSIS

When a patient has had recurrent fever episodes for more than 2 years, it is increasingly unlikely that these are caused by an infection or a malignant disorder. The differential diagnosis at that time may include numerous inflammatory disorders, such as juvenile rheumatoid arthritis, adult-onset Still's disease, inflammatory bowel disease, Schnitzler syndrome, and Behçet's disease, in addition to the hereditary periodic fever syndromes (Table 113-2). Because the hereditary syndromes are rare (except for familial Mediterranean fever [FMF] in individuals with a distinct ethnic background), the more common diagnoses should be excluded first.

The mainstay of the diagnosis of hereditary periodic fever is clinical assessment, with a detailed medical and family history, and preferably at least one observation of the patient during a fever episode because physical examination of the patient in a period of remission is seldom abnormal. Another helpful clue, although not pathognomonic, in differentiating the familial autoinflammatory syndromes is often gained from knowing the patient's ethnic origin. This clinical assessment often yields enough information to build a differential diagnosis of the specific familial autoinflammatory syndromes (see Table 113-1), to determine the direction of genetic testing (Fig. 113-2).

FAMILIAL MEDITERRANEAN FEVER

EPIDEMIOLOGY

FMF (Mendelian Inheritance in Men [MIM] 249100) is the most prevalent disorder among the hereditary autoinflammatory syndromes, with more than 10,000 patients affected worldwide. It occurs primarily in people originating from the Mediterranean basin, including Armenians, Sephardic Jews, Arabs, and Turks. FMF is an autosomal recessively inherited disorder. Most families reported with an apparent autosomal dominant inheritance pattern of FMF[5] represent

Table 113-1 Differential Diagnosis of Familial Autoinflammatory Syndromes

	Familial Mediterranean Fever (FMF)	Mevalonate Kinase Deficiencies			Tumor Necrosis Factor Receptor–Associated Periodic Syndrome (TRAPS)	Cryopyrin Diseases		
		Classic Hyper-immunoglobulin D syndrome (HIDS)	Mevalonic Aciduria	Variant HIDS		Familial Cold Autoinflammatory Syndrome (FCAS)	Muckle-Wells Syndrome (MWS)	Chronic Infantile Neurologic Cutaneous and Articular Syndrome (CINCA)
Mode of Inheritance	Autosomal recessive	Autosomal recessive	Autosomal recessive	?	Autosomal dominant	Autosomal dominant	Autosomal dominant	Autosomal dominant
Age at Onset (yr)	<20	<1	<1	<10	<20	<1	<20	<1
Duration of attack (days)*	<2	4-6	4-5	6-8	>14	<2	1-2	?
Cutaneous Involvement	Erysipelas-like erythema	Maculopapular rash	Morbilliform rash	Maculopapular rash	Migratory rash, overlying area of myalgia	Cold-induced urticaria-like lesions	Urticaria-like rash	Urticaria-like lesions
Musculoskeletal Involvement	Monarthritis common	Arthralgia, occasional oligoarthritis	Arthralgia common	Arthralgia	Severe myalgia common; occasional frank monarthritis	Arthralgia common; occasional mild myalgia	Lancing limb pain, arthralgia common; arthritis can occur	Epiphyseal bone formation
Abdominal Involvement	Sterile peritonitis common	Splenomegaly, severe pain common	Splenomegaly, pain may occur	May occur	Severe pain very common	None	May occur	Hepatosplenomegaly
Eye Involvement	Uncommon	Uncommon	Uncommon	Uncommon	Conjunctivitis and periorbital edema very common	Conjunctivitis	Conjunctivitis; sometimes optic nerve elevation	Papilledema with possible loss of vision, uveitis
Distinguishing Clinical Symptoms	Erysipelas-like erythema	Prominent cervical lymphadenopathy	Dysmorphic features, neurologic symptoms	Lymphadenopathy may occur	Migratory nature of myalgia and rash, periorbital edema	Cold-induced urticaria-like lesions	Sensorineural hearing loss	Chronic aseptic meningitis, sensorineural hearing loss, arthropathy
Gene Involved	MEFV	MVK	MVK	?	TNFRSF1A	CIAS1	CIAS1	CIAS1
Protein Involved	Pyrin (marenostrin)	Mevalonate kinase	Mevalonate kinase	?	Type 1 tumor necrosis factor receptor	Cryopyrin	Cryopyrin	Cryopyrin

Note. For details on Blau syndrome and pyogenic sterile arthritis, pyoderma gangrenosum, and acne (PAPA) syndrome, see text.
*Duration may vary; this is a typical duration.
Adapted from Hull KM, Shoham N, Chae JJ, et al: The expanding spectrum of systemic autoinflammatory disorders and their rheumatic manifestations. Curr Opin Rheumatol 15:61-69, 2003.

Peritonitis, vomiting, arthritis, erysipelas-like
skin lesions

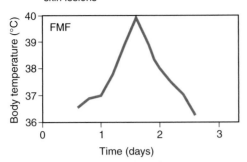

Cervical lymphadenopathy, erythematous
macules, abdominal pain, vomiting, arthralgia

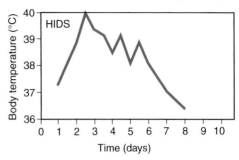

Conjunctivitis, erythematous skin lesions,
myalgia/arthralgia, abdominal pain

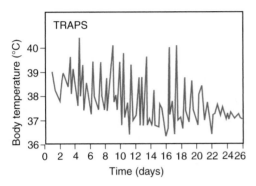

Rash, chills, polyarthralgias, conjunctivitis

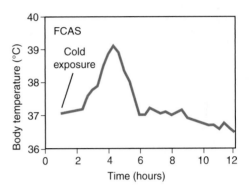

Chills, arthralgias, erythematous rash,
conjunctivitis

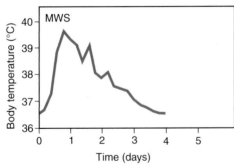

Deformative arthropathy, chronic meningitis

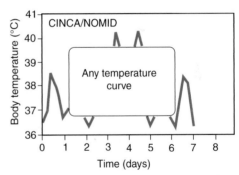

Figure 113-1 Characteristic patterns of body temperature during inflammatory attacks in the familial autoinflammatory syndromes. There is considerable interindividual variability for each syndrome, and even for the individual patient, the fever pattern may vary greatly from episode to episode. Note the different time scales on the x-axes. See text for abbreviations.

examples of pseudodominant inheritance owing to consanguinity combined with the high carrier frequency of FMF mutations in certain populations[5-7]; however, at least three families studied do seem to show a true dominant inheritance, even after extensive genetic analysis.[7]

ETIOLOGY

In 1997, two groups independently traced the genetic background of FMF to a hitherto unknown gene on the short arm of chromosome 16, dubbed the MEditteranean FeVer (MEFV) gene.[8,9] At least 67 disease-linked mutations in the MEFV gene have been described so far, most of which are clustered in the 10th exon of this gene (for details see the online mutation database at http://fmf.igh.cnrs.fr/

infevers/). Most are missense mutations that produce a single amino acid change in the protein (Fig. 113-3). There are six common mutations, accounting for almost 99% of all FMF chromosomes: M694V (occurring in 20% to 65% of cases, depending on the population examined[10]), V726A (in 7% to 35%), M680I, M694I, V694I, and E148Q. For the first three mutations mentioned here, a founder effect has been established,[9] pointing to common ancestors at least 2500 years ago. The high frequency of the mutated MEFV gene in more than one Middle Eastern population has led to the hypothesis that heterozygous carriers have an as-yet-unknown advantage, possibly a heightened (inflammatory) resistance to an as-yet-unidentified endemic pathogen of the Mediterranean basin.[9] In about 30% of patients, only one or no mutations in the MEFV gene can

Table 113-2 Differential Diagnosis of Periodic Fever

1. Hereditary (see Table 113-1)

2. Nonhereditary
   a. Infectious
      i. Hidden infectious focus (e.g., aortoenteric fistula, Caroli's disease)
      ii. Recurrent reinfection (e.g., chronic meningococcemia, host defense defect)
      iii. Specific infection (e.g., Whipple's disease, malaria)
   b. Noninfectious inflammatory disorder
      i. Adult-onset Still's disease
      ii. Juvenile chronic rheumatoid arthritis
      iii. Periodic fever, aphthous stomatitis, pharyngitis, and adenitis (PFAPA)
      iv. Schnitzler syndrome
      v. Behçet's syndrome
      vi. Crohn's disease
      vii. Sarcoidosis
      viii. Extrinsic alveolitis
      ix. Humidifier lung, polymer fume fever
   c. Neoplastic
      i. Lymphoma (e.g., Hodgkin's disease, angioimmunoblastic lymphoma)
      ii. Solid tumor (e.g., pheochromocytoma, myxoma, colon carcinoma)
   d. Vascular
      i. Recurrent pulmonary embolism
   e. Hypothalamic
   f. Psychogenic periodic fever
   g. Factitious or fraudulent

be detected; the etiology in these patients still needs to be determined.

PATHOGENESIS

The *MEFV* gene encodes for a protein of 781 amino acids, known as pyrin or marenostrin. Pyrin is expressed as a cytoplasmic protein in mature monocytes in association with microtubules,[11] but is predominantly found in the nucleus in granulocytes, dendritic cells, and synovial fibroblasts.[12] The expression of pyrin is induced by inflammatory mediators such as interferon-α and tumor necrosis factor (TNF).[13] The pyrin domain is shared by many proteins involved in apoptosis and inflammation and is a member of the death-domain superfamily that includes death domains, death-effector domains, and caspase-recruitment domains. Pyrin binds specifically to other proteins that contain a pyrin domain, which include the adapter protein "apoptosis-associated specklike-like protein with a CARD" (ASC).

The proinflammatory cytokine interleukin (IL)-1β is central in the pathogenesis of FMF. This cytokine is expressed as an inactive precursor, which is cleaved by caspase-1 to yield the active IL-1β. Caspase-1 itself first needs to be activated through the interaction with a protein complex termed an *inflammasome*. Several inflammasomes have been described so far. The major inflammasome complex involved in the activation of caspase-1 and IL-1β is the cryopyrin or NALP3 inflammasome.[14,15] Two hypotheses have been proposed regarding the effect of pyrin on IL-1β processing. The "sequestration hypothesis" holds that pyrin has an inhibitory effect on caspase-1-mediated activation of IL-1β, through its prevention of the formation of the cryopyrin inflammasome by competitive binding of

the adapter protein ASC and procaspase-1 and binding caspase-1.[16,17] Under this hypothesis, FMF mutations are thought to interfere with the inhibiting interactions of pyrin, resulting in decreased regulation of IL-1β activation.[17] The second hypothesis, proposed by Yu and coworkers,[18] suggests that pyrin can form its own specific inflammasome for activation of IL-1β, although not all the components of this proposed inflammasome have been specified so far. The FMF mutations would increase the sensitivity of this putative pyrin inflammasome. Apart from its role in regulation of IL-1β, there also is conflicting evidence for the effect of pyrin on regulation of nuclear factor κB (NFκB) or apoptosis, varying from inhibition to stimulation.[14]

CLINICAL FEATURES

In approximately 90% of FMF patients, symptoms start before age 20 years.[19] The inflammatory attacks of FMF usually last only 1 to 3 days, and their frequency can vary widely; 2 to 4 weeks is the most common interval (see Fig. 113-1). Fever is the principal symptom in FMF and is usually accompanied by symptoms of serositis (peritonitis, pleuritis, or synovitis). Abdominal pain of 1 or 2 days' duration occurs in 95% of patients, varying in severity from severe peritonitis resembling an acute abdomen to only mild abdominal pain without overt peritonitis.[20] Arthritis (rarely destructive) is often confined to one large joint, such as the knee, ankle, or wrist, and may be the only symptom. Chest pain resulting from pleuritis is usually unilateral and associated with a friction rub or transient pleural effusion. Skin involvement occurs in approximately 30% of patients, most often as erysipelas-like skin lesions on the shins or feet (Fig. 113-4).[21] Other, more uncommon, symptoms are pericarditis, occurring in less than 1%[22]; acute scrotal swelling and tenderness[23]; aseptic meningitis; and severe protracted myalgia, especially of the legs.

Fertility problems are encountered in FMF. For a variety of reasons, including peritoneal adhesions and ovulatory dysfunction, subfertility in women is common.[24] In men, subfertility secondary to azoospermia (sometimes secondary to testicular amyloidosis) or impairment of sperm penetration has been found.[25]

DIAGNOSIS AND DIAGNOSTIC TESTS

FMF is still primarily a clinical diagnosis. There is a set of validated diagnostic criteria with a reported sensitivity and specificity of 96% to 99% (Table 113-3).[26] These criteria were validated in a population with a very high prevalence of FMF and low prevalence of the other autoinflammatory disorders, however, and the ethnic origin of the patient needs to be taken into account.

Because the location of FMF mutations is known, it is possible to establish a molecular diagnosis of FMF. Genetic laboratories usually screen for the five most common mutations, and rare mutations are missed. *MEFV* mutations occur on both alleles in only 70% of typical cases,[27] whereas in the remaining 30%, only one or no mutation can be detected, even after sequencing. There also is evidence of reduced penetrance. Despite these limitations, molecular testing can be used as a confirmatory test in cases in which there is a high

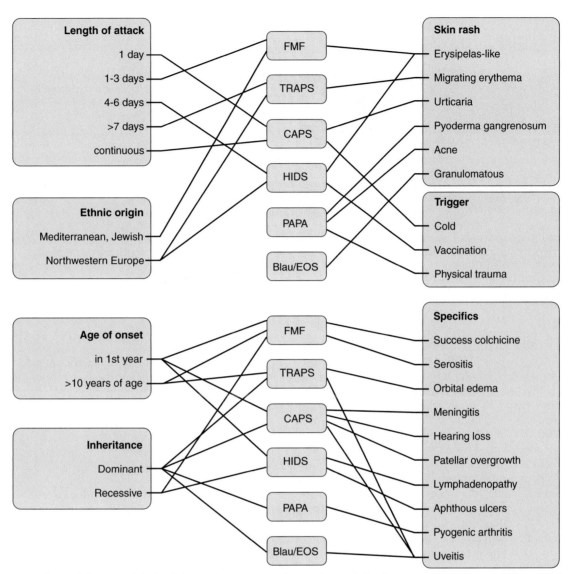

Figure 113-2 Differential diagnosis of the familial autoinflammatory syndromes. First exclude other, more common causes of fever and inflammation in the patient. When a familial autoinflammatory syndrome seems likely, check the clinical characteristics found in the patient on the right and left of the diagram, and assign one point to each syndrome that is linked to these characteristics by a line (one characteristic could lead to or point to more than one syndrome). The final combined score assigns a rank for the likelihood of the disorders in this patient and offers help in deciding on the correct subsequent diagnostic tests. This algorithm is not evidence-based, but is solely derived from expert opinion. See text for abbreviations.

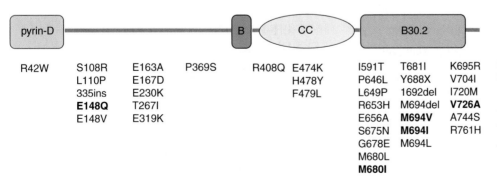

Figure 113-3 Schematic representation of pyrin (marenostrin) protein, with four conserved domains, including a pyrin domain, a B-box (B), coiled-coil domain (CC), and a B30.2 domain. Indicated are mutations as found in familial Mediterranean fever (FMF), with the five most common missense mutations in bold type.

index of suspicion. Whether or not the results are positive, treatment with colchicine is warranted in symptomatic cases of fitting ethnic origin fulfilling the diagnostic criteria.[28,29]

No specific biologic marker is available to distinguish an inflammatory FMF attack from an infectious fever or appendicitis. During an inflammatory attack, there is an acute-phase response, which includes elevation of SAA, CRP, and plasma fibrinogen and polymorphonuclear leukocytosis. Proteinuria in patients with FMF is highly suggestive of renal amyloidosis.

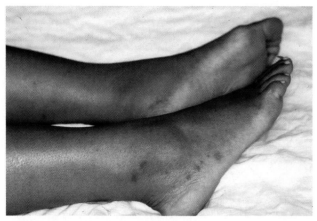

Figure 113-4 Erysipelas-like eruption in a patient with a familial Mediterranean fever attack. *(Courtesy of Professor A. Livneh, Heller Institute of Medical Research, Tel Hashomer, Israel.)*

Table 113-3 Diagnostic Criteria for Familial Mediterranean Fever*

Major Criteria
Typical attacks[†] with peritonitis (generalized)
Typical attacks with pleuritis (unilateral) or pericarditis
Typical attacks with monarthritis (hip, knee, ankle)
Typical attacks with fever alone
Incomplete abdominal attack

Minor Criteria
Incomplete attacks[‡] involving chest pain
Incomplete attacks involving monarthritis
Exertional leg pain
Favorable response to colchicine

*Requirements for diagnosis of familial Mediterranean fever are ≥1 major criteria or ≥2 minor criteria.
†Typical attacks are defined as recurrent (≥3 of the same type), febrile (≥38°C), and short (lasting between 12 hours and 3 days).
‡Incomplete attacks are defined as painful and recurrent attacks not fulfilling the criteria for a typical attack.
From Livneh A, Langevitz P, Zemer D, et al: Criteria for the diagnosis of familial Mediterranean fever. Arthritis Rheum 40:1879-1885, 1997.

TREATMENT

Colchicine is the first-line of treatment for patients with FMF. Its efficacy was established in three controlled clinical trials in 1974.[30-32] Colchicine prevents inflammatory attacks in 60% of patients, and it significantly reduces the number of attacks in an additional 20% to 30%.[25] The average dose in adults is 1 mg daily, but this may be increased to 3 mg in cases in which no response is seen at the lower dose. This regimen is usually well tolerated; gastrointestinal side effects, including diarrhea and abdominal pain, generally resolve with dose reduction. More serious side effects, such as myopathy, neuropathy, and leukopenia, are rare and occur primarily in patients with renal or liver impairment. During a fever attack, oral or intramuscular nonsteroidal anti-inflammatory drugs (NSAIDs) can be used for pain relief. Glucocorticoids have limited efficacy.

Compliance with colchicine use is important because colchicine has been shown to prevent the occurrence of amyloidosis. Since the introduction of colchicine therapy, the incidence of amyloidosis in FMF has decreased dramatically, whereas in areas with a high prevalence of FMF where colchicine is not routinely available, such as Armenia, amyloidosis is still common.

Colchicine's principal effect at the cellular level is to depolymerize microtubules by interacting with tubulin, inhibiting motility and exostosis of intracellular granules. It has a powerful antimitotic effect, causing metaphase arrest. It has been speculated, in cases of infertility in patients treated with colchicine, that this medication causes azoospermia. Colchicine does not have a significant adverse effect on sperm production or function, however.[33] Unfounded fear of teratogenic effects of colchicine often wrongly leads to cessation of this drug in young women who wish to get pregnant, with a subsequent increased frequency and severity of attacks, which enhances problems with fertility and pregnancy. Colchicine has proved to be safe, even in early pregnancy, and treatment should not be interrupted for this reason.[24,34] It also can be used while breastfeeding.[25]

Not all patients respond well to colchicine, in some cases because of poor intestinal resorption of the drug. Lidar and colleagues[35] used parenteral colchicine in such refractory cases. We have observed that the IL-1β inhibitor anakinra worked in such a patient (unpublished observation). Chae and coworkers[17] reported the successful use of anakinra in an FMF patient with amyloidosis who could not tolerate colchicine because of side effects.

OUTCOME AND PROGNOSIS

Recurrent attacks of peritonitis may lead to intra-abdominal or pelvic adhesions, resulting in complications such as small bowel obstruction or reduced fertility in female patients. Another serious long-term complication of FMF is amyloid A (AA) amyloidosis. This amyloidosis is primarily found in the kidneys, resulting in renal failure, but also can occur in the gastrointestinal tract, liver, and spleen, and eventually in the heart, testes, and thyroid. The prevalence of amyloidosis varies, especially depending on the ethnic origin, but is high in untreated patients. It is common among Sephardic Jews, but rare in Ashkenazi Jews.[36]

HYPER–IMMUNOGLOBULIN D SYNDROME

EPIDEMIOLOGY

Hyper-IgD syndrome (HIDS) (MIM 260920) also is an autosomal recessively inherited disorder, but it is far less prevalent than FMF. The International Hyper-IgD Syndrome Registry, based in Nijmegen, the Netherlands, in which clinical information is actively collected from physicians worldwide, currently holds data on approximately 220 patients. Approximately 75% of these patients are from Western Europe, and 50% are from the Netherlands and France. Most HIDS patients are white. These observations can be explained partly by a founder effect.[37] In the Netherlands, the carrier frequency of a hyper-IgD mutation is estimated to be 1:530.[38] Men and women are affected in equal numbers.

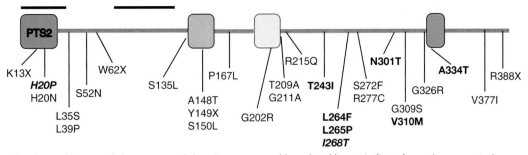

Figure 113-5 Mevalonate kinase, with four conserved domains represented by colored boxes. Indicated are missense mutations, nonsense mutations, and two deletions, which have been identified in mevalonate kinase deficiency. In bold are mutations found in mevalonic aciduria patients; in bold and italic are mutations found in classic hyper-IgD syndrome (HIDS) and mevalonic aciduria.

ETIOLOGY

HIDS in its classic form is caused by mutations in the gene encoding for the enzyme mevalonate kinase, located on the long arm of chromosome 12 (for details, see the online mutation database available at http://fmf.igh.cnrs.fr/infevers/).[39-41] Patients with classic HIDS are most often compound heterozygotes for two different missense mutations in the mevalonate kinase gene (Fig. 113-5). Two mutations (leading to a valine-to-isoleucine change, V377I, and to a isoleucine-to-tyrosine change, I268T) account for greater than 85% of the patients described to date.[42,43] Not all patients with HIDS have a gene defect of mevalonate kinase. We have designated these patients as variant HIDS (see Table 113-1).[41]

PATHOGENESIS

Mevalonate kinase is part of the isoprenoid pathway; it is involved in the next step after 3-hydroxy-3-methyl-glutaryl–coenzyme A (HMG-CoA) reductase by phosphorylating mevalonic acid. The isoprenoid pathway has many diverse end products that include cholesterol, dolichol, and ubiquinone, and it leads to isoprenylation of proteins, with a post-translational modification directing these proteins, such as Rho and Ras, to the cell membrane.[44]

The HIDS mutations lead to a constantly diminished activity of mevalonate kinase to about 5% to 15% of normal levels, and these levels decrease further during a fever attack.[45] Because of this reduced enzyme activity, the substrate mevalonic acid accumulates in serum and urine. Higher levels are found during the episodes of fever. There does not seem to be a dramatic shortage of any specific end product; concentrations of cholesterol, ubiquinone, and dolichol in patients are normal to slightly decreased.[14]

Another syndrome already was linked to mutations in the mevalonate kinase gene before the discovery of HIDS[46]—classic mevalonic aciduria. Patients with mevalonic aciduria carry specific mutations that cause a more severe reduction of mevalonate kinase enzyme activity, often reducing it to undetectable levels. These patients constantly produce large amounts of mevalonic acid and often have more than 1000 times as much mevalonic acid in their urine than do HIDS patients.[47] Patients with mevalonic aciduria also have a more severe phenotype, which is described in the next section. Classic mevalonic aciduria and HIDS seem to be two extremes of a continuous spectrum of disease related to mevalonate kinase deficiency.[48]

The pathogenetic link between mevalonate kinase deficiency and inflammation is still unclear, but there is increasing evidence for a connection between the isoprenoid pathway and inflammation. Inhibition of the isoprenoid pathway by statins, the inhibitors of HMG-CoA reductase (the enzymatic step before that of mevalonate kinase) can have anti-inflammatory effects, ranging from increased apoptosis of inflammatory cells to reduction of expression of cytokines.[49,50] In other settings, statins seem to be proinflammatory, most notably in a study in which stimulation with *Mycobacterium tuberculosis* or mitogens in combination with statins increased caspase-1 activation and IL-1β secretion by monocytes, through a decrease of geranilgeraniol.[14]

The ex vivo production of IL-1β is increased in HIDS,[51-53] whereas treatment with the IL-1 blocker anakinra is beneficial.[54] This links HIDS to the autoinflammatory disorders with a direct defect of inflammasome function.

A defect in apoptosis also may contribute to the pathogenesis of HIDS. Lymphocytes from HIDS patients (who had no fever at the time of blood sampling) showed a decrease in apoptosis when stimulated with anisomycin, which was not found in patients with TNF receptor–associated periodic syndrome (TRAPS) or FMF patients.[55] Such a decrease in apoptosis would result in increased survival of lymphocytes and may delay the resolution of the inflammatory response. An ordinarily innocuous stimulus in HIDS patients would more easily lead to a full-blown fever episode.

Whether the pathophysiologic effects of mevalonate kinase deficiency are due to a transient deficiency of one or more isoprenoid end products or toxicity of mevalonate accumulation still needs to be clarified. The cause of the characteristic high serum concentrations of IgD in this syndrome, which have led to its name, also is still unexplained.

CLINICAL FEATURES

Ninety percent of patients with classic HIDS experience their first fever episode in the first year of life,[40] and these episodes become most frequent in childhood and adolescence. The high fevers may lead to seizures, especially in young children. Vaccination, minor trauma, surgery, and physical or emotional stress are factors that provoke a fever episode, although often a triggering factor is not obvious. The fevers often begin with cold chills and a sharp increase in body temperature.[1] They are almost always accompanied by (cervical) lymphadenopathy and abdominal pain with vomiting

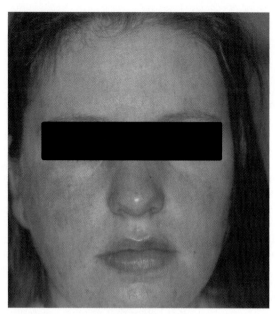

Figure 113-6   Facial erythematous macules and papules in a hyper-IgD syndrome patient during an attack.

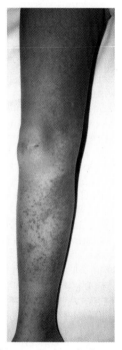

Figure 113-7   Petechiae on the leg of a hyper-IgD syndrome patient during a febrile attack.

and diarrhea. Other frequent symptoms are headache, myalgia, and arthralgia. Apart from the lymphadenopathy, physical signs frequently consist of splenomegaly and a skin rash with erythematous macules and papules (Fig. 113-6) or petechiae (Fig. 113-7).[56] Sometimes there are also signs of frank arthritis (principally large joints) and hepatomegaly. About 40% of patients report painful aphthous ulcers in the mouth, vagina, or scrotum (Fig. 113-8). The fever disappears spontaneously after 3 to 5 days, although it may take longer before the symptoms in joints or skin disappear completely. These inflammatory attacks occur, on average, once

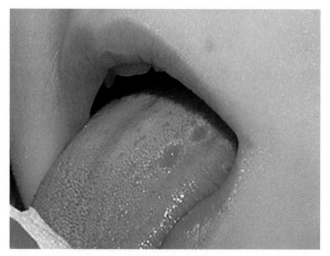

Figure 113-8   Aphthous ulceration detected on the tongue of a patient with hyper-IgD syndrome. *(Courtesy of Dr. K. Antila, North Carelian Central Hospital, Joensuu, Finland.)*

every 4 to 6 weeks, although this may vary from patient to patient or in an individual patient. The phenotype of variant HIDS differs slightly from and is milder than that of classic HIDS.[41]

Patients with mevalonic aciduria, the metabolic disorder that also is caused by mevalonate kinase gene mutations, experience similar inflammatory episodes as HIDS patients, but these are often of less importance compared with the severity of the rest of the phenotype, which consists of psychomotor retardation, ataxia, failure to thrive, cataracts, and dysmorphic facies. These patients usually die in early childhood.[47] An intermediary clinical phenotype between classic mevalonic aciduria and HIDS has been described.[48]

DIAGNOSIS AND DIAGNOSTIC TESTS

HIDS is diagnosed based on a combination of characteristic clinical findings and continuously elevated IgD concentrations (>100 IU/mL) (Table 113-4). There are numerous caveats concerning IgD serum concentration, however: Values may be normal in very young patients (especially patients <3 years old),[57] persistently normal levels have been reported in a few patients with classic HIDS,[39] and patients with other familial autoinflammatory syndromes also may have elevated IgD concentrations, although these are usually only slightly elevated. More than 80% of HIDS patients combine a high concentration of IgD with high IgA levels.[57,58] During fever attacks, a brisk acute-phase response is observed, including leukocytosis, high levels of SAA and CRP, and activation of the cytokine network.[52,59]

The diagnosis of classic HIDS can be confirmed by DNA analysis of the mevalonate kinase gene. The best approach is to start with screening for the two most prevalent mutations, V377I and I268T. If this screening is negative, but the clinical suspicion remains high, sequencing of the entire gene can be considered. A good alternative is the measurement of urinary mevalonic acid concentrations during an attack, which are slightly elevated. Gas chromatography–mass spectroscopy is necessary to detect this slight increase,

Table 113-4 Diagnostic Indicators of Hyper–Immunoglobulin D Syndrome

At Time of Attacks
Elevated erythrocyte sedimentation rate and leukocytosis
Abrupt onset of fever (≥38.5°C)
Recurrent attacks
Lymphadenopathy (cervical)
Abdominal distress (e.g., vomiting, diarrhea, pain)
Skin manifestations (e.g., erythematous macules and papules)
Arthralgias and arthritis
Splenomegaly
Constantly Present
Elevated IgD (≥100 U/mL) measured on 2 occasions at least 1 mo apart*
Elevated IgA (≥2.6 g/L)
Classic Hyper–Immunoglobulin D Syndrome Only
Mutations in mevalonate kinase gene
Decreased mevalonate kinase enzyme activity

*Extremely high serum concentrations of IgD are characteristic, but not obligatory.

however.[60] The measurement of mevalonate kinase enzyme activity is complicated and time-consuming and should be reserved for research purposes.

TREATMENT

There is no established treatment regimen for HIDS. A double-blind, placebo-controlled, crossover trial of the HMG-CoA reductase inhibitor simvastatin showed a beneficial effect of this drug, with a reduction in number of days of illness in five out of six patients.[61] Takada and associates[62] reported a favorable preliminary experience with the TNF antagonist etanercept.[54] In one report, use of the IL-1β inhibitor anakinra curtailed the fever episode in a HIDS patient.[54]

Some individual patients have been reported to have benefited from treatment with corticosteroids, colchicine, intravenous immunoglobulin, or cyclosporine, but these results have not been repeated in most patients.[56] Thalidomide did not have an effect on disease activity in a placebo-controlled trial.[63]

OUTCOME AND PROGNOSIS

The long-term outcome in classic and variant HIDS is relatively benign in most patients. In many patients, the fever episodes occur less frequently and become less severe later in life, starting from late adolescence. Joint destruction is rare, but abdominal adhesions are seen, resulting from repeated abdominal inflammation or (unnecessary) diagnostic laparotomy because of suspected acute abdomen.

Until more recently, no cases of amyloidosis had been seen in HIDS patients since its first description in 1984. Since 2004, four HIDS patients 19 to 27 years old have been reported who developed renal failure because of AA amyloidosis.[64-66] Regular screening for proteinuria also may be advisable in HIDS patients, especially patients with frequent and severe fever episodes.

TUMOR NECROSIS FACTOR RECEPTOR–ASSOCIATED PERIODIC SYNDROME

EPIDEMIOLOGY

TRAPS (MIM 142680) has an autosomal dominant inheritance pattern. It was originally described in a large family from Irish and Scottish descent as "familial Hibernian fever."[67] It is found primarily in patients from northwestern Europe, but also has been described in families from Australia, Mexico, Puerto Rico, Portugal, and the Czech Republic.[68] Any ethnic group may be affected. Other previous nomenclature for this syndrome includes "autosomal dominant familial periodic fever"[69] and "familial perireticular amyloidosis."[70]

ETIOLOGY

Mutations are found in the gene for the type I TNF receptor (*TNFRSF1A*), which is located on the short arm of chromosome 12.[4] These are mainly single-nucleotide missense substitutions, located in exons 2, 3, and 4, which encode for the extracellular domain of *TNFRSF1A*. Many of these mutations disrupt one of the highly conserved cysteine residues involved in extracellular disulfide bonds of the 55-kD type I TNF receptor protein (Fig. 113-9) (for details, see the online mutation database available at http://fmf.igh.cnrs.fr/infevers/).

There are some general genotype-phenotype correlations, especially when mutations are grouped in cysteine and noncysteine mutations. Noncysteine mutations have, overall, a lower penetrance than cysteine mutations, and amyloidosis is seen far more often in association with cysteine mutations.[71] Two missense mutations in *TNFRSF1A*, P46L and R92Q, have a particularly low penetrance and are found in approximately 1% to 10% of control chromosomes.[71-73] R92Q has been observed in higher prevalence in a group of patients with arthritis. It is thought that the clinical manifestations of patients with an R92Q mutation depend on other so-far-unidentified modifying genes, environmental factors, or both.[71]

PATHOGENESIS

The TRAPS mutations are supposed to be gain-of-function mutations, leading to increased TNF-α signaling. TNF-α is a pleiotropic molecule, which induces cytokine secretion, activation of leukocytes, fever, and cachexia. Activation of the receptor by TNF-α causes cleavage and shedding of its extracellular part into the circulation, where it acts as an inhibitor of TNF-α. When an in vitro shedding defect was shown for numerous TRAPS mutations, the "shedding hypothesis" was postulated for the pathogenesis of TRAPS. Reduced shedding of the type I TNF receptor would lead to prolonged TNF-α signaling and uncontrolled inflammation. Not all TRAPS mutations cause decreased shedding, however, and although serum concentrations of the shedded soluble *TNFRSF1A* in TRAPS patients during periods without symptoms are often found to be significantly reduced compared with normal subjects, this is not always the case.[14] The hypothesis of reduced shedding, although

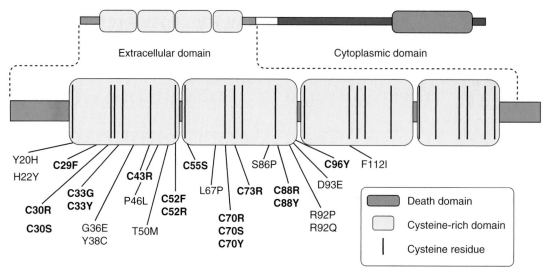

Figure 113-9 Schematic representation of the tumor necrosis factor (TNF) receptor type 1 protein (TNFRSF1A), depicting mutations found in TNF receptor–associated periodic syndrome (TRAPS) up to this time (except for one intron mutation affecting a splice site). Mutations disrupting cysteine residues are in boldface type.

attractive by its simplicity, is not supported as the sole cause of the fever attacks in TRAPS, and additional mechanisms seem to be at work.

A new hypothesis suggests that the increased inflammation in TRAPS is independent of the TNF-signaling function of the mutated type I receptor.[74,75] It has been shown that there is less binding of TNF-α to the mutated receptor,[76,77] less cell surface expression,[77-79] and decreased TNF-induced NFκB-activation.[78,80] The mutated *TNFRSF1A* is retained intracellularly, pooled in the endoplasmic reticulum.[74,77,81] Mutant *TNFR1* cannot associate with the wild-type version, but can form aggregates by self-interaction.[74,75] Either this cytoplasmic receptor aggregation results in ligand-independent signaling,[75] or accumulation of the misfolded mutant protein in the endoplasmic reticulum turns on an exaggerated unfolded protein response leading to induction of cytokines such as IL-1β.[74] This new hypothesis also might offer an explanation for the observation that blocking IL-1β works better in some TRAPS patients than blocking TNF.[82]

CLINICAL FEATURES

The clinical features can vary much more between individual TRAPS patients than is generally seen in FMF or HIDS.[68] The age of onset can vary, even within the same family, with a documented range of 2 weeks to 53 years old.[68,83] There also is a large variation in duration and frequency of the fever episodes in TRAPS. On average, attacks last 3 to 4 weeks and recur two to six times each year, but episodes also may be limited to a few days (see Fig. 113-1). Although the index patient, through whom the diagnosis is made, often displays well-defined inflammatory attacks, affected family members may have less typical symptoms, such as episodic mild arthritis.

During inflammatory attacks, a high, spiking fever can be accompanied by skin lesions, myalgia and arthralgia, abdominal distress, and ocular symptoms. The most common cutaneous manifestation is a centrifugal, migratory, erythematous patch, which may overlie a local area of

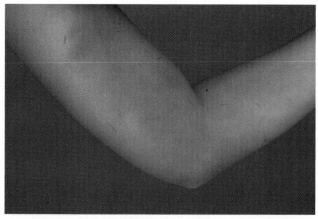

Figure 113-10 Migrating erythematous rash during a tumor necrosis factor receptor–associated periodic syndrome attack. *(Courtesy of Dr. T. Fiselier, University Medical Center St. Radboud, Nijmegen, The Netherlands.)*

myalgia (Fig. 113-10),[84] but urticarial plaques also may be seen. Myalgia is often located primarily in the muscles of the thighs, but it may migrate during the fever episode, affecting all of the limbs and the torso, face, and neck.[68] Arthralgia primarily affects large joints, including hips, knees, and ankles. Frank synovitis is rarer, and when it does occur it is nonerosive, asymmetric, and monarticular.[68] Abdominal pain occurs in 92% of TRAPS patients during inflammatory attacks; other gastrointestinal symptoms often seen include vomiting and constipation. Ocular involvement is characteristic in TRAPS, and it may involve conjunctivitis, periorbital edema, or periorbital pain in one or both eyes. Severe uveitis and iritis have been described, and any TRAPS patient with ocular pain should be examined for these complications.[68,84] Other, less frequently observed symptoms during fever attacks in TRAPS are chest pain, breathlessness, pericarditis, and testicular and scrotal pain, which may be caused by inflammation of the tunica vaginalis.[68,83] One case report described a patient who presented with psychosis without fever.[85] It has been suggested from

Table 113-5 Diagnostic Indicators of Tumor Necrosis Factor Receptor–Associated Periodic Syndrome

1. Recurrent episodes of inflammatory symptoms spanning >6 mo duration (several symptoms generally occur simultaneously)
   a. Fever
   b. Abdominal pain
   c. Myalgia (migratory)
   d. Rash (erythematous macular rash occurs with myalgia)
   e. Conjunctivitis or periorbital edema
   f. Chest pain
   g. Arthralgia or monarticular synovitis
2. Episodes last >5 days on average (although variable)
3. Responsive to glucocorticosteroids, but not colchicine
4. Affects family members in autosomal dominant pattern (although may not always be present)
5. Any ethnicity may be affected

From Hull KM, Drewe E, Aksentijevich I, et al: The TNF receptor-associated periodic syndrome (TRAPS): Emerging concepts of an autoinflammatory disorder. Medicine (Balt) 81:349-368, 2002.

observation in one of the first families with TRAPS that this disorder is associated with an increased incidence of indirect inguinal hernias,[86] but this has not been shown in other patients. Lymphadenopathy is rare in TRAPS.

DIAGNOSIS AND DIAGNOSTIC TESTS

As in the other familial autoinflammatory syndromes, laboratory investigations during inflammatory attacks show a clear acute-phase response, and even in between fever attacks, such an inflammatory response may be measured. Autoantibodies generally are not detected in TRAPS. The IgD level may be elevated, but the value is almost always less than 100 IU/mL.[83,86] Most patients exhibit a significantly lower concentration of soluble *TNFRSF1A*, most prominently in symptom-free intervals, compared with appropriate controls,[86] although this does not seem to be a universal rule.[68] Also, because soluble *TNFRSF1A* is cleared by the kidneys, TRAPS patients with renal insufficiency (e.g., owing to renal amyloidosis) may have normal or elevated plasma concentrations of this protein.[87]

Hull and colleagues[68] proposed a set of clinical diagnostic criteria for TRAPS (Table 113-5). These criteria are not validated by epidemiologic measures, but they may be used as a first step in evaluation of patients. TRAPS is ultimately a genetic diagnosis, defined by a missense mutation in the gene for *TNFRSF1A*. Clinical penetrance of TRAPS mutations is not 100%, however, even for cysteine mutations, and asymptomatic carriers are common. Also, the finding of a R92Q or P46L variant in this gene would pose a difficulty. Because they have many characteristics of a polymorphism rather than a direct disease-causing mutation (see etiology), it is debatable whether such a finding should lead to a diagnosis of TRAPS.

TREATMENT

NSAIDs and glucocorticoids in high doses (>20 mg/day of oral prednisone) alleviate the symptoms of fever and inflammation in most TRAPS patients, although they do not alter the frequency of attacks. They can be used beneficially at

times of attack, and glucocorticoids usually can be tapered in the course of 1 or 2 weeks, as tolerated. In mild cases of TRAPS, NSAIDs are often sufficient.

Intravenous infusion of a synthetic TNFRSF1A fusion protein was tried in one patient by Drewe and coworkers,[88] but this seemed to provoke a severe attack. Use of etanercept, a fusion product of TNFRSF1B (the receptor that is not defective) has been more successful.[68,71,88,89] A study with twice-weekly administration of etanercept (25 mg for adults or 0.4 mg/kg for children) in nine TRAPS patients with various mutations revealed an overall 66% response rate as determined by decreased number of attacks over a 6-month period.[68] Another study with the same dosage of etanercept for 24 weeks in seven TRAPS patients also showed a clear beneficial effect without serious adverse events.[88] A similar regimen of etanercept reversed the nephrotic syndrome in a patient with amyloidosis.[90]

Drewe and colleagues[91] described one patient whose symptoms were resistant to administration of etanercept, who responded favorably to use of oral sirolimus (4 to 6 mg daily). Infliximab, a monoclonal antibody against TNF, has been shown to be less effective than etanercept in TRAPS and seems to cause increased symptoms.[88,91,92] In one patient with severe inflammatory attacks of TRAPS resistant to etanercept, we have seen a good response to the IL-1β inhibitor anakinra.[82] There is no response to colchicine or immunosuppressive drugs, such as azathioprine, cyclosporine, thalidomide, or cyclophosphamide.[68]

OUTCOME AND PROGNOSIS

Reactive AA amyloidosis is the principal systemic complication of TRAPS. It occurs in about 15% to 25% of patients[4,71] and generally leads to renal impairment. Amyloidosis in a patient with TRAPS places other affected family members at high risk for this complication. It is principally associated with *TNFRSF1A* mutations affecting cysteine residues.[71] Because proteinuria is the initial manifestation of renal amyloidosis, it is advisable to screen urine samples from TRAPS patients regularly by dipstick examination, especially affected family members of a TRAPS patient with amyloidosis.

CRYOPYRIN-ASSOCIATED PERIODIC SYNDROME

Cryopyrin-associated periodic syndrome (CAPS) encompasses three clinical syndromes that all have been traced to mutations in one common gene: Muckle-Wells syndrome (MWS), familial cold autoinflammatory syndrome (FCAS), and chronic infantile neurologic cutaneous and articular syndrome (CINCA), also known as neonatal-onset multisystemic inflammatory disease (NOMID). After the recognition of the genetic defect, it became clear that there is considerable overlap between these three disorders. Most notably, families have been described with features of MWS and FCAS.[93] FCAS, MWS, and CINCA/NOMID might represent a spectrum of disease, with FCAS the mildest and CINCA the most severe form. Given their common genotype, they are discussed under one heading here, but clinical features and outcomes are dealt with separately.

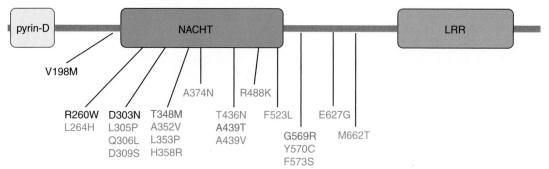

Figure 113-11 Cryopyrin protein, containing an N-terminal pyrin domain, a nucleotide binding site (NACHT), and a leucine-rich repeat (LRR) domain. Indicated are missense mutations identified in patients with familial cold autoinflammatory syndrome (FCAS) *(red)*, Muckle-Wells syndrome (MWS) *(green)*, or chronic infantile neurologic cutaneous and articular syndrome (CINCA/NOMID) *(blue)*, and mutations found in common in two or all of these clinical syndromes *(black)*.

EPIDEMIOLOGY

All three syndromes are rare, autosomal dominantly inherited syndromes. Most articles on FCAS, first described in 1940, describe large families from Europe and North America with extensive pedigrees, but sporadic cases have been described. There seems to be a founder effect in American families of Northern European extraction.[94] MWS was first described in 1962 and has since been described in large families, although it does occur in isolated cases and small nuclear families. Most affected families come from France and the United Kingdom.[95] CINCA is rare, and, to date, some 70 cases and only a few families have been described. Most patients come from France and Argentina, but cases also are seen in other European countries and the United States.[96,97]

ETIOLOGY

The first indications that MWS and FCAS are allelic stem from early linkage studies showing that FCAS and MWS were linked to the same region on the long arm of chromosome 1 (1q44).[95,98] In 2001, the gene for FCAS and MWS was identified. In a large-scale, positional cloning effort using three families with FCAS and one family with MWS, missense mutations in a new gene were found. This gene, *CIAS1* (synonyms are NALP3 and PYPAF), encodes for a protein denoted cryopyrin. Later studies showed that *CIAS1* mutations also were associated with CINCA.[97,99] Practically all mutations are missense mutations found in exon 3 of the *CIAS1* gene, which encodes for the NOD domain of cryopyrin.[100] Some mutations occur in MWS and FCAS (R260W) or in MWS and CINCA (D303N) (Fig. 113-11) (for details, see the online mutation database available at http://fmf.igh.cnrs.fr/infevers/).[97]

PATHOGENESIS

Cryopyrin was a previously unknown protein at the time of the discovery of the mutations involved in these syndromes. Since that time, it has become the focus of numerous studies, which have led to a new concept—the inflammasome.[101] Cryopyrin is a member of the NOD-LRR protein family.[102] Alternative names include NALP3 (Nacht domain–, leucine-rich repeat– and PYD-containing protein) and PYPAF1 (Pyrin domain-containing APAF-like protein). It consists

of a pyrin domain (PYD), a NOD (also known as NACHT domain), and a LRR domain. Cryopyrin is mainly expressed in monocytes and neutrophils, but also is found in human chondrocytes.[99,103,104]

Cryopyrin is thought to be an intracellular sensor of pathogens or danger signals, regulating innate immunity. On stimulation with various ligands, which include bacterial RNA, imidazoquinolone compounds,[105] gram-positive bacterial toxins nigericin and maitotoxin, adenosine triphosphate,[106,107] and uric acid crystals,[108] cryopyrin forms interactions with adapter proteins ASC and cardinal, which results in a multiprotein complex termed the *cryopyrin inflammasome*.[101] The cryopyrin inflammasome activates caspase-1, which subsequently cleaves pro-IL-1β to the active IL-1β.[109,110]

There is conflicting evidence for a role of cryopyrin in regulation of transcription factor NFκB.[14] Possibly, the ultimate effect on NFκB is determined by interaction of multiple proteins. Four more recent publications by independent groups that each developed a cryopyrin-deficient mouse showed no effect, however, on NFκB activation in these mice, whereas they did show a clear deficiency in caspase-1-mediated IL-1β activation.[105-108]

Monocytes from patients with mutations in the NOD of cryopyrin show increased activation of caspase-1 and subsequently increased release of IL-1β.[110,111] The key role of IL-1β in CAPS is confirmed by the success of treatment with the IL-1 blocker anakinra in all three clinical syndromes (see treatment section).

The exact effect of the cryopyrin mutations is still unclear. An attractive hypothesis involves a possible autoinhibitory loop of cryopyrin.[110] Mutations in the NOD could interfere with this autoinhibitory mechanism of cryopyrin, leading to undue and excessive activation of caspase-1 and IL-1β.

CLINICAL FEATURES AND OUTCOME

Familial Cold Autoinflammatory Syndrome

FCAS (MIM 120100) is characterized by episodes of rash, fever, and arthralgia after generalized exposure to cold (see Fig. 113-1). The disease occurs in large families as an autosomal dominant inherited disorder with an almost complete penetrance.[94] The rash usually starts on the exposed extremities and, in most episodes, extends to the remainder of the body. It consists of erythematous macules and plaques

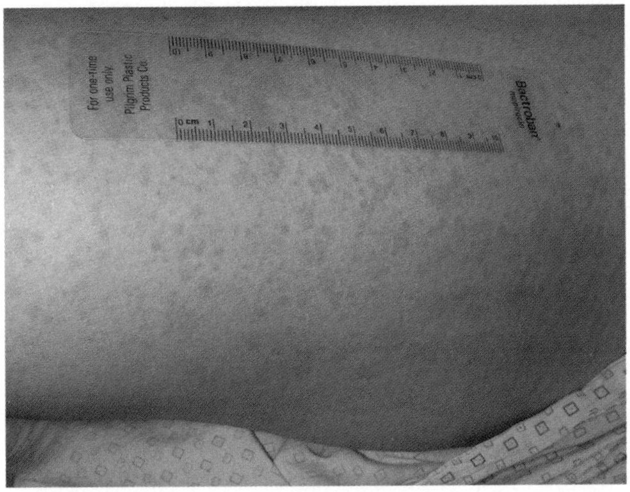

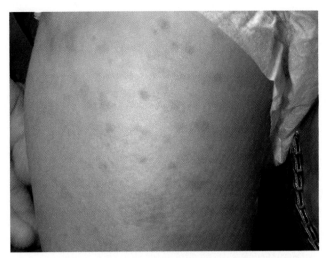

Figure 113-12 Fine, confluent, erythematous macules on the upper leg of a patient with familial cold autoinflammatory syndrome. *(Courtesy of Dr. Johnstone, Medical College of Georgia, Augusta, Ga.)*

Figure 113-13 Detail of upper leg with fine, confluent, erythematous macules in familial cold autoinflammatory syndrome. *(Courtesy of Dr. Johnstone, Medical College of Georgia, Augusta, Ga.)*

(Figs. 113-12 and 113-13), urticarial lesions, and sometimes petechiae,[112] and can cause a burning or itchy sensation. In one case report, FCAS was associated with Raynaud's disease.[113] In some cases, localized edematous swelling of extremities is reported. The arthralgias, present in 93% of cases, most often affect the hands, knees, and ankles, but also can involve feet, wrists, and elbows.[114] Frank arthritis is not seen. Most patients (84%) also report conjunctivitis during a fever episode. Other symptoms include myalgia, profuse sweating, drowsiness, headache, extreme thirst, and nausea.

A typical feature of FCAS is the requirement of cold exposure to trigger the symptoms. The delay between cold and onset of symptoms varies from 10 minutes to 8 hours.[114] When Hoffman and colleagues[115] provoked an inflammatory attack in FCAS patients by generalized cold exposure in a cold room, they saw that patients developed rash, fever, and arthralgias within 1 to 4 hours. The occurrence of these symptoms could be blocked by pretreatment with the IL-1β inhibitor anakinra.[115]

The subsequent fever attack varies in length, depending on the degree of cold exposure; generally it lasts a few hours to a maximum of 3 days. These episodes start at an early age, with 95% of patients having had their first fever episode in the first year of life—60% even within the first days of life. The symptoms tend to become less severe with advancing age.[112] Type AA amyloidosis complicated by renal insufficiency has been described in three FCAS families.[114]

Muckle-Wells Syndrome

MWS (MIM 191900) is a rare autosomal dominant inflammatory disorder with incomplete penetrance. Patients have recurrent episodes of fever, abdominal pain, myalgia, urticarial rash (Figs. 113-14 and 113-15), and conjunctivitis, frequently accompanied by arthralgias, arthritis with limb pain, or both. Attacks start in adolescence and can be provoked by hunger, by tiredness, and sometimes by exposure to cold.[116] The inflammatory episodes generally last 24 to 48 hours (see Fig. 113-1) and start with ill-defined malaise and transient chills and rigor, followed by aching or lancinating

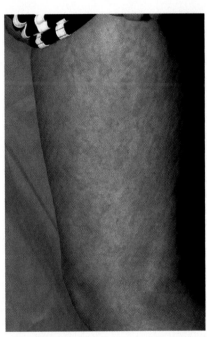

Figure 113-14 Urticarial skin rash in a patient with Muckle-Wells syndrome. *(Courtesy of Dr. D.L. Kastner, National Institute of Health, Bethesda, Md.)*

pains in the distal limbs and larger joints. Arthralgia is a common feature of the attacks, but synovitis of the large joints is less common.[117] The rash consists of usually aching and sometimes pruritic erythematous papules 1 to 7 cm in diameter. In a few cases, genital and buccal aphthous ulcers have been seen.[118] Ocular symptoms include uveitis and conjunctivitis. Symptoms typically start in adolescence, although they have been reported at an earlier age. Late-onset development of perceptive deafness is common in MWS. Bone involvement, such as clubbing of nails and pes cavus, can be seen as well. Most often, patients have a positive family history for the disease, which is indicative of autosomal dominant inheritance, but isolated cases have been reported. The most feared complication of the inflammatory attacks is type AA amyloidosis, which affects the

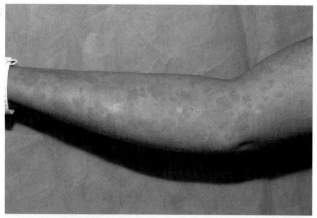

Figure 113-15   Urticarial skin rash on the arm of a patient with Muckle-Wells syndrome. *(Courtesy of Dr. D.L. Kastner, National Institute of Health, Bethesda, Md.)*

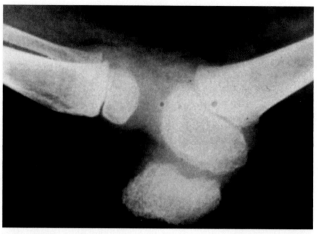

Figure 113-17   Radiograph of the knee in a patient with chronic infantile neurologic cutaneous and articular syndrome showing greatly enlarged epiphyses and patella with punctate increased density. *(Courtesy of Dr. A.M. Prieur, Hôpital Necker-Enfants Malades, Paris, France.)*

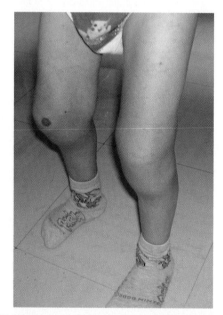

Figure 113-16   Severe deformational arthropathy of the knees in a patient with chronic infantile neurologic cutaneous and articular syndrome. *(Courtesy of Dr. A.M. Prieur, Hôpital Necker-Enfants Malades, Paris, France.)*

kidneys first, leading to proteinuria and subsequent rapid progression to renal failure.

Chronic Infantile Neurologic Cutaneous and Articular Syndrome

CINCA or NOMID (MIM 607115) is a rare congenital disorder defined by the presence of the triad of (1) neonatal-onset skin lesions, (2) chronic aseptic meningitis, and (3) recurrent fever along with joint symptoms.[119] CINCA is an autosomal dominant inherited disorder.[97] The key clinical feature of CINCA is a skin rash accompanied by peculiar joint manifestations and central nervous system involvement. The symptoms in CINCA begin right after birth or in the first months of life with a generalized skin rash. The disease follows an unpredictable course with persistent nonpruritic sind migratory rash with fever, hepatosplenomegaly, and lymphadenopathies. Central nervous system

involvement is not obvious from the outset, although occasional patients present with seizures, spasticity, or transient episodes of hemiplegia. In most patients, there are signs of chronic persistent aseptic meningitis.[120] Cerebrospinal fluid analysis may show mild pleiocytosis, and there may be an increased intracranial pressure. Brain imaging shows mild ventricular dilation, prominent sulci, central atrophy, and, in long-standing cases, calcifications of fauces and dura.

In older children, headache is often a prominent feature as a sign of chronic meningitis. Mental retardation is present in almost all cases. Progressive sensorineural impairment leading to high-frequency hearing loss can be seen in a few cases. Ocular manifestations are prominent, with optic disk changes, such as optic disk edema, pseudopapilledema, and optic atrophy, and anterior segment manifestations, such as chronic anterior uveitis.[96] These symptoms may lead to visual impairment. Hoarseness, especially in older children, is typical. Joint and bone symptoms are a prominent feature of CINCA, and these manifest as bone inflammation, which gives rise to major arthropathies secondary to epiphyseal and metaphyseal disorganization. Growth cartilage alterations, such as enlarged epiphyses and patellar overgrowth, can be an impressive feature of the disease (Figs. 113-16 and 113-17). Erosive changes occur, especially in the phalanges of hands and feet. There are typical dysmorphic features, such as frontal bossing and a saddle nose. These common physical features are the reason CINCA patients give the impression that (totally) unrelated patients are siblings. The prognosis of these patients is grave; 20% die in childhood because of infections, vasculitis, and amyloidosis.[119]

DIAGNOSIS AND DIAGNOSTIC TESTS

Diagnosis starts with a thorough patient and family history (see Table 113-1). Hoffman and coworkers[114] suggested a set of diagnostic criteria for FCAS after studying six large families with this syndrome (Table 113-6), but these have not been validated in an independent cohort. Laboratory examination during a fever episode in CAPS shows an acute-phase response with polymorphonuclear leukocytosis

Table 113-6 Diagnostic Criteria for Familial Cold Autoinflammatory Syndrome

1. Recurrent intermittent episodes of fever and rash that primarily follow generalized cold exposures
2. Autosomal dominant pattern of disease inheritance
3. Age of onset <6 mo
4. Duration of most attacks <24 hr
5. Presence of conjunctivitis associated with attacks
6. Absence of deafness, periorbital edema, lymphadenopathy, and serositis

From Hoffman HM, Wanderer AA, Broide DH: Familial cold autoinflammatory syndrome: Phenotype and genotype of an autosomal dominant periodic fever. J Allergy Clin Immunol 108:615-620, 2001.

and increased erythrocyte sedimentation rate, but this does not differentiate among the periodic fever disorders. Symptoms such as an urticarial rash after cold exposure highly favor a diagnosis of FCAS. The ice cube test (i.e., holding an ice cube to a patch of skin to provoke urticaria), which is diagnostic in acquired cold urticaria, is negative in FCAS. Typical facial features, such as frontal bossing, and a long pediatric history, including chronic aseptic meningitis, point to CINCA/NOMID.

Genetic testing of the CIAS1 gene can subsequently help to establish the genetic diagnosis. Usually, exon 3 of this gene is screened for mutations. There seems to be genetic heterogeneity in CINCA because not all patients have CIAS1 mutations.

TREATMENT

In recent years, daily treatment with the IL-1 inhibitor anakinra has emerged as beneficial for patients with any of the cryopyrin-associated periodic syndromes.[51,113,115,121-126] Most of these studies were close observations of single patients or small groups of patients, which is inevitable because of the rarity of these syndromes, but the results have since been confirmed in clinical practice. The largest study was by Goldbach-Mansky and colleagues,[126] who studied 18 patients with CINCA/NOMID, 12 of whom had mutations in the cryopyrin gene. All of them had a rapid and sustained response to daily subcutaneous injection of anakinra (1 to 2 mg/kg body weight), with decrease of symptoms, acute-phase response and leptomeningeal lesions as seen on MRI.[126] Withdrawal of the drug in 11 patients after 3 months resulted in a disease flare within days; subsequent retreatment with anakinra led to rapid improvement. No serious adverse events were observed.[126] Mirault and associates[127] described improvement of sensorineural deafness in a patient with MWS on treatment with anakinra. Promising new inhibitors of IL-1, such as IL1-trap from Regeneron (Tarrytown, NY), are presently being developed for therapeutic use.

Since the advent of IL-1 inhibition, it is the treatment of choice for patients with severe forms of cryopyrin-associated periodic syndrome. Previously, high-dose oral corticosteroids were often used and found to be beneficial in some patients.[114,116,128] NSAIDs, disease-modifying antirheumatic drugs, and cytotoxic drugs generally do not help.

BLAU SYNDROME/EARLY-ONSET SARCOIDOSIS

EPIDEMIOLOGY

Blau syndrome,[129] also known as familial granulomatous arthritis (OMIM 186580), and early-onset sarcoidosis (OMIM 609464) (BS/EOS) are now recognized as the same disorder.[130,131] "Pediatric granulomatous arthritis" has been suggested as a new name to describe this syndrome,[132] although this might, erroneously, give the impression that the disease occurs only in children. Little is known about its epidemiology, although it is thought to occur worldwide.[130]

ETIOLOGY

The inheritance pattern of BS/EOS is autosomal dominant. In many cases, a de novo mutation is found, which explains the relatively high incidence of sporadic cases. These sporadic cases were often classified as early-onset sarcoidosis precisely because of the absence of affected relatives, but Blau syndrome and early-onset sarcoidosis have now been shown to be caused by mutations in the nucleotide-binding oligomerization domain 2/caspase recruitment domain 15 gene (NOD2/CARD15).[131,133,134] Nine different mutations have been described, all located in exon 4 of NOD2/CARD15. The predominant mutations are two missense mutations at position 334 (R334Q and R334W).[132]

PATHOGENESIS

The NOD2/CARD15 protein is considered to be an intracellular sensor for pathogenic components, analogous to the Toll-like receptors. Activation of NOD2/CARD15 results in a wide array of downstream effects that are still not well understood, including activation of NFκB and mitogen-activated protein kinase pathways, turning on an innate immune response of diverse cytokines (e.g., IL-1β) and defensins.[135]

Seven of the nine different mutations of NOD2/CARD15 linked to BS/EOS are located in the NOD domain of the protein, similar to the mutations in cryopyrin in the cryopyrin-associated syndromes. The two most common mutations affect a codon at a homologous position in the NOD domain to the location of the cryopyrin R260W mutation.[136] This suggests a similar pathophysiologic effect on the function of the protein.

Polymorphisms in another part of this same NOD2/CARD15 gene on chromosome 16 are associated with increased susceptibility to Crohn's disease[137]; the risk of developing Crohn's disease is increased 40-fold in individuals homozygous for these polymorphisms. Whether these polymorphisms result in a gain or loss of function of this protein is debated.[137] There are some shared features between the two diseases: Both are characterized by granulomatous inflammation, and although bowel inflammation is not seen in Blau syndrome, Crohn's disease can manifest with uveitis, arthritis, and skin rash.

CLINICAL FEATURES AND OUTCOME

The clinical phenotype of BS/EOS consists of recurrent granulomatous inflammations. The three typical sites affected are joints, eyes, and skin. The granulomatous arthritis is most often polyarticular, with a synovitis or tenosynovitis.[130] The uveitis associated with this disorder tends to follow a chronic, persistent course. It can be an acute anterior uveitis, but it often extends to a panuveitis.[132] Cataracts, secondary glaucoma, and significant visual impairment can result. Involvement of the skin results in a papular, erythematous skin rash with associated dermal granulomas, usually generalized and intermittent, on trunk and extremities.[138] Other symptoms include campylodactyly (contracture of multiple interphalangeal joints), cranial neuropathies, fever, and arteritis.[133] In some severely affected patients, granulomatous inflammation can disseminate at an advanced stage into a systemic disease, with granulomas in liver, lung, and kidney.[132] Age of onset is generally before age 5. In familial cases, genetic anticipation is often observed (i.e., the course of disease tends to be more severe in later generations). The major long-term complications are joint deformity and visual impairment.[130]

DIAGNOSIS

The most important aspect of diagnosis is the histologic evidence of granulomas at the site of inflammation. This evidence can be obtained by biopsy of any involved site, of which skin is least invasive. A study showed that skin biopsy was diagnostic in all cases with the typical skin rash, whereas synovial biopsy was not positive in all patients, perhaps owing to sampling error.[132] Genetic testing is available for *NOD2/CARD15* mutations, but in some series, not all patients with a typical clinical phenotype carried a mutation in this gene.[133]

TREATMENT

There are no controlled studies of management of BS/EOS patients. There tends to be a poor response to NSAIDs. A good response to the TNF inhibitor infliximab (5 to 10 mg/kg every 4 to 8 weeks) was published in abstract form,[139] although some degree of synovitis always remained, and the response of the uveitis is more dubious.[130] The panuveitis usually is managed by topical, subconjunctival, or systemic corticosteroids.[130]

PYOGENIC STERILE ARTHRITIS, PYODERMA GANGRENOSUM, AND ACNE SYNDROME

EPIDEMIOLOGY

Pyogenic sterile arthritis, pyoderma gangrenosum, and acne (PAPA) syndrome (MIM 604416) is an autosomal dominant disorder first described by Lindor and colleagues.[140] So far, it is the rarest disorder described here; less than 10 families have been reported. These reports have come from the United States, Italy, the Netherlands, and New Zealand.

ETIOLOGY

Wise and coworkers[141] identified mutations in the CD2-binding protein 1 (*CD2BP1*) gene as the cause of PAPA syndrome. *CD2BP1*, also known as proline-serine-threonine phosphatase interacting protein 1 (PSTPIP1), is highly expressed in neutrophils.[100] At this time, three missense

mutations within one domain of this gene are known (see the online mutation database available at http://fmf.igh.cnrs.fr/infevers/).

PATHOGENESIS

PSTPIP1 can form interactions with pyrin, the protein mutated in FMF.[142] The mutations in PAPA syndrome result in hyperphosphorylation of PSTPIP1,[142-144] which increases the strength of the interaction between PSTPIP1 and pyrin.[142] This increased interaction of PSTPIP1 and pyrin leads to increased IL-1β production. This activity correlated with a higher IL-1β production in response to lipopolysaccharide stimulation of peripheral blood leukocytes from a PAPA patient ex vivo compared with a healthy control.[142] It places PAPA syndrome in the same pathogenic pathway as FMF. Other studies report an increased production of TNF-α.[145,146] Dysregulated apoptosis also may be involved.[147]

CLINICAL FEATURES AND OUTCOME

The episodic inflammation in this syndrome includes, as the name aptly indicates, symptoms of pyogenic sterile arthritis, pyoderma gangrenosum, and severe cystic acne. Lesions generally occur at the site of mild physical trauma, but sometimes no obvious trigger can be discerned.[140] The inflammation can be severe and eventually may lead to destruction of joints, muscle, and skin. Fever is not prominent in this syndrome. Age of onset has been reported as 1 to 16 years of age.[140,148] The acne generally starts early in puberty and persists in adulthood.

DIAGNOSIS

No specific diagnostic test exists. Diagnosis is based on a finding of the typical constellation of symptoms and a positive family history. A specialized DNA diagnostics department would be able to perform the genetic test for PAPA syndrome. At this time, it is unknown whether this genetic test would detect all patients, or whether other genes could be involved.

TREATMENT

Diverse anecdotal evidence only is available on treatment options in PAPA syndrome. High-dose steroids generally have a positive effect on the pyoderma gangrenosum, but may be associated with increased acne.[140] Pyogenic arthritis is often responsive to glucocortoids intra-articularly and orally.[148] Varying results have been reported with anticytokine treatment. The TNF inhibitor etanercept was beneficial in one report,[145] whereas the IL-1 inhibitor anakinra was successful in two other reports.[142,149] Stichweh and colleagues[150] reported on a patient with severe pyoderma gangrenosum, however, who did not respond to either etanercept or anakinra, but in whom the other TNF inhibitor infliximab did prove very successful.

CONCLUSION

The familial autoinflammatory syndromes are characterized by recurrent episodes of fever and inflammation. This group of disorders should be considered in a patient with a history

Table 113-7 Summary of Treatment Options

Disorder	Treatment Options
FMF	Colchicine In refractory cases or intolerance of colchicine: intravenous colchicine; IL-1 inhibition (anakinra)
HIDS	Simvastatin; etanercept; IL-1 inhibition (anakinra)
TRAPS	NSAIDs; etanercept; IL-1 inhibition (anakinra)
CAPS	IL-1 inhibition (anakinra)
BS/EOS	Corticosteroids; infliximab?
PAPA	High-dose steroids; IL-1 inhibition (anakinra); etanercept; infliximab

See text for details.
IL, interleukin; NSAIDs, nonsteroidal anti-inflammatory drugs.

of years of such inflammatory attacks with symptom-free intervals in between (except for CINCA/NOMID, in which some symptoms and morphologic features persist). Dysregulation of the IL-1β pathway is central to many familial autoinflammatory syndromes, especially CAPS and FMF.

The discovery of the causative genes has had an enormous impact in the field of periodic fevers. This discovery has been made possible because of the accurate phenotypic characterization of patients with periodic fever. Careful analysis and proper clustering of these patients is indispensable to allow the elucidation of the genetic background and the evaluation of possible treatment options (Table 113-7). Central periodic fever registries have afforded the opportunity to appreciate previously unrecognized symptoms, to give insight into the long-term prognosis, and to allow better evaluation of drug regimens. Despite these efforts at classification, however, many patients with periodic fever do not fall in one of the previously mentioned disease categories. It is to be expected that in the future other periodic fever syndromes and corresponding genes will be discovered.

REFERENCES

1. Drenth JPH, van der Meer JWM: Hereditary periodic fever. N Engl J Med 345:1748-1757, 2001.
2. Knockaert DC, Vanneste LJ, Bobbaers HJ: Recurrent or episodic fever of unknown origin: Review of 45 cases and survey of the literature. Medicine (Balt) 72:184-196, 1993.
3. de Kleijn EM, Vandenbroucke JP, van der Meer JWM: Fever of unknown origin (FUO), I: A prospective multicenter study of 167 patients with FUO, using fixed epidemiologic entry criteria. The Netherlands FUO Study Group. Medicine (Balt) 76:392-400, 1997.
4. McDermott MF, Aksentijevich I, Galon J, et al: Germline mutations in the extracellular domains of the 55 kDa TNF receptor, TNFR1, define a family of dominantly inherited autoinflammatory syndromes. Cell 97:133-144, 1999.
5. Yuval Y, Hemo-Zisser M, Zemer D, et al: Dominant inheritance in two families with familial Mediterranean fever (FMF). Am J Med Genet 57:455-457, 1995.
6. Aksentijevich I, Torosyan Y, Samuels J, et al: Mutation and haplotype studies of familial Mediterranean fever reveal new ancestral relationships and evidence for a high carrier frequency with reduced penetrance in the Ashkenazi Jewish population. Am J Hum Genet 64:949-962, 1999.
7. Booth DR, Gillmore JD, Lachmann HJ, et al: The genetic basis of autosomal dominant familial Mediterranean fever. QJM 93:217-221, 2000.
8. French FMF Consortium: A candidate gene for familial Mediterranean fever. Nat Genet 17:25-31, 1997.
9. International FMF Consortium: Ancient missense mutations in a new member of the RoRet gene family are likely to cause familial Mediterranean fever. Cell 90:797-807, 1997.
10. Touitou I: The spectrum of familial Mediterranean fever (FMF) mutations. Eur J Hum Genet 9:473-483, 2001.
11. Mansfield E, Chae JJ, Komarow HD, et al: The familial Mediterranean fever protein, pyrin, associates with microtubules and colocalizes with actin filaments. Blood 98:851-859, 2001.
12. Diaz A, Hu C, Kastner DL, et al: Lipopolysaccharide-induced expression of multiple alternatively spliced MEFV transcripts in human synovial fibroblasts: A prominent splice isoform lacks the C-terminal domain that is highly mutated in familial Mediterranean fever. Arthritis Rheum 50:3679-3689, 2004.
13. Centola M, Wood G, Frucht DM, et al: The gene for familial Mediterranean fever, MEFV, is expressed in early leukocyte development and is regulated in response to inflammatory mediators. Blood 95:3223-3231, 2000.
14. Simon A, van der Meer JW: Pathogenesis of familial periodic fever syndromes or hereditary autoinflammatory syndromes. Am J Physiol Regul Integr Comp Physiol 292:R86-R98, 2006.
15. Drenth JP, van der Meer JW: The inflammasome—a linebacker of innate defense. N Engl J Med 355:730-732, 2006.
16. Chae JJ, Komarow HD, Cheng J, et al: Targeted disruption of pyrin, the FMF protein, causes heightened sensitivity to endotoxin and a defect in macrophage apoptosis. Mol Cell 11:591-604, 2003.
17. Chae JJ, Wood G, Masters SL, et al: The B30.2 domain of pyrin, the familial Mediterranean fever protein, interacts directly with caspase-1 to modulate IL-1beta production. Proc Natl Acad Sci U S A 103:9982-9987, 2006.
18. Yu JW, Wu J, Zhang Z, et al: Cryopyrin and pyrin activate caspase-1, but not NF-kappaB, via ASC oligomerization. Cell Death Differ 13:236-249, 2006.
19. Ben Chetrit E, Levy M: Familial Mediterranean fever. Lancet 351:659-664, 1998.
20. Simon A, van der Meer JW, Drenth JP: Familial Mediterranean fever—a not so unusual cause of abdominal pain. Best Pract Res Clin Gastroenterol 19:199-213, 2005.
21. Majeed HA, Quabazard Z, Hijazi Z, et al: The cutaneous manifestations in children with familial Mediterranean fever (recurrent hereditary polyserositis): A six-year study. QJM 75:607-616, 1990.
22. Kees S, Langevitz P, Zemer D, et al: Attacks of pericarditis as a manifestation of familial Mediterranean fever (FMF). QJM 90:643-647, 1997.
23. Eshel G, Vinograd I, Barr J, et al: Acute scrotal pain complicating familial Mediterranean fever in children. Br J Surg 81:894-896, 1994.
24. Ehrenfeld M, Brzezinski A, Levy M, et al: Fertility and obstetric history in patients with familial Mediterranean fever on long-term colchicine therapy. Br J Obstet Gynaecol 94:1186-1191, 1987.
25. Ben Chetrit E, Levy M: Colchicine: 1998 update. Semin Arthritis Rheum 28:48-59, 1998.
26. Livneh A, Langevitz P, Zemer D, et al: Criteria for the diagnosis of familial Mediterranean fever. Arthritis Rheum 40:1879-1885, 1997.
27. Chen X, Fischel-Ghodsian N, Cercek A, et al: Assessment of pyrin gene mutations in Turks with familial Mediterranean fever (FMF). Hum Mutat 11:456-460, 1998.
28. Livneh A, Langevitz P, Shinar Y, et al: MEFV mutation analysis in patients suffering from amyloidosis of familial Mediterranean fever. Amyloid 6:1-6, 1999.
29. Shohat M, Magal N, Shohat T, et al: Phenotype-genotype correlation in familial Mediterranean fever: Evidence for an association between Met694Val and amyloidosis. Eur J Hum Genet 7:287-292, 1999.
30. Zemer D, Revach M, Pras M, et al: A controlled trial of colchicine in preventing attacks of familial mediterranean fever. N Engl J Med 291:932-934, 1974.
31. Dinarello CA, Wolff SM, Goldfinger SE, et al: Colchicine therapy for familial Mediterranean fever: A double-blind trial. N Engl J Med 291:934-937, 1974.
32. Goldstein RC, Schwabe AD: Prophylactic colchicine therapy in familial Mediterranean fever: A controlled, double-blind study. Ann Intern Med 81:792-794, 1974.

33. Haimov-Kochman R, Ben Chetrit E: The effect of colchicine treatment on sperm production and function: A review. Hum Reprod 13:360-362, 1998.

34. Rabinovitch O, Zemer D, Kukia E, et al: Colchicine treatment in conception and pregnancy: Two hundred thirty- one pregnancies in patients with familial Mediterranean fever. Am J Reprod Immunol 28:245-246, 1992.

35. Lidar M, Kedem R, Langevitz P, et al: Intravenous colchicine for treatment of patients with familial Mediterranean fever unresponsive to oral colchicine. J Rheumatol 30:2620-2623, 2003.

36. Grateau G: The relation between familial Mediterranean fever and amyloidosis. Curr Opin Rheumatol 12:61-64, 2000.

37. Simon A, Mariman EC, van der Meer JWM, et al: A founder effect in the hyperimmunoglobulinemia D and periodic fever syndrome. Am J Med 114:148-152, 2003.

38. Houten SM, Van Woerden CS, Wijburg FA, et al: Carrier frequency of the V377I (1129G>A) MVK mutation, associated with Hyper-IgD and periodic fever syndrome, in the Netherlands. Eur J Hum Genet 11:196-200, 2003.

39. **Houten SM, Kuis W, Duran M, et al: Mutations in MVK, encoding mevalonate kinase, cause hyperimmunoglobulinemia D and periodic fever syndrome. Nat Genet 22:175-177, 1999.**

40. **Drenth JPH, Cuisset L, Grateau G, et al: Mutations in the gene encoding mevalonate kinase cause hyper-IgD and periodic fever syndrome. International Hyper-IgD Study Group. Nat Genet 22:178-181, 1999.**

41. Simon A, Cuisset L, Vincent MF, et al: Molecular analysis of the mevalonate kinase gene in a cohort of patients with the hyper-IgD and periodic fever syndrome: Its application as a diagnostic tool. Ann Intern Med 135:338-343, 2001.

42. Houten SM, Frenkel J, Kuis W, et al: Molecular basis of classical mevalonic aciduria and the hyperimmunoglobulinaemia D and periodic fever syndrome: High frequency of 3 mutations in the mevalonate kinase gene. J Inherit Metab Dis 23:367-370, 2000.

43. Cuisset L, Drenth JPH, Simon A, et al: Molecular analysis of MVK mutations and enzymatic activity in hyper-IgD and periodic fever syndrome. Eur J Hum Genet 9:260-266, 2001.

44. Houten SM, Wanders RJ, Waterham HR: Biochemical and genetic aspects of mevalonate kinase and its deficiency. Biochim Biophys Acta 1529:19-32, 2000.

45. Houten SM, Frenkel J, Rijkers GT, et al: Temperature dependence of mutant mevalonate kinase activity as a pathogenic factor in hyper-IgD and periodic fever syndrome. Hum Mol Genet 11:3115-3124, 2002.

46. Schafer BL, Bishop RW, Kratunis VJ, et al: Molecular cloning of human mevalonate kinase and identification of a missense mutation in the genetic disease mevalonic aciduria. J Biol Chem 267: 13229-13238, 1992.

47. Hoffmann GF, Charpentier C, Mayatepek E, et al: Clinical and biochemical phenotype in 11 patients with mevalonic aciduria. Pediatrics 91:915-921, 1993.

48. Simon A, Kremer HP, Wevers RA, et al: Mevalonate kinase deficiency: Evidence for a phenotypic continuum. Neurology 62:994-997, 2004.

49. Jain MK, Ridker PM: Anti-inflammatory effects of statins: Clinical evidence and basic mechanisms. Nat Rev Drug Discov 4:977-987, 2005.

50. Abeles AM, Pillinger MH: Statins as antiinflammatory and immunomodulatory agents: A future in rheumatologic therapy? Arthritis Rheum 54:393-407, 2006.

51. Frenkel J, Wulffraat NM, Kuis W: Anakinra in mutation-negative NOMID/CINCA syndrome: Comment on the articles by Hawkins, et al and Hoffman and Patel. Arthritis Rheum 50:3738-3739, 2004.

52. Drenth JPH, van Deuren M, van der Ven-Jongekrijg J, et al: Cytokine activation during attacks of the hyperimmunoglobulinemia D and periodic fever syndrome. Blood 85:3586-3593, 1995.

53. Drenth JPH, van der Meer JWM, Kushner I: Unstimulated peripheral blood mononuclear cells from patients with the hyper-IgD syndrome produce cytokines capable of potent induction of C-reactive protein and serum amyloid A in Hep3B cells. J Immunol 157:400-404, 1996.

54. Bodar EJ, van der Hilst JC, Drenth JP, et al: Effect of etanercept and anakinra on inflammatory attacks in the hyper-IgD syndrome: Introducing a vaccination provocation model. Neth J Med 63:260-264, 2005.

55. Bodar EJ, van der Hilst JC, van Heerde WL, et al: Defective apoptosis of peripheral blood lymphocytes in hyper-IgD and periodic fever syndrome. Blood 109:2416-2418, 2007.

56. Drenth JPH, Haagsma CJ, van der Meer JWM: Hyperimmunoglobulinemia D and periodic fever syndrome: The clinical spectrum in a series of 50 patients. International Hyper-IgD Study Group. Medicine (Balt) 73:133-144, 1994.

57. Haraldsson A, Weemaes CM, de Boer AW, et al: Immunological studies in the hyper-immunoglobulin D syndrome. J Clin Immunol 12:424-428, 1992.

58. Klasen IS, Goertz JH, van de Wiel GA, et al: Hyper-immunoglobulin A in the hyperimmunoglobulinemia D syndrome. Clin Diagn Lab Immunol 8:58-61, 2001.

59. Simon A, Bijzet J, Voorbij HA, et al: Effect of inflammatory attacks in the classical type hyper-IgD syndrome on immunoglobulin D, cholesterol and parameters of the acute phase response. J Intern Med 256:247-253, 2004.

60. Kelley RI, Herman GE: Inborn errors of sterol biosynthesis. Annu Rev Genomics Hum Genet 2:299-341, 2001.

61. Simon A, Drewe E, van der Meer JW, et al: Simvastatin treatment for inflammatory attacks of the hyperimmunoglobulinemia D and periodic fever syndrome. Clin Pharmacol Ther 75:476-483, 2004.

62. Takada K, Aksentijevich I, Mahadevan V, et al: Favorable preliminary experience with etanercept in two patients with the hyperimmunoglobulinemia D and periodic fever syndrome. Arthritis Rheum 48:2645-2651, 2003.

63. Drenth JPH, Vonk AG, Simon A, et al: Limited efficacy of thalidomide in the treatment of febrile attacks of the hyper-IgD and periodic fever syndrome: A randomized, double-blind, placebo-controlled trial. J Pharmacol Exp Ther 298:1221-1226, 2001.

64. Obici L, Manno C, Muda AO, et al: First report of systemic reactive (AA) amyloidosis in a patient with the hyperimmunoglobulinemia D with periodic fever syndrome. Arthritis Rheum 50:2966-2969, 2004.

65. Lachmann HJ, Goodman HJ, Andrews PA, et al: AA amyloidosis complicating hyperimmunoglobulinemia D with periodic fever syndrome: A report of two cases. Arthritis Rheum 54:2010-2014, 2006.

66. Siewert R, Ferber J, Horstmann RD, et al: Hereditary periodic fever with systemic amyloidosis: Is hyper-IgD syndrome really a benign disease? Am J Kidney Dis 48:e41-e45, 2006.

67. Williamson LM, Hull D, Mehta R, et al: Familial Hibernian fever. QJM 51:469-480, 1982.

68. Hull KM, Drewe E, Aksentijevich I, et al: The TNF receptor-associated periodic syndrome (TRAPS): Emerging concepts of an autoinflammatory disorder. Medicine (Balt) 81:349-368, 2002.

69. Mulley J, Saar K, Hewitt G, et al: Gene localization for an autosomal dominant familial periodic fever to 12p13. Am J Hum Genet 62: 884-889, 1998.

70. Bergman F, Warmenius S: Familial perireticular amyloidosis in a Swedish family. Am J Med 45:601-606, 1968.

71. Aksentijevich I, Galon J, Soares M, et al: The tumor-necrosis-factor receptor-associated periodic syndrome: New mutations in TNFRSF1A, ancestral origins, genotype-phenotype studies, and evidence for further genetic heterogeneity of periodic fevers. Am J Hum Genet 69:301-314, 2001.

72. Tchernitchko D, Chiminqgi M, Galacteros F, et al: Unexpected high frequency of P46L TNFRSF1A allele in sub-Saharan West African populations. Eur J Hum Genet 13:513-515, 2005.

73. Ravet N, Rouaghe S, Dode C, et al: Clinical significance of P46L and R92Q substitutions in the tumor necrosis factor superfamily 1A gene. Ann Rheum Dis 65:1158-1162, 2006.

74. Lobito AA, Kimberley FC, Muppidi JR, et al: Abnormal disulfide-linked oligomerization results in ER retention and altered signaling by TNFR1 mutants in the TNFR1 associated periodic fever syndrome (TRAPS). Blood 108:1320-1327, 2006.

75. Todd I, Tighe PJ, Powell RJ: TNF and TNF receptors in TRAPS. Curr Med Chem Anti-Inflammatory Anti-Allergy Agents 4:577-585, 2005.

76. Galon J, Aksentijevich I, McDermott MF, et al: TNFRSF1A mutations and autoinflammatory syndromes. Curr Opin Immunol 12: 479-486, 2000.

77. Todd I, Radford PM, Draper-Morgan KA, et al: Mutant forms of tumour necrosis factor receptor I that occur in TNF-receptor-associated periodic syndrome retain signalling functions but show abnormal behaviour. Immunology 113:65-79, 2004.

78. Siebert S, Fielding CA, Williams BD, et al: Mutation of the extra-cellular domain of tumour necrosis factor receptor 1 causes reduced NF-kappaB activation due to decreased surface expression. FEBS Lett 579:5193-5198, 2005.

79. Huggins ML, Radford PM, McIntosh RS, et al: Shedding of mutant tumor necrosis factor receptor superfamily 1A associated with tumor necrosis factor receptor-associated periodic syndrome: Differences between cell types. Arthritis Rheum 50:2651-2659, 2004.

80. Siebert S, Amos N, Fielding CA, et al: Reduced tumor necrosis factor signaling in primary human fibroblasts containing a tumor necrosis factor receptor superfamily 1A mutant. Arthritis Rheum 52:1287-1292, 2005.

81. Rebelo SL, Bainbridge SE, Amel-Kashipaz MR, et al: Modeling of tumor necrosis factor receptor superfamily 1A mutants associated with tumor necrosis factor receptor-associated periodic syndrome indicates misfolding consistent with abnormal function. Arthritis Rheum 54:2674-2687, 2006.

82. Simon A, Bodar EJ, van der Hilst JC, et al: Beneficial response to interleukin 1 receptor antagonist in TRAPS. Am J Med 117:208-210, 2004.

83. Dode C, Andre M, Bienvenu T, et al: The enlarging clinical, genetic, and population spectrum of tumor necrosis factor receptor-associated periodic syndrome. Arthritis Rheum 46:2181-2188, 2002.

84. Toro JR, Aksentijevich I, Hull K, et al: Tumor necrosis factor receptor-associated periodic syndrome: A novel syndrome with cutaneous manifestations. Arch Dermatol 136:1487-1494, 2000.

85. Hurst M, Hull K, Nicholls D, et al: Hereditary periodic fever syndrome sans fever or distinct periodicity presenting with psychosis. J Clin Rheumatol 11:329-330, 2005.

86. McDermott EM, Smillie DM, Powell RJ: Clinical spectrum of familial Hibernian fever: A 14-year follow-up study of the index case and extended family. Mayo Clin Proc 72:806-817, 1997.

87. Simon A, Dode C, van der Meer JWM, et al: Familial periodic fever and amyloidosis due to a new mutation in the TNFRSF1A gene. Am J Med 110:313-316, 2001.

88. Drewe E, McDermott EM, Powell PT, et al: Prospective study of anti-tumour necrosis factor receptor superfamily 1B fusion protein, and case study of anti-tumour necrosis factor receptor superfamily 1A fusion protein, in tumour necrosis factor associated periodic syndrome (TRAPS): Clinical and laboratory findings in a series of seven patients. Rheumatology (Oxf) 42:235-239, 2003.

89. Simon A, van Deuren M, Tighe PJ, et al: Genetic analysis as a valuable key to diagnosis and treatment of periodic fever. Arch Intern Med 161:2491-2493, 2001.

90. Drewe E, McDermott EM, Powell RJ: Treatment of the nephrotic syndrome with etanercept in patients with the tumor necrosis factor receptor-associated periodic syndrome. N Engl J Med 343:1044-1045, 2000.

91. Drewe E, Powell RJ: Novel treatment for tumour necrosis factor receptor associated periodic syndrome (TRAPS): Case history of experience with infliximab and sirolimus post etanercept. Clin Exp Rheumatol 20(Suppl 26):S71, 2002.

92. Jacobelli S, Andre M, Alexandra JF, et al: Failure of anti-TNF therapy in TNF-receptor-1-associated periodic syndrome (TRAPS). Rheumatology (Oxf) 46:1211-1212, 2007.

93. Aganna E, Martinon F, Hawkins PN, et al: Association of mutations in the NALP3/CIAS1/PYPAF1 gene with a broad phenotype including recurrent fever, cold sensitivity, sensorineural deafness, and AA amyloidosis. Arthritis Rheum 46:2445-2452, 2002.

94. Hoffman HM, Gregory SG, Mueller JL, et al: Fine structure mapping of CIAS1: Identification of an ancestral haplotype and a common FCAS mutation, L353P. Hum Genet 112:209-216, 2003.

95. Cuisset L, Drenth JPH, Berthelot JM, et al: Genetic linkage of the Muckle-Wells syndrome to chromosome 1q44. Am J Hum Genet 65:1054-1059, 1999.

96. Dollfus H, Hafner R, Hofmann HM, et al: Chronic infantile neurological cutaneous and articular/neonatal onset multisystem inflammatory disease syndrome: Ocular manifestations in a recently recognized chronic inflammatory disease of childhood. Arch Ophthalmol 118:1386-1392, 2000.

97. Aksentijevich I, Nowak M, Mallah M, et al: De novo CIAS1 mutations, cytokine activation, and evidence for genetic heterogeneity in patients with neonatal-onset multisystem inflammatory disease (NOMID): A new member of the expanding family of pyrin-associated autoinflammatory diseases. Arthritis Rheum 46:3340-3348, 2002.

98. Hoffman HM, Wright FA, Broide DH, et al: Identification of a locus on chromosome 1q44 for familial cold urticaria. Am J Hum Genet 66:1693-1698, 2000.

99. Feldmann J, Prieur AM, Quartier P, et al: Chronic infantile neurological cutaneous and articular syndrome is caused by mutations in CIAS1, a gene highly expressed in polymorphonuclear cells and chondrocytes. Am J Hum Genet 71:198-203, 2002.

100. Hull KM, Shoham N, Chae JJ, et al: The expanding spectrum of systemic autoinflammatory disorders and their rheumatic manifestations. Curr Opin Rheumatol 15:61-69, 2003.

101. Martinon F, Tschopp J: Inflammatory caspases: Linking an intracellular innate immune system to autoinflammatory diseases. Cell 117:561-574, 2004.

102. Ting JP, Kastner DL, Hoffman HM: CATERPILLERs, pyrin and hereditary immunological disorders. Nat Rev Immunol 6:183-195, 2006.

103. Hoffman HM, Mueller JL, Broide DH, et al: Mutation of a new gene encoding a putative pyrin-like protein causes familial cold autoinflammatory syndrome and Muckle-Wells syndrome. Nat Genet 29:301-305, 2001.

104. Manji GA, Wang L, Geddes BJ, et al: PYPAF1, a PYRIN-containing Apaf1-like protein that assembles with ASC and regulates activation of NF-kappa B. J Biol Chem 277:11570-11575, 2002.

105. Kanneganti TD, Ozoren N, Body-Malapel M, et al: Bacterial RNA and small antiviral compounds activate caspase-1 through cryopyrin/Nalp3. Nature 440:233-236, 2006.

106. Mariathasan S, Weiss DS, Newton K, et al: Cryopyrin activates the inflammasome in response to toxins and ATP. Nature 440:228-232, 2006.

107. Sutterwala FS, Ogura Y, Szczepanik M, et al: Critical role for NALP3/CIAS1/Cryopyrin in innate and adaptive immunity through its regulation of caspase-1. Immunity 24:317-327, 2006.

108. Martinon F, Petrilli V, Mayor A, et al: Gout-associated uric acid crystals activate the NALP3 inflammasome. Nature 440:237-241, 2006.

109. Martinon F, Burns K, Tschopp J: The inflammasome: A molecular platform triggering activation of inflammatory caspases and processing of proIL-beta. Mol Cell 10:417-426, 2002.

110. Agostini L, Martinon F, Burns K, et al: NALP3 forms an IL-1beta-processing inflammasome with increased activity in Muckle-Wells autoinflammatory disorder. Immunity 20:319-325, 2004.

111. Dowds TA, Masumoto J, Zhu L, et al: Cryopyrin-induced interleukin 1beta secretion in monocytic cells: Enhanced activity of disease-associated mutants and requirement for ASC. J Biol Chem 279:21924-21928, 2004.

112. Doeglas HM, Bleumink E: Familial cold urticaria: Clinical findings. Arch Dermatol 110:382-388, 1974.

113. Metyas SK, Hoffman HM: Anakinra prevents symptoms of familial cold autoinflammatory syndrome and Raynaud's disease. J Rheumatol 33:2085-2087, 2006.

114. Hoffman HM, Wanderer AA, Broide DH: Familial cold autoinflammatory syndrome: Phenotype and genotype of an autosomal dominant periodic fever. J Allergy Clin Immunol 108:615-620, 2001.

115. Hoffman HM, Rosengren S, Boyle DL, et al: Prevention of cold-associated acute inflammation in familial cold autoinflammatory syndrome by interleukin-1 receptor antagonist. Lancet 364:1779-1785, 2004.

116. Watts RA, Nicholls A, Scott DG: The arthropathy of the Muckle-Wells syndrome. Br J Rheumatol 33:1184-1187, 1994.

117. Schwarz RE, Dralle H, Linke RP, et al: Amyloid goiter and arthritides after kidney transplantation in a patient with systemic amyloidosis and Muckle-Wells syndrome. Am J Clin Pathol 92:821-825, 1989.

118. Berthelot JM, Maugars Y, Robillard N, et al: Autosomal dominant Muckle-Wells syndrome associated with cystinuria, ichthyosis, and aphthosis in a four-generation family. Am J Med Genet 53:72-74, 1994.

119. Prieur AM: A recently recognised chronic inflammatory disease of early onset characterised by the triad of rash, central nervous system involvement and arthropathy. Clin Exp Rheumatol 19:103-106, 2001.

120. Prieur AM, Griscelli C, Lampert F, et al: A chronic, infantile, neurological, cutaneous and articular (CINCA) syndrome: A specific entity analysed in 30 patients. Scand J Rheumatol Suppl 66:57-68, 1987.

121. Hawkins PN, Lachmann HJ, Aganna E, et al: Spectrum of clinical features in Muckle-Wells syndrome and response to anakinra. Arthritis Rheum 50:607-612, 2004.

122. Hawkins PN, Bybee A, Aganna E, et al: Response to anakinra in a de novo case of neonatal-onset multisystem inflammatory disease. Arthritis Rheum 50:2708-2709, 2004.

123. Dailey NJ, Aksentijevich I, Chae JJ, et al: Interleukin-1 receptor antagonist anakinra in the treatment of neonatal onset multisystem inflammatory disease. Arthritis Rheum 50:S440, 2004.

124. Ramos E, Arostegui JI, Campuzano S, et al: Positive clinical and biochemical responses to anakinra in a 3-yr-old patient with cryo-pyrin-associated periodic syndrome (CAPS). Rheumatology (Oxf) 44:1072-1073, 2005.

125. Boschan C, Witt O, Lohse P, et al: Neonatal-onset multisystem inflammatory disease (NOMID) due to a novel S331R mutation of the CIAS1 gene and response to interleukin-1 receptor antagonist treatment. Am J Med Genet A 140:883-886, 2006.

126. Goldbach-Mansky R, Dailey NJ, Canna SW, et al: Neonatal-onset multisystem inflammatory disease responsive to interleukin-1beta inhibition. N Engl J Med 355:581-592, 2006.

127. Mirault T, Launay D, Cuisset L, et al: Recovery from deafness in a patient with Muckle-Wells syndrome treated with anakinra. Arthritis Rheum 54:1697-1700, 2006.

128. Fuger K, Fleischmann E, Weber M, et al: Complications in the course of the Muckle-Wells syndrome. Dtsch Med Wochenschr 117:256-260, 1992.

129. Blau EB: Familial granulomatous arthritis, iritis, and rash. J Pediatr 107:689-693, 1985.

130. Becker ML, Rose CD: Blau syndrome and related genetic disorders causing childhood arthritis. Curr Rheumatol Rep 7:427-433, 2005.

131. Kanazawa N, Okafuji I, Kambe N, et al: Early-onset sarcoidosis and CARD15 mutations with constitutive nuclear factor-kappaB activation: Common genetic etiology with Blau syndrome. Blood 105:1195-1197, 2005.

132. Rose CD, Wouters CH, Meiorin S, et al: Pediatric granulomatous arthritis: An international registry. Arthritis Rheum 54:3337-3344, 2006.

133. Wang X, Kuivaniemi H, Bonavita G, et al: CARD15 mutations in familial granulomatosis syndromes: A study of the original Blau syndrome kindred and other families with large-vessel arteritis and cranial neuropathy. Arthritis Rheum 46:3041-3045, 2002.

134. Miceli-Richard C, Lesage S, Rybojad M, et al: CARD15 mutations in Blau syndrome. Nat Genet 29:19-20, 2001.

135. Abraham C, Cho JH: Functional consequences of NOD2 (CARD15) mutations. Inflamm Bowel Dis 12:641-650, 2006.

136. Chamaillard M, Girardin SE, Viala J, et al: Nods, Nalps and Naip: Intracellular regulators of bacterial-induced inflammation. Cell Microbiol 5:581-592, 2003.

137. Eckmann L, Karin M: NOD2 and Crohn's disease: Loss or gain of function? Immunity 22:661-667, 2005.

138. Alonso D, Elgart GW, Schachner LA: Blau syndrome: A new kindred. J Am Acad Dermatol 49:299-302, 2003.

139. Brescia AC, McIlvain-Simpson G, Rose CD: Infliximab therapy for steroid-dependent early onset sarcoid arthritis and Blau syndrome. Arthritis Rheum 46:S313, 2002 (abstract).

140. Lindor NM, Arsenault TM, Solomon H, et al: A new autosomal dominant disorder of pyogenic sterile arthritis, pyoderma gangrenosum, and acne: PAPA syndrome. Mayo Clin Proc 72:611-615, 1997.

141. Wise CA, Gillum JD, Seidman CE, et al: Mutations in CD2BP1 disrupt binding to PTP PEST and are responsible for PAPA syndrome, an autoinflammatory disorder. Hum Mol Genet 11:961-969, 2002.

142. Shoham NG, Centola M, Mansfield E, et al: Pyrin binds the PST-PIP1/CD2BP1 protein, defining familial Mediterranean fever and PAPA syndrome as disorders in the same pathway. Proc Natl Acad Sci U S A 100:13501-13506, 2003.

143. Cote JF, Chung PL, Theberge JF, et al: PSTPIP is a substrate of PTP-PEST and serves as a scaffold guiding PTP-PEST toward a specific dephosphorylation of WASP. J Biol Chem 277:2973-2986, 2002.

144. Badour K, Zhang J, Shi F, et al: Fyn and PTP-PEST-mediated regulation of Wiskott-Aldrich syndrome protein (WASp) tyrosine phosphorylation is required for coupling T cell antigen receptor engagement to WASp effector function and T cell activation. J Exp Med 199:99-112, 2004.

145. Cortis E, De Benedetti F, Insalaco A, et al: Abnormal production of tumor necrosis factor (TNF)-alpha and clinical efficacy of the TNF inhibitor etanercept in a patient with PAPA syndrome [corrected]. J Pediatr 145:851-855, 2004.

146. Edrees AF, Kaplan DL, Abdou NI: Pyogenic arthritis, pyoderma gangrenosum, and acne syndrome (PAPA syndrome) associated with hypogammaglobulinemia and elevated serum tumor necrosis factor-alpha levels. J Clin Rheumatol 8:273-275, 2002.

147. Baum W, Kirkin V, Fernandez SB, et al: Binding of the intracellular Fas ligand (FasL) domain to the adaptor protein PSTPIP results in a cytoplasmic localization of FasL. J Biol Chem 280:40012-40024, 2005.

148. Tallon B, Corkill M: Peculiarities of PAPA syndrome. Rheumatology (Oxf) 45:1140-1143, 2006.

149. Dierselhuis MP, Frenkel J, Wulffraat NM, et al: Anakinra for flares of pyogenic arthritis in PAPA syndrome. Rheumatology (Oxf) 44:406-408, 2005.

150. Stichweh DS, Punaro M, Pascual V: Dramatic improvement of pyoderma gangrenosum with infliximab in a patient with PAPA syndrome. Pediatr Dermatol 22:262-265, 2005.

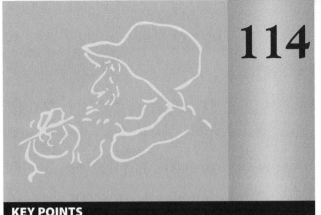

114

Tumors and Tumor-like Lesions of Joints and Related Structures 📹

ANDREW E. ROSENBERG

KEY POINTS

Most mass lesions in and around joints are benign, with synovial cysts being the most common. These are not true cysts because they lack an epithelial lining. They may involve joints (Baker's cyst) or tendon sheaths (ganglion cysts). Treatment depends on the symptoms, with many ganglion cysts better left alone.

Synovial chondromatosis is an uncommon benign condition characterized by nodules of hyaline cartilage, often ossified, within the subsynovial connective tissue, most frequently involving the knee. Treatment is removal of nodules.

Tenosynovial giant cell tumor of joints and tendon sheaths, previously known as pigmented villonodular synovitis, affects both sexes equally, usually in the third or fourth decade. Lesions are most often monarticular, with the knee being involved in 80% of cases. Studies have shown that the disease is due to a translocation resulting in overexpression of colony-stimulating factor-1. Although they can be locally destructive, the tumors do not metastasize; treatment is removal.

The most common primary malignant tumor of joints is synovial sarcoma, which usually affects children and young adults. The disease has an aggressive course, with a long-term survival of around 50%.

Lymphoproliferative diseases may involve joints, especially acute leukemia. Joint involvement is most common in children, where the reported incidence of joint involvement ranges from 12% to 65%. Arthritis can occur at any time in the course of the disease and can be the presenting complaint. It is due to leukemic infiltration into the synovium.

Joints and periarticular structures are often involved by non-neoplastic, mass-forming lesions, such as synovial cysts and loose bodies. These structures are affected infrequently, however, by benign or malignant neoplasms. Joint neoplasms can be divided into tumors that are primary or arise de novo within the joint and tumors that are secondary and access the joint by invading from neighboring bones and soft tissues or spreading from distant sites via the vascular system. Primary joint neoplasms are more common and tend to recapitulate the phenotype of tissues that normally construct the joint—synovium, fat, blood vessels, fibrous tissue, and cartilage. Regardless of the histologic type, the benign variants greatly outnumber their malignant counterparts, and as a group these tumors tend to develop in the synovium and not the other periarticular structures. These biologically and morphologically diverse lesions often pose significant challenges in diagnosis and treatment, and their clinicopathologic features are the focus of this chapter.

NON-NEOPLASTIC LESIONS

SYNOVIAL AND GANGLION CYSTS

Cysts are defined as closed compartments or sacs that are lined by epithelium and frequently filled with fluid. Neither the synovial cyst nor the ganglion cyst is considered a true cyst because each lacks an epithelial lining.

Synovial cysts are common and form from the synovial lining of a joint, tendon, or bursa. They are non-neoplastic lesions and are caused by herniation of the synovium through the joint capsule or tendon sheath into the neighboring tissues or expansion of a preexisting bursa. In adults, synovial cysts frequently develop in association with a variety of joint disorders, including trauma, osteoarthritis, crystal arthropathies, infection, and rheumatoid arthritis or one of its variants. Most synovial cysts have an anatomic relationship to a joint, and most originate in the posterior aspect of the knee, where they are known as a popliteal or Baker's cyst, followed in frequency by the shoulder and hip. The posteromedial region of the knee may be prone to the development of synovial cysts because the synovial-lined joint capsule in this anatomic site may not provide adequate structural support.[1] Synovial cysts of the posterior knee joint are purported to affect 2.4% of children, who, in contrast to adults, are usually asymptomatic and have an otherwise normal knee joint.[2]

Synovial cysts can enlarge as they become increasingly distended with synovial fluid.[1-4] Consequently, they may manifest as a periarticular mass, produce progressive joint pain and swelling, limit joint mobility, and compress adjacent neurovascular structures. An example of the last-mentioned occurs in the spine, where synovial cysts that arise from facet joints may impinge on spinal nerves and cause radicular pain.[5] Other complications of synovial cysts, which sometimes can produce dramatic clinical findings, are acute rupture and secondary infection.

A variety of radiographic techniques have been used to image synovial cysts. The imaging modalities that provide the most diagnostic information are arthrography, ultrasonography, computed tomography (CT), and magnetic resonance imaging (MRI).[1-4] All of these modalities reveal synovial cysts to be simple or septated thin-walled structures associated with joints and periarticular structures and filled with fluid whose density is similar to that of water (Fig. 114-1).

Grossly, synovial cysts usually range in size from 1 to 10 cm. Their inner surface is smooth, glistening, and translucent; however, prior hemorrhage or secondary infection may distort this surface by virtue of attached blood clot and inflammatory debris or the generation of granulation tissue. The cyst wall comprises an inner surface lined by flattened or plump cuboidal synoviocytes arranged one or several

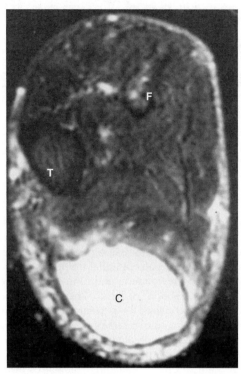

Figure 114-1 MR image shows high T2 signal intensity, large, oval-shaped synovial cyst that extends from the knee joint into the posterior calf. C, synovial cyst; F, fibula; T, tibia.

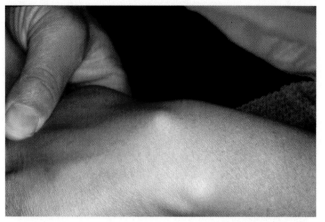

Figure 114-3 Round, firm ganglion cyst bulging from the dorsal aspect of the hand.

cell layers thick, which are surrounded by an outer sheath of fibrous tissue (Fig. 114-2). Sometimes the synovial lining cells may be hyperplastic and form papillary fronds, and occasionally there are scattered subsynovial collections of hemosiderin-laden macrophages, which are indicative of previous hemorrhage.

The treatment of synovial cysts varies and depends on their location and associated symptoms. These cysts may be managed successfully with conservative therapy; however, in certain situations surgical excision is required.[1-5]

Ganglion cysts have been recognized for centuries; Hippocrates described them as being composed of "mucoid flesh."[6] They are more common than synovial cysts and arise from tendon sheaths, ligaments, menisci, joint capsules, and bursae.[6] Occasionally, they develop de novo in the subchondral areas of bone, and rarely they arise within skeletal muscle and lack communication with a joint. Ganglion cysts are distinguished from synovial cysts by virtue of the fact that they lack a surface lining and do not communicate directly with a joint cavity or synovial lining. A variety of hypotheses have been proposed to explain their pathogenesis, but none have been proven.[6] The most accepted theory is that ganglia develop from mucoid cystic degeneration of periarticular structures. They are commonly associated with repetitive motion activities, inflammatory arthritides, and trauma.

Most ganglia arise along the dorsal and volar aspects of the wrists and fingers, and the dorsum of the feet.[6,7] They are usually asymptomatic and typically manifest as a slowly growing, mobile, firm mass that moves with the structure from which it has arisen (Fig. 114-3). Ganglia may be painful if traumatized and can compress adjacent neurovascular structures producing a variety of symptoms. The radiographic characteristics of ganglia are similar to those of synovial cysts, and they appear on images as small, fluid-filled cystic structures.[1,7]

Macroscopically, most ganglia are round, but they may form elongate cylindrical structures if they track along a tendon sheath. Ganglia are uniloculated or multiloculated, have thin walls, and are filled with translucent mucoid fluid (Fig. 114-4). The cyst lacks an inner cell lining, and the bulk of the wall consists of dense fibrous tissue, which is usually surrounded by areolar tissue (Fig. 114-5). In many instances, the cyst wall is distorted by variable amounts of reactive myxoid tissue and muciphages, which result from small ruptures and extravasation of fluid.

When ganglion cysts form, they may remain stable for years or spontaneously resolve, and ganglia that disappear may subsequently redevelop. Treatment is frequently conservative because of their innocuous nature. Ganglia occasionally require aspiration or surgical excision, however, especially if they are symptomatic.

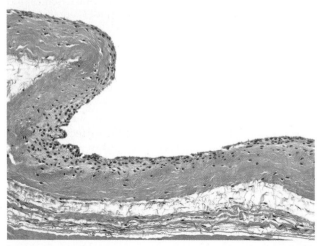

Figure 114-2 Wall of synovial cyst, composed of an inner lining of synoviocytes overlaying a layer of dense, fibrous tissue.

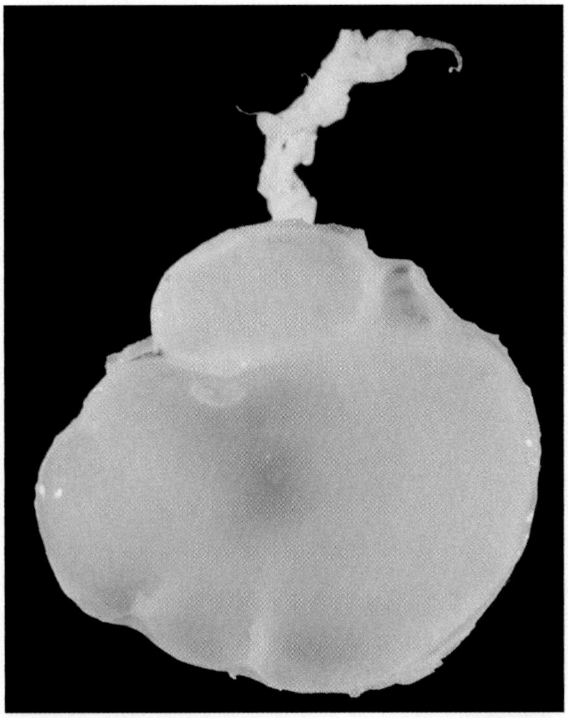

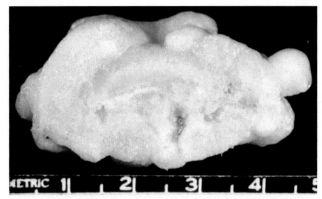

Figure 114-6 Large nodular loose body formed from a semilunar-shaped piece of articular cartilage that is surrounded by newly formed cartilage.

Osteoarticular loose bodies are a secondary complication of a variety of conditions, including trauma, osteochondritis dissecans, and arthritides of various etiologies. When dislodged, the sloughed articular cartilage remains viable because it receives its nourishment from the synovial fluid, but the bone dies because it derives its nutrition solely from blood vessels. Over time, as the loose body tumbles in the joint, its edges become rounded and smooth; however, it eventually becomes embedded within the synovium. When the synovium encompasses the loose body, either it digests and resorbs it, or adjacent subsynovial connective tissue cells undergo a proliferative and metaplastic response.

These cells produce layers of newly formed fibrocartilage and hyaline cartilage, which may undergo enchondral ossification and which are deposited on the surface of the loose body (Fig. 114-6). These layers of newly formed tissue surround the centrally located loose body similar to the cambium layers of a tree and provide a mechanism for the whole structure to increase gradually in size and become significantly larger than the initial osteochondral defect from which it originated (Figs. 114-7 and 114-8). As the loose body enlarges, the innermost portion of original articular cartilage cannot be supported adequately by diffusion of

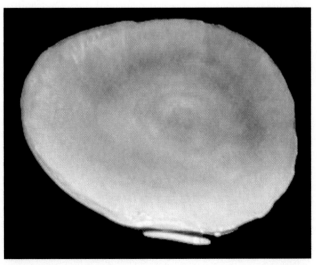

Figure 114-7 Loose body with visible layers of newly formed tissue.

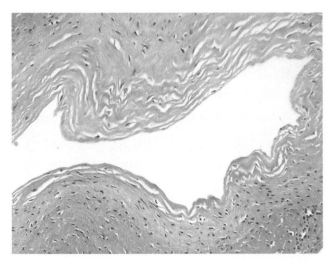

Figure 114-4 Intact ganglion cyst with threadlike pedicle that attaches to a periarticular structure.

LOOSE BODIES

Loose bodies and *joint mice* are generic terms for free-floating structures within a joint cavity. They are the most common tumor-like lesion of joints and may be exogenous, such as fragments of a bullet, or endogenous, such as pieces of articular cartilage, osteophytes, menisci, ligaments, or bone.[8,9] When not otherwise specified, the term *loose bodies* refers to detached pieces of articular cartilage or subchondral bone (osteoarticular loose bodies) or both that lie free within the joint or that have become secondarily embedded in the synovium. Loose bodies can cause pain, crepitance, and locking, and they can limit joint range of motion.

Figure 114-5 Ganglion cyst wall composed of scattered flattened fibroblasts on the luminal surface and a well-formed layer of fibrous tissue.

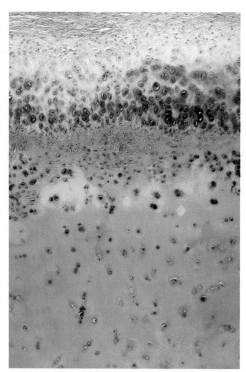

Figure 114-8 Loose body composed of sloughed articular hyaline cartilage (bottom) covered by consecutive layers of newly formed metaplastic hyaline cartilage and bone.

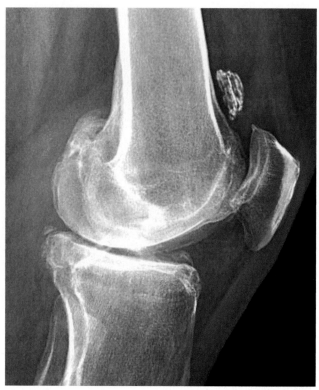

Figure 114-9 Knee with an osteoarticular loose body in the suprapatellar region.

synovial fluid, and it dies and calcifies. This combination of events causes the loose body to appear as dense speckled and ringlike calcifications on x-rays (Fig. 114-9). Radiographically and histologically, the differential diagnosis includes synovial chondromatosis. Treatment is simple excision, which can be done arthroscopically.[9]

INTRA-ARTICULAR OSSICLES

Small bony nodules normally occur in the knees of some rodents[10] and other mammals and may rarely occur in humans.[11,12] In rodents, they are constantly found in the anterior portions of the joint and frequently in the posterior portions as well. In humans, these nodules develop within the substance of the meniscus of the knee joint adjacent to its attachments to the tibia.

The exact etiology of such structures is unknown, although they probably either are true sesamoid bones, as seen in rodents, or represent ossification secondary to local injury. This latter possibility is supported by the fact that previous knee trauma has been noted in numerous reported cases. The main symptom of meniscal ossicles is pain after exertion, such as walking or prolonged standing, with relief when the knee is at rest. Radiographs may reveal an intra-articular calcification that can be confused with a loose body.[12] MRI shows the ossicle to be a corticated marrow-containing structure that has increased signal intensity on T1-weighted images and decreased signal intensity on T2-weighted images.[11,12] The ossicle is located within either the lateral or the medial meniscus and appears as a small (approximately 1 cm in diameter), palpable bony nodule (Fig. 114-10). If the ossicle is symptomatic, it should

be excised; however, if it is an incidental finding, it can be managed conservatively.[11]

NEOPLASMS

FATTY LESIONS OF THE SYNOVIUM

Although the subsynovial connective tissue of diarthrodial joints is rich in fat, a true lipoma of the synovium is rare. When these rare tumors develop, they most frequently affect the knee joint and the synovial sheaths of tendons

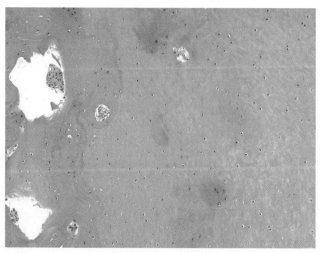

Figure 114-10 Intra-articular ossicle embedded in the fibrocartilage of the meniscus.

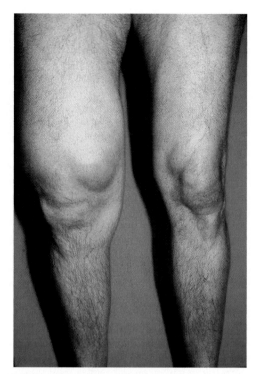

Figure 114-11 Lipoma arborescens manifesting as a suprapatellar mass.

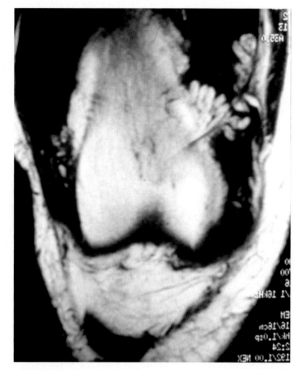

Figure 114-12 MR image of lipoma arborescens shows villonodular mass in the knee joint

of the hands, ankles, and feet, where they are more common in the extensor than the flexor synovial sheaths.[13,14] Synovial lipomas can be sessile or pedunculated, and when pedunculated they may produce pain if they twist on their stalks and become secondarily ischemic. Synovial lipoma, similar to its subcutaneous counterpart, comprises lobules of mature white adipocytes that are delineated by a thin fibrous capsule.

A more common but still unusual fatty lesion of the joint is lipoma arborescens, also known as villous lipomatous proliferation of the synovium.[15,16] This disorder is characterized by a diffuse increase in the quantity of subsynovial fat, which bulges into the overlying synovial lining producing a villous architecture. It is uncertain whether the proliferating fat is neoplastic (lipomatosis) or a manifestation of a hyperplastic or reactive process. Affected patients are usually adults because the lesion infrequently develops during childhood.[17] Lipoma arborescens causes chronic effusions, pain, and swelling, and restricts joint motion.[16] The duration of symptoms is often long, and symptoms may be present for 30 years; however, acute onset also has been documented.

Lipoma arborescens most commonly arises in the knee (Fig. 114-11), especially the suprapatellar portion, although it also has been observed in the hip, ankle, and wrist joints. It is typically localized to one joint, but several cases of bilateral knee involvement have been described.[16] Laboratory studies are unremarkable, and the joint fluid is clear and yellow.[16] Plain films show joint fullness, and findings of osteoarthritis are often present. Arthrography reveals multiple lobulated filling defects, which on CT represent a villonodular mass of low signal intensity that on MRI has the density of fat (Fig. 114-12).[18] At surgery, the affected synovium has a prominent villous or villonodular architecture and is tan-yellow (Fig. 114-13). Histologically, the lesion comprises

sheets of mature adipocytes admixed with nutrient blood vessels, all of which are partially compartmentalized by fibrous septa, and is covered on its intra-articular surface by several layers of synovial cells (Fig. 114-14). Synovectomy may relieve the symptoms and prevent effusions, but the associated osteoarthritis may be progressive.[16]

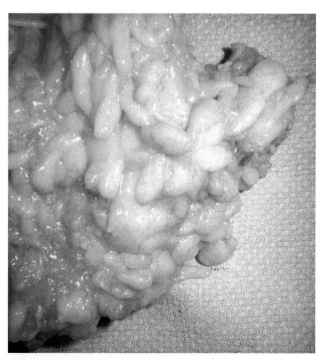

Figure 114-13 Lipoma arborescens composed of a villonodular mass of fatty tissue covered by glistening synovium.

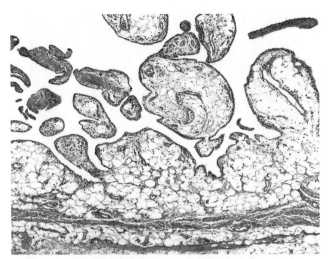

Figure 114-14 Lipoma arborescens with subsynovial compartment filled with mature adipocytes and covered by synoviocytes.

The clinicopathologic differential diagnosis includes diffuse tenosynovial giant cell tumor, synovial chondromatosis, and synovial hemangioma. These lesions can be distinguished easily from lipoma arborescens by their distinct histologic features. Another disorder that should be included in the differential diagnosis is Hoffa's disease, a condition of irritation, inflammation, and hyperplasia of the synovial lining in regions where fat is normally present, such as adjacent to the patella or patellar ligament.[19]

VASCULAR LESIONS OF THE SYNOVIUM

Benign vascular tumors of the synovium are rare. They are subclassified according to their growth pattern into localized and diffuse variants. Both tend to predominate in adolescence and young adulthood, but symptoms frequently can be traced back to childhood.[20] The joint most commonly involved is the knee, but hemangiomas also have been described in the elbow, ankle, tarsometatarsal, and temporomandibular joints, and the tendon sheaths of the wrist and ankle.[21] Unusual complications of synovial hemangiomas include a secondary destructive arthritis and Kasabach-Merritt syndrome.

Synovial hemangiomas produce a variety of symptoms, including unilateral, intermittent, joint pain and enlargement, which may result in limitation of motion, locking, buckling, and hemarthrosis, especially after minimal trauma.[21] Classically, the affected joint diminishes in size if sufficiently elevated to allow the blood to drain out of the lesion. On physical examination, the joint is swollen and doughy, and nearby cutaneous hemangiomas may be evident. Joint aspiration frequently yields bloody fluid. Preoperative diagnosis of localized hemangioma is difficult, and the differential diagnosis includes localized tenosynovial giant cell tumor, and in the knee includes discoid meniscus, meniscal tears, cysts, and ossicles.[22] The diffuse hemangioma is more easily identified, but it can mimic diffuse tenosynovial giant cell tumor and hemophilic arthropathy.

Radiographic evaluation may show nothing more than a vague soft tissue shadow indicative of a swollen synovium and distended joint capsule or regional osteoporosis in patients who have had long-term symptoms and recurrent hemarthrosis. Rarely, calcified phleboliths are apparent; however, they are associated more often with a soft tissue arteriovenous malformation with secondary joint involvement than an isolated intra-articular hemangioma (Fig. 114-15). Arthrography may show an intra-articular filling defect, and arteriography may be negative in small localized capillary hemangiomas, but contrast material may collect in the more diffuse lesions that contain cavernous or large ectatic vascular spaces (Fig. 114-16). CT reveals a lobulated soft tissue mass with mild enhancement after contrast injection.[22,23] MRI may show the tumor to have a low signal on T1-weighted images and high signal intensity on T2-weighted images.[24]

Macroscopically, the localized hemangioma tends to be small, but larger lesions (8 cm) have been documented. It may be sessile or stalked, is well circumscribed, and ranges in color from red to dark blue-purple. Microscopically, the hemangioma is usually of the cavernous or venous type with large dilated blood-filled vessels lined by cytologically benign endothelial cells. In the diffuse form, the entire synovium may be edematous and beefy red or stained brown by hemosiderin, and consists of prominent tortuous, congested vessels that may penetrate the joint capsule and extend into the neighboring soft tissues. Histologically, the vessels recapitulate architecturally abnormal arteries, veins, and capillaries; have abnormal interconnections; and are arranged in a disorganized tangle.[23]

Therapy for a localized hemangioma is marginal surgical excision, which usually is curative. Diffuse lesions frequently are difficult to eradicate because of their extensive nature.

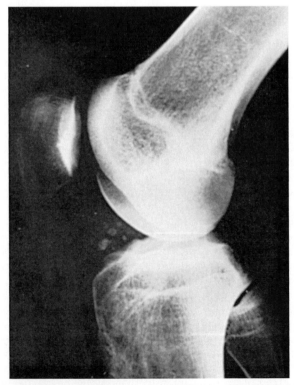

Figure 114-15 Localized synovial hemangioma with phleboliths prominently seen in the joint. The patient is 16 years old with many years' history of painful swelling when standing and relief of this pain when the knee is flexed.

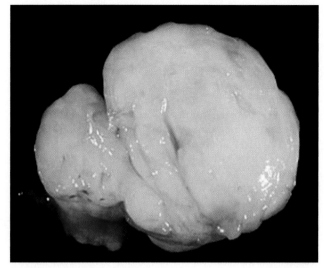

Figure 114-17 Fibroma of tendon sheath manifests as a well-circumscribed, tan-white mass.

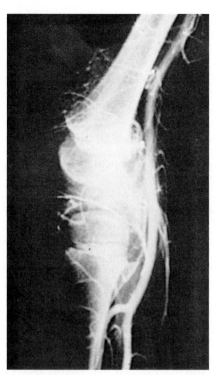

Figure 114-16 Arteriogram of an arteriovenous malformation in the soft tissues of the thigh and leg with involvement of the knee joint. The extensive vascular blush in the knee indicates aberrant synovial and capsular vasculature.

Incomplete excision or debulking may be the only surgical option. Radiation therapy is not indicated.

FIBROMA OF TENDON SHEATH

Fibroma of tendon sheath is an uncommon benign lesion that clinically mimics giant cell tumor of tendon sheath, but is morphologically distinct. Fibroma of tendon sheath first was identified as a clinicopathologic entity in 1936, and since that time more than 220 cases have been reported.[24,25] Although it is uncertain whether this lesion is some sort of reactive process, hyperplasia, or a benign neoplasm, the more recently identified translocation involving chromosomes 2 and 11 in this tumor support the concept that it is neoplastic.

Fibroma of tendon sheath usually arises from the tendons and sheaths of the flexor surfaces of the distal extremities; approximately 70% involve the fingers or hand. Of the fingers, the thumb is affected most frequently followed in descending order by the index and middle fingers.[24] Less commonly, large diarthrodial joints such as the knee and rarely the elbow and ankle are sites of origin.[24,25] Patients range in age from infants to the elderly, but the median is in the early fourth decade of life.[24,25] Most series report a male predominance, with the largest study of 138 cases having a male-to-female ratio of 3:1.[24] Patients present with a slow-growing, painless mass that usually has been noted for several months to a year.[25] In 6% to 10% of cases, there is a history of antecedent trauma.

Plain x-rays show soft tissue fullness; rarely is there evidence of bony erosion.[24] CT or MRI shows a solid well-circumscribed mass of soft tissue density. At surgery, the tumors usually are attached directly to the tendon or tendon sheath. They are rubbery, oblong, well circumscribed, or encapsulated; average 1.5 to 1.8 cm in greatest dimension; and have a tan-white cut surface (Fig. 114-17).[24,25]

Microscopically, fibroma of tendon sheath is multilobular with clefts interposed between adjacent lobules. The lobules are composed of spindle and stellate fibroblasts enmeshed in a collagenous and sometimes myxoid stroma (Fig. 114-18). Immunohistochemically, the tumor cells have the staining profile of myofibroblasts, and ultrastructurally, the cells have features of fibroblasts and myofibroblasts.[26]

The natural history of fibroma of tendon sheath is a slow growth that eventually ceases. The treatment of choice is surgical excision, but there is a 24% recurrence rate.[24]

SYNOVIAL CHONDROMATOSIS

Synovial chondromatosis is an uncommon condition characterized by the formation of multiple nodules of hyaline cartilage within the subsynovial connective tissue. If the cartilage nodules undergo enchondral ossification, the term *synovial osteochondromatosis* is appropriate. It is unclear

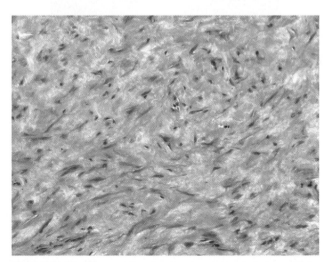

Figure 114-18 Fibroma of tendon sheath composed of a hypocellular collagenous mass.

whether the proliferating cartilage is metaplastic or neoplastic; however, more recent cytogenetic abnormalities involving chromosome 6 found in the cartilage of these lesions support a neoplastic process.[27] Regardless, synovial chondromatosis is benign and does not metastasize.

Synovial chondromatosis most commonly affects middle-aged men with an average age in the fifth decade of life.[28] Middle-aged women are more likely to develop the disease in the temporomandibular joint. The genders are equally affected with regards to hand and foot involvement, and patients with hand and foot involvement are usually in their sixth decade.

Patients commonly complain of joint pain, swelling, stiffness, crepitance, and limitation of motion with a locking or grating sensation on movement.[28] The symptoms usually are long-standing, recurrent, and progressive.

Synovial chondromatosis typically arises in large diarthrodial joints. The knee is affected in more than 50% of the cases, usually as a monarticular condition.[28] Other common sites include the hip, elbow, shoulder, and ankle. Infrequently, synovial chondromatosis arises in the small joints of the hands and feet[29] and the temporomandibular joint.[30] When the cartilage nodules develop in the synovial lining of bursae, tendons, and ligaments, it is known as extra-articular synovial chondromatosis.[31] The extra-articular variant most commonly affects the fingers, followed by the toes, hand, wrist, foot, and ankle, and more than one synovial sheath may be involved.[31]

The plain x-ray findings largely depend on whether the cartilage nodules are calcified or ossified, and if they erode the adjacent bony structures. Visible calcifications are absent in 5% to 33% of cases; however, in most there are multiple oval intra-articular radiodensities that range in size from a few millimeters to several centimeters (Fig. 114-19).[32] The pattern of

mineralization varies and may appear as irregular flecks that represent calcified cartilage or show a trabecular architecture, which is a manifestation of enchondral ossification. Lesions that are not mineralized can be seen on an arthrogram because they produce multiple filling defects.[32] In approximately 11% of cases, the nodules erode the neighboring skeleton, especially along the anterior aspect of the distal femur.

CT may show masslike nodules in the synovium that have a density similar to skeletal muscle. CT also can detect small calcifications and erosions before they are apparent on plain films. MRI shows that the nodules of cartilage have low signal intensity on T1-weighted sequences and high intensity on T2-weighted sequences, which reflects the high water content of the hyaline cartilage.[32] Areas of calcification or mineralized bone have a low signal intensity on T1-weighted and T2-weighted sequences. CT and MRI scans are helpful in identifying the intra-articular source of the lesion and its anatomic extent. In long-standing disease, the involved joints also may be osteoporotic and show changes of secondary osteoarthritis.

The cartilage in extra-articular synovial chondromatosis has similar radiographic changes. The nodules of cartilage are more frequently mineralized and may appear as a linear arrangement of small calcific densities that are aligned along the sheath and that can span many joints (Fig. 114-20).

The radiographic differential diagnosis of synovial chondromatosis includes osteochondritis dissecans, osteoarthritis with loose bodies, tuberculosis, hemopathic arthropathies, pseudogout with extensive synovial calcification, and synovial tumors. In many instances, the clinical presentation and radiographic picture should lead to the correct diagnosis. There are many cases, however, in which the x-rays and clinical picture are vague so that only a biopsy specimen can remove all doubts about the diagnosis.

Characteristic of synovial chondromatosis is a thickened synovium containing numerous opalescent firm nodules of cartilage that bulge from the surface in a cobblestone pattern (Fig. 114-21). The nodules are usually less than 5 cm in size and may lose their attachment to the synovium and form loose bodies, sometimes hundreds of them. The calcified cartilage is white, and areas of ossification manifest as gritty tan trabeculae, which may house fatty marrow. The synovium adjacent to the cartilage may show reactive changes, such as edema, hyperemia, hyperplasia, and villous transformation.

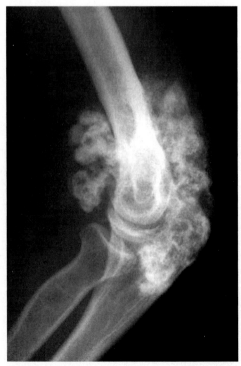

Figure 114-19 Synovial chondromatosis of the elbow. Multiple large calcified bodies fill the joint space and are adjacent to bone.

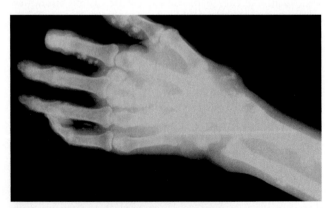

Figure 114-20 Synovial chondromatosis of the hand and forearm. There are multiple calcified nodules of varying size in the soft tissues of the fingers, wrist, and forearm.

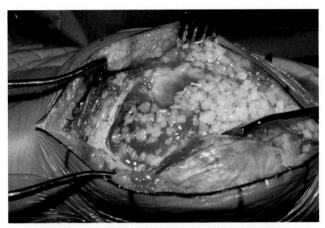

Figure 114-21 Intraoperative appearance of synovial chondromatosis. Innumerable nodules of cartilage fill the joint.

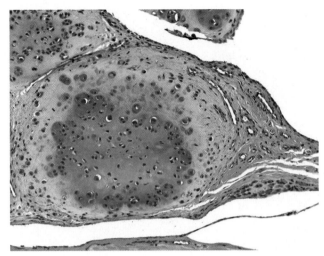

Figure 114-23 Nodules of hyaline cartilage merging with the surrounding connective tissue in synovial chondromatosis.

The cartilage develops in the connective tissue of the subsynovial compartment (Fig. 114-22). The mesenchymal cells give rise to uniformly small round chondrocytes, which produce the hyaline matrix and eventually form individual nodules that blend peripherally with the surrounding tissues (Fig. 114-23). In some cases, the cartilage is hypercellular, and the chondrocytes are large, binucleate, and hyperchromatic similar to the chondrocytes in intraosseous chondrosarcoma (Fig. 114-24). Despite these ominous histologic findings, experience has shown that these hypercellular lesions with atypical chondrocytes usually behave in a benign fashion. Infrequently, the disease manifests as a single, extremely large nodule of cartilage, which may undergo partial enchondral ossification. This giant intraarticular osteochondroma can severely limit joint motion and be confused clinically with other types of neoplasms.[33]

Over time, the nodules of cartilage attached to the synovium are invaded by blood vessels. This invasion results in enchondral ossification with woven and lamellar bone formation and the development of a medullary cavity with fatty marrow (Fig. 114-25). If these nodules lose their synovial attachments and become free-floating, they may continue to increase in size because the cartilage derives its

nourishment from synovial fluid, although the osseous portion and marrow die.

The treatment of choice for synovial chondromatosis is excision of the involved synovium and removal of all loose bodies. The prognosis is good, although there may be recurrences if removal is incomplete. Most recurrences develop in the setting of diffuse involvement of the synovium.

Synovial chondromatosis rarely undergoes malignant transformation into chondrosarcoma, although in one series this phenomenon occurred in 5% of cases. A significant percentage of the few reported cases of synovial chondrosarcomas has shown evidence of underlying synovial chondromatosis, however.[34-36]

CHONDROMA OF TENDON SHEATH AND PERIARTICULAR STRUCTURES

A solitary soft tissue chondroma is considered to be a benign neoplasm. It commonly arises in tendon sheaths and infrequently involves joint capsules or other periarticular structures.

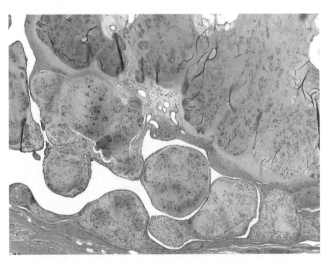

Figure 114-22 Synovial chondromatosis with nodules of hyaline cartilage in the synovium.

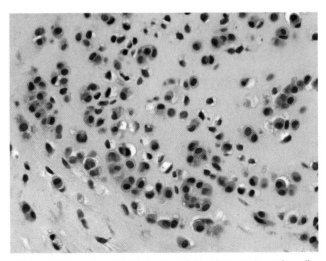

Figure 114-24 The cartilage in synovial chondromatosis can be cellular, and the chondrocytes may exhibit limited cytologic atypia.

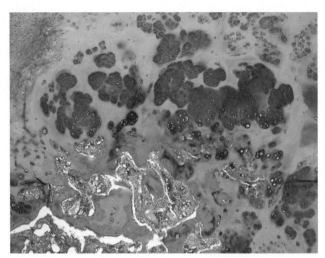

Figure 114-25   Nodules of cartilage in synovial chondromatosis undergoing enchondral ossification.

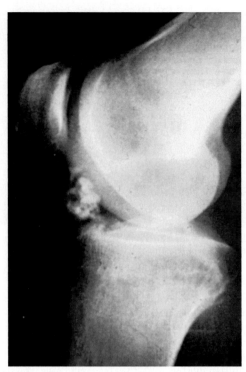

Figure 114-26   Intra-articular solitary chondroma of the knee in the infrapatellar region; it is a well-delineated mass with amorphous dense calcification, suggesting mineralized cartilage. *(Courtesy of Dr. C. Campbell.)*

Tendon sheath chondromas usually arise in the flexor tendon sheaths of the distal extremities and are about three times more common in the hands than in the feet.[37-39] They affect the sexes equally and are detected in early to mid adulthood as they present as a painless, slowly growing firm mass. Radiographically, tendon sheath chondromas appear as an extraosseous, well-delineated soft tissue mass that contains calcifications that are either punctate or ringlike in 33% to 70% of cases.[42,43] Grossly, the tumors are ovoid, firm, blue-white, well-circumscribed masses of hyaline cartilage that are usually 1 to 2 cm in dimension, and, in contrast to synovial chondromatosis, are solitary. Histologically, the hyaline cartilage is well formed with occasional small foci of myxoid change. The cartilage can be cellular, and the chondrocytes may show cytologic atypia, which causes confusion with chondrosarcoma.[40] The treatment of choice is simple excision. Although these tumors may recur in a few cases, they are benign and do not metastasize.[38-40]

The intracapsular and periarticular regions are uncommon sites for soft tissue chondromas. When they occur, they usually originate in the anterior infrapatellar region of the knee (Fig. 114-26).[41] In this location, the chondroma can achieve a large size (8 cm) and mechanically interfere with knee motion. Morphology and biologic behavior are similar to soft tissue chondromas that arise elsewhere. Intracapsular chondromas have been reported in knees of three members of a family with familial dysplasia epiphysealis hemimelica.[42] Two other cases have been described in which cartilaginous hamartomas of the volar plates of the proximal and distal interphalangeal joints of the hands and feet were associated with peculiar hypertrophic skin lesions of the hand and hemihypertrophy of the limb. It is possible that these peculiar cartilaginous lesions represent an abnormality in which primitive cartilage tissue persists in joint sites similar to the involvement of bones in multiple enchondromatosis (Ollier's disease).

TENOSYNOVIAL GIANT CELL TUMOR

Tenosynovial giant cell tumor comprises a group of benign tumors that affect the synovial lining of joints, tendon sheaths, and bursae.[43] These lesions have been previously known as giant cell tumor of tendon sheath and pigmented villonodular synovitis. Tenosynovial giant cell tumor may be localized or diffuse and may be locally aggressive in that it may invade into bone, grow through joint capsules, extend along tendons, and infiltrate into adjacent soft tissues. Despite their destructive potential, they do not have the capacity to metastasize.

The common histologic denominator of these lesions is the neoplastic proliferation of synovial-like cells that may form a localized mass or spread along the synovial surface and invade downward into the subsynovial connective tissue. The growing cells expand the subsynovial compartment producing finger-like extensions, villi, and redundant folds. These projections often fuse into nodules and form convoluted lobulated masses admixed with a tangle of hair-like villi. The process may be a local phenomenon involving only part of the synovial lining, or it may be extensive with the whole synovial surface affected.

Until more recently, the etiology of tenosynovial giant cell tumor was unknown. Previously considered a reactive process, possibly in response to repeated hemorrhage, many tenosynovial giant cell tumors now have been shown to result from a translocation between chromosomes 1p13 and 2q35 in which the gene encoding colony-stimulating factor-1 is fused to collagen VI alpha-3 (*COL6A3*) gene.[43,44] Consequently, there is overexpression of colony-stimulating factor-1 in the neoplastic cells, which account for only 2% to 16% of the cells in mass.[44] The remaining cells largely represent non-neoplastic inflammatory cells that are recruited into the tumor because they contain the receptor for colony-stimulating factor.[44,45] This phenomenon has been termed a *landscape effect*; it also is observed in certain types of lymphomas.

Tenosynovial Giant Cell Tumor of Joints and Tendon Sheaths—Diffuse Type (Synonym: Pigmented Villonodular Synovitis)

The diffuse type of tenosynovial giant cell type of the joint involves large areas of the synovial lining, although uninvolved areas are invariably present. Its incidence is approximately 1.8 per 1 million. Although it may occur in all age groups spanning children to the elderly, most affect young adults in the third to fourth decades of life.[46] The sexes tend to be equally affected, although some series have reported a predominance of either males or females.[46-48]

Diffuse tenosynovial giant cell tumor of the joint usually manifests as monarticular arthritis. Bilaterality or involvement of multiple separate sites has been infrequently reported. Some patients with polyarticular disease also have had significant congenital anomalies. The main complaints include pain and mild intermittent or repeated bouts of swelling. The symptoms develop insidiously and progress slowly over a long time ranging from months to years.[46,48] The involved area may be stiff, swollen, and warm, and a palpable mass sometimes can be appreciated. Point tenderness can be detected in approximately 50% of patients. Anatomic instability of the involved joint is uncommon.

The knee joint is affected most commonly and is involved in about 80% of cases.[46,48] The next most frequent sites are the hip, ankle, calcaneocuboid joints, elbow, and tendon sheaths of fingers and sometimes toes. Occasionally, the palm, the sole of the foot, and unusual locations such as the temporomandibular joint and posterior elements of the spine are involved. Bursal involvement is rare, but if it happens, it usually occurs in the popliteal and iliopectineal bursae and the bursa anserina. Infrequently, the disease affects large tendon sheaths proximal to the ankle and wrist and produces a periarticular soft tissue mass.[49,50] It is thought that some of these lesions dissect through either a joint capsule or a tendon sheath and extend along fascial planes to produce a soft tissue mass.[49]

Invasion of bone on either side of a joint can be seen with intra-articular, bursal, or tendon sheath involvement. This most frequently occurs when the tumor involves "tight" joints, such as the hip, elbow, wrist, and feet, or when tendon sheaths are closely opposed to neighboring bones (Fig. 114-27).[51,52] Rarely, only one bone may be invaded by an intra-articular lesion, and in this situation it may be difficult to distinguish from a primary bone tumor (Fig. 114-28).[53]

Joint aspiration frequently yields blood-tinged brown fluid that lacks diagnostic abnormalities.[54] Synovial fluid analysis may show a low glucose content, minimally elevated protein level, and a fair mucin clot. The inflammatory cell count is usually low, but may be elevated. Similar findings also can be seen in trauma, Charcot joint, bleeding disorders, sickle cell disease, and Ehlers-Danlos syndrome.

In at least two thirds of cases, a soft tissue density, which is due to the tumor or effusion or both, can be visualized on a plain film.[58] Joint narrowing or calcification is uncommon. Arthrography may show numerous nodular filling defects that extend into an expanded joint space. Arteriograms are unusually striking owing to the prominent vascularity of the tumor. There tends to be an inverse correlation between the degree of vascularity and the amount of fibrosis or scarring of the lesion.

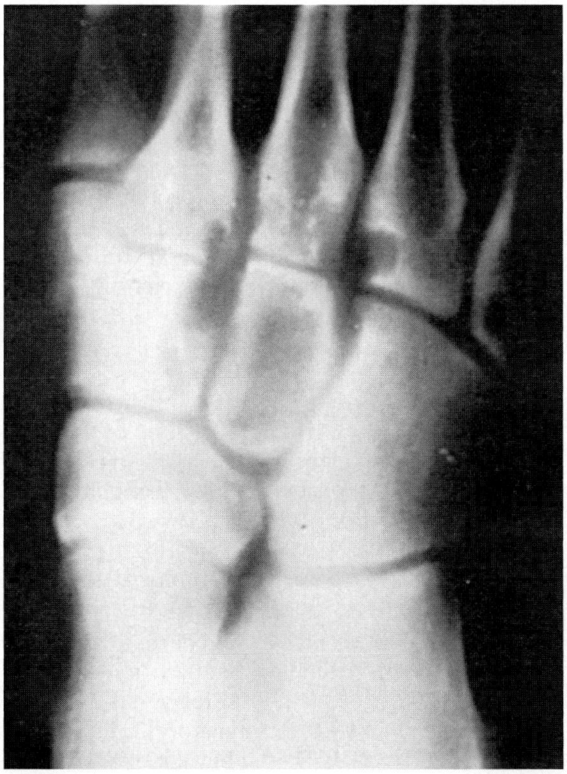

Figure 114-27 Pigmented villonodular synovitis involving the small joints of the foot with multiple bone erosions. No calcification is present in the lesion.

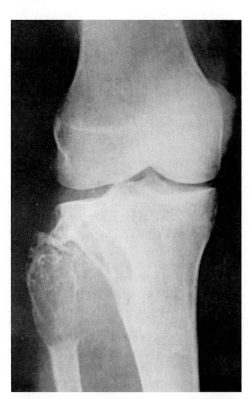

Figure 114-28 Pigmented villonodular synovitis involving the tibiofibular joint with an adjacent extensive soft tissue mass and eccentric erosion of the both bones, simulating a primary bone tumor. The knee joint is normal.

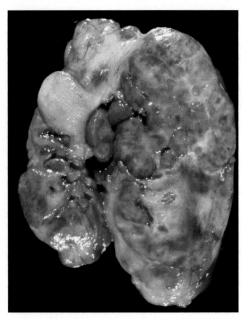

Figure 114-29 Diffuse type of tenosynovial giant cell tumor consisting of mottled brown-yellow-red villonodular mass.

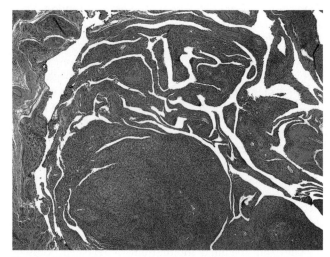

Figure 114-30 Diffuse type of tenosynovial giant cell tumor growing with a villonodular architecture. Invading cells produce the nodular configuration.

CT and MRI are useful in delineating the extent of disease and can detect intralesional lipid and hemosiderin deposits that are important diagnostic features.[55-57] Extension into the bone manifests radiographically as multiple, well-marginated, subchondral cystlike lucencies or juxtacortical oval pressure erosions (see Figs. 114-27 and 114-28).[52,53] In the knee, the femoral area adjacent to the intercondylar region is the site most frequently invaded as the tumor grows along the cruciate ligamentous insertions. Periarticular osteopenia, periosteal reactions, and joint destruction are unusual because the joint space is preserved until late in the course of the disease.[56,57] The radiographic differential diagnosis of a given case includes (1) tuberculosis, which generally has more osteopenia and joint destruction; (2) hemophilia, which also is associated with more extensive joint destruction; (3) synovial chondromatosis, which frequently has calcified radiopaque bodies; and (4) rheumatoid arthritis, which shows more severe osteopenia and joint narrowing.

Grossly, the synovium in diffuse tenosynovial giant cell tumor is red-brown to mottled orange-yellow and looks like a plush angora rug (Fig. 114-29). Matted masses of villous projections and synovial folds are prominent and are admixed with sessile or pedunculated, rubbery-to-soft nodules (0.5 to 2 cm in diameter). The synovial membrane is thick and succulent, and is often coated with a fibrinous exudate. Red-brown or golden brown tissue may extend deep into subsynovial structures or invade the joint capsule. If a tendon sheath is involved, a sausage-shaped mass may be evident as the sheath is distended by the proliferating tumor. If the joint capsule is invaded, adjacent soft tissue structures, including nerves and vessels, may be covered by wispy, red-brown tissue. If soft tissue invasion is extensive, the lesion may appear as a soft-to-rubbery, red-brown mass with foci of hemorrhagic cysts. Similar tissue may be present near the chondro-osseous junction or wrapped around vascular and ligamentous attachments to bone surfaces, which represent entrance points into the interior of the bone. Although other conditions, such as hemochromatosis and hemosiderosis, also may discolor the synovium brown, the nodular component is usually absent; in addition, microscopic features are definitive for separating these entities (see later).

Microscopic examination reveals marked synovial cell hyperplasia with surface proliferation and, more important, subsynovial invasion by masses of mitotically active polygonal or round cells with moderate amounts of eosinophilic cytoplasm and round nuclei (Figs. 114-30 and 114-31). Included among the invading synovial cells are scattered lymphocytes, multinucleated giant cells (osteoclast, Touton, or foreign body type), hemosiderin-laden macrophages, and fibroblasts. Hemosiderin also can be seen between cells and in synovial lining cells and polygonal cells. Foci of hemorrhage are common and are surrounded peripherally by giant cells and macrophages (Fig. 114-32). Scattered collections of foamy macrophages (xanthoma cells) filled with lipid also

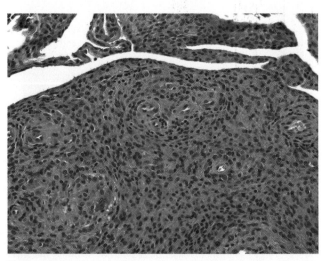

Figure 114-31 Synovial lining cells covering the mass of proliferating polyhedral cells admixed with multinucleated giant cells.

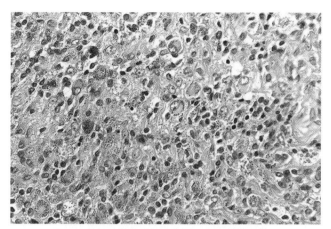

Figure 114-32 Sheets of macrophages containing abundant hemosiderin.

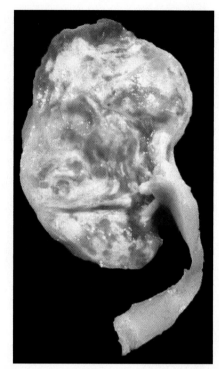

Figure 114-33 Localized tenosynovial giant cell tumor of the joint with attached pedicle. The mass is well circumscribed and brown-yellow.

are a frequent finding. These different cell populations fill and distend the synovial villi and cause them to fuse with adjacent ones, forming nodules. In some nodules, there may be abundant collagen deposition with hyalinization causing confusion with neoplastic bone.

Immunohistochemical studies of these tumors have not yielded consistent results and have been interpreted to support a synovial cell or fibrohistiocytic phenotype.[26,58] Importantly, the cells that harbor the translocation express colony-stimulating factor-1. Flow cytometric analyses have shown that some of these tumors, especially tumors that have large extra-articular soft tissue components, may be aneuploid and have high proliferative indices.[50] Although these flow cytometric findings may help predict which cases would be more locally aggressive, examples of diffuse tenosynovial cell tumors with these attributes have not been shown to metastasize.[50]

The treatment of diffuse tenosynovial giant cell tumor of the joint is not standardized and has included radiation therapy, total synovectomy, arthrodesis, bone grafting, and primary arthroplasty.[59] Although no single therapy has been consistently successful, currently, wide synovectomy is the recommended treatment.[46,48] It is difficult to perform an actual complete synovectomy, however; residual involved synovium frequently remains causing a local recurrence rate of 16% to 48%.[60-62] Tumors arising in the knee have a higher rate of recurrence compared with tumors arising in other joints.[63] Rarely, recurrent disease or tumors with large extra-articular components may require more radical surgery, such as ray resection or amputation.[50] More recent studies have shown that moderate doses of radiation may control and even cure patients with such extensive disease, possibly obviating the need for radical surgery or amputation.

Malignant Diffuse Tenosynovial Giant Cell Tumor

Malignant tenosynovial giant cell tumor is a rare lesion with only a handful of cases having been reported.[64,65] The knee has been the joint most commonly affected, and in many cases there was coexisting benign-appearing, diffuse tenosynovial giant cell tumor. In the malignant variant, the neoplastic mononuclear polyhedral cells are cytologically malignant. These tumors have the capacity to behave aggressively; almost 50% of patients have died from metastatic disease.[64]

Localized Tenosynovial Giant Cell Tumor of the Joint (Synonyms: Benign Giant Cell Synovioma, Benign Synovioma, Localized Nodular Synovitis)

Localized tenosynovial giant cell tumor of the joint manifests as a solitary, well-circumscribed mass. It usually consists of a single sessile or pedunculated, sometimes lobulated, mass that ranges from 1 to 8 cm in diameter (Fig. 114-33). Most commonly, it is unilateral, arises in the knee, and is equally distributed between the sexes.[66]

Symptoms are similar to those of diffuse tenosynovial giant cell tumor except that in the localized variant there is a higher frequency of joint locking because the mass interferes with motion.[66] A few patients may present with acute severe joint pain caused by torsion and infarction of the tumor. Effusions are common, but the synovial fluid tends to be less bloody than in pigmented villonodular synovitis and may be clear.

Imaging studies show a heterogeneous nodular mass that contains lipid and hemosiderin deposits (Fig. 114-34). In the knee joint, the tumor frequently arises in the suprapatellar notch, in the femoral notch, and between the meniscus and joint capsule.[66] There is usually no bone invasion. Marginal excision is usually curative.[67] Small lesions can be extirpated arthroscopically.[66]

Histologically, localized tenosynovial giant cell tumor of the joint is identical to the nodules of the diffuse variant. The main difference is that the prominent synovial villi present in the diffuse variant are absent or sparse.

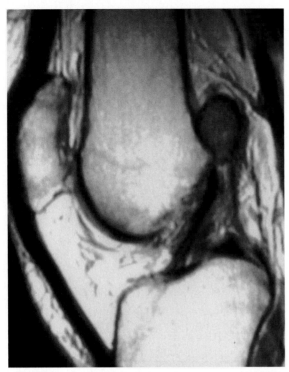

Figure 114-34   MR image shows well-delineated dark mass in posterior knee joint.

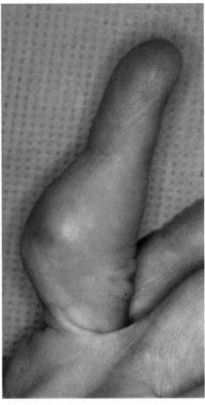

Figure 114-35   Tenosynovial giant cell tumor manifesting as a mobile, solid, firm mass.

Localized Tenosynovial Giant Cell Tumor of the Tendon Sheath (Synonyms: Giant Cell Tumor of Tendon Sheath, Fibroxanthoma of Tendon Sheath)

Localized tenosynovial giant cell tumor of the tendon sheath usually involves the hand or wrist, and less frequently the foot or ankle.[47] Localized tenosynovial giant cell tumor of the tendon sheath is the most common soft tissue tumor of the hand. It usually arises from the flexor tendon sheaths of the fingers; the index finger is affected most frequently, followed in descending order of frequency by the middle finger, ring finger, little finger, and thumb.

Finger tumors predominate in females with a ratio of at least 2:1,[47,68] and tumors of the toes have an equal sex distribution.[47] On average, patients are in the third to fifth decades and present with a painless, palpable, firm, mobile mass.

Clinically, the mass is usually solitary and located on the flexor surface, but it may bulge into the extensor or lateral aspects of the digits (Fig. 114-35). The tumors are slow growing, and the intervals between detection and surgical treatment have ranged from several weeks to greater than a decade with an average of slightly more than 2 years.[47,68]

Radiographically, tumors appear as well-circumscribed soft tissue masses, and in about 25% of cases, there is adjacent extrinsic excavation of the cortical bone that has a sclerotic margin (Fig. 114-36).[47,68] MRI reveals the lesions to have a hypointense signal on T1-weighted images and either a hypointense or a hyperintense signal on T2-weighted images. These findings are helpful in distinguishing giant cell tumor of tendon sheath from other soft tissue tumors.[69]

The gross pathology is that of a well-circumscribed, multinodular, round, rubbery mass, generally not larger than 5 cm in diameter, which is firmly attached but easily peeled off the involved tendon (Fig. 114-37). Sometimes at surgery, the variegated red-brown-tan lesion may "pop out" of the

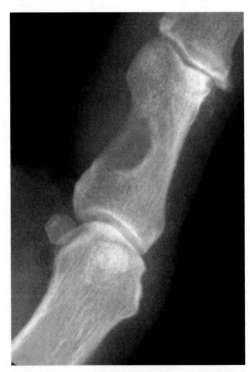

Figure 114-36   The cortex of the phalanx is eroded by the tenosynovial giant cell tumor.

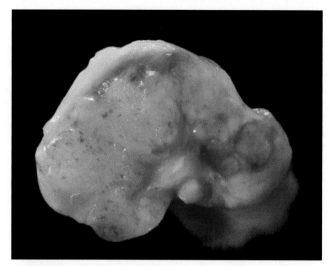

Figure 114-37 Well-delineated, white-yellow and focally brown tenosynovial giant cell tumor.

incision. The cut surface reveals a solid mass that ranges from hues of yellow to orange-brown, depending on the amount of lipid and blood pigments present. Often there are bands or septa of white fibrous tissue that subcompartmentalize the lesion. Microscopically, the cell types present are identical to those in the diffuse variant (Fig. 114-38).[70] Ultrastructurally, the proliferating cells have features similar to type A and type B synovial lining cells.[68-71] Their antigenic and enzymatic profiles have suggested a synovial or monocyte/macrophage lineage, the latter being similar to osteoclasts.[72] Flow cytometry has been performed on a few cases, and all have been diploid.[50] Cytogenetics show that many of these tumors have a translocation between 1p13 and 2q35.[44,45,73]

These tumors are benign and do not metastasize. Rarely have malignant giant cell tumors of tendon sheath been reported.[64,74] The treatment of choice is conservative surgical excision, which is usually curative. There may be local recurrence if excision is incomplete.[47,68]

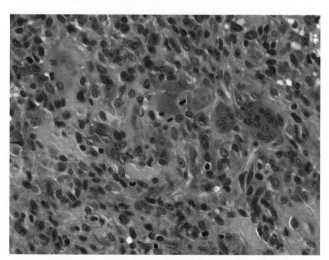

Figure 114-38 Mitotically active polyhedral cells and scattered osteoclast-type giant cells in tenosynovial giant cell tumor.

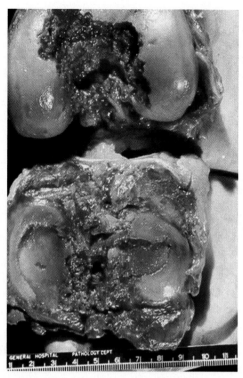

Figure 114-39 Angiosarcoma of synovium of the knee joint. The hemorrhagic tumor erodes into the distal femur and proximal tibia.

MALIGNANT TUMORS OF THE JOINT

Malignant tumors of joints are uncommon and are classified into primary and secondary types. Primary malignancies are virtually always sarcomas and usually arise within the synovium of large diarthrodial joints, especially the knee. The patients are adults who present with the chronic symptoms of pain, swelling, and effusion, and most of the tumors are either chondrosarcomas or synovial sarcomas. Rarely, other sarcomas originate within a joint; we have experience with intra-articular myxoinflammatory fibroblastic sarcoma, pleomorphic fibrosarcoma, extraskeletal myxoid chondrosarcoma, conventional chondrosarcoma, malignant tenosynovial giant cell tumor, and angiosarcoma (Fig. 114-39). Secondary malignant tumors of joints, by definition, originate beyond the confines of the joint, and most are sarcomas that extend from neighboring bones or surrounding soft tissues. Although synovial tissue is very vascular, metastases or involvement of the synovium by carcinoma, lymphoma, or leukemia is uncommon.

PRIMARY SARCOMAS OF JOINTS

Conventional Chondrosarcoma

Conventional chondrosarcoma arising in the synovium is unusual, and less than 50 cases have been reported in the English language.[34-36,65,75] In approximately 50% of these cases, the chondrosarcoma arose in association with preexisting synovial chondromatosis.[36,37,76,77] The patients are usually in the fifth to seventh decade and have an equal sex distribution.[77] Typically, they present with a progressively enlarging mass in the joint that may cause mechanical dysfunction, pain, and stiffness. In patients who have preexisting synovial chondromatosis, the duration of symptoms is usually long, and in some instances, symptoms may be present for 25 years.[77] Most chondrosarcomas arise in the knee joint, followed by the hip and elbow joints.

Radiographic studies usually show a periarticular soft tissue mass that may have dense irregular or ringlike calcifications. Occasionally, invasion into the medullary cavity of adjacent bone is present. The radiographic differential diagnosis varies according to the presence of calcification and includes synovial chondromatosis, synovial sarcoma, diffuse tenosynovial giant cell tumor, and chronic synovitis.[77]

Grossly, the involved joint is filled with synovium massively thickened by innumerable nodules of opalescent blue-white cartilage. The nodules of cartilage vary in size and may be free-floating in the joint cavity. In several cases, the tumor has extended into the adjacent soft tissue and bone.

Microscopically, the tumor usually is composed of malignant hyaline and myxoid cartilage. Rarely, the matrix is entirely myxoid and has the features of extraskeletal myxoid chondrosarcoma.[76] The neoplastic cartilage is cellular and contains cytologically atypical chondrocytes. The periphery of the lobules of cartilage is typically the most cellular, and in this region some of the tumor cells are spindled. Other findings include necrosis and permeation of invaded bone.[77] Coexisting synovial chondromatosis can be identified by its well-formed nodules of hyaline cartilage that are less cellular, containing cytologically banal-appearing chondrocytes and a matrix that is frequently mineralized.

Treatment is usually surgical extirpation with consideration given for chemotherapy in high-grade lesions or lesions that have metastasized. Inadequate surgical removal virtually ensures local recurrence, which may necessitate subsequent radical excision. Metastases have occurred in approximately one third of the reported patients, with the lung being the most common site for systemic spread.[77]

Synovial Sarcoma

Synovial sarcoma is a common sarcoma and accounts for approximately 6% to 10% of soft tissue sarcomas. It usually develops in the deep soft tissues and rarely arises in joints (Fig. 114-40), but may secondarily invade articular synovium from neighboring soft tissues. Earlier descriptions of this tumor attest to its wide spectrum of morphology because such names as adenosarcoma and synovial fibrosarcoma were used until the term *synovial sarcoma*, first introduced in 1936, became commonplace. The morphology of synovial sarcoma mimics a joint in its early stage of development in that it contains cleftlike spaces and glands delineated by large polygonal (epithelioid) cells that are surrounded by fascicles of spindle cells. The clefts and glands simulate a microscopic "joint space" that is bounded by synovial lining cells and supported by subsynovial mesenchymal cells. Because either the epithelioid or the spindle cells may predominate, synovial sarcoma has been subtyped into biphasic and monophasic spindle cell and epithelioid types.

Synovial sarcoma commonly affects adolescents and young adults. In a series of 121 cases, the age range was 9 to 74 years with a median of 34 years; however, it occurs in children with significant frequency.[77,78]

Although the term *synovial sarcoma* implies that the tumor originates from the synovium, less than 10% of cases are intra-articular or in continuity with a synovial lining.[79,80] The fact that many synovial sarcomas arise near

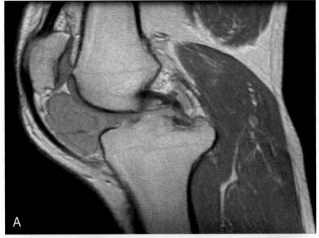

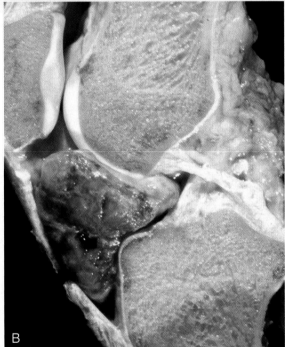

Figure 114-40 **A,** MR image of a rare example of intra-articular synovial sarcoma. The infrapatellar tumor is well circumscribed and has a focal inhomogeneous appearance. **B,** The gross specimen shows that the tan, hemorrhagic tumor bulges into the joint, but is covered by synovium.

joints also was misconstrued as supporting its synovial origin.[81] Approximately 60% to 70% of synovial sarcomas arise in the extremities, especially the lower limb, in the vicinity of large joints, particularly the popliteal area of the knee and foot.[82] Regions of the thigh, hand, leg, and digits may be affected, and in the distal extremities, the tumors often are adjacent to joint capsules or tendon sheaths or both. Tumors also have been reported in the neck, torso, craniofacial region, retroperitoneum, orbit, tongue, mediastinum, soft palate, kidney, lung, pleura, and prostate.

There are no clinical features specific to synovial sarcoma that distinguishes it from other sarcomas. The most common complaint is the development of a slowly enlarging, deep-seated palpable mass that is painful in about 50% of the cases.[78,82] Symptoms may be present for an unusually long time before medical evaluation is sought, ranging from months to 25 years with an average of about 6 months to

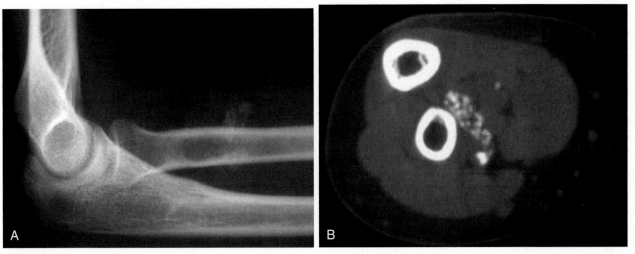

Figure 114-41 **A,** Focally mineralized synovial sarcoma in the deep soft tissues in the vicinity of the elbow joint. **B,** Axial CT scan shows intratumoral calcification.

2.5 years.[78,82] Delay in diagnosis is more frequent with tumors that are located in the deep soft tissues compared with tumors based in the more superficial and clinically noticeable regions. In some cases involving the knee region, vague mild pain over several months may occur before a mass is appreciated, and if the tumor reaches a large size, limitation of motion finally may occur. Head and neck lesions produce symptoms related to their specific sites, such as hoarseness and breathing or swallowing difficulties. Rarely, a patient may present with symptoms secondary to pulmonary metastases such as hemoptysis.[82]

Classically, the plain film findings of synovial sarcoma are a well-circumscribed, deep-seated soft tissue mass. Synovial sarcoma is one of the few primary soft tissue tumors that frequently calcifies. Approximately 30% to 50% of cases have radiographically detectable calcifications that can have a fine, stippled, or dense appearance (Fig. 114-41).[83] The calcification may be focal or present throughout most of the tumor.[84] Periosteal reaction of the adjacent bone is elicited in approximately 20% of cases, but the bone is rarely invaded by the tumor.

CT is more sensitive than plain radiographs in showing calcification or periosteal reaction. MRI is important in delineating the anatomic extent of the tumor and usually shows a large inhomogeneous mass with areas of hemorrhage. The radiographic differential diagnosis includes hemangioma, lipoma, synovial chondromatosis, soft tissue chondrosarcoma or osteosarcoma, myositis ossificans, aneurysms, and other sarcomas.

The gross pathology of synovial sarcoma reveals a well-demarcated, pink-tan, fleshy mass that easily detaches or "shells out" from its tumor bed (see Fig. 114-40B). The cut surface is usually uniform, gray-yellow, and rubbery. The calcified areas are gritty and hard. In larger tumors, areas of hemorrhage or necrosis or both with cystification and gelatinous breakdown of tissue also may be seen. Synovial sarcoma sometimes grows between tendons, muscle, and fascial planes or wraps around neurovascular bundles.

Synovial sarcoma is subtyped into three patterns on the basis of predominant microscopic findings: monophasic spindle cell, monophasic epithelioid, and biphasic variants. There is some subjectivity in the use of such a classification

system because many of these tumors have a variable histologic picture. A useful differential observation is that marked cellular pleomorphism and atypia are usually not present in synovial sarcoma, and when present, tend to point to some other type of neoplasm, such as pleomorphic fibrosarcoma.

Microscopically, the hallmark of the more common biphasic synovial sarcoma is the two different populations of neoplastic cells consisting of epithelioid and spindle cells (Fig. 114-42). The epithelioid cells may be cuboidal or columnar and similar to true epithelium have well-defined cytoplasmic borders. These cells may form glandlike spaces, line papillae, or cleftlike spaces, or grow in cohesive groups (see Fig. 114-42). The epithelioid cells usually are surrounded by fascicles of uniform small and plump spindle cells. The spindle cell fascicles are densely cellular and frequently are arranged in a "herringbone" pattern. In most biphasic synovial sarcomas, the spindle cell component predominates, and it is in the spindle cell regions in which calcification of hyalinized stroma most frequently occurs. Some tumors may have bone formation, which may be present in the spindle or epithelioid areas. In the monophasic variants, either the spindle or the epithelioid cells predominate

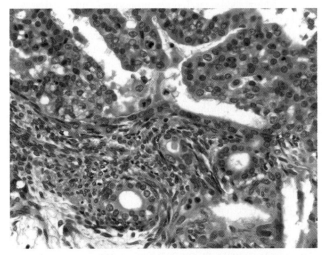

Figure 114-42 Biphasic synovial sarcoma with epithelial cells forming glands and papillary structures. The spindle cell component surrounds the glands.

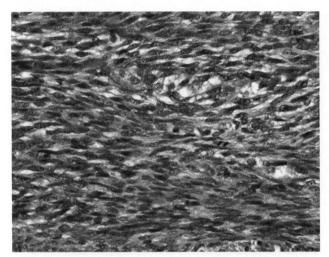

Figure 114-43 Monophasic spindle cell variant of synovial sarcoma with the fascicles of tumor cells forming a herringbone pattern.

(Fig. 114-43; see Fig. 114-42). Pure epithelioid synovial sarcomas are extraordinarily rare.

Immunohistochemistry has shown that the epithelioid and the spindle cell components frequently stain with antibodies to keratin and epithelial membrane antigen, which usually are associated with epithelial neoplasms.[85-87] This pattern of reactivity has helped make it possible to separate synovial sarcoma from other morphologically similar tumors, such as fibrosarcoma and malignant peripheral nerve sheath tumor.[87] Also, it has provided evidence that synovial sarcoma does not arise from or recapitulate the synovium because normal synovial cells do not stain with these antibodies.[88]

Cytogenetic studies of synovial sarcomas have detected a consistent translocation t(X;18)(p11.2;q11.2) in almost all cases regardless of whether the tumor is biphasic or monophasic.[89] This finding provides insight into the genesis of synovial sarcoma and can be used as a diagnostic feature. There is no consensus regarding its utility in providing prognostic information.

The prognosis of synovial sarcoma is poor. In one study of 150 patients with nonmetastatic disease, the 5-year, 10-year, and 15-year disease-free survival rates were 59%, 52%, and 52%.[90] Many factors influence prognosis. Tumors that are small (<5 cm), that arise in patients younger than 25 years old, and that lack poorly differentiated areas have a high rate of cure.[78] In contrast, large tumors (≥5 cm) that arise in patients 25 years old or older and that contain poorly differentiated areas have a dismal outcome.[78] The impact of histologic subtype has been controversial. Some studies have indicated that the monophasic spindle cell variant behaves the most aggressively, and tumors that are heavily calcified do the best.[84]

The natural history of synovial sarcoma is local recurrence, which may be repetitive. Most recurrences manifest within 2 years after initial treatment, but intervals longer than 10 years are not exceptional. Ultimately, metastases develop in many patients with the most common site being the lungs; regional lymph node involvement has been reported in a few patients.[90] About 10% of patients die within 1 year after diagnosis with metastatic disease, 90% of whom have massive pulmonary metastases.

Treatment must contend with issues involved with local and systemic therapy. Successful local control usually can be achieved by limb salvage surgery combined with radiation.[90,91] Because the regional lymph nodes may be involved, their status should be evaluated carefully, and they should be treated if enlarged. Systemic treatment consists of various chemotherapy regimens, which have been of questionable benefit, although adjuvant chemotherapy usually is recommended for patients who are at high risk—patients with tumors larger than 5 cm.[90,91]

SECONDARY MALIGNANT TUMORS OF THE JOINT

Sarcomas

Primary sarcomas of bone, such as osteosarcoma and chondrosarcoma, infrequently involve a joint because intact articular cartilage usually acts as a barrier to direct tumor extension. When joint invasion does occur, however, it is usually via a pathway created by a transarticular fracture, via growth along tendoligamentous structures, or through capsule insertion sites. This circumstance may make it difficult to distinguish on histologic grounds alone some forms of synovial chondromatosis from a low-grade intraosseous chondrosarcoma that has secondarily spread into the joint.

Similarly, primary soft tissue sarcomas gain access into the interior of a joint by growing through the joint capsule in conduits occupied by preexisting vascular structures or along tendons and ligaments. This complication can make adequate therapy challenging because treatment may require en bloc resection of the joint.

Metastatic Carcinoma

The synovium, in contrast to other richly vascular tissues, is rarely the site of metastatic carcinoma; this may reflect the fact that only clinical cases in which joint symptoms prevail are reported because at autopsy joints are not routinely examined. Most carcinomas that metastasize to the synovium originate in the lung, followed by the gastrointestinal tract and breast.[92,93] Affected patients are usually elderly, and the knee is the most frequently involved joint. In many reported cases, the underlying bone also contains metastatic deposits.

Malignant Lymphoproliferative Disease

The various types of malignant lymphoproliferative diseases, including leukemia, lymphoma, and myeloma, can involve the synovium and produce osteoarticular symptoms.[94-96] This complication occurs most frequently in leukemia and is seen in the acute and chronic forms.[96] Joint symptoms have been observed in 12% to 65% of children and in 4% to 13% of adults with leukemia.[96] The arthritis can develop at any time during the disease course and can be the presenting complaint. Large joints are affected more commonly than small joints, and the arthritis is often pauciarticular, asymmetric, migratory, and severe. The symptoms may result from leukemic infiltration of the synovium or irritation of the neighboring periosteum. When arthritis is the major presenting symptom, it may cause confusion with septic arthritis, rheumatic fever, subacute bacterial endocarditis, or rheumatoid arthritis.

REFERENCES

1. **Fritschy D, Fasel J, Imbert JC, et al: The popliteal cyst. Knee Surg Sports Traumatol Arthrosc 14:623, 2006.**
2. Seil R, Rupp S, Jochum P, et al: Prevalence of popliteal cysts in children: A sonographic study and review of the literature. Arch Orthop Trauma Surg 119:73, 1999.
3. Labropoulos N, Shifrin DA, Paxinos O: New insights into the development of popliteal cysts. Br J Surg 91:1313, 2004.
4. Beaman FD, Peterson JJ: MR imaging of cysts, ganglia, and bursae about the knee. Magn Reson Imaging Clin N Am 15:39, 2007.
5. Choudhri HF, Perling LH: Diagnosis and management of juxtafacet cysts. Neurosurg Focus 20:E1, 2006.
6. McEvedy BV: Simple ganglia. Br J Surg 49:40, 1962.
7. Nahra ME, Bucchieri JS: Ganglion cysts and other tumor related conditions of the hand and wrist. Hand Clin 20:249, 2004.
8. **Milgram JW: The classification of loose bodies in human joints. Clin Orthop 124:282, 1977.**
9. Clarke HD, Scott WN: The role of debridement: through small portals. J Arthroplasty 18:10, 2003.
10. Cooper G, Schiller AL: Anatomy of the Guinea Pig. Cambridge, Harvard University Press, 1975.
11. Kato Y, Oshida M, Saito A, et al: Meniscal ossicles. J Orthop Sci 12:375, 2007.
12. Van Breuseghem I, Geusens E, Pans S, et al: The meniscal ossicle revisited. JBR-BTR 86:276, 2003.
13. Hirano K, Deguchi M, Kanamono T: Intra-articular synovial lipoma of the knee joint (located in the lateral recess): A case report and review of the literature. Knee 14:63, 2007.
14. Sonoda H, Takasita M, Taira H, et al: Carpal tunnel syndrome and trigger wrist caused by a lipoma arising from flexor tenosynovium: A case report. J Hand Surg Am 27:1056, 2002.
15. Allen PW: Lipoma arborescens. In: Tumors and Proliferations of Adipose Tissue. Chicago, Year Book Medical Publishers, 1981, p 129.
16. Kloen P, Keel SB, Chandler HP, et al: Lipoma arborescens of the knee. J Bone Joint Surg Br 80:298, 1998.
17. Cil A, Atay OA, Aydingoz U, et al: Bilateral lipoma arborescens of the knee in a child: A case report. Knee Surg Sports Traumatol Arthrosc 13:463, 2005.
18. Davies AP, Blewitt N: Lipoma arborescens of the knee. Knee 12:394, 2005.
19. Hoffa A: The influence of the adipose tissue with regard to the pathology of the knee joint. JAMA 43:795, 1904.
20. **Devaney K, Vinh TN, Sweet DE: Synovial hemangioma: A report of 20 cases with differential diagnostic considerations. Hum Pathol 24:737, 1993.**
21. Lichtenstein L: Tumors of synovial joints, bursae, and tendon sheaths. Cancer 8:816, 1955.
22. Greenspan A, Azouz EM, Matthews J 2nd, et al: Synovial hemangioma: Imaging features in eight histologically proven cases, review of the literature, and differential diagnosis. Skeletal Radiol 24:583, 1995.
23. Cotten A, Flipo RM, Herbaux B, et al: Synovial haemangioma of the knee: A frequently misdiagnosed lesion. Skeletal Radiol 24:257, 1995.
24. **Chung EB, Enzinger FM: Fibroma of tendon sheath. Cancer 44:1979, 1945.**
25. Pulitzer DR, Martin PC, Reed RJ: Fibroma of tendon sheath: A clinicopathologic study of 32 cases. Am J Surg Pathol 13:472, 1989.
26. Maluf HM, DeYoung BR, Swanson PE, et al: Fibroma and giant cell tumor of tendon sheath: A comparative histological and immunohistological study. Mod Pathol 8:155, 1995.
27. Buddingh EP, Naumann S, Nelson M, et al: Cytogenetic findings in benign cartilaginous neoplasms. Cancer Genet Cytogenet 141:164, 2003.
28. Davis RI, Hamilton A, Biggart JD: Primary synovial chondromatosis: A clinicopathologic review and assessment of malignant potential. Hum Pathol 29:683, 1998.
29. Hettiaratchy SP, Nanchahal J: Synovial chondromatosis of the metacarpophalangeal joint. J Hand Surg Br 27:104, 2002.
30. Mandrioli S, Polito J, Denes SA, et al: Synovial chondromatosis of the temporomandibular joint. J Craniofac Surg 18:1486, 2007.
31. Sim FH, Dahlin DC, Ivins JC: Extra-articular synovial chondromatosis. J Bone Joint Surg Am 59:492, 1977.
32. Murphey MD, Vidal JA, Fanburg-Smith JC, et al: Imaging of synovial chondromatosis with radiologic-pathologic correlation. RadioGraphics 27:1465, 2007.
33. Edeiken J, Edeiken BS, Ayala AG, et al: Giant solitary synovial chondromatosis. Skeletal Radiol 23:23, 1994.
34. Sah AP, Geller DS, Mankin HJ, et al: Malignant transformation of synovial chondromatosis of the shoulder to chondrosarcoma: A case report. J Bone Joint Surg 89:1321, 2007.
35. Taconis WK, van der Heul RO, Taminiau AM: Synovial chondrosarcoma: Report of a case and review of the literature. Skeletal Radiol 26:682, 1997.
36. Ontell F, Greenspan A: Chondrosarcoma complicating synovial chondromatosis: Findings with magnetic resonance imaging. Can Assoc Radiol J 45:318, 1994.
37. Dahlin DC, Salvador AH: Cartilaginous tumors of the soft tissues of the hands and feet. Mayo Clin Proc 49:721, 1974.
38. **Chung EB, Enzinger FM: Chondroma of soft parts. Cancer 41:1414, 1978.**
39. Lichtenstein L, Goldman RL: Cartilage tumors in soft tissues, particularly in the hand and foot. Cancer 17:1203, 1964.
40. Jones WA, Ghorbal MS: Benign tendon sheath chondroma. J Hand Surg Br 11:276, 1986.
41. Gonzalez-Lois C, Garcia-de-la-Torre P, SantosBriz-Terron A, et al: Intracapsular and para-articular chondroma adjacent to large joints: Report of three cases and review of the literature. Skeletal Radiol 30:672, 2001.
42. Hensinger RN, Cowell HR, Ramsey PL, et al: Familial dysplasia epiphysealis hemimelica, associated with chondromas and osteochondromas: Report of a kindred with variable presentations. J Bone Joint Surg 56:1513, 1974.
43. **Rubin BP: Tenosynovial giant cell tumor and pigmented villonodular synovitis: A proposal for unification of these clinically distinct but histologically and genetically identical lesions. Skeletal Radiol 36:267, 2007.**
44. **West RB, Rubin BP, Miller MA, et al: A landscape effect in tenosynovial giant-cell tumor from activation of CSF1 expression by a translocation in a minority of tumor cells. Proc Natl Acad Sci U S A 103:690, 2006.**
45. Moller E, Mandahl N, Mertens F, et al: Molecular identification of COL6A3-CSF1 fusion transcripts in tenosynovial giant cell tumors. Genes Chromosomes Cancer 47:21, 2008.
46. Tyler WK, Vidal AF, Williams RJ, et al: Pigmented villonodular synovitis. J Am Acad Orthop Surg 14:376, 2006.
47. Rao AS, Vigorita VJ: Pigmented villonodular synovitis (giant-cell tumor of the tendon sheath and synovial membrane): A review of eighty-one cases. J Bone Joint Surg Am 66:76, 1984.
48. Mendenhall WM, Mendenhall CM, Reith JD, et al: Pigmented villonodular synovitis. Am J Clin Oncol 29:548, 2006.
49. Somerhausen NS, Fletcher CD: Diffuse-type giant cell tumor: Clinicopathologic and immunohistochemical analysis of 50 cases with extraarticular disease. Am J Surg Pathol 24:479, 2000.
50. Abdul-Karim FW, el-Naggar AK, Joyce MJ, et al: Diffuse and localized tenosynovial giant cell tumor and pigmented villonodular synovitis: A clinicopathologic and flow cytometric DNA analysis. Hum Pathol 23:729, 1992.
51. Carpintero P, Gascon E, Mesa M, et al: Clinical and radiologic features of pigmented villonodular synovitis of the foot: Report of eight cases. J Am Podiatr Med Assoc 97:415, 2007.
52. De Schepper AM, Hogendoorn PC, Bloem JL: Giant cell tumors of the tendon sheath may present radiologically as intrinsic osseous lesions. Eur Radiol 17:499, 2007.
53. Jergesen HE, Mankin HJ, Schiller AL: Diffuse pigmented villonodular synovitis of the knee mimicking primary bone neoplasms: A report of two cases. J Bone Joint Surg 60:825, 1978.
54. Myers BW, Masi AT: Pigmented villonodular synovitis and tenosynovitis: A clinical epidemiologic study of 166 cases and literature review. Medicine (Balt) 59:223, 1980.
55. Lin J, Jacobson JA, Jamadar DA, et al: Pigmented villonodular synovitis and related lesions: The spectrum of imaging findings. AJR Am J Roentgenol 172:191, 1999.
56. Al-Nakshabandi NA, Ryan AG, Choudur H, et al: Pigmented villonodular synovitis. Clin Radiol 59:414, 2004.
57. Masih S, Antebi A: Imaging of pigmented villonodular synovitis. Semin Musculoskel Radiol 7:205, 2003.
58. O'Connell JX, Fanburg JC, Rosenberg AE: Giant cell tumor of tendon sheath and pigmented villonodular synovitis: Immunophenotype suggests a synovial cell origin. Hum Pathol 26:771, 1995.
59. Flandry F, Hughston JC: Pigmented villonodular synovitis. J Bone Joint Surg 69:183, 1987.

60. Sharma H, Rana B, Mahendra A, et al: Outcome of 17 pigmented villonodular synovitis (PVNS) of the knee at 6 years mean follow-up. Knee 14:390, 2007.

61. Chiari C, Pirich C, Brannath W, et al: What affects the recurrence and clinical outcome of pigmented villonodular synovitis? Clin Orthop 450:172, 2006.

62. Flandry FC, Hughston JC, Jacobson KE, et al: Surgical treatment of diffuse pigmented villonodular synovitis of the knee. Clin Orthop 300:183, 1994.

63. Adem C, Sebo TJ, Riehle DL, et al: Recurrent and non-recurrent pigmented villonodular synovitis. Ann Pathol 22:448, 2002.

64. Bertoni F, Unni KK, Beabout JW, et al: Malignant giant cell tumor of the tendon sheaths and joints (malignant pigmented villonodular synovitis). Am J Surg Pathol 21:153, 1997.

65. Bhadra AK, Pollock R, Tirabosco RP, et al: Primary tumours of the synovium: A report of four cases of malignant tumour. J Bone Joint Surg Br 89:1504, 2007.

66. Dines JS, DeBerardino TM, Wells JL, et al: Long-term follow-up of surgically treated localized pigmented villonodular synovitis of the knee. Arthroscopy 23:930, 2007.

67. Rydholm U: Pigmented villonodular synovitis. Acta Orthop Scand 69:203, 1998.

68. Ushijima M, Hashimoto H, Tsuneyoshi M, et al: Giant cell tumor of the tendon sheath (nodular tenosynovitis): A study of 207 cases to compare the large joint group with the common digit group. Cancer 57:875, 1986.

69. Kitagawa Y, Ito H, Amano Y, et al: MR imaging for preoperative diagnosis and assessment of local tumor extent on localized giant cell tumor of tendon sheath. Skeletal Radiol 32:633, 2003.

70. Monaghan H, Salter DM, Al-Nafussi A: Giant cell tumour of tendon sheath (localised nodular tenosynovitis): Clinicopathological features of 71 cases. J Clin Pathol 54:404, 2001.

71. Alguacil-Garcia A, Unni KK, Goellner JR: Giant cell tumor of tendon sheath and pigmented villonodular synovitis: An ultrastructural study. Am J Clin Pathol 69:6, 1978.

72. Wood GS, Beckstead JH, Medeiros LJ, et al: The cells of giant cell tumor of tendon sheath resemble osteoclasts. Am J Surg Pathol 12:444, 1988.

73. Nilsson M, Hoglund M, Panagopoulos I, et al: Molecular cytogenetic mapping of recurrent chromosomal breakpoints in tenosynovial giant cell tumors. Virchows Arch 441:475, 2002.

74. Wu NL, Hsiao PF, Chen BF, et al: Malignant giant cell tumor of the tendon sheath. Int J Dermatol 4:543, 2004.

75. Bertoni F, Unni KK, Beabout JW, et al: Chondrosarcomas of the synovium. Cancer 67:155, 1991.

76. Gebhardt MC, Parekh SG, Rosenberg AE, et al: Extraskeletal myxoid chondrosarcoma of the knee. Skeletal Radiol 28:354, 1999.

77. Okcu MF, Munsell M, Treuner J, et al: Synovial sarcoma of childhood and adolescence: A multicenter, multivariate analysis of outcome. J Clin Oncol 21:1602, 2003.

78. Bergh P, Meis-Kindblom JM, Gherlinzoni F, et al: Synovial sarcoma: Identification of low and high risk groups. Cancer 85:2596, 1999.

79. Dardick I, O'Brien PK, Jeans MT, et al: Synovial sarcoma arising in an anatomical bursa. Virchows Arch A Pathol Anat Histol 397:93, 1982.

80. McKinney CD, Mills SE, Fechner RE: Intraarticular synovial sarcoma. Am J Surg Pathol 16:1017, 1992.

81. DeSanto DA, Tennant R, Rosahn P: Synovial sarcomas in joints, bursae, and tendon sheaths. Surg Gynecol Obstet 72:72, 1961.

82. Cadman NL, Soule EH, Kelly PJ: Synovial sarcoma: An analysis of 134 tumors. Cancer 18:613, 1965.

83. Milchgrub S, Ghandur-Mnaymneh L, Dorfman HD, et al: Synovial sarcoma with extensive osteoid and bone formation. Am J Surg Pathol 17:357, 1993.

84. Varela-Duran J, Enzinger FM: Calcifying synovial sarcoma. Cancer 50:345, 1982.

85. Corson JM, Weiss LM, Banks-Schlegel SP, et al: Keratin proteins and carcinoembryonic antigen in synovial sarcomas: An immunohistochemical study of 24 cases. Hum Pathol 15:615, 1984.

86. Fisher C: Synovial sarcoma. Diag Pathol 1:13, 1994.

87. Olsen SH, Thomas DG, Lucas DR: Cluster analysis of immunohistochemical profiles in synovial sarcoma, malignant peripheral nerve sheath tumor, and Ewing sarcoma. Mod Pathol 19:659, 2006.

88. Miettinen M, Virtanen I: Synovial sarcoma—a misnomer. Am J Pathol 117:18, 1984.

89. Amary MF, Berisha F, Bernardi F, et al: Detection of SS18-SSX fusion transcripts in formalin-fixed paraffin-embedded neoplasms: Analysis of conventional RT-PCR, qRT-PCR and dual color FISH as diagnostic tools for synovial sarcoma. Mod Pathol 20:482, 2007.

90. Guadagnolo BA, Zagars GK, Ballo MT, et al: Long-term outcomes for synovial sarcoma treated with conservation surgery and radiotherapy. Int J Radiat Oncol Biol Phys 69:1173, 2007.

91. Brecht IB, Ferrari A, Int-Veen C, et al: Grossly-resected synovial sarcoma treated by the German and Italian Pediatric Soft Tissue Sarcoma Cooperative Groups: Discussion on the role of adjuvant therapies. Pediatr Blood Cancer 46:11, 2006.

92. Younes M, Hayem G, Brissaud P, et al: Monoarthritis secondary to joint metastasis: Two case reports and literature review. Joint Bone Spine 69:495, 2002.

93. Capovilla M., Durlach A., Fourati E., et al: Chronic monoarthritis and previous history of cancer: Think about synovial metastasis. Clin Rheumatol 26:60, 2007.

94. Ehrenfeld M, Gur H, Shoenfeld Y: Rheumatologic features of hematologic disorders. Curr Opin Rheumatol 11:62, 1999.

95. Gur H, Koren V, Ehrenfeld M, Ben-Bassat I, et al: Rheumatic manifestations preceding adult acute leukemia: Characteristics and implication in course and prognosis. Acta Haematol 101:1, 1999.

96. Evans TI, Nercessian BM, Sanders KM: Leukemic arthritis. Semin Arthritis Rheum 24:48, 1994.

INDEX

A

AA. *See* Adjuvant arthritis.
α_1-Antichymotrypsin, as proteinase inhibitor, 122, 124t
α_2-Antiplasmin, as proteinase inhibitor, 122, 124t
Abatacept, 1131
  for rheumatoid arthritis, 954–958
    clinical studies of, 954–957, 955t, 956f
    current role of, 957
    pathogenesis of rheumatoid arthritis and, 958
    safety issues with, 957
Abatacept in Inadequate Responders to Methotrexate trial, 955, 955t, 1131
Abatacept Study of Safety in Use with Other RA Therapies trial, 957
Abatacept Trial in Treatment of Anti-TNF Inadequate Responders, 955, 955t, 956, 956f, 1131
Abdomen, acute, in systemic lupus erythematosus, 1292
Abdominal pain
  in acute rheumatic fever, 1779
  in polyarteritis nodosa, 1455
  in systemic lupus erythematosus, 1278
Abdominal reflex, in neck pain, 582
ACA. *See* Acrodermatitis chronica atrophicans.
ACCESS study, 1796
Accessory nerve testing, in neck pain, 580t
ACE. *See* Angiotensin-converting enzyme.
Acetabular joint, arthrocentesis technique for, 732–733, 733f
Acetaminophen, 19
  analgesic actions of, 846
  cyclooxygenase inhibition by, 347
  for fibromyalgia, 564
  for low back pain, 621t
  for osteoarthritis, 1566–1567
  for rheumatoid arthritis, 1134
Acetylcholine receptor, in skeletal muscle, 96t
Acetylsalicylic acid, 842t, 843–844
  action of, molecular basis of, 840
  for antiphospholipid syndrome, in pregnancy, 1290
  cardiovascular benefits of, 850
  in cartilage, 40t, 41
  combined with nonsteroidal anti-inflammatory drugs and coxibs, 850–851
  creation of, 834
  cyclooxygenase inhibition by, 840
  for fibromyalgia, 564
  for giant cell arteritis, 1419
  for Kawasaki disease, in children, 1693
  for systemic lupus erythematosus, in pregnancy, 1289
  for thrombosis, in antiphospholipid syndrome, 1307
  thromboxane inhibition by, 348
Achilles bursitis, therapeutic injection in, 724
Achilles tendinitis, therapeutic injection in, 724
Achilles tendinosis, 647

Achilles tendon, 530
  ankle pain and, 645–646, 645t
  arthrocentesis technique for, 734
  enthesitis of insertion, 530, 530f
  in rheumatoid arthritis, 1096
Achondroplasia, 1641–1642
  fibroblast growth factor in, 76
Acid maltase deficiency, differential diagnosis of, 1371t, 1372
ACLE. *See* Acute cutaneous lupus erythematosus.
ACR20 response criteria, 456, 459, 470–471
ACR70 response criteria, 456
Acrodermatitis chronica atrophicans, 696, 697
Acromegaly, 1836–1837
  polyarthritis secondary to, 551
Acromioclavicular joint
  arthrocentesis technique for, 729
  disorders of, shoulder pain due to, 604–605, 605f
  examination of, 519
ACTH. *See* Adrenocorticotropic hormone.
Actin
  α-actin as, in skeletal muscle, 96t
  neutrophil chemotaxis and, 221
  in skeletal muscle, 96t, 99
Activation fragment assays, 330t, 331, 331t
Activation-induced cell death, 170
Activation-induced cytidine deaminase
  as antigen-activated B cell marker, 191t
  B cell maturation and, 190
Activator protein-1, in rheumatoid arthritis, 1069
Activities of daily living
  modification of, in osteoarthritis, 1564
  in rheumatoid arthritis, 1138
Acupuncture, 508
  for osteoarthritis, 1566
Acute abdomen, in systemic lupus erythematosus, 1292
Acute cutaneous lupus erythematosus, 688–689, 689f
Acute hemorrhagic edema of childhood, 695
Acute rheumatic fever. *See* Rheumatic fever.
Acute-phase reactants, 767–773
  in acute rheumatic fever, 1780
  acute-phase response and, 768–770, 768f
    C-reactive protein and, 768–769, 769f, 769t
    cytokines and, 770, 770t
    ferritin and, 769–770
    serum amyloid A and, 769
  erythrocyte sedimentation rate and, 770, 771t
  practical use of, 772
  in rheumatic disease management, 770–772
    adult-onset Still's disease as, 772
    ankylosing spondylitis as, 772
    giant cell arteritis as, 771–772
    osteoarthritis as, 772
    polymyalgia rheumatica as, 771–772
    rheumatoid arthritis as, 770–771
    systemic lupus erythematosus as, 771
AD. *See* Alzheimer's disease.
Adalimumab, 935–936, 1129. *See also* Tumor necrosis factor inhibitors; TNF-α.
  for ankylosing spondylitis, 1183–1184, 1185t

Adalimumab (*Continued*)
  clinical trials with, 932
  dose for, 936
  efficacy of, 936
  pharmacokinetics of, 935
  structure of, 935
ADAM gene family, matrix degradation and, 119t, 121–122, 123t
  in rheumatoid arthritis, 130
ADAM proteinases, in cartilage degradation, 53, 53t
ADAMTS gene family
  as biomarkers, 480
  joint destruction and, in rheumatoid arthritis, 1077
  matrix degradation and, 118, 119t, 121–122
    in osteoarthritis, 131
    in rheumatoid arthritis, 130
  in osteoarthritis, 1530, 1536
ADAPT. *See* Arthritis, Diet, and Activity Promotion Trial.
Adapter proteins, T lymphocyte activation and, 161–162
Adaptive immunity, 277, 291–300, 292t
  complement system in, 329
  effector T cell types and, 300
  innate immunity compared with, 277, 278t
  innate mechanisms' influence on, 285–286, 285f
  lymphocyte migration paradigms and, 291–294
    egress from lymph nodes and, 294
    for extravasation, 291–293
    immunologic synapses maintaining antigen-specific interactions with dendritic cells and, 293–294
    interstitial, tissue organization and, 293
    thymus-sphingosine-1-phosphate and, 294
  lymphoid tissues and
    primary, 294–295
    secondary, 295–299
    tertiary, 299–300
Addison's disease, 1836
  as autoimmune disease, 261t
  eosinophils and, 230–231
Adenoma Prevention with Celecoxib trial, 849
Adenomatous Polyp Prevention On Vioxx trial, 846, 849, 856
Adenosine, 883
  transmethylation reaction inhibition by, 884–885
Adenosine triphosphate, concentration of, buffering of, in muscle, 102–103
Adenovirus arthritis, 1768
Adhesion molecules. *See* Cell adhesion molecules; Intercellular adhesion molecule(s); Vascular cell adhesion molecule-1.
Adhesive capsulitis
  of shoulder, in diabetes mellitus, 1834
  shoulder pain due to, 607–608
Adipokines, in cartilage destruction, 56
Adiponectin, in cartilage destruction, 56
Adjuvant arthritis, animal models of, 397, 398t, 399, 400t
ADLs. *See* Activities of daily living.

Note: Page numbers followed by b indicate boxed material; those followed by f indicate figures; those followed by t indicate tables

i

Antinuclear antibodies *(Continued)*
  myositis-specific autoantibodies and, 749–750
  in juvenile rheumatoid arthritis, 751
  mixed connective tissue disease associated with, 751
  overlap syndromes associated with, 751
  in polyarthritis, 546t
  in Raynaud's phenomenon, 751
  scleroderma associated with, 748–749, 749t
    antikinetochore and anti-topoisomerase I and, 748
    anti-polymyositis-scleroderma and, 749
    anti-RNA-polymerases and, 748
    Sjögren's syndrome associated with, 750–751, 751t
  in systemic lupus erythematosus, 1279
  systemic lupus erythematosus associated with, 746–748, 747t
    antiribosomes and, 748
    chromatin-associated antigens and, 746–747
    ribonucleoproteins and, 747–748
Antiphospholipid antibodies, paraneoplastic, 1842t, 1845
Antiphospholipid Antibody in Stroke Study, 1307
Antiphospholipid syndrome, 1301–1309
  animal model of, 334
  antinuclear antibodies in, 751–752
  catastrophic, 1304, 1305t, 1306–1307
    treatment of, 1308
  cause of, 1301–1302
  clinical features of, 1304
  definition of, 1301, 1302t
  diagnosis of, 1304–1307
    differential diagnosis and, 1306–1307
    laboratory studies in, 1304–1305, 1306f
    magnetic resonance imaging in, 1305
    pathology and, 1305
  epidemiology of, 1301
  pathogenesis of, 1302–1304, 1303f
  in pregnancy, 1304, 1306–1307, 1307–1308
    treatment of, 1290, 1307–1308
  prognosis of, 1309
  in systemic lupus erythematosus, 1290
  treatment of, 1307–1309
    antimalarials for, 898–899
    in antiphospholipid antibody-negative patients with clinical events, 1308–1309
    in antiphospholipid antibody-positive patients with ambiguous events, 1308
    in asymptomatic patients, 1308
    in catastrophic antiphospholipid syndrome, 1308
    in pregnancy, 1290, 1307–1308
    for thrombosis, 1307, 1307t
Anti-polymyositis-scleroderma antibodies, in scleroderma, 749, 749t
Antipyretic drugs, cyclooxygenase inhibition by, 841
Antirheumatic therapy. *See also specific drugs and drug types.*
  angiogenesis inhibition in, 362–363
  cell adhesion inhibition in, 362–363
  chemokine inhibition in, 362–363
  neutrophil functions and, 227
Antiribosomal antibodies, in systemic lupus erythematosus, 1279
Antiribosomes, in systemic lupus erythematosus, 748
Anti-RNA-polymerases, in scleroderma, 748, 749t
Anti-Ro/SS-A, in systemic lupus erythematosus, 748

Anti-Smith (anti-Sm) antibodies, in systemic lupus erythematosus, 1235
Anti-ssDNA antibodies, in systemic lupus erythematosus, 1234, 1279
Antistreptolysin O, in polyarthritis, 546t
Antisynthetase syndrome, 1363
Anti-TNF Trial in Rheumatoid Arthritis with Concomitant Therapy trial, 930t, 932, 1128
Anti-TNF-α therapy. *See* Tumor necrosis factor inhibitors, TNF-α.
Anti-topoisomerase, in scleroderma, 748, 749t
Anti-tRNA synthetases, in inflammatory muscle diseases, 750t
Antiviral protein regulation, in rheumatoid arthritis, 1069–1070
Aortic regurgitation, in Takayasu's arteritis, 1422
Aortitis, granulomatous, in rheumatoid arthritis, 1104
AP₅₀. *See* Alternative pathway equivalent.
APASS. *See* Antiphospholipid Antibody in Stroke Study.
APC trial. *See* Adenoma Prevention with Celecoxib trial.
APECED. *See* Autoimmune polyendocrine syndrome 1.
Apheresis, for Wegener's granulomatosis, 1442
Aphthae, in Behçet's disease, 1476, 1476f
Aphthous ulcers, in hyper-IgD syndrome, 1870, 1870f
Apical ectodermal ridge, 5
Apley compression test, 631–632
Apley grind test, 529
Apolipoprotein H, in antiphospholipid syndrome, 1301–1302
Apolipoproteins, secreted by macrophages, 150t
Apoptosis, 379, 380f
  accelerated, in degenerative rheumatic disorders, 390
  antiapoptotic proteins and, 384–385
  biochemistry of, 382, 382t
  biologics and, 391
  Caenorhabditis elegans paradigm of, 379, 380f
  caspases and, 385–386
  defective, of immune cells, 388
  defective uptake and processing of apoptotic cells and, 388–389
  detection of, 387–388
    caspase activation and, 387–388
    cell membrane alterations and, 387
    chromatin condensation and DNA fragmentation and, 388
    loss of mitochondrial membrane potential and, 387
  in diffuse connective tissue diseases, 1385
  drugs affecting apoptotic pathways and, 390–391
  endoplasmic reticulum stress and, 384
  genotoxic injury and, 384
  glandular destruction and, in Sjögren's syndrome, 1151–1152
  mitochondrial pathways of, in rheumatoid arthritis, 206–207
  mitochondrial stress and, 384
  neutrophils and, 217
  prolonged exposure to growth factors and, 389, 389f
  receptor-mediated, in rheumatoid arthritis, 207
  regulation of, 852–853
  removal and degradation of apoptotic cells and, 386–387, 387f
  in rheumatoid arthritis, 1070–1071
    fibroblast-like synoviocytes and, 206–207

Apoptosis *(Continued)*
  genes regulating, 1070–1071
  therapeutic interventions increasing, 1071
  signal transduction in, 339–341
    Bcl-2 family signaling and, 340–341
    death receptor signaling and, 340
    p53 and cell cycle arrest and, 341
  systemic lupus erythematosus and, 1244
  therapeutic induction of, 391
  therapeutic intervention and, 391–392, 391f
  tissue injury in organ-specific autoimmunity and, 389–390
Apprehension test, in patellofemoral pain, 633, 633f
APPROVe trial. *See* Adenomatous Polyp Prevention On Vioxx trial.
APRIL, in rheumatoid diseases, 370t
APS. *See* Antiphospholipid syndrome.
Aquatic exercise, in physical medicine and rehabilitation, 1027–1028
Arachidonic acid
  intake of, 505
  metabolism of, cyclooxygenase pathway of, 344, 346f
  metabolites of
    neutrophil production of, 222–223, 223f
    in synovial fluid, in rheumatoid arthritis, 1056
Arachidonic acid cascade, 836
Arachnodactyly, contractural, congenital, 1652
ARAMIS database, 871–872
ARF. *See* Rheumatic fever.
Arginine-rich end leucine-rich repeat protein, in cartilage, 40t, 41
Arm abduction test, in neck pain, 582
Arm syndrome, in rubella arthritis, 1763–1764
ARMADA trial, 932t, 936
Aromatase inhibitors, osteoporosis induced by, 1595–1596
Arteritis. *See also* Giant cell arteritis; Polyarteritis nodosa; Takayasu's arteritis.
  coronary, in rheumatoid arthritis, 1104
Arthralgia
  arthritis vs., 551, 552t
  HIV-related, 1747, 1748t
  in Sjögren's syndrome, 1154
  in systemic sclerosis, 1332
Arthritis. *See also specific types of arthritis.*
  of acute rheumatic fever, 1777
  arthralgia vs., 551, 552t
  autoimmune, mononuclear phagocytes and, 149
  in Behçet's disease, 1477
  collagen-induced, 264
  in dermatomyositis, 1363
  destructive, apatite-associated, 1516
  in Henoch-Schönlein purpura, in children, 1694
  HIV-related, 1747–1749, 1749t
  mast cells in, 242–243, 242f, 242t
    in acute arthritis, 242, 243f
    in chronic arthritis, 242–243
  mononuclear phagocytes and, 149
  in polymyositis, 1363
  self-management of, 993–996
    assistive devices for, 994
    cognitive coping for, 994
    exercise for, 993–994
    fatigue management for, 994
    program effectiveness and, 994–995
    tips for clinicians about, 995–996
  in sickle cell disease, 1828
  susceptibility to, regulation of, 407, 407f
  in systemic lupus erythematosus, 1269, 1269f

Cartilage, articular (*Continued*)
  cell density in, 38
  collagens of, 37, 38, 39, 41
  craniofacial, development of, 8
  destruction of
    animal models of, 407–408, 408f
    pannus-cartilage junction and,
      1074–1075, 1075f
    in psoriatic arthritis, matrix
      metalloproteinases and, 1213
    in rheumatoid arthritis, 37, 52,
      1074–1075, 1075f
  development of, 8
  embryonic, 8
  endochondral ossification of, 37
  extracellular matrix of
    components of, 13, 13t
    degradation and turnover in, markers of, 59
    structure-function relationships of
      components of, 39, 40t, 41
  fibrillation of, 58
  fibroblast-like synoviocyte attachment to, in
    rheumatoid arthritis, 207–208
  formation of, 5–7
  inflammatory molecules produced by, in
    osteoarthritis, 1535–1537
  interface with synovium, immunohistology
    of, 715–716, 716f
  mature, 13, 13t, 14f
  mechanical injury of, osteoarthritis and,
    1533–1534
  metabolism of, 48–52
    bone morphogenetic protein in, 50, 50t
    cytokine signaling pathways involved in,
      57–58, 57f
    fibroblast growth factor in, 49
    insulin-like growth factor-1 in, 48–49
    transforming growth factor in, 49–50, 50t
  morphogenesis of, 6
  movement of, synovial facilitation of, 30
  in osteoarthritis, imaging of, 794
  physical properties of, 39
  proteinase destruction of
    extracellular matrix degradation and,
      128–129, 129f
    in osteoarthritis, 128–129, 131
    in rheumatoid arthritis, 129–130, 130f
  regions of, 38, 38f
  repair of, 58–60
    cartilage aging and, 58
    cartilage matrix degradation and turnover
      markers and, 59
    chondrocyte aging and, 58
  structure of, 37–39, 38f, 39f, 1636
  subchondral bone interactions with, 13
Cartilage explant cultures, 45
Cartilage intermediate layer protein, 40t
Cartilage matrix protein, 40t
Cartilage oligomeric matrix protein, 1642, 1643f
  as biomarker, 477t, 480–481
  in cartilage, 40t, 41
  matrix metalloproteinase degradation of, 129
  as osteoarthritis biomarker, 1539
Cartilage-specific antigens, autoimmunity to,
  rheumatoid arthritis and, 1045
Cartilaginous joints, 107
Case-control studies, 435t, 436
CASPAR trial. *See* Classification of Psoriatic
  Arthritis trial.
Caspase(s), 385–386
  activation of, apoptotic cell detection using,
    387–388
  apoptosis and, 386
  functional subgroups of, 386
  regulation of, 386
  T lymphocyte activation and, 162

Caspase activation and recruitment domain
  proteins, as pattern-recognition receptors,
    282, 283, 286
CAT. *See* Computer adaptive testing.
Catabolin, 54
Cataracts, glucocorticoid-induced, 876
Catcher's crouch syndrome, in rubella arthritis,
  1763–1764, 1764f
Cathepsin(s)
  cathepsin B
    in cartilage degradation, 53t
    gene expression of, 125–126
    matrix degradation and, 116t, 117
    in osteoarthritis, 1530
    in rheumatoid arthritis, 209
    in synovial macrophages, 24
  cathepsin D
    in cartilage degradation, 53t
    matrix degradation and, 115, 116t
    in synovial macrophages, 24
  cathepsin G
    in cartilage degradation, 53t
    link protein degradation by, 129
    matrix degradation and, 116t, 117
  cathepsin K
    in cartilage degradation, 53t
    gene expression of, 125, 126
    matrix degradation and, 116t, 117
    in rheumatoid arthritis, 209
  cathepsin L
    in cartilage degradation, 53t
    gene expression of, 125, 126
    matrix degradation and, 116t, 117
    in rheumatoid arthritis, 209
    in synovial macrophages, 24
  cathepsin S
    in cartilage degradation, 53t
    matrix degradation and, 116t, 117
  joint destruction and, in rheumatoid
    arthritis, 1076–1077
Cationic peptides, secreted by macrophages,
  150t
Cat's claw, for osteoarthritis, 1571
Cauda equina syndrome, mobility of, 1176
Causalgia. See Reflex sympathetic dystrophy.
Cbfa 1. See Runt-domain transcription factor.
C4-binding protein, complement regulation
  by, 326t
CCL19, B cell homing and, 185
CCL20, B cell homing and, 185
CCL21, B cell homing and, 185
CCN2. See Connective tissue growth factor.
CCR5, as dendritic cell maturation marker,
  141t
CCR6, as dendritic cell maturation marker,
  141t
CCR7, as dendritic cell maturation marker, 141t
CD1a, as dendritic cell maturation marker,
  141t
CD2, as surface marker on T cells, 167t
CD3 complex, T lymphocyte activation and,
  160, 160f
CD3, as surface marker on T cells, 167t
CD4⁺ cells, 300
  Borrelia burgdorferi and, 1716
  functions of, 165
  inadequate downregulation by, in systemic
    lupus erythematosus, 1251–1252
  inflammation and, 171
  in organ-specific autoimmunity, 390
  T helper, in sarcoidosis, 1796–1797
  T lymphocyte activation and, 161
CD4, T lymphocyte development and, 156,
  158–159
CD4⁺CD25⁺ cells, T lymphocyte activation
  and, 164–165

CD5, B cell activation and, 188
CD5-1C, 958
CD7, as surface marker on T cells, 167t
CD8
  T lymphocyte activation and, 161
  T lymphocyte development and, 156,
    158–159
CD8⁺ cells, 300
  Borrelia burgdorferi and, 1716
  functions of, 165
  inadequate downregulation by, in systemic
    lupus erythematosus, 1251–1252
  inflammation and, 171
CD10
  as B cell maturation marker, 183t
  surface, as antigen-activated B cell marker,
    191t
CD11a, in synovial macrophages, 24
CD11a/CD18, as surface marker on T cells,
  167t
CD11b
  in synovial lining, 9
  in synovial macrophages, 24
CD11c, in synovial macrophages, 24
CD14
  as dendritic cell maturation marker, 141t
  in synovial lining, 9
CD16. See FcτRIII.
CD18, in synovial macrophages, 24
CD19
  B cell activation and, 187
  as B cell maturation marker, 183t
CD20
  as B cell maturation marker, 183t
  surface, as antigen-activated B cell marker,
    191t
CD21
  B cell activation and, 187
  as B cell maturation marker, 183t
CD22
  B cell activation and, 187
  as B cell maturation marker, 183t
CD23, as B cell maturation marker, 183t
CD26, as surface marker on T cells, 167t
CD28, T lymphocyte activation and, 162–163,
  164
CD29, as surface marker on T cells, 167t
CD31, in synovial vascular endothelial lining
  cells, 28, 29f
CD34
  as B cell maturation marker, 183t
  in synovial vascular endothelial lining cells,
    28, 29f
CD36, 145t
CD38
  as B cell maturation marker, 183t
  surface, as antigen-activated B cell marker,
    191t
CD40
  as B cell maturation marker, 183t
  as dendritic cell maturation marker, 141t
  platelets and, 252
CD44
  in cartilage, 40t
  chondrocyte interactions with, 47, 48
  as surface marker on T cells, 167t
  in synovial lining, 9–10
  in synovial subintimal layer, 27
CD45
  B cell activation and, 186–187
  as B cell maturation marker, 183t
  in synovial macrophages, 24, 26f
CD45RA, as surface marker on T cells, 167t
CD45RO, as surface marker on T cells,
  167t
CD47. See Integrin-associated protein.

CD54
as surface marker on T cells, 167t
in synovial subintimal layer, 27
CD55. *See* Decay-accelerating factor.
in synovial lining, 9
CD58, as surface marker on T cells, 167t
CD59, complement regulation by, 326t
CD68
in synovial lining, 9
in synovial macrophages, 24, 26f
CD72, B cell activation and, 188
CD77, surface, as antigen-activated B cell marker, 191t
CD80
as dendritic cell maturation marker, 141t
T lymphocyte activation and, 162–163
CD83, as dendritic cell maturation marker, 141t
CD86
as dendritic cell maturation marker, 141t
T lymphocyte activation and, 162–163
CD95. *See* Fas.
CD97, in synovial macrophages, 24, 26f
CD99, neutrophil diapedesis and, 221
CD123, as dendritic cell maturation marker, 141t
CD163
in synovial lining, 9
in synovial macrophages, 24, 26f
CDAI, 1135
Cefazolin, for bacterial arthritis, 1708t, 1709t
Cefepime, for bacterial arthritis, 1708t
Cefotaxime, for bacterial arthritis, 1708t, 1709t
Ceftriaxone
for bacterial arthritis, 1708t, 1709t
for Lyme disease, 1723
Celecoxib, 840, 843t, 845–846
adverse effects of, 848, 849, 850
development of, 834
for osteoarthritis, 1567
Celecoxib Long-Term Arthritis Safety Study, 845–846, 848
Celiac disease, 1227–1228
Celiac sprue, as autoimmune disease, 261t
Cell adhesion, inhibition of, in antirheumatic therapy, 362–363
Cell adhesion molecules, 138. *See also* Intercellular adhesion molecule(s).
in angiogenesis, 362
glucocorticoid effects on, 868
neural cell, condensation and, 5
platelet-endothelial cell, angiogenesis and, 359, 359t
vascular. *See* Vascular cell adhesion molecule-1.
Cell cycle arrest, p53 and, 341
Cell death
apoptotic. *See* Apoptosis.
intrinsic pathways of, 384–385
nonapoptotic, 380
Cell-mediated immune response, myositis and, 1356–1358, 1357f, 1358f
Cellular debris, removal of, by complement system, 330
Central nervous system
angiitis of. *See* Vasculitis, of central nervous system.
pain projection to brain and, 971, 972f, 972t
spinal cord and, 573–574, 573f
pain transmission to, 970–971, 970f
sensitization at, 971
Central nervous system disorders
in Behçet's disease, 1477
painful, 976
Centroblasts, 190
Centrocytes, 190, 191t

Centromere, in scleroderma, 748, 749t
Cervical cancer, in systemic lupus erythematosus, 1851
Cervical radiculopathy, shoulder pain due to, 609
Cervical spine
arthrocentesis technique for, 728
rheumatoid arthritis of, 1090–1091, 1091f, 1092f
Cervicogenic headache, 575, 577
Cevimeline, for Sjögren's syndrome, 1161, 1161t
CGRP. *See* Calcitonin gene-related peptide.
CH50. *See* Whole complement assay.
Charcot-Leyden crystals, eosinophils and, 228, 230
Charcot's joints. *See* Neuropathic arthropathy.
CHD. *See* Coronary heart disease.
Chédiak-Higashi syndrome, 224–225, 224t
Cheilectomy, 649
Cheirarthropathy, diabetic, 1833, 1834t
Chemoattractants, neutrophils and, 217–218
Chemokines, 357, 359–360, 360t. *See also specific chemokines.*
in angiogenesis, 360–362, 361f, 361t
B cell homing and, 185
C, 360, 360t
in cartilage destruction, 56, 56t
CC, 359–360, 360t
in angiogenesis, 361
regulation during leukocyte recruitment, 362
classification of, 359, 360t
CXC, 359, 360, 360t
in angiogenesis, 360–361
regulation during leukocyte recruitment, 362
inhibition of, in antirheumatic therapy, 362–363
as mast cell mediators, 239
in osteoarthritis, 1535
production of
during leukocyte recruitment, regulation of, 362
regulation during leukocyte recruitment, 362
receptor signaling by, T cell extravasation and, 292
receptors for, 360
in rheumatoid arthritis, 1064
secreted by macrophages, 150t
T lymphocyte homing and, 159–160
Chemotaxis
deficiency of, 224–225, 224t
neutrophils and, 221
Chest expansion, in ankylosing spondylitis, 1177
Chest pain
in ankylosing spondylitis, 1175
in Sjögren's syndrome, 1154
in systemic lupus erythematosus, 1276t
in Takayasu's arteritis, 1422
Chest wall, anterior, arthrocentesis technique for, 728
CHF. *See* Congestive heart failure.
Chikungunya virus arthritis, 1764–1765, 1764t
Chilblain lupus, 690
Childhood, mixed connective tissue disease in, 1394
Children. *See also* Juvenile *entries.*
bacterial arthritis in, treatment of, 1709t
dermatomyositis in. *See* Dermatomyositis, juvenile.
diffuse cutaneous systemic scleroderma in, 1686–1688
cause and pathogenesis of, 1686, 1686f

Children (*Continued*)
clinical features of, 1686–1687, 1687f, 1687t
diagnosis of, 1687–1688, 1688f
epidemiology of, 1686
outcome of, 1688
treatment of, 1688
eosinophilic fasciitis in, 1689
localized scleroderma in, 1688–1689, 1689f
mixed connective tissue disease in, 1689–1690
systemic lupus erythematosus in. *See* Systemic lupus erythematosus, in children.
vasculitis in, 1690–1696, 1690t
giant cell, 1695–1696, 1696f
necrotizing, of medium and small arteries, 1690–1693
of small vessels, 1693–1695
Chitinase 3-like protein, in cartilage, 40t, 41
CH3L. *See* Chitinase 3-like protein.
Chlamydia, rheumatoid arthritis and, 1042
Chlorambucil, 913–914
dosage for, 914
drug interactions of, 913
mechanism of action of, 910t, 913
pharmacology of, 913–914
for polyarteritis nodosa, 1456t
structure of, 913
toxicity of, 913
Chloroquine. *See also* Antimalarials.
chemical structure of, 897, 897f
for sarcoidosis, 1804
Cholesterol, structure of, 864f
Cholestyramine, drug interactions of, 893
Chondritis
costal, 519
in relapsing polychondritis, 1630
in relapsing polychondritis, 1629–1630, 1630f, 1631f
Chondroadherin, in cartilage, 40t, 41
Chondrocalcinosis
familial, 1516
imaging in, 798
Chondrocytes, 37
aging of, 58
autologous, transplantation of, 59
in cartilage pathology, 52–58, 52f
cartilage matrix-degrading proteinases and, 52–53, 53t
cytokine signaling pathways and, 57–58, 57f
cytokines and, 53–56, 54f, 54t
cartilage repair and, 58–60
cartilage aging and, 58
cartilage matrix degradation and turnover markers and, 59
chondrocyte aging and, 58
cell lines of, 46
cell origin of, 42
classification of, 42–43, 44f
cultures of
cartilage explant, 45
monolayer, 45
three-dimensional, 46
differentiation of, 42–43, 44f
function of
normal, adult, 17
synthetic, 43–44
hypertrophic, 46
interactions with extracellular matrix, 46–48
cell surface receptors and, 47–48
integrins and, 47
mechanotransduction of, osteoarthritis and, 1534
metabolism of
in articular chondrocytes, 45–46
culture models for study of, 44–46, 45f

Metastatic disease, 1852–1853, 1853t, 1900
Metatarsalgia, 646
Metatarsophalangeal joints, arthrocentesis technique for, 735
Methadone, for chronic pain, 985–986
Methemoglobinemia, with dapsone, 922
Methotrexate, 883–890
   actions of, 883–886, 884f, 885f
   for ankylosing spondylitis, 1183
   apoptosis and, 391
   for Behçet's disease, 1478
   chemical structure of, 883, 884f
   contraindications to, 890
   dose and administration of, 887–888
      for geriatric patients, 887–888, 888t
   drug interactions of, 890, 893
   efficacy of, 895t
   for giant cell arteritis, 1419
   indications for, 886–887
   for juvenile idiopathic arthritis, 1669, 1670
   malignancy associated with, 1849–1850, 1855
   mechanism of action of, 895t
   neutrophil functions and, 227
   pharmacology of, 886
   for polyarteritis nodosa, 1456t
   for polymyalgia rheumatica, 1420
   in pregnancy, 1288
   for psoriatic arthritis, 1215
   for reactive arthritis, in HIV infection, 1750
   to reduce inflammation, lessening vascular risk in rheumatoid arthritis via, 426
   for relapsing polychondritis, 1632
   for rheumatoid arthritis, 871, 1121–1122
      combination disease-modifying antirheumatic drug therapy for patients with active disease despite, 900–901, 901f
   for sarcoidosis, 1804
   special considerations with, 888t
   for systemic lupus erythematosus, 1284t, 1286
   for Takayasu's arteritis, 1424–1425
   toxicity of, 888–890, 895t
   for Wegener's granulomatosis, 1441
N-Methyl-D-aspartate, inflammation and, 413
Methylprednisolone
   drug interactions of, 866
   effects on hypothalamic-pituitary-adrenal axis, 869–870
   for giant cell arteritis, 1418
   for injection, 725t
   for juvenile idiopathic arthritis, 1666
   pharmacodynamics of, 865t
   for polyarteritis nodosa, 4, 1456t
   during pregnancy, 866
   pulse therapy using, 874
   structure of, 864f
   for systemic lupus erythematosus, 1282
      in children, 1680
   for Wegener's granulomatosis, 1439
Met-RANTES, leukocyte infiltration and, 363
Mevalonic aciduria, 1864t, 1869
Mexiletine, for chronic pain, 989t
MHC. See Major histocompatibility complex.
Mi-2, in inflammatory muscle diseases, 750t
Microsatellites, 314
Microscopic colitis, 1228–1229
Microscopic polyangiitis, 1403, 1404, 1443–1444, 1465
   antineutrophil cytoplasmic antibodies and. See Antineutrophil cytoplasmic antibody.
   clinical features of, 1443–1444
   diagnosis of, 1444
   differential diagnosis of, 1444, 1446t
   treatment and prognosis of, 1444

Microvasculature, synovial, immunohistology of, 715
MIF. See Macrophage inhibitory factor.
Migratory polyarthritis, 545
Milnacipran, for fibromyalgia, 564
Milwaukee shoulder, 606–607, 1516, 1518
Mimecan/osteoglycin, in cartilage, 41
Mind/body interventions, 509–510
   definition of, 502t
Mineralocorticoids actions, of glucocorticoids, 876
Minimally clinical important difference, 454
Minocycline
   for osteoarthritis, 1571
   for rheumatoid arthritis, 1123
MIP-1α. See Macrophage inhibitory protein-1α.
MIP-1β. See Macrophage inhibitory protein-1β.
Misoprostol, for ulcer prevention, 855
Mitochondria
   loss of membrane potential by, apoptotic cell detection using, 387
   stress of, apoptosis and, 384
Mitochondrial myopathy, differential diagnosis of, 1371t, 1373
Mitogen-activated protein kinases
   in rheumatoid arthritis, 1067–1069, 1068f
   signal transduction and, 337–338
Mixed connective tissue disease, 1382, 1388–1394
   antinuclear antibodies in, 751
   in children, 1689–1690
   clinical features and diagnosis of, 1388–1394, 1389t
      blood and, 1393–1394
      blood vessels and, 1393, 1393f
      early symptoms and, 1389–1390, 1390f
      fever and, 1390
      gastrointestinal tract and, 1392–1393
      heart and, 1390–1391
      joints and, 1390, 1391f
      kidneys and, 1392
      lungs and, 1392, 1392f
      muscle and, 1390, 1391f
      nervous system and, 1393
      skin and mucous membranes and, 1390
   glucocorticoid therapy for, 870t
   juvenile, 1394
   in pregnancy, 1394
   serologic features of, 1388
Mixed cryoglobulinemia, 1470
   essential, 1405
   paraneoplastic, 1842t, 1843
MM creating phosphokinase, in skeletal muscle, 96t
MMPs. See Matrix metalloproteinases.
MMR. See Macrophage mannose receptor.
Mobility devices, in physical medicine and rehabilitation, 1030
Molecular mimicry, 170
   B cell autoimmunity and, 193–194, 194t, 195f
   in diffuse connective tissue diseases, 1385
Monarticular arthritis, 533–543
   diagnostic studies in, 542–543
      bone biopsy as, 543
      cultures as, 542
      laboratory studies as, 542–543
      magnetic resonance imaging as, 543
      nuclear medicine as, 543
      radiography as, 543
      synovial biopsy as, 543
      synovial fluid analysis as, 542
      ultrasonography as, 543
   differential diagnosis of, 533–534, 534f, 535t, 536–537, 536t

Monarticular arthritis (Continued)
      bone pain and, 534
      internal derangement and, 533
      muscular pain syndromes and, 537
      neuropathic pain and, 536
      soft tissue infection and, 536
      tendinitis and bursitis and, 534, 536
   history taking in, 537
   inflammatory, acute, 537, 539–540, 539f
      crystal-induced, 540
      infectious, 537, 539–540
      with systemic manifestations, 540–541
      without systemic manifestations, 540–541
   inflammatory, chronic, 541, 542f
   noninflammatory, 541–542
   synovial histopathology in, 710–711, 710f
Monocyte(s), 135
   in gout, 1497
   systemic sclerosis pathogenesis and, 1323
Monocyte chemoattractant protein-1
   in cartilage destruction, 56, 56t
   fibrosis and, in systemic sclerosis, 1326–1327
Monolayer chondrocyte cultures, 45
Mononeuritis multiplex, in polyarteritis nodosa, 1454–1455
Mononeuropathies, pain generation with, 975
Mononuclear phagocytes, 135–151, 136f, 137t
   future research directions for, 150–151
   gene expression and secretion and, 146, 148–149, 150t, 151t
   heterogeneity of, 136–138, 138f, 139f, 139t
   life history of, 136–138, 138f, 139f, 139t
   mobilization of, 139, 140f, 141–142, 141f, 141t
   phagocytosis and endocytosis and, 144–145, 148f, 149f
   recognition and, 142–144
      complement receptors and, 143, 147t
      Fc receptors and, 143–144, 148f
      NOD-like receptors and, 144
      non-toll-like receptors and, 143, 143f, 144f, 145t, 146f, 147f
      toll-like receptors and, 142–143, 142f
   rheumatic diseases and, 149–150
   signaling responses in, 145–146
Monosodium urate crystals, 540
Monounsaturated oils, 506t
Mood disturbances, glucocorticoid-induced, 877–878
Morphea, 1341–1342, 1342t
   generalized, 1342t
   plaque, 1342t
   skin lesions in, 692–693, 693f
Morphine, for chronic pain, 985
Mortality. See also Death.
   in mixed connective tissue disease, 1394
   in rheumatoid arthritis, 1113–1114
   in systemic lupus erythematosus, 1293
Morton's neuroma
   arthrocentesis technique for, 735, 735f
   foot pain and, 646
   therapeutic injection in, 724
Motion. See also Range of motion entries.
   limitation of
      examination for, 517–518
      history taking and, 516
Motion against resistance testing, in neck pain, 581
Motoneuron disease, differential diagnosis of, 1372, 1372t
Mouth
   dry, in Sjögren's syndrome, 1153–1154, 1153f, 1155
      treatment of, 1161
   in systemic sclerosis, 1331

R

RA. *See* Rheumatoid arthritis.
RA 33, in rheumatoid arthritis, 762
"Raccoon-eyes" sign, in AM amyloidosis, 1789, 1789f
Radial nerve, testing of, in neck pain, 580t
Radiation, systemic sclerosis and, 1314
Radiation therapy, malignancy associated with, 1856
Radiculopathy, cervical, 575–576, 583
Radiocarpal joint, arthrocentesis technique for, 730, 730f
Radiofrequency ablation, for low back pain, 622
Radiographic Patient Outcomes trial, 931t, 935, 1128
Radiography, conventional. *See* Conventional radiography; *under specific conditions.*
Radionuclide scintigraphy, 781–782
  clinical application of, 781–782
RAG(s). *See* Recombination-activating genes.
Ragged red fibers, in myopathy associated with HIV treatment, 1752
RA-HAQ, 1025
Raloxifene, for osteoporosis, 1587
Randomization, in clinical trials, 453–454
Randomized clinical trials. *See* Clinical trials.
Randomized Evaluation of Long-term Efficacy of Rituximab in RA trial, 949t, 950, 951, 952
Range of motion, of joint degrees of freedom, 108–109
Range of motion exercise, in physical medicine and rehabilitation, 1027
Range of motion testing, in neck pain, 580–581
RANK, in rheumatoid diseases, 370t
RANKL. *See* Receptor activator of NFκB.
RANTES, in cartilage destruction, 56, 56t
Rapamycin. *See* Sirolimus.
Rashes
  with antimalarials, 899
  with azathioprine, 916
  in dermatomyositis, 1360–1362, 1361f, 1362f
    juvenile, 1682–1683, 1683f
  in human T-cell leukemia virus type 1 infection, 1767–1768, 1768f
  in hyper-IgD syndrome, 1870, 1870f
  with leflunomide, 893
  in Muckle-Wells syndrome, 1875, 1875f, 1876f
  with sulfasalazine, 896
  in systemic lupus erythematosus, 1266–1268
    acute, 1266–1267, 1267f
    chronic, 1267, 1268f
    subacute, 1267, 1268f
Raynaud's phenomenon
  antinuclear antibodies in, 751
  in diffuse cutaneous systemic scleroderma, 1688
  imaging of, 807, 808f
  in mixed connective tissue disease, 1393
  occupation-related, 494t
  in Sjögren's syndrome, 1156
  in systemic sclerosis, 1329–1330, 1330f, 1330t
  treatment of, 1340, 1340t
RCIs. *See* Clinical trials.
Reactive arthritis, 1196–1199
  cause of, 1196, 1196t
  clinical features of, 1196–1197, 1197f, 1197t
  definition of, 1196
  enteric, 1225–1227
    causes of, 1225–1226, 1226t
    diagnosis of, 1226
    epidemiology of, 1225

Reactive arthritis (*Continued*)
    outcome of, 1227
    pathogenesis of, 1226
    treatment of, 1226–1227
  epidemiology of, 1196
  genetics of, 1196
  glucocorticoid therapy for, 870t
  in HIV infection, 1749–1750, 1749f
    treatment of, 1749–1750
  imaging in, 791
  laboratory tests in, 1197
  natural history of, 1197–1198, 1198t
  pathogenesis of, 1196
  polyarthritis in, 550
  polyarticular, 549
  poststreptococcal, 1777–1778
  rheumatoid arthritis *vs.*, 1107
  skin lesions in, 686–687, 686f
  synovial fluid in, 705t
  synovial histopathology in, 712
  treatment of, 1198–1199
    in HIV infection, 1749–1750
    sulfasalazine for, 896
  uveitis in, 679
Reactive oxygen species
  platelets and, 253
  in rheumatoid arthritis, synovium and, 1070
Reading level, psychosocial management and, 1003–1004, 1003t
Recall bias, in cohort studies, 436
Receptor activator of NFκB
  bone destruction regulation by, 1078, 1078f
  osteoclasts and, 74, 75
  osteoporosis and, 1580
  in psoriatic arthritis, 1213
  in rheumatoid arthritis, osteoclastogenesis and, 210
Receptor editing, 271
RECK, as MMP inhibitor, 10t, 125
Recombination-activating genes
  gene 1
    as B cell maturation marker, 183t
    VDJ gene rearrangement and, 180
  gene 2
    as B cell maturation marker, 183t
    VDJ gene rearrangement and, 180
Recreation-related musculoskeletal disorders, 494–497, 495t, 496t
REFLEX. *See* Randomized Evaluation of Long-term Efficacy of Rituximab in RA trial.
Reflex sympathetic dystrophy
  occupation-related, 494t
  pain generation with, 975
  paraneoplastic, 1842t, 1844
  shoulder pain due to, 611
Regression toward the mean, 455
Rehabilitation
  goals of, 1023
  interdisciplinary *vs.* multidisciplinary, 1023
  International Classification of Functioning, Disability and Health and.
    See International Classification of Functioning, Disability and Health.
Reiter's syndrome. *See* Reactive arthritis.
Relapsing polychondritis, 1629–1633
  clinical features of, 1629–1631, 1630t
  course of, 1632
  criteria for, 1629, 1630t
  definition of, 1629
  differential diagnosis of, 1632
  epidemiology of, 1629
  evaluation in, 1632
  laboratory findings in, 1631–1632, 1631f
  pathophysiology of, 1629
  polyarthritis in, 549

Relapsing polychondritis (*Continued*)
  prognosis of, 1632
  skin lesions in, 698
  treatment of, 1632–1633
  uveitis in, 679
Relapsing seronegative symmetric synovitis, rheumatoid arthritis *vs.*, 1112
Reliability, test-retest, 470
Renal biopsy, in systemic lupus erythematosus, 1271–1272
  evaluation and interpretation of specimens and, 1272, 1272f, 1273f
  indications for, 1271–1272
Renal disorders. *See also specific disorders.*
  in amyloidosis, 1791t
  in ankylosing spondylitis, 1176
  of Behçet's disease, 1477
  in Churg-Strauss syndrome, 1445
  in hyperuricemia, 1487–1488, 1487f, 1488t
  in microscopic polyangiitis, 1443
  in mixed connective tissue disease, 1392
  in polyarteritis nodosa, 1455
  in relapsing polychondritis, 1631
  in rheumatoid arthritis, 1102
  in Sjögren's syndrome, 1155
  in systemic lupus erythematosus, 1270–1274
  in systemic sclerosis, 1336–1338
  in Wegener's granulomatosis, 1435
Renal fibrosis, in systemic sclerosis, 1317
Renal toxicity
  of coxibs, 851
  of cyclophosphamide, 910–911
  of nonsteroidal anti-inflammatory drugs, 847t, 851
Renal transplantation
  in systemic lupus erythematosus, 1291–1292
  in systemic sclerosis, 1338
Renal tubular acidosis, in Sjögren's syndrome, 1155
  treatment of, 1162
Reproductive toxicity, of nonsteroidal anti-inflammatory drugs, 847t
Rest
  in physical medicine and rehabilitation, 1026
  for rheumatoid arthritis, 1137
Reticulohistiocytosis, multicentric
  paraneoplastic, 1842t, 1845
  rheumatoid arthritis *vs.*, 1110
  skin lesions in, 699–700
  synovial histopathology in, 712
Retinacular cysts, 659
Retinal vasculitis, 679
Retinopathy, with antimalarials, 899
Retropatellar pain, 528
Retrospective cohort studies, 435t, 437
Retroviral infection, rheumatoid arthritis and, 1042–1043
Revascularization procedures, for Takayasu's arteritis, 1425
Reynold's syndrome, 1386
RFs. *See* Rheumatoid factors.
Rhabdomyolysis, HIV-associated, 1752
RHD. *See* Rheumatic heart disease.
Rheumatic fever, 1771–1782
  adult, polyarticular arthritis in, 549
  clinical course of, 1780–1781
  clinical features of, 1776–1779, 1777t
    arthritis as, 1777
    carditis as, 1778, 1778t
    chorea as, 1778–1779
    erythema marginatum as, 1779
    minor, 1779
    reactive arthritis as, 1777–1778
    rheumatic heart disease as, 1778
    subcutaneous nodules as, 1779

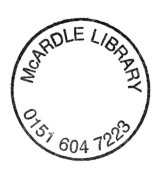

McARDLE LIBRARY

0151 604 7223